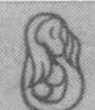

PREGNANCY SAFETY

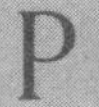

PEDIATRIC IMPLICATIONS

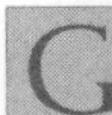

GERIATRIC IMPLICATIONS

MOSBY'S

Pharmacology in Nursing

MOSBY'S

Pharmacology in Nursing

20th Edition

Leda M. McKenry
PhD, RN, CS, FNP

Associate Professor,
School of Nursing,
University of Massachusetts
Amherst, Massachusetts

Evelyn Salerno
RPh, BS, PharmD, FASCP

Courtesy Professor,
School of Nursing,
Florida International University;
Clinical Assistant Professor,
Nova-Southeastern College of
Pharmacy
Miami, Florida

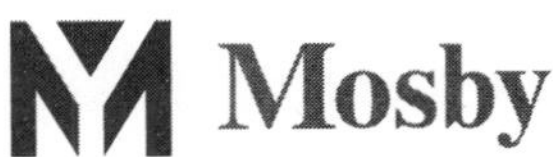

St. Louis Baltimore Boston Carlsbad Chicago Minneapolis New York Philadelphia Portland
London Milan Sydney Tokyo Toronto

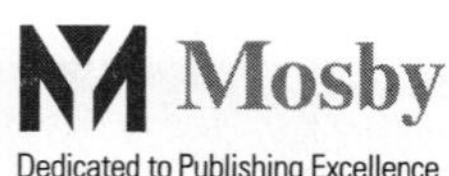

Dedicated to Publishing Excellence

A Times Mirror Company

Publisher: Sally Schrefer
Editor: Michael S. Ledbetter
Managing Editor: Jeanne Allison
Developmental Editor: Laurie K. Muench
Project Manager: Dana Peick
Senior Production Editor: Stavra Demetrulias
Designer: Yael Kats
Manufacturing Supervisor: Karen Boehme

TWENTIETH EDITION

A NOTE TO THE READER

The authors and publisher have made every attempt to check dosages and nursing content for accuracy. Because the science of pharmacology is continually advancing, our knowledge base continues to expand. Therefore, we recommend that the reader always check product information for changes in dosage or administration before administering any medication. This is particularly important with new or rarely used drugs.

Printed in the United States of America
Composition by Accu-color, Inc.
Illustrations by DesignPointe Communications, Inc.
Printing/binding by Word Color, Inc.

Mosby-Year Book, Inc.
11830 Westline Industrial Drive
St. Louis, Missouri 63146

International Standard Book Number
0-8151-4515-2

97 98 99 00 01/9 8 7 6 5 4 3 2 1

Consultants

BARBARA BROOME, RN, MSN, CNS
Assistant Professor of Nursing
Kent State University
Kent, Ohio

SUSAN COLE, RN, MSN, CS
Assistant Professor
Cardinal Stritch College
Milwaukee, Wisconsin

CRIS DUNBAR, BScN
Nurse Professor
Fanshawe College
London, Ontario

LINDA FELVER, RN, PhD
Associate Professor, School of Nursing
Oregon Health Sciences University
Portland, Oregon

JOAN PARKER FRIZZELL, RN, PhD
Assistant Professor, School of Nursing
LaSalle University
Philadelphia, Pennsylvania

LINDA LANE LILLEY, RN, MS
Associate Professor, School of Nursing
Old Dominion University
Norfolk, Virginia

EDWINA McCONNELL, RN, PhD, FRCNA
Independent Nurse Consultant, Madison, Wisconsin
Professor, Texas Tech University Health Sciences Center
School of Nursing
Lubbock, Texas

DIANA MELANCON, RN, MSN, CPN
Assistant Professor of Nursing Education
College of Mainland
Texas City, Texas

BETSY TODD, RN, BSN, MPH
Adjunct Faculty, Hunter-Bellevue School of Nursing
City University of New York
New York, New York

Preface

Mosby's Pharmacology in Nursing, twentieth edition, continues the long tradition of providing nurses with a sound basis for the clinical application of pharmacology. The book has enjoyed tremendous success as a textbook for students who, when confronted with some of the rigorous content of their pharmacology course work, find our organization and presentation both accessible and helpful. *Mosby's Pharmacology in Nursing* has additional appeal as a pharmacology reference because of its thorough coverage of pharmacologic principles and its emphasis on clinical nursing management. This makes the book useful both as a primary textbook and as a clinical reference for later use.

ORGANIZATION

Text Organization

The book is divided into **two major parts.** Part One, Basic Concepts, includes four units, *Unit 1: Principles of Pharmacology; Unit 2: The Nursing Process and Pharmacology; Unit 3: Biopsychosocial Aspects of Pharmacology;* and a **new** *Unit 4: Current Issues in Pharmacology.* In the new Unit 4 there are two new chapters, *Chapter 11: Over-the-Counter (OTC) Medications,* and *Chapter 12: Alternative and Complementary Pharmacology,* both addressing the latest issues in pharmacology. Part Two, Clinical Aspects, consists of the broad pharmacologic units that make up the largest portion of the book. Its sixteen units focus on major drug categories and body system reviews. Thoroughly updated coverage of **approximately 140 new drugs** has been incorporated through Part Two. The twentieth edition also features a **new** Appendix that includes an additional **50 new drugs** approved through July of 1997.

Our **focus** is on basic concepts of pharmacology, with special emphasis on the role of the nurse in developing a comprehensive approach to the clinical application of drug therapy through use of the **nursing process.** With the increasing importance of pharmacology for the professional nurse, many nursing programs now offer specialized course work as a separate part of the curriculum. In this context, our goal remains to update and expand the scientific foundation that will provide the learner with rationales for clinical practice. Examples of **care plans** based on **nursing diagnoses** are given for major drug classifications to provide guidance for the reader.

Chapter Organization

Each chapter begins with **chapter focus, learning objectives,** and a list of **key terms** and **key drugs** to help students focus on important material in the upcoming chapter. **Summary tables** and **boxes** are included throughout to supplement, reinforce, or help the student make comparisons among similar drugs. Pediatric and geriatric implications and pregnancy safety boxes have been retained to highlight important considerations for these specific clients.

The majority of the chapters, the drug chapters, begin with a discussion of a drug group. Then, individual drugs are discussed using a clinically oriented **drug monograph format** of mechanism of action, indications, pharmacokinetics, side effects/adverse reactions, significant drug interactions (when appropriate), and dosage and administration, and conclude with nursing management. The nursing management section uses the following **nursing process format:** assessment, including management of drug interactions; nursing diagnoses; implementation with, when appropriate, subheads for monitoring, intervention, and education; and evaluation.

More coverage is given to representative or prototypical drugs in each drug class. These **key drugs** are identified with a special icon ▲, which makes it easy to integrate the study of drug classifications into medical-surgical study or other course work in integrated programs.

Each chapter concludes with a **chapter summary** that provides students with a succinct overview of the chapter material. Following the summary, **critical thinking questions** present "real-life" scenarios to help students apply the chapter material they just read. **Collaborative learning activities** is a new feature designed to encourage students to work in groups and apply their knowledge to specific situations.

FEATURES

Creating a learning atmosphere that encourages discussion and critical thinking is a constant challenge. Every chapter of

Mosby's Pharmacology in Nursing has been extensively updated. Listed below are both classic features retained from the previous edition and new features for the twentieth edition, all designed to enhance learning and highlight important areas pertaining to the role of pharmacology in nursing management:

- New • **Design:** An attractive new design provides improved visual presentation with special icons to identify new and existing features. More than 180 illustrations have been redrawn to further enhance the visual presentation.
- New • **Two new chapters:** Over-the-Counter (OTC) Medications (Chapter 11) and Alternative and Complementary Pharmacology (Chapter 12) present important discussions concerning these current issues in pharmacology.
- **Key drugs:** These representative or prototype drugs are given more thorough treatment and highlighted with a special icon ▲ in the narrative for quick identification.
- New • **Serious drug interactions:** Highlighted within the drug interactions tables, these interactions alert the student to those drug interactions that the nurse must take special care to prevent. These are drugs that should be avoided or a potentially serious drug interaction may occur.
- **Drug name pronunciations:** Precede the discussion of each drug.
- **Cultural Aspects boxes:** Include issues and considerations related to pharmacology and culture, gender, or race.
- New • **Management of Drug Overdose boxes:** Alert the nurse to important information and guidelines regarding overdoses for specific medications.
- **Home Health boxes:** Feature nursing care related to pharmacology in the home setting.
- **Case studies:** Provide clinical situations and questions designed to test knowledge and promote critical thinking.
- **Research boxes:** Present a synopsis of recent research in nursing or pharmacology, followed by a series of critical thinking questions.
- **Critical thinking questions:** These questions test student's analytical and problem solving skills.
- New • **Collaborative learning activities:** At the end of each chapter, these activities encourage students to work in groups to apply critical thinking skills to problems.
- New • **Appendix G:** New appendix includes 50 new drugs approved up through July of 1997.
- **Disorders index:** A separate index that provides an alphabetical reference to disorders, conditions, and diseases in the text. The disorders index facilitates use of the book in programs where pharmacology is integrated into the curriculum and not offered as a separate course.
- New • **Patient Teaching disk:** Packaged in the back of the book, this innovative disk helps students provide patient teaching for more than 30 generic drugs.

ANCILLARIES

A carefully prepared and expanded ancillary package has been developed to provide a complete teaching resource for faculty in either integrated or separate pharmacology courses. This ancillary package includes the following:

An innovative **Instructor's Resource Kit** in a binder format with nine tabbed section dividers for the following:

- Section I: Suggested lecture outlines, including learning objectives, key terms, and chapter outlines in a unique three-column format with teaching strategies and collaborative learning activities
- Section II: Review sheets
- Section III: Printed test bank
- Section IV: "How to Teach Pharmacology in an Integrated Curriculum," with descriptions for integrated and separate courses
- Section V: Answer guidelines for the text's Critical Thinking Questions
- Section VI: Transparency acetates
- Section VII: Transparency masters
- Section VIII: Pharmacology newsletter, including the latest issues of *Mosby's Pharmacology Update*
- Section IX: Videos—explanation on available medication administration and intravenous therapy videos, with worksheets!

Computerized test bank: This computerized version of the printed test bank is available in both Windows and Macintosh formats.

Mosby's Pharmacology Transparency Acetates: 36 full-color transparencies feature illustrations of how drugs work in the body plus approximately 10 medication administration illustrations.

Student Learning Guide: Includes review sheets found in the Instructor's Resource Kit for those instructors who would prefer not to use photocopies or would like their students to have a separate study guide.

Quick Medication Administration Reference: Packaged with every copy of the text, this handy reference has been widely expanded with new information on dosage calculations, lifespan considerations, client assessment, home health, and more!

Lecture Video: Demonstrates the Five Rights of Medication Administration.

Mosby's Medication & IV Therapy Videos: Series of videos that provide a thorough review of medication administration techniques and intravenous therapy from Mosby's Nursing Skills Video Series.

We have done our best to provide instructors with the best teaching tools to make the most effective use of their time both inside and outside the classroom. This ancillary package is also geared to encourage student involvement and to facilitate comprehension of key content related to pharmacology for nurses.

ACKNOWLEDGMENTS

We would like to thank the many people who have contributed to the development of the twentieth edition of *Mosby's Pharmacology in Nursing*. Students, classroom instructors, and reviewers have provided us with suggestions and constructive comments that were most helpful in guiding us through this revision. In addition, all the editorial staff and associates at Mosby were outstanding in their professional support of this project. We are especially grateful to our Editor, Michael Ledbetter; Developmental Editor, Laurie Muench; Project Manager, Dana Peick; Senior Production Editor, Stavra Demetrulias; and to Robin Carter and Jeanne Allison, who helped with the early development of the book.

Last, but not least, we would like to thank our families, friends, and colleagues for their patience and encouragement. Without your support, this edition would not have been possible.

Leda M. McKenry
Evelyn Salerno

PUBLISHER'S HISTORICAL PERSPECTIVE

Mosby's Pharmacology in Nursing has a tradition of providing the nursing student, educator, and practicing nurse with thorough and up-to-date pharmacology and nursing management.

In all of its previous editions, the book has sold over 2,000,000 copies, making it the most most widely used and successful nursing pharmacology textbook ever published.

Currently in its twentieth edition, *Mosby's Pharmacology in Nursing* has its roots in *A Textbook of Materia Medica for Nurses* by A.L. Muirhead, published in 1919. In 1936 Hugh Alister McGuigan became the primary author, at which time the book was renamed *Materia Medica and Pharmacology*. In 1940 Elsie E. Krug joined McGuigan as coauthor, a role she was to hold until 1948 when she became the primary author. The book was renamed *Pharmacology in Nursing* in 1955 after 10 successful editions.

In recognition of the book's long history, each unit's chapter opening page displays a graceful photograph by Jim Leick of historical medicinal items from the private collection of Evelyn Salerno. We are grateful for her generosity in allowing us to include some of her personal treasures in the twentieth edition. These photographs are depicted below.

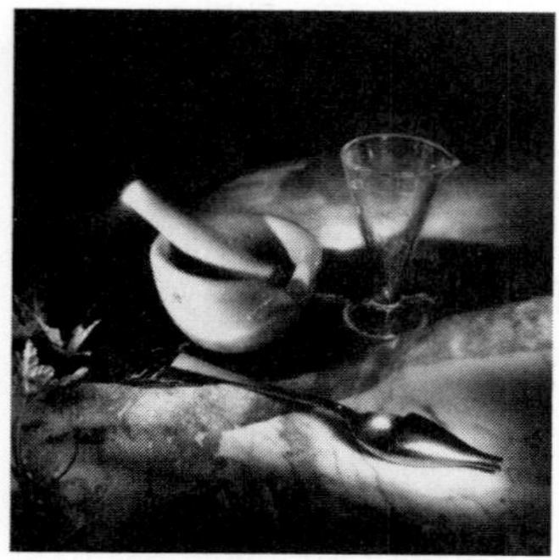

UNIT 1
Principles of Pharmacology

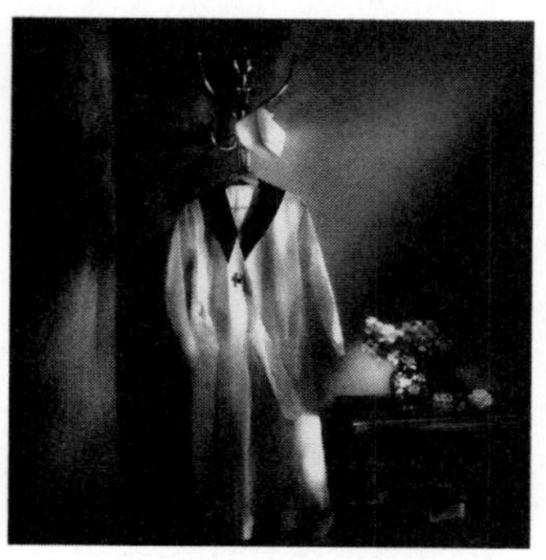

UNIT 2
The Nursing Process and Pharmacology

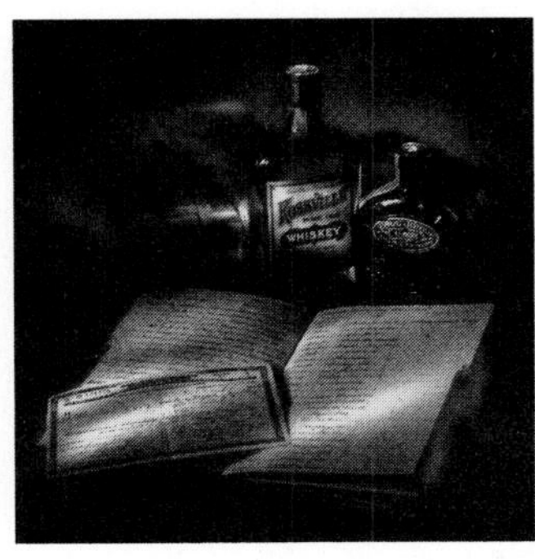

UNIT 3
Biopsychosocial Aspects of Pharmacology

The National Prohibition Act (1919 to 1933) restricted the sale of beverage alcohol but permitted the legal distribution of alcohol by prescription for treatment of a known ailment. Physicians and pharmacists had to have a federal permit to prescribe or dispense medicinal spirits or whiskey. Physicians were required to write their alcohol orders on an official U.S. Internal Revenue form and also had to record each prescription in a government-issued Physician's Record book. The whiskey bottles dispensed had a warning on the label: "For Medicinal Purposes Only." The physician's record book had columns for the patient's name and address type and quantity of liquor prescribed, ailment, and directions.

The items displayed in this photograph are original. The entries for pints of whiskey indicate alcohol was prescribed for ailments that included slight colds, acute gastritis, bronchitis, and pneumonia. Pharmacologically, alcohol has little if any effect in these conditions, and in fact it is reported to cause gastritis.

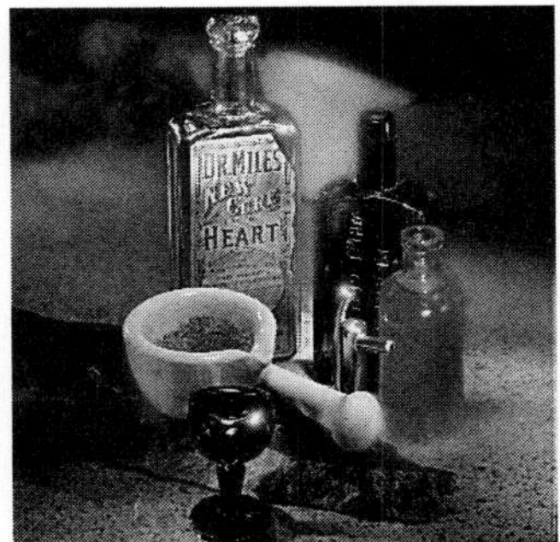

UNIT 4
Current Issues in Pharmacology

Before the twentieth century, diseases and illnesses were treated primarily with home remedies, vegetable concoctions, or narcotic-laced nostrums. At that time, trained medical professionals were few and drug legislation limited. Today, public interest in self-care management is at an all-time high. Thus the nurse should be knowledgeable about the major categories of over-the-counter drugs and the alternative natural remedies available for self-treatment.

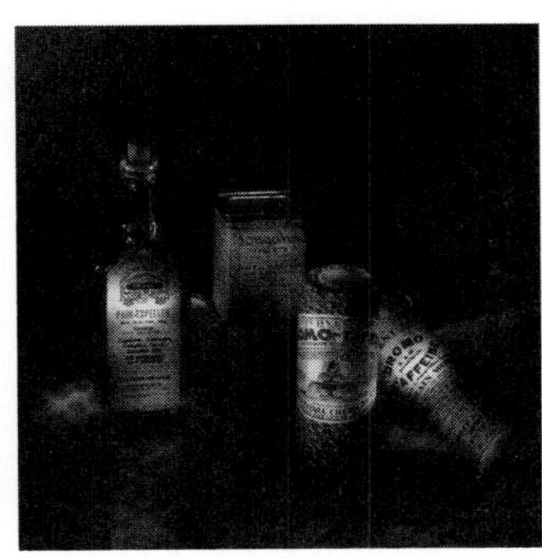

UNIT 5
Drugs Affecting the Central Nervous System

The old medications featured here include the Pain-Expeller, a preparation containing 49% alcohol that was promoted as a liniment and inhaler. The Tongaline tablet container states it is "a thorough eliminative for the various forms of Rheumatism and Neuralgia, as also La Grippe, Nervous Headache, Gout and Sciatica or wherever the salicylates are indicated." Ingredients are not listed.

Bromo-Lithia Effervescent was acetanilide combined with caffeine citrate, lithium bitartrate and sodium bromide in a pure fruit acid. The indications for Bromo-Lithia were headache, biliousness, and rheumatism, whereas the Bromo Caffeine for Brain Workers contained effervescent hydrobromate of caffeine, a "remedy for relief of the nervous headache resulting from overtaxed mental energy or excitement, acute attacks of indigestion, the depression following alcoholic excesses, the supra-sensitiveness of chloral, morphia and opium habituates and with ladies, the headache and backache of neurasthenia, hysteria, dysmenorrhea and kindred disorders" (from label).

Several of the drugs in the previous preparations are still in use today—for example, lithium for the treatment of mania and caffeine with aspirin. Bromides and acetanilide have been replaced with safer products.

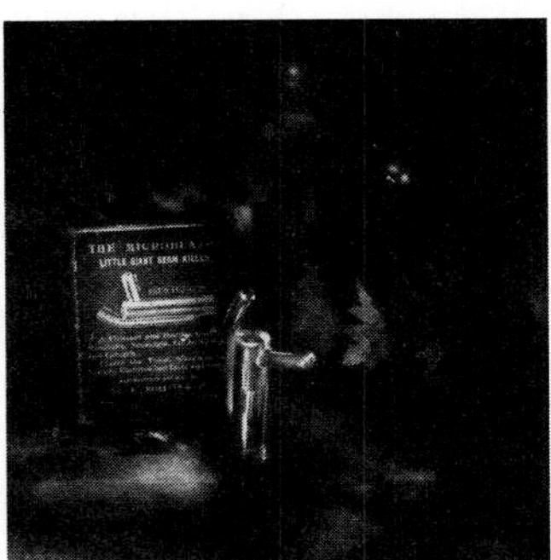

UNIT 6
Drugs Affecting the Autonomic Nervous System

The Microbeater was an early version of a nasal inhaler; the patient inserted one metal arm in the mouth and the second curved arm in the nose and blew. This product was promoted as a cure to headache, neuralgia, colds, coughs, and catarrh. This device was probably a precursor to the inhalers in use today.

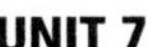

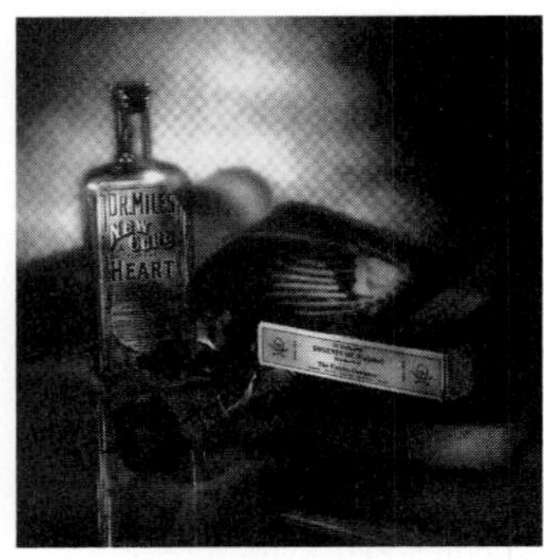

UNIT 7
Drugs Affecting the Cardiovascular System

The preparations on display are illustrative of medicines used in the late 1800s to early 1900s for treatment of heart disease. Dr. Franklin Miles, a physician who began marketing his remedies, such as Dr. Miles New Cure for the Heart (and stomach, lungs, kidneys, etc.), in 1885. The law then did not require patent medicines to list their ingredients, but the testimonials used in their advertising implied the ingredients were digitalis and cactus. However, laboratory analysis revealed this cure only contained a small amount of iron, phosphate, glycerin and alcohol colored with caramel and no digitalis. This bottle dates between 1888 and 1920, when the name of the product changed to Heart Treatment. It was taken off the market in 1938.

Diginfuse contains tablets of Digitalis purpurea leaves. To prepare an infusion, a tablet is crushed, boiling water is poured over it, and this mixture is allowed to stand for one hour. The mixture is then strained and dispensed to the patient. (Date on this package is 1935.)

The two active cardiac glycosides isolated from digitalis leaves are digoxin and digitoxin. These glycosides are more stable and reliable and have replaced the early products.

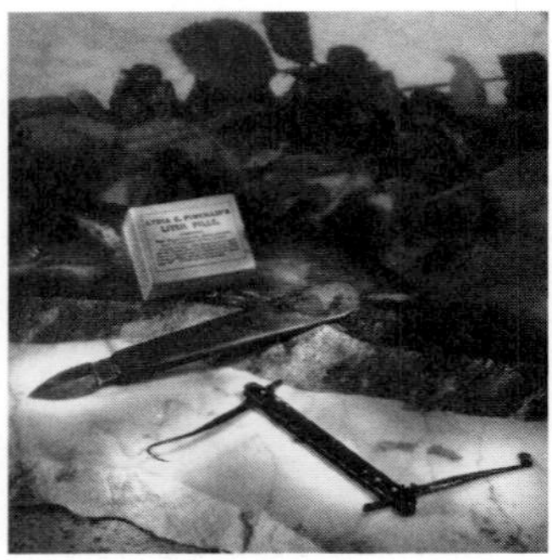

UNIT 8
Drugs Affecting the Blood

This photograph shows two types of Civil War–era bleeding devices and Pinkham's Liver Pills. The center device is a venisection knife, while the bottom instrument is a combination tenaculum and lancet. Such devices were used to bleed patients to remove excesses from the blood. Overzealous physicians may have hastened death in their patients by utilizing this procedure. It has been reported that George Washington had 9 pints of blood removed in 24 hours for the treatment of an infected throat. He died from this "throat infection."

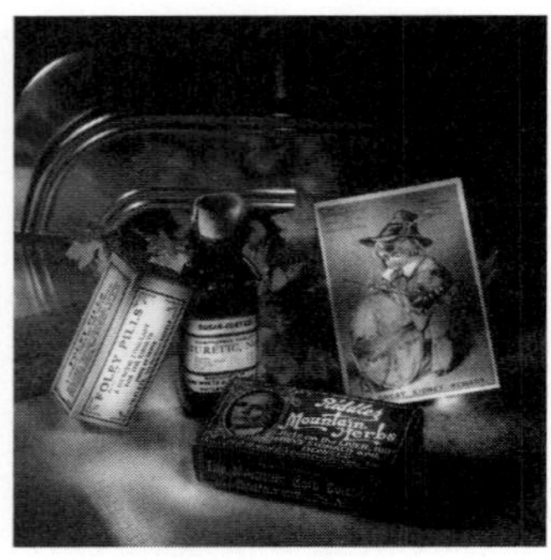

UNIT 9
Drugs Affecting the Urinary System

This photo shows an advertising card and a variety of turn-of-the-century medications used to treat kidney disease. The Mountain Herbs product lists about 30 disease states, along with a number of testimonials. All three products contain herbs or plant ingredients, with the Diuretic product also containing digitalis. This is an interesting assortment of early kidney medications.

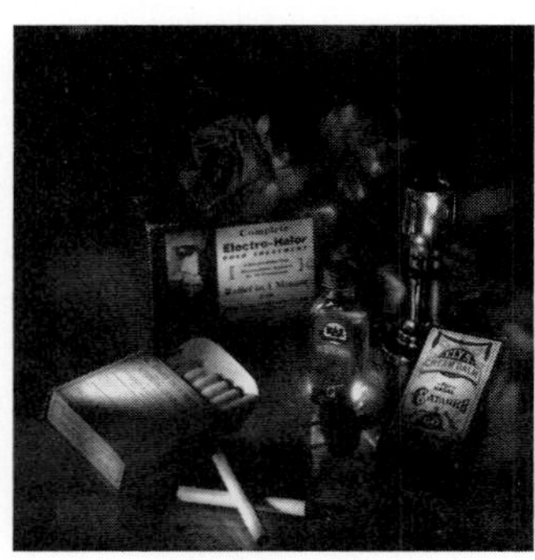

UNIT 10
Drugs Affecting the Respiratory System

The equipment and products pictured here were used to treat respiratory illnesses—for example, Dr. Guild's Green Mountain Asthmatic Cigarettes to relieve attacks and paroxysms of asthma. Ingredients included stramonium and belladonna with directions to "put tube end into mouth and light closed end, same as ordinary cigarettes, but the smoke should be inhaled deeply. . . . An adult should not exceed 6 cigarettes or a child 3 cigarettes per 24 hours."

The Electro-Halor Cold Treatment gave relief in 1 minute from head colds, lung colds, coughs, and hay fever. The contents of the box are next to it: the Kaz inhalant and the electrical cup for inhalation. Ely's Cream Balm was for nasal catarrh or cold in the head. A government analysis of this preparation stated it contained mainly liquid petrolatum (mineral oil) with small amounts of thymol and menthol. The chemist reported that a 69 cent bottle of Ely's contained about a half-cent's worth of liquid petrolatum.

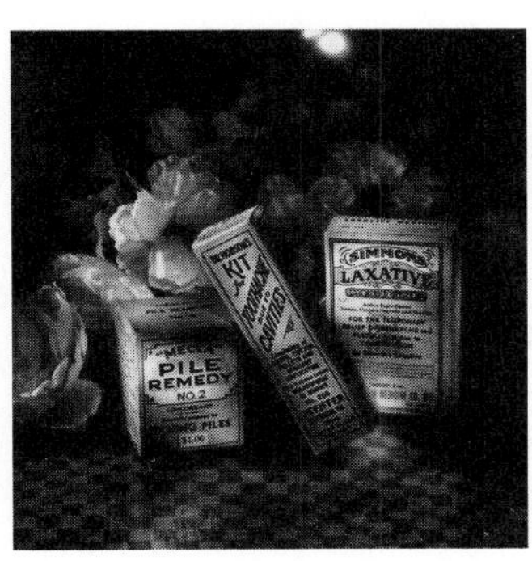

UNIT 11
Drugs Affecting the Gastrointestinal System

The three drug packages pictured include Mecca Pile Remedy No. 2 "for blind bleeding and protruding piles . . . " It contained carbolic acid. Dr. Hobson's Kit for Toothache Due to Cavities contained bottle, cotton pellets, and tweezers. The liquid in the bottle contained chloroform, creosote, oil of cloves, oil of camphor, and phenol. Simmons Laxative Medicine was for temporary relief of headache and flatulence due to constipation. This powder contained senna, cáscara sagrada, and gentian.

Carbolic acid or phenol was used in the Mecca package, as an antiseptic for hemorrhoids, but today, both the safety and the efficacy of this use are questionable. Phenol has been approved by the FDA for relief of teething in infants 4 months of age and older. Currently the FDA states there is no effective OTC product that can be placed in the tooth cavity to relieve toothache.

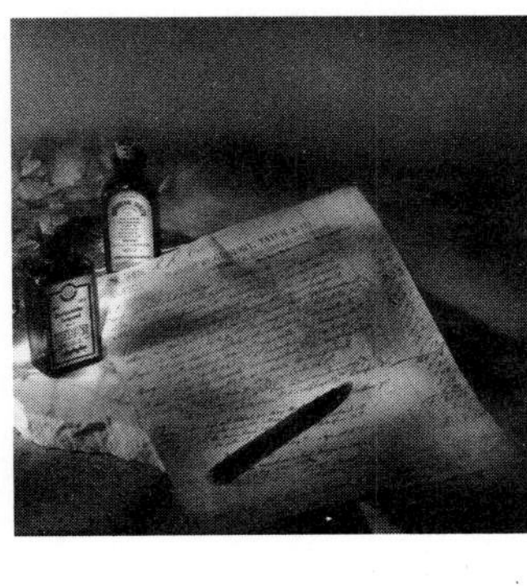

UNIT 12
Drugs Affecting the Visual and Auditory Systems

The two large eye cups have patent dates of 1917 on the bottom, while the Dearco Eye Water is advertised as "excellent for automobiles and others subjected to dust and winds" (1928).

Dr. Dickey's Painless Eye Water has a copyright date of 1908. According to Nostrums and Quackery (1912), Dr. Pettit's Eye Salve contained morphine, an unusual ingredient for an eye preparation. Many of these products were astringents or eye washes.

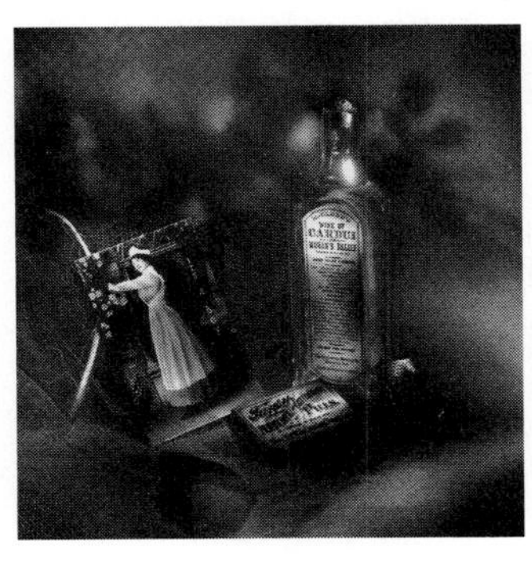

UNIT 13
Drugs Affecting the Endocrine System

The photograph shows two turn-of-the-century glandular products, an original druggist's bill dated 1863, and an instrument. The bottles contained suprarenal gland, with the Pluriglandular Compound also containing thyroid and ovarian residue. The druggist's bill was from Tallahassee, Florida, listing items purchased by General R.K. Call from 1861 to 1862. (An R.K. Call was governor of territorial Florida in 1836 and 1841.)

UNIT 14
Drugs Affecting the Reproductive System

The "It's a Boy" postcard is an early example of an announcement of the birth of a baby boy, while McElree's Wine of Cardui or Woman's Relief was promoted as a remedy for the treatment of female diseases. The label indications include "suppressed or delayed menses, painful menstruation, profuse or too frequent flow of menses, whites, falling of the womb, change of life and as a general restorative for delicate women." The label states it contains 20% alcohol.

The tin contains Tansy Pennyroyal and Cotton Root Pills, a Reliable, Female Regulating Pills. Dated 1896, the insert states, "It is best, in beginning the use of these pills, that the bowels should be thoroughly opened by some good cathartic. . . . It is also well, while using these pills, to make use of a warm foot bath every night, which may be made further efficient by the addition of a small quantity of mustard, salt or salsoda. . . . "

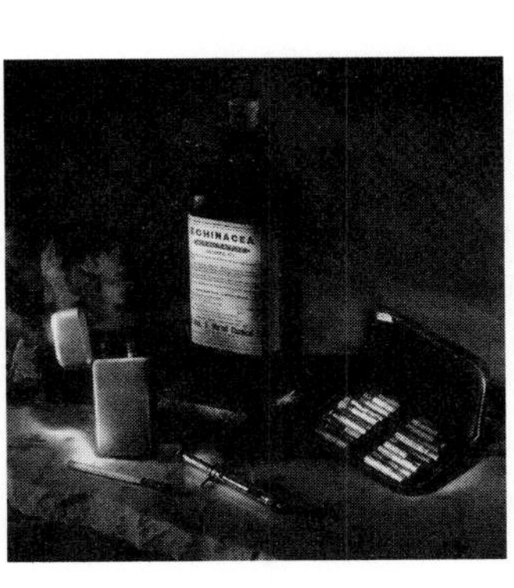

UNIT 15
Drugs Used in Neoplastic Diseases

The photograph shows a turn of the century bottle of Echinacea, a substance used to treat cancer, blood poisoning, syphilis, rabies, bites of reptiles, and many other disease states. The two small doctor kits contain vials of hypodermic tablets (strychnine, morphine, atropine, etc.). The kit on the left also contained a syringe (pictured in front) and needles. Note that the syringe barrel is similar to an injector unit in common use today. The items date from the nineteenth century to the early twentieth century.

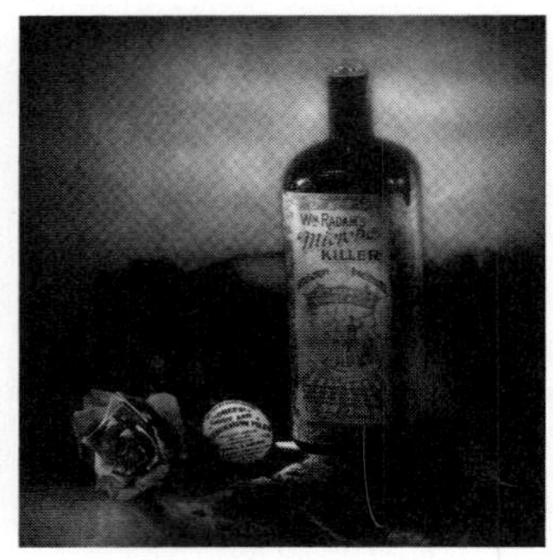

UNIT 16

Drugs Used in Infectious Diseases and Inflammation

William Radam, a gardener, made a concoction of muriatic acid, sulphurous acid, red wine, and water and sold it as a cure for cancer, consumption, diabetes, diphtheria, yellow fever, paralysis, and men's diseases. The government charged the company with quackery, and then seized and destroyed cases of this product. On analysis, this product contained 99.381% water. Note embossment on label and back of bottle that pictures a man clubbing a skeleton. The trademark is registered 1887 and 1893 on label.

The Dref's Gout and Rheumatism Pill tin is dated 1916 and has explicit instructions: "One pill at night when required. Cannot be given to children." Ingredients unknown.

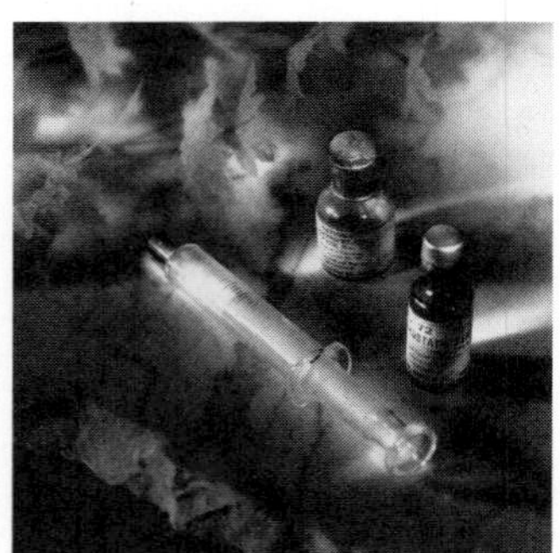

UNIT 17

Drugs Affecting the Immunologic System

A glass syringe lies next to two early injectable vials. The Hemostatic (Hemoplastin) labeled vial has a U.S. License No. 1 on the label, while the second vial is Erysipelas Vaccine, a bacterial vaccine made from streptococcus.

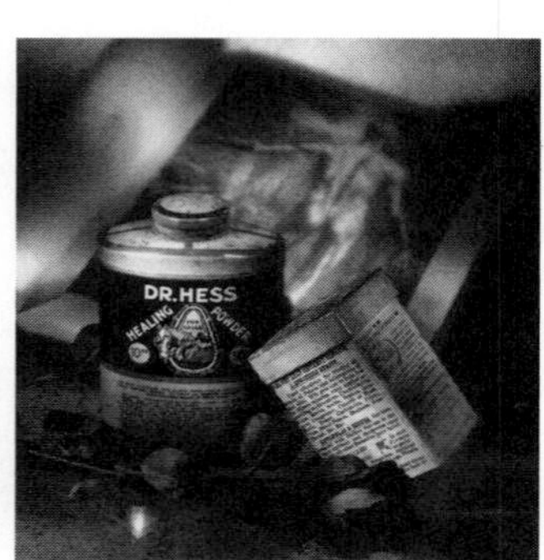

UNIT 18

Drugs Affecting the Integumentary System

Dr. Hess Healing Powder is a good example of a product for multiple uses, a patent medicine good for man and beast. The front of this tin lists all the human reasons for using the product while the back lists a variety of animal conditions. Mail order medicines were common on the frontier—a product that could service all in a household was preferred.

The second item is Velvet Leaf Ointment Compound, a substance promoted as treating all diseases of the rectum (piles, hemorrhoids, tumors, fissures, and rectal ulcers), blood poison, rattlesnake bite, eczema, abscesses, lumps and tumors, cuts, burns, scalds, congestion of the head, deafness, sore throat, etc. This product has the 1906 Food and Drugs Act Guarantee.

During the twentieth century, legislation and marketing of drug products have changed. Therefore, while similar drugs may still be commonly used in humans and animals, veterinary medicine generally has developed as a separate specialty.

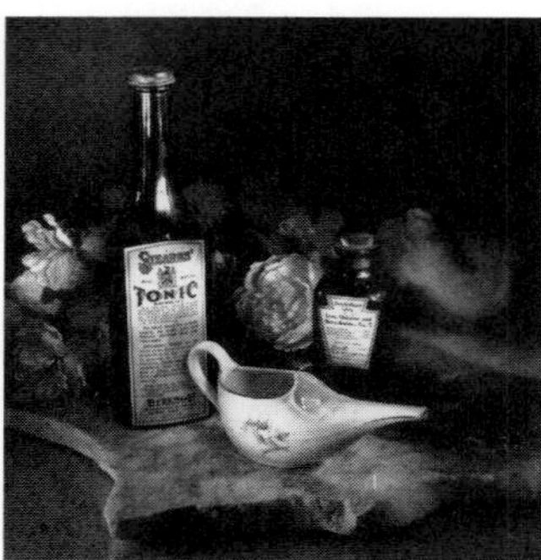

UNIT 19

Intravenous and Nutritional Therapy

An invalid or sick feeder is shown with Stearns' Tonic and Iron, Quinine and Strychnine No. 2 tablets. The latter product was used as a hematinic and bitter tonic. Strychinine was used in tonics because of its bitter taste, which was believed to stimulate gastric secretion and appetite.

Stearns' Tonic came in a triangular bottle and contained beef and cod liver peptones, calcium, iron, and ammonium citrate. It was promoted as the ideal tonic for the elderly, for weak, pale, and delicate children, and for convalescents.

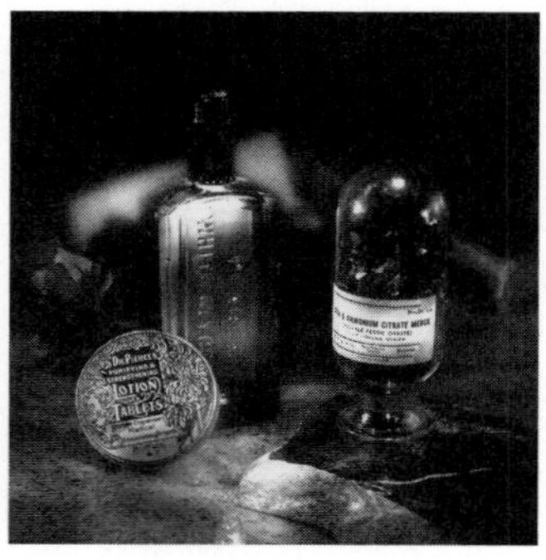

UNIT 20

Miscellaneous Agents

The items in this photograph include Dr. Pierces Lotion Tablets, a cobalt bottle of Pearl's White Glycerine, and a pharmacy display bottle. Dr. Pierces tablets were crushed and dissolved in hot water to make an antiseptic lotion. The Iron & Ammonium Citrate Merck pharmacy bottle is an inverted show bottle that was used to display chemicals. At the turn of the century, many pharmacists displayed these bottles in their prescription areas.

Detailed Contents

Chapter 1

Orientation to Pharmacology

Chapter Focus

To safely administer medications and educate clients and caregivers to effectively manage a therapeutic drug regimen nurses need to understand and apply the principles of pharmacology. The chapter will focus on the historical development of pharmacology as a science for the improvement of health, its terminology, and the scope of nursing practice associated with pharmacology. The following objectives and key terms are important for a good understanding of the chapter.

Key Terms

chemical name (p. 3)
collaborative problems (p. 8)
dosage (p. 8)
drug (p. 3)
generic name (p. 3)
indications (p. 8)
mechanism of action (p. 8)
nonprescription or over-the-counter (OTC) drug (p. 3)
pharmacokinetics (p. 8)
pharmacopeia (p. 2)
pregnancy safety (p. 8)
prescription drug or legend drug (p. 3)
side effects/adverse reactions (p. 8)
trade name or brand name (p. 3)

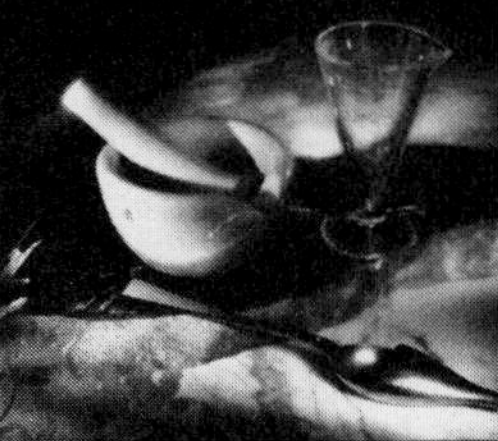

Objectives

1. Define key terms used in pharmacology.
2. Cite significant historical events in the development of pharmacology.
3. Describe the difference between chemical, generic, and trade names of drug products.
4. Differentiate between alkaloid, glycoside, gum, resin, and oil.
5. Name four main sources of drug and biologic products.
6. Identify authoritative sources for drug information.
7. Identify the scope of nursing responsibilities related to pharmacology.
8. Correlate the steps of the nursing process with the study of pharmacology.

Pharmacology is a science that studies drug effects within a living system. It deals with all drugs used in society today, legal or illegal, including street, prescription, and nonprescription or over-the-counter medications. The pharmacologic agents available today have controlled, prevented, cured, and in a few instances, eradicated disease. The result has been an improved quality of life and, perhaps, extension of the life span.

But medications can also potentially harm the client, which is reflected by the fact that the term "pharmaceutical" is actually derived from the Greek word for poison (Siler et al, 1982). Therefore the nurse should understand thoroughly any medication before giving it to a client. The nurse must know the usual dose; route of administration; indication(s); significant side effects and adverse reactions; major drug interactions; contraindications; and appropriate nursing assessment, planning, implementation, and evaluation techniques necessary to safely administer the drug.

A number of terms are fundamental to the knowledge base of nurses. The lists of key terms that are essential for nurses to understand are at the beginning of this chapter and future chapters along with the pages on which the definitions may be found.

HISTORICAL TRENDS

Since the beginning of time, people have searched for substances to treat illness and cure disease. The oldest prescriptions known were found on a clay tablet written by a Sumerian physician about 3000 BC, or nearly 5000 years ago.

Primitive people through the Egyptian period believed that disease was caused by evil spirits living in the body. Asclepias, who lived between 600 and 700 BC, was considered to be the principal Greek god of healing. He combined religion and healing in a temple setting, and his large family represented health or medical ideology. For example, his wife Epione soothed pain; daughter Hygeia, the goddess of health, represented the prevention of disease; and Panacea, another daughter, represented treatment. His large temple settings were used to treat both the rich and poor to cure their illnesses.

Hippocrates (fifth century BC) advanced the idea that disease resulted from natural causes and could only be understood through a study of natural laws. He believed the body had recuperative powers and saw the health care provider's role as assisting the recuperative process. Called the Father of Medicine, Hippocrates influenced the principles that control the practice of medicine today.

The fall of the Roman Empire marked the beginning of the medieval period (400 to 1580 AD). Germanic barbarians overran Western Europe, which reverted to a medicine of folklore and tradition similar to that of the Greeks before Hippocrates. At the same time, Christian religious orders built monasteries that became sites for all learning, including pharmacy and medicine. They aided the sick and needy with food, rest, and medicinals from their monastery gardens. The Arabs' interest in medicine, pharmacy, and chemistry was reflected in the hospitals and schools they built, the many new drugs they contributed, and their formulation of the first set of drug standards.

In 1240 AD Emperor Frederick II declared pharmacy to be separate from medicine but pharmacy was not truly established separately until the sixteenth century, when Valerius Cordus wrote the first pharmacopeia as an authoritative standard. A **pharmacopeia** is the total of all authorized drugs available within a country, containing descriptions, recipes, strengths, standards of purity, and dosage forms for the drugs.

Paracelsus (1493 to 1541), professor of physics and surgery at Basel, denounced "humoral pathology" and substituted the idea that diseases were actual entities to be combated with specific remedies. He improved pharmacy and therapeutics for succeeding centuries, introducing new remedies and reducing the overdosing so prevalent in that period.

In the seventeenth and eighteenth centuries great progress was made in pharmacy and chemistry. The first London pharmacopeia appeared in 1618 and many preparations introduced then are still in use today, including opium tincture, coca, and ipecac. The first important national pharmacopeia was the French *Codex* (1818), followed by the *United States' Pharmacopeia* in 1820, Great Britain in 1864, and Germany in 1872. See Box 1-1 for a summary of major drug discoveries.

The study of accurate dosages in the nineteenth century led to the establishment of large-scale manufacturing plants to produce drugs. Drug dosages and knowledge of their expected action became more precise. Rational medicine had begun to replace empiricism. As we approach the twenty-first century, dramatic changes are occurring to reform the health care systems in the United States and Canada. The emphasis on providing quality health care in a more cost-effective manner is leading to a redefinition of professional roles and decision-making responsibilities among health professionals (Blumengold, 1995; McCombs, et al, 1995). An integrated health care delivery team is evolving, a team that centers on client-focused care that at a minimum includes assessment, planning, monitoring, client counseling, accountability for therapeutic outcomes, and client advocacy. A health promotion focus and managed care approaches will require changes in professional education. As drug therapy is the mainstay in the application of restorative and rehabilitative care, the nurse needs to have a solid foundation in pharmacology.

As a result of the current and projected trends, the health care consumer will be asking for more information; one of the persons most often questioned is the nurse. Nurses in all practice roles and settings need to understand the therapeutic uses and potential for injury of prescription, over-the-counter, and illicit drugs. Nursing roles, which include the administration of medications in health care agencies, community, and home care settings, client teaching for safe and effective self-administration of medications, and the detection of drug-related problems require nurses to be well prepared with comprehensive and current knowledge (Naegle, 1994). Nurses will take on greater responsibility for profes-

BOX 1-1

Summary of Major Drug Discoveries

Drug	Time period	Comments
opium tincture, coca (cocaine), and ipecac	17th century	Important drugs, still used today
digitalis	1785	Cardiac medication, source of cardiac glycosides (digoxin, digitoxin)
smallpox vaccine	1796	Important vaccine in its time; now smallpox has been eradicated worldwide
morphine	1815	Most important analgesic derived from opium; used to treat severe pain
quinine, atropine, and codeine	19th century	Still available for use today
ether and chloroform	1840s	First general anesthetics; rare or obsolete today
insulin	1922	Most important discovery for treatment of diabetes mellitus
penicillin	mid-1940s	Revolutionized treatment of microbial infections; precursor of many other antibiotics
cortisone	1949	Important hormone from adrenal gland cortex; also synthetically prepared
polio vaccines	1955, 1961	Discovery of inactivated and live oral poliovirus vaccine were very significant in eliminating polio epidemics
oral contraceptives	late 1950s	Chemicals similar to natural estrogen or progesterone hormones that have been used by millions of women worldwide
antivirals	mid-1970s	Useful for the prophylaxis and treatment of viral diseases

sional judgment in the administration and supervision of drug therapy, and in advanced roles, prescriptive authority. Therefore, nurses must know about and use drug information to better care for their clients. This nursing activity is made more complex by the knowledge that a single drug may bear many names.

NAMES OF DRUGS

A **drug** is any substance used in the diagnosis, cure, treatment, or prevention of a disease or condition. As a drug passes through the investigational stages before it is approved and marketed, it collects three different types of names. The first is the chemical name, second is the generic or nonproprietary name, and the third is the trade or proprietary name.

The **chemical name** is a precise description of the drug's chemical composition and molecular structure. It is particularly meaningful to the chemist. For example, the chemical name of a popular analgesic is *N*-(4-hydroxyphenyl) acetamide. Its generic name is acetaminophen, and it is also sold under a number of brand or trade names—Tylenol, Tempra, and Datril, among others.

The **generic** or **nonproprietary name** is often assigned by the manufacturer with the approval of the United States Adopted Name Council (USAN). Since the generic name is simpler than the chemical name, it is the official name listed in official compendiums, such as *The United States Pharmacopeia.* When drug companies market a particular drug product, they often select and copyright a **trade, brand,** or **proprietary name** for their drug. This copyright restricts the use of the name to only the individual drug company. Since numerous brand names may exist for the same ingredient, such as for acetaminophen, prescribers are encouraged to use the generic name. The use of generic names is also widely advocated to avoid confusion between trade names that are similar.

With some exceptions, the majority of generic drug products sold are considered therapeutically equivalent to the brand name product. In addition, such generic products are often much less expensive than the brand name drug.

To encourage physician prescribing and promote sales of the trade name drug, extensive advertising is usually necessary. This expense is borne mainly by the consumer. However, much of the research in new drugs is done in laboratories of reputable drug firms. To realize a legitimate return for the cost of research, drug companies need to patent their products and have exclusive rights to their manufacture and sale for a specified time period.

The brand, trade, or proprietary name of drugs discussed in this book will be found enclosed in parentheses following the generic name.

In addition, a drug may be considered a **prescription drug** or a **legend drug,** which means it requires a legal prescription in order to be dispensed; or it may be a **nonprescription** or **over-the-counter** (**OTC**) **drug,** a drug which may be purchased without a prescription. Some prescription drugs may be purchased in lower dosages that are considered to be relatively safe for sale, over the counter. Such a drug is ibuprofen. It is sold as an OTC in its 200 mg strength as Advil or Motrin IB, but requires a prescription for the 300, 400, 600, or 800 mg tablet.

SOURCES OF DRUGS

Drugs and biologic products have been identified or derived from four main sources: (1) plants, examples of which are digitalis, vincristine, and colchicine; (2) animals and humans, from which drugs such as epinephrine, insulin, and ACTH are obtained; (3) minerals or mineral products, such as iron, iodine, and Epsom salts; and (4) synthetic or chemical substances made in the laboratory. The drugs made of chemical substances are pure drugs, and some of them are simple substances, such as sodium bicarbonate and magnesium hydroxide. Others are products of complex synthesis, such as the sulfonamides and the adrenocorticosteroids.

Active constituents of plant drugs. The leaves, roots, seeds, and other parts of plants may be dried or otherwise processed for use as a medicine and, as such, are known as crude drugs. Their therapeutic effect is produced by the chemical substances they contain. When the pharmacologically active constituents are separated from the crude preparation, the resulting substances are more potent and usually produce effects more reliably than does the crude drug. Some of the types of pharmacologically active compounds found in plants, grouped according to their physical and chemical properties, are alkaloids, glycosides, gums, and oils.

1. *Alkaloids* are organic compounds that are alkaline in nature and are chemically combined with acids in the laboratory to form water-soluble salts, such as morphine sulfate and atropine sulfate. Synthetic alkaloids formulated in the laboratory have activity similar to that of plant alkaloids.
2. *Glycosides* are active plant substances that, on hydrolysis, yield a sugar plus one or more additional active substances. The sugar is believed to increase the solubility, absorption, permeability, and cellular distribution of the glycoside. An important cardiac glycoside used in medicine is digoxin.
3. *Gums* are plant exudates. When water is added, some of them will swell and form gelatinous masses. Others remain unchanged in the gastrointestinal tract, where they act as hydrophilic (water-attracting) colloids; they absorb water, form watery bulk, and exert a laxative effect. Agar and psyllium seeds are examples of natural laxative gums, while methylcellulose and sodium carboxymethylcellulose are synthetic colloids. Gums are also used to soothe irritated skin and mucous membranes.
4. *Oils* are highly viscous liquids and are generally of two kinds, volatile or fixed. A volatile oil imparts an aroma to a plant; because of their pleasant odor and taste, these oils were frequently used as flavoring agents. Peppermint and clove oil are examples of volatile oils occasionally used in medicine. Fixed oils are generally greasy and do not evaporate easily, unlike volatile oils. Olive oil is a fixed oil used in cooking, while castor oil is an example of a fixed oil used in medicine.

DRUG CLASSIFICATION

Drug classification can be approached from two perspectives, by clinical indication or by body system. This book uses both approaches where appropriate. Examples of drugs classified by clinical indication include:

- Chapter 38—Mucokinetic and Bronchodilator Drugs
- Chapter 60—Antifungal and Antiviral Drugs

An example of drugs classified by body system is:

- Unit Five—Drugs Affecting the Central Nervous System

These drug groupings can assist the nurse to understand and learn about the individual agents available for drug therapy. Pharmacology becomes easier when one understands the common characteristics of each drug classification and when a *key* or *prototype* drug within each group is studied thoroughly. When a new drug becomes available, the nurse will then be able to associate it with its drug classification and make inferences about many of its basic qualities before reading about its specific properties. Learning which of its qualities are different from those of the prototype drug and its dosage is extremely helpful.

The basic information to be learned about each major drug includes its generic name and original trade name, the category to which it belongs, its clinical uses, its mechanism of action, side/adverse effects, and other specifics associated with the nurse's role in administration of, evaluation of, and client teaching about that drug. "Looking it up" should become second nature to the nursing student as well as the practicing nurse. *Nurses are professionally, morally, legally, and personally responsible for every dose of medication they administer.*

Sources of Drug Data

Any nursing process will be only as effective as the knowledge base and the analytic thought that go into it. Logic and judgment improve as the nurse's information base is perfected, partly as experience is tested against knowledge. Nowhere is ongoing self-learning more essential than in nursing pharmacotherapeutics. The "need to know" escalates, for example, when a nurse who is responsible for administering medications is confronted with an order for an unfamiliar drug or by an unexpected client symptom not usually associated with the diagnosis.

Realistically it is not possible to know everything about all medications on the market, even those that nurses use frequently. Therefore, knowing where to get essential information as it is required is important. Various reference sources exist, each with its own emphasis, yet most are not completely adequate alone to meet the specialized needs of nursing pharmacotherapeutics. See Table 1-1 for drug information resources.

TABLE 1-1 Drug information resources

Reference	Comments
American Hospital Formulary Service (AHFS) Drug Information (Bethesda, MD: American Society of Hospital Pharmacists, Inc.)	Objective overview in monograph form Comprehensive source of comparative, unbiased drug information on nearly every available drug in U.S. Issues supplements; updated annually Widely used drug information source for all health care professionals
United States Pharmacopeia Dispensing Information (USP DI) (Rockville, MD: U.S. Pharmacopeial Convention)	Available in several volumes; Volume I for health care professionals, Volume II offers advice for patient in lay language Consists of extensive drug monographs with practical information Highlights clinically significant information to reduce drug risks Issues monthly updates; updated annually Highly recommended drug reference for all health care professionals
Physicians' Desk Reference (PDR) (Oradell, NJ: Medical Economics)	Widely used source for physicians Pharmaceutical industry finances the book Drug information same as drug package insert Lacks comparative information on safety and efficacy Lacks nursing information Has drug product identification section and manufacturers' addresses and phone numbers
Physicians GenRx (St Louis, MO: Mosby)	Comprehensive drug information Contains drug product identification charts Includes product ratings (equivalent, not equivalent classifications) from FDA Has drug costs comparisons Published annually
Drug Facts and Comparisons (St Louis, MO: Facts and Comparisons, Inc.)	Loose leaf edition updated monthly Comprehensive drug information arranged to facilitate comparisons and evaluations Contains package sizes and strengths plus cost index information Has manufacturers' addresses and phone numbers Has section for orphan drugs, diagnostic aids, radiopaque agents, antidotes, and drugs in development Widely used reference source, especially for pharmacists
Drug Newsletter The Medical Letter (New York: The Medical Letter, Inc.)	Biweekly newsletter with evaluation of the efficacy, safety, rationale, and price comparison of current medications Objective summaries Valuable newsletter, highly recommended
Handbook of Nonprescription Drugs (Washington, DC: American Pharmaceutical Association)	Comprehensive over-the-counter (OTC) drug information Each chapter reviews physiology, the primary minor illnesses, and the drugs used in treatment Has tables with specific OTC drug information
Various drug handbooks for nurses	Gives brief overviews of drugs in outline format Helpful as a quick refresher on the unit to remind nurse of important points once nurse has had a course in pharmacology Drug information is formatted according to the nursing process; give nursing considerations
Computerized pharmacology databases	Available in some health agencies Allow for drug information to be printed for clients to have for personal use Some systems allow for individualization of information for clients

Other Drug Information Sources

Drug information centers are located throughout the United States to disseminate information about the clinical uses of drugs and related equipment. Both general and specific information can be obtained, with advice based on scientific literature. These centers are often located within large medical center settings. Many difficult pharmacologic questions related to client care can be dealt with quickly by contacting the nearest drug information center. In addition, drug manufacturers, package inserts, and pharmacists are usually available to provide similar information.

Agencies frequently furnish similar sources of information. The area or unit where a nurse works often has a card file of package inserts; ideally, a nursing library shelf on each floor contains pharmacology information and other material of interest. Any nurse can initiate the development of such material and request funds or supplies. The agency's nursing staff development department is responsible for promoting ongoing and updated learning and can facilitate audiovisual aids, references, or a seminar program. Building a personal library and maintaining its currency are also important professional activities.

No text is a complete source of all the pharmacology information necessary for nursing practice. The nurse must gather reliable information from various sources to meet clinical needs.

THE SCOPE OF NURSING MANAGEMENT OF DRUG THERAPY

Drugs can help or harm. Nurses, physicians, and clinical pharmacists are held legally responsible for safe and therapeutically effective drug administration. Specifically, nurses are liable for their actions and omissions and for those duties they delegate to others, who may include medication technicians, pharmacy technicians, practical nurses, or even physicians. They are personally responsible—legally, morally, and ethically—for every drug they administer or have administered, no matter who actually prescribed it. Indeed, all members of a health team may be held liable for a single injury to a client. The increase in litigation against nurses and physicians indicates that society tolerates only a minimal margin of error in relation to human injury and life. Claims have been brought against health professionals for drug errors that caused loss of life and permanent injury. When claims against health professionals are supported with evidence that the conduct of one or more health professionals helped to bring about the loss or injury, those parties may be held liable. The law, a legal and social norm, requires health professionals to be safe and competent practitioners and permits compensation to those harmed or injured.

However, the law is a protective force for the knowledgeable, competent, and responsible nurse. Nurses who are determined to safeguard clients from drug-induced harm will, for example:

- Use correct techniques and precautions
- Observe and chart drug effects explicitly
- Keep their knowledge base current
- Refer to authoritative sources in professional literature and to physicians, pharmacists, and other colleagues
- Question a drug order that is unclear or that appears to contain an error
- Refuse to administer or refuse to allow others to order or administer a drug if there is reason to believe it will be harmful

The law, in turn, protects such nurses from unfair litigation. Chapter 2 discusses the legal role of the nurse related to drug therapy in greater detail.

Much remains to be learned about the actual mode of action of many commonly prescribed drugs, as well as effects from prolonged use. Furthermore, there is increasing concern about drug-induced disease. Fortunately, drug therapy for most conditions or for illness prevention is temporary. However, some diseases require lifelong use of drugs to sustain life (such as insulin for diabetes mellitus) or prolonged use to maintain relatively normal physiologic or psychologic functioning (such as phenobarbital for seizure disorders).

Nurses are entrusted with potent and habit-forming drugs, and they must not abuse or misuse this trust. Used respectfully and intelligently, drugs are comforting and lifesaving. Used unwisely or with undue dependence, they can lead to tragedy. The nurse who combines diligent and intelligent observation with moral integrity and factual knowledge is a safe and competent practitioner and a credit to the nursing profession.

In addition, the nurse must establish with the client a "therapeutic alliance," a respectful and trusting relationship to facilitate the highest level of self-care attainable. The client is the most important participant in the team effort for safe and effective drug administration. Clients are not expected to be submissive, acquiescent, and unquestioning followers of the health team's instructions, but must be motivated to assume responsibility for their own care; nurses must recognize that the willingness to participate is ultimately the client's. All the nurse's knowledge, skill, and ability are brought to bear on the establishment of a therapeutic alliance to facilitate the most appropriate level of self-care related to medications.

Close attention to all drugs the nurse administers helps the nurse learn to identify them, tailor their application, and spot errors before they occur. Expertise is built in just this fashion. Learning names of drugs, their formulations, and their pharmacologic actions is best done in small increments and in a systematic way by making associations between information about a known drug in a classification, its close analogues, and clients for whom the nurse has provided care. The learning value of analysis and synthesis of these data in actual practice far outweighs that of memorizing long lists of unrelated drugs and their properties.

Nurses in emergency departments and in community health practices are frequently challenged to identify medications from clients' personal unlabeled pill boxes or containers. Often many varieties of drugs and pieces of tablets are mixed together. Clients are often unable to assist in identification of their drugs, having never been properly educated by health care providers. The *Physicians' Desk Reference,* the *USP DI,* and the *Physicians GenRx* provide actual photographs of drugs, which will assist the nurse in making visual identification. In addition, manufacturers often place letters or numbers constituting an identification code on their solid oral dosage forms. Although these markings may not be meaningful to the practicing nurse, pharmacists and local drug information centers can provide assistance in the identification of generic and trade products from them. Difficult identification problems may be referred to the FDA Drug Listing Branch or the FDA Division of Poison Control, both in Rockville, Maryland.

Pharmacology applies knowledge from many different disciplines, including anatomy and physiology, pathology, microbiology, organic chemistry and biochemistry, mathematics, anthropology, psychology, and sociology. Thus clinical drug therapy can be considered an applied science. The thousands of drugs available would present a formidable study if they had to be approached as individual agents. Fortunately drugs can be systematically classified into a reasonable number of drug groups based on chemical, pharmacologic, or therapeutic relatedness.

Understanding the characteristic effects of a particular class of drugs at the subcellular, tissue, organ, and functional system levels permits a student or practitioner to extrapolate information to a wide variety of drugs. A typical representative drug can be selected and studied and its specific characteristics compared with those of others in the same class. Gradually the individual builds a knowledge base.

Lists of drugs, dosages, and their indications should not be regarded as dogma. Laboratory research and new scientific methods of evaluation are constantly generating new information. Occasionally there are reports that a drug, even an old and trusted one, is suspected of causing mutations, birth defects, cancer, or less serious secondary effects. Not only nursing students but also practicing nurses are challenged by the proliferation of drugs; most of the drugs on the market today were developed recently. Change is the only constant in pharmacology.

Pharmacology books must be kept up-to-date in the nurse's library. In addition, official current literature on drugs must be followed carefully, since new drugs only slowly make their way into more permanent literature. For the nurse working in a hospital or home health service, physicians, instructors, in-service educators, and pharmacists will be on hand to help. In a more isolated practice, greater personal effort will be required to maintain currency. In any case, nurses must pay close attention to the drug therapy of their clients.

Learning is an active process. Therefore clinical experience with drugs is invaluable, for it enables the student to:

- Note which drugs are most commonly used to treat certain diseases or specific signs and symptoms
- Note the frequency with which certain drugs are administered
- Observe which drugs are most effective in relieving particular signs and symptoms
- Witness individual differences in clients' reactions to a specific drug
- Relate knowledge obtained from authoritative sources to real-life situations

Regardless of what is to be learned, reasoning and the ability to analyze and synthesize information are prerequisites to understanding. These cognitive skills, along with perceptual skills, permit a student to see meaningful relationships, make comparisons, and determine significance, all of which are essential for sound decision making in nursing.

THE NURSING PROCESS AND DRUG ADMINISTRATION

The *nursing process* is a systematic method for identifying actual or potential health care problems or impediments to the activities of daily living. It points the way to rational nursing actions and objective evaluation of care.

The direction of the nursing process is fairly universal in the field, although its structure may vary from the widely used pattern of four phases or steps: (1) assessment of data (which may culminate in a nursing diagnosis), (2) planning, (3) implementation, and (4) evaluation.

To apply the nursing process to drug therapy, nurses *assess* the medication needs of their clients partly in terms of how these needs are matched by the prescriber's orders. The result of this assessment by the nurse is the nursing diagnosis. Nurses make *plans,* which include goals that directly relate to the client's *nursing diagnoses* and specific outcome criteria. The stage is then set for *implementation* of the goals, using specific, rationale-based nursing actions. Such actions may include: *monitoring* the client for therapeutic and nontherapeutic effects of the drug and ability to manage the therapeutic regimen; *intervention* related to the preparation and administration of a medication as ordered, or they might include steps to withhold a dose and obtain a change in the medication order, as well as *client education,* for the safe and accurate self-administration of the drug. The final step is the *evaluation* of the nursing care provided based upon the level of achievement of the outcome criteria for which the client and nurse have planned. Each time nursing care is evaluated, nurses' knowledge bases increase and become more valuable. The nursing process is discussed in more detail in Unit 2, The Nursing Process and Pharmacology.

GOALS OF THIS TEXT

This text orients the reader to nursing pharmacology and therapeutics by presenting a firm theoretic foundation and a practical approach to drug therapy applicable in many settings—the home, the clinic, the extended care facility, the office, the classroom, and the hospital.

Part One provides general principles, theories, and facts about drugs and their administration. Practical information is presented on the integration of the nursing process with pharmacology, and general principles of action are given to facilitate a student nurse's learning in both academic and clinical environments. The rest of the book presents specific drug information about clinical applications and nursing management. Thus this book can be used both as a text and as a reference.

To find information about a particular drug in this book:

1. Look it up in the index.
2. When you find the information about the drug, refer back to the beginning of the chapter or unit and read the material that precedes the specific discussion.

Reading only the pages listed in the index for the drug will illuminate only the drug's specifics, out of context and without necessary fundamental information about that class of drugs. Reading the background information offers an overall view and places the drug information into an understandable framework.

One of the more effective ways to study pharmacology is to understand the pharmacologic characteristics of a classification of drugs: its major uses; mechanisms of action; absorption, distribution, metabolism, and excretion; onset and duration of action; and adverse reactions. Throughout the book, key drugs are highlighted with the symbol ▲. These drugs can be studied as representatives of the drug classification under discussion. Other drugs within the classification can be identified then in the manner in which they differ from the prototype. This approach will enhance learning rather than the rote memorization of a multiplicity of facts about each and every drug.

The specific drug information in the text summarizes what is needed to administer drugs safely and competently. Each discussion is titled with some of the common names by which the particular drug is known. The trade names of drugs that are available in Canada but not in the United States are followed by a maple leaf symbol (🍁).

The **mechanism of action** section explains how the drug acts at the biochemical or cellular level to produce its therapeutic effects. The officially approved therapeutic purpose of the drug or the conditions for which it is used are detailed as **indications.** The **pharmacokinetics** section specifies how the drug is absorbed, distributed, associated with tissue, biotransformed or metabolized, and excreted. The section titled **side effects/adverse reactions** details most of the common secondary effects that may be experienced when the drug is administered. The **dosage** presents currently approved regimen governing the size, frequency, and number of doses of a therapeutic agent. It must be noted that not all drugs have been tested for safety and efficacy in administration to the elderly, pregnant women, women who are breastfeeding, or children. Routes and special techniques for drug preparation are also listed here in each monograph. The **pregnancy safety** section in each monograph lists the FDA pregnancy safety category that indicates the documented problems with the use of a drug during pregnancy.

Nursing Management Sections

The nursing management sections describe distinctive nursing measures:

Assessment: data gathering about an individual's experience with medications, identifying preexisting medical conditions that might influence the choice of dosage of drug, and/or concurrent drugs that might cause significant interactions, as well as baseline observations that are essential by which to measure changes in the client's health status during the medication regimen or determine whether administration of the drug is appropriate.

Nursing diagnoses: identification of selected nursing diagnoses that nurses, by virtue of their education and experience, are able and licensed to treat, as well as **collaborative problems,** which are physiologic complications that nurses monitor to detect their onset or changes in status (Carpenito, 1995).

Planning is an important step in the nursing process. However, to prevent redundancies within each drug monograph, modifications to administration of the drug will be found in the intervention section and the outcome criteria will be discussed in the evaluation section.

Implementation: incorporates nursing activities of monitoring, intervention, and education, which need to be planned in order to safely and accurately administer a specific drug.

Monitoring: significant observations relative to the client's health status, including diagnostic and laboratory tests, that ensure a safe and effective drug regimen.

Intervention: special handling, timing of doses, and other significant aspects of the actual administration of a drug.

Education: client teaching to enable the client and/or caregiver to effectively manage the therapeutic medication regimen at home.

Evaluation: provides the planned outcome criteria for reviewing care of the client in regard to safe and effective drug therapy.

Safe, therapeutically effective drug administration is a major responsibility of nurses. It depends on sound, current knowledge of medications and careful monitoring of their effects on clients. With increasingly shorter lengths of stay by clients in acute care settings, nurses have an increasing responsibility to ensure that clients and caregivers can effectively manage the medication regimen at home. Ongoing laboratory and clinical research modifies and enlarges available drug information, necessitating continual effort to keep one's knowledge up-to-date. The modes of action of many commonly prescribed drugs, effects of their prolonged use, and the possibility of drug-induced disease are yet to be completely understood. There are many sources of current drug information, but even the most diligent student of these sources requires clinical experience to develop competence in drug administration. Few areas of nursing demand more intellectual curiosity, integrity, factual knowledge, and motivation to use reference sources.

SUMMARY

Pharmacology, the study of drug effects within a living system, has held importance for humanity through the ages, since it has always been linked to our concept of health and illness.

Each drug is identified by three names: chemical; generic (nonproprietary), generally a simplification of the chemical name; and trade, brand, or proprietary name, under which the pharmaceutical company markets the drug. Because generic drugs are less expensive than trade name drugs, most states allow pharmacists to substitute them for trade name drugs within limitations.

Plants, animals and humans, minerals, and chemical substances are the four sources of drugs. Pharmacologically active compounds derived from plants are alkaloids, glycosides, gums, resins, and oils.

Drugs are classified either by clinical indication or by body system. Drug classifications facilitate the nurse's understanding of pharmacology by allowing the conceptualization of the common characteristics of each grouping and prototype drug and the association of new drugs with a classification as these drugs become available.

Pharmacology is a field of ever-increasing importance for nursing. Because nurses are held by law to be responsible for the drugs that they administer, they should maintain a current knowledge base and be competent in the assessment, planning, implementation, and evaluation of the client's nursing care. The goal of this text is to assist the learner to achieve that knowledge and competence within pharmacology.

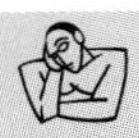

Critical Thinking

1. Why is the study of pharmacology important for nurses? Think of three clinical examples that would indicate its importance to the care of clients.
2. Review the structure of one of the later chapters in the text that discusses a classification of drugs. Consider how you might go about studying for an exam on that chapter.
3. A nurse in the process of administering medications is confronted with a prescriber's order for a drug with which he or she is not familiar. What sources of drug information could he or she utilize?

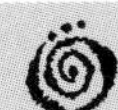

Collaborative Learning Activities

1. Each student will be assigned a different drug by its generic name. Each student will seek information about that drug using the resources for drug information available to them within the health agency in which they are practicing. Compare and contrast the advantages and disadvantages of the various resources and discuss clinical situations for which each of the resources might be the best to consult.

BIBLIOGRAPHY

Anderson KL, et al. (Eds.) (1994). *Mosby's medical, nursing, & allied health dictionary* (4th ed.). St Louis: Mosby.

Atkinson LD & Murray ME (1995). *Clinical guide to care planning: Data to diagnosis*. New York: McGraw-Hill.

Blumengold JG (1995). Strategic and financial considerations for integrated health care delivery, *Medical Interface* 8 (5):77-79,83,85.

Carpenito LJ (1995). *Nursing care plans and documentation: Nursing diagnoses and collaborative problems* (2nd ed.). Philadelphia: JB Lippincott.

Carpenito LJ (1995). *Nursing diagnosis: Application to clinical practice* (6th ed.). Philadelphia: JB Lippincott.

Leake CD (1975). *An historical account of pharmacology to the twentieth century*. Springfield, IL: Charles C Thomas.

Lyons AS & Petrucelli RJ II (1978). *Medicine: An illustrated history*. New York: Harry N Abrams.

McCombs JS, Nichol MB, Johnson KA, et al. (1995). Is pharmacy's vision of the future too narrow? *Am J Health-Syst Pharm* 52(11): 1208-1214.

Naegle MA (1994). Prescription drugs and nursing education: Knowledge gaps and implications for role performance, *J Law Med & Ethics* 22(3):257-261.

O'Donnell J (1994). Drug therapy: 20 ways your role will change, *Nursing* 24 (3):46-48.

Olin BR (Ed.) (1996). *Facts and comparisons*. Philadelphia: JB Lippincott.

Roger FB (1972). *A syllabus of medical history*. Boston: Little, Brown.

Siler WA, et al. (1982). *Death by prescription*. Tallahassee, FL: Rose Publishing.

United States Pharmacopeial Convention (1996). *USP DI: Drug information for the health care professional* (16th ed.). Rockville, MD: The Convention.

Chapter 2

Legal and Ethical Aspects of Medication Administration

Chapter Focus

As the professional role has grown in nursing, nurses have become more autonomous in their practice. With autonomy has come a growing legal accountability. Nurses need to consider this responsibility as they practice. But even the law and the technologic advances in health care are not sufficient to cope with many of the ethical dilemmas facing nurses. This chapter will discuss the legal foundations and ethical considerations for the use of drugs. The following objectives and key terms are important for a good understanding of this chapter.

Key Terms

assay (p. 18)
beneficence (p. 26)
bioassay (p. 18)
controlled substances (p. 12)
Controlled Substances Act (p. 12)
Five Rights of Medication Administration (p. 25)
informed consent (p. 20)
International Narcotics Control Board (p. 19)
LD_{50} (p. 19)
negative drug formulary (p. 15)
nonmalfeasance (p. 26)
Nuremburg Code (p. 20)
product liability (p. 14)
Pure Food and Drug Act (p. 11)
therapeutic index (p. 19)

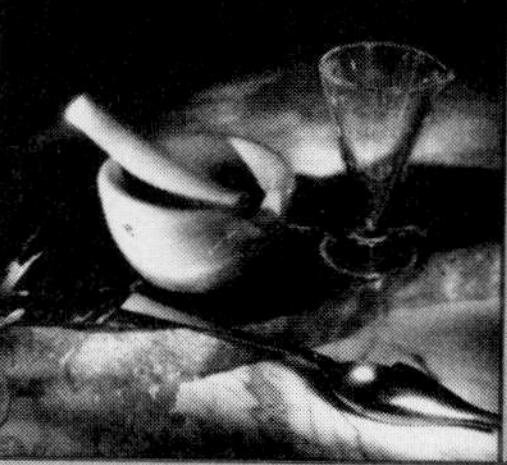

Objectives

1. Identify the process used in the development and evaluation of a new drug before marketing.
2. Differentiate between over-the-counter (OTC) and prescription drugs.
3. Describe the procedure for evaluation of OTC drugs and prescription drugs for safety and effectiveness.
4. Identify legislative or authoritative source(s) for drug standards.
5. Describe the difference between permissive and mandatory drug substitution in the United States.
6. Describe the FDA pregnancy categories for drugs.
7. Discuss the nurse's role in drug research.
8. Discuss the changing nursing roles related to drug administration.
9. Discuss ethical issues involved in the administration of medications.

Many remedies of the past lacked the information we take for granted today, such as the strength of the substance in a preparation or even the ingredients themselves. This type of medical practice, although not always ineffective, extended well into the nineteenth century. Not until the twentieth century were standards for drug identification, drug preparation, and proof of drug effectiveness and safety required.

UNITED STATES DRUG LEGISLATION

Before 1906 patent medicines and remedies were sold by medicine men in traveling wagon shows, in drugstores, by mail order, and by doctors, real or self-titled. Such products were not required to list ingredients on the label, so many contained potent and dangerous drugs such as opium, morphine, heroin, chloral hydrate, and alcohol. Many persons (especially infants) were reportedly injured, became addicted, or died as a result of the ingredients contained in these preparations.

In 1906 the first U.S. law, the federal **Pure Food and Drug Act,** was passed to protect the public from adulterated or mislabeled drugs. The law required the drug company to declare on the package label the presence of any of 11 identified dangerous and perhaps addictive drugs (some of which were in the list just mentioned). This first law had loopholes that were used by the patent medicine dealers for their own gain. For example:

1. False and misleading claims about the curative value of the product were not allowed *on the package*, which was described as a bottle, label, or wrapper that encircled the bottle. Claims made in advertisements, newspapers, or drug almanacs, by word of mouth, or on signs in store windows were not covered under the law. Unscrupulous nostrum dealers took full advantage of this oversight.
2. Serial numbers were required for products containing any of the 11 dangerous drugs, and each label was to bear the words "Guaranteed under the Food and Drugs Act." This meant that the dealer had registered his product and was legally responsible for it if it was improperly sold under this act. However, many patent medicine dealers implied that this was the government seal of approval. In response to this abuse, this clause was abolished in 1919.
3. Only drugs sold in interstate commerce (made in one state and sold to persons living in other states) were covered. Drugs made and sold within the same state did not fall under the jurisdiction of this law.

The Food and Drug Act of 1906 designated *The United States Pharmacopeia* and the *National Formulary* as official standards and empowered the federal government to enforce them. Drugs were required to comply with the standards of strength and purity professed for them, and labels had to indicate the kind and amount of morphine or other narcotic ingredients present. In 1912 Congress passed the Sherley Amendment, prohibiting use of fraudulent therapeutic claims.

A further update of the drug legislation occurred in 1938 with the passage of the federal Food, Drug, and Cosmetic Act. More than 100 deaths occurred in 1937 as a result of ingestion of a diethylene glycol solution of sulfanilamide. This preparation had been marketed as an "elixir of sulfanilamide" without investigation of its toxicity. Under the 1906 law the only charge that could be made against the drug company was mislabeling, since it was labeled an "elixir" and the drug failed to meet the definition of an elixir as an alcoholic solution. The 1938 act prevented the marketing of new drugs before they had been properly tested for safety.

The Durham-Humphrey Amendment of 1952 further changed the 1938 drug act as it specified how legend, or prescription, drugs and refills could be ordered and dispensed (Box 2-1). This amendment also recognized a second class of drugs, over-the-counter drugs (OTCs), for which prescriptions are not required.

In 1958 a U.S. Senate investigation into the drug industry was begun when it became known that drug companies were making huge profits and that some drug promotion was false or misleading. This investigation received little support until given impetus by the thalidomide tragedy, although for the United States it was more a might-have-been catastrophe than a real one. Thalidomide, a hypnotic marketed in Europe, was found to be responsible for severe deformities in babies whose mothers had taken the drug during the early stages of pregnancy. These events led to passage of the Kefauver-Harris Amendment in 1962.

The Kefauver-Harris Amendment required proof of both safety and efficacy before a new drug could be approved for use. This meant that all drugs introduced under the safety-only criteria in effect from 1938 to 1962 had to be evaluated. To do this the FDA signed a contract in 1966 with the National Academy of Sciences and the National Research Council (NAS/NRC) to study all supporting data for all therapeutic claims. This program of study was called the Drug Efficacy Study Implementation (DESI).

BOX 2-1

Prescription (Legend) Drugs

Legend drugs must bear the legend "Caution: Federal law prohibits dispensing without prescription." These include all drugs given by injection as well as the following:

1. Hypnotic, narcotic, or habit-forming drugs or derivatives thereof as specified in the law
2. Drugs that because of their toxicity or method of use, are not safe unless they are administered under the supervision of a licensed practitioner (physician, dentist, or nurse practitioner)
3. New drugs that are limited to investigational use or new drugs that are not considered safe for indiscriminate use by the public

Thousands of drugs and therapeutic claims have been evaluated and many ineffective drugs have been withdrawn from the market. Those rated as "possibly effective" or "probably effective" are being withdrawn or reformulated, although a drug may remain on the market while claims are being modified and scientific data collected to substantiate the claims. However, an approved drug can be prescribed for a disorder for which the drug has not been FDA approved. Informed consent for this nonresearch application of the drug is generally not required. (See Box 2-2 below for a summary of important legislation.)

Over-the-Counter Drug Review

Of the estimated 400,000 drug products marketed in the United States, more than 300,000 are OTC drugs (Covington, 1996). The 300,000 individual drug products contain approximately 700 to 1000 active ingredients. In 1972 the FDA assembled an advisory review panel to perform an ingredient review, asking primarily the following questions: are the ingredients safe and effective for consumers to self-medicate, and are the labeling, indications, dosage instructions, and warnings provided sufficient? If they were found lacking, appropriate recommendations had to be developed.

BOX 2-2

Important Drug Legislation (U.S.)

Food, Drug, and Cosmetic Act of 1938	Mandated that drug manufacturers must test all drugs for harmful effects and that drug labels must be accurate and complete
Wheeler-Lea Act of 1938	Defined criteria for nonfraudulent advertising
Durkham-Humphrey Amendment of 1952	Distinguished more clearly between drugs that can be sold with or without a prescription and those that cannot be refilled
Drug Amendment of 1962 (Kefauver-Harris Act)	Tightened controls over drug safety and statements about adverse reactions and contraindications; drug testing methods; and drug effectiveness criteria
Controlled Substances Act of 1970 (Comprehensive Drug Abuse Prevention and Control Act of 1970)	Categorized controlled substances based on their relative potential for abuse
Drug Regulation Reform Act of 1978	Shortened the drug investigation process to release drugs sooner to the public

This study, completed in 1983, found that approximately one third of the ingredients reviewed were safe and effective for labeled indications. Ingredients found particularly or potentially dangerous were either transferred to prescription status only (such as hexachlorophene, an antibacterial topical with a potential for inducing neurologic toxicities) or removed entirely from the market (such as camphorated oil or camphor liniment). See Chapter 11 for a discussion of OTC medications.

Prescription Drugs Switched to OTC Drug Status

The OTC review panels are primarily responsible for switching a number of prescription drugs to nonprescription or OTC status. These drug products are considered to be safe for self-treatment by consumers without professional guidance. Cimetidine (Tagamet HB), famotidine (Pepcid AC), diphenhydramine (Benadryl) and topical hydrocortisone, are examples of products switched from prescription to over-the-counter status.

Control of Opioids (Narcotics) and Other Dangerous Drugs

Narcotic and drug abuse laws. The Harrison Narcotic Act (1914) was the first federal law aimed at curbing drug addiction or dependence. This law not only established the word "narcotic" as a legal term but also regulated the importation, manufacture, sale, and use of opium and cocaine and all their compounds and derivatives. Marijuana and its derivatives were also included in this act, as were many synthetic analgesic drugs that proved to produce or sustain either physical or psychologic dependence.

This act and other drug abuse amendments now have only historical import, since they have been superseded by the Comprehensive Drug Abuse Prevention and Control Act of 1970*, also called the **Controlled Substances Act** (CSA), which became effective May 1, 1971. This law was designed to provide increased research into, and prevention of, drug abuse and drug dependence; to provide for treatment and rehabilitation of drug abusers and drug dependent persons; and to improve the administration and regulation of the manufacturing, distributing, and dispensing of **controlled substances** (drugs covered by this act, which are classified according to their use and abuse potential) by legitimate handlers of these drugs to help reduce their widespread dispersion into illicit markets.

The CSA classifies controlled substances solely according to their use and abuse potential. Drugs are classified into numbered levels, or schedules, from Schedule I to Schedule V (Table 2-1). Drugs with the highest abuse potential are placed in Schedule I; those with the lowest po-

*Current regulations can be obtained from the nearest Regional Director, Drug Enforcement Administration, or from the Drug Enforcement Administration, Department of Justice, Washington, DC, 20004.

TABLE 2-1 Schedule of controlled substances

Schedule	Characteristics	Dispensing restrictions	Examples
I	High abuse potential No accepted medical use—for research, analysis, or instruction only May lead to severe dependence	Approved protocol necessary	Heroin, marijuana (cannabis), tetrahydrocannabinols, LSD, mescaline, peyote, psilocybin, methaqualone
II	High abuse potential Accepted medical uses May lead to severe physical and/or psychologic dependence	Written Rx necessary (signed by the practitioner)—emergency verbal prescriptions must be confirmed in writing within 72 hours No Rx refills allowed Container must have warning label*	Opium, morphine, hydromorphone, meperidine, codeine, oxycodone, methadone, secobarbital, pentobarbital, dextroamphetamine, methylphenidate, cocaine, and others
III	Less abuse potential than Schedules I and II Accepted medical uses May lead to moderate/low physical dependence or high psychologic dependence	Written or oral Rx required Rx expires in 6 months No more than 5 Rx refills allowed within a 6-month period Container must have warning label*	Preparations containing limited opioid quantities, or combined with one or more active ingredients that are noncontrolled substances: acetaminophen with codeine, aspirin with codeine, etc. Also, paregoric, nandrolone, stanozolol, testosterone, etc.
IV	Lower abuse potential than Schedule III Accepted medical uses May lead to limited physical or psychologic dependence	Written or oral Rx required Rx expires in 6 months with no more than 5 Rx refills allowed Container must have warning label*	Phenobarbital, chloral hydrate, meprobamate, fenfluramine, chlordiazepoxide, diazepam, oxazepam, clorazepate, flurazepam, lorazepam, propoxyphene, pentazocine, mazindol, alprazolam, and others
V	Lower abuse potential than Schedule IV Accepted medical uses May lead to limited physical or psychologic dependence	May require written Rx or be sold without Rx (check state law)	Medications, generally for relief of coughs or diarrhea, containing limited quantities of certain opioid controlled substances Examples: terpin hydrate with codeine, etc.

From DEA pharmacist's manual—an informational outline of the Controlled Substances Act of 1970, U.S. Dept. of Justice, Washington, DC; Red Book, 1996.

*Caution: Federal law prohibits the transfer of this drug to any person other than the patient for whom it was prescribed.

tential for abuse are in Schedule V. These classifications are flexible because drugs may occasionally be added or changed from one schedule to another without new legislation. It might be anticipated, for example, that marijuana will be changed to another schedule if and when it is accepted for use in treating nausea associated with cancer chemotherapy or for treatment of glaucoma. Some drugs with potential for dependence, such as ethanol and certain analgesics, are not listed as controlled substances. Anyone handling controlled substances must follow the more inclusive or stringent requirements of the laws, federal or state.

In July 1973 the Drug Enforcement Administration (DEA), in the Department of Justice, became the nation's sole legal drug enforcement agency.

Possession of controlled substances. It is unlawful for any person to possess a controlled substance unless it has been obtained by a valid prescription or order or unless its possession is pursuant to actions in the course of professional practice. It is a federal offense to transfer a drug listed in Schedule II, III, or IV to any person other than the individual for whom the drug was ordered.

Drug suppliers and hospitals—as well as physicians, pharmacists, and nurses—are individually and collectively responsible for accounting for inventory and management of the flow and distribution of controlled substances. Institutional control of the flow of controlled substances is maintained by carefully recorded checks of the balance on hand, supplies added, and doses administered. The nurse responsible for stock supplies of controlled substances, the one who carries the keys to the "narcotics box," is required to perform actual counts of the doses of each controlled substance in the unit's stock at the beginning and end of each shift or workday. Completed documentation and high accountability are demanded of the nurses who do this counting as well as all who handle controlled substances during the work period. Thus each dose is accounted for as it is administered, discarded, wasted, or withheld. All doses of controlled substances should be kept in double-locked cabinets or other secure areas, with the keys in the custody of a designated nurse. Although these protocols may seem to entail a needless waste of time, they are necessary to safeguard the control of drug flow.

Additional Regulatory Bodies or Services

Food and Drug Administration. The Food and Drug Administration (FDA) is charged with the enforcement of the federal Food, Drug, and Cosmetic Act. Seizure of offending (improperly manufactured or packaged) goods and criminal prosecution of responsible persons or firms in federal courts are among the methods used to enforce the Act. In addition, pharmaceutical firms must report at regular intervals to the FDA all adverse effects associated with their new drugs.

The FDA also has an adverse-reaction reporting program. All health professionals are encouraged to relate an unusual occurrence or unusually high number of occurrences associated with a drug, its formulation, or packaging, and so forth. Communication may be made directly to the FDA by telephone or by completing a Drug Experience Report form. A response from the FDA will follow. The purpose of this program is to detect reactions that have not been revealed by previous clinical or pharmaceutical studies. Changes in the drug package insert may result, or in some instances the drug may be withdrawn from the market.

Public Health Service. The Public Health Service is part of the U.S. Department of Health and Human Services. One of this agency's many functions is the regulation of biologic products. This refers to viral preparations, serums, antitoxins, or analogous products that are used for the prevention, treatment, or cure of diseases. The Public Health Service exercises control over these products by inspecting and licensing the establishments that manufacture them and by examining and licensing the products as well.

Product liability. In a majority of the states the rule of strict manufacturer's liability has been adopted. This doctrine holds manufacturers liable for injuries caused by defects in their products, drugs, or devices. **Product liability** exists (1) if a product is defective or not fit for its reasonably foreseeable uses, (2) if the defect arose before the product left the control of the manufacturer, and (3) if the defect caused some person harm. If these three criteria are met, the manufacturer must pay money damages for harm unless the liability can be shifted to some other party. Anyone harmed by a defective product has the right to sue the manufacturer for compensation.

Manufacturers are legally responsible for knowing the effects of their products. If an unknown risk could have been discovered through a reasonable amount of research, the manufacturer will be held liable for any resulting harm. Since nurses are accountable, they will want to stay alert to defects in the drugs they administer. Despite manufacturers' quality assurance programs, drug products are susceptible to errors in the manufacturing, packaging, and delivery processes. Although detection of chemical defects is usually outside the nurse's province, detection of observable physical defects is not. Nurses should learn to be keenly aware of physical characteristics of the drugs they administer and make comparisons before administering them. For example, unusual discoloration, precipitates, other inconsistencies, or foreign bodies in parenteral fluids should be considered suspect. Such observations warrant withholding the drug and contacting the pharmacy department or other authoritative source. Recall of defective drugs is necessary to prevent client harm.

Occasionally, human error can be expected to cause the wrong medication to be dispensed from the pharmacy. Again, the nurse is responsible for every medication administered. In this case the nurse who administers the wrong drug and the pharmacist who labeled it may both be held liable for any resulting client harm. This liability has been sustained in the courts on several occasions. Helpful color photographs of many drug formulations can be found in the *Physicians' Desk Reference* and the *USP DI: Drug Information for the Health Care Professional.* Contact the pharmacist for verification and assistance or verification of any questionable medication.

Drug Substitution

Nearly every state has a drug substitution law that either permits or mandates substitution on the part of the pharmacist, although the prescriber retains the prerogative to require the dispensing of a particular brand of drug. In permissive states the prescriber must give express permission for substitution by either signing a special section on the prescription form or by checking the correct phrase on the prescription. If substitution is not wanted, the prescriber may note this by writing "dispense as written," "brand necessary," or "medically necessary."

In states with a mandatory law, the pharmacist is required to dispense approved, less expensive, generic drugs to the client. Several exceptions apply in such situations; for example, the consent of the client may be required before substitution, or the prescriber may mark the individual prescription with a term that prohibits substitution, such as "medically necessary." Some states, such as Florida, have enacted a **negative drug formulary,** a list of drugs that have a proven potential for different bioavailabilities or therapeutic problems and that may not be substituted for trade name drugs (see Box 2-3). If the prescriber orders a brand name for these products, then only that specific brand may be dispensed. If the prescriber orders any of these products by a generic name, then the pharmacist may select a generic drug product that is FDA approved—that is, a drug with an approved new drug application (NDA) or abbreviated new drug application (ANDA).

CANADIAN DRUG LEGISLATION

In Canada the Health Protection Branch (HPB) of the Department of National Health and Welfare is responsible for administration and enforcement of the Food and Drugs Act as well as the Proprietary or Patent Medicine Act and the Narcotic Control Act. These acts are designed to protect the consumer from health hazards and fraud or deception in the sale and use of foods, drugs, cosmetics, and medical devices. Canadian drug legislation began in 1875 when the Parliament of Canada passed an act to prevent the sale of adulterated food, drink, and drugs. Since that time foods and drugs have been controlled on a national basis.

Canadian Food and Drugs Act. In 1953 the present Canadian Food and Drugs Act was passed by the Senate and House of Commons of Canada. Since that time the law has been amended often. The Act stipulates that no food, drug, cosmetic, or device is to be advertised or sold to the general public as a treatment, preventive, or cure for certain diseases listed in Schedule A of the Act. Among the diseases included in the list are alcoholism, arteriosclerosis, and cancer. When it is necessary to provide adequate directions for the safe use of a drug used to treat or prevent diseases mentioned in Schedule A, that disease or disorder may be mentioned on the labels and inserts accompanying the drug. In addition, the Act prohibits the sale of drugs that are contaminated, adulterated, or unsafe for use and those whose labels are false, misleading, or deceptive. According to the Act, drugs must comply with prescribed standards as stated in recognized pharmacopeias and formularies listed in Schedule B of the Act, or with the professed standards under which the drug is sold. Recognized pharmacopeias and formularies include the following:

- *Pharmacopoeia Internationalis*
- *The British Pharmacopoeia*
- *The United States Pharmacopeia*
- *Pharmacopée Française*
- *The Canadian Formulary*
- *British Pharmaceutical Codex*

The legend "Canadian standard drug" or the abbreviation CSD must appear on the inner and outer labels of a drug to signify that it meets the standards prescribed for it.

Sale of certain drugs is prohibited unless the premises where the drug was manufactured and the process and conditions of manufacture have been approved by the Minister of National Health and Welfare. These drugs are listed in Schedules C and D and include injectable liver extracts, all insulin preparations, anterior pituitary extracts, radioactive isotopes, antibiotics for parenteral use, serums and drugs other than antibiotics prepared from microorganisms or viruses, and live vaccines. Distribution of samples of drugs is also prohibited, with the exception of distribution to duly licensed individuals such as physicians, dentists, or pharmacists. Schedule F of the Act contains a list of drugs that can be sold and refilled only on prescription. Refills may be permitted at specified intervals but cannot exceed 6 months. Drugs listed in Schedule F include the antibiotics, hormones, and tranquilizers. They must always be properly and clearly labeled and include directions for use. Labels on containers of Schedule F drugs must be marked with the symbol Pr (prescription required). These drugs cannot be advertised to the general public other than giving the name, price, and quantity of the drug. (See Box 2-4 for a summary of Canadian prescription [Schedules F and G] and restricted [Schedule H] drugs.)

Controlled drugs are those listed in Schedule G of the Act and include amphetamines, barbituric acid and its derivatives (barbiturates), and phenmetrazine. Controlled drugs must be marked with the symbol Ⓒ in a clear and conspicuous color and size on the upper left quarter of the label. The proper name of the drug must appear on the labels, either immediately preceding or following the proprietary or trade name. Controlled drugs can be dispensed only on prescription.

When a controlled drug is dispensed by prescription, the labels must carry the following:

1. Name and address of the pharmacy or pharmacist
2. Date and number of the prescription
3. Name of the person for whom the controlled drug is dispensed
4. Name of the practitioner
5. Directions for use
6. Any other information that the prescription requires be shown on the label

BOX 2-3

Florida Negative Drug Formulary List (as of September, 1996)

1. digoxin
2. digitoxin
3. quinidine gluconate
4. theophylline (controlled release)
5. warfarin (coumadin)
6. conjugated estrogens
7. chlorpromazine (solid oral dosage forms)
8. dicumarol
9. phenytoin
10. levothyroxine sodium
11. pancrelipase (oral dosage forms)

*This list may change in response to the publication of new information or evidence that can alter previous reviewed data.

BOX 2-4

Canadian Prescription and Restricted Drugs

Category	Description
Prescription drugs	
Schedule F	May be used only after professional consultation; includes over 200 drugs, identified by Pr on the label
Schedule G (also called "controlled drugs")	Affect the central nervous system (stimulants, sedatives); identified by Ⓒ on the label
Restricted drugs	
Schedule H	Available only to institutions for research; they present dangerous physiologic and psychologic side effects and have no recognized medical use

Prescriptions for controlled drugs cannot be refilled unless at the time the prescription was issued the practitioner so directed in writing and specified the number of times it could be refilled and the dates for or intervals between refilling. All information on the labels must be clearly and prominently displayed and readily discernible. Controlled drugs cannot be advertised to the general public.

Designated drugs are the following controlled drugs: (1) amphetamines, (2) methamphetamines, (3) phenmetrazine, and (4) phendimetrazine. Physicians may prescribe a designated drug for the following conditions: (1) narcolepsy, (2) hyperkinetic disorders in children, (3) mental retardation (minimal brain dysfunction), (4) epilepsy, (5) parkinsonism, and (6) hypotensive states associated with anesthesia. Permission can be obtained to prescribe amphetamines for clients with diagnoses other than those listed.

Restricted drugs are those listed in Schedule H of the Act and include the hallucinogenic drugs lysergic acid diethylamide (LSD), diethyltryptamine (DET), dimethyltryptamine (DMT), and dimethoxyamphetamine (STP, DOM). Sale of these drugs is prohibited. These drugs may be obtained for research by a qualified investigator if authorized by the Minister of National Health and Welfare. Precautions must be taken to ensure against loss or theft of a restricted drug.

Following are some of the additional requirements to be found in the Canadian food and Drugs Act:

1. Labels of drugs must show:
   a. Proper name of the drug immediately preceding or following the proprietary or brand name
   b. Name and address of the manufacturer or distributor
   c. Lot number of the drug
   d. Adequate directions for use
   e. Quantitative list of medicinal ingredients and their proper or common names
   f. Net amount of drug
   g. Common or proper name and proportion of any preservatives used in parenteral drugs
   h. Expiration date if the drug does not maintain its potency, purity, and physical characteristics for at least 3 years from the date of manufacture
   i. Recommended single and daily adult dose; if the drug is for children, the label must state "Children: As directed by physician" or:

Age in Years	Proportion of Adult Dose
10-14	One-half
5-9	One-fourth
2-4	One-sixth
Under 2	As directed by physician

   j. A warning that the drug be kept out of the reach of children and any precautions to be taken (e.g., "*Caution:* May be injurious if taken in large doses for a long time. Do not exceed the recommended dose without consulting a physician." Warning is to be preceded by a symbol—octagonal in shape, red in color, and on a white background)
   k. Contraindications and side effects of nonprescription drugs
   l. On and after July 1, 1974, the drug identification number assigned to the drug, preceded by the words "Drug Identification Number" or the abbreviation "D.I.N."; to be shown on the main labels of a drug sold in dosage form (i.e., one ready for use by the consumer)
2. Other specific regulations, such as:
   a. Manufacturers must be able to demonstrate that a drug in oral dosage form represented as releasing the drug at time intervals actually is released and available as represented.
   b. Oral tablets must disintegrate within 45 minutes. Enteric-coated tablets must not disintegrate for 60 minutes when exposed to gastric juice but must disintegrate within an additional 60 minutes when exposed to intestinal juices.
   c. Drugs containing boric acid or sodium borate as a medicinal ingredient must carry a statement that the drug should not be administered to infants or children under 3 years of age.
   d. Safety factors such as sterility and absence of pyrogens must be assured in parenteral drugs.

The regulations allow the government to withdraw from the market drugs found to be unduly toxic. New drugs introduced to the market must have shown effectiveness and safety in human clinical studies to the satisfaction of the manufacturer and the government.*

*For more specific information, see *Health Protection and Drug Laws* from Supply and Services Canada, Canadian Government Publishing Centre, Ottawa, Canada, KIA 0S9.

Canadian Narcotic Control Act. The regulations of the Canadian Narcotic Control Act govern the possession, sale, manufacture, production, and distribution of narcotics. The Canadian Narcotic Control Act was passed in 1961 and revoked the Canadian Opium and Narcotic Act of 1952. The 1961 Act has been amended a number of times.

Only authorized persons can be in possession of a narcotic. Authorized persons include a licensed dealer, pharmacist, practitioner, person in charge of a hospital, or a person acting as an agent for a practitioner. A licensed dealer is one who has been given permission to manufacture, produce, import, export, or distribute a narcotic. Practitioners include persons registered under the laws of a province to practice the profession of medicine, dentistry, or veterinary medicine. However, persons other than these may be licensed by the Minister of National Health and Welfare to cultivate and produce opium poppy or marijuana or to purchase and possess a narcotic for scientific purposes. Members of the Royal Canadian Mounted Police and members of technical or scientific departments of the government of Canada or of a province or university may possess narcotics in connection with their employment. A person who is undergoing treatment by a medical practitioner and who requires a narcotic may possess a narcotic obtained on prescription. This person may not knowingly obtain a narcotic from any other medical practitioner without notifying that practitioner that he or she is already undergoing treatment and obtaining a narcotic on prescription.

All persons authorized to be in possession of narcotics must keep a record of the name and quantity of all narcotics received, from whom narcotics were obtained, and to whom narcotics were supplied (including quantity, form, and dates of all transactions). In addition, they must ensure the safekeeping of all narcotics, keep full and complete records on all narcotics for at least 2 years, and report any loss or theft within 10 days of discovery.

The schedule of the Act lists those drugs, as well as their preparations, derivatives, alkaloids, and salts, that are subject to the Canadian Narcotic Control Act. Included in the schedule are opium, coca, and marijuana. Before a pharmacist may legally dispense a drug included in the schedule or a medication containing such a drug, he or she must receive a prescription from a physician. A signed and dated prescription issued by a duly authorized physician is essential in the case of any narcotic medication prescribed as such or any preparation containing a narcotic in a form intended for parenteral administration. Medications containing a narcotic and two or more nonnarcotic ingredients may be dispensed by a pharmacist on the strength of a verbal prescription received from a physician who is known to the pharmacist or whose identity is established. Prescriptions of any narcotic drug may not be refilled.

There is one exception to the prescription requirement. Certain codeine compounds with a small codeine content may be sold to the public by a pharmacist without a prescription. In such instances the narcotic content cannot exceed 8 mg per tablet or 20 mg/28 ml. In products of this kind, codeine must be in combination with two or more nonnarcotic substances and in recognized therapeutic doses.

Additionally, items of this nature are required to be labeled in such a fashion as to show the true formula of the medicinal ingredients and a caution to the following effect: "This preparation contains codeine and should not be administered to children except on the advice of a physician." These preparations cannot be advertised or displayed in a pharmacy. It is also unlawful to publish any narcotic advertisement for the general public.

Labels of containers of narcotics must legibly and conspicuously bear the proprietary and proper or common names of the narcotic, the names of the manufacturer and distributor, the symbol "*N*" in the upper left-hand quarter, and the net contents of the container and of each tablet, capsule, or ampule.

Although the administration of the Canadian Narcotic Control Act is legally the responsibility of the Department of National Health and Welfare, the enforcement of the law has been made largely the responsibility of the Royal Canadian Mounted Police. Prosecution of offenses under the Act is handled through the Department of National Health and Welfare by legal agents specially appointed by the Department of Justice.

The Narcotic Control Act defines a narcotic addict as "a person who through the use of narcotics has developed a desire or need to continue to take a narcotic, or has developed a psychological or physical dependence upon the effect of a narcotic." A person brought into court for a narcotic offense may be placed in custody by the court for observation and examination. If the person is convicted of the offense and found to be a narcotic addict, the court can sentence him or her to custody for treatment for an indefinite period.

Amendments to this Act place special restrictions on methadone. No practitioner can administer, prescribe, give, sell, or furnish methadone to any person unless the practitioner has been issued an authorization by the Minister of National Health and Welfare.

Application to nursing. A nurse may be in violation of the Canadian Narcotic Control Act if he or she is guilty of illegal possession of narcotics. Ignorance of the content of a drug in the nurse's possession is not considered a justifiable excuse. Proof of possession is sufficient to constitute an offense. Legal possession of narcotics by a nurse is limited to times when a drug is administered to a client on the order of a physician, when the nurse is acting as the official custodian of narcotics in a department of a hospital or clinic, or when the nurse is a client for whom a physician has prescribed narcotics. A nurse engaged in illegal distribution or transportation of narcotic drugs may be held liable, and heavy penalties are imposed for violation of the Canadian Narcotic Control Act.

Certain rules for controlled drugs, apart from general rules for prescription drugs, apply in most health agencies:

1. A PRN order (an "as required for pain" order) for narcotics must be rewritten every 72 hours.

2. A standing order (i.e., drug dose administered by the nurse for the physician without obtaining a signed order) is not permitted for narcotic drugs.
3. In an emergency situation a verbal order is permitted if the nurse documents the nature of the emergency in the chart and validates the order within 24 hours.
4. When a narcotic drug is administered to a client, the nurse must record the date, time of administration, client's name, and physician's name, and must sign the entry.
5. When a client refuses a dose of narcotic, it should be placed in the sewage system in the presence of a witness. If a dose of the drug is contaminated or wasted, the nurse should make an entry in the records book explaining how the dose was disposed of; a witness should then sign the entry.
6. All controlled substances stored on nursing units must be kept in locked cabinets so that only authorized personnel have access to them.

STANDARDIZATION OF DRUGS

Drugs may vary considerably in strength and activity. Drugs obtained from plants, such as opium and digitalis, may fluctuate in strength from plant to plant depending on where the plants are grown, the age at which they are harvested, and how they are preserved. Since accurate dosage and reliability of a drug's effect depend on uniformity of strength and purity, standardization is necessary.

The technique, either chemical or biologic, by which the strength and purity of a drug are measured is known as **assay.** Chemical assay is a chemical analysis to determine the ingredients present and their amounts. For example, opium is known to contain certain alkaloids and these may vary greatly in different preparations. The United States official standard demands that opium must contain not less than 9.5% and not more than 10.5% of anhydrous morphine. Opium of a higher morphine content may be reduced to the official standard by admixture with opium of a lower percentage or with certain other pharmacologically inactive diluents such as sucrose, lactose, glycyrrhiza, or magnesium carbonate.

In the case of some drugs, either the active ingredients are not known or there are no available methods of analyzing and standardizing them. These drugs may be standardized by biologic methods—**bioassay.** Bioassay is performed by determining the amount of a preparation required to produce a defined effect on a suitable laboratory animal under certain standard conditions. For example, the potency of a certain sample of insulin is measured by its ability to lower the blood sugar of rabbits.

Drug standards in the United States. Since 1980 the only official book of drug standards in the United States has been *The United States Pharmacopeia (USP)*. Any drug included in this book has met high standards of quality, purity, and strength. Drugs meeting these criteria can be identified by the letters U.S.P. following the official name. The *National Formulary (NF)*, was established in 1888 by the American Pharmaceutical Association, and through the years it has been the project of pharmacists. In 1906 when the first Food and Drug Act was passed, both of these privately issued compendia, the *USP* (revised primarily by physicians) and the *NF*, were established as the official standards by the United States government. Since 1980 the only official book of drug substances and dosage forms in the United States has been *The United States Pharmacopeia* (Cowen and Helfand, 1990).

Although numerous additional reference books and guides are available on the market, two very valuable resources for drug information in a clinical setting are *USP DI: Drug Information for the Health Care Professional* and the *AHFS Drug Information*. The *USP DI* contains information for both the health care provider and the client. Drug information resources are reviewed in Chapter 1.

Drug standards in Great Britain and Canada. *The British Pharmacopoeia (BP)* is similar to the *USP* in scope and purpose. Drugs listed in the *BP* are considered official and subject to legal control in the United Kingdom and those parts of the British Commonwealth in which *The British Pharmacopoeia* has statutory force. *The United States Pharmacopeia* is used a great deal in Canada, and some preparations used in Canada conform to the *USP* instead of the *BP* because many of the drugs used in Canada are manufactured in the United States.

The *British Pharmaceutical Codex* is published by the Pharmaceutical Society of Great Britain. In general, it resembles the *National Formulary*. The Canadian formulary contains formulas for preparations used extensively in Canada. It also contains standards for new drugs prescribed in Canada but not included in *The British Pharmacopoeia*. The publication has been given official status by the Canadian Food and Drugs Act.

The Physician's Formulary contains formulas for preparations that are representative of the needs of medical practice in Canada. It is published by the Canadian Medical Association.

INTERNATIONAL DRUG CONTROL

International control of drugs legally began in 1912 when the first "Opium Conference" was held at The Hague. International treaties were drawn up legally obligating governments to (1) limit to medical and scientific needs the manufacturing of and trade in medicinal opium, (2) control the production and distribution of raw opium, and (3) establish a system of governmental licensing to control the manufacture of and trade in drugs covered by the convention.

In 1961 government representatives formulated the "Single Convention on Narcotic Drugs," which became effective in 1964. This act consolidated all existing treaties into one document for the control of all narcotic substances by:

1. Outlawing their production, manufacture, trade, and use for nonmedicinal purposes
2. Limiting possession of all narcotic substances to authorized persons for medical and scientific purposes

3. Providing for international control of all opium transactions by the national monopolies (countries designated to produce opium, such as Turkey) and authorizing production only by licensed farmers in areas and on plots designated by these monopolies
4. Requiring import certificates and export authorizations

An **International Narcotics Control Board** was established to enforce this law. This Board is an international organization of governmental representatives established to enforce the "Single Convention on Narcotic Drugs." Since enforcement is an immense task, it is impossible to prevent illicit trafficking in drugs. For example, during a 1-year period it was estimated that 1200 tons of opium were circulated in the illicit market when 800 tons were considered sufficient for world medical needs. Laws need to be frequently updated and strictly enforced, but the unfortunate fact is that financial support for regulation and enforcement is sometimes not equal to the task.

INVESTIGATIONAL DRUGS

The multibillion dollar pharmaceutical industry is constantly screening substances with potential to market as new drugs. Prospective drugs may take years and huge amounts of capital to progress through the following FDA-required testing sequence:

A. Animal studies, to ascertain:
   1. Toxicity
      a. Acute toxicity—as represented by the LD_{50} (the median lethal dose; the dose that is lethal to 50% of the laboratory animals tested). This is also known as the median lethal dose.
      b. Subacute toxicity
      c. Chronic toxicity
   2. **Therapeutic index**—a quantitative measure of the relative safety of a drug; the ratio of the median lethal dose to the median effective dose
   3. Modes of absorption, distribution, metabolism (biotransformation), and excretion

B. Human studies
   1. Phase I—initial pharmacologic evaluation
   2. Phase II—limited controlled evaluation
   3. Phase III—extended clinical evaluation

A noteworthy lack of correlation exists between levels of toxicity in animals and adverse effects in humans. In addition, many symptoms of adverse effects in humans simply cannot be determined in animals. A partial list of common human symptoms that are not measurably distinguishable in animals includes such effects as dizziness, nausea, drowsiness, nervousness, indigestion, headache, and weakness.

FDA approval process. The FDA approval process and specifications are as follows:

1. Investigational New Drug (IND)—if a pharmaceutical company or individual desires to investigate a new drug substance or an old drug for a new indication or at a different, unapproved dosage in humans, an IND application must be completed and submitted to the FDA. The IND will include evidence of drug safety by providing animal or clinical information, proof of the investigator's qualifications to perform this research, and evidence of the drug product's proven quality and strength. The investigation covered under the IND is divided into three phases:

   Phase I—initial pharmacologic evaluation. A small number of normal individuals (usually volunteers) will take the drug so that the investigators can determine the pharmacokinetics of the agent (absorption, distribution, metabolism, routes of elimination or excretion). Blood tests, urine analysis, vital signs, and specific monitoring tests are performed during this phase.

   Phase II—limited controlled evaluation. Now the drug will be administered at gradually increasing dosages to selected individuals with the targeted disease. For example, if the product is believed to have antihypertensive properties, individuals with documented hypertension would be chosen for this phase. During this phase, the individual will be closely monitored for drug effectiveness and for side effects. If no serious side or adverse effects occur, the study will progress to phase III.

   Phase III—extended clinical evaluation. The drug is now ready for testing in various centers in the United States in larger numbers of individuals. Standards (protocols) have been developed and are to be followed at all investigative sites. The three objectives for this phase are: (1) determination of clinical effectiveness, (2) drug safety determination, and (3) establishment of tolerated dosage or dosage range.

   Several other factors are involved with this program. First, the investigator reports to the FDA after completion of each phase and needs its approval before progressing to the following phases. Second, a double-blind study may be instituted, usually in phase II or phase III. A double-blind study involves the administration of the research drug or a placebo (such as lactose) and/or a marketed drug with the same pharmacologic effects as the drug being studied. All of the products are formulated to look the same and then packaged, usually by code numbers. Generally no one involved with the study knows which bottle of medicine the client is taking, the study drug (the active drug) or the placebo. Therefore bias will be eliminated and the evaluation will be done accurately, on the basis of therapeutic response.
2. New Drug Application (NDA)—after the completion of phase II of the IND and assuming the data collected indicate that the new drug is very promising, investigators will submit all the collected data to the FDA. After careful review of the information, the FDA may approve or reject the NDA. If the NDA is approved, the drug product can be marketed for the selected indication in the dosing schedules as studied. If the NDA is rejected, the FDA may require additional studies or information before reconsideration.
3. Abbreviated New Drug Application (ANDA) (for generic drug approval)—Generic formulations of currently marketed medications are not usually required to repeat all the

previous steps before marketing. A company is required to prove that its product can produce the same therapeutic effects as the already marketed drug. Although nearly all generic drugs require the ANDA, the FDA may require different methods to prove generic equivalency, depending on the drug. For example, chlordiazepoxide (Librium) and amitriptyline (Elavil) require in vivo studies—that is, the generic drug must be given to humans, and blood and urine studies data should be equivalent to data obtained when the name brand product is given, according to statistical analysis. Other drug products, such as chlorpheniramine (Chlor-Trimeton) and dexamethasone (Decadron) only need to prove that the manufacturing process is in compliance with Good Manufacturing Practice guidelines and that their quality control standards are equivalent. Thus the FDA establishes the criteria according to the drug product, the possibility of bioequivalency problems, or the lack of such problems. Drugs marketed before 1938, such as chloral hydrate and phenobarbital, do not require an approved ANDA before marketing.

The nurse should be aware of several of the limitations of the testing and marketing process. The number of persons studied and the time allotted for the study are limited. Also, certain types of individuals are excluded from the study, such as children, pregnant women, persons with multiple disease states, and the elderly. If a drug is considered safe and effective during the time of study, with the previously mentioned limitations, it is marketed. Once marketed, the drug will be used in much greater numbers of clients, probably for longer periods; thus it is inevitable that the drug will be reported to produce additional effects (possibly therapeutic but often adverse) that were not noted during the trial studies.

Therefore, a phase IV, or postmarketing surveillance period, has been advocated to monitor and tabulate information about new drugs in order to disseminate it to health care professionals and consumers. This is a more difficult phase to supervise, since it depends on the voluntary reports of persons in the medical field. The importance of this phase should not be underestimated, since it will affect many more people than the previous three phases combined. (See Box 2-5 on classifications for newly approved drugs.)

In 1993 the FDA initiated MedWatch, a voluntary program to enhance the reporting by health care professionals of adverse effects they suspect are related to medications and medical devices. The nurse need not verify the cause of an adverse effect, but to inform the agency of medication or medical device related events that are suspected to have resulted in death or the risk of death, hospitalization, persistent or permanent disability, birth defect, or the need for medical intervention to prevent permanent impairment. The FDA is requesting that nurses provide information about products even if clients are not involved such as contaminated products or product labeling which might be confusing. Nurse and client confidentiality are maintained in the reporting. The paperwork is a one-page form that can be obtained from the hospital's risk manager. The American Nurses Association was involved in the development of MedWatch and supports the program for providing another way in which nurses can advocate for client safety.

Informed consent. All participants in experimental drug studies should be true volunteers and not subjected to any coercion. **Informed consent** must be obtained from the participants. This is the written consent to an experimental procedure by an individual after he or she has been given a careful explanation of the purpose of the study, procedure to be used, the expected effects, and the risks involved. New drug studies in children require special consideration. Beginning in 1983, new rules stipulated that both children's and parents' consent are required for research involving children if it is funded by the Department of Health and Human Services. In addition, these researchers must follow more rigorous guidelines to protect a child's rights. The rights of human participants in medical research have come to be protected under the umbrella of the **Nuremberg Code.** This code was developed under the aegis of American physicians as a result of the post-World War II trials at Nuremberg of Nazi physicians who had conducted experiments on political prisoners without their consent. The Code states essentially that:

1. Truly voluntary consent of the human subject is critical.
2. The experiment must be proved to be valid or made possible only through the use of human subjects.
3. The results and risks are justified by the study.
4. Unnecessary suffering, death, or disability will be avoided.
5. The experiment will be conducted in a careful and professional manner by scientifically qualified persons.
6. The subject or the investigator may terminate the experiment at any point that it is felt unendurable or impossible.

Additionally, any experimental drug trials using humans, if they are supported by the U.S. Department of Health and Human Services, must also meet federal guidelines for the protection of participants. Institutions supporting such investigational research have review boards that evaluate aspects of the research as it affects human subjects and that formally approve or disapprove research proposals accordingly.

Pregnancy safety categories. Before using any drug during pregnancy, the expected benefits should be considered against the possible risks to the fetus. While the FDA has established the following scale to indicate drugs that may have documented problems in animals and/or humans during pregnancy, for many drugs this information is unknown. For drugs with published classifications, though, the prescriber, nurse and client should carefully review any precautionary information before using the drug product.

Category A—Adequate and well-controlled studies indicate no risk to the fetus in the first trimester of pregnancy (and there is no evidence of risk in later trimesters).

Category B—Animal reproduction studies indicate no risk to the fetus and there are no well-controlled studies in pregnant women.

BOX 2-5

FDA Classifications for Newly Approved Drugs

To assist the professional in immediately classifying new drug entities, the FDA has developed the following method of drug classification. A number and a letter are assigned to each new drug at the IND phase or at the NDA review by the FDA. The manufacturer has a right to contest this classification and have it changed before the final classification is established.

Numerical classification

1. A new molecular drug.
2. A new salt of a marketed drug.
3. A new formulation or dosage form not previously marketed.
4. A new combination not previously marketed.
5. A drug that is already on the market, a generic duplication.
6. A product already marketed by the same company. (This designation is used for new indications for a marketed drug.)

Letter classification

A —Drug offers an important therapeutic gain.
B —Medication offers a modest therapeutic gain over drugs already on the market.
C —Drug offers little or no therapeutic gain over other marketed drugs.
M—Drug marketed in a foreign country.
R —Drug has individual unique conditions for approval that are outlined in NDA approval letter.
T —Drug has toxicity problem (such as carcinogenicity in animals).
U—Drug is apt to be used for treatment of children.
D —Drug has less safety or is less effective as compared with marketed drugs but has a compensating virtue (such as being available for persons who have not responded to or are unable to tolerate the alternative available drugs on the market).
P —The important feature of the product is the container or package, not the drug.

New FDA classification system

In January 1992 the FDA added a new system for classifying drugs that will eventually replace the A, B, and C ratings. Drugs will now be rated *P* for priority—a new therapeutic advance—or *S* for standard—a drug that is similar to drugs already on the market. This rating is issued by the FDA when a New Drug Application is received. Drugs approved in 1991 or before will have the A, B, or C rating.

The above classification is available by request from the Freedom of Information Staff at the Bureau of Drugs (Food and Drug Administration, 5600 Fishers Lane, Rockville, MD., 20857).

Category C—Animal reproduction studies have reported adverse effects on the fetus; and there are no well-controlled studies in humans, but potential benefits may indicate use of the drug in pregnant women despite potential risks.

Category D—Positive human fetal risk has been reported in data from investigational or marketing experience, or human studies. Considering potential benefit versus risk may, in selected cases, warrant the use of these drugs in pregnant women.

Category X—Fetal abnormalities reported and positive evidence of fetal risk in humans is available from animal and/or human studies. The risks involved clearly outweigh the potential benefits. These drugs should not be used in pregnant women.

NURSES AND DRUG RESEARCH

Nurses involved in research projects concerning human subjects must be knowledgeable about the precepts of the Nuremberg Code and must protect clients by being ever alert to the possibility of subtle slipups in protocol or oversights in adherence to the tenets of the Code. The most important elements of the Code relate to subjects' rights to informed consent and to participation that is without coercion and fully voluntary.

Informed consent must be obtained in writing. This particular consent is heir to the flaws of other client consents: the information conveyed may be incomplete or not delivered in nonmedical language or perhaps presented at a time when the individual is sleepy or sedated and not fully cognizant of the ramifications of what is being signed. It is the nurse's obligation to ensure that this does not happen and that it is the researcher or the physician, not the nurse, who gives full explanation and answers pertinent questions.

Expanding roles in nursing often include nurses on the team researching experimental drug development. Indeed, more nurses than ever before are conducting research of their own, much of it clinical even if not directly related to investigational drugs, using human subjects. Because of a healthy professional commitment to client well-being, nurses may find themselves caught in an ethical conflict. They likely may feel ambivalent about clients' right to know (vis-a-vis the Patient's Bill of Rights) and yet be uncomfortably aware that too much information may unduly influence a person's behavior or condition in some way and thereby adversely influence the variable under study. This area of ethics awaits further study.

Nurses involved in clinical drug studies should be fully informed about the study and the drug under investigation. All information available to the prescriber, researcher, or pharmacist should also be available to the nurse. Ethical and legal responsibilities mandate that a nurse's actions be based on adequate knowledge and skill and that clients be protected from foreseeable harm. This necessitates that the nurse know the recommended dosage range and route of administration, the desired therapeutic effect, and the undesired and toxic effects. Throughout the entire investigation the nurse must strictly adhere to the protocols of the study. Recordings of all observations should be as precise as possible, for they will have a direct influence on the study outcome.

NURSING LEGISLATION

Nursing practice is regulated not only by the previous drug standards and legislation but also by individual state nurse practice acts; joint policy statements among the state nursing associations, medical associations, and hospital associations; and institutional and agency policies. Institutions and agencies may set policies that interpret more specifically those actions allowable under state nursing practice acts, but they may not modify, expand, or restrict the intent of such acts. Personal and professional ethical standards further govern actual nursing decisions and judgments in practice.

The nurse practice acts of individual states define conditions under which nurses may be licensed to practice professionally. One of their functions is to protect the public from unskilled, undereducated, or unlicensed nurses and to delineate clearly the scope of nursing as a health care profession. Another function is to protect nurses by defining clearly their responsibilities and freedoms. Every state nurse practice act includes laws and regulations on reciprocity and suspension or revocation of nurse licenses.

Changing nursing roles. Clearly the traditional roles of the nurse are changing and expanding along with newer techniques and approaches to drug therapy. These expanding roles often find the nurse in activities beyond traditionally accepted nursing practices, which challenge the judgment and accountability of the nurse legally. Two such areas are prescription writing and certain modes of drug administration.

Prescribing medications has been, in the past, a purely medical function as determined by state law, while medication administration has usually been delegated to nurses and occasionally to licensed pharmacists and other trained personnel. In reality, astute nurses have been indirectly prescribing for many years, using diplomatic ploys with physicians to attend to changing patient needs: "Will you write an order for Dulcolax for Mrs. Rommel? She hasn't had a bowel movement for 3 days." Now, certain expanding roles in nursing, along with increased education and expertise (e.g., certification as nurse practitioner by the American Nurses' Association), have legalized the prescribing function of nurse practitioners.

Two reports acknowledged this need, one from the American Medical Association in 1970 and the other from the Department of Health, Education, and Welfare in 1971. Both clearly state that the prescribing of medications "may be the practice of medicine when carried out by a physician and the practice of nursing when carried out by the nurse." Many states as a result of this change have amended their nurse practice acts. These amendments have predominantly given authorization to the nurse practitioner to write prescriptions according to established protocols or under physician supervision or collaboration. In 49 states and Washington, DC, nurse practitioners have legislative authority to prescribe as of January 1997 (Pearson, 1997), although within these states there is a wide disparity; some states have almost no prescription barriers to nurse practitioner practice, while in other states the barriers are still significant (see Box 2-6).

Other states have nurse-prescribing bills pending. Many states and institutions therein have developed protocols for designating the types of clients to be treated by nurse practitioners. They have also developed formularies to aid in their selection of prescribed drugs and to provide reviews of their prescribing activities, usually by periodic chart audits. One evaluative study of 1000 nurse practitioner-generated prescriptions demonstrated high levels of accuracy, accountability, and legibility. Of these prescriptions 25% were for relief of discomfort, 25% were for contraceptive purposes (one fourth of these were for diaphragms), 40% were for antibiotics, 6% were written to treat chronic stabilized disorders, and a small number were written in consultation with a physician for controlled substances. Nonprescription preparations such as Pepto-Bismol, aspirin, and vitamin supplements were also recommended by nurse practitioners. Of the drugs ordered 99% were consistent with the related protocol. There was no evidence of any complications arising from the medication prescribed, and all were deemed appropriate in terms of safety and therapeutic usefulness. It is of interest to note that the ratio of

BOX 2-6

Prescriptive Authority for Nurse Practitioners within the United States

States with independent nurse practitioner prescribing authority*

Including controlled substances:

Alaska	Montana	South Carolina†
Arizona	Nebraska	South Dakota
Colorado	New Hampshire*	Vermont
Delaware	New Mexico	Washington (Schedule V)
District of Columbia	Oklahoma	Wisconsin
Iowa	Oregon	Wyoming
Maine		

States with dependent nurse practitioner prescribing authority

Including controlled substances:

Arkansas	Louisiana†	North Carolina
California	Maryland	North Dakota
Connecticut	Massachusetts	Pennsylvania
Georgia	Minnesota	Rhode Island
Indiana	Mississippi†	Utah
Kansas†	New York	West Virginia

Excluding controlled substances:

Alabama	Michigan	Ohio†
Florida	Missouri	Tennessee
Hawaii	New Jersey	Texas
Idaho	Nevada	Virginia
Kentucky		

Within Illinois there was no legislative authority for nurse practitioners to prescribe as of January 1997.

Adapted from Pearson LJ (1997). Annual update of how each state stands on legislative issues affecting advanced nursing practice, *Nurse Practitioner* 22 (1):18-25.

*Independent prescribing means that prescribing is defined by the State Board of Nursing of a state as an activity within the actual practice of a nurse practitioner. It is not statutorily defined as a delegated medical act and so does not require physician collaboration or supervision.

†In narrowly specified situations.

drug prescriptions to clients was lower among the nurse practitioners than among the physicians (Nichols, 1992).

The AMA Socioeconomic Monitoring System has ascertained that physicians who employ nurse practitioners or physicians' assistants are able to charge less for visits and to manage about 20% more client visits per week than those who do not. Physicians who employ nurse practitioners report that they are generally pleased. Those physicians who were polled stated that they fully expected that more nurse practitioners would be part of the health care delivery system in the future and that this would be for the better. The plethora of studies attesting to the nurse practitioner's functional effectiveness, safety, and acceptance by the client may offer one solution to the high costs, long waits, and depersonalization in health care today.

Drug administration was, for a very long period in health care history, a function of physicians only. In fact, nurses were kept ignorant of the medications the client might be receiving. Gradually, medication administration became an interdependent function. Now nurses find that they are increasingly taking responsibility for suggesting and selecting drugs, their dosages, and regulation. For example, in specialty units of some acute care hospitals, nurses assume responsibility for titrating the infusion rates and the dosages of potent antihypertensive medications against blood pressure parameters. They frequently are responsible for titrating intravenous (IV) fluids to replace gastrointestinal drainage milliliter for milliliter. In the past, nurses were authorized to administer large-volume continuous IV infusions. Nurses now also administer medications by small-volume intermittent IV infusion (by "piggyback" or "rider"). Many hospitals, particularly in their specialized care units, authorize nurses to give very small-volume, undiluted medications either directly into a vein by IV "push" or into IV tubing.

Generally, changing roles and functions and the laws that govern them are not enacted simultaneously. Usually a time lag exists between the adoption of a new function and official approval. Thus nurses who fill drug reservoirs for epidural administration of analgesia and inject medications intravenously are breaking new legal ground. Such procedures are potentially more risky than other medication procedures, and nurses who perform them are probably placing themselves in a tenuous legal position unless (1) they are qualified by virtue of adequate training, education, and experience; and (2) there exists written sanction. Health agency policy provides solid grounding for the nurse to follow in the interpretation of role responsibilities (*Treinis v. Deepdale General Hosp.*—570 N.Y.S. 2d 185, 1991). Policies should be drawn up jointly by the administration of the hospital or agency and nursing representatives. These policy statements should carefully delineate the roles of nurses and physicians and present guidelines for these procedures. They should include a list of drugs and routes to be used only by physicians and a list of criteria for permitting nurses to give medications by an IV route or other system. Currently a trend exists for pharmacy department personnel to draw up and prepare admixtures in large-volume IV solutions before delivering the medication to the nursing area. This procedure is done under controlled conditions in agency pharmacies, with the goal of reducing IV solution contamination.

At the implementation stage, three conditions should be met before a nurse may legally begin to administer a medication by any mode:

1. The medication order must be valid.
2. The physician/prescriber and the nurse must be licensed. The nonphysician prescriber is prescribing within the regulations of the state.
3. The nurse must know the purpose, actions, effects, and major side effects and toxic effects of the drug, and the teaching required to enable the client or caregiver to safely and accurately self-administer the drug.

A valid order is one that leaves no room for doubt as to the medication prescribed, its dose and route, the dosing interval, and the prescriber's name/signature. Moreover, the drug must also be deemed appropriate for that specific client. Since nurses are legally, morally, and ethically responsible for their actions, they must assess the medication order for its preciseness, accuracy, and appropriateness.

The medication order must be written and worded in such a way that it is correct, complete, legible, and clearly understandable. If it is not, clarification must be sought from the prescriber. Creating a healthy, open, questioning atmosphere in the prescriber-nurse relationship avoids the very real hazard lurking behind "guessing," "assuming," and "not wanting to bother the doctor."

Although not every medication given in error results in actual client harm, the potential always exists. It is wise to avoid such incidents by clarifying the prescribing situation in the following ways.

Verbal order. A physician's order may be given verbally (often at a client's bedside), such as "Just give her a little Mylanta." It is then appropriate to remind the prescriber that nurses cannot give medication unless the order is in writing. If the order is not written at that time, it is often forgotten. If the medication has already been given and it has not been "signed for" by the prescriber, it is illegal until the order is written and signed. Managing this before the prescriber leaves the area is often not possible.

Telephone order. An order given over the telephone can easily be miscommunicated, misinterpreted, or not clearly heard, and such an order often remains too long unsigned by the prescriber. Many institutions have a specific policy that limits acceptance of verbal or telephone orders to emergency situations only. In any event, the prescriber should sign all orders as soon as possible. Nursing students should not be held responsible for following or transcribing *any* unsigned telephone or verbal orders.

Incomplete order. Orders that are not complete in medication name, dose, route, time, or signature must be clarified and completed before administration. Orders for medications to be given by the IV route are the ones most often found incomplete; frequently the rate of infusion is the part missing from the order.

Incorrect or inappropriate order. The order may be judged by the nurse to be incorrect or inappropriate for the client (for example, a dose too high for a client of low body weight or impaired renal function as evidenced by low creatinine clearance, or a medication ordered for a client with a recent myocardial infarction that is noted to have secondary effects of tachycardia or dysrhythmias). Here, the situation may be quite intimidating to the nurse, who is now in the position of challenging the judgment of the prescriber at the risk of incurring embarrassment, job threat, or both. Of course, such intimidation is not justifiable. It is the nurse's or nursing student's absolute right and responsibility to question *any* proposed action that is potentially harmful to a client. Often prescribers and some nurses (and many consumers) are under the mistaken impression that nurses who merely act by following a prescriber's order are absolved from any untoward results of that act. Medications are written by the prescriber at a given time in the treatment of the client. But the condition of the client may change, so the nurse must exercise critical judgment as to the appropriateness of each dose for that client before it is administered. Actually, *no one can relieve a nurse of responsibility for his or her actions;* to carry out an order that the nurse knows to be incorrect constitutes negligence. To change an order by modifying any part of it, if done without consultation with the prescriber, is similarly illegal.

If an order is believed to be in error, some suggested actions are as follows:

1. Validate the order by consulting an authoritative reference source, such as *USP DI: Drug Information for the Health Care Professional* or *AHFS Drug Information.*
2. If the order is apparently incorrect, objectively report the conflicting facts and discuss it with the prescriber in a factual, nonblaming manner.
3. If the prescriber still wants the medication given as ordered after the nurse's objections have been raised, can the nurse give the medication if the prescriber takes full responsibility? Again, *no one* can release nurses from full responsibility for every medication they give just because they are acting under a prescriber's order. To do so is to court a lawsuit for negligence. This fact must be made clear to the prescriber as the rationale for the nurse's refusal to medicate.

If the prescriber chooses to administer the medication personally after the nurse refuses to do so in the belief that it could be potentially harmful to the client, the nurse should see that the facts of the situation are made known to the immediate supervisors, and consultation should be sought if necessary. Every hospital should have in place a mechanism for such reporting (*Campbell v. Pitt County Mem. Hosp.*—352 S.E. 2d 902-N.C., 1991). If the drug is given, the medication record should reflect that it was the prescriber who gave it.

Invalid order. Orders signed by medical students, physicians' assistants, and in some states, nurse practitioners are not legally accepted as having been signed by a duly licensed physician (this is the wording of many nursing practice acts) and should not be until a physician actually signs it (unless the law is changed). Nurses should be aware of their health agency's policy and state regulation. Validity of orders written and signed by an unlicensed intern or resident may be equivocal, depending on local law or policy.

Order for unfamiliar drug. Orders for a medication that is unfamiliar to the administering nurse must stimulate a nearly reflex reaction to "look it up" or to "ask the pharmacist." Administration of an unfamiliar drug while remaining in ignorance of its actions, its intended effects and side effects, and its adverse reactions (at the very minimum) is considered nursing negligence if it results in harm to the client. For instance, a nurse was found liable when a 3-month-old infant died after being given an injectable form of digoxin instead of the pediatric elixir. In another instance, hospital staff members were found negligent when prolonged infiltration of a dopamine infusion went unobserved, causing permanent injury (*Macon-Bibb Hosp. Authority v. Ross*—335 S.E. 2nd 633-GA) (see Box 2-7).

Safeguards. Astute nurses are alert not only to the set limits of functioning but also to the quality of functioning within those limits. Although lawsuits can be initiated when a nurse exceeds the limits of accepted practice, few have actually been instituted. However, more can be anticipated in the near future as the public becomes more aware of nurses' liability. Most suits, however, are brought by clients or their families who feel they have been subjected to behavior or to a procedure that was not of the quality of practice reasonably expected of someone with a nurse's professional education and experience and under the particular circumstances. This is identified legally as malpractice. The nurse can take precautions against malpractice resulting from errors of medication administration by observing the **Five Rights of Medication Administration**:

BOX 2-7

Legal Aspects

How often do nurses encounter an infiltrating IV in the routine care of clients? The assessment and action taken by the nurse can be significant for the client, as in the case of *Macon-Bibb Hosp. Authority v. Ross* (335 S.E. 2d 633-GA).

Ms. Ross was brought to the emergency department of the hospital with dyspnea, bradycardia, and a blood pressure of 250/150. She went into respiratory arrest at 2:55 PM; she was intubated with an endotracheal tube, and nitroprusside was administered IV to decrease her blood pressure. Because of the rapid drop in blood pressure, an IV administration of dopamine was then started at 3:28 PM in her right wrist to increase her blood pressure. When her BP was stable, she was transferred to the cardiac care unit at 4:30 PM. At midnight, a nurse noted that the IV site had a "bruise bluish in color." The next notation was at 11:00 AM the following day, in which it was recorded that the client's right arm was swollen and painful with a large blistered area around the IV site. The same notation was made at 4:00 PM. It was not until 6:50 PM that a note indicated that a physician was informed of the infiltration. As a result of the extravasation of dopamine, the client's lower right arm was permanently scarred. On a jury verdict, the court entered judgment for the client. The hospital appealed.

The court of appeals affirmed the judgment of the lower court. It was noted that although an infiltration may result from an improper technique, it may also be due to the size of the needle, the status of the client's veins, or a particular intolerance to an IV. However, according to the expert nurse's testimony, supported by suitable references, dopamine should be infused into a "large vein," such as in the antecubital fossa, to minimize the risk of extravasation. In addition, dopamine should be monitored continuously for free flow. If extravasation of dopamine occurs, the recommended treatment of the site is infiltration with a saline solution of phentolamine (Regitine) within 12 hours.

The nurses were criticized for not being sufficiently knowledgeable regarding dopamine, which resulted in their failure to notify a physician of the client's impaired tissue integrity.

Critical thinking questions

- How could the emergency department nurse caring for Ms. Ross have prevented this incident?
- What action should have been taken by Ms. Ross's admitting nurse in the ICU to prevent this incident?
- What action should have been taken by the nurse who noted that the IV site had a "bruise bluish in color"?
- In what way could this hospital prevent a similar occurrence in the future?

1. The *right medication* (the one that was prescribed and one that is not contraindicated)
2. The *right client* (not someone else's medication by mistake, or someone in the next bed)
3. The *right dosage* as prescribed and appropriate (it may involve simple mathematical computations)
4. The *route, form of the drug, and administration technique* as prescribed
5. The drug at the *right time* (usually within half an hour of the time indicated and at beneficial intervals as ordered)

The following are examples of nursing actions that support and facilitate the meeting of these expectations:

- Refusing to allow administration of a drug against good nursing judgment
- Preparing medications in a quiet, undisturbed environment conducive to thoughtfulness and accuracy
- Comparing the information on the medication Kardex or the computer printout sheet with the prescriber's order and medication chart to prevent wrong dosage, double-dosing, or the like
- Looking up information about all new or unfamiliar drugs before administering them
- Reading medication labels three times—when taking the drug container from its storage place, when preparing the dose, and when returning the drug container to its storage place
- Carefully calculating the dosage as necessary, especially when working with decimals
- Administering only drug doses that were self-prepared
- Positively identifying the client by comparing the arm band with the name on the medication administration record
- Listening intently to clients when they question the administration of a particular drug, its color, size, dosage, or a possible allergy; clients frequently give nurses crucial data in this manner
- Recording the administration of each dose as soon as possible
- Observing carefully for side effects and adverse effects, reporting them, and documenting actions taken

For the nurse's part, *accountability* is a term that has gained increasing import, particularly as related to pharmacotherapeutics. Nurses are no longer considered to be merely "physicians' handmaidens" or to be accorded "umbrella protection from litigation" by the prescriber and the institution. Nurses are increasingly expected to take the responsibility for and be answerable for the service they provide or make available.

In summary, basic guidelines to litigation-free, professional nursing practice and to medication administration in particular include:

1. Knowing the limitations of nursing practice in the community through awareness of agency policies, joint medical and nursing practice statements, nursing practice acts, and state and federal laws, and then abiding by them
2. Knowing the limitations of one's own skills, expertise, knowledge, and experience and never exceeding them
3. Informing involved personnel of and documenting thoroughly and carefully all happenings related to client care, especially those with potential legal implications
4. Maintaining a professional, caring, and collaborative relationship with clients and their families. Aside from this approach being proper, it can act to dissolve potential dissatisfaction of clients with health care, with the institution, or with its policies.

ETHICAL CONSIDERATIONS

Conflicts in values for nurses occur as a result of the changing legislation governing many of the activities of nurses in relation to the administration of medications and the increasing role of nurses in clinical research in pharmacotherapeutics, as well as day-to-day practice when nurse, client, and prescriber have differing opinions as to what measures to take in a specific situation.

Probably the most powerful fundamental force at work in the actual implementation of right and proper nursing practice is the nurse's own concept of ethical and moral correctness and responsibility. The American Nurses' Association (1985), the Canadian Nurses' Association (1980), and the International Council of Nurses (1973) have adopted similar codes of ethics for nurses, which can serve as guides to standards of conduct, relationships, and practice. The nurse's responsibilities to clients as defined by these codes of ethics are to promote health, prevent illness, restore health, and alleviate suffering. At the core of any such professional code is that its precepts spring from the reality that the client is a person with rights and dignity not to be subsumed under the needs or rights of any other person or the machinations of an institution or society at large. Thus nurses are obligated to respect the wishes of clients and to treat them with dignity. For example, a client has every right to know necessary information about a drug he or she is receiving and to refuse to take it after having been given an explanation, no matter what the consequences. The client's right to respect from the nurse is independent of nationality, race, creed, color, age, sex, politics, or physical or social status.

When ethical dilemmas occur, nurses may experience conflicting loyalties to their profession, colleagues, clients, agencies, and society. But nursing ethics, which provide guidance for nursing action, are based on the principles of **nonmalfeasance** (the duty to do no harm), **beneficence** (the duty to do good), client autonomy, truthfulness, justice, fidelity (faithfulness to one's obligations), and integrity (being true to one's word). These issues are essential to the bond of trust in the nurse-client relationship and demonstrate the caring perspective that is the heart of nursing practice. The tenets of the codes of practice for nurses assure the client that the nurse will act in the client's best interest.

This obligation of the nurse to the client includes respecting the client's values whether or not the nurse agrees with the client's decision in relation to his or her health care. For example, some clients might value remaining mentally alert and in control of their experiences over taking medications that would offer pain relief but that might also alter their thought processes. The responsibility of the nurse is to assist the client in the decision-making process by ensuring that the client is informed of the risks and benefits of the therapy and can make a knowledgeable decision.

NURSING PRACTICE

Early in a nursing career, the study of legal issues related to the administration of medications can seem a somewhat less than fascinating exercise. However, as the nurse builds practical experience, this study will prove its worth time and time again. Laws, acts, codes, and regulations shaping pharmacologic practice provide the boundaries for safe practice. Experience proves that knowing the accepted scope of nursing practice of one's nation, state, locale, and institutional community provides security and support for the nurse who aspires to provide harm-free care. Legal statutes only guide; nurses have to translate these guides into action. Often what guides best within legal constraints is the individual nurse's judgment based on his or her own code of ethics, professionalism, and sense of accountability. A fundamental precept is that what is best for the client usually turns out to be best for the nurse.

There are few hard and fast rules in nursing practice. Many specific questions about legalities in drug administration must be answered, and the answer is often "It depends . . . ." This should not immobilize nurses and prevent them from acting in healthy, assertive ways. If they function within the accepted boundaries of practice, continue to stretch for new knowledge, and act accountably for the benefit of their clients, little exists that can harm their clients, themselves, their professional reputations, or their jobs. The sureness that comes with experience flourishes as they exercise these skills. And exercising these skills often demands that they stand up for what is right in client care despite pressures in the situation generated by time constraints or by others who want them to "just get on with it." Being human, nurses will occasionally fail to use the best judgment or to be perfect. This is reasonable, but it is also reasonable for nurses to aspire to structure their practice in ways that make it difficult to fail.

The neophyte nurse may be somewhat shaken by the wealth of background information necessary to safe practice. The more experienced nurse will probably grapple with the temptation to become complacent and to make dangerous assumptions about the limits of his or her practice. Both need equally to continue to read and question in order to improve the quality of their decisions, whether the issues stem from legal, ethical, or moral considerations.

The art of drug development, evaluation, and prescribing, although sophisticated and well regulated in theory, may in practice be sometimes inadequate. Moreover, since all chemical substances such as drugs create side effects, adverse reactions, and interactions and many have been identified as having questionable efficacy, it becomes increasingly compelling to avoid medicating, when feasible, and to substitute rational nursing measures. For example, nursing interventions to promote comfort, if instituted effectively and early in the pain cycle, can often substantially reduce pain so that "as necessary" medications become less necessary.

SUMMARY

Although substances to treat illness and cure disease have always existed, it was not until the twentieth century that the need to standardize and regulate such substances became apparent. In the United States the Pure Food and Drug Act of 1906 was the first to limit false and misleading claims for drugs, but only those for interstate commerce. It also established *The United States Pharmacopeia* and the *National Formulary* as official standards for drugs. Further legislation in 1938 required the testing of drugs for safety, and in 1952 the requirements for distinction between legend drugs and OTCs were established. Since that time, both types of preparations have proliferated and there has been constant review to ensure their safety and efficacy.

The Harrison Narcotic Act of 1914 was the first law passed by any nation to regulate opium and other substances producing drug dependence. Currently such drugs are governed by the Controlled Substances Act, which in addition to other regulation, classifies controlled substances into their compared use and abuse potential. This law influences the daily routine of many nurses, since the controlled substances count is performed at the beginning and end of every shift in settings where supplies of these drugs are maintained. Other protection in effect for consumers includes the reporting of drug reactions by clinicians to the FDA, the regulation of biologic products by the Public Health Service, and the legislation of product liability by many states.

In Canada similar legislation exists for the protection of its citizens. Although often amended, the Canadian Food and Drugs Act of 1953 stipulates the standards for drugs through a variety of pharmacopeias and formularies; prohibits the sale of unsafe drugs and those with misleading labels; and, in general, regulates biologic, legend, controlled, and designated drugs. The Canadian Narcotic Control Act of 1961 governs the possession, sale, manufacture, production, and distribution of narcotics. By this Act a nurse can be in legal possession of a narcotic only when administering a drug on the order of a physician, acting as the official custodian of narcotics in a hospital or clinic, or being a client for whom a physician has prescribed a drug.

Because drugs vary in strength and activity, standardization is necessary to ensure uniformity of strength and purity by either chemical or biologic assay. The only official book of drug standards in the United States is *The United States Pharmacopeia (USP)*, whereas Canada uses the *USP*, *The Canadian Formulary*, and *The British Pharmacopoeia*.

The progress of any drug from concept to acceptance in general practice is a lengthy and costly one. The FDA approval process ensures that each drug progresses sequentially after being classified as an Investigational New Drug, with an initial pharmacologic evaluation, a limited controlled evaluation, and an extended clinical evaluation. If the drug is promising, a New Drug Application is submitted to the FDA for approval. If the NDA is approved, then a postmarketing surveillance period follows. All participants in the experimental studies of this process should have given informed consent. Because nurses have increasing contact with clinical drug studies, they need to understand the precepts of the Nuremberg Code and be alert to the protection of clients' rights.

Nurses in their practice are regulated not only by the legislation previously discussed but also by the nurse practice acts of the individual state in which they practice. These statutes define the scope of nursing practice as a health care profession within that state. As the roles of nurses are changing and expanding in drug therapy, most states are allowing nurse practitioners to prescribe within limitations. But even for nurses without a practitioner qualification, medication administration has become more of an interdependent function. Three conditions are essential for the administration of any drug by a nurse: (1) the physician and the nurse must be licensed; (2) the medication order must be valid; and (3) the nurse must be knowledgeable about the drug. In addition, nurses can safeguard themselves from errors of medication administration by observing the Five Rights of Medication Administration. With increasing accountability for their role in pharmacotherapeutics, nurses should be aware of guides to litigation-free, professional nursing practice.

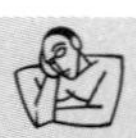

Critical Thinking

1. A nurse is working with a client with advanced cancer for whom the physician orders chemotherapy. The client has reservations about starting the chemotherapy regimen and asks numerous questions about the benefits and risks associated with it. The nurse has been told that the client's condition is terminal and knows that the chemotherapy may alter the client's comfort with severe nausea and vomiting. Although the nurse realizes that the physician recommends the chemotherapy, she feels a conflict with her role as client advocate. What action should the nurse take?
2. A nurse is preparing to administer medications to a client when she notices that the container for one of the medications, instead of having a drug name, bears a number as an experimental drug with instructions to be given "one tablet three times a day." What action should the nurse take?

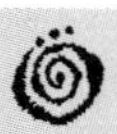

Collaborative Learning Activities

1. Student teams will be preassigned to bring copies of journal articles on current drug studies. Each team will present their perception of the study in relation to its stage of the FDA approval process. How were study participants protected? Would they be willing to participate as a researcher on this study?
2. The students will form groups of 5-6 to discuss critical thinking question #1. The groups will report back to the class.

BIBLIOGRAPHY

American Nurses' Association (1985). *Code for nurses with interpretive statements*. Kansas City, MO: The Association.

Anderson KN, et al. (Ed.) (1994). *Mosby's medical, nursing, & allied health dictionary* (4th ed.). St Louis: Mosby.

Benjamin M & Curtis J (1992). *Ethics in nursing* (3rd ed.). New York: Oxford University Press.

Blake JB (Ed.) (1968). *Safeguarding the public: Historical aspects of medicinal drug control*. Baltimore: The Johns Hopkins University Press.

Canadian Nurses' Association (1980). *CNA code of ethics: An ethical basis for nursing in Canada*. Ottawa: The Association.

Couig MP & Merkatz RB (1993). MedWatch: The new medical products reporting program, *Am J Nurs* 93(8):66.

Covington TR (Ed.) (1996). *Handbook of nonprescription drugs* (10th ed.). Washington, DC: American Pharmaceutical Association.

Cowen DL & Helfand WH (1990). *Pharmacy: An illustrated history*. New York: Harry N Abrams.

Dippel JVH (1993). Legally speaking: Reporting to the FDA, *RN* 56(12):61-2.

Drug Enforcement Administration (1990). *Pharmacist's manual: An informational outline of the Controlled Substance Act of 1970*. Washington, DC: U.S. Department of Justice.

Farley D (1987/1988). Getting outside advice for the "close calls"... advise FDA about the safety and effectiveness of drugs and biological products, *FDA Consum* 21 (10):14.

Farley D (1987/1988). How FDA approves new drugs, *FDA Consum* 21 (10):6.

Florida negative drug formulary (1994). *Florida Board of Pharmacy* 11 (2):3.

Gift AG (1993). Informed consent and vulnerable subjects, *Clin Nurs Spec* 7 (4):183.

Johnson JM (1986). Clinical trials: New responsibilities and roles for nurses *Nurs Outlook* 34(3):149.

Kallet A & Schlink FJ (1933). *100,000 guinea pigs: Dangers in everyday foods, drugs, and cosmetics*. New York: The Vanguard Press.

Mahoney DF (1994). Appropriateness of geriatric prescribing decisions made by nurse practitioners and physicians, *Image* 26 (1):41-5.

Modell W & Lansing A (1967). *Drugs*. New York: Life Science Library, Time.

New FDA classification system (1992). *Am Pharm NS*32(4):11.

Nichols LM (1992). Estimating the cost of underusing advanced practice nurses, *Nurs Economics* 10 (5):343.

Pearson LJ (1997). Annual update of how each state stands on legislative issues affecting advanced nursing practice, *Nurse Pract* 22 (1):18-25.

Shapiro RS (1994). Legal bases for the control of analgesic drugs, *J Pain & Sympt Manag* 9 (3):153-159.

Tabak N (1995). Decision making in consenting to experimental cancer therapy, *Cancer Nursing* 18 (2):89-96.

United States Pharmacopeial Convention (1996). *USP DI: Drug information for the health care professional* (16th ed.). Rockville, MD: The Convention.

Young JH (1961). *The toadstool millionaires: A social history of patent medicines in America before federal regulation*. Princeton, NJ: Princeton University Press.

Chapter 3
Principles of Drug Action

Chapter Focus

Since the number of drugs used therapeutically is increasing tremendously, the nurse's responsibilities concerning these agents have also expanded. To approach the level of knowledge needed to meet these increased responsibilities, all health professionals must develop a fundamental theoretical framework within which to study and apply an understanding of drug therapy. This chapter presents theories of drug action, physiologic processes mediating drug action, variables affecting drug action, and unusual and adverse responses to drug therapy. The nurse can transfer this knowledge to care of the unique problems of individual clients. The following objectives and key terms are important for a good understanding of the chapter.

Key Terms

absorption (p. 31)
bioavailability (p. 36)
biotransformation (p. 37)
dissolution (p. 30)
distribution (p. 36)
excretion (p. 38)
half-life (p. 41)
iatrogenic (p. 44)
loading or priming dose (p. 33)
maintenance dose (p. 33)
receptor (p. 40)

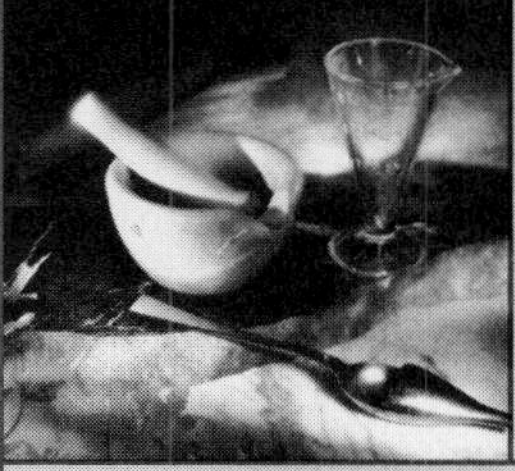

Objectives

1. Discuss the three general properties of drugs.
2. Describe the three phases of drug activity: pharmaceutical, pharmacokinetic, and pharmacodynamic.
3. Cite examples of drug properties that influence pharmacokinetics.
4. Describe the physiochemical processes mediating drug action.
5. Discuss the variables that influence the rate and extent of absorption.
6. Explain current theories of drug action: drug-receptor interaction, drug-enzyme interaction, and nonspecific drug interaction.
7. Discuss conditions that can alter the body's response to drugs.
8. Utilize nursing assessments that can identify unusual and adverse responses to drug therapy.
9. Implement nursing management of drug therapy related to client variables that alter drug responses.

Nurses have traditionally administered drugs to clients. Today, in many health care delivery settings, the nurse's responsibility has shifted to ensuring safe administration of drugs by a variety of specially educated health workers and to observing and interpreting the client's response to drug therapy. Because the moral, ethical, and legal responsibilities remain the nurse's, an understanding of the principles of drug action, or pharmacokinetics, is essential.

GENERAL PROPERTIES OF DRUGS

As stated earlier, a drug is a chemical that interacts with a living organism to produce a biologic response. This text deals with drugs administered in doses that obtain therapeutic, prophylactic, or diagnostic effects. These effects are achieved by some underlying biochemical and/or physiologic interaction between the drug and a functionally important tissue component (usually a receptor) in the body. Thus it is important to recognize the following general properties of drugs:

1. *Drugs do not confer any new functions on a tissue or organ in the body; they only modify existing functions.* Therefore the effects of drugs can be recognized only by alterations of a known physiologic function or process such as, replacing, interrupting, or potentiating a physiologic process in specialized tissues. The following are examples: Drugs used to treat anemia can replace iron to restore the adequate production of red blood cells. Atropine, on the other hand, reduces the rate of salivation in preoperative clients, which is an essentially abnormal state but a necessary one to decrease the surgical risk of aspiration. Finally, the administration of a cathartic can potentiate the rate of evacuation of the large intestine.
2. *Drugs in general exert multiple actions rather than a single effect.* Consequently, drugs may in varying degrees produce undesirable responses because of their potential to modify more than one function of the body. These unwanted effects may be avoided somewhat by administering more specific or more selective drugs. For example, metaproterenol is a selective beta$_2$-adrenergic agent used to produce bronchodilation. Yet a common side effect is beta$_2$-mediated muscle tremors.
3. *Drug action results from a physicochemical interaction between the drug and a functionally important molecule in the body.* Some drugs act by combining with a small molecule (e.g., antacids neutralize gastric acid) or producing alteration of cell membrane activity (e.g., local anesthetics). However, the major mechanism by which drugs interact is by combining with macromolecular components of tissues, such as receptors.

MECHANISMS OF DRUG ACTION

To produce its optimal effect, a drug must reach appropriate concentrations at its site of action. This means that the molecules of the chemical compound must proceed from their point of entry into the body to the tissues with which they react. In addition, the magnitude of the response depends on the dosage and the frequency of doses of the drug in the body. Therefore the concentration of the drug at its site of action is influenced by various processes, which may be divided into three phases of drug activity: pharmaceutical, pharmacokinetic, and pharmacodynamic. The sequential order of these phases is depicted in Figure 3-1.

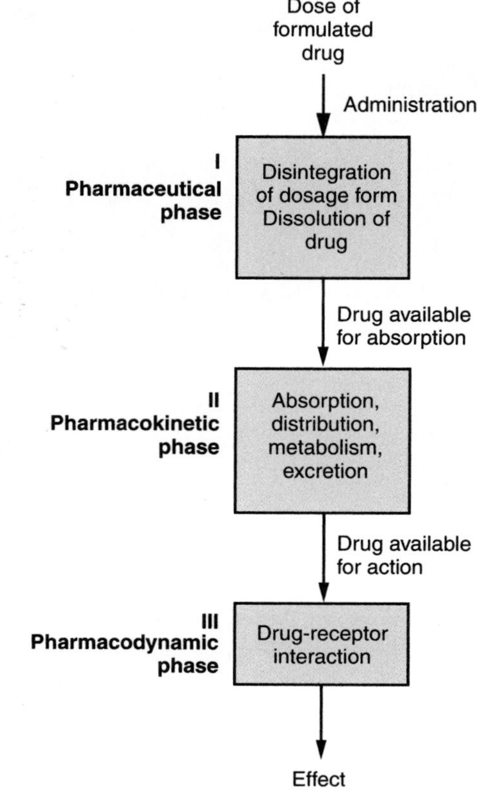

FIGURE 3-1 Phases affecting drug activity.

Pharmaceutical Phase

Pharmaceutics is the study of the ways in which various drug forms influence pharmacokinetic and pharmacodynamic activities. A drug may appear in solid form (tablet, capsule, or powder) or in liquid form (solution or suspension).

Disintegration of solid dosage forms must occur before **dissolution**, the process by which a drug goes into solution and becomes available for absorption, occurs. The drug dosage form is important, for the more rapid the rate of dissolution, the more readily the compound crosses the cell membrane to achieve absorption. Obviously, oral drugs in liquid form are more rapidly available for gastrointestinal absorption than those in solid form (Figure 3-2 and Box 3-1).

Pharmacokinetic Phase

Pharmacokinetics is the study of the concentration of a drug during the processes of absorption, distribution, biotransformation, and excretion. The concentration that a drug attains

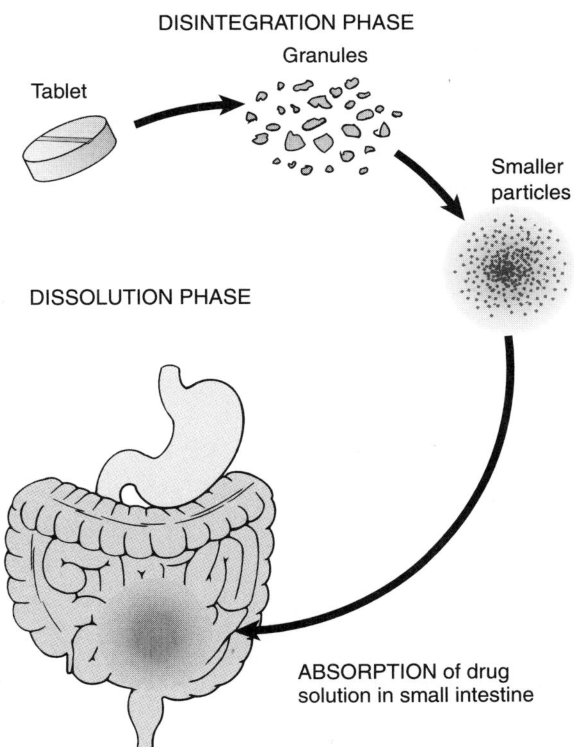

FIGURE 3-2 Pharmaceutical phase.

BOX 3-1

Absorption of Preparations

Preparation	Rate
Liquids, elixirs, syrups	Fastest
Suspension solutions	↓
Powders	↓
Capsules	↓
Tablets	↓
Coated tablets	↓
Enteric-coated tablets	Slowest

at its site of action is influenced by four primary factors: the rate and extent to which a drug is (1) absorbed into body fluids, (2) distributed to sites of action or storage areas, (3) biotransformed or metabolized to breakdown or active metabolites, and (4) excreted from the body by various routes (Figure 3-3; see Figure 3-1).

Properties That Influence Pharmacokinetic Activity

Physiochemical Properties of Drugs

In general, drugs exist as weak acids or weak bases and in body fluids they appear in either ionized or nonionized forms. The ionized (polar) form is usually water soluble (lipid insoluble) and does not diffuse readily through the cell membranes of the body. By contrast, the nonionized (nonpolar) form is more lipid soluble (less water soluble) and is more apt to cross the cell membranes. The influence of pH on these compounds is discussed under Absorption in this chapter.

Physiochemical Properties of Cell Membranes

The extent to which a drug attains pharmacokinetic activity (absorption, distribution, biotransformation, and excretion) depends on the rate at which it crosses the cell membrane. The membrane consists of a bimolecular layer of lipids that contain protein molecules, which are irregularly dispersed throughout the lipid bilayer. The protein molecule itself may act as a carrier, an enzyme, a receptor, or an antigenic site. The drugs that are lipid (fat) soluble can easily pass through the lipid membrane, while ionized or water-soluble drugs have difficulty crossing cell membranes. The membrane, which appears to contain pores, permits the passage of small water-soluble substances such as urea, alcohol, electrolytes, and water itself.

Drug molecules, when free to move to sites of action, are transported from one body compartment to another by way of the plasma. However, free movement can be somewhat limited because these various sites are enclosed by membranes. Barriers to drug transport may consist of a single layer of cells, such as the villus in intestinal epithelium, or several layers of cells, such as skin. Nevertheless, in order for a drug to gain access to the interior of a cell or a body compartment, it has to penetrate cell membranes. All the physiologic processes mediating drug action—absorption, distribution, metabolism, and excretion—are predicated on two physiochemical properties: passive transport and active transport.

Passive transport. Passive transport of drugs occurs when the membrane is not required to generate energy to carry out the process.

Passive transport or diffusion is the random movement of a substance from a region of higher concentration to a region of lower concentration until equilibrium is established at the membrane. The vast majority of drugs are transported via this mechanism.

Carrier or active transport. Moderate-sized ions and water-soluble molecules, including the ionic forms of most drugs, do not readily enter cells but require some means of transport. Carrier or active transport is believed to be conducted by "carriers" that form complexes with drug molecules on the membrane surface, carry them through the membrane, and then dissociate from them. The dynamics of active transport are similar to those of facilitated diffusion except that in this type of transfer an energy source is required. Active transport involves the movement of drug molecules against the concentration gradient (from areas of low concentration to areas of high concentration) or, in the case of ions, against the electrochemical potential gradient such as occurs with the "sodium pump." Active transport is usually more rapid than passive diffusion.

Pharmacokinetic Activities

Absorption

Absorption is a process involving the movement of drug molecules from the site of entry into the body to the circu-

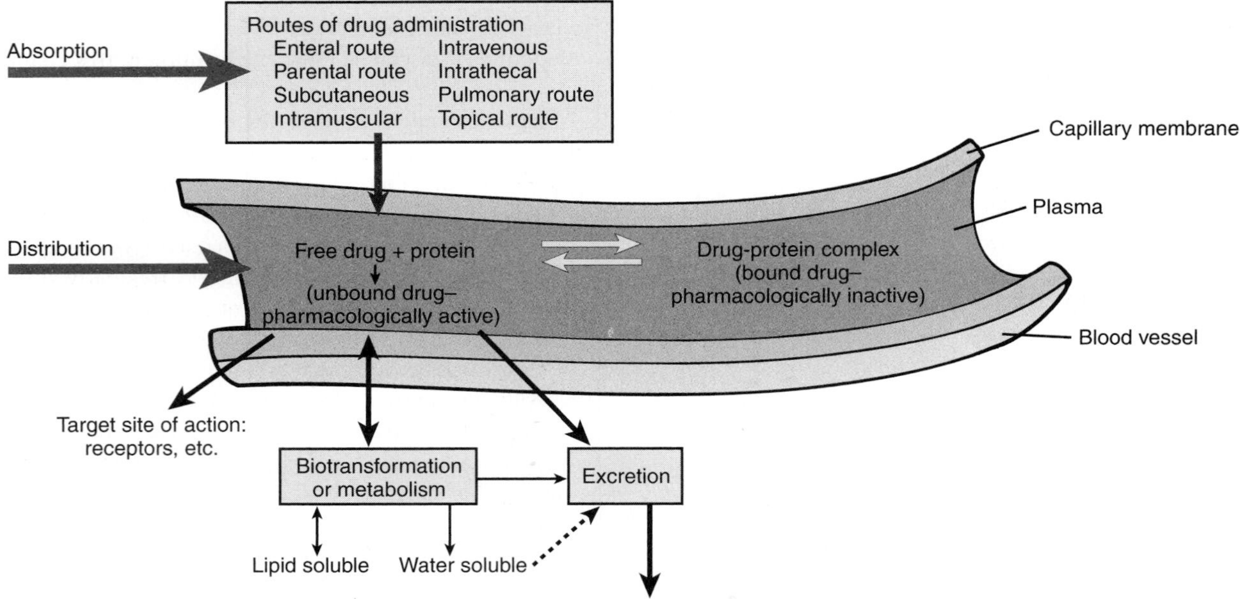

FIGURE 3-3 Schema of pharmacokinetic phase of drug action, showing absorption, distribution, biotransformation, and excretion of drugs. Note that only free drug is capable of movement for absorption, distribution to the target site of action, biotransformation, and excretion; the drug-protein complex represents bound drugs; and because the molecule is large, it is trapped in the blood vessel and serves as a storage site for the drug.

lating fluids. Absorption begins at the site of administration and is essential to the three subsequent processes—distribution, metabolism, and excretion. The rate of drug absorption is significant because it determines when a drug becomes pharmacologically available to exert its action. Of importance is that both the duration and the intensity of drug action are greatly influenced by the rate of this process. Accordingly, this type of response depends on the selection of the *route* of administration, the *dose* of the drug, and the *dosage form* (tablet, capsule, or liquid) of the agent administered.

Variables that affect drug absorption. The rate and extent to which a drug is absorbed are influenced by the following:

1. Nature of the absorbing surface (cell membrane) through which the drug must traverse. The drug molecule may pass through a single layer of cells (intestinal epithelium), in which case transport is faster than when it traverses several layers of cells (skin). In addition, the size of the surface area of the absorbing site is an important determinant of drug absorption. Generally, the more extensive the absorbing surface, the greater the drug absorption and the more rapid its effects. Anesthetics are absorbed immediately from the pulmonary epithelium because of the vast surface area. Absorption from the small intestine, which offers a massive absorbing area, is more rapid than from a smaller absorbing surface, such as the stomach.
2. Blood flow to the site of administration. Circulation to the site of administration is a significant factor in the absorption of drugs. A rich blood supply (sublingual route) enhances absorption, whereas a poor vascular site (subcutaneous route) delays it. An individual in shock, for example, may not respond to intramuscularly administered drugs because of poor peripheral circulation. Drugs injected intravenously, on the other hand, are placed directly into the circulatory system and are totally available. Intravenous administration is desirable when speedy drug effects are necessary, but it carries the potential danger of achieving temporarily toxic responses in vital organs such as the heart or the brain. Therefore, to prevent deleterious effects, some drugs must be injected slowly. In addition, the decreased peripheral blood flow in clients with congestive heart failure or circulatory shock may cause a significant reduction in the rate of transport of injected drugs to the target tissues, thereby considerably altering their efficacy.
3. Solubility of the drug. To be absorbed, a drug must be in solution; the more soluble the drug, the more rapidly it will be absorbed. Because cell membranes contain a fatty acid layer, lipid solubility is a valuable attribute of drugs to be absorbed from certain areas—for example, the alimentary tract and the placental barrier. Chemicals and minerals that form insoluble precipitates in the gastrointestinal tract, such as barium salts, or drugs that are not soluble in water or lipids cannot be absorbed. Parenterally administered drugs prepared in oily vehicles, such as streptomycin, will be absorbed more slowly than drugs dissolved in water or isotonic sodium chloride.

4. pH. When in solution, drugs are a mixture of ionized and nonionized forms. The nonionized drug is lipid soluble and readily diffuses across the cell membrane; the ionized drug is lipid insoluble and nondiffusible. An acidic drug (e.g., aspirin) becomes relatively undissociated in an acid environment such as the stomach and therefore can readily diffuse across the membranes into the circulation. In contrast, a basic drug tends to ionize in the same acid environment and is not absorbed through the gastric membrane. Absorption is enhanced in the less acidic or more basic sites, such as the small intestine. The reverse occurs when a drug is in an alkaline medium (Figure 3-4).

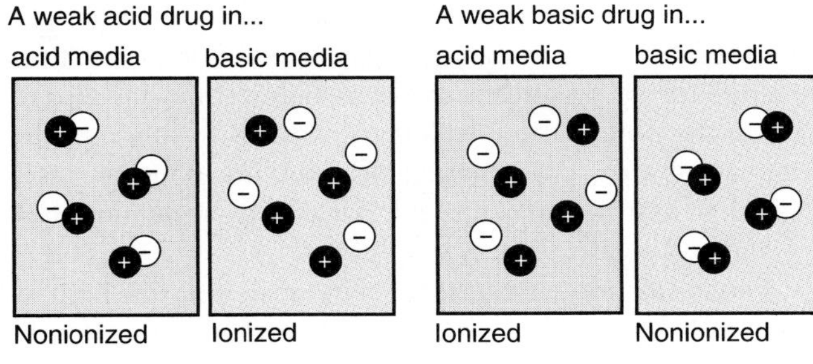

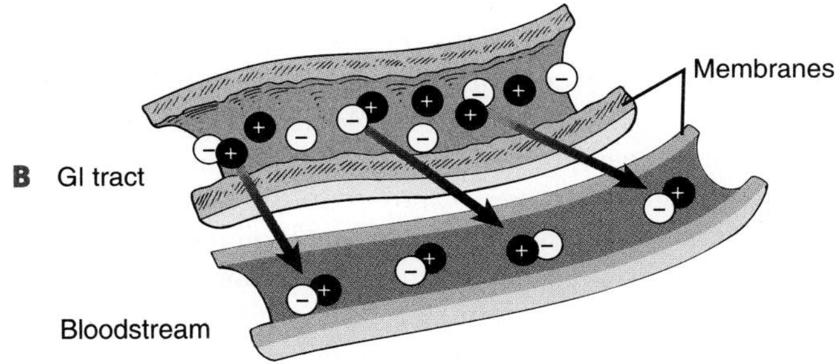

FIGURE 3-4 Effect of pH on drug ionization and transport. **A**, Effects of pH on drug molecules. **B**, Effects of pH on the transport of drug molecules through membranes.

5. Drug concentration. Drugs administered in high concentrations tend to be more rapidly absorbed than drugs administered in low concentrations. In certain situations, a drug may be initially administered in large doses that temporarily exceed the body's capacity for excretion of the drug. In this way, active drug levels are rapidly reached at the receptor site. Once an active drug level is established, smaller daily doses of the drug can be administered to replace only the amount of the drug excreted since the previous dose. The initial, temporary large doses of the drug are **loading,** or **priming doses,** used to rapidly reach a therapeutic drug response, while the smaller daily doses are **maintenance doses,** used to maintain a therapeutic drug response (Figure 3-5). Such manipulation of drug dosage is frequently used, for example, with digitalis and steroid preparations in acute situations.
6. Dosage form. Drug concentration can be manipulated by pharmaceutical processing. It is possible to combine an active drug with a resin or another substance from which it is slowly released or to prepare a drug in a vehicle that offers relative resistance to the digestive action of stomach contents (enteric coating). Enteric coatings on drugs are used: (1) to prevent decomposition of chemically sensitive drugs by gastric secretions (penicillin G and erythromycin are unstable in an acid pH), (2) to prevent dilution of the drug before it reaches the intestine, (3) to prevent nausea and vomiting induced by the drug's effect in the stomach, and (4) to provide delayed action of the drug.

Routes of drug administration. The mode of drug administration affects both the rate at which onset of action occurs and the magnitude of the therapeutic response that results. Therefore the choice of the route of administration is crucial in determining the suitability of a drug for an individual client. For example, a client who is vomiting will have little or no appreciable gastrointestinal absorption of a drug when it is administered orally. Obviously, rectal or parenteral

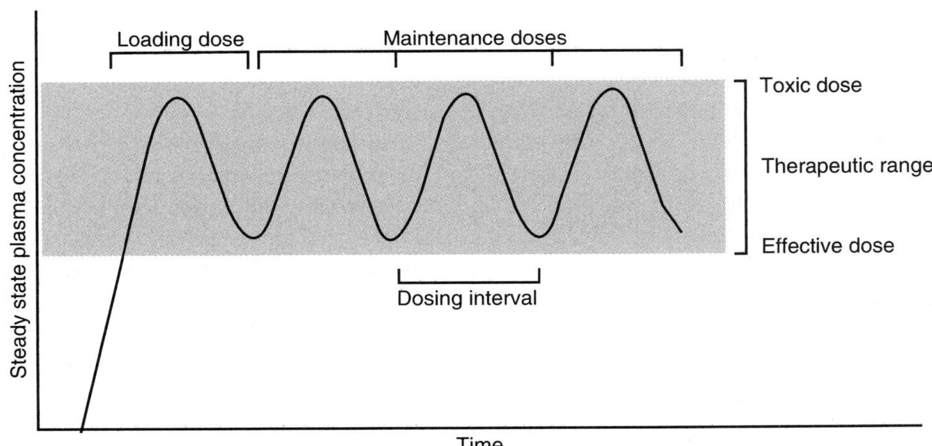

FIGURE 3-5 A loading dose is administered to reach a therapeutic response level rapidly. Maintenance doses are administered at prescribed intervals to maintain a therapeutic drug response.

administration would be more beneficial in obtaining a therapeutic drug response.

Drugs are given for either local or systemic effects. The local effect of a drug usually occurs at the immediate site of application, in which case absorption is a disadvantage. When a drug is given for a systemic effect, absorption is an essential first step before the agent appears in the circulation and is distributed to a location distant from the site of administration.

A drug may enter the circulation either by being injected there directly—intravenously—or by absorption from depots in which it has been placed. The routes of drug administration can be classified into the following categories: (1) enteral (drugs administered along any portion of the gastrointestinal tract), (2) parenteral—subcutaneous, intramuscular, intravenous, intrathecal, (3) pulmonary, and (4) topical (see Figure 3-3).

Enteral route. Generally, the oral or enteral ingestion is the most commonly used method of giving drugs. It is also the safest (because drug may be retrieved), most convenient, and most economical route of administration. However, the frequent changes of the gastrointestinal environment produced by food, emotion, and physical activity may make it the most unreliable and slowest of the commonly used routes. Drugs are absorbed from several sites along the gastrointestinal tract.

Oral absorption. The oral cavity is lined with mucous membranes that consist of epithelial cells; these cells secrete saliva to begin digestion of food. Although the oral cavity possesses a thin lining, a rich blood supply, and a slightly acidic pH, little absorption occurs in the mouth. On the other hand, despite its small surface area, the oral mucosa is capable of absorbing certain drugs as long as they dissolve rapidly in the salivary secretions. The oral mucosa absorbs drugs given by the sublingual and buccal routes. In sublingual administration the drug is placed under the tongue to permit tablet dissolution in salivary secretions. Nitroglycerin is administered in this manner, and the client is advised to refrain as long as possible from swallowing the saliva containing the tablet form of the drug. Because nitroglycerin is nonionic with a high lipid solubility, the drug readily diffuses through the lipid mucosal membranes. After absorption it enters the systemic circulation without preliminary passage through the liver. Accordingly, absorption is rapid, and the effects of the drug may become apparent within 2 minutes. In buccal administration the drug (tablet) is placed between the teeth and the mucous membrane of the cheek. Some hormones and enzyme preparations are administered by this route and are rapidly absorbed. Both sublingual and buccal routes avoid drug destruction by gastrointestinal fluids and the first pass effect of the liver by avoiding the portal circulation.

Gastric absorption. Although the stomach has a rich blood supply and a large surface area, which provide excellent potential for drug absorption, it is not an important absorption site. The length of time a substance remains in the stomach is a significant variable in determining the extent of gastric absorption. This is governed by the pH of the drug and gastric motility.

In the stomach the pH is low (about 1.4), and drugs such as the barbiturates, which are slightly acidic, tend to remain nonionized and thus are readily absorbed into the circulation. Morphine and quinine are slightly basic; they ionize in the stomach and thus are poorly absorbed. A large majority of drugs are weak bases and on entry into the small intestine are absorbed because of the alkaline pH of the environment.

Generally, slowing the gastric emptying rate decreases drug absorption and vice versa. This is the reason so many drugs are administered on an empty stomach with sufficient water (8 ounces) to ensure dissolution, rapid passage into the small intestine, and drug absorption in the larger surface area. Since some drugs cause gastric irritation, they are usually given with food. In addition, after solid-dose drug administration, the client should be encouraged to sit upright for at least 30 minutes to hasten gastric emptying time (time required for the drug to reach the small intestine) and also to reduce the potential for tablets or capsules to lodge in the esophageal area. Prolongation of emptying time increases the risk of destruction of unstable drugs (e.g., acetaminophen [Tylenol]) by gastric juices.

Small intestine absorption. The small intestine with its many villi has a larger absorption area than the stomach. Also, it is highly vascularized. Drugs that are poorly soluble in the stomach pass into this region and are absorbed primarily in the upper part of the small intestine. The pH of the intestinal fluid is alkaline (7 to 8), which strongly influences the rate of absorption of the nonionized basic drugs. Increased intestinal motility caused, for example, by diarrhea or cathartics may decrease exposure to the intestinal membrane and thereby diminish absorption. Prolonged exposure, on the other hand, allows more time for absorption.

Rectal absorption. The surface area of the rectum is not very large, but drug absorption does occur because of extensive vascularity. In addition, drugs administered rectally are not subjected to hepatic alteration, since the blood that perfuses this region bypasses the liver. Disadvantages to rectal drug administration include erratic absorption because of rectal contents, local drug irritation with some medications, and uncertainty of drug retention.

Parenteral route. The parenteral route refers to the administration of drugs by injection. It is the most rapid form of systemic therapy.

Subcutaneous. A subcutaneous injection means a drug is given beneath the skin into the connective tissue or fat immediately underlying the dermis. This site can be used only for drugs that are not irritating to the tissue; otherwise severe pain, necrosis, and sloughing of tissue may occur. The rate of absorption is slow and can provide a sustained effect.

Intramuscular. Intramuscular administration means a drug is injected into skeletal muscle. Absorption occurs more rapidly than with subcutaneous injection because of greater tissue blood flow.

Intravenous. The intravenous route produces an immediate pharmacologic response because the desired concentration of drug is injected directly into the bloodstream, thereby circumventing the absorption process. Intravenous drugs should be administered slowly to prevent adverse effects.

Intrathecal. Intrathecal administration means that a drug is injected directly into the spinal subarachnoid space, bypassing the blood-brain barrier. Many compounds cannot enter the cerebrospinal fluid or are absorbed in this region very slowly. When rapid effects of drugs are desired, as in spinal anesthesia or in treatment of acute infection of the central nervous system, this route may be used.

Epidural. Epidural administration of a drug means that it is injected via a small catheter into the epidural space, the space outside of the dura mater, of the spinal column. This route is increasingly being used with opioids for pain management.

Other parenteral routes. Drugs may be injected into other cavities of the body. Intraarticular administration of a drug delivers the medication into the synovial cavity of a joint, usually to relieve pain, reduce inflammation, and maintain joint mobility. Intraosseous drug administration delivers drugs or blood into the bone marrow when IV access is difficult. Intraperitoneal and intrapleural administration of antineoplastic agents allows for these drugs to be delivered directly to the tumor sites.

Pulmonary route. To ensure that normal gas exchange of oxygen and carbon dioxide is continuous in the lungs, drugs must be in the form of gases or fine mists (aerosols) when they are administered by inhalation. The lungs provide a large surface area for absorption, and the rich capillary network adjacent to the alveolar membrane tends to promote ready entry of medication into the bloodstream. Drugs such as bronchodilators, mucolytics, and antibiotics are administered by various inhalation devices (nebulizers, pressure tanks) that propel the agents into the alveolar sacs and produce primarily local effects and at times unwanted systemic effects. Additionally, epinephrine may be administered into the intratracheal tube to restore cardiac rhythm in cardiac arrest.

Topical route. Absorption of drugs applied topically to the skin and mucous membranes of various structures in the body is generally rapid (see Nursing Research box below).

Skin. Drugs applied to the skin are employed to produce a local or systemic effect through ointments or transdermal patches. Only lipid-soluble compounds are absorbed through the skin, which acts as a lipid barrier. To prevent adverse effects from systemic absorption of toxic chemicals, only an intact skin surface should be used. Massaging the skin enhances absorption of the drug because capillaries become dilated and local blood flow is increased as a result of the warmth created by the friction of rubbing.

Transdermal. Usually a disk or patch that contains a day to a week's supply of medication. After application to the skin the medication is absorbed at a steady rate. Examples of drugs that are applied transdermally are nitroglycerin (Nitrodisc) and scopolamine (Transderm-Scop).

Eyes. Administration of drugs in the eye produces a local effect on the conjunctiva or anterior chamber. Eyeball movements promote the distribution of drug over the surface of the eye.

Ears. Administration of drops into the auditory canal may be chosen to treat local infection, inflammatory conditions, or wax in the external ear.

Nasal mucosa. Drugs may be instilled in droplet form or in a prepackaged specific-dose swab intended for direct in-

Nursing Research

Perspectives on new drug delivery approaches

Recent developments in both applied dermal physiology and in pharmaceutical technology are expanding the more nontraditional routes of drug administration, which will have an effect on nursing practice. Among these approaches, transdermal and transmucosal applications appear particularly promising because of the accessibility, noninvasiveness, compliance, safety, and efficacy associated with the techniques.

Under normal clinical conditions, the transdermal patch delivers the drug at a rate below the absorbing capacity of the skin. Uptake of the drug by local blood flow then lowers the concentration of the drug in the skin, maintaining the concentration gradient between the transdermal reservoir and the skin. Fentanyl, the prototypical opioid for transdermal applications, is available for general clinical use in the pain management of clients with cancer.

Also newly developed for transmucosal administration is a fentanyl lozenge that allows for the comfortable premedication, anxiolysis, and sedation of both children and adults within 20 to 40 minutes. Although the drug in a candy matrix was readily accepted, provided a rapid onset of action, and a high rate of "good to excellent" induction conditions, it was also noted that dose-related respiratory depression, facial pruritus, nausea, and vomiting occurred.

The potent synthetic opioid sufentanil and the tranquilizer midazolam have established therapeutic efficacy with intranasal instillation. Despite some limitations, practitioners have developed great skill at administering carefully titrated amounts of premedicant drugs to children and adults.

Nontraditional approaches to the administration of medications are currently under extensive investigation. As these technologies become refined, the ability to achieve and control therapeutic concentrations of drugs within the body will be realized.

Critical thinking questions

- With a client wearing a transdermal patch, what might occur if the client experienced very low cutaneous blood flow from, for example, hypothermia or low cardiac output?
- What might be of ethical concern with fentanyl lozenges?

tranasal application for systemic absorption or to facilitate shrinkage of the mucosa to enhance breathing or to insert a nasotracheal tube.

Bioavailability. **Bioavailability** refers to the percentage of active drug substances absorbed and available to target tissues, following administration. Thus drugs are biologically equivalent if they attain similar concentrations in blood and tissues at similar times; they are therapeutically equivalent if they provide equal therapeutic effectiveness in clinical trials. Of importance is the similarity of the absorption and therapeutic performances of drugs, which can be altered markedly by the ingredients and method of drug manufacture. Furthermore, different brands of the same drug can vary, and even different lots from a single manufacturer may show different levels of effectiveness. Thus the FDA is paying more attention to drug preparation and trying to ensure that the bioavailability of a drug conforms to uniform standards. Both the proportion of active drug and the percentage of its absorption are essential to attain therapeutic equivalence among all chemically similar drugs.

Distribution

Once absorbed a drug is immediately distributed throughout the body by blood circulation. **Distribution** is defined as the transport of a drug in body fluids from the bloodstream to various tissues of the body and ultimately to its site of action (see Figure 3-3). The rate at which a drug enters the different areas of the body depends on the permeability of capillaries for the drug's molecules. As already discussed, lipid-soluble drugs can readily cross capillary membranes to enter most tissues and fluid compartments, whereas lipid-insoluble drugs require more time to arrive at their point of action. However, cardiac functions also affect the rate and extent of distribution of a drug; specifically, cardiac output (the amount of blood pumped by the heart each minute) and regional blood flow (the amount of blood supplied to a specific organ or tissue) determine how much time is required. Most of the drug is first distributed to organs that have a rich blood supply: heart, liver, kidney, and brain. Afterward, the drug enters organs with a poor blood supply, which include muscles and fat.

Drug reservoirs. Storage reservoirs allow a drug to accumulate by binding to specific tissues in the body. This sustains the pharmacologic effect of a drug at its point of action. The body's storage reservoirs involve two general types of drug pooling: plasma protein binding and tissue binding.

Plasma protein binding. On entry into the circulatory system, drugs may become attached to proteins, mainly albumin contained in the blood. Thus, as free drug enters the plasma, it binds to the protein to form a drug-protein complex. This combination can also be reversed:

Free drug + Protein = Drug-protein complex

The formula indicates that equilibrium is established between the amount of free drug and the amount of drug that is bound to protein (drug-protein complex). Protein binding decreases the concentration of free drug in the circulation, thereby limiting the amount that travels to the site of action. The drug-albumin molecule is too large to diffuse through the membrane of the blood vessel, so the bound molecule is trapped in the bloodstream and pharmacologically inactive. It becomes a circulating drug reservoir or storage depot (see Figure 3-3).

The equilibrium process is dynamic. As free drug is eliminated from the body, the drug-protein complex begins to dissociate so that more free drug is released to replace what is lost. As a result, the fact that the body temporarily stores the drug molecules in the drug-protein complex allows the drug to be available for a longer period of time. For example, a sulfonamide is highly bound to protein; and because free drug molecules are released slowly from the bound form, the antiinfective action of the antibiotic is long-lasting.

Degree of drug binding. Plasma protein binding is expressed as a percentage, which represents the percent of total drug that is bound. Among the *highly protein-bound* drugs are warfarin (Coumadin), which is 99% protein bound, and propranolol, which is 93% protein bound. Accordingly, a ratio exists between free and bound drug. In the case of propranolol this means that in a given period of time, 93% is bound to plasma proteins and only 7% of free drug is available for therapeutic use, eventual biotransformation, and excretion. Therefore if more than 7% of the drug is free to act within this same period of time, toxicity may occur. In the literature, protein binding is expressed in general terms with ranges as follows, rather than in terms of specific percentages:

- Very high: >90%
- High: 65% to 90%
- Moderate: 35% to 64%
- Low: 10% to 34%
- Very low: <10%

Competition for binding sites. Since albumin and other plasma proteins provide a number of binding sites, two drugs can compete with one another for the same site and displace each other. This competition may have dangerous consequences if particular combinations of drugs are administered. For example, serious problems can arise when a client who is satisfactorily stabilized on maintenance doses of warfarin, an anticoagulant, is simultaneously given aspirin, an analgesic. The aspirin may displace some of the protein-bound warfarin, thereby increasing the free drug level and causing severe hemorrhage. Because warfarin is normally highly protein bound, its continued administration may raise the concentration of free drug, causing further severe adverse reactions. Therefore the nurse must be alert to the potential dangers of drug interactions occurring when multiple agents are prescribed concurrently.

Hypoalbuminemia. Hypoalbuminemia is characterized by low levels of albumin in the blood. Either hepatic damage, such as cirrhosis of the liver, or some type of body cavity drainage may cause hypoalbuminemia. Furthermore, failure of the liver to synthesize enough of the plasma proteins needed to bind drugs means that more free drug is available for distribution to tissue sites. Therefore when a client is given the normal dosage of a drug that normally has plasma protein binding, more of the free form of drug is allowed into the circulation, resulting in possible overdosage and toxicity. The drug dosage should be adjusted (reduced) until a normal level of plasma protein is reported.

Tissue binding

Fat tissue. Lipid-soluble drugs have a high affinity for adipose tissue, which is where these drugs are stored. Moreover, the relatively low blood flow in fat tissue makes it a stable reservoir for drugs. As an example, a lipid-soluble drug such as thiopental (Pentothal) may stay in low concentrations in body fat for as long as 3 hours after administration. If this drug is given again before it is all excreted, it can produce a cumulative effect, since an additional amount of the agent will be stored in the fat tissue.

Bone. Some drugs have an unusual affinity for bone; for example, the antibiotic tetracycline accumulates in bone after being absorbed onto the bone-crystal surface. Tetracycline can interfere with the growth of bones when it accumulates in skeletal tissues of the fetus (by crossing the placenta from the mother) or young children. When the drug is distributed to unerupted teeth in a fetus or young child, discoloration of teeth results. Brownish pigmentation of permanent teeth also may result if this drug is given during the prenatal period or early childhood. See Box 3-3 for specific actions of drugs in fetal tissues.

Barriers to drug distribution. Specialized structures made up of biologic membranes can serve as barriers to the passage of drugs at certain sites in the body. These include the blood-brain barrier and the placental barrier.

Blood-brain barrier. The blood-brain barrier is a special anatomic arrangement that allows distribution of only lipid-soluble drugs (e.g., general anesthetics, barbiturates) into the brain and cerebrospinal fluid. Actually the barrier is made up of a row of capillary endothelial cells covered by a fatty sheath of glial cells joined by continuous tight intercellular junctions. Consequently, compounds that are strongly ionized and poorly soluble in fat cannot enter the brain. Thus antibiotics that cross the blood-brain barrier with difficulty cannot be used to treat infections of the central nervous system. However, if a drug is instilled intrathecally, it bypasses the blood-brain barrier and directly treats the bacterial infection.

Placental barrier. The membrane layers that separate the blood vessels of the mother and the fetus constitute the placental barrier. In addition, tissue enzymes in the placenta can metabolize some agents (e.g., catecholamines) by inactivating them as they travel from the maternal circulation to the embryo. Despite the thickness of the structure, it does not afford complete protection to the fetus. Unlike the blood-brain barrier, the nonselective passage of drugs across the placenta to the fetus is a well-established fact. Although lipid-soluble substances preferentially diffuse across the placenta, the barrier is also permeable to a great number of lipid-insoluble drugs. Consequently, many agents intended to produce a therapeutic response in the mother also may cross the placental barrier and exert harmful effects on the developing embryo. Among the drugs easily transported across the placenta are steroids, narcotics, anesthetics, and some antibiotics (Box 3-2).

Biotransformation or Metabolism

After drug absorption and distribution, the body eliminates the drug by biotransformation and excretion. **Biotransformation** (metabolism) chemically inactivates a drug by converting it into a more water-soluble compound, or metabolite, that can be excreted from the body (see Figure 3-3). The liver is the primary site of metabolism of drugs, but other tissues also may be involved in this process, namely the plasma, kidneys, lungs, and intestinal mucosa.

Hepatic biotransformation. After distribution to their sites of action, most drugs undergo metabolic changes, or

BOX 3-2

Fetal Drug Effects

Two major types of drug effects occur in the fetus. When given during the first trimester of pregnancy, some drugs induce aberrant development of organs and systems during the formation of these structures. This type is known as a teratogenic drug, which is defined as an agent that causes physical defects in a developing embryo. Many drugs that cause anomalies are known to cross the placenta and exhibit teratogenicity.

The second type of drug affects the second half of pregnancy as well as delivery, causing respiratory depression in the newborn because of the underdeveloped capacity of the infant to biotransform the drug and excrete it.

The rate of maternal blood flow to the placenta limits the availability of the drug to the fetus. Because passage of drugs is delayed, drugs take action in the mother more rapidly than in the fetus. This fact explains why an alert infant can be delivered to an anesthetized mother, provided that delivery occurs within 10 to 15 minutes of the time the drug is administered to the mother. Long-term administration of drugs to the mother, however, may produce adverse effects on the fetus. For example, infants born to mothers dependent on narcotics or cocaine manifest withdrawal symptoms after delivery and removal from the flow of the products through the mother.

Unfortunately the teratogenic effects of many drugs have not been adequately studied. Also, a potentially dangerous drug may be administered to a woman who is not aware of her pregnancy. It should be assumed that any drug will be able to pass the placental barrier, and the nurse must advise pregnant women not to take any drug without consulting the physician. Drugs should be administered during pregnancy only when the advantages greatly outweigh the potential risks to the fetus.

biotransformation. The chemical alterations are produced by microsomal enzyme systems, located largely in the liver, which consist of endoplasmic reticula, a series of membranes that appear as a network of canals within the cells. The microsomal enzymes usually affect biotransformation of lipid-soluble, nonpolar drugs. To increase polarity, they undergo one or both of two general types of chemical reactions. One type of transformation consists of oxidation, hydrolysis, or reduction. These chemical reactions increase the water solubility of drug molecules (increased polarity). The second type, called conjugation, involves the union of the polar group of a drug with another substance in the body—glucuronide, glycine, methyl, or other alkyl groups. The conjugated molecule also becomes more polar or more water soluble and therefore more excretable. These responses generally produce a loss in pharmacologic activity and occasionally are referred to as *detoxication reactions.*

Individuals vary considerably in the rates at which they metabolize drugs. The microsomal enzyme system can be depressed by conditions that affect hepatic function, such as starvation and obstructive jaundice. Individuals with liver disease, severe cardiovascular dysfunction, or renal problems may be expected to have prolonged or decreased drug metabolism. Infants with immature metabolizing enzyme systems and the aged with degenerative enzyme function are major groups that experience depressed biotransformation. Genetically determined differences also affect metabolism. Some drugs (e.g., procainamide, hydralazine, and isoniazid) are metabolized by the acetyltransferase system. This system divides the population into "rapid acetylators" and "slow acetylators." The rapid acetylators metabolize a greater proportion of a drug dose than do the slow acetylators. The rapid acetylators may develop reactions caused by the metabolic products of a drug, whereas the slow acetylators may appear more sensitive to a drug by experiencing severe toxic effects. For example, an individual who is a slow acetylator and who is receiving procainamide (Pronestyl) is apt to develop a lupus-like syndrome, which is a serious adverse response. If drug metabolism is delayed, cumulative drug effects may be expected and may be manifested as excessive or prolonged responses to ordinary doses of drugs. If drug metabolism is stimulated, a state of apparent drug tolerance is produced. A number of substances cause increased activity by hepatic microsomal enzymes, including CNS depressants, xanthines, pesticides, food preservatives, and dyes. Repeated administration of some drugs may stimulate the formation of new microsomal enzymes. This is thought to be the case with some hypnotic drugs, whose effect diminishes with prolonged administration.

Hepatic first-pass effect. Orally administered drugs absorbed from the gastrointestinal tract normally travel first to the portal system and the liver before entering the general circulation. However, some drugs may first be taken up by the hepatic microsomal enzyme system, so that a significant amount is metabolized before the drug ever reaches the systemic circulation. Consequently, only a small fraction of the dose is available for distribution to produce a pharmacologic effect. Thus the hepatic first-pass effect is defined as an initial biotransformation of drug (on passage through the liver from the portal vein) that produces a loss of pharmacologically active molecules. In some cases, the hepatic first-pass effect may result in complete elimination of the drug without the production of any pharmacologic activity. Hence a drug with an extensive hepatic first-pass effect may require an increase in dosage to produce a therapeutic effect. Alternatively, the drug may be administered parenterally to bypass the liver, thereby preventing initial biotransformation.

Excretion

A drug continues to act in the body until it is biotransformed or excreted. Drug molecules (intact, changed, or inactivated) ultimately must be removed from their sites of action by physiologic channels involving mechanisms of excretion. **Excretion** is a process whereby drugs and pharmacologically active or inactive metabolites are eliminated from the body, primarily through the kidneys.

Organs of excretion

Kidneys. Drug excretion via the kidneys is the most important route for elimination. Some drugs are excreted unchanged in the urine, while other drugs are so extensively metabolized that only a small fraction of the original chemical substance is excreted intact.

Excretion is accomplished through passive glomerular filtration, active tubular secretion, and partial reabsorption (Figure 3-6). The availability of a drug for glomerular filtration depends on its concentration in unbound form in plasma. Free, unbound drugs and water-soluble metabolites are filtered by the glomeruli, whereas protein-bound substances do not pass through this structure. After filtration, lipid-soluble compounds are not excreted; instead, they are reabsorbed by the tubular nephron and reenter the systemic circulation. The water-soluble compounds, on the other hand, fail to be reabsorbed and therefore are eliminated from the body.

Urinary pH varies between 4.6 and 8.2 and affects the amount of drug reabsorbed in the renal tubule by passive diffusion. Weak acids are excreted more readily in alkaline urine and more slowly in acidic urine; the reverse is true for weak bases. In cases of poisoning by weak organic acids such as aspirin or phenobarbital, alkalinizing the urine can result in increased urinary drug excretion. Raising the pH of the urine causes weak acids to become ionized, and subsequently these agents are excreted.

Urine may be alkalinized by administering sodium bicarbonate or tromethamine (Tham-E). By contrast, high doses of vitamin C or ammonium chloride acidify the urine and promote the excretion of basic drugs. By altering the pH of urine, increased elimination of certain drugs can be facilitated, thus preventing prolonged action or overdosage of a toxic compound.

Another technique to alter the rate of excretion of a drug is to produce a competitively blocking effect. For example, probenecid may be used to block the renal excretion of penicillin. This prolongs the effect of the antibiotic by maintaining a higher therapeutic plasma level.

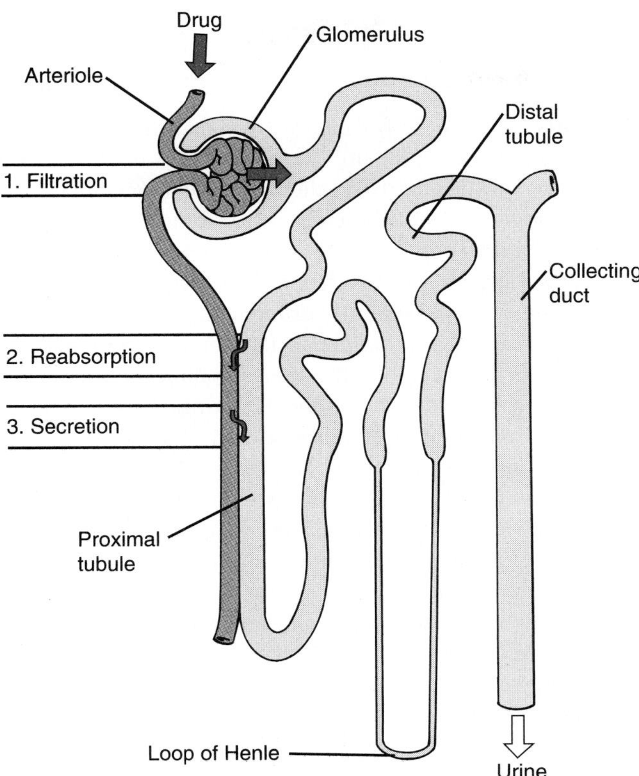

FIGURE 3-6 The drug excretion process.

Drugs may also be eliminated through the use of extracorporeal dialysis, which was originally designed to substitute for renal function in cases of severe but temporary renal shutdown. Overdosage of drugs may lead to just such a situation. By an artificial process resembling glomerular filtration, dialysis can achieve rapid reduction of high plasma levels of a drug. As a general rule, substances that are completely or almost completely excreted by the normal kidney can be removed by hemodialysis. Such substances include some central nervous system (CNS) stimulants and depressants, some nonnarcotic analgesics, and metals.

Intestine. Some medications are eliminated through the intestine by biliary excretion. After metabolism by the liver, the metabolite is secreted into the bile, passed into the duodenum and eliminated with feces. Certain drugs such as fat-soluble agents may be reabsorbed by the bloodstream and returned to the liver. This is the enterohepatic cycle. These compounds are later excreted by the kidney.

Lungs. Most drugs removed by the pulmonary route are generally intact and not metabolites. Agents such as gases and volatile liquids (general anesthetics) that are administered through the respiratory system usually are eliminated by the same route. On inspiration, these agents enter the bloodstream and, after crossing the alveolar membrane, are distributed by the general circulation. The rate of gas loss depends on the rate of respiration. Therefore exercise or deep breathing, which causes a rise in cardiac output and a subsequent increase in pulmonary blood flow, promotes excretion. By contrast, decreased cardiac output, such as that occurring in shock, prolongs the period of time for drug elimination. Other volatile substances such as ethyl alcohol and paraldehyde, which are highly soluble in blood, are excreted in limited amounts by the lungs. Remaining quantities are largely metabolized in the liver and excreted in urine. However, these compounds can be easily detected because the individual expires the gases into the atmosphere.

Sweat and salivary glands. Drug excretion through sweat and saliva is relatively unimportant because this process depends on diffusion of lipid-soluble drugs through the epithelial cells of the glands. The elimination of drugs and metabolites in sweat may be responsible for side effects such as dermatitis and several other skin reactions. Drugs excreted in the saliva are usually swallowed and undergo the same fate as other orally administered agents. Furthermore, certain compounds that are given intravenously also may be excreted into saliva and cause the individual to complain of the "taste of the drug."

Mammary glands. Many drugs or their metabolites cross the epithelium of the mammary glands and are excreted in breast milk. Breast milk is acidic (pH 6.5), and therefore basic compounds such as narcotics (e.g., morphine and codeine) achieve high concentrations in this fluid. On the other hand, weak acids (diuretics, barbiturates, and others) are less concentrated in breast milk. A major concern arises over the transfer of drugs from mothers to their breast-fed babies. Although small quantities of any drug may be obtained in this manner, a cumulative effect can occur because of the undeveloped metabolizing system of the infant. Thus the nursing mother should be warned against taking the drugs because of their potential for reaching her infant.

Pharmacodynamic Phase

Pharmacodynamics is the study of the mechanism of drug action on living tissue, the response of tissues to specific chemical agents at various sites in the body. The effects of drugs can be recognized only by alterations of a known physiologic function; that is, drugs modify physiologic activity but do not confer any new function on a tissue or organ in the body. They may increase, decrease, or replace enzymes, hormones, or body metabolic functions. Some drugs inhibit or destroy foreign organisms or malignant cells in the body while other drug substances may protect cells from foreign agents. The goal of drug therapy is to attain a therapeutic effect in an individual. Therefore, in this context, some drugs are used for the treatment of symptoms and cure of disease while others are used for diagnosis or prevention of disease.

Essentially *pharmacokinetics* refers to the way the body processes or handles the drug while *pharmacodynamics* is the effect the drug has on the body (Katzung, 1992).

Theories of Drug Action

The means by which drugs produce an alteration in function at their sites of action is known as the mechanism of action. The mechanism of action of most compounds is believed to involve a chemical interaction between the drug and a functionally important component of the living system. Most drugs produce their effects by one of the following ways: a drug-receptor, a drug-enzyme, or a nonspecific drug interaction.

Drug-receptor interaction. Structural specificity is an essential postulate of the receptor theory of drug action. This theory hypothesizes that drugs are selectively active substances that have a high affinity for a specific chemical group or a particular constituent of a cell. In essence the drug-receptor interaction theory states that a certain portion (active site) of the drug molecule selectively combines or interacts with some molecular structure (a reactive site on the cell surface or within the cell) to produce a biologic effect. Thus a **receptor** is a reactive cellular site with which a drug interacts to produce a pharmacologic response. The relationship of a drug to its receptor has often been likened to that of the fit of a key in a lock. The drug represents the key that fits into the lock, or receptor. Thus some sort of reciprocal or complementary relationship exists between a certain portion of the drug molecule and the receptor site of the cell.

It has been postulated that the drug molecule with the best fit to the receptor will produce the greatest response from the cell. It has been suggested that there must be some force that attracts a receptor and holds it in combination with a specific drug long enough to produce a pharmacologic response. Following absorption, a drug gains access to the receptor after it leaves the bloodstream and is distributed to tissues that contain receptor sites. (Box 3-3 lists terms used in this theory of drug action.)

Drug-enzyme interaction. An interaction between drug and cellular enzyme is the second way by which drugs produce their effects. Enzymes are indispensable biologic catalysts that control all biochemical reactions of the cell. Drugs can inhibit the action of a specific enzyme and alter a physiologic response. For example, neostigmine (Prostigmin), an agent used to manage the muscle weakness caused by myasthenia gravis, acts chemically by combining with acetylcholinesterase, preventing the inactivation of acetylcholine at the neuromuscular junction.

Drugs that combine with enzymes are thought to do so by virtue of their structural resemblance to an enzyme's substrate molecule (the substance acted on by an enzyme). A drug may resemble an enzyme's substrate so closely that it can combine with the enzyme instead of with the normal substrate. Drugs resembling enzyme substrates are termed "antimetabolites" and can either block normal enzymatic action or result in the production of other substances with unique biochemical properties. The antimetabolites, then, become the receptors for the drug. However, although enzymes may be receptors, not all receptors are enzymes. An example of an antimetabolite is the anticancer drug methotrexate.

Nonspecific drug interaction. Some drugs demonstrate no structural specificity and presumably act by more general effects on cell membranes and cellular processes. These drugs may penetrate into cells or accumulate in cellular membranes, where they interfere, by physical or chemical means, with some cell function or some fundamental metabolic processes.

BOX 3-3

Drug-Receptor Interaction Terms

affinity the propensity of a drug to bind or attach itself to a given receptor site.

efficacy (intrinsic activity) the drug's ability to initiate biologic activity as a result of such binding.

agonist a drug that combines with receptors and initiates a sequence of biochemical and physiologic changes; possesses both affinity and efficacy.

antagonist an agent designed to inhibit or counteract effects produced by other drugs or undesired effects caused by cellular components during illness.

competitive antagonist an agent with an affinity for the same receptor site as an agonist; the competition with the agonist for the site inhibits the action of the agonist; increasing the concentration of the agonist tends to overcome the inhibition. Competitive inhibition responses are usually reversible.

noncompetitive antagonist an agent that combines with different parts of the receptor mechanism and inactivates the receptor so that the agonist cannot be effective regardless of its concentration. Noncompetitive antagonist effects are considered to be irreversible or nearly so.

partial agonist an agent that has affinity and some efficacy but that may antagonize the action of other drugs that have greater efficacy. Not infrequently, antagonists share some structural similarities with their agonists.

Cell membranes are complex lipoprotein structures that regulate the flow of ions and metabolites in a highly selective manner, thereby maintaining an electrochemical gradient between the interior and exterior surfaces of the cell. Structurally nonspecific drugs are exemplified by the general anesthetics, which are lipid-soluble compounds of unrelated chemical structure but with similar properties. It is believed that general anesthetics alter the properties of lipids in cell membranes of nerves rather than act on specific receptors.

Other structurally nonspecific drugs may act by biophysical means that do not affect cellular or enzymatic functions. Drugs acting as a result of their obvious physical properties include the ointments and emollients. Hydrophilic indigestible substances exert a cathartic effect because of their physical action on the bowel. Examples of true chemical reactions that produce biologic effects are the interaction of a molecule such as lead with an antidotal drug and the neutralization by antacid drugs of hydrochloric acid present in gastric juice. Neither is considered a receptor interaction because no macromolecular tissue elements are involved. Detergents, alcohol, hydrogen peroxide, and phenol derivatives, such as Lysol, are also structurally nonspecific and act by irreversibly destroying the functional integrity of the living cell.

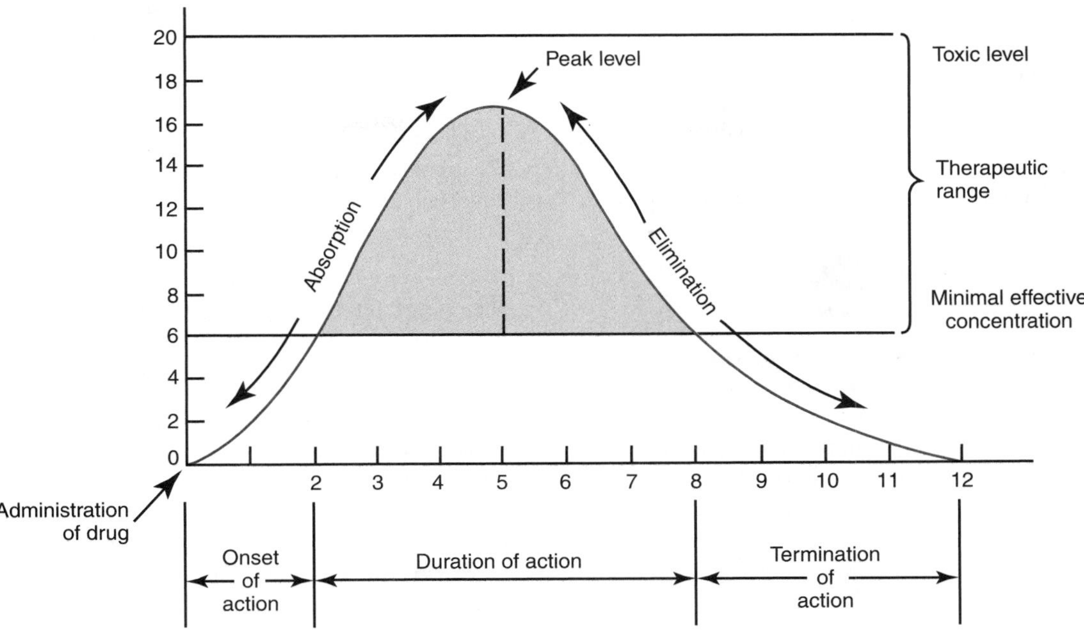

FIGURE 3-7 Plasma level profile of a drug.

Drug-Response Relationship

After administration, each drug has its own characteristic pharmacokinetics, which can be analyzed by performing a plasma level profile. In many instances nurses are required to monitor serum drug levels to help the prescriber determine the dose, scheduling, and route of administration for an individual client. These data also provide information concerning the degree of therapeutic effectiveness so that potential adverse reactions can be predicted, thereby preventing serious clinical problems.

Plasma level profile of a drug. The plasma or serum level profile graphically demonstrates the relationship between the plasma drug concentration and the level of therapeutic effectiveness over a course of time. After one dose is administered, the time course of the amount of drug in the body depends on the rates of absorption, distribution, metabolism, and elimination. For example, the drug in Figure 3-7 has an onset of action of approximately 2 hours, peak level at 5 hours, and a 6-hour duration of action or effect. By monitoring the plasma level of a compound, the efficacy and safety of drug therapy can be more closely controlled. Box 3-4 lists important terms used in plasma level profiles and explains their interrelationships.

Biologic half-life. The rate of biotransformation and excretion of a drug determines its biologic **half-life** (t $^1/_2$), the time required to reduce by one half the amount of unchanged drug that is in the body at the time equilibrium is established. Moreover, the duration of a dose can be demonstrated by the biologic half-life. The half-life of each drug is different. One with a short t $^1/_2$, such as 2 or 3 hours, will need to be administered more often than one with a long t $^1/_2$, such as 12 hours.

BOX 3-4

Plasma Level Profile Terms

onset of action or latent period interval between the time a drug is administered and the first sign of its effect

termination of action point at which a drug effect is no longer seen

duration of action period from onset of drug action to the time when response is no longer perceptible

minimal effective concentration lowest plasma concentration that produces the desired drug effect

peak plasma level highest plasma concentration attained from a dose

toxic level plasma concentration at which a drug produces serious adverse effects

therapeutic range range of plasma concentrations that produce the desired drug effect without toxicity (the range between minimal effective concentration and toxic level)

The half-life does not change with the drug dose; it always takes the same amount of time to eliminate one half of the drug present in the body. If, for example, 10,000 units of a drug are administered and that drug has a half-life of 4 hours, then 5000 units of the drug will be excreted in 4 hours. In the next 4 hours, 2500 units will be excreted, with 1250 units more being excreted in the third 4-hour period. In hepatic dysfunction and in renal disorders, drug elimination may be prolonged and drug half-life lengthened, which usually necessitates reduction of drug dosage.

Therapeutic index. The therapeutic index (TI) provides a quantitative measure of the relative safety of a drug. It represents a ratio between two factors: (1) lethal dose (LD_{50}), which is the dose of a drug that is lethal in 50% of laboratory animals tested, and (2) effective dose (ED_{50}), which is the dose required to produce a therapeutic effect in 50% of a similar population. The therapeutic index is calculated as follows:

$$TI = \frac{LD_{50}}{ED_{50}}$$

The closer the ratio is to 1, the greater the danger involved in administration of that drug to human beings. Obviously, in humans the dose that promotes a side effect or the first sign of a toxic response is of greater importance than the therapeutic index of the drug, since the prescriber's major concern is avoiding even an isolated fatality caused by drug toxicity.

SIDE/ADVERSE DRUG RESPONSES

In addition to producing therapeutic effects, drugs have the potential of causing undesirable responses, such as side effects or adverse reactions. Side effects are usually predictable, and in many instances, an unavoidable secondary effect(s) produced by the drug at usual therapeutic drug dosages. For example, a drug such as an opioid analgesic often causes the side effects of drowsiness and constipation. These effects occur at the usual prescribed dose but drowsiness may occur soon after drug administration while constipation is often a delayed side effect that occurs later in therapy. The intensity of the side effects, though, is often dose-dependent.

The most commonly reported side effects are nausea, vomiting, dizziness, drowsiness, dry mouth, abdominal gas or distress, constipation, and diarrhea. For some side effects, health care providers may provide nonpharmacologic advice such as advising the individual to use caution when getting up suddenly from a lying or sitting position (to reduce the potential for dizziness or hypotension); to use sugarless gum or candy or ice chips for relief of dry mouth; or to not drive or use dangerous machinery until the individual's response to the medication can be assessed. Persistent or troublesome side effects, though, may require pharmacologic interventions such as laxatives, antiemetics, and antidiarrheals for constipation, vomiting, and diarrhea. In general, however, side effects are manageable, and in some instances tolerance may develop to the side effect. Clients should be taught the most common side effects reported with a particular medication and also how to avoid or self-manage it when possible and when to report the especially persistent effects to the prescriber.

Adverse effects or reactions are unintended, undesirable and often unpredictable drug effects. Every medication has a potential for causing harm and sometimes these effects are immediately apparent while at other times they may take weeks or months to develop. Because only up to several thousand persons are exposed to each drug before release, all potential adverse effects may not be detected before the drug is marketed. Therefore the nurse should be alert to any unusual individual responses to drugs, especially to newly released medications.

Adverse reactions can range from mild to fatal but with the increasing numbers of drugs being used, the incidence of adverse reactions has increased and is presently a significant problem in clinical practice (Nies & Spielberg, 1996).

Predictable Adverse Responses

Some factors such as age, body mass, sex, environment, time of administration, pathology, genetic factors, and psychologic characteristics can alter the response to drug therapy. Deviant drug reactions can frequently be traced to the predictable influence of such variables. The nurse must be cognizant of characteristics that modify cell conditions and, therefore, the activity of a drug (Table 3-1).

Age. Young children and the elderly are usually highly responsive to medications. Infants often have immature hepatic and renal systems and, therefore, incomplete metabolic and excretory mechanisms. Elderly persons may demonstrate different responses to drug therapy because of a decline in hepatic and renal function, which is often accompanied by a concurrent disease process.

Body mass. The relationship between body mass and amount of drug administered influences the distribution and concentration of a drug. To maintain a desired drug concentration in individuals of various sizes, drug dosage must be adjusted in proportion to body mass. For a given dose of drug, the greater the volume of distribution, the lower the concentration of drug reached in various body compartments. Since the volume of interstitial and intracellular water is related to body mass, weight has a marked influence on the quantitative effects produced by drugs. The average adult drug dose is calculated on the basis of the drug quantity that will produce a particular effect in 50% of persons who are between the ages of 18 and 65 and weigh about 150 pounds (70 kg). Therefore, particularly for children and for very lean and very obese individuals, drug dosage is frequently determined on the basis of amount of drug per kilogram of body weight or body surface area.

Sex. Differences in drug effects related to the variable of sex result, in part, from size differences between men and women. Women are usually smaller than men, which will lead to high drug concentrations if dosage is prescribed indifferently. Demonstrable differences also exist in relative proportions of fat and water in the bodies of men and women, and some drugs may be more soluble in one or the other. Since drugs taken by a pregnant woman might affect the fetus as a result of placental transfer, the use of drugs is best avoided during pregnancy unless an absolute necessity exists.

Environmental milieu. Drugs affecting mood and behavior are particularly susceptible to the influence of the individual's environment. With such drugs one has to consider effects of: (1) the drug itself, (2) the personality of the user,

TABLE 3-1 Factors altering drug responses

Factor and pertinent description	Nursing considerations
Age	
infants—immature body systems children—dosage adjustment usually necessary elderly—depressed hepatic and renal systems	Modify dosages. Children have a different physiologic profile and body mass distribution. Thus, dose per kilogram is individualized. It could be more or less than in an adult. Elderly clients may also have concomitant physical conditions that alter drug effects; altered excretion mechanism may also require less drug or different scheduling of medication.
Body mass	
the greater the drug's volume of distribution in body mass, the lower the concentration of drug in the body compartments calculation: average adult dose based on drug quantity that will produce a particular effect in 50% of population between the ages of 18 and 65 and weighing about 150 pounds (70 kg)	Adjust dosage in proportion to body mass. For children, dosage frequently is determined on the basis of amount of drug per kilogram of body weight or body surface area.
Sex	
women—smaller than men; definite differences during pregnancy and in relative proportions of fat and water; drugs vary by water or fat solubility	Allow for size differential and whether a drug is water or lipid soluble. Avoid drugs during pregnancy unless an absolute necessity exists.
Environmental milieu	
mood and behavior modified by (1) drug itself, (2) personality of the user, (3) environment of the user, and (4) interaction of these three factors; other factors: sensory—deprivation or overload; physical environment—cold vs heat, oxygen deprivation (altitude)	Be aware of the physical situation of the client with regard to heat and cold, interactions with other individuals, drug effects, and the way the client generally reacts to situations.
Time of administration	
food—presence or absence	Give irritating drugs when food is in the client's stomach. Follow manufacturer's recommendations.
biologic rhythms—sleep-wake cycle, drug-metabolizing enzyme rhythms, corticosteroid secretion rhythm, blood pressure rhythms, circadian (24-hour) cycle in absorption and urinary excretion; also rhythm of drug receptor susceptibility	Make every effort to understand the client's normal and abnormal rhythms, and seek possible relationships between the client's biologic rhythms and reactions to drug therapy.
insufficient fluid intake with solid dosage forms	Administer drugs at same time of day with a full glass of water. Altered body cycles (shift workers) may result in altered response to a drug.
Pathologic state	
presence and severity of pathologic state—pain intensifies need for opioids; anxiety may produce resistance to large doses of tranquilizing drugs; presence of circulatory, hepatic, and/or renal dysfunctions interferes with physiologic processes of drug action	Take into account any pain, disease, or altered metabolic state of the client and adjust dosage accordingly.
Genetic factors	
genetically determined abnormal susceptibility to a chemical, or "idiosyncratic response"	Be aware that any client may show an idiosyncratic response. Always monitor closely, especially when beginning therapy, for abnormal susceptibility. Be aware of common drug idiosyncrasies.
Psychologic factors	
symbolic investment in drugs and faith in their efficacy placebo effect hostility toward or mistrust of medicine or health personnel	Be aware of the attitude and the impression the nurse creates at the time of drug administration, and use them to enhance the drug's effects.

(3) the environment of the user, and (4) the interaction of these three components. Sensory deprivation and sensory overload may also affect responses to drugs. Physical environment can modify drug effects. For example, temperature affects drug activity: heat relaxes peripheral vessels and thus intensifies the actions of vasodilators, while cold has the opposite effect. The relative oxygen deprivation at high altitudes may increase sensitivity to some drugs.

Time of administration. It is well known that drugs are absorbed more rapidly if the gastrointestinal tract is free of food and that irritating drugs are more readily tolerated if there is food in the stomach. Research has indicated that the time of drug administration in relation to human biologic rhythms can significantly affect the response to certain medications. It seems quite plausible that in humans the sleep-wake rhythm, drug-metabolizing enzyme rhythms, and circadian (24-hour) variations contribute to the effective, ineffective, adverse, or toxic response to particular drugs. For example, cyclophosphamide, an antineoplastic agent, should be administered in the morning to reduce the risk of hemorrhagic cystitis (blood in the urine) (*USP DI,* 1996). Chronopharmacology and chronotoxicology are new areas that health care professionals are monitoring with great interest.

Pathologic state. The presence of a pathologic condition and the severity of symptoms may call for careful consideration of the type of drug administered and for adjustment in dosage. For example, the presence of severe pain tends to increase a client's requirement for an analgesic, and an extremely anxious individual can prove resistant to very large doses of tranquilizing and sedating drugs. Aspirin administered to a client with a fever will produce a decrease in temperature, whereas a client taking the drug for its analgesic effects will show no temperature change at all. In addition, it bears repeating that the presence of circulatory, hepatic, or renal dysfunctions will interfere with the physiologic processes of drug action.

Genetic factors. Genetic differences may affect an individual's response to a number of drugs. Such differences may arise from genetically conditioned deficiencies in drug metabolism or in receptor sensitivity. These pharmacogenetic abnormalities often manifest themselves as "idiosyncrasies" and may be mistakenly diagnosed as drug allergies. For example, some individuals may lack pseudocholinesterase activity in their plasma. If they receive an injection of succinylcholine, which is normally hydrolyzed by plasma cholinesterase, they may become paralyzed and remain that way for a long time. The field of pharmacogenetics is of great interest, since it may provide a rational explanation for many so-called drug idiosyncrasies.

Psychologic factors. The client's symbolic investment in drugs and faith in their effects strongly influence and usually potentiate drug effects. The placebo effect is an outstanding example of how strong motivation can influence the emergence of desired drug effects, whereas hostility and mistrust of medicine and health personnel can diminish drug effects. It is important for nurses to realize that their attitudes and the impressions created at the time of drug administration may influence the therapeutic result.

Iatrogenic Responses

An **iatrogenic** condition is any adverse mental or physical condition induced in a client by a prescribed treatment or diagnostic procedure. Because these often involve prescribed medications, this term has also been used to define a disease caused by a physician, for example, the use of phenothiazines in psychotic persons, which results in drug-induced Parkinson's disease. Other drug-induced diseases may include blood dyscrasias, hepatotoxicity, nephrotoxicity, and teratogenicity. With careful prescribing and monitoring, iatrogenic conditions are usually avoidable. The nurse, by careful evaluation of a client's response to a drug, may be able to avoid or limit an iatrogenic disease.

Unpredictable Adverse Responses

Adverse drug reactions are one way of characterizing unpredictable and sometimes unexplainable drug responses that have not been clearly and distinctly defined. The most common and best-defined adverse drug reactions are the following.

Allergic Drug Reactions

A drug allergy is an altered state of reaction to a drug, resulting from previous sensitizing exposure and the development of an immunologic mechanism. Substances foreign to the body act as antigens to stimulate the production of antibodies or immunoglobulins (IgE, IgG, IgM). Later, when a previously sensitized individual is again exposed to the foreign substance, the antigen reacts with the antibodies to release substances such as histamine, which then provoke allergic symptoms. *Hypersensitivity, drug allergy,* and *chemical allergy* are all terms used to describe an allergic drug reaction (Klaassen, 1996). There are four different types of allergic drug reactions:

Type I (anaphylactic reaction) is an immediate reaction that occurs within minutes of exposure to the chemical in a previously sensitized person. This reaction is mediated by IgE antibodies located on the surface of mast cells and basophils. An immediate, severe reaction results, which may be fatal if not recognized and treated quickly. The most dramatic form of anaphylaxis is sudden, severe bronchospasm, vasospasm, severe hypotension, and rapid death. Signs and symptoms are largely caused by contraction of smooth muscles and may begin with irritability, extreme weakness, nausea, and vomiting and may proceed to dyspnea, cyanosis, convulsions, and cardiac arrest. Drugs associated with this type of reaction include penicillins and cephalosporins. Antihistamines, epinephrine, and bronchodilators are indispensable in the treatment of anaphylactic shock.

Type II (cytotoxic reaction) involves a drug and IgG or IgM; it has sometimes been called an autoimmune response. This reaction manifests as hemolytic anemia (methyldopa or penicillin induced), thrombocytopenia (quinidine induced), or lupus erythematosus (procainamide induced). Removal of the medication usually results in improvement, although it may take several months for the reaction to subside.

Type III (or Arthus, an immune complex reaction) is sometimes called "serum sickness." With this reaction the drug forms a complex with IgG antibodies in the blood vessel, resulting in angioedema, arthralgia, fever, swollen lymph nodes (lymphadenopathy), and splenomegaly in approximately 1 to 3 weeks after drug exposure. Penicillins, sulfonamides, and phenytoin can cause this type of delayed reaction.

Type IV is a cell-mediated or delayed hypersensitivity reaction. For example, direct skin contact between the drug and sensitized cells results in an inflammatory reaction, such as contact dermatitis from poison ivy. This type of reaction involves sensitized T lymphocytes and macrophages (Klaassen, 1996).

Drug-Induced Reactions

An individual who has had a mild allergic response to a particular drug should avoid reexposure to that drug and, optimally, should have skin tests performed in order to more definitively diagnose the response. Mild allergic reactions may be characterized by the development of a rash, angioedema, rhinitis, fever, asthma, and pruritus.

Reinstitution of therapy with the same drug in a client who manifests allergic reactions is always dangerous, since an anaphylactic reaction may occur.

Idiosyncrasy is any abnormal or peculiar response to a drug, which may manifest itself by (1) overresponse or abnormal susceptibility to a drug; (2) underresponse, demonstrating abnormal tolerance; (3) a qualitatively different effect from the one expected, such as excitation after the administration of a sedative; or (4) unpredictable and unexplainable symptoms. Idiosyncratic reactions are generally thought to result from genetic enzymatic deficiencies that lead to an abnormal mechanism of drug metabolism. This term has been used rather vaguely to describe drug reactions that are qualitatively different from the usual effects obtained in the majority of patients and that cannot be attributed to drug allergy.

Tolerance refers to a decreased physiologic response after repeated administration of a drug or a chemically related substance. It is a reaction that necessitates an increase in dosage to maintain a given therapeutic effect. Drugs well known for their propensity to produce tolerance are tobacco, opium alkaloids, nitrites, and ethyl alcohol. The actual mechanism of tolerance is unknown. In some instances, prolonged administration of some drugs somehow induces the synthesis of extra drug-metabolizing enzymes in the liver, which may account for the client's increased ability to tolerate larger drug doses than previously.

Cross tolerance between related chemicals (such as between alcohol and some anesthetics) is a well-documented phenomenon. It is quite clear, however, that not all cases of tolerance are attributable to a drug's increased rate of metabolism. For example, the remarkable tolerance to morphine cannot be the result of its more rapid metabolic degradation.

Tachyphylaxis refers to a quickly developing tolerance after repeated administration of a drug. It is rapid in onset, and the client's initial response to the drug cannot be reproduced, even with larger doses of the drug.

A *cumulative effect* occurs when the body cannot metabolize one dose of a drug before another dose is administered. In other words, when drugs are excreted more slowly than they are absorbed, each new dose adds more to the total quantity in the blood and organs than is lost in the same amount of time by excretion. Unless drug administration is adjusted, high concentrations can be reached, producing toxic effects. Cumulative toxicity can occur rapidly, as dramatically illustrated in ethyl alcohol intoxication, or it can occur insidiously, as is the case in poisoning with heavy metals, such as lead. Lead is stored in many body tissues and deposited in bones, therefore having prolonged effects on the body while accumulation continues.

Drug dependence is the term preferred over the previous terminology of "habituation" and "addiction." The World Health Organization has suggested the use of the term *dependence* in conjunction with the drug being described (e.g., barbiturate dependence or opiate dependence). Dependence can be physical or psychologic. Physical dependence refers to a state of physiologic drug adaptation that manifests itself by intense physical disturbance when the drug is withdrawn. Psychologic dependence is a state of emotional reliance on a drug to maintain an effect. Its manifestations may range from a mild desire for a drug to craving to compulsive use of the drug. Drug dependence is explored in greater detail in Chapter 9.

Drug interaction occurs when the effects of one drug are modified by the prior or concurrent administration of another drug, thereby increasing or decreasing the pharmacologic action of each. Drug interactions may be either beneficial (e.g., probenecid prolongs the action of penicillins) or detrimental (e.g., aspirin increases the action of anticoagulants, causing hemorrhage).

Drug antagonism occurs when the combination effect of two drugs is less than the sum of the drugs acting separately.

Summation (addition or additive effect) occurs when the combined effect of two drugs produces a result that equals the sum of the individual effects of each agent. The mathematical equivalent is $1 + 1 = 2$. For example, codeine and aspirin both act as analgesics and when given together they provide an additive or greater pain relief than when either one is used alone. This combination allows the administration of a lower dosage of each drug, with a resultant decrease in adverse reactions.

Synergism describes a drug interaction in which the combined effect of drugs is greater than the sum of each individual agent acting independently. Mathematically the response can be written as $1 + 1 = 3$ or more. This can be exemplified by the use of a combination of drugs in treating hypertension. Each of the drugs lowers blood pressure but in a different way; however, the combined effect produces a greater decrease in hypertension than if either drug were given alone.

Potentiation refers to the concurrent administration of two drugs in which one drug increases the effect of the other drug.

NURSING MANAGEMENT OF DRUG THERAPY

The nurse's responsibilities in the administration of drugs require more than memorization of specific drugs, their actions, and their dosages. Rather, effective implementation depends on a sound comprehension of the theories of drug action, constituting clinical judgment that the nurse can apply to the individual client, each with a specific diagnosis and definable individual needs. Such a background necessitates the understanding of theories of drug action, physiologic processes mediating drug action, variables effecting drug action, and unusual and adverse responses to drug therapy.

The application of critical thinking in the nursing management of a client's therapeutic regimen is essential. A prescriber's order for a specific medication for an individual client is written at a particular time when such a pharmacologic intervention is determined to be appropriate. However, circumstances change and a client may respond differently to a medication than was intended. The nurse must assess whether each dose is appropriate for that client each time it is to be administered. An analogy would be that the prescriber's order exists in time and space much like a pedestrian sign flashing "walk" or "don't walk" regardless of what is occurring in the environment. It is the judgment taken as to whether it is safe to cross the street at any given time—that the traffic has really stopped—that is important, regardless of what the sign indicates. So the nurse monitors for the therapeutic and nontherapeutic effects of the client's medications on an ongoing basis with every dose to ensure safe administration of the drug therapy.

On entry into the body, a drug initiates a series of physiologic events before it reaches its site of action. The extent of drug absorption depends on the form of the drug. Assessment of the client's ability to tolerate a particular form or route is essential—for example, testing the client's ability to swallow before an oral medication is administered. Tablets or capsules must first disintegrate and then be dissolved before absorption through the intestinal membrane can occur. However, the nurse should never crush an enteric-coated tablet, because the coating protects it from destruction by the acid pH of the stomach. To maintain its effectiveness, the drug is produced in this form so it can disintegrate and dissolve in the alkaline pH of the intestine. Drugs that irritate the gastric mucosa must also be coated.

The time of administration is another important concern of the nurse. To obtain the maximal pharmacokinetic benefit, oral drugs should be given with a glass of water (8 oz) $^1/_2$ hour to 1 hour before meals. It is important to remember that the presence of food, which delays stomach emptying, tends to diminish the therapeutic effect of the drug. Occasionally, an agent must be administered with meals to prevent gastrointestinal irritation. The nurse should anticipate a rapid response when a drug is given intravenously, because the full dose is placed directly into the bloodstream, thus bypassing the need for absorption.

Individuals with hepatic dysfunction are susceptible to drug overdosage, especially if the drug is highly bound to plasma proteins. In addition, the nurse should be alert to the client's response to a drug if there is renal dysfunction. Since most agents are excreted by the kidneys, the client should be observed for a cumulative effect that may result from the continued administration of the drug. Usually drug dosage is adjusted in individuals with hepatic or renal disorders so that adverse effects will be prevented.

In instances when the nurse is required to monitor serum drug levels, careful observations of the client's response to the drug provide information that aids the prescriber in determining the dosage of a drug, the frequency of administration, and the route of administration. The data are essential for promoting the optimal therapeutic benefit to the client and at the same time preventing potential adverse reactions.

Finally, the nurse should advise a pregnant woman about the danger of taking medications and, to prevent teratogenic effects, instruct her to check with her prescriber or licensed nurse midwife before taking any drug. In addition, if a medication is required, the lowest possible dose of the prescribed drug should be administered.

Unit 2, The Nursing Process and Pharmacology, which follows, will provide the principles upon which the nursing judgment necessary for the safe and accurate administration of medications can be developed.

SUMMARY

Drugs, as chemicals that interact with a living organism to produce biologic responses, do so according to certain theories of drug action, physiologic processes mediating drug action, variables affecting drug action, and unusual and adverse responses to drug therapy. Drugs modify only existing functions and exert multiple actions rather than a single effect. These actions result from a physiochemical interaction between the drug and a functionally important molecule in the body.

To produce the desired effect, a drug must have an appropriate concentration at its site of action. This concentration is influenced by a number of processes, which can be divided into three phases: pharmaceutical, pharmacokinetic, and pharmacodynamic. The pharmaceutical phase focuses on the form of the drug, solid or liquid, and its dissolution to achieve absorption. The pharmacokinetic phase is concerned with the concentration of the drug during the processes of absorption, distribution, biotransformation, and excretion. Absorption involves the movement of drug molecules from the site of entry into the body to the circulating fluids. The following factors influence absorption: the nature of the absorbing surface through which the drug must pass, blood flow to the site of administration, solubility of the drug, pH, drug concentration, and dosage form. Drugs may be given for their local or systemic effect. The routes of drug administration are classified as enteral, parenteral, pulmonary, and topical. Distribution is the transport of a drug in body fluids to various tissues of the body and ultimately to the site of action. It is influenced by the body's storage reservoirs for drugs—plasma protein binding and tissue binding—as well as by barriers to drug distribution, such as the blood-brain barrier and the placental barrier. In biotransformation the liver, as the primary site for drug metabolism, inactivates the drug by converting it to a metabolite that can be excreted from the body. Excretion, elimination of the pharmacologically active or inactive metabolites from the body, occurs primarily through the kidneys, with some elimination through the intestine, lungs, mammary glands, and sweat and salivary glands.

The pharmacodynamic phase is concerned with the response of tissues to specific chemical agents at various sites in the body. The mechanism for action between the drug and a functionally important component of the living system may be a drug-receptor interaction, a drug-enzyme interaction, or a nonspecific drug interaction. Because each drug has its own characteristic pharmacokinetic activity, it may be necessary to monitor a client by obtaining a plasma level of a drug. The biologic half-life and the therapeutic index of a drug also provide information to assist the prescriber in determining the dose, scheduling, and route of administration for an individual client.

No drug is totally safe; it can sometimes react in the body to produce unpredictable and harmful effects. However, some identifiable factors do alter the response to drug therapy: age, body mass, sex, environmental milieu, time of administration, pathologic states, genetic factors, and psychologic factors. The adverse effects caused unintentionally by treatment are known as iatrogenic disease. With drug therapy, iatrogenic diseases may be manifested in five major effects: blood dyscrasias, hepatic toxicity, renal damage, teratogenic effects, and dermatologic effects. Other, and somewhat unpredictable, adverse effects may be evidenced as drug allergy, idiosyncrasy, tolerance, tachyphylaxis, cumulation, drug dependence, drug interaction, drug antagonism, summation, synergism, potentiation, or immediate reactions, such as anaphylaxis.

It is important that the nurse understand the principles involved in drug action and their influence on nursing practice in order to make possible the administration of medication with the greatest safety and efficacy.

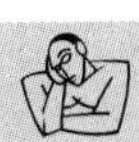

Critical Thinking

1. If you were administering a medication with a long half-life, what types of clients would be more at risk for the cumulative effects of the drug?
2. If you were administering diazepam (Valium), an anxiolytic drug, and warfarin (Coumadin), an oral anticoagulant, both of which are highly protein bound, to the same client, what assessments of the client would be particularly important?
3. How can a drug that has CNS activity but cannot cross the blood-brain barrier be administered for effectiveness?

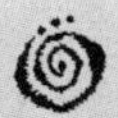

Collaborative Learning Activities

1. The students will form small groups and determine the answers to the following questions related to Figure 3-7. If the administration of this drug were at 8:00 A.M., what would be the earliest that the nurse could expect to observe a therapeutic effect? At what time would a drug plasma level be drawn if the prescriber were concerned about drug toxicity?

BIBLIOGRAPHY

DiPiro JT, et al. (Eds.) (1993). *Pharmacotherapy: A pathophysiological approach* (2nd ed.). New York: Elsevier.

Hardman JG & Limbird LE (Eds.). (1995). *Goodman & Gilman's the pharmacological basis of therapeutics* (9th ed.). New York: McGraw-Hill.

Katzung BG (1992). *Basic & clinical pharmacology* (5th ed.). Norwalk, CT: Appleton & Lange.

Keen JH (1994). Drug update: Giving medications to different age groups, *J Emerg Nursing* 20(6):549-551.

Klaassen CD (1996). Principles of toxicology and treatment of poisoning. In Hardman JG & Limbird (Eds.). *Goodman & Gilman's the pharmacological basis of therapeutics* (9th ed.). New York: McGraw-Hill.

Mallet L (1992). Counseling in special populations: The elderly patient, *Am Pharm NS* 32(10):71.

Miller SW & Strom JG Jr. (1990). Drug-product selection: Implications for the geriatric patient, *Consult Pharmacist* 5(1):30.

Morrissey MR, et al. (1991). Prospective review of dosing of renally eliminated medications for nursing home residents, *Consult Pharmacist* 6(8):623.

Nies AS & Spielberg (1996). Principles of therapeutics. In Hardman JG & Limbird LE (Eds.). *Goodman & Gilman's the pharmacological basis of therapeutics* (9th ed.). New York: McGraw-Hill.

United States Pharmacopeial Convention (1996). *USP DI: Drug information for the health care professional* (16th ed.). Rockville, MD: The Convention.

Young LY & Koda-Kimble MA (Eds.) (1995). *Applied therapeutics: The clinical use of drugs* (6th ed.). Vancouver, WA: Applied Therapeutics.

Weinstein E, et al. (1993). *Giving drugs by advanced techniques*. Springhouse, PA: Springhouse.

Chapter 4

Assessment, Nursing Diagnosis, and Planning

Chapter Focus

Whether the nurse has contact with a client in the home, ambulatory care setting, extended care facility, or hospital, the nurse uses the nursing process to work with clients in relation to drug therapy. When its five components—assessment, diagnosis, planning, implementation, and evaluation—are applied to drug therapy, the nurse develops a systematic, organized approach to handling the wealth of data about clients and their drugs. This chapter discusses the first three components: assessment, diagnosis, and planning. Consider the key terms and the following objectives for a good understanding of this chapter.

Key Terms

analysis (p. 58)
collaborative domain (p. 63)
collaborative problems (p. 59)
contraindications (p. 55)
dependent domain (p. 63)
drug history (p. 49)
incompatibilities (p. 58)
independent domain (p. 63)
nursing diagnosis (p. 59)
nursing process (p. 49)
outcome criteria (p. 63)
prn order (p. 53)
protocol (p. 54)
routine order (p. 53)
single order (p. 54)
stat order (p. 54)

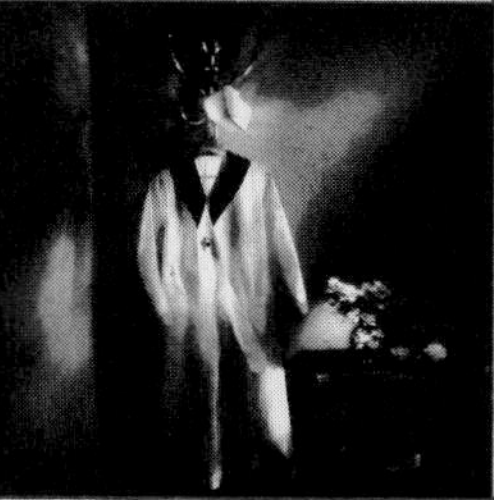

Objectives

1. Obtain an accurate and thorough drug history from a client.
2. Articulate the components and types of drug orders essential for safe, effective drug administration.
3. Assess contraindications to the administration of a drug and take appropriate action.
4. Identify the variables influencing drug interactions, and common drug interactions and incompatibilities.
5. Describe the components and purpose of the nursing diagnosis.
6. Identify the most common nursing diagnoses for any medication.
7. Discuss the three domains of nursing interventions.
8. Explain the importance of setting goals or outcome criteria for nursing care related to drug therapy.
9. Apply the nursing process steps of assessment and planning as it relates to drug therapy of a client.

The **nursing process** applied to drug therapy provides the nurse with a systematic observational and problem-solving technique to collaborate with the client on appropriate medication-related interventions and evaluation of the effectiveness of these interventions. It provides direction for rational nursing actions to manage problems related to drug therapies. Its process and phases are analogous to scientific and problem-solving methods. Although other variations exist, it is described here in four phases: (1) assessment, culminating in nursing diagnoses and collaborative problems, (2) planning, (3) implementation, and (4) evaluation. Figure 4-1 diagrams these phases or steps, which are discussed in this chapter and in Chapter 5. It should be kept in mind that the steps of the nursing process have an ongoing, cyclic nature—no step should be considered complete or static.

ASSESSMENT

The assessment phase of the nursing process is both the first phase and a continuous phase that ends only on discharge of the client. During assessment of data, all the facts relating to clients and their drug therapy, relationships with others, health history, and environment are collected and organized so that the nurse can begin to make inferences about the client's drug therapy. The data that are collected and analyzed form the basis for development of nursing diagnoses and/or collaborative problems.

The client's status and the assessment data derived from these indicated sources are constantly changing. Nursing diagnostic statements will change as well. In collaboration with the prescriber, these changes may result in revision of the treatment plan, such as drug deletions, additions, or dosage changes.

Nurses must have a sound base of knowledge about a client's disorder and drugs being administered, as well as the skill to use references to answer questions that arise. The ability to ask questions and seek answers about the data collected will form a solid foundation for the planning, implementation, and evaluation phases of the nursing process.

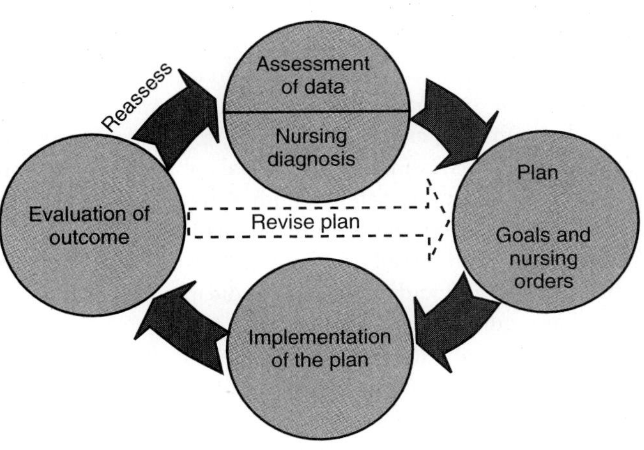

Figure 4-1 The nursing process.

Drug History Guidelines

Taking a **drug history,** the process of gathering information that is relevant to the management of a client's medication regimen, is essential for planning nursing interventions and client education. Obtaining a comprehensive drug history requires a combination of nursing knowledge, interviewing skills, and a review of specific drug reference resources whenever necessary. A drug history should explore the client's usage of prescription medications, usage of over-the-counter (OTC) drugs, self-treatment with herbal or home remedies, general and specific health history, and, when possible, specific cultural factors that influence individual drug therapies. Assess the client's readiness and ability to provide information. Explain the purpose of a drug history so the client understands why some questions are asked that may sound personal. Figure 4-2 shows a sample drug history form.

A thorough drug history can provide extremely useful information for the entire health care team. For example, it can:

1. Explain a mysterious new symptom reported in the client.
2. Provide clues about unreported chronic disorders.
3. Reveal learning needs or concerns regarding the client's effective management of a therapeutic regimen.
4. Provide information crucial to prevent drug interactions, allergies, or side/adverse effects.
5. Help interpret laboratory tests reliably.
6. Identify the risk for drug-drug and drug-food interactions.

When a nurse is taking a drug history, it is important to communicate at the level of understanding appropriate for the client. Medical terminology may be confusing to the nonmedically trained person; therefore the nurse should be familiar with local observances and, when applicable, ethnic or cultural terms for specific diseases, illnesses, symptoms, and other information. Rapport must be established if transfer of relevant information is to be made freely.

Open-ended questioning is preferred to direct "yes" or "no" questions during an interview. For example, to obtain information about a client's use of analgesics, a "yes" or "no" question would be: "Do you take analgesics? If 'yes,' name them." If the person is unsure of the meaning of the term *analgesia,* a "no" answer might be the natural response. The question can be reworded to ask, "What do you take when you have pain, such as a headache, backache, muscle sprain, or other type of ache or pain?" and the more descriptive information the nurse is seeking may then be forthcoming. Questions concerning over-the-counter drugs must often be accompanied by reminders from the interviewer. Commonly used product names or currently advertised brands may be suggested to jog the memory of the client. For example, aspirin is an ingredient in hundreds of OTC preparations; therefore simply asking the client if he or she consumes aspirin may limit the answer to only products labeled as aspirin. Suggesting trade name products, such as Anacin, Bufferin, or Alka-Seltzer, would expand the possibility of obtaining a more thorough drug history.

DRUG HISTORY

Client's name ________________ Sex ________ Age ______ Date of interview ________________

Occupation Physician

Diagnosis and past history (if relevant)

Frequency of meals? Special diet, prescribed or self-imposed:

Allergies/drug reactions (food and/or drugs; describe reaction, approximate date, and action taken or outcome):

Close family members with drug allergies (relationship, drug, and reaction):

Caffeine intake: (type & amount) Type/daily consumption of alcohol: Smoking (type and amount):

Over-the-counter medications:
(List medications, dose, frequency, and when last dose was taken for following:)
Constipation (laxatives):
Diarrhea (antidiarrheal):
Gastric upset/heartburn (antacids):
Pain, headache (analgesics):
Cold medication (antihistamine, decongestants):
Cough medicine (syrups/other forms):
Drugs for sleep:
Drugs to stay awake:
Drugs for menstrual conditions in premenopausal women:
Drugs for nerves:
Drugs for fluid retention:
Do you use any salt substitutes (obtain brand name; Morton Lite Salt, CoSalt, etc.)
Do you use any food supplements? Name and quantity per day:
Do you buy herbal teas or health food store products? Obtain complete listing and daily consumption.

Do you take vitamins/minerals/iron? Note type, strength, and amount per day:

Current prescribed medications; include name, strength, daily dosage, indication, and therapeutic/nontherapeutic responses:
(Note client's knowledge about medications and the need for teaching.)

Prescription medications taken during the previous three months:

Nurse ________________________

Figure 4-2 Sample drug history.

If the interview is performed in the client's living quarters, the nurse should ask to see the medications. In an ambulatory care setting, request that the client bring all his or her medications into the clinic so that they may be reviewed. Many individuals, especially the elderly, forget to report all the medications they have on hand for self-medicating purposes. Also the storage place for medications should be noted, since this may be important information if a potentially hazardous site is used. Storage in a bathroom cabinet or over a kitchen sink or stove may adversely affect many medications. Areas of heat and moisture are not recommended as proper storage areas for most drugs. Almost all medications, unless they are to be refrigerated, are to be stored below 40° C (104° F), preferably between 15° and 30° C (59° and 86° F) and are to be protected from freezing.

Evaluating the client's knowledge about proper disposal of drugs (via the sink or toilet), ability to read and understand the labels on medication, and ability to locate expiration dates is part of assessing the individual's ability to store and consume medications safely. Studies have indicated that many persons (from one third to one half of various elderly populations) cannot read or do not understand drug package labels. This high incidence clearly indicates an area of concern that requires nursing assessment.

Information should also be obtained on the individual's general lifestyle, consumption of alcohol, use of caffeine-containing products, and smoking habits. All these factors may affect or modify a typical drug response. (See the section on drug interactions in this chapter for further information.)

Client and Environmental Data

Client and environmental data are collected from clients, their friends, or their relatives by subjective and objective observations. In addition to observation of clients and their environment, interactions of clients with others and notes from the history and physical examination sections of the clinical record are used as sources. At the initial interview the practitioner notes a client's past health history and does a physical examination to assess the client's current status. The resulting prioritized problem list directs the therapeutic approach. Information obtained in the client's history and physical examination should be reviewed to select pertinent data. The nurse needs to gather data in certain areas to assess the appropriateness of the planned drug therapy. If drug dosage and route of administration are not carefully selected, alterations in the various systems may result in either an increased or exaggerated drug effect or a decrease in drug response. Table 4-1 lists the major factors to be evaluated and pertinent data to be obtained.

Current Client Drug Data

Drug data include information derived from a prescriber's orders or prescription and that gained from assessment of the drugs' effects on the client, based on observation, vital signs, and laboratory reports. The characteristics of the drugs administered and the way the prescriber orders them have an impact on the client's nursing care.

Drug Orders and Prescriptions

"Medicating" a client begins when the medication is suggested and authorized by a legally sanctioned prescriber, usually a licensed physician or dentist. These two professionals are currently the only ones legally allowed to initiate medication plans in all states. In many states, nurse practitioners, pharmacists, or physicians' assistants have also been given that function legally within specified limitations; in other states this is under consideration. The practicing nurse should be aware of and follow the limitations outlined in the state nurse practice act in the state in which they practice.

TABLE 4-1 Client and environmental data

Factor	Questions for evaluation	Rationale
Medical diagnosis	Are the drugs ordered clinically indicated and corroborated by the best judgments according to authoritative literature?	The client must be protected from wrongful harm; the administering nurse may be held legally accountable.
Age	Has the client's age been considered? Have drug reactions occurred in the past?	The very young and the elderly are subject to a wide range and great intensity of side and adverse effects because of reduced functioning of body systems that absorb, transport, affect the metabolism of, and excrete drugs (see also Chapters 7 and 8).
Body mass	Was the dosage assessed in relation to total body weight, body surface area (weight-to-height ratio), and lean body mass?	For prescribing purposes, the person up to 12 years old is usually considered a child and given a pediatric dosage. The dose is based on the different physiologic and pharmacokinetic factors in the neonate, infant, or older child. The average weight of a 12-year-old child is about 90 pounds; an "average" adult weighs 150 pounds. An adult at or near the weight of 90 pounds who receives the "average adult dose" may exhibit signs of overdosage.
Inherited factors	Have genetic differences (pharmacogenetic variations) in enzyme production or destruction, which may cause apparent therapeutic failure or secondary effects when a drug is metabolized too rapidly, too slowly, or incompletely, been considered?	Many aberrant reactions (termed *idiosyncrasy*) are often acutely caused by genetic abnormalities. An example is the lack of the enzyme glucose-6-phosphate dehydrogenase, found in a small percentage of people of Mediterranean descent (Italians, Greeks, Arabs, and Sephardic Jews) and in about 10% of American black males, less often in black females. Fava beans and medications such as aspirin, antimalarials, and sulfonamides, if taken by these susceptible people, may cause hemolytic anemia. Also, hypersensitivity (allergy) to specific medications often correlates with a tendency to other common allergies to certain foods, grasses, trees, molds, or animal dander.

Continued

TABLE 4-1 Client and environmental data—cont'd

Factor	Questions for evaluation	Rationale
Coexisting conditions	Are there disorders that affect any of the major body systems, especially those of the gastrointestinal tract or the circulatory, hepatic, or renal system, that will interfere with normal digestion, absorption, transport, metabolism, degradation, and detoxification or excretion of the drugs prescribed?	Impaired capacity for biotransformation may alter drug action and increase the possibility of toxic effects or therapeutic failure. Pregnancy or breastfeeding precludes administration of all but essential medications (see Chapter 7).
Management of therapeutic regimen	Is there a past history or other factors indicating that the client, if self-medicating, will not follow medication instructions? (See Chapter 6 for full discussion of client management of therapeutic regimen.)	Attitudes and behavior conducive to positive health behavior depend on psychosocial, cultural, economic, cognitive, and physical factors—how the client views and values health and illness; how the client understands or accepts illness; what he or she knows about the drug in question; how he or she relates to the health care surroundings, system, and practitioners; how the client assigns control and decision making; whether the client communicates and thinks logically; how he or she has been educated; and whether he or she has manipulative skills, among others. Studies show that having faith in a therapy has a decidedly favorable effect on its outcome. A subtle approach is needed to evaluate these parameters.

The prescriber's orders are meant for the one who dispenses the medication. There are two different formats, the prescription blank and the order sheet. The prescription blank is given to clients in an ambulatory care setting or upon discharge from the health care agency and is to be filled by a community pharmacist; it may look similar to Figure 4-3. For clients in an institutional setting, the order is written on an order sheet found in the client's chart (Figure 4-4). It is filled by the pharmacy within the institution or contracted for by the institution and sent to the medication area on the client's unit for access by the client's medication nurse. The process of ordering medications for clients has been computerized in some health care settings, but the principles remain the same and frequently the computer printouts resemble the former noncomputerized hospital stationery for medication administration.

The prescriber's order has seven elements that should be present and identifiable. These elements and the associated "Five Rights" of medication administration are included in Box 4-1. All parts of the order should be legible and clearly expressed. If there is any doubt, the prescriber must be contacted to validate or clarify. Obviously, to administer a drug under questionable instructions is to risk harm to the client in an area with a high potential for error (see Chapter 5).

Safe nursing practice is to follow approved procedures in the particular work environment and to administer only drugs that are ordered in writing. Nursing students should be

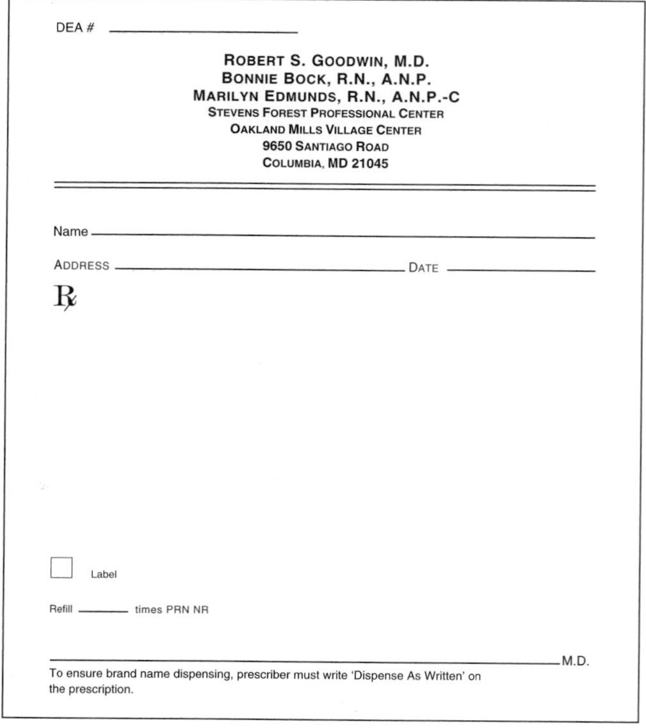
DEA # ____________

ROBERT S. GOODWIN, M.D.
BONNIE BOCK, R.N., A.N.P.
MARILYN EDMUNDS, R.N., A.N.P.-C
STEVENS FOREST PROFESSIONAL CENTER
OAKLAND MILLS VILLAGE CENTER
9650 SANTIAGO ROAD
COLUMBIA, MD 21045

Name ____________

ADDRESS ____________ DATE ____________

℞

☐ Label

Refill ______ times PRN NR

____________ M.D.

To ensure brand name dispensing, prescriber must write 'Dispense As Written' on the prescription.

Figure 4-3 Example of a prescription pad order form. (From Edmunds MW [1995]. *Introduction to clinical pharmacology*. St Louis: Mosby.)

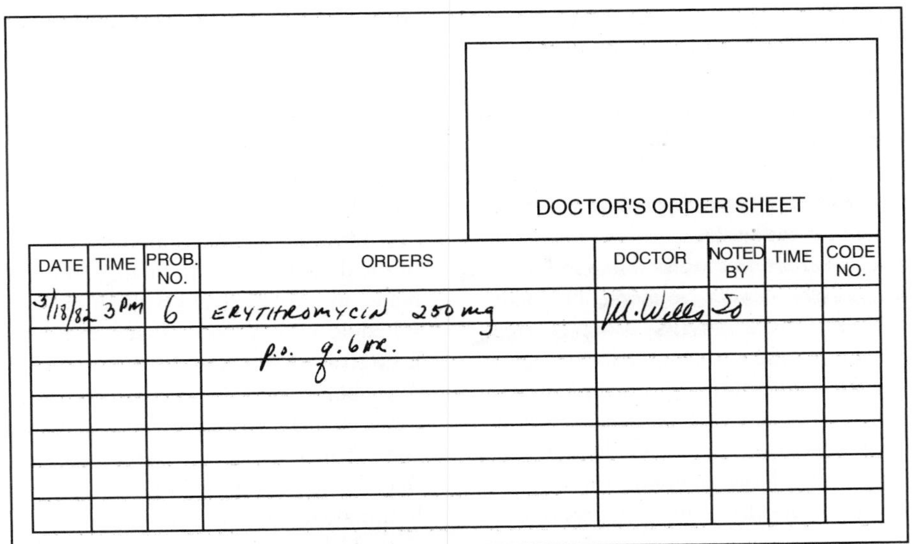

DOCTOR'S ORDER SHEET

DATE	TIME	PROB. NO.	ORDERS	DOCTOR	NOTED BY	TIME	CODE NO.
3/18/82	3 PM	6	ERYTHROMYCIN 250 mg	M. Wells	Jo		
			p.o. q.6hr.				

Figure 4-4 Example of an order sheet.

BOX 4-1

Elements Essential For Medication Administration

Five rights	Elements of medication order
Right client	1. Client's name
	2. Date order written
Right drug	3. Medication name
Right dose	4. Dosage
Right route	5. Route
Right time	6. Frequency
	7. Prescriber signature

aware of special limitations imposed on their actions by the educational and/or clinical institution. In particular, they should be advised to follow only written orders. However, sometimes a verbal or telephoned order from a prescriber, often in response to the nurse's telephoned request, is unavoidable. When this occurs it is best for the nurse to copy the order as it is being given, then verify it by repeating it back to the prescriber. Verbal or telephoned orders should be rare, involving circumstances of some urgency rather than convenience. Such an order must be clearly communicated and noted on the client's chart by the nurse. The prescriber must countersign it, usually within 24 hours in most institutions, in order for it *to be legal*. Allowing the order to remain unsigned is careless and negligent because it violates both the law and institutional policy. This allows a precarious period of nursing vulnerability to malpractice charges (see Chapter 2).

Types of Drug Orders

It is probably obvious by now that although outpatients are free to medicate themselves with any medication accessible, once an individual is admitted to a clinical institution, usually neither the client nor the nurse may legally administer any medication without a written order. Contents of the prescriber's orders dictate the conditions under which the ordered drug may be administered. Several types of orders follow.

Routine order. The most common type is the **routine order,** which means that the drug as ordered is to be regularly administered until a formal discontinuation order is written or until a specified termination date is reached. Automatic termination or "automatic stops" may be explicit in agency policy. Automatic stop policies may be mandated for institutional accreditation or licensure requirements, or they may be applied variously by institutions. Such policies act as a stimulus to the prescriber to reevaluate the continued need for those drugs that require especially close attention.

Prn order. A prn order is an order for drugs to be administered according to client need. Within the other criteria specified by the order, the decision of when to medicate is left to the nurse's judgment. This type has implications for nursing autonomy similar to protocol orders.

Medications to reduce the perception of pain make up the bulk of **prn orders.** Keen nursing assessments of pain are required to carry out these prn orders appropriately. (See Chapter 14 for specifics for the evaluation of pain.) It is sufficient to note that pain is a very complex phenomenon, influenced by factors of subjectivity, emotions, and age, among others. The most dependable guide is that the pain is what and when the client says it is; assumptions by the nurse are not as reliable. Research has demonstrated that clients are frequently undermedicated for pain. Children especially are frequently left to suffer, undermedicated for pain, under the assumption that their pain is less severe than it seems.

Single order. A **single order** is an order for a drug to be administered only once at the time indicated. An example is an order for a preoperative medication.

Stat order. A **stat order** is an order for a drug to be administered as a single dose immediately.

Protocol. A **protocol** is a set of criteria that serves as a directive under which medication may be given. Protocols may typically be one of two types: standing orders or flow diagram protocols. Standing orders are officially accepted sets of orders (not only for medications) to be applied routinely by nurses to the care of clients with certain conditions or under certain circumstances (e.g., as part of admission orders in some critical care units). Flow diagram protocols are criteria that give nurses guidelines for administration of certain treatments and medications on the basis of client variables. These protocols provide the widest scope for application of nursing judgment and decision making of all the types of orders. Criteria and direction may be either very specific, for those with limited expertise or responsibility, or less specific and allow for greater latitude, self-reliance, and sophistication in decision making.

Assessment of Medication Orders

Client. Every possible effort should be made to ensure that the client receives the intended medication in the manner planned by the prescriber. Toward this end, clients with similar names should be widely separated in the health care setting, and all their paperwork must be clearly distinguishable. An identifying arm band must be kept on every client and compared with identifying information that accompanies each dose of medication.

Date. The date that a medication order was written must be checked against other information for accuracy or for confirmation of when the last dose is to be given.

Medication. The medication's name may be written either in generic or trade form. The client should know the name of the medication. If this practice is not yet agency policy, nurses in the agency should be actively working with administrative leaders to reverse the policy. Clients should be told the names of their drugs while hospitalized so they can reasonably be expected to follow self-administration orders successfully at home. It is dangerous to keep clients ignorant of their medications. Exact names and dosages are crucial information for health care providers to know if, for example, emergency treatment is needed.

Dosage and frequency. Drug dosages should be given as prescribed in the medication order unless nursing judgment detects, for example, that the size of the dose ordered falls outside the range of usual limits or that there are intervening factors in the client-dosage, its frequency, or the route of administration. The drug would then not be administered and would be held until the nurse consults the prescriber.

During the development of a drug the manufacturer makes determinations in regard to optimal range of dosage, frequency, and effective route for administration for most people. These are based on the known pharmacokinetics of the drug. For example, a drug that routinely undergoes biotransformation slowly may remain in the body system longer and produce more prolonged effects than another drug. This drug, therefore, may be given effectively on a once-a-day basis; however, a drug that is excreted rapidly may need to be given every 4 hours around the clock if effective serum levels of the drug are to be maintained. Nursing judgments must be made in order to align an individual client's medication schedule with agency policy at appropriate intervals or to keep to a single schedule to meet a specific drug requirement (e.g., before or after meals) or a special need of the client. Some reasons to individualize administration time include client convenience and avoiding disturbing the client's rest, sleep, meals, visiting hours, other activities, or treatments. Rationale for other modifications in the therapeutic regimen should be discussed with the prescriber.

Route. Every medication order should include a specified route for administration. Making assumptions in this area is negligent. However, choice of the actual *site* of administration of injectables is a nursing or nurse-client decision. For example, subcutaneous, intramuscular, and intravenous sites to avoid include any areas of obvious injury, disease, or lesions, even if minor; any that are noticeably erythematous (reddened), vesicular (blistered), open and weeping or pustular, ecchymotic (bruised), or scarred; and those previously overused for injection. Such areas may have impaired circulation or may be adversely affected by the injection itself or by the material injected. Injection sites are rotated to avoid tissue damage from injections. (Details may be found in Chapter 5.)

The ordered route of administration should routinely be assessed for efficacy, feasibility, or practicality. For example, the oral route would naturally be precluded for the client who is nauseated or vomiting. Prior consultation with the prescriber must be made before administering a drug by a different route, because dosage or other factors may have to be readjusted if bioavailability is affected by such changes.

Evaluation of Primary and Secondary Effects

The ultimate effects of drugs on the body can be divided into two types. The main purpose of administering a medication is to use its primary or therapeutic effect. All other consequences can be considered secondary effects, largely unintended and often nontherapeutic. Figure 4-5 illustrates the association between common terms that are used to describe the relative severity of secondary effects.

Drugs are developed and formulated to promote special effects; therefore the appearance of secondary effects demonstrates a continuing challenge to drug manufacturers. The crux of this problem is that most drugs are not selective enough to target only one body system, organ, tissue, or cell. When the drug is circulated or distributed to other areas, reactions may range in severity from merely inconvenient or annoying side effects to very serious adverse effects. On the other hand, a side effect may actually be the sought-after pri-

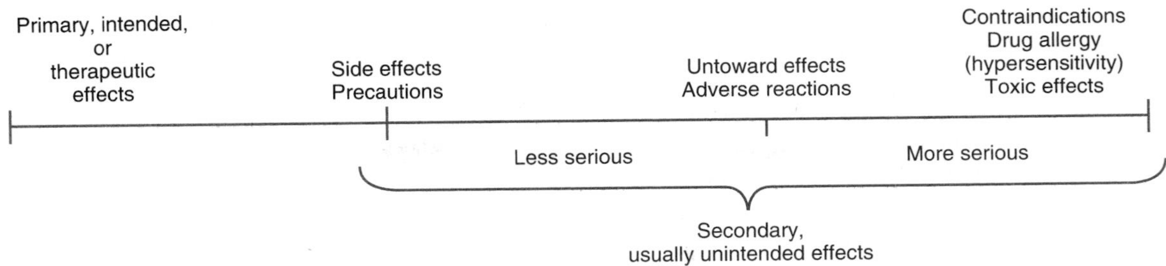

Figure 4-5 Terms indicating relative severity of medication effects—a continuum.

mary effect under certain circumstances or may be exploited by the prescriber as a therapeutic effect along with the primary effects. For example, diphenhydramine (Benadryl) is an antihistamine that produces a high incidence of drowsiness or sedation-type side effects. If this antihistamine is prescribed for an irritable child afflicted with an itching, poison ivy rash, the effect of sedation becomes a desired secondary effect. In fact, diphenhydramine is commonly prescribed as a sleep medication for the elderly. But if diphenhydramine is prescribed for an allergic reaction in a person who handles dangerous machinery or drives a commercial vehicle for a living, this side effect is undesired. In such instances, the prescriber should probably select an antihistamine without a significant sedative side effect.

Primary and secondary effects are often dose related—directly related to increases in dosage—or they may be related to the duration of that specific therapy.

In the assessment phase of the nursing process, it is essential to discover any **contraindications** to a drug's administration. Contraindications are conditions that would preclude the administration of a drug. A contraindication to administration of a drug has potential to be more harmful than do side effects and adverse reactions, which may be discerned only in the evaluation phase (see Chapter 5), after the administration of the drug. It is essential that the medicating process be assessed with regard to each medication's clinical indications and potential efficacy and any contraindications, especially any allergy to the drug or any pathologic condition that would preclude its administration (Box 4-2).

An allergy history of any sort, even if unrelated to the medication, must be explored to rule out and prevent any possible allergic reaction. The occurrence of drug allergy reactions is extremely individualized, unpredictable except for history, and not usually closely dose related. The reaction may result in a very serious and life-threatening situation; consequently the drug must not be given. Reactions may vary from mild rash to severe exfoliative dermatitis and from asthma to anaphylactic shock. They may include urticaria, angioneurotic edema, and drug fever.

An allergic drug response is caused by a specific reaction between a drug and the immune system. Most drugs are organic molecules with molecular weights of less than 1000 daltons, a dalton being an arbitrary unit of mass equivalent to 1.657×10^{-24} g. Such small molecules act as haptens; that is, they take on the ability to act as an allergen (to cause allergic reactions) only if they become bound to a carrier protein. This happens when the drug or its metabolite combines with tissue or plasma proteins to form the drug-protein complex, the complete allergen, necessary to stimulate the immune response and provoke an allergic response. At initial exposure to the drug, sensitive persons may exhibit a latent period of 10 to 20 days before the allergic reaction occurs. Reactions upon reexposure to the drug may occur sooner, even immediately.

It is essential to place alerting stickers or notations regarding the client's allergic history in the clinical record, computerized information system, Kardex, or other places according to agency policy. These locations need to be checked before any medications are given. Records may denote "no known allergy" (NKA), but usually this refers to drugs. Because a correlation often exists between one allergic response and the development of another, the client's description of *any* past allergic manifestations—to drugs, in-

BOX 4-2

Medications Frequently Implicated in Allergic Reactions

Antibiotics: penicillin (the most common cause of drug-induced anaphylaxis), cephalosporins, tetracyclines, streptomycin, erythromycin, neomycin, nitrofurantoin, and sulfa drugs (very frequently)

Other drugs: aspirin, hydantoins, acetaminophen, tolbutamide, gold salts, phenylbutazone, phenothiazines, histamines, aminopyrine, iodides, iron dextran, methylergonovine, quinidine, dipyrone, aminosalicylic acid, thiouracil, tranquilizers, anesthetics such as benzocaine (particularly troublesome because they are frequently used for application topically to irritated or delicate mucous membranes), tetracaine, procaine, lidocaine, and cocaine

Diagnostic agents such as iodinated contrast media (e.g., dye for intravenous pyelogram [IVP]), iopanoic acid (Telepaque), dehydrocholic acid (Decholin), Congo red dye

Biologicals such as antitoxins, vaccines, gamma globulin, insulin, ACTH, enzymes, and their preservatives such as thimerosal, parabens, and antibiotics

halants, foods (typically include eggs, orange juice, chocolate, shellfish, or strawberries), or whatever—must be clarified and evaluated. Often the client erroneously defines an unexpected response as an allergic one. For example, the nausea following a meperidine (Demerol) injection may be labeled an allergic reaction by the client, when in actuality it is likely to be only a normal, if exaggerated, side effect. Correcting such misinformation with the client and in the records may become important because it makes that drug available for therapy when necessary. Before any questionable medications are administered, nurses should specifically inquire about previous experiences with these agents and, if necessary for a client who has many allergies, discuss with the prescriber the need for a test dose. Special methods for those who must take medication to which they are allergic (e.g., aspirin, local anesthetics, or contrast media in diagnostic agents) include pretreatment medication in the form of antihistamines, prednisone, and ephedrine or cautiously increasing dosages of the allergy-provoking drug under supervision. Clients may also have allergies to additives found in foods and drug products (Box 4-3).

Other contraindications to drug therapy must be assessed before administration. Clients may have medical problems that contraindicate a given drug or, if the drug is deemed necessary, that the risk-benefit ratio be carefully considered and caution taken to carefully monitor the client. For example, opioid analgesics are contraindicated in clients with acute respiratory depression, since the condition would be exacerbated by the drug's respiratory depressive effects. On the other hand, most drugs, including opioid analgesics, would be administered with caution, and probably with dosage modifications, to clients with hepatic or renal function impairment because they are metabolized in the liver and excreted by the kidneys. Assessment for and planning of the pharmacologic therapeutic regimen to minimize adverse effects and provide for client safety are essential.

Drug Interactions

The complexity of modern pharmacotherapy is nowhere more obvious than in the ever-growing list of drugs that interact nontherapeutically with one another, with foods, and with fluids and that distort laboratory test results. That these chemical substances will interact with or potentiate one another is not surprising. This fact should always be kept in mind when medications appear either ineffective or harmful or when the accuracy of laboratory tests is crucial.

Variables influencing drug interaction include (1) intestinal absorption, (2) competition for plasma binding, (3) drug metabolism or biotransformation, (4) action at the receptor site, (5) renal excretion, and (6) alteration of electrolyte balance. The following are examples of these variables' effects that interact nontherapeutically with other drugs, food, juices, and other liquids and distort many laboratory test results:

1. Intestinal absorption: foods or antacids that contain calcium, magnesium, or aluminum, such as antacids, may form a complex with or bind tetracycline, resulting in reduced absorption of the antibiotic.
2. Competition for plasma protein binding: tolbutamide (Orinase), an oral antihyperglycemic agent, can be displaced from its binding on plasma proteins by sulfonamides, resulting in severe hypoglycemia. Many drugs are weak acids that are bound largely to plasma proteins. These weak acids may compete for binding sites on plasma proteins, thus increasing the free, active drug, which may have potent effects.
3. Drug metabolism or biotransformation: the monoamine oxidase inhibitors prevent the biotransformation of tyramine, which is present in aged cheese, liver, overripe fruit, and preserved meat (sausage, bologna, pepperoni, salami) and may provoke a hypertensive crisis, a rapid and severe increase in blood pressure.
4. Action at the receptor site: numerous examples exist of one drug intensifying or antagonizing the action of another drug at the receptor site. For example, the antihistaminics decrease many effects of histamine, while cocaine increases the actions of epinephrine.
5. Renal excretion: probenecid (Benemid) inhibits the renal clearance of penicillin because it inhibits the active renal tubular secretion of many weak organic acids, of which penicillin is one.
6. Alteration of electrolyte balance: the thiazide diuretics may cause hypokalemia, which predisposes to digitalis toxicity, because there is increased renal secretion of potassium with their use.

In addition to the drug interactions discussed above, the nurse should also consider drugs that have a pharmacodynamic interaction. These interactions are caused by the concurrent administration of two drugs that have the opposite effect or drugs having similar effects. Interactions with drugs having similar effects, such as alcohol and sedatives, or drugs having hypotensive effects may be easier to identify than those drugs having opposite effects. An example of such an interaction is a client with asthma who is being treated with a beta adrenergic drug such as albuterol (Proventil, Ventolin) for its bronchodilating effects, being administered a beta adrenergic blocking drug as an antihypertensive agent (Hussar, 1993).

BOX 4-3

Allergic Reactions to Food Additives

Allergic reactions have been reported after ingestion of food additives, such as monosodium glutamate (MSG), tartrazine, and sulfites. Tartrazine and sulfites are also used as additives, preservatives, and antioxidants in various medications. The most serious adverse reaction, resulting in some reported deaths, occurred most often in asthmatic patients. Current lists of foods and drug products containing tartrazine and sulfites should be reviewed in assessing reported allergic reactions.

Not all drug interactions are dangerous; some are relatively insignificant or even beneficial. Tables listing known drug interactions should be posted in the medication area as a reference for nurses.

Drug-Drug Interactions

Some drugs commonly involved in clinically significant drug-drug interactions include antacids, warfarin, aspirin, tricyclic antidepressants (MAO inhibitors), aminoglycosides, amphetamines, corticosteroids, digitalis glycosides, diuretics, sulfonamides, alcohol, phenytoin, quinidine, antihypertensives, beta blockers, and theophylline. Before any such medication is given, an appropriate source should be consulted to assess the drug, its mechanism, and any other medications given concurrently to determine the probability of interactions developing. This text gives this information in the context of specific drug monographs.

Other Drug Interactions

Drug-induced malabsorption of foods and nutrients. Drugs that change gastric or intestinal motility can alter the digestion or absorption of certain nutrients. Important drugs that affect these changes are stimulant cathartics and mineral oil, which increase bowel motility and, at the other extreme, anticholinergics and narcotics, which inhibit it. Cholestyramine (Questran), a drug indicated for hypercholesteremia, adsorbs and combines with bile acids to form an insoluble complex that is excreted through the feces. Such loss of bile acids lowers blood cholesterol levels. However, the drug also adsorbs the fat soluble vitamins, A, D, E, and K, which are then excreted rather than absorbed into the body. Some oral contraceptives impair folic acid absorption in undernourished clients.

Food-induced malabsorption of drugs. Fatty foods or foods low in fiber will delay stomach emptying by up to 2 hours, which may result in delayed and/or reduced drug absorption. However, several medications, such as griseofulvin and possibly spironolactone, exhibit enhanced bioavailability (absorption) following a high-fat meal. Many tetracyclines can form insoluble complexes in the gastrointestinal tract if given at the same time as foods or drugs containing ions of calcium, aluminum, magnesium, or iron. Thus administering tetracycline medication along with milk-based tube feedings or common antacids should be avoided. Ascorbic acid from citrus fruits or juices enhances the absorption of iron, but carbonated soft drinks or acid juices (fruit or vegetable) can cause drugs to dissolve more quickly in the stomach than in the intestine or can neutralize them, thereby changing the intended rate or completeness of absorption.

Milk, coffee, eggs, tea, whole-grain breads and cereals, dietary fiber, and foods containing bicarbonates, carbonates, phosphates, or oxalates may all reduce iron absorption if given concurrently. Iron products should be ingested no sooner than 1 hour before or 2 hours after the mentioned food substances are given.

Alteration of enzymes. Enzyme alterations, either induction or inhibition, may affect the metabolism of a food or drug. The natural extract of black licorice is chemically similar to that of steroids; therefore if taken in excess, licorice can cause hypokalemia, retention of sodium and water with resultant hypertension, and alkalosis. Ingestion of large amounts would be contraindicated for clients who are concurrently taking potassium-losing diuretics or those who have cardiovascular disease.

Similarly, consumption of large amounts of foods high in vitamin K (such as liver and green leafy vegetables) may reduce or antagonize the effectiveness of oral anticoagulants. Difficulty in maintaining the desired anticoagulant response with appropriately prescribed dosages indicates the need for an assessment of food and drug consumption.

Monoamine oxidase inhibitors (tricyclic antidepressants) act by inhibiting the breakdown of norepinephrine, a vasopressor substance. This excess norepinephrine is then stored in the neurons. The ingestion of certain tyramine-containing foods (aged cheeses, beef and chicken liver, pickled herring, broad beans, canned figs, bananas, avocados, soy sauce, active yeast preparations, beer, sherry in large quantities, Chianti wine, chocolate, anchovies, caffeine, mushrooms, raisins, sausages, dried fish, tuna fish, cola drinks, and many fermented foods) may elevate the quantity of norepinephrine to toxic levels, thereby precipitating hypertensive crises. Over-the-counter cold remedies containing ephedrine, phenylephrine, and phenylpropanolamine, and amphetamines in general can act similarly, releasing stored quantities of norepinephrine. The net effect can be a headache, a sudden climb in blood pressure to dangerous levels, cardiac arrhythmias, or intracranial bleeding.

Alcohol consumption. Of the more than 100 most frequently prescribed drugs, more than half contain at least one ingredient known to interact adversely with imbibed alcohol. An interaction is probable if the drug is known to affect the central nervous system or is metabolized by the liver. The effects are dose-related, and whether quantities of alcohol are used habitually, chronically, or only occasionally often makes a distinct difference in the direction of interactive effects. Patterns of alcohol consumption are likely to have a bearing on the client's concurrence with drug treatment and follow-through as well. Alcohol consumption should be limited or totally avoided if a client is taking narcotics, tranquilizers, sedatives, and other CNS depressant-type drugs, which may cause additive or synergistic respiratory and CNS depression. Thus it is obvious that it is important to elicit information about patterns of alcohol consumption when a history is being taken.

The fact that many elixirs and tinctures are liquid formulations of drugs dissolved in alcohol is significant, especially in the assessment of pharmacotherapy for children. These preparations must be reassessed and cannot be assumed to have the same rates and degrees of absorption as the same drugs in aqueous solution, since bioavailability may be altered.

Cigarette smoking. The main pharmacokinetic effect of heavy cigarette smoking is the lowering of drug plasma levels by induction of microsomal enzyme systems responsible for increased drug metabolism or excretion. The rate of theophylline (Theo-Dur) breakdown is increased, necessitating an increase in dosage of from 1½ times to twice the average dose. The usual doses of other drugs have diminished effectiveness in the heavy cigarette smoker—for example, the antidepressant imipramine; analgesics such as pentazocine (Talwin) and propoxyphene (Darvon); vitamins C, B_{12}, and B_6; and the influenza vaccine. The absorption rate of insulin by the subcutaneous route is twice as slow as usual. Smoking also interacts with glutethimide, furosemide (Lasix), and propranolol (Inderal). Depression of the CNS and drowsiness are less frequent with diazepam (Valium), and drowsiness is reduced with chlorpromazine (Thorazine). When smoking is combined with use of estrogens, the risk of heart attack, stroke, and other circulatory disorders increases. Laboratory test results may also be somewhat outside the range of normal, depending on the duration of smoking history and inhalation practices. The white cell count is increased (in the absence of clinical infection); hemoglobin concentration, hematocrit, and red blood cell size are increased; and clotting time is reduced. Some investigators of cigarette smoking have found an abnormal increase in cholesterol, and others have found carcinoembryonic antigen levels as high as for persons with colon cancer, yet without other evidence of it. Therefore smokers sometimes can be expected to exhibit more numerous drug therapy "failures" or adverse effects, or they may even have fewer or different reactions to drugs than do nonsmoking clients. Certain laboratory test results must be interpreted in light of cigarette smoking history.

Caffeine consumption. Caffeinated beverages present a medical problem in that many people consume enough caffeine to produce substantial effects on a number of organ systems. Caffeine stimulates the central nervous system and cardiac muscle, and acts on the kidney to produce diuresis. Individuals ingesting caffeine or caffeinated beverages usually experience less drowsiness and fatigue, and a more rapid and clearer flow of thought. However, as the dose is increased, signs of progressive CNS stimulation occur, including nervousness, anxiety, restlessness, insomnia, and tremors. Caffeine will produce tachycardia and in higher doses arrhythmias. Increases in blood pressure with caffeine ingestion are the result of an increase in systemic vascular resistance. Caffeine causes secretion of both pepsin and gastric acid from parietal cells of the stomach. The use of caffeine by an individual taking beta-adrenergic blockers may inhibit their therapeutic effect. Excessive CNS stimulation may occur with the concurrent use of caffeine and other CNS stimulating medications, progressing from nervousness to possibly convulsions or cardiac arrhythmias. Caffeine inhibits the absorption of calcium and promotes the excretion of lithium and other drugs. Combined with monoamine oxidase (MAO) inhibitors, caffeine may produce severe hypertension.

Food-initiated alteration of drug excretion. Changes in the pH of urine caused by food (making the urine overly acidic or alkaline) can have a significant effect on the excretion rates of some drugs, since pH influences the ionization of weak acids and bases. A drug will diffuse more easily from the urine back into the blood in its nondissociated state, thereby prolonging drug action. Thus action of acidic drugs is prolonged when urine is acidic. Although it is quite difficult to override the kidneys' ability to regulate urine pH, an alkaline-ash or acid-ash diet, whether by purpose or not, can drive urinary pH above 8 or below 5, creating a medium for potential drug reactions. Continued taking of many antacid tablets each day in concert with quinidine administration was seen in one instance to create quinidine intoxication by shifting urinary pH toward the base and causing a serious arrhythmia necessitating hospitalization.

Drug Incompatibilities

Drug interactions occurring when drugs are mixed before administration, as in a single syringe or in intravenous fluids, are termed drug **incompatibilities**. Drugs that are physically incompatible may produce unwanted changes through processes such as liquefaction, deliquescence, or precipitation. Chemical incompatibilities may result when ingredients interact to form new compounds or are neutralized (see Nursing Research box at right). If drug incompatibilities are anticipated, separate administration routes should be sought. Some drugs are highly incompatible in solution with many other drugs. Because solution incompatibilities are frequently time dependent, fewer difficulties may be associated with mixing drugs in one syringe than in IV solutions; both drugs should be administered as soon after mixing as possible. Examples of drugs that are noted for interacting incompatibly with many other drugs in a syringe and that therefore should be administered alone include chlordiazepoxide (Librium), diazepam (Valium), pentobarbital (Nembutal), phenobarbital (Luminal), phenytoin (Dilantin), secobarbital (Seconal), and sodium bicarbonate. See the **inside of the back cover** of this text for the compatibility of selected medications in a syringe.

Many drugs have explicit manufacturer's instructions for preparation (dilution and method of adding to selected parenteral solutions), which should be closely followed. A check for drug compatibility is indicated before two or more drugs are added to the same IV solution. Standard IV parenteral drug charts and guides are available for reference use. Many hospital pharmacies provide an IV preparation service that screens for incompatibilities before preparation and delivery to the nursing area.

With the increase in the number of potent drugs and the variety of combinations, use of the pharmacist's expertise in a controlled environment is probably a wise policy. If the nurse is required to prepare IV solutions on the nursing unit, then adequate references, including a list of incompatibilities, should be posted in the area where the nurses perform this duty. Open communication on a regular basis with the pharmacy department is necessary in order to obtain new or additional information and assistance whenever necessary.

ANALYSIS OF DATA

When data from the nursing assessment have been collected, the next phase is **analysis**—the critical evaluation of infor-

Nursing Research

Incompatible drug infusions via multilumen catheters

Nurses have long been alert to the occurrence of incompatibilities when mixing multiple medications in the same syringe. But with the increase in the use of multilumen catheters to maintain long-term, reliable central venous access for frequent administration of multiple drugs and hyperalimentation solutions and blood sampling and transfusions, consideration needs to be given to the possibility of such incompatibilities occurring in vivo. To examine the physicochemical phenomena that occur when two incompatible drugs (phenytoin and total parenteral nutrition) are simultaneously administered through multilumen catheters, Collins and Lutz* used an in vitro model venous flow system in which flow conditions and drug infusions mimicked the in vivo clinical situations to evaluate two central venous catheter types, a double- and a triple-lumen catheter. Video recordings were made of drug interactions, and assays of phenytoin concentration were performed on samples of the circulating fluid. White clouds of phenytoin precipitation were observed near the tip of the double-lumen catheter but not the triple-lumen catheter. Infusion through the double-lumen catheter resulted in an average loss of phenytoin of 6%, the precipitate of which, on microscopic examination, appeared as spindle-shaped crystals 25 to 50 μm in length and 5 to 10 μm wide. In some instances, millimeter-sized fragments of phenytoin were seen to dislodge from the tip of the double-lumen catheter. The adjacent orifices at the tip of the double-lumen catheter appeared to permit interaction of the two effusing streams of the incompatible drugs, whereas the staggered orifices of the triple-lumen catheter minimized this interaction. Although the clinical significance of in vivo precipitate incompatibility has yet to be determined, theoretically possible complications would include reduced bioavailability of the drug, thrombophlebitis from particulate matter, pulmonary emboli from larger precipitate fragments, and occlusion of the catheter.

Critical thinking questions

- In what way do you think this research could effect the utilization of central venous catheters with clients on multidrug regimens?
- If you were administering precipitate-incompatible drugs to a client with a double-lumen central venous catheter, how would you modify your nursing care?

*Collins JL & Lutz RJ (1991). In vitro study of simultaneous infusion of incompatible drugs in multilumen catheters, *Heart Lung* 20(3):271.

mation to determine its meaning and importance. As with all phases of the nursing process, analysis is continuous. It is the process of interpreting data based on sound pharmacologic and nursing principles.

To facilitate analysis the nurse may follow several steps. Initially, data are organized into categories. Categorization is accomplished by use of a planned systematic assessment, and gaps in data are noted. Once identified, missing information can be obtained to complete the assessment. Accepted standards and norms are then applied to determine discrepancies between what is and what should or could be, and conclusions are drawn regarding what actual problems may be present and those for which the client may be at high risk. The culmination of analysis is the diagnostic statement, which includes nursing diagnoses and collaborative problems toward which nursing care may be directed.

NURSING DIAGNOSIS/ COLLABORATIVE PROBLEM

The North American Nursing Diagnosis Association (NANDA) has defined a **nursing diagnosis** as a clinical judgment about individual, family, or community responses to actual or potential health problems/life processes. Nursing diagnosis provides the basis for selection of nursing interventions to achieve outcomes for which the nurse is accountable (NANDA, 1995). NANDA is the formal organization sanctioned by the American Nurses' Association (ANA) to govern the development of a classification system for nursing diagnoses. Proposed nursing diagnoses are submitted to NANDA for official acceptance.

Until 1992 the phrase "potential for" was used if the client was at risk of developing a particular nursing diagnosis. Since then, "high risk for" or "risk for" has been the appropriate terminology, defined by NANDA to indicate "a clinical judgment that an individual, family, or community is more vulnerable to develop the problem than others in the same or similar situation."

Collaborative problems are "certain physiologic complications that nurses monitor to detect onset or changes of status. Nurses manage collaborative problems utilizing physician-prescribed and nursing-prescribed interventions to minimize the complications of the events" (Carpenito, 1995). Whereas for nursing diagnosis the assessment of the client involves the detection of signs and symptoms of actual problems and risk factors for high-risk nursing diagnoses, the assessment for collaborative problems focuses on determining the status of the collaborative problem, that is, that certain conditions are present that increase the client's vulnerability to the complication, or that the client has experienced the complication. The nurse's responsibility is to monitor the client's physiologic status, perform specific activities to manage and minimize the severity of the situation, and consult with a physician to obtain orders for appropriate interventions. Collaborative problems can be written "Potential Complication: (Specify)." An example of a collaborative problem with the administration of a nonsteroidal anti-inflammatory analgesic would be "Potential complication (PC): gastrointestinal bleeding," or with methotrexate, an antineoplastic agent, "PC: hepatoxicity."

The nurse makes independent decisions for both nursing diagnoses and collaborative problems. The difference is that in nursing diagnoses, nursing prescribes the definitive treatment, whereas with collaborative problems both nursing and medicine prescribe for the definitive treatment to achieve desired outcomes for care of the client.

The nursing profession is working actively toward a classification for nursing practice. Standardization of terminology facilitates communication among practitioners. An aim is to classify groups of nursing diagnoses so that patterns will emerge, leading to categories of diagnoses. NANDA has endorsed a classification of nursing diagnoses by human response patterns with approved terminology (McCourt & Carroll-Johnson, 1992). Whenever possible, diagnostic statements used in this book are drawn from the list of NANDA-approved nursing diagnoses. The NANDA list and other widely circulated lists are not considered complete, but rather nurses are encouraged to test nursing diagnoses and develop new ones. See Box 4-4 for a current list of NANDA-approved nursing diagnoses.

Several examples of nursing diagnoses follow. Note that there could be countless ways to convey the same thoughts, all equally correct; variations can arise from differences among individuals constructing the diagnoses and from the wording chosen. A nursing diagnosis includes two main components: a description of altered health status and an inferred reason for it. If the nursing diagnosis is an actual one rather than one for which the client is at high risk, the symptoms by which the client evidences the problem may also be included in the statement. The following list presents some sample nursing diagnoses:

- Risk for alteration in urinary elimination: urinary retention related to history of benign prostatic hypertrophy and concurrent anticholinergic therapy
- Risk for constipation related to morphine sulfate administration
- Fluid volume excess: edema related to steroid therapy evidenced by 2+ pitting edema of ankles and weight gain of 4 pounds over 3 days
- Ineffective individual management of therapeutic regimen: failure to refill prescriptions related to inadequate financial resources to buy drugs evidenced by client statement "I wish I could afford my heart pills"

Box 4-4 contains the NANDA-approved nursing diagnoses, with the ones more commonly resulting from drug therapy noted by asterisks; however, the nurse should consider the full range of nursing diagnoses during assessment.

For each medication, there is a combination of nursing diagnoses and collaborative problems that should be anticipated or for which the client needs to be assessed, in addi-

BOX 4-4

North American Nursing Diagnosis Association (NANDA) Approved Nursing Diagnoses

*Activity intolerance
*Activity intolerance, risk for
Adaptive capacity, decreased: intracranial
Adjustment, impaired
Airway clearance, ineffective
*Anxiety
*Aspiration, risk for
Body image disturbance
Body temperature, altered, risk for
Bowel incontinence
*Breastfeeding, effective
Breastfeeding, ineffective
Breastfeeding, interrupted
*Breathing pattern, ineffective
Cardiac output, decreased
Caregiver role strain
Caregiver role strain, risk for
Communication, impaired verbal
Community coping, potential for enhanced
Community coping, ineffective
Confusion, acute
Confusion, chronic
*Constipation
Constipation, colonic
Constipation, perceived
Coping, defensive
Coping, family: potential for growth
Coping, ineffective family: compromised
Coping, ineffective family: disabling
*Coping, ineffective individual
Decisional conflict (specify)
Denial, ineffective
*Diarrhea
Disuse syndrome, risk for

*Nursing diagnoses more commonly seen with drug therapy.

BOX 4-4

North American Nursing Diagnosis Association (NANDA) Approved Nursing Diagnoses—cont'd

Diversional activity deficit
Dysreflexia
Energy field disturbance
Environmental interpretation syndrome, impaired
Family processes, altered: alcoholism
Family processes, altered
*Fatigue
Fear
Fluid volume deficit
*Fluid volume deficit, risk for
*Fluid volume excess
*Gas exchange, impaired
Grieving, anticipatory
Grieving, dysfunctional
Growth and development, altered
*Health maintenance, altered
*Health-seeking behaviors (specify)
*Home maintenance management, impaired
Hopelessness
Hyperthermia
Hypothermia
Incontinence, functional
Incontinence, reflex
Incontinence, stress
Incontinence, total
Incontinence, urge
Infant behavior, disorganized
Infant behavior, disorganized: risk for
Infant behavior, organized: potential for enhanced
Infant feeding pattern, ineffective
*Infection, risk for
Injury, perioperative positioning: risk for
*Injury, risk for
*Knowledge deficit (specify)
Loneliness, risk for
Management of therapeutic regimen, community: ineffective
Management of therapeutic regimen, families: ineffective
Management of therapeutic regimen, individual: effective
*Management of therapeutic regimen, individuals: ineffective
Memory, impaired
Mobility, impaired physical
*Noncompliance (specify)
*Nutrition, altered: less than body requirements
Nutrition, altered: more than body requirements
Nutrition, altered: risk for more than body requirements
*Oral mucous membrane, altered
Pain
Pain, chronic
Parent/infant/child attachment, altered: risk for
Parental role conflict
Parenting, altered
Parenting, altered, risk for
Peripheral neurovascular dysfunction, risk for
Personal identity disturbance
*Poisoning, risk for
Post-trauma response
Powerlessness
*Protection, altered
Rape-trauma syndrome
Rape-trauma syndrome: compound reaction
Rape-trauma syndrome: silent reaction
Relocation stress syndrome
Role performance, altered
Self-care deficit, bathing/hygiene
Self-care deficit, dressing/grooming
Self-care deficit, feeding
Self-care deficit, toileting
Self-esteem disturbance
Self-esteem, chronic low
Self-esteem, situational low
Self-mutilation, risk for
*Sensory/perceptual alterations (specify) (visual, auditory, kinesthetic, gustatory, tactile, olfactory)
*Sexual dysfunction
*Sexuality patterns, altered
*Skin integrity, impaired
*Skin integrity, impaired, risk for
*Sleep pattern disturbance
Social interaction, impaired
Social isolation
Spiritual distress (distress of the human spirit)
Spiritual well-being, potential for enhanced
Suffocation, risk for
*Swallowing, impaired
Thermoregulation, ineffective
*Thought processes, altered
Tissue integrity, impaired
*Tissue perfusion, altered (specify type) (renal, cerebral, cardiopulmonary, gastrointestinal, peripheral)
Trauma, risk for
Unilateral neglect
Urinary elimination, altered
*Urinary retention
Ventilation, inability to sustain spontaneous
Ventilatory weaning response, dysfunction (DVWR)
Violence, risk for: directed at others
Violence, risk for: self-directed

*Nursing diagnoses more commonly seen with drug therapy.

tion to quite specific ones that may be particular to the individual client.

1. Client issues related to the client's preexisting health status. These may be stated as "Potential complication (PC): (specify the physiologic complication related to the client's preexisting medical conditions, age, and childbearing status)" such as with morphine—"PC: acute respiratory depression related to client's preexisting chronic obstructive pulmonary disease and the administration of morphine." On the other hand, a number of nursing diagnoses might also relate to the client's preexisting health status and the administration of morphine, i.e., "Risk for constipation related to the client's age (76 years), low fiber intake, and the administration of morphine" or "Risk for urinary retention related to client's history of benign prostatic hypertrophy and the administration of morphine."
2. Client issues related to concurrent drug therapy. "PC: (specify the physiologic complication related to concurrent drug therapy)," such as "PC: digoxin toxicity related to the concurrent administration of digoxin and diuretic therapy." An appropriate nursing diagnosis related to concurrent drug therapy might be: "Risk for injury related to postural hypotension secondary to the concurrent administration of propranolol (Inderal) and diuretic therapy."
3. Client issues related to the ineffectiveness of the drug. "PC: (specify the physiologic complication of the client's underlying condition related to the ineffectiveness of the drug)," such as "PC: sepsis related to the ineffectiveness of antibiotic therapy." A nursing diagnosis related to the ineffectiveness of therapy might be "Chronic pain related to ineffective pain management program." The assessment of the effectiveness of the client's drug regimen is essential. If the outcome criteria for the client's drug therapy are not met, the drug is considered to be ineffective and the prescriber will need to alter the client's medications.
4. Client issues related to the drug's side effects/adverse reactions. "PC: (specify the physiologic complication related to the side effects/adverse reactions of the administered drug)," such as "PC: thrombocytopenia related to heparin therapy" or "PC: GI bleeding related to aspirin therapy." An appropriate nursing diagnosis related to drug side effects might be "Sleep pattern disturbance related to caffeine ingestion." Carpenito (1995) has described "Potential Complication: Medication Therapy Adverse Effects" as well as specific potential complications for anticoagulant, antianxiety, adrenocorticosteroid, antineoplastic, anticonvulsant, antidepressant, antiarrhythmic, antipsychotic, and antihypertensive therapy.
5. Risk for poisoning: drug toxicity, which is the accentuated risk of accidental exposure to or ingestion of drugs or dangerous products in doses sufficient to cause poisoning. The elderly are particularly prone to this nursing diagnosis because of reduced vision, forgetfulness, polypharmacy, and the effects of drugs in the aging body.
6. Knowledge deficit related to initiation of or change in the medication regimen. Although knowledge deficit, the state in which an individual or group experiences a deficiency in cognitive knowledge or psychomotor skills concerning the condition or treatment plan, is listed as a nursing diagnosis, it does not represent a human response, alteration, or a pattern of dysfunction (Jenny, 1987). However, each client must be assessed for the level of knowledge related to his or her health condition and medication regimen. If the client requests information or expresses an inadequate knowledge of his or her health condition or medications to self-administer the prescribed drugs accurately and safely, client education is necessary.
7. Noncompliance, the state in which an individual or group desires to comply but is prevented from doing so by factors that deter adherence to health-related advice given by health professionals, is another nursing diagnosis that should be considered in the client's assessment. Indicators that noncompliance may be an issue are that the client is not participating in therapy, if symptoms persist, the disease progresses, and drug therapy outcome criteria are not met. The nursing diagnosis "noncompliance" is not used to describe a client who has made an informed autonomous decision not to comply (Cassells & Redman, 1989).
8. Ineffective management of the therapeutic regimen related to (specify) is a pattern in which the individual experiences or is at high risk to experience difficulty integrating into daily living a program for treatment of illness and the sequelae of illness that meets specific health goals (NANDA, 1996). Factors that contribute to ineffective management may be a lack of trust in health care providers, insufficient confidence, knowledge, or resources.

In the interests of producing a textbook that is still manageable in size, the reader should keep all of these eight client issues in mind when the client assessment is discussed for each drug, because they will not be listed with every drug. They are considered to be universal and are relevant to every medication.

The nursing diagnoses and collaborative problems form the basis for the design of the subsequent phases of the nursing process: planning, implementation, and evaluation. The diagnosis differentiates between actual problems, possible problems, and those that the client has a high risk of developing. Table 4-2 defines each type and the corresponding focus of the interventions.

Nature of Nursing Actions

Nursing interventions may be categorized into three domains: dependent (or delegated), collaborative, and independent. Medicine diagnoses and treats pathologic or cellular responses, whereas nursing diagnoses and treats the

TABLE 4-2 Nursing diagnoses and related interventions

Type	Definition	Focus of nursing interventions
actual (is present)	validated major signs and symptoms	to reduce or eliminate or promote positive diagnoses
risk (may happen)	presence of risk factors	to prevent onset
potential (may be present)	suspected to be present	to obtain additional data to rule out or confirm

Modified from North American Nursing Diagnosis Association (NANDA) taxonomy, 1996.

human response. Activities that legally require a physician directive are considered to be within the **dependent domain** of nursing interventions and constitute a significant portion of nursing practice related to pharmacology. A significant number of interventions within the **collaborative domain** involve interdependent activity between nurses and other health care providers. Client conditions require differing ratios of medical (or other health care provider) and nursing input (Figure 4-6). Neither nurses nor other health care providers possess exclusive responsibility for diagnosis and treatment of collaborative problems. Each group maintains its own responsibility throughout its involvement with the client. The **independent domain** involves the diagnosis and treatment of problems that are primarily nursing in nature. The nurse identifies these problems and assumes primary responsibility for ordering needed interventions.

Utility of Nursing Diagnosis

By describing human responses, nursing diagnosis distinguishes nursing from other health care disciplines. Nursing diagnoses are most useful in the independent domain. Their use provides a focus for goals and interventions: a nursing diagnosis is a clear, concise description of a problem that is uniquely addressed by nurses. The development of nursing diagnoses has added much to the refinement and description of nursing care by providing structure, focus, and language for clear communication.

Because of the continuing development of nursing diagnosis, implementation of nursing diagnoses is hampered by divergent views, conceptual controversies, and confusing terminology. The nursing profession's health-related, client-strength–oriented emphases are not easily addressed by currently accepted nursing diagnoses, and it may be unrealistic to expect nursing diagnoses to describe all of nursing practice. Much of the nurse's role in pharmacotherapeutics encompasses the dependent and collaborative domains, areas that are not thoroughly addressed by nursing diagnoses but are more appropriately addressed by the identification of collaborative problems as potential complications. Throughout this textbook the use of nursing diagnosis is encouraged but not forced upon situations in which it is inappropriate. As the evolution of nursing diagnosis continues, application to pharmacotherapeutics will become increasingly appropriate and useful.

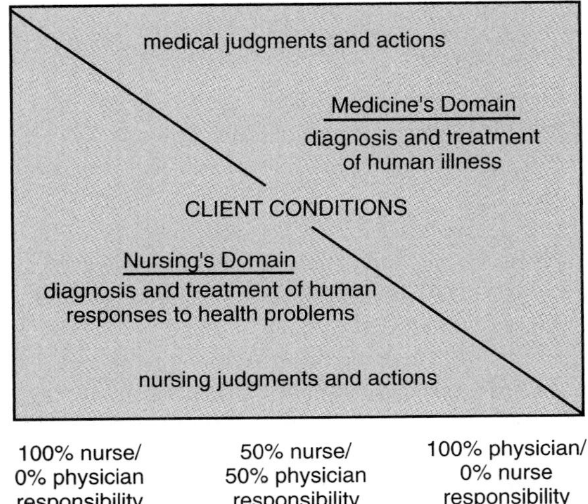

Figure 4-6 Nursing and medical responsibilities. (From McLane AM [Ed.]. [1987]. *Classification of nursing diagnoses: Proceedings of the Seventh Conference.* St Louis: Mosby.)

PLANNING FOR DRUG THERAPY

The planning phase of the nursing process has two parts, setting goals and specific plans for interventions that will implement the goals. Goals are usually stated as **outcome criteria,** statements of observable or measurable results that should occur as the result of nursing and other health service activities. The planning to meet the pharmacotherapeutic nursing needs of clients should be characterized by an orientation to (1) the client, (2) resources in the environment, and (3) the future. The goals are to be established in collaboration with the client and others on the health care team, and in turn should be characterized by a balance between the real and the ideal.

Goals associated with medication needs of clients may be stated in many ways to encompass these three orientations. They must actually be stated (e.g., in the nursing care plan) to provide communication with the rest of the staff and to give clear direction for the subsequent implementation and evaluation phases. Otherwise, the implementation and evaluation of nursing care will be based on vague events and partially remembered and incomplete actions.

Goals are objectives to be met sometime in the future. Therefore the use of the words "will be" in the goal statement is appropriate. An approximation of time limits for the goal to be accomplished should be included in the statement to provide a way of measuring progress toward the goal, whether short term, intermediate, or long term: "by date of discharge," "in 3 days," "by 2 PM today," and so forth. The time limit should be the best estimate, not an edict carved in stone. The goal should be client oriented in that it *should describe what the client's condition or behavior will be at the outcome of nursing care,* not what the nurse intends to *do* for the client. For example, a goal is best stated as "Client will demonstrate the safe and accurate self-administration of insulin in 3 days," rather than "To promote understanding of the drug regimen by the time of discharge from the hospital." The sample nursing care plan below illustrates client-oriented outcome criteria. If the goal describes only what nurses do, they could work diligently to promote a client's understanding of a drug regimen and success would merely be measured in the evaluation of what procedures were performed, yet the client may never have actually learned, which is the intent of the goal.

The nurse can prevent the blurring of the distinction between goals and interventions—two entirely different phases of the nursing process—by stating outcome criteria in terms of behavioral objectives for the client. If criteria are stated in words that depict nursing interventions or actions, such as "prevent," "provide," "promote," or "maintain," then the evaluation of care becomes more an appraisal of what the nurse did by intervening than of the client's condition.

Finally, outcome criteria related to each nursing problem or diagnosis identified earlier may be ranked in priority to meet the client's needs.

The rest of the planning phase lays the ground work for carrying out specific actions in the implementation phase. Such plans for nursing actions should be supportable by applicable principles from the arts, sciences, and humanities, which are the foundations of nursing.

Development of a positive, accountable attitude through goal setting and planning for each nursing action strengthens what nurses do for clients and why. The completed abbreviated nursing care plan, as a blueprint for action, can be entered in writing in the Kardex, the computerized nursing information system, or on the client's chart and makes up the plan for nursing management. The outcome criteria related to drug therapy may also be incorporated into interdisciplinary protocols for care, such as critical paths for client care. Outcome criteria and specific planning provide documentation for peers and preclude legal challenge, while first and foremost guiding the selection of appropriate caring actions.

SUMMARY

Although its structure and terminology may change, the nursing process remains an extremely useful clinical tool. It should be approached as a framework for organizing client care in creative and satisfying ways.

Professional nurses enhance their decision-making skills by critically reviewing their clients' medication plans and maintaining a strong knowledge base about medications, including their indications, mechanisms, pharmacokinetics, and dosages.

The quality of nursing assessment relies on the nurse's ability to observe significant cues, to make sound inferences, and to recognize the client's individuality and establish rapport. Thus a nurse can develop a valid diagnosis, establish realistic goals with the client, and shape an effective nursing plan.

Medication administration is a highly visible, legal function of nurses. Because it depends heavily on the structure and content of prescriber's orders, conscientious assessment of the drug order becomes a very healthy habit. Professional accountability for all disciplines demands open collaboration on questions about clients' medication orders and plans. Underlying the routine of assessing medication therapy is the major goal of preventing harm. Assessment should empha-

Nursing Care Plan

Selected Nursing Diagnoses Related to Client-Oriented Outcome Criteria

Nursing diagnosis	Goals/expected outcomes	Nursing interventions
Knowledge deficit related to her new drug regimen of digoxin, furosemide, and potassium chloride	Before discharge Ms. Strauss will: State the action of each drug and how it relates to her cardiac status. Identify at least three untoward reactions that should be reported to her health care provider. Weigh herself accurately and report results to nurse. Demonstrate the ability to take her own pulse accurately.	1. Discuss with Ms. Strauss the action of each drug and how it relates to her cardiac status. 2. Instruct her about possible side/adverse effects of each drug. 3. Instruct her to report to her health care provider symptoms such as palpitations, resting pulse rate of <60 or >100, sudden change in weight, anorexia, nausea, or lethargy. 4. Discuss the importance of weighing daily and reporting a weight gain of 2 pounds or more. 5. Instruct in pulse-taking, using daily practice. 6. Include her significant other/caretaker in the teaching, if possible. 7. Provide her with written instructions concerning all of her care as a guide for her use at home.

size protecting the client from receiving drugs that will interact, be incompatible, or evoke an allergic response; drugs that will not be degraded or excreted adequately; or drugs that will be transferred to a nursing infant or fetus. Creative nursing consists of finding ways to reschedule or space intervals between dosages of interactive drugs. If there is any question about pregnancy or breastfeeding, administration of a drug should be suspended and the prescriber contacted for consultation. Allergic reactions, if anticipated, are usually grounds for a prescriber's decision to change drugs. However, a nurse is often the one who notes the offending allergenic substance via a client's history and other data. Again, effective nursing assessment can improve compliance, enhance therapeutic outcomes, and avoid negative secondary effects.

The nursing assessment culminates in the identification of nursing diagnoses (actual, possible, or risk for) and collaborative problems as potential complications. Although there is the possibility of any number of issues within nursing pharmacotherapeutics, there are eight that must be considered with every medication to be administered:

1. Client issues related to the client's preexisting medical conditions, age, and childbearing status.
2. Client issues related to concurrent drug therapy.
3. Client issues related to the physiologic complication of the client's underlying condition related to the ineffectiveness of the drug.
4. Client issues related to the physiologic complication related to the side effects/adverse reactions of the administered drug.
5. Risk for poisoning: drug toxicity.
6. Knowledge deficit related to initiation of or change in the medication regimen.
7. Noncompliance (specify).
8. Ineffective management of the therapeutic regimen.

Interventions by the nurse to address identified problems may involve collaborative interventions with physicians and other health care providers or interventions that are solely the domain of nurses. Problems falling within the independent nursing domain are best described by the nursing diagnosis, which is a concise statement of a problem that is uniquely addressed by nurses. The potential complications of the pharmacotherapeutic regimen are seen as collaborative problems.

After the identification of problems and the formulation of nursing diagnoses and collaborative problems, goals in the form of outcome criteria are established. A specific plan is developed to direct nursing care toward meeting the goals. The development of goals and clear planning form the basis for implementing and evaluating nursing care.

Critical Thinking

1. If a history of a client's medications and medication-taking behaviors were not taken or were inadequate, what might be the possible consequences to the client?
2. What nursing actions could be taken to minimize the different types of drug interactions discussed in the text?
3. Using information from the drug history of a client, discuss the potential for each of the eight problems within the nursing diagnoses that could be applied to the medications that might be prescribed for that client.

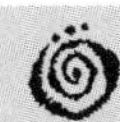

Collaborative Learning Activities

1. Each student will complete a drug history on a client, analyzing the data in relation to the client's preexisting medical condition, age and childbearing status, concurrent drug therapy, potential for physiologic complications of the client's underlying condition for which the drug is being administered, the side effects/adverse reactions of the client's drugs, and the client's risk for drug toxicity. Discuss in class.

BIBLIOGRAPHY

American Hospital Formulary Service (1996). *AHFS drug information '96*. Bethesda, MD: American Society of Hospital Pharmacists.

Anderson KN, et al. (1994). *Mosby's medical nursing, and allied health dictionary*. (4th ed.). St Louis: Mosby.

Carpenito LJ. (1995). *Nursing diagnosis: Application to clinical practice*. (6th ed.). Philadelphia: JB Lippincott Co.

Cassells JM & Redman BK (1989). Preparing students to be moral agents in clinical nursing practice, *Nurs Clin North Amer* 24(2):463-473.

Craig C (1995). Teaching food-drug interactions, *J Psychosoc Nurs* 33(2):44-46.

Hardman JG & Limbird LE (Eds.) (1996). *Goodman and Gilman's the pharmacological basis of therapeutics*. (9th ed.). New York: Macmillan.

Hussar DA (1993). Reviewing drug interactions, *Nursing* 23(9):50-57.

Jenny J (1987). Knowledge deficit: Not a nursing diagnosis, *Image* 19(4):184-185.

Kim MJ, McFarland GK, & McLane AM (1995). *Pocket guide to nursing diagnoses*. (6th ed.). St Louis: Mosby.

McCourt A & Carroll-Johnson RM (Eds.). (1992). *Classification of nursing diagnosis: Proceedings of the ninth NANDA national conference*. Philadelphia: JB Lippincott.

McPherson ML (1996). Taking an accurate medication history, *Home Health Care Prac* 5(4):35-40.

NANDA (1995). *Nursing diagnoses: Definitions and classification 1997-1998*. Philadelphia: NANDA.

United States Pharmacopeial Convention (1996). *USP DI: Drug information for the health care professional*. (16th ed.). Rockville, MD: The Convention.

Chapter 5

Implementation and Evaluation

Chapter Focus

The last two components of the nursing process—implementation and evaluation—involve the monitoring of the client's health status, nurse- or physician-prescribed interventions, and client education as well as the determination of the effectiveness of the therapeutic regimen. This chapter will focus on the nursing management of these last nursing process components as they relate to drug therapy. Consider the key terms and the following objectives for a good understanding of this chapter.

Key Terms

apothecary system (p. 76)
drug potency (p. 74)
duration of action (p. 74)
household system (p. 76)
infiltration (p. 88)
infusion (p. 88)
injection (p. 88)
latency (p. 74)
maximum effect (p. 74)
metric system (p. 75)
therapeutic index (p. 74)
Z-track method (p. 86)

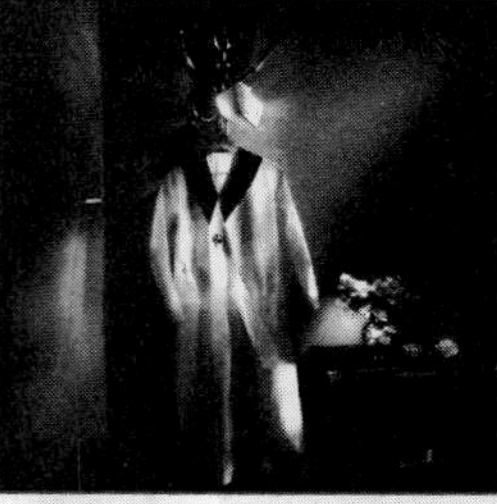

Objectives

1. Identify common pharmaceutical preparations and dosage forms.
2. Identify nursing activities related to proper drug storage and distribution.
3. Describe the factors considered in establishing the dosage, dosing intervals, and scheduling of medication.
4. Cite methods used to measure the correct dosage or rate of administration.
5. Differentiate between systemic effects and local effects of medications.
6. Cite the advantages and disadvantages of the various routes of medication administration.
7. Identify the landmarks for the administration of medications via the intramuscular route.
8. Identify specific procedures used to maintain client safety during the preparation and administration of medications.
9. Evaluate the effectiveness of a client's drug therapy.

IMPLEMENTATION

The implementation phase of the nursing process consists of putting goals into action. It is the actual giving of care as prescribed by the nursing care plan or nursing orders. The nurse, guided by the nursing care plan (formal or informal), with goals clearly in focus, can initiate proposed actions in an orderly way. The best chance for success lies in clear, frequent communication and collaboration with the client, since any goal or action not viewed by clients as congruent with their own goals will decrease participation.

The implementation phase in drug therapy comprises all the steps of the act of the administration of medications. It includes collaborating with the prescriber and medicating clients according to prescribers' orders using nursing judgment, preparing drugs (including any necessary mathematical calculations), techniques and procedures with modifications for individual clients, alertness to errors, recording medications given, and teaching clients about their drugs. Evaluation of goals follows and, depending on the specific goal, most often relates to some aspect of drug effects. For individual clients, outcomes are measured and compared with the criteria established in the goals during the planning phase. Broader evaluation is done by nursing audit committees that critique the quality of nursing care administered to groups of clients as well as individuals. To perform all the functions of the nursing process, nurses must have strong interpersonal, cognitive, and psychomotor skills. Nursing actions are the product of foundational work in the psychosocial as well as the biologic and physical sciences.

Drug Administration

The nursing function that is most closely identified with nursing by the public, and the one carrying the most legal vulnerability, is that of administering medications. It requires much preparation, a solid knowledge base, skilled decision-making abilities, and close attention to the "Five Rights" (see Chapter 4).

Pharmaceutical Preparations

Pharmaceutical preparations are the formulations that make a drug suited to various methods of administration. They may be made up by the pharmacist but more often are prepared by the pharmaceutical company from which they are purchased. The nurse who is informed about various preparations can make more astute judgments about their individual applications and appropriate recommendations to the prescriber when necessary. Box 5-1 details common preparations and their various applications.

Drug Storage

The appropriate storage of drugs on the nursing unit is a nursing responsibility, usually with the guidance and supervision of pharmacy staff.

The potency (the strength per milligram of drug) and efficacy (the maximum ability of a drug to produce a result) of drugs are affected by the way they are handled and stored. Proper storage of a drug is necessary to maintain drug stability. Most drugs can be stored on the stock supply shelves or in the medication cart, but some must be stored according to specific manufacturer's directions (on the label or package insert) to retard deterioration (e.g., live vaccines, most reconstituted drugs, and most suppositories). Many drugs change composition or potency when exposed to light, heat, moisture, or gases in the environment. The *USP* has defined the nomenclature used in instructions for prevention of changes from heat:

- Freeze: store below 0° C (32° F)
- Store in a cold place: temperature no higher than 15° C (59° F)
- Refrigerate: 2° to 15° C (36° to 59° F)
- Avoid excessive heat: temperature no higher than 40° C (104° F)
- Most drugs may be stored at room temperature, which is considered to be between 15° and 30° C (59° to 86° F).

Medication refrigerators should be used solely for the storage of drugs and related necessities and should be cleaned out regularly; expired drugs or drugs belonging to discharged clients should be returned to the pharmacy. Medications should be stored within the refrigerator, not on the door shelves or within the freezer compartment, to ensure a more constant cool temperature. At least one thermometer should be kept inside to monitor temperature maintenance.

The use of amber-colored containers protects some medications (such as furosemide [Lasix] and nitroglycerin) against deterioration by light. This fact and its significance should be pointed out to clients who are self-medicating and who might otherwise transfer medications to a different container (to take to work, on vacation, and the like). Storage in a closed cabinet or other dark place should also be advised. If it is feasible, clients should be given information about how to tell if their medication has deteriorated and they should be told that the medication may need replacement if storage requirements have not been maintained or if the medication's appearance or effects have changed.

Certain drugs given intravenously are significantly light-sensitive: amphotericin B (Fungizone), B-complex vitamins, cisplatin (Platinol), daunorubicin (Cerubidine), doxorubicin (Adriamycin), and nitroprusside (Nitropress). These should be checked for visible signs of deterioration, such as color change, precipitation, or gas formation. Deterioration may neutralize the drugs or make them toxic, and this can occur without any warning signs. Thus nitroprusside (Nitropress) and amphotericin (Fungizone) solutions for infusions should be kept covered with foil or an amber plastic bag (not a brown paper bag, which is not light-protective). Unless freshly prepared, all the other solutions should also be kept covered.

Tight lids can prevent degradation or change of the drug form or its active constituents by preventing exchange of moisture or gases within the container.

BOX 5-1

Various Forms of Drug Preparations

Preparations for oral use

Liquids

Aqueous solutions (substances dissolved in water and syrups)

Aqueous suspensions (solid particles suspended in liquid)

Emulsions (fats or oils suspended in liquid with an emulsifier

Spirits (alcohol solution)

Elixirs (aromatic, sweetened alcohol and water solution)

Tinctures (alcohol extract of plant or vegetable substance)

Fluidextracts (concentrated alcoholic liquid extract of plant or vegetables)

Extracts (syrup or dried form of pharmacologically active drug, usually prepared by evaporating solution)

Solid

Capsules (soluble case [usually gelatin] that contains liquid, dry, or beaded drug particles)

Tablets (compressed, powdered drug(s) in small disk)

Troches/lozenges (medicated tablets that dissolve slowly in mouth)

Powders/granules (loose or molded drug substance for drug administration, with or without liquids)

Preparations for parenteral use

Ampules (sealed glass container for liquid injectable medication)

Vials (glass container with rubber stopper for liquid or powdered medication)

Cartridge/Tubex (single-dose unit of parenteral medication to be used with a specific injecting device)

Intravenous infusions (suspended on hanger at bedside)

Glass bottles, flexible collapsible plastic bags, and semirigid plastic containers in sizes from 150 to 1000 ml used for continuous infusion of fluid replacement with or without medications

Intermittent intravenous infusions—usually a secondary IV setup of a small plastic or glass bottle (volume between 50 to 250 ml) to which medication is added. It runs as a "piggyback," hung separately from the primary IV infusion via a secondary administration tubing set usually for a period of 20 to 120 minutes. The primary IV solution is run during the time between medication doses.

Heparin lock or angiocath—a port site for direct administration or intermittent IV medications without the need for a primary IV solution.

Preparations for topical use

Liniments (liquid suspensions for lubrication that are applied by rubbing)

Lotions (liquid suspensions that can be protective, emollient, cooling, astringent, antipruritic, cleansing, etc.)

Ointment (semisolid medicine in a base for local protective, soothing, astringent, or transdermal application for systemic effects [such as nitoglycerin, scopolamine, estrogen])

Paste (thick ointment primarily used for skin protection)

Plasters (solid preparations that are adhesive, protective, or soothing)

Creams (emulsions that contain an aqueous and an oily base)

Aerosols (fine powders or solutions in volatile liquids that contain a propellant)

Transdermal patches (patches containing medication that is absorbed continuously through the skin and acts systemically)

Preparations for use on mucous membranes

Drops are aqueous solutions with or without gelling agent to increase retention time in the eye. Drops used for eyes, ears, or nose

Topical instillation of an aqueous solution of medications usually for topical action but occasionally used for systemic effects, including enemas, douches, mouthwashes, throat sprays, and gargles

Aerosol sprays, nebulizers, and inhalers deliver aqueous solutions of medication in droplet form to the target membrane, such as bronchial tree (e.g., bronchodilators)

Foams are powders or solutions of medication in volatile liquids with a propellant, such as vaginal foams for contraception

Suppositories usually contain medicinal substances mixed in a firm but malleable base (cocoa butter) to facilitate insertion into a body cavity (e.g., rectal or vaginal)

Miscellaneous drug delivery systems

Intradermal implants are pellets containing a small deposit of medication that are inserted in a dermal pocket. Designed to allow medication to leach slowly into tissue. Usually used to administer hormones such as testosterone or estradiol

Micropump system is a small, external pump attached by belt or implanted that delivers medication via a needle in a continuous steady dose. Insulin, anticancer chemotherapy, and opioids are examples

Membrane delivery systems are drug-laden membranes that are instilled in the eye to deliver a steady flow of medications, such as pilocarpine or corticosteroids

The expiration dates printed on drug labels mean simply that the drug contained is probably at its peak effectiveness until some point in time around that date. Because quality controls in drug production are subject to error rates similar to all other control programs, pharmaceutical companies tend to estimate these expiration dates somewhat conservatively. Thus the drug is not instantly rendered useless or harmful by that date, but the effectiveness of the therapy may be gradually diminished and the drug may produce inadequate or occasionally even toxic results some time after the printed date. The nurse should not administer doses from an outdated lot of drug or container; a fresh supply must be obtained.

Certain precepts should guide the way clients' drugs are stored, distributed, and managed. Health care agencies have developed policies that, with some variations, support these precepts as rules for client protection and prevent nurses from making errors. In addition, rational nursing judgments must enter into decision making, allowing departure from these rules as a wise and necessary choice, but this should never be undertaken lightly. It should also be a practice to consult other expert personnel or authorities.

The following guidelines are not necessarily listed in order of importance.

1. All medicines should be kept in a special place, which may be a cart or room. The area should not be freely accessible to the public.
2. Narcotic drugs and those dispensed under special legal regulations must be kept in a locked box or compartment (many states require double locks) and accounted for at the end of each shift. Any dose that is wasted or discarded must be attested to by another nurse by initialing of such a notation.
3. Each client's medicines are kept in a designated place on a shelf or compartment of the medicine room or in a drawer of the medication cart. Such an arrangement means that the nurse must be careful to keep the client's medicines in the right area and to make certain that when the client leaves the hospital the medicines are returned to the pharmacy.
4. If stock supplies are maintained, they should be arranged in an orderly manner. Preparations for internal use should be kept separate from those used externally.
5. Some preparations, such as serums, vaccines, certain suppositories, certain antibiotics, and insulin, may need to be refrigerated.
6. Labels of all medicines should be clean and legible. If they are not, they should be sent to the pharmacist for relabeling. *Nurses should not label or relabel medicines.*
7. Bottles of medicines should always be stoppered and protected from light, heat, and high humidity as necessary.

Many intravenous drugs require a diluent to dissolve the medication, which then can be added to a larger-volume solution for administration. The storage times for such medications can vary, depending on the following:

1. The expiration date on the package for the fresh package of medication stored under the specific instructions of the manufacturer
2. The expiration time period allotted for the dissolved medication
3. The expiration time period allotted for the dissolved medication added to a larger volume of solution

To obtain accurate information for an individual drug, refer to the drug's package insert or the *USP DI.* Table 5-1 illustrates differing storage requirements and expiration times within the same drug classification (cephalosporin antibiotics).

Preparation of the Dosage

Technically, written medical orders are the only legal means for the administration of medications by nurses. Written orders constitute permanent legal records of the prescriber's plans and can be submitted as evidence in case of litigation. Thus nurses must routinely ensure that (1) each order is appropriate, accurate, and complete and (2) the order is followed unerringly to completion or that the prescriber is consulted as to why it was not completed, because nurses are held legally accountable for every dose of medication they

TABLE 5-1 Storage requirements of selected intravenous drugs

	Stability after reconstitution at		
Drug	Room temperature*	Refrigeration	If frozen
cefamandole (Mandol)	24 hr	96 hr	6 mo
cefazolin sodium (Ancef, Kefzol)	24 hr	10 days	12 wk
cefoperazone sodium (Cefobid)	24 hr	5 days	3-5 wk, depending on concentration and parenteral solution used
sterile cefoxitin sodium (Mefoxin)	24 hr	10 days	At least 13 wk, depending on method of preparation
cephalothin sodium (Keflin, Ceporacin)	12 hr	96 hr	12 wk

Data from *USP DI,* Volume I, 1997.
*Recommended temperatures: room temperature: 25° C (77° F); refrigeration temperature 5° C (41° F); frozen: −20° C (−4° F).

administer. Free flow of communication between prescriber and nurse is crucial to fulfillment of this responsibility. Nurses must be ready to consult with the prescriber as necessary to clarify, understand, or suggest medication therapy as needed. Assertiveness is a quality that must be developed by professional nurses if they are to deal from an appropriate position of strength within the health care system to promote their clients' best interests while achieving equity for their own contributions.

What is the process by which a prescriber's order is translated into the administration of a medication? It is first transcribed by a unit secretary, nurse manager (or nursing care coordinator), or primary nurse from an order sheet onto the Kardex, medication administration record (MAR) (Figure 5-1), or the whole process may be computerized. In many health agencies the physician places the medication order into a computer that requisitions the drug from the pharmacy, and the order is automatically transcribed directly onto a computerized MAR from which the nurse prepares the medication. Accuracy in transcription of the medication order to the medication administration record is essential. If a handwritten order has been processed by a unit secretary, it should be verified by a nurse, who can then better relate the medication to the client and the diagnosis. The nurse must check the dosage of the medication and the age of the client, check for drug interaction possibilities and for allergies, and ensure the completeness and clarity of the order to prevent error (Box 5-2). Whatever the question concerning the prescriber's order, legally it can only be clarified with the prescriber who has written the order. Verifying an order with physician or nursing colleague who happens to be present does not suffice.

BOX 5-2

Checking Transcription

Which medication?

Is it quinine sulfate (a medication for leg cramps) or quinidine sulfate (a cardiac depressant)? Pentobarbital or phenobarbital? Digoxin or digitoxin? Ornade or Orinase? Decadron or Doriden?

Which dose?

Is it a loop of an *f*, *g*, or *q*, or another zero?

Vital signs q 4 h
Gentamycin 600 mg IV 6 h

Anything missing?

Does Halcion i HS mean 0.125 mg or 0.25 mg?

The drug is supplied by the institution's pharmacy department. When the supply arrives, it is appropriately stored in an individual client's own medication box or the drawer of a medication cart. The nurse then may administer the medication per schedule. Because of space limitation, physicians, pharmacists, and nurses rely on pharmacologic abbreviations or symbols for communication. These are often from the Latin and are universally used. Table 5-2 includes the most commonly used abbreviations, along with some symbols common to clinical practice. Although apothecary symbols are sometimes used, they are frequently misinterpreted and may be used incorrectly. The nurse should convert the apothecary measure to a metric measure when transcribing the medication order. In addition, prescribers should be encouraged to use the metric system to avoid errors. Abbreviations are a key to communication in the busy health field and should be learned. In addition, a number of prescribers also use abbreviations for ordering specific medications (Table 5-3). Because of the danger of misinterpretation, variant or nonstandard abbreviations should not be used. The nurse should review the approved abbreviation listing for the specific health agency.

When transcribed, the prescriber's order must contain all the elements described in Chapter 4. It must contain the *full name* of the client (and bed location—e.g., Room 212, Bed A); the *date* the order was written; the *medication name, dosage, route,* and *frequency*; and, according to agency policy, the *name* or *initials* of the nurse responsible for the transcription or computer entry.

Types of Drug Delivery Systems

There are several approaches to distributing and dispensing drugs to clients in an institutional setting: the floor stock system, individual client prescription orders, unit dose drug distribution, and a combination of these. In the floor stock system, all medications except those infrequently used are stored in bulk on the nursing unit in the medication room. The use of this system is rare because of the increased potential for medication errors caused by the large array of stock medications to choose from, the financial loss caused by misplaced or forgotten charges and expired drugs to be returned, the need for frequent total drug inventorying, and the storage problems inherent in crowded medication rooms. Thus this system is more costly and less safe for the client. The national norm is unit dose dispensing of the majority if not all of the prescribed medications.

Single-dose packages of drugs are dispensed in the unit dose drug distribution method. Each oral dose, for example, may be a tablet encased in a blister pack or a paper tear-off strip of tablets. This packaging is said to be the safest and most economical method of drug distribution. However, drug wastage with unit dose distribution systems occurs in many instances in long-term care settings where the drugs are issued in 30-day blister packages that have to be discarded when the drug is discontinued for the client, even if only a few of the total doses have been administered. The regulations governing this practice are being reviewed in many states.

Lorenzo, Joseph
M144444 8/15/55
Dr. Powell

MEDICATION RECORD

INIT	DO / SD	RD / NSD	MEDICATION DOSE, ROUTE, FREQUENCY	TOUR	TIME INTERVAL	DATE 3/10	DATE 3/11	DATE 3/12	DATE 3/13	DATE 3/14	DATE 3/15	DATE 3/16
L	3/9		Erythomycin	N	12 - 6	12 6	12 6		D/C	X	X	X
M			enteric coated	D	12	12	12					
M	3/13		250 mg q6hr. p.o.	E	6	6						
				N								
				D								
				E								
				N								
				D								
				E								
				N								
				D								
				E								
				N								
				D								
				E								
				N								
				D								
				E								
				N								
				D								
				E								
				N								
				D								
				E								
				N								
				D								
				E								
				N								
				D								
				E								

RECOPIED BY: DATE:

	—Medication given
O	—Medication Omitted— Explanation on Nurses' Notes.
D/C	—Medication Discontinued. In addition to this record, anticoagulant and Diabetic records are also maintained
D.O.	—Date ordered
S.D.	—Stop date
N.S.D.	—New stop date

ALLERGIES:

Penicillin

SIGNATURES	J. Jones R.N.	M. Whitehead RN	T. Ivey R.N	J. Jones RN	M. Whitehead RN																
	N	D	E	N	D	E	N	D	E	N	D	E	N	D	E	N	D	E	N	D	E

Figure 5-1 Sample medication administration record (MAR). In many health care agencies, this form has been computerized.

TABLE 5-2 Common abbreviations and symbols related to medication administration*

Abbreviation	Unabbreviated form	Meaning
ac	ante cibum	before meals
ad lib	ad libitum	freely
AM	ante meridiem	morning
bid	bis in die	twice each day
c̄	cum	with
caps	capsule	capsule
cc, cm^3	cubic centimeter	cubic centimeter (ml)
clt	client	client
D/C or DC	discontinue	terminate
elix	elixir	elixir
g, gm	gram	1000 milligrams
gr	grain	60 milligrams
gtt	gutta	drop
h, hr	hora	hour
hs	hora somni	at bedtime
IM	intramuscular	into a muscle
IV	intravenous	into a vein
IVPB	IV piggyback	secondary IV line
kg	kilogram	2.2 lb
KVO	keep vein open	very slow infusion rate
Ⓛ	left	left
L	liter	liter
µg, mcg	microgram	one millionth of a gram
mg	milligram	one thousandth of a gram
mEq	milliequivalent	the number of grams of solute dissolved in one milliliter of a *normal* solution
min or m	minim	minim (1/15 or 1/16 ml)
ml, mL	milliliter	one thousandth of a liter
ng	nanogram	one billionth of a gram
ō	no or none	no or none
OD	oculus dexter	right eye
OS	oculus sinister	left eye
os	os	mouth
OTC	over-the-counter	nonprescription drug
OU	oculus uterque	each eye
pc	post cibum	after meals
PM	post meridiem	after noon
PO	per os	by mouth, orally
prn	pro re nata	according to necessity
pt	patient	patient
q	quaque	every
qd	quaque die	every day
qh	quaque hora	every hour
q4h, q4°	every 4 hours	every 4 hours around the clock
qid	quater in die	four times each day
qod	quaque aliem die	every other day
qs	quantum satis	sufficient quantity
®	right	right
℞	receipt	take
s̄	sine	without
SL	sub linguam	under the tongue
SOS	si opus sit	if necessary, one dose only
ss	semis	a half
stat	statim	at once
SC, SQ	subcutaneous	into subcutaneous tissue
tbsp	tablespoon	tablespoon (15 ml)
tid	ter in die	three times a day
TO	telephone order	order received over the telephone
tsp	teaspoon	teaspoon (4 or 5 ml)
U	unit	a dosage measure for insulin, penicillin, heparin
VO	verbal order	order received verbally
i, ii	one, two	one, two (as in "gr i," "gr ii,")
ʒ	dram	4 or 5 ml
℥	ounce or fluid-ounce	ounce (30 milliliters)
×	times	as in two times a week
>	greater than	greater than
<	less than	less than
=	equal to	equal to
↑, ↗	increase or increasing	increase or increasing
↓, ↙	decrease or decreasing	decrease or decreasing

*It is recommended that certain abbreviations be abandoned if they are found to be confusing.

TABLE 5-3 Drug abbreviations

Abbreviation	Definition
ACTH	adrenocorticotropic hormone
ASA	acetylsalicylic acid (aspirin)
DES	diethylstilbestrol
DM	dextromethorphan
D_5W	5% dextrose in water
D_5S	5% dextrose in normal saline
DSS or DOSS	dioctyl sodium sulfosuccinate
DW	distilled water
EC	enteric coated
ETH & C	elixer terpin hydrate with codeine
Fe	iron
5-FU	5-fluorouracil
FUD	floxuridine
HC	hydrocortisone
HCTZ	hydrochlorothiazide
INH	isoniazid
K	potassium
KCl	potassium chloride
LOC	laxative of choice
MOM	milk of magnesia
6-MP	6-mercaptopurine
MS	morphine sulfate
Na	sodium
NS	normal saline
NSAID	nonsteroidal antiinflammatory drug
NTG	nitroglycerin
PAS	para-aminosalicyclic acid
PB	phenobarbital
PCN	penicillin

However, the advantages of using the unit dose system far outweigh the disadvantages. The most important advantages are increased medication safety and decreased errors, since drug computations are largely eliminated. The drug is already properly labeled and does not have to be prepared. All the nurse needs to do is deliver the package to the client; it is opened at the bedside and administered. This may permit clients to check on their own drugs and be assured of proper medication and dosage. Unit dose packaging also decreases chances of deterioration and, in most instances, clients can be given financial credit for drugs that are not used. Disadvantages include increased cost to set up the system and the need for additional pharmacy personnel to fill new orders and resupply the client's units each 24 hours. The administration of new and stat medication orders may be delayed while the medication order is sent to the pharmacy, filled, and then delivered back to the nurse rather than being immediately available on the unit. But the safety features of the unit dose system far outweigh any temporary inconvenience it may cause.

Strip packages make narcotic counting more convenient for nurses, since all packages in the strip are numbered. This also prevents contamination caused by pouring narcotic tablets into the hands for counting, which is a grossly improper technique. Prefilled unit dose disposable syringes are also available.

Unit dose dispensing systems in hospitals may be centralized, decentralized, or a combination of both. In the centralized system the pharmacist and the pharmacy are located in a central area from which drugs are distributed to client care areas. In the decentralized system, clinical pharmacists and satellite pharmacies are located in client care areas and drugs are prepared and distributed to clients from those particular areas. In the combined system, medications are prepared in a central area, with clinical pharmacists assigned to various client care areas to oversee drug therapy, thus providing safer and more controlled drug ordering and drug distribution.

Role of the Clinical Pharmacist

A present trend in drug delivery is toward more extensive use of clinical pharmacists stationed in nursing areas to work closely with physicians, nurses, therapists, and dietitians. Because pharmacists are educated in the compounding, dispensing, and control of drugs, they can be an invaluable resource for assistance in solving pharmacologic problems. Nurses frequently consult them about medication administration methods, dosages, drug identification, and secondary effects. Clinical pharmacists are consulted by health care personnel from all disciplines with questions relating to drug therapy. The health care system today demands more of this kind of interdisciplinary collaboration and shared expertise for the benefit of all, especially the client.

Hospital pharmacies can have special "clean rooms" and specially filtered air for compounding various parenteral solutions. A pharmacist or supervised designee may be responsible for putting all additives into intravenous solutions and checking all such solutions for compatibility reactions.

Role of the Nurse

Regardless of any changes in ordering, distributing, or administering drugs, nurses are responsible for their clients' care 24 hours a day. Advanced technology and the release of more potent drugs on the market make it crucial for the nurse to be better informed on drugs and their actions. Nurses must observe clients and their response to drug therapy, determine whether prn orders are to be given, and consult with prescribers about withholding, discontinuing, or changing drugs. They continue to take histories, to teach clients about medications and their effects, to work collaboratively with pharmacists, and to work with clients to plan the management of their drug therapy after returning home.

Preparing to Administer Drugs

Doses, Dosing Intervals, and Scheduling

Understanding the rationale for selection of a particular dose and frequency of administration requires a basic understanding of the drug in question. Within limits, increasing a drug's dose or frequency of administration increases its pharmacologic effect but can also increase the risk of side and adverse effects. The various relationships involved can be represented as follows:

Optimal dosages → Dose-response relationship

Optimal frequencies → Time-response relationship

The variables to deal with in *dose-response* relationships are defined as follows:

- **Drug potency**: absolute amount of drug required to produce a desired effect
- **Therapeutic index**: relative margin of safety; the ratio of lethal dose to effective dose
- **Maximum effect**: greatest response possible regardless of dose given

Time-response relationships deal with these variables:

- **Latency**: time necessary for therapeutic effect
- **Time for maximum effect**: time after administration for the drug's effect to peak
- **Duration of action**: length of time of a drug effect

These last variables are affected by route used, pharmacokinetics involved, and individual client biorhythms.

To avoid wide fluctuations in the serum concentration of a drug, doses are given at appropriate intervals to avoid drug accumulation and toxicity. If the dosage interval is too short, drug accumulation with potential for toxicity will occur. If it is too long, serum concentration will drop because the drug will continue to be excreted and not replaced. Drugs with very short half-lives will not accumulate but they need to be given frequently to achieve a steady state (see Chapter 3 for a discussion of drug half-life). Drugs with very long half-lives are often given once a day. These dosing relationships are interpreted on the basis of a normal curve in drug studies. Dosages and dosing intervals are derived for treating the ideal "average" person in a population. Although dosing intervals have been studied statistically, drug therapy regimens must continually be reassessed for individual needs. Some people will always fall outside the "average" range in responding to a drug. In addition, dosing intervals may be modified in consideration of client convenience and their effect on the client's management of the therapeutic regimen.

Times to administer routine medications may be determined by agency policy. For example, qid drugs may routinely be given at 10 AM, 2 PM, 6 PM, and 10 PM, or at 9 AM, 1 PM, 5 PM, and 9 PM, and so forth. Special units, such as pediatrics, have other medication hours to coincide with the special needs of their clients. Based on the drug's pharmacokinetics, client convenience, and the need to avoid mealtimes or other activities that might interfere with drug administration, nurses may choose autonomously to vary the times (but not the intervals) if the decision is based on solid rationale (Box 5-3). For example, calcium supplements might be given at bedtime rather than 9 AM on a daily schedule because calcium is better absorbed at night. Drugs administered once daily can usually be given according to a flexible schedule, perhaps just before or after a treatment that would interfere with a dosing time, such as a client's trip off the nursing unit to the physical therapy department or the radiology department. Drugs should be administered as close to the time indicated as possible, but obviously a nurse cannot medicate each of a group of assigned clients at exactly the same time. Agency policies may vary, but usually they stipulate administration within ½ hour before or after the indicated time. Exempt from this flexibility are stat or one-time-only drug orders, such as those given before diagnostic procedures or surgery, and those medications administered at the more frequent intervals, such as q2h or q4h.

BOX 5-3

Examples of Clinical Implications of Drug Dosing

Blood levels of steroids administered between 7:30 AM and 8:30 AM may most closely match levels as they would occur normally. Permanent night shift workers would be exceptions.

Antibiotics should be administered around the clock to achieve a steady state in the bloodstream.

Anticoagulant dosages should be titrated with tests of the client's own partial thromboplastin time or a similar determination.

Diuretics should not be administered late in the day or before appointments, when urinary urgency would be inconvenient for the client.

Drug effects are monitored by the prescriber and the nurse according to either *direct assessment* (subjective, by observation for clinical responses) or *indirect assessment* (objective, by laboratory values or serum concentrations of the drug). Because of their unique presence and expertise, nurses are most capable of assisting the prescriber in making keen assessments of clients' responses.

Dosage Measurement

If the drug is formulated in units that are multiples of the dosage ordered, whether tablet or liquid, the computation to determine the correct dose is simple. If, however, the drug does not come in units that are multiples of the dose prescribed, if the drug must be dissolved in water, or if the order is written in the apothecary system and the drug is available only in metric units, dosage calculations will be necessary.

Flow rate calculations are necessary for certain therapies in order to set the proper amount for the desired dose effect. Intravenous infusions necessitate careful flow rate calculation. These therapies should be ordered by the prescriber in definitive amounts and rates. Intravenous fluids can be adjusted to deliver the number of drops per minute that will provide the prescribed total amount over the prescribed time. Given the total volume of solution to be infused, the total number of minutes the solution is to be infused, and the drop factor (number of drops per milliliter that the tubing set-up delivers—a number that varies among tubing manufacturers and is found on the back of the tubing box), the prescribed drops per minute can be calculated and the set regulated by counting drops in the drip chamber of the tubing. A simple formula for IV flow rate calculation can be found in Exercise 9 later in this chapter. Details of regulating by manual clamps, the most common mode, may be found in a basic nursing text such as Potter and Perry (1996) (see Bibliography.) Infusion controllers and pumps will be discussed later in this chapter.

Most dosage calculations, however, deal with computing numbers of tablets to give or with changing from one unit of measurement to another. A dosage problem may be as simple as giving 400 mg of ibuprofen (Motrin) from a container of 200 mg tablets. It is almost as easy to figure out how many milliliters of morphine sulfate one must give if the container is labeled "15 mg = 1 ml" and the order reads "10 mg morphine sulfate SC." Calculating dosage becomes more complex when the units of measurement in the medication order must be converted to a different type of unit in which the drug is available.

Currently three systems of measurement are in use for administering medications: the metric system (the most widely adopted and the most convenient), the apothecary system (which has nearly been phased out), and the household system (the least accurate and not widely used except in the home setting).

Metric system. The **metric system** of weights and measures was invented by the French at the end of the eighteenth century, and toward the end of the nineteenth century the Bureau of Weights and Measures was formed and given the challenge to develop metric standards for international use. The United States joined the worldwide trend toward adoption of the metric system with the enactment of the Metric Conversion Act of 1975. The basic metric units of measurement are the meter, the liter, and the gram. The *meter* is the unit for linear measurement, the *liter* for capacity or volume, and the *gram* for weight. A meter is a little longer than a yard; a liter is a little more than a quart; and a gram is a little more than the weight of a steel paper clip.

The metric system is a decimal system; the basic units can be divided or multiplied by 10, 100, or 1000 parts to form secondary units that differ from each other by 10 or some multiple of 10. The names of the secondary units are formed by joining Greek or Latin prefixes to the names of the primary units (Table 5-4). Subdivisions of the basic units are made by moving the decimal point to the left, and multiples of the basic units are indicated by moving the decimal point to the right.

The meter is the unit from which the other metric units are derived. Centimeters and millimeters are the chief linear measures used in health-related work. Measurement of the size of body organs is made in centimeters and millimeters, and the sphygmomanometer used to measure blood pressure is calibrated in millimeters of mercury. There are approximately 2.5 cm (25 mm) in 1 inch.

The liter is the unit of capacity or volume and is equal to approximately 1000 cc or 1000 ml. Fractional parts of a liter are usually expressed in milliliters or cubic centimeters. For example, 0.6 liter would be expressed as 600 ml or 600 cc. Multiples of a liter are similarly expressed; 2.4 liters would be 2400 ml or cc. The abbreviation cc is in the process of being dropped and is considered obsolete; either ml or mL may be used, according to the National Bureau of Standards.

TABLE 5-4 Metric prefixes, meanings, and relationships

Prefix	Meaning
Giga	Billions
Kilo*	Thousands
Hecto	Hundreds
Deka	Tens
Base units of water, liter, gram	One unit
Deci	Tenths
Centi*	Hundredths
Milli*	Thousandths
Micro*	Millionths
Nano*	Billionths

*Prefixes most commonly encountered in nursing.

The gram is the metric unit of weight that is used in weighing drugs and various pharmaceutical preparations. The approved abbreviation for gram is g; G as the abbreviation for gram is no longer approved because it conflicts with the abbreviation for the prefix giga. Gm is also not approved by the National Bureau of Standards.

As a review of Table 5-4 indicates, a decigram is 10 times greater than a centigram and 100 times greater than a milligram. To change decigrams to centigrams, one multiplies by 10; to change decigrams to milligrams, one multiplies by 100. To change milligrams to centigrams, one divides by 10; to change milligrams to decigrams, one divides by 100; to change milligrams to grams, one divides by 1000; and so forth.

The style of notation proposed as the International System of Units from the National Bureau of Standards is recommended except when it conflicts with proper English language norms:

- Units are not capitalized (gram, not Gram).
- No period should be used with abbreviations of units (ml, not m.l. or ml.).
- A single space should be left between the quantity and the symbol (24 kg, not 24kg).
- Except in the apothecary system, only decimal notation should be used, not fractions (0.25 kg, not ¼ kg).
- Numerical quantities less than 1 should have a zero placed to the left of the decimal point (0.75 mg, not .75 mg).
- Abbreviations should not be pluralized (kg, not kgs).

Nurses need the foregoing as part of their knowledge base not only to use in preparing medications but also to interpret laboratory data (some are reported in milliliters, others in deciliters or nanograms, and so forth), to weigh clients (kilograms instead of pounds), and to figure flow rates of IV infusions. (Refer to the table of abbreviations and symbols, Table 5-2, as necessary.)

Until the metric system is fully accepted in clinical practice, nurses may need to deal with all three systems of measurement: metric, apothecary, and household (Table 5-5). The nurse can memorize a few crucial relationships. These data can then be readily inserted where applicable as part of a formula or as half of a ratio-and-proportion equation often used for dosage calculation. A suggested practical list of equivalents that nurses should know is presented in Table 5-5.

Apothecary system. Only a few medications are now available in units of the **apothecary system.** It is less convenient and less precise than the metric system. In a recent poll most nurses responding said they rarely (42%) or never (19%) see a drug ordered in the apothecary system (Cohen, 1993). However, unfamiliarity with the apothecary system may lead to dosage errors. The basic unit of weight is the *grain,* which is derived from the age-old standard of weight of a single grain of wheat, a weight now variously accepted as approximately equivalent to 60 or 65 mg (60 mg is the more widely accepted of the two). Other units of weight commonly used in the apothecary system are the fluidram, the fluidounce, and the pound.

The basic unit of fluid volume is the *minim,* approximately equal to the volume of water that would weigh a grain, a very small amount, about 0.05 or 0.06 ml. Other volume measures, which may also be considered household measures, are the pint and the quart.

In written prescriptions the placement of abbreviations and the type of numerals used in the apothecary system follow a more complex arrangement than in the metric system. In the apothecary system the abbreviation is placed before the numeral. Whole numerical quantities usually are expressed in Roman numerals (e.g., gr X for 10 grains). Fractional quantities are usually expressed by Arabic numerals rather than by decimals (e.g., gr ¼, not gr 0.25, for one-quarter grain).

Household systems. Measures of the **household system** include the glass, cup, tablespoon, teaspoon, and drops; pints and quarts are often included in this system as well as in the apothecary system. Shortened hospital stays and correspondingly lengthened convalescence at home and the increasing geriatric population have expanded the numbers of people receiving their care at home. Because standardized measurements of household equipment usually do not exist in the home, the community health nurse may not have access to accurately calibrated measuring devices in the home. For example, the average teacup or coffee cup can hold from 5 to 9 ounces or more, not the accepted 8 ounces or half pint. The average household teaspoon can hold 4 to 5 ml or more of liquid medication rather than the standard 5 ml. A drop and a minim *cannot* be considered equivalents, since drop size will vary with the viscosity of the medication even when measured by an approved dropper. Therefore any listing of household measurements on a table of equivalent measures must be considered only an approximation.

Depending on the situation (e.g., medicating infants) and the need for precise dosage, such measures may or may not be adequate. Clients may need to obtain precise measuring instruments from the local pharmacy or the visiting nurse for medication administration at home.

Dosage Calculation

Challenges to the mathematical skills of nurses occur infrequently in the administration of medications. An equation can be set up to apply what the nurse has learned about a few

TABLE 5-5 Common approximate equivalents of weights and measures

Metric	Apothecary	Household
Weight		
1 kg*	2.2 pounds	
1000 mg = 1 gram*	gr xv	
60 mg* (occasionally seen as 65 mg)	gr i̇	
30 mg	gr ss (one half)	
1 μg (mcg) = 0.001 mg		
Volume		
	4 quarts	1 gallon
1000 ml* = approx 1 liter = 1000 cc	Approx 1 qt	1 quart
500 ml	Approx 1 pint (½ qt)	16 ounces
240 or 250 ml	℥ viii (8 fluidounces)† = approx ½ pint	1 cup or 1 glass
30 ml* = approx 30 cc	℥ i̇ (1 fluidounce)	2 tbsp
Approx 16 ml = approx 16 cc	ʒ iv (4 fluidrams)	1 tbsp
Approx 8 ml	ʒ i̇i̇ (2 fluidrams)	2 tsp
4 to 5 ml	ʒ i̇ (1 fluidram)	1 tsp
1 ml* = approx 1 cc	Minims xv or xvi	Minims cannot be compared with drops

*These equivalents may be committed to memory for ready application to dosage problems.
†Note the small difference in the symbols for fluidounce and fluidram.

crucial equivalents and how that relates to what needs to be solved—all in a logical sequence or relationship. Calculators may not be appropriate in the nursing unit for they tend to have exasperating battery failures or to "disappear" from busy hospital units and nursing homes. It is more reliable to develop and maintain a basic competence in mathematical calculations. Following are some typical exercises to do, accompanied by explanations and answers. These exercises assume a working knowledge of decimals, fractions, and a ratio-and-proportion approach to problem solving. Again, if you are used to working with another method that works as well, use it instead—just check your answers and rationale with the following.

Exercises

1. If a drug is ordered in units different from the units on hand, the order must be mathematically translated into the units available. Thus if the medication order is written in terms of milligrams and the client's drug is supplied in grams, you must translate the needed dose into grams.
Question: A drug is ordered to be given in the amount of 1500 mg. How many grams would you give?
Answer: Knowing that there are 1000 mg in a gram, set up the ratio in logical sequence. The logic of the relationships ("this is to this as that is to that") remains constant in a ratio-and-proportion approach, but which of the relationships is set down first in the equation does not matter. Some people set down first, on the left side of the equation, the relationship between what has been ordered or what information is wanted in the problem and the unknown quantity, or x. Then on the right side of the equation they set down the known equivalents, the conversion factors, or the "givens." Once set up, the equation is solved by multiplying the means (middle adjacent numbers) by the extremes (numbers on each end):

$$1500\text{ mg}: x = 1000\text{ mg}: 1\text{ g}$$
$$1000\,x = 1500$$
$$x = 1.5\text{ g}$$

Or an alternate arrangement is

$$\frac{1500\text{ mg}}{x} = \frac{1000\text{ mg}}{1\text{g}}$$

Then cross multiply so that

$$1000\,x = 1500 \times 1$$
$$1000\,x = 1500$$
$$x = \frac{1500}{1000}$$
$$x = 1.5\text{ g}$$

Question: A dosage of 30 ml of cough syrup is ordered to be given qid. The label on the bottle of medication states that it contains a total of 240 ml. How many doses of medication are available?
Answer: 30 ml: 1 dose:: 240 ml: x doses

$$\frac{240}{30} = 8\text{ doses or a 2-day supply}$$

Question: 10 mEq of potassium chloride (KCl) is to be added to an IV infusion solution. KCl is available for this application in vials of 40 mEq/20 ml. How many milliliters would you give?
Answer: Again set up the equation in logical sequence, possibly starting with the desired ingredient and the unknown quantity.

$$10\text{ mEq}:x = 40\text{ mEq}:20\text{ml}$$
$$40x = 200$$
$$x = \frac{200}{40} = 5\text{ ml}$$

2. Sometimes medication for injection comes in powdered or concentrated liquid form and must be dissolved (reconstituted) or diluted before it can be injected. Most often directions as to how much diluent (dissolving or diluting solution) and what kind should be added by needle and syringe are on the label of the container of the drug. All that the nurse needs to know to determine the amount to give is on the label.
Question: A certain antibiotic has been ordered "750 mg IV." The drug comes in a 10-g multiple-dose vial (there is more than enough of the drug in the vial for one dose) in powdered form. The label reads, "Add 7.2 ml sterile water or sodium chloride solution for injection to yield 10 ml of reconstituted drug." After the diluent has been added, how many milliliters would you give?
Answer: 10 ml now contains 10 g; thus 1 ml equals 1 g. You should already know or be able to refer to a listing of standard equivalents to find out that 1 g equals 1000 mg. You may then start the equation by setting down the relationship between what you want to give and the volume that contains it. Then follow the same sequence of relationship on the other side of the equation, which indicates what is available in which volume.

$$750\text{ mg}:x = 1000\text{ mg}:1\text{ ml}$$
$$1000x = 750$$
$$x = \frac{750}{1000} = 0.75\text{ ml}$$

Whenever a drug appears in concentrated form (powder or liquid), after the appropriate diluent has been added and well dispersed or dissolved the same mathematical approach can be used no matter what the volume of the finished solution. NB: Do not fall into the trap of including the amount of ***diluent*** anywhere in your equation.

3. *Question:* The quantity of a certain medication is ordered as "gr XV," and the tablets on hand are in gr V dosage. How many tablets should be given?
Answer:

$$\text{gr }15:x = \text{gr }5:1\text{ tablet}$$
$$5x = 15$$
$$x = \frac{15}{5} = 3\text{ tablets}$$

4. *Question:* A client's medication has been ordered based on body weight. If the client weighs 150 pounds, how many kilograms is that?
Answer: You need to know that 1 kg is equal to 2.2 pounds.

$$150\text{ lb}:x = 2.2\text{ lb}:1\text{ kg}$$
$$2.2x = 150$$
$$x = \frac{150}{2.2} = 68.2\text{ kg}$$

5. *Question:* Atropine sulfate gr $^1/_{150}$ is ordered. How many tablets would you give if the available supply is in tablets of 0.2 mg?
Answer: First you need to known that 1 grain is equivalent to 60 mg; then you can find how many milligrams are equivalent to gr $^1/_{150}$. Second, you need to find out how many tablets will provide the milligram equivalent of gr $^1/_{150}$.

$$\text{gr }^1/_{150}:x(\text{mg}) = \text{gr }1:60\text{mg}$$
$$x = 60(^1/_{150})$$
$$x = \frac{60}{150} = 0.4\text{ mg}$$

The second step may certainly be done without pencil and paper, but it is more likely to be accurate if not calculated in the head.

$$0.4 \text{ mg}:x = 0.2 \text{ mg}:1$$
$$0.2x = 0.4$$
$$x = \frac{0.4}{0.2} = 2 \text{ tablets}$$

6. *Question:* You may also be confronted with the reverse of the preceding question. How many grains would you give if 0.6 mg scopolamine has been ordered?
Answer:

$$0.6 \text{ mg}:x \text{ (gr)} = 60 \text{ mg}:\text{gr } 1$$
$$60x = \frac{0.6}{60}$$
$$x = \text{gr } 0.01 = \text{gr } {}^{1}\!/_{100}$$

7. *Question:* Codeine gr ss is ordered; how many milligrams would you give?
Answer: You need to know that the symbol "ss" indicates the quantity one half.

$$\text{gr } 1/2:x \text{ (mg)} = \text{gr } 1:60 \text{ mg}$$
$$x = 60\ ({}^{1}\!/_{2})$$
$$x = {}^{60}\!/_{2} = 30 \text{ mg}$$

8. *Question:* The client is to take 6 ounces of magnesium sulfate solution, and the calibrations on the available measuring device are in milliliters. How many milliliters would you give?
Answer: You need to know that 1 ounce is equivalent to 30 ml.

$$6 \text{ oz}:x \text{ (ml)} = 1 \text{ oz}:30 \text{ ml}$$
$$x = 60 \times 30$$
$$x = 180 \text{ ml}$$

9. Although some practitioners may not technically consider IV infusions to be medications, we will practice figuring IV infusion rates here.

The amount of IV solution to be infused during a given length of time is the IV flow rate. It is dictated by the prescriber's order, which should give the total amount of fluid and the number of milliliters that should be infused over each 1-hour period or less, *or* the number of drops per minute that should be infused. However, some prescribers write IV orders that give only the total volume of solution to be infused (e.g., 1000 ml) over a longer period (e.g., 8 hours).

If the order does not specify the rate of flow in drops per minute, the following formula may be used to figure this out:

$$\frac{\text{Total number of milliliters to be infused}}{\text{Total number of minutes infusion is to run}} \times \text{Drop factor}$$
$$= \text{Rate in drops per minute}$$

Question: If an order is given for 1000 ml D_5W to run for 8 hours and the drop factor is 10 drops per milliliter for the particular tubing used (other types deliver 15 drops or 60 drops—often used to infuse children), how fast should the IV infusion be set to run?
Answer:

$$\frac{1000 \text{ ml}}{480 \text{ min}} \times 10 = \frac{100}{48} \times 10$$
$$= 20.8 \text{ drops (gtt)/min}$$
$$= 21 \text{ gtt/min}$$

A bit more challenging are some of the calculations involved with IV rates for infusion pumps. These pumps are often used for giving drugs whose dosages must be calculated more closely.
Question: Dopamine 400 mg is ordered to be added to 250 cc D_5W to be infused at a rate of 350 µg/min. It is to be regulated by a volumetric infusion pump that is calibrated to deliver the fluid in units of milliliters per hour. At how many milliliters per hour should the pump be set?
Answer: Here you are asked to convert the "language" of one flow rate to the language of another. First, you need to know that 1 µg is equal to 0.001 mg, so:

$$350\ \mu\text{g}:x = 1 \text{ mg}: 0.001 \text{ mg}$$
$$x = 0.350 \text{ mg or } 0.35 \text{ mg}$$

Thus 0.350 mg is being infused every minute. Now you need to calculate the rate per hour. That is, if 0.35 mg is infused every minute, how many milligrams will be infused per hour?

$$x: 60 \text{ min} = 0.35 \text{ mg}: 1 \text{ min}$$
$$x = 60 \times 0.35$$
$$x = 21 \text{ mg}$$

Now convert to milliliters per hour:

$$21 \text{ mg}: x \text{ (ml)} = 400 \text{ mg}: 250 \text{ ml}$$
$$400x = 21 \times 250 = 5250$$
$$x = 13.125 \text{ or } 13 \text{ ml/hr}$$

10. *Question:* 30 mg of a drug for three-times-a-day dosing has been ordered for a child who weighs 15 kg and is 90 cm tall. The recommended 24-hour total pediatric dosage is 90 to 150 mg/m^2. Is the ordered dose safe or unsafe for this child? Refer to the West nomogram (see Figure 7-1).
Answer: According to the nomogram, a line drawn from points indicating 90 cm and 15 kg crosses the body surface area (BSA) column at the 0.62 point. This means that the child's body surface area is about 0.62 m^2. Multiply 0.62 by each of the numbers indicating the drug's range of safety to see if the ordered 24-hour dosage is within that range.

Some rules of thumb will become more important as the metric system predominates.

- Place a zero to the left of the decimal point when there is no integer in the decimal.
- Carry out problems to the hundredths place, and then round off only in the final answer.
- Use judgment in rounding off numbers. The smaller the answer (the lower the number), the more significant the relative change in the answer made by rounding off.

Many excellent nursing texts are available that one can use to develop and practice arithmetic skills necessary in the administration of medications. (See the references at the end of this chapter.) Much more practice is necessary than is presented here for introductory purposes.

Procedures and Techniques of Administration

Accurate and full identification of the client before each dose of medication is given ensures that the right person gets the right medication. Using the client's full name on all paperwork and in all references helps prevent mixups, as does being alert to similarities in names and geographically separating people with similar names. Nurses should not rely on memory to identify clients. *Checking the client's name on the arm band or name tag* against the name on the accompanying medication sheet is the *most reliable* mode of identification. Asking the client his or her name and comparing it with the name on the medication Kardex, computer sheet, or MAR is not foolproof. For example, a client may give his name as "James" or "Santiago" (first name), and then be given medication intended for "Mr. James" or "Mr. Santiago" (last name). Checking the client's name by calling it out and waiting for a corroborating answer is particularly risky; in a sleepy state, clients have been known to answer to almost any name. Reliance on names on bed tags or labels is dangerous because clients are often away from their beds; a bed can be inadvertently occupied by another client who is in a groggy state after returning, for example, from a laboratory test. Asking a family member is not foolproof either; a distraught family member may respond inappropriately. Again, the *surest* way to identify a client before giving medication is to *check the wrist band* or *identifying tag*. In an institutional setting, medications should not be administered to any client not wearing an identification band or tag. Each institution has a policy for the replacement of identification bands or tags inadvertently removed or lost, and this policy should be complied with and the band or tag restored before any medications are administered. One exception might be in the case of an emergency, in which a delay might be detrimental. Even in an emergency the client's identity should be verified by some method before drug administration.

Before administering medications, the nurse must also make sure that the drug order has not been changed in any way (e.g., discontinued or dosage changed) from what appears on the medication sheet or MAR. It is also wise to check the medication administration record to see that the dose about to be given has not already been given by someone else caring for the client (such as another nurse or nursing student). Individual agency policies spell out the checking procedure to be used; these policies should be followed routinely to avoid error.

The following are recommended guidelines for distributing or administering drugs to clients.

1. When preparing or giving medicines, concentrate your whole attention on what you are doing. Do not permit yourself to be distracted while working with medicines.
2. Make certain that you have a written order for every medication for which you assume the responsibility of administration. (Verbal and telephone orders should be written out and signed by the prescriber as soon as possible. These orders should be used only in limited circumstances and not for the convenience of the prescriber.)
3. Make certain that the data on the medication computer sheet or MAR corresponds exactly with the prescriber's written order and with the label on the client's medicine. Do not decipher illegible orders or make assumptions. Do not accept incomplete orders. Question the use of nonstandard abbreviations and symbols; do not use them yourself.
4. Make a habit of reading the label on the medicine and comparing it with the MAR carefully at least three times: first, when removing the drug from the supply drawer or medication cart; second, when placing the medication in a souffle cup, ounce cup, or syringe; and third, just before administering it to the client, before the container is discarded. Never give a medicine from an unlabeled container or from one on which the label is not legible.
5. Look up information on all new or unfamiliar drugs before administering them. Read the package insert carefully for specific instructions when giving a drug for the first time.
6. If you must in some way calculate the dosage for a client from the preparation on hand and you are uncertain of your calculation, verify your work on paper by having some other responsible person—an instructor, nurse in charge, or pharmacist—check it. In some hospitals certain drug dosages (e.g., insulin) are routinely verified by another nurse. Whenever the result of a calculation calls for more than two units (tablets, vials, etc.) of a drug to make a dose, double check the calculation. It is highly unusual for more than two units of a single drug to be administered in a single dose.
7. Measure quantities as ordered, using the proper equipment: graduated containers for milliliters, fluidounces, or fluidrams; minim glasses or calibrated syringes for minims; and droppers for drops. When measuring liquids, hold the container so that the line indicating the desired quantity is on a level with the eye. The quantity is read when the lowest part of the concave surface of the fluid (meniscus) is on this line.
8. Dosage forms such as tablets, capsules, and pills should be handled so that the fingers do not come into contact with the medicine. Use the cap of the container to guide or lift the medicine into the medicine glass or container you will be taking to the bedside of the client. Administer with water (8 oz).
9. Avoid waste of medicines. Medicines tend to be expensive; in some instances a single capsule may cost the client several dollars. Dropping medicine on the floor is one way of being wasteful. Prepare medications while working over a counter work space.
10. When pouring liquid medicines, hold the bottle so that the liquid does not run over the side and obscure the label. This is known as "palming the label." Wipe the rim of the bottle with a clean piece of paper tissue before replacing the stopper or cover.
11. Always prepare an IV admixture before you label the container, and verify the dosage on the emptied additive container when labeling the IV container.
12. When preparing an injection, always label the syringe immediately. Keep the vial with the syringe, and do not rely on memory to determine what solution is in which syringe.
13. Never administer medication prepared by another person. In doing so, you accept the responsibility for accuracy, dose, correct medication, and so forth. If the person who prepared the medication has made an error, you are accountable for any harm done to the client.
14. Positively identify the client by comparing the wrist band and the name on the medication administration record.
15. If a client expresses doubt or concern about a medication or the dosage of a medication, reassure the client as well as yourself by rechecking to make certain that there is no error, *before* administering the medication. You may need to recheck the order, the label on the medicine container, or the client's chart. The astute and caring nurse also recognizes that a client who refuses medication has the right to do so and that this behavior is giving a message about expressed or unexpressed feelings. The understanding nurse is not content to simply chart that the client refused his or her 10 AM medication. Clients should be able to talk about whatever feelings caused the behavior or their concerns about the medication. This will help clients feel that their concern is important and understood and, depending on the reasons, will be appropriately addressed.
16. Assist weak or impaired clients to take their medications. Do so as patiently and unhurriedly as possible.
17. Many liquid medicines should be diluted with water or other liquid. This is especially desirable when medicines have a bad taste. Exceptions to this rule include cough medicines that are

given for a local effect in the throat. The client (in the sitting position) should be supplied with *at least 240 ml (glassful) of water* for swallowing solid forms such as tablets or capsules, unless the individual is allowed only limited amounts of fluid. This will facilitate dissolution and reduce gastric irritation, if any. Esophageal erosion caused by an adherent tablet or pill has been reported when inadequate amounts of water were given.

18. *Remain with the client until the medicine has been taken.* Most clients are very cooperative about taking medicines when the nurse brings them. However, sometimes clients are more ill than they appear and have been known to hoard medicines until they have accumulated a lethal amount and then take the entire amount, with fatal results. In some instances, however, clients may be permitted to keep medicines at their bedsides (with a prescriber's order) and take them as necessary, such as nitroglycerin and antacids.
19. Stay, for at least 5 minutes with a client who is receiving the first dose of an IV medication, especially antibiotics, and monitor closely for adverse effects.
20. Do not leave a tray or cart of medicines unattended. If you are in a client's room and must leave, take the tray of medicines with you. Similarly, do not leave the medication cart unattended in the hall; either lock the cart in the hallway or take it into the client's room with you.
21. Record the administration of each dose as soon as possible. Never chart a medicine as having been given until it has been administered. Nursing students should check the chart before giving a medication. MARs should document all medications, including prn ones, one-time-only medications, and special drugs (e.g., heparin), in one place to allow the nurse to consider incompatibilities and/or duplications of similar drugs. The name of the drug, the dosage, the time of administration, and the route of administration should be noted on the medication record in the chart. In the recording of parenteral medications, the site of injection is always included. The client's response, adverse as well as intended, to the medication should be recorded in the progress notes or nursing notes.
22. Always verify a drug's route of administration. Sometimes preparations for a specific route of administration may be used for another route. For example, Mycostatin suppositories developed for vaginal use may be used as an oral troche for an oral yeast infection, or some parenteral preparations may be diluted for oral use, such as vancomycin when indicated for pseudomembranous colitis. In this latter example and with other drugs, do not put oral drugs in syringes used for injection. Oral syringes that cannot accommodate a needle should be used to prevent accidental parenteral injection of an oral preparation.
23. Within an institutional setting, any unused medication should be returned to the pharmacy. According to institutional policy and in some states the law requires the unused portion to be credited to the client's account. If it can be used for another client, the pharmacy will verify that it has been stored correctly and relabel it.
24. Borrowing medications from one client's supply for another client is not appropriate and leads to dosing errors. Only medications issued by the pharmacy and labeled for a specific client should be used for that client, except in the case of a stock medication kept on the nursing unit. If the facility has a unit-dose system, never administer "loose" medications. Medications brought into the hospital by a client should be sent back home with a family member or, if they are to be used in the institutional setting, sent to the hospital pharmacy to be verified and relabeled.

All medicine containers and trays should be scrupulously clean, and water supplied to the client with the medicine should be fresh. Carelessly prepared medicines and lack of consideration in the way a medicine is handed to a client can convey a demeaning or insulting message, whether intended or not.

When a medicine with an unpleasant taste is given, it is better to admit that it may be unpleasant than to make a client feel that his or her reaction is grossly exaggerated or silly. The nurse can attempt to improve the taste by diluting the medicine (if possible) or by offering chewing gum or hard candy immediately after the medicine.

If an injection is likely to sting or hurt, it is honest to tell the client beforehand. The client who is told is also more likely to deal with the pain more effectively than one who is not told. It is better to tell a child just before the injection rather than much beforehand, so that there is little time for the child to anticipate and grow anxious, thereby actually increasing the pain.

The route of administration of a drug is determined by its physical and chemical properties, the condition or status of the client, the desired action of the drug, its speed of absorption, and the rapidity of response desired. As a rule, drugs are administered for either local or systemic effects (see Chapter 3). Some drugs given locally may produce both local and systemic effects if they are partly or entirely absorbed; some drugs are applied for local absorption, i.e., transdermally, yet are targeted solely for systemic effect, such as nitroglycerin, fentanyl, and scopolamine. There has been an increasing awareness that many more substances are absorbed through the skin than was previously believed. Incidents of toxicity in infants exposed to topically applied dermal medication are increasing. Some of these drugs are boric acid, iodides, hexachlorophene, corticosteroids, and rubbing alcohol. Care is advised in use of any topically applied drug on infants' skin. Yet a drug may be injected into a joint cavity and have little or no effect beyond the tissues of that structure.

Administration for Local Effects

Application to skin. Medications are applied to the skin primarily for the following effects:

1. *Astringent*: constricts; draws together; a substance that may result in vasoconstriction, tissue contraction, and decreased secretions and sensitivity
2. *Antiseptic or bacteriostatic*: inhibits growth and development of microorganisms
3. *Emollient*: soothing and softening effect to overcome dryness and hardness
4. *Cleansing*: for the removal of dirt, debris, secretions, or crusts

These medications may be applied in the form of a lotion, tincture, ointment or cream, foam, wet dressing, bath, or soak. The effectiveness of medicinals applied to the skin for local effect is limited by the fact that highly specialized layers of skin resist penetration of many (but not all) foreign substances to protect the internal body environment. Topical absorption is increased when the skin is thin or macerated, when there is increased drug concentration, when there is prolonged contact of the drug with the skin, or when the drug is combined with a solvent-penetrant (e.g., dimethyl sulfoxide [DMSO] and acyclovir are under study for topical use in this way). See information presented in Chapter 43 on ophthalmic drugs, Chapter 45 on otic drugs, Chapter 66 on dermatologic drugs, and Chapter 67 on debriding agents.

Application to mucous membranes. Drugs are well absorbed across mucosal surfaces, and therapeutic effects are easily obtained. However, mucous membranes are highly selective in their absorptive capacity and vary in sensitivity. To produce the same effects, a drug applied to oral (buccal or sublingual) mucosa may be twice as concentrated as that applied to nasal mucosa, whereas its concentration may be reduced one fourth to one half for application to delicate membranes of the eye or urethra. Aqueous solutions are quickly absorbed from mucous membranes; oily liquids are not. Oily preparations should not be applied to nasal or respiratory mucosa by sprays or nebulae because the droplets of oil may be carried to terminal portions of the respiratory tract and retained there, causing lipoid pneumonia.

Respiratory mucosa may be medicated by means of inhalation or insufflation. The inhalation method uses sprays or nebulae, whereby the drug is sprayed in the nose or throat by a nebulizer; aerosols are delivered by a flow of air or oxygen under pressure to disperse the drug throughout the lower respiratory tract. In the insufflation method a fine powder is blown or sprayed. Drugs so administered tend to have both a local respiratory and a systemic effect. The respiratory mucosa offers an enormous surface of absorbing epithelium. If the drug is volatile and can be absorbed chemically and if there is more in the inspired air than in the blood, the drug is instantaneously absorbed. This fact is of significance in emergencies. Amyl nitrite and oxygen are examples of volatile and gaseous agents that are given by inhalation.

Drugs in suppository form can be used for their local effects on the mucous membranes of the vagina, urethra, or rectum. Packs and tampons may be impregnated with a drug and placed in a body cavity; these are used particularly in the nose, ears, and vagina. Drugs may also be painted or swabbed on a mucosal surface, instilled (e.g., a vaginal douche), or administered via irrigation.

Administration for Systemic Effects

Drugs that produce a systemic effect must be absorbed into the bloodstream and carried to the cells or tissues capable of responding to them. The route of administration used depends on the nature and amount of drug to be given, the desired rapidity of effect, and the general condition of the client. Routes selected for systemic effect include the following: dermal, oral, sublingual, rectal, and parenteral (injection). Routes of parenteral administration include the intradermal (or intracutaneous), subcutaneous, intramuscular, intravenous, intraspinal (or intrathecal), and sometimes intraarticular, intracardiac, intrapericardiac, intraosseous, and intraperitoneal.

Application to skin. Topical applications of some medications in patch form are administered for systemic effects, now that microquantitative assay capabilities make possible precise unit dosages using transdermal modes. For example, nitroglycerin, which is used to treat anginal pain, is available in small unit-dose adhesive bandages that slowly release the medication over a 24-hour period. Some of them employ a semipermeable, rate-controlling membrane placed next to the skin; others disperse the nitroglycerin evenly throughout a gel matrix. Nitrodisc, Nitro-Dur, and Transderm-Nitro are some trade name products. See Figure 29-1 for diagram of some transdermal patches. Similarly, motion sickness is treated with scopolamine (Transderm-V); duration of effects of one application behind the ear is about 3 days. Fentanyl (Duragesic), an analgesic, is also available in a transdermal system that provides continuous release of the potent opioid for 72 hours. Clonidine, estrogen, and nicotine are other medications available in patch form. The nurse should apply the patch over a clean, dry, and hair-free area, rotating the application sites.

Oral administration. Oral administration is the safest, most economical, and most convenient way of giving medicines. Therefore it is the preferred route unless some distinct advantage is to be gained by using another way. Most drugs are absorbed from the small intestine; only a few are absorbed from the stomach and colon. This explains the ineffectiveness of cathartics and enemas in removing most toxins and overdoses in cases of poisoning.

The drug effects of orally administered drugs are *slower* in onset and *more prolonged* but *less potent* than those of parenterally administered drugs. Thus when a steady state in pharmacokinetics is desired, it is often more closely approached with oral than with parenteral administration. When rapid, high dosages are needed as loading doses or in emergencies, the parenteral route may be used. Strategies for wise pain care, if carefully tailored to individual needs, can exploit these characteristics of oral and parenteral routes for analgesics. For the client who has low-level or chronic pain, the oral route for analgesics can be more successful than other routes in promoting a steady state (fewer oscillations) in pain relief. Acute pain may submit to an initial dose of analgesic by the parenteral route, followed by oral doses. Altered effects from oral administration may result from (1) variation in absorption as a result of drug composition, gastric or intestinal pH and motility, food content, or a pathologic condition within the gastrointestinal tract, or (2) alteration of the drug resulting from its retention, inactivation, or biotransformation in the liver.

Disadvantages of the oral administration of certain drugs are that (1) they may have an objectional odor or taste or be bulky to swallow, (2) they may irritate the gastric mucosa, causing nausea and vomiting, (3) they may be aspirated by a seriously ill or uncooperative individual, (4) some may be destroyed by digestive enzymes, and (5) they may be inappropriate for some clients, such as those who must be given nothing by mouth.

Sublingual administration. Drugs given sublingually are placed under the tongue, where they should be retained until dissolved and absorbed. The thin epithelium and rich network of capillaries on the underside of the tongue permit both rapid absorption and rapid drug action. In addition, there is greater potency than with oral administration, since the drug gains access to the general circulation without entering the portal circulation of the liver or being affected by gastric and intestinal enzymes. Many of the same effects apply also to buccal administration, whereby a tablet is held in the mouth in the pocket between gums and cheek for local dissolution and absorption.

The number of drugs that can be given sublingually is limited (e.g., nitroglycerin tablets). The drug must dissolve readily and the client must be able to cooperate; the client must understand that the drug is not to be swallowed and that taking a drink must be avoided until the drug has been absorbed. However, usually little harm is done if a sublingual drug is inadvertently swallowed; effects may be neutralized or delayed slightly.

Rectal administration. Rectal administration of certain preparations can be used advantageously when the stomach is nonretentive or traumatized, when the medicine has an objectionable taste or odor, or when it can be changed by digestive enzymes. It is also a reasonably convenient and safe method of giving drugs when the oral method is unsuitable, as when the individual is either a small child (or infant) or is unconscious. Rectal administration is contraindicated, however, if the anal area is irritated, or if diarrhea, rectal bleeding, or hemorrhoids are present.

Use of the rectal route avoids irritation of the upper gastrointestinal tract (however, aminophylline suppositories often irritate the rectal mucosa) and may promote higher bloodstream drug titers because venous blood from the lower part of the rectum does not traverse the liver. The suppository as a drug vehicle is often superior to the retention enema because the drug is released at a slow but steady rate to ensure a protracted effect. One disadvantage of the retention enema is unpredictable retention of the drug; another is that some of the fluid may pass above the lower rectum and be absorbed into the portal circulation. An evacuant enema before administration of rectal medication is usually advisable to ensure that there is no fecal bulk in the rectum to obstruct free flow of the medicated enema or the action of a suppository. The amount of solution that can be given rectally is usually small.

Refrigerated suppositories will soften and cannot be inserted if they are handled or carried in the pocket for even a brief period. Cold running water will restore rigidity to suppositories. To be retained for effective therapy, suppositories and enema tubing must be inserted beyond the internal anal sphincter (2 to 3 inches). The dose of a drug in suppository form cannot be divided by cutting the suppository in sections because the active drug constituent may not be evenly distributed.

Parenteral administration. Strictly speaking, parenteral administration means administration by any route other than oral; thus technically it could be defined to include topical or inhalation administration. In practical usage, however, parenteral usually means administration by the use of a needle (Table 5-6).

Parenteral administration of drugs includes all forms of drug injection into body tissues or fluids using a syringe and needle or catheter and container (Figures 5-2 and 5-3). Drugs given parenterally must be sterile, readily soluble and absorbable, and relatively nonirritating. Because the parenteral administration of drugs can be hazardous, precautions are required: (1) aseptic technique must be used to avoid infection and (2) accurate drug dosage, proper rate of injection, and proper site of injection are essential to avoid harm such as lipodystrophy (atrophy or hypertrophy of subcutaneous fat tissue), abscesses, necrosis, skin slough, nerve injuries, prolonged pain, or periostitis. *An injected drug is irretrievable,* and an error in dosage or method or site of injection is not easily corrected.

With drugs given parenterally (as compared with orally): (1) the onset of drug action is more rapid (except as noted previously), (2) the dosage is often similar, since drug potency remains unaltered, and (3) the cost of drug therapy may be greater. Parenteral administration of drugs requires specialized knowledge, aseptic technique, and manual skill to ensure safety and therapeutic effectiveness. Most methods of parenteral administration may be performed by the nurse, but some are usually done only by a physician or other health care providers with advanced educational preparation. The nurse should know and adhere to agency policy. Clients and family members may also learn to administer injections.

Intradermal. Intradermal or intracutaneous injection means that the injection is made into the upper layers of the skin, almost parallel to the skin surface (Figure 5-4). The amount of drug given is small, and absorption is slow. This method is used to advantage in testing for allergic reactions and for giving small amounts of a local anesthetic. In a test for allergic reactions, minute amounts of the solution to be tested are injected just under the outer layers of the skin. The medial surface of the forearm and the skin of the back are the sites frequently used. These injections are best made with a fine, short needle (26- or 27-gauge) and a small-barrel syringe (such as a tuberculin syringe) (Figure 5-5).

Subcutaneous (SC). Small amounts of drug in solution are given subcutaneously usually by means of a 25-gauge (or thinner) needle and syringe. The needle is inserted through the skin with a quick movement, but the injection is made slowly and steadily (Figure 5-6). The nurse should slightly withdraw the plunger of the syringe before injecting the drug, to make sure that a blood vessel has not been entered. The angle of insertion should usually be 45 to 60 degrees (but can be any angle from 30 to 90 degrees, depending on needle length and depth of fat pads), and insertion should be made on the fat pads of the abdomen, the outer surface of the upper arm, the anterior surface of the thigh, or occasionally the lower abdominal surface (heparin). In these locations there are fewer large blood vessels, and sensation is less keen than on the medial surfaces of the extremities. Massage of the part after injection tends to increase the rate of absorption but should be avoided after injection of some drugs, such as heparin, to minimize bruising as the drug spreads through the tissues. Disposable syringes and needles contribute to aseptic safety of the procedure but also to cost and problems of storage and disposal. Subcutaneously injected medicines are limited to drugs that are highly soluble and nonirritating and to solutions of limited volume (ideally no more than 1 ml).

TABLE 5-6 Suggested injection guides

Route	Common areas	Region	Needle sizes*	Volume injected (ml) Average	Range†	Examples of medication by this route
Intradermal (intracutaneous)	Skin (corium)	Inner aspect of mid-forearm or scapula	26 or 27 gauge × 3/8 in	0.1	0.001 to 1.0	Tuberculin, allergens, local anesthetics
Subcutaneous	Beneath the skin	Lateral upper arms; thighs; abdominal fat pads except the 1-in area around umbilicus and tissue over bone; upper back; upper hips	25 to 27 gauge × 1/2 to 5/8 in‡	0.5	0.5 to 1.5	Epinephrine (non-oily), insulin, some narcotics, tetanus toxoid, vaccines, vitamin B_{12}, heparin
Intramuscular	Gluteus medius	Dorsogluteal	20 to 23 gauge × 1½ to 3 in‡	2 to 4	1 to 5	Most intramuscular and Z-track injections
	Gluteus minimus	Ventrogluteal	20 to 23 gauge × 1½ to 3 in‡	1 to 4	1 to 5	All intramuscular medications
	Vastus lateralis	Anterolateral midthigh	22 to 25 gauge × 5/8 to 1 in‡	1 to 4	1 to 5	Almost all intramuscular medications
	Deltoid	Upper arm below shoulder	23 to 25 gauge × 5/8 to 1 in‡	0.5	0.5 to 2	Vaccines, absorbed tetanus toxoid, most narcotics, epinephrine, sedatives, vitamin B_{12}, lidocaine
Intravenous bolus	Cephalic and basilic veins	Dorsum of hand and forearm; antecubital fossa	18 to 23 gauge × 1 to 1½ in	1 to 10	0.5 to 50 (or more by continuous infusion	Antibiotics, vitamins, fluids and electrolytes, antineoplastics, vasopressors, corticosteroids, aminophylline, blood products

*Needles used for withdrawing medication from a container should be changed before injecting medication drawn (1) from ampules, because irritating medication may cling to needle (filter-needles should be used to withdraw medication from ampules) and (2) from vials, because needles are dulled after insertion through rubber tops; disposable needles are thus labeled "for one-time use only."

†Administration of the largest volumes listed here should be avoided if possible by dividing the dose and using different sites or by using another route in consultation with prescriber.

‡See text for discussion of factors influencing choice of needle length.

Irritating drugs given subcutaneously can result in the formation of sterile abscesses and necrotic tissue, especially if injections are made repeatedly in the same site. Care should be exercised to avoid contamination and to rotate sites. Subcutaneous injections are not effective in individuals with sluggish peripheral circulation (i.e., the client in shock).

Intramuscular (IM). Deeper injections are made into muscular tissue, through the skin and subcutaneous tissue, when a drug is too irritating to be given subcutaneously. However, irritation may also occur with some drugs given intramuscularly. Larger doses can be given by intramuscular injection—up to 5 ml—than by subcutaneous injection. Subcutaneous or intramuscular absorption is delayed in circulatory collapse (i.e., shock states); the intravenous route should then be chosen.

A drug may be given intramuscularly in an aqueous solution, an aqueous suspension, or a solution or suspension of oil. Suspensions form a depot of drug in the tissue, and slow,

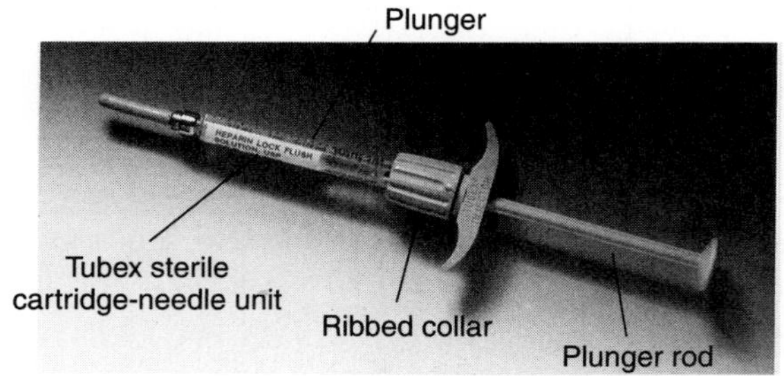

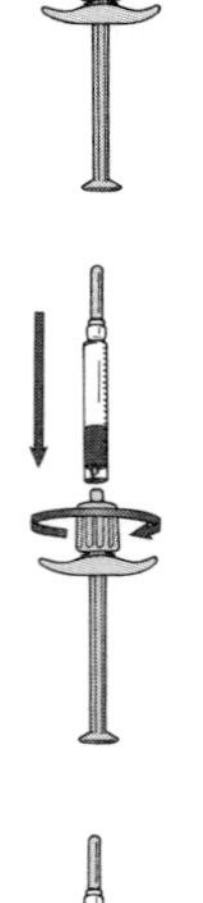

How to load

1. Turn the ribbed collar to the "open" position until it stops.

2. Hold injector with the open end up and fully insert the Tubex sterile cartridge-needle unit.

   Firmly tighten the ribbed collar in the direction of the "close" arrow.

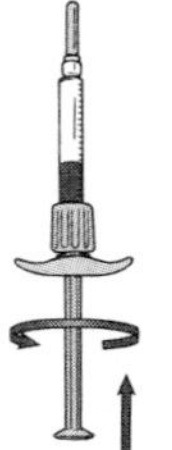

Thread the plunger rod into the plunger of the Tubex sterile cartridge-needle unit until slight resistance is felt.

The injector is now ready for use in the usual manner.

How to administer

Method of administration is the same as with conventional syringe. Remove needle cover by grasping it securely; twist and pull. Introduce needle into patient, aspirate by pulling back slightly on the plunger, and inject.

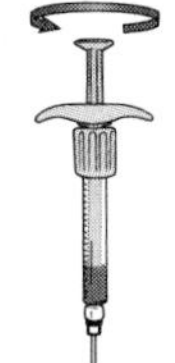

How to unload and discard used unit

1. Do not recap the needle. Disengage the plunger rod.

2. Hold the injector, needle down, over a needle disposal container and loosen the ribbed collar. Tubex cartridge-needle unit will drop into the container.

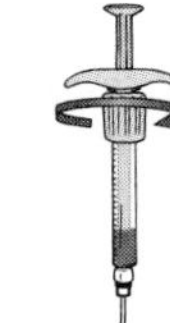

Discard the needle cover.

The Tubex injector is reusable; do not discard.

Figure 5-2 Directions for use of Tubex closed-injection system. (Courtesy Wyeth-Ayerst Laboratories, Philadelphia, PA)

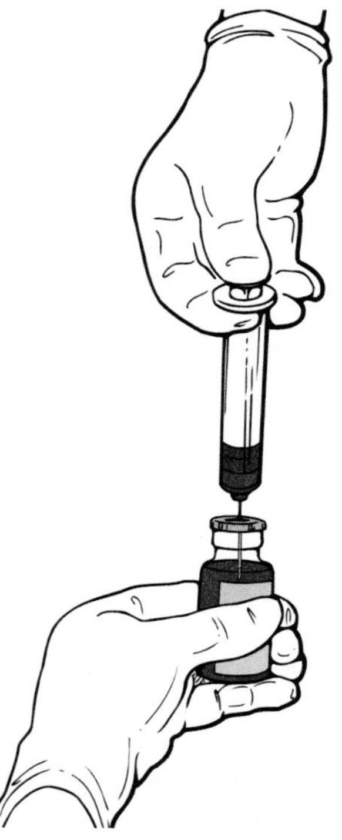

Figure 5-3 Withdrawing medication from a rubber-topped vial. To prevent a vacuum, the vial is inverted to inject a volume of air equivalent to the volume of medication to be withdrawn. If a large amount is to be withdrawn, it may be necessary (in order to be able to withdraw the liquid) to alternate actions (while the needle remains inserted) of instilling air and withdrawing medication. Another method is to use a second needle as an airway in the vial top, maintaining the tip of the medication needle within the liquid; otherwise, only air will be drawn up. Current literature is equivocal about the procedure of drawing an additional 0.1 to 0.3 ml bubble of air into the syringe after the precise medication dosage has been drawn up. This bubble will rise to the top of the medication dose in the syringe when injected, to form an absorbable plug so that irritating medication will not back up the skin track made by the needle.

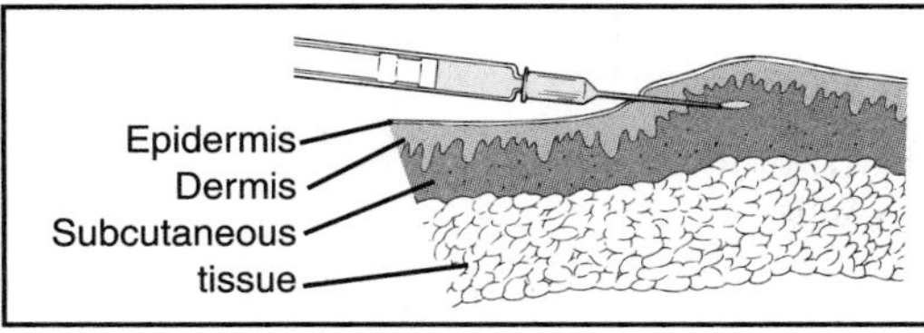

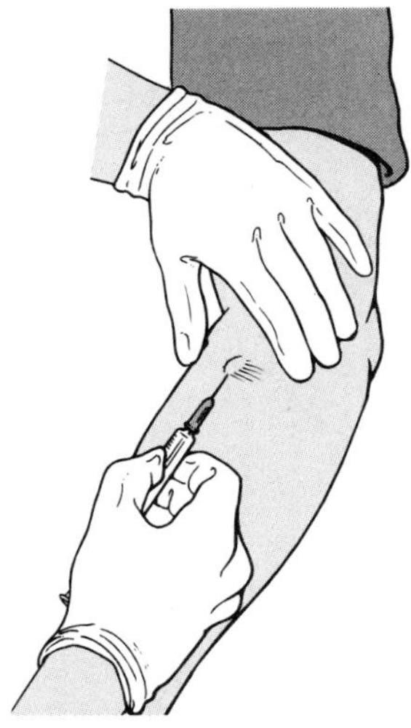

Figure 5-4 Intradermal injection. The needle penetrates epidermis and goes into dermis but not subcutaneous tissue. (Note that the skin is not pinched up.)

gradual absorption usually results allowing for the drug to act over a longer period of time. Two disadvantages are sometimes encountered when preparations in oil are used: the client may be sensitive to the oil, or the oil may not be absorbed. In the latter case, incision and drainage of the oil may be necessary. However, few drugs are formulated in oil.

Criteria for selection of a safe intramuscular injection site include distance from large, vulnerable nerves, bones, and blood vessels and from bruised, scarred, or swollen sites of previous injection or infusion. The type of needle used for intramuscular injection depends on the site of the injection, the condition of the tissues, the size of the client, and the nature of the drug to be injected. Needles from 1 to 1½ inches in length are common. The usual gauge is 21 to 23 (*the larger the number, the finer the needle*). Fine needles can be used for thin solutions, and heavier needles for suspensions and oils. Needles for injection into the deltoid area should be ⅝ to 1 inch in length, the gauge again depending on the material to be injected. The deltoid can readily absorb up to 2 ml of drug. For many intramuscular injections the gluteals are preferred because of fewer nerve endings and less discomfort at this site. The needle must be long enough to avoid depositing the solution of drug into the subcutaneous or fatty tissue. The depth of insertion depends on the amount of subcutaneous tissue and will vary with the weight of the client.

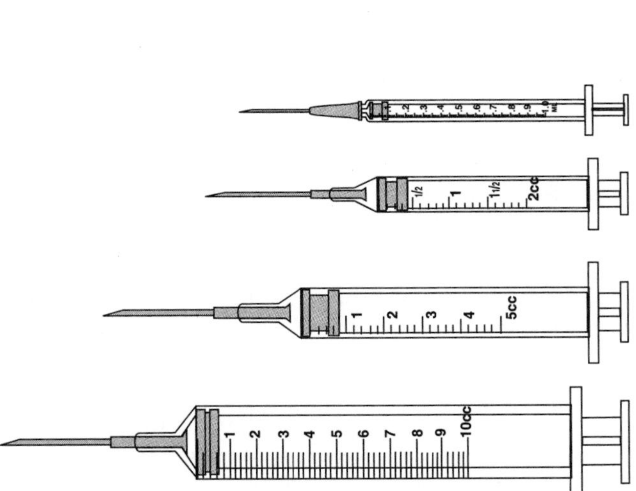

Figure 5-5 These syringes are used to accurately measure varying amounts of liquids and liquid medications. The uppermost syringe is known as a tuberculin syringe and is graduated in 0.01 cc (ml). It is a syringe of choice for administration of very small amounts. The 2-cc syringe is the one commonly used to give a drug subcutaneously or intramuscularly or intravenously; for withdrawing blood for laboratory testing; or for obtaining urine specimens from urinary catheters (20-cc syringes may be preferred for the last two uses). These syringes and needles are not drawn to scale (e.g., the tuberculin syringe is much thinner and shorter than the others).

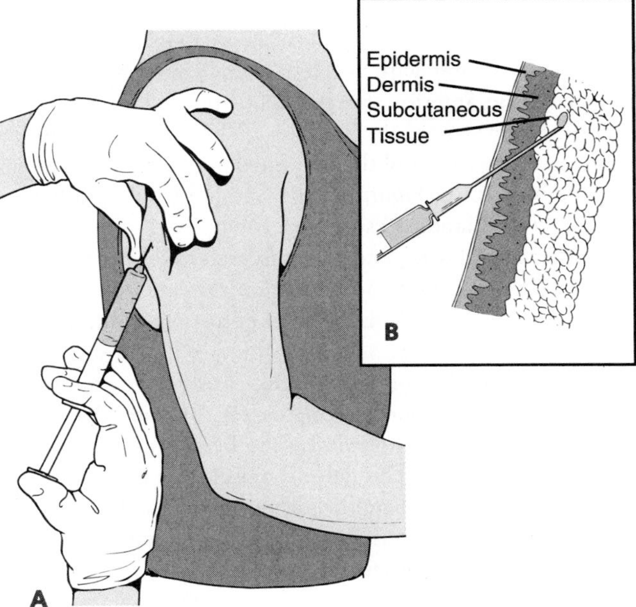

Figure 5-6 Subcutaneous injection. The skin surface has been cleansed, and the syringe is held at the angle at which the needle will penetrate subcutaneous tissue. The left hand is used to pinch the arm gently but firmly. When the needle has been inserted into the subcutaneous tissue, the tissue of the arm is released and the solution is steadily injected. Based on the client's condition or the medication to be injected, nursing judgment may dictate a different angle or an approach different from pinching up the skin.

It is essential to locate the appropriate landmarks to limit the areas safe for injections (see Figure 5-7; Table 5-6). Intramuscular injections may be given into such clearly defined areas of musculature as the gluteal region of the lower back (provides slowest absorption), the deltoid area, and the anterolateral thigh. At first it seems to most nursing students that the fleshy part of the buttock is a logical intramuscular site. It is not, since underneath, centrally, and running diagonally is the sciatic nerve, which if damaged can result in permanent leg paralysis. Every attempt must be made to avoid this area.

There are now two acceptable ways to map appropriate intramuscular sites in the gluteal region. The formerly used method of dividing the gluteus medius into imaginary quadrants and injecting into the upper outer quadrant is out of favor because it does not necessarily prevent an injection into the sciatic nerve, especially if the nerve's course runs abnormally in an individual.

The nurse can best locate the *dorsogluteal site* (the muscle underneath is the gluteus medius) by asking the client to lie face down and exposing the entire area so that the landmarks and injection site can be clearly located. The proper site for this injection is outlined by an imaginary diagonal line drawn from the area of the greater trochanter of the femur to the posterior iliac spine. The injection should be given at any point between that imaginary straight line and below the curve of the iliac crest (hipbone; see Figure 5-7, *A*).

The *ventrogluteal site* can be made accessible with the client in a supine, prone (which is awkward), or sidelying position. This site is used for intramuscular injections in either children or adults and could be used more often than it is. To locate it on the right side, the nurse should palpate for the right greater trochanter with the left palm, point the left index finger to the anterior superior iliac spine, and extend the middle finger toward the iliac crest. The injection should be made into the center of the V formed between the index and middle fingers (see Figure 5-7, *B*). Similarly, the right hand is used to detect landmarks in the left hip.

Either of the two gluteal sites is preferred for the Z-**track method**, an injection method useful for administration of medication known to cause pain or permanent staining of superficial tissues (Figure 5-8).

The *mid-deltoid area* is the muscular area in the arm formed by the rectangle bounded on the top by the edge of the shoulder and on the bottom by the beginning of the axilla (see Figure 5-8, *D*). The deltoid muscle has a considerably higher blood flow than the other intramuscular injection sites and, for rapid onset, is the area of choice for many small-volume (2 ml or less) medications.

The *vastus lateralis* is a muscular area in the upper outer leg. The potential site for injection is within a long rectangular area just lateral to the frontal plane of the thigh. Its top boundary is found about one handsbreadth below the greater trochanter, and the bottom boundary is about one handsbreadth above the knee (see Figure 5-7, C). This area can accommodate volumes of medication the same size as the gluteus medius and is distant from any major blood vessels or nerves, but injection here may be more painful than in the buttocks.

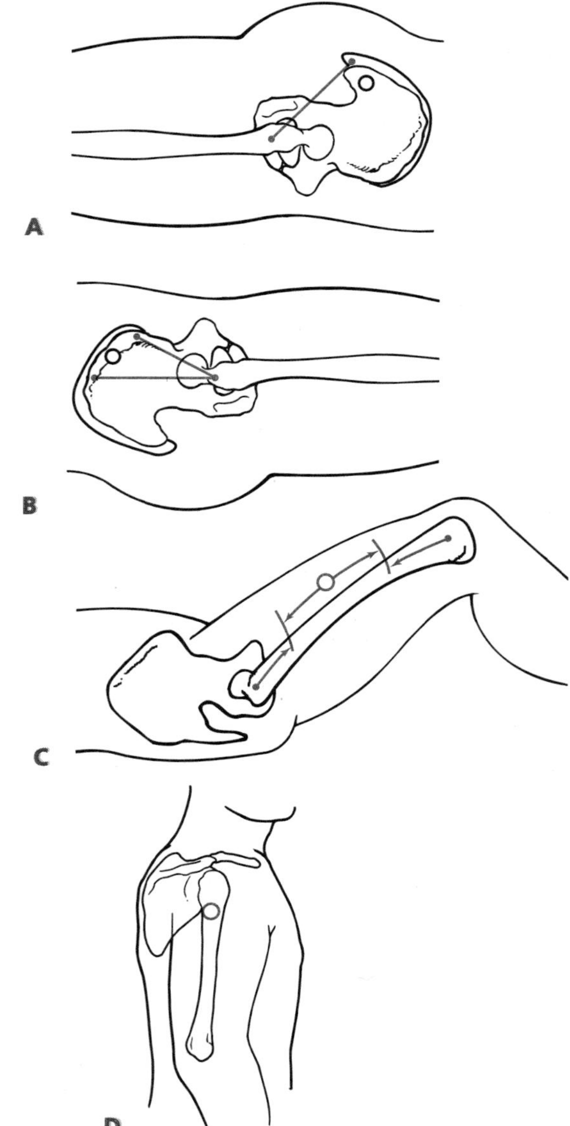

Figure 5-7 Intramuscular injection. A, Dorsogluteal site, located anterior to the diagonal line from the trochanter to the posterior iliac spine. An injection near the middle of the buttocks may result in an injury to the sciatic nerve. The needle is inserted with a quick firm movement, entering perpendicular to the skin. After aspiration to make certain the needle is not in a blood vessel, the solution is injected slowly and steadily. B, Ventrogluteal intramuscular injection site. The V fans out from the greater trochanter between the anterior iliac spine and iliac crest. The injection site *(X)* is centered at the base of the triangle. C, Vastus lateralis (midlateral thigh) intramuscular injection—a handsbreadth below the greater trochanter and a handsbreadth above the knee and halfway between the front and side of the thigh. D, Mid-deltoid intramuscular injection site—below the acromion and lateral to the axilla.

Relaxation and comfort may be enhanced during an intramuscular injection into the gluteal muscles if the client lies in a prone position with a pillow under the legs just below the

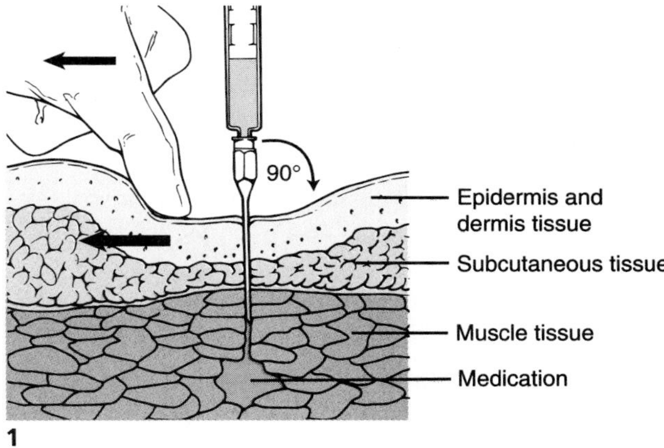

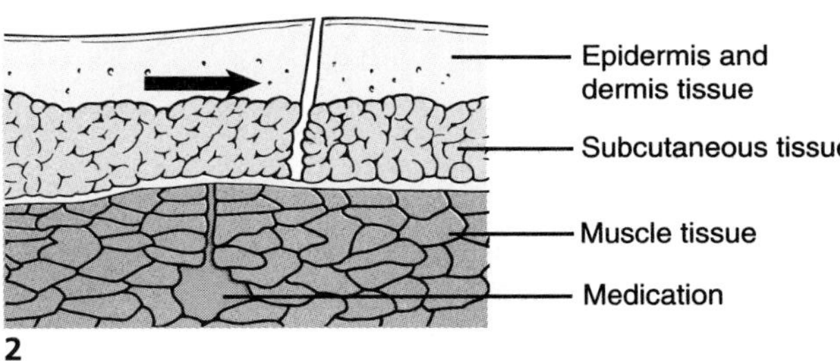

Figure 5-8 Z-track intramuscular injection method, which is useful for administration of medication known to cause pain or permanent staining of superficial tissues. **1**, The skin is stretched to one side and medication injected as usual, perpendicular to the skin surface. **2**, Needle is then removed and the skin allowed to return to resting position, sealing off the deposited medication from the track made by the needle. The site is not massaged in this method.

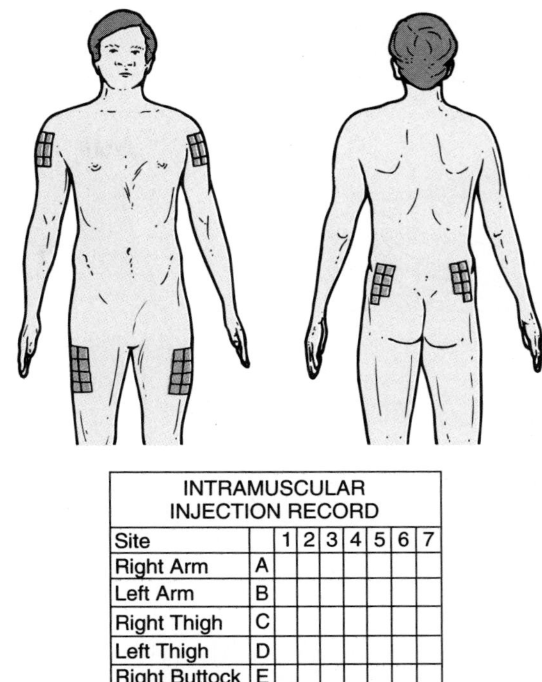

INTRAMUSCULAR INJECTION RECORD								
Site		1	2	3	4	5	6	7
Right Arm	A							
Left Arm	B							
Right Thigh	C							
Left Thigh	D							
Right Buttock	E							
Left Buttock	F							

Figure 5-9 Anatomic chart for the rotation of intramuscular injections. The chart may be kept with the MAR, nursing Kardex, or care plan to provide a reference for the nurse administering medication.

knees, and in a toes-in position (to relax the buttocks) or by having the client put the toes of both feet together. The side-lying position is an alternative. To prevent local postinjection complications (such as discomfort, scars, abscesses), no two injections should be made in the same spot during a course of treatment. Injection sites should be rotated and the site for each intramuscular injection should be recorded on the clinical record (Figure 5-9).

For intramuscular injection the needle and syringe assembly is held as if it were a dart while the other hand stretches taut the skin of the injection site. The nurse can test sensitivity of the area by tapping it with the fingers. If the muscle mass underlying the injection site is inadequate to accommodate the length of the needle, the flesh may instead be pinched up before needle insertion. The injection should be made *perpendicular to the skin surface,* from a distance of about 2 inches, in one quick motion. If possible, the needle should not be inserted to its full depth; a small portion of it should be left accessible above the skin so that it can be retrieved should it break, a very rare event. It is necessary to make certain that the needle is not in a blood vessel, thus causing the unintended deposit of medication into the bloodstream instead of muscle tissue (also very unusual). This is ascertained by pulling out the plunger *slightly* after the needle is in place in tissue (termed "aspiration"). The medication may have a slight pinkish tinge close to the needle hub, or a small amount of blood may enter the barrel of the syringe if the needle is in a blood vessel rather than in tissue. If this is the case, the needle and the medication-filled syringe should be withdrawn and discarded before continuing. In certain instances injection of oily or particulate medicines or killed bacteria by such an inadvertent intravessel administration could result in a serious emergency.

Contrary to popular belief, needle puncture of the skin is not always the prime source of discomfort associated with injections, although a dull needle such as one inserted through a vial's rubber stopper will certainly contribute to pain. Also, it is not the length of the needle that causes pain, but the diameter; a 3-inch needle will hurt no more than a $^5/_8$-inch one if the diameter is similar. Except for the psychologic aspect of anxiety about needles, most injection pain is thought to occur from stretching of tissue (pain receptors in the skin) as it accommodates the volume of the drug; from irritation from the drug itself; from unsteadiness in the injector's technique, which results in jiggling of the needle during overly slow insertions; during aspiration; while the injector is reaching for

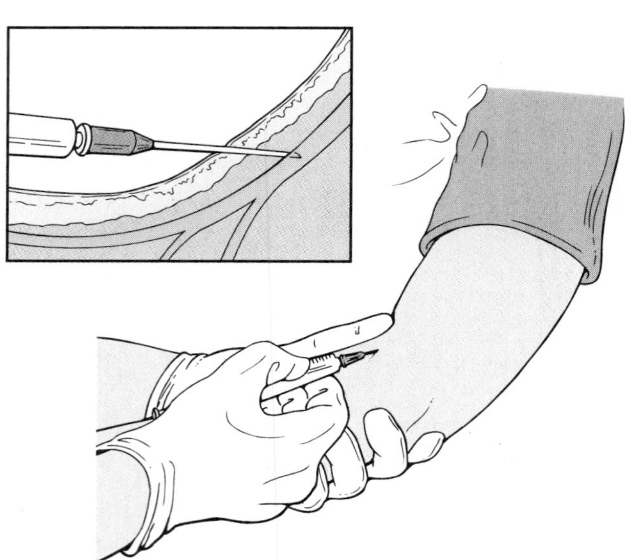

Figure 5-10 Intravenous injection. The skin has been cleansed with a solution of alcohol. Thumb of left hand holds the skin taut. Withdrawal of blood indicates needle is in the vein. Solution is injected slowly and steadily.

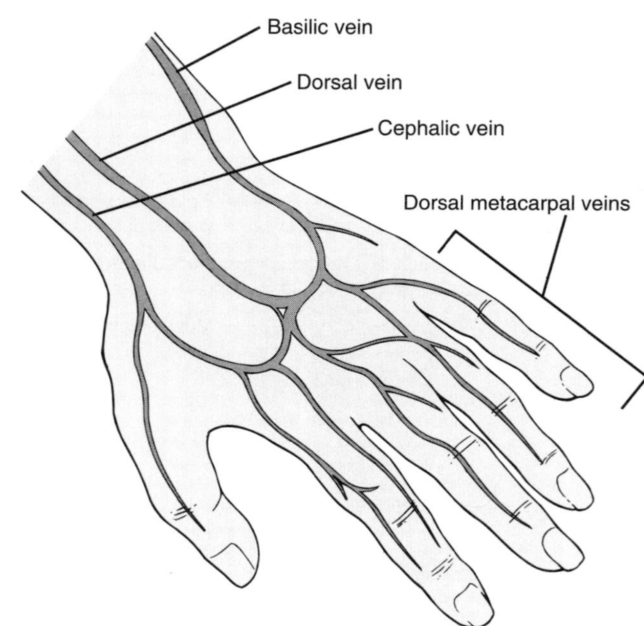

Figure 5-11 The major sites for IV injection in the hand include the basilic, dorsal metacarpal, cephalic veins. These vessels are fairly easy to locate. As the cephalic and basilic veins traverse the forearm, they branch into other vessels that also are easily accessible for IV injections.

the antiseptic swab at completion; or from wet antiseptic on the skin during insertion. Quick withdrawal of the needle in the same angle as insertion with firm pressure applied to the injection site with an antiseptic swab will prevent discomfort as the injection is completed. Massaging the site (except after heparin, iron dextran products, and others) acts to disperse the medication and may also reduce any discomfort.

Intravenous (IV). When an immediate effect is desired, when for any reason a drug cannot be injected into other tissues, or when absorption may be inhibited by poor circulation, the drug may be given directly into a vein as an **injection** (the act of forcing a liquid into the body by means of a syringe) or as an **infusion** (the introduction of a substance directly into a vein by means of gravity flow). The terms *injection* and *infusion* also refer to the substances so administered. These methods require skill and asepsis, and the drug must be highly soluble and capable of withstanding sterilization. This method is of great value in emergencies. The dose and amount of absorption can be determined with accuracy. However, the rapidity of absorption and the fact that there is no recall once the drug has been given constitute dangers worthy of consideration. From this standpoint it is one of the least safe methods of administration. Precautions must be taken to prevent extravasation, or leakage, of drug or fluids into surrounding tissue (**infiltration**).

In IV injection ("IV push") a comparatively small amount of solution (also referred to as a bolus) is given by means of a syringe into IV tubing, into a heparin lock, or directly into a vein over a 1- to 7-minute period. The drug is dissolved in a suitable amount of normal (physiologic) saline solution or some other isotonic solution. The injection may be made into the median basilic or median cephalic vein at the bend of the elbow (Figure 5-10), or the basilic, dorsal metacarpal, and cephalic veins of the forearm and dorsal surface of the hand (Figure 5-11). Factors that determine the choice of vein for IV therapy are related to the thickness of the skin over the vein, the closeness of the vein to the surface, the presence of a firm support (bone) under the vein, and the need to use a larger vein for concentrated or irritating substances. The veins in the antecubital fossa are readily accessible, although the veins of the back of the hand are also sometimes used for infusions. Leg veins are avoided because of their potential for phlebitis.

A vein that is normally distended with blood is much easier to enter than a partially collapsed one. A tourniquet is drawn tightly around the extremity proximal to the IV site to distend the vein, the air is expelled from the syringe, and the needle is introduced pointing proximally, bevel up. A few drops of blood aspirated into the syringe indicate that the needle is in the vein; the tourniquet is then removed and the solution is injected slowly. As in all types of injections, the needle, syringe, and solution must be sterile; hands must be scrupulously washed; and antiseptic must be applied to the insertion site and allowed to dry. An IV bolus dose is the method of choice for rapidly administering drugs in an emergency because it is a reliable way to achieve optimal drug blood levels rapidly. It is also the way to administer certain IV medications that may be incompatible in solution;

digoxin (Lanoxin), diazepam (Valium), furosemide (Lasix), diazoxide (Hyperstat), certain anticancer drugs, and diagnostic agents in dye form. A 20-gauge needle is commonly used for IV push or bolus doses.

Many drugs given intravenously must be given slowly to avoid cardiac, neurologic, or respiratory changes. It is necessary for the nurse to know the dosage rate that should be given IV to avoid a potentially fatal problem.

In IV infusion a larger amount of fluid is given, usually with adults, starting with 1 L. The solution flows by gravity from a graduated glass bottle or plastic bag through tubing, connecting tip, and needle or catheter into a vein, or it may be infused with an IV controller or pump.

The rate of replacement fluids with or without other additives by IV infusion may be regulated in one of two basic ways. One is by a simple *roller clamp* on the tubing, which can be manually adjusted to deliver the number of drops per minute that will provide the prescribed total amount over the prescribed time. Given the total volume of solution to be infused, the total number of minutes the solution is to be infused, and the drop factor (number of drops per milliliter that the tubing set-up delivers—a number that varies among tubing manufacturers and is found on the back of the tubing box), the prescribed drops per minute can be calculated and the set regulated by counting drops in the drip chamber of the tubing. See the formula for IV flow rate calculation discussed in Exercise 9 earlier in this chapter. Details of regulating by manual clamps, the most common mode, may be found in a basic nursing text such as Potter and Perry (1996); (see Bibliography.)

Another way that infusions can be made to run more precisely is by the use of instrumentation such as IV controllers and pumps. These can be used in situations that require more accurate titration of infusion fluids or nutrients than is provided by hand-adjusted roller clamps, which can allow up to a 5% error in flow rate within the first 15 minutes of flow and other variations thereafter. Most of the instrumentation to regulate infusions consists of various applications of either infusion controllers or infusion pumps. These small, boxlike devices are attached to IV poles. The infusion tubing is strung for regulation of rate to ensure automatic delivery of solutions at preselected rates or volumes. CAUTION: For instruments that can accommodate either macrodrip or microdrip tubing, the tubing must be appropriate for the drop factor used to calculate drop rate. A rate calculated on the basis of microdrip tubing but accidentally administered by macrodrip could seriously overdose or overhydrate a client.

Infusion controllers work simply by utilizing the force of gravity. Controllers are not capable of delivering rates with the accuracy of infusion pumps (which may be more useful in special situations in which rises in back pressure are transmitted to the fluid in the tubing; such is the situation in arterial infusions or when the client is a restless child or a woman in labor). However, unlike infusion pumps, IV controllers will not pump fluid into interstitial tissue if the infusion needle infiltrates. Controllers are useful in 80% to 85% of cases calling for intravenous therapy. There are many infusion pumps and controllers on the market, and manufacturers produce new models frequently.

Infusion pumps are of at least two kinds, both delivering infusion fluids under positive pressure: (1) nonvolumetric ("infusion pumps"), which measure fluid volume delivery by drop rate (not as accurate because drop volume may vary), and (2) volumetric ("volume pumps," which can measure very precisely even smaller volumes of infusion solution by milliliter per hour. This latter pump is especially useful for small children, total parenteral nutrition, and the administration of potent drugs by continuous IV infusion (such as streptokinase, dopamine, or nitroglycerin). Alarm readout messages (e.g., "fix me") may be displayed on the front panel of the instrument.

Similar instrumentation is made by several different manufacturers, which use various physical principles to sense pressures and amount of pump fluid and read out the flow-rate settings and the like. Their capabilities include greater accuracy than other modes of infusion delivery systems and alarms to warn of blocked tubing, air in the tubing, or empty solution containers. These features sound ideal but, like all mechanical devices, infusion pumps are subject to malfunction and therefore nurses need to be continually watchful to ensure reliability. They also need to maintain personal contact with the purpose of it all—the client. Currently there is a growing body of literature on this type of equipment. Its intricacy presents nurses with still another challenge, although not an insurmountable one. The reader is referred to the excellent references at the end of this chapter to learn more.

Infusions are most commonly given to relieve tissue dehydration, to restore depleted blood volumes, to dilute toxic substances in the blood and tissue fluids, to supply electrolytes or drugs, to provide an IV line if an emergency is anticipated, or to provide a fluid challenge to evaluate kidney function.

The fluid is usually given slowly to prevent a reaction or fluid overload, which may impair cardiac or pulmonary function, especially in elderly clients or those with cardiac disease. Ordinarily 8 hours are required for every 1000 ml of fluid, depending on the condition of the client and the nature of and reason for the solution. For children the rate will be slower and is determined by age, weight, and urinary output.

See Unit 19 for a discussion of various IV infusion solutions and parenteral nutrition, and Chapter 31 for a discussion of blood products.

A number of commercial solutions are used in IV replacement therapy. Some solutions contain not only salts of sodium and potassium but also salts of calcium and magnesium. Vitamins are also added to IV fluids when necessary.

Total parenteral nutrition (TPN) or hyperalimentation is the infusion of an individual's total basic nutritional need via an infusion catheter into a large central vein and/or into a peripheral one. The choice of site depends partly on the phlebitis-causing potential of the medium. Fat emulsions have a much lower potential for causing phlebitis than hypertonic dextrose solutions used for TPN.

Whole blood and blood products are likewise given intravenously to restore depleted blood volume as well as constituents of the blood. Blood products should be introduced through IV tubing that has been primed with a normal saline infusion solution rather than dextrose solution, which would cause "stickiness" of red blood cells, causing them to clump artificially, possibly clogging the needle or causing hemolysis. Insertion of an 18-gauge or larger needle when blood products are expected to be infused will help minimize trauma to blood cells. Tubing should also be of the sort that incorporates a filter to trap cell particles and clumped cells to prevent them from circulating or clogging the needle.

Some drugs, such as antibiotics, are administered by intermittent infusion (known as "IV piggyback" [IVPB] or "IV rider" in some parts of the United States). They are given via a setup that is secondary to the primary IV infusion and that is hung in tandem and connected to the primary setup.

Most intermittent diluted drug infusions are meant to have a total infusion time of 20 or 30 minutes to 1 hour, depending on factors such as the amount of diluent required and the potential for vein wall irritation by the drug.

The presence of particulate matter (which can consist of tiny chunks of rubber stoppers or glass slivers from ampules) in IV infusion solutions is disturbingly common. It can be introduced during manufacture, during changing of the solution bottle, or during administration of a medication. The resulting potential for phlebitis is high. It is recommended that in-line filtering devices be used for all IV therapy. Optimal filtration is provided by 0.22-μm filters; most organisms, except certain strains of *Pseudomonas* and the viruses, are filtered out by 0.45-μm in-line filters. To prevent injection of larger particles, disposable needles with 5-μm filters can be used to draw medication up.

Stainless steel scalp-vein needles ("butterfly needles") produce lower rates of infection and phlebitis, but plastic catheters (over-needle catheters) or cannulas (through-the-needle catheters) tend to decrease the incidence of infiltration and work best when an infusion needle will be in place for a long period (Figure 5-12). Advantages and disadvantages must be weighed at the time of insertion (Table 5-7).

Intravenous devices that are inserted only by a physician are the subclavian through-the-needle catheter and the Hickman catheter. The subclavian through-the-needle catheter (12 inches or 30 cm) is used when poor venous access prohibits the use of peripheral veins or when irritating solutions must be infused directly into a large central vein to avoid phlebitis. The Hickman catheter is implanted surgically and is used for long-term IV therapy.

Although starting infusions and drawing blood were traditionally the responsibility of physicians, most nurses today

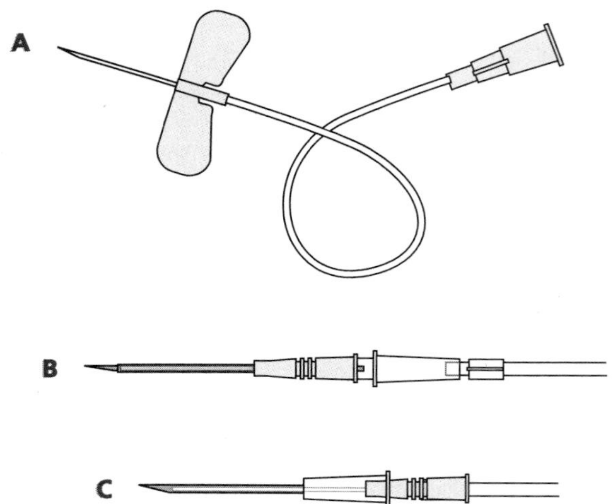

Figure 5-12 IV needles. **A**, Butterfly needle. **B**, Over-needle catheter. **C**, Cannula (through the needle catheter).

TABLE 5-7 Intravenous needles in common use by nurses

IV needle	Length of needle	Length of tubing	Indication
Wing-tip or scalp-vein needle (E-Z Set or butterfly	½ to 1¼ in (1.3 to 3.1 cm)	3 to 12 in (7.5 to 30 cm)	Client in stable condition; IV fluids or medications of short duration; intermittent IV push injections, indefinite period of time; pediatric scalp vein (see Figure 5-12)
Over-the-needle catheter (Abbocath, Jelco, or Angiocath)	Varies	1¼ to 5½ in (3.1 to 13.8 cm); 1¼ to 2 in (3.1 to 5 cm) most commonly used	Client in unstable condition (needs large volume replacement); only available veins are poor; caustic medications to be administered
Through-the-needle catheter (Intracath)	1½ to 2 in (3.8 to 5 cm)	8 to 36 in (20 to 90 cm)	Client has poor venous access; long-term IV therapy; extremely caustic medications (continuous chemotherapy, total parenteral nutrition)

perform these functions, especially in critical care areas. Probably one of the most effective approaches is the preparation of IV teams whose sole job is to maintain, remove, and replace IV needles, catheters, and so forth. However, such teams may prove to be a mixed blessing; even though they become very proficient at their job, they also may serve to further fragment a client's care.

Table 5-8 lists data to assess for IV needle site complications and suggests concomitant nursing interventions.

Epidural: Epidural analgesia is being used increasingly for the management of acute and chronic pain. For this route of drug administration, the physician implants an epidural catheter beneath the client's skin with its tip in the epidural space, which lies just outside the subarachnoid space in which cerebrospinal fluid (CSF) circulates. The drug diffuses into the CSF bypassing the blood-brain barrier. Narcotic analgesics such as morphine, fentanyl (Sublimaze), and hydromorphone (Dilaudid), administered either by IV bolus dose or by continuous infusion, work well because opiate receptors are found along the spinal cord allowing the drugs to produce localized analgesia without loss of motor function. Once the catheter is in place, the nurse is responsible for monitoring the infusion and the client's status relative to it.

Follow the manufacturer's instructions and your health care agency's policies to prepare the infusion device, checking the drug concentration and infusion rate against the prescriber's order. Ensure that the client understands the procedure and that an appropriate consent form has been completed. Assist with the epidural catheter insertion and label the tubing as "epidural infusion" to avoid confusion with other infusion lines in which drugs might be administered. To prevent migration of the catheter, tape it securely and monitor the symbols on the catheter that indicate length. Have oxygen, an intubation set, resuscitation equipment, naloxone (Narcan) 0.4 mg IV, and ephedrine 50 mg IV on hand for emergency use. The client should have peripheral IV access (IV infusion or heparin lock) to permit immediate access for the administration of emergency drugs. Instruct the client to report pain using a pain scale from 0 to 10; see Chapter 14, Analgesics, for the nursing management of pain.

Assess the client's respiratory rate and blood pressure every 2 hours for 8 hours, every 4 hours for 8 hours for the first 24 hours, and then once a shift according to the client's condition, or as prescribed. Notify the prescriber if the client's respiratory rate is less than 10/minute or if the systolic blood pressure is less than 90 mm Hg. Assess the client's level of sedation, mental status, and pain relief every hour initially until the client reports adequate pain control, then every 2 to 4 hours. Notify the prescriber if the client becomes extremely drowsy or experiences other adverse effects such as nausea and vomiting, pruritus, urinary retention, or unrelieved pain. Assess lower extremity strength and sensation every 2 to 4 hours. If deficits occur, the dosage may need to be decreased. Because drugs administered by the epidural route diffuse slowly, monitor the client for adverse effects for 12 hours after the infusion has been discontinued.

Change the dressing over the catheter site every 24 to 48 hours, and the infusion tubing every 48 hours or as needed, or according to the health care agency's policies. Observe the catheter insertion site for redness and swelling. Minimize headache as a complication by having the client lie flat and maintain an adequate fluid intake. If epidural analgesia is to

TABLE 5-8 Common intravenous needle site complications

Needle site data	Infiltration	Clot over needle opening or obstruction	Phlebitis	Infection at site of needle insertion
Color	Pale	No change	Red	Red over site
Temperature	Cool to cold	No change	Warm to hot	Warm at site
Swelling	Rounded	None	Cordlike vein path	Small amount at site
Pain	Yes, usually	None	Yes	None usually
Flow	Slowed or stopped	Slowed or stopped	No change or may be slowed	No change
Nursing actions	Tourniquet proximally (flow continues—infiltration) Lower bottle (blood in tubing—no infiltration Discontinue IV Restart IV at another site or call IV team	Check for infiltration Reposition arm Raise IV container, close clamp, coil tubing, release quickly Restart IV at another site or call IV team	Discontinue IV *usually* Contact prescriber Resite IV to another area/call IV team Note irritating solution (Valuim, Keflin, KCl running too fast) Warm compresses; elevate and immobilize part	Do not discontinue IV until IV team advice has been sought or physician has been notified (it may be the only vein available for essential infusion)

be used at home, the client/caregiver must be willing and capable of managing the therapy. Alcohol and street drug use must be avoided by the client as these substances potentiate the effects of the opiates.

Intrathecal. Intrathecal (into a sheath) injection is also known as intraspinal, subdural, subarachnoid, or lumbar injection. The technique is the same as that required for a lumbar puncture. Nurses do not usually directly administer drugs intraspinally. However, filling the drug reservoir of an implanted intraspinal delivery system may be required. The nurse needs to be specially trained, and the manufacturer's instructions should be followed closely.

■ ■ ■

In addition, drugs are occasionally administered by intracardiac, intrapericardiac, intraventricular, intraperitoneal, intraarticular, and intraosseous injections; however, state regulation and institutional policy may not allow nurses to administer drugs by these routes.

Special situations

Swallowing difficulty. The following suggestions are for clients who have difficulty swallowing oral medications. If the cause is a diminished swallow reflex, however, the drug should be given by another route after consultation with the prescriber.

1. Have the client drink some water *just before* taking the medication and drink only a small amount *with* the medication. After the drug, at least 240 ml of liquid should be taken. Clients are capable of taking fluids more easily if they are in Fowler's position (upright sitting position).
2. Instruct the client to place the tablet at the midpoint of the tongue and toss it back to the throat with the water. For the hemiplegic client, place the tablet on the unaffected side of the tongue for swallowing.

If the head is tipped slightly forward, the act of swallowing follows more naturally; choking is more likely when the head is tilted back. Initiation of the mechanical act of swallowing may be facilitated by massaging the laryngeal prominence (Adam's apple) or the area just under the chin.

Medications may be crushed, except enteric-coated or sustained-action forms (Box 5-4 lists medications that should not be crushed), or capsules may be opened and contents sprinkled on a small portion of easy-to-swallow food such as applesauce or a gelatin dessert. The client should be told about this procedure and instructed to eat the medicated contents first so that very little remains unadministered if the rest is refused. This approach should be used cautiously on children because the particular food may be rendered distasteful and be rejected by the child in the future.

Medications may be liquefied for drinking by the addition of water, or they may be administered by instillation into the mouth next to the cheek by a large syringe with or without a short tubing attached.

Suggestions for clients with a tracheostomy tube in place. The tube should have a cuff, and it should be inflated whenever any substance is taken by mouth, in order to prevent it from accidentally entering the lungs. If there is an

BOX 5-4

Medications That Should Not Be Crushed

The following is a partial listing of drugs that should not be crushed.* Whenever possible, it is suggested that if a liquid dosage form of the medication is available, it should be used instead of a crushed tablet. Coated tablets generally should not be crushed because the coating was applied for a specific reason, such as (1) to prevent stomach irritation (e.g., Dulcolax Tablet); (2) to prevent destruction by stomach acids (e.g., Ananase); (3) to produce a prolonged or extended effect (e.g., Dimetapp); or (4) to avoid an unwanted reaction (e.g., chloral hydrate in capsule has a very bitter taste and Povan tablet will stain the mouth red; Kaon tablets may produce a burning effect on sensitive mucosa).

Afrinol Repetabs	Diamox Sequel	Feosol Spansule	Quinaglute Duratab
Allerest Capsule	Donnatol Extentab	Ferro Grad-500 Tab	Quinidex Extentab
Aminodur Duratab	Drixoral tablet	Inderal LA	Slow K tablet
Artane Sequel	Dulcolax tablet	Isordil Sublingual	Sudafed SA Capsule
ASA Enseals	Ecotrin tablet	Kaon tablet	Theo-Dur tablet
Azulfadine Entab	E-Mycin tablet	Nitroglycerin tab	Teldrin Capsule
Betaphen-VK	Entozyme tablet	Nitrospan capsule	Trental
Compazine Spansule	Feosol tablet	Ornade Spansule	

Although pharmaceutical manufacturers develop new drugs and reformulate existing ones, some common terms attached to a drug name may indicate a sustained-release form of a drug which should not be crushed.

Bid: Lithobid, Pavabid
Dur: K-Dur, Theo-Dur
LA (long-acting): Inderal LA, Inderide LA
SA (sustained-action): Peritrate SA
SR (sustained-release): Pronestyl SR, Ritalin SR (*USP DI*, 1995)

*From Mitchell and Pawlicki, 1992.

external attachment in place to allow the client to talk, a T-piece should be substituted. After the medication has been swallowed, the cuff is deflated after suctioning is performed.

Suggestions for administering medications to clients with a nasogastric (NG) or gastrostomy tube. Follow the procedure for administering tube feedings, with these additional precautions:

1. Check placement of the tube before giving medications or tube feedings.
2. Give medications and tube feedings at separate intervals to avoid potential drug-food interactions.
3. Assess for potential drug-food interactions (penicillin G and most tetracyclines) if you must administer drugs with a feeding, just as you would with any oral drugs. Also administer medications before the tube feeding.
4. Check with the pharmacy for availability of liquid preparations of the client's medications. Liquids are always preferable to crushing tablets, but if tablets must be crushed, flush the tubing before and after the medication to prevent the drug from sticking to the inside of the tube. See Box 5-4 for cautions about tablet crushing.
5. Afterward, position the client upright and turned slightly to the left if the medication is for local effect in the stomach (e.g., antacids), and have the client remain there for a time.

Alternative Drug Delivery Systems

Innovative advances in scientific technology and computerization provide impetus for the development of increasingly sophisticated drug delivery systems, particularly in the treatment of diabetes mellitus and cancer. Some examples of these technologies include implanted drug deposits and needle-syringe pump assemblies.

Implanted capsules of a progestin hormone, called the Norplant method, are being used for contraceptive efficacy. Implantation takes 15 minutes and is immediately effective. Contraceptive effects are said to last 5 to 7 years.

Small pumps weighing about half a pound are now available as portable infusion systems for continuous drug treatment of certain clients with type I diabetes or cancer. The systems currently approved and in use usually consist of a battery, a programmable electronic "brain," an electric motor and pump, and a syringe, all of which are detachable as a unit from the small needle kept in place either in subcutaneous abdominal or thigh tissue (for diabetes), or by Silastic catheter inserted into an artery supplying the malignant tumor. These programmable pumps allow for various flow rates and have an on-off feature. For clients with varying clinical needs such a device appears to be quite efficient. Some systems are designed to be worn externally over clothing, stored in a pocket, or suspended from a belt or a neck chain (Figures 5-13 and 5-14). See also Figure 5-15 for Sof-set cannula procedure.

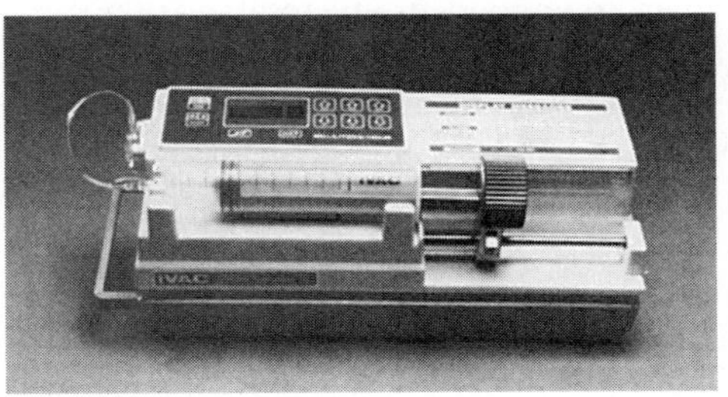

Figure 5-13 Microcomputer-controlled larger-volume syringe pump for use when medication or fluids of up to 50 ml need to be administered with accuracy and at a constant rate.

Preventing and Reporting Errors

It may help to be aware of some of the pitfalls with regard to medication administration. Box 5-5 recounts actual errors related to medication administration to call attention to some common but careless nursing acts.

To prevent errors in medication administration as described in Box 5-5, follow the recommended guidelines presented on pp. 79-80. Refuse to allow the administration of a drug against good nursing judgment. Mistakes seem to breed other errors. It is axiomatic that when one thing goes wrong in a client's care, other mishaps generally follow. No one knows why. Stay alert! Question! Learn!

Drug-related malpractice in the United States accounts for approximately 10% of all cases (Trout, 1991). Most successful litigation against nurses concerns the administration of medications. Although there are many types of medication errors, such as omission, unauthorized dose, wrong dose, wrong route, wrong rate, wrong dosage form, wrong time, wrong preparation of a dose, and incorrect administration technique, wrong dosage heads the list. Many computer programs for updating dosage calculation skills now exist,

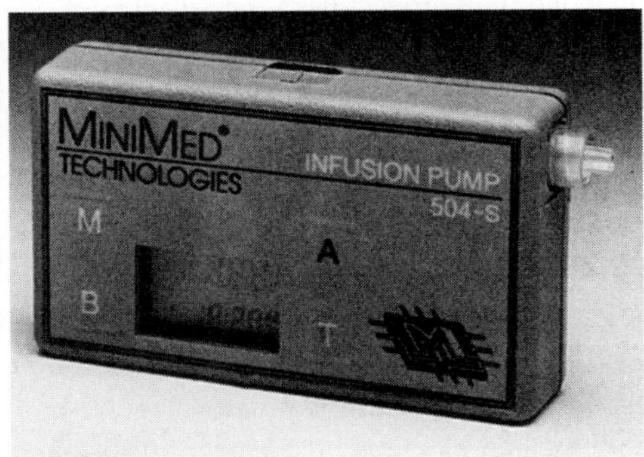

Figure 5-14 MiniMed Insulin Syringe. This pump (Infusion Pump 504-S) is one of the smallest and lightest available—it weighs only 3.1 ounces. The pump is easy to wear under clothing, carry in pockets, or attach to belts. Its features include a water-resistant package, long battery life (monthly change of batteries), and an alarm system to warn the user of an occlusion, an empty syringe, a runaway infusion, or a low or depleted battery. The unit can be programmed for four basal variation rates in 24 hours, thus providing flexibility for the user. A 24-hour hotline is available to answer any questions on diabetes and the pump battery. (Courtesy MiniMed Technologies, Sylmar, California.)

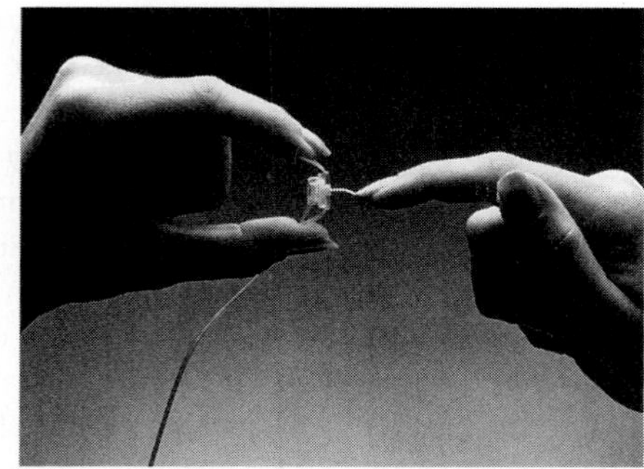

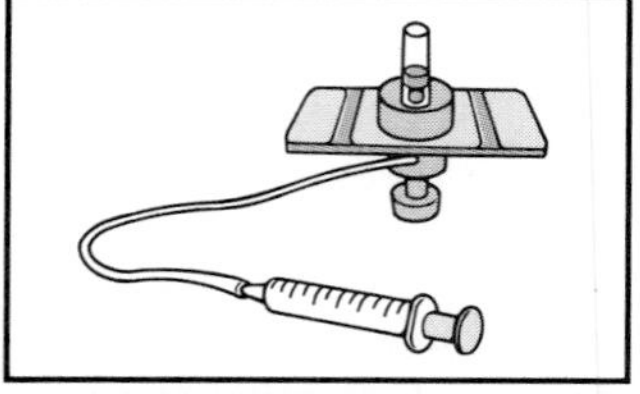

1. Fill syringe and Sof-set™

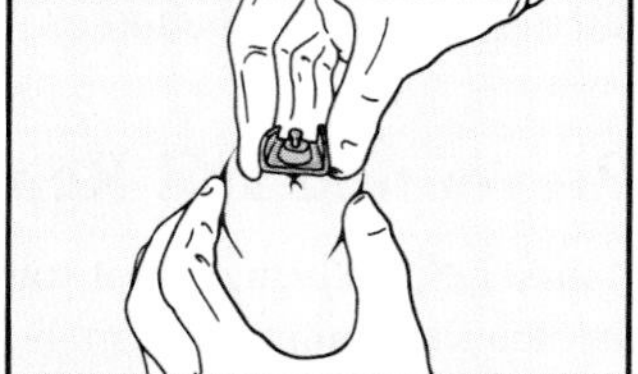

2. Cleanse and pinch skin

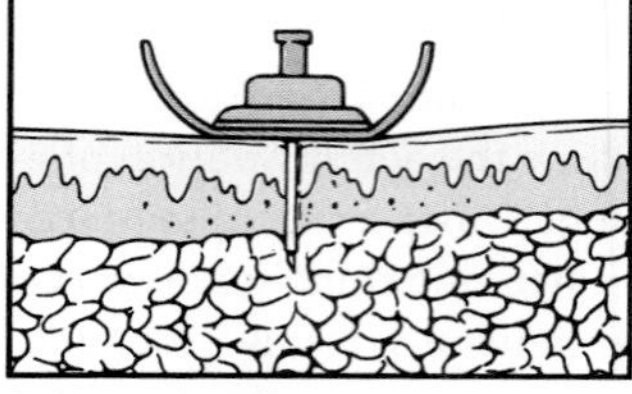

3. Insert needle

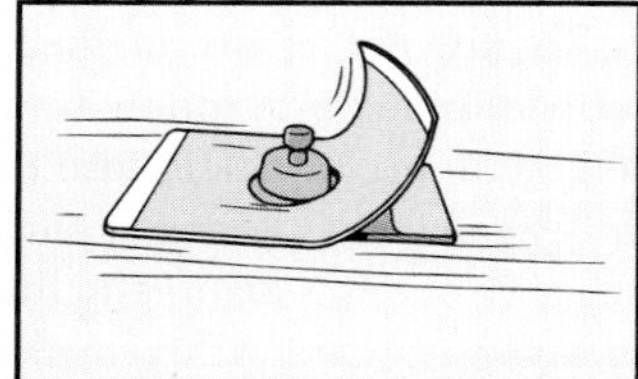

4. Place tape over Sof-set™

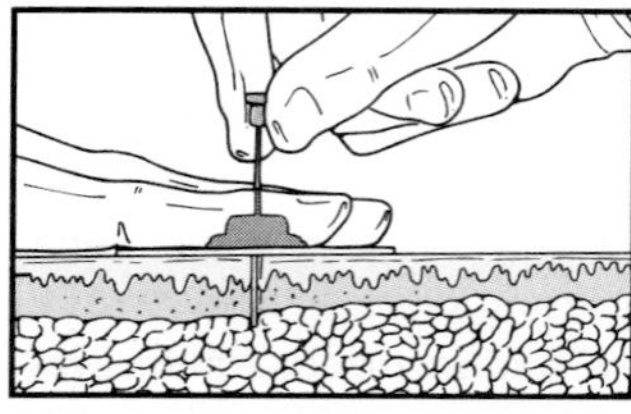

5. Remove introducer needle

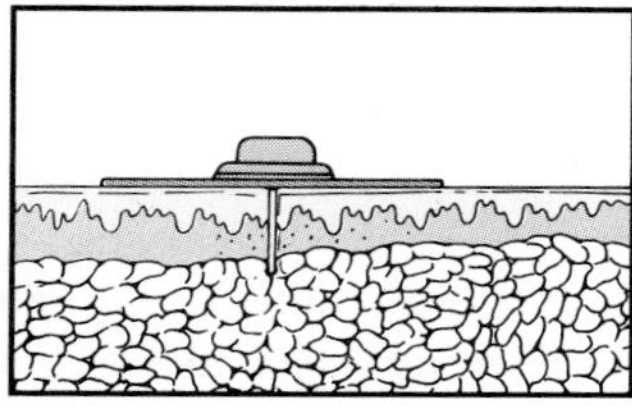

6. Begin pumping

Figure 5-15 Sof-set, a soft teflon cannula and tubing that is inserted by needle, which is then withdrawn so the pump can operate without one. This product has a special adhesive dressing that inhibits bacterial growth. (Courtesy MiniMed Technologies, Sylmar, California.)

and more are on the way. Innumerable helpful instructional materials, including programmed learning texts, are available; some are listed at the end of the chapter. All personnel who as part of their jobs must calculate dosages should be alert for gaps in their mathematical competence. To double-check calculations with others when uncertain and to maintain proficiency by practice are practical, professionally necessary actions.

To err is human. However, to admit the possibility of error and one's susceptibility is essential. To safeguard one's client as well as one's reputation and psyche, the first step in a suspected medication error is to backtrack to double-check one's actions or computations to see if an error occurred. Next is the step requiring the most accountability: to consult one's instructor or superior to inform him or her and to gain perspective and objective support. The client's prescriber should also be informed. Actions to correct drug effects and to normalize the client's condition follow. Precise, objective documentation of the event and the circumstances is made both on the chart and on a special form called the incident report. This report is an intraagency communication that is analyzed by the agency's risk management personnel to develop procedures for preventing the same or similar incidents.

Monitoring

Although evaluation is considered to be the final step of the nursing process, this text presents within the implementation activities of the nursing process related to drug therapy a cluster of nursing actions to be included in monitoring the client for therapeutic effect and the occurrence of adverse drug reactions. Given that approximately 30% of hospitalized clients experience an adverse drug reaction and that as many as 1.5 million persons are hospitalized because of an adverse drug reaction, this monitoring takes on additional importance. These adverse reactions might be related to an underlying condition of the client (medical condition, age, child-bearing status), other drugs that the client might be taking, and side and/or adverse effects of the drug itself.

BOX 5-5

Errors in Medication Administration

1. Not knowing why a medication was to be administered caused one nurse to irrigate a client's bladder with a topical astringent-antiinflammatory agent, Burow's solution, instead of the genitourinary antibiotic irrigant distributed by a manufacturer of a similar name. In another instance this caused another nurse to delay giving a dose of medication essential to recuperation after cancer chemotherapy because she believed it to be "just a vitamin" instead of folinic acid.
2. Not identifying clients by their arm bands caused several nurses to give medication to the wrong individual in the right beds. One of the nurses even asked a client his name, which turned out to be similar to another client's. One nurse called out her client's name, and the wrong person responded. The result was the same—they all got the wrong medication.
3. Not checking with the prescriber caused one nurse to give her client 30 ml of milk of magnesia every hour rather than every night because she misinterpreted the "qn" (an unacceptable abbreviation) order for "qh." Another nurse gave 2.5 mg of digoxin instead of 0.25 mg; although the order was wrong, the nurse did not recognize that it was excessive. The result was that the client received a toxic dose of medication.

O'Donnell (1992) divides these reactions into two broad categories. The first of these, type A, has predictability; if you know the drug's properties, you have a fair idea of the type of reaction that may occur. Most of these reactions relate to the mechanism of action of the drug and often they are dose-dependent. Examples of Type A reactions are the orthostatic hypotension with volume depletion that can occur with furosemide (Lasix), a powerful diuretic, or the overgrowth of nonsusceptible organisms that can occur with ampicillin, an antibiotic. Type B reactions are not as predictable as Type A reactions. Anaphylaxis is a classic example of a Type B reaction; it is unusual, unexpected, life-threatening, and occurs even when a normal therapeutic dose is administered.

Early recognition of adverse drug reactions is important so that therapy can be altered as quickly as possible to prevent or minimize injury to the client, by decreasing the dosage or discontinuing the drug, administering an antidote or symptomatic treatment, or both. In addition, other caregivers should be alerted by the nurse documenting the reaction in the clinical records and advising the client to alert future caregivers and carry a card or wear a bracelet warning others that the client has had an adverse reaction to a specific drug.

The nurse should be alert for adverse drug effects if the client evidences clinical or laboratory findings that are not typical of the client's disease, if a pathologic sign or symptom occurs at a site that is not involved with the condition being treated, or if a pathologic process occurs that is not in keeping with the condition being treated. If the client exhibits any of these, the nurse should review the medication record to see if the signs and symptoms are related to one or more of the client's drugs. Issues to be considered in determining causality are: (1) *temporal relationship* (Did the reaction occur at a reasonable time after the drug was administered?); (2) presence of a positive *dechallenge* (Did the client's reaction diminish or resolve after the drug was discontinued?); (3) presence of a positive *rechallenge* (Did the client's reaction return when the drug was administered again?); and (4) lack of a confounding effect (Can the reaction be explained by a concurrently administered drug or the client's clinical condition?).

Therapeutic drug monitoring requires that the nurse understand the mechanism of action of the drug in relation to the client's health status in order to clinically determine whether the drug is effective. Clinical indicators should be monitored at appropriate intervals to assess drug efficacy. For example, in an acute asthmatic episode, the nurse would monitor vital signs, breath sounds, skin color, sputum, and signs of respiratory dysfunction, such as irritability, stridor, nasal flaring, and retractions. If a $beta_2$ agonist drug administered as a bronchodilator were to be evaluated as effective, the respiratory and pulse rate would decrease towards a more normal rate; the client would experience less wheezing and irritability, be more relaxed, and expend less effort with the respiratory process. Other signs of respiratory dysfunction would also diminish within minutes. However, with a client who is not actively bleeding, the hemoglobin concentration should increase by approximately 0.1 g/dl daily within 2 weeks after starting oral iron therapy for iron deficiency anemia.

Therapeutic drug monitoring may entail determining blood drug levels to determine effective drug dosages and to prevent adverse effects related to toxicity. This is particularly important with drugs such as cardiotonics, anticonvulsants, and others, in which the margin of safety within the therapeutic range is narrow. Blood samples may be taken at the drug's peak level (the highest concentration) and/or at the trough/residual level (the lowest concentration) after a steady state of the drug has been reached in the client. Steady state is generally reached after 4 to 5 half-lives of a drug. Peak levels are useful when testing for toxicity, and trough levels are useful to demonstrate a satisfactory therapeutic level. Different laboratories use different units for reporting test results and normal ranges.

Some drugs have organ- or system-specific adverse or toxic effects, or potential complications, to which the nurse can be particularly alert. For example, clients receiving drugs having the potential complication of hepatotoxicity need to be monitored for symptoms of hepatic dysfunction such as anorexia, indigestion, malaise, jaundice, petechiae, ecchymoses, dark urine, clay-colored stools, and increased bleeding tendencies. There is little evidence that drug-induced liver damage can be diagnosed routinely by performing frequent liver function studies before symptoms develop (AMA, 1995). However, liver function tests (serum bilirubin, alkaline phosphatase [ALP], alanine aminotransferase [ALT or SGPT], lactic dehydrogenase [LDH]) or a prothrombin time test may be ordered as part of a baseline assessment before the drug regimen is started or if clinical symptoms of hepatic dysfunction appear.

On the other hand, drug-induced nephrotoxicity usually develops subtly and kidney damage may occur before symptoms such as insufficient urine output (>30 ml/hr), elevated blood pressure, and dependent edema, are evident. In this case, when a nephrotoxic drug is given in higher doses or for prolonged periods of time, routine urinalyses and serum creatinine determinations are helpful in early detection of toxicity.

The nurse needs to remain vigilant in the ongoing monitoring of the client's health status by direct observation, and evaluation of laboratory and diagnostic tests in relation to drug therapy.

Client Teaching

Updating clients and keeping them informed about their treatment and providing other necessary information should be an ongoing activity that occurs naturally during any interaction with clients. Teaching should be a part of the plan in any nursing process. It may be a formal plan (e.g., a diabetic teaching program), or it may be a simple impromptu discussion based on a question the client raises.

Although teaching-learning interactions between client and nurse are among the most necessary and professionally demanding, teaching clients is not as visible as bathing them, taking their vital signs, or giving them injections. When it is done, it may not be seen important enough to be noted in nursing progress notes. However, successful client learning has a direct bearing on successful convalescence at home. A strong rationale for teaching clients comes from the many state nurse practice acts that define teaching as a necessary part of nursing, thereby giving it the power of a state mandate: one could be sued for not teaching clients. Accreditation agencies recognize the importance of client teaching and look for documentation during their inspection visits when evaluating agencies that provide health care.

Clients need to learn the following about their medications: the names of the medications (write them down), what they are for and how to recognize the proper effects (in very specific ways), some of the major secondary effects (expected and tolerable, and those representing toxicity), what to do if they miss a dose, how to store the medication, how to take it (e.g., with meals), and whom to call if there is a problem. Clients can be expected to forget many of the instructions; a printed fact sheet or checklist to take home will be helpful to many clients and should augment the verbal explanation. Chapter 10, Client Teaching for Self-Administration of Medications, discusses this essential role of nursing in greater detail.

Recording Drug Administration

Recording the administration of each dose of medication as soon as possible after it is given provides a documented record if there is any question as to whether the client received the dose. Otherwise the client may inadvertently receive a second dose from another nurse or nursing student. The busy nurse who "double-pours" (prepares two doses at one time—a "sloppy" practice) may also be tempted to record the second dose at the same time the first dose is recorded. Medications should not be recorded (charted) before they are actually given because something may come up to prevent that dose from being administered. Then the medication record, which is a legal document, will have to be corrected carefully and perhaps an incident report filed.

Several different forms are used to record medications for each client. These forms usually include areas to note each medication's name, date, dose, route, time of administration, and the administering nurse's initials (see Figure 5-1). Extra notations may be added in certain instances. For example, when digitalis is given, the apical and radial pulses taken just before administration may be noted ("AP, 78; RP, 76"). If the pulses are found to be outside the normal limits established by that agency, the medication should not be given, the record should be marked "held" and initialed, and the prescriber should be consulted. Clients also have the right to refuse treatment, including medications, and sometimes do, despite explanations. "Refused" is then noted in the appropriate spot on the medication record, with the reason for the client's refusal. Medication may also be recorded as "discarded" or "wasted" if only part of it was administered and the rest had to be discarded (as in a prefilled syringe), or if the medication was dropped or contaminated. If the medication is a controlled substance, its reason for disposal must be documented and fully witnessed with the signatures of two nurses required on the narcotic record.

Routine (or continuous) daily medications are recorded on the MAR. Once-only, loading doses, prn medications, and stat medications should be recorded on the same MAR. Administration of a controlled substance is recorded both on the MAR and on that particular drug's control sheet in the "narcotic book", which includes a running tally of the balance of the controlled substance. A notation is usually made in the progress notes on the client's chart relating to the assessment of the need for the administration of any prn medication and the client's response (noted in an hour or so) as to its effects.

Potential for error in drug administration is almost limitless. Some significant mistakes can be rectified if discovered and acted on quickly. Also, if an error is properly reported and appropriate actions are taken, courts tend to look more kindly on the nurse than if these were not done. Courts generally recognize that nurses are human and that there is potential for error in clinical practice.

Evaluation

Evaluation is the final step in the nursing process, which facilitates the delivery of high-quality nursing care in regard to pharmacotherapeutics. While planning nursing care and establishing goals, the nurse determines what kind of evaluation will take place and when and how it will be done. Clear and specifically stated goals or outcome criteria make it easy to determine whether the intended outcomes have been achieved, or to what degree they have been achieved. Evaluation includes both subjective and objective data. When evaluating the nursing care for a client undergoing drug therapy, the nurse looks at the outcome criteria for the specific nursing diagnoses/collaborative problems. But in general an evaluation of drug therapy includes the following areas:

1. Therapeutic response to the drug
2. Nontherapeutic responses to the drug, such as side effects, or adverse reactions related to the administered drug itself, the client's health status, or concurrent drug therapy
3. Level of client's knowledge related to the medication regimen
4. The client's ability to manage the therapeutic regimen (self-medication)

In evaluating therapeutic response, the nurse must have a clear understanding of the therapeutic goals. Evaluation may center on a reduction of symptoms, decreased frequency of attacks, enhanced organ function, elimination of infection, or a multitude of other goals. Clinical observation of the client as well as monitoring of appropriate laboratory studies is essential. Evaluation examines a drug's therapeutic response, but it is also directed toward detection of *any* response that may be attributed to the drug. The outcome criteria to be evaluated may also relate to the absence of any adverse side effects or adverse reactions. An awareness of the pharmacology of the drug used and any potential effects guides this evaluation. For example, outcome criteria related to the therapeutic response for the anticonvulsant phenytoin (Dilantin) would be that the client will demonstrate: (1) an absence of or decrease in the frequency or severity of seizures; (2) therapeutic serum levels of the drug; and (3) an absence of side effects/adverse reactions such as ataxia, slurred speech, mental confusion, drowsiness, nystagmus, diplopia, or gingival hyperplasia.

The nurse will have to determine if educational goals are being met. Often, clients can report back what they have been told yet be unable to apply this knowledge. Asking hypothetical questions and observing return demonstrations are helpful techniques for evaluating learning. Examples of outcome criteria for client teaching are:

The client will:

State the effect of each drug.

Identify at least three adverse reactions to the drug for which consultation should be immediately sought with the prescriber or other health care professional.

Demonstrate any monitoring techniques associated with the drug, for example, daily weights, pulse, and blood pressure measurements.

In addition, the nurse needs to evaluate whether the client can effectively manage the therapeutic medication regimen in the home environment. This means that in addition to the outcome criteria given above for the educational goals, the client will:

Describe in his or her own words an appropriate description of the condition for which the drug was prescribed

Describe the relationship between drug regimen and health condition

Explain the importance of taking the prescribed drug as ordered

Describe the difference between adverse reactions to the drug and the signs and symptoms of health condition

Identify signs and symptoms of either adverse reactions of the drug and/or the health condition that need to be reported to the prescriber or other health professional

Demonstrate the safe and accurate self-administration of the drug

Effective management of the therapeutic regimen refers to following the prescribed regimen correctly. The inability to accomplish any of the above mentioned outcome criteria would indicate ineffective management of the therapeutic regimen. Other behaviors might also be indicators. Does the client or family/caregiver continue to speak of nonparticipation in the regimen, have partially used or unused prescriptions been observed, or is there persistence or progression of the underlying condition given that the regimen prescribed is an appropriate one? Have undesired effects of the drug gone unreported to the health care provider? Research indicates that at least one fourth of all outpatients fail to follow prescribed drug therapy correctly.

In addition to the evaluation by the individual nurse or nursing team of the client's progress toward the goals and expected outcomes of nursing care, health care agencies also evaluate the process of medication administration, in general, as an important aspect of nursing care provided by that agency. Standards by which to evaluate care are developed from within the health care organization and may also be suggested by external organizations. The Joint Commission on Accreditation of Healthcare Organizations (JCAHO) is an organization that offers voluntary accreditation to health care agencies throughout the United States based on standards that are "recognized as representing a contemporary national consensus on quality patient care that reflects changing health care practices and current health care delivery trends" (JCAHO, 1990). Within the JCAHO standards for nursing services regarding policies and procedures, guidelines are set forth concerning medication administration in an effort to ensure safe nursing practice. They stipulate that the nursing department or service of a health care organization have policies and procedures to govern medication administration, and that these "should specify, in accordance with applicable law and regulation and pertinent medical staff rules and regulations, who may give orders for drugs; who may accept verbal orders for drugs and when the orders must be authenticated by the prescribing practitioner; who may verify orders for drugs and how this must occur; who may supervise the administration of medications; and who may administer these medications, which medications they may administer, and how these individuals are to be supervised, if necessary (JCAHO, 1986). These policies and procedures serve to protect both client and nurse by stating the roles and responsibilities of all the members of the health care team for the administration of medications. Nursing practice can then be evaluated to determine whether the care provided to clients was in keeping with the agency's policies and procedures.

The following are suggested indicators for evaluating the administration of medications as part of the nursing quality assurance process, which may also be known as Total Quality Management (TQM) or Continuous Quality Improvement (CQI).

1. The drug is administered in the ordered dose.
2. The drug is administered by the ordered route.
3. The drug is administered by the ordered site.
4. The drug is administered at the ordered rate.
5. The drug is administered in the ordered drug form.
6. The drug is administered by the ordered schedule.
7. The drug is administered using the correct technique.

These indicators may be incorporated into a process of monitoring and evaluation by which nursing professionals examine the care they provide, determine possibilities for improvement of their practice, and take necessary action.

SUMMARY

The implementation phase of the nursing process with regard to drug therapy begins when the nurse acts to attain the goals established as described in Chapter 4. Nursing interventions are directed at the actual administration of drugs, which includes the preparatory steps as well as the subsequent recording of drug administration.

The traditional Five Rights—to ensure the right client, the right medication, the right route, the right dose, and the right time—continue to be reliable criteria for competent, safe, and individualized medication administration. So that nurses who are eager to provide high-quality care might have some of their penetrating questions answered, some of the theoretical bases for selection of drug dosages and dosing intervals have been included in this chapter. Examples have been presented of typical kinds of dosage calculations that sometimes challenge nurses, even ones who have been practicing for a long time. Answers and explanations have also been included. Common drug routes and sites have been detailed and illustrated.

Evaluation of nursing functions in medication administration includes a critique of one's own techniques, but it is not limited to that. The environment should be made conducive to high-quality care by the nurse's efforts toward thoughtful and safe medication administration. Enough time must be set aside, and double-checking of calculations should be routine. Careful identification of clients is essential to ensure that the right person receives the medication as intended. Because nurses are in the position of being on the client care scene and of taking care of clients as no one else does, they are uniquely placed to detect even subtle secondary drug effects, interactions, or incompatibilities.

Prevention of errors in medication administration is crucially important to nurses because it is an area fraught with much potential for irreversible harm to clients. Alert attention to all the details of medication administration, including client comments, must be maintained so that safety is not compromised and clients obtain the most beneficial effects of their drug therapy. Recording a drug dose is the final act of communication; it signifies that the drug was given and assures accountability by the nurse who "signs for it."

In short, the actual act of administering medications—the implementation or intervention phase of the nursing process—demands a solid knowledge base, well-practiced skills, commitment to continuous learning, and intense, unremitting concentration to sustain the best interests of the client. Potential for error is rife; medication administration cannot be a casual act or the risk will escalate.

Evaluation of therapeutic effects, secondary effects, effective management of the prescribed regimen, and client learning follows the implementation phase of the nursing process. It allows the nurse to determine if goals were met and measures the effectiveness of nursing care.

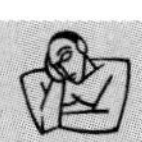

Critical Thinking

1. As a student what restrictions are placed upon your role in the administration of medications? How will you respond to a prescriber who gives you a verbal order for a medication at the client's bedside?
2. You are preparing a client medication with which you are not familiar. After searching through the drug references on the unit, information about the drug cannot be found. What actions should be taken?
3. A hospitalized client expresses curiosity after observing that his medications are administered "in little packages" rather than the "child-proof" containers that he is used to receiving from his pharmacy. How would you compare the advantages and disadvantages of the medication delivery systems for your client?
4. If one of the adverse effects of the drug you were administering was bone marrow depression, what laboratory results would you monitor to evaluate your client's drug therapy?

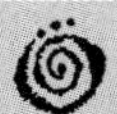

Collaborative Learning Activities

1. Have the students complete a nursing care plan based on the analysis of the drug history that they completed as part of the Chapter 4 collaborative learning activities. Limit the care plan to the three nursing diagnoses of highest priority given the specific client and the client's drug therapy. An evaluation of the client's drug therapy according to the planned outcome criteria should be included.

BIBLIOGRAPHY

American Medical Association (1995). *Drug evaluations: Annual 1995.* Chicago: The Association.

Anderson KN, et al. (Eds.) (1994). *Mosby's medical, nursing, & allied health dictionary* (4th ed.). St Louis: Mosby.

Carpenito LJ (1995). *Nursing diagnosis: Application to clinical practice* (6th ed.). Philadelphia: JB Lippincott.

Cohen MR (1993). What you said about the apothecary system, *Nursing* 23(7):56-8.

Hardman JG & Limbird LE (1996). *Goodman & Gilman's the pharmacological basis of therapeutics* (8th ed.). New York: McGraw Hill.

Hicks W (1995). Taking the right approach to a drug error, *Nursing* 25(3):72.

Joint Commission on Accreditation of Healthcare Organizations (1990). *Committed to quality: An introduction to the joint accreditation of Healthcare Organizations.* Oakbrook Terrace, IL: The Commission.

Joint Commission on Accreditation of Hospitals (1986). *A guide to JCAH nursing services standards.* Chicago: The Commission.

Lilley LL & Guanci R (1994). Getting back to basics, *Amer J Nurs* 94(9):15-6.

Loeb S (Ed.) (1993). *Giving drugs by advanced techniques.* Springhouse, PA: Springhouse.

Medication errors: Help new nurses avoid making errors. (1993). *Nursing* 23(3):66.

Mitchell JF & Pawlicki KS (1992). Oral dosage forms that should not be crushed: 1992 revision, *Hosp Pharm* 27(8):690.

National Bureau of Standards, US Department of Commerce (1977). *The international system of units (SI).* Special Pub No 330.

O'Donnell J (1992). Understanding adverse drug reactions, *Nursing* 22(12):48.

Potter PA & Perry AG (1997). *Fundamentals of nursing: Concepts, process and practice.* (4th ed.). St Louis: Mosby.

Chapter 6

Cultural and Psychologic Aspects of Drug Therapy

Chapter Focus

Health beliefs and treatment outcome are strongly influenced by a client's cultural background, ethnic practices, psychologic beliefs, and traditions. Effective caring for clients from different cultural groups requires an understanding of the predominant ethnic-specific influences and an assessment of the individual client to determine how those cultural influences affect health needs. Because nearly 2000 cultures and subcultures exist, it is impossible for the nurse to have a working knowledge of all of them. Instead, nurses and other health care professionals should study the predominant cultural groups in their communities. This chapter will focus on some health beliefs and practices related to pharmacology. The following objectives and key terms are necessary for a good understanding of this chapter.

Key Terms

cultural background (p. 100)
health beliefs (p. 100)
placebo (p. 109)

Objectives

1. Discuss the influence of culture and psychologic beliefs on drug therapy.
2. Discuss on a symbolic level what drugs mean to clients.
3. Identify situations in which placebos are appropriately used.
4. Differentiate between the advantages and disadvantages of self-treatment using nonprescription medication.

The **cultural background** of a client, the set of learned values, beliefs, customs, and behavior of the client, influences health beliefs and various practices that relate to pharmacology. **Health beliefs** are perceptions of susceptibility to disease or condition, the consequences of contracting the disease or condition, the benefits of care and barriers to preventive behavior, and the internal or external stimuli that result in appropriate health behavior by the person. Health beliefs of an individual influence their management and response to their drug therapy. Some similarities exist across cultures in the way the use of drugs is perceived; a primary goal of the appropriate use of medications is to achieve optimal health. Although most individuals share common views regarding life patterns, significant differences occur in values, beliefs, and attitudes. Clients bring to health settings cultural and psychologic differences in perceptions of masculine and feminine roles, in rural and urban backgrounds, in ethnic groups, and in social classes that influence drug use. The literature from transcultural nursing and anthropology (see Bibliography) provides valuable insights into various health care beliefs and practices.

In addition, there is a fundamental difference between the health beliefs of health care providers and clients. Although each person enters the health professions with culture-bound definitions of health and illness, these ideas change as the person is socialized into the "health care provider culture." A schism is then created between the provider and the recipient of health care. Only if providers become more sensitive to the traditional health beliefs and practices of clients can comprehensive and appropriate health care be provided (Spector, 1991).

Increased cultural awareness is of even greater importance when the demographic changes occurring in North America are considered. According to the 1990 census, Whites comprised 80.3% of the population. The ethnic/racial minorities constituted 16.8% of the population in 1980 and 19.7% in 1990. The distribution of those minorities by percentage are: Black, 12%; Spanish origin, 8.9%; Asian and Pacific Islander, 2.9%; American Indian, Eskimo, and Aleut, 0.8%; other races, 4%. The numbers of the adult and elderly populations have increased the most, with the 25-to-44 age group growing from 63 million in 1980 to 80.8 million in 1990. The 65-and-over population has increased from 26.3 million to 31.2 million persons, or from 11.4% to 12.6% of the total population. The median age of the total population increased from 30.0 years in 1980 to 32.9 years in 1990. In Canada, according to the 1986 census, the total population was 23,941,000, with 11% being age 65 or over. The dominant ethnic groups at that time were the British (34%) and the French (24%), with 5% of the population being a British-French mixture. Sixteen percent were Asian, 3% Black, and 6% aboriginal Canadians (Communication Division of Statistics, 1992). Canadians are living longer and having fewer children. As we approach the twenty-first century significant changes are occurring in the population of the United States and Canada. The white majority is shrinking and aging; the Black, Hispanic, Asian, and Native American populations are young and growing.

Because of these demographic changes the nurse's practice will be increasingly concerned with the care of aged and ethnic populations. To meet this challenge the nurse needs to better understand the different health and illness perspectives of these groups. This chapter examines the cultural and psychologic aspects of drug therapy; the special needs of older clients will be addressed in greater detail in Chapter 8. To administer medications effectively and to teach clients self-administration require an understanding of the predominant cultural influences within the community, a knowledge base of the psychologic aspects, and an assessment of the individual client to determine how these factors influence health needs.

CULTURAL INFLUENCES ON HEALTH CARE

Published anthropologic and transcultural studies have offered nurses extensive information on how to assess cultural influences on their clients. Creative cultural measures for improved therapeutics and comfort are available in numerous books and research articles (Andrew & Boyle, 1995; Bullough & Bullough, 1982; Geissler, 1994; Henderson & Primeaux, 1981; Shubin, 1980; Spector, 1991). But the nurse needs to remember that although each cultural group has different cultural attitudes towards health, health care, and illness, within each of these groups there exist widely varying health and illness beliefs and practices.

Dr. M.L. Leininger (1978), a nurse-educator credited as the major voice of the transcultural impetus in nursing, has suggested asking questions such as the following to assess a client's cultural influences: "Could you tell me about yourself and your family?" "How do you keep well?" "What made you become ill?" If the nurse has gained the confidence of the client and family, feelings and beliefs will be more openly discussed. If the nurse treats this information with respect and incorporates some of its important aspects into the nursing care plan, the client is likely to respond more readily to therapy. See Box 6-1 for a comprehensive guide for the assessment of cultural manifestations.

If an illness is mild, the person self-treats the symptoms or, as is often the case, does nothing, and gradually the symptoms disappear. If the illness is more severe or is of longer duration, the assistance of a healer of one type or another, usually a physician, will be sought. Many cultural groups avoid standard Western medicine until herbal or home remedies are totally ineffective or the illness becomes acute. Such groups may also use traditional remedies and Western ones concurrently to validate each other or to enhance the therapy. Haitian, Hispanic, Cuban, Vietnamese, Samoan, Jamaican, Chinese, Native American, and other clients generally follow this practice. Nurses should be aware of any reluctance to seek standard medical care. When the need arises such individuals should be counseled on appropriate ways in which to seek health care.

BOX 6-1

Guide for the Assessment of Cultural Manifestations

- I. Brief history of the origins of the cultural group, including location
- II. Value orientations
  - A. World view
  - B. Code of ethics
  - C. Norms and standards of behavior (authority, responsibility, dependability, competition)
  - D. Attitudes toward:
    1. Time
    2. Work versus play/leisure
    3. Money
    4. Education
    5. Physical standards of beauty, strength
    6. Change
- III. Interpersonal relationships
  - A. Family
    1. Courtship and marriage patterns
    2. Kinship patterns
    3. Childrearing patterns
    4. Family function
       - a. Organization
       - b. Roles and activities (sex roles, division of labor)
       - c. Special traditions, customs, ceremonies
       - d. Authority and decision making
    5. Relationship to community
  - B. Demeanor
    1. Respect and courtesy
    2. Politeness, kindness
    3. Caring
    4. Assertiveness versus submissiveness
    5. Independence versus dependence
  - C. Roles and relationships
    1. Number and types
    2. Functions
- IV. Communication
  - A. Language patterns
    1. Verbal
    2. Nonverbal
    3. Use of time
    4. Use of space
    5. Special usage: titles and epithets, forms of courtesy in speech, formality of greetings, degree of volubility versus reticence, proper subjects of conversation, impolite speech
  - B. Arts and music
  - C. Literature
- V. Religion and magic
  - A. Type (modern versus traditional)
  - B. Tenets and practices
  - C. Rituals and taboos (e.g., fertility, birth, death)
- VI. Social systems
  - A. Economics
    1. Occupational status and esteem
    2. Measures of success
    3. Value and use of material goods
  - B. Politics
    1. Type of system
    2. Degree of influence in daily lives of populace
    3. Level of individual/group participation
  - C. Education
    1. Structure
    2. Subjects
    3. Policies
- VII. Diet and food habits
  - A. Values (symbolism) and beliefs about foods
  - B. Rituals and practices
- VIII. Health and illness belief systems
  - A. Values, attitudes, and beliefs
  - B. Use of health facilities (popular versus folk versus professional sectors)
  - C. Effects of illness on the family
  - D. Health/illness behaviors and decision making
  - E. Relationships with health practitioners
  - F. Biologic variations

From Andrews MM & Boyle JS (1995). *Transcultural concepts in nursing care* (2nd ed.). Philadelphia: JB Lippincott.

African Americans

Although a number of blacks have emigrated voluntarily from Africa and the various islands of the West Indies this century, the majority of African Americans are descendants of Africans brought to America as slaves. Brought to this continent against their will, those of African heritage endured overwhelming hardships and inhumane treatment during slavery but in most circumstances maintained a family and community awareness (Gutman, 1976). After the Civil War, those in the South were overtly segregated and lived in conditions of hardship and poverty; the people who migrated to the North were subjected to the poverty, racism, and covert segregation of urban life (Bullough & Bullough, 1982). The nurse who wants to integrate traditional health and illness beliefs with modern practice needs to appreciate the historic problems of the African American community (Spector, 1991).

Traditional beliefs about health and illness stem from the African origins of Blacks. Life was considered a process rather than a state, and could be influenced by other forces. When one was healthy one was in harmony with nature; illness was a state of disharmony. In traditional black belief, there was no separation of mind, body, and spirit (Jacques, 1976). Disharmony or illness was the result of the activity of demons and evil spirits, so the goal of prevention was to ward them off and the goal of therapy was to remove them from the body of the ill person. Several traditional practices were used to meet these goals. Voodoo, a belief system evolved from ancient West African practices, reached its height in Louisiana in the mid-1800s. Although there may be little evidence that voodoo is practiced today, many people continue to fear voodoo and believe in it to some extent. In this belief system many illnesses were the result of a "hex" placed on a person. Gris-gris, usually oils or powders, were used as symbols of voodoo to prevent illness or to cause illness in others (Hughes & Bontemps, 1958). Gris-gris are available today and can be purchased in many American cities, particularly cities with significant Haitian populations, such as Miami.

Many African Americans believe in the power of healers. These healers may rely on the strong religious faith of the people and use prayer and the laying on of hands, or they may be more traditional healers using herbs and roots in the treatment of illness. (See Table 6-1 for additional cultural values and culture care meanings and action modes for African-American culture.) Advertisements for both types of practitioners are commonly found in African American community newspapers.

Some Blacks are practicing Muslims and maintain a highly structured lifestyle based on religious beliefs. Muslims believe in self-help, the need for self-discipline, and highly value life and good health. This belief system fosters the effective management of a therapeutic regimen. Dietary restrictions are similar to a kosher diet, that is, abstinence from pork or pork products is required, and from beans, such as black-eyed, kidney, and lima beans, which are considered to be for animal consumption (Spector, 1991). Alcohol intake is not permitted because it is believed to cause illness. Because pork consumption is prohibited a Muslim who has diabetes should not be administered pork insulin. Like other religions, Islam has various sects that differ in the strictness of their practices.

The practices for health promotion and the treatment of illness in the black community are varied and abundant. Proper diet, rest, and a clean environment are believed to be important for health maintenance. Herb teas and laxatives may be used to keep the body working well. Amulets or bracelets may be worn to protect the wearer from harm, so precautions should be taken during nursing care that these items not be removed. In addition to prayer and the laying on of hands, "rooting" may be used as folk medicine. In "rooting" the healer or "rootman" determines the cause of the illness and then prescribes a therapeutic regimen of substances and practices. Because "rooting" is a practice derived from voodoo, it is essential to obtain a healer who is stronger than the originator of the "hex" or the cause of illness; the more prestigious the healer, the stronger the medicine. In addition, there are a variety of home remedies. For example, just a few of the remedies for colds and congestion are: hot lemon water with honey; hot toddies of tea, honey, lemon, and an alcoholic beverage; the ingestion of Vicks Vaporub mixed with sugar; and a body rub with white high-proof rum. Home remedies have been passed from one generation to the next. The health practices of each client should be determined so that the prescribed therapeutic regimen can be individualized to meet that client's needs.

For a number of reasons folk medicine continues to be used even when African Americans live close to local health services. According to Spector (1991) African Americans may perceive their interaction with the health care system as a degrading and humiliating experience. Although a health care provider may not intend to be patronizing or demeaning, the client may feel insulted. Those who use clinics may have long waits and lose time at work and those who are indigent cannot afford health insurance or the high cost of health care. Although these issues could apply to any health care recipient, "the inherent racism within the health system cannot be denied" (Spector, 1991).

Hispanic Americans

Hispanic Americans have their origins in Cuba, Mexico, Puerto Rico, any Central or South American country, or Spain. Mexican Americans constitute the largest group of Hispanic Americans, and their number is rapidly rising because of high birth rates and immigration.

Some Mexican Americans consider health to be the consequence of good luck, whereas others see it as being the result of good behavior. One is expected to maintain health by acting, eating, and working appropriately. Prayer, the wearing of amulets, and herbs and spices are all employed for the prevention of illness. Poor health is perceived as a change of luck, an imbalance in the body, or the result of some misdeed (Table 6-1).

According to Spector (1991) the causes of illness can be grouped into five major categories: imbalance in the body, dislocation of parts of the body, magic causes outside the body, strong emotional states, and "envidia" (envy). The imbalance in the body relates to the four aspects of the body: blood, which is hot and wet; yellow bile, which is hot and dry; phlegm, which is cold and wet; and black bile, which is cold and dry. According to this "imbalance" theory of ill health, equilibrium can be regained if cold remedies or foods are taken for "hot" illnesses and vice versa. However, perceptions of what foods or medications are hot or cold may vary from client to client because these terms do not refer to temperature but are qualities assigned to particular substances. It is best to consult with the client for specifics once it is determined that this imbalance theory is part of the client's health belief system. "Empacho" is an example of a dislocation of a part of the body as being a cause of illness. The symptoms of abdominal discomfort, pain and cramping, are thought to be caused by a ball of food clinging to the wall of the stomach. It is treated by massaging the spine while prayers are spoken.

TABLE 6-1 Cultural values and culture care meanings and action modes for selected groups

Cultural values	Culture care meanings and action modes
Anglo-American culture (mainly U.S. middle and upper classes) 1. Individualism—focus on a self-reliant person 2. Independence and freedom 3. Competition and achievement 4. Materialism (things and money) 5. Technology dependent 6. Instant time and actions 7. Youth and beauty 8. Equal sex rights 9. Leisure time highly valued possible 10. Reliance on scientific facts and numbers 11. Less respect for authority and the elderly 12. Generosity in time of crisis	1. Stress alleviation by ▪ Physical means ▪ Emotional means 2. Personalized acts ▪ Doing special things ▪ Giving individual attention 3. Self-reliance (individualism) by ▪ Reliance on self ▪ Reliance on self (self-care) ▪ Becoming as independent as possible ▪ Reliance on technology 4. Health instruction ▪ Teach us how "to do" this care for self ▪ Give us the "medical" facts
Mexican-American culture[*] 1. Extended family valued 2. Interdependence with kin and social activities 3. Patriarchal (machismo) 4. Exact time less valued 5. High respect for authority and the elderly 6. Religion valued (many Roman Catholics) 7. Native foods for well-being 8. Traditional folk-care healers for folk illnesses 9. Belief in hot-cold theory	1. Succorance (direct family aid) 2. Involvement with extended family ("other care") 3. Filial love/loving 4. Respect for authority 5. Mother as care decision maker 6. Protective (external) male care 7. Acceptance of God's will 8. Use of folk-care practices 9. Healing with foods 10. Touching
Haitian-American culture[†] 1. Extended family as support system 2. Religion—God's will must prevail 3. Reliance on folk foods and treatments 4. Belief in hot-cold theory 5. Male decision maker and direct caregivers 6. Reliance on native language	1. Involve family for support (other care) 2. Respect 3. Trust 4. Succorance 5. Touching (body closeness) 6. Reassurance 7. Spiritual healing 8. Use of folk food, care rituals 9. Avoid evil eye and witches 10. Speak the language
African-American culture[‡] 1. Extended family networks 2. Religion valued (many are Baptists) 3. Interdependence with "blacks" 4. Daily survival 5. Technology valued, e.g., radio, car, etc. 6. Folk (soul) foods 7. Folk healing modes 8. Music and physical activities	1. Concern for my "brothers and sisters" 2. Being involved with 3. Giving presence (physical) 4. Family support and "get togethers" 5. Touching appropriately 6. Reliance on folk home remedies 7. Rely on "Jesus to save us" with prayers and songs

Modified from Leininger MM (1991). *Culture care diversity and universality: A theory of nursing.* New York: National League for Nursing Press.

[*] These findings were from Leininger's transcultural nurse studies (1970, 1984) and other transcultural nurse studies in the United States during the past two decades.

[†] These data were from Haitians living in the United States during the past decade (1981-1991).

[‡] These findings were from Leininger's study of two southern U.S. villages (1980-1981) and from a study of one large northern urban city (1982-1991) along with other studies by transcultural nurses.

Continued

TABLE 6-1 Cultural values and culture care meanings and action modes for selected groups—cont'd

Cultural values	Culture care meanings and action modes
North-American Indian culture[§]	
1. Harmony between land, people, and environment	1. Establishing harmony between people and environment with reciprocity
2. Reciprocity with "Mother Earth"	2. Actively listening
3. Spiritual inspiration (spirit guidance)	3. Using periods of silence ("Great Spirit" guidance)
4. Folk healers (shamans) (the circle and four directions)	4. Rhythmic timing (nature, land and people) in harmony
5. Practice culture rituals and taboos	5. Respect for native folk healer, carers, and curers (use of circle)
6. Rhythmicity of life with nature	6. Maintaining reciprocity (replenish what is taken from Mother Earth)
7. Authority of tribal elders	7. Preserving cultural rituals and taboos
8. Pride in cultural heritage and "nations"	8. Respect for elders and children
9. Respect and value for children	

[§]These findings were collected by Leininger and other contributors in the United States and Canada during the past three decades. Cultural variations among all nations exist, and so these data are some general commonalities about values, care meanings, and actions.

Although helpful in many cases, like many folk practices it may delay the client from seeking medical attention for serious illnesses. "Mal ojo," an example of an illness caused by magic, has symptoms of malaise, lethargy, and headaches and is thought to be the result of being excessively admired by another. The remedy is to locate the admirer to provide care for the affected individual. "Susto" is a state of depression caused by a strong emotional state of fright. This illness involves the loss of soul—the soul leaves the body and wanders freely. A "curandero," or folk healer, is required to coax the soul back into the person's body. "Envidia," or envy, as a cause of illness is part of a more universally held belief in peasant cultures of "limited good," that if there is material wealth or achievement it comes at the expense of the rest of the community, because there is only a certain amount of "good" available. Misfortune, or ill health, then, may be the result of the envy and resentment of neighbors.

The services of a curandero may be sought and religious rituals may be practiced, such as lighting candles, praying, and visiting shrines. Curanderismo is a relatively well-documented form of holistic folk medicine (Kiev, 1968; Saunders, 1958). Kay (1977) reported that a third of her interviewees used the services of a curandero, as well as local health services. Curanderos prescribe specific herbs to take in teas, usually determined by the content of the affected individual's dreams. Therapies by the curandero include support for the religious practices, massage, and "cleansings" such as the passing of an unbroken egg or small bundles of herbs over the body of the client. Curanderos are well respected within the Mexican-American community and usually maintain a personal relationship with the client. Mexican Americans may expect to have such a relationship with their health care providers, which may not be met within the established health care system (Spector, 1991). This may account for the continued popularity of curanderismo as a health care modality.

Barriers for many Hispanic Americans to receive appropriate health care continue to be language and poverty. There still are inadequate numbers of Spanish-speaking health care providers, despite the fact that Spanish-speaking individuals are one of the largest minority groups. This will be remedied when more Hispanic Americans are recruited into the health field and when more health care providers learn to speak Spanish (Spector, 1991).

Asian Americans

Although the Asian American community includes people whose origins are in Japan, Korea, Hawaii, Vietnam, and the Philippines, this discussion will focus on the Chinese, who constitute the majority of Asian Americans.

Medicine has been a recorded science in China since the Emperor Huang-ti's writings, *Huang-ti Nei Ching* (The Yellow Emperor's Book of Internal Medicine), in 1628. Within these writings the universe is seen as an indivisible entity in which man must adapt to the order of nature. This universe has two basic components, yin and yang, which are in opposition as well as in unison. Yang is the male force, a positive energy that creates light, warmth, and fullness. Yin is female, a negative energy representing darkness, cold, and emptiness. Illness is caused by an imbalance of yin and yang. If yin is too strong, one is nervous, apprehensive, and catches colds easily. Yang must be nurtured because it protects the body against outside forces. The inside of the body is yin, the outside yang. The five solid organs, which collect and store secretions—the liver, heart, spleen, lungs, and kidneys—are yin. The six hollow organs, which excrete—the gallbladder, stomach, large intestine, small intestine, bladder, and lymph nodes—are yang. The organs have a complex interrelationship that maintains the balance and harmony of the body (Chang, 1991).

Traditionally illness was prevented by wearing amulets to ward off evil spirits, or jade charms, which were believed to bring health. The individual is expected to practice moderation, balancing the yin and yang aspects of the body and taking foods and herbs as supplements to maintain that balance (Louie, 1990). The healer in Chinese medicine is the physician, who in ancient times was responsible not only for curing disease but also for preventing it. In fact, physicians were paid only when the client was healthy. In the event of illness physicians were not paid and had to provide the necessary medicines. The traditional Chinese physician uses inspection, particularly of the tongue, from which more than 100 conditions can be determined, and palpation of many different pulse types, which there are 15 ways of characterizing (Spector, 1991).

The three primary methods of traditional Chinese healing are acupuncture, moxibustion, and herbal remedies, the purpose of which is to restore the balance of yin and yang. Acupuncture is a method of producing analgesia or altering the function of a system of the body by inserting fine, wire-thin needles into the skin at specific sites on the body along a series of lines called meridians. Precise puncture points along the meridians are identified in terms of yin and yang, as well as for specific symptoms and diseases. Whereas acupuncture is perceived as a cold treatment, moxibustion is based on the therapeutic value of heat and is used for an excess of yin. In moxibustion, pulverized wormwood is heated and placed on the skin over specific meridian points (Spector, 1991).

Herbal remedies are prepared by Chinese herbalists according to specific prescriptions, the purpose of which is to restore yin-yang balance. In China these folk remedies usually consist of a single dose of a liquid preparation, so taking tablets or capsules on a regular schedule could be confusing to the older Chinese client. This may be why this group prefers teas and topical remedies.

Barriers to health care for the Chinese relate to language difficulties and poverty as for other minorities, but may also include their beliefs regarding medical practices. Although immunization and the use of x-rays are accepted, intrusive practices such as the drawing of blood and surgical procedures are seen as contrary to having respect for an intact body (Spector, 1991).

Hospital food is seen as alien and increases the client's sense of social isolation. Even the common practice of leaving ice water at the client's bedside for the administration of medications is questionable because many Chinese and Chinese-Americans believe that cold drinks are unhealthy for the sick; they may therefore avoid this fluid intake. This preference, as well as any food preferences, should be discussed with the individual and, if medically acceptable, hot tea or other substitutes should be provided. If appropriate the family should be encouraged to bring in the client's preferred foods.

Native Americans

Culturally the American Indians' belief system of being in harmony with nature or of maintaining a balance between the body, the mind, and the environment is crucial to health maintenance. Illness is perceived as being out of balance because of ill spirits, not following traditional beliefs, or a disruption in nature (see Table 6-1). Because Native Americans do not ascribe to the germ theory, the cause of the illness must be traced back to an action or lack of action on the part of the client, which may not be known to the individual (Wauneka, 1990). Recovery therefore is based on diagnosing the problem and reestablishing the harmony or balance with nature. Although these are some beliefs that are held by Native Americans, each tribe (there are well over 200) has specific ideas and practices related to health and illness (Primeaux, 1977).

The medicine man is the traditional healer of Native Americans and is considered to be wise in the ways of nature and able to seek out the spiritual causes of illness. For diagnosis, the medicine man may use meditation or, in the case of the Navaho, sandpainting, in which the shape of the painting determines the illness and its treatment; stargazing, in which the color emanating from the star determines cause and prognosis of the illness; and listening, in which the divination is heard rather than seen (Wyman, 1966).

Treatments used by medicine men include massage, the application of heat, sweatbaths, total immersion in water as an act of purification, and the use of herbal remedies. Because of the belief in harmony with nature, herbs are specifically prescribed and carefully prepared, with meticulous attention being given to the timing and the procedures used for gathering them (Spector, 1991). Again, the personal bond between the healer and client is strong, which is why folk medicine continues to be popular.

The difference between what the health care provider and the Native American client believe is the cause of the illness can constitute a barrier to health care for Native Americans. In addition, differences in communication styles may lead to misunderstanding. The questioning involved in taking a health history may be seen as intrusive as well as a demonstration of incompetence because Native Americans believe that the diagnosis should be arrived at through observation of nonverbal communication. Because Native Americans have maintained their rich history through an oral tradition, note taking is not viewed favorably and the nurse should rely on memory rather than notes when in the client's presence.

■ ■ ■

In addition to the various cultural groups briefly discussed, there are white ethnic communities to be served by the health care delivery system. To describe the health beliefs and practices of all the various cultures is beyond the scope of this text. The student is advised to seek additional information from the current journals and references cited in the bibliography of this chapter. The nurse should gain knowledge of the various cultural groups within the local area of clinical practice. Local hospitals and other health care settings frequently hold conferences and maintain reference sources of relevant cultural material for the local communities.

One major way that many private and some public hospitals have recognized the cultural differences in health care is to offer ethnic meals as alternatives to the standard fare. This is because dietary concerns are also strongly intertwined with cultural beliefs. For example, many ethnic groups (Italian, Mexican, Cuban, and others) believe that their own foods hasten the recovery process. Discussing food preferences and preferred methods of preparation with clients is often very important for the well-being of the client.

Additionally, the nurse should be aware of possible cultural influences on medicating behaviors of clients. Such information may be used to guide the nurse to ask the right questions during the initial history, to be aware of possible reasons for ineffective management of a therapeutic drug regimen, and to help identify specific areas needing additional client teaching.

The client is always the ultimate source of information on the specific ways in which culture affects the client's participation in health care. Nurses need to be sensitive to the client's life experiences and adapt their nursing care accordingly. The nurse should be aware of two dangers: ethnocentrism or the belief that the health care provider's ethnic group is superior to other cultures or ethnic groups; and client stereotyping, or the assumption that all persons from a particular culture or ethnic group will have the same response to the same or similar situation. These are mistaken beliefs. Ethnocentrism can interfere with the provision of health care to individuals from groups other than the provider while client stereotyping may limit the provider's objectivity and ability to provide nursing care.

A wide range of different responses to the administration of medications and the management of the therapeutic regimen is possible within each cultural or ethnic group. An understanding of the potential cultural or ethnic patterns of a client is helpful as a starting point in caring for the individual, as long as stereotypical conclusions are avoided (Salerno, 1995).

ETHNIC AND RACIAL DIFFERENCES IN DRUG RESPONSE

In addition to differences in health beliefs, values, and attitudes, pharmacologic research in the last 15 years has uncovered significant differences among racial and ethnic groups in their metabolism rates, clinical drug responses, and side effects to drugs. A new field of clinical study has evolved, pharmacogenetics, or the genetic influence on drug response that may occur from inherited metabolic defects or deficiencies. This emerging area of clinical investigation is leading to new, clinically relevant information about drug responses in ethnic and racial minorities (Levy, 1993). Nurses need to be aware of these differences so as to better monitor the drug therapy of clients from culturally diverse populations. These differences where documented by research will be discussed throughout the text.

Analgesics

Some individuals will have an inadequate analgesic response to codeine because of a genetic alteration in debrisoquine-sparteine polymorphism, an enzyme responsible for metabolizing codeine to morphine. About 5% to 10% of the population are poor metabolizers. When Chinese participants were compared with Caucasians in a study utilizing codeine as the analgesic for pain, the Chinese population was found to be less able to metabolize codeine. To achieve analgesia the Chinese required increased dosage adjustments to achieve a therapeutic effect (Levy, 1993).

The debrisoquine-sparteine metabolic path is important for the metabolism of cardiac antidysrhythmics, antidepressants, beta-blocking agents, neuroleptics, and opioids. Therefore persons that are extensive metabolizers (metabolize at a high rate) may produce multiple chemical substances at the enzyme site that clinically may result in an increase in drug interactions. Drugs that are capable of producing this type effect in extensive metabolizers include quinidine, propafenone (Rythmol), flecainide (Tambocor) and metoprolol (Lopressor). Alternately, poor metabolizers may have a variety of drug responses such as prolonged drug effects or toxicity to phenformin, thioridazine (Mellaril), isoniazid, sulfapyridine, and codeine (Meyer, 1992).

Cardiovascular Medications

The debrisoquine-sparteine polymorphism is also an important pathway for a number of cardiac medications. It was reported that blacks are less responsive to beta-blocking agents, especially propranolol (Inderal), nadolol (Corgard), and atenolol (Tenormin). Labetalol (Normodyne), a combination drug with alpha- and beta-blocking properties, is equally effective in blacks and white individuals.

In general, individuals of African descent respond better to diuretics than to beta-blockers if only one agent is used. Even among the beta-blocking agents, responses vary widely between racial or ethnic groups. For example, Chinese clients are considerably more sensitive than Caucasians to the effects of the beta-blocker propranolol (Inderal) (Zhou et al, 1990). It was reported that Chinese persons may be twice as responsive to propranolol's effects on blood pressure and heart rate and also have a greater atropine-induced increase in heart rate than the white population in comparative studies (Levy, 1993).

Plasma renin levels may also be important in determining a person's response to the beta-blocking agents and, because Caucasians usually have higher levels than Blacks, this may also contribute to the racial difference in drug response (Levy, 1993).

Central Nervous System Agents

A comparative study between Chinese and Caucasian subjects indicated that the Chinese group required lower dosages of benzodiazepines (diazepam [Valium]; alprazolam [Xanax]), tricyclic antidepressants, atropine, and propran-

BOX 6-2

Ethnic and Racial Differences in Response to CNS Agents

Comparison groups	Drug class example	Clinical response
Chinese/whites	Benzodiazepines (diazepam, alprazolam)	Chinese require lower doses; more sensitive to sedative effects
Chinese/whites Hispanics/Anglos	Antidepressants (imipramine, desipramine, amitriptyline, clomipramine)	Chinese and Hispanics require lower doses; side effects greater in Hispanics
Asians/whites	Neuroleptics (e.g., haloperidol)	Asians require lower doses
Asian Indians/whites	Analgesics (e.g., acetaminophen, codeine)	Asian Indians have greater clearances rates
Chinese/whites	Analgesics (e.g., morphine)	Chinese less sensitive to cardiovascular and respiratory effects, but more sensitive to GI side effects
Asians/whites	Alcohol	Asians more sensitive to side effects
Native Americans/whites	Alcohol	Native Americans have faster metabolism and less tolerance

From Levy RA (1993). *Ethnic and racial differences in response to medicines: Preserving individualized therapy in managed care pharmaceutical programs.* Reston, VA: National Pharmaceutical Council.

olol (Inderal) (Levy, 1993). When dosages administered were comparable to those given to the Caucasians, an increase in side effects occurred in the Chinese subjects. Box 6-2 gives a summary of ethnic and racial differences in response to CNS agents.

■ ■ ■

As a result of the pharmacologic research conducted over the last two decades, more consideration is being given to the need to individualize drug therapy for special population groups. The vast majority of drug manufacturers now test and evaluate new drugs so as to include ethnic and racial minorities within the clinical trial groups. A survey by the Pharmaceutical Manufacturers Association (Edwards, 1991) revealed that 79% of pharmaceutical companies collect data on race, and the majority (67%) are making extra efforts to include racial minorities in their clinical trials. Almost all of the companies (100) responding to the survey include African Americans in their trials, while over three quarters include Asians (84) or Hispanics as well (Figure 6-1). This effort is likely to reveal additional drug actions and side effects specific to minority groups and may also lead to the discovery of therapies that are of specific advantage to minorities (Levy, 1993).

PSYCHOLOGIC ASPECTS

Every drug administered to a client has a symbolic meaning and a potential psychologic effect in addition to its pharmacodynamic action. A drug not only alters the function or structure of some part of the body, but it may also influence the behavior, sense of well-being, and mental state of the client. Psychologic responses of clients to symbolism may mimic pharmacologic reactions, adverse effects, or even allergic reactions to drugs. A profound reaction may be observed in clients receiving placebos.

Medications tend to be more effective when individuals believe in their capacity to get well, when they have a strong desire to get well, and when they believe that the health personnel expect the medication to be effective and say so. Clients' past and present conditioning to drugs, illness, hospitals, nurses, and other health personnel as well as their health goals are determinant factors in the response to drugs. Nurses must remember that among the major deterrents to successful drug therapy are divergent goals of the client and the health personnel. An accurate appraisal of the client's goal in seeking health advice and therapy is important to planning and implementing an effective plan of care.

Symbolic Meaning of Drugs to Clients

Medications may be a symbol of help to the client. This meaning is strengthened and drug effectiveness enhanced when prescribers and nurses suggest to a client that a partic-

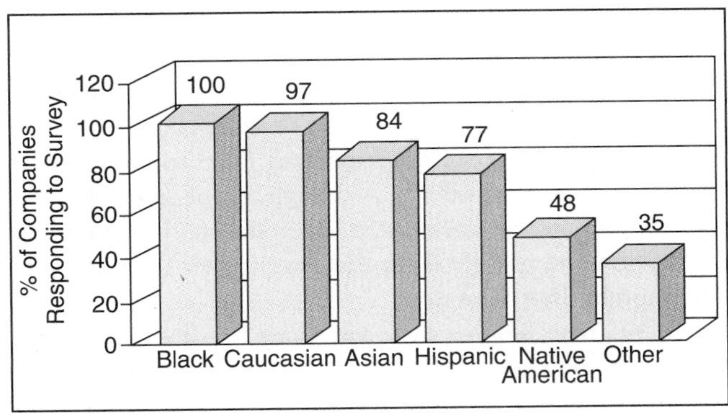

Figure 6-1 Percentage of companies that responded to the Pharmaceutical Manufacturers Association survey that include different racial groups in their drug trials.

ular drug will be of benefit or help. Repeated suggestions to the client that the drug is beneficial further reinforce the therapeutic value. This is similar to the relief a mother's kiss gives to her child's pain; the assurance it gives makes the child feel better. Investigation of the effects of drugs on the mind has resulted in the conclusion that some drugs are effective only in the presence of an appropriate mental state.

Drugs may also be viewed as symbols of danger. Clients may interpret cure as a serious threat to their emotional security if they are using their illness to meet a need for dependence. Taking medication may also be objectionable if there is a strong need to exhibit an image of independence; adverse reactions may even result. The client may complain of dry mouth, nausea, vomiting, palpitation, fatigue, and other vague feelings of discomfort. The individual may resist taking the medication, refuse to have the prescription refilled, or even throw the drug away.

Many people have ambivalent feelings about taking medications. An expressed desire to regain health may coexist with an unconscious reluctance to give up the secondary gains of the sick role. These gains can include freedom from responsibilities and extra attention. Individuals may report secondary drug effects or find reasons why they cannot take the medication to retain these benefits.

Clients may harbor unsubstantiated notions about medications. Some believe a medication is too strong or not needed any longer and therefore may refuse to take the drug, decrease its amount at any one time, or decrease the number of times it is taken. This behavior may be suspected when a drug known to be effective for a specific condition is ineffective in a particular client with that condition.

A client who believes the drug is too weak may take the drug too often, request the drug more often than prescribed, or continue drug therapy for longer than prescribed. However, the drug therapy itself should be reviewed first to eliminate the possibility of undertreatment by the professional staff. For example, analgesics may be inadequately prescribed or administered, thus resulting in the type of behavior described here. In self-medication some clients will increase the amount of drug taken, believing that "if one dose is good, two will be better," and overdose themselves. When the therapeutics are determined to be appropriate, the reasons for this behavior should be sought and addressed.

Some fantasies concerning resistance evolve from fears. Individuals tend to fear radioactive drugs such as ^{32}P or ^{131}I and to fear dependence on drugs that have antidepressant, analgesic, or sedative effects. Although few people today believe in cure-all remedies, some have blind faith in a certain medication and prefer taking that drug rather than make an alteration in their lifestyle.

Clients who believe they are allergic to a certain drug, for real or imagined reasons, are likely to react with fear or panic when administration of that drug is contemplated. A detailed personal history and (when possible) tests for drug allergy should be used to corroborate or refute the client's belief. Rejecting a client's claim of an allergic response without evidence is an unwise assessment of data and negligent to say the least.

The route of administration of a drug and the financial cost of treatment as well as a client's conscious and unconscious attitudes toward illness, drugs, physicians, nurses, other health care providers, and so on influence the extent, duration, and intensity of the client's response to medication. When a client is angry, resentful, or hostile, some medications used in usual doses may not be effective.

A client's illness may affect the emotional response to a drug. When the illness is short, recovery complete, and medical and drug expense not too great, the client tends to have a positive reaction to drugs, hospitals, and health and nursing personnel. Strong negative reactions toward drugs or health personnel result when clients are falsely reassured that they will make a quick and complete recovery, when drugs are both ineffective and expensive, or when symptoms of allergy, side or toxic effects, or overdosage occur. Preparing clients for the realistic limitations of drugs, for side and adverse effects, and for drug expense tends to create reasonable expectations.

In any chronic illness a client may suddenly rebel against ill health and resist therapy with life-sustaining medications. When this occurs, clients may be testing to see if they are really dependent on the drugs, or they may be attempting a real or symbolic act of self-destruction. A stressful event or decision may be the root cause. Exploring the client's underlying fears and concerns is essential. Support, caring, and objective assistance in coping will be necessary.

To avoid causing the client unnecessary concern or to deflect time-consuming questions, many health care providers are reluctant to present any negative aspects when teaching clients about drugs. A clear, nonthreatening explanation about the purpose of the medication and its effects (including the most common side effects reported) is only the most basic of explanations required by the client. On the whole, most clients prefer knowing the potential risks of drug therapy. This knowledge also tends to increase their participation and to engender trust. Litigation could also ensue if clients suffer harm from unrecognized secondary effects of a drug because they were not informed. The nurse should be aware that some people do not want to know the details of their treatment and that some are very suggestible.

It is important to *listen intently to what the client says* about the medication, the feelings associated with it, and the condition for which it has been prescribed. Then the health care provider can begin to see the situation from the client's point of view and develop an understanding of the client's motivation to seek health care. Does the individual see the treated condition as a physical threat? How much of a threat? How susceptible to treatment? How much control does the client want to exert over the condition? How probable is it that such control will reduce the threat adequately? Until these concerns and other personal factors are at least briefly explored, the success of treatment is uncertain.

Effects of Drugs on the Mind

Many common drugs have a secondary effect on the client's central nervous system (CNS) and result in altered thought processes and sensory/perceptual alterations. Drugs may interfere with judgment, mood, sense of values, motor ability, and coordination. Certain antihistamines used to treat allergies may decrease alertness and cause drowsiness, depression, and predisposition to accidents. Antihypertensive agents may cause depression. Barbiturates and tranquilizers may induce inattentiveness and confusion and reduce initiative. Drug-induced depression calls for discontinuance or for decreasing the dosage of the offending drug. Clients should be monitored for self-destructive tendencies—pharmacologic literature has abundant examples of clients with drug-induced depression who have attempted suicide.

Placebo Therapy

In the past when a physician had no medicine to offer a client who expected treatment, a "sugar pill," or **placebo**, was given to placate the sick individual. A placebo is any treatment—medication, surgical or diagnostic procedure, or nursing action—that elicits a client's response simply because of its intent rather than its known active properties. A placebo is most often a formulation of a pharmacodynamically inert substance such as lactose or sugar, distilled water, normal saline, or a very small drug dose of a substance such as a vitamin. In medicine placebos are employed in one of two ways: in experimental drug studies as a simulated medication given to a control group (e.g., before the drug's approval by the FDA) or, much more rarely, to satisfy a client's demand for a particular medication when in the considered judgment of the prescriber withholding a dose will impede psychologic or physical health.

The nurse should be aware that pain relief with administration of a placebo does not mean the client did not have real pain. Studies on effective clinical responses of pain to a placebo indicate that a physiologic response occurs; endogenous substances called endorphins are stimulated and released by the brain, which interact with the opioid receptors in the body to reduce pain. Thus the effect produced is similar to the effect achieved by an opioid analgesic. Various other stimuli such as vigorous exercising, jogging, etc., may also increase release of these chemicals in the brain. Such evidence indicates that a client's response to a placebo is therefore physical and not mental, as previously believed.

The placebo response may result from objective physiologic and biochemical changes in the body as well as a change in the client's subjective complaints. This response can vary considerably from one client to another, but in published studies it is reported to be fairly consistent, about 20% to 40% of clients have a placebo response (Katzung, 1992).

"The use of a placebo for the treatment of pain to distinguish psychic and real pain is a deceptive practice that should be avoided" (Salerno & Willens, 1996). The American Pain Society guidelines (1992) discourage the use of placebos in the assessment of pain and state "The deceptive use of placebos and the misinterpretation of the placebo response to discredit the patient's pain report are unethical and should be avoided."

SELF-TREATMENT

Public interest in self-care management is at an all-time high, as exemplified by the numerous self-care books and clinics that now abound. One of the most effective and inexpensive ways to counteract rising health care costs may be through expanded, educated self-care management. Many people visiting a physician have already started a self-treatment plan. If these people were also helped to learn when to seek medical supervision and how to follow treatment advice wisely, they would have a still greater potential for regaining good health.

Nurses, with their commitment to collaboration with the client to further health, can educate clients, as can pharmacists, physicians, and many other health care professionals. Consumer information pamphlets abound; they are printed by the FDA and others in large type for the visually impaired, or in various languages, and offer valuable advice about drug interactions, health foods, and nonprescription pain relievers.

Development of the science of public health has led to the realization that the state of a nation's health does not depend exclusively on the interplay between professional medical practice on the one hand and bacteria, malignancy, and other causes of disease on the other. The influence on community health of the individual's personal attempts at self-treatment or at lifestyle alterations has frequently been ignored or underestimated.

Drugs sold without prescription can induce sleep or wakefulness, relieve pain or tension, or supply the body with vitamins and minerals. Remedies can be purchased for symptoms affecting any part of the body. Sales of prescription and nonprescription (OTC) drugs have made the pharmaceutical industry a continually growing multi-billion dollar industry. Concern over the use of home remedies and self-medication is not new but continues to be a controversial subject. See Chapter 11, Over-the Counter Medications.

Self-Treatment Using Herbal Remedies

Treating illness with a natural remedy, such as herbal products, dates back to the earliest records of mankind and is common to many cultures. The idea that a simple herbal or folk medicine can cure or prevent many health problems is believed and practiced in many societies today. Although some of the prominent medications used today originated from plant sources (such as digitalis from foxglove and vincristine or vinblastine from periwinkle), home brewing of such plants can be extremely dangerous.

Use of herbals, or the back-to-nature movement, has largely evolved from the frequent warnings issued about food additives, preservatives, or products that are said to have cancer-causing substances in them. This movement has spawned a multi-million dollar enterprise that no longer only appeals to specific cultural or ethnic groups but is widespread in the general population. The proliferation of health food stores, natural organic vegetables, and pharmacies and other outlets that sell organic vitamins, cosmetics, etc., are indicative of this trend. Chapter 12, Alternative Medications, will examine self-medication with nontraditional remedies in greater detail.

Self-Treatment Using Nonprescription Drugs

Advantages. The individual has a right to practice self-medication. Throughout history the public has searched for medicines to relieve ailments and has tried almost every natural material known in the battle against pain, discomfort, and disease. That the public is health conscious is evident by the number of OTC and nonprescription drugs available. Many ailments are minor and temporary, and the client wants to eliminate discomfort as quickly as possible. Minor ailments do not always require the expertise of a physician, but because many nonprescription drugs can interact with prescription drugs, it is best to check with a prescriber or pharmacist. Minor complaints can be successfully treated by nonphysicians. Indeed, if individuals sought medical advice for every minor ailment (colds, headaches, minor wounds, temporary gastrointestinal upsets, or minor burns), health care providers would be unable to attend to individuals who need professional health care. However, self-medication, if misused or abused, can be harmful. Box 6-3 lists the general benefits and risks of OTC medications. Risks associated with the use of nonprescription drugs can be reduced by professionally implemented client teaching.

Disadvantages. Most preparations that were available before the twentieth century were either harmless vegetable concoctions or narcotic-laced nostrums. Modern chemistry and pharmacology produced literally thousands of preparations for self-medication. Some are quite effective for certain minor ailments, some are potentially dangerous, and some are worthless. Generally speaking, Americans are overmedicated. Americans have developed a casual attitude toward drug use and often believe every discomfort or disorder requires chemical treatment.

Today, OTC drugs can be bought in drugstores, supermarkets, restaurants, and vending machines. Widespread sales promotion via the media encourages self-medication. Because the hazards are generally insufficiently detailed in advertisements and commercials, persistent abuse of medications, and the resultant toxic effects, are fairly common. Many drugs tested and found to be harmless can actually

BOX 6-3

General Benefits and Risks of Over-the-Counter Medications

Benefits

- Occasional use of certain simple preparations can be highly effective for specified minor, usually self-limiting conditions.
- Cost is low in relation to prescription drugs, and the cost of a physician's visit is eliminated.
- The client regains some control over personal health care.
- Directions and some possible secondary effects are listed on the label.
- Condition is immediately treatable. OTC medications are as accessible as the nearest store supply, and a wait for a physician's appointment is eliminated.

Risks

- Treatment depends on client judgment in differentiating a minor condition from a major, more complex one and in selecting appropriate medication.
- Signs and symptoms of a serious condition may be masked by the medication.
- Costs in the long run may be higher if a serious condition progresses while improperly treated.
- Substances taken as OTC drugs are not always viewed as "drugs" with potential for harm, and dosing may be exceedingly casual.
- Available combination preparations very often contain useless or harmful stimulants or depressants (caffeine or alcohol) and allergy-producing preservatives in addition to the active ingredient.
- Professional advice to integrate the drug into an overall plan (e.g. to prevent interactions) is absent unless all drugs are obtained from one source that keeps a drug profile on clients.
- Dosage may be too low to be effective, risking decisions by the client to overdose or delay needed professional treatment.
- Many do not read labels, and most label print is too small for easy reading, even with glasses, by those with failing eyesight.
- Professional follow-up for other conditions may be avoided unknowingly.
- OTC drug self-treatment promotes the idea that there is a "magic bullet" for every ailment, major or minor, and that no discomfort should be tolerated.
- OTC drug containers are especially vulnerable to criminal package tampering if they are kept accessible on shelves or are not in tamper-proof containers.

cause serious secondary effects. Aspirin may upset the gastrointestinal tract or cause bleeding; one 325-mg tablet of aspirin impairs platelet aggregation to some extent for up to 1 week.

Serious, complex problems can develop from vitamin and mineral overuse (e.g., vitamin A or D overdosage). Habitual use of mineral oil may prevent absorption of fat-soluble vitamins or cause colon atony so that the treatment perpetuates constipation. Few established dosage limits exist for the use of OTCs by the pregnant or breast-feeding woman, and effects on the fetus and neonate may be extremely harmful. Therefore *no drug of any sort should be taken by a pregnant or breast-feeding woman until a health care provider is consulted.* Many OTC drugs are intended only for adults, not for children; the dosage should not simply be altered for administration to children.

Additionally, *a health care provider should be consulted before the client takes any drug that may have caused a previous allergic reaction.* Often a surprising lack of critical judgment is employed when evaluating a newly marketed drug. Typically there is an initial overreaction, especially to a new OTC or a well-marketed prescription drug: a "honeymoon phase" occurs—the agent is introduced with fanfare and used and prescribed somewhat casually for a time. Then when longer-term results are apparent and newly discovered secondary reactions are reported, its reputation suffers for a while, and its use may be overcautiously controlled. After another time period, use again builds to a more moderate level as the prescribers and the public recognize that judicious use under specified circumstances is the rational approach.

Habitual self-medication with nonprescription drugs may mask a serious condition, prevent diagnosis, endanger the individual's life, or create long-term, expensive medical problems. Health care providers have an obligation to understand how taking medication "fits" with clients' understandings, attitudes, and lifestyles. Box 6-3 outlines how to understand and explore the risk-to-benefit ratio when consumers are contemplating the use of nonprescription drugs. An additional factor for consideration are the cultural influences on self-treatment behaviors.

Cultural Influences on Self-Treatment Behaviors

Although research on the use of medications in various ethnic-cultural groups is limited, awareness of the meaning of specific terminology or health care perceptions from an individual cultural group is crucial in the health care setting. For example, Gaston-Johansson et al (1990) studied the use of language or pain terms commonly used by Hispanic Americans, Native Americans, African Americans, and others and concluded that the word descriptors used (e.g., pain, ache, and hurt) were similar in clients with different cultural backgrounds.

DeSantis (1989) performed a descriptive survey of 30 Cuban and 30 Haitian immigrant mothers to study their health care orientations; that is, their different concerns about types of illnesses, meanings attached to signs and symptoms, typical therapy management groups, and their use of the biomedical health care system. For a sick child, home remedies such as teas, herbs, warm oil rubs, castor oil, etc., were generally tried first. A sick child with an illness believed to be caused by a supernatural power (spells or evil spirits) would be taken to a voodoo priest or priestess; the traditional physician would be consulted for treatment of natural disease states (fever, bronchitis, impetigo). DeSantis reported that unlike the Cuban mothers in the study, the Haitians did not mention OTC medications nor did they identify any prescribed medications by name that were used for their children. This finding was similar to the results reported by Salerno et al (1985).

Salerno et al (1985) performed a descriptive survey study of the four predominant cultural groups in Miami (i.e., Hispanics, Haitians, African Americans, and Caucasian Americans). This study reviewed the factors that influenced the elderly of these groups when choosing and using OTC substances. An added feature was the development of a Self-Medicating Behavior Safety Scale (SMBSS), which included a numerical value for safety. The pharmacist investigator reviewed all questionnaires and extracted data to answer the question "Was there any difference between the cultures in regard to potential for misuse or abuse of OTC medications?" The following data were extracted from this study:

1. The Haitian elderly reported the highest number of health problems, but the greatest number of OTC products used was reported by the Caucasian subjects. The mean OTC product usage per group was Caucasian, 7.4; African American, 4.4; Haitian, 5.8; and Hispanic, 2.4.

   One should be cautious in applying self-reported health information, however. The nurse should be aware of the "yea-saying" tendencies of minority groups when they are asked about their health or health care attitudes; their answer is often an effort to please a member of the dominant group and/or health care provider. This behavior is much more likely in minorities of Spanish heritage than in others. Lopez-Aquires et al (1984) advise using the traditional measure of self-reported health perception among Hispanics cautiously because their findings indicate that Hispanics significantly underestimate their objective health problems and conditions.
2. The ability to read and understand the label of a typical OTC cold medicine was tested on all individuals. The findings here were particularly alarming. Over 50% of the subjects could not read or comprehend the package label. This high incidence has explicit implications for all health care personnel working with the elderly. Many geriatric clients may need help in choosing an appropriate OTC medication and specific instructions concerning the proper way to take the medication.
3. The influencing factors reported to affect the selection of OTC products were significantly different in

the four groups. Whereas all relied highly on the suggestions of others, including professionals, the Caucasians reported a high reliance on reading materials, television, radio, and self-knowledge influencing their choice of OTC products.

4. The most common types of OTC products used by all groups were gastrointestinal (antacids, antidiarrheals, and laxatives) and analgesics (aspirin and acetaminophen products). The Caucasian subjects reported a high usage of vitamins whereas the Haitians reported a high usage of herbals and teas. The latter was not a major report from the other groups. However, this finding is not surprising, since Scott (1978) reported that many Haitians self-treat with herbs and home remedies before orthodox health care is sought.
5. Statistics concerning forgetfulness in taking medications were also significant among all four groups. Each group reported that memory was the most common system used to remember to take medication.
6. The evaluation of abuse and misuse of nonprescribed medications was largely dependent on the items listed in the Self-Medicating Behavior Safety Scale. Although the researchers reported no differences among the four groups studied, the group mean was only 8.4. (The scale ranged from 1 to 15 with 15 [100%] being the highest and safest score possible.) The lowest score for safety, 7.6 (51%), was reported by the Haitian group; 8.03 by Caucasians; 8.63 by Hispanics; and 10.9 (73%) by African Americans. The overall findings were in the low to low-average range for safety for all four groups.

   Approximately 56% of all subjects in the study used OTC medications inappropriately. The Caucasian group, at 81% inappropriate usage, was the highest. The latter was mainly demonstrated in inappropriate use of vitamins and health food products, with dosages in excess of U.S. RDAs* and in some instances approaching megadosages. Examples quoted from the article (Salerno, 1985) include:

   > One individual believed all OTC substances were "foods"; and she not only consumed large amounts of such products, but also advised all her friends to do the same. Another interviewee reported taking vitamin K tablets to treat "blood spots" or "skin bruises." All four groups interviewed offered many unapproved indications as reasons for consuming nonprescribed substances. Examples included taking vitamin C "to help the eyes" or "whenever it rains"; Milk of Magnesia tablets "whenever dizzy"; Pepto Bismol for "hard stools"; Alka-Seltzer for "throat allergies"; Bufferin for "indigestion or greasy food"; and aspirin "to clean out the stomach" or "for heat in the stomach." Although some expressions were endemic to a specific culture, the basic need for guidance and valid professional advice was evident.

7. Other potentially dangerous situations noted included a number of drug-drug interactions, the use of an OTC sympathomimetic in hypertensive persons; and the use of alcohol by clients taking aspirin, nitrates, antihypertensives, and CNS depressants. Many participants were not aware of the possible interactions or the alternate methods (spacing drugs apart with antacids) employed when using such medications. Foreign drugs were being taken along with American medications, and in several instances, duplicate consumption of the same medications under different names was identified. For additional information on over-the-counter medications see Chapter 11.

*U.S. Recommended Daily Allowances published by the FDA (Covington, 1996).

SUMMARY

Medications tend to be more effective when clients believe in their own capacity to get well and in the drug itself. An accurate assessment of clients' past and present experiences with drugs, illness, hospitals, nurses, and other health care personnel, as well as their own health beliefs and practices, all influence their response to drug therapy. This assessment is most important in planning and implementing an effective care plan.

Health beliefs and treatment outcome are strongly influenced by a client's cultural background, ethnic practices, beliefs, and tradition. Caring effectively for clients from different cultural groups requires an understanding of the predominant ethnic-specific influences and an assessment of individual clients to determine how those cultural influences affect health needs. There are also significant differences among racial and ethnic populations in their metabolism rates of drugs, clinical drug responses, and side effects to drugs.

Because many clients avoid standard American medicine until either their home remedies or OTC self-treatments are totally ineffective or they become acutely ill, it is essential that the nurse be aware of these practices and be prepared to counsel and support clients on appropriate methods to use in seeking health care. Although self-treatment using nonprescription drugs has its advantages for the treatment of minor complaints, consumers need a greater awareness of the risks of such medications. Clients should be reminded that nonprescription drugs are not curative but offer only symptomatic relief and that a health care provider should be seen when treated conditions are persistent or recurrent or when unusual reactions occur.

Critical Thinking

1. What personal experiences or client experiences with drug therapy can you think of that relate to the expectations of a drug's effect on symptoms?
2. What do you think are your health beliefs related to the use of medications?
3. Under what circumstances would it be appropriate to administer a placebo? What would you say to a client if you were about to administer a placebo and he or she asked what the medication was?
4. How would you respond to a client requesting information on the advisability of self-medicating with OTC preparations?

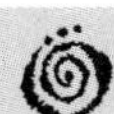

Collaborative Learning Activities

1. The students will explore the health beliefs of the different ethnic groups within their community by research, interview, collection of ethnic community newspapers, etc. The class will discuss their findings. Discuss how these health beliefs might be incorporated into teaching clients about their medications.

BIBLIOGRAPHY

American Nurses Association (1991). *Position statement on cultural diversity in nursing practice.* Kansas City, MO: The Association.

American Pain Society (1992). *Principles of analgesic use in the treatment of acute pain and cancer pain* (3rd ed.). Skokie, IL: American Pain Society.

Anderson KN, et al. (Eds.) (1994). *Mosby's medical, nursing, & allied health dictionary* (4th ed.). St Louis: Mosby.

Andrews MM & Boyle JS (1995). *Transcultural concepts in nursing care* (2nd ed.). Philadelphia: JB Lippincott.

Brink PJ (Ed.). (1990). *Transcultural nursing.* Prospect Heights, IL: Waveland Press.

Bullough VL & Bullough B (1982). *Health care for other Americans.* New York: Appleton-Century-Crofts.

Caudle P (1993). Providing culturally sensitive health care to Hispanic clients, *Nurse Pract 18*(12):40, 43-44, 46.

Chang K (1991). Chinese Americans. In Giger JN & Davidhizar RE (Eds.). *Transcultural nursing: Assessment and intervention.* St Louis: Mosby.

Communication Division of Statistics (1992). *Canada Year Book 1992.* Ottawa: Publications Division, Statistics Canada.

Covington TR (Ed.). (1996). *Handbook of nonprescription drugs* (11th ed.). Washington DC: American Pharmaceutical Association.

Edwards L (1991). Most major companies test medicines in women, monitor data for gender differences. In *New medicines in development for women.* Pharmaceutical Manufacturers Association.

Gaston-Johansson F et al. (1990). Similarities in pain descriptions of four different ethnic-culture groups, *J Pain Sympt Manage 5*(2):94.

Gaut DA (Ed.). *A global agenda for caring.* New York: National League for Nursing.

Geissler EM (1994). *Pocket guide to cultural assessment.* St Louis: Mosby.

Germain CP (1992). Cultural care: A bridge between sickness, illness, disease, *Holist Nurs Pract 6*(3):1-9.

Giger JN & Davidhizar RE (Eds.) (1995). *Transcultural nursing: Assessment and intervention* (2nd ed.). St Louis: Mosby.

Gordon SM (1994). Hispanic cultural health beliefs and folk remedies, *J Holist Nurs 12*(3):307-22.

Gutman HG (1976). *The black family in slavery and freedom, 1925-1975.* New York: Pantheon.

Henderson G & Primeaux M (1981). *Transcultural health care.* Menlo Park, CA: Addison-Wesley Publishing.

Hughes L & Bontemps A (Eds.). (1958). *The book of Negro folklore.* New York: Dodd Mead.

Jacques G (1976). Cultural health traditions: A black perspective. In Branch M & Paxton PP (Eds.). *Providing safe nursing care for ethnic people of color.* New York: Appleton-Century-Crofts.

Katzung BG (1992). *Basic and clinical pharmacology* (5th ed.). Norwalk, CT: Appleton & Lange.

Kay MA (1977). Health and illness in a Mexican American barrio. In Spicer EH (Ed.). *Ethnic medicine in the Southwest.* Tucson: University of Arizona Press.

Kiev A (1968). *Curanderismo: Mexican-American folk psychiatry.* New York: The Free Press.

Koerner J (1992). Culturally competent nursing, *Qual Assessment Q* (Summer):2.

Leininger M (1978). *Transcultural nursing: Concepts, theories and practices.* New York: John Wiley & Sons.

Leininger M (1979). *Transcultural nursing '79.* New York: Masson Publishing USA.

Leininger M (1991). *Culture care diversity and universality: Theory for nursing.* New York: National League for Nursing.

Levy RA (1993). *Ethnic and racial differences in response to medicines: Preserving individualized therapy in managed care pharmaceutical programs.* Reston, VA: National Pharmaceutical Council.

Lopez-Aquires W et al. (1984). Health needs of the Hispanic elderly, *J Amer Geriatr Soc,* p 191.

Louie TT (1990). Explanatory thinking in Chinese Americans. In Brink PJ (Ed.). *Transcultural nursing.* Prospect Heights, IL: Waveland Press.

Lynch EW (1992). The importance of cross-cultural effectiveness, *Caring 11*(10):14-19.

Martinez RA (1978). *Hispanic culture and health care: Fact, fiction, folklore.* St Louis:Mosby.

Meyer UA (1992). Drugs in special patient groups: Clinical importance of genetics in drug effects. In Melmon KL, et al. (Eds.). *Clinical Pharmacology.* New York: McGraw-Hill.

Moore LG et al. (1980). *The biocultural basis of health: Expanding views of medical anthropology.* Prospect Heights, IL:Waveland Press.

Orque MS et al. (1983). *Ethnic nursing care: A multicultural approach.* St Louis:Mosby.

Primeaux H (1977). American Indian health care practices: A cross-cultural perspective, *Nurs Clin North Amer 12*(1):57.

Robertson MHB (1987). Folk health beliefs of health professionals, *West J Nurs Res 9*(2):257.

Rawl SM (1992). Perspectives on nursing care of Chinese Americans, *J Holist Nurs 10*(1):6-17.

Salerno E et al. (1985). Self-medicating behaviors, *Fla J Hosp Pharm 5*(3):13.

Salerno E (1995). Drug update: Race, culture and medications. *J Emerg Nurs 21*(6):560-562.

Salerno E & Willens JS (1996). *Pain management handbook.* St Louis: Mosby.

Saunders L (1958). Healing ways in the Spanish Southwest. In Jaco EG (Ed.). *Patients, physicians, and illness.* Glencoe, IL: Free Press.

Scott CS (1978). Health and healing practices among five ethnic groups in Miami, Florida. In Bauwens E. *The anthropology of health.* St Louis:Mosby.

Shubin S (1980). Nursing patients from different cultures, *Nursing 10*(6):78.

Spector RE (1991). *Cultural diversity in health and illness.* (3rd ed.). Norwalk, CT: Appleton & Lange.

United States Department of Commerce, Bureau of the Census (1992). *Population profile of the United States.* Washington, DC: U.S. Government Printing Office.

Wallnofer H & von Rottauscher A (1972). *Chinese folk medicine.* New York: American Library.

Wauneka AD (1990). Helping a people to understand. In Brink PJ (Ed.). *Transcultural nursing.* Prospect Heights, IL:Waveland Press.

Wood CS (1979). *Human sickness and health: A biocultural view.* Palo Alto, CA: Mayfield Publishing.

Wyman LC (1966). Navaho diagnosticians. In Scott WR & Volkart EH (Eds.). *Medical care.* New York: Wiley.

Zhou HH et al. (1990). Differences in plasma binding of drugs between Caucasians and Chinese subjects, *Clin Pharmacol Ther 48*:10.

Chapter 7

Maternal and Child Drug Therapy

Chapter Focus

The effects of pharmaceutical agents vary in clients of different ages. The reasons for these variations are complex. Understanding the rationale behind these effects will help the nurse administer medications safely and evaluate the responses to these drugs appropriately. In addition, the client's age might also determine special techniques of administering medication to provide greater safety for the client.

In this and the following chapter special factors relating to dosing and administration of medications in the childbearing client, the neonate (birth to about 1 month of age), infants (1 month to 2 years), children, and the elderly are discussed. Medication use in the adult is discussed throughout this book, so a special chapter devoted to this topic is unnecessary. The following objectives and key terms are necessary for a good understanding of maternal and child drug therapy.

Key Terms

carcinogenic (p. 116)

fetal alcohol syndrome (p. 118)

mutagenic (p. 116)

teratogenic (p. 116)

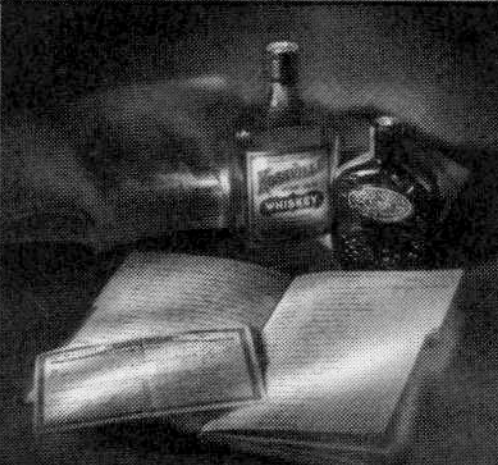

Objectives

1. Discuss special considerations for drug administration to childbearing or breastfeeding women.
2. Calculate pediatric dosages using body weight and body surface area methods.
3. Identify the preferred intramuscular injection sites in the infant or child.
4. Describe pharmacokinetic alterations related to the childbearing, breastfeeding, or pediatric client.
5. Administer medications safely and accurately to the childbearing, breastfeeding, or pediatric client.

A human life span is a continuum in which development, maturity, and then degeneration occur without any distinct demarcation. However, individuals mature and decline and/or have special needs at different ages, at different rates, and under different circumstances. These factors affect the client's response to drug therapy in characteristic ways. Therefore nursing management of drug therapy needs to be based on both physiologic and psychosocial development levels.

CHILDBEARING CLIENTS

Any substance ingested or absorbed by a pregnant woman is likely to reach the fetus by way of maternal circulation or to be transferred to the breastfed neonate by way of breast milk if the substance is in sufficient concentration and is well distributed. Thus drugs taken by the mother can cause serious harm to the fetus or neonate. No drug is known to be *absolutely* safe for the developing embryo, but some oral medications that are inactivated in the mother's stomach or not absorbed by the maternal gastrointestinal tract are assumed to be relatively safe. However, the effects of many drugs and other substances on the fetus are unknown.

Considerations for drug therapy in the childbearing client center on the risk-benefit ratio. This ratio is evaluated based on the mother's condition and the effect of the drug(s) on the mother and the developing fetus or nursing infant. Prescription and over-the-counter (OTC) drugs taken during pregnancy have, in some instances, resulted in fetal drug toxicity and teratogenicity (the ability to cause fetal abnormalities). Although the possible effect of some medications taken during pregnancy is known, new medications, different drug combinations, or a deficiency in metabolism in the fetus may change a drug previously known to be safe into a hazardous one. The period of greatest danger for drug-induced developmental defects is during the first trimester of pregnancy. Therefore, self-treatment of minor illnesses is discouraged during pregnancy and women should be instructed to keep a complete record of all medications consumed during pregnancy (Bobak & Jensen, 1991).

The childbearing client takes an average of four or more drugs (other than vitamins) during pregnancy, and the fetal effects of these drugs are unknown. Thus this topic is of utmost concern during the parenting stage of life. Nurses are commonly required to provide accurate information with rationale, discuss the health care options available, and support parents' decisions during the childbearing process. Health care providers and parents alike may have to make difficult choices based on the benefit-to-risk ratio based on maternal medication regimens, the benefits to the mother, and the risks to the fetus or neonate. This dilemma illustrates the absolute necessity for nurses to be knowledgeable about medications and highly skilled at retrieving information from reliable sources. Parents should make the final decisions regarding care based on informed, sensitive input from all appropriate health professionals.

Drug Transfer to the Fetus

Pharmacokinetics

There are multiple physiologic changes related to pregnancy that affect pharmacokinetics. Pregnancy does not seem to have much effect on drug absorption from the gastrointestinal tract, but protein binding is decreased for some substances, which increases the amount of drug available for placental transfer. Biotransformation of drugs in the liver is probably delayed in pregnancy, but renal excretion may be more rapid because renal blood flow dramatically increases glomerular filtration rate. (See Chapter 3, Principles of Drug Action.)

At the placental interface, the transfer of drugs and other substances is primarily by simple diffusion and partly by active transport. Transfer across the placenta depends on the chemical properties of the drug: its molecular weight, protein-binding capabilities, chemical configuration, and lipid solubility. The potential for transfer to the fetus is proportional to the period of time the drug remains in the maternal bloodstream. Transfer is greater during late gestation because of enhanced uteroplacental blood flow, increased placental surface at the interface, thinner membranes separating maternal blood flow and placental capillaries, and an increased proportion of free drug available to the circulation. Pathologic processes in the placenta, such as inflammation, degeneration, or partial separation, can alter blood flow and thus drug transfer. By whichever mechanism, drug transfer can result in significant fetal drug effects (see section on fetal drug effects).

Many drugs are transferred across the placenta but not all are dangerous. Thus the traditional concept of the placenta being a completely protective barrier to circulating substances must be discarded. Most drugs that cross the placenta stabilize in the fetus at a level between 50% and 100% of the maternal level. Some (such as diazepam and local anesthetics) stabilize at levels even higher than those of the mother's. However, continued exposure of the fetus to a drug is more important than the rate of placental transport. See Box 7-1 for drugs associated with neonatal withdrawal symptoms (Levy & Spino, 1993).

Fetal Drug Effects

Fetal drug effects may be more significant and prolonged than in the mother because of (1) probable immature enzyme drug metabolizing systems or absence of such systems and (2) slower excretion rates. Drug excretion by the fetus is accomplished by the kidneys. Waste products are excreted into the amniotic fluid, which is reabsorbed by the mother or swallowed by the fetus. Thus the fetus's immature or underdeveloped physiologic mechanisms may result in altered drug responses and perhaps toxicity.

Occasionally, various fetal complications such as anemia and syphilis exposure have been actively treated by drugs in utero. The drug delivery routes chosen have been either the passive, transplacental approach or direct instillation into the amniotic fluid. Use of these drug delivery routes is still controversial.

It continues to be well documented, however, that various drugs administered before delivery or the continued use of abuse drugs throughout pregnancy may have toxic and harmful effects on the newborn. The embryo or fetus runs the risk of developing the usual side or toxic effects, just as the mother does. For example, if the mother consumes alcohol, barbiturates, or narcotics, the neonate at birth may have withdrawal symptoms: hyperactivity, crying, irritability, seizures, and perhaps sudden death. Box 7-1 lists drugs that can cause symptoms of withdrawal.

Medications may be lethal or **teratogenic** (causing fetal defects), **mutagenic** (causing genetic mutation), or **carcinogenic** (causing or accelerating the development of cancer). An example of the last is the precancerous or cancerous cell changes discovered in youths whose mothers took the hormone diethylstilbestrol (DES) during pregnancy.

Every embryo undergoes a series of precisely programmed steps from cell proliferation, differentiation, and migration to organogenesis. The critical periods for drug effects on the fetus are the first 2 weeks of rapid cell proliferation, when exposure to drugs can be lethal to the embryo, and the third through the tenth weeks of pregnancy, when the axial skeleton, muscles, limbs, and organs are developing most rapidly.

An unfortunate example of teratogenic effect is the hypnotic drug thalidomide, which caused abnormal limb development (phocomelia) in many children whose mothers received the drug during pregnancy. When it was administered beyond the tenth week of pregnancy, physiologic or behavioral alterations and delays in growth were more likely.

Cocaine abuse by pregnant women has resulted in frequent miscarriages, fetal hypoxia, and low-birth-weight in-

BOX 7-1

Drugs Associated with Neonatal Withdrawal Symptoms*

	Symptoms	
	General	CNS
Alcohol	Irritability, poor sleep pattern, diaphoresis	Crying, hyperactivity, increased sensitivity to sound, hypertonicity, tremor, seizures
Cocaine	Tremulousness, poor sleep pattern	Hypotonia, hyperreflexia
Antihistamines		
diphenhydramine (Benadryl)	Tremulousness	
hydroxyzine (Atarax, Vistaril)	Irritability	Hyperactivity, tremor, jitteriness, shrill cry, hypotonia, seizures
Barbiturates		
amobarbital (Amytal) ethchlorvynol (Placidyl) phenobarbital, secobarbital (Seconal)	Irritability, poor sleep pattern, diaphoresis, skin abrasions	Excessive crying, hyperreflexia, increased sensitivity to sound, hypertonicity, tremor, seizures
Benzodiazepines		
chlordiazepoxide (Librium)	Irritability	Tremors
diazepam (Valium)	Hypothermia	Hyperactivity, hypotonia, hypertonia, apnea/tremor, hyperreflexia
Opiates		
codeine heroin meperidine (Demerol)	Irritability, wakefulness, yawning, tearing, fever, diaphoresis Skin excoriations, voracious sucking	Coarse tremors, seizures, twitching Hyperactivity (high-pitched cry), hypertonicity
methadone morphine pentazocine (Talwin)	Poor sleep pattern Hypothermia Respiratory (stuffy, runny nose, sneezing, tachypnea, respiratory alkalosis), gastrointestinal (hiccups, salivation, vomiting, diarrhea, failure to thrive)	Hyperreflexia, increased sensitivity to sound, photophobia, apneic spells
propoxyphene (Darvon)	Irritability, fever	Hyperactivity, tremor, high pitched cry

*Modified from Levy M & Spino M (1993). Neonatal withdrawal syndrome: Associated drugs and pharmacologic management, *Pharmacotherapy* 13(3):202-211.

fants. Cocaine exposure in utero has caused fetal tremors, strokes, and an increase in stillbirth rates. Exposed infants are also at high risk for developing congenital heart disease, skull defects, and other congenital malformations. At birth the newborn may exhibit symptoms of withdrawal: increased irritability, increased respiratory and heart rates, diarrhea, irregular sleeping patterns, and poor appetite. It has been reported that long-term behavioral patterns of infants born to cocaine-abusing women may occur, such as poor attention spans and a decrease in organizational skills (Hall et al, 1990). In a number of instances the courts or legal system have intervened to protect the unborn fetus, or to punish the mother of a child born with medical complications resulting from cocaine abuse.

In certain situations drugs are necessary during pregnancy and breastfeeding. Some maternal conditions (e.g., hypertension, epilepsy, diabetes, and infection) seriously jeopardize both mother and fetus if untreated. Although authoritative literature and drug package inserts routinely warn that drugs have not been tested for use in pregnancy, during breastfeeding, or for infants, much empiric and some research data are accumulating. The FDA now rates drugs as to their safety for use during pregnancy. This rating is discussed in Chapter 2 and is used throughout this textbook.

A major issue regarding drugs used during pregnancy and the neonatal period involves the legal and ethical problems that are associated with drug research experiments during pregnancy, which contributes to the lack of information in this area. Well-controlled research, although fraught with ethical dilemmas, is undeniably needed. Nurses are in a good position to participate in this important research, and they should do so.

Certain categories of drugs are expressly contraindicated during pregnancy or are used only when the risk-benefit situation has been carefully considered and thoroughly discussed with the client. See Box 7-2 for drugs with reported teratogenic effects. Some drugs considered relatively safe during pregnancy, depending on the situation, are listed in Table 7-1.

However, drug use should be severely curtailed, being limited to only those pregnant women whose life or that of the fetus would be in jeopardy without drug treatment. If necessary to administer drug therapy, the following variables should be considered:

1. The dose that reaches the embryo or fetus depends on the maternal dosage, the maternal volume of distribution, and the metabolic clearance rate of the mother

BOX 7-2

Drugs and Potential Teratogenic Effects

Drug	Critical time period	Potential defect
angiotensin-converting enzyme (ACE) inhibitors	2nd-3rd trimester	renal dysgenesis, defects in skull ossification
alcohol, chronic use	<12 weeks	heart defects, CNS abnormalities
	>24 weeks	delay in development, low birth weight
aminopterin	<14 weeks	spontaneous abortion
	1st trimester	limb, craniofacial, and neural tube defects
androgens	>10 weeks	external female genitalia masculinization
carbamazepine	<30 days after conception	spina bifida
cigarette smoking	<20 weeks	miscarriage
	>20 weeks	low birth weight and perhaps delay in development
cocaine	2nd-3rd trimester	abruptio placentae
	3rd trimester	premature labor and delivery; intracranial bleeding
diethylstilbestrol (DES)	<12 weeks	vaginal adenosis, vaginal carcinoma, uterine abnormalities, male infertility
isotretinoin (Accutane)	>15 days after conception	hydrocephalus, CNS abnormalities, fetal death
lithium	<2 months	Ebstein's anomaly
methotrexate	6-9 weeks after conception	skull ossification defect, limb and craniofacial defects
phenytoin (Dilantin)	1st trimester	craniofacial defects, phalanges/nails underdevelopment
tetracycline	>20 weeks	stained teeth, bone growth defect
valproic acid	<1 month after conception	spina bifida
	1st trimester	craniofacial defects
vaccines (measles, mumps, rubella)	1st trimester	spontaneous abortions, premature births, possibly congenital defects
vitamin A (high doses & parenteral)	—	fetal abnormalities including urinary tract malformations, growth retardation

Modified from Jennings, 1996.

TABLE 7-1 Some drugs considered relatively safe for use in pregnancy

Agent	Recommendations and cautions*
Analgesics	
acetaminophen	Considered safest analgesic during pregnancy
Antiasthmatics	
cromolyn sodium	Relatively safe
metaproterenol (aerosol)	Relatively safe for mild, intermittent episodes: avoid oral form
theophylline	Relatively safe if blood levels are closely monitored
Anticoagulants	
heparin	For use during first trimester; use caution if given during last trimester
Anticonvulsants	
phenobarbital	Can cause malformations: for use only if necessary to maintain seizure control; if given during pregnancy, monitor neonate during first 24 hours for neonatal coagulation defect (bleeding)
Antidiabetics	
insulin	Relatively safe; drug of choice
Antiemetics	
pyridoxine	Relatively safe for morning sickness
doxylamine	For use as necessary for severe nausea or vomiting
prochlorperazine	
trimethobenzamide	
cyclizine	
meclizine	
Antihypertensives	
methyldopa	Safest of antihypertensives during pregnancy (especially as substitute for diuretics in pregnancy for diastolic blood pressure >110 mm Hg in the third trimester)
hydralazine	Safest for hypertensive crises in pregnancy
Antiinfectives	
cephalosporins	Safe during pregnancy
erythromycin	For use as substitute for penicillin hypersensitivity
metronidazole	Not to be used during the first trimester
miconazole	Relatively safe
penicillin and derivatives	Relatively safe
Antituberculosis drugs	
rifampin	Relatively safe
ethambutol	
Cardiac glycosides	
digoxin	Relatively safe; maternal plasma levels should be closely monitored

*Recommendations are likely to change; therefore, manufacturers' package inserts should always be consulted. No drugs are known to be *absolutely* safe during pregnancy. The use of many substances, including most drugs not on this list, should be carefully considered by the obstetrician as to risks and benefits. See drug monographs for specific drug information; see also bibliography. Consult references for sources of information about drugs in this table.

2. The fetal gestational age at time of exposure
3. Duration of therapy planned
4. Fetal and maternal genotypes
5. Any other drugs administered concurrently

Dosages, dosing intervals, and duration of treatment should be adjusted carefully to avoid harmful effects.

Excessive maternal intake of alcohol, especially at or near time of conception, is associated with **fetal alcohol syndrome**, which produces congenital anomalies, and both growth and mental retardation (Box 7-3). Other very common substances that are potentially dangerous during pregnancy include extended release aspirin (pregnancy category D), parenteral vitamin A (category X), and nicotine chewing gum and nicotine transdermal systems (category X and category D respectively) (*USP DI*, 1996).

A problem with drug use is that the effects on the embryo may occur before the woman is aware that she is pregnant. Women of childbearing age who are not using contraceptives and who are sexually active should be prescribed drugs carefully and should be instructed to use over-the-counter medications cautiously. Education and prevention are considered the best therapy.

Nursing Management

Medication Administration with Childbearing Clients

Most nursing goals related to medication administration should be aimed at ensuring that parents know that any foreign substance absorbed by the mother may have lifelong effects on the child and family. A balance must be maintained between protecting the individual while promoting the role and formation of the family. Essential to these goals, the nurse should be an advocate for the client, establish an environment conducive to the exchange of information, and minimize parental feelings of guilt or fear associated with

BOX 7-3

Alcohol and the Childbearing Client: Fetal Alcohol Syndrome

Many people do not consider alcohol to be a drug; thus it may be overlooked as being hazardous if used during pregnancy. The teratogenic effects of intrauterine alcohol exposure on the fetus are well documented. Heavy use of alcohol by the childbearing client has been associated with the following effects:

Facial: ptosis, strabismus, myopia, cleft lip or palate
CNS: retardation, impaired coordination, increased irritability during infancy, hyperactivity in childhood
Growth: retarded
Cardiac: murmurs, tetralogy of Fallot
Muscular: hernias of the groin, umbilicus, or diaphragm

While a direct relationship between the quantity of alcohol consumed and the severity of fetal alcohol syndrome (FAS) has not been identified, it appears alcohol consumption in excess of the liver's capability to detoxify it places the fetus at greatest risk.

Although the exact mechanism of FAS has not been identified, studies indicate that counseling to eliminate maternal alcohol intake has a beneficial effect on the health of both the mother and infant. It has been suggested that women discontinue alcohol use at least 3 months before becoming pregnant (Wong, 1993).

The nurse must be aware of clients who are at risk of FAS and be prepared to provide client education, counseling, and referral (Briggs, 1992; Wong, 1993).

drug administration and the potential impact on the unborn. The following information should be conveyed to the family:

1. Potential harm to the unborn child resulting directly from substances to which the mother is exposed and potential risks and benefits to both mother and child if treatment is not begun must both be weighed. These decisions must be made with the prescriber whenever exposure to an unfamiliar substance or drug is contemplated.
2. Over-the-counter medications and other common substances such as aspirin, high-dose or multiple vitamin supplements, alcohol, caffeine, and nicotine may also have detrimental effects on the fetus.
3. Any prescription written by a professional who is not a specialist in the care of pregnant women or nursing mothers should be evaluated by an obstetrician or pediatrician. The prescription may need to be changed by the specialist to a safer drug or dosage.
4. If the mother is exposed to a questionable substance, close health care supervision is essential. If there is high risk for fetal or infant injury, the parents need ongoing support as they endure the sometimes long wait for effects to be manifested. If birth defects or toxic effects are present or if invasive diagnostic tests or a therapeutic abortion is to be performed, objective psychologic intervention may help the parents endure this critical period.

PEDIATRIC CLIENTS

Neonates

Because newborns lack many of the protective mechanisms that allow older children and adults to be relatively resistant to stressors of all kinds, they require special considerations. Their skin is thin and permeable, their stomachs lack acid, and their lungs lack much of the mucous barrier. Neonates regulate body temperature poorly and become dehydrated easily. Their liver and kidneys are immature and cannot manage foreign substances as well as older children and adults. Specific factors affecting medication use in neonates are covered in Table 7-2.

Breastfed Infants

Almost *all* forms of drugs in maternal circulation can be readily transferred to the colostrum and breast milk. Because drugs or their biotransformed products are handled by different pathways in the infant and the fetus, the impact of maternal medications on the infant probably differs (is probably less) than that on the fetus. This difference can guide in prescribing medications for the breastfeeding woman. Typical nontherapeutic outcomes in the breastfed infant are signs of the drug's usual side or toxic effects.

Adverse effects may also occur, such as allergic sensitization to penicillin, or gray-brown stains of the later-erupting teeth as a result of tetracycline therapy of more than 10 days duration. Most drug products that reach the neonate via breast milk have undergone maternal biotransformation and are probably less than the original dose. However, immaturity of the neonate's hepatic and renal systems may limit the infant's capacity for further metabolism and excretion.

Data about an infant's capabilities for drug absorption, digestion, distribution, metabolism, and excretion are scant and conflicting. In general the proved benefits of continuing breastfeeding must be weighed on an individual basis against the risks of maternal medication to the infant. Although the mammary glands are a relatively insignificant route for maternal drug excretion and the drug level in breast milk is usually less than the actual maternal dose, the infant's actual dose depends largely on the volume of milk consumed. Thus a single measurement of a drug in human milk will not accurately reflect the total dose the infant receives.

The concentration of the drug in maternal circulation depends on the relationship of several factors: dosing and route of administration, the drug's distribution, its protein binding, and maternal metabolism and excretion. The mammary alveolar epithelium consists of a lipid barrier with water-filled pores; thus it is more permeable to drugs during the colostrum stage of milk production—during the first week of life.

Drug factors that enhance drug excretion into milk are nonionization, low molecular weight, fat solubility, and concentration. The absorptive processes of the infant's gastrointestinal tract and drug distribution are estimated to be similar to those in the adult, which means that lipid-soluble substances are well absorbed. The infant's age (thus the amount of drug-containing milk consumed) and the relative immaturity of the infant's important organs bear greatly on the outcome. The following factors are also relevant: (1) if the drug is fat soluble, it may be more highly concentrated in breast milk at the end of feedings and at midday; (2) because the infant's total serum protein is lower in comparison to the adult's, more free drug may be available to the circulation; (3) metabolic reactions in the infant's liver are slower than in the older child's, consequently, drug biotransformation may likewise be delayed; and (4) drug excretion is delayed in the neonate because it is largely via the kidneys, where immature glomerular filtration rates and tubular functioning are maintained for several months. The extreme variability among drug effects and infants' capabilities makes it difficult to decide whether the mother should take a drug and whether or not she should breastfeed.

If human milk contains small, fixed amounts of substances absorbed by the mother, it is usually recommended that breast-feeding be temporarily interrupted (usually for 24 to 72 hours) and the breasts pumped to remove drug-containing milk. Less often, it is advisable to cease breastfeeding altogether. Dosages and routes may also be changed. It is recommended that certain drugs be avoided while breastfeeding (Box 7-4).

Drug effects may be minimized by substituting formula for the midday breastfeeding, since that is the feeding highest in fat content and thus more likely to contain higher

TABLE 7-2 Pharmacokinetics that influence drug dosing in neonates

Physiologic process	Neonate	Type of drugs affected
Absorption		
Gastric pH	Increased to 6 to 8 for first 24 hours; then usually a 10- to 15-day achlorhydria	Acid-labile drugs, such as oral penicillin, better absorbed Oral forms of phenobarbital or phenytoin: reduced bioavailability
Gastric emptying time	Prolonged, usually 6 to 8 hours	Oral absorption of penicillin increased; phenytoin, phenobarbital decreased
Distribution		
Total body water (TBW) content	75% to 79%	Average adults have about 60% TBW and 25% to 45% fat
Adipose (fat) content	5% to 12%	Vast differences in drug distribution across the age span Water-soluble drugs have a larger volume of distribution in newborns, fat-soluble drugs have considerably less Drug dosage adjustments largely based on this factor
Protein binding	Decreased	Highly protein-bound drugs require dose adjustment to avoid toxicity
Metabolism		
Liver metabolism	Decreased	Potent or potentially toxic drugs requiring liver metabolism are slowly metabolized; lower doses are necessary for such drugs (especially chloramphenicol and theophylline, among others)
Microsomal enzymes	Low	
Excretion		
Glomerular filtration	Decreased	Drugs excreted by filtration or secretion will accumulate in the neonate; dose adjustments necessary (especially aminoglycosides and digoxin)
Tubular secretion	Decreased	

BOX 7-4

Drugs Contraindicated During Breastfeeding

The American Academy of Pediatrics committee on drugs has suggested the following drugs be avoided by the woman who is breastfeeding:

amphetamines	gold salts
bromocriptine	heroin
cocaine	lithium
cyclophosphamide	marijuana
cyclosporine	methotrexate
doxorubicin	nicotine (smoking)
ergotamine	phenindione

amounts of fat-soluble drug products. In addition, breastfeeding mothers who must take medications can take the medication immediately *after* breastfeeding so as much time as possible elapses and the drug can reach a relatively low concentration before the next feeding (Table 7-3).

With radioactive substances, therapy is of short duration, or if merely a diagnostic radioisotope test is to be done, breastfeeding is interrupted until all radiation is absent from milk samples. Breastfeeding will probably be terminated at any time when the drug is so potent that minute amounts may profoundly affect the infant, when the drug has high allergenic potential, when the mother's renal function decreases (which augments drug excretion into breast milk), or when serious pathologic conditions require prolonged administration of high doses of the drug.

TABLE 7-3 Some drugs considered relatively safe during breastfeeding

Agent	Recommendations and precautions*
Analgesics	
acetaminophen	Relatively safe
aspirin	
mefenamic acid	
propoxyphene	
meperidine	
Antiinfectives	
cephalexin	Safe; not found in breast milk
cephalothin	
oxacillin	
penicillin	Relatively safe after 1 mo, but may sensitize the infant
erythromycin	Safe after 1 mo
isoniazid	Safe
ethambutol	Safe
Cardiovascular drugs	
digoxin	Safe if maternal serum levels are closely monitored
guanethidine	Safe in recommended dosages
methyldopa	Safe
propranolol	Relatively safe at lower maternal dosages (higher drug levels in breast milk than in maternal bloodstream because of high lipid solubility of drug)
Diuretics	
spironolactone	Safe
thiazides and furosemide	May suppress lactation; avoid in first month of lactation
Sedative-hypnotics	
lorazepam	Excreted in milk; monitor for drug accumulation in infant, lethargy
prazepam	
oxazepam	
Anticonvulsants	
primidone	Relatively safe with close observation
phenytoin	
Bronchodilators	
ephedrine	Safe; destroyed in infant's GI tract
cromolyn sodium	Observe for infant irritability or insomnia
theophylline	
Psychotropic drugs	
chlorpromazine	Appear safe, although found in milk; may cause drowsiness in baby. All classified as "use cautiously" may have cause for concern†
phenothiazine	
tricyclic antidepressants	
Antidiabetics	
insulin	Safe; destroyed in the GI tract
Thyroid drugs	
thyroid hormones	Relatively safe if monitored for thyroid function and response
Gastrointestinal drugs	
antacids	Safe; electrolytes should be monitored
metoclopramide	
laxatives (except cascara and danthron)	
Pesticides	Under usual conditions found less in human milk than in cow's milk
Air pollutants	Have not been found in human milk
Vaccines	
RhoGAM	Considered safe

*Over time recommendations may change; therefore manufacturer's package inserts should always be consulted by pediatricians and nurses. Most substances should be avoided during the period of breastfeeding. (Details about specific drugs are located under relevant chapter headings in this text.) Consult bibliography for sources of information.

†By American Academy of Pediatrics.

Changes in the activity levels of the fetus or nursing infant signal dangerous effects resulting from drug administration. Parents should be taught how to assess and report unusual fetal inactivity or infant apathy.

Alternatives to drug therapy. Both health professionals and clients place a high value on the use of pharmaceuticals to treat minor illnesses. However, many illnesses are self-limited or cause only minor discomforts that end or decrease without medication or with nondrug alternatives, for example, relaxation techniques rather than tranquilizers. The risk-to-benefit effect of any medication should consider physiologic, physical, and psychologic effects of the therapy on both the mother and the child.

Another consideration for the breastfeeding woman is to delay the mother's pharmacologic therapy until the infant is weaned or to select another drug to meet the therapeutic goal without interfering with breastfeeding. The age and maturity of the child must be considered also. As the infant develops physiologically the drug's ability to cause harmful effects will diminish. The frequency of feedings should also be considered. An infant dependent on breast milk for total nutrition will receive higher doses of drugs than an infant breastfeeding only once or twice a day and receiving other forms of nourishment.

Nonbreastfed Infants

Infant formula feeding is used when the mother:

- chooses not to breastfeed *or*
- is advised not to breastfeed because of illness or disease *or*
- has an infant with special formulation needs.

Commercially available preparations are available prepared from nonfat cow's milk and are generally divided into two categories: general purpose and special purpose infant formulas (see Box 7-5 for selected formulas from each category).

Infant formulas contain essential and minor trace elements as found in human breast milk, plus the three sources of calories (protein, carbohydrate, and lipids) in a balanced proportion to promote growth. Many of the formulas contain vitamins and minerals and usually the vitamin K in these formulas is more than is contained in breast milk. Vitamin K is included because it reduces the risk of hemorrhagic disease in the infant.

Cow's milk differs from human milk in protein content. The protein (80%) in cow's milk is casein, whereas human milk contains whey protein (70%). Human milk protein (whey) is richer in immunoglobulins, albumin, lysozyme, amylase, transaminase, protease, and lipases. Casein provides lesser amounts of these ingredients. Although the protein in many of the formulations is of a higher quality than cow's milk, some infant formulas may contain bovine whey, a protein that contains beta-lactoglobulin. This substance contributes to the development of cow milk allergies.

Infants can absorb 20% to 50% of the iron they need from breast milk, whereas iron from infant formulations is only minimally absorbed (4% to 7%). The reason for this difference in absorption is unknown. The Committee on Nutrition of the American Academy of Pediatrics checked the iron content in formulas and found that as many as 20% of infants receive a formula with a low-iron content (1.5 mg/L). The possible reason for the use of these products is prescribers believing that iron is responsible for colic, con-

BOX 7-5

Selected Examples of Infant Formulations

Product name/manufacturer	Indications/special features
General purpose	
Enfamil (Mead Johnson)	Supplement to breastfeeding
Good-Start (Carnation)	
PediaSure (Ross)	
Special purpose	
Alimentum Liquid (Ross)	Severe food allergies, protein sensitivity or maldigestion, or fat malabsorption; corn and lactose free
Isomil Liquid & Powder (Ross)	Infants and children allergic to cow's milk, lactose deficient, or are galactosemic; lactose free
Phenex-1 Powder (Ross)	Infants with phenylketonuria (PKU)
Pregestrimil Powder (Mead Johnson)	Severe malabsorption disorders
ProSobee (Mead Johnson)	Infants with family history of allergies; lactose, milk, and sucrose free
Infant formulas with iron	
Enfamil with Iron (Mead Johnson)	
Similac w/Iron (Ross)	
SMA Iron Fortified (Mead Johnson)	
Lofenalac Powder (Mead Johnson)	Low phenylalanine plus iron

stipation, diarrhea, and regurgitation, and thus recommending the lower iron formulations. Research indicates this belief is unfounded; thus the Committee has recommended that these formulations be removed from the market and iron-fortified formulas be exclusively utilized (Pray, 1993).

Pediatric Drug Administration

Administering medications to pediatric clients requires special knowledge and approaches. The dosage of a medication may be prescribed, but it is the nurse's responsibility to know the safe dosage range of any medication administered to children. A standard medication dosage is nearly nonexistent in pediatrics (Box 7-6); therefore medications are usually ordered according to the weight or body surface area of the child. Some pharmaceutical companies continue to supply medications in a standard adult dosage strength, and the nurse must be able to calculate the correct pediatric dosage before administering the medication.

A nurse calculating dosages of digitalis, insulin, barbiturates, and narcotics should have the calculations as well as the prepared medication dosage checked by a nurse or pharmacist before the drug is administered. Pediatric dosages are often minute, and a slight calculation error may result in a greater proportional error.

BOX 7-6

Pediatric Drug Labels

In 1979 the FDA proposed that drug manufacturers add more complete pediatric dosing information on their drug products. However, a survey conducted by the American Academy of Pediatrics reported that 80% of all products released from 1984 to 1989 lacked pediatric dose information. In 1992 the FDA again indicated that more complete information related to pediatric dosing needs to be included on drug labeling. This latest FDA proposal does not specifically require data from well-designed, controlled studies; thus whatever is known about drug use in children should be submitted by health care providers for review. But even under these circumstances, physicians and pharmacists are fearful that useful drug information for pediatric use will be lacking (Chi, 1992).

Critical questions that need answers before safe pediatric drug use include:

- Was the drug used in children? If so, what were the dosage and method of administration?
- What was the age of the youngest child or infant who received the drug?
- Were any side or adverse effects reported: Frequency of such effect?
- Should the FDA require these data before marketing the drug?

Weight as a basis. The following is a formula for calculating estimated safe dosages based on weight alone (Clark's rule). Because this formula is based on weight alone, it is often considered an imprecise calculation for children.

$$\frac{\text{Average adult dose} \times \text{Weight of child in pounds}}{150}$$

Example: How much acetaminophen (Tylenol) should a 1-year-old child weighing 21 pounds receive if the average adult dose is 10 grains?

Answer:

$$\frac{10\text{ (grains)} \times 21\text{ (weight in pounds)}}{150} = \text{gr } 1^2/_5$$

Calculating the pediatric dose on the basis of weight alone implies that the pediatric client is a small adult, which is not true. Physiologic differences in an infant as compared with an adult definitely affect the amount of drug needed to produce a therapeutic effect.

For example, an infant's body composition is approximately 75% water (adults have 50% to 60%) and they have less fat content than the adult. Therefore, water-soluble drugs are generally administered in larger doses to infants and children in proportion to body weight than to adults. A good example of this is the water-soluble drug gentamicin, an intravenous antibiotic. Recommended dosages from *USP DI* (1996) are: older neonates and infants, 2.5 mg/kg every 8 to 16 hours; children, 2 to 2.5 mg/kg every 8 hours; and adults under 60 kg, 1.5 mg/kg every 12 hours.

Rules based on weight, such as Clark's rule, are generally taught and used by students in clinical areas to assess pediatric dosages. Although it has limited usefulness as a guide, using Clark's rule for a number of drugs is questionable and may yield inaccurate results. Determining pediatric drug dosages by body surface area (BSA) is considered more accurate.

Body surface area as a basis. It was suggested years ago that drug dosages be calculated on size or the proportional amount of body surface area (BSA) to weight. While prescribers continue to use weight as the basis for calculating drug dosages and body surface area for calculating fluid requirements, most clinicians advocate using body surface area for determining drug dosage for adults as well as children. Prescribers usually carry a simple slide rule or nomogram, such as the West nomogram (Figure 7-1) to make rapid BSA conversions from weight and height. It is believed that the larger amount of total body water (TBW) in children, as well as the percentage of water in body weight and the part of that percentage formed by extracellular water, accounts for the fact that children tolerate or require larger doses of some drugs on a mg/m^2 basis.

For the approximately 75% of drugs that have no established dosage for children, calculating the pediatric dosage as a fraction of the average adult dose using Clark's rule is really too imprecise for most applications, yet it may be used (mg/kg) when the dosage according to body surface area has not been established. The surface area rule is the most accu-

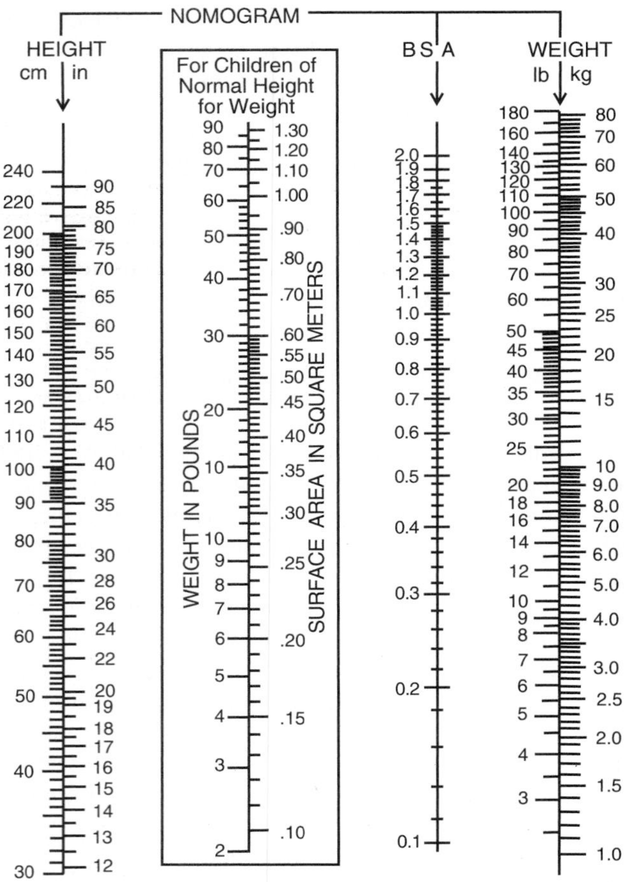

Figure 7-1 BSA is indicated where straight line that connects height (on the left) and weight (on the right) levels intersects BSA column or, if client is above average size, from weight alone (enclosed area). (Modified from data of E Boyd by CD West.)

rate. As a relationship between height and weight, it can provide a more precise guide to the maturity of the child's organs and metabolic rate of functioning for effective pharmacokinetics. The dosage should be tailored to the individual child according to the amount of medication per square meter of body surface area. The BSA rule for pediatric dosages follows:

Approximate pediatric dose =

$$\frac{\text{Child's BSA in square meters (from nomogram)} \times \text{Adult dose}}{1.73}$$

For example, using Figure 7-1, a child with a height of 34 inches weighing 10 kg would be considered to have a body surface area (m^2) of 0.5. The dosage calculation then would be:

$$\text{Child's approximate dose} = \frac{0.5 \times \text{Adult dose}}{1.73}$$

If the student is uncertain about dosage, the following sources are recommended: the drug monograph in a package insert, *USP DI, AHFS,* pediatric drug handbooks, or consultation with a pharmacist.

■Nursing Management

Medication Administration in Pediatric Clients

Although these rules have been devised for converting adult dosage schedules to infants and children, it must be emphasized that *no rules or charts are adequate to guarantee safety of dosage at any age,* particularly in the neonate. No method takes into account all variables, particularly individual tolerance differences. Astute, accurate nursing observations of how individual children react to drugs can assist in monitoring drugs and dosages.

Administering medications to infants and children is both challenging and frustrating. Giving injections skillfully will enhance safety and help to gain a child's cooperation. A sound knowledge of growth and development also provides the nurse with information about how a child might be approached, whether reasoning will help or hinder the process, and whether assistance will be needed. The principles of safe administration of medication apply to all age groups, but children differ from adults, and the nurse has added responsibilities (Box 7-7).

Ideally, a child will cooperate more readily with a nurse once a positive relationship has been established. The child may also more easily accept the discomforts of injections and of some oral medications from a nurse who is associated with daily hygiene, feeding, holding, play, and happy times. In addition, the nurse will feel less guilty when the child associates the nurse with pleasure and comfort most of the time and with discomfort only when it is necessary in order for the child to get well.

When a child is afraid or anxious, the natural response is to strike out at the frustration or avoid it. By accepting this behavior as a natural response, the nurse will be able to deal with it and to be honest when a medication or procedure will be unpleasant or painful.

Truthful explanations are essential with children. They have a right to an explanation of any procedure that concerns them. The timing and type of explanation should be geared to the child's ability to perceive and understand. For the child 2 years of age or younger very simple explanations such as "I have some medicine for you to drink" or "I have an injection to give you, and it will hurt a little" are sufficient. Young children may be less resistant to injectable medications if a parent holds and comforts them. In an ambulatory care setting, it is best to have the child all dressed and ready to leave before administering immunizations and other injectables. With just brief exposure of the appropriate injection site to determine landmarks, a quick injection and then exit from the facility will decrease the child's association of the discomfort of an injection with the clinical setting.

Long explanations to children under 5 years of age do little more than prolong the anticipation and increase anxiety or fear. Telling 4-year-olds to stop kicking, hitting, or performing any other avoidance behavior only conveys to them that they are not understood and that they will receive little or no help with their feelings of frustration about being med-

BOX 7-7

Pediatric Drug Administration Guidelines

1. Parents are frequently good sources of information about successful methods or vehicles of giving medications to their children.
2. Try to avoid putting medications in essential foods such as milk, cereal, or orange juice, since the child may refuse to accept that food in the future.
3. Never underestimate children's reactions. The taste of medication may not need to be disguised.
4. A sip of cold fruit juice, ice chips, a frozen fruit-bar, or a mint-flavored substance before and after the administration of an unpalatable medicine may effectively dull its taste.
5. Sugarless vehicles should be used to disguise the taste of medications given to diabetic children or those on a ketogenic diet.
6. Jam and syrup are ideal for suspending drugs that do not dissolve easily in water.
7. Because fruit syrups are usually acid, they should not be used for medicines that react in an acid medium (e.g., sodium bicarbonate, soluble barbiturates, and penicillin).
8. Elixirs have an alcohol base that when undiluted may cause the child either to refuse them or to cough and choke; they may also cause a drug-drug interaction. Small amounts of water added to elixirs of phenobarbital or chloral hydrate occasionally help.
9. Nursing time can be saved by recording the most successful method of administering medications and pertinent nursing orders on the child's care plan. This notation also saves the child frustration, fear, and anxiety.

icated. Providing the preschool-age child opportunities at play (e.g., to give a doll an "injection" [empty syringe without a needle] or "drops") affords an important outlet and allows the child to work through the trauma of the experience.

Many children are courageous, or like to be considered so, and appealing to their courage is sometimes effective. Children 4 years old or over may choose to hold their own medicine cup or drink unassisted, and to take pills from the container without any assistance from the nurse. Children of this age are motivated by social reinforcers, such as being praised for their cooperation, or "your job is to stay very still," which enhance their self-esteem and feelings of competence. Helping the child identify what they can do during the procedure will assist the child to cope. Because of the sense of achievement that follows, they may want to save the medicine cups to show their parents (Box 7-8).

Oral medications. Success in administering oral medications usually requires a kind but firm approach and a positive attitude. Certainty that the child will take the medicine should be reflected in choice of words and tone of voice. The nurse might say, "Jimmy, it's time to take your yellow medicine" or "Do you want to take your pill now or with your Jell-O?" This indicates that Jimmy is expected to cooperate. It also allows the child some control over the situation. An unwise approach that conveys doubt on the nurse's part might be: "I have your yellow pill, Jimmy. Will you take it for me, please?"

Nurses should be aware of how a medicine tastes so that they can answer such questions as, "Does it taste bad? Will it burn my mouth?" A helpful reply would be, "It tastes like cherry to me. Tell me what it tastes like to you." Often the child will accept the suggestion to taste and find out. However, if the medication has an unpleasant taste, attempting to deceive or lying to the child is as futile and destructive as it is to an adult.

Medications that have a disagreeable taste should be disguised if at all possible. Small amounts of syrup, jam, fruit, and some fruit juices are suitable sweet vehicles for less palatable drugs. Some pills can be crushed and suspended in small amounts of these substances as long as the two are compatible. Infants and children swallow many liquid medications more readily if mixed with a sweet substance or diluted with a small amount of water. (However, if large amounts of water or other substances are used and the child refuses to take all of the mixture, it is difficult to estimate how much medication the child received.) Fortunately, many drugs are available as palatable syrups or in suspension form well suited for administration to infants and children. Suspensions, however, should be thoroughly agitated to ensure that doses are not offered in unequal concentrations.

Exercise caution when giving oral medications to children so as to prevent aspiration. Medications must be given to infants slowly and in small amounts to avoid choking. Liquid medications may be administered via a nipple, plastic medicine cup, plastic dropper, or plastic syringe without the needle. Water should be rinsed through the inside of these *first* to prevent medication from sticking, which can cause an inaccurate dose. Glass cups, droppers, or syringes should be avoided because of the obvious danger of them breaking in the child's mouth. A dropper or syringe is best suited for placing a liquid medication along one side of an infant's tongue. Older infants and toddlers seem to prefer to take their medications from a plastic medicine cup. If children are held or placed in a sitting position, they are less likely to aspirate the medication than if lying on their backs.

When administering a medication with a dropper or syringe, the nurse may purse the infant's lips with one hand to keep the medicine from running out of the mouth. Droppers and syringes used for medication should be kept clean, they should be reserved for only one client's use, and they should be rinsed or washed before being returned to the medication bottle.

If the child refuses to cooperate even after explanations and encouragement, the nurse may have to ask whether the child will take the medication alone or will need the nurse to give it. Physical coercion is seldom necessary, but if used, it

BOX 7-8

A Developmental Perspective for Administering Medications

General interventions

Always come prepared for procedure with all equipment and assistance necessary.

Ask the parent and/or child if parent should or should not remain for procedure (for in-hospital administration).

Assess comfort methods appropriate pre- and postadministration.

Infants

Perform procedure swiftly, then offer comfort measures (e.g., parent holding, rocking, cuddling, soothing).

Allow self-comforting measures (e.g., use of pacifier, fingers in mouth, self-movement).

Toddlers

Offer brief, concrete explanation of procedure, then perform it.

Accept aggressive behavior within reasonable limits as a healthy response.

Provide comfort measures immediately after procedure (e.g., touch, holding)

Help child understand the treatment and his feelings through puppet play or play with hospital equipment, such as a syringe and water.

Provide for ways to release aggression with such play as hammering or water play.

Preschoolers

Offer brief, concrete explanation.

Provide comfort measures after procedure (e.g., touch, holding).

Accept aggressive responses and provide outlets for them.

Make use of magical thinking—use "ointments" or "special medicines" to make discomfort go away.

Role of parent very important for comfort and understanding.

School-aged children

Explain procedure, allowing for some control over body and situation.

Provide comfort measures.

Explore feelings and concepts by therapeutic play, drawings of own body and self in hospital; use books and realistic hospital equipment.

Set appropriate behavior limits (e.g., okay to cry or scream but not bite).

Provide activities for releasing aggression and anger.

Use opportunity to teach about relation of medication to body function and structure (e.g., what a seizure is and how medication helps prevent the seizure).

Offer the complete picture (e.g., need to take medication, relax with deep breaths, medication will help prevent pain).

Adolescents

Prepare in advance for procedure.

Allow for expression in a way that doesn't cause "losing face," such as giving the adolescent time alone after the procedure and giving him time to discuss his discomfort if he wants to verbalize his feelings.

Explore current concepts of self, hospitalization, and illness and correct any misconceptions.

Encourage self-expression, individuality, and self-care.

Encourage participation in procedure to a preagreed-upon extent. Increased participation should be discussed after procedure.

Modified from Blaber M (1990). Related to nursing intervention in pain. *Newington Children's Hospital Manual for Global Pediatric Nursing Assessment* (unpublished).

should be mild and used with dispatch and firmness, since aspiration is a danger. The nurse must not combine force with anger or resort to force when one nurse has been unable to administer the medication. Careful consideration should be given to such factors as: Why does the child resist? Does the child disapprove only of one nurse? Have past experiences with medications given at home or in the hospital frightened the child? Will forcing a medication cause a struggle that will negate the effects of a drug given for sedation? If mild restraint is necessary, the nurse should explain to the child that this form of treatment is necessary. The child will not cooperate if force is seen as a punishment for inability to cooperate; often the child loses confidence in all personnel.

Topical medications. Children have a large skin surface area in proportion to total body weight. Their skin, especially neonates' skin, is particularly thin and permeable and has limited protective oil.

Although adults absorb much more medication through intact skin than was previously believed, the child is at increased risk for systemic medication administration. The discovery that hexachlorophene can cause encephalopathy in newborns and that topically applied boric acid can cause systemic poisoning testifies to the hazard of applying drugs to children's skin, especially for prolonged contact or over broken skin areas. Plain soap and water, not medicated dressings, may be the preferred treatment for abrasions or open lesions.

Subcutaneous injections. There are wide variations in the amounts of subcutaneous fat during childhood years. Neonates have a proportionately smaller amount; body fat increases slightly to 23% by 1 year of age. From 1 to 5 years of age the amount of body fat drops to between 8% and 12%. Then the amount of body fat climbs to about 20% when the child reaches the age of 10. Lipid-soluble drugs have an affinity for fat tissue; less subcutaneous fat means that lower doses of fat-soluble drugs, such as diazepam and barbiturates, are necessary to maintain blood levels. In addition, less subcutaneous tissue for injections may be available. An alternate route may need to be selected—oral, intramuscular, or intravenous.

Intramuscular injections. The principles and techniques of administrating intramuscular injections in children are similar to those for adults.

Most authorities believe that the risk of sciatic nerve injury is too great to warrant the use of the gluteal site for administration. The sciatic nerve is the largest nerve in the body; its normal pathway is the hollow midway between the ischial tuberosity and the greater trochanter, covered by the gluteus maximus muscle. This pathway, however, varies a great deal from individual to individual. In addition, the small size of the gluteal mass in the infant or neonate and the potential neurotoxicity of many drugs enhance the possibility of iatrogenic trauma secondary to IM injections. Trauma of this kind is the leading cause of sciatic neuropathy in infancy. A lesion at this level of the sciatic nerve is usually tragically associated with marked permanent disability.

The younger the child, the less the muscle tissue available for IM injections. If repeated injections are necessary, the available sites may become overused, inflamed, or dystrophic, requiring concerted efforts by the nurse to develop systematic plans for rotating sites and informing the rest of the staff about them. The vastus lateralis muscle is the site of choice for IM injections in children under 3 years of age since it is well developed at birth (see text in Chapter 5 and Figure 5-10, *C*). The ventrogluteal site is preferred for the child over 3 years old who has been walking for a year or two (see Figure 5-10, *B*). The dorsogluteal muscles should not be used for injections in the child under 4 to 6 years old if other IM sites are available. These muscles should not be used for injections at all until the younger child has been walking for at least 1 year.

For injection into the left gluteals, the thumb is placed on the trochanter and the middle finger on the iliac crest. The index finger placed midway between the thumb and middle finger will indicate a safe injection area. Infants should receive no more than 0.5 ml in each injection site. Small children can tolerate a volume of 1 ml at each site. Similarly, the deltoid muscle is not used for children under 5 years of age because of its underdevelopment. Rather than the skin being held taut, as for adults, the muscle mass should instead be pinched up. The needle will thus avoid striking deeper-lying structures such as nerves, bones, or blood vessels. The IM injection is still made at a 90-degree angle to the top of the massed flesh. Preferred needle sizes for pediatric IM injections are 25- to 27-gauge and 1/2 to 1 inch in length. A 21- or 22-gauge needle may be preferred if a viscous medication such as procaine penicillin is to be given. In the interest of safety, the child should usually be restrained for an injection and the injection given rapidly. Two or more persons should be available for children over 4 years of age, even those who promise to "hold still." An extra sterile needle may be carried in a pocket in case a needle becomes contaminated when a child moves unexpectedly. A child's attention may be distracted from the injection by asking the youngster to wiggle the toes. Because children enjoy trying out each other's beds, the identifying armband must be checked to ensure proper client identification before giving each medication.

Rectal administration. When oral administration is difficult or contraindicated, the rectal route is often advised. Many children perceive use of the rectal route as an extreme invasion of their bodies or anticipate pain as a result. It may help to let them participate, for example, to insert the suppository. Several drugs, such as sedatives, aspirin, and antiemetics, are available in suppository form. Suppositories made with a cocoa butter base will melt rapidly at normal body temperature, releasing the drug for absorption. After a suppository is inserted in an infant, the buttocks should be held or taped together for 5 to 10 minutes to relieve pressure on the anal sphincter and thereby help ensure retention and absorption of the medication. Infants and children with diarrhea, however, may easily expel suppositories with explosive stools. Similarly, a suppository inserted into a child who has constipation problem or a rectum full of stool will be surrounded with stool and will have little chance of being absorbed.

Health care professionals often divide suppository doses by cutting them to obtain correct doses. This is dangerous practice because all the medication might be contained in one area of the suppository. If divided doses must be administered, the pharmacist should be contacted for alternate product advice and guidance.

Nose drops, eardrops, and eye drops. Aqueous preparations of nose drops are the only safe preparations to use, because of the danger of aspiration. Many nose drop preparations contain vasoconstrictors, and prolonged or excessive use may be harmful. Infants are nose breathers, and nasal congestion will inhibit their sucking. For this reason, nose drops, if necessary, should be instilled 20 minutes to 1/2 hour before feedings.

To instill *nose drops* (Figure 7-2):

1. Hold the infant in your arm, allowing the head to fall back over the edge of your arm, or place a small pillow under the shoulders and allow the head to fall back over the edge of the pillow.
2. Place your free arm so that the forearm is around the far side of the child's head, stabilizing the head between your forearm and your body. Use your hand to stabilize the arms and hands.
3. With your free hand you can then instill the prescribed drops with minimum struggle and maximum accuracy.

Before the initial administration of a course of therapy with *eardrops*, the nurse should assess whether the child has

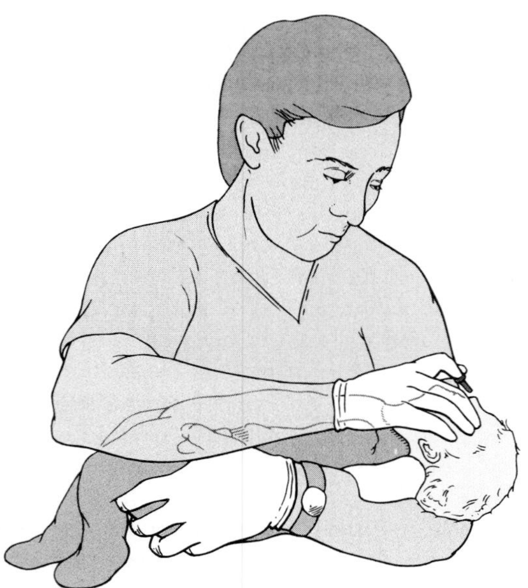

Figure 7-2 Administration of nose drops.

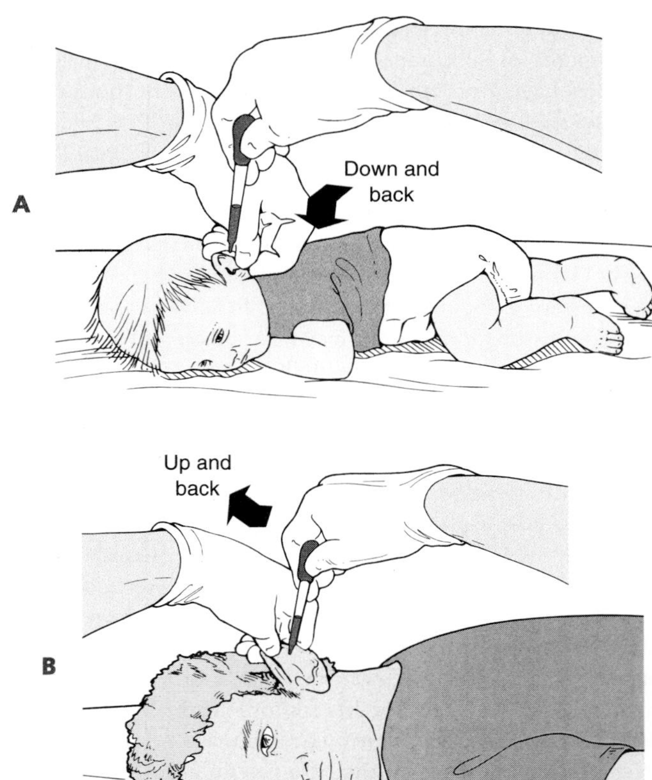

Figure 7-3 Administration of eardrops. The infant or child is positioned on the side of the unaffected ear. **A,** The nurse pulls the pinna down and back to administer eardrops to infants and children under 3 years of age. **B,** When administering eardrops to children older than 3 years and adults, the nurse gently pulls the pinna up and back. The nurse should stabilize his or her hand on the client's head for safety and instill the prescibed number of drops. The drops are directed toward the ear canal to avoid hitting the tympanic membrane, which can cause pain. The client should remain in the position for 5 to 10 minutes. Otic drugs should be warmed before they are instilled, to prevent nausea or vertigo.

excessive cerumen. If so, it may be necessary to consult with the prescriber about its removal with cerumen softeners or irrigation before instilling the eardrops. The instillation of eardrops requires knowledge of anatomic structure, because the shape of the auditory canal of a young child is different from that of an adult. (Figure 7-3 illustrates the administration of eardrops.) Gentle massage of the area immediately anterior to the ear will facilitate the entry of the drops deeper into the ear canal after their instillation.

Eye drop instillation is done in the same way with children as with adults except that the head may be stabilized by an assistant. Depending on the child's age, he or she may be asked to look up so that the cornea reflex is diminished, and the dropper should be introduced from the side. The lower lid is retracted, and the drops are instilled into the conjunctival sac. Many eye drops cause a burning sensation for a few seconds, so if both eyes are to be medicated it is wise to do the second instillation quickly before the child begins to blink and tear as a reaction to the burning sensation occurring in the first eye medicated. Mild pressure for 30 seconds over the inner canthus next to the nose will prevent premature drainage of the medication away from the eye (see Figure 43-1).

Aqueous preparations of nose, ear, and eye drops may support the growth of bacteria and fungi. For this reason small volumes of such medications are ordered and should be used for only *one* individual (not shared by family members). The dropper (especially eye droppers) should not be permitted to become contaminated by touching anything but the medication. The dropper should never be inverted so that medication or water runs into the rubber bulb to form a medium for microbiologic growth. A dropper from one medication should not be used to measure and administer another type of medication because droppers are not standardized—all droppers are not manufactured to deliver drops of the same volume. Viscosity of drugs also varies, affecting the drop size.

Eye drops and eardrops are more comfortably tolerated if they are warmed (if not contraindicated) before instillation. Run warm water over the side of the bottle without the label or immerse the bottle in some warm water in a medicine cup. Even carrying the bottle in a pocket for half an hour or so will take the chill off the drops.

Intravenous medications. Use of IV drug therapy is widespread on most pediatric services for several reasons. In children with vomiting and diarrhea, medications given by mouth may be vomited, losing precious time in drug management. These children may have poor absorption of drugs and fluids as a result of dehydration or peripheral vascular collapse, so drugs administered via the IM route may be equally ineffective. (See the case study on p. 129.) It may be

Case Study

Timmy, a 4-year-old child with reversible obstructive airway disease, is admitted to the emergency room with bilateral wheezing and moderate respiratory distress. He has received two aerosol treatments yet continues to be in moderate distress with continued wheezing. An IV bolus of aminophylline has been ordered to be followed by a continuous IV infusion of aminophylline.

1. What factors should be considered in selecting the intravenous route for drug administration in the child?
2. What measures should the nurse use to maintain the integrity of the intravenous infusion?
3. Timmy is to be discharged on oral theophylline. The appropriate dose of oral theophylline for a child Timmy's age is 16 mg/kg. Calculate the dose for Timmy, who weighs 42 pounds. Convert weight in pounds to kilograms.
4. Given that Timmy is developmentally appropriate for his chronologic age, what should the nurse teach Timmy's parents about administering this oral medication?

preferable to give premature or physiologically distressed neonates certain high-osmolality drugs by IV rather than giving the syrup or elixir forms by the oral route. Premature infants are at risk for necrotizing enterocolitis (NEC) and death when administered feedings or oral drugs that have an osmolality greater than that of body fluids. Although elixirs of theophylline, phenobarbital, calcium, digoxin, and dexamethasone all have osmolalities 10 times greater than body fluids and have been implicated in causing NEC, analysis shows that the contained additives actually raise the medication's osmolality. Related studies continue.

The pediatric nurse responsible for the administration of IV drugs may find the suggestions in Box 7-9 helpful (see also Chapter 5). Most older children may be given fluids or drugs intravenously following the same principles and techniques used for adults. The younger and smaller the child, the narrower the margin for error.

Neonates, infants, and children must be adequately restrained so as not to dislodge or pull out an infusion needle or catheter once it is in place. The following hints may be helpful to the nurse caring for a client receiving IV therapy (Figure 7-4):

1. The needle or catheter should be fixed with plastic tape.
2. When a loop of tubing directly above the needle is secured to the tape, tension is relieved from the needle should it be pulled by sudden movement.
3. Because most children move about or are restless, it is necessary, if the IV site is in the arm, to support the limb with a padded arm board and immobilize the site of IV therapy. Support should extend to the joints above and below the site (with arm boards or IV boards).
4. If the infusion bottle is too high, the pressure in the vein will increase, causing fluid to seep into the surrounding tissues.

BOX 7-9

Pediatric IV Drug Administration

1. IV drug therapy should be used only if other channels of drug administration are impractical. Pediatric nurses skilled in giving medications to children via other routes may be able to influence prescribers' decisions regarding successful routes of drug administration.
2. For small infants a scalp vein or a superficial vein of the wrist, hand, foot, or arm may be most convenient and most easily stabilized. Scalp veins have no valves and thus infusions may be in either direction. They are the most frequent sites for infant infusions. Older children may receive infusions through any accessible vein.
3. A too-rapid IV infusion or injection may cause "speed shock": rapid fall in blood pressure, respiratory irregularity, blood incoagulability, and even death. Preventive measures include use of the minidropper (note that the milliliter per hour in the order translates to the drops per minute with this tubing), calibrated volume control chambers, and infusion pumps.
4. Total parenteral nutrition (TPN) solutions are usually infused into the vena cava or innominate or subclavian veins approached via the external or internal jugular veins. Occasionally, the inferior vena cava is entered via the femoral vein.
5. Once a drug is injected intravenously, the drug's action is relatively irreversible.
6. Drugs must be properly diluted. Too much emphasis cannot be placed on this caution: GIVE THE SMALLEST POSSIBLE DOSE AT THE SLOWEST POSSIBLE RATE.

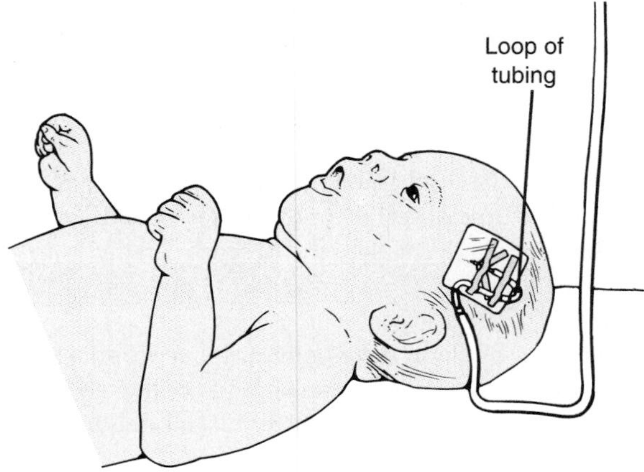

Figure 7-4 Securing a scalp vein infusion for infants.

5. Specific classifications of medications must be administered over a specific time period and require the use of an electronic medication pump or infusion device.

Other factors influencing drug dosages. Again, the dosage of most agents is related to the child's age, weight, and height. A child's body systems grow and develop at varying rates, which makes for unpredictable primary and secondary effects in pediatric medication administration. One example of secondary effects specific to children is discoloration of teeth and depression of enamel growth with administration of tetracycline liquid medications in children under 8 years of age. (This adverse reaction is well-documented, but the drug is still being prescribed for this age group, according to the FDA.) The skeletal growth of children receiving long-term adrenocortical steroids is also impaired.

Individual variations are noted in children's responses to digitalis, insulin, opiates, and oral enzyme products; doses require careful titration. Paradoxical responses are noted with a few drugs; responses may be directly opposite to those could be expected in the adult. Excessive reactivity to atropine by infants may be related to immaturity of the central nervous system. In addition, many drugs that are safe and effective for adults have not been tested for use with children, nor have doses been established, because of the complex medicolegal issues involved in experimentation on children.

SUMMARY

Nursing management of the administration of medications to clients of different age groups requires that the nurse be knowledgeable about growth and development as well as the various effects of pharmaceutical agents on clients of different ages. Understanding the rationale behind these effects will help the nurse to administer medications safely and to evaluate client responses appropriately, regardless of the client's age. Childbearing clients, neonates, infants, and children all have unique needs related to the accurate and safe administration of medications, which are based on their unique physiologic and psychosocial developmental needs.

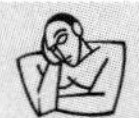

Critical Thinking

1. Select one drug, such as phenytoin or warfarin, and discuss the potential risks to the fetus or breastfeeding child in relation to needed benefits to the mother.
2. Ms. Leverett, a nursing student, is assigned to care for Sally, a 3-year-old, and Loretta, an 8-year-old, who are sharing the same hospital room. From a developmental perspective, how will her approach to the two children differ when it comes to administering medications?

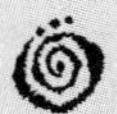

Collaborative Learning Activities

1. Preassign student teams to discuss each of the questions of the case study of the pediatric client. For the team answering #2, would it make any difference if Timmy were small for his age at 37¾ inches or if he were lanky for his age at 43⅓ inches? Have the team use different methods for calculating the dosage.

BIBLIOGRAPHY

American Hospital Formulary Service (1996). *AHFS drug information '96*. Bethesda, MD: American Society of Hospital Pharmacists.

Anderson KN, et al. (Eds.) (1994). *Mosby's medical, nursing, & allied health dictionary* (4th ed.). St Louis: Mosby.

Bobak IM, Lowdermilk DL & Jensen MD. (1995). *Essentials of maternity nursing* (4th ed.). St Louis: Mosby.

Briggs GG (1995). Teratogenicity and drugs in breast milk. In Young LY & Koda-Kimble MA (Eds.). *Applied therapeutics* (6th ed.). Vancouver: Applied Therapeutics.

Chi J (1992). FDA tries again for improved pediatric labels: Will it work? *Hosp Pharm Report* 6(12):9.

Hall WC, et al. (1990). Cocaine abuse and its treatment, *Pharmacotherapy* 10(1):47.

Jennings JC (1996). Guide to medication use in pregnant and breastfeeding women, *Pharm Pract News* 23(4):10.

Keene EF (1993). Another way to administer antiepileptic medications in infants and children, *MCN* 18(6):270.

Levy M & Spino M (1993). Neonatal withdrawal syndrome: Associated drugs and pharmacologic management, *Pharmacotherapy* 13(3):202-211.

Olin BR (1996). *Facts and comparisons*. St Louis: Facts and Comparisons.

Pray WS (1993). Infant formulas and nutrition, *US Pharmacist* 18(3):29.

United States Pharmacopeial Convention. (1996). *USP DI: Drug information for the health care professional* (16th ed.). Rockville, MD: The Convention.

Wong DL (1997). *Whaley & Wong's essentials of pediatric nursing* (5th ed.). St Louis: Mosby.

Chapter 8

Drug Therapy for the Elderly

Chapter Focus

The elderly represent the fastest growing population in the United States and Canada. Thus an understanding of the physiologic changes that occur with the aging process will help the health care provider to safely prescribe and monitor drug regimens. The goal of drug treatment is to develop strategies to treat or alter a disease process and if possible restore function to the elderly. Because many of the medication-related problems reported in the elderly are preventable, the nurse and all health care professionals have a vital role in this area. The following objectives and key terms are necessary for a good understanding of this chapter.

Key Terms

polypharmacy (p. 132)

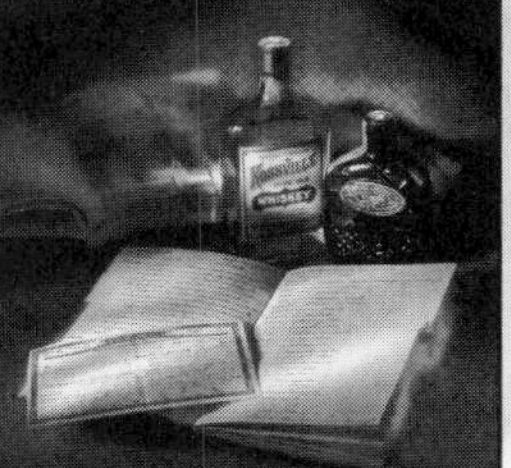

Objectives

1. Discuss factors that promote drug misuse in the elderly.
2. Describe alterations in pharmacokinetics and pharmacodynamics related to aging.
3. Identify the risk factors for ineffective management of the medication regimen by the geriatric client.
4. Manage effectively the administration of medications for geriatric clients.

While the geriatric population represents approximately 12% of the population in the United States and Canada today, it has been reported that they:

- consume 30% of all prescribed drugs and 50% of all over-the-counter (OTC) medications in the United States
- are admitted to hospitals for adverse drug reactions (ADRs) three times more frequently than younger adults
- represent 51% of the deaths and 39% of hospitalizations from ADRs (persons over 60 years)
- experience more drug-related incidents than other aged populations (25% of all admissions from a nursing home setting to a hospital are drug-related) (Trends & Analysis, 1995)

By the year 2030 it has been projected that more than 20% of the population will be 65 years or older (Trends & Analysis, 1995). Because the elderly are the most rapidly increasing segment of the U.S. population, an understanding of age-related alterations in pharmacokinetics and pharmacodynamics is necessary. Also the increased incidence of chronic diseases in the elderly often results in an increase in the number of prescriptions, OTC medications, and home remedies prescribed or self-selected. Pollow et al (1994) determined that almost two-thirds of the community-dwelling elderly in their study were at risk for at least one drug-drug or drug-alcohol combination associated with a possible adverse reaction. To minimize the risks associated with use of multiple medications and adverse drug reactions in this population, the health care provider needs to provide continuous drug regimen monitoring, with a primary goal of reducing or eliminating inappropriate medications and improving the client's quality of life.

The age of specialization has in some ways added to this problem; multiple health care providers may prescribe a variety of medications, often without discontinuing any previous drugs the client is taking. The result is **polypharmacy,** which is usually defined as the consumption of four or five medications (Kovach, 1992). Polypharmacy can be a dangerous practice that may increase the risk of drug interactions and adverse reactions and the need for or prolonging of hospitalization. Jinks and Fuerst (1992) report that adverse drug reactions in the elderly in 1985 resulted in 243,000 hospitalizations, 32,000 hip fractures, and 163,000 cases of drug-induced mental alterations or impairments. Although the magnitude of problems caused by polypharmacy is enormous, it is frequently overlooked as being the causative factor. It is important that health care providers realize that the vast majority of undesirable drug effects resulting from polypharmacy are *preventable.*

PHYSIOLOGIC CHANGES OF AGING

Aging persons undergo a variety of physiologic changes that may increase their sensitivity to drugs and drug-induced disease (Figure 8-1). The loss in body weight in many elderly clients may require initiating therapy at a lower adult dose or reevaluation of dosages of medications already in use. The criterion for dosage should be shifted from age to weight. Some older clients weigh no more than the average large child and some weigh a lot less, yet they are prescribed the larger "adult" doses.

Pharmacokinetics (Box 8-1) are altered in the aging client because of reduced gastric acid and slowed gastric motility, resulting in unpredictable rates of dissolution and absorption of drugs. Changes in absorption may occur when acid production decreases, altering the absorption of weakly acidic drugs such as barbiturates. However, few studies of drug absorption have shown clinically significant changes occurring with advanced age.

Changes in body composition, such as increased proportion of body fat and decreased total body water, plasma volume, and extracellular fluid, have been noted in the elderly. The increased proportion of body fat increases the body's ability to store fat-soluble compounds such as phenothiazines and barbiturates and thus increases the accumulation of those drugs. The reduced lean body mass affects drug distribution by decreasing the volume in which the drug circulates, thereby causing higher peak levels. The risk of toxicity with hydrophilic or water-soluble drugs increases as total body water decreases. Digoxin (Lanoxin), theophylline (Theo-Dur) and the aminoglycosides are examples of hydrophilic drugs that may accumulate and result in an adverse reaction or toxicity.

Decreased serum albumin for highly protein-bound drugs may lead to increased amounts of free drug in the circulation.

BOX 8-1

Potential Altered Pharmacokinetics in the Elderly

Absorption

Increase in gastric pH
Altered gastric emptying and intestinal blood flow
Decrease in first-pass metabolism in the liver

Distribution

Altered body composition (decrease in lean body mass, increase in adipose [fat] stores)
Decrease in total body water
Decrease in serum albumin
Decrease in blood flow and cardiac output

Metabolism

Phase I metabolic reactions decrease with age
Decrease in enzymatic activity with age (P-450 system)
Decrease in hepatic blood flow and drug metabolism

Excretion

Decrease in renal function; most persons lose 10% renal function per decade after age 50

Modified from Trends & Analysis, 1995.

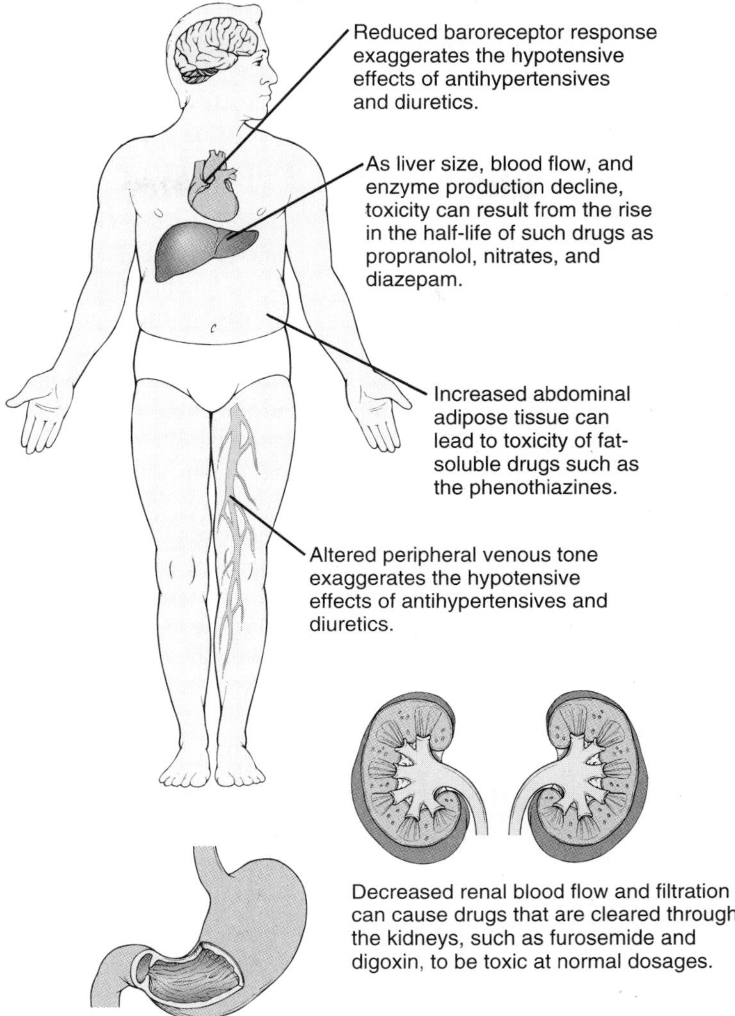

Figure 8-1 How pharmacokinetics change with age.

Warfarin (Coumadin), phenytoin (Dilantin) and diazepam (Valium) are a few examples of highly bound drugs.

Liver drug metabolism is also affected by aging. Medications that undergo phase I metabolism (reduction, oxidation, hydroxylation, or demethylation) may have a decreased metabolism while phase II (glucuronidation, acetylation, conjugation, etc.) is not affected by aging. Thus drugs that may have a decrease in hepatic metabolism in the elderly are the nitrates, barbiturates, propranolol (Inderal) and lidocaine (Jinks & Fuerst, 1995).

Disorders common to the aging person, such as congestive heart failure (CHF), may impair liver function and influence biotransformation by decreasing the metabolism of drugs and increasing the risk of drug accumulation and toxicity. Renal function may be impaired because of loss of nephrons, decreased blood flow, and decreased glomerular filtration rate. A reduction in renal function is also secondary to CHF. Decreased renal clearance may cause increased plasma drug concentrations and longer half-lives of drugs and active metabolites that the kidney usually excretes. Drugs that are highly dependent on the kidneys for excretion include the aminoglycosides, ciprofloxin (Cipro), digoxin (Lanoxin), lithium (Eskalith), and numerous other drugs (Jinks & Fuerst, 1995).

Thus careful monitoring of drug regimens is crucial, especially for the elderly client. Box 8-2 describes how to assess the at-risk geriatric client.

BOX 8-2

How to Assess the "At-Risk" Geriatric Client

1. Interview client to obtain a complete drug history. Carefully question him or her about disease states, illnesses, current use of medications (prescribed, over-the-counter, home remedies, herbals, vitamins, etc.), drug allergies (obtain description of allergy, time it occurred, intervention used, outcome), and any troubling side or adverse effects.
2. Make list of name, strength, and directions of each medication (prescribed and OTC) the person takes. Include prn medications, especially if person reports taking them one or more times per week.
3. Identify all prescribers for this client. This information may be obtained by client interview and should be verified by checking prescription labels.
4. Prescription bottles may also provide additional information to review, for example, check name(s) of pharmacies that have dispensed medications to the person. If more than one pharmacy is involved, determine the reason why.
5. Check all prescription and OTC drug containers for expiration dates. Ask the client for permission to destroy any expired medications because they have the potential of being ineffective or causing harm.
6. Question clients on their self-medication practices: how do they remember to take their scheduled medications; do they ever forget to take a dose and if so, what do they do; have they ever deliberately stopped their medication—if yes, obtain an explanation why, etc? Such information will help in evaluating compliance and if the medications are being consumed safely according to the prescribed schedule.
7. Discover whether the client has any limitations that may impair safe, self-administration of medication. Examples include physical impairment, memory loss, health or cultural beliefs, financial constraints, and lack of social support.

ALTERATIONS IN PHARMACOKINETICS

It has been estimated that 70% to 80% of all adverse drug reactions in the elderly are dose-related. The physiologic changes previously discussed may result in a decrease in drug metabolism, distribution in the body, and renal excretion. Therefore higher blood and tissue levels of potent medications may result in an increased incidence of adverse drug reactions. Diazepam's (Valium's) half-life increases from 20 hours in a 20-year-old to 90 hours in individuals in their 80s, because of the increase in volume of drug in the body of the elderly person. Although reduced or impaired renal function of drugs primarily excreted by the kidneys may result in drug accumulation and perhaps toxicity, up to one third of the elderly have little or no "age-related renal insufficiency" (McCue et al, 1993). Thus the previously described aging process does not necessarily affect all elderly people.

ALTERATIONS IN PHARMACODYNAMICS

Changes in target organ or receptor sensitivity in the elderly may result in a greater or lesser drug effect at these sites. The reason for this alteration is unknown, but it may be due to a decrease in the number of receptors at the site or an altered receptor response to the medication. The elderly often exhibit a decreased response to beta agonists and antagonists, but they have a greater response (CNS depression) with diazepam (Valium) (Erwin, 1993). It has also been reported that the muscarinic receptors in the cortex tend to decrease with aging so the elderly are often very sensitive to anticholinergic medications. Anticholinergic side effects of confusion, dry mouth, blurred vision, constipation, and urinary retention are frequently noted (Lucas, Noyes, & Stratton, 1995). See Chapter 21 for additional information on anticholinergic drugs.

There is also believed to be a loss in responsiveness or an age-related decline in beta-adrenergic receptors and dopamine receptors in the elderly. The number of receptors may vary or the alteration may be in different areas of the aging body, which may result in altered drug responses or an increased risk for drug-induced Parkinson's disease (Lucas, Noyes, & Stratton, 1995).

In summary, the elderly are perceived to have a greater sensitivity to drugs, especially to CNS-acting medications. If monitoring and dosage adjustments are not instituted, they may encounter more adverse reactions than younger persons.

INEFFECTIVE MANAGEMENT OF THE SELF-MEDICATION REGIMEN

The numerous factors that complicate drug therapy regimens (Box 8-3) may result in improper self-medication, errors in administration, and therapeutic failure. Detecting medication misuse is an important function of the health care provider, because appropriate interventions may reverse this outcome. A variety of situations may result in medication misuse, leading one to ask the following questions:

1. Does the risk or cost of one or more of the drugs in the client's drug regimen outweigh the benefits? Benefits may be viewed as physiologic response or as psychologic and economic considerations.
2. What is the elderly person or the primary caregiver's knowledge of the prescribed therapy? Does the client follow a specific medication schedule (by times or hours), keeping track of all medications taken daily? Does the client or primary caregiver know the name of and use for each of the medications? Can they ex-

BOX 8-3

Factors That May Complicate Drug Therapy in the Elderly

The elderly
- are living longer
- may have one or more chronic diseases
- may receive prescriptions from two or more prescribers
- undergo physiologic changes that may result in:
  altered pharmacokinetics
  altered pharmacodynamics
- may have altered thought processes such as confusion, memory loss
- may have impaired physical mobility related to arthritis, fatigue
- may have sensory-perceptual alterations such as impaired vision or hearing
- may have limited income, which may affect continuity of drug therapy
- on an average use more prescription and OTC drugs than general population
- may experience polypharmacy, which has resulted in increase in reports of drug interactions, side effects, and adverse reactions

plain the instructions from the label on each bottle? (Read Chapter 10 for a detailed discussion of client education.)

3. Can the client open the child-resistant caps on his or her medications? Is the client aware that he or she can receive regular caps if requested from the pharmacist?
4. Is the client having any difficulty taking the medication, perhaps needing a change in dosage form, such as from tablet to liquid, to more easily facilitate swallowing?
5. Is the client exhibiting drug side effects or adverse reactions? These are often overlooked, and the prescriber may prescribe a new medication for the symptoms rather than discontinuing the offending medication.

The health care provider should constantly compare the person's current function with his or her past performance because behavioral and mental changes are very common symptoms of medication misuse. Consultation with a family member or caregiver is essential. Confusion, increased irritability, disorientation, and agitation are just a few of the changes noted that are often caused by medications (Miller, 1995). Physical problems such as increased weakness, falls, and a decrease in physical activity may also be caused by a variety of prescribed medications. Although most individuals can identify an acute drug reaction if it occurs after the start of a new medication, the slower-evolving side effects are often more difficult to identify. At times the prescriber may discontinue a potential offending drug and observe the client for signs of alleviation of the side effects. The prescriber may discontinue a drug that has a long duration of action, substituting a drug that has a shorter duration of action. This too will help avoid the cumulative or additive effects of medications, especially the CNS-acting drugs (i.e., hypnotics, antianxiety agents, antidepressants, narcotics, and tranquilizers).

BOX 8-4

Inappropriate Drugs for the Elderly

Category	Drug examples
analgesics	propoxyphene (Darvon) pentazocine (Talwin)
antidiabetic	chlorpropamide (Diabinese)
antidepressant	amitriptyline (Elavil)
antiemetic	trimethobenzamide (Tigan)
antihypertensives	propranolol (Inderal) methyldopa (Aldomet) reserpine (Serpasil)
hypnotic/sedative	diazepam (Valium) chlordiazepoxide (Librium) flurazepam (Dalmane) meprobamate (Miltown) pentobarbital (Nembutal) secobarbital (Seconal)
muscle relaxants	cyclobenzaprine (Flexeril) methocarbamol (Robaxin) carisoprodol (Soma) orphenadrine (Norflex)
nonsteroidal anti-inflammatory agents (NSAIDs)	indomethacin (Indocin) phenylbutazone (Butazolidin)
platelet inhibitor	dipyridamole (Persantine)
peripheral vasodilators (dementia therapy)	cyclandelate (Cyclospasmol) isoxsuprine (Vasodilan)

MEDICATIONS IN THE ELDERLY

Potent medications available to treat the elderly often have a narrow index between effectiveness and toxicity. A study of more than 6,000 persons 65 years or older living in the community indicated that physicians prescribe inappropriate medications for at least 25% of that elderly population (Willcox, Himmelstein, & Woolhandler, 1994). Box 8-4 lists inappropriate drugs for the elderly. This list of potentially inappropriate medications was derived from a previously published list (Beers et al, 1991) and was limited to drugs that should be avoided entirely in the geriatric client. For example, the three long-acting benzodiazepines (diazepam [Valium], chlordiazepoxide [Librium], and flurazepam [Dalmane]) have been associated with daytime sedation and an increased risk of falls while the antidepressant amitriptyline (Elavil), has been reported to cause the most anticholinergic and orthostatic hypotension side effects as compared with other drugs in this category. Therefore the prescribing of such medications in the aged client increases the risk of inducing side effects, adverse drug reactions, and perhaps injury.

Table 8-1 is a list of commonly prescribed medications for the elderly with the most common side or adverse effects reported. "Although all systems are altered by the aging process, the central nervous system and the cardiovascular system appear to be the most affected" (Lucas, Noyes, & Stratton, 1995). To reduce the potential for adverse effects, it has been recommended that CNS-acting medications be reduced to approximately 50% of the usual adult recommended dose (Lucas, Noyes, & Stratton, 1995). If the prescriber titrates slowly to the therapeutic effect, the potential of drug-induced adverse effects declines.

Avorn & Gurwitz (1995) report that nursing home residents receive more medications than noninstitutionalized elderly persons. The use of inappropriate prescribed medications (see Box 8-4) was also documented in this setting. In addition, the prolonged use of oral antibiotics, short-acting benzodiazepines, and histamine-2 antagonists and high drug dosages of iron products, histamine-2 antagonists, and the antipsychotic medications were also reported. Inappropriate prescribing of psychotropic medications in long-term facilities has resulted in federal legislation (OBRA) that established guidelines for the proper use of such medications in the elderly. See Chapter 19, Psychotherapeutic Drugs, for additional information.

Responsibility of health care providers. The primary responsibility of a health care provider is to reduce or eliminate the potentially adverse risk factors associated with various drug regimens. This can be accomplished by a thorough assessment of the client's health status, current medication regimen, environmental factors that would influence the accurate and safe administration of medication by the client or the client's caregivers, and the implementation of the appropriate interventions, client education, and counseling. More information is presented in Chapters 4, 5, 6, and 10.

A study involving assessment and monitoring of an elderly hospital population by a multidisciplinary team (physician, geriatric nurse specialist, home care nurse, pharmacist, social worker, dietician, and physical therapist) reported a significant decrease in hospital readmissions and mortality rates as compared with a control group of participants (62 persons in study group, 58 persons in control group). Each team member evaluated each person in the experimental group, made recommendations in the chart, forwarded the recommendations to the client's primary physician, and continued to monitor each person throughout the study. The control group did not receive recommendations or any subsequent visits. After 6 months, the study group reported a reduced mortality rate (21% of controls died, compared with 6% of the persons in the study), and this group was more actively involved in daily activities necessary for independence (Practice Trends, 1993). This indicates the benefits of a thorough assessment and close monitoring of the elderly client.

Ideally the prescriber will individualize and simplify drug therapy for the client (Gambert, Grossberg, & Morley, 1994).

TABLE 8-1 Commonly prescribed medications in the elderly

Medication	Common side/adverse effects
aminoglycoside antibiotics (gentamycin, etc.)	Ototoxicity (hearing impairment or loss), renal impairment, or failure
analgesics, opioid	Confusion, constipation, urinary retention, (morphine and others) nausea, vomiting, respiratory depression
anticholinergics, antispasmodics, esp. antihistamines, anti-Parkinson's drugs, atropine, etc.	Blurred vision, dry mouth, constipation, confusion, urinary retention, nausea, delirium
anticoagulants (heparin, warfarin)	Bleeding episodes, hemorrhage, increase in drug-interaction potential
antihypertensive medications	Sedation, orthostatic hypotension, sexual dysfunction, CNS alterations, nausea
aspirin, aspirin-containing products	Tinnitus, gastric distress, ulcers, GI bleeding
digoxin, digitalis preparations, especially at higher dosages	Nausea, vomiting, cardiac arrhythmias, visual disorders, mental-status changes, hallucinations
diuretics (thiazides, furosemide, etc.)	Electrolyte disorders, rash, fatigue, leg cramps, dehydration
hypnotics/sedatives (flurazepam, triazolam, etc.)	Confusion, daytime sedation, gait disturbances, lethargy, increased forgetfulness, depression, delirium
H_2 receptor antagonists (cimetidine, ranitidine, etc.)	Confusion, depression, mental status alterations
nonsteroidal anti-inflammatory agents (NSAIDs)	Gastric distress, GI bleeding, ulceration
psychotropics (neuroleptic agents)	Sedation, confusion, hypotension, drug-induced parkinsonian effects, tardive dyskinesia
tricyclic antidepressants (amitriptyline, doxepin, and others)	Confusion, cardiac arrhythmias, seizures, agitation, anticholinergic effects, tachycardia, etc.

The nurse should be an advocate for the simplification of the client's medication regimen (see the Case Study on p. 137). Keeping medications to a minimum with the least frequent dosage administration necessary will help to reduce the potential for drug interactions and also improve the client's ability to manage the drug regimen effectively (Box 8-5).

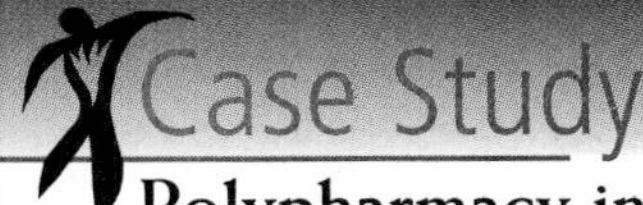

Case Study: Polypharmacy in the Elderly

Walter Smith is an 86-year-old divorced man who lives alone in a public housing project for the elderly. He describes himself as a loner and expresses a great deal of pride at being independent for his entire life.

Mr. Smith was admitted to the hospital after a fall from which he received scalp lacerations. He was alert, well read, but quite suspicious of the health care givers. He weighed 138 pounds and was 5'10". He had very poor vision and hearing.

Mr. Smith was diagnosed with hypertension, arteriosclerotic heart disease, atrial fibrillation, eczematous dermatitis of his legs, and a urinary tract infection. He spent 3 days in the hospital and was discharged on the following medications:

Valisone cream 0.1% to legs twice daily	Feosol spansule 1 bid
digoxin 0.125 mg daily	Vitamin C 1 capsule daily
Lasix 20 mg daily	Dicloxacillin 500 mg qid for 10 days
Aldomet 250 mg bid	Darvocet-N 100 mg qid as needed
Isordil 5 mg qid	

Before this hospitalization, Mr. Smith had relied heavily on self-care and self-medication, which he resumed upon discharge. He consumed large quantities of natural vitamin and mineral supplements. He used Corn Huskers Lotion on his legs. One week after discharge, the visiting nurse found that Mr. Smith had fallen twice during the week but had sustained only minor bruises. He was weak, and although he was oriented to place and person, he was uncertain as to time and showed memory loss and some incoherence in thought processes. He had trouble describing his medications but complained that they were expensive and caused him to experience incontinence. His blood pressure was 98/64.

The nurse convinced Mr. Smith to visit a physician he knew and liked. The physician was tolerant of Mr. Smith's need to remain in his home and of his health practices. Mr. Smith insisted on using the Corn Huskers Lotion instead of the "too expensive" cream. The physician agreed to this change and in addition was able to reduce Mr. Smith's medications to digoxin 0.125 mg daily, Isordil 5 mg qid, and Dyazide 1 capsule daily. Mr. Smith agreed to take his heart medications and to use fewer of his nonprescription vitamins and minerals.

1. Why is polypharmacy a common problem with elderly clients?
2. What assessment data should the nurse obtain to understand the client's beliefs and practices regarding medications?
3. How might the following have contributed to the confusion Mr. Smith experienced?
   a. Effects of age-related changes in circulatory, renal, and hepatic function on the drugs taken.
   b. The specific actions or adverse effects of the following drugs:
      digoxin
      Lasix
      Aldomet
      Darvocet-N
4. What factors affected Mr. Smith's ability and willingness to carry out the medication regimen?

Nursing Management

Medication Administration for Geriatric Clients

In view of the effects just outlined and the multiplicity of drugs prescribed for elderly clients, the older person's potential for occasionally unreliable memories and senses, inadequate financial status, and propensity for developing adverse secondary effects to drugs, nurses must make every attempt to simplify the geriatric drug therapy plan. Suspect medications as the cause whenever you note a change in an elderly client's behavior, particularly restlessness, irritability, and confusion. These alterations of thought processes may be the earliest signs of drug toxicity. Elderly clients are at risk for toxicity because of the effects of drugs in the aging body, variables of drug administration, and the effects of polypharmacy. Encourage others, such as nursing assistants and family caregivers to report to a nurse any changes they notice in the client's behavior. Often what passes for senility is drug-induced lethargy or confusion.

In the administration of medications, the geriatric client may have special needs as discussed in Chapter 5. Older persons frequently have dry mucous membranes, which impede swallowing, so offer water before and after oral medications if the client's condition permits. Position the elderly client so that gravity will assist the drug through the esophagus and minimize the possibility of aspiration. Because of diminished sensation, the client may be unaware that the tablet is stuck between the lip and gum, so ask the client if you can examine his or her mouth to ensure that the medication has been swallowed. Some geriatric clients may have slowed reflexes and reduced understanding of treatment. It helps to organize the dispensing of medication so that enough time is allowed for clients who require more time and assistance with medications, possibly by medicating them last so as not to be rushed.

Selection of sites for injectable medications in elderly clients may present the nurse with a challenge. Because muscle mass declines with age, suitable sites for intramuscular injection may be fewer than in younger individuals, and

BOX 8-5

Over-the-Counter Drug Use by the Rural Elderly

A study to examine the OTC drug-taking practices of the noninstitutionalized elderly was conducted with 100 rural and 100 urban adults over the age of 65, using a multiple-choice/fill-in-the-blank questionnaire. Participants answered questions about the number and names of OTC drugs used, the frequency with which the drugs were taken, the degree of their dependence on these drugs for daily functioning, and the occurrence of side effects related to their use.

Although both the urban and rural elderly used OTC drugs daily, 14% of the urban elderly and 27.3% of the rural elderly used four or more. Individuals in both groups also took prescription drugs every day, with 62% of the rural and 50% of the urban subjects responding that they combined them with OTC drugs on a daily basis. Thirty-nine percent of the rural and 18% of the urban participants said that they could not perform their daily living activities without the OTC drugs.

The findings of Moore and Johnson (1993) indicate that the rural aged are more likely to engage in self-diagnosis and treatment of their health problems. This self-treatment may be the consequence of geographic and physical isolation, and the fact that many rural areas are medically underserved. However, the implications for nursing are that elderly clients, particularly those in rural areas, require additional education regarding responsible drug use and that nurses need to maintain an awareness that the elderly may be using multiple medications.

Critical thinking questions

- What ways could be used to disseminate information regarding the safe use of OTC medications to the elderly population of a rural community?
- As a community health nurse, what steps would you take with your individual clients in their home settings to ensure that they take their medications safely and accurately?

From Moore and Johnson (1993).

palpating to detect muscles of adequate body and size will require more skill and effort. On the other hand, decreased sensory perception, including perception of pain, may make injections less painful.

Physical problems may often interfere with the ability of the older client to comply with prescribed drug regimens. Some older clients may be unable to read labels or locate drugs because of failing eyesight; others, such as arthritic clients, may have difficulty opening bottles (particularly child-proof containers) or handling small pills, and the hearing-impaired client may not hear all of the instructions. The logistics of obtaining drugs and the economic cost may be a deterrent to complying with therapy. Multiple-drug therapy may simply be too complex for the client to manage without assistance. The nurse can simplify drug administration and scheduling as much as possible. Dosage schedules and calendars often help the forgetful client. Drug packaging that is easy to use and clearly labeled, as well as printed directions and drug information, help to ensure compliance in the older client.

BOX 8-6

Client Education for Medication Administration

- Review all medications with the client or caregiver to determine drug effectiveness and side/adverse effects.
- Have the client (or the caregiver) repeat the name and use for each medication plus the dosing instructions. If necessary, clarify the information.
- Perform a functional assessment to determine if client needs a compliance aid or a memory cue to take medications. If a caregiver is not available, determine if one is necessary.
- Provide a written medication schedule in large print for the client to refer to to enhance independent, effective management of therapeutic regimen.
- If the drug regimen is complicated, discuss possible changes (simplification) with the prescriber. Then recommend ways the client may be able to manage the drug regimen.

The elderly client's functional capabilities must be assessed to determine the educational requirements for safe and accurate self-administration of medications in the home (Isaac, et al, 1993) (Box 8-6). The nurse's creativity and skill are essential in devising teaching plans to enhance client compliance with the home medication regimen (see Chapter 10, Client Teaching for Self-Administration of Medications). Discuss prescription and OTC medications with clients and their family and friends, and have them describe in detail how and when they take all medications. Nurses should frequently reassess the effectiveness of the management of the therapeutic regimen as the older adult's functional capacity changes (Cohn, Taylor, & Messina, 1995).

The most important part of the nursing process for aging clients may be the nurse's ability to communicate patience, warmth, and understanding, and to treat the elderly as persons having dignity and the ability to reason, to feel, and to contribute.

SUMMARY

As the aged population within the Western world increases, proportionately as well as in numbers, it becomes of greater importance to ensure their well-being. In addition, the tendency towards polypharmacy in this population requires more astute assessment, intervention, teaching, and counseling on the part of the nurse. The nursing management of the administration of medications to geriatric clients requires that the nurse be knowledgeable about the various pharmacokinetic and pharmacodynamic effects of pharmaceutical agents in this population. Understanding the rationales behind these effects will help the nurse to administer medications safely and to evaluate client responses appropriately, regardless of the client's age. All geriatric clients have unique physiologic and psychosocial needs.

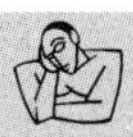

Critical Thinking

1. In the Moore and Johnson (1993) study of OTC medication use by the rural elderly, one of the participants stated "I've been taking care of myself, wife, and kids all of my life. I ran this ranch year-round, even when snow was everywhere and the wind blew so hard a body could hardly stand. Why would I drive 112 miles just to see a doctor and get some pills when I can go to the store 20 miles down the road and get some that do the trick just as good?" What approach would you use to provide information about the safe use of OTC medications with this client?
2. Mr. Holmes is an 81-year-old client of a home health agency in a rural area of western Massachusetts. He lives alone and still drives himself for shopping, health care provider visits, and other errands. Describe the assessment required to determine if Mr. Holmes is at risk for ineffective management of his medication regimen.

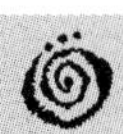

Collaborative Learning Activities

1. Have each of the students contact an elder in the community. If the student does not have ready access to an elder, a pharmacy is a good location to ask an individual about medications. Have the students do a survey on the number of medications each elder takes, OTC and prescription. Have the class discuss their findings.

BIBLIOGRAPHY

American Hospital Formulary Service (1996). *AHFS drug information '96*. Bethesda, MD: American Society of Hospital Pharmacists.

Anderson KN, et al (Eds.) (1994). *Mosby's medical, nursing, & allied health dictionary* (4th ed.). St Louis: Mosby.

Avorn J & Gurwitz JH (1995). Drug use in the nursing home, *Ann Intern Med 123*(3):195-204.

Beers MH, Ouslander JG, & Rollingher I, et al. (1991). Explicit criteria for determining inappropriate medication use in nursing homes, *Arch Intern Med 151*:1825-1832.

Conn VS, Taylor SG, & Messina CJ (1995). Older adults and their caregivers: The transition to medication assistance, *J Geront Nurs 21*(5): 33-38.

Erwin WG (1993). Geriatrics. In DiPiro JT, et al. *Pharmacotherapy* (2nd ed.). Norwalk, CT: Appleton & Lange.

Isaac LM, Tamblyn RM, & the McGill-Calgary Drug Research Team (1993). Compliance and cognitive function: A methodological approach to measuring unintentional errors in medication compliance in the elderly, *Geront 33*(6):772-781.

Gambert SR, Grossberg GT, & Morley JE (1994). How many drugs does your aged patient need?, *Patient Care 28*(6):61-6, 69-72.

Jinks MJ & Fuerst RH (1995). Geriatric drug use and rehabilitation. In Young LY & Koda-Kimble MA. *Applied Therapeutics* (6th ed.). Vancouver, WA: Applied Therapeutics.

Kovach LJ (1992). Polypharmacy in the elderly, *P & T Journal 17*(11):1709.

Lucas DS, Noyes MA, & Stratton MA (1995). Principles of geriatric pharmacotherapy, *Clin Consult 14*(5):1-8.

McCue JD, et al. (1993). *Geriatric drug handbook for long term care*. Baltimore: Williams & Wilkins.

Melmon KL (Ed.). (1992). *Clinical pharmacology* (3rd ed.). New York: McGraw-Hill.

Miller CA (1995). Medications that may cause cognitive impairment in older adults, *Geriatr Nurs 16*(1):47.

Moore JF & Johnson JE (1993). Over-the-counter drug use by the rural elderly, *Geriatr Nurs 14*(4):190.

Pollow RL, Stoller EP, Forster LE, & Duniho TS (1994). Drug combinations and potential for risk of adverse drug reaction among community-dwelling elderly, *Nurs Research 43*(1):44-49.

Practice Trends (1993). Geriatric assessment reduces mortality, *Amer Pharm NS33*(7):10.

Santo-Novak D & Edwards RM (1989). Rx: Take caution with drugs for elders, *Geriatr Nurs 10*(2):72.

Trends & Analysis (1995). Long-term care of elderly patients: Chronic disease comorbidity and other considerations, *Consult Pharm 10*(6):583-593.

United States Pharmacopeial Convention (1996). *USP DI: Drug information for the health care professional* (16th ed.). Rockville, MD: The Convention.

Willcox SM, Himmelstein DU, & Woolhandler S (1994). Inappropriate drug prescribing for the community-dwelling elderly, *JAMA 272*(4):292-6.

Chapter 9

Substance Misuse and Abuse

Chapter Focus

The misuse and abuse of drugs and alcohol in North American society are widespread, despite concerted efforts to educate the public and to curb their use. Because of the scope of the problem, the issue has moved to the forefront of health care. No matter what the health care delivery setting, the nurse must be able to recognize and assist clients with substance abuse problems. The following objectives and key terms are necessary for a good understanding of this chapter.

Key Terms

abstinence or withdrawal syndrome (p. 147)
Drug Abuse Warning Network (DAWN) (p. 143)
drug abuse (p. 141)
drug misuse (p. 141)
hallucinogen (p. 146)
metabolic (pharmacologic) tolerance (p. 143)
physical dependence (p. 143)
pK_a (p. 158)
psychologic dependence or addiction (p. 141)
receptor site (tissue) tolerance (p. 143)

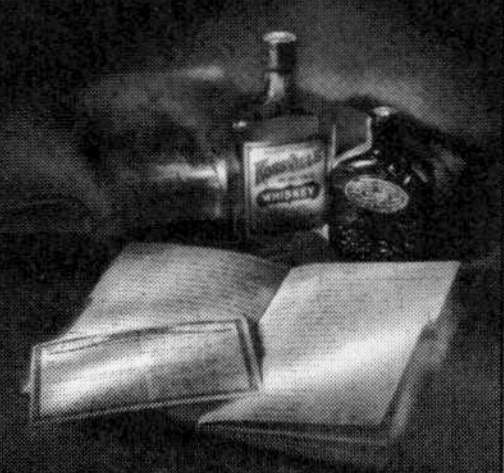

Objectives

1. Describe the scope of substance and drug abuse in the United States.
2. Cite etiologic factors of drug abuse.
3. Identify the pharmacologic basis of physical drug dependence and tolerance.
4. Describe the pathophysiologic changes characteristic of chronic drug abuse.
5. Identify the signs, symptoms, and treatment for overdose of drugs commonly abused.
6. List street names for drugs commonly used.
7. Discuss nursing management of the care of clients who abuse drugs and other substances.

All drugs prescribed or self-administered have the potential to be misused or abused. The prescribing of drugs without adequate exploration of the client's presenting complaint, for example, represents drug misuse by a prescriber. Prolonged and unsupervised administration of drugs for symptomatic relief is another example. In general, **drug misuse** refers to nonspecific or indiscriminate use of drugs, including alcohol. **Drug abuse** refers to self-medication or self-administration of a drug in chronically excessive quantities, resulting in physical and/or psychologic dependence, functional impairment, and deviation from approved social norms.

Psychologic dependence or addiction is a behavioral pattern characterized by drug craving, out of control drug usage, overwhelming concern with obtaining a drug supply, drug use causing personal and legal problems, denial, and continuing to use despite personal and legal difficulties. Most importantly, the use of the drug does not improve the person's quality of life (Sees & Clark, 1993).

Drug abuse is neither a new nor a recent phenomenon. It has been known throughout history as one expression of an individual's search for relief of physical, psychologic, social, and economic problems. Contemporary drug abuse has attained prominence as an issue with moral, legal, religious, social, psychologic, and medical implications. Drug abuse is not a problem confined to any particular socioeconomic, cultural, or ethnic group.

Drug and alcohol abuse in the workplace has been estimated to cost businesses up to $100 billion a year in the United States (Malatestinic, 1991). The impact on society of alcohol and drug abuse is tremendous. For example, alcohol played a role in the following societal problems:

- 40% of assaults reported and at least one-third of all rape and child abuse cases are alcohol-related
- nearly 50% of prisoners state they were under the influence of alcohol when they committed their crimes
- half of all U.S. traffic accidents and nearly 80% of accident fatalities that occur between 8 PM and 4 AM involve alcohol-impaired drivers
- in one rural state, alcohol was present in 35% of suicides, 63% of homicide victims, and 49% of unintentional injury fatalities (Baldwin & Cook, 1995).

Substance abuse is a major medical, social, economic, and interpersonal problem affecting individuals from all economic backgrounds and across the life span.

SUBSTANCE ABUSE AND PROFESSIONALS

In 1984 Bissell and Haberman studied alcoholism and the use of other drugs with alcohol in professionals, including doctors, nurses, dentists, attorneys, social workers, and college women. After following a group of approximately 400 professionals for 5 to 7 years, they found that alcoholism or alcohol abuse with other drugs was usually identified as a problem during the first 15 years of professional practice. The combination of alcohol and other drugs was quite prevalent, especially with physicians and nurses. This group reported the greatest addiction to hard narcotics. Their narcotic of choice was meperidine (Demerol) because it was readily available in their settings and also because it produced less pupillary constriction than the other opioids. Most physicians and nurses stated that they obtained their drugs through professional channels. Many started with a painful condition, such as back pain, or stress for which legitimate drugs were prescribed. One study of nearly 2000 chemically dependent health care professionals found that those who abused medications generally used more than four substances (Gallegos et al, 1988).

Although many nurses find it difficult to believe colleagues may be drug abusers, the American Nursing Association has publicly recognized substance abuse as a problem among nurses (ANA, 1984). Drug abuse is estimated to involve 6% to 8% of the 1.9 million nurses in the United States (Stammer, 1988).

While health care professionals most commonly abuse prescription drugs (opioids and benzodiazepines), alcohol, and tobacco, the choice of drug and route of administration may vary by profession. Nurses and physicians are more apt to abuse injectable drugs, pharmacists often use multiple oral drugs, dentists have a problem with nitrous oxide addiction, and anesthesiologists and nurse anesthetists commonly abuse fentanyl (Sublimaze) or similar products (Baldwin & Cook, 1995).

Career pressures and easy accessibility to drugs place health care professionals at greater risk for drug abuse. Unfortunately, impaired health professionals constitute a hazard to their clients' well-being and to themselves, so they cannot be ignored, overlooked, or left unreported. It is vital that health agencies be alert to suspected drug abusers on their staffs. Many agencies and most states have mandatory reporting of, and active rehabilitation programs for, impaired health professionals.

Substance abuse (alcohol and drugs) is considered a "handicap," and such employees may be protected by state and federal employment discrimination laws. The Rehabilitation Act (29 USC, Section 706[7][B]) states that employers are required to employ these individuals if they can properly perform their job functions and are not a threat to safety or property (Malatestinic, 1991). Many health care facilities and other businesses have established employee assistance programs to help impaired employees with rehabilitation.

DRUG TESTING

In an effort to identify persons with alcohol and drug-related problems, many businesses, government agencies, and health-related facilities are performing drug analysis or urine drug tests under specified conditions on their employees. Drug screens may also be part of a pre-employment physical examination. While a number of testing procedures are available, it is important to know the analytic techniques used and the purpose and limitations of any tests performed. Also, initial positive tests should be confirmed with more specific and

BOX 9-1

Time Versus Drug Detection in Urine

Drug	Detection in urine (days)*
alcohol	less than 1 day
amphetamines	up to 1 day
barbiturates	up to 1 day
benzodiazepines	up to 2 days
cocaine	up to 2 days
methadone	up to 3 days
marijuana	
single use	up to 6 days
chronic use	up to 29 days
opioids	
short acting	up to 1 day
phencyclidine	up to 6 days
phenobarbital	up to 6 days

From Baldwin & Cook, 1995.
*Chronic high doses may extend the time intervals.

BOX 9-2

Drug Abuse Characteristics

The four characteristics of drugs of abuse are:

1. Altered state of consciousness
2. Development of tolerance
3. Rapid onset of action of desired effects
4. Possibly abstinence syndrome if drug is discontinued abruptly after extended period of use

accurate tests because false-positive and false-negative results may occur. To ensure accuracy, a second test specific for the agent reported in the screening test is necessary. Health care providers interpreting the tests should be familiar with drugs known to cross-react or give a false-positive result with the test in use. For example, diphenhydramine (Benadryl) may test positive in urine for methadone, and phenylpropanolamine has been reported to test positive for amphetamines (Buchanan, et al, 1992). If the individual reports taking such medications, an alternate, more specific drug test could then be ordered.

Urine testing for specific drugs may detect substances used days or even a week before the test (Box 9-1). Such tests only give evidence of use or prior exposure to a drug and are not indicative of the individual's pattern of drug abuse or degree of drug dependency.

It is beyond the scope of this chapter to explore all aspects of drug abuse in depth. Rather the focus is on drug actions and the treatment of drug abuse. However, the nurse is urged to investigate independently other aspects of the complex phenomenon of drug abuse to achieve a more holistic frame of reference.

ETIOLOGIC FACTORS

A characteristic common to most drugs that cause dependence is that they are initially taken because the individual believes that a desirable pharmacologic effect will result. The person who is dependent on a drug has found something that provides relief from personal problems, and the drug generally is used as a maladjustive coping mechanism or, as evidence of the nursing diagnosis, ineffective individual coping. Since very few drugs or substances without CNS effects are abused, one of the predominant factors contributing to drug abuse appears to be intrapsychic—a desire to alter one's state of mind. This desire may arise from a number of factors, such as curiosity, boredom, peer pressure, multiple and diverse alienation, hedonism (pleasure-seeking behavior), affluence, and the attention paid to drug abuse by the mass media. All or any combination may lead to misuse of drugs and substances. More individual or subjective reasons are personal inadequacy or failure, conflicts terminating in tension, feelings of shame, and a predisposition to depression, which may lead to emotional and behavioral problems. The characteristics of drug abuse are listed in Box 9-2.

More specifically, some psychologic hypotheses have been advanced in relation to persons prone to use drugs as escape mechanisms. Persons with potentially drug-dependent predispositions are described as having strong psychologic dependence, low threshold of frustration, fear of failure, and feelings of inadequacy. Other authorities dispute the "addiction-prone" personality hypothesis, maintaining that everyone has the potential to become dependent on something.

"In 1990 alcoholism and other chemical dependencies were described by the American Society of Addiction Medicine (ASAM) as primary, chronic, relapsing diseases with genetic, psychosocial, and environmental factors influencing their development and manifestations" (Baldwin & Cook, 1995, p 81-1). Thus treatment centers have evolved to address the biopsychosocial factors associated with substance abuse.

Types of Drugs and Substances Abused

Although all drugs have some abuse potential, the more frequently abused chemically active substances are the xanthines and caffeine, found in coffee, tea, chocolate, and colas (see Chapter 18). Although these substances rarely are perceived as drugs by the lay public, they produce mild stimulant and euphoric effects, and their use may lead to physical dependence. Nicotine and ethyl alcohol (ethanol) are the most frequently misused and abused drugs, with consequent physical and psychologic dependence. Other CNS drugs such as anticholinergics, steroids, amphetamines, pentazocine, and L-dopa are examples of agents that may induce altered states of perception, thought, and feelings and drug-induced psychoses as a result of prolonged and concentrated therapeutic use or abuse. Few drugs without CNS effects are misused or abused.

This chapter will review the drugs most commonly reported to the **Drug Abuse Warning Network (DAWN)** as being involved in drug-abuse–related emergency room episodes. DAWN is a federal agency that monitors data on medical and psychologic problems associated with drug use and changing patterns of drug abuse. Box 9-3 lists the top 15 drugs misused or abused in 1993. See Table 9-1 for selected drugs commonly abused and symptoms of abuse.

Drug abuse may take several forms. (1) *Experimental abuse* occurs when individuals use drugs in an exploratory way and after which they accept or reject continuing use of the drugs. (2) *Social-recreational drug abuse* may occur only in social contexts; drugs that are frequently abused in social situations are alcohol, marijuana, cocaine, nicotine, and caffeine. (3) *Episodic drug abuse* refers to the periodic abuse of a drug. (4) *Compulsive drug abuse* is characterized by irrational, irresistible, or compelling abuse of a drug. (5) *Ritualistic drug abuse* may be related to religious practices. Polydrug or multiple drug abuse is common. Marijuana, alcohol, and other depressants frequently are used together and in conjunction with CNS stimulants. Heroin may be used with cocaine, and pentazocine (Talwin) with tripelennamine (PBZ), alcohol, or other depressants.

In the 1980s cocaine (especially crack cocaine) became popular and its abuse was seen fairly often but initially was somewhat curtailed by its high cost. In the 1990s, cocaine usage increased as reported in emergency department statistics; its use was reported in 37% of emergency room episodes that involved men and in 18% of drug episodes involving women.

The 1980s also documented the development of synthetic "designer drugs" produced by illegal laboratories or chemists. The molecular structure of a controlled substance is modified to produce a new variant that mimics the effects of the original drug. The types of drugs most commonly modified and sold are analogs of meperidine (Demerol), fentanyl (Sublimaze), and MDMA (3,4-methylenedioxymethamphetamine) from the illicit psychedelic agent MDA (methylenedioxyphenylethylamine). When "designer drugs" are identified, the Drug Enforcement Agency (DEA) enacts regulations to ban them. Until it is banned, such a substance is legal to make, sell, or use. Once outlawed, though, the underground chemists often make a new, legal variation of the product, and it will be sold until a ban against it is established. Thus "designer drugs" are constantly changing and should be considered potentially dangerous substances. Contaminants have been identified in these products, and overdoses and deaths have been reported with their use.

BOX 9-3

Leading Drugs Resulting in Emergency Department Visits in U.S.*

Males	Females
1. alcohol in combination	1. alcohol in combination
2. cocaine	2. cocaine
3. heroin/morphine	3. acetaminophen
4. marijuana/hashish	4. heroin/morphine
5. acetaminophen (Tylenol)	5. aspirin
6. methamphetamine/speed	6. alprazolam (Xanax)
7. aspirin	7. ibuprofen (Motrin)
8. ibuprofen (Motrin)	8. marijuana/hashish
9. diazepam (Valium)	9. diazepam (Valium)
10. PCP/PCP combinations	10. lorazepam (Ativan)
11. benzodiazepine (unspecified)	11. clonazepam (Klonopin)
12. alprazolam (Xanax)	12. amitriptyline (Elavil)
13. clonazepam (Klonopin)	13. d-propoxyphene (Darvon products)
14. amitriptyline (Elavil)	14. acetaminophen with codeine
15. amphetamine	15. diphenhydramine (Benadryl)

*Trade names are in parentheses; many of these products are also available under other trade or generic names. Statistics are based on drug episodes caused by an illegal drug or nonmedical use of a legal drug resulting in emergency department visits.
From 1993 Emergency Department Data (DAWN, 1996)

PHARMACOLOGIC BASIS OF DEPENDENCE AND TOLERANCE

Psychologic and **physical dependence** on a drug can exist independently or simultaneously. In contrast to psychologic dependence (defined earlier), physical dependence is an adaptive state, occurring after prolonged use of a drug, in which discontinuation of the drug causes physical symptoms that are relieved by readministering the same drug or a pharmacologically related drug. Both types of dependence can potentially lead to compulsive patterns of drug use in which the user's lifestyle is focused on procurement and administration of the drug. Several hypotheses attempt to explain the pharmacologic basis of the physiologic adaptation that occurs in tolerance and physical drug dependence.

Tolerance may exist with either psychologic or physical dependence and may be viewed in two ways. **Receptor site (tissue) tolerance** is a form of adaptation in which the effect produced depends both on the concentration of the drug and on the duration of the exposure. In this type of tolerance the clinical effect of the drug is reduced as the duration of exposure continues.

The second type of tolerance is **metabolic (pharmacologic) tolerance**, which refers to an aspect of drug disposition. Prolonged exposure to a drug can change the body's metabolic response to the drug, increasing drug clearance with repeated ingestion. For example, with prolonged exposure to barbiturates, the steady-state blood concentrations will fall progressively with continued administration of the

TABLE 9-1 Selected drugs commonly abused and symptoms of abuse

Drug category	Street names	Methods of use	Symptoms of use	Hazards of use
MARIJUANA/ HASHISH	Pot, grass, reefer, weed, Columbian, hash, hash oil, sinsemilla, joint	Most often smoked; can also be swallowed in solid form	Sweet, burnt odor Neglect of appearance Loss of interest, motivation Possible weight loss	Impaired memory, perception Interference with psychologic maturation Possible damage to lungs, heart, and reproduction and immune systems Psychologic dependence
ALCOHOL	Booze, hooch, juice, brew	Swallowed in liquid form	Impaired muscle coordination, judgment	Heart and liver damage Death from overdose Death from car accidents Addiction
STIMULANTS				
Amphetamines* Amphetamine Dextroamphetamine Methamphetamine	Speed, uppers, pep pills Bennies Dexies Moth, crystal Black beauties	Swallowed in pill or capsule form, or injected into veins	Excess activity Irritability; nervousness Mood swings Needle marks	Loss of appetite Hallucinations; paranoia Convulsions; coma Brain damage Death from overdose
Cocaine	Coke, snow, toot, white lady, crack, ready rock	Most often inhaled (snorted); also injected or swallowed in powder form, smoked	Restlessness, anxiety Intense, short-term high followed by dysphoria	Intense psychologic dependence Sleeplessness; anxiety Nasal passage damage Lung damage Death from overdose
Nicotine	Coffin nail, butt, smoke	Smoked in cigarettes, cigars and pipes, snuff, chewing tobacco	Smell of tobacco High carbon monoxide blood levels Stained teeth	Cancers of the lung, throat, mouth, esophagus Heart disease; emphysema

DEPRESSANTS				
Barbiturates	Barbs, downers	Swallowed in pill form or injected into veins	Drowsiness Confusion Impaired judgment Slurred speech Needle marks Constricted pupils	Infection after parenteral use Addiction with severe life-threatening withdrawal symptoms Loss of appetite Death from overdose Nausea
Pentobarbital	Yellow jackets			
Secobarbital	Red devils			
Amobarbital	Blue devils			
Opioids		Swallowed in pill or liquid form, injected	Drowsiness Lethargy	Addiction with severe withdrawal symptoms Loss of appetite Death from overdose
Dilaudid, Percodan				
Demerol, Methadone				
Morphine	Dreamer, junk	Injected into veins, smoked	Needle marks	
Heroin	Smack, horse			
Codeine	School boy	Swallowed in pill or liquid form		
HALLUCINOGENS				
PCP (phencyclidine)	Angel dust, killer weed, supergrass, hog, PeaCe pill	Most often smoked; can also be inhaled (snorted), injected or swallowed in tablets	Slurred speech; blurred vision, uncoordination Confusion, agitation Aggression	Anxiety, depression Impaired memory, perception Death from accidents Death from overdose
LSD	Acid, cubes, purple haze	Injected or swallowed in tablets		
Mescaline	Mesc, cactus	Usually ingested in their natural form	Dilated pupils Delusions; hallucinations Mood swings	Breaks from reality Emotional breakdown Flashback
Psilocybin	Magic mushrooms			
INHALANTS				
Gasoline		Inhaled or sniffed, often with use of paper or plastic bag or rag	Poor motor coordination Impaired vision, memory and thought processes Abusive, violent behavior	High risk of sudden death Drastic weight loss Brain, liver, and bone marrow damage
Airplane glue				
Paint thinner				
Nitrites	Poppers, locker room, rush, snappers	Inhaled or sniffed from gauze or ampules	Slowed thought Headache	Anemia, death by anoxia
Amyl				
Butyl				

From Blue Cross & Blue Shield Association, Chicago, Ill.
*Includes lookalike drugs resembling amphetamines that contain caffeine, phenylpropanolamine (PPA), and ephedrine.

same dose. This may be attributed to barbiturates' inducing effect on hepatic microsomal enzymes, which increases barbiturate metabolism.

PATHOPHYSIOLOGIC CHANGES

Physical and psychologic dependence on drugs is frequently associated with debilitated physical states caused by the user's extensive abuse of the drug, which often results in malnutrition, dehydration, and hypovitaminosis. Respiratory complications such as pneumonia, pulmonary emboli, and abscesses frequently are associated with neglect, debilitation, and the respiratory depression produced by CNS depressants. The intravenous administration of illicit drugs often leads to a high incidence of sepsis, hepatitis, infective endocarditis, and AIDS as a result of the use of contaminated equipment. In addition, cellulitis, sclerosis of the veins, phlebitis, and skin abscesses may occur. Death from accidental overdose is common. Overdosage is a particularly significant potential danger because illegal drugs are notoriously unreliable in regard to the potency of their active ingredient. The drugs are frequently adulterated (mixed) with various substances such as active (amphetamines, benzodiazepines, hallucinogens, etc.) and inactive substances (lactose, sugars) by the time they reach the user. If an individual who has been using such drugs unknowingly receives pure or stronger drugs, the risk of toxicity and death exists. Overdosage also may occur when an individual who has been withdrawn from drugs for some time (thereby having lost accumulated tolerance) injects the previous usual dose, which now is in excess of the tolerance level.

As a consequence of all these factors, the life expectancy of persons who are psychologically dependent on drugs is generally lower than that of nondependent individuals. Table 9-2 presents common drug groups that are abused, along with signs and symptoms of acute intoxication.

CULTURAL ASPECTS OF DRUG ABUSE

Various societies accept certain drugs as legal and useful, while other drugs may be banned or considered illicit. For example, in the United States and parts of Western Europe, alcohol, caffeine, and nicotine are widely accepted and commonly used substances. Amphetamines are the major drug of abuse in Japan, where increases in personal productivity are desired. In the Middle East cannabis is considered a legal drug, whereas alcohol is usually forbidden. Some Native American tribes use peyote, a **hallucinogen** (a drug that causes auditory or visual hallucinations), for religious services, but in general such hallucinogens have no accepted therapeutic usage in the United States. In the high-altitude South American Andes and other mountainous areas (e.g., Peru), coca leaves are brewed as a tea or chewed to decrease the sensation of hunger, increase work performance, and increase a sense of well-being. Thus the use and acceptance or rejection of a substance depend on the society and its subgroups. When drug substances are considered illicit or illegal and are in short supply, non–law-abiding persons may be motivated to produce and/or sell the banned substances. This activity is usually extremely profitable.

TYPES OF DRUGS MOST COMMONLY ABUSED

Opioids (Heroin/Morphine and Other Agonist Opioids)

Opioids are one of the most abused drug categories, often listed in the top five for drug-related emergency room episodes. The pharmacologic types of drugs from natural sources (opiate) include the opium alkaloids (heroin, morphine), the semisynthetic group (hydromorphone [Dilaudid], oxymorphone [Numorphan]), and the synthetic

TABLE 9-2 Signs and symptoms of acute drug intoxication

Drug(s) abused	Signs and symptoms
cannabis drugs	Tachycardia and postural hypotension, conjunctival vascular congestion, distortions of perception, dryness of mouth and throat, possible panic
cocaine	Increased stimulation, euphoria, increased blood pressure and heart rate, anorexia, insomnia, agitation; in overdose, increased body temperature, hallucinations, seizures, death
opiates	Depressed blood pressure and respiration; fixed, pinpoint pupils; depressed sensorium; coma; pulmonary edema
barbiturates and other general CNS depressants	Depressed blood pressure and respirations; ataxia, slurred speech, confusion, depressed tendon reflexes, coma, shock
amphetamines	Elevated blood pressure, tachycardia, other cardiac dysrhythmias, hyperactive tendon reflexes, pupils dilated and reactive to light, hyperpyrexia, perspiration, shallow respirations, circulatory collapse, clear or confused sensorium, possible hallucinations, paranoid feelings
hallucinogenic agents	Elevated blood pressure, hyperactive tendon reflexes, piloerection, perspiration, pupils dilated and reactive to light, anxiety, distortion of body image and perception, delusions, hallucinations

group (meperidine [Demerol], levorphanol [Levo-Dromoran], methadone [Dolophine]). Heroin, d-propoxyphene (Darvon), oxycodone (Percodan, Percocet), and morphine are the most often abused. The term *opioid* is preferred because it refers to both natural and synthetic products that have morphine-like effects.

Mode of administration. The opium derivatives generally can be administered percutaneously (absorbed through the mucous membranes) by sniffing *(snorting)*, by subcutaneous injection *(skin popping)*, or by direct IV injection *(mainlining)*. The rate of absorption is correspondingly increased, with mainlining producing almost immediate drug effects.

Mechanism of action and effects. Opium derivatives are CNS depressants that probably act on the sensory cortex or higher centers, and thalami. Because they can relieve pain, change or elevate mood, relieve tension, fear, and anxiety, and produce feelings of peace, euphoria, and tranquility, they are particularly likely to lead to physical and psychologic dependence. Rapid intravenous injection of these drugs produces warm, flushing sensations described as being similar to sexual orgasm followed by a soothing state that seems to be best characterized as a state of complete drive satiation. The individual "high" on opioids feels no need to satisfy drives for basic biologic needs and is often described as being "on the nod"—drowsy, content, and euphoric. The drugs do not produce hallucinogenic or psychotomimetic effects.

Acute overdosage. Acute overdosage of opioid substances may result in severe pulmonary edema and respiratory depression. These outcomes are dose dependent and are related to the degree of individual tolerance. What constitutes a lethal dose depends on the individual's tolerance for the drug. Symptoms occur rapidly in most clients (see Table 9-2, Signs and Symptoms of Acute Drug Intoxication).

Opioid toxicity is manifested in various ways, such as slow, shallow breathing; cold, clammy skin; miosis (pinpoint pupils, common with most opioids; however, mydriasis may occur in meperidine overdose); severe hypoxia (*AHFS*, 1996); mixed overdose conditions; or severe acidosis. Bradycardia, hypotension, muscle spasm, lethargy, respiratory depression, and urinary retention may also occur, although meperidine's toxic effects may be more excitatory, causing significant tachycardia (Sinatra & Savarese, 1992). The presence of thrombophlebitis, scarred veins, and puckered scars from subcutaneous injections may help identify the client with opioid toxicity. Opioids tend to delay motility and gastric emptying time, so that the revival of the client may increase peristalsis and thus further increase absorption of the drug, producing a coma cycle. Chronic abuse may result in abscesses, cellulitis, endocarditis, glomerulonephritis, encephalopathy, tetanus, and thrombophlebitis. These are caused by a spectrum of factors ranging from injection technique to adulterants in the substance of abuse.

The treatment of choice for acute overdosage is administration of an antagonist (e.g., naloxone) and respiratory support. The box at right describes management of an opioid overdose.

Physical dependence and acute abstinence syndrome. In a client physically dependent on opioids, an abrupt and complete reversal of narcotic effects with naloxone may precipitate an acute **abstinence or withdrawal syndrome,** symptoms experienced by a chemically dependent person who is suddenly deprived of their intake of their substance of abuse.

! MANAGEMENT OF DRUG OVERDOSE

Opioids

General approach

Provide symptomatic and basic supportive care of airway, breathing, and circulation (the "ABCs"). Maintain cardiac output, blood pressure, urinary output, and peripheral perfusion.

If oral opioids were consumed and client is not lethargic or unresponsive, empty stomach by emesis or gastric lavage.

Specific approach

If apnea is present, maintain a patent airway, using assisted or controlled respiration and oxygen as necessary.

When the triad of miotic pupils, coma or stupor, and bradypnea (respirations slowed to a rate of four to six per minute) appears, the administration of naloxone (Narcan) is indicated and will help to differentiate narcotic poisoning from other conditions.

Naloxone, a pure narcotic antagonist, reverses opioid toxicity. The usual adult dose is 0.4 to 2 mg given intravenously, which may be repeated at 2- to 3-minute intervals if necessary. Larger doses may be required to treat acute overdoses of butorphanol (Stadol), nalbuphine (Nubain), propoxyphene (Darvon and Darvocet products), and pentazocine (Talwin). Failure to respond to high doses of a narcotic antagonism may indicate a mixed substance overdose or involvement of a nonopiate substance.

Support blood pressure and maintain respiration after response to naloxone (Narcan). Blood and urine samples should be examined with a multiple drug screen to aid in diagnosis. A positive response to naloxone is characterized by dilation of the pupils (if previously miotic) and an increase in respiratory function, blood pressure, and cardiac rate.

Children with a known or suspected narcotic overdose may receive 0.01 mg/kg of naloxone (Narcan) as the first dose. (Dilute naloxone with sterile water for injection.) If the child does not respond to the first dose, additional intravenous doses at 2- to 3-minute intervals may be administered.

Naloxone reverses apnea and coma within minutes and should be titrated to the client's arousal with a respiratory rate in a range of 10 to 20 breaths per minute. Continued client monitoring is necessary because additional naloxone (IV bolus or by intravenous infusion) is often necessary to prevent the reemergence of opioid toxicity.

Although opioid abstinence syndrome may be reversed by administration of an opioid, to do so in a drug-dependent client is prohibited by law except if the person is an inpatient who was admitted for an emergency procedure or is being detoxified or maintained in an approved federal drug-treatment program. Methadone usually is considered the drug of choice in the treatment of this clinical condition.

Physical dependence on opiates usually is described in relation to heroin or morphine, but the other derivatives manifest similar symptoms. Physical dependence is evident in the withdrawal syndrome that develops if the drug is withheld and in the marked tolerance that develops with continued use of the drug. Also, because persons dependent on heroin or morphine so frequently feel satiated, physical, emotional, and social deterioration often occurs. The individual may feel little need for food and become grossly malnourished and weak. Preoccupation with obtaining the drug makes participation in the usual social and vocational aspects of life difficult if not impossible. As the drug craving grows, tolerance to the drug also increases, and eventually the motivation for using the drug becomes oriented more to the avoidance of withdrawal symptoms and less to the achievement of euphoria.

Withdrawal symptoms. The initial withdrawal symptoms are related to the half-life of the opioid being used. Symptoms of withdrawal from heroin are autonomic in origin and appear within 8 hours after the last dose in physically dependent individuals. These symptoms are less life-threatening than with other substances of abuse and manifest as restlessness, chills and hot flashes, restless sleep, piloerection on the skin (which gives rise to the term *cold turkey*), rhinorrhea, drowsiness, lacrimation, and mydriasis during the first 24 hours. As withdrawal progresses, these symptoms are more severe and additional symptoms may include sneezing, yawning, generalized anxiety, abdominal cramps, lower back pain, lower extremity cramps, vomiting and diarrhea, anorexia, diaphoresis, muscular twitching, insomnia, elevated pulse rate, blood pressure, and temperature, and a craving for the drug. Depending on the drug used, abstinence syndrome develops within 2 to 48 hours and peaks at 72 hours.

Occasionally withdrawal symptoms are severe enough to result in cardiovascular collapse. If withdrawal is untreated, it may continue for up to 7 to 10 days, after which the physical dependence of the body on the presence of opioids is eventually lost. Psychological dependence continues for a longer period; some authorities claim it continues forever.

Treatment of opioid dependence

Withdrawal programs. Generally, opioid withdrawal is difficult, and repeated relapses may be expected. Abrupt and complete withdrawal (*cold turkey*) can be accomplished but should generally be avoided because this procedure is a dangerous (especially in clients with a co-existing medical illness) and inhumane approach. Therapeutic withdrawal from an opioid may be somewhat more comfortably achieved by successively tapering the drug's dosage over a period of several days.

The choice of withdrawal program is partly influenced by the following factors: the client's physical condition, the duration of drug dependence, the type and amount of drug being taken, motivations for drug abuse and withdrawal, and whether the individual is also dependent on other drugs, such as alcohol. In some instances, depending on these factors, opioid withdrawal may need to be accomplished in a hospital with close medical supervision.

In identifying criteria for evaluating opioid withdrawal, one should note that recovery from morphine-type dependence is not equated with cure. Regardless of repeated relapses to drug abuse, therapeutic programs should continue. Progress in withdrawal may be indicated by progressively longer periods of abstinence from opioids without resort to the use of other psychoactive drugs or alcohol and by the client's growing confidence in the ability to function effectively without drugs.

Therapeutic community programs. The ultimate goal of using any medication to treat dependency is to provide relief from the compulsive craving for the drug of abuse. To achieve rehabilitation, the abuser needs to turn to more than another medication, prescribed or illicit. The individual also needs human dignity, sincerity, compassion, warmth, self-respect, and hope with positive reinforcement. To achieve independence and become a self-sustaining, productive member of the community, the abuser must be provided with emotional and social support. These human resources have not been effectively addressed by many treatment programs, and failures have resulted.

Because persons withdrawing from drugs frequently cannot make the transition easily, groups of persons who have decided to abstain from drug use can meet or live together in an attempt to support and guide one another. Such therapeutic community programs as Phoenix House and halfway houses have been established that include group psychotherapy and self-help approaches. Ultimately an individual should emerge from such a program with sufficient personal growth and appropriate support systems to be able to manage life satisfactorily without resorting to drug abuse.

Methadone detoxification and withdrawal. A currently preferred method of withdrawal is substitution of methadone. Methadone is a synthetic opioid analgesic that, by virtue of cross-tolerance, permits effective substitution of methadone dependence for heroin dependence. Its effectiveness against heroin dependence results from its ability to forestall the euphoriant effects of heroin and the craving for the drug without producing heroin's deleterious physical and mental effects. When properly administered, methadone allows the individual to function adequately, without intellectual or emotional impairment.

For adults in detoxification, methadone is taken orally in 15- to 40-mg doses per day, titrated according to client response, until withdrawal symptoms are controlled. Methadone therapy is initiated empirically based on client symptoms. As a general guide, 1 mg methadone is substituted for 20 mg meperidine, 4 mg morphine, or 2 mg heroin (Baldwin & Benson, 1995). For a review of recommended dosages and dosage adjustments, refer to current drug abuse references or references cited in this section.

Regular administration results in the development of tolerance to methadone and cross-tolerance to heroin. The client will not experience the opioid-induced "rush" and euphoria unless higher doses than tolerance is exceeded. Because of this, the nurse should be aware that some clients might exaggerate their withdrawal symptoms to obtain more methadone. When the abuser is being treated with methadone, supportive psychologic or psychiatric counseling may relieve some of the burdens that led to drug dependence. During this phase the methadone may be gradually withdrawn, usually at a rate of 20% reduction or 5 mg in daily dosage. However, methadone maintenance programs are controversial and are not always successful. Previous opioid abusers who are unable to negotiate life in a drug-free state may revert to their former dependence or alternative substance abuse or may return to the methadone therapy detoxification.

Methadone maintenance. In the United States, maintenance methadone treatment programs require both FDA and state licensing and approval. The ultimate goal of these programs is complete withdrawal from drug dependency for the participant, although some clients continue on methadone for an extended time. Methadone programs can include psychologic, vocational, and rehabilitation services in addition to medical support. Approved methadone programs are required to comply with all the requirements in the Federal Methadone Regulations.

Admittance to a methadone maintenance program usually requires evidence of current dependence on morphine-type drugs and at least a 1-year history of opioid dependence. Nurses should be aware that addicts hospitalized with medical conditions other than addiction may require pharmacologic support with methadone or opioids during their stay. Be aware also that a cross tolerance to opioids is common, and thus these clients usually require higher analgesic doses to control pain. Usually verification of enrollment in an approved methadone maintenance program is required in order to continue methadone during the hospital stay. The hospital pharmacist should be consulted on the regulations and for assistance in such matters.

The nurse should also be aware that treatment centers vary in their methods and drugs used for opioid withdrawal. Some treatment centers report having accomplished withdrawal from methadone through the use of clonidine, whereas others maintain that methadone is the drug of choice.

Methadone dependence does occur, but withdrawal symptoms are less severe although they last for a longer period. Methadone withdrawal programs generally include supplemental rehabilitation techniques such as vocational and social rehabilitation. After individuals have functioned free from heroin for a sufficient period, secured steady employment, and readjusted their lifestyle, theoretically they can be withdrawn from methadone maintenance.

Levomethadyl acetate (Orlaam) is a longer-acting alternative to methadone for use only in approved opioid treatment programs. It is similar to methadone with a longer duration of action; it is usually given three times a week. The federal regulations do not allow take-home dosages of levomethadyl (Orlaam), so clients that are ill or require hospitalization usually are transferred to methadone on a temporary basis (Baldwin & Benson, 1995).

Heroin maintenance. Diacetylmorphine (heroin), a Schedule I drug (see Chapter 2), is a substance with no accepted medical use in the United States. It was banned because of its high potential for abuse and the increasing number of heroin addicts. Today it is still one of the top drugs abused in the United States and often is used in combination with cocaine.

While most countries have banned heroin use, it is a legal drug in Belgium, Canada, and England, although it is rarely used in Belgium and Canada. Physicians are permitted to prescribe heroin and other opioids for persons who have a history of intractable dependence, thereby maintaining them and preventing withdrawal symptoms. Prescriptions are issued through designated hospitals or clinics.

The approval of heroin as an analgesic for intractable pain has been proposed and denied numerous times in the United States. Pharmacologically, heroin is a prodrug—when it is administered it is converted in the liver to morphine—and thus opponents of heroin legislation state that legalized heroin is unnecessary because morphine and other opioids are available in the United States (Lipman, 1993).

Clonidine treatment. Clonidine (Catapres), a sympatholytic antihypertensive, stimulates $alpha_2$ receptors in the brain, which decreases sympathetic outflow from the CNS. This effect produces a decrease in peripheral resistance, heart rate, and blood pressure. It is also under investigation for relieving the symptoms of acute drug withdrawal (e.g., opioids, nicotine, alcohol) and aid in the detoxification process. Withdrawal symptoms may be caused by the hyperactivity of the locus ceruleus, a major noradrenergic nucleus of the brain. When clonidine transdermal patches are used, the nurse should be aware that it takes 2 to 3 days to reach a peak effect, which is often too late to treat the worst effects seen with opioid withdrawal. The tablet dosage form offers a quicker and a more easily titratable method of preventing or reducing unwanted effects.

A clonidine dosage of 5 µg/kg/day increasing to 17 µg/kg/day as necessary, has been used to prevent withdrawal syndrome. The dose is individualized according to the client's tolerance and quantity and type of opioid agonist used. The daily dosage is administered in equally divided doses over a 24-hour period for approximately 10 days. Then the dosage is reduced by 50% on days 11, 12, and 13 and discontinued on day 14 (*USP DI,* 1996).

The clinical usefulness of clonidine is limited by the drug's sedative and hypotensive effects, and extremely close supervision of the client is necessary to monitor side effects, adverse effects, and any manipulation of the dose by the client. The nurse should hold the dose of clonidine and consult the prescriber if blood pressure is less than 90 systolic or 60 diastolic. Physical dependence on opioids is eliminated by this detoxification process, and nonpharmacologic intervention can be used to address the remaining psychologic dependence.

Other Analgesics

pentazocine [pen taz' oh seen] (Talwin)
Pentazocine (Talwin) 60 mg IM is considered approximately equivalent as an analgesic to 10 mg IM of morphine. Sharp increases in the incidence of pentazocine drug abuse led the Drug Enforcement Administration to place this drug in Class IV under the Controlled Substances Act. Pentazocine's potential for producing psychologic and physical dependence is significant even in low doses, and infants born to pentazocine-dependent women experience withdrawal immediately postpartum. Pentazocine can also cause psychotomimetic reactions such as visual hallucinations, feelings of depersonalization, and nightmares.

The CNS effects of pentazocine are similar to those of the opioids, including analgesia, sedation, and respiratory depression (reversed by naloxone [Narcan]). In high doses pentazocine causes increases in blood pressure and heart rate. Lung problems have been reported when tablets are crushed, dissolved, and administered intravenously. This may be due to the talc binders and other particulate matter in tablet dosage forms. The use and reuse of cotton as a filter may result in "cotton fevers," a type of allergic reaction caused by tiny cotton fibers. This syndrome occurs within 30 minutes of the injection, and the client experiences increased heart rate, hypotension, increased sweating, shaking chills, and fever. Often these symptoms resolve in approximately 4 to 24 hours without treatment although the health care provider should be aware that sepsis, embolism, and other complications are also possible. Other potential effects include seizures and ulceration and severe sclerosis of the skin and subcutaneous tissue and muscles, caused by subcutaneous or intramuscular injections. The combination of pentazocine with other CNS depressants such as barbiturates and alcohol may be lethal.

Pentazocine (Talwin) and tripelennamine (PBZ) abuse first appeared in the late 1960s to early 1970s as a result of shortages or the high cost of heroin in large metropolitan areas. This combination is known as *Ts and blues* (*T* for Talwin and *blue* for the color of the generic tablet of tripelennamine). Ts and blues are oral tablets crushed together, dissolved, and injected either through a cotton filter intravenously, like heroin, or subcutaneously. Abscesses and necrotic tissue have resulted, which require hospitalization and grafting. Drug abusers report that tripelennamine is used to increase the onset of action and prolong the duration of euphoria produced by pentazocine.

To discourage abuse, oral pentazocine now contains naloxone (Talwin-Nx). The addition of naloxone has no effect on the analgesic properties of oral pentazocine but if this combination is administered intravenously, the naloxone will nullify or cancel the rush effect of the injected Ts and blues combination.

The treatment of pentazocine dependence is gradual reduction of the drug itself in a controlled environment. The psychotomimetic effects should be observed closely in a controlled environment because they may persist for 5 to 7 days.

propoxyphene [pro pox' i feen] (Darvon, Novopropoxyn🍁)
Use of propoxyphene products in excessive doses, either alone or in combination with other CNS depressants including alcohol, is a significant cause of drug-related deaths. Since an overdose of propoxyphene may result in fatality, intensive supportive and symptomatic therapy must be instituted immediately.

Propoxyphene should not be taken in doses higher than those recommended by the manufacturer and clients should be so warned. The judicious prescribing of propoxyphene is essential for safe use of this drug. With clients who are depressed or suicidal, consideration should be given to the use of nonnarcotic analgesics.

Because of its depressant effects, propoxyphene should be prescribed with caution for individuals whose medical condition requires the concomitant administration of sedatives, tranquilizers, muscle relaxants, antidepressants, or other CNS depressant drugs. Clients should be cautioned against the concomitant use of propoxyphene products and alcohol because of potentially serious CNS additive effects of these agents. Some deaths have occurred as a consequence of the accidental ingestion of excessive quantities of propoxyphene alone or in combination with other drugs. Propoxyphene-related deaths have occurred in individuals with previous histories of emotional disturbances or of misuse of tranquilizers, alcohol, and other CNS-depressant drugs.

The clinical effects of an acute propoxyphene overdose are similar to an acute opioid toxicity—coma, respiratory arrest, pulmonary edema, circulatory collapse, and death. Grand mal seizures have also been reported. Propoxyphene is metabolized in the liver to norpropoxyphene, which may be responsible for some of its toxicity. Toxic propoxyphene serum levels are between 0.6 and 10 μg/ml; lethal levels reportedly are more than 10 μg/ml (*AHFS*, 1996).

Norpropoxyphene has less CNS depressant effect than propoxyphene but it has a greater anesthetic effect on the myocardium, similar to that of amitriptyline and antidysrhythmic drugs such as lidocaine and quinidine. Electrocardiographic monitoring is essential in management of overdose. The manufacturer recommends that in all suspected overdose cases, a poison control center should be contacted for the most current treatment of the overdose.

This drug has also been abused by parenteral administration of the oral dosage form. Propoxyphene napsylate (Darvon-N, Darvocet-N) is considered a less toxic propoxyphene formulation because of its delayed absorption orally and its relative insolubility in water. Thus the napsylate dosage form has less abuse potential than propoxyphene hydrochloride.

Propoxyphene is pharmacologically related to the opioids, so naloxone, may reverse the signs of toxicity. Overdose may be accompanied by seizures requiring anticonvulsants, and emergence from a coma may require restraints before administration of naloxone because of the client's disorientation, agitation, and confusion. Clients need psychologic and emotional support during this time. A quiet, calm environment with reduced sensory stimulation may reduce the incidence of disorientation and agitation. The nurse should use a simple, direct approach and communicate with reality orientation and reassurance.

Alcohol

Although there are many different kinds of alcohols, the term *alcohol* usually refers to ethyl alcohol. Methyl, propyl, butyl, and amyl alcohols are examples of other alcohols that are very toxic when taken orally.

ethyl alcohol (Ethanol)

Ethyl alcohol is the only alcohol used extensively in medicine and in alcoholic beverages. Many OTC "night-time" cough and cold remedies may be abused because of their considerable sedative potential because as they contain alcohol (up to 25%, or 50-proof) with antihistamines. Table 9-3 lists the ethyl alcohol content of various OTC preparations. Ethyl alcohol is a colorless liquid that mixes readily with water and because it lowers surface tension, it is a good solvent for a number of substances. Ethyl alcohol, also referred to as grain alcohol, is the product of the fermentation of a sugar by yeast.

Therapeutically, ethyl alcohol has been used as a cardiac disease preventative, an appetite stimulant for clients with poor appetite during periods of convalescence and debility, and as a hypnotic for older persons who do not tolerate other hypnotics.

Mechanism of action. Ethyl alcohol may have either a local or a systemic action.

Local effect. Ethyl alcohol denatures proteins by precipitation and dehydration, which may be the basis for its germicidal, irritant, and astringent effects. It irritates denuded skin, mucous membranes, and subcutaneous tissue. Subcutaneous injection of alcohol may cause considerable pain and sloughing of the tissues. When it is injected into or near a nerve, alcohol may cause nerve degeneration and anesthesia.

Systemic effect. Contrary to popular belief, alcohol is not a stimulant but a CNS depressant. What sometimes appears to be stimulation results from the depression of the higher faculties of the brain and represents the loss of inhibitions acquired by socialization.

Alcohol is thought to interfere with the transmission of nerve impulses at synaptic connections, but how this is accomplished is not known. It causes progressive and continuous depression of the central nervous system, the sequence being cerebrum, cerebellum, spinal cord, and medulla. Its action is comparable to that of the general anesthetics. The excitement stage, however, is longer, and when the anesthetic stage is reached, definite toxic symptoms are present. The margin between the anesthetic stage and the fatal dose is a narrow one.

TABLE 9-3 Content of ethyl alcohol in OTC products

Medicinals	Alcohol content (%)	Alcohol proof
Cough-cold preparations		
Ambenyl-D	9.5	19
Comtrex Maximum	10	20
Vicks 44	10	20
Vicks NyQuil	10	20
Benadryl	0	0
Benylin Expectorant	0	0
Naldecon DX and EX	0	0
Triaminic	0	0
Mouthwash preparations		
Cepacol	14.5	29
Listerine	26.9	53.8

Modified from *Nonprescription products: formulations & features '97-'98* (1997). Washington, DC: American Pharmaceutical Association.

The action of alcohol varies with the individual's tolerance, the presence or absence of extraneous stimuli, the rate of ingestion, and the gastric contents. Small or moderate quantities produce a feeling of well-being, talkativeness, greater vivacity, and increased confidence in one's mental and physical power. There is a general loss of inhibitions. The finer powers of discrimination, insight, concentration, judgment, and memory are gradually dulled and lost. Large quantities may cause excitement, impulsive speech and behavior, laughter, hilarity, and in some persons, pugnaciousness, while others may become melancholy or unduly sentimental. Table 9-4 lists the content of ethyl alcohol in various beverages.

The effects of large quantities of alcohol may become apparent when the individual attempts to operate machinery such as an automobile. Visual acuity (especially peripheral vision) is diminished, reaction time is slowed, judgment and self-control are impaired, and the individual tends to be complacent and pleased with themselves. Many drivers will take chances when under the influence of alcohol that they would never take ordinarily. This leads to disaster, as accident statistics reveal.

The intoxicated individual usually becomes ataxic, mutters incoherently, has disturbance of the special senses, is often nauseated, may vomit, and eventually may lapse into stupor or coma. The respiratory neurons are usually not depressed except by large doses of alcohol.

Cardiovascular. Alcohol depresses the vasomotor neurons in the medulla and causes dilation of the peripheral blood vessels, especially those of the skin. This causes a feeling of warmth. Heat is also lost from the interior,

TABLE 9-4 Content of ethyl alcohol in various beverages

Beverages	Alcohol content (%)	Alcohol proof
Beer	4	8
Wine (red/white)	12	24
Brandy	30-45	60-90
Whiskey, vodka	45	90
Martini, Manhattan	30	60
Daiquiri, Alexander	15	30

Data from Hinds, 1985.

which accounts for the fact that an intoxicated person may freeze to death more quickly than a nonintoxicated person. Alcohol also depresses the heat-regulating mechanism.

Small doses (10 to 25 ml) produce an insignificant increase in the pulse rate, caused mainly by the excitement and the reflex effect on the gastrointestinal tract. Larger doses (over 25 ml) produce the same effect but may be followed by lowered blood pressure caused by the effect on the vasoconstrictor neurons. Chronic alcoholism may result in cardiomyopathy, hypertension, and a variety of cardiac arrhythmias, especially atrial fibrillation and flutter. Epidemiology studies, though, report light to moderate consumption of alcohol (up to 2 drinks per day) reduces the risk for myocardial infarction and cardiac death (Jungnickel & Hunnicutt, 1995).

Gastrointestinal. The effect of alcohol on the function of the digestive organs depends on the presence or absence of gastrointestinal disease, the degree of alcohol tolerance, the concentration of the alcohol, and the type and amount of food present. Small doses of alcohol will stimulate the secretion of gastric juice rich in acid. Salivary secretion is also reflexively stimulated. Large and concentrated doses of alcohol tend to inhibit secretion and enzyme activity in the stomach, although the effect in the intestine seems to be negligible. Chronic alcohol ingestion causes pancreatitis and hepatic cellular damage, which results in fibrosis and scarring, cirrhosis, and/or hepatitis. In addition, when large quantities of alcohol are taken over a prolonged period, gastritis, nutritional deficiencies, and other untoward results have been observed.

Pharmacokinetics. Alcohol does not require digestion before absorption. A small amount is absorbed in the stomach while most is absorbed in the small intestine. Approximately 90% of the alcohol is metabolized in the liver. The liver enzyme, alcohol dehydrogenase, oxidizes alcohol (ethanol) to acetaldehyde; acetaldehyde oxidizes to acetic acid, which is buffered to an acetate that eventually oxidizes to carbon dioxide and water. Approximately 90% to 98% of ethanol is metabolized (oxidized) in the liver with the remainder primarily excreted by way of the lungs and kidneys. As plasma ethanol levels increase, though, the hepatic alcohol dehydrogenase pathway becomes saturated, resulting in an increase in the unmetabolized alcohol ratio. Chronic alcohol use may result in hyperlipidemia, fatty deposits in the liver, and ultimately alcoholic cirrhosis.

Alcohol produces an increased flow of urine because of the increase in fluid intake. Alcohol also acts as a diuretic through CNS depression and inhibition of antidiuretic hormone (ADH) release. If the individual has preexisting renal disease, the kidney may be further damaged. Large and concentrated doses of alcohol are thought to injure the renal epithelium.

After absorption, alcohol is distributed in every tissue of the body in approximately the same ratio as its water content. Therefore a rough estimate of the quantity consumed may be obtained from an analysis of the blood (Table 9-5).

Health care professionals should be aware of the approximate total amount of alcohol in different beverages: 12 oz of beer = 4 oz of wine = 1 oz of whiskey. Therefore alcohol abuse can occur with any of the beverages, depending on the quantity consumed.

TABLE 9-5 Concentration of alcohol in blood and related clinical observations

Stage	Blood alcohol mg/dl	Clinical observations
Subclinical	30-100	Slight evidence of performance deterioration possible, such as motor function, coordination, personality or mood and mental acuity
Emotional instability	100-200	Decreased inhibitions; emotional instability; slight muscular incoordination; slowing of responses to stimuli
Confusion	200-300	Disturbance of sensation; decreased pain sense; staggering gait; slurred speech
Stupor	300-400	Marked decrease in response to stimuli; muscular incoordination approaching paralysis
Coma, death	Over 400	Complete unconsciousness; depressed reflexes; subnormal temperature; anesthesia; impairment of circulation; possible death

Drug interactions. The most commonly used and abused drug in North America is alcohol. It interacts with many prescription and OTC drugs, resulting in serious adverse effects leading to emergency room admission or even death. The magnitude of this potential interaction is enormous. Most people, professionals and lay persons alike, may not be fully cognizant of some of the most significant alcohol-drug interactions (Table 9-6).

Alcohol Abuse

Signs of alcohol abuse typically are these: changes in drinking patterns, such as the need for early morning drinking, drinking alone, hiding partial or full liquor bottles, or the need to have a drink before performing a potentially stressful event (e.g., job interview, keeping an appointment); personality changes; family discord; job absenteeism; personal appearance neglect; poor eating habits; memory lapses; and blackouts. Sudden abstinence from alcohol in a heavy drinker can be very dangerous because alcoholic withdrawal syndrome may occur (Box 9-5).

The major objectives for treatment of ethyl alcohol withdrawal include a quiet environment, monitoring of health status, symptom relief, prevention or treatment of complications and the development of long-term rehabilitation plans. Supportive care includes fluid and electrolyte replacement, adequate nutrition, thiamine to prevent development of Wernicke encephalopathy, and anticonvulsant medications if necessary. A sedative drug such as a long-acting benzodiazepine may be necessary for severe withdrawal reactions; its dosage can then be tapered and discontinued. In selected persons, beta-adrenergic blocking agents or clonidine may be used to reduce the sympathetic manifestations of alcohol withdrawal, such as increased anxiety, tachycardia, hypertension, and tremors.

Toxic Alcohols

Isopropyl alcohol and methyl or wood alcohol are toxic when taken internally. When some alcoholic individuals are unable to purchase ethanol (ethyl alcohol), they substitute agents such as isopropyl (rubbing) alcohol, methyl alcohol (antifreeze), or any available substance that might prevent al-

TABLE 9-6 Selected significant alcohol-drug interactions

Substances interacting with alcohol	Mechanism	Possible effect(s)
I. antihistamines antidepressants opioid analgesics sedative-hypnotics antianxiety agents antipsychotic drugs	Additive	Enhanced CNS depressant effects
II. disulfiram (Antabuse) cefamandole and some other second and third generation cephalosporins chlorpropamide (Diabinese) other oral antidiabetic agents to varying degrees griseofulvin (Fulvicin) metronidazole (Flagyl) procarbazine (Matulane)	Inhibition of aldehyde dehydrogenase in metabolism of alcohol, leading to acetaldehyde accumulation (disulfiram or a "disulfiram-type reaction")	Most severe effects seen with disulfiram and alcohol: flushing, stomach pain, head throbbing, increased heart rate, hypotension, sweating, nausea, and vomiting With antidiabetic agents: mild to severe hypoglycemia
III. phenytoin (Dilantin)	Increase or decrease in liver metabolism	In chronic alcohol abuse: possible decrease in anticonvulsant effect caused by increased metabolism In acute alcohol use: a possible decrease in metabolism, causing increased serum level of phenytoin and toxicity
IV. salicylates	Additive	Increased gastrointestinal irritability and bleeding
V. nitrates nitroglycerin	Additive	Vasodilation leading to hypotension, syncope

cohol withdrawal. This is a dangerous practice that can cause severe poisoning and death.

isopropyl alcohol

A clear, colorless liquid with a characteristic odor, isopropyl alcohol compares favorably with ethyl alcohol in its antiseptic action. It has been recommended for skin disinfection and for rubbing compounds and lotions used on the skin. Its bactericidal effects are said to increase as its concentration approaches 100%.

methyl alcohol (Wood Alcohol, Methanol)

Methyl alcohol, if taken orally, is a central nervous system toxin. However, intoxication does not occur as readily as with ethyl alcohol unless large amounts are consumed. Methyl alcohol is oxidized in the tissues to formic acid, which is poorly metabolized, the basis for the development of a severe acidosis.

Symptoms of poisoning include nausea and vomiting, abdominal pain, headache, dyspnea, blurred vision, and cold, clammy skin. Symptoms may progress to delirium, convulsions, coma, and death. In nonfatal cases the individual may become blind or suffer from impaired vision. Treatment is directed toward the relief of acidosis since this seems to be related to the severity of the visual symptoms. Large amounts of sodium bicarbonate may be needed to treat acidosis successfully. One dose of 60 ml of methyl alcohol has been known to cause permanent blindness. Fluids containing methyl alcohol usually bear a "Poison" label.

BOX 9-5

Clinical Stages of Alcohol Withdrawal*

Stage	Description	Time from last dose
Minimal	Mild expressed anxiety, fidgets, mentally clear, pulse and temperature normal	12 hours
Mild	Clear hyperactivity, appears anxious, sweaty, pulse rate up, mentally alert, restless	12-24 hrs
Moderate	Momentary mental lapses, marked agitation, sweaty, rapid pulse, fearful, severely restless, fairly cooperative	24-48 hrs
Severe	Hallucinations, mental lapses markedly interfering with communication, severe agitation, sweaty, tachycardia, unable to cooperate, may have convulsion	24-48 hrs

From Iber (1991).

*Remember that these symptoms may be delayed until the third or fourth day in trauma clients or those operated on in an emergency situation who have subsequently received analgesia.

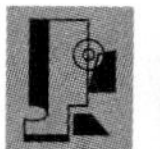

Ethical Considerations

Organ Transplantation in People with Unhealthy Lifestyles

Organ transplantation is a widely accepted treatment option in the United States for individuals with end-stage renal, heart, or liver disease. Success rates for transplantation are reported as the percentage of functioning grafts 1 year after transplant because most grafts fail in the first year. The success for heart transplants is between 80% and 85% and for liver transplants between 70% and 80%. With kidney transplants, about 75% are functioning after 5 years.

However, with rising health care costs, the economics of transplantation has been called into question. The cost analysis for kidney transplantation can be calculated by comparing the cost of transplantation with the cost of 5 years of hemodialysis, the alternative to transplantation, and transplantation is seen as more cost effective. Such calculations are not possible for heart and liver transplantation because there is no other treatment available for end-stage heart and liver disease and the alternative is death. In addition, transplantation is seen as economically viable because of the costs of repeated and extensive hospital stays of people in end-stage disease, and because of the possibility that the organ recipient can return to a productive life.

With organ transplantation established as a cost effective and desirable treatment for people with end-stage disease, how will these limited resources be allocated? The debate over the rationing of health care is on-going and increasing. To allocate scarce donor organs is to make judgments about the worthiness of the potential recipients. It would seem that rationing of donor livers already exists as evidenced by the data that only 10% of liver transplants are performed on recovering alcoholics although alcoholism is the leading cause of liver failure in the United States. The position taken to limit transplantation for alcoholics (even those who are "dry") is that the donor organ is a nonrenewable resource that should be reserved for those whose disease was not a result of their behavior. The argument that survival rates will be lower in recovering alcoholics has been disproved.

1. What other factors might be involved in the selection process for liver transplantation in recovering alcoholics?
2. Would the situation be different for heart transplantation to individuals with unhealthy lifestyles of smoking, overeating, and not exercising?
3. What is the nurse's role in providing comprehensive and individualized care for people in stigmatized groups?

From Thomas (1993).

Drugs Used in Treatment of Chronic Alcoholism

disulfiram [dye sul' fi ram] (Antabuse)

Disulfiram is used to sensitize an individual to alcohol by inducing an unpleasant alcohol-disulfiram reaction. This disulfiram reaction begins with flushing of the face and develops into intense vasodilation of the face, neck, and upper part of the body. Hyperventilation and increased pulse rate may occur. Nausea occurs in 30 to 60 minutes along with facial pallor, hypotension, and copious vomiting. There is usually an intense feeling of discomfort, pulsating headache, palpitations, dyspnea, syncope, and a constrictive feeling in the neck. The reaction lasts from 30 minutes to several hours, as long as alcohol is being metabolized; it is then followed by drowsiness and sleep. Other drugs have been reported to cause a disulfiram-type reaction when taken with alcohol (Table 9-6 lists these drugs).

Mechanism of action. Disulfiram inhibits the enzyme aldehyde dehydrogenase, which converts acetaldehyde to acetate. This permits acetaldehyde to accumulate and cause the unpleasant toxic effects. Disulfiram has few effects unless the person ingests alcohol.

Pharmacokinetics. Metabolism is hepatic and initial effect may be delayed from 3 to 12 hours because of drug storage in adipose tissue. Studies indicate that up to 20% of a dose remains in the body for up to 6 days. Elimination is via the kidneys with smaller amounts excreted in feces and lungs. Because of slow and incomplete absorption and elimination, effects persist for up to 2 weeks after therapy is discontinued. Clients should be instructed not to ingest any alcohol-containing substance during this time.

Dosage and administration. Initially the client is given up to 500 mg orally daily for 7 to 14 days; maintenance dose is 250 mg orally daily.

■ Nursing Management
Disulfiram Therapy

Assessment. The client's history should be reviewed for conditions in which particular caution should be used with disulfiram therapy, such as allergic eczematous contact dermatitis, cardiovascular disease, diabetes mellitus, epilepsy, hypothyroidism, and severe pulmonary insufficiency because a disulfiram-alcohol reaction may worsen these conditions. In clients with psychosis or depression, behavioral toxicity may be precipitated. There is a higher rate of hepatotoxicity in clients with existing hepatic dysfunction. Sensitivity to disulfiram, rubber, pesticides, and fungicides should be ascertained. The use of disulfiram should be carefully considered during pregnancy. It must be ascertained that the client has not ingested alcohol in any form (i.e., beverages, sauces, OTC preparations, as well as liniments, colognes, and aftershave lotions) or been treated with paraldehyde in the 12 hours before beginning a disulfiram regimen.

Before treatment commences, the client's level of understanding of the purpose, procedure, and consequences of disulfiram therapy should be determined because of the unpleasant reaction the client will experience with the ingestion of alcohol. Written client consent should be obtained before beginning disulfiram therapy.

The client's medications should be assessed for significant drug interactions. When disulfiram is given with:

Drug	Possible effect and management
alcohol	Will result in a disulfiram-alcohol reaction if alcohol is consumed during or within 2 weeks of disulfiram therapy
alfentanil (Alfenta)	May prolong the action of alfentanil
anticoagulants	Increased anticoagulant effects; dosage adjustments may be necessary; monitor closely for untoward bleeding
anticonvulsants, especially phenytoin (Dilantin), hydantoins	Increased serum levels of hydantoins; monitor serum levels before and during concurrent drug therapy because dosage adjustments may be necessary
isoniazid (INH)	Increased CNS side effects; disulfiram dosage may need to be reduced or stopped; monitor closely for ataxia, insomnia, dizziness, irritability
metronidazole (Flagyl)	Confusion and psychotic episodes; this combination should be avoided. Metronidazole should not be administered concurrently or during the 2 weeks after disulfiram therapy
paraldehyde	Inhibition of acetaldehyde dehydrogenase may occur, resulting in increased blood levels of paraldehyde and acetaldehyde

A complete blood count (CBC), blood chemistry profile, and liver function studies should be done as a baseline assessment before therapy begins. The nature of the client's support services should also be determined.

Nursing diagnosis. The following selected nursing diagnoses may be identified with a client receiving disulfiram:

- risk for injury related to a preexisting condition that contraindicates or requires the cautious use of disulfiram; adverse drug reactions; and occurrence of disulfiram-alcohol reaction (nausea and vomiting, blurred vision, confusion, dizziness, tachycardia, flushing of the face, diaphoresis, headache, dyspnea, and rarely, seizures, chest pain, loss of consciousness, or death)
- altered sleep patterns related to the drug's CNS effects (drowsiness)
- altered comfort (headache, rash, stomach discomfort)
- altered nutrition less than body requirements related to gustatory alterations (metallic or garlic-like taste in the mouth)
- altered thought processes related to a psychotic reaction (mood or mental changes)
- altered sexuality patterns related to decreased sexual ability in men
- potential complications of peripheral neuritis (numbness, tingling, or weakness in hands and feet), optic neuritis (change in vision), encephalopathy (mental changes), and hepatitis (abdominal discomfort, jaundice, dark urine, light stools)

Implementation

Monitoring. The effectiveness of the disulfiram therapy is monitored by assessing the client's abstinence from alcohol use. Clinically the client should be observed for visual disturbances and eye pain, which might indicate an optic neuritis. Peripheral neuritis may be developing if the client has tingling or numbness of the hands or feet. Jaundice may indicate a drug-induced hepatotoxicity.

A transaminase test for liver function evaluation is recommended 10 to 14 days into disulfiram therapy and every 6 months during therapy, along with a CBC and blood chemistry profile to monitor for adverse effects of the drug. Serum cholesterol concentrations may increase with disulfiram doses of 500 mg a day.

Intervention. Provide support to assist the client to achieve the goal of abstinence. Psychotherapy aimed at mental and social rehabilitation should accompany disulfiram therapy. Refer to an appropriate support group in planning for discharge.

Supportive measures will need to be instituted in instances of a severe alcohol-disulfiram reaction to restore the blood pressure and treat the client for shock. The reaction usually lasts 30 minutes to several hours until the alcohol is metabolized, depending on the amount of alcohol ingested, the dose of disulfiram, and the time since its last administration. Administer oxygen and monitor potassium levels and ECG tracings. Large IV doses of ascorbic acid, iron, and antihistamines have been used, but these are of questionable value (*AHFS*, 1996).

Ensure safety precautions such as assistance with transferring and ambulation if the client has the CNS effect of drowsiness.

Education. Caution the client that the ingestion of any form of alcohol while taking disulfiram, and for up to 14 days after the last dose, will cause a very unpleasant response—dizziness, syncope, nausea and vomiting, headache, chest pain, dyspnea, palpitations, tachycardia, profuse sweating, facial flushing, blurred vision—and if the response is severe, seizures, unconsciousness, heart attack, and death could result. The extent of the reaction will depend on the dose of the drug and the amount of alcohol ingested.

All foods and liquid medications should be checked for the presence of alcohol. Alcohol is available in prescription drugs, OTC drugs, liquid cough-cold analgesic products, foods, flavoring, mouthwashes, salad dressings, and the like, and the individual should be warned of the possible interaction and the need to check all liquids for alcohol. Lotions with a high alcohol content that are liberally applied topically should also be used cautiously.

It is advisable for the client to wear a Medic Alert identification while taking the drug and to alert any health care professionals providing care. Identification cards describing the most common symptoms of the alcohol-disulfiram reaction are available from the manufacturer.

Caution the client against driving or operating any hazardous equipment if drowsiness resulting from the drug occurs. A slight metallic or garlic-like taste may occur for the first few weeks of therapy. Alert the client that many drug-induced reactions subside after about 2 weeks of therapy. The client should consult with the health care provider at 6-month intervals for blood studies or if any of the following occur: chest pain, respiratory difficulty, jaundice, or the ingestion of alcohol.

Evaluation. The client will: abstain from alcohol; experience no disulfiram-alcohol reactions; demonstrate no adverse effects of disulfiram; verbalize content taught about the drug; and self-administer the drug safely and accurately when managing his or her own medication regimen.

CNS Stimulants

The primary CNS stimulants abused in the United States include cocaine and amphetamine products, especially methamphetamine.

Cocaine

Cocaine, while classified as a controlled substance, is an alkaloid related to the belladonna alkaloids. Topically it has local anesthetic and vasoconstriction therapeutic effects; thus it has a limited use in a few selected surgical procedures, such as nasal surgery. Cocaine abuse has reached epidemic levels. In the United States it is one of the most frequently mentioned drugs resulting in emergency room visits, second only to alcohol in combination with other substances (DAWN, 1996).

It has been estimated that 3 million Americans are regular users of cocaine (Scott & Gabel, 1995). Cocaine is a very potent CNS stimulant that is highly addicting and also a potentially lethal drug. As a social-recreational drug of abuse it is popular for its euphoric effects. It also produces increased energy like the amphetamines and may lead to a similar psychotic state with strong elements of paranoia.

The purity of the illicitly produced drug varies greatly because this short-lived CNS stimulant is often diluted or cut with agents such as amphetamines, boric acid, quinine, mannitol, procaine, and lidocaine. The vasoconstricting effect of cocaine may be responsible for limiting its own absorption. Multiple drugs are often taken with or after cocaine, such as alcohol (84% of users), marijuana (98% of cocaine addicts), heroin, barbiturates, benzodiazepines, and phencyclidine (PCP) (Scott & Gabel, 1995). Cocaine is a very dangerous substance with a high financial, psychologic, and physical control over the user.

Routes of administration. Cocaine may be taken by sniffing (snorting) the white, fluffy crystalline powder (which resembles snow, hence its street name), by direct IV injection, or by smoking (transalveolar route) the converted base form, "freebase" or crack. In the United States, cocaine is usually found as the hydrochloride (HCl) salt or in the base form. Cocaine HCl is water soluble, and thus it can be snorted or injected intravenously. Freebase and crack cocaine (minus the HCl salt) are essentially the same free alkaloidal base; the difference between them is that different solvents are used in the manufacturing process (Scott & Gabel, 1995). Freebase is dangerous to make (ether and ammonia are involved) and dangerous to use. The freebase form is heat resistant, lending itself to smoking in any form including "coke pipes." Smoking freebase cocaine produces a more intense effect and is dangerous because of the possibility of an excessive dose being administered. The freebase solvents are flammable and may explode during the process, causing further harm to the user.

Freebase cocaine has largely been replaced by "crack" or "rock" cocaine. Crack cocaine is also a freebase, but it is made without any volatile chemicals. It became popular because of its availability in smaller amounts at a much lower cost than freebase cocaine and because its use does not require any elaborate paraphernalia. The cocaine market has thus become affordable to all economic groups. Freebase cocaine when dried looks like rocks and when smoked makes a cracking sound. Therefore the street names of freebase cocaine include rock, crack, gravel, and readyrock. Crack cocaine also produces a fast and very intense effect.

Cocaine HCl may be inhaled (snorted) from a small spoon, rolled dollar bills, a lengthened finger nail, or various other inhalation devices. Sniffing causes vasoconstriction, which limits the amount of cocaine absorbed from the nasal mucosa into systemic circulation; thus more intense effects are derived from the freebase or crack cocaine.

Pharmacokinetics. Cocaine is rapidly metabolized in the liver, and the cocaine abuser may need to use the drug every half hour or less to maintain the high. Cocaine serum levels are not proportional to toxicity, and the elimination half-lives by oral, intranasal, and intravenous routes are similar (50, 80, and 60 minutes, respectively). Cocaine stimulation of the CNS initially affects the intellect (cognition) and behavior (affective domain).

At this time there is no absolute level known to be lethal. The rapidity of the increase in blood level may be as important in determining fatal reactions as the peak blood concentration. Factors other than blood concentration of cocaine must be examined. These factors include tolerance, reverse tolerance, previous history of cocaine abuse, individual susceptibility, presence of other drugs and the medical problems associated with cocaine abuse.

Initial symptoms of cocaine use are restlessness, mydriasis, hyperreflexia, vasoconstriction, tachycardia, hypertension, hallucinations, nausea, vomiting, and muscle spasms, which may be followed by respiratory failure, convulsions, coma, and circulatory collapse. In chronic abusers, a toxic cocaine psychosis (similar to paranoid schizophrenia) is often found, characterized by hallucinations and paranoid delusions. Skin eruptions (with itching and compulsive scratching) caused by self-inflicted skin irritation are also frequently observed. The energetic client may be prone to outbursts of violent behavior. Blood in the nose and a perforated nasal septum are frequently seen in those who chronically snort cocaine.

Medical complications associated with cocaine abuse effect many body systems, including cardiovascular (hypertension, tachycardia, myocardial infarction, arrhythmias, thrombosis, and sudden death); respiratory (pulmonary abscesses, lung infections, pulmonary edema and hemorrhage, and pneumonitis); renal (rhabdomyolysis [the release of skeletal muscle contents into the plasma] which results in generalized muscle aches and pains and, in one third of the reports, acute renal failure); neurologic (seizures, stroke, and intracranial hemorrhage); psychiatric (psychosis, suicide, delirium, and clinical depression). Miscellaneous other conditions may also occur, including septicemia, hepatitis, and HIV. The medical complications are numerous and vary with the type cocaine used and the route of administration.

Cocaine is particularly dangerous in pregnant women. It has been associated with an increased risk of stillbirth, preterm labor, and neonatal complications such as congenital malformations, cerebral infarction and hemorrhage, and sudden infant death syndrome. Neonatal complications include acute withdrawal symptoms (increased irritability, tremors, abnormal reflexes, tachypnea, and poor eating and sleeping patterns) and neurobehavioral delays during the first year of life. They may also be susceptible to cocaine-induced seizures, cerebral infarction, and potentially a variety of other complications (Young, Vosper & Phillips, 1992). Such effects have resulted in child-abuse convictions of mothers that used cocaine while pregnant (Schydlower, 1990). See the box below for Management of a Cocaine Overdose.

MANAGEMENT OF DRUG OVERDOSE

Cocaine

General approach

Provide symptomatic and basic supportive care of airway, breathing, and circulation.

Establish an intravenous line using an isotonic or hypotonic solution for administration of medications necessary to treat the adverse effects induced by cocaine.

Continuously monitor client's vital signs and core body temperature.

Avoid or reduce sensory stimulation as it may provoke or worsen agitation and paranoid behavior.

Specific approach

Treat medical complications as necessary, for example, for:

- metabolic acidosis, administer sodium bicarbonate.
- hyperthermia, utilize external cooling measures such as sponging with cold water or use a cooling blanket.
- seizure, intravenously administer diazepam (Valium), lorazepam (Ativan), phenobarbital (Luminal), phenytoin (Dilantin), or thiopental (Pentothal) as necessary.
- cardiac arrhythmias, administer propranolol (Inderal), labetalol (Normodyne), phentolamine (Regitine), or lidocaine as necessary.
- hypertension, administer phentolamine (Regitine), labetalol (Normodyne), verapamil (Isoptin), or nitroprusside as indicated

Monitor and treat other side/adverse effects as necessary.

Amphetamine Products

Amphetamine abuse has been reported for more than 50 years and while it declined for a while, its use now has increased, as noted in Box 9-3. It was estimated that 3 million Americans used these drugs for nonmedical purposes in 1992 (Scott & Gabel, 1995) (see Table 9-1 for street names and additional information).

Chemically, amphetamines are similar to the natural catecholamines, epinephrine, norepinephrine, and dopamine. They can activate catecholamine receptor sites to increase stimulation; therefore, they have been classified as sympathomimetic agents. In addition, they also increase release of natural catecholamines and block their reuptake into the neurons, which results in the induction of an artificial "fight or flight" response (Scott & Gabel, 1995).

Oral amphetamine is absorbed from the GI tract and concentrates in the brain, kidneys, and lungs. It is metabolized in the liver and excreted via the kidneys. Amphetamine is a basic drug with a **pK_a** (the point at which half the drug amount in the body is ionized and half nonionized) of 9.9; therefore, a urine pH of 7 or more extends the half-life of amphetamine to approximately 20 hours. A pH of 5, however, reduces the half-life to 5 to 6 hours. Persons that abuse this drug are usually aware of the prolonged effect they can achieve by alkalizing their urine. Prescribers are also aware that acidifying the urine to a pH of 4.5 to 5.5, will enhance amphetamine excretion.

Effects. The amphetamines are usually abused because they produce mood elevation, reduction of fatigue, and a sense of increased alertness. They do not create extra physical or mental energy; instead, they promote expenditure of present resources, often to the point of hazardous fatigue. Intravenous amphetamine injection results in marked euphoria, an orgasmic feeling knows as a "rush" that is accompanied by a sense of great physical strength and clear thinking. The person feels little or no need for rest, sleep, or food and may continually engage in vigorous activity that may be perceived as exhilarating and creative. To an observer, however, they are inefficient and performing repetitious type behaviors, which is common during an amphetamine high.

Termination of the drug's effect may result from exhaustion, fright, or inability to obtain more drug. Drug withdrawal is followed by long periods of sleep, and on awakening the individual often feels hungry, extremely lethargic, and profoundly depressed, a phenomenon known as "crashing." Suicide risk is quite possible during this period.

The stimulant properties of amphetamines can cause dramatic cardiorespiratory effects, such as tachycardia, dyspnea, chest pain, and hypertension. The person may panic because these signs and symptoms are those of a myocardial infarction. To deal with these disturbing symptoms, amphetamine users often use depressants or "downers" such as large amounts of alcohol, marijuana, benzodiazepines, barbiturates, or heroin (Scott & Gabel, 1995) to offset the overstimulation effect.

Acute toxic amphetamine effects can be very serious and, in addition to the signs and symptoms mentioned previously, seizures and circulatory collapse have been reported. "Fatal intoxication usually is preceded by hyperpyrexia, convulsion, and shock" (Scott & Gabel, 1995). Detoxification and use of conventional therapies for medical complications are necessary in the treatment of the acute toxicity.

Amphetamines are also said to be psychotomimetic although there is conflicting evidence as to the cause of amphetamine psychosis. The questions asked include: Is the psychosis caused by heavy use of amphetamines or is the user perhaps also mentally ill? Or are some of the symptoms (paranoia, aggression, delusions of persecution, hallucinations) secondary to the insomnia (sleep deprivation) induced by prolonged amphetamine abuse?

The health care professional should be aware that amphetamines (especially methamphetamine) usage is on the increase, with much of it being made by illicit laboratories in the United States. Crystal methamphetamine (known as ice or crystal meth) is gaining popularity because a high results in usually less than a minute when these crystals are heated and the vapor inhaled (Scott & Gabel, 1995). In some instances oral amphetamine users are also smoking methamphetamine concurrently to vastly increase the intensity of effect. Methamphetamine serum levels after smoking produce elevated plasma levels and a high that can persist for 12 hours (with a half-life of approximately 12 hours), whereas the smoking of freebase cocaine rapidly peaks and is eliminated because it has a half-life of about an hour. The toxicity resulting from the combination of smoking and oral administration of the drug produces an enhanced and potentially dangerous effect.

Preparations. Chemically there are three types of amphetamines—salts of racemic amphetamines, dextroamphetamines, and methamphetamines—all of which vary in degree of potency and peripheral effects. Dextroamphetamine is said to have fewest peripheral effects, such as hypertension and tachycardia.

Treatment of toxicity. No specific antidote is available to treat amphetamine overdose. Psychotic symptoms usually occur within 36 to 48 hours after a single large overdose, which usually clear in approximately 1 week. Treatment is mainly supportive and symptomatic. If a large overdose is discovered within an hour in a conscious, nonconvulsant client, vomiting or gastric lavage may be utilized, followed with a saline cathartic. The person should be closely monitored because of the potential for hypertension, hyperpyrexia, and seizures. To increase renal excretion of amphetamines, an osmotic diuretic such as mannitol with a urinary acidifier (ammonium chloride) may be necessary. After the acute episode, the amphetamine abuser will need intensive counseling, and perhaps desensitization techniques, on a long-term basis to overcome the craving and relapses common with abuse of this stimulant drug.

Cannabis Drugs (Marijuana/Hashish)

The cannabis drugs are derived from the leaves, stems, fruiting tops, and resin of both female and male hemp plants (*Cannabis sativa*). The potency of the active ingredient, tetrahydrocannabinol (THC), is greatest in the flowering tops of the plant and seems to vary according to the climatic conditions under which the plant is grown. In the United States the plants grow wild or are illegally cultivated and thus potency varies. The only legal cultivation is that by the federal government for research purposes.

Both the availability of more potent species and varieties of marijuana and the increase in use among young teenagers (12 to 14 years of age) require a new attitude of concern toward the substance. The potency of THC in marijuana varies, with the typical leaf containing 3%. Imported marijuana, when carefully cultivated, may contain 6% to 10% THC (Jungnickel, 1995). Marijuana grown under scientifically controlled conditions is often much more potent than the domestic variety smoked in the past.

Preparations. Marijuana and hashish are the most common forms of cannabis in use. *Hashish* refers to the powdered form of the plant's resin, which contains 7% to 12% THC (Jungnickel, 1995). Other forms of cannabis, used in such countries as Jamaica, Mexico, Africa, India, and the Middle East, include *banji, ganga,* and *charas*, which correspond, respectively, to American marijuana, hashish, and unadulterated resin. In Morocco *kif* is used, whereas in South America a cannabis drug called *dagga* is often used.

Mode of administration. Cannabis drugs may be absorbed when administered by oral, subcutaneous, or pulmonary routes, but they are most potent when inhaled. Either the pure resin or the dried leaves of the cannabis plant may be smoked in pipes or cigarettes. Because the smoke is acrid and irritating, some users prefer to smoke marijuana through a water pipe. The smoke is inhaled deeply and retained in the lungs as long as possible to achieve maximal saturation of the absorbing surface. Powdered hashish and marijuana may also be mixed with foods, a mode of administration that delays the drug's absorption. The effects sought by users are mental relaxation and euphoria. The sedative-hypnotic effects of smoking are rapid and generally last 2 to 3 hours, while the effects of the orally ingested drugs may not begin for several hours. Hashish oil injected intravenously has a high incidence of mortality.

Marijuana plants contain hundreds of different chemicals. Approximately 100 chemicals have been isolated and are generally termed *cannabinoids*. Of these, only THC (delta-9-tetrahydrocannabinol) and CBD (cannabidiol) have been studied in humans to identify their pharmacologic effects. While many questions are still unanswered, it is believed the major psychoactive ingredient in cannabis is THC.

Dronabinol (Marinol or THC) and nabilone (Cesamet) are synthetic cannabinoids available for the treatment of nausea and vomiting induced by cancer chemotherapy that are not responsive to standard therapies. Both products have a high potential for abuse, so they are closely regulated under the Federal Control Substances Act (Schedule II).

Mechanism of action. All the cannabis drugs seem to act as CNS depressants. They depress higher brain centers and consequently release lower centers from inhibitory influences. Although some controversy exists regarding their classification, the cannabis drugs are not narcotic derivatives but are legally classified as controlled substances. They are more frequently classified as sedative-hypnotic-anesthetics or psychedelic (capable of altering perception, thought, and feeling) drugs. Like the sedative-hypnotics, they appear to depress the ascending reticular activating system. As dosage increases, their effects proceed from relief of anxiety, disinhibition, and excitement to anesthesia. If dosage is high enough, respiratory and vasomotor depression and collapse may occur.

Pharmacokinetics. The peak plasma level of THC after smoking one marijuana cigarette is reported to occur within minutes. It is metabolized in the liver and the major route of elimination of THC is bile and feces. Only trace amounts of the unmetabolized THC are detected in the urine.

Marijuana may affect the metabolism of other drugs in the liver or compete with other drugs for protein-binding sites in the plasma; ethyl alcohol, barbiturates, amphetamines, cocaine, opiates, and atropine are some of the reportedly affected drugs.

Effects. Marijuana cigarettes (joints) are illicitly used in the United States. While potency varies with plant strain and cultivation, the cigarettes usually produce moderate to intense psychopharmacologic effects that reach a peak in 15 minutes and last 1 to 4 hours. The drug has intoxicating, mind-altering properties. It induces an anxiety-free state characterized by a feeling of well-being. Perceptions of time and space are distorted. Ideas flow freely and disconnectedly; interruptions in thought that are blanks or gaps similar to epileptic absence may occur. The individual may experience palpitations, loss of concentration, lightheadedness, floating sensations followed by weakness, tremors, postural hypotension, incoordination, and ataxia. Hallucination can occur with high doses of the drug.

Dissociative phenomena also are reported; research suggests that impaired decision making and psychometric performance are related to the use of marijuana. The drug experience is highly subjective; the presence of an altered state of consciousness may be perceived by the novice until sensitized to it by colleagues. Some factors that influence the psychologic and behavioral effects of marijuana are drug dose, the user's personality, the user's expectations of the effects of the drug, environment, social influences, and life experiences.

Side effects include immediate tachycardia and delayed bradycardia, delayed hypotension, conjunctival vascular congestion (red eyes), dry mouth and throat, delayed gastrointestinal disturbances, possible vasovagal syncope, and enhanced appetite and flavor appreciation. More serious side effects are psychologic and include fear, panic (especially among first-time or naive users), paranoia, disorientation, memory loss, confusion, and a variety of perceptual alterations. Marijuana has been known to precipitate acute psychotic reactions and toxic psychoses in poorly organized personalities. The incidence of adverse effects appears to be highest in novice users of the drugs.

Withdrawal symptoms. Physiologic withdrawal symptoms have been reported on discontinuance of marijuana.

Minor discomfort may pass in several days but insomnia, anxiety, irritability, and restlessness may persist for weeks. Craving for the drug can recur intermittently for months after the drug is stopped. Generally, nonpharmacologic interventions and an exercise program are preferred over substitution of another drug product.

CNS Depressants

Barbiturates and Nonbarbiturates

Barbiturates and nonbarbiturate sedative-hypnotics usage and abuse reports have declined greatly in recent years, probably as a result of newer agents available with greater safety and effectiveness profiles. It has been suggested that treatment of abuse and addiction to these agents should be familiar to the interventions reviewed for alcohol and benzodiazepine abuse (O'Brien, 1996) (see Table 9-1 for barbiturate information).

Benzodiazepines (Diazepam, Alprazolam, Lorazepam)

Benzodiazepines are commonly prescribed medications for anxiety or insomnia. Although they are not considered street or illegal drugs, misuse, abuse, and drug dependency have been reported, especially with diazepam (Valium), alprazolam (Xanax), and lorazepam (Ativan).

Benzodiazepine withdrawal syndrome is more likely to occur if the drug was taken regularly for more than 3 months; if the drug dose consumed was higher than recommended; if clients have a history of substance abuse or passive and dependent personality traits; or if the drug is discontinued abruptly. Withdrawal symptoms from short-acting benzodiazepines occur within 1 to 2 days and from long-acting benzodiazepines in 5 to 7 days. Symptoms include increased anxiety and irritability, twitching, aching, muscle weakness, tremors, headache, nausea, anorexia, depression, lethargy, blurred vision, sleep disturbance, hypersensitivity to stimuli (light, touch, sound), and hyperreflexia. Delirium, psychosis, and convulsions are rare but have been reported.

Management of benzodiazepine dependence should include gradual drug withdrawal. If the individual is dependent on a short-acting benzodiazepine, switching them to a long-acting benzodiazepine is recommended for the withdrawal process. The symptoms occur more frequently and are more severe in individuals who suddenly withdraw from the short-acting benzodiazepines, while use of a long-acting benzodiazepine is associated with less prominent withdrawal symptoms (Box 9-6). Generally a 10% to 25% reduction in benzodiazepine dose every 1 to 2 weeks is recommended. While titration schedules and dose reduction may vary, the time frame is usually within 1 to 4 months. In very difficult withdrawals, the addition of carbamazepine (Tegretol), an anticonvulsant, or propranolol (Inderal), a beta-adrenergic blocker, may help reduce withdrawal symptoms (Grimsley, 1995).

Flumazepil (Romazicon) is a benzodiazepine receptor antagonist that is administered intravenously for the treatment of benzodiazepine toxicity. Although it appears to have no pharmacologic effects of its own, it has been reported to be associated with seizures, cardiac dysrhythmias, and other serious adverse effects in clients receiving benzodiazepines, or those with mixed drug overdoses (particularly with tricyclic antidepressants). Therefore, in high-risk clients the smallest effective dose should be used with close monitoring (Olin, 1996).

See Chapter 16 for benzodiazepine pharmacokinetics, additional pharmacologic information, treatment of benzodiazepine overdose, and nursing management of benzodiazepine therapy.

BOX 9-6

Benzodiazepine Classifications

Short-acting (half-life less than 24 hours)
alprazolam (Xanax)
bromazepam (Lectopam 🍁)
clonazepam (Klonopin)
lorazepam (Ativan, Apo-Lorazepam 🍁)
nitrazepam (Mogadon 🍁)
oxazepam (Serax, Ox-Pam 🍁)
temazepam (Restoril)
triazolam (Halcion)

Long-acting (half-life longer than 24 hours)
chloriazepoxide (Librium, Apo-Chlorax 🍁)
clorazepate (Tranxene)
diazepam (Valium, Apo-Diazepam 🍁)
flurazepam (Dalmane, Novoflupam 🍁)
halazepam (Paxipam)
ketazolam (Loftran 🍁)
prazepam (Centrax)
quazepam (Doral)

Nonopioid Analgesics (Acetaminophen, Aspirin, Ibuprofen)

Acetaminophen (Tylenol), aspirin, and ibuprofen (Motrin) are OTC drugs readily available in many outlets in the United States and Canada. These same ingredients may also be contained in additional combination formulations and sold with or without a prescription. Thus the potential for intentional and nonintentional drug overdose exists with this category of drugs.

Overdoses from nonopioid analgesics are commonly seen in emergency departments. Covington (1996) reports that 66% of OTC analgesic overdose reports in the United States are associated with acetaminophen, while ibuprofen and aspirin account for 19% and 15% respectively. Also, approximately 58% of the overdoses occur in children under the age of 6 years old.

See Chapter 11, Over-the-Counter Drugs, for additional information on this drug category.

Hallucinogens

Classifications of the most common hallucinogenic agents include lysergic acid diethylamide or lysergide (LSD) and its variants, mescaline, psilocybin, and phencyclidine (PCP). *Entactogen* is a term used today that refers to substances that have mind-altering effects (Jungnickel, 1995). A number of psychoactive hallucinogenic drugs have been used as adjuncts to religious services or were used experimentally on college campuses in the 1960s and are now experiencing a resurgence in popularity. LSD, dimethyltryptamine (DMT), PCP, mescaline, psilocybin, and MDMA (5-methoxy-3,4-methylene dioxyamphetamine), known as ecstasy (Box 9-7) are examples of the drugs that can produce distortions in perception or thinking at very low doses.

The use of most of these drugs declined in the 1970s to 1980s, with the exception of PCP, but use is increasing again in the 1990s (Kaufman & McNaul, 1992).

BOX 9-7

Other Hallucinogens

MDA an amphetamine type drug, similar in structure to MDMA. Destroys serotonin-producing neurons in the brain

MDMA (ecstasy, Adam, XTC) a stimulant-hallucinogenic used largely by college students. Evidence indicates it can destroy brain dopamine neurons. High dose or chronic use may lead to Parkinson's symptoms and eventually paralysis

MPPP (meperidine analog) synthesis usually produces a toxic byproduct, MPTP, which has caused permanent, irreversible Parkinson's disease in users (Hall, 1989)

LSD (lysergide)

LSD is a very potent hallucinogenic drug that illicitly is usually available in doses of approximately 200 µg. After oral administration it will cause a central sympathomimetic effect within 20 minutes—hypertension, dilated pupils, hyperthermia, tachycardia, and enhanced alertness. The psychoactive effects occur in about 1 to 2 hours and have been described as heightened perceptions, distortions of the body, and visual hallucinations. The effect on mood is unpredictable, ranging from euphoria to severe depression and panic.

Unpleasant experiences with LSD are rather frequent. Clinically, evidence of impaired judgment in the toxic state is frequent and examples of such behavior are well known, as demonstrated, for example, by LSD users attempting to stop traffic with their bodies. Altered states of consciousness may cause psychosis to develop or trigger a latent psychosis into activity. Feelings of acute panic and paranoia during a toxic LSD psychosis can result in homicidal thoughts and actions. Toxic delirium, with altering and alternating levels of consciousness, follows toxic psychosis, and the experience generally resolves in a stage of exhaustion in which the user feels "empty," unable to coordinate thoughts, and depressed. During this time suicide is a definite risk.

Significant unfavorable reactions induced by LSD include prolonged, delayed, and recurrent reactions such as depression and long-term schizophrenic or psychotic reactions. The recurrent reactions have been described as flashback phenomena, referring to the transient, spontaneous repetition of a previous LSD-induced experience that is unrelated to renewed administration of the drug. Flashbacks occur in 15% to 77% of LSD users. Moreover, a bad trip (anxiety or panic reaction) on LSD is likely to be a paranoid experience, and tendencies toward violence can be characteristic of LSD intoxication.

Treatment for bad trips has not changed over the years. A "talk-down" approach in a quiet, relaxed environment is often used. This helps to reassure the individual they are safe and that the drug effects will dissipate in a few hours. If the panic cannot be helped by talking down, then drug therapy with an oral benzodiazepine such as diazepam (Valium) might be considered. Avoid the use of phenothiazines, especially chlorpromazine (Thorazine) as such agents can potentiate the panic reaction, induce postural hypotension, and perhaps induce anticholinergic toxicity. In any case, the administration of medication is recommended only as an adjunct to crisis intervention psychotherapy, which consists of directing the person's attention away from perceptions that produce panic and providing reassurance that the experience will dissipate and that no permanent harm has been done. Flashbacks are treated as acute drug-induced episodes (Jungnickel, 1995).

The practice of administering massive doses of tranquilizers, applying restraints, and isolating such individuals should be avoided. The client's dramatically heightened awareness of the environment and distorted perceptions may render these measures traumatic rather than therapeutic.

Pregnant women should be especially cautioned against taking LSD. Because lysergic acid is the base of all ergot alkaloids, it has uterine stimulant properties that can adversely affect a pregnancy.

mescaline

Mescaline is the chief alkaloid extracted from mescal buttons (flowering heads) of the peyote cactus, and it produces subjective hallucinogenic effects similar to those produced by LSD. It is usually ingested in the form of a soluble crystalline powder that is either dissolved into teas or capsulated. The usual dose of mescaline is 300 to 500 mg.

The effects of mescaline doses up to 500 mg are characterized by prodromal abdominal pain, nausea, vomiting, and diarrhea, which are followed by vivid and colorful visual hallucinations. After oral ingestion, a syndrome of sympathomimetic effects including anxiety, hyperreflexia, static tremors, and psychic disturbances with vivid visual hallucinations is encountered. The half-life of mescaline is about 6 hours, and it is excreted in the urine.

psilocybin

Psilocybin is a drug derived from Mexican mushrooms and it produces subjective hallucinogenic effects similar to those produced by mescaline but of shorter duration. Within ½ to 1 hour after ingestion of 5 to 15 mg psilocybin a hallucinogenic dysphoric state begins. A dose of 20 to 60 mg may produce effects lasting 5 or 6 hours. The mood is pleasant to some users and others experience apprehension. The user has poor critical judgment capacities and impaired performance ability. Also seen are hyperkinetic compulsive movements, laughter, mydriasis, vertigo, ataxia, paresthesia, muscle weakness, drowsiness, and sleep.

PCP (phencyclidine)

PCP is an hallucinogen with a history of the most serious adverse effects; more suicides, assaults, and murders appear to result from its usage. It was developed in the late 1950s as an anesthetic for dissociative anesthesia, a cataleptic state in which the person appears to be awake but is detached from the surroundings and unresponsive to pain. As hallucinogenic effects were noted in clients emerging from this anesthetic, the drug was withdrawn from human use. It is, however, used in veterinary practice and this use is the origin of one of its street names, "hog" (Katzung, 1992).

Pharmacokinetics. PCP is rapidly metabolized in the liver to inactive metabolites, and ingestion of large amounts results in high concentrations of the unmetabolized drug in urine. PCP is lipophilic and has a half-life of ½ to 1 hour in small doses and from 1 to 4 days in larger doses. The pK_a of the drug is 8.5. The "ion trapping" of the drug into extravascular areas, which are more acidic than the serum, is thought to be a major cause of prolonged toxicity. The recirculation of the drug, secretion into the acidic gastric fluid, and reabsorption in the small intestine may also account for the prolonged toxicity and offer a key to the management of the toxicity of overdosage. These observations have led to treatment using urine acidification with diuresis and continuous gastric drainage in severe intoxication to enhance elimination. Urinary excretion is enhanced when the urine is acidified to 5.5 pH or less with ascorbic acid. The fact that PCP may be found in adipose tissue may indicate that the long-term effects are related to its lipophilic nature. Possibly during a nutritional fast PCP is released, and resulting symptoms are interpreted as a flashback.

Effects. In humans, common peripheral signs include flushing, profuse sweating, nystagmus, diplopia, ptosis, analgesia, and sedation. Other effects of PCP are as follows:

- A state similar to alcohol intoxication with ataxia and generalized numbness of extremities
- Psychologic effects that usually proceed in three stages:
  1. Change in body image and feelings of depersonalization
  2. Perceptual distortions (visual or auditory)
  3. Discomforting feelings of apathy, estrangement, or alienation
- Disorganization of thought and derealization that is greater than with LSD
- Impairment of attention span, motor skills, and sense of body boundaries, movement, and position
- Hallucinations that can recur unpredictably for days, weeks, or months

PCP is similar to ketamine in producing stages of anesthesia. In addition, excitation, paranoid behavior, self-destructive acts (because sensation or feeling of pain is absent), horizontal and vertical nystagmus, tachycardia, hypertension, seizures, increased reflexes, muscle rigidity, respiratory depression, and coma with open eyes may ensue. PCP is a strong sympathomimetic and hallucinogenic dissociative anesthetic agent. Since the drug is now classified as a controlled substance, penalties for illegal manufacture have been enacted and enforced.

Effects of PCP are claimed by some investigators to mimic schizophrenia more accurately than those of other psychotomimetics or hallucinogenics. Like the symptoms of schizophrenia, the effects of PCP are reduced by sensory deprivation. Currently no chemical antidote exists for inhibiting the effects of PCP. Keeping the user quiet and away from sensory stimuli may decrease the intensity of some of the effects.

Toxic effects. The pressor effects of PCP may cause hypertensive crisis, intracerebral hemorrhage, convulsions, coma, and death.

Intoxication and treatment. The clinical symptoms and signs of PCP intoxication are dose related. The waxing and waning of the intoxicative signs may be related to the pharmacokinetics of enteric reabsorption for the alkalized (nonionized) PCP with the recirculation and redistribution of the agent, as described earlier.

The nurse should be aware of these signs since this time period will constitute the greatest threat for both the client and health care provider. The client often has alternating periods of paranoia, assaultiveness, terror, and hyperactivity followed by a calm demeanor, blank stare, or withdrawn period. For the first 10 days after ingestion the nurse should never assume that the calm states are permanent. During an acute intoxication phase the client is unable to process incoming sensory stimuli; therefore the nurse should plan client interventions accordingly.

Treatment is primarily symptomatic. The client should be kept in a dark room with minimal sensory stimulation and protected from self-inflicted injury. The nurse should not attempt to talk down the PCP-anxious individual because it may provoke more serious anxiety or agitation. Diazepam (Valium) or haloperidol (Haldol) have been used for their antianxiety and antipsychotic effects, respectively. Urine acidification will enhance the excretion rate of PCP. Cranberry juice is frequently used to acidify the urine for this purpose.

The use of PCP causes a wide range of subjective effects requiring careful observations of the overdosed client. The prolonged and severe behavioral disturbances may progress to respiratory and cardiovascular emergencies as serum levels of the drug change.

Inhalants

Volatile hydrocarbons and aerosols are other substances of abuse. Representatives of this group are toluene, xylene, benzene, gasoline, paint thinner, typewriter correction fluid, lighter fluid, airplane glue, and nitrous oxide.

Volatile hydrocarbons are often used as propellants in aerosol products. When sniffed (inhaled), these agents may produce a rapid general CNS depression with marked inebriation, dizziness, floating sensations, exhilaration, and intense feelings of well-being that are at times exhibited as reckless abandonment, disinhibition, and feelings of increased power and aggressiveness similar to those seen with alcohol intoxication. Inhalation may result in bronchial and laryngeal irritation, transient euphoria, headache, giddiness, vertigo, ataxia, and renal tubular acidosis, especially with glue sniffing. At high doses, confusion and coma occur as well as blood dyscrasia. Depression may follow these early excitatory effects.

Chronic toluene abuse will lead to hepatic and renal toxicity, and death from cardiac dysrhythmia and respiratory failure has been reported. Recovery from lower doses may be seen in 15 minutes to a few hours. Inhalants are used mainly by young children and preteens (6 to 15 year olds). The nurse in the pediatric setting may be the first health professional to become aware of a child's problem with inhalants.

Butyl nitrite is a clear, yellow liquid sold as a room deodorizer under trade names such as Rush, Bolt, and Bullet. The substance is sold in drug paraphernalia shops and adult book stores and by mail order. The opened container is placed under the nose; and the individual inhales deeply and becomes dizzy, feels faint, and possibly loses consciousness. This rush lasts less than 1 minute and may include a headache, perspiration, and flushing, all caused by rapid vasodilation. It strongly resembles the effects achieved from amyl nitrite (a prescription smooth muscle relaxant and vasodilator).

Amyl nitrite is sometimes abused to heighten a sexual orgasm in both partners. Both butyl nitrite and amyl nitrite lower blood pressure and reduce the heart's oxygen consumption. They diminish sexual inhibition and by their physiologic action, may prolong sexual intercourse (Katzung, 1992).

Inhaled nitrite abuse has been implicated as being associated with or as being a contributory factor in the development of opportunistic infections and Kaposi's sarcoma in immunosuppressed homosexuals. Nitrites themselves are not considered a major risk factor, but as amyl nitrite (and other nitrite products) users tend to have more sexual partners, they could be at a higher risk of developing such infections (*AHFS*, 1996).

The development of tolerance also occurs with inhalants. For example, persons starting with one tube of sniffing glue per day may eventually increase to three, four, or more tubes per day to maintain the effect. In economically depressed populations inhalants are often the first drug of abuse used.

Anabolic (Androgenic) Steroids

Anabolic-androgenic steroids are synthetic formulations produced from testosterone, the male hormone. Young people are taking these agents to increase strength and body weight, to look good, and to improve their chances of winning in sports (Box 9-8). The Council on Scientific Affairs (1990) reported that anabolic steroids are used by men and women of all ages who are involved in athletic activity. Use is estimated in up to 80% of weight lifters and body builders while its use overall in competitors is approximately 50%. The abuse of these drugs is widespread and has been documented in young school-age students and in older persons and in both males and females.

BOX 9-8

Major Effects Associated with Anabolic Steroids

Androgen-type effects
- Increased growth and development of the seminal vesicles and prostate gland
- Increased body and facial hair
- Increased production of oil from the sebaceous glands
- Deepening of the voice
- Increased sexual interest and desire
- Enhancement of abstract and spatial dimension thinking ability
- Increased aggression

Anabolic-type effects
- Increased organ and skeletal muscle mass
- Increased calcium in bones
- Increased retention of total body nitrogen
- Increased hemoglobin concentration
- Increased protein synthesis

Data from Council on Scientific Affairs, 1990.

Since 1984, many organizations have publicly denounced or banned the use of anabolic steroids, including the American College of Sports Medicine, the American Medical Association, the National Collegiate Athletic Association, the International Olympic Committee, and the U.S. Powerlifting Federation. Many states have also passed laws to ban or limit the selling of such products (Council on Scientific Affairs, 1990).

Nevertheless the debate continues over the use of steroids. Anabolic steroids have been prescribed, especially for underweight persons and for athletes seeking an edge in the competitive field. Many steroidal preparations are available and are used orally and parenterally. Athletes often use the drugs in amounts far in excess of the recommended dosages. This misuse led to the withdrawal of anabolic steroid products from the market in 1982. "Stacking" of drugs or taking multiple anabolic steroids at one time is a practice employed by a number of athletes. This usually includes taking very large dosages of the steroids on an 8-week cycle schedule while following a regular strenuous exercise program (perhaps on isolated muscle groups) and consuming a high-protein diet. The long-term effects of such a schedule have not been studied, but documented short-term effects include increased aggressive behavior and some masculinization in females.

The disqualification of Olympic athletes for using steroids, along with the many undesirable and harmful effects reported from their usage, has led to an increase in regulation of this category of drugs. In 1991 all anabolic steroids were placed in the Schedule III controlled substances category. Some states have or are considering placing these substances in the Schedule II category to further restrict the availability of these drugs for nontherapeutic usage (Surface, 1991). The general public should be informed of the serious health problems associated with short-term and long-term consumption of anabolic steroids (Box 9-9).

BOX 9-9

Major Adverse Effects of Anabolic Steroids

Females

Oily skin; acne

Decrease in breast size, ovulation, lactation, or menstruation

Hoarse and deep voice tone (usually irreversible)

Clitoral enlargement

Unusual hair growth and/or male type baldness (usually irreversible)

Males

Prepuberty

Increased size of penis, number of erections, and secondary male characteristics

Postpuberty

Priapism (continuing erections), difficult/increased urination

Increase in breast size (gynecomastia)

Testicular atrophy, oligospermia, impotence

Both Sexes

Hypercalcemia

Edema of feet or legs

Jaundice, liver impairment

Liver carcinoma (rare)

Urinary calculi

Hypersensitivity

Insomnia

Iron deficiency anemia

Nausea, vomiting, anorexia, stomach pains

Nursing Management

Substance Misuse and Abuse

Great diversity exists both among substances that may be abused and the manner of the abuse. The role of the nurse may involve prevention, detection, treatment, and rehabilitation. Preventive nursing roles both inside and outside the health agency environment include (American Nurses' Association, 1987):

- Education on addiction as it is manifested in relation to a substance or behavior, including recreational misuse of such substances as alcohol and drugs
- Identification of individuals at high risk for the development of addictions, e.g., children of alcoholics and individuals who have been involved in a wide range of drug experimentation
- Identification of early signs and symptoms of addiction
- Activities to effect social change, such as networking and support of legislation and policy directed toward reducing the incidence of addiction and its consequences to society
- Use of knowledge about alcohol, tobacco, food, and drug use and abuse in comprehensive health teaching of clients receiving nursing care
- Use of knowledge of compulsive and dependent behaviors as the basis for health maintenance teaching

Health care providers, including nurses, have a high rate of substance abuse and related problems. Nurses must be aware of the potential for drug or substance abuse among themselves and other health care providers and be alert to recognize and deal with this problem should it arise.

Although the nurse plays an essential role in the prevention of drug abuse, many times the initial contact with the client may be in the acute setting during acute drug intoxication and withdrawal. Signs of acute intoxication differ according to the drug abused and may manifest themselves variably. In addition, identification of the problem may be complex if multiple drugs are used. Drug overdose and intoxication, including alcohol, may be life threatening. Immediate goals are to stabilize and maintain vital functions and minimize damage. Supportive treatment is combined with specific treatment once the drug has been identified. This is a time of acute psychologic stress for the client, and the nurse must remember to treat the whole client, not just a physiologic system. It is also a crisis during which the client and family may be especially receptive to intervention and long-term treatment of the problem.

Each nurse must evaluate his or her own feelings and responses to drug abuse. Some nurses tend to react with disgust or disdain, behavior that often increases a client's low self-esteem and results in ineffective lectures and scare tactics. Another common response of the nurse is that of "enabler": someone who shields the client from the consequences of substance abuse or unintentionally encourages continued substance abuse. The most effective response is to recognize and confront the problem directly. Nurses must acknowledge that if left untreated, substance abuse often results in death. However, appropriate treatment can often help these individuals overcome their problems and restore them to productive lives without dependence on harmful substances or drugs. Often simply addressing the problem and providing an avenue for assistance can begin the process of recovery, which might not start then but months or years later.

Since substance abuse transcends the boundaries of economics, social class, race, and ethnic background, all clients have the potential to abuse substances or be affected by someone who does.

In 1978 the National Nurses Society on Addictions (NNSA) developed a position statement on the role of the nurse in alcoholism treatment that can be used to consider concerns related to substance abuse in general. The five areas of nursing interventions addressed were identification of the problem with alcohol; communication about the problem; education regarding alcohol use, abuse, and alcoholism; counseling the alcoholic individual, family, and significant others; and referral for treatment and aftercare (Bennett & Woolf, 1991). This approach is not limited to alcohol abuse but is also useful for intervention with clients abusing other substances.

Assessment. Assessment includes both physical and psychologic signs and symptoms of substance abuse. The nurse should closely observe both verbal and nonverbal responses to questions since an element of denial may often be ascertained in clients who abuse substances. The nonverbal response may provide additional information, contradict, or reinforce what is verbally stated.

Physical assessment includes vital signs, pupillary signs, skin (especially for needle marks or "tracks" and abscesses that are often seen with injected drug abuse), and collecting data on nutrition, elimination, and sleep patterns. Diagnostic tests may be used to detect drugs or their metabolites in the blood or urine. The nurse should be aware of the possibility of falsely positive results.

Past medical history of the client may include prior treatment of drug abuse or history of drug-related illness such as hepatitis, abscesses, or bacterial endocarditis. Alcohol-related problems should be considered in clients with any of the following medical diagnoses: cellulitis, gastritis, ulcers, pancreatitis, cirrhosis, pneumonia, tuberculosis, peripheral neuropathy, seizure disorders, cerebellar degeneration, depression, suicide attempt, injuries from accidents or victimization, anemia, or malnutrition (Zahourek, 1986). A thorough drug history for current or past use of OTC, prescribed, or social/recreational drugs should be taken and should include the frequency, magnitude, and circumstances of drug use and abuse, as well as the development of withdrawal symptoms if the drug was stopped.

Box 9-10 provides examples of selected clinical data that may indicate substance abuse upon a general nursing assessment using Gordon's Function Health Patterns (Gordon, 1987). A cluster of data that might indicate substance abuse needs further assessment.

One of the simplest and most widely used screening tools is the CAGE questionnaire (Mayfield et al, 1974; Zahourek, 1986; Iber, 1991). It was designed for use with alcoholics but can be modified for substance abuse. It can be verbally incorporated into the process of taking every client's history by asking, "Have you:

- ever felt the need to Cut down your drinking (use of drugs)?
- ever felt Annoyed by criticism of your drinking (drug use)?
- ever had Guilt feelings about drinking (drug use)?
- ever taken a morning Eye opener (required a drug fix to get on with your day's activities)?"

This assessment addresses common reactions to abuse, including concern for harm, hypersensitivity to criticism, perception of guilt in the harm the abuse does to others, and the occurrence of habituation or tolerance requiring a repeated dose to prevent early withdrawal symptoms (Iber, 1991).

Nursing diagnosis. The following selected nursing diagnoses may be identified in a client with substance abuse problems:

- knowledge deficit related to denial of problem, misinformation from associates, or no experience with substance abuse
- ineffective individual coping related to lack of supportive others, inadequately learned coping behaviors, or social life revolving around substance use
- risk for self-directed/other-directed violence related to social isolation, hopelessness, or depression
- altered health maintenance related to substance dependency, inadequate diet, poor lifestyle habits, impaired perception, poverty, inability to communicate needs, or denial of need for change
- ineffective management of therapeutic regimen related to lack of resources (financial, social, personal), knowledge deficit, denial of substance abuse, mistrust of health personnel, or powerlessness
- potential complication of withdrawal syndrome.

Implementation

Monitoring. Assessment of the effectiveness of the client's therapy is focused on how the client has tolerated the withdrawal period and developed new coping strategies. After the withdrawal period, the client must decide to remain drug free and maintain a healthy lifestyle. Relapses may occur and should not be viewed as the nurse's failure, for the goal of treatment is longer and longer periods of sobriety/substance-free status and shorter and less frequent relapses. Participation by the client in long-term support from the appropriate agencies is essential in helping the client remain drug free. Ultimately the decision to use and abuse drugs remains with the client.

Intervention. Physical and/or psychologic withdrawal symptoms may follow abrupt cessation of drug or substance use. Interventions include monitoring of vital signs, administering medications (if prescribed for treatment of withdrawal), and providing supportive nursing care. Clients abusing substances often have nutrition deficiencies and other health problems, which should be corrected. Promotion of adequate nutrition, safety, rest, and orientation are areas of general nursing interventions during this time. Medications may be administered to reduce the withdrawal symptoms. Rehabilitation begins during the withdrawal period and is continued in an attempt to avoid relapse.

The nurse should use a straightforward and receptive approach with clients abusing substances. Therapeutic communication should be focused on increasing self-esteem and confronting manipulative behavior while teaching effective

BOX 9-10

Nursing Assessment for Substance Abuse

Functional health pattern	Client data that may indicate substance abuse
Health perception–health management	Choices of daily living ineffective for meeting the goals of a treatment or prevention program
	Leaving the hospital against medical advice after a few days
	Stating a desire to decrease substance use
	Boasting of ability to tolerate large amounts of substances
	Frequent change of health care provider
	Appearing older than stated age
Nutritional-metabolic pattern	Malnutrition
	Irregular meal pattern
	Poor dental hygiene
	Frequent heartburn, anorexia, nausea
	Skin lesions (rash, ulcers, bruises, needle marks)
Elimination pattern	Recurrent diarrhea
	Chronic constipation
Activity-exercise pattern	Fatigue, decreased energy
	Loss of interest in non–substance seeking activities
	Poor hygiene
	Smelling of alcohol or other substances
	Heavy smoking
Sleep-rest pattern	Insomnia
	Diminished response to sleep or pain medication
Cognitive-perceptual pattern	Mental confusion
	Memory loss
	Poor judgment
	Diminished reality testing
	Blackouts
	Hallucinations
	Seizures
Self-perception–self-concept pattern	Denial of problem
Role-relationship pattern	Social life revolves around substance use
	Poor fiscal management
	Marital problems
	Vulnerable individuals in home neglected
	Verbalized inability to meet role expectations
	Unemployed or excessive absenteeism from work
	Repeated minor injuries on and off the job
Sexuality-reproductive pattern	Impotence
Coping-stress tolerance pattern	Binge drinking/drug binging
	Negative behaviors: hostility, aggression, lying, paranoia
	Depression
	Chronic complaints of anxiety/stress
	Frequent hospitalization
	Suicide attempts
Values-belief pattern	Lack of belief in future
	Lack of realistic goals
	Lack of belief system (religious or philosophical)

Adapted from Bennett and Woolf, 1991.

coping mechanisms and problem solving. A client cannot restructure a manner of thinking, feeling, and acting until he or she achieves a new image. Many abusers suffer from deprivation of basic needs such as physical closeness and emotional openness, which may in part be caused by the dissolution of basic family relationships. Such deprivation affects individual needs and the expectations of what one is entitled to in these meaningful relationships. Lack of fulfillment of these needs leads to a pronounced disequilibrium. On the other hand, substance abuse affects all members of the family. Commonly, family members enable the alcoholic or drug abuser to continue an abuse pattern by denying the problem. An open, caring, nonjudgmental discussion of the problem with the client and family members can have a positive effect on client outcomes.

A multidisciplinary approach often serves these clients best since they frequently have many health, personal, and social problems that must be addressed. Referral to appropriate agencies (e.g., Alcoholics Anonymous, Alateen, Cocaine Anonymous, Narcotics Anonymous, Al-Anon, Rational Recovery, and Adult Children of Alcoholics) will assist in the follow-up care of these clients and their family members and provide much needed support and encouragement.

Education. The nurse should assist the client to develop effective coping mechanisms and "nondrug strategies" to deal with stress. Information should be provided in a factual, nonjudgmental way. Education of the client and family should include content about drugs and abused substances, such as signs and symptoms, effects upon the body, progression of the condition, health problems associated with substance abuse, and psychosocial effects of substance abuse. General treatment options and the types and location of specific treatment facilities within the community should be discussed.

Evaluation. The client will experience minimal or no effects of withdrawal, verbalize an understanding of substance abuse and treatment, evidence positive coping without abused substances, not experience violent behaviors, demonstrate improvements in health maintenance, and successfully manage the therapeutic regimen.

SUMMARY

Although drug abuse is not a new phenomenon, the dimension of the problem for society is great. Substance abuse is a common denominator across cultural, ethnic, and socioeconomic populations and affects every aspect of the abuser's life. As a consequence, the nurse needs to be familiar with drugs with the potential for abuse, not only in their therapeutic use but also in their street forms. This knowledge will enhance the nursing role for the prevention, detection, treatment, and rehabilitation of the drug abuser.

The etiology of substance abuse for any given client may vary, but the drug must produce a desired effect for it to cause dependence. Currently the commonly abused drugs are opioids and related compounds; antianxiety agents; amphetamines, cocaine, and other CNS stimulants; cannabis; hallucinogens and other mood modifiers; inhalants; and anabolic steroids. In addition, multiple drug use is common, and psychic and physical dependence can exist independently or simultaneously.

Opioids are some of the most abused drugs. For that reason the nurse should be alert to opioid abuse in the general population, as well as in the health professions. The "high" from opioids is characterized by complete drive satiation, so the client may exhibit malnutrition and other signs of neglect from ignoring basic biologic needs. Acute overdosage of opioids with miotic pupils, stupor, and respiratory depression is considered to be a medical emergency, but symptoms may be reversed by adequate amounts of naloxone (Narcan), a narcotic antagonist. Treatment of opioid dependence may be withdrawal with supportive therapy, methadone detoxification and withdrawal, or clonidine treatment followed by either a methadone maintenance program or a therapeutic community program.

Other forms of analgesics such as pentazocine and propoxyphene tend to be abused based on access, fashion, and availability of other substances on the street.

Alcohol is the most common substance of abuse and the ingestion of alcohol does not carry with it the social stigma as does the abuse of other drugs. However, the chronic abuse of alcohol causes physiologic damage to every body system; its therapeutic use is quite limited. Disulfiram (Antabuse) is used to sensitize the individual to alcohol by causing such an unpleasant response—nausea, headache, palpitations, dyspnea, and intense discomfort—that the use of alcohol is no longer desired.

Benzodiazepines are the antianxiety agents most abused, generally as the result of over-prescribing to women and the elderly.

Amphetamines and cocaine are the most commonly abused CNS stimulants. Because cocaine is available as "crack" at a much lower cost than other drugs, it is becoming increasingly popular and much more of a health problem with its strong physical and psychologic dependence.

Cannabis drugs are increasingly used by young teenagers for recreation to produce an anxiety-free state of relaxation and sense of well-being. Studies indicate that impaired decision making, apathy, and memory loss are related to cannabis use. Psychic and physical dependence develop with chronic use.

Psychedelic drugs and inhalants are also substances for abuse for their mind-altering properties, whereas anabolic steroids are abused by individuals who want to improve their appearance or performance in sports.

The nurse has an important role in the prevention of drug abuse because of his or her knowledge and extent of contact with the public of all ages and circumstances. Assessment for the detection of drug abuse and intervening in an acute overdose or withdrawal situation are performed in a straightforward and receptive approach with the client abusing substances. Because of the multiplicity of the drug abuser's problems, the nurse may be part of a multidisciplinary team in the provision of support to these clients.

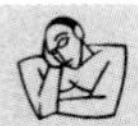

Critical Thinking

1. Jane Parker is a receptionist for the executive office suite of a large manufacturing firm. She is single, attractive, and enjoys an active social life. A few months ago she began attending parties at which cocaine was being used. She began using cocaine to "fit in" with the crowd. Her co-workers have noticed that she has become edgy, lost weight, and been unable to concentrate on her work. One of the executives sends Jane to the company nurse because she "does not look well." As the company's occupational nurse, how could you intervene with Ms. Parker? What activities could the company undertake as part of a drug abuse prevention program?
2. Ronald Taylor, age 72, is brought to the hospital after falling off his roof while doing home repairs. He is taken to surgery for an open reduction of a fractured femur. On the third day of hospitalization, Mr. Taylor becomes increasingly irritable and refuses to participate in his physical therapy. He indicates that he wishes to sign himself out of the hospital. The nurse notes from Mr. Taylor's past medical history that he has sustained multiple injuries as the result of minor automobile and home accidents. The nurse begins to consider that Mr. Taylor might abuse alcohol. Why would that be a consideration at this time? As the nurse in question, how will you intervene?

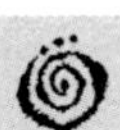

Collaborative Learning Activities

1. Invite a speaker from a local substance abuse treatment center to discuss: (1) the most current commonly abused substances and street names within the local community; (2) a few case studies of clients generally treated at the center; and (3) local community resources available for client referral.
2. Have the students discuss the availability of drugs with abuse potential that they have encountered in the past and present social spheres.

BIBLIOGRAPHY

American Hospital Formulary Service (1996). *AHFS drug information '96.* Bethesda, MD: American Society of Hospital Pharmacists.

American Medical Association (1995). *Drug evaluations annual 1995.* Chicago: The Association.

American Nurses Association (1984). *ANA cabinet on nursing practice: Statement on scope of addiction nursing practice.* Kansas City: The Association.

American Nurses Association, Drug and Alcohol Nursing Association, and National Nurses Society on Addictions (1987). *The care of clients with addictions: Dimensions of nursing practice.* Kansas City: The Association.

Anderson KN, et al. (Eds.). (1994). *Mosby's medical, nursing, & allied health dictionary* (4th ed.). St Louis: Mosby.

Antai-Otong D (1995). Helping the alcoholic patient recover, *Amer J Nurs 95*(8):22-9.

Baldwin JN & Benson B (1995). Depressant and inhalant use. In Young LY & Koda-Kimble MA (Eds.). *Applied therapeutics: The clinical use of drugs* (6th ed.). Vancouver: Applied Therapeutics.

Baldwin JN & Cook MD (1995). Issues: Psychoactive substance use disorders. In Young LY & Koda-Kimble MA (Eds.). *Applied therapeutics: The clinical use of drugs* (6th ed.). Vancouver: Applied Therapeutics.

Balkon J & Balkon N (1990). Drug testing in the workplace, *US Pharm 15*(6):44.

Bennett EG & Woolf DS (1991). *Substance abuse: Pharmacologic, developmental and clinical perspectives* (2nd ed.). Albany: Delmar Publishers.

Bissell C & Haberman PW (1984). *Alcoholism in the professions.* Oxford: Oxford University Press.

Buchanan JF, et al. (1995). Drug abuse. In Koda-Kimble MA & Young LY (Eds.). *Applied therapeutics: The clinical use of drugs* (6th ed.). Vancouver: Applied Therapeutics.

Burns CM (1993). Assessment and screening for substance abuse: Guidelines for the primary care nurse practitioner, *Nurse Pract Forum 4*(4):199-206.

Caulker-Burnett I (1994). Primary care screening for substance abuse, *Nurse Pract 19*(4):42, 44-8.

Council on Scientific Affairs (1990). Medical and nonmedical uses of anabolic-androgenic steroids, *JAMA 264*(22):2923.

Covington TR (Ed.) (1996). *Handbook of nonprescription drugs* (11th ed.). Washington, DC: American Pharmaceutical Association.

DAWN (1996). *Data from Drug Abuse Warning Network. Statistical series: Annual emergency department data for 1993.* Rockville, MD: US Department of Health and Human Services.

Gallegos K, et al. (1988). Substance abuse among health professionals, *Maryland Med J 37*(3):191-6.

Gordon M (1987). *Manual of nursing diagnosis 1986-1987.* New York: McGraw-Hill.

Grimsley SR (1995). Anxiety disorders. In Young LY & Koda-Kimble MA (Eds.). *Applied therapeutics: The clinical use of drugs* (6th ed.). Vancouver: Applied Therapeutics.

Group for the Advancement of Psychiatry Committee on Alcohol and the Addictions (1991). Substance abuse disorders: A psychiatric priority, *Am J Psychiatry 148*(10):1291.

Hall IN (1989). US illicit drug production booming, *Street Pharmacol 12* (Spring):4.

Henderson GL, et al. (1992). Street and designer drugs, *Patient Care 26*(18):118-24, 129-32, 135-6, 143-4, 146, 148-50,153-4, 157.

Hinds M (Ed.) (1985). How much blood alcohol content per drink? *Informed Families of Dade County 2*(6):1.

Hughes TL & Smith LL (1994). Is your colleague chemically dependent? *Amer J Nurs 94*(9):31-5.

Iber FL (Ed.). (1991). *Alcohol and drug abuse as encountered in office practice.* Boca Raton, FL: CRC Press.

Jungnickel PW (1995). Entactogen and phencyclidine abuse. In Young LY & Koda-Kimble MA (Eds.). *Applied therapeutics: The clinical use of drugs* (6th ed.). Vancouver: Applied Therapeutics.

Jungnickel PW & Hunnicutt DM (1995). Alcohol abuse. In Young LY & Koda-Kimble MA (Eds.). *Applied therapeutics: The clinical use of drugs* (6th ed.). Vancouver: Applied Therapeutics.

Katzung BG (1992). *Basic & clinical pharmacology* (5th ed.). Norwalk, CT: Appleton & Lange.

Kaufman E & McNaul JP (1992). Recent developments in understanding and treating drug abuse and dependence, *Hosp Comm Psychiat 43*(3):223-36.

Lipman AG (1993). The argument against therapeutic use of heroin in pain management, *Am J Hosp Pharm 50*(5):996-8.

Long MC (1993). Overview of substance abuse: Implications for the primary care nurse practitioner, *Nurse Pract Forum 4*(4):191-8.

Malatestinic WN & Jorgenson JA (1991). Dealing with substance abuse in the workplace, *Hosp Pharm 26*(1):102-5.

Mayfield D, et al. (1974). The CAGE questionnaire: Validation of a new alcoholism screening instrument, *Am J Psychiatry 131*:1121.

Milzman DP & Soderstrom CA (1994). Substance use disorders in trauma patients: Diagnosis, treatment, and outcome, *Crit Care Clin 10*(3):595-611.

Navarra T (1995). Enabling behavior: The tender trap, *Amer J Nurs* 95(1):50-2.

Neafsey PJ, Fisk NB, & Williams CA (1993). Updating the critical care nurse on alcohol and other drug abuse, *Crit Care Nurse* 13(5):98-101, 103-7.

O'Brien CP (1996). Drug addiction and drug abuse. In Hardman JG & Limbird LE (Eds.). *Goodman & Gilman's the pharmacological basis of therapeutics* (9th ed.). New York: McGraw-Hill.

Olin BR (Ed.). (1996). *Facts and comparisons.* St Louis: JB Lippincott.

Schydlower M (1990). Current issues affecting drug-exposed infants and their mothers, *Healthcare Executive Currents, Special Issue* 34(1):2.

Scott DM & Gabel TL (1995). Central nervous system (CNS) stimulant abuse. In Young LY & Koda-Kimble MA (Eds.). *Applied therapeutics: The clinical use of drugs.* Vancouver: Applied Therapeutics.

Sees KL & Clark HW (1993). Opioid use in the treatment of chronic pain: Assessment of addiction, *J Pain & Sympt Manag* 8(5):257-64.

Sinatra RS & Savarese A (1992). Parenteral analgesic therapy and patient-controlled analgesia for pediatric pain management. In Sinatra RS, et al. (Eds.). *Acute pain: Mechanism & management.* St Louis: Mosby.

Stammer ME (1988). Understanding alcoholism and drug dependency in nurses, *Qual Rev Bull* 14(3):75-80.

Surface RE (Ed.) (1991). Drug information: Anabolic steroids now Schedule III, *The White Sheet* 25(3):3.

Thomas DJ (1993). Organ transplantation in people with unhealthy lifestyles, *AACN Clin Issues* 4(4):665-8.

United States Pharmacopeial Convention (1996). *USP DI: Drug information for the health care professional* (16th ed.). Rockville, MD: The Convention.

Wadler GI (1994). Drug use update, *Med Clin North Amer* 78(2):439-55.

Watling SM, et al. (1995). Nursing-based protocol for treatment of alcohol withdrawal in the intensive care unit, *Amer J Crit Care* 4(1):66-70.

Young SL, Vosper HJ, & Phillips SA (1992). Cocaine: Its effects on maternal and child health, *Pharmacotherapy* 12(1):2-17.

Zahourek RP (1986). Identification of the alcoholic in the acute care setting, *Crit Care Q* 8(4):1-10.

Chapter 10

Client Education for Self-Administration of Medication

Chapter Focus

Effective management of a therapeutic regimen requires a major commitment by the client and the family or caregiver. A well-planned teaching program can provide information needed to accurately self-manage medications in the home setting. It can also decrease the number of complications arising from medications by preparing the client to recognize early signs and symptoms of adverse effects of drugs and to report them to the prescriber. The nurse, then, needs to be not only knowledgeable in pharmacologic content, but also skilled in client education. The following objectives and key terms are important for a good understanding of this chapter.

Key Terms

compliance (p. 175)
ineffective management of therapeutic regimen (p. 174)
knowledge deficit (p. 174)
locus of control (p. 173)
noncompliance (p. 174)
therapeutic seeding (p. 179)

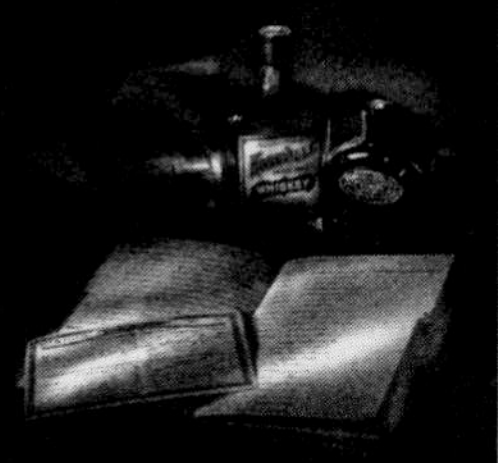

Objectives

1. Assess a client and family regarding the need and readiness to learn to administer medications.
2. Write measurable objectives for the client who is learning to self-administer medications.
3. Discuss at least three teaching techniques that may increase a client's knowledge of medications.
4. Identify four or more safety precautions necessary for clients in self-administering medications.
5. Document the client's and the family's learning, including content, method, and progress toward learning goals.
6. Identify the nursing diagnoses of knowledge deficit, noncompliance, and ineffective management of the therapeutic regimen relating to self-administration of medications.
7. Identify factors that affect client compliance in self-administration of medications.

Nurses have been teaching their clients since the discipline's beginnings. In the last three decades, however, an increasing emphasis has been placed on the role of nurses in supporting clients' abilities for self-care, adaptation to illness, and high-level wellness. Various factors are responsible for this change in emphasis. A growing consumer awareness of health issues and services has made the client much more of a participant in his or her own health care than in the past. The client is more apt to request information. Nurses have responded by promoting the client's active involvement in planning and implementing nursing care. In 1972 the American Hospital Association published "A Patient's Bill of Rights," which gave formal recognition to the client's right to know about his or her health status, treatments, alternative methods of treatment, and continuing care requirements. In addition, client education is being recognized as one way of making possible a shorter length of hospital stay. This is an important factor in the present economic climate since the development in 1983 by the U.S. Health Care Financing Administration of a prospective payment system for health care, the advent of DRGS, which continues to shorten lengths of stay.

Technology has extended life expectancy and increased the numbers of the chronically ill. Many of these elderly or debilitated clients require health teaching to enable them to remain independent. Since 1976 the Joint Commission for the Accreditation of Healthcare Organizations (JCAHO) has required that there be evidence in the client's clinical record of specific instructions provided to the client and his or her family regarding medications, diet, and follow-up care. Nurse practice acts have set guidelines and developed standards for the nurse's role in health education. In addition, there have been successful lawsuits alleging that nurses provided less than adequate health teaching. All of these factors have reinforced the nurse's participation in client education.

Client education, then, is a process assisting people to learn and incorporate health-related behaviors into everyday life. Because learning is defined as a change in behavior, nurses then assist individuals to change behavior. Nurses provide health-related information and teach in such a way as to ensure the client's compliance with a therapeutic regimen. Nowhere is that more important than in the area of client education for self-administration of prescription medications. Misuse and noncompliance with drug regimens have been well documented (Charonko, 1992; Gullickson, 1993; Proos, 1992; Shea et al, 1992). Although a number of factors determine whether or not clients adhere to a medication regimen, they must be provided with accurate information upon which to base their behaviors.

The teaching-learning process may be structured along the lines of the nursing process with the first step being assessment, the gathering of facts and information that will assist the nurse to meet the client and family's needs for learning. Planning, the next step in the process, begins as soon as a learning need has been identified, with goals being written as outcomes for the client's learning. The implementation phase is the actual communication of information. And evaluation focuses on the client's behaviors and attitudes as a measure of whether the client has achieved the learning objectives.

ASSESSMENT

A thorough assessment of the client is essential to the provision of health teaching about medications in the most efficient and effective way. The nurse should conduct a comprehensive assessment regarding the client's response to illness. A comprehensive assessment includes determining the client's competence in self-care and mobility, nutritional status, sleep patterns, and social support mechanisms. Data collected should describe factors influencing the client's ability, motivation, and interest in following health advice. The client's cultural perspectives, health beliefs, and attitudes need to be included in the assessment. All of these factors will influence the teaching-learning process for the self-administration of medications. Not all clients will need to know everything about their medications, nor will all clients be ready to learn about them. Realistic goals for clients' medicating behaviors are the result of the nurse's accurate assessment.

Assessing learning needs means ascertaining what the client already knows. "What medications are you presently taking? What is each medication for? How often and how much of each medication should you be taking? What are the side effects of each drug? Which of these side effects should you report to your prescriber if it occurs?" (See Chapter 4 for a medication history form.) If the client knows the answers to these questions, the objective for learning may have been met.

The nurse also needs to determine a point of reference for learning by validating the client's present level of knowledge. New information is easier to absorb when it can be related to what the client already knows. For example, when teaching about nitroglycerin, the nurse might ask the client what he or she understands the diagnosis of angina to be. By using the words the client used to describe his or her condition, the nurse can discuss the therapeutic action of the nitroglycerin. In addition, a baseline of data must be determined to evaluate what knowledge the client has gained, by comparing what was known before and after the learning process.

The nurse needs to be aware of any incorrect knowledge or misunderstanding the client may have. The client's health information may be a collection of folklore, hearsay, handed-down family experience, advertising claims, and misconceptions. Incorrect information needs to be identified and dealt with before the teaching of the correct material can be initiated. The Cultural Aspects box on p. 172 describes a study by Lile and Hoffman (1991) that provides examples of medication-taking beliefs and behaviors.

Sometimes, because of the shortened length of stay, instruction has to be limited to survival content—only the most important information (Proos et al, 1992). What will the client need to know about what to do when he or she returns home? What must the client learn to survive until additional information can be obtained? Does the client know whom to call if additional information is needed? Although

Cultural Aspects — Medication-Taking by the Frail Elderly in Two Ethnic Groups

A complex and dangerous area of medical intervention with the elderly population is drug therapy. Many elderly use large quantities of both prescription and OTC medications with little understanding of the potential health risk. A study demonstrating this was undertaken, investigating the medication-taking behaviors of Hispanic and Anglo noninstitutionalized frail elderly in the Las Cruces, New Mexico area.

The purposeful sample of 20 (10 Anglo, 10 Hispanic) consisted of subjects attending senior citizen community centers, those waiting to see doctors in the office, and some individuals at home. The participants were six men and 14 women. The age range was from 70 to 90 years with the median age of the Anglo group being 81 years, and the Hispanic group, 85.5 years. The educational level ranged from less than high school (55%) to college graduates (5%). The majority of the Anglos had an income between $10,000-$20,000 annually, while the majority of the Hispanics had income less than $10,000.

An interview schedule containing 20 items was used to facilitate data collection related to medication-taking behaviors of the participants. The tool focused on prescription and OTC medications, home remedies currently used, factors influencing the purchase of OTC drugs, difficulties experienced taking the medications, adverse reactions to the drugs, methods of record keeping, and money spent on medications. The tool was translated into Spanish for Hispanic subjects and then retranslated back into English to determine accuracy. The interview was administered by a trained bilingual registered nurse.

The findings revealed that the subjects used cardiovascular drugs, Anglos 80% and Hispanics 90%; diuretics, Anglos 40% and Hispanics 10%; and antianxiety drugs, both groups, 40%. Thirty percent of the Hispanic group used drugs for the treatment of diabetes, which is prevalent in their ethnic group, versus none in the Anglo group. Both groups used respiratory drugs (20%) and laxatives (40%). OTC acetaminophen and aspirin were used by 70% of the Anglos and 80% of the Hispanics. A variety of other prescription and nonprescription drugs were used by both groups. Anglo participants used home remedies such as warm milk, beer, and bourbon for sleep and raspberry tea for hypertension. Hispanic subjects used prunes as a laxative, mustard weed for upset stomach, and herbal teas for sleep and as diuretics.

The investigators reported that Hispanic subjects were three times more likely to be influenced by television in OTC drug purchases, whereas 60% of the Anglo group were influenced by family in their OTC purchases. Interestingly, 70% of the Hispanics shared or gave their medications to others and 20% borrowed drugs from others as opposed to 10% of the Anglos.

Both groups expressed a concern for the difficulty involved in taking their medications. Although the drug labels were written in English, 90% of the Hispanics and 50% of the Anglos had difficulty reading them. Forty percent of the Hispanics and 10% of the Anglos admitted to having difficulty understanding the labels. Fifty percent of the Anglo participants had difficulty opening the drug containers. Most were able to administer their own medications (90% of the Anglos, 60% of the Hispanics); the rest depended on family members or others to assist.

These findings indicate that noninstitutionalized frail elders of both ethnic groups studied are at risk for injury because of their medication-taking behaviors.

1. What are the implications of the results of this study for the community?
2. What are the implications for nursing?

Data from Lile J & Hoffman R, 1991.

many nurses would prefer to teach some pharmacokinetics of the client's drug as a foundation for the self-administration of medications, sometimes the client's anxiety and health status preclude that depth of explanation. With the increases in ambulatory surgery, clients are discharged after receiving an array of medications before and during their surgical procedures, which may lessen their ability to understand and process information (Jones, 1995). Common classifications of agents used in these settings, such as benzodiazepines, opioid analgesics, and anticholinergics, have been shown to impair the ability of clients to process and recall information (Kerr et al, 1991; Barbee, 1993).

A client can become easily overwhelmed by highly technical content and lose the essential information needed to take the drug safely and accurately. However, some may ask for additional technical information. Hospitalized clients tend to focus on issues related to hospitalization, such as how to administer the insulin injection, rather than long-term dietary management for their diabetes mellitus. Clients in ambulatory care may have difficulty absorbing all they need to understand about their medications in the brief time of a typically scheduled visit.

Not all clients are ready to learn. During an assessment, the nurse needs to consider the client's current emotional state, adaptation to the illness, level of maturity, and expectations. A client's emotional state influences his or her perspective on the world and readiness to learn. Smith (1989) found that clients' feelings of satisfaction not only correlated with current compliance but also predicted future compliance, indicating a readiness to participate in their own care. Mild anxiety may stimulate the client to learn, whereas severe anxiety may shorten the attention span so as to be incapacitating.

A client goes through various stages in the adaptation to illness or injury, including developing awareness, reorganization, resolution, and identity change. During the assessment the nurse should be aware of the client's stage of adaptation. Understanding the client's coping strategies will keep the nurse from attempting to teach information that the client is not ready to learn. Anger, fear, and mistrust of health care personnel may also impede readiness for learning. Many factors affect the client's readiness to learn (Table 10-1).

Attitude and the client's beliefs about himself and the illness often affect the level of adherence to a medication regimen. According to Becker (1979), a client is more apt to comply with the therapy when he believes the physician is correct, the illness can cause him harm, the prescribed treatment will reduce the risk of complication or death, or his health will improve. Individuals lacking functional literacy (lacking the ability to read well enough to understand and

TABLE 10-1 Some factors affecting educational readiness

Pathophysiologic	Severity of illness, pain, fatigue, sensory deprivation, physical disabilities
Treatment-related	Complexity of regimen
Situational	Illiteracy, language differences, ineffective coping patterns, financial concerns, home environment
Maturational	Family roles and relationships, health maintenance practices

use information as it was intended), as well as those with a language barrier, are also at risk for not following a medication regimen. Language barriers exist not only when there are differences in the primary language spoken by the health care provider and the client, but also when health care providers use unfamiliar medical terminology with clients when describing disease processes and medical interventions. When questioned about understanding, the person will most likely indicate that the material was understood even if it was not. This response may be due to an inadequate vocabulary or inability to problem-solve in order to explain what is not understood (Hussey, 1991). In addition, clients from other cultures may indicate understanding as a sign of respect. For example, in Asian cultures it is respectful to smile and nod one's head to a person of authority, regardless of the level of understanding. In these instances the nurse may enlist the assistance of the client's support system, the individuals or group that provide him with comfort, aid, and information to help him cope with life—family, friends, and members of the community and church or religious groups.

Whenever possible, learn the language of the clients with whom you interact. If that is not practical, learn key phrases related to greetings and the health care services you provide. Interpreters can also be used, but they should understand health care terminology, have training in transcultural interpretation, know the language of both the health care provider and the client, and respect both cultures (Wenger, 1993).

In addition, Tripp-Reimer et al (1989) offer the following guidance for working with clients having a language barrier:

- Speak slowly (plan the teaching session to last at least twice as long as a typical session).
- Make the sentence structure simple (use active, not passive, voice; use a straightforward subject-verb pattern).
- Avoid technical terms (for example, use "heart" rather than "cardiac"), professional jargon, and American idioms ("red tape").
- Provide instructional material in the same sequence in which the client should carry out the plan.
- Do not assume you have been understood. Ask the client to explain the protocol; optimally, if appropriate, obtain a return demonstration.

Although these guidelines are suggested for clients with a language barrier, they hold true for most clients.

If at all possible, avoid using family members or visitors as interpreters because the shared information sometimes includes sensitive material. Also, the interpreter may modify the interpretation to protect the client from information they believe will cause cultural strain or difficulty for the client and family (Wenger, 1993).

Nonverbal communication is also important in teaching across cultures. Unspoken cues such as eye contact, distance between speakers, body movements, touch, and silence have cultural components. Generally, Caucasian Americans value direct eye contact when speaking. It provides feedback to ensure understanding of what has been communicated. In some other cultures, such as Native American, Asian, and African, direct eye contact is considered disrespectful. Diverting the eyes downward and to one side of the speaker indicates that a person is listening intently. Nurses need to be observers of nonverbal communication and learn what these cues mean from the client's cultural perspective (Wenger, 1993).

A cultural assessment should be conducted to elicit the client's beliefs, values, and attitudes about health, illness, medications, and the client role (see Chapter 6). Care should then be negotiated between client and nurse until an agreement is reached for a culturally appropriate and acceptable intervention. Only then will culturally appropriate teaching and learning have taken place (Wenger, 1993).

The manner in which a client perceives the ability to change or control his or her life has an impact on his or her willingness or ability to adhere to a medication regimen. **Locus of control** is the concept concerning how a client perceives his or her ability to influence or control his or her life along an internal-external continuum. At one end of the continuum, a client can be internally (self-) oriented and at the other end, externally (others- or fate-) oriented about his or her health behaviors. Clients with an internal locus of control are more apt to be health-oriented and adhere to a medication regimen. The locus of control may be assessed by listening to the client making statements such as, "I forgot to take my medication" (internal locus) rather than, "My husband didn't remind me to take my medicine" (external locus). In one instance the client assumes accountability for the actions, and in the other the responsibility is placed elsewhere.

The nurse should assess the client's level of development since this will affect the ability to make decisions, assume the responsibility for the result of those decisions, and the ability to manage life. The physical, emotional, and psychologic stages of development and related developmental tasks have been described by Erickson and others (Box 10-1 describes Erickson's stages of development). All individuals pass through the same predictable life stages; however, passage through these predictable stages occurs at different rates. Some are ready to accept adult responsibilities at age 18;

BOX 10-1

Erickson's Stages of Development

Infant (birth to 1 year of age): Trust vs mistrust. Infant learns to trust himself, others, and the environment; learns to love and be loved.

Toddler (1 to 3 years of age): Autonomy vs shame and doubt. Toddler learns independence; learns to master the physical environment and maintain self-esteem.

Preschooler (3 to 6 years of age): Initiative vs guilt. Preschooler learns basic problem-solving; develops conscience and sexual identity; initiates activities as well as imitates.

School-age child (6 to 12 years of age): Industry vs inferiority. School-age child learns to do things well; develops a sense of self-worth.

Adolescent (12 to 18 years of age): Identity vs role confusion. Adolescent integrates many roles into self-identity through role models and peer pressure.

Young adult (18 to 45 years of age): Intimacy vs isolation. Young adult establishes deep and lasting relationships; learns to make commitment as spouse, parent, partner.

Middle-aged adult (45 to 65 years of age): Generativity vs stagnation. Adult learns commitment to community and world; is productive in career, family, civic interests.

Older adult (over 65 years of age): Integrity vs despair. Older adult appreciates life role and status; deals with loss and prepares for death.

others may be well past 35 before they are ready to accept responsibility for themselves and others. Although people move sequentially through stages, they fluctuate among stages, often in response to stress. Stressors, such as illness and hospitalization, may cause the client to regress temporarily to an earlier stage. The client needs to be addressed at his or her current developmental stage, rather than the developmental stage that one would expect for the client's chronologic age. If the client's developmental stage is not accurately assessed, the nurse may misdirect goals and inhibit client learning (Box 10-2). The aging changes are important in deciding whether the client can self-administer medications accurately (Drake & Romano, 1995). In some instances, the administration of medications may need to be delegated to a caregiver.

The nurse needs also to consider modification of the teaching plan for clients with vision and hearing impairments. Instructions in large print and pill containers with the days of the week in braille are two modifications that may be considered for the visually impaired client. Written instructions are imperative for the hearing impaired; try to keep all written communication simple and straightforward. If the client with a hearing impairment can lip or speech read, ensure you are facing the client to support this activity.

The assessment phase can be used to establish rapport and gain the mutual respect of nurse and client necessary for the teaching-learning process. Because nurses are seen as having a position of power in relation to the client, they need to recognize the need to initiate the educational process. When the client perceives an attitude of sincerity, integrity, and warmth in the nurse, the milieu is set for the client to feel free to ask questions and to discuss all matters, regardless of how personal those issues may be.

The assessment for teaching-learning is similar to other types of nursing assessment; it is continuous and involves observation, listening and questioning, and other communication skills.

NURSING DIAGNOSES RELATED TO SELF-ADMINISTRATION OF MEDICATIONS

Three of the most common nursing diagnoses determined in relation to clients and the self-administration of medications are *knowledge deficit, noncompliance,* and *ineffective management of the therapeutic regimen.* **Knowledge deficit** is the state in which the individual has a deficiency in cognitive knowledge or psychomotor skills regarding the condition or treatment plan, which is somewhat different from noncompliance. **Noncompliance** is the state in which an individual or group desires to comply but is prevented from doing so by factors that deter adherence to health-related advice given by health professionals (Carpenito, 1995). **Ineffective management of therapeutic regimen** is a pattern of regulating and integrating into daily living a program for treatment of illness and the sequelae of illness that is unsatisfactory for meeting specific health goals (Carpenito, 1995). *All clients having drug therapy, whether administered by the client or a health care provider, should be assessed for the nursing diagnoses of risk for knowledge deficit, noncompliance, and ineffective management of therapeutic regimen.* Because this is so, these three nursing diagnoses are not always listed for each drug as it is discussed in the text.

Intervention to enhance compliance and effective management of the therapeutic regimen is focused on client concerns or health beliefs, such as concern over possible adverse effects or the cost of the drug, and is distinctly different than teaching for knowledge deficit. Teaching for knowledge deficit is appropriate when the assessment clearly identifies that the client does not have sufficient or accurate information about the medication regimen and that the deficit is interfering with the client's ability to self-administer medications. Any of these nursing diagnoses might appear in the same fashion, that is, with the client's inability to administer medications safely and accurately; return of the client's symptoms or the occurrence of complications; or inappropriate behavior related to the therapeutic regimen. However, in the case of knowledge deficit, the client may request information, verbalize a misconception, or state the problem,

BOX 10-2

Selected Aging Changes and Educational Strategies Appropriate to Pharmacology Content

Changes associated with aging that may influence learning	Nursing interventions
Altered thought processes	
Slowed cognitive functioning	Slow pace of presentation
Decreased short-term memory	Provide smaller amounts of information at one time
Decreased ability to think abstractly	Repeat information frequently
Decreased ability to concentrate	Use examples to illustrate information
Increased reaction time (slower to respond)	Decrease external stimuli as much as possible
	Allow more time for feedback from elderly learners
	Use a variety of methods—audiovisuals and practice sessions
	Provide written instructions for home use
Altered sensory-perceptual status	
Hearing	
Decreased ability to distinguish sounds, e.g., words beginning with S, Z, T, D, F, and G	Speak distinctly
	Sit on side of learner's "best" ear
Decreased conduction of sound	Do not shout; speak in a normal voice, but lower its pitch
Loss of ability to hear high frequency sounds	Face the client so that lip reading is possible
	Use visual aids to reinforce verbal instruction
	Reinforce teaching with easy-to-read materials
	Decrease extraneous noise
Vision	
Decreased visual acuity	Ensure glasses are clean and in place
Decreased ability to read fine detail	Use printed material with large print
Decreased ability to discriminate between blue, violet, and green; all colors tend to fade, with red fading the least	Use high-contrast materials, i.e., black on white
	Avoid use of blue, violet, and green in type or graphics; use red instead
Lens become thicker and yellower with decreased accommodation	Use nonglare lighting and avoid contrasts of light, e.g., darkened room with single light
Pupil smaller; decreased amount of light reaching retina	
Decreased depth perception	Adjust teaching to allow for the use of touch to gauge depth
Peripheral vision decreased	
Touch and vibration	
Sense of touch decreased	Increase time for the teaching of psychomotor skills, repetitions, and return demonstration
Decreased sense of vibration	Teach to palpate more prominent pulse sites, e.g., carotid and radial

Modified from Weinrich SP, et al. (1989). Continuing education: adapting strategies to teach the elderly. *J Gerontol Nurs 15*(11):17.

"I don't understand. . . ." With noncompliance or ineffective management of the therapeutic regimen, the client may also fail to keep appointments or evidence an inability to set or keep mutually agreed upon goals. The nurse may be aware of previous appropriate health education from the clinical record or may even have done the teaching and determine that the client did not seem to integrate the content into health-related behaviors. Then the issue is a matter of noncompliance or ineffective management rather than a lack of knowledge.

Compliance is the degree to which clients take medication instructions seriously, concur with them, and follow through. It is a term that can have an offensively controlling ring to it, implying that the prescriber directs the client, who must follow those directions. Some practitioners prefer the term *adherence* or, most recently, *effective management of the thera-*

peutic regimen. When care is mutually planned by nurse and client, noncompliance is minimized. However, since compliance is the standard accepted term, it is used here; but "concurrence with therapy" and "adherence to instructions" are synonymous.

Why do clients seek medical care and then not follow through on the suggested medication plan at home? There are many reasons, some personal, some social, some psychologic, some cultural. Everyone is potentially noncompliant, whether intentionally or not. Medication compliance has been estimated to vary between 13% and 93% (Bond & Hussar, 1991; Harvey & Plumridge, 1991). Some clients never fill the prescription, most take them at unscheduled times, and many stop taking the medication early.

The consequences include inexplicable medication failures with continuing symptoms or overdoses. Medication not used may be kept and taken inappropriately later when its potency and chemical activities may have changed. Prescribers tend simply to increase the drug dosage or change medications when confronted with apparent medication failures instead of investigating for noncompliance with the therapeutic plan.

The following are examples of situations known to foster ineffective management of the therapeutic regimen or noncompliance.

1. The client is chronically ill or on prolonged therapy. The symptoms in chronic illness tend to grow worse, then improve in a cyclic fashion. Clients, therefore, do not often see any clear causal relationship between taking or not taking the prescribed medication methodically and the waxing and waning of symptoms. It has been shown that the routine action of reviewing medications with clients and inquiring how they are taken at home dramatically increases compliance. It should be stressed when appropriate that medication will have to be taken indefinitely and should not be precipitously discontinued.
2. The client is relatively asymptomatic or feels better. Reasons for needing to take the drug completely should be explained. Many people are not aware that organisms mutate, for example, and that to ensure their eradication in the first place, antibiotic medications should be completed as prescribed.
3. The medication is expensive or inconvenient to obtain. Prescriptions purchased by generic name and further explanations of the medications importance, i.e., the consequences of not taking the drug, may be effective in remotivating this client.
4. The medication instructions are complex and not easily understood. "Take with meals" may mean twice a day to the person who always skips breakfast or before or after meals for others. Written instructions with a sample of the drug taped to them may assist as a reminder when the client is home and has forgotten what was heard in the office or in the hospital when being discharged.
5. The medication is unwieldy to take because the bottle cap is difficult for arthritic hands or there are complicated mixing or measuring directions. Measuring cups or droppers can be offered, and the client should be told that easy-to-remove caps can be requested when the medicine is purchased.
6. The medicine tastes unpleasant or must be taken at inconvenient times (during sleep hours, at work) or too many times a day to be feasible. Medication can be mixed with or taken with various liquids that are both pleasant and compatible. Medication prescriptions can often be changed after consultation with the prescriber to higher doses given less frequently or to a sustained-action form if available and if feasible.
7. The therapeutic plan contains many different medications, so the drug-taking schedule is complicated. Occasional systematic review of the medications by the prescriber and the nurse, especially in home health care, is necessary to see if the client still needs all of them and to simplify the care plan (Drake & Romano, 1995). Confrontation of the client's habits is necessary when medication containers remain full when they should be empty. Written schedules with sample drugs attached are helpful. Also, small medication boxes with separate compartments for each dosing time are available at pharmacies. The nurse may suggest that the client keep the medication near equipment used at a specific time each day (such as a coffee cup or the kitchen table) or associate taking the medication with a specific routine activity, such as walking the dog or watching the television news.
8. Most people wait more than an hour to be seen by their prescriber in the office or clinic setting. Waiting longer than this has been correlated with a distinct drop in following the prescriber's medication instructions. Often the wait is unavoidable, but the situation can be improved if the practitioner is empathic.
9. The client does not understand or accept the illness or disorder, or the explanation of the illness or treatment plan does not fit the client's concepts of illness, health care, or health. Typical of the factors that influence attitudes toward treatment are the extent to which clients believe (a) themselves to be susceptible to the illness, (b) the illness to be serious, and (c) that they will benefit from taking action. *Giving information, therefore, is not the entire answer.* It helps to seek the active participation of the client in the health and nursing process and to show interest in and respect for client ideas, feelings, and beliefs.
10. The client and health care practitioners perceive the clients' problems or goals in divergent ways, yet do not effectively communicate this.
11. The medication is seen as an artificial additive or contaminant to the body or as a crutch on which dependence should be limited.

12. Side effects are severe or interfere with functioning in daily activities.
13. The client has problems with memory or confusion or is visually or hearing impaired.

The specific nursing diagnosis selected for a particular client will depend upon the nurse's astute assessment of the individual situation with the client and family.

PLANNING

The next part of the teaching-learning process is planning, which begins once a learning need has been identified. The learning needs are discussed; and the planning of objectives is a mutual undertaking between the nurse, the client, and, where appropriate, the family. The learning objectives for the client's ability to self-medicate are goals or expected outcomes that should result from the teaching-learning interactions. However, whether the teaching plan is a standardized one generated as part of a protocol, or a unique one developed specifically for a client with complex learning needs, it needs to be included in the written plan of care. The written plan should include: the topic, who initiates teaching and when, who reinforces teaching and when, educational materials given, and a comments section for documenting client/caregiver response (Weaver, 1995).

In order for the teaching plan objectives to clarify what is to be learned and how that learning will be evaluated, the objective should contain a verb that is measurable (Box 10-3). Although the nurse would like the client to "know" about his medications, "understand" how the medication relates to the illness, and "comprehend" what action to take if an adverse effect occurs, these verbs are not appropriate for writing goals, since they are neither easily interpreted nor measurable. On the other hand, terms such as "define," "list," "identify," and "state" are measurable, have fewer interpretations, and are therefore more useful in evaluating achievement of goals for learning. The following are examples:

The client will:

- state the major action of digoxin.
- identify at least three adverse effects of digoxin that should be reported to the prescriber.
- list the signs and symptoms of hypoglycemia, such as tachycardia; palpitations; cool, clammy skin; diaphoresis; irritability; tiredness; hunger; numbness; and blurred vision.

In addition, goals need to be realistic with regard to the client's achievements. Goals can be determined only by assessing with the client his or her ability to achieve the expected outcomes.

BOX 10-3

Examples of Measurable and Nonmeasurable Verbs

Measurable verbs

describe	administer	stand
discuss	demonstrate	walk
identify	perform	has an increase in
list	self-administer	has a decrease in
relate	exercise	has an absence of
state	cough	
verbalize	sit	

Nonmeasurable verbs

accept	feel	think
appreciate	know	understand

How will you know that the client understands? What behaviors need to be evident for you to observe that he or she appreciates (or accepts, etc.)?

IMPLEMENTATION

Once a learning need has been identified and the expected outcome agreed on by the client and the nurse, the most difficult steps of the teaching-learning process have been completed. The implementation phase consists of conveying the specific information required by the objectives.

Instructional sessions about medications should be integrated throughout the extent of nurse-client interactions and not saved for the day of discharge from the health agency. Short encounters staggered over the course of the client's length of stay enhance learning because it takes place in small incremental steps, rather than one overwhelming session. For example, one of the most appropriate times to teach the client about medications is as they are being administered. This dialogue will assist the client to cue in specific medications at certain times of the day and at particular dosage intervals.

The practice of manual skills is rather straightforward, such as the manipulation of a syringe and vial to self-administer insulin. Nurses are familiar with the practices of demonstration and return demonstration, but variations exist that can conserve time. A nurse may draw up the insulin and ask the client to complete the injection, the nurse may ask the client to direct her through the procedure, or the nurse may coach the client through the procedure. Equipment may be left with the client to allow for practice time without the nurse being present before a return demonstration is scheduled. Such equipment should be labeled as "practice equipment," and the client should be instructed that this material is contaminated and should not be used on himself or herself.

The communication of ideas is more complex but just as necessary. Ideas are more easily understood if they are organized in a logical order and if they move from simple to complex. For example, it is helpful for clients to know the therapeutic effect of a drug before learning about its side and adverse effects. Ideas need to be practiced, too. Application of information is important for clients. "What will you do if you take your pulse and the rate is below 60 beats per minute?" Knowing what to do is more helpful than reciting the symptoms of digoxin toxicity. Providing the client with scenarios in which decisions must be made regarding lifestyle and medications is beneficial. Ask a client who takes disulfiram (Antabuse), a drug that causes vomiting when alcohol is taken, "Suppose you're having dinner at a friend's home and you're asked to have a drink, how will you respond?" The client can demonstrate commitment if able to state to nurse and family how he or she intends to manage administration of a medication that needs to be taken four times a day within a schedule that includes home, office, and business travel. Coudreaut-Quinn and others (1992) report a self-medication program while the client is still in the hospital to be an approach to increase adherence to a medication regimen.

The client should be encouraged to plan for the administration of medications and the incorporation of this activity into his or her lifestyle. Written instructions are particularly helpful for the client to refer to once discharged from the health care setting (Figure 10-1). Medication schedules have proven to be particularly helpful to assist clients with adherence to a medication regimen (see Nursing Research box on p. 179). A medication calendar may be made by obtaining a calendar with space enough to write in the names of the drugs and the times of the day they should be taken. In this fashion they can be checked off when taken and the client will have a home medication record. This method is particularly helpful with clients who are concerned that they may forget or for those clients trying to establish a routine for taking their medications. Having an alarm clock next to the calendar so that the alarm may be reset for the next dose assists to decrease the anxiety related to forgetting a dose. Written information for each client should be available concerning the medication and including its name, purpose, appearance, directions for taking, time to take it, what action to take if a dose is missed, and any special precautions related to the drug. The side/adverse effects of the drug should also be written, along with those symptoms that should be reported and to whom they should be reported. In addition to information regarding the client's specific medication regimen, the nurse should take the opportunity to educate the client as a consumer of drugs (Box 10-4).

The nurse should develop a repertoire of approaches and materials to be used for client teaching. A nurse who relies solely on the hearing of the client is not encouraging the op-

MEDICATION CAUTIONS

- ☐ 1. Avoid alcoholic beverages while taking this medication.
- ☐ 2. Swallow these tablets. Do not chew them. Do not take if coating is cracked.
- ☐ 3. Do not drive a car or operate machinery if this medication makes you drowsy. If you have to drive home, wait until you get home to take your first dose.
- ☐ 4. Do not allow this medication to contact the skin, eyes, or clothing.
- ☐ 5. Take this medication on an empty stomach either 1 hour before meals or 2 hours after meals. You may drink water.
- ☐ 6. Do not take this medication with fruit juice.
- ☐ 7. Take this medication ________ hour(s) before meals.
- ☐ 8. Limit caffeine use.
- ☐ 9. Do not take this medication with milk or milk products. You may drink water or juice.
- ☐ 10. Take this medication with at least 8 ounces of water.
- ☐ 11. Take this medication with food to avoid upset stomach.
- ☐ 12. This medication may discolor the urine or stools.
- ☐ 13. Do not take this medication with antacids.
- ☐ 14. Do not take aspirin with this medication.
- ☐ 15. Do not take mineral oil with this medication.
- ☐ 16. Take orange juice, bananas, and other foods high in potassium while taking this medication.
- ☐ 17. Avoid tyramine-rich foods such as cheese, pickled herring, and wine while taking this medication.
- ☐ 18. Count your pulse (by feeling at the wrist) each time before taking this medication. If it is less than 60 beats a minute, do not take the dose. Contact the prescriber.
- ☐ 19. Check with your prescriber before taking any other medications (even over-the-counter medications).
- ☐ 20. Do not take this medication if pregnant or breast-feeding or if you have ever had an allergic reaction to it. Instead, contact prescriber for instructions.
- ☐ 21. Do not take this medication if you have the following medical problems or symptoms:

Figure 10-1 Example of a general medication instruction sheet for the client, which may be individualized by indicating specific instructions appropriate to the client's therapeutic regimen.

timal learning experience. The nurse should include as many of the client's senses in the learning experience as possible. For example, in teaching about medications while administering them within the hospital setting, the nurse allows the client to hear the reason the drug is indicated for the condition. The pill can also be seen and felt by the client and tasted while taken. During recent years the amount of health teaching materials in a variety of media has proliferated. Audiovisual and other materials such as pamphlets and videotapes can show the client settings and situations that are beyond the ability of the nurse to present at the bedside, in the clinic, or in the home setting. Computer-generated instructions as part of a standard teaching plan has demonstrated success (Weaver, 1995) as well as computer-assisted instruction for some clients (Tibbles et al, 1992). These are useful supplements and should be used by the nurse teacher to enhance the teaching process. With increasingly short lengths of stay in hospitals or brief encounters in the office, clinic, or home, these adjuncts become more important to include in the nurse's scope of teaching techniques. These materials should be selected according to the appropriateness of content, accuracy, simplicity, and appeal for the client. They should, however, never replace individualized instruction, since the client may overlook needed information or be overwhelmed by a comprehensive audiovisual presentation. These various media techniques should facilitate the nurse's role as teacher rather than act as substitutes.

Bille (1981) recommends the process of **therapeutic seeding** as a teaching approach when clients have not been able to express learning needs or concerns. This technique is one of mentioning ideas to clients, allowing time to pass so the client has a chance to think about the idea, then reintroducing the idea. On the second opportunity the client may more easily identify the concept and see it as a learning need. For example, if an older female client had been prescribed conjugated estrogens on a previous clinic visit, she may not

Nursing Research

The effects of medication education on adherence to medication regimens in an elderly population

With the population of individuals over 65 rapidly increasing and a third of all prescriptions being written for this population, the numbers of elderly that are hospitalized annually related to adverse drug reactions are increasing. Improving the effective management of the therapeutic regimen by the elderly would decrease the cost and increase the quality of health care by decreasing the risk of hospitalization for such reactions. The purpose of this study was to evaluate educational protocols to see which would be more effective in increasing medication compliance rates within an elderly population.

Clients participating in the study were age 65 or older; hospitalized for at least 24 hours; oriented to time, place and person; discharged to home; able to self-administer medications or take them with minimal assistance; and able to complete a mini-mental test with a score of 23 or higher as a screening test for dementia and to determine cognitive functioning. The participants were randomized into four intervention groups.

The intervention groups were as follows: Group 1 (n=11) received the medication information usually distributed by the study site institution, which included a medication fact sheet and a discharge instruction sheet indicating the date of return visit, any special instructions related to diet, activity, dressings and treatments, when to call the doctor, and medications prescribed by the doctor (name, dose, and frequency of dosage). Group 2 (n=8) received the medication fact sheet and 30 minutes of verbal instruction. Group 3 (n=10) received a medication schedule written in large dark lettering, which included the name of the medicine, color of the pill, dose, a list of side effects, a dosage schedule, and the reason for each medication. Group 4 (n=14) received the same medication schedule and 30 minutes of verbal instruction. Visits were then made to the clients' homes 2 weeks, 1 month, and 2 months after discharge. All visits were conducted using the following process: pill counts were done and compared with medication orders; clients gave self-reports on how they administered their medications and any missed or increased doses; reasons for noncompliance were recorded; and it was determined if the client had received any other medication education other than that from the investigator.

In the evaluation of the results from the three follow-up visits, clients in groups 3 and 4 had fewer medication errors than in groups 1 and 2. Adherence scores in groups 1 and 2 exhibited increased changes in the follow-up visits when compared with groups 3 and 4. Mini-mental test scores, education levels and age were similar in all groups. Involvement in home health services did not seem to effect the rate of error in the medication regimen. The individuals in this study reported forgetting to take their medication as the primary reason for noncompliance.

The groups with the medication schedule did have decreased incidence of medication error compared with those in groups without a schedule. However, given the sample size of this study, 42 participants, further research is needed to provide more evidence of the benefits of the medication schedule compared with other education protocols.

1. The clients in group 1, which had the highest error rate, also had a slightly higher medication complexity index. How might this contribute to higher error rates?
2. Given the rationale cited by these participants for noncompliance, what advantage would a medication schedule have for them?
3. What could you generalize from these results?

*Esposito L (1995). The effects of medication education on adherence to medication regimens in an elderly population, *J Adv Nursing* 21:935-943.

BOX 10-4

Consumer Education Topics

1. Awareness that OTC medications are truly drugs, just as are prescription drugs, and deserve the same care in use.
2. Identification of some types of medications that are considered useful for home treatment (see Chapter 11).
3. Advising client about safety precautions:
   a. Make sure all medications, including OTCs, have clear and understandable labels.
   b. Heed instructions and explain warnings on labels—for example, "Do not drive or operate machinery while taking this medication" or "Discontinue use if rapid pulse, dizziness, or blurring of vision occurs" (see Figure 10-1).
   c. Take water, 1 to 2 ounces before taking solid dosage forms to hasten their movement to the stomach. Whenever possible, drink a full glass of water to assist in their dissolution.
   d. Check all medications periodically for expiration dates and for deterioration. Discard outdated or deteriorated medications.
   e. Discard unused portions of drugs and do not share these with friends or family even if they appear to have symptoms like your own. Do not even save them for yourself without asking a prescriber.
   f. Keep all medications out of children's reach, and never refer to medications as "candy" to induce children to take the medication. A childproof cap may serve only to slow a child down.
   g. Do not take any medication in the dark.
   h. Do not mix medications in one container. Store drugs in the original container with the original label. Keep tightly capped.
   i. If you suspect a mistake or overdose, call your local Poison Control Center, prescriber, or pharmacist. Have the medication container at hand.
   j. Learn both the generic and brand or trade names of prescribed drugs. Learn the appearances of your drugs.
   k. Tell the prescriber and pharmacist about any allergies or other conditions you have as well as any previous unusual reactions, current pregnancy, or if you are breastfeeding.
   l. Take the medication precisely as directed and for the length of time prescribed. Ask the health practitioner or consult the *USP DI* about what to do if one dose of the medication is omitted. Do not just stop the medication on your own.
4. Instruction that nonprescription drugs do not usually cure a condition but rather just make the symptoms bearable. Treated conditions that persist, recur, or produce unusual reactions should be seen by a health care provider.
5. Counseling and instruction, when appropriate, about alternate nursing therapies or therapies that accompany drug taking (e.g., instruct about increasing fluids, activity, and roughage to reduce a laxative habit).
6. Warnings about certain drugs that can produce physical and psychologic dependence (e.g., analgesics, stimulants, and laxatives).

have identified any drug-related learning needs at that time. The nurse on the next visit may use therapeutic seeding by a statement such as, "Ms. Ackerman, many women who take this medication have expressed concerns about its adverse effects. What concerns do you have about the medication?" If she states "I'm not concerned about that," she may be saying "I'm not ready to hear that information yet." Reference to the comment on the next visit may prepare the way for the nurse to discuss possible adverse effects and what symptoms should be reported to the prescriber if they occur. Therapeutic seeding allows the client more of an opportunity to negotiate the teaching-learning program.

Practical information about prescription drugs is available to consumers from the American Medical Association, package inserts produced by the pharmaceutical houses, some health care providers, or within the *USP DI: Advice for the Patient* volume. Most available printed information includes the drug's purpose, possible side and adverse effects, and the best way to take the drug. More than 1000 common drugs are listed annually in the *U.S. Pharmacopeia Dispensing Information,* which is geared partly to those who dispense or administer prescriptions and partly to those who take them. Volume II, *Advice for the Patient,* offers jargon-free guidelines for safe and informed self-administration of prescription drugs by generic name. The *USP DI* is available to consumers by health practitioners or pharmacists who can reproduce for distribution a limited number of pages from the Advice section.*

The client and family need to be active members of the team, especially since much of the convalescent care is shifting from hospital to home. They need to be encouraged to participate when and wherever possible in all aspects of the client's care. Family members may be responsible for the changing of dressings, taking care of drains and intravenous lines, and running complex equipment, as well as the administration of intramuscular and intravenous medications. The client's family may be of great support not only in providing assistance but also in easing the transition to home.

*The *USP DI* is available for purchase from United States Pharmacopeia, Customer Service Department, 12601 Twinbrook Parkway, Rockville, MD 20852; or use the toll-free number, 1-(800) 227-8772. Students receive a 40% discount.

The nurse needs to identify which family members are supportive and can assume the ongoing responsibility for care, including the administration of medications. In a crisis, family members tend to gather around the client but may normally live at some distance or return to a daily work schedule when the client is ready to return home. The nurse must ensure that the appropriate family members are taught to provide the ongoing care. If the family will not be in attendance at home, it may be more appropriate to provide information to the client's friends, neighbors, or paid care providers regarding the medications.

Although there may be many opportunities to teach family members, the nurse may have to schedule an appointment with them to ensure that they are present to learn the medication regimen and other discharge instructions. The assistance of family members needs to be actively sought and encouraged, since some may be hesitant because they are unsure of the part they are to play in the client's care.

Teaching programs with clients and families about medications that tend to be successful include the following: (1) positive reinforcement or praise for desired behaviors; (2) feedback about progress toward goals; (3) individualization, whereby learning needs are determined for the specific client and the pace of teaching is mutually negotiated; (4) facilitation, in which the nurse assists the client to take action, such as making personalized medication schedules; and (5) relevance, making sure that the content and teaching-learning methods are meaningful for the client. The nurse should attempt to incorporate these issues into each of the teaching sessions.

There is no single best way to educate clients to self-administer medications. Using the same approach each time does not take into account the data gathered from the client in the assessment phase of the teaching-learning process. Assessing each individual's learning needs in order to develop the best teaching approach results in the most effective use of nursing resources.

EVALUATION

Evaluation of whether client education has taken place is essential. Some nurses may consider the process of teaching to be a brochure handed out or a videotape shown and then consider the task of education to be complete. But the emphasis should be on the client's response—behavioral changes, knowledge, and skills gained as a result of the methodology and content of the teaching-learning process. The evaluation process should involve an assessment of the client's progress toward the specific goals for self-administration of medication within the teaching plan, as well as the response to the teaching-learning process.

DOCUMENTATION

Documentation is the final step in the process of client teaching for the self-administration of medications. Unfortunately, the JCAHO has found that the lack of documentation of the client's and family's knowledge of self-care is one of the most common nursing deficiencies cited during accreditation audits. Documentation relating to the teaching about medications should minimally contain three items: the specific content, the method of teaching, and the evaluation of learning.

Although the nursing care plan contains the specific learning goals agreed on by the nursing team and the client, the narrative documentation following the teaching-learning process should indicate the specific content that was covered. This information needs to be recorded in such a way that any other nurse will know enough about what was taught to be able to continue the teaching from that point. The following are appropriate examples: "the need for taking a pulse before a digoxin dose was discussed," "the client was cautioned not to take antacids with the tetracycline," or "the side effect of furosemide, low potassium, was discussed." A common error of documentation is the statement "medications taught," particularly in a setting where the client may have a polydrug regimen such as in home health care. The following questions are raised: What medications? What about them? What dosing schedule? What side/adverse effects? What special precautions? Such vague documentation does not support the provision of skilled nursing care and in the home health care setting may provide justification for nonreimbursement for nursing care. Because clients are transitioned from one health care setting to another more frequently in today's health care environment, documentation becomes even more important. It provides data for the nurse within the client's next health care setting to provide continuity of instruction without repetition of previous information and omission of essential learning.

Documenting the method of instruction allows the next nurse to know which teaching techniques were successful for the client's learning. Although "taught" is the most common verb used, it does not explain what or how the material was covered. More appropriate words are "discussed," "demonstrated," or "a specific piece of literature was reviewed and given to the client." These may also include the client's characteristics as a learner and any barriers to learning that the nurse may have determined. Recording the "teaching" part of the teaching-learning process leads then to the most important part, recording the "learning" of that process.

Many health care agencies that utilize a clinical pathway approach to the provision of care and its documentation have also developed teaching pathways to provide a comprehensive approach to client education for specific disease or procedure populations. These teaching pathways serve as a guide to teaching and identifying learning objectives along a designated time line, as well as providing for consistent documentation (Sciartelli, 1995).

The recording of an evaluation of the client and/or family's learning indicates the achievement of, or progress toward, the learning goals originally established by client and nurse. The evaluation documentation includes a description of what occurred; the client's response to the teaching-learning encounter, using his or her own words and behaviors; and the observable or measurable activities of the client and family that would indicate that the instructions were understood. Documentation, as the final step of the teaching-learning process, is essential to record the client's progress.

SUMMARY

Medications tend to be more effective when clients believe in their capacity to get well and in the drug itself. Clients' past and present conditioning to drugs, illness, hospitals, nurses, and other health care personnel, as well as their own health beliefs and practices, influence their response to drug therapy. An accurate assessment of these factors is most important in order to plan and implement an effective care plan.

Three of the most common nursing diagnoses related to the self-administration of medications for which the client is at risk are knowledge deficit, ineffective management of the therapeutic regimen, and noncompliance. These problems need to be resolved so that the client may accurately and safely self-administer medications.

From the onset of drug therapy the client should be advised of the purpose of the medication and any possible side or adverse effects. All information should be presented in a nonthreatening and straightforward manner. It is important to listen to what the client has to say about the medication, the feelings associated with the drug and whether they are based on fear or anxiety, and the perception of the condition for which the drug has been prescribed.

Client education plays an important role when, at discharge, the individual needs to follow a prescribed medication plan. Routinely reviewing medications with clients and inquiring about how medications are taken at home have been shown to increase compliance with a medication plan.

The nurse should make sure that the client thoroughly understands the medication instructions. Written schedules and instructions will remind clients when they are at home and may have forgotten what they heard in the office or on discharge from the hospital.

Documentation of the teaching-learning process for self-administration of medications needs to include content, method, and client and family's progress in relation to the planned objectives for learning.

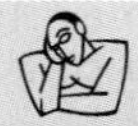

Critical Thinking

1. What kind of strategies would you use to determine the educational needs of a client who will eventually self-administer medications at home?
2. If your contact time with a client is limited, as in an emergency room setting, what are the most essential elements to get across to the client?
3. How would you differentiate between the nursing diagnoses of knowledge deficit and ineffective management of the therapeutic regimen if you ascertained that the client was not taking medications as prescribed?
4. How would you go about assessing the learning needs and developing a teaching plan for an elderly client? a client with a language barrier?

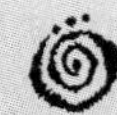

Collaborative Learning Activities

1. The students will discuss their own experiences with self-administering medications. Did they complete all of their prescription? What were the issues that supported their compliance? What were the issues that made it difficult for them to be compliant with the drug therapy? What support/counseling would have assisted them to maintain their own drug regimen?
2. The students will be divided into teams and each will create a quick mini-skit on assessment and intervention strategies for the following special clients: an alert, elderly Hispanic woman who insists her sister's prescription is helping her; a young nursing student who is angry and grieving about her diagnosis of multiple sclerosis; a middle-aged man who expresses doubts about the limiting prognosis of his ailment; an elderly man who "swears by" his Danish grandmother's tea recipe for treating his hypertension; a Vietnamese woman who smiles and nods but does not comply with instructions; and a Native American woman who will not make eye contact with the nurse.

BIBLIOGRAPHY

Barbee JG (1993). Memory, benzodiazepines, and anxiety: Integration of theoretical and clinical perspectives, *J Clin Psychiatry 54* (suppl):86-97.

Becker M (1979). Patient perceptions and compliance. In Haynes R, et al. (Eds.). *Compliance in health care.* Baltimore: Johns Hopkins University Press.

Bille DA (Ed.). (1981). *Practical approaches to patient teaching.* Boston: Little, Brown & Co.

Bond WS & Hussar DA (1991). Detection methods and strategies for improving medication compliance, *Am J Hosp Pharm 48*:1978-1988.

Carpenito LJ (1995). *Nursing diagnosis: Application to clinical practice* (6th ed.). Philadelphia: JB Lippincott.

Charonko CV (1992). Cultural influences in "noncompliant" behavior and decision making, *Holist Nurs Pract 6*(3):73-8.

Coudreaut-Quinn EA, et al. (1992). Self-medication during inpatient psychiatric treatment, *J Psychosoc Nurs 30*(12):32-6.

Craig C (1995). Teaching food-drug interactions, *J Psychosoc Nurs 33*(2):44-6.

Drake AC & Romano E (1995). Protect your older patient from the hazards of polypharmacy, *Nursing95 25*(6):34-9.

Gullickson C (1993). Client-centered drug choice: An alternative approach to managing hypertension, *Nurs Pract 18*(2):30-41.

Harvey LJ & Plumridge RJ (1991). Comparative attitudes to verbal and written medication information among hospital outpatients, *DICP 25*:925-8.

Hussey LC (1991). Overcoming the clinical barriers of low literacy and medication noncompliance among the elderly, *J Gerontol Nurs 17*(3):27.

Jones LA (1995). Patient information issues in the ambulatory surgery setting, *Today's OR Nurs 17*(2):9-12.

Kerr B, et al. (1991). Concentration-related effects on morphine on cognition and motor control in human subjects, *Neuropsychopharmacol 5*:157-66.

Lile JL & Hoffman R (1991). Medication-taking by the frail elderly in two ethnic groups, *Nurs Forum 26*(4):19-24.

Proos M, et al. (1992). A study of the effects of self-medication on patients' knowledge of and compliance with their medication regimen, *J Nurs Care Qual (Special Report)*:18-26.

Redman BK (1993). *The process of patient education.* (7th ed.). St. Louis: Mosby.

Sciartelli CH (1995). Using a clinical pathway approach to document patient teaching for breast cancer surgical procedures, *Oncol Nur Forum* 22(1):131-7.

Shea S, et al. (1992). Correlates of nonadherence to hypertension treatment in an inner-city minority population, *Am J Publ Health* 82(12):1607.

Smith CE (1987). Overview of patient education: opportunities and challenges for the twenty-first century, *Nurs Clin North Am* 24(3):583.

Tibbles L, et al. (1992). Computer assisted instruction for preoperative and postoperative patient education in joint replacement surgery, *Computers Nurs* 10(5):208.

Tripp-Reimer T, et al. (1989). Cross-cultural perspectives on patient teaching, *Nurs Clin North Am* 24(3):613.

Weaver J (1995). Patient education: An innovative computer approach, *Nurs Manag* 26(7):78-83.

Wenger AZ (1993). Teaching families from diverse cultural backgrounds, *Neonat Netw* 12(1):69-70.

Chapter 11

Over-the-counter (OTC) Medications

Chapter Focus

Over-the-counter (OTC) or nonprescription drugs are medications that can safely be used to self-treat minor illnesses without the supervision of a licensed health care practitioner, providing consumers follow the directions on the package. Because OTC drugs are widely available and frequently used by clients, nurses need to be aware to elicit information about their use as part of every drug history. The nurse's knowledge of nonprescription drugs should be as thorough as with prescription drugs for the nurse to provide client education for potential drug-drug interactions, expected outcomes of their use, and other issues related to OTC drugs. Collaboration with a pharmacist is recommended. The following objectives will assist you with an understanding of this chapter.

Key Terms

analgesic (p. 187)
antacid (p. 192)
antihistamine (p. 204)
constipation (p. 193)
diarrhea (p. 200)
laxative (p. 193)
perceived constipation (p. 194)

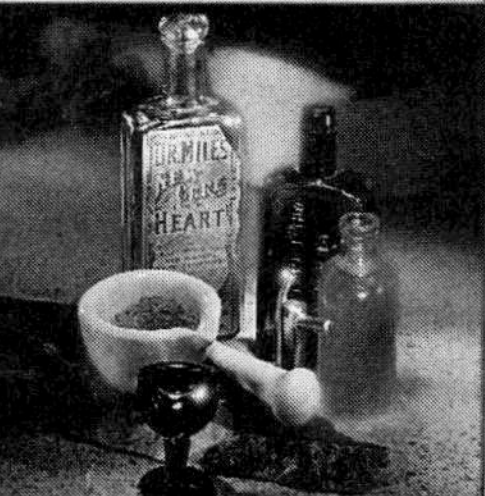

Key Drugs [▲]

acetaminophen
aspirin

Objectives

1. Compare and contrast strength, dosing, and other recommendations for prescription and over-the-counter (nonprescription) drugs.
2. Discuss issues related to drug marketing, safety, selection, storage, and administration of over-the-counter medications by the client.
3. Advise the client on the safe self-administration of selected over-the-counter preparations, e.g., analgesics, antacids, laxatives, cough-cold preparations, and other OTC agents, as they become available.

Over-the-counter (nonprescription) medications are utilized by the general public to self-treat minor illnesses. Such preparations are readily available in pharmacies, supermarkets, and other nonpharmacy outlets for selection by individuals that want to avoid the time and expense associated with going to a prescriber. The Nonprescription Drug Manufacturers' Association reports that Americans visit their physicians for only 10% of their illnesses and injuries, while the Health Care Financing Administration (HCFA) states that 6 out of every 10 medications purchased are OTC medications. Over-the-counter drugs are a tremendous market; it has been estimated that there are over 300,000 such products available in the United States. These products contain from 700 to 1000 active ingredients (Burns, 1991; Zimmerman, 1993). When used wisely, they result in time and money savings for the individual, and ultimately a reduction in overall health care costs. A good example of these cost savings is hydrocortisone cream, a product commonly used to treat rash and pruritus. When the cream became available as an OTC preparation, it was estimated to have saved Americans more than one billion dollars over a 3-year period as compared with the medical model of physician visits, prescriptions, and other related costs (Burns, 1991).

While OTC medications are generally considered to be safe and effective for consumer use, it is apparent that problems can result from their usage. For example, self-medication requires self-diagnosis of the signs and symptoms of a clinical condition. Generally the public may consider most illnesses to be minor. However, if a potentially serious condition is self-treated with OTC medications, the condition may be masked and the seeking of professional help for appropriate treatment delayed (Covington, 1996). Also, OTC drugs may contain potent chemicals, many of which were prescription drugs previously. The biggest trend in the 1990s is to transfer more and more prescription medications to OTC status. Thus the health care professional should be aware that many OTC products (new and old) are capable of producing both desired and undesirable effects, drug interactions and drug toxicity. This potential problem has been recognized by a current pharmacy law (Omnibus Budget Reconciliation Act or OBRA), which mandates that OTC drugs be considered an important part of the individual's medical record (Fitzgerald, 1994).

Although the Food and Drug Administration (FDA) issued regulations that require OTC package labeling be stated in terms that are likely to be read and understood by the average consumer, many consumers believe the labels are confusing and often the print is too small to read. Approximately 35% of Americans read at a 6th to 10th grade level while an estimated 20% are considered functionally illiterate (that is, they have a reading level below 5th grade) (Covington, 1996). Therefore, OTC labeling that is difficult to understand and apply may result in unsafe and possibly improper use of the medications.

This chapter will review the regulatory difference between a prescription and nonprescription drug and discuss the process of a drug being changed from prescription to OTC status, general considerations on drug marketing, consumer education for safe administration of OTC drugs, and selected major OTC drug categories.

DIFFERENCE BETWEEN A PRESCRIPTION AND NONPRESCRIPTION DRUG

The Food and Drug Administration (FDA) regulates and makes decisions about the safety and effectiveness of drugs, the classification of a product as a prescription or OTC drug, and the information printed on the drug labels. Thus drug substances are subjected to regulation, review, and various study requirements before being released and to a limited extent may be monitored afterward. Medications not considered safe enough for the general public to use without medical supervision are restricted to prescription status only. Nonprescription drugs are defined as safe and effective drugs for self-treatment by the public, assuming good manufacturing practices are followed by the manufacturer and the label directions are followed by the consumer.

Because many drugs were marketed without the more current standards of proof of documented safety and effectiveness, the FDA in 1972 established a number of OTC expert advisory panels to review drug categories and make recommendations to the FDA. As a result of this review, many ingredients used in such products were removed from the market, mainly because they lacked proof of effectiveness for their claims. Examples include aphrodisiacs, hair growers, hexachlorophene products, and others. These drugs were found to be either ineffective, dangerous, or both. In 1991 the FDA established an OTC Drugs Advisory Committee to assist in the review and evaluation and to advise the FDA Commissioner on its findings and recommendations. The Committee may also suggest prescription drugs to change to OTC status based on expert findings that the medication is safe and effective for general public usage.

The definitions for OTC drug safety and effectiveness include:

- **safety:** the drug product has a low incidence of severe side effects and a low potential for harm assuming proper instructions and adequate warnings are given on the label.
- **effectiveness:** the drug ingredient when properly used will provide relief of the minor symptom or illness in a significant portion of the population.

CHANGE OF A DRUG FROM PRESCRIPTION TO OTC STATUS

In the past few years the FDA has approved a number of ingredients in prescription drugs to be sold as OTC medications, including 17 new products in 1995 (Newton, Pray, & Popovich, 1996). With some products a lower strength of the active ingredient in the OTC product was required while with others the same prescription strength was released

TABLE 11-1 Prescription drugs changed to OTC status

Ingredient prescription name	OTC name	Principal use
brompheniramine (Dimetane, etc.)	Dimetane, Bromphen, etc.	antihistamine
clemastine (Tavist)	Tavist, etc.	antihistamine
chlorpheniramine (Chlor-Trimeton, etc.)	Chlor-Trimeton, Aller-chlor, etc.	antihistamine
cimetidine (Tagamet)	Tagamet HB	heartburn, acid indigestion
clotrimazole (Lotrimin, etc.)	Lotrimin AF, Zeasorb-AF, etc.	antifungal
diphenhydramine (Benadryl)	Benylin Cough, Diphen Cough, etc.	cough
diphenhydramine (Benadryl)	Nytol, Sominex, etc.	sleeping aid
famotidine (Pepcid)	Pepcid AC	heartburn, acid indigestion
hydrocortisone (Cort Dome, etc.)	Cortizone, Dermolate, etc.	topical for itching and rash
ibuprofen (Motrin)	Advil, Nuprin, etc.	analgesic
loperamide (Imodium, etc.)	Imodium A-D, Kaopectate II, etc.	antidiarrheal
miconazole (Monistat)	Micatin, etc.	antifungal
pyrantel (Antiminth)	Reese's Pinworm, etc.	pinworm remedy
sodium fluoride	Fluorigard, ACT, etc.	dental rinse
triprolidine (Myidyl, etc.)	Actidil, etc.	antihistamine

OTC. For example, ibuprofen (Motrin) was released in a 200 mg strength as an OTC drug while the higher dose tablet strengths, 400 or 800 mg, still require a prescription. The lower strength of ibuprofen is considered to be safe and effective for self-treatment of a minor illness, if the label instructions are followed. Use of higher strength ibuprofen requires medical supervision and a prescription because it has the potential of causing serious side/adverse effects. See Table 11-1 for examples of prescription to OTC drugs.

DRUG MARKETING

In contrast to prescription drugs, OTC medications may be marketed without FDA approval. Monographs of information developed by the OTC drug review identified specific drugs "generally recognized as safe and effective" (GRASE). Therefore, any drug manufacturer may produce such products for market without prior government approval. The manufacturer, however, has flexibility in package labeling. While it is required to use certain approved terminology (e.g., heartburn, acid indigestion, and sour stomach for antacids) other terms may also be used that have not been approved as long as they are not false or misleading.

In contrast to prescription medications, no regulations require the reporting of OTC adverse reactions. Also the manufacturer may substitute a GRASE ingredient in an OTC preparation for another GRASE ingredient without changing the name of the OTC drug and without indicating the change to the public by placing a warning on the package or label. The only method of determining a product's ingredients is to check the label for the listing of ingredients before each purchase (Covington, 1996).

Another important concept to understand is the difference between drug potency and drug effectiveness. As defined in Chapter 5, drug potency is the amount of drug required to produce a desired effect. When drug manufacturers claim their product is more potent than another product, this usually means that less quantity of the drug is necessary to produce the same effect as the comparison drug. This does not mean the *more potent drug is also the more effective drug* (unless greater effectiveness has been proven and clearly stated)—it only refers to amount of drug necessary to produce a desired effect. This terminology is often used and may be misleading if the difference between potency and effectiveness is not understood by health care providers or consumers.

Over-the-counter analgesics have a number of extra strength dosage forms that imply greater potency than the regular strength of the same brand or the competitor's usual adult strength (usually 500 mg compared with 325 mg of analgesic) product. However, if a more potent drug does not have documented proof of greater effectiveness when compared with an equivalent dose of the second drug, then there is no advantage to a "more potent" medication. When the only difference is drug strength, the therapeutic effect expected with either drug is the same and the potential disadvantages in using a more potent drug may increase costs and side effects and have unknown long-term effects.

CONSUMER EDUCATION FOR OVER-THE-COUNTER DRUGS

Nurses have a major role in the education of consumers for the accurate and safe self-administration of over-the-counter medications. Although many of these medications are also found in care settings where the role of the nurse is to administer such drugs, it is important to maintain a familiarity with OTC medications to best advise clients for safe self-treatment of minor illnesses. The following information about OTC preparations should be shared with clients as an aspect of health promotion, in both formal and informal instructional situations. Such teaching would be applicable in almost any setting in which the nurse has interaction with clients.

Over-the-counter drugs have the image of being very safe and thus not requiring the special precautions necessary to take a prescription drug safely. Nothing could be farther than the truth. These products also have the potential for being misused, abused, and inducing side/adverse effects. They also may be very dangerous if taken in certain concurrent disease states, or if taken concurrently with other drugs, food or alcohol. The health care professional needs to be aware of this information before administering or advising on an OTC preparation.

Product ingredients have either proven or questionable effectiveness; therefore a careful check of ingredients is necessary to select the appropriate product in a specific drug category. Encourage the consumer to select the proper ingredient for treatment of the specific symptom the consumer is experiencing. Combination products may contain substances that are not necessary for the person's symptoms. If the individual has an adverse reaction to the combination drug, it would be difficult to determine the responsible ingredient.

In addition, many different products may also have the same active ingredients that may or may not differ in strength, dosage forms (liquid, tablet, capsule), or with other ingredients in combination. If the ingredients are not carefully checked, accidental overdosing is possible by taking the same ingredient in a number of different products. Another aspect of having the same ingredients is that it may allow for product substitution. For example, thousands of antacid products are available throughout the United States that primarily contain only four or five recognized active ingredients. Thus many OTC antacids are duplicate preparations. The generic product is often as effective as the advertised product; therefore, there is usually little if any advantage in purchasing the more expensive item.

Consumers should check the selected product for tampering. Most products are now packaged in tamper-resistant packaging or tampering-evident packaging, which allows the consumer to detect signs of tampering. If the package is suspect, take it to the pharmacist or store manager. The expiration date should also be checked to ensure that it has not passed.

Consumers should read labels very carefully if they have ever had an allergic or unusual response to any medication, food, or other substance, such as yellow dye or sulfites, to ensure such an ingredient is not included. Caution should be used if the individual is on a special diet, such as low-sugar or low-sodium, because many OTC drugs contain more than their active ingredients, and many liquid preparations contain alcohol. The woman who is pregnant or breastfeeding should not take OTC medications without first consulting her health care provider. Individuals with underlying medical conditions, such as hypertension or diabetes, should read labels carefully to assess whether the medication may be contraindicated with their condition.

Over-the-counter medications are just that, medications. They should be reported to any health care provider when a drug history is being taken. Instructions and warnings on the label are to be followed carefully. If the instructions seem unclear, ask the pharmacist for clarification. If the symptoms for which the OTC drug is being taken are not relieved in an appropriate time interval as indicated on the label, a health care provider should be consulted.

Unless instructed otherwise, store both prescription and OTC medications in closed containers in a cool, dry place, out of the reach of children. Do not store in the bathroom, near sinks, or in damp places because heat, moisture and strong light may cause deterioration or loss of medication potency.

All solid-dose medications (tablets and capsules) should be taken with a full glass of water (8 oz). The individual should be advised to sit up for approximately 15 to 30 minutes after taking the solid-dose medication to help reduce the potential for esophageal irritation or injury. If the person has a problem with dry mouth or minor problems in swallowing, taking a small amount of water before taking a tablet or capsule is very helpful. If the drug is a long-acting medication, it should be swallowed whole. If the medication is in a liquid form, utilize the specially marked measuring spoon or other device provided by the manufacturer to measure each dose accurately.

SELECTED OTC DRUG CATEGORIES

The following is a review of the most commonly purchased OTC drug categories: analgesics, antacids, laxatives, antidiarrheals, and cold-cough preparations. The information will include a review of the ingredients in each category, mechanism of action, indications, pharmacokinetics, warnings, drug interactions, and specific tips on the proper and safe use of the individual product. This information should assist the nurse in identifying and evaluating the multitude of OTC medications on the market. By understanding the basic information presented in this chapter and checking package ingredients, a safer and more logical approach to product selection can be made. However, the nursing management of the client receiving any of these OTC medications will be discussed in the chapters presenting these same drugs in their prescription status.

Analgesics

Pain is one of the most common and feared symptoms known to man. For minor pain such as headache, toothache, muscle and joint aches, swelling (inflammation), and fever, many people can obtain relief fairly inexpensively with an over-the-counter (OTC) medication. **Analgesic** is the term used to describe a drug that relieves pain.

Since OTC analgesics have different therapeutic effects, side effects, drug interactions, and other characteristics, they will be divided into the three major categories available over-the-counter, acetaminophen, aspirin, and the nonsteroidal antiinflammatory drugs (NSAIDs).

acetaminophen (a seat a min' oh fen)
Many brand name products of acetaminophen are available, including Tylenol, Anacin-3, Feverall Sprinkle, Liquiprin, Panadol, and Tempra, to name a few. The mechanism of action for acetaminophen is primarily inhibition of prostaglandin synthesis in the CNS and to a lesser degree blocking the generation of peripheral pain impulses. Acetaminophen is equivalent to aspirin as an analgesic and antipyretic agent but it does not have antiinflammatory effects. Acetaminophen has been used to treat mild forms of arthritis (osteoarthritis), but aspirin or the nonsteroidal antiinflammatory drugs (NSAIDs) are preferred in moderate to severe arthritis, especially rheumatoid arthritis (Box 11-1).

Acetaminophen offers several advantages over aspirin, which include that it may:

- be used by people allergic to aspirin
- rarely cause abdominal upset, tinnitus, or gastric bleeding (inhibition of platelet aggregation) as reported more often with aspirin
- be used by clients taking anticoagulant medications
- be used by children with colds and flu symptoms because it has not been associated with Reye's syndrome as reported with aspirin (see Box 11-2)

Pharmacokinetically, acetaminophen, taken orally, is rapidly absorbed, reaching peak serum levels in 1/2 to 1 hour and its half-life in 2 to 3 hours. It is metabolized in the liver and excreted by the kidneys. Side/adverse effects are rare with acetaminophen, although in some instances nausea and rash have occurred. However, the drug should be discontinued and a health care provider contacted immediately if an allergic type reaction (hives, pruritus, respiratory difficulties); or blood in the urine or stool; or a severe pain in the side or lower back, or unusual bleeding, bruising, weakness or tiredness occur.

Acetaminophen overdose can cause serious damage to the liver and kidneys. See Chapter 14 for management of an acetaminophen overdose. The maximum acetaminophen dose per day for adults is 4 g/day; for children, the single dose is 40 to 480 mg depending on age and weight but no more than 5 doses should be given in 24 hours (Insel, 1996).

Prescription and nonprescription drug interactions with acetaminophen include:

Drug	Possible effect and management
alcohol	Increased possibility of hepatotoxicity, especially in persons who regularly drink large amounts of alcoholic beverages, or if more acetaminophen is taken than recommended on the label, or if acetaminophen is taken over a long period. Avoid alcoholic beverages when taking acetaminophen.
anticoagulants such as warfarin (Coumadin) and heparin	High doses and frequent use of acetaminophen may increase anticoagulant action of these drugs, increasing the risk of bleeding. Occasional use of acetaminophen in persons taking anticoagulants is usually not a problem.
prescription drugs containing acetaminophen, such as Tylenol with codeine, Darvocet, Percocet, and others	Combined use may result in an acetaminophen overdose. See Chapter 14 for symptoms and treatment of an acetaminophen overdose.
other OTC drugs that contain acetaminophen	Use of two or more OTC products containing acetaminophen may result in acetaminophen overdose.

Box 11-2 describes acetaminophen and aspirin OTC warnings.

Over-the-counter acetaminophen is available in powder, tablet, chewable tablet, liquid, drops, and suppository dosage forms. The usual adult dose is 325 to 650 mg every 4 hours, or 325 to 500 mg every 3 hours, or 650 to 1000 mg every 6 hours when needed. The usual pediatric dose is 10 to 15 mg/kg every 4 to 6 hours as needed.

BOX 11-1

Common Types of Arthritis

Osteoarthritis or degenerative joint disease affects 85% of persons over 70 years old, although symptoms may start in the fifth or sixth decade of life. This common form of arthritis is the result of deformation or mismatched joint surfaces rather than an inflammatory disease as in rheumatoid arthritis. Symptoms include joint stiffness that usually lasts only a few minutes after initiating joint movement, and perhaps an aching pain in weight-bearing joints. Early disease stages may respond to local heat and nonprescription analgesics. Later stages may require orthopedic or other interventions.

Rheumatoid arthritis usually occurs between 30 to 70 years of age, more often in women than men. Early symptoms may include feelings of fatigue and weakness, joint pain and stiffness, and several weeks later, joint swelling. Joints are inflamed (warm, red, swollen) and often are limited in range of motion. This is a progressive disease that leads to joint deformity. Aspirin and aspirin type products (NSAIDs) are usually necessary to reduce the inflammation around the joints. Heat therapy, weight control, and exercise may also be helpful.

Acetaminophen Combinations

Analgesic combinations of acetaminophen with other ingredients are also available over-the-counter. At one time, combination products were thought to be stronger because of the extra ingredients, and also to have fewer side effects because the dose of each ingredient was usually less than the full dose of a single ingredient alone. This reasoning is outdated and highly questionable today. Most combination products offer little advantage over acetaminophen or aspirin alone.

The more common combinations include acetaminophen with salicylates (aspirin, salicylamide); combined with a salicylate and caffeine; or with an antacid (sodium bicarbonate, calcium carbonate, or "buffered"). Box 11-3 lists acetaminophen and aspirin formulations.

Salicylates, salicylamide, and aspirin are from the salicylate drug family, thus they have analgesic, antipyretic, and antiinflammatory effects. The antiinflammatory effect depends on the amount of salicylates in the product, but because the combination dosages of aspirin are usually low, they are not recommended to treat severe inflammation or severe arthritic pain.

BOX 11-2

Acetaminophen and Aspirin OTC Warnings

General precautions for both analgesics

Consult with prescriber before taking any analgesic if the person reports they are allergic to an analgesic or have had a severe allergic analgesic reaction such as asthma, swelling, hives, rash, and other symptoms.

Avoid taking analgesics if the individual has kidney disease, liver damage, is pregnant or breastfeeding, has taken the analgesics for more than 10 days for pain in an adult or 5 days in a child or 3 days for fever, if pain increases or painful site is inflamed, if new symptoms develop, or sore throat is very painful or lasts more than 2 days.

If stomach distress occurs, take analgesic after meals or with food.

Aspirin

Special dosing information

- Children and teenagers (under age of 17 years old) should avoid aspirin use for fever or symptoms of a viral infection, especially flu or chickenpox, without prescriber approval. The use of aspirin in viral illnesses may cause a very serious condition known as Reye's syndrome in children. Symptoms include severe vomiting, weakness, stupor that may progress into coma, convulsions, and even death.
- Stop aspirin use at least 5 to 7 days before a scheduled surgery.
- Never put aspirin products directly on a tooth or gum surface, as they can burn the tissues and cause injury.
- Avoid consumption of aspirin that has a strong, vinegar-like odor, because the odor indicates the aspirin is deteriorating.

The prescriber should be informed about an individual who has aspirin or salicylate allergy, asthma, nasal polyps, anemia, gout, ulcers or ulcer symptoms, or hemophilia or other bleeding problems.

Salicylamide is also considered to be much less effective than either acetaminophen or aspirin. In addition, the Food and Drug Administration (FDA) has stated that salicylamide lacks documented proof of being effective as an analgesic or antipyretic.

Caffeine and analgesic combinations may enhance or produce a better pain relief effect than the individual analgesic

BOX 11-3

Acetaminophen and/or Aspirin Formulations*

- Acetaminophen with salicylates
  - acetaminophen with salicylates (Gemnisyn)
  - acetaminophen and salicylamide (Duoprin)
- Acetaminophen with aspirin/salicylate and caffeine
  - acetaminophen, aspirin, salicylamide, and caffeine (Saleto; Tri-pain)
  - acetaminophen, aspirin, and caffeine (Goody's Extra Strength Tablets; Duradyne; Excedrin Extra-strength)
  - acetaminophen, salicylamide, and caffeine (Rid-A-Pain Compound; S-A-C)
- Aspirin/salicylates combined with caffeine
  - aspirin and caffeine (Anacin, Instantine, Nervine, 217 Strong, McNess Pain Tablets)
- Acetaminophen combinations with antacid
  - buffered acetaminophen, aspirin, and caffeine (Gelpirin; Supac; Buffets; Vanquish)
  - buffered acetaminophen, aspirin, and salicylamide (Presalin)
  - acetaminophen, sodium bicarbonate, and citric acid (Bromo-Seltzer)
  - acetaminophen with calcium carbonate (Extra Strength Tylenol)
- Aspirin/salicylates with antacid (buffering agents)
  - aspirin, sodium bicarbonate, citric acid (Alka-Seltzer Original, Alka-Seltzer Flavored, Alka-Seltzer Extra Strength†)
  - aspirin, aluminum hydroxide, magnesium hydroxide (Arthritis Pain Formula, Magnaprin, Maprin)
  - aspirin, calcium carbonate, magnesium carbonate, magnesium oxide (Bayer Plus Buffered Aspirin and Bayer Plus, Extra Strength Buffered Aspirin)
  - aspirin, magnesium oxide (Buffaprin, Buffaprin Extra, Buffasal, Buffasal Max, Buffinol)
  - aspirin, calcium carbonate, magnesium oxide, magnesium carbonate (Bufferin Tri-Buffered, Bufferin Arthritis Extra Strength, Tri-Buffered)
- Enteric-coated or delayed-release aspirin (Ecotrin, Bayer 8-hour, Extra Strength Bayer Caplets, etc.)

*Extra strength usually refers to 500 mg analgesic as compared with 325 mg in regular strength products.
†Primary difference between the Alka-Seltzer products is taste and 500 mg aspirin in the extra strength product compared with 325 mg in the other two products.

alone. Although some studies report the caffeine-analgesic combination may provide better pain relieving effects, the FDA indicates that sufficient proof is lacking for this effect (*USP DI*, 1996).

The addition of an antacid buffer to acetaminophen or aspirin is also of questionable benefit. If acetaminophen causes little if any stomach upset then the addition of an antacid is unnecessary. If the purpose is to avoid gastric distress caused by the other ingredients (aspirin or salicylates), this is also questionable because studies have indicated that there is no difference between buffered and unbuffered tablets in the production of gastric damage. It appears that the amount of antacid or buffering agent added in the tablets may not be in sufficient quantities to produce this effect.

If the buffer hastens drug dissolution, then a more rapid absorption of the analgesic may occur, which is why the effervescent antacid preparations (Alka Seltzer, Bromo Seltzer, etc.) are more rapidly absorbed. In general, liquid dosage forms of medication are faster and better absorbed. Evidence is lacking, however, that such products produce a more rapid or more effective analgesia than the tablet dosage form, especially when the tablets or capsules are taken with a full glass of water (8 oz). The nurse should also be aware that effervescent medications usually contain a large amount of sodium, which must be avoided in persons with cardiac problems or renal failure (Lipman, 1996).

In summary, combination analgesic products are no more effective and are often more expensive than taking either acetaminophen or aspirin alone. The health care provider should also be aware that acetaminophen is often included in numerous products that contain more than one ingredient, such as cold, cough, allergy, menstrual or premenstrual, and sleeping aid products.

▲ **aspirin** (as' pir in)

Aspirin available over the counter includes ASA, acetylsalicylic acid, Bayer, Ecotrin, Norwich, St Joseph, and many other commercial products. The mechanism of action for aspirin and the NSAIDs is inhibition of prostaglandin synthesis in both the CNS and periphery. See Chapter 14 for additional analgesic and NSAID information.

Aspirin has analgesic, antipyretic, antiplatelet and antiinflammatory effects. It is indicated for the treatment of pain, fever, rheumatic fever, rheumatoid arthritis and osteoarthritis, and for the prevention of myocardial infarction or reinfarction and prevention of platelet aggregation in ischemia and thromboembolism. The advantages of aspirin over acetaminophen include its antiinflammatory effects and its effectiveness in preventing myocardial infarction and thrombi.

Pharmacokinetically, aspirin in tablets for oral administration is rapidly absorbed, reaching peak serum level within 1 to 2 hours or more rapidly with liquid preparations; the peak antirheumatic effect occurs in 2 to 3 weeks. Tissue and blood esterases hydrolyze aspirin to acetic acid and salicylate; salicylates are then metabolized in the liver and excreted primarily by the kidneys.

Common side/adverse effects include stomach irritation, cramps or discomfort, heartburn or indigestion, and nausea or vomiting. Taking aspirin with a full glass of water helps to reduce these effects. Less common or rare adverse effects include severe abdominal pain, blood in stools, tinnitus, hematemesis, allergic reaction, confusion, weakness, flushing, visual disturbances, severe nausea or vomiting, and gastric ulcers. See the box on p. 260 in Chapter 14 for clinical management of aspirin overdose. Prescription and OTC drug interactions with aspirin include:

Drug	Possible effect and management
alcohol, NSAIDs, and corticosteroids	Increased risk of GI side effects, such as irritation, bleeding and ulceration. Avoid taking aspirin concurrently with these substances.
anticoagulants, such as warfarin (Coumadin), heparin; thrombolytic agents such as carbenicillin (Geopen), cefamandole (Mandol), cefoperazone (Cefobid), cefotetan (Cefotan), plicamycin (Mithracin), ticarcillin (Ticar), and anticonvulsants, such as divalproex (Depakote), valproic acid (Depakene)	Can increase anticoagulant effects, resulting in increased risk of bleeding and hemorrhage. Avoid taking aspirin concurrently with these drugs.
antidiabetic drugs, oral	May increase therapeutic and side effects of the antidiabetic agents, especially when large doses of aspirin/salicylates are taken. Avoid taking aspirin/salicylates concurrently.
furosemide (Lasix)	Increased risk for hearing loss, especially if high doses of aspirin or salicylates are consumed routinely. Limited, in termittent use may not be problematic.
methotrexate (Mexate)	May increase methotrexate plasma levels, leading to severe systemic toxic effects. Avoid taking salicylates while taking this drug.
probenecid (Benemid), sulfinpyrazone (Anturan)	Concurrent administration de creases the effect of antigout medications. Avoid use of aspirin or salicylates if taking these medications.
vancomycin (Vancocin)	Increased potential for hearing loss, which can progress to deafness. Avoid taking aspirin/salicylates concurrently with vancomycin.
Antacid analgesic combinations: The same drug interactions as listed above plus:	
bismuth subsalicylate (Pepto Bismol)	Taking large, repeated dosages of this product with frequent use of aspirin products increases the risk of toxicity (overdose). If taking this product for traveler's diarrhea or chronic diarrhea, be careful or avoid taking additional aspirin-containing products.

Drug	Possible effect and management
Antacid analgesic combinations—cont'd	
bulk-forming laxatives (Metamucil, Perdiem, and others)	If taken with aspirin/salicylate products, they may reduce the absorption and effect of aspirin/salicylates. Take these products 2 hours apart.
ketoconazole (Nizoral)	Antacids or buffering agents may increase stomach acidity, which reduces the absorption and effectiveness of keto conazole. Buffered aspirin products should be taken at least 3 hours before or after ketoconazole.
oral tetracycline (Achromycin V)	Antacids and the magnesium in some salicylate medications can interfere with absorption of the tetracyclines. To re duce this effect, take the as pirin/salicylate preparation 3 to 4 hours apart from the tetracycline.
Enteric-coated aspirin products, in addition to the interactions noted above, may also interact with:	
antacids or H_2-blocking agents such as cimetidine (Tagamet), ranitidine (Zantac), nizatidine (Axid), and famotidine (Pepcid)	The increase in gastric pH pro duced by these drugs may cause enteric-coated tablets to dissolve early, thus losing the benefit of the enteric coating in the stomach.
Caffeine in analgesic medications, in addition to the interactions noted above, the following may occur:	
other caffeine products, appetite suppressants, theophylline, pemoline (Cylert), selegiline (Eldepryl), tranylcy-promine (Parnate), fluox-etine (Prozac), methyl-phenidate (Ritalin), sertra-line (Zoloft), and sympatho-mimetics in oral, inhaler, and injectable dosage forms	An increase in CNS stimulation effects occur, such as nervousness, tremors, increased irritability, insomnia, and possibly cardiac arrhythmias. Reducing or avoiding caffeine-containing products can reduce this effect.
lithium	Caffeine may increase lithium excretion from the body, which results in a reduction of lithium effects. Reduce or avoid use of caffeine-containing products.
monoamine oxidase inhibitors (MAO) such as tranylcy-promine (Parnate), procar-bazine (Matulane), and possibly selegiline (Eldepryl)	May result in an increase in CNS stimulating effects (see above), hypertension, and dangerous cardiac arrhythmias. Avoid use of large amounts of caffeine-containing products.

Aspirin products are available in tablet, chewable tablets, chewing gum tablets, extended-release tablets, and suppository dosage forms. The usual adult dose is one to two regular strength tablets (325 to 650 mg) every 4 hours or 500 to 1000 mg (extra-strength) every 6 hours as needed. The adult maximum OTC aspirin dose per day is 4 g/day. The pediatric dose is 1.5 g/m^2/daily, in 4 to 6 divided doses. Check package labels for further dosing information.

Aspirin Combinations

Pain-relieving combinations of aspirin with other ingredients are available without a prescription. Aspirin/salicylates have been combined with acetaminophen, caffeine, and antacids (buffering agents) like acetaminophen, and therefore the same comments from acetaminophen apply to aspirin. For examples of acetaminophen and aspirin formulations see Box 11-3.

Nonsteroidal Antiinflammatory Drugs (NSAIDs)

Nonsteroidal antiinflammatory drugs (NSAIDS) and aspirin have analgesic, antipyretic, and antiinflammatory effects. Unlike aspirin, NSAIDS were all prescription drugs before approval by the FDA for the change to OTC status. Currently, ibuprofen (Advil, Motrin IB, etc.), naproxen (Aleve), and ketoprofen (Actron, Orudis KT) are available over-the-counter, with manufacturers of other NSAIDs expected to seek OTC approval in the near future.

The difference between the prescription and OTC medication is the strength of the product. For example, prescription strengths for ibuprofen are 300 mg, 600 mg, and 800 mg tablets, while the OTC product is 200 mg. Naproxen prescription strengths are 250 mg, 375 mg, and 500 mg tablets, while the OTC product is 200 mg. Ketoprofen prescription strengths are 25 mg, 50 mg, 75 mg, and a 200 mg extended release dosage form, while the OTC product is 12.5 mg. As mentioned previously, OTC strengths are considered to be safe and effective for consumer use without professional supervision, assuming the label instructions and warnings are closely followed. The higher strength products are prescription medications in the United States because of their potential side/adverse effects.

The mechanism of action for NSAIDs is inhibition of cyclooxygenase, which results in a decrease synthesis of prostaglandins. The decrease in prostaglandins may be responsible for both therapeutic and adverse effects associated with this drug category. For additional information see Chapter 14, Analgesics.

Pharmacokinetics. Ibuprofen, naproxen, and ketoprofen are well absorbed orally, although concurrent food and antacids may decrease absorption. The onset of action is ½ hour for ibuprofen, 1 hour for naproxen, and unknown for ketoprofen. The peak effect for ibuprofen is 1 to 2 hours; ketoprofen, ½ to 2 hours; and naproxen 2 to 4 hrs. The duration of action is 6 hours for ibuprofen, up to 7 hours for naproxen, and not available for ketoprofen (Olin, 1996; *USP DI,* 1996). Metabolism of NSAIDs is primarily hepatic with excretion by the kidneys.

The side/adverse effects of NSAIDs are primarily GI distress (nausea, vomiting, diarrhea, cramps, gas), gastric ulcers, and bleeding. For additional side/adverse effects and drug interactions, see Chapter 14, Analgesics. Box 11-4 describes over-the-counter NSAID warnings.

The usual adult ibuprofen dose is one (200 mg) tablet every 4 to 6 hours when necessary. If the pain or fever does not respond to one tablet, two may be taken but the maximum is 6 tablets in 24 hours without prescriber approval.

BOX 11-4

Nonsteroidal Antiinflammatory OTC Drug Warnings

General precautions

With NSAIDs, contact the prescriber if the person reports they had a severe allergic reaction to any analgesic, such as asthma, swelling, hives, rash, or any other reaction, since the NSAIDs are capable of causing similar reactions.

- Avoid taking NSAIDs with any other OTC analgesics (acetaminophen, aspirin, or other NSAIDs).
- Avoid taking these products for more than 10 days for pain, 3 days for fever, if painful area is inflamed, if pregnant or breastfeeding, if new symptoms occur or current symptoms worsen, or if abdominal pain occurs. Contact prescriber for advice.
- Do not use NSAIDs during the last 3 months of pregnancy because it may adversely affect the fetus or result in complications during delivery.
- Alcohol (especially 3 or more drinks daily) and many other medications may result in adverse drug interactions. Review all medications with the prescriber or pharmacist before taking an NSAID.

The usual adult ketoprofen dose is one (12.5 mg) tablet every 4 to 6 hours. If pain or fever is not improved within an hour, a second dose may be taken. Do not take more than 2 tablets in any 4-to-6 hour period nor more than 6 doses in 24 hours. Do not administer to children under 16 years of age.

The usual adult naproxen dose is one (200 mg) tablet every 8 to 12 hours when necessary. Some persons may need 2 tablets initially and then one 12 hours later. Do not take more than 3 tablets in 24 hours. The elderly should not take more than 2 tablets in 12 hours and children under 12 should not take this product.

ANTACIDS

Various medical conditions, overeating, or eating certain foods may result in stomach upset, gas, heartburn, and indigestion. **Antacids,** drugs that buffer, neutralize, or absorb hydrochloric acid in the stomach, are commonly used for these conditions. Americans have been estimated to spend one billion dollars annually on antacids (Cornacchia & Barrett, 1993). For additional information on antacids, see Chapter 41. Antacids buffer or neutralize hydrochloric acid in the stomach, increasing gastric pH. The major ingredients in antacids include aluminum salts, calcium carbonate, magnesium salts, magaldrate (aluminum-magnesium combination), and sodium bicarbonate. Simethicone may be added to these preparations as a defoaming or antigas agent.

Antacids generally have a rapid onset of action. A small amount of absorbable antacid is absorbed systemically (15% to 30%), but the remainder is broken down via the digestive process and excreted in feces. Table 11-2 lists side effects/adverse reactions. Long-term use of antacids or their use in the presence of impaired renal function may result in increased adverse effects from metal ion absorption, especially of calcium carbonate or magnesium hydroxide.

Dosage and administration. The amount of antacid necessary to neutralize hydrochloric acid depends on the individual, the condition being treated, and the buffering capability of the preparation used. The acid-neutralizing property of antacids varies for the individual client. Antacids taken before meals have a duration of action of approximately 30 minutes. If the antacid is taken after meals, the duration may be prolonged up to 3 hours. Duodenal ulcer, Zollinger-Ellison syndrome, and other hypersecretory conditions may require 80 to 160 mEq of acid-neutralizing effect per dose (*USP DI,* 1996); for pain relief, the dose of antacids should provide 40 to 80 mEq neutralizing effect (Table 11-3) (Pinson & Weart, 1996). Antacids are not very effective for the treatment of gastric ulcers (Brunton, 1996).

Liquid and powder dosage forms have been found to be more effective antacids than the tablet dosage formulations. Most tablets require chewing before swallowing to be effective. The majority of antacids contain 10 mg or less of sodium per recommended adult dose. Clients on sodium restricted diets should read ingredient listings carefully. Examples of antacids containing more than 10 mg per recommended adult dose (Pinson & Weart, 1996) include:

Alka-Seltzer Extra Strength	588 mg sodium/tablet
Alka-Seltzer Original	567 mg sodium/tablet
Bell/ans	144 mg/tablet

The maximum dosages listed on antacid packages should be followed. Many individuals exceed the (FDA) recommendations, thus increasing the potential for producing many of the potential side effects or adverse reactions.

Pregnancy safety. Antacids are generally considered safe for use in pregnancy if prolonged or high doses are avoided.

Antacid Combinations

While there are numerous antacid preparations on the market, the magnesium-aluminum combinations are the most common antacids selected by individuals and health care professionals alike, e.g., Gelusil, Maalox and Mylanta. Antacid recommendation should be based on its ingredients relative to the client's health status. Combination antacids have been formulated to reduce the risk of diarrhea or constipation as a side effect. However, the antacid combination Gaviscon deserves particular attention because of its uniqueness and widespread use.

antacid combination plus alginic acid (Gaviscon)
Gaviscon forms a viscous cohesive foam that floats on the surface of the stomach contents, neutralizing stomach acid. This helps to protect the sensitive mucosa from irritation, because the foam precedes the stomach contents into the lower esophagus when reflux occurs. The foam is caused by

TABLE 11-2 Antacid side effects/adverse reactions

Name	Side effects/adverse reactions*
Aluminum	Constipation (combination products with magnesium reduce this)
aluminum carbonate (Basaljel)	Phosphate depletion via feces (including weakness, apnea, hemolytic anemia, tetany)
aluminum hydroxide (AlternaGEL, Alu-Cap, Amphojel)	Delay in gastric emptying
	Concretions (intestinal and renal)
	Encephalopathy from aluminum intoxication
aluminum/magnesium compounds (Aludrox, Gaviscon, Maalox, Mylanta)	Bone demineralization (osteomalacia, osteoporosis)
Bicarbonate	Systemic alkalosis or sodium overload (elevated plasma pH and carbon dioxide, anorexia, mental confusion)
sodium bicarbonate (Alka-Seltzer, Instant Metamucil)	Gastric acid hypersecretion ("acid rebound")
	Enhanced effects of amphetamines, quinidine, quinine
Calcium	Milk-alkali syndrome (including metabolic alkalosis, anorexia, nausea, vomiting, confusion, hypercalcemia, possibly renal impairment)
calcium carbonate (Tums)	Increased potential for calcium stone formation
	Nephrocalcinosis
	Gastric acid hypersecretion ("acid rebound")
	Antagonism of digitalis preparations
	Elevated serum and urine calcium levels
	Kidney failure
	Constipation
	Decreased phosphate levels (if dietary phosphate intake low)
Magnesium	Diarrhea (combination products with aluminum reduce this)
magnesium hydroxide (Milk of Magnesia)	Decreased potassium levels (hypokalemia)
magnesium trisilicate	Increased magnesum levels (hypermagnesemia) in clients with renal failure or severe kidney impairment (causing low blood pressure, nausea, vomiting, respiratory depression, CNS depression, coma)
Sodium	Sodium overload or systemic alkalosis
sodium bicarbonate	Salt and water retention (causing edema, ascites, effusion, hypertension)
	Metabolic alkalosis
	Milk-alkali syndrome (see under calcium)
	Gastric acid hypersecretion ("acid rebound")

*Chronic, high-dose usage.

the alginic acid contained in the product; the other ingredients are aluminum hydroxide, magnesium trisilicate, and sodium bicarbonate.

Antiflatulents

simethicone [si meth' i kone] (Mylicon, Silain, Orol♣)
Simethicone, a defoaming agent, relieves flatulence by dispersing and preventing the formation of mucus-surrounded gas pockets in the gastrointestinal tract. Gas retention is a problem in conditions such as air swallowing, diverticulitis, functional dyspepsia, peptic ulcer, postoperative gaseous distention, and spastic or irritable colon.

The tablets are taken four times daily, chewed thoroughly after meals and at bedtime, and as needed for flatulence. Antacid liquid combination products also often contain simethicone.

LAXATIVES

Laxatives, drugs given to induce defecation, may be classified according to their source, site of action, degree of action, or mechanism of action. Figure 11-1 and Table 11-4 summarize the traditional laxatives that can be bought without a prescription.

One of the major indications for the use of laxatives is constipation. **Constipation** is difficult fecal evacuation as a result of hard stool and perhaps infrequent movements. The primary causes of constipation are reviewed in Chapter 41. Failure to respond to the normal defecation impulse, insufficient time to permit the bowel to produce an evacuation, inadequate fluid and dietary fiber intake, sedentary habits and insufficient exercise may be factors. Constipation is also a side effect of many medications, such as antacids, diuretics,

TABLE 11-3 Antacids: acid-neutralizing capacity

Antacid	Primary ingredients	Acid neutralizing capacity	Dose to neutralize 80 mEq HCl
Liquid Preprations		**mEq/5 ml**	**ml needed**
Gelusil	aluminum hydroxide, magnesium hydroxide, simethicone	12	33
Maalox	aluminum hydroxide, magnesium hydroxide	13.3	30
Maalox Plus			
Extra Strength	aluminum hydroxide, magnesium hydroxide, simethicone	29	14
Mylanta	aluminum hydroxide, magnesium hydroxide, simethicone	12.7	31
Mylanta Double Strength	aluminum hydroxide, magnesium hydroxide, simethicone	25.4	16
Riopan Plus Susp	magaldrate, simethicone	15	27
Tablet Preparations		**mEq/tablet**	**Tablets approx. needed**
Gelusil	aluminum hydroxide, magnesium hydroxide, simethicone	11	7
Maalox	aluminum hydroxide, magnesium hydroxide	8.5	9
Maalox Plus	same as Maalox plus simethicone	10.6	7
Mylanta	aluminum hydroxide, magnesium hydroxide, simethicone	11.5	7
Mylanta Gelcaps	same as above, double strength	23	3.5
Riopan Plus	magaldrate, simethicone	13.5	6
Rolaids	calcium carbonate, magnesium hydroxide	7.5	10.5
Tums	calcium carbonate	10	8

From *USP DI*, 1996.

morphine, tricyclic antidepressants, codeine, aluminum hydroxide, and anticholinergics.

In addition to constipation, laxatives may be administered within a health care agency setting for a variety of purposes, such as preparation for surgery, in cases of food and drug poisoning, and to promote the elimination of an offending substance from the gastrointestinal tract. Saline cathartics are considered useful for this purpose. **Perceived constipation** is a nursing diagnosis, the state in which an individual makes a self-diagnosis of constipation and ensures a daily bowel movement through use of laxatives, enemas, and suppositories. In this instance, laxatives may be misused and abused to meet the client's perception of a normal bowel elimination pattern. Consumer education should be focused on the lifestyle changes necessary to promote a normal bowel elimination pattern for those with constipation and perceived constipation.

Laxatives are also used to keep the stool soft when it is essential to avoid the irritation or straining that accompanies the passage of a hardened stool. This indication might include: rectal disorders, irritated polyps in the bowel, hemorrhoidectomy, and perianal abscess; or the recovery phase of a myocardial infarction, cerebrovascular accident, or the repair of a hernia. Saline laxatives are routinely used to expel parasites and toxic anthelmintics and to secure a stool specimen to be examined for parasites.

Laxatives should not be taken if the individual is experiencing undiagnosed abdominal pain because this may be due to an inflammatory disorder of the alimentary tract, such as appendicitis, typhoid fever, and chronic ulcerative colitis. If the pain is caused by an inflamed appendix, a laxative may bring about a rupture of the appendix by increasing intestinal peristalsis. Laxatives should be taken with caution after some operations, such as repair of the perineum or rectum (at least for a time); during pregnancy and breastfeeding; by clients with severe anemia, and by debilitated clients. Other conditions in which caution is needed include chronic and spastic constipation.

Because constipation is common in children, parents need to be informed about problems associated with indiscriminate use of laxatives (Box 11-5). In children, emotions, environmental changes (new home, new school, new friends), dietary changes, and febrile illnesses may all contribute to or cause constipation. Adding or increasing fluids, vegetables, fruits, and bran products may be very helpful. Malt soup extract is often suggested for infants up to 2 months old. For older children, glycerin suppositories or docusate sodium may be appropriate.

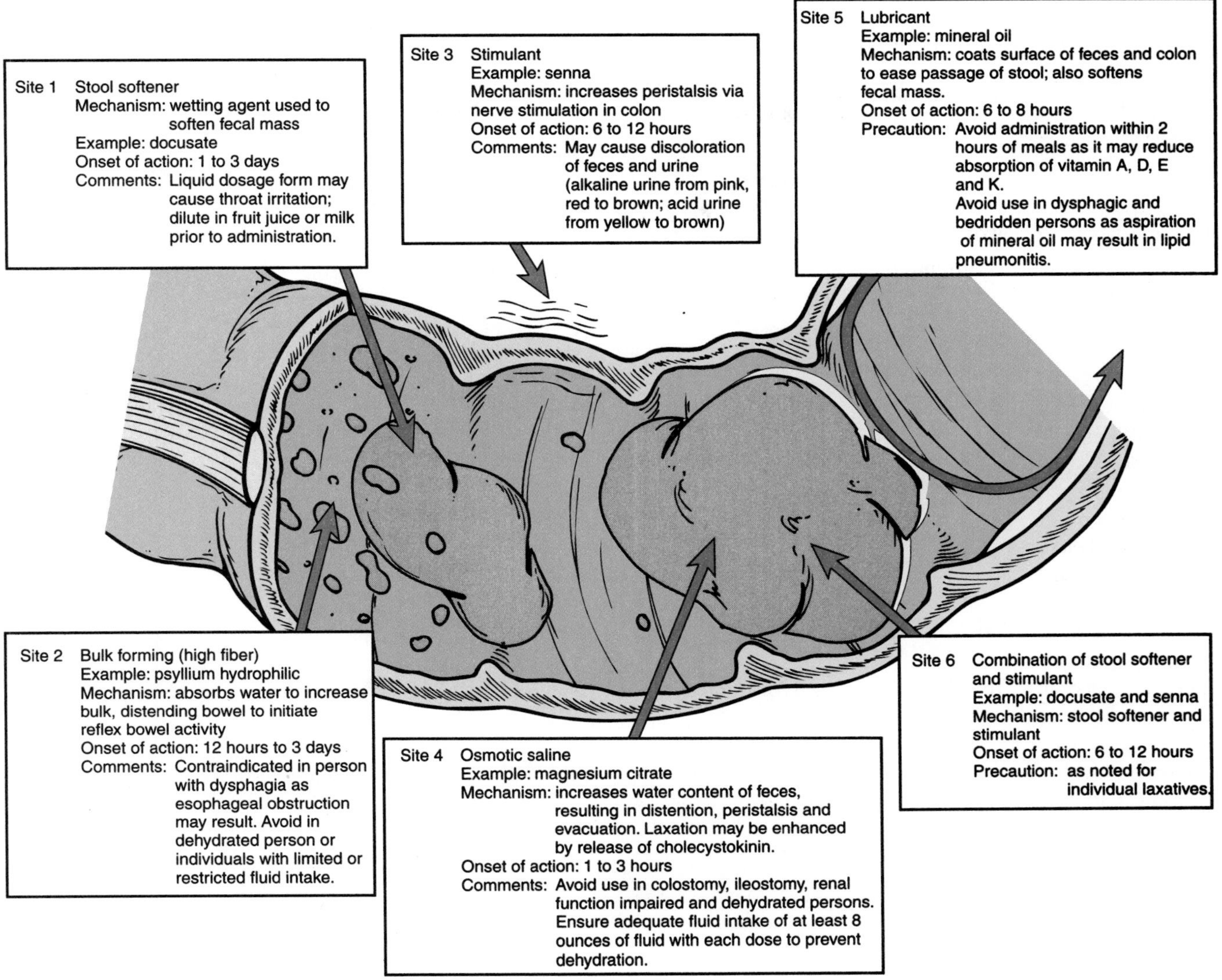

Figure 11-1 Classification of laxatives according to site of action.

The elderly may have an increased incidence of constipation because of multiple illnesses that require a variety of medications, the aging process with its associated decline in physiologic functions, plus a progressive decrease in physical activity (see the box on Geriatric Implications on p. 197). An increase in fluid intake, a moderate exercise program if permitted, and an increase in intake of bran products, vegetables, and fruit will help to correct this problem. Laxative abuse is often reported with this age group (see Box 11-5). Because there may be many factors contributing to constipation, a complete and thorough history by the health care professional is necessary.

Constipation is commonly reported during pregnancy. It is usually caused by colon compression as a result of the increase in the size of the uterus or a decrease in muscle tone and peristalsis. Vitamins containing iron and calcium are often prescribed for pregnant women, and such products also tend to be constipating. Laxatives used in pregnancy should be limited to emollients or bulk-forming laxatives. Most of the other laxatives have the potential for undesirable effects; for example, castor oil may induce premature labor, mineral oil may decrease absorption of fat-soluble vitamins, and osmotic agents may induce dangerous electrolyte alterations. Advise the childbearing woman about proper diet, adequate fluid intake, appropriate exercise programs, and the importance of discussing the problem with her nurse-midwife or physician.

For additional information on the nursing management of laxative therapy, see Chapter 41.

Saline Laxatives

The saline laxatives are soluble salts that are only slightly absorbed from the alimentary canal. Because of their osmotic effect of drawing water in the small intestine, they retain and

TABLE 11-4 Laxatives: over-the-counter varieties

	Stimulant (contact)	Osmotic saline	Stool softener surfactant or wetting agent	High-fiber and bulk-forming	Lubricant
Disadvantages with repeated frequent (long-term) administration	Watery stools, gripping	Watery stools, cramps	Unreliable results, may contribute to liver toxicity	Obstruction of narrowed lumen, some difficulty in chewing and swallowing	Anal leakage, lipid pneumonia
Increases rate of transit in small bowel	Yes	Yes	Yes	Yes	Unknown
Causes net secretion of water and electrolytes in small bowel	Yes	Yes	Yes	Yes	No
Inhibits absorption in small bowel	Yes	Yes	Yes	Yes	Yes
Increases mucosal permeability in small bowel	Yes	Not studied	Yes	Not reported	Not reported
Causes mucosal damage in small bowel	Yes	Not studied	Yes	Not reported	Not reported
Acts only in colon (not small bowel)	No	No	No	No	Yes
Indicated for long-term treatment	No	No	No	Probably	No
Examples of type	anthraquinone, bisacodyl, phenolphthalein, castor oil, danthron	magnesium salts, MOM, sodium salts, glycerin	DSS, DCS Polomaxer 188	methylcellulose, karaya gum, sodium CMC, malt soup extract, psyllium seed, agar, plantago bran (unprocessed), polycarbophil	mineral oil
Physical or chemical property responsible for action	Mucosal surface irritation to stimulate or increase intestinal motor function or activity	Hyperosmolar ingredients trap water in intestinal lumen; hypertonicity of colon increases liquid in colon; hyperosmotic or saline	Changes surface tension of fecal mass, provides increased penetration of colonic water; penetrates and softens fecal mass by wetting agents	Absorbs water on surface, increases soft fecal mass, adds bulk and moisture to feces causing distention and elimination	Coats over fecal mass, passes with ease, lubricates gastrointestinal tract and softens feces

BOX 11-5

Laxative Abuse

Regular or excessive use of laxatives usually leads to laxative abuse. This syndrome takes several years to develop and is often undiagnosed. It is often reported among the elderly. Laxative abuse may occur in conjunction with eating disorders, such as bulimia or anorexia. Symptoms are similar to other disease states, such as nephritis, diabetes insipidus, ulcerative colitis, or Addison's disease. The major complaints on hospital admission are diarrhea and abdominal cramps. More often than not, clients deny excessive laxative usage.

If chronic laxative abuse is not detected and the client is not weaned off the laxative, permanent bowel damage, osteomalacia, and electrolyte imbalance may occur.

increase the water content of feces. The water in the intestinal lumen produces fluid accumulation and distention, leading to peristalsis and eventual evacuation of bowel contents. The result is a fecal mass of liquid or semiliquid stools. The laxative effect may be enhanced by the intestinal release of cholecystokinin (CCK). Diarrhea is created in the small intestine to overcome constipation in the colon. Laxation may result in 30 minutes to 3 hours.

The saline laxatives are the laxative of choice for securing a stool specimen for examination, for fecal impaction, for use with certain anthelmintics, and in some cases of food and drug poisoning.

Phosphate enemas are useful as preparations for a barium enema. When the object is merely to empty the intestine, magnesium sulfate, sodium phosphate, or milk of magnesia is effective. Milk of magnesia (magnesium hydroxide) is the mildest of the salines and is often the cathartic of choice for children. The sodium salts are contraindicated for those on a sodium restricted diet. The magnesium and potassium salts are contraindicated in clients with renal disease.

The intestinal membrane is not entirely impermeable to the passage of saline laxatives. Electrolyte disturbances have been reported with their long-term daily use. Some saline laxatives find their way into the general circulation only to be excreted by the kidney, in which case they act as saline diuretics. Hypertonic saline solutions in the bowel may result in so much fluid loss that little or no diuretic effect will be possible. Some saline laxatives contain up to 1 g or more of sodium per dose. Some ions may have a toxic effect in impaired renal function if they accumulate in the blood in sufficient quantity. This may occur with magnesium ions if a solution is retained in the intestine for a long time or if the client suffers from renal impairment. Magnesium acts as a depressant of the central nervous system and neuromuscular activity.

Dosage and administration. The following salts, when taken for their laxative effect, are usually taken orally. Some of them may be given rectally as an enema. The salts tend to

Geriatric Implications

Nonpharmacologic laxative therapy

The elderly often use and/or abuse laxatives because they believe that regularity implies a daily bowel movement (Ahronheim, 1992). The nursing diagnosis of perceived constipation is a common finding in the elderly.

To reduce the potential for chronic laxative use and/or dependency, the client should be taught nonpharmacologic measures, such as encouraging an increase in fluid intake to 6 to 8 glasses of water/day if permitted and tolerated. Also recommended is a regular exercise routine, such as a daily walk or active and passive exercise for bedridden clients.

The nurse should obtain a dietary and laxative history from the client. Consistent intake of low-fiber diets or a regular intake of foods that tends to harden stools, such as processed cheese, hard-boiled eggs, liver, cottage cheese, high sugar content foods and rice, may result in constipation.

High-fiber or high-residue diets along with adequate fluid intake serves to accelerate food transport time in the gastrointestinal tract and exert a mild laxative effect.

High-fiber foods include orange juice with pulp or a fresh orange, bran or whole grain cereals, whole grain or bran breads, leafy vegetables, and fresh fruits. While prunes, bananas, figs, and dates are high in dietary fiber, prunes also contain a laxative substance that stimulates intestinal motility pharmacologically.

Avoid fiber supplements in nonambulatory clients or those who are on restricted or limited fluid intake. Bulk or fiber laxatives are also contraindicated in fecal impaction.

have a rapid action, especially if ingested before breakfast. They may be taken at bedtime with food for early morning evacuation (food delays the effect). Clients sometimes complain of gaseous distention after taking saline laxatives. All preparations should be dissolved and accompanied by a liberal (8-oz) intake of water, since the salts do not readily leave the stomach and may cause vomiting if not well diluted.

When a salt such as magnesium sulfate is taken, it should not only be dissolved in an adequate amount of water and taken on an empty stomach but it should also be disguised in fruit juice, plain water (chilled), citrus-flavored carbonate beverage, or chipped ice to increase palatability.

Magnesium sulfate [mag nee' zhum] (Epsom salt). Magnesium sulfate occurs as a crystal or white powder that is readily soluble in water. It has a bitter saline taste. The usual dose for laxative effect is 15 g in 8 oz of water. Children over 6 are given 5 to 10 g in 4 oz of water.

Magnesium hydroxide (Milk of Magnesia; MOM). Magnesium hydroxide is also used as an antacid. In the stomach the magnesium hydroxide reacts with hydrochloric acid to form magnesium chloride, which is responsible for the laxative effect. The usual dose for adults is 30 to 60 ml with additional liquids; children 1 to 12 years receive 7.5 to 30 ml.

Magnesium citrate solution. Magnesium citrate solution is not very soluble, hence the need for a relatively large dose. It is not unpleasant to take because it is carbonated and flavored. The usual adult dose is 240 ml, and the usual dose for children 6 to 12 years old is 50 to 100 ml.

Effervescent sodium phosphate. This is made effervescent by the addition of sodium bicarbonate, citric and tartaric acids. The usual dose is 10 g. A concentrated aqueous solution of sodium biphosphate and sodium phosphate is available under the name of Fleet Phospho-Soda as a laxative. The usual oral adult dose is 20 to 45 ml mixed with ½ glass of cold water. Children 6 to 9 years are given 5 ml while children over 10 years receive 10 ml, diluted in 4 oz of water. It is also marketed in a disposable enema unit for rectal administration.

Stimulant (Contact) Laxatives

With the exception of bisacodyl, the principal members of the stimulant laxatives (cascara, senna, rhubarb, and aloe) are botanical glycoside drugs obtained from the bark, seed pods, leaves, and roots of a number of plants. These laxatives are absorbed and later secreted to produce stimulation and peristalsis in the intestines. Their exact mechanism of action is unknown.

The stimulant laxatives usually act in 6 to 8 hours. Their primary effect is on the small and large intestines, which explains their tendency to produce cramping. Aloe and rhubarb are almost obsolete because of their irritating properties.

Stimulant laxatives are used in preparation for barium enemas, in some cases of acute constipation, and before a proctologic examination.

Side effects of stimulant laxatives include abdominal cramping, nausea, diarrhea, and flatulence. Adverse reactions that should be reported to a health care provider if they occur include allergic reactions, esophageal or intestinal obstruction, change in heart rate, disorientation, cramping of muscles, increased weakness, and skin rash. Senna, cascara sagrada, and aloe are passed through the breast milk, initiating laxation in the nursing infant. Their occasional use should be restricted to 1 week because long-term abuse may lead to a poorly functioning large intestine. The contact stimulant laxatives may also lead to mucus secretion and fluid evacuation.

Table 11-5 compares the stimulant laxatives in use today. Laxatives are habit forming; they should be used judiciously.

bisacodyl [bis a koe' dill] (Dulcolax)

Bisacodyl is a relatively nontoxic laxative agent that reflexively stimulates peristalsis on contact with the mucosa of the colon. Bisacodyl has been successful in the treatment of various types of constipation. In larger doses, it is also widely used for cleansing the bowel before some surgeries and before proctoscopic and roentgenographic examinations.

Bisacodyl has an insoluble coating that was formulated to dissolve in intestinal fluids and, when released, produces its stimulating effects on the colon. It should not be chewed, crushed, or taken with milk or antacids because it can have an irritating effect on the stomach that might manifest as severe abdominal cramps. If antacids are to be taken, they should be taken at least several hours apart from the bisacodyl.

Oral adult dosage is 2 to 3 tablets (10 to 15 mg). While the tablets produce evacuation of the bowel in 6 to 8 hours; suppositories and enemas act within 15 to 60 minutes. The suppositories may cause a burning sensation and proctitis.

TABLE 11-5 Stimulant laxatives

Name	Therapeutic effect (hrs)	Stool consistency	Remarks
bisacodyl (Dulcolax)	6-10	Soft	Not to be taken with or within 1 hr after ingestion of milk or antacids to prevent premature dissolving of enteric coating and gastrointestinal irritation
castor oil (Neoloid emulsion, Castor Oil)	2-6	Watery	Chilling, mixing with fruit juice or carbonated drinks increases palatability
cascara sagrada	6-10	Soft, formed	Gives a yellowish brown color to acid urine; reddish color to alkaline urine
phenolphthalein (Ex-Lax, Feen-A-Mint, Phenolax, Doxidan)	6-10	Semifluid	Gives pink color to alkaline urine or feces; action may persist for 3-4 days; may cause skin eruptions as dermatitis
senna (X-prep, Senokot)	6-12	Soft	Crude senna may cause urine discoloration like cascara

cascara sagrada [kas' kar a]
Cascara sagrada was one of the most extensively used laxatives in the past. It is considered to be the mildest laxative belonging to this group. Its action is mainly on the small and large bowel. The active ingredients reach the large bowel by way of the bloodstream, as well as by passage along the alimentary tract. Bowel evacuation occurs in about 8 hours. Cascara may discolor urine to pink, red, violet or brown depending on the urinary pH. The client should be alerted to this possibility.

Aromatic cascara fluid-extract contains 18% to 20% alcohol. Each milliliter represents 1 g cascara sagrada. The usual dose is 5 ml (range 5 to 15 ml). For infants up to 2 years the dose is 1 to 3 ml. Cascara is also available in tablets.

senna [sen' a] (Senexon, Senokot)
Senna is obtained from the dried leaves of the *Cassia* plant. It produces a thorough bowel evacuation in 6 to 12 hours, which may be accompanied by abdominal pain or gripping. Senna resembles cascara but is more powerful. It is also found in proprietary remedies, such as Fletcher's Castoria and Black Draught. Senna tea is an infusion of senna leaves made from adding a teaspoonful of leaves to a cup of hot water.

A powdered concentrate of senna (X Prep Liquid) is said to contain the desirable laxative components but to be free of the impurities that cause cramping. This compound is sold under the name of Senokot (tablets, syrup, granules, and suppositories). The usual adult dose of Senokot is two tablets, 10 to 15 ml of the syrup or 1 teaspoon of the granules twice daily. For children over 6 years of age, the dose is one tablet twice daily.

castor oil [kas' tor]
Castor oil is obtained from the seeds of the castor bean. It is a bland, colorless, emollient glyceride that passes through the stomach unchanged, but like other fatty substances, it retards the emptying of the stomach. For this reason it is usually given when the stomach is empty. In the small intestine the oil is hydrolyzed by pancreatic lipase to glycerol and a hydroxy fatty acid, ricinoleic acid. This hydroxy fatty acid is responsible for irritation of the bowel, especially the small intestine. Its irritating effect causes a rapid propulsion of contents from the small intestine, including any of the oil that may have escaped hydrolysis.

A therapeutic dose will produce several copious semiliquid stools in 2 to 6 hours, so it should not be taken at bedtime. The fluid nature of the stool is caused by the rapid passage of the fecal content rather than by a diffusion of fluid into the bowel. The drug is excreted into the milk of nursing mothers.

Castor oil is used much less often today than it was formerly, although it may be used in the preparation of certain clients scheduled for a roentgenographic examination of abdominal viscera. The usual adult dose of castor oil is 15 to 60 ml orally. The dose for children 2 years and older is 5 to 15 ml.

phenolphthalein [fee nole thay' leen]
(Ex-Lax, Phenolax)
Phenolphthalein is a synthetic substance with an action similar to the stimulant laxatives. Evacuation of a semi-fluid stool occurs in 6 to 8 hours, unaccompanied by cramping. It acts on both the small and the large bowels, particularly the latter. When given orally, part (15%) of the drug is absorbed and secreted in bile, which may cause a prolonged laxative action for up to 3 days, in some individuals.

Repeated large doses may cause cardiac and respiratory distress, nausea, and in some susceptible individuals an allergic skin rash (pink-purple color). In other cases a prolonged and excessive purgative effect may indicate individual idiosyncrasy. The usual adult dose is 90 to 180 mg orally at bedtime. Phenolphthalein is the active ingredient of a number of commonly used OTC laxatives, including Evac-U-Gen, Ex-Lax, Feen-a-Mint and others.

Bulk-Forming Laxatives
The laxatives constituting this group are polycarbophil (Mitrolan) and other natural or semisynthetic cellulose derivatives such as psyllium and methylcellulose. Hydrophilic colloids stimulate peristalsis by swelling, increasing bulk and modifying the consistency of the stool. This mechanism of laxative action is normal stimulus and is one of the least harmful. These drugs do not interfere with absorption of food, but if not administered with sufficient fluids (8 oz of water or juice), they can cause esophageal obstruction, fecal impaction or obstruction.

The effect of these laxatives may not be apparent for 12 to 24 hours, and their full effect may not be achieved until the second or third day after administration. Some prescribers maintain that bran and dried fruits (e.g., prunes, prune juice, and figs) exert the same effect, and they prefer to suggest these foods rather than the bulk-forming laxatives. Bulk-forming laxatives are used in irritable bowel syndrome, diverticular disease, and postpartum constipation. Because of the altered bulk consistency, they have also been found to be useful in the treatment of diarrhea. Side effects are minimal; most commonly reported are flatulence and bulky stools.

polycarbophil calcium [pol i kar' boe fil] (Mitrolan)
Polycarbophil is used to normalize stools both in diarrhea and in constipation by restoring the normal moisture level and providing bulk in the intestinal tract. In diarrheal conditions the intestinal mucosa is unable to absorb the excess fecal water. This agent absorbs water (up to 60 times its weight) by forming a gel in the intestinal lumen, thus creating formed stools. In constipation the agent retains water in the lumen.

Polycarbophil has a low sodium content; each tablet contains 150 mg of calcium. The maximum dosage of calcium recommended by the FDA is much higher than the 1800 mg a patient would receive by taking the maximum dosage of 12 tablets per day. Nevertheless, clients with hypercalcemia or those susceptible to hypercalcemia should not take this product without prior consultation with their prescriber (Curry, Jr & Tatum-Butler, 1996).

psyllium [sill' i yum] (Metamucil, Konsyl)
Psyllium hydrophilic mucilloid is a powder that contains about 50% powdered mucilaginous portion (outer epidermis) of psyllium seeds and about 50% dextrose or sucrose. This mixture is used to treat constipation because it promotes the formation of a soft, water-retaining gelatinous residue in the lower bowel within 12 to 72 hours. In addition, it has a demulcent effect on inflamed mucosa. The dosage is 4 to 7 g, administered one to three times daily.

Sugar-free Metamucil contains aspartame (Nutra-Sweet). Products containing aspartame should not be taken by clients on a phenylalanine-restricted diet.

Lubricant Laxatives

mineral oil

Mineral oil (liquid petrolatum, MO) a mixture of liquid hydrocarbons obtained from petroleum, is not digested, and absorption is minimal. Mineral oil penetrates and coats the fecal mass and also prevents excessive absorption of water.

Mineral oil is especially useful when it is desirable to keep feces soft and when straining at stool must be reduced, as after abdominal surgery, rectal operations, prevention of hemorrhoidal tearing, repair of hernias, eye surgery, aneurysm, or myocardial infarction. It is also indicated for clients who have chronic constipation because of prolonged inactivity, as in the case of clients with orthopedic conditions.

Some health care providers object to the use of mineral oil on the basis that it impairs the absorption of fat-soluble vitamins A, D, E, and K. If mineral oil is taken with meals, gastric emptying time will be delayed. Another objection to its use is that in large doses it tends to leak or seep from the rectum, which may cause anal pruritus and interfere with healing of postoperative wounds in the region of the anus and perineum. This leakage is often an embarrassment to the client.

Although absorption of mineral oil is limited, after prolonged use it may cause a chronic inflammatory reaction in tissues where it is found. Indiscriminate use by elderly or weak individuals should be discouraged because of the increased potential for aspiration leading to lipid pneumonia.

Concurrent use with fecal moistening agents should be avoided because they increase absorption of mineral oil. The adult dose ranges from 15 to 45 ml. For children over 6 years, doses range from 5 to 15 ml.

Emollient or Fecal Moistening Agents

Emollient or fecal moistening agents include stool softeners and surfactants. They decrease the consistency of stools by reducing surface tension, this allows water to penetrate feces. They are commonly used for the treatment of hard or dry stools.

docusate or dioctyl sodium sulfosuccinate
[dok' yoo sate] (Colace, Doxinate)

Docusate acts like a detergent; it permits water and fatty substances to penetrate and be well mixed with the fecal material. It may also inhibit water absorption from the bowel and stimulate water secretion into the GI tract. Thus this agent promotes the formation of soft-formed stool and is useful in the treatment of constipation. Formed stools are usually excreted in 1 to 3 days. Docusate is available in three different salt formulations: calcium (Surfak), potassium (Dialose, Diocto-K), and sodium (Colace, Regulex, DSS, Modane Soft).

These agents are indicated for clients with rectal impaction, hemorrhoids, chronic constipation, postpartum constipation, painful conditions of the rectum and anus and for persons who should avoid straining (e.g., after rectal surgery or myocardial infarction) at time of defecation. Docusate may be useful for immobile clients, especially children. It is said to have a wide margin of safety and few potential adverse reactions. All the following dosages should be given with a full glass of water.

- *sodium docusate:* For adults and children over 12 years, 50 to 500 mg daily orally. Children 6 to 12 years, 40 to 120 mg daily.
- *calcium docusate (Surfak):* For adults, one capsule daily, 50 to 240 mg daily orally.
- *docusate potassium (Dialose):* For adults, 100 to 300 mg daily. Children over 6 years, give 100 mg at bedtime.

hyperosmotic suppository
Glycerin suppositories are available in adult, child, and infant sizes. The suppositories are osmotic agents that absorb water, lubricate and increase stool bulk. They may also promote peristalsis through local irritation of the mucous membrane of the rectum. Evacuation occurs in 15 to 60 minutes after insertion. The adult dose is 3 g; for children under 6 years of age the dose is 1 to 1.5 g held high in the rectum for 15 minutes. Effects are achieved in 15 minutes to 1 hour.

Antidiarrheal Agents

The term **diarrhea** describes the abnormal passage of stools with increased frequency, increased fluidity, or increased weight and increase in stool water excretion. Diarrhea is acute when it is of sudden onset in a previously healthy individual, lasts about 3 days to 1 to 2 weeks, is self-limiting, and resolves without sequelae. Morbid and mortal consequences are seen in malnourished populations, the elderly, infants, and debilitated persons.

Chronic diarrhea lasts for more than 3 to 4 weeks, with the recurring passage of diarrheal stools, fever, anorexia, nausea, vomiting, weight reduction, and chronic weakness. It is the result of multiple causative factors, as seen in Box 11-6. Chronic diarrhea necessitates definitive treatment directed to the organic cause or causes. The causes vary from psychogenic to neoplastic origins.

This section focuses on the OTC drugs with a direct pharmacologic effect on the gastrointestinal tract. The drugs providing symptomatic therapy do not alter the pathophys-

BOX 11-6

Causes of Acute and Chronic Diarrhea

Causes of acute diarrhea

Bacterial

1. Invasive organisms
   a. *Campylobacter fetus (jejuni)*
   b. *Clostridium difficile*
   c. *Escherichia coli* (enteropathogenic)
   d. *Salmonella*
   e. *Shigella dysenteriae*
   f. Staphylococci
2. Noninvasive toxigenic organisms
   a. Cholera (*Vibrio cholerae*) enterotxin
   b. *Escherichia coli* (enterotoxigenic) toxin
3. Food poisoning as toxin mediated
   a. *Bacillus cereus*
   b. *Clostridium perfringens*
   c. *Salmonella*
   d. *Staphylococcus aureus*

Viral

1. Adenoviruses
2. Coxsackievirus
3. Coronaviruses
4. Eshoviruses
5. Norwalk agent
6. Rotavirus

Protozoal

1. Amebic dysentery (*Entamoeba histolytica*), amebiasis
2. Giardiasis (*Giardia lamblia*)

Nutritional

1. Allergy
2. Ingestion without discretion (spices, fats, roughage, seeds, preformed toxin)
3. Enteral nutrition

Other

1. Bile acids
2. Carcinoma
3. Diverticulitis
4. Fatty acids
5. Neurogenic
6. Psychogenic
7. Radiation therapy
8. Regional and ulcerative colitis
9. Stress

Causes of chronic diarrhea

1. Addison's disease
2. Diabetic enteropathy/neuropathy
3. Iatrogenic
   a. Bacterial overgrowth
   b. Postsurgical
4. Inflammatory bowel disease
   a. Chronic ulcerative and granulomatous colitis
   b. Crohn's enteritis
5. Irritable bowel syndrome
6. Malabsorption syndrome
7. Pancreatic adenoma—nongastrin secreting, such as syndrome of watery diarrhea-hypokalemia-achlorhydria (WDHA)
8. Pancreatic insufficiency
9. Thyroid—hyperthyroidism
10. Tumors
    a. Carcinoma of colon and rectum
    b. Intestinal
    c. Lymphoma
    d. Polyposis
    e. Villous adenoma
11. Other
    a. Blind loops, ileostomy, colostomy
    b. Carcinoid syndrome
    c. Enteritis
    d. Gardner's syndrome
    e. Gastrointestinal hormones
    f. Gluten enteropathy
    g. Zollinger-Ellison syndrome
    h. Many other conditions

iology of diarrhea and do not prevent electrolyte and fluid loss. The antidiarrheal agents diminish stool water by inhibiting intestinal fluid secretion or by increasing intestinal fluid absorption. Although these drugs decrease the number, consistency, and fluidity of the stool, there is no absolute clinical evidence that an effective antidiarrheal therapeutic benefit accrues to the client. However, there is a relief of the bothersome symptoms that interrupt daily routines.

For additional information on the nursing management of antidiarrheal therapy, see Chapter 41.

Adsorbents

Adsorbents act by coating the walls of the gastrointestinal tract, absorbing the bacteria or toxins causing the diarrhea, and passing them out with the stools. Examples of drugs in this class not requiring a prescription are activated charcoal, aluminum hydroxide, bismuth salts, attapulgite, kaolin, and pectin. Attapulgite, activated charcoal, polycarbophil, and bismuth salts are the GI adsorbents in clinical use today. The bismuth salts are used as adsorbent, astringent, and protective.

The adsorbent preparations are usually taken after each loose bowel movement until the diarrhea has been controlled. Constipation may develop because of the large amounts of the adsorbent products that must be used. A caution with all the adsorbents is they may interfere with the absorption of medications given concurrently (e.g., digoxin, clindamycin, and others).

The drugs and nutrients adsorbed include a wide range of ingested substances. These may be decreased by administering the adsorbent 2 hours or more before or after a drug (except when used to inactivate a drug or for a specific poison in overdose situations).

bismuth subsalicylate [bis' meth] (Pepto-Bismol)
Bismuth subsalicylate is an antidiarrheal, antacid (weak) and antiulcer medication. It has several actions including: (1) inhibition of GI secretions, i.e., it stimulates absorption of fluid and electrolytes in the intestine, (2) inhibition of synthesis of prostaglandins that produce intestinal inflammation and hypermotility, and (3) suppression of the growth of *H. pylori*. It is the only bismuth preparation available in the United States (Pinson & Weart, 1996; *USP DI*, 1996).

Administered orally, more than 90% of dose is absorbed; it is bound to plasma proteins and excreted by the kidneys. Because bismuth subsalicylate is a salicylate and may be taken in large amounts to control the diarrhea, it will enhance the effects of oral anticoagulants (i.e., increased bleeding time, bruising). Methotrexate may be displaced from its protein binding sites, thus causing toxicity. Probenecid, an antigout agent, promotes the renal excretion of uric acid. When combined with bismuth subsalicylate the uricosuric effects of probenecid can be inhibited by the salicylate.

Bismuth salicylate may antagonize the effects of hypoglycemic agents and could require a change in the dosage of the hypoglycemic agent. Be aware of possible salicylate toxicity when the drug is taken in large doses by persons taking large amounts of aspirin daily. Bismuth salicylate also has the potential for drug interactions if taken with oral anticoagulants, methotrexate, or any other drug that interacts with aspirin. The suspension of bismuth salicylate contains 130 mg of salicylate in 15 ml; the original tablet contains 102 mg while the caplets and cherry flavored tablets contain 99 mg of salicylate (Longe, 1996).

The usual adult dose of bismuth subsalicylate is 30 ml or two tablets chewed or dissolved every 30 to 60 minutes (up to eight doses in 24 hours).

activated charcoal
(Charcocaps, Charcodote♣, charcoal)
Activated charcoal is used for the relief of intestinal gas, diarrhea and for GI distress associated with indigestion. It acts as an adsorbent; it adsorbs toxic substances, irritants, and gas. It may also adsorb medication, nutrients, and enzymes.

The activated charcoal is administered as two capsules repeated every 30 to 60 minutes as needed up to eight doses (16 Charcocaps) for treatment of diarrhea symptoms. Tablets may be chewed or dissolved in the mouth and followed by water.

attapulgite (Kaopectate)
Attapulgite, a hydrated magnesium aluminum silicate, is a GI adsorbent and protective agent that has replaced the kaolin-pectin in Kaopectate. Kaolin and pectin are being reviewed by the FDA, and currently the evidence for kaolin is better that the combination of kaolin and pectin for treatment of acute, nonspecific diarrhea (Longe, 1996). Attapulgite is also being reviewed for both safety and efficacy. Therefore the health care professional should carefully watch for labeling changes on these products in the future.

Synthetic Opioids

loperamide [loe per' a mide] (Imodium)
Loperamide is a synthetic OTC opioid that decreases gastrointestinal motility by inhibiting propulsive movements in the gut. It produces a direct musculotropic effect that decreases hyperperistalsis, slows passage of intestinal contents, and allows reabsorption of water and electrolytes, resulting in a reduction in stool frequency.

Loperamide is indicated for the treatment of acute nonspecific and chronic diarrhea. Peak plasma levels after administration is 5 hours with the capsule dosage form or 2.5 hours for the oral liquid; half-life ranges from 9 to 14 hours with duration of action up to 24 hours. Loperamide is metabolized in the liver and excreted both fecally and by the kidneys.

Side effects are usually minimal, including dizziness, dry mouth, and skin rash. Drug-induced gastrointestinal side effects are difficult to separate from those of diarrhea itself (epigastric pain, abdominal cramps, nausea, vomiting, anorexia).

The usual adult OTC dose is 4 mg (2 tablets) initially, followed by 2 mg after each loose stool, not exceeding 8 mg per day for more than 2 days.

Cough-Cold Preparations

In 1990, it was estimated that more than $10 billion was spent on OTC medications; nearly 3 billion of this amount was used to buy cough, cold, and flu preparations (Popovich, Newton, & Pray, 1992). Box 11-7 describes the major differences between cold, allergic rhinitis, and influenza (flu). This section will be devoted to a description of the symptoms of these conditions and the medications used to treat coughs and colds, such as antitussives, antihistamines, expectorants, and decongestants. Many cough-cold products contain a combination of ingredients, some of which are subtherapeutic dose combinations or are unnecessary for the particular symptoms they are purported to treat. Such preparations are not considered rational and may not be safe and effective.

While some combination products are very useful, they should be carefully selected according to the presenting

BOX 11-7

Colds, Allergic Rhinitis, and Influenza: Signs or Symptoms

Signs or symptoms	Common cold	Allergic rhinitis	Influenza
Fever	Rare	Absent	Common—sudden onset, may range 102-104° F
Aches and pains	Slight	Absent	May be severe
Sneezing	Usual	Common	Infrequent
Pruritus	Absent or rare	Common	Absent
Cough	Mild-moderate	Uncommon	Common
Headaches	Rare	Can occur	Prominent
Causative	Usually viruses	Usually allergens	Usually viruses
Occurrence	Anytime	Usually seasonal	Anytime
Complications	Sinus congestion, earache	Uncommon	Bronchitis, pneumonia

symptoms. Generally cough-cold preparations that contain analgesic and antipyretic agents should be avoided. Routine use of such products may mask a fever secondary to a bacterial infection, and if side/adverse effects occur, it would be difficult to determine the causative ingredient. In fact, the American Academy of Pediatrics Committee on Drugs has recommended against the use of combination cold-cough preparations (Tietze, 1996).

Products that do not provide full information on the label, such as the strength and/or amount of each ingredient should also be avoided. It is difficult to evaluate such products when essential information is missing. Information on how to select a combination product will be provided later in this chapter.

Cough

Coughing is defined as protective reflex for clearing the respiratory tract of environmental irritants, foreign bodies, or accumulated secretions and thus should not be depressed indiscriminately. The afferent impulses that arise from irritated pharyngeal and laryngeal tissues initiate the central cough reflex. A productive cough occurs when irritants or secretions are removed from the respiratory tract and generally should not be suppressed because it is helping to clear the airways. If a nonproductive cough is dry, irritating, frequent and prolonged, it should be treated, since it can be exhausting, painful, and taxing to the circulatory system and the elastic tissue of the respiratory system, particularly in the elderly and young children.

Treatment of the cough is secondary to treatment of the underlying disorder. Antitussives should not be taken in situations in which retention of respiratory secretions or exudates may be harmful. The therapeutic objective is to decrease the intensity and frequency of the cough yet permit adequate elimination of tracheobronchial secretions and exudates.

Drugs act either by suppressing the cough center in the medulla or by lessening irritation of the respiratory tract peripherally. Intake of fluids and inhalation of fully water-saturated vapors (steam) should be stressed as one of the most important means of producing increased amounts of mucus and thinning such secretions.

Antitussives

The primary OTC cough suppressant agents that affect the cough center centrally are codeine and dextromethorphan. Diphenhydramine (Benadryl), an antihistamine, and benzonatate (Tessalon) also have antitussive effects. Benzonatate is a prescription drug in the United States so it will be reviewed in Chapter 39, while diphenhydramine will be reviewed in the antihistamine section of this chapter.

While codeine is included in selected combination products, dextromethorphan is the preferred antitussive agent in OTC preparations. Codeine is an effective antitussive but as an opioid many laws govern its use as a nonprescription drug. The amount of codeine permitted in OTC products is also limited because codeine has a higher potential for misuse and abuse than the other products. Dextromethorphan has no addictive properties and works centrally to raise the coughing threshold. It also has fewer side effects (drowsiness and gastric distress) than codeine. As an antitussive, 8 to 15 mg of codeine is considered equivalent to 15 to 30 mg of dextromethorphan (Olin, 1996).

dextromethorphan [dex troe meth or′ fan] (Sucrets Cough Control and others)
dextromethorphan in combination with cough syrups, antihistamines, expectorants, and benzocaine (Pertussin ES, Benylin DM, and others)

Dextromethorphan is well absorbed orally with an onset of action between 15 and 30 minutes and a duration of activity up to 6 hours. In usually recommended doses, side effects are minimal. Nausea, mild dizziness, and drowsiness have been reported.

Significant drug interactions have been reported with central nervous system (CNS) depressant and monoamine oxidase (MAO) inhibitor medications. The former may result in enhanced CNS depressant effects while concurrent use with MAO inhibitors may result in increased excitability, tremors, sedation, severe hypertension, intracranial bleeding, hyperpyrexia, and psychosis. Dextromethorphan should not be taken by persons taking an MAO inhibitor.

The dosage of adults and children 12 years and older is 10 to 20 mg orally every 4 hours or 30 mg every 6 to 8 hours, up to a maximum of 120 mg per day. For children 6 to 12 years, the recommended dosage is 5 to 10 mg every 4 hours up to a maximum of 60 mg per day; 2 to 6 years old, 2.5 to 5 mg every 4 hours to a maximum of 30 mg per day. Dextromethorphan is not recommended for use in children under 2 years old. Pregnancy safety is not established.

Many other products have been used as antitussive agents in various preparations, but the FDA advisory review panel on nonprescription cold, cough, allergy, bronchodilator, and antiasthmatic products has indicated that more evidence is needed to prove their effectiveness. Some of the products in this category include noscapine, beechwood creosote, elm bark, cod liver oil, horehound, and others.

Antihistamines

Antihistamines are drugs that compete with histamine for its receptor sites. With the discovery of two histamine receptors, H_1 and H_2, the antihistamines related to cold and allergy symptoms, such as diphenhydramine (Benadryl), chlorpheniramine (Chlor-Trimeton), and others, are H_1 receptor antagonists while the H_2 receptor antagonists related to the symptoms of gastric hyperacidity, such as cimetidine (Tagamet), ranitidine (Zantac), and others, are discussed in Chapter 41.

Receptor Antagonists

Antihistamines prevent the physiologic histamine effects of sneezing, increased nasal secretions, and itching, watering eyes by preventing histamine from reaching its site of action. The antihistamines of the H_1 type have the greatest therapeutic effect on nasal allergies, particularly on seasonal hay fever and colds with histamine-like symptoms. In allergies, they relieve symptoms better at the beginning of the hay fever season than during its height but fail to relieve asthma that may frequently accompany hay fever. Antihistamines are palliative agents. Their action is comparatively short-lived and provides only symptomatic relief.

Many OTC preparations contain antihistamines; some contain two or more different ones. Antihistamines may be used in a variety of over-the-counter medications including antitussive, cough-cold products, sleep-inducing products, oral analgesic products, menstrual formulations, and many others. For example, diphenhydramine depresses the cough center in the medulla of the brain (antitussive effect), has antihistamine effects (blocks H_1 receptors), central antimuscarinic effects (antiparkinson action), sedative-hypnotic effects, and is used to prevent or treat nausea and vomiting associated with motion sickness. The consumer should check ingredients of all medications they buy, consume, or administer. Often individuals have unwanted side effects or are accidently overdosed by the same product available in several different medications they are consuming, which unfortunately is often overlooked in a community setting.

The antihistamines currently available OTC include:

- brompheniramine [brome fen air' uh meen] (Dimetane, generics)
- chlorpheniramine [klor fen air' uh meen] (Allerchlor, Chlor-Trimeton, and others)
- diphenhydramine hydrochloride [dye fen hye' dra meen] (AllerMac, Benadryl 25, and others]
- phenindamine [fen in' da meen] (Nolahist)
- pyrilamine [peer il' uh meen] (generics available)

The primary difference between the OTC and prescription antihistamines is the strength of the product. For example OTC chlorpheniramine is 4 mg while prescription products are 8 mg, 12 mg time-release, and injectable dosage forms.

Absorption of oral doses of antihistamines is good, with onset of action within 15 to 60 minutes. Time to peak effect can vary with each individual preparation. For example, brompheniramine has a peak effect in 3 to 9 hours, chlorpheniramine within 6 hours, and diphenhydramine 1 to 4 hours. Duration of action is also variable with brompheniramine 4 to 8 hours, chlorpheniramine 4 to 8 hours, diphenhydramine 6 to 8 hours, and pyrilamine at 8 hours. These agents are primarily metabolized in the liver and excreted in the kidneys.

The most frequently reported OTC antihistamine side effects include: constipation, a decrease in sweating, difficulty in initiating urinary stream in elderly males, sedation, visual disturbances, photosensitivity, nausea or vomiting, and dry mouth, nose, or throat. Less often reported effects are orthostatic hypotension, headaches, anxiety, weak hands or feet, sore mouth and tongue, abdominal pain or increased excitability, and muscle cramps. Rarely reported adverse effects include glaucoma or eye pain in susceptible persons (individuals with predisposition to angle-closure glaucoma), skin rash, and confusion, especially in elderly having taken high doses. Figure 11-2 shows a comparison of selected antihistamines, efficacy, and side effects.

Expectorants

Expectorants are substances that reduce the viscosity of secretions thus promoting the ejection of mucus or other exudates from the lungs, bronchi, and trachea. In OTC preparations the only expectorant with evidence of safety and effectiveness is guaifenesin. Many other expectorants such as ammonium chloride, iodides, and terpin hydrate are listed as Category III; i.e., safe but not proven to be effective (Tietze, 1996).

Decongestants

Decongestant agents are vasoconstricting agents used to shrink engorged nasal mucous membranes in mild upper respiratory tract infections. In OTC products, they are available in oral and nasal preparations.

The oral agents are sympathomimetic amines and their vasoconstricting properties are not limited to the nasal mucosa. They can also elevate blood pressure in individuals with hypertension, induce cardiac stimulation and arrhythmias in some people, and depending on the sympathomimetic, may increase blood glucose in those with diabetes. For this reason, warnings on the labels instruct the consumer with hypertension, hyperthyroidism, diabetes mellitus, or ischemic heart disease to contact their prescriber before using the product. Reported side/adverse effects include CNS stimulation or nervousness, insomnia, restlessness, dizziness, headaches, and increased irritability.

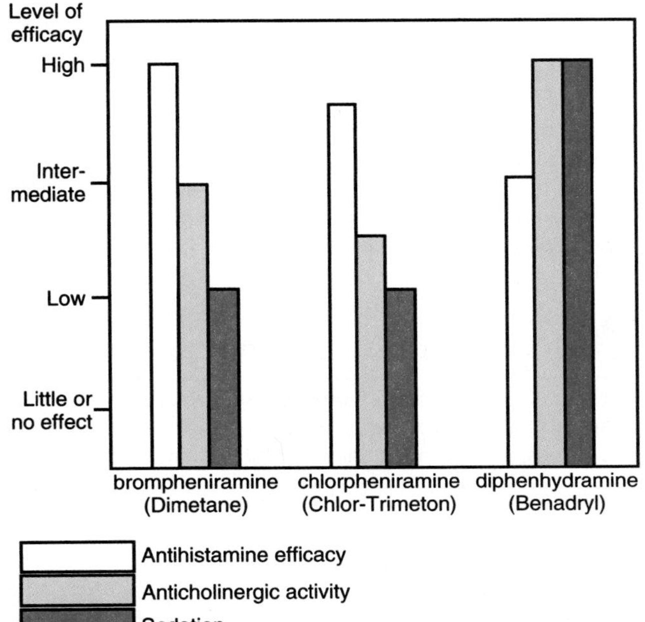

Figure 11-2 Comparison of efficacy and side effects of selected antihistamines.

Three agents (phenylephrine, phenylpropanolamine, and pseudoephedrine) have been classified as Category I, safe and effective if label instructions are followed. These ingredients are often incorporated in combination products for their decongestant effects.

Many drugs are used exclusively as nasal vasoconstrictors or topical decongestants. Because of their wide popular use and lack of serious hazard (when used topically), a large number of preparations have been provided by the pharmaceutical industry for direct sale to the public.

The FDA advisory review panel has recommended the following products as safe and effective topical nasal decongestant products: ephedrine 0.5%; naphazoline (Privine) 0.05%, 0.025%; oxymetazoline (Afrin, Dristan) 0.05%, 0.025%; phenylephrine (Neo-Synephrine) 0.125%, 0.25%, 1%; and xylometazoline (Otrivin) 0.1%, 0.05%. Table 11-6 lists recommended dosages for topical nasal decongestant products and oral decongestant products. These drugs are adrenergic agents that act on alpha receptors of blood vessels in the nasal mucosa to produce vasoconstriction and so a decrease in mucosal swelling. Some nasal decongestant products (those containing ephedrine, epinephrine, metaproterenol, and others) also possess beta-stimulating effects, which may cause the CNS stimulation and perhaps the adverse effect of vasodilation after vasoconstriction.

Nasal decongestant drugs are used to shrink engorged mucous membranes of the nose and to relieve nasal stuffiness. However, there is a tendency on the part of the public to misuse them by using them excessively or too frequently. Excessive use may result in "rebound" engorgement or swelling of the mucous membranes and a paradoxical bronchospasm. If an infection is present, there is always the possibility of spreading the infection deeper into the sinuses or to the middle ear with the use of nasal sprays or drops.

TABLE 11-6 Topical/oral nasal decongestants: dosage

Drug/strength	Adults	Children (6 to 12 years old)
ephedrine, 0.5% (in Va-Tro-Nol and others)	2-3 drops every 4 hr	1-2 drops every 4 hr
naphazoline (Privine and others)		
0.05%	1-2 drops/spray, every 6 hr	Not recommended
0.025%	—	1-2 drops every 6 hr
oxymetazoline (Afrin, Allerest, Dristan Long-Lasting and others)		
0.05%	2-3 drops twice daily	Same as adults
phenylephrine (Neo-Synephrine and others)		
1%	1-2 drops/spray every 4 hr	Not recommended
0.25%	Same as 1%	1-2 drops every 4 hr
xylometazoline (Otrivin)		
0.1%	2-3 drops/spray every 8-10 hr	Not recommended
0.05%	Same as 0.1%	2-3 drops/spray every 8-10 hr
Oral nasal decongestants (usually combined with other drug products)		
phenylephrine	10 mg every 4 hr	5 mg every 4 hr
phenylpropanolamine	25 mg every 4 hr	12.5 mg every 4 hr
pseudoephedrine	60 mg every 6 hr	30 mg every 6 hr

Additives such as preservatives, antihistamines, detergents, etc. are sometimes included in a decongestant preparation. In some cases, reactions may be caused by the additive rather than by the decongestant. Sprays and nose drops are beneficial when used judiciously. Table 11-6 lists topical and oral dosage of nasal decongestants.

Selection of Combination Cough-Cold Preparations

Combination OTC products require careful selection because some of these multi-drug formulations contain unnecessary drugs for the individual. As previously mentioned, combinations that contain an analgesic or antipyretic agent should be avoided for several reasons. First, there is the risk of masking a bacterial infection. Second, a fixed amount of analgesic or antipyretic is taken with other ingredients on a regular basis, whether needed or not. And third, if a side/adverse effect occurs, it would be difficult to identify the offending agent. If an analgesic/ antipyretic is necessary, the proper dose should be selected and administered separately.

When only one drug effect is necessary, such as a nasal decongestant, expectorant, or an antihistamine effect, a therapeutic dose of that single drug entity should be taken. If the individual has several symptoms that need to be addressed, selection of a combination product should be limited to addressing just those symptoms with few if any additional substances. For example, for a cough suppressant and expectorant, an OTC product that contains guiafenisen and dextromethorphan (Robitussin DM and many others) may be selected. To treat allergy, nasal congestion, sneezing, and rhinorrhea, an antihistamine and decongestant combination is used, such as triprolidine and pseudoephedrine (Actifed) or chlorpheniramine and phenylpropanolamine (Allerest, etc.) or many others. With nasal or sinus congestion alone, an oral or a nasal decongestant may be selected (pseudoephedrine) [Sudafed] or oxymetazoline [Afrin, Allerest]).

SUMMARY

Over-the-counter drugs or nonprescription drugs are medications that may safely be used to self-treat the symptoms of minor self-limiting illnesses without the supervision of a health care practitioner. Because these drugs are widely used and readily available, the nurse should be knowledgeable about clients' OTC drug practices and the drugs themselves. In addition to acquiring the skill to elicit information about such practices during the client's drug history, the nurse's knowledge of OTCs will assist in the guidance of clients on the safe self-administration of these medications. The most commonly used types of OTCs are analgesics, antacids, laxatives, cough-cold preparations, and antidiarrheals.

Clients should be instructed to carefully review the labels of OTC medications before selection to assure the ingredients have proven safety and effectiveness and are also safe for use in the individual (check warnings and contraindications). Advise the client to follow dosing instructions carefully and to be aware that many OTC medications do not contain a list of possible drug interactions. Clients taking prescription drugs should consult with their prescriber before taking any OTC medication. Over-the-counter preparations wisely used can effectively treat many client symptoms at a savings to the individual and the health care delivery system.

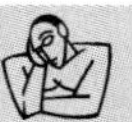

Critical Thinking

1. One of the home health aides at the health care agency comes to you and indicates that her two children are home from school with colds. She asks your advice about treating them with OTC preparations. How will you respond?
2. Paul Taylor, aged 55, comes to the health center for symptoms of an upper respiratory infection. Mr. Taylor, a client with moderate hypertension, has had his blood pressure well controlled with his antihypertensive drug regimen for more than 3 years, but on this visit you find it to be elevated above his usual BP determination. What information should be elicited from Mr. Taylor?

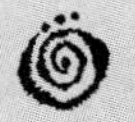

Collaborative Learning Activities

1. The students will form teams to explore OTC medications available in the community. Assign each team a classification of drugs, such as analgesics or laxatives, and a specific setting, such as a local pharmacy, super market, or convenience store. Discuss in class the variety of OTCs available, the most common active ingredients, and the quality of instructional material that accompanied some of the drugs. What concerns for client safety would the students have as a result of this experience?

BIBLIOGRAPHY

Anderson KN, et al. (Eds.) (1994). *Mosby's medical, nursing, & allied health dictionary* (4th ed.). St Louis: Mosby.

Burns J (Ed.) (1991). OTC drugs can be a low-cost alternative; The value of pharmaceuticals, *Business & Health Special Report.* Montvale, NJ: Medical Economics Publishing.

Brunton LL (1996). Agents for control of gastric acidity and treatment of peptic ulcers. In Hardman JF & Limbird LE (Eds.). *Goodman & Gilman's the pharmacological basis of therapeutics* (9th ed.). New York: McGraw-Hill.

Covington TR (1996). Self-care and nonprescription pharmacotherapy. In Covington TR (Ed.). *Handbook of nonprescription drugs* (11th ed.). Washington, DC: American Pharmaceutical Association.

Carpenito LJ (1995). *Nursing diagnosis: Application to clinical practice* (6th ed.). Philadelphia: JB Lippincott.

Cornacchia HJ & Barrett S (1993). *Consumer health: A guide to intelligent decisions.* St. Louis: Mosby.

Curry Jr CE & Tatum-Butler D (1996). Laxative products. In Covington TR (Ed.). *Handbook of nonprescription drugs* (11th ed.). Washington, DC: American Pharmaceutical Association.

Fitzgerald WL (1994). Legal control of pharmacy services. In *OBRA '90: A practical guide to effecting pharmaceutical care.* Washington, DC: American Pharmaceutical Association.

Insel PA (1996). Analgesic-antipyretic and antiinflammatory agents and drugs employed in the treatment of gout. In Hardman JG & Limbird LE (Eds.). *Goodman & Gilman's the pharmacological basis of therapeutics* (9th ed.). New York: McGraw-Hill.

Lipman AG (1996). Internal analgesic and antipyretic products. In Covington TR (Ed.). *Handbook of nonprescription drugs* (11th ed.). Washington, DC: American Pharmaceutical Association.

Longe RL (1996). Antidiarrheal products. In Covington TR (Ed.). *Handbook of nonprescription drugs* (11th ed.). Washington, DC: American Pharmaceutical Association.

Newton GD, Pray WS, & Popovich NG (1996). New OTC drugs and devices: a selected review, *J Amer Pharmaceut Assoc* S36(2): 108-116.

Olin BR (Ed.) (1996). *Facts and comparisons.* Philadelphia: Lippincott.

Pinson JB & Weart CW (1996). Acid-peptic products. In Covington TR (Ed.). *Handbook of nonprescription drugs* (11th ed.). Washington, DC: American Pharmaceutical Association.

Popovich MG, Newton GD, & Pray WS (1992). New OTC drugs: A selected review, *Amer Pharmacy NS*32(2):26-38.

Tietze KJ (1996). Cold, cough, and allergy products. In Covington TR (Ed.). *Handbook of nonprescription drugs* (11th ed.). Washington, DC: American Pharmaceutical Association.

United States Pharmacopeial Convention. (1996). *USP DI: Drug information for the health care professional,* Vol I, & *Advice for the patient,* Vol II, (16th ed.). Rockville, MD: The Convention.

Zimmerman DR (1993). *Complete guide to nonprescription drugs* (2nd ed.). Detroit: Gale Research Inc.

Chapter 12
Alternative and Complementary Pharmacology

Chapter Focus

Today, one in three clients within the "mainstream" health care delivery system is using an alternative therapy. In 1993, there were more than 400 million visits to providers of alternative modalities. The public is increasingly taking a proactive approach to their own health promotion and treatment of medical conditions. Of the many clients that utilize alternative therapies, seven of ten such individuals do so without the physician's knowledge (Anderson, 1996). Health professionals should be knowledgeable about alternative options to help guide the client through the array of alternative options and utilize those that may be of benefit (Liebert, 1994). This chapter will provide an understanding of the most common alternative, or complementary substances taken to prevent and/or treat disease. The following key terms will assist in your understanding of this chapter.

Key Terms

allopathic medicine (p. 209)
alternative/complementary medicine (p. 209)

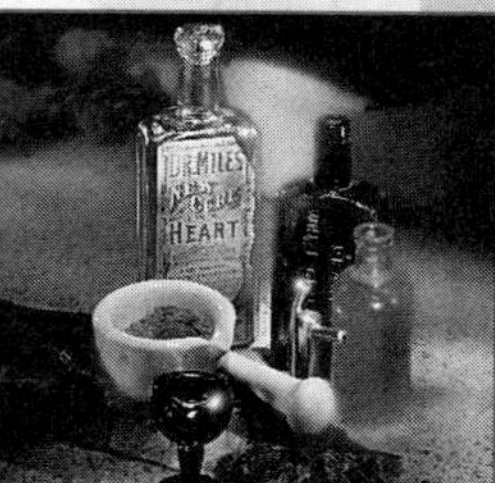

Objectives

1. Differentiate between allopathic medicine and alternative/complemetary medicine.
2. Describe the role of the Office of Alternative Medicine (OAM) in evaluation of alternative/complementary medicine.
3. Discuss the advantages and disadvantages of alternative/complementary remedies.
4. Discuss specific alternative/complementary remedies that might help or harm.
5. Provide consumer information for clients taking alternative/complementary remedies.

Treating illness with a natural remedy, such as herbal products, dates back to the earliest records of mankind. All cultures have long folk medicine histories that include the use of plants and other substances. Through history, people have methodically and scientifically collected information on herbs and other medicinal materials and maintained well-defined pharmacopeias. Well into the twentieth century, many remedies of scientific medicine were derived from the herbal lore of native people. As medicine evolved in North America, plants continued as a mainstay of rural medicine. Until the 1940s, textbooks of pharmacognosy—books that characterize plants as proven-by-use medication—contained hundreds of medically useful comments on barks, roots, berries, twigs, and flowers. Many drugs used today, such as aspirin, vincristine, curare, and ergot, are of herbal origin. But as twentieth century technology advanced and created an increasing admiration for technology, simple plant and water mixtures and other folk remedies were discarded by allopathic medicine. **Allopathic medicine** is the dominant medical culture of the Western world, a system of medical therapy in which a disease or abnormal condition is treated with active interventions, such as medical or surgical treatment, intended to bring about effects opposite from those produced by the disease or condition. Many therapies that fall outside of this scientific type of medicine are now considered alternative therapies. **Alternative/complementary medicine** is considered to be all health systems, modalities, and practices that are not intrinsic to the politically dominant health system. Although many modalities, are considered alternative or complementary, such as massage, acupressure, bioelectromagnetic applications, etc., the content of this chapter will focus on herbs and other substances taken to promote health, prevent illness, relieve symptoms, and cure disease.

The U.S. Food and Drug Administration (FDA) generally considers herbal remedies to be worthless or potentially dangerous (Snider, 1991) and allows their marketing only as food supplements. However, a growing number of Americans are again becoming interested in herbal and other remedies. This may be due to the increasing availability of herbs and other remedies in health food stores, the increasing cost of pharmaceutical drugs, and the increasing willingness of people to self-treat or supplement allopathic medicine.

Most of these alternative medicines have little scientific data to support their claims. Until recently, the research that has been done has been performed in Europe, India, China, and Japan, where herbal and other alternative medicines are more widely accepted.

In France, 32% of all physicians regularly prescribe homeopathic remedies, and 68% of all French citizens believe the medications work (*NARD J,* 1992). Homeopathy is a system of therapeutics based on the theory that "like cures like," that if a large amount of medicine produced symptoms of a disease then a moderate amount may reduce those symptoms. Only the smallest amount of the drug necessary to control the symptoms, is prescribed and only one drug is prescribed at a time. One in five German physicians and 42% of all United Kingdom physicians also use remedies that would be considered alternative (*NARD J,* 1992).

Mainstream medical practitioners in North America are trained to prescribe medicines whose composition is well defined and whose safety and effectiveness have been established in scientifically designed tests and trials. Physicians who have spent years studying physiology and biochemistry tend at best to be uneasy about substances like herbs, enzymes, and extracts from plant and animal sources. While many have been administered for years to hundred of thousands of sick people by traditional healers, homeopathic physicians, and non-Western medical practitioners, the composition of these substances can vary enormously and they may not be as effective for some individuals as for others (Kriegel, White, & Sculti, 1994).

In the last 20 years, considerable interest has been growing in alternative or complementary approaches to mainstream medicine. As public interest has grown, some allopathic prescribers are beginning to be interested in learning about alternative treatments in order to determine what alternative/complementary treatment entails, what benefits are claimed, the potential risks, and the physiologic effects of the ingredients. Some are attempting to submit such substances to the same rigorous study as other pharmaceutical agents.

To support this interest, the Office of Alternative Medicine (OAM) was established at the National Institutes of Health in 1992. The role of the OAM is "to facilitate the evaluation of alternative medical treatment modalities for the purpose of determining their effectiveness and to help integrate effective treatments into the mainstream medical practice" (McDowell, 1994). Part of the problem, however, is to determine which therapies are considered alternative. These would include any health practice "that does not have sufficient documentation in the United States to show that (1) it is safe and effective against specific diseases and conditions; (2) it is not generally taught in medical schools; and (3) it is generally not reimbursable for third party insurance billing" (McDowell, 1994). The OAM is attempting not to be exclusionary in nature. It is considering a broad interpretation of alternative therapies including "approaches from nutritional and lifestyle changes to hypnotherapy, acupressure, chelation therapy, and bioelectromagnetic applications such as magnetoresonance spectroscopy and blue light treatment" (McDowell, 1994). Of the 1993 and 1994 grant awards, approximately $30,000 each, the topic of modality and frequency of 43 grant awards are as follows: acupuncture (4); massage therapy (4); Chinese herbal/medical therapy (4); imagery (4); hypnosis (3); electrical therapy (3); homeopathy (2); Ayurvedic therapy (2); biofeedback (2); yoga (2); and one each of the following; enzyme therapy, anti-hepatitis plants, music therapy, energetic therapy, dance movement, tai chi, manual palpation, macrobiotic, acumoxa, therapeutic touch, antioxidants, intercessory prayer, and qi gong.

The OAM will serve as a clearinghouse of information for the alternative health community by sponsoring research as well as programs for grant writing and clinical research and maintaining a network within the NIH and other government agencies for collaboration. Although the OAM cannot serve as a referral agency or advise individual clients, it does provide information about specific therapies. It provides contact names for organizations that represent different types of treatments and individual fact sheets on issues and events.

As a result of the establishment of the Office of Alternative Medicine, the allopathic medical community is reconsidering its position toward understanding the alternative therapies and their benefits. According to Daly (1995), 28 medical schools in the United States now offer 45 courses in alternative medicine and both Harvard and Columbia University have established centers for the study of alternative/complementary therapies. Nurses should also have an understanding of these alternative modalities to be able to respond to clients' questions or be able to direct clients to appropriate sources of information. However, given the range of alternative therapies, this chapter will consider only alternative pharmacology and only the most commonly used substances will be discussed.

Clients who do wish to take alternative medicine need to be aware that at present there is no guarantee about those medications. Under the Dietary Supplement and Health Education Act of 1994, a new category of substances has been created distinct from food or drugs. This new category includes vitamins, herbs, amino acids, and any other substance that had been sold as a supplement before October 15, 1994. As a result, manufacturers of these remedies are not required to test for standardization, safety, or efficacy, which is routine for regular drugs. As a consequence, there is no way to be sure that: (1) any active ingredients, whatever they might be, have actually ended up in the pills or other dosage form; (2) an ingredient is in a form that is usable by the body; (3) the dosage is appropriate; (4) there are not other ingredients in the pills; (5) the pills are safe; or (6) the next bottle of pills will have the same ingredients. Figure 12-1 illustrates the lack of standardization of one of these products, ginseng.

This lack of standardization also applies to home preparation of herbal remedies. Efficacy of herbal preparations depends on the ailment and the quality and dose of the preparation used. Efficacy cannot be determined with home preparation of herbs because the quality and dose of the preparation is unknown.

There is also concern that alternative/complementary therapies may be harmful. Their use may delay the individual from seeking medical consultation for a condition that warrants allopathic medicine. There is also concern that the preparations have no efficacy and so are a waste of the client's effort and money, or that they may actually be toxic. Some Chinese herbal medications have been found to be contaminated with a variety of substances: undeclared prescription drugs, such as nonsteroidal antiinflammatory drugs (mefenamic acid, phenylbutazone), benzodiazepines, anticholinergics, corticosteriods, ephedrine (Gertner et al, 1995; Nelson, Shih, & Hoffman, 1995; Goldman & Myerson, 1991); aconitine (a family of plants that have medicinal and poisonous properties); heavy metals (lead) (Chan et al, 1993); benzaldehyde (a solvent used in the synthesis of dyes and perfumes); and other deleterious substances (Gorey, Wahlqvist, & Boyce, 1992). Table 12-1 lists the 20 most popular Asian patent medicines that contain toxic ingredients.

REMEDIES THAT MIGHT HELP

The following substances have reasonably strong evidence of beneficial physiologic effects and are the subject of further research. This information is not a recommendation for their use. Some, like ginger, are considered innocuous, but none should be relied on for regular medical therapy. All clients should discuss their use of alternative/complementary therapies with their prescriber. These substances should also be discussed within the context of a health history as would any other drug.

Astragalus (Astragalus membraneous [huanqi]). This herb is used as a tonic and for the treatment of colds and flus.

Product (listed alphabetically)	Ginseng per capsule*	Ginsenosides per capsule†	Concentration† (percentage ginsenoside)
American Ginseng	250 mg	12.8 mg	
Ginsana (extract)	100	3.0	
Herbal Choice Ginseng-7 (extract)	100	6.5	
KRG Korean Red Ginseng	518	11.5	
Natural Brand Korean Ginseng	648	23.2	
Naturally Korean Ginseng	648	2.3	
Nature's Resource Ginseng	560	10.7	
Rite Aid Imperial Ginseng	250	0.4	
Solgar Korean Ginseng (extract)	520	10.5	
Walgreen's Gin-zing (extract)	100	7.6	

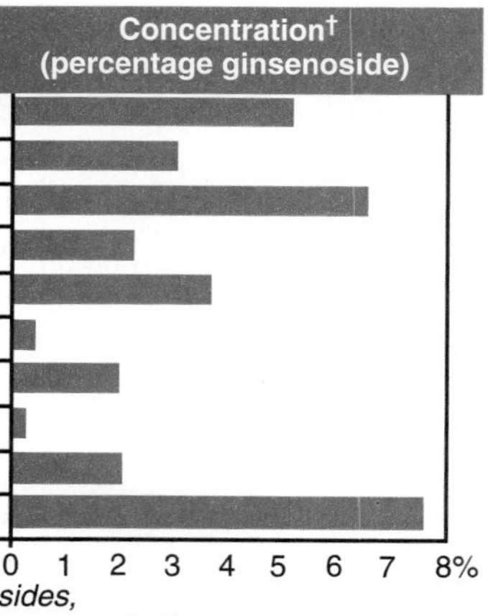

* According to label
† Based on six major ginsenosides. Estimates for two other ginsenosides, if added, would boost totals only slightly and not change variation in concentrations.

Figure 12-1 Variations of total "ginsenoside" in 10 brands of ginseng. (Modified from Consumer Reports, November 1995.)

TABLE 12-1 The 20 most popular Asian patent medicines that contain toxic ingredients

Product name	Manufacturer	Toxic ingredients
Ansenpunaw Tablets	Chung Lien Drugs Works Hankow, China	cinnabar (mercury chloride)
Bezoar Sedative Pills	Lanzhou Fo Ci Pharmaceutical Factory Lanzhou, China	cinnabar 2% or 10%
Compound Kangweiling	Wo Zhou Pharmaceutical Factory Zhe Jiang, China	centipede (scolopendra) 10%
Dahuo Luodan	Beijing Tung Jen Tang Beijing, China	centipede (scolopendra)
Danshen Tabletoco	Shanghai Chinese Medicine Works Shanghai, China	borneol
Fructus Persica Compound Pills	Lanzhou Fo Ci Pharmaceutical Factory Lanzhou, China	cannabis indica seed*
Fuchingsung-N Cream	Tianjin Pharmaceutical Corp. Tianjin, China	fluocinolone acetanide* (topical corticosteroid)
Kwei Ling Chi	Changchun Chinese Medicines & Drugs Manufactory Chang Chun, China	cinnabar
Kyushin Heart Tonic	Kyushin Seiyaki Co., Ltd. Tokyo, Japan	toad venom, borneol
Laryngitis Pills	China Dzechuan Provincial Pharmaceutical Factory Chenhtu Branch	borax 30%, toad-cake 10%
Leung Pui Kee Cough Pills	Leung Pui Kee Medical Factory Hong Kong	dover's powder (opium powder)*
Lu-Shen-Wan	Shanghai Chinese Medicine Works Shanghai, China	toad secretion
Nasalin	Kwangchow Pharmaceutical Industry Co. Kwangchow, China	centipede 5%
Nui Huang Chieh Tu Pien	Tung Jen Tang Beijing, China	borneo camphor
Nui Huang Xiao Yan Wan Bezoar Antiphlogistic Pills	Soochow Chinese Medicine Works Kiangsu, China	realgar 19.23% (arsenic disulfide, used in pyrotechnics)
Pak Yuen Tong Hou Tsao Powder	Kwan Tung Pak Yuen Tong Main Factory, Hong Kong	scorpion 10%
PoYing Tan Baby Protector	Po Che Tong Poon Mo Um Hong Kong	camphor 20%
Superior Tabellae Berberini HCl	Min-Kang Drug Manufactory I-Chang, China	berberini HCl*
Watson's Flower Pagoda Cakes	A.S. Watson & Co., Ltd. Hong Kong	piperazine phosphate*
Xiao Huo Luo Dan	Lanzhou Fo Ci Pharmaceutical Factory Lanzhou, China	aconite 42%

*Requires a prescription.
Modified from Oriental Herb Association, State of California Department of Health Services, January 28, 1992.

The herbal medicine is derived from the root of the nontoxic Chinese species. Traditional Chinese physicians consider this plant to be a true tonic that helps strengthen debilitated people and increases resistance to disease. In contemporary Chinese medicine astragalus is a chief component of combination therapy to restore immune function in oncology patients undergoing chemotherapy and radiation (Oubre, 1995). Pharmacologic studies in the West support the immune system–enhancing effects of astragalus (Weil, 1995). In vitro and in vivo studies of *Astragalus membraneous* show that it contains active compounds that increase phagocytic activity, stimulate interferon production, and potentiate the effects of biologic response modifiers such as recombinant interleukin (Chu et al, 1988a). In addition, in vivo animal studies have demonstrated that substances isolated from this herb can reverse immune suppression (Chu et al, 1988b). Chu and his colleagues at M.D. Anderson Medical Center isolated an important immune-enhancing fraction that they labeled fraction 3 (F3), composed largely of polysaccarides (Oubre, 1995). At present, more research is being done in relation to *Astralgalus'* therapeutic effects.

***Echinacea* (purple cornflower).** This herb is used as a general immunity booster. In Europe, clinicians use *Echinacea* preparations as preventatives and treatments for colds and flu. In more than 350 studies, most conducted in Europe, *Echinacea* seems to stimulate the immune system nonspecifically rather than against specific organisms (Jacobs et al, 1992). A critical review of these studies by Melchart and others (1994) identified only three randomized placebo-controlled clinical trials of monopreparations, i.e., preparations in which *Echinacea* was not combined with other substances. Two of these studies determined that an extract of the root of the plant had a positive effect on the symptoms of upper respiratory tract infections (Braunig et al, 1992; Braunig & Knick, 1993), and the other demonstrated a slight reduction in the risk of infection (Schoneberger, 1992). There are an additional 15 randomized trials (13 claiming positive results) of the treatment and prevention of infections or on the reduction in undesirable effects of antineoplastic therapies (Melchart et al, 1995). Melchart (1995) felt that until the problems of dose-response relationships and the influence of application schedules are resolved, the use of *Echinacea* will continue to be based on subjective experience.

In laboratory tests, *Echinacea* increased the number of immune system cells and developing cells in bone marrow and lymphatic tissue, and it seemed to speed their development into immunocompetent cells (Stimpel et al, 1984). It speeds release of these cells into circulation, so more are present in blood and lymph, and increases their phagocytosis rate (Coeugniet & Elek, 1987). *Echinacea* also inhibits the enzyme hyaluronidase, which bacteria use to enter tissues and cause infection (Jacobs et al, 1992). A few controlled studies suggest that it can increase resistance to upper respiratory infections, probably by stimulating white blood cells.

Feverfew *(Tanacetum parthenium).* Feverfew has been used for the treatment of headaches since the first century. Parthenolide is considered as the active component of feverfew for the treatment for migraines. However, depending on geographic location, the parthenolide content of feverfew has been found to be highly variable or absent (Awang, 1989). To ensure uniformity of dosage, the Canadian government requires a minimal level of 0.2% parthenolide for feverfew products when they are submitted for a Drug Identification Number, along with certification of botanical identity; the French require 0.1%. However, in the United States, all herb products sold before the passage of the Dietary Supplement Health and Education Act of 1994 are "grandfathered" in as dietary supplements (Foster, 1995). Heptinstall and others (1992) found that none of the North American products tested contained as much as 0.1% parthenolide, if it was detected at all. It is essential that only products in which the parthenolide has been assayed or standardized be used. The recommended daily dosage is 125 mg of dried leaves containing a minimum parenthenolide content of 0.2%.

When drug trials are conducted to demonstrate the efficacy of feverfew, only feverfew capsules of known parthenolide content are utilized. In a 1988 study conducted at the University Hospital in Nottingham, England, treatment with feverfew was clearly associated with a reduction in migraines and associated vomiting attacks, with a trend toward a reduction in migraine severity (Murphy, Heptinstall, & Mitchell, 1989). Mouth ulcers and digestive disturbances have been reported with the use of feverfew, particularly with those that chew the leaves of the plant for the prevention or treatment of migraine (Johnson et al, 1985).

Garlic *(allium sativum [da suan]).* Garlic has long been used as a flavoring in many of the world cuisines and as a substance with healing properties in many folk medicine traditions. Recent research indicates that garlic may have a wide range of health benefits, enough to justify its use as a general tonic (Weil, 1995).

Garlic has far reaching effects on the cardiovascular system. It is used primarily to decrease serum cholesterol levels. A meta-analysis, reported in the *Annals of Internal Medicine,* of the controlled trials of garlic to reduce hypercholesteremia showed a significant reduction in total cholesterol levels. The best available evidence suggests that garlic, in an amount approximating 1/2 to 1 clove per day, decreased total serum cholesterol levels by about 9% in the groups of individuals studied (Warshafsky, Kamer, & Sivak, 1993). It lowers blood pressure like antihypertensive drugs but without causing impotence, headache, and other effects that these drugs may have (Brody, 1994). In addition, one of the therapeutic actions of garlic includes inhibition of platelet aggregation, which reduces the clotting tendency of blood and may prevent heart attacks and stroke. Das, Khan, & Sooranna (1995) found this effect to be dose-dependent. However, this effect may account for the many reports in the literature related to garlic and an increased risk of bleeding in persons undergoing surgery (German, Kumar, & Blackford, 1995; Burnham, 1995; Petry, 1995). Clients on anticoagulants should be cautioned about garlic dietary supplements.

Garlic also acts as a antiinfective, counteracting the growth of many kinds of bacteria that cause disease in humans (Farbman, 1993). There is also interest in garlic for its antiviral activity. In one study, the in vitro antiviral activity of garlic extract on human cytomegalovirus (HCMV) was evaluated by Guo et al (1993), and a dose-dependent inhibitory effect was evident. The effect was stronger with pretreatment with garlic extract and persisted after the extract had been removed. Their recommendation for clinical use of garlic extract against HCMV was that it be used persistently and that prophylactic use is preferable in immunocompromised individuals. Again, further research is required before garlic's antiviral activity can be substantiated.

In the recent literature there have been studies to test the chemical constituents of garlic, using in vitro and in vivo models, for their inhibiting effects on carcinogenesis, with varying results. It appears in some of the studies that garlic, in addition to stimulating the immune system, blocks the formation of carcinogens in the gut and protects DNA from damage by other carcinogens (Weil, 1995). After reviewing the strengths and weaknesses of 60 of these studies, Dorant et al (1993) concluded in the *British Journal of Cancer* that, at this time, evidence from laboratory experiments and epidemiologic studies is not conclusive as to the preventive activity of garlic. However, the data that are available warrant further research into the possible role of garlic in the prevention of cancer in humans.

Ginger *(Zingiber officinale [sheng jiang]).* Ginger, like garlic, is a culinary spice. However, it has been used as a medicinal since ancient times. Ginger is recommended to stimulate digestion, relieve nausea, and aches and pains. It improves the digestion of protein, strengthens the mucosal lining of the upper gastrointestinal tract, and so protects against ulcers, and has a wide range of action against intestinal parasites (Weil, 1995). Phillips, Ruggier, & Hutchinson (1993) found the incidence of nausea and vomiting was similar in patients given metoclopramide (Reglan) and ginger (27% and 21%) and less than in those who received placebo (41%) without any difference in the requirements for postoperative analgesia, recovery time, and time until discharge in 120 women presenting for elective laproscopic gynecologic surgery on a day-stay basis. These antiemetic effects, however, are not associated with gastric emptying (Phillips, Hutchinson, & Ruggier, 1994). No side effects have been noted with therapeutic dosages, but the potential exists to inhibit clotting (Lumb, 1994). There is evidence that ginger modulates eicosanoid (prostaglandins, thromboxanes, and leukotrienes) synthesis in ways that reduce abnormal inflammation and clotting. It may be as effective as some of the nonsteroidal antiinflammatory drugs while protecting the lining of the stomach rather than damaging it as the NSAIDs may. Ginger comes in a variety of forms, from the fresh rhizome to candied pieces to encapsulated dried, powdered ginger. It is considered to be nontoxic, but some may experience heartburn if large amounts of raw ginger are taken on an empty stomach; advise taking it with food.

Ginseng root *(Panax ginseng [ren shen]).* The Chinese have used ginseng for more than 3000 years as a tonic, restorative, and a specific treatment for several ailments (Jacobs et al). In recent years, ginseng has been subjected to extensive study. In a review of recent advances on ginseng research, Liu and Xiao (1992) indicated that ginseng has a wide range of pharmacologic actions: it acts on the central nervous system, cardiovascular system (Kim, Chen & Gillis, 1992), and endocrine secretion, promotes immune function and metabolism, possesses biomodulation action (Watanabe et al, 1991), and antistress activity (Bhattacharya & Mitra, 1991). Yun and Choi (1995) examined the preventive effect of ginseng intake against various types of cancers using a case-control study on 1987 pairs. Ginseng intakers had a decreased risk for most cancers compared with nonintakers, which was dose related, i.e., there was a decrease in risk with increasing frequency and duration of ginseng intake. In 1993, Saita and others isolated an antitumor substance, panaxynol, from ginseng and found that it inhibited the growth of various kinds of cultured tumor cell lines in a dose-dependent manner. Other derivatives of ginseng were found to have immunologic activity by Tomoda et al (1993). Others have also documented the cancer inhibiting effects of ginseng (Sohn et al, 1993; Tode et al, 1993) as well as its antiulcer effects (Sun, Matsumoto, & Yamada, 1992).

Green tea (Camellia simensis). Tea, in general, is one of the most popular beverages consumed worldwide. Green tea is taken by many as a refreshing beverage as well as a tonic. Studies in Japan, where green tea is the national beverage, indicate that there is an inverse association between consumption of green tea and various serum markers, which shows that green tea may act protectively against cardiovascular disease and disorders of the liver (Imai & Nakachi, 1995). Many laboratory studies have demonstrated inhibitory effects of green tea preparations and tea polyphenols against tumor formation and growth; skin carcinogenesis and tumor progression (Wang et al, 1994; Katiyar, Agarwal & Mukhtar, 1993; Wang et al, 1992a); lung tumorigenesis (Xu et al, 1992; Wang et al, 1992b); and small bowel and liver cancers (Khan et al, 1992). This inhibitory activity is believed to be mainly due to the antioxidative and possible antiproliferative effects of polyphenolic compounds in green tea. These polyphenolics suppress the activation of carcinogens and trap genotoxic agents. A large population-based, case-control study of esophageal cancer in urban Shanghai suggested a protective effect of green tea consumption (Gao et al, 1994). The effect of tea consumption on cancer is likely to depend on the causative factors of the specific cancer. Further laboratory and epidemiologic study is required to determine the relationship between green tea consumption and human cancer risk (Yang, 1993).

Hawthorn *(Crataegus oxyacantha).* Hawthorn grows as a spiny tree or shrub with thorny, branching stems. Both its blossoms and berries are used for their therapeutic properties. Hawthorn had a long history of use in Europe before it was introduced to this country in the nineteenth century. Since then, it has been used as a folk remedy, primarily as a cardiac tonic and a mild diuretic. Its therapeutic properties have long been recognized in Europe. This acceptance has been supported by a 4-year study of hawthorn commissioned by the German Federal Ministry of Health. The study concluded that hawthorn increases cardiac contractility and the rate of blood flow. It was also found to increase both coronary and myocardial circulation by its dilation effect on the coronary arteries. After taking hawthorn, individuals report a reduction in the number of angina attacks as well as symptom relief (Popping et al, 1994). In the United Kingdom, clinicians use hawthorn for its mild antihypertensive effect in clients with hypertension (Hoffman, 1995). In these individuals, hawthorn inhibits angiotensin converting enzyme (ACE), increases the contractility of the heart, and confers a mild diuretic action. If clients also take beta blockers for their hypertension, which reduce cardiac output, the inotropic effects of hawthorn may cause a slight increase in their blood pressure.

Hawthorn has been used in combination with digitalis, enhancing the effects of the cardiac glycosides found in digitalis. The dose of digitalis may be decreased if used in conjunction with hawthorn. Those with mild to moderate congestive heart failure may benefit from hawthorn alone. While hawthorn, because of a lack of data, cannot be seen as a substitute for the more powerful prescription drugs, it may complement them, enhancing their activity. For this reason, clients currently on cardiac drugs should discuss the use of hawthorn with their prescriber before taking the drug.

Milk thistle *(Silybum marianum).* This plant is used to prevent liver damage against a variety of toxins. Standardized extracts concentrate silymarin, a substance that apparently prevents the membrane of undamaged liver cells from letting toxins enter. Human trials for the treatment of hepatitis and cirrhosis have been "encouraging" (Weil, 1995).

Shark cartilage. This substance is one of the most controversial subjects of current medical debate. Although it has been suggested that it has antineoplastic properties and is presently in clinical trials by the Food and Drug Administration (FDA) on terminally ill individuals in New Jersey, shark cartilage is becoming more widely known as a treatment for osteoarthritis and rheumatoid arthritis. Researchers have been unable to determine the exact therapeutic agent in shark cartilage, however, most agree that the primary antiinflammatory component is the complex carbohydrates, mucopolysaccharides. Two of these mucopolysaccarides, condroitin sulfates A and C, have long been used by nutrition medicine practitioners to fight inflammation and enteritis. The naturally occurring forms of these compounds in shark cartilage are more effective than the synthetically refined mucopolysaccharides. When combined with the angiogenesis inhibition properties that are attributed to these proteins, shark cartilage may provide not only inflammation relief, but also inhibit the vascularization of cartilage in joints, which is also associated with advanced cases of osteoarthritis and rheumatoid arthritis. This action, inhibiting the formation of new blood vessels, is the basis for shark cartilage's alleged anticancer activity (Sculti, 1994).

Shark cartilage has been deemed nontoxic by the FDA and is sold as a food supplement in the United States There are major differences in the available forms of shark cartilage—tablets, capsules, caplets, soft gel caps, powders, and liquids. There are more than 40 different brand name products of shark cartilage sold directly to consumers in the United States and Canada. Many manufacturers claim their products have advantages in terms of purity, source, or manufacture but there is no industry standard. Many formulations contain binders or fillers; consumers should seek a product that is 100% pure shark cartilage. Even at that, bioavailability studies of shark cartilage components are lacking and the recommended dose is unsubstantiated. Pure shark cartilage generally contains about 35% protein, 50% minerals (60% of which is calcium and phosphorus in a 2:1 ratio), 8% carbohydrates (mainly present as mucopolysaccharides), 7% water, and less than 1% fat. The protein strands are thought to contain the active antiangiogenic components (Holt, 1995).

Although the dosage is unsubstantiated, most physicians familiar with shark cartilage agree that it is effective when the daily dosage is taken orally, three times a day, in equal amounts, about 15 to 30 minutes before meals. Each gram of dried powdered shark cartilage may be mixed in a blender with 2 oz of nonacidic fruit juice or nectar to make it more palatable. Capsules can be taken with water. Side effects seem to be limited to nausea related to its fishy taste. However, because of the material's antiangiogenetic effect, children, pregnant women, and those who have experienced a recent myocardial infarction should not be taking shark cartilage. It should be discontinued 3 months before and after any surgical procedure (Sculti, 1994).

Valerian *(Valeriana officinalis).* This herb is used for sleep problems and probably has mild sedating and tranquilizing effects. The plant's medicinal use has been recorded since ancient Greek and Roman times. Although it is an attractive plant with pink and white flowers, even the Roman physician Galen noted its objectionable odor. Valerian is used extensively in Europe, where it is accepted by allopathic medicine (Ravitzky, 1994).

The root and the rhizome of the plant are used for therapeutic effect. The root contains the volatile oils, valepotrits, valeranic acid, valeranone, and valereal, which are said to have a calming effect (Pedersed, 1987). Valerian not only eases the trouble of falling asleep but also improves the quality of sleep during the night. It seems to offer the benefit of a good night's sleep without the grogginess that accompanies some OTC sleep medications. Unlike some other sedatives, valerian seems to have none of the dependency risk; there is no synergistic effect when it is taken concurrently with alcohol or prescription drugs.

It is recommended that the root, chopped into small pieces, be steeped until cool before drinking, 1 teaspoon of root for each cup of liquid. One to three cups may be taken each day. It is also prepared in capsule and tincture forms for dosing. Valerian is considered to be nontoxic even when taken over long periods.

REMEDIES THAT MIGHT HARM

Because some herbal remedies can be harmful, the nurse should be familiar with the more toxic agents. Table 12-2 lists selected, unsafe herbs that should not be formulated and used as food, beverage, or medication. Table 12-3 lists herbal teas and the potential harmful effects associated with their usage.

The following are other remedies that might be harmful.

Chaparral. This desert shrub is sold as a tea, tablet, and capsule for its antioxidant properties. Chaparral was removed from the FDA's "generally recognized as safe" list in

TABLE 12-2 Selected unsafe herbals

Botanical name	Common names	Comments
Arnica montana	arnica flowers, Wolfsbane, mountain tobacco, *Flores Arnicae*	Substances extracted affect the heart and vascular systems. Arnica is extremely irritating and can induce a toxic gastroenteritis, nervous system disturbances, extreme muscle weakness, collapse, and perhaps, death
Artemisia absinthium	wormwood, absinthe, madderwort, absinthium, Mugwort	Contains a narcotic poison (oil of wormwood); can cause nervous system damage and mental impairment
Atropa belladonna	belladonna, deadly nightshade	Considered a poisonous plant that contains the toxic alkaloids of atropine, hyoscyamine, and hyoscine. Anticholinergic symptoms range from blurred vision, dry mouth, and inability to urinate to unusual behaviors and hallucinations
Aesculus hippocasteranum	buckeyes, horse chestnut, aesculus	Contains coumarin glycoside, aesculin; may interfere with normal blood clotting; a toxic plant
Conium maculatum	hemlock, conium, spotted hemlock, spotted parsley, St. Bennet's herb, spotted cowbane, fool's parsley	Contains toxic alkaloid coniine and perhaps, four other related alkaloids
Lobelia inflata	lobelia, Indian tobacco, wild tobacco, asthma weed, emetic weed	Toxic plant that contains lobeline plus other alkaloids; excessive use of plant or its leaves or fruit extracts can result in severe vomiting, pain, sweating, paralysis, decreased temperature, collapse, coma, and death
Vinca major *Vinca minor*	periwinkle, vinca, greater or lesser periwinkle	Contain toxic alkaloids (vinblastine, vincristine) that are cytotoxic and may cause liver, kidney, and neurologic damage

From Tyler (1993).

1970 after animal studies revealed damage to kidney and lymph organs. Four reports of liver toxicity occurred in 1992, which prompted the FDA to warn against the use of any product containing chaparral (News you can use, 1995). In addition to these U.S. cases, three cases have been reported in Canada (FDA, 1993).The National Nutritional Foods Association has asked its member companies not to carry these products; however, chaparral is still being sold and sometimes is an ingredient in combination products.

Comfrey. This herb is sold as a tea, tablet, capsule, tincture, poultice and lotion. Comfrey has been linked to a number of cases of liver impairment. Studies with animals demonstrate injury to lung, kidney, and gastrointestinal tissue. Australia, Canada, Germany, and the United Kingdom restrict the availability of comfrey.

Ephedra *[ma huang].* This substance is promoted for energy-boosting and weight control. Ephedra contains the sympathomimetic drugs ephedrine and pseudoephedrine, both of which cause vasoconstriction and may increase blood pressure, may cause cardiac arrhythmias, and are contraindicated for clients with angle-closure glaucoma, thyroid disorders, diabetes, hypertension, and angina. Ohio has restricted OTC ephedrine products, including ma huang, and a number of state drug regulators have requested the FDA to limit its use to prescription use only.

Lobelia *(Lobelia inflata [Indian tobacco]).* This leaf yields lobeline sulfate, which acts like nicotine and so may be used as antitobacco therapy. It acts as an agonist at nicotine receptors peripherally and centrally. Lobelia produces behavioral stimulation and depression, cardiac acceleration, peripheral vasoconstriction, and elevated blood pressure. It is contraindicated for use in individuals with unstable cardiovascular conditions such as angina, arrhythmias, postmyocardial infarct, and hypertension.

Yohimbe. Yohimbe is a plant product made from the bark of an African tree and is generally touted as a aphrodisiac for men. Its active ingredient, yohimbine, is used for the treatment of erectile impotence; however, neither the United States or Canada include that as an indication for its use in its package labeling. In some individuals it has caused

TABLE 12-3 Herbal teas and toxic reactions

Herbal tea	Proposed usage	Potential toxic effect
chamomile	appetite stimulant, anodyne, carminative, antispasmodic	With persons allergic to ragweed, chrysanthemums, etc., it can cause skin rash and severe hypersensitivity reactions, including anaphylaxis
hydrangea	kidney stones, diuretic	Some species contain cyanide-producing compounds, especially when smoked; may make users very ill (Tyler, 1993)
mistletoe	parasitic; American mistletoe stimulates smooth muscles, increasing blood pressure and GI contractions; European mistletoe has opposite effect, lowers blood pressure and is antispasmotic	Over 200 species available with toxic proteins; can be poisonous, avoid use
rue	antispasmotic, calmative, abortifacient, insect repellent	Contains coumadin deratives; external use can cause skin blisters and photosensitization; internal use can cause gastric upset and toxicity (Tyler, 1993)
shave grass or horsetail plants	diuretic	Contains silica and glycosides (when consumed by horses and other grazing animals, anorexia, loss of muscle control, excitability, diarrhea, seizures, coma, and death may occur)

Adapted from Tyler (1993); Nightingale (1993).

increased blood pressure and heart rate, dizziness, headache, irritability, or nervousness. According to the *AMA Drug Evaluations* (1995), the documentation of yohimbine's usefulness to treat impotence is inconclusive.

CONSUMER EDUCATION FOR ALTERNATIVE/COMPLEMENTARY REMEDIES

Alternative/complementary remedies will continue to be used because of the strong traditions and the desire to increase a sense of control on the part of clients to improve their well being.

The nurse must recognize and clarify his or her own values. This awareness will assist the nurse not to impose his or her own health beliefs onto the client and family. The nurse can then assist the client and family to explore their values and beliefs. This will assist the client to make the "right" decisions and help the nurse to better understand and support the client's choices. Nurses may then incorporate the reasonable components of the alternative therapy into the client's therapeutic regimen.

If a client takes or wishes to take an alternative/complementary remedy the following recommendations should be helpful.

The client should consult with his or her primary health care provider as to the benefit or harm that might occur as a result of taking these substances. This would prevent the client from delaying contact with a caregiver because of the use of an alternative therapy. The prescriber could also provide information on the efficacy of the particular remedy. This consultation would be especially important if the client is taking prescription medications. Any of the alternative/complementary medications may interact with the client's current medication regimen, either by enhancing its effects or inhibiting them, or by combining for a toxic effect. Alternative/complementary remedies, just like OTC drugs, should be considered as medications, and information related to their use should be shared as a part of the client's health history as current medications. Pregnant and breastfeeding women should not take any alternative remedies without the prescriber's approval.

Providers should proactively question clients about the use of alternative/complementary remedies and the answers should be documented in their health record.

Counsel the client as to lifestyle changes that may be more effective than the use of alternative/complementary remedies to accomplish the client's therapeutic goals. For example, if the client wishes to lower serum cholesterol levels, a low fat, high fiber diet and exercise may be more effective and less expensive then taking garlic supplements. Just as with allopathic medications, the therapeutic outcome is enhanced by supportive behavioral changes.

Just as with OTC medications, the client should use single-agent products. This provides for more effective evaluation of the remedy's therapeutic effect, as well as minimizing adverse responses that may occur as a result of ingesting multiple substances. Also, if the client experiences an adverse effect, determination of the causative agent is easier. Evaluate the product for standardization. This increases the chance of the contents of the remedy of being consistent from dose to dose.

If a serious toxicity is suspected, the client should be able to provide a sample of the remedy for chemical analysis. Health care providers should report serious adverse reactions involving herbal remedies to the FDA MedWatch Program (800-332-1088).

Labels should be well read and warnings on the package heeded. Parents need to be cautioned to keep these substances out of the reach of children. The client needs to be knowledgeable about the expected actions of the medication, and if they do not occur in a reasonable time, the drug should be discontinued. Objective criteria should be determined with the client so that measurable progress or lack of progress can be documented to decrease the power of suggestion as to the drug's therapeutic effects, e.g., weekly weights in the case of weight loss medications. Adverse effects of the drug should also be known and the client should discontinue the drug if there's a problem and notify a physician.

Caution clients that commercially available alternative medications may be adulterated because they do not undergo standardized testing for safety and efficacy by the FDA. The role of the nurse is to educate clients regarding the appropriate use of or possibly hazardous misuse of alternative/complementary remedies.

SUMMARY

Many alternative/complementary remedies have been promoted on the basis of anecdotal accounts—sometimes for hundreds of years—from people who have indicated that a particular substance has kept them well or cured their illness. There is no way of knowing what might have been the result if the individual had not taken the remedy; many illnesses are self-limiting. The placebo effect also can not be discounted. Many of these remedies show promise for further research. But until the same rigorousness of randomized, double-blind trials is applied to alternative/complementary remedies as is applied to allopathic medicines, one needs to remain cautious about their use.

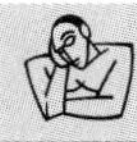

Critical Thinking

1. Given all the cautions previously discussed regarding alternative/complementary remedies, how would these cautions differ from the adverse effects of allopathic medicines?

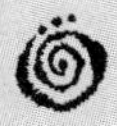

Collaborative Learning Activities

1. Visit a pharmacy or health foods store. Assign each student team a health product that would seem to have a positive health value, such as the ones listed in the chapter. Determine the annual cost of such a product. Discuss the cost/benefits of the health products.

BIBLIOGRAPHY

American Medical Association (1995). *Drug evaluations annual.* Chicago: The Association.

Anderson LA (1996). Concern regarding herbal toxicities: Case reports and counseling tips, *Annal Pharmacother* 30:79-80.

Awang DVC (1989). Feverfew, *Can Pharm J* 122(5):266-70.

Bhattacharya SK & Mitra SK (1991). Anxiolytic activity of Panax ginseng roots: An experimental study, *J Ethnopharmacol* 34(1): 87-92.

Brody JE (1994, July 27). Personal health: Modern doctors confirm the ancient wisdom that garlic has many benefits, *New York Times*.

Burnham BE (1995). Garlic as a possible risk for postoperative bleeding, *Plast Reconstr Surg* 96(2):483-4.

Chan TY, et al. (1993). Chinese herbal medicines revisited: A Hong Kong perspective, *Lancet* 342 (8886-8887):1532-4.

Chu DT, Wong WK, & Mavaligit GM (1988a). Immunotherapy with Chinese medicinal herbs. II. Reversal of cyclophosphamide-induced immune induced suppression by administration of fractionated *Artragalus membranaceous* in vivo, *J Clin Lab Immunol* 25:125-9.

Chu DT, Wong WK, & Mavaligit GM (1988b). Immunotherapy with Chinese medicinal herbs. I. Immune restoration of local xenogeneic graft-versus-host reaction in cancer patients by fractionated *Atragalus membranaceous* in vitro, *J Clin Lab Immunol* 25:119-23.

Coeugniet EG & Elek E (1987). Immunomodulation with *Viscum album* and *Echinacea purpurea* extracts, *Onkologie* 10(3 Suppl.): 27-33.

Das I, Khan NS, & Sooranna SR (1995). Potent activation of nitric oxide synthase by garlic: A basis for its therapeutic applications, *Curr Med Research & Opinion* 13(5):257-63.

Dorant E, et al. (1993). Garlic and its significance for the prevention of cancer in humans: A critical review, *Brit J Cancer* 67(3):424-9.

Eisenberg DM, et al (1993). Unconventional medicine in the United States: Prevalence, costs, and patterns of use, *New Engl J Med* 328(8):246-52.

Farbman KS, et al. (1993). Antibacterial activity of garlic and onions: A historical perspective, *Pediatr Infect Disease J* 12(7):613-4.

Fletcher DM (1992). Unconventional cancer treatments: Professional, legal, and ethical issues, *Oncol Nurs Forum* 19(9):1351-4.

Food and Drug Administration (FDA) (1993). From the Food and Drug Administration, *JAMA* 269(3):328.

Foster S (1995). Feverfew: When the head hurts, *Alternat & Complement Therap* 1(5):335-7.

Gao YT, et al. (1994). Reduced risk of esophageal cancer associated with green tea consumption, *J National Cancer Institut* 86(11):855-8.

German K, Kumar U, & Blackford HN (1995). Garlic and the risk of TURP bleeding, *Brit J Urol* 76(4):518.

Gertner E, et al. (1995). Complications resulting from the use of Chinese herbal medications containing undeclared prescription drugs, *Arthrit & Rheum* 38(5):614-7.

Goldman JA & Myerson G (1991). Chinese herbal medicine: Camouflaged prescription antiinflammatory drugs, corticosteriods, and lead, *Arthrit & Rheum* 34(9):1207.

Gorey JD, Wahlqvist ML, & Boyce NW (1992). Adverse reaction to a Chinese herbal remedy, *Med J Australia* 157(7):484-6.

Guo NL, et al. (1993). Demonstration of the antiviral activity of garlic extract against human cytomegalovirus in vitro, *Chin Med J* 106(2):93-6.

Heptinstall S, et al. (1991). Parthenolide content and bioactivity of feverfew. Estimation of commercial and authenticated feverfew products, *J Pharm Pharmacol* 44:391-5.

Herbal roulette. (1995). *Consumer Reports* 60(11):698-705.

Hoffman D (1995). Hawthorn: The heart helper, *Alternat & Complement Therap* 1(3):191-2.

Holt S (1995). Shark cartilage and nutriceutical update, *Alternat & Complement Therap* 1(6):414-6.

Imai K & Nakachi K (1995). Cross sectional study of effects of drinking green tea on cardiovascular and liver diseases, *BMJ 310* (6981):693-6.

Johnson ES, et al. (1985). Efficacy of feverfew as a prophylactic treatment of migraine, *Brit Med J 291*:569-573.

Khan SG, Katiyar SK, Agarwal R, & Mukhtar H (1992). Enhancement of antioxidant and phase II enzymes by oral feeding of green tea polyphenols in drinking water to SKH-1 hairless mice: Possible role in cancer prevention, *Cancer Research 52*(14): 4050-2.

Katiyar SK, Agarwal R, & Mukhtar H (1993). Protection against malignant conversion of chemically induced benign skin papillomas to squamous cell carcinomas in SENCAR mice by a polyphenolic fraction isolated from green tea, *Cancer Research 53*(22):5409-12.

Kim H, Chen X, & Gillis CN (1992). Ginsenosides protect pulmonary vascular endothelium against free radical-induced injury, *Biochem & Biophys Res Commun 189*(2):670-6.

Liebert MA (1994). From the publisher: Introducing alternative & complementary therapies, *Altern & Complement Therap 1*(1):ix.

Liu CX & Xiao PG (1992). Recent advances on ginseng research in China, *J Ethnopharmacol* 36(1):27-38.

Lumb AB (1994). Effect of dried ginger on human platelet function, *Thromb & Haemosta 71*(1):110-1.

McDowell B (1994). Institutional profile: The National Institutes of Health Office of Alternative Medicine: Evaluating research outcomes, *Alternat & Complement Therap 1*(1):17-25.

Murphy J, Heptinstall S, & Mitchell JRA (1989). Randomized, double-blind, placebo-controlled trial of feverfew in migraine prevention, *Lancet* July 23:189-192.

Nelson L, Shih R, & Hoffman R (1995). Aplastic anemia induced by an adulterated herbal medication, *J Toxicol - Clin Toxicol 33* (5): 467-70.

NARD J (1992). Real medicine or snake oil?, *NARD J 115*(2):17-20.

News you can use. (1995). *Alternat & Complement Therap* 1(5):342.

Nightingale SL (1993). From the Food and Drug Administration: Public warning about herbal products, *JAMA 269*(3):328.

Oubre A (1995). Social context of complementary medicine in Western society, part II: Traditional Chinese medicine and HIV illness, *J Alternat & Complement Med 1*(2):161-85.

Petry JJ (1995). Garlic and postoperative bleeding, *Plast Reconstr Surg 95*(1):213.

Phillips S, Hutchinson S, & Ruggier R: Zingiber officinale does not affect gastric emptying rate: A randomised, placebo-controlled, crossover trial, *Anaesthesia 48*(5):393-5.

Phillips S, Ruggier R, & Hutchinson S (1993). Zingiber officinale (ginger)—an antiemetic for day case surgery, *Anaesthesia 48*(8):715-7.

Popping J, et al. (1994). Effect of crataegus extract on the contraction and the consumption of oxygen of isolated cardiac muscle cells, *Med Wschr 136*:39-46.

Ravitzky M (1994). Valerian: Nature's antianxiety agent, *Alternat & Complement Therap* 1(1):48-9.

Saita T, et al. (1993). The first specific antibody against cytotoxic polyacetylenic alcohol, panaxynol, *Chem & Pharmaceut Bull 41*(3):549-52.

Sculti L (1994). Arthritis benefits from shark cartilage therapy, *Alternat & Complement Therap 1*(1):35-7.

Snider S (1991). Beware the unknown brew: Herbal teas and toxicity, *FDA Consumer* (May):31-33.

Sohn HO, et al. (1993). Effect of subchronic administration of antioxidants against cigarette smoke exposure in rats, *Arch Toxicol 67*(10):667-73.

Stimpel MA, et al. (1984). Macrophage activation and induction of macrophage cytotoxicity by purified polysaccharide fractions from the plant Echinacea purpurea, *Infect Immun 46*(3):845-9.

Sun XB, Matsumoto T, & Yamada H (1992). Anti-ulcer activity and mode of action of the polysaccharide fraction from the leaves of Panax ginseng, *Planta Medica 58*(5):432-5.

Tode T, et al. (1993). Inhibitory effects by oral administration of ginsenoside Rh2 on the growth of human ovarian cancer cells in nude mice, *J Cancer Res & Clin Oncol 120*(1-2):24-6.

Tomoda M, et al. (1993). Characterization of two acidic polysaccharides having immunological activities from the root of Panax ginseng, *Biol & Pharmaceut Bull 16*(1):22-5.

Tyler VE (1993). *The honest herbal* (3rd ed.). New York: Pharmaceutical Products Press.

Wang ZY, et al. (1994). Inhibitory effects of black tea, green tea, decaffeinated black tea, and decaffeinated green tea on ultraviolet B light-induced skin carcinogenesis in 7,12-dimethylbenz[a]anthracene-initiated SKH-1 mice, *Cancer Research 54*(13):3428-35.

Wang ZY, et al. (1992a). Inhibitory effect of green tea on the growth of established skin papillomas in mice, *Cancer Research 52*(23):6657-65.

Wang ZY, et al. (1992b). Inhibition of N-nitrosodiethylamine- and 4-(methynitroamino)-1-(3-pyridyl)-1-butanone-induced tumorigenesis in A/J mice by green tea and black tea, *Cancer Research 52*(7):1943-7.

Warshafsky S, Kamer RS, & Sivak SL (1993). Effect of garlic on total serum cholesterol: A meta-analysis, *Ann Intern Med 119*(7 Pt 1):599-605.

Watanabe H, et al. (1991). Effect of Panax ginseng on age-related changes in the spontaneous motor activity and dopaminergic nervous system in the rat, *Japan J Pharmacol 55*(1):51-6.

Weil A (1995). *Spontaneous healing: How to discover and enhance your body's natural ability to maintain and heal itself.* New York: Alfred A. Knopf.

Xu Y, et al. (1992). Inhibition of tobacco-specific nitrosamine-induced lung tumorigenesis in A/J mice by green tea and its major polyphenol as antioxidants, *Cancer Research 52*(14):3875-9.

Yang CS & Wang ZY (1993). Tea and cancer, *J National Cancer Inst 85*(13):1038-49.

Yun TK & Choi SY (1995). Preventive effect of ginseng intake against various human cancers: a case-control study on 1987 pairs, *Cancer Epidemiol Biomarkers & Prev 4*(4):401-8.

Chapter 13

Overview of the Central Nervous System

Chapter Focus

The nervous system coordinates all body functions, and its activities allow the individual to adapt to the internal and external environment. Because of the complexity of this system, the monitoring of pharmacologic interventions can be challenging. Knowledge of the anatomy and physiology of the central nervous system provides a foundation for sound clinical decision making in this area. The following objectives and key terms are important for a good understanding of this chapter.

Key Terms

acetylcholine (p. 225)
blood-brain barrier (p. 223)
brainstem (p. 221)
catecholamines (p. 226)
cerebellum (p. 221)
cerebrum (p. 220)
endorphins (p. 226)
extrapyramidal system (p. 225)
hypothalamus (p. 221)
limbic system (p. 225)
midbrain (p. 221)
pons (p. 221)
reticular activating system (RAS) (p. 224)
synapse (p. 225)
thalamus (p. 221)

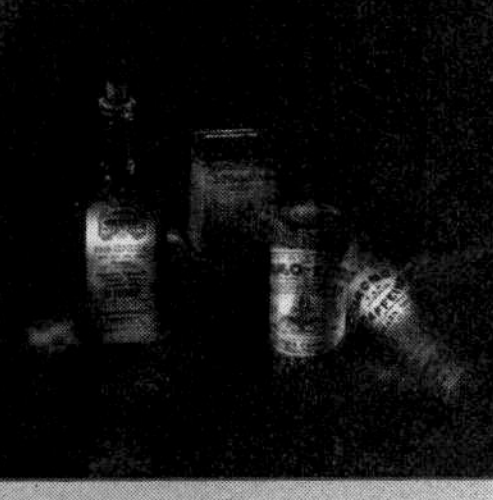

Objectives

1. Identify the major components of the CNS.
2. Describe the functions of the components of the CNS.
3. Identify the structure and function of the blood-brain barrier.
4. Describe three major functional systems of the CNS.
5. Describe the function of the common neurotransmitter substances.

The nervous system consists of the central nervous system (CNS) and the peripheral nervous system (PNS) (Figure 13-1). The PNS is discussed in Chapter 20. This chapter reviews the primary areas of the CNS, focusing on the specific areas affected by drug therapy.

The CNS, composed of the brain and spinal cord, essentially controls all functions in the body. The PNS is the network that transmits information to and from the CNS, thus alerting the CNS to internal and external changes, such as muscle tension, blood vessel alterations, pain, fever, sound, smell, taste, touch, and sight. This information is integrated, and instructions are then relayed to appropriate cells or tissues to produce the necessary actions and environmental adjustments. Information concerning these actions and adjustments is again fed back into the CNS. The constant feeding of information into the CNS permits continuous adjustments to be made in the instructions sent to various tissues to ensure effective control of body functions.

BRAIN

The brain can be physically divided in various ways. A simplified approach is to divide it into major components—cerebrum, parietal lobe, frontal lobe, thalamus, occipital lobe, temporal lobe, cerebellum, midbrain, pons, and medulla oblongata (Figure 13-2). The following are the major areas of the brain affected by specific drug therapies.

Cerebrum. The **cerebrum,** the largest and uppermost section of the brain, is the highest functional area of the brain, where memory storage and sensory, integrative, emotional, language, and motor functions are controlled. The cerebrum consists of two hemispheres (right and left) connected by fibrous tracts. The outer surface of the cerebrum is called the cerebral cortex or gray matter of the brain, and it covers the four lobes into which each hemisphere is divided. These lobes are named for the bones of the skull under which they lie—frontal, parietal, occipital, and temporal. The frontal lobe contains the motor and speech areas. The sensory cortex is located in the parietal lobe, the visual cortex in the occipital lobe, and the auditory cortex in the temporal lobe. Association areas lie near these lobes and act in conjunction with them. In addition, large parts of the cortex are concerned with higher mental activity—reasoning, creative thought, judgment, memory—those attributes that are unique to humans and separate them from other animals.

Drugs that depress cortical activity may decrease acuity of sensation and perception, inhibit motor activity, decrease alertness and concentration, and even promote drowsiness and sleep. Drugs that stimulate the cortical areas may cause more vivid impulses to be received and greater awareness of the surrounding environment. In addition, increased muscle activity and restlessness may occur. The specific response brought forth by a drug depends to a large extent on the personality of the individual, the emotional and physiologic

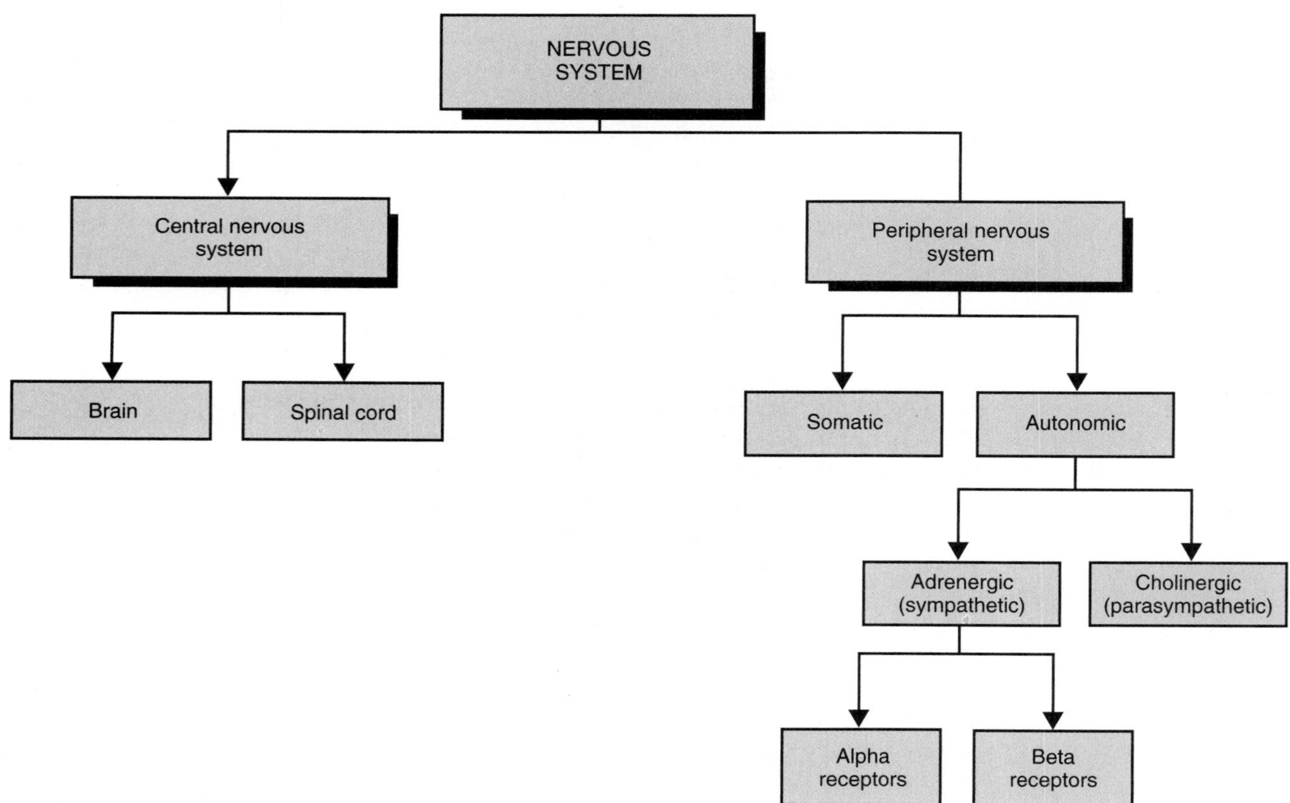

Figure 13-1 Overview of the nervous system.

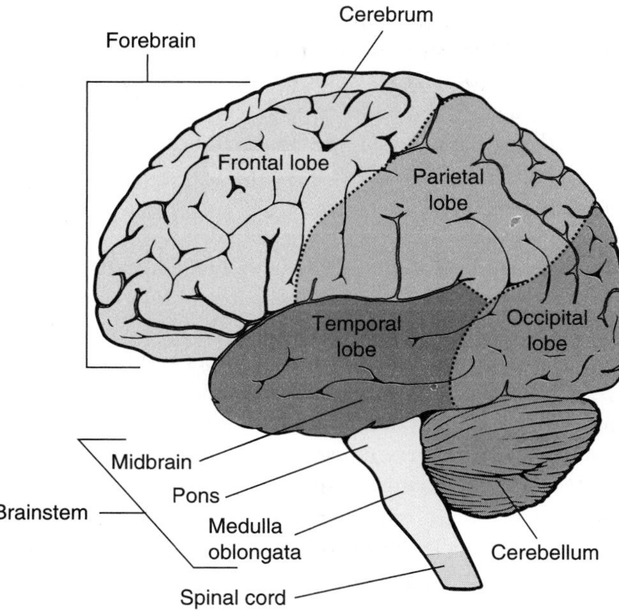

Figure 13-2 The human brain.

state, the specific attributes of the drug, and a host of other factors.

Thalamus. The **thalamus** is composed of sensory nuclei and serves as the major relay center for impulses to and from the cerebral cortex. It also registers such sensations as pain, temperature, touch, and other sensory impulses and relays this information to the cerebrum.

The thalamus enables the individual to have impressions of pleasantness or unpleasantness, and it also appears to play a part (with the reticular activating system) in arousal or alerting signals. (See Reticular Activating System [RAS] later in this chapter for a further description.) Drugs that depress cells in the various portions of the thalamus may interrupt the free flow of impulses to the cerebral cortex. This is one way in which pain may be relieved.

Hypothalamus. The **hypothalamus** lies below the thalamus and is vital for maintaining many body functions and for the well-being of the individual. It is a major link between the mind and the body, and it also regulates the release of anterior pituitary gland hormones. Functions of the hypothalamus include regulation of body temperature, carbohydrate and fat metabolism, and water balance; the appetite center and pleasure or reward centers are also believed to be located here. There is evidence that a center for sleep and wakefulness also exists within the hypothalamus. Some of the sleep-producing drugs are thought to depress hypothalamic centers.

As part of its integrative role in neurohormonal regulation, neurons in the hypothalamus release hormones that affect the anterior pituitary gland. Growth hormone, hormones that affect sexual glands or functions, and thyroid and the adrenal cortex hormones are under the control of the hypothalamus.

The hypothalamus, along with other specific areas of the brain, is also involved with the control of emotions. These functions of the hypothalamus may be affected by drugs. An example is the use of antidepressants to treat the symptoms of depression. The action of tricyclic antidepressants on the hypothalamus often reverses the symptoms of weight loss, anorexia, decreased libido, and insomnia associated with depression. Other psychotherapeutic agents may cause a number of hypothalamic side effects, including breast engorgement, lactation, amenorrhea, appetite stimulation, and alterations in temperature regulation.

Brainstem. The **brainstem** is composed of the midbrain, pons, and medulla oblongata and is the source of 10 of the 12 cranial nerves (Table 13-1); the exceptions are the olfactory and optic nerves. The **midbrain** contains nerve tracts to and from the cerebrum. It is also the source of the third (oculomotor) and fourth (trochlear) cranial nerves; some optic fibers are also located here. The midbrain serves as a relay station from higher areas of the brain to lower centers. The source of the fifth, sixth, seventh, and eighth cranial nerves is the **pons**. It also contains a center that controls involuntary respiratory regulation. The midbrain and pons are affected by drugs as they stimulate or depress the reticular activating system. The medulla oblongata contains the vital centers: the respiratory, vasomotor, and cardiac centers. Such centers are referred to as vital because they are necessary for survival. Other essential functions also originate here, such as vomiting, hiccuping, sneezing, coughing, and swallowing reflexes.

If the respiratory center is stimulated by drugs, it will discharge an increased number of nerve impulses over nerve pathways to the muscles of respiration. If it is depressed, it will discharge fewer impulses, and respiration will be correspondingly affected. Other centers in the medulla that respond to certain drugs are the cough center and the vomiting center. The medulla, pons, and midbrain contain many important correlation centers (gray matter), as well as ascending and descending pathways (white matter).

Cerebellum. The **cerebellum**, located in the posterior cranial fossa behind the brainstem, contains centers for muscle coordination, equilibrium, and muscle tone. It receives afferent impulses from the vestibular nuclei, as well as the cerebrum, and plays an important role in the maintenance of posture and voluntary muscular activity. Drugs that disturb the cerebellum or vestibular branch of the eighth cranial nerve cause dizziness and loss of equilibrium.

SPINAL CORD

The spinal cord, a center for reflex activity, also functions in the transmission of impulses to and from the higher centers in the brain and may be affected by the action of drugs. Ascending sensory tracts conduct impulses up from peripheral nerves to the brain, and descending motor tracts conduct impulses down from the brain to peripheral nerves.

A cross-section of the spinal cord reveals an internal mass of gray matter enclosed by white matter (Figure 13-3). The butterfly-shaped gray matter is divided into horns; the afferent (sensory) nerve fibers are located in the dorsal or posterior section, whereas the efferent (motor) nerve fibers exit from the ventral or anterior horns. For example, when a pain impulse reaches the dorsal horn, the impulse will be transmitted along special tracts (lateral spinothalamic tract) to the thalamus, which then distributes the message to other areas of the brain. The brain responds by means of the descending efferent fiber pathways to inhibit or modify other incoming pain stimuli. (See the discussion of the gate theory of pain in Chapter 14.) Small doses of spinal stimulants may increase reflex excitability; larger doses may cause convulsions.

When a drug is described as having a central action, it means that it has an action on the brain or the spinal cord.

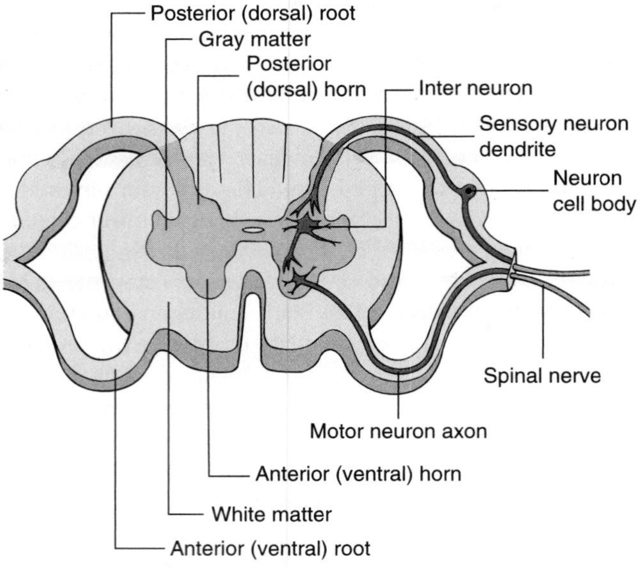

Figure 13-3 Cross-section of the spinal cord.

CELL TYPES

The two major cell types in the CNS are glial cells and neurons. The functions of the glial cells are not fully understood, although recent studies indicate that they are composed of many types of neurotransmitter receptors and ion channels. It is possible that this type of network might serve to support and assist neurons in the transfer and integration of information in the central nervous system (Wingard, 1991).

Neurons have four basic parts: dendrites, cell body, axon, and axon or nerve terminals (Figure 13-4). The cell body contains the nucleus (genetic information) and the ribosomes, Nissl substance, and endoplasmic reticulum necessary for protein synthesis. The Golgi complex stores, processes, and concentrates the protein while the mitochondria in the cell body and dendrites provide the production of energy necessary for protein synthesis and lipid metabolism.

Dendrites also contain some neurotransmitter vesicles; thus incoming messages from other neurons are received in the dendrites, processed in the cell body, transported in the axon, and exit via the axon terminal. This process of conveying messages from one cell body to another usually involves electrical or chemical transport of the message across a synapse. Most information transmitted in the central nervous system is due to alterations in electrical currents; the

TABLE 13-1 Cranial nerves

Cranial nerve	Type of nerve	Function
I Olfactory	Sensory	Smell
II Optic	Sensory	Sight
III Oculomotor	Motor	Movement of eye and eyelid muscles, pupillary constriction
IV Trochlear	Motor	Eye muscle for downward and inward motion of eye
V Trigeminal	Motor	Chewing, lateral jaw movement
	Sensory	Sensations of the face, scalp, oral cavity, teeth, and tongue
VI Abducens	Motor	Eye movements
VII Facial	Motor	Facial expressions
	Sensory	Taste
VIII Acoustic	Sensory	Hearing, equilibrium
IX Glossopharyngeal	Motor	Swallowing, salivation
	Sensory	Taste, throat sensations
X Vagus	Motor	Voice production, decrease in heartbeat, swallowing, increased peristalsis
	Sensory	Gag reflex; sensations of throat, larynx, and abdominal viscera
XI Spinal accessory	Motor	Head and shoulder movements
XII Hypoglossal	Motor	Tongue movements

Drug effects, toxicity, or both have been reported to affect various cranial nerve functions. For example, ototoxicity, or eighth cranial nerve damage, has been reported with aminoglycoside antibiotics. Vincristine, an antineoplastic agent, may produce ptosis (cranial nerve III), trigeminal neuralgia (cranial nerve VII), facial palsy (cranial nerve V), and jaw pain. Since various medications have the potential for affecting the cranial nerves adversely, the student should be familiar with the functions of the cranial nerves.

following is a brief summary of this process. For more detailed information, refer to a current anatomy and physiology textbook.

The electrical properties of nerve cells are generated by various ions, pumps, and channels located in the cell membrane. A nerve cell in the resting state is illustrated in Figure 13-5. A membrane difference or potential is caused by changes in ion concentration of sodium, potassium, and chloride. Pumps are capable of actively moving charged ions from one side of the membrane to the other side, and channels are membrane pores that allow the movement of specific ions to pass.

In the resting state, sodium and chloride are found in large amounts outside the cell while potassium is in high concentration in the cell. The concentration gradients are stabilized by the sodium-potassium ATPase pump, which trades three sodium ions from the intracellular fluid for two potassium ions from the extracellular fluid. This helps to maintain the resting membrane potential. The movement and concentration of these ions in and around the cell are the primary determinants affecting the membrane potential of the nerve cells.

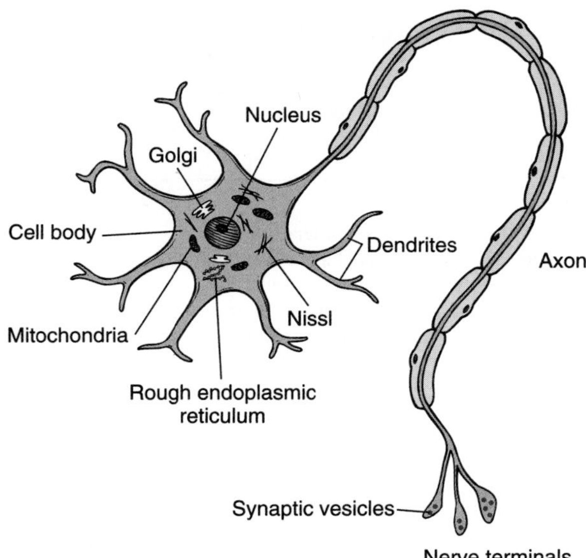

Figure 13-4 Structural components of nerve cells.

During rest or after an electrical potential, potassium ions selectively flow to outside the nerve cell, which allows sodium (positive ions) to enter the nerve cell. This action alters or reduces the membrane potential, and as the sodium influx increases, the cell depolarizes. Depolarization will result in the opening of more sodium channels, thus allowing more sodium to flow into the cell, which causes further depolarization of the nerve cell. This reduction in membrane potential generates an action potential as a result of the changes illustrated in Figure 13-6.

Drugs can act directly on the ion channel or via receptors that affect ion channels. For example, general anesthetics and ethanol bind to specific receptors, which effectively reduces sodium influx, preventing regeneration of the action potentials and conduction of nerve impulses. The action of the sodium-potassium pump on cardiac cells will be discussed in the cardiac glycoside section in Chapter 25.

BLOOD-BRAIN BARRIER

The **blood-brain barrier** is actually a covering of nerve cells (astrocytes) that encircle the brain's capillary walls. This covering prevents the passage of many drugs or large molecules into the brain, but it will allow small molecules (such as water, alcohol, oxygen, and carbon dioxide), glucose, gases, and lipid-soluble substances to penetrate. Such selective processing allows the brain a degree of security against the toxic

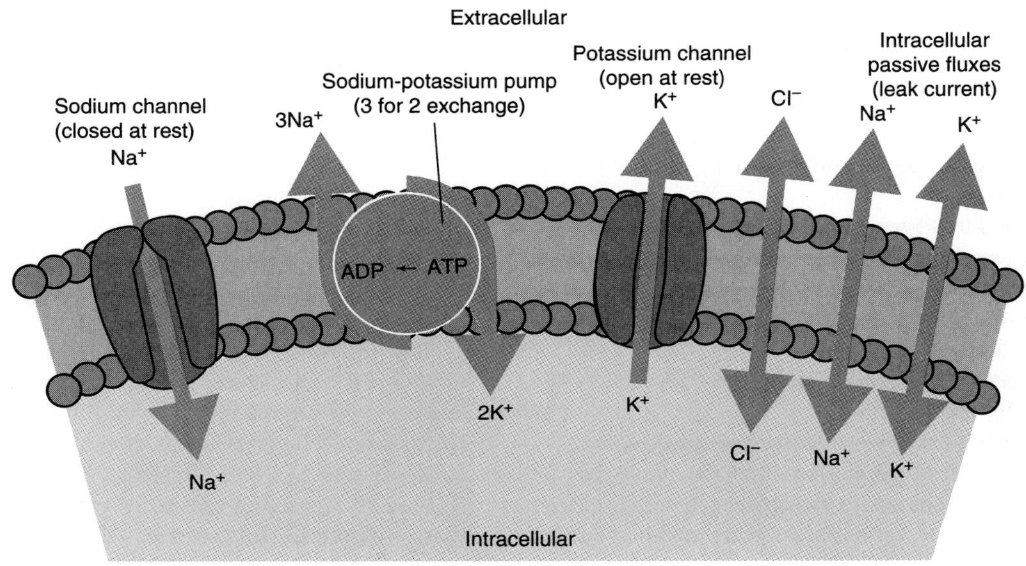

Figure 13-5 Primary determinants of resting membrane potential in nerve cells.

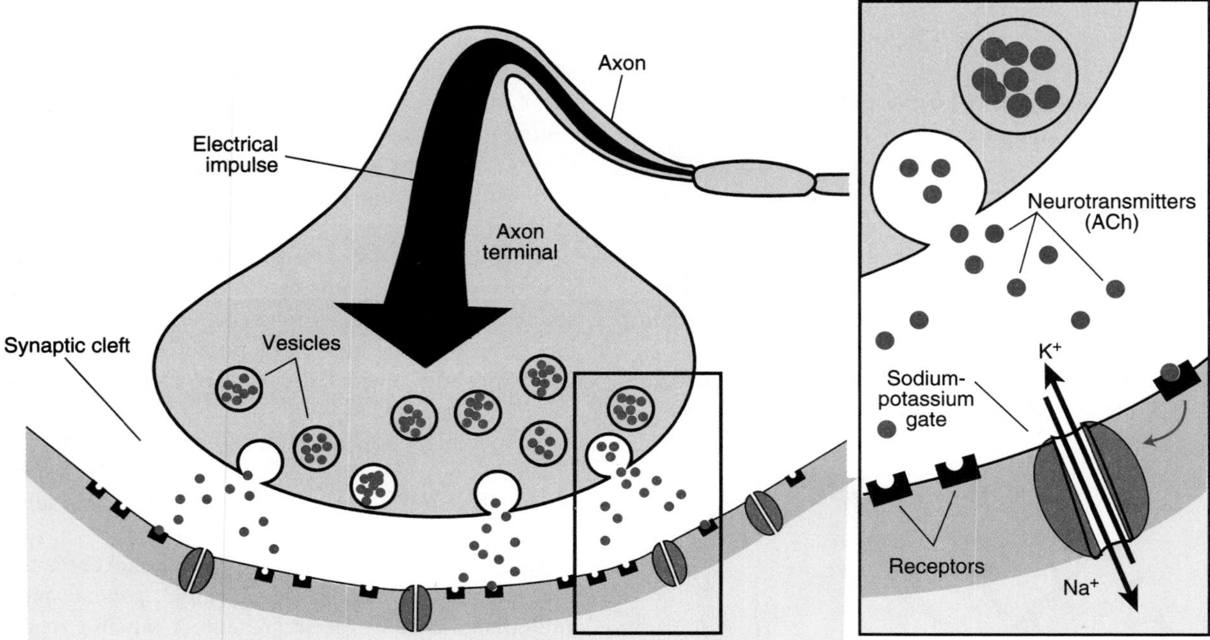

Figure 13-6 Nerve cell depolarization. Intracellular sodium is lower than extracellular sodium concentration in the resting state, which is regulated by the sodium-potassium ATPase pump. Electrical impulses release neurotransmitters that alter the membrane potential of the nerve cell. The sodium-potassium gate opens during cell depolarization, resulting in an increased Na^+ influx into the cell. Then the sodium channels are inactivated (gate closes) to start the beginning of the repolarization phase. See text for further information.

effects of some drugs on the CNS. However, in large doses or in instances of meningeal inflammation the permeation of such substances across the blood-brain barrier will increase. Current research is studying methods to increase the permeability of the blood-brain barrier to specific therapeutic agents, such as antibiotics or antineoplastic agents, needed to treat a localized brain infection or brain tumors.

CNS FUNCTIONAL SYSTEMS

The three major CNS functional systems affected by selected drug or chemical administration include (1) the reticular activating system, (2) the limbic system, and (3) the extrapyramidal system.

Reticular activating system. The **reticular activating system** (RAS) is a diffuse system of nuclei in the brainstem that permits a two-way communication among the spinal cord, thalamus, and the cerebral cortex. The primary functions of the RAS are:

1. Consciousness and arousal effect
2. An alerting mechanism
3. A filter process that allows for concentration

When stimulated, the gray matter of the pons and the midbrain transmits impulses to the thalamus, which further transmits the impulse to various areas of the cerebral cortex. This results in consciousness or awakening and possibly an arousal effect. Arousal reactions require an external signal, such as a pain stimulus, an alarm clock, or bright lights. The cerebral cortex may signal the RAS or vice versa, but the end result is activation of both areas that may lead to additional transmission of impulses throughout the body (e.g., skeletal muscle activation). Inactivation of the RAS results in sleep, whereas injury or disease may produce a lack of consciousness or comatose state.

The alerting mechanism's primary function is self-preservation—for example, waking up at night because of a chilly sensation. Once awakened, the individual can assess the situation and discover the reason for awakening, such as the blanket on the bed having fallen to the floor. The sensation of feeling chilly activated the RAS and caused the awakening, but the situation had to be assessed to determine why the chilliness occurred.

The filter mechanism allows the individual to decrease the perception of monotonous stimuli that usually surround us. It permits us to concentrate on a specific stimulus at a given time. For example, imagine attending a large party where nearly everyone is talking at the same time. A functioning RAS will allow us to focus on the single conversation or person we are interested in by filtering out all the other conversations. In other words, it permits us to have selective concentration.

Many drugs act on the RAS. Anesthetics dampen its activity and induce sleep, whereas amphetamines stimulate or activate the system. LSD and some of the other hallucinogenic agents may act on the RAS by interfering with its ability to filter out stimuli; therefore the person taking this substance is bombarded by all kinds of wanted and sometimes unwanted stimuli. In contrast, it is a proposed theory that chlorpromazine stimulates the activity of the RAS and reinstates the activity of the filtering process, thus making it useful in reducing hallucinations in the psychotic client and in individuals experiencing an untoward reaction to LSD, a hallucinogenic drug.

Limbic system. The **limbic system** is a border of subcortical structures that surround the corpus callosum (Figure 13-7). This system forms a ring around the top of the brainstem that consists of the portions of the brain remaining after the cerebral hemispheres and cerebellum have been removed.

The emotions of anger, fear, anxiety, sexual feelings, pleasure, and sorrow are related to this system. Learning and memory have been associated with the hippocampus, a component of the limbic system.

The limbic system is extremely complex in its functioning. It may work with or inhibit other parts of the brain such as the cerebral cortex, brainstem, or hypothalamus to normalize expressions of emotions, influence their ultimate expression to other than normal, or affect the biologic rhythms, sexual behavior, and motivation of an individual.

Drugs that affect the limbic system are the benzodiazepines, meprobamate, and morphine. The benzodiazepines and meprobamate are believed to suppress the limbic system, preventing it from activating the reticular formation, thus resulting in drowsiness and sleep, especially in clients with anxiety. Morphine is thought to alter the subjective reactions of the individual to pain in addition to abolishing pain stimuli received by special areas within the limbic system.

Extrapyramidal system. The **extrapyramidal system** is a somatic motor pathway located in the CNS that affects skeletal muscles. This system is associated with coordination of muscle group movements and posture. Antipsychotic agents that block dopamine receptors may produce side effects or adverse effects related to this system. For further discussion of these effects see Chapter 19.

SYNAPTIC TRANSMISSION IN THE CNS

The **synapse** is the junction point between two neurons or between a neuron and an effector organ. There is evidence that transmission of impulses at synapses in the CNS is humoral, through a neurotransmitter secretion. When the neurotransmitter is released, it either stimulates or inhibits the activity of the postsynaptic neurons.

Inhibition of motor neuron activity may be presynaptic or postsynaptic. Studies indicate that presynaptic inhibition occurs in the brain and is widespread at the spinal level, affecting transmission in afferent fibers from skin and muscle. The function of presynaptic inhibition is probably to suppress weak inputs that would otherwise cause unnecessary responses. This modulation of nerve impulses results in less transmitter substance being liberated. The net effect is a limiting or "inhibiting" of impulses to postsynaptic nerve fibers. Inhibition is important for orderly function.

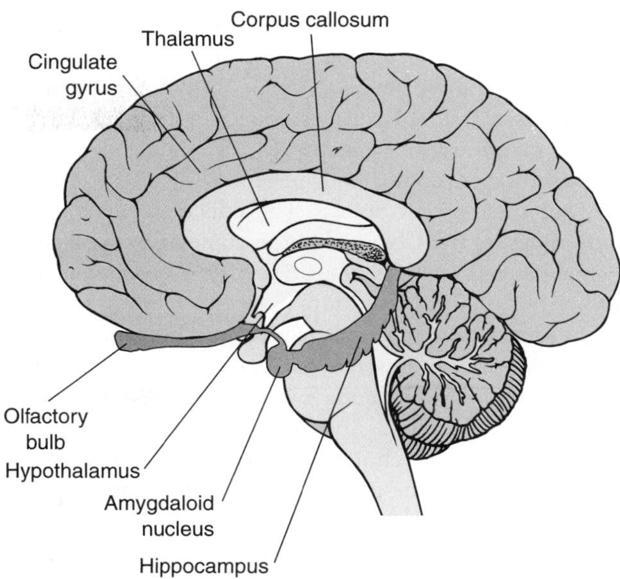

Figure 13-7 The limbic system.

Postsynaptic inhibition may be the result of changes in the membrane permeability of the postsynaptic cells caused by release of chemical transmitters from presynaptic nerve endings. Upper motor neurons are scattered throughout the cerebral cortex; a number of them are located in the motor cortex. About three fourths of the nerve fibers from these motor neurons cross to the opposite side at the level of the medulla, descend to the spinal cord, and synapse with interneurons, which in turn synapse with the lower motor neurons. Almost all motor neurons of one side are controlled by the motor cortex of the other side. Therefore injury to the motor cortex of the right side of the brain causes paralysis on the left side of the body (left hemiplegia). Systems other than the upper and lower motor neuron systems are concerned with voluntary movement, but lower motor neurons form the common final pathway for stimuli for voluntary movement.

Some of the neurotransmitters that will be discussed are acetylcholine, the catecholamines (dopamine, norepinephrine, and epinephrine), serotonin, and neuroactive peptides (enkephalins, endorphins, and dynorphins).

Acetylcholine. **Acetylcholine** is the best known chemical transmitter of nerve impulses. Not all parts of the CNS contain acetylcholine. Those areas that have high concentrations are the motor cortex, thalamus, hypothalamus, and anterior spinal roots; very low concentrations are found in the cerebellum, optic nerves, and dorsal roots of the spine. Acetylcholine can cause cardiac inhibition, vasodilation, gastrointestinal peristalsis, and other parasympathetic effects.

Lower motor neurons release acetylcholine at the neuromuscular junction, causing contraction in striated (voluntary) muscle. The concentration of acetylcholine must be high, since a large number of muscle fibers must respond synchronously for striated muscle contraction to occur and also because acetylcholine is very rapidly destroyed by the enzyme cholinesterase.

Catecholamines and related substances. Dopamine, norepinephrine, and epinephrine, a group of sympathetic compounds, and the amine serotonin (5-hydroxytryptamine) are synthesized, stored, and metabolized in the brain. They act directly on sympathetic effector cells by binding to receptors. These substances do not easily penetrate the blood-brain barrier, but their precursors do. The effect of injected catecholamines on the CNS is slight in comparison with the effect on the autonomic nervous system. However, an increase in catecholamines and serotonin causes cerebral stimulation. Drugs such as reserpine that release catecholamines and reduce amine concentration in the brain have a depressing or sedative action. Methyldopa lowers the serotonin and norepinephrine levels and this, too, has a cerebral depressing effect.

Special staining techniques indicate that there are adrenergic (sympathomimetic) and serotoninergic tracts within the CNS. Dopamine, a catecholamine, is especially concentrated in the basal ganglia. The low level of dopamine at this site in individuals suffering from Parkinson's disease led to the therapeutic approach of using its precursor, L-dopa, with good results in many cases.

Neuroactive peptides. Neuroactive peptides may be considered neuromodulators, neurohormones, or neurotransmitters. Studies indicate that a peptide may affect neuronal activity by increasing or decreasing the synthesis, release, or breakdown of neurotransmitters, neurohormones, or neuromodulators. The parenteral or intracerebral injection of these components causes potent behavioral effects. A number of these peptides exist in tissues other than the CNS, primarily in the gastrointestinal tract cells.

Enkephalins, endorphins, and dynorphins are three major polypeptides found in the brain that have opioid activity. Enkephalins may block opiate receptors in the dorsal horn of the spinal cord by blocking the release of substance P. Substance P, a transmitter of pain impulses in the nerve fibers, has been proposed to be a transmitter for the primary afferent sensory fibers. Enkephalins behave as inhibitory neurotransmitters, decreasing the perception and emotional aspect of pain. Studies indicated that enkephalins may bind to the same neuroreceptor membranes as morphine, and the concept of internal opiates or natural pain killers developed. The enkephalins allow modification and control of the perception of pain.

Endorphins (from "endogenous morphine") is a general term that includes many peptides in the brain that suppress pain. These peptides are also found in the pituitary gland, intermediate lobe, and the corticotrophin cells of the adenohypophysis. Subgroups of endorphins have been isolated and identified, including beta-endorphin, an analgesic substance that is much more potent than enkephalin.

Technology has shown that the brain, pituitary gland, and gastrointestinal tract each have enkephalins and beta-endorphins. These peptides are not found in the same cells. Further, the brain cells containing beta-endorphin are different from those that contain enkephalins.

Dynorphin is an endorphin found in the pituitary gland, hypothalamus, and spinal cord. This is the most potent pain-relieving substance discovered; dynorphin is 50 times more potent than beta-endorphin and 200 times more potent than morphine.

Naloxone, a potent opioid antagonist, reverses the analgesic effect of narcotics. Animal studies demonstrate that if naloxone is administered after enkephalins or endorphins are given, it will reverse the analgesic effect produced by the polypeptides.

Endorphin release in the body is higher after acupuncture and transcutaneous electrical nerve stimulation, and both effects may be reversed by the use of naloxone. It has been proposed that the analgesic response associated with the use of a placebo may result from an increased release of endorphins in the body. From peptide research may come pain relievers with fewer side effects and minimal to no addiction potential. We may also gain an increased understanding of mental disorders and addiction mechanisms from this research.

SUMMARY

The central nervous system (CNS) is composed of the brain and the spinal cord and essentially controls all of the functions of the body. The CNS integrates information received from the peripheral nervous system concerning the body's internal and external environment and then sends messages out again to produce the necessary adjustments to maintain homeostasis.

The cerebrum is the highest functional area of the brain. Drugs that affect the cerebral cortex may decrease mental acuity, consciousness, and motor function by their depressive action or increase muscle activity and restlessness through their stimulating effects. The thalamus relays impulses to the cerebral cortex, as well as registering pain, temperature, touch, and other sensory impulses. The hypothalamus is a major link between the nervous and the endocrine systems. The origins of 10 of the 12 cranial nerves and the involuntary respiratory center are found in the brainstem.

The respiratory center, as well as the centers for coughing and vomiting in the brainstem, are highly sensitive to drugs. Medications that disturb the cerebellum cause dizziness and loss of balance. The spinal cord, which transmits impulses to and from the brain, may also be affected by drugs. The passage of many drugs into the brain is prohibited by the blood-brain barrier.

The reticular activating system, the limbic system, and the extrapyramidal system are the three major CNS functional systems. They are responsible, respectively, for the following: consciousness, filtering, and alerting to stimuli; the emotions of anger, fear, anxiety, pleasure, and sorrow and learning and memory; and muscle coordination. All of these may be affected by medications.

Neurotransmitters affect the postsynaptic neurons to increase or decrease their activity. The most important of these are acetylcholine, the catecholamines, serotonin, and the neuroactive peptides. Currently neurobiologic research is demonstrating the increasing importance of understanding more about these substances and, in general, the central nervous system.

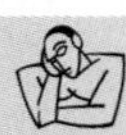

Critical Thinking

1. Harry Green was accidentally struck on the head with a golf club and became unconscious. When he regained consciousness, he was unable to recall what had occurred during approximately the 15 minutes before he was struck. Why could that occur?
2. Delores Lightfoot sustained a head injury in an automobile accident. The physician suspects that there may be injury to the cerebellum. What symptoms would Delores most likely exhibit to indicate cerebellar involvement?
3. How do neurotransmitters function in synaptic transmission?

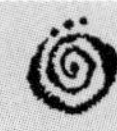

Collaborative Learning Activities

1. Three teams of students are to role play examples of everyday situations in which each of the CNS functional systems (the reticular activating system, the limbic system, and the extrapyramidal system) comes into play. The presenting group should then present examples of specific drugs that affect their system and indicate how the system would be affected.
2. Students will be separated into groups of four, with half of the groups discussing the first Critical Thinking question and the other half the second question. The groups will briefly report back to the class.

BIBLIOGRAPHY

Anderson KN, et al. (Eds.) (1994). *Mosby's medical, nursing, & allied health dictionary* (4th ed.). St Louis: Mosby.

Barker E (1994). *Neuroscience nursing*. St Louis: Mosby.

Katzung BG (1992). *Basic & clinical pharmacology* (5th ed.). Norwalk, CT: Appleton & Lange.

Martini F, et al. (1992). *Fundamentals of anatomy and physiology* (2nd ed.). Englewood Cliffs, NJ: Prentice Hall.

Melmon KL, et al. (Eds.) (1992). *Melmon and Morrelli's clinical pharmacology: Basic principles in therapeutics* (3rd ed.). New York: McGraw-Hill.

Seeley RR, Stephens TD, & Tate P (1996). *Anatomy & physiology* (3rd ed.). St Louis: Mosby.

Thibodeau GA & Patton K (1995). *Anatomy and physiology* (3rd ed.). St Louis: Mosby.

Van Wynsberghe D, Noback CR, & Carola R (1995). *Human anatomy and physiology* (3rd ed.). New York: McGraw-Hill.

Wingard LB, et al. (1991). *Human pharmacology*. St Louis: Mosby.

Chapter 14

Analgesics

Chapter Focus

Pain is a paradox. It is a sufficiently universal occurrence so that everyone experiences pain occasionally in a lifetime, but everyone's experience is unique and subjective. Only the client is an expert on his or her pain. Because the pain experience is so common with clients with whom we come into contact, nurses need to be knowledgeable about pain and skillful in interventions to prevent and relieve it. The following objectives and key terms are necessary for a good understanding of this chapter.

Key Terms

abstinence syndrome (p. 246)
acute pain (p. 231)
analgesic (p. 229)
chronic pain (p. 231)
equianalgesic (p. 232)
gate control theory (p. 232)
neuropathic (deafferentation) pain (p. 231)
nociceptive pain (p. 231)
opioid (p. 240)
opioid agonist-antagonist (p. 240)
prostaglandin (p. 231)
selective tolerance (p. 229)
somatic pain (p. 231)
step system approach (p. 241)
visceral pain (p. 231)

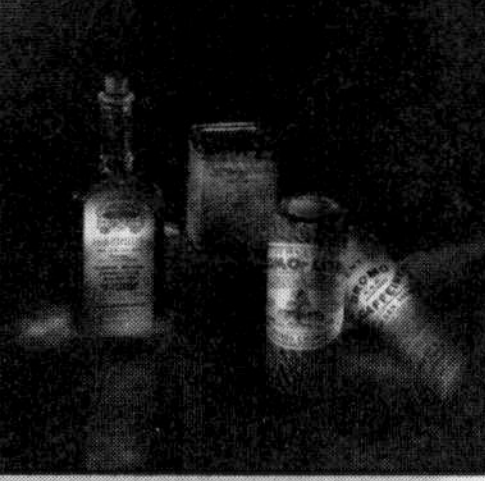

Key Drugs [▲]

morphine
naloxone
pentazocine

Objectives

1. Describe the physiology, characteristics, and types of pain.
2. Explain the effect of opioid binding with the four major opioid receptors.
3. Discuss special considerations for use of CNS analgesics and antagonists for pediatric and geriatric clients.
4. Describe the nurse's role in opioid therapy.
5. Differentiate among the opioid analgesics, antagonists, and agonist-antagonist agents.
6. Describe the relationship between prostaglandin synthesis and NSAID effects in inflammation.
7. Discuss the pharmacokinetics, side effects/adverse reactions, and drug interactions of NSAIDs.
8. Implement a plan of care for individual clients who require the administration of opioid analgesics, opioid antagonists, and NSAIDs.

Pain, is one of the most common problems afflicting human beings. It is more distressing and disabling than nearly any other client symptom (Salerno, 1996). This is unfortunate, since the potent **analgesics** (pain relieving drugs) currently available are both safe and effective when health care providers properly select an analgesic, and apply pain management techniques based on the pharmacokinetics of the drug and the individual client's response. This chapter will review the primary fears or myths that interfere with pain management, pain components and concepts, and analgesic pharmacology (opioid and nonopioid).

FEARS OR MYTHS THAT INTERFERE WITH PAIN MANAGEMENT

Addiction or Tolerance

The greatest abuse with opioid analgesics is not inducing addiction but the *fear* of inducing addiction. This "pseudoaddiction" (Weissman & Haddox, 1989) refers to clients that are inadequately treated for pain and as a result, develop a pattern of drug-seeking behaviors to achieve pain control. This pattern is often mistaken for opioid addiction (Jacox et al, 1994).

Health care providers and the general public are overly concerned about the potential of inducing addiction with the use of opioid analgesics for the treatment of pain. This is unfortunate because addiction is very rare in clinical practice, and fear of inducing addiction or even respiratory depression in a client with severe pain is not an acceptable reason for undertreatment (Salerno, 1996).

Studies have reported the risk of addiction in hospitalized persons receiving opioids at regular intervals is minimal. Porter and Jick (1980) reviewed approximately 40,000 hospital charts and reported that nearly 12,000 clients had received opioid analgesics. Of this group only four cases of addiction were documented in clients with no previous history of drug abuse. Another study of more than 10,000 hospitalized burn patients reported no cases of opioid or iatrogenic-induced addiction (Watt-Watson & Donovan, 1992). Thus psychologic dependence (addiction) is a rare complication of opioids.

Tolerance, or the need to increase the dose of an analgesic to maintain the desired effect, is another concern in practice. Tolerance is not usually seen in opioid-naive clients with severe acute or chronic pain for which there is a physical cause, such as trauma, tumor growth, and postsurgical pain. Usually an increase in pain in such individuals is due to disease progression or complications. Persons in pain respond differently to an analgesic than drug-seeking individuals that crave opioids for a euphoric effect. One should not confuse physical or psychologic dependence with tolerance (Jacox et al, 1994).

Physical dependence is an altered physiologic condition in a long-term drug user that requires consistent use of the drug to avoid withdrawal symptoms. Clients with cancer may be titrated to large amounts of opioids to control pain without producing the adverse effects of respiratory depression or excessive sedation. Pain specialists believe this is the result of **selective tolerance,** tolerance to some of the effects of the drug without interfering with the drug's analgesic effect (Jacox et al, 1994; Foley, 1991).

Fear of Inducing Respiratory Depression

An additional fear of health care professionals is the risk of inducing respiratory depression with the use of opioids. With careful assessment, prescribing, and monitoring, the potential for this adverse effect is low (Box 14-1). In clients with advanced cancer or terminally ill clients, very large amounts of opioids are often necessary to control pain. In such instances, tolerance develops to the respiratory depression effect but not to the analgesia. Therefore the client in true pain may have opioid doses increased until pain control is achieved (Gossel & Wuest, 1993). Significant respiratory depression is rarely seen in this population because the dose of medication has been titrated to meet an individual's requirement.

Health Care Professionals' Biases

Another area of concern is the influence of personal biases on the administration of pain medications. Cohen (1980) and McCaffery and Ferrell (1992) have raised the question of gender effect and bias in pain management. It was reported that nurses generally believe there is a difference between male and female pain sensitivity, pain tolerance, and distress, which then influences the nurse's assessment of the client's pain and the amount of drug used in treatment. The result is women are usually undertreated for pain.

Cleeland et al (1994) studied pain treatment in approximately 1300 outpatients with metastatic cancer from 54 cancer treatment centers that ranged from university cancer centers to community based hospitals and oncology programs. The study outcome indicated undertreatment with medication for pain: (1) women were at a greater risk for being undermedicated for pain, especially those under the age of 50; (2) the elderly over 70 years old (both sexes) often received less potent pain medication, even with reports of significant pain; (3) clinics that service predominantly minority populations were nearly three times more likely to undertreat pain compared with nonminority centers; (4) there

BOX 14-1

Time Required to Produce Maximal Respiratory Depression Effects with Opioid Analgesics

Route of administration	Approximate times
IV	Within 7 minutes
IM	Within 30 minutes
SC	Within 90 minutes

was a vast discrepancy between the physician's and the individual cancer patient's estimate of pain severity; and (5) over half the patients in this study had pain, with 62% reporting pain interfered with their daily functioning.

Studies and research have identified the problems associated with inadequate cancer pain management and the Agency for Health Care Policy and Research (AHCPR) issued Clinical Practice Guidelines for Acute Pain Management and Cancer Pain Management (Carr et al, 1992; Jacox et al, 1994) to help correct this problem.* However, additional studies are needed in the area of sex, age, and ethnic and cultural biases in pain management (see the Cultural Aspects box at right).

Fear of Legal Regulation of Opioids

Opioids have the potential for abuse and illegal diversion; therefore federal and state laws strictly monitor and regulate the availability, prescription, and use of these medications. The intent of federal law is not to interfere with a health care provider's appropriate prescribing of these substances, but many states have enacted laws or regulations that limit, restrict, or so closely monitor opioid prescribing that prescribers are reluctant to prescribe opioids for fear of prosecution and suspension or loss of their professional licenses. Such regulations have resulted in undertreatment of pain, even in clients with severe pain from cancer (Jacox et al, 1994).

Need for More Potent Analgesics

During the past decade or two, congressional legislation for the approval of diacetylmorphine (heroin) for intractable pain has been proposed and denied. The proponents for this bill have used the argument that heroin is an alternate therapy comparable to other opioids and that it might be useful for persons in intolerable pain because of its analgesic and euphoric effects. Some advocates believe it is more potent, faster acting, and produces a more prolonged analgesic and euphoric effect than other analgesics (McCarthy & Montagne, 1993).

The opponents of heroin in the United States state heroin is unnecessary because the opioids available, if properly prescribed, are sufficient for the treatment of intractable pain. Pharmacologically heroin is a prodrug; that is, when it is administered orally or intravenously, it is converted in the liver to morphine and morphine metabolites. While rapid IV injection of heroin crosses the blood-brain barrier faster than morphine to cause the euphoric or high effect, a potentially clouded sensorium is generally undesirable clinically. Most seriously ill persons want pain relief and also want to be able to communicate with their health care providers, friends, and family.

Although heroin is legitimately available in Belgium, Canada, and England, it is rarely used in Belgium and Canada. Heroin is a popular illegal drug of abuse, so an additional fear in legalizing it is that it may result in an increased risk for drug diversion, pharmacy burglaries, and crime. If heroin offers few (if any) advantages over the already marketed opioids, then, as Dr. A. Lipman (1993, p 998) has succinctly stated, ". . . legalization of heroin is not in the public interest."

*AHCPR Publications Clearinghouse, P.O. Box 8547, Silver Spring, Md 20907. (Available in professional and consumer versions in English and Spanish.)

Cultural Aspects — Culture and Pain: A Mesoamerican Perspective

Culture has been identified as a factor that influences a person's reaction to pain. Research in the area of pain and culture has not established a clear link between cultural meanings and attitudes associated with pain and pain behaviors. The purpose of this ethnohistoric study was to explore the beliefs related to the experience of pain within ancient Mesoamerica. Six themes regarding the cultural meaning of pain emerged from this study that have relevance in contemporary Mesoamerican cultures, specifically Mexican-Americans.

1. Pain was an accepted, anticipated, and necessary part of human life.
2. Humans had an obligation to the gods, and to the community of man, to endure pain in relation to the performance of duties.
3. The ability to endure pain and suffering stoically was valued.
4. The type and amount of pain a person experienced was in part predetermined by the gods.
5. Pain and suffering were viewed as a consequence of immoral behavior.
6. Specific methods of pain alleviation were directed toward maintaining balance within the person and the surrounding environment.

These findings serve as a benchmark from which to understand Mexican-American meanings, expressions, and care associated with pain. The authors indicate that previous studies have identified specific Mexican-American cultural responses to pain that fall within the themes emerging from this study. However, additional research is needed to determine how these ancient beliefs have evolved and are more specifically expressed in contemporary cultures.

1. How transferable are findings of ethnohistoric study to contemporary times? Can you identify other historic beliefs about illness that have contemporary relevance?
2. Given the six themes identified above, how might these beliefs influence the behavior of a client experiencing pain?

From Villarruel AM & Ortiz de Montellano B (1992). Culture and pain: A Mesoamerican perspective. *Adv Nurs Sci 15*(1):21.

PAIN COMPONENTS AND CONCEPTS

Because of its highly subjective nature, pain is difficult to define. Pain can be viewed as having two components: the physical component or the sensation of pain, which involves the nerve pathways and the brain; and the psychologic component or the emotional response to pain, which is the product of such factors as the individual's anxiety level, previous pain experience, age, sex, and culture.

A relatively constant pain threshold exists in all persons under normal circumstances. For example, heat applied to the skin at an intensity of 45° to 48° C will initiate the sensation of pain in almost all individuals. However, pain tolerance—the point beyond which pain becomes unbearable—varies widely among individuals and in a single individual under different circumstances. Figure 14-1 shows factors affecting the pain threshold.

Welk (1991) described an educational model that illustrates pain and suffering and the various issues that influence suffering in a terminally ill client (Figure 14-2). As noted from this model, physical pain is only part of the suffering model and is not interchangeable with suffering. A person may be suffering without physical pain or may have physical pain without suffering. Suffering then is described as multiple issues that prevent a person from living without fear such as physical pain, emotional fear (fear of the unknown, fear of dying, fear of dying alone, etc.), social conflict (resolution of conflicts with family and friends, etc.), and spiritual despair (not necessarily religious, a spiritual dimension to meet an individual client's need). Other persons in persistent, chronic pain may also have factors other than physical pain involved. Such concerns are often addressed by interdisciplinary teams in hospices and pain management programs.

Pain Classification

Pain can be classified in various ways; for instance it may be acute or chronic. **Acute pain,** a state in which an individual experiences the presence of severe discomfort or an uncomfortable sensation, has a sudden onset and usually subsides with treatment. Examples of acute pain include the pain of myocardial infarction, appendicitis, and kidney stones. **Chronic pain,** such as accompanies cancer and rheumatoid arthritis, is a persistent or recurring pain that continues for more than 6 months; chronic pain can be difficult to treat (Table 14-1).

Pain may also be classified as visceral, somatic (nociceptive), or neuropathic (deafferentation). **Visceral pain** has its origin in smooth musculature or sympathetically innervated organ systems. This pain is often difficult to localize since it is dull and aching and may also be referred, that is, felt at a site distant from its origin (such as the pain of a myocardial infarction that is felt initially in the arm). **Somatic pain** arises from activation of nociceptors in the skeletal muscles, fascia, ligaments, vessels, or joints. This pain is usually localized, constant, and may be described as aching or throbbing (Patt, 1993). Direct cancerous infiltration of the bone causes a somatic pain mediated by prostaglandins. **Prostaglandins** are hormone-like unsaturated fatty acids that act on local target organs to affect vasomotor tone, capillary permeability, smooth muscle tone, platelet aggregation, endocrine and exocrine functions, and the autonomic and central nervous systems. This somatic pain may present as a persistent ache that diffuses widely over the affected areas, usually unrelated to position or activity. In some persons it may appear as an intermittent piercing pain localized to a small area, which may be related to position, weight-bearing, and activity (Kinzbrunner & Salerno, 1994). Somatic pain responds best to the nonsteroidal antiinflammatory agents, whereas visceral pain usually responds well to opioid analgesics.

Whereas **nociceptive,** or **somatic pain** is usually the result of direct stimulation of intact afferent nerve endings, **neuropathic (deafferentation) pain** is caused by peripheral nerve injury and not stimulation. This pain has been described as burning, shooting, and/or tingling, and it is often associated with paresthesia or dysesthesia. This type of pain caused by cancer tumor invasion or treatment-induced nerve damage, may be accompanied by sympathetic nervous system dysfunction. Neuropathic pain responds less well to opioid analgesics and often requires the addition of adjunct medication (anticonvulsant, tricyclic antidepressant, etc.) to the client's drug regimen.

Pain may also have psychogenic origins. Psychiatric illness or psychosocial issues, including anxiety and depression, fear of dying, etc., have been known to cause severe somatic pain. In such cases, drug therapy alone does not usually bring relief; psychotherapy is indicated.

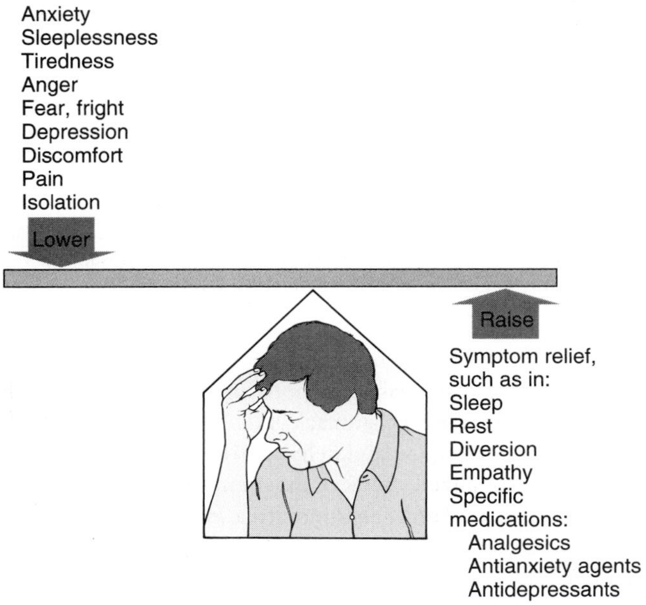

Anxiety
Sleeplessness
Tiredness
Anger
Fear, fright
Depression
Discomfort
Pain
Isolation
Lower
Raise
Symptom relief, such as in:
Sleep
Rest
Diversion
Empathy
Specific medications:
Analgesics
Antianxiety agents
Antidepressants

Figure 14-1 Factors affecting the pain threshold.

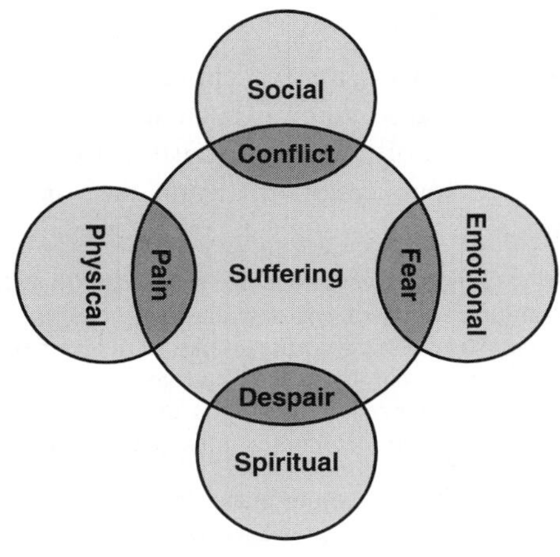

Figure 14-2 Education model illustrating pain and suffering.

TABLE 14-1 Pain: acute vs chronic

	Acute pain	Chronic pain
Onset	Usually sudden	Longer duration
Characteristics	Generally sharp, localized, may radiate	Dull, aching, persistent, diffuse
Signs and symptoms	Physiologic response: increased blood pressure and heart rate, sweating, pallor	Physiologic response: often absent
	Emotional response: increased anxiety and restlessness	Emotional response: client may be depressed, withdrawn, expressionless, and exhausted
Therapeutic goals	Relief of pain Sedation often desirable	Prevention of pain Sedation *not* desirable
Drug administration		
Timing	As needed or upon request often adequate	Regular preventive schedule
Dose	Standard dosages often adequate	Individualized according to client response
Route	Parenteral	Oral

The great variation in the pain experience has prompted research and led to the proposal of several theories of pain transmission and pain relief. The **gate control theory,** proposed by Melzack and Wall in 1965, attempts to explain the modulations in the pain experience (Figure 14-3). This theory proposes that a mechanism in the dorsal horn of the spinal cord (the "spinal gate") can alter the transmission of painful sensations from the peripheral nerve fibers to the thalamus and cortex of the brain, where they are recognized as pain. The "spinal gate" is closed by large diameter low-threshold afferent fibers (the fast-acting A-delta fibers) and opened by small-diameter high-threshold afferent fibers (the slower-acting C fibers). The "gate" is further influenced by descending control inhibition from the brain. Thus stimulation of large-diameter fibers will "close the gate" to stop perception of slower-acting painful stimuli (Warfield, 1993). It is on this theory that many nondrug regimens for pain relief are based, including massages or use of counterirritants. It is also a foundation of the Lamaze theory of "natural childbirth."

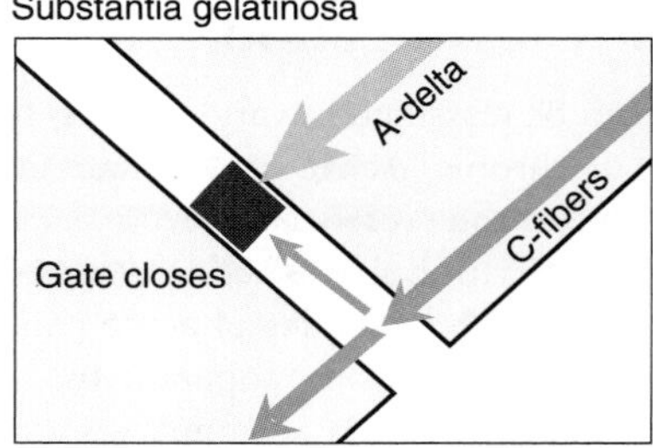

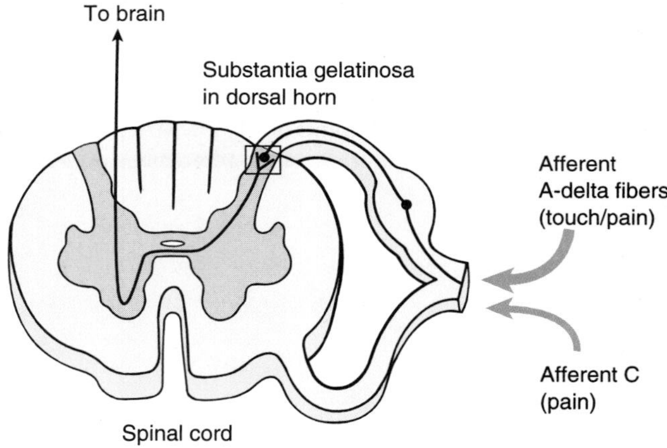

Figure 14-3 Gate control theory. Activity from A-delta (large afferent) fibers excites activity in the substantia gelantinosa, thus closing the gate to C, the pain-stimulating carrying fibers.

Pain Management

While proper pain management techniques are available, the wide institution or application of such approaches has been slow. The foreword of the U.S. Department of Health and Human Services publication on acute pain management (1992) states:

> Unfortunately, clinical surveys continue to indicate that routine orders for intramuscular injections of opioid "as needed"—the standard practice in many clinical settings—fail to relieve pain in about half of postoperative clients. Postoperative pain contributes to client discomfort, longer recovery periods, and greater use of scarce health care resources and may compromise patient outcomes.

In the United States, cancer annually is diagnosed in over a million persons and is the reason for 20% of all reported deaths (Jacox et al, 1994). Pain is a common symptom identified in persons with cancer with 20% to 50% reporting pain at the time of diagnosis and approximately 33% reporting pain during therapy (Hammack & Loprinzi, 1994). In the general population, Gu and Belgrade (1993) reported nearly 35% of hospitalized medical inpatients identified pain as their major complaint. The undertreatment with analgesics of clients in pain is well documented in the literature (Cleeland et al, 1994; Zhukovsky et al, 1995).

Although several major reasons for such undertreatment were reviewed earlier in this chapter, the nurse should be

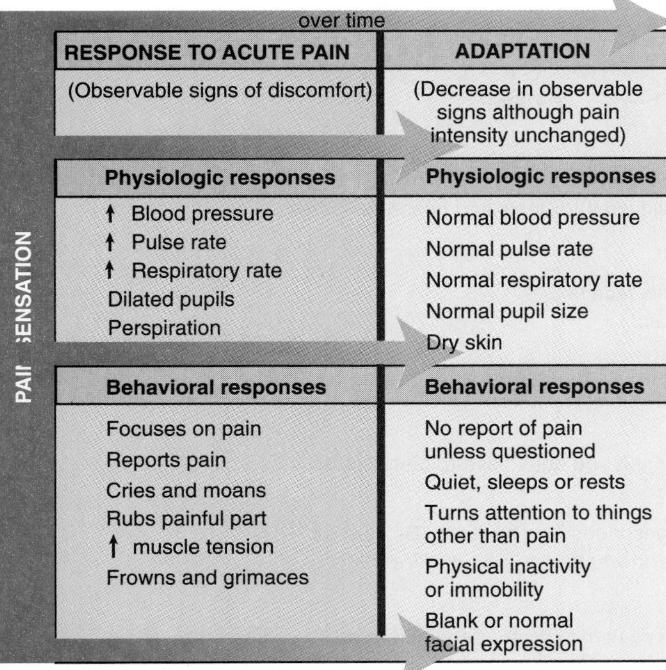

Figure 14-4 Acute pain model versus adaptation. (Modified from McCaffery M & Beebe A (1989). *Pain: Clinical manual for nursing practice.* St Louis: Mosby.)

aware that a major difference exists in the expression of pain in clients with acute pain as compared with the person with chronic, severe pain. The latter person experiences an adaptation process; thus there may be a decrease or absence of the observable signs and symptoms even in clients with very severe pain. McCaffery and Beebe (1989) have described the differences in both behavioral and physiologic responses (Figure 14-4).

The undertreatment of pain has resulted in a court awarding a multimillion dollar settlement to the family of a nursing home resident because his pain was mismanaged by the nurses and he died an unnecessarily painful death (Cushing, 1992). Despite health care providers being legally as well as morally responsible for pain relief, undertreatment or improper use of analgesics continues to be a major problem in both acute and chronic pain settings. Extensive information about the proper treatment of pain is available and should be utilized in practice today (Salerno & Willens, 1996).

Opioid Use in Pregnancy, Labor, and Delivery

Opioid analgesics cross the placenta, so that routine use of such drugs in the mother may lead to physical drug dependence in the fetus, causing severe withdrawal reactions in the neonate after birth. Pregnant women in methadone maintenance programs may demonstrate fetal distress syndrome in utero and usually deliver an underweight baby at birth.

Since the opioid analgesics cross the placenta to enter fetal circulation, the potential for inducing respiratory depression in the fetus must be considered. If at all possible, such drugs should be avoided in the delivery of a premature infant because the respiratory depressant effect is enhanced. Because of its extended duration of action, methadone should not be used in obstetrics. Morphine, codeine, and perhaps other opioids may prolong labor.

Meperidine (Demerol) IM or IV is the most commonly used opioid for the relief of pain for women in labor. Administered intravenously, the effect is rapid, reaching a peak effect in 5 to 10 minutes. The peak effect after an IM injection is between 40 to 50 minutes (Bobak, Lowdermilk, & Jensen, 1995). Meperidine should be used with caution in women with cardiac disease because it may induce tachycardia. Morphine has also been utilized in dosages of 1 to 2 mg IV but neonatal respiratory depression is greater with morphine than with meperidine. Naloxone (Narcan) should be available to treat the mother or neonate if excessive CNS depression occurs. If an opioid is administered to a woman who is nursing, it should be 4-6 hours before the next scheduled feeding to minimize the amount of drug passed on to the infant.

Opioid Use in Children

Children are also untreated or inadequately treated for pain. They suffer needlessly because of the many myths and misconceptions about pain and pain management in this population. Assessment of pain in young children is more difficult and should be based on a thorough knowledge of the procedure or event causing the pain and the child's nonverbal behavior. Even when children have the ability to verbalize their feelings, they are often reluctant to express pain, fearing the results (diagnostic test, examination, or injection) may be more painful. Young children are unable to make the connection between an immediate pain from the injection and the pain relief experienced later. Their reaction to the injection may interfere with nursing judgment, resulting in no medication and unnecessary pain for the child (Waters, 1992).

The health care provider should consider giving medication to the pediatric client for pain in the same circumstances as the adult client would be given medication. In children under 2 years of age with observably increased irritability, anorexia, loss of interest in play and in whom the assessment of whether the problem is "merely" irritability or pain is unclear, the decision to medicate appropriately is justified. Medicating in this instance should lead to a more comfortable, less anxiety-ridden child. In the child over 2 years old, the health care provider should know how the child's age and stage of development will influence the ability to perceive and communicate the experience. The approach to the child should be individualized, using the child's words and gestures for communication. Figure drawings may be helpful for the child to point out "where it hurts." More graphic scales may be used with children to rate the intensity of their pain (Figure 14-5). Other signs of discomfort, such as restlessness, decreased activity, anorexia, whining, and crying, should be assessed. The parents are to be consulted regarding the child's pain status, since they are most familiar with the child.

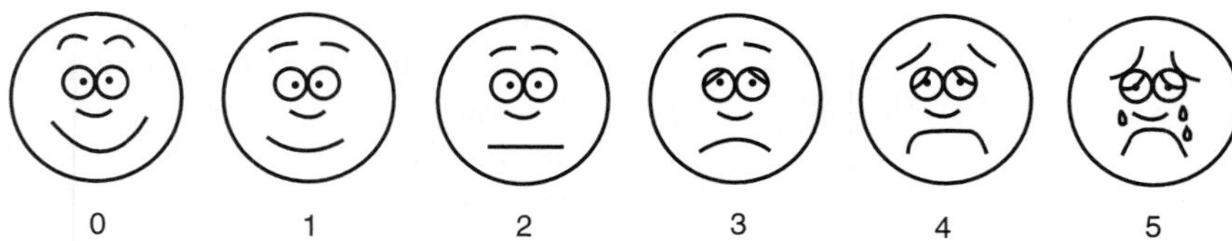

1. Explain to the child that each face is for a person who feels happy because he has no pain (hurt, or whatever word the child uses) or feels sad because he has some or a lot of pain.

2. Point to the appropriate face and state, "This face is ..."
   0-"very happy because he doesn't hurt at all."
   1-"hurts just a little bit."
   2-"hurts a little more."
   3-"hurts even more."
   4-"hurts a whole lot."
   5-"hurts as much as you can imagine, although you don't have to be crying to feel this bad."

3. Ask the child to choose the face that best describes how he feels. Be specific about which pain (e.g., "shot" or incision) and what time (e.g., now? earlier? before lunch?).

Figure 14-5 Scale for rating the intensity of pain with pediatric clients. (Modified from Wong D [1995]. *Whaley & Wong's Nursing care of infants and children* [5th ed.]. St Louis: Mosby.)

As with adults, pain is best managed if the child is given medication early rather than when the pain becomes severe. To decrease the possibility of the child denying pain to avoid an injection, the nurse may administer analgesics by an alternative route. Children find suppositories and liquid formulations more acceptable than injections. The nurse can assist the child in associating the medication with the relief from pain by indicating that it will make him or her "feel better." The nurse must check to see if the medication has been effective and remind the child that he or she probably "feels better" because of the medication. Guidelines for administration of injections to the child are found in Chapter 7. Table 14-2 lists dosing data for opioid analgesics for infants, children, and adolescents.

Opioid Use in the Elderly

Analgesic dosing in the elderly usually requires dosage and dosing interval adjustments according to the client's therapeutic response and development of undesirable side effects (increased pain, confusion, excessive untoward CNS effects, respiratory depression). The elderly reportedly have enhanced medication responses and may not tolerate side or adverse drug effects as well as younger clients. Elderly persons often have multiple medical problems and may have additional medications prescribed for them (polypharmacy). Thus it is important to carefully assess, evaluate, and closely monitor the geriatric client to reduce the potential for undertreatment or overtreatment and adverse effects. Height, weight, and body surface area are not accurate measurements for dosing analgesics in the elderly.

The elderly often report pain differently than younger persons, frequently because of physiologic, psychologic, and cultural differences (Carr et al, 1992). Cognitive impairment, dementia, and confusion may add to the barriers for pain assessment in this population. As traditional approaches are limited, pain assessment and management in this population require close supervision and monitoring of daily functioning and quality of life as outcomes. In the past, lower dosages of analgesics were often recommended for the aged, but this approach should not be the rule. Age is not a significant factor in determining analgesic dosage, but it is important in establishing the frequency of drug dosing. Because liver or kidney impairment may reduce drug clearance, less frequent drug dosing may be necessary. Both dosage and drug frequency should be carefully titrated to the individual's response to the analgesic medication. The presence of adverse effects would influence drug dosage and drug frequency.

Specific analgesics that may be considered inappropriate for use in the elderly include propoxyphene (Darvon products), pentazocine (Talwin) (Beers, et al, 1992; Wallace, 1994; Willcox, et al, 1994), and meperidine (Demerol) (Wallace, 1994). It is generally believed that these agents are more toxic in the elderly and much safer analgesics are available.

The intramuscular and subcutaneous routes of analgesic administration may also be influenced by the aging process. The elderly may have a diminished circulatory process, which results in slower absorption of drugs administered by these parenteral routes. Administering additional dosages in such a situation may result in unpredictable or increased drug absorption, which increases the potential for adverse effects.

The elderly client may be less likely to ask for pain medication because of an acceptance of pain as a part of old age, not wanting to be a "bother," or denying discomfort as a cul-

TABLE 14-2 Dosing data for opioid analgesics for infants, children, and adolescents

Drug	Approximate equianalgesic oral dose	Approximate equianalgesic parenteral dose	Recommended starting dose (adults more than 50 kg body weight)		Recommended starting dose (children and adults less than 50 kg body weight)*	
			Oral	Parenteral	Oral	Parenteral
Opioid agonist						
Morphine†	30 mg q3-4h (around-the-clock dosing) 60 mg q3-4h (single dose or intermittent dosing)	10 mg q3-4h	30 mg q3-4h	10 mg q3-4h	0.3 mg/kg q3-4h	0.1 mg/kg q3-4h
Codeine‡	130 mg q3-4h	75 mg q3-4h	60 mg q3-4h	60 mg q2h (intramuscular/subcutaneous)	1 mg/kg q3-4 h§	Not recommended
Hydromophone† (Dilaudid)	7.5 mg q3-4h	1.5 mg q3-4h	6 mg q3-4h	1.5 mg q3-4h	0.06 mg/kg q3-4h	0.015 mg/kg q3-4h
Hydrocodone (in Lorcet, Lortab, Vicodin, others)	30 mg q3-4h	Not available	10 mg q3-4h	Not available	0.2 mg/kg q3-4h§	Not available
Levorphanol (Levo-Dromoran)	4 mg q6-8h	2 mg q6-8h	4 mg q6-8h	2 mg q6-8h	0.04 mg/kg q6-8h	0.02 mg/kg q6-8h
Meperidine (Demerol)	300 mg q2-3h	100 mg q3h	Not recommended	100 mg q3h	Not recommended	0.75 mg/kg q2-3h
Methadone (Dolophine, others)	20 mg q6-8h	10 mg q6-8h	20 mg q6-8h	10 mg q6-8h	0.2 mg/kg q6-8h	0.1 mg/kg q6-8h

From Acute Pain Management Guideline Panel. Acute Pain Management in Infants, Children, and Adolescents: Operative and Medical Procedures. Quick Reference Guide for Clinicians. AHCPR Pub. No. 92-0020. Rockville, Md: Agency for Health Care Policy and Research, Public Health Service, U.S. Department of Health and Human Services.

Note: Published tables vary in the suggested doses that are equianalgesic to morphine. Clinical response is the criterion that must be applied for each patient; titration to clinical response is necessary. Because there is not complete cross tolerance among these drugs, it is usually necessary to use a lower than equianalgesic dose when changing drugs and to retitrate to response.

Caution: Recommended doses do not apply to patients with renal or hepatic insufficiency or other conditions affecting drug metabolism and kinetics.

***Caution:** Doses listed for patients with body weight less than 50 kg cannot be used as initial starting doses in babies less than 6 months of age. Consult the *Clinical Practice Guideline for Acute Pain Management: Operative or Medical Procedures and Trauma* section on management of pain in neonates for recommendations.

†For morphine, hydromorphone, and oxymorphone, rectal administration is an alternate route for patients unable to take oral medications, but equianalgesic doses may differ from oral and parenteral doses because of pharmacokinetic differences.

‡**Caution:** Codeine doses above 65 mg often are not appropriate due to diminishing incremental analgesia with increasing doses but continually increasing constipation and other side effects.

§**Caution:** Doses of aspirin and acetaminophen in combination opioid/NSAID preparations must also be adjusted to the patient's body weight.

Continued

TABLE 14-2 Dosing data for opioid analgesics for infants, children, and adolescents—cont'd

Drug	Approximate equianalgesic oral dose	Approximate equianalgesic parenteral dose	Recommended starting dose (adults more than 50 kg body weight)		Recommended starting dose (children and adults less than 50 kg body weight)*	
			Oral	Parenteral	Oral	Parenteral
Oxycodone (Roxicodone, also in Percocet, Percodan, Tylox, others)	30 mg q3-4h	Not available	10 mg q3-4h	Not available	0.2 mg/kg q3-4h§	Not available
Oxymorphone† (Numorphan)	Not available	1 mg q3-4h	Not available	1 mg q3-4h	Not recommended	Not recommended
Opioid agonist-antagonist and partial agonist						
Buprenorphine (Buprenex)	Not available	0.3-0.4 mg q6-8h	Not available	0.4 mg q6-8h	Not available	0.004 mg/kg q6-8h
Butorphanol (Stadol)	Not available	2 mg q3-4h	Not available	2 mg q3-4h	Not available	Not recommended
Nalbuphine (Nubain)	Not available	10 mg q3-4h	Not available	10 mg q3-4h	Not available	0.1 mg/kg q3-4h
Pentazocine (Talwin, others)	150 mg q3-4h	60 mg q3-4h	50 mg q4-6h	Not recommended	Not recommended	Not recommended

tural and ethnic issue. Nonverbal communication, such as irritability, anorexia, decreased activity, crying easily, or gripping an object, should be carefully assessed. The decreased activity resulting from pain increases the risk of complications of immobility. The stress of the pain experience leads to fatigue and anxiety, reducing the elderly client's diminished physical and psychologic resources. Because the elderly client may be taking many drugs concurrently, health care providers should be aware of specific drug interactions with analgesic therapy. Careful nursing care should be used in working with the elderly client experiencing pain.

■ Nursing Management

Pain Therapy

Nurses must use all of their skills to successfully manage the care of clients who are experiencing pain. The nurse often initiates or coordinates the implementation of pain management.

Assessment. Accurate assessment of pain is based on both subjective and objective information. Since "pain" cannot be observed (pain is a perception, not an object), the nurse must assess the client's physical and psychologic signs and symptoms. Each person perceives and reacts to pain differently based on physical, emotional, and cultural influences. In particular, a client's cultural background affects the manner in which pain is communicated. In addition, the perception of pain is individual; there is the capacity to respond differently to the same noxious stimulus. A pain stimulus will not necessarily produce the same amount of pain for all clients. For example, when children receiving injections use a simple coping strategy, such as squeezing a hand in proportion to the pain they feel, or when they are actively involved in preparing an injection site, such as selecting the site or cleaning the site with an alcohol swab, they will generally experience less pain (McGrath, 1990). Nurses should not assess pain by the presence or absence of any individual behavior such as crying or moaning but evaluate the totality of signs and symptoms that the client presents and evaluate each episode of pain as unique.

The assessment of pain requires careful documentation as a baseline for the nurse to select appropriate nursing interventions and to evaluate the effectiveness of nursing care. Figure 14-6 is an example of a tool developed by McCaffery and Beebe (1989), which illustrates the essential components for the assessment of pain. It is necessary to determine the location of the client's pain. For example, all postoperative discomfort cannot be assumed to be "incisional" pain when there is the possibility that the client may be experiencing pain related to other conditions such as deep vein thrombosis or myocardial infarction. It is vital that assessment related to the quality of the pain (sharp, dull, burning, radiating, stabbing, or cramping), as well as what seems to intensify or relieve it, be described in the client's own words. The nurse can then determine the client's manner of expressing pain and its effects.

Although a complete pain assessment tool such as the one in Figure 14-6 may not be available in all health care agencies, many agencies use scales to rate the intensity of pain. Figure 14-7 illustrates a number of these scales. If printed scales are not available, the nurse should ask the client to rate the pain on a scale of 0 (no pain) to 10 (unbearable pain), to provide consistency for the assessment of the client's perception of the pain. In addition, having the client rate the pain at an appropriate time interval after the administration of an analgesic allows for evaluation of the effectiveness of the medication and titration of the dosage to achieve adequate pain relief without adverse effects.

Pain may bring forth many emotions from the client, such as fear, anger, or impatience. There are a number of physiologic responses, usually sympathetic in nature, to pain; these include increased blood pressure, pulse, or respirations; sweating; pallor; restlessness or agitation.

Nursing diagnosis. The client should be assessed for the following nursing diagnoses: anxiety, disturbed sleep pattern, activity intolerance, fear, fatigue, self-care deficits, social isolation, ineffective individual coping, and altered comfort: acute or chronic pain.

Implementation

Monitoring. The nurse should observe the client's response to the analgesic and record the degree and duration of pain relief and any adverse effects that may occur.

Intervention. All clients in pain should receive nursing care directed toward reducing the perception of and reaction to pain and to enhance the analgesic effect of medications. The nurse often has significant influence over pain medication through prn (when needed) prescribing of analgesic medications. As previously mentioned, the greatest abuse of analgesics is under-utilization, which results in failure to adequately relieve or control pain. Analgesics should be used *before* the pain reaches peak intensity and painful events occur. A prn order can be used preventively if the nurse meticulously assesses the client's needs. For acute, intermittent pain, the appropriate dose of analgesic with a rapid onset of action should be used, with dosing on an as-needed or prn basis. If the order is for "q4h prn" and the nurse determines that the pain will be fairly constant for the next 24 hours, the drug may be given at 4-hour intervals and documented in the medication record to be given every 4 hours around the clock. This regimen in no way exceeds what the prescriber has specified as long as the nurse monitors the client for signs that the frequency or the dose should be decreased, such as respiratory depression or confusion. Because the blood levels of the analgesic remain steady, there should be no pain breakthrough. An alternate method of maintaining serum levels is the use of a patient-controlled analgesic (PCA) infusion pump. The consistent pain relief allows the client to participate more freely in his or her care, and, it is hoped, to recover more quickly. The client's anxiety level should be reduced, knowing when the next dose is being administered. For chronic, continuous pain, the appropriate dose of analgesic is titrated to the client's needs. The analgesic should have as long a duration as feasible and be given on an around-the-clock basis to prevent the return of pain. Breakthrough

Date ____________

Client's Name ____________ Age ______ Room ______

Diagnosis ____________ Physician ____________

Nurse ____________

I. Location: Client or nurse mark drawing

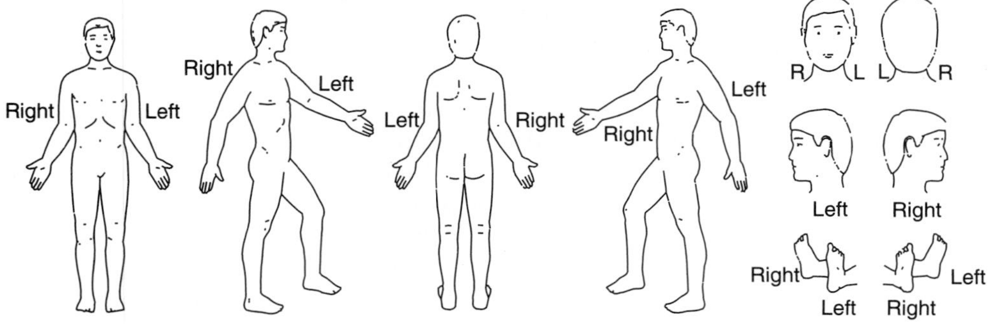

Right Left Right Left Left Right Right Left

R L L R

Left Right

Right Left

Left Right

II. Intensity: Client rates the pain. Scale used ____________

Present: ____________

Worst pain gets: ____________

Best pain gets: ____________

Acceptable level of pain: ____________

III. Quality: (Use client's own words, e.g., prick, ache, burn, throb, pull, sharp) ____________

IV. Onset, duration variations, rhythms: ____________

V. Manner of expressing pain: ____________

VI. What relieves the pain? ____________

VII. What causes or increases the pain? ____________

VIII. Effects of pain: (Note decreased function, decreased quality of life.

Accompanying symptoms (e.g., nausea) ____________

Sleep ____________

Appetite ____________

Physical activity ____________

Relationship with others (e.g., irriability) ____________

Emotions (e.g., anger, suicidal, crying) ____________

Concentration ____________

Other ____________

IX. Other comments: ____________

X. Plan: ____________

Figure 14-6 Pain assessment tool developed by M. McCaffery and A. Beebe.

pain should be medicated using appropriate medications on a prn basis.

In addition, nonpharmacologic forms of interventions can serve as adjuncts to analgesic therapy. It is well known that anxiety exacerbates pain and causes muscle tension. Relaxation techniques can be effective in reducing the amount of pain experienced. Simple methods that promote comfort, such as a quiet, pleasant environment or proper body position, may prove very effective. Rhythmic breathing, counting, and purposeful relaxation of muscle groups are among the techniques nurses can teach clients. More advanced methods include guided imagery, therapeutic touch, biofeedback, and hypnosis. An example of a highly successful relaxation technique for pain control is the psychoprophylactic or "Lamaze" method of rhythmical breathing and focusing to blunt the perception of pain during labor and delivery. The same techniques also are useful for the management of many other types of acute pain.

Shifting the client's focus of attention away from the painful stimulus is known as distraction. This technique greatly improves the client's ability to cope with chronic pain. Clients may even find that they have developed the ability to distract themselves without realizing it. Watching television, visiting with friends, walking, or working on a project can be effective distractions.

Stimulating the client's skin to relieve pain (cutaneous stimulation) has been found to be very effective in pain management. Transcutaneous electrical nerve stimulation (TENS) is a method of applying a small electrical current to skin areas over nerves or around surgical incisions; it works very well in selected situations. TENS has been shown to cause both the re-

I. Pain Intensity Scales

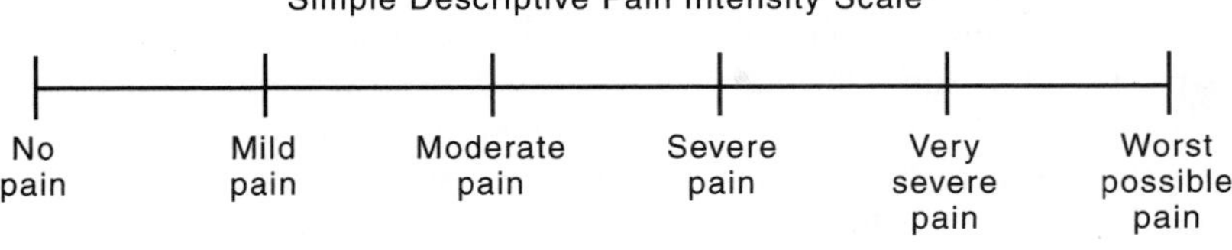

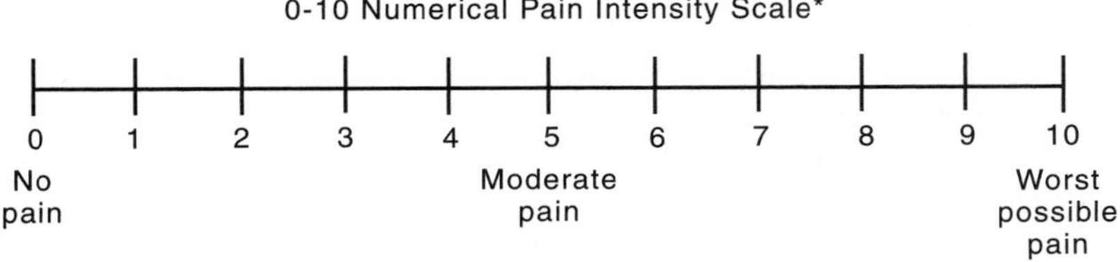

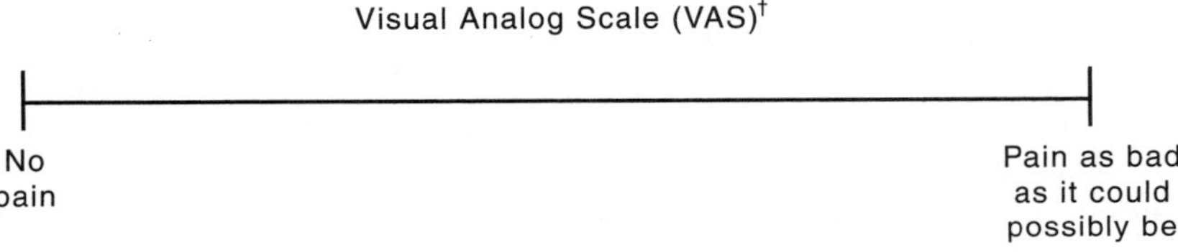

II. Pain Distress Scales

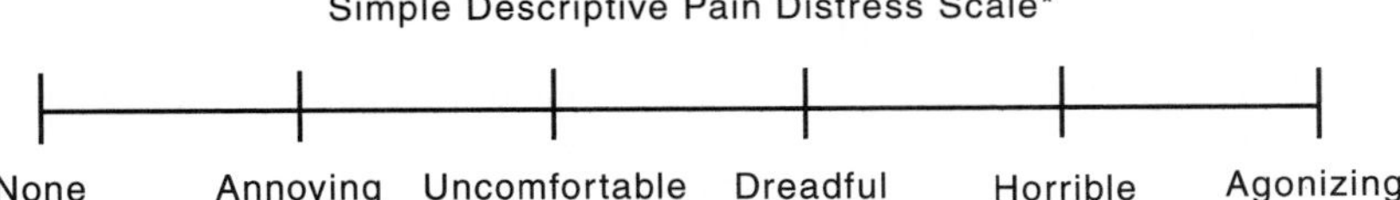

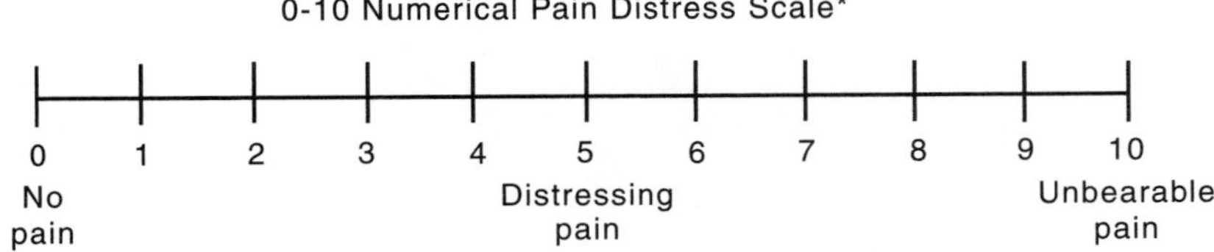

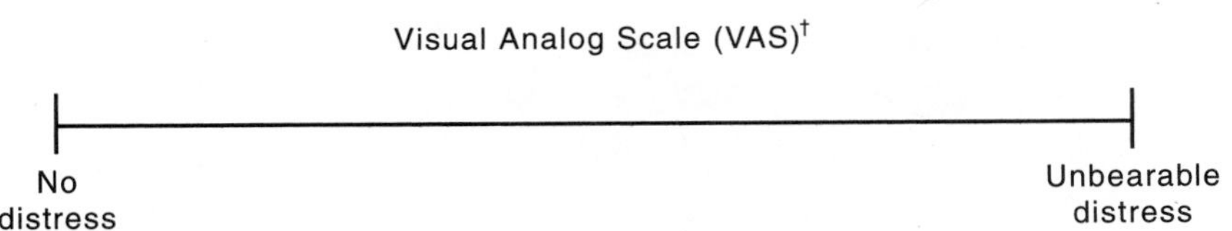

Figure 14-7 Scales for rating the intensity and distress of pain. *If used as a graphic rating scale, a 10-cm baseline is recommended.† A 10-cm, baseline is recommended for VASs. (From Acute Pain Management Guideline Panel [1992]. *Acute pain management: Operative or medical procedures and trauma. Clinical practice guideline.* AHCPR Pub. No. 92-0032. Rockville, MD: Agency for Health Care Policy and Research, Public Health Service, U.S. Department of Health and Human Services.)

lease of natural analgesic substances (endorphins) and interference with pain impulse conduction (see gate control theory, p. 232). Nurses have used cutaneous stimulation for years in the form of massage, stroking, and application of heat and cold.

The nurse should always remember to question the client about pain relief methods they have used in the past. Reinforcing these methods and supplementing them with new techniques often reduces the need for pain-relieving medications.

Education. Instructing the clients in various self–pain-relief techniques is an important part of pain therapy, especially in chronic pain. The nurse can work with the client to determine a method of dealing with pain. The nurse may know many techniques for dealing with painful situations that can be taught to the client, such as splinting an abdominal incision with a pillow to reduce the discomfort of coughing. Clients given drugs for relief of pain should be informed of the medication's purpose. Analgesic effects may be enhanced by positive suggestion. Clients who self-administer pain-relieving medications should be taught adverse effects, proper dosage, drug or food interactions, correct administration, and safe storage of medications.

Evaluation. After the implementation of pain relief therapy, an evaluation of effectiveness must be made. Assessment once again evaluates the physiologic responses and the client's perception of pain. Rating the pain using a pain scale before and after treatment serves to document the response to treatment. In evaluation of analgesic drug therapy, the nurse also looks at several parameters. These areas include compliance with therapy and the development of addiction, dependence, tolerance, or adverse effects.

ANALGESIC PHARMACOLOGY

OPIOID (AGONIST) ANALGESICS

Receptor Classification

The term *agonist* means "to do", and the term *antagonist* means "to block." **Opioids,** natural or synthetic agents that have a morphine-like effect, have been classified as agonist, partial agonist, or mixed agonist-antagonist medications. An agonist drug binds with the receptor(s) to activate and produce the maximum response of the individual receptor, whereas a partial agonist produces a partial response. A mixed **opioid agonist-antagonist** drug will produce mixed effects; it is a drug that acts as an agonist at one type of receptor and as a competitive antagonist at another receptor (Figure 14-8). A review of selected examples of opioid receptor response are listed in Table 14-3.

The mechanism of action for opioids is related to their binding to specific opioid receptors in and outside of the central nervous system (CNS) (Jacox et al, 1994). The primary opioid receptors concentrated in the CNS are mu (μ), kappa (κ), delta (δ) and sigma (σ) receptors. Analgesia has been associated with the first three receptors, with research limited on the delta receptor. Therefore the primary analgesic receptors at this time are the mu and kappa receptors. The sigma receptors are primarily associated with psychotomimetic or unwanted effects, such as dysphoria, hallucinations, and confusion.

The agonist analgesics (morphine, hydromorphone, etc.) activate both the mu and kappa receptors while the agonist-antagonist agents (butorphanol, nalbuphine, pentazocine)

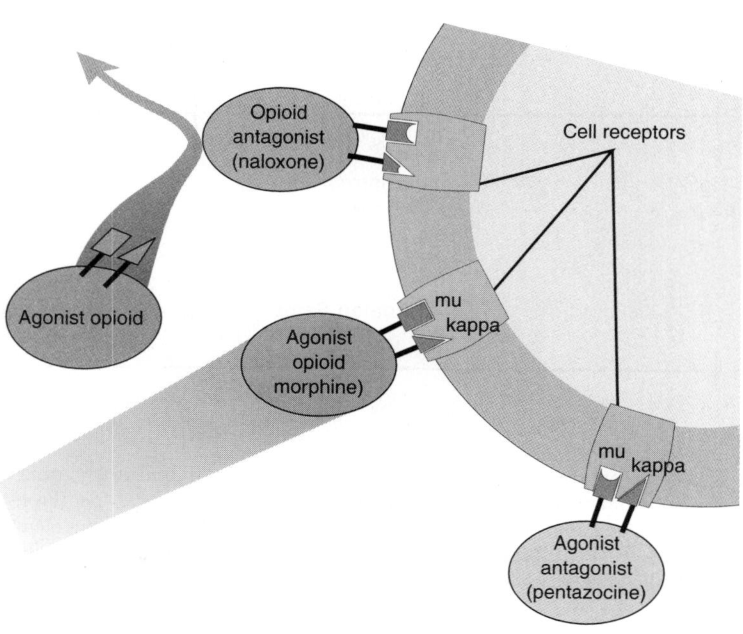

Figure 14-8 Receptor interactions of opioids.

TABLE 14-3 Selected opioid receptor responses

Receptor	Medication examples	Response
mu	Strong agonist: morphine, hydromorphone Partial agonist: buprenorphine Weak agonist: meperidine	Supraspinal analgesia, euphoria, respiratory depression, sedation, constipation, urinary retention, drug dependence
	Antagonist: naloxone, opioid agonist-antagonist	Reverses opioid effects, induces acute withdrawal in opioid dependency
kappa	Agonist: pentazocine, morphine, nalbuphine, butorphanol Little or no activity: levorphanol, methadone, meperidine	Spinal analgesia, sedation
	Antagonist: naloxone, buprenorphine	Reverses opioid effects, induces acute withdrawal in opioid dependency

activate kappa receptors (agonist) and block or have minimal effects on the mu receptors (antagonist). The agonist-antagonist drugs (especially pentazocine) may induce the undesirable effects associated with sigma receptor activity.

In addition to analgesia, opioids are capable of altering perception and emotional responses to pain because the receptors are widely distributed in the CNS, especially in the spinal and medullary dorsal horn, limbic system, thalamus, hypothalamus, and midbrain. When these areas are stimulated, pain perception is inhibited (Willens, 1996), which enhances the analgesic effect of morphine.

Agonist Opioids

▲ **morphine** [mor' feen]

Morphine is the prototype agonist opioid. It is still obtained from opium poppy because of the difficulty encountered in synthesizing morphine in the laboratory. Many analgesics are available now, but none has been proved to be clinically superior with morphine. In fact, all new analgesics are compared with morphine, which is the standard, for potency and for side or adverse effects. The World Health Organization (WHO) recommends a three-**step approach** to the management of cancer pain, using nonopioid analgesics initially and progressing to stronger analgesics in the second and third steps (1990). Morphine and other agonist opioids are used to treat step three, the treatment of severe pain. See Figure 14-9 for pharmacologic flow chart for the management of pain.

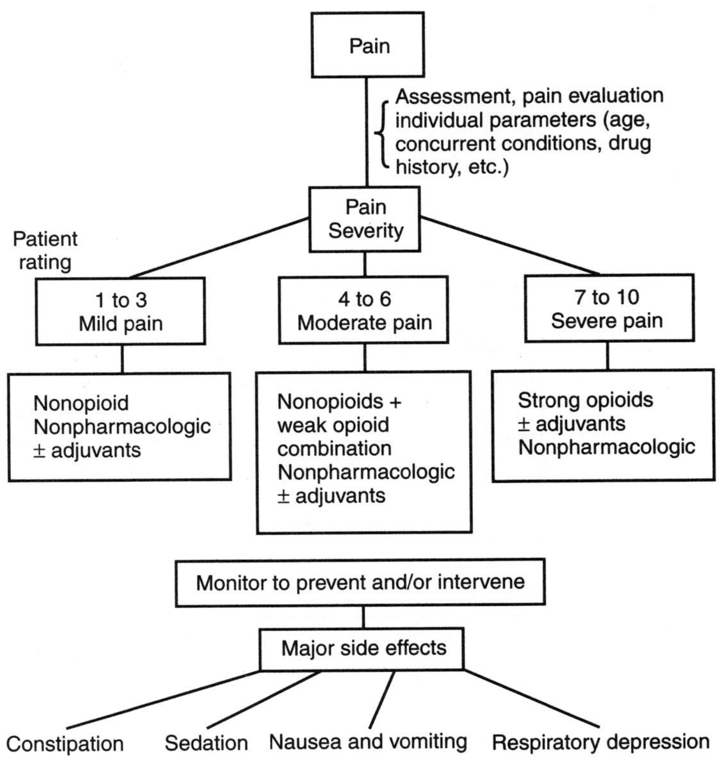

Figure 14-9 Pharmacologic flow chart for the management of pain.(From Salerno E, Willens JS (1996). *Pain management handbook: An interdisciplinary approach.* St. Louis: Mosby.)

TABLE 14-4 Selected opioid dosage forms: pharmacokinetic overview

Drug/dosage form	Onset of action (min)	Peak effect (min)	Duration of action (hr)
codeine			
Oral	30-45	60-120	4
IM	10-30	30-60	4
SC	10-30		4
hydrocodone (Hycodan)			
Oral	10-30	30-60	4-6
hydromorphone (Dilaudid)			
Oral	30	90-120	4
IM	15	30-60	4-5
IV	10-15	15-30	2-3
SC	15	30-90	4
Rectal	Not available	Not available	6-8
levorphanol (Levo-Dromoran)			
Oral	10-60	90-120	4-5
IM	Not available	60	4-5
IV	Not available	Within 20	4-5
SC	Not available	60-90	4-5
meperidine (Demerol)			
Oral	15	60-90	2-4 (usually 3)
IM	10-15	30-50	2-4 (usually 3)
IV	1	5-7	2-4 (usually 3)
SC	10-15	30-50	2-4 (usually 3)
methadone			
Oral	30-60	90-120	4-6*
IM	10-20	60-120	4-5*
IV		15-30	3-4
morphine			
Oral			
Solution,† syrup,‡ tablets	10-30	60-120	4-5
Extended-release tablets§	—	—	8-12
IM	10-30	30-60	4-5
IV		20	4-5
SC	10-30	50-90	4-5
Epidural‖	15-60	—	Up to 24
Intrathecal‖	15-60	—	Up to 24
Rectal**	20-60	—	4-5
oxycodone			
Oral	Not available	60	3-4
Controlled release	Not available	3-4	12
oxymorphone (Numorphan)			
IM	10-15	30-90	3-6
IV	5-10	15-30	3-4
SC	10-20	Not available	3-6
Rectal	15-30	120	3-6
propoxyphene (Darvon)			
Oral	15-60	120	4-6

*With active metabolites and continuous dosing, half-life and duration of action may increase to 22 to 48 hours.
†Roxanol, M.O.S., MSIR.
‡Morphite, Morphitex-1, Morphitec-5, (not commercially available in United States).
§MS Contin, Roxanol SR.
‖Duramorph (preservative-free).
**RMS suppositories.

Mechanism of action. As mentioned previously, morphine produces its potent analgesic effects by combining with receptor sites in the brain called opioid receptors (see previous discussion of opioid receptors).

Although morphine is considered the drug of choice for cancer pain (Jacox et al, 1994), it has additional pharmacologic effects that are useful in treating symptoms other than pain. For example, morphine may be used in the treatment of clients with lung cancer, to treat pain aggravated by coughing, or an unproductive nagging cough. Small doses of morphine may depress the cough center; this secondary effect is useful in selected situations. For persons with a cough caused by a cold, less potent and potentially safer medications should be utilized (such as the nonopioid antitussive dextromethorphan).

Another indication for morphine therapy is in the treatment of acute pulmonary edema secondary to left ventricular heart failure. Morphine's peripheral vasodilation effect on veins and arteries can be very useful in decreasing heart workload, resulting in enhanced cardiac function and a reduction of lung fluid. Morphine's effectiveness in treating myocardial infarction is due to the fact that it does not significantly alter heart rate and blood pressure at usual doses, as well as its calming effect along with the peripheral vasodilation effect, which may result in a decrease in cardiac workload (Salerno & Willens, 1996).

The opioid drugs also act centrally and locally to alter intestinal motility (antidiarrheal effect). Morphine's gastrointestinal effects include a decrease in peristalsis and glandular secretions, which usually result in the side effect of constipation.

Indications. The analgesic effect of morphine is indicated for the treatment of severe pain.

Pharmacokinetics. Morphine may be administered orally, intramuscularly, intravenously, subcutaneously, epidurally, intrathecally, and rectally. Tables 14-4 and 14-5 describe the pharmacokinetics and dosage and administration of morphine. Morphine is distributed widely in body tissues. It is metabolized in the liver primarily to morphine 3-glucuronide (M3G) and morphine 6-glucuronide (M6G), an active metabolite, and is excreted primarily via the kidneys.

Side effects/adverse reactions. Most frequently reported side effects of morphine and the other opioids include vertigo, faintness, and lightheadedness, which occur most often in ambulatory clients. Fatigue, sleepiness, nausea and vomiting, increased sweating, constipation, and hypotension may also occur. Less frequently seen side effects include dry mouth, headache, anorexia, abdominal cramping, nervousness, increased anxiety, mental confusion, urinary retention or painful urination, visual disturbances, and nightmares.

Among the more serious adverse reactions reported are seizures (particularly with meperidine and propoxyphene), tinnitus, jaundice (hepatic toxicity), pruritus, skin rash or facial edema (allergic reaction), breathing difficulties, respiratory depression, excitability (paradoxical reaction seen mainly in children), confusion, and tachycardia (*USP DI*, 1996).

TABLE 14-5 Morphine analgesic dosage and administration

Route	Adult dosage
IV	4-10 mg diluted in 4-5 ml sterile water administered slowly
IM	5-20 mg every 4 hr
SC	5-20 mg every 4 hr
Epidural	1-5 mg initially; assess in 1 hr; if inadequate for pain relief, 1-2 mg increments may be administered; 10 mg in 24 hr maximum
Intrathecal	0.2-1 mg as single dose only; repeated dosage by this route not recommended
Oral (individualized)	Initially 10-30 mg every 4 hr for morphine sulfate syrup, oral solution, and tablets; may be increased according to pain severity and client's response
Rectal suppositories	20-30 mg rectally every 4-6 hr

Continuous Infusion of Opioids

Continuous infusion of opioids may be used when traditional routes of administration are inappropriate or have failed to provide satisfactory pain relief, as with the client with intractable vomiting or severe local bruising following IM or SC injection, or the client with severe pain unrelieved by oral, rectal, or intermittent parenteral opioid dosing, or for pain management in the postoperative period. Intravenous opioids are helpful for short-term treatment of severe pain.

Before starting the pump infusion, the nurse should obtain a baseline blood pressure and respiratory rate, rhythm, and depth. All previous medication orders for pain are discontinued. The solution is administered using a microdrip infusion set and infusion control pump. Figure 14-10, *A*, shows a portable wrist model of a PCA (patient-controlled analgesia) unit commonly used in a hospital setting, most often after surgery. This pump also allows the client to receive a predetermined IV bolus (a quantity of drug introduced into a vein at one time) of an analgesic (usually morphine) by striking the syringe pump mechanism. Thus the client can control the administration of the analgesia. The prescriber orders the predetermined analgesic dose and a set lockout interval of 5 to 20 minutes. The pump then is calibrated to deliver the ordered dose whenever the client activates the button. The lockout mechanism prevents an inadvertent overdosage or excessive analgesic administration by the client. This pump can also record the number of times the button is struck and the total cumulative dose delivered. Figure 14-10, *B*, illustrates the CADD-PCA pump that may be programmed for continuous administration, client-activated, or clinician-activated delivery. The pump also records all bolus attempts, successful and unsuccessful, made by the client. Thus the nurse and the prescriber are able to evaluate the appropriateness of the medication therapy and determine when the client is not receiving adequate medi-

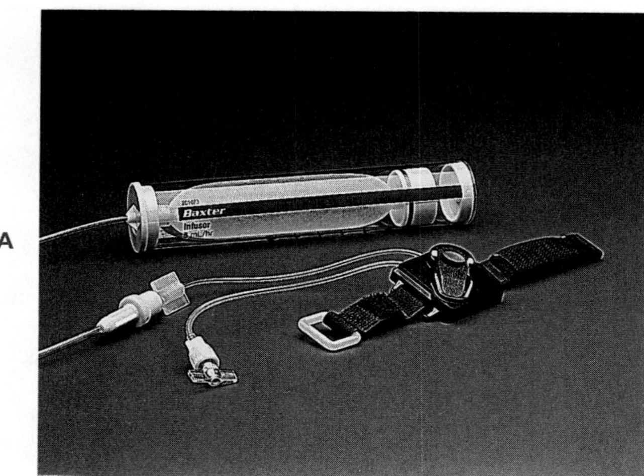

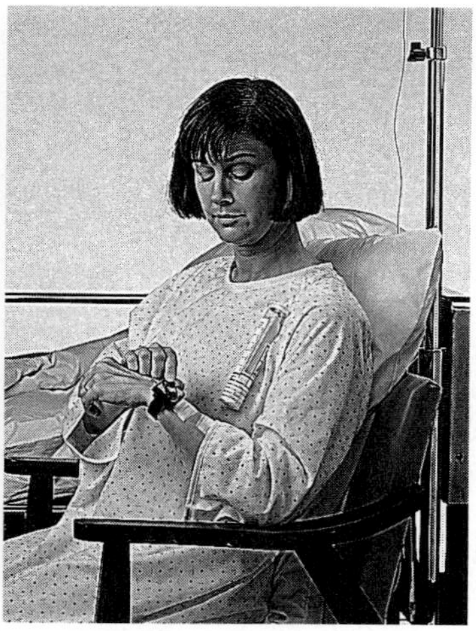

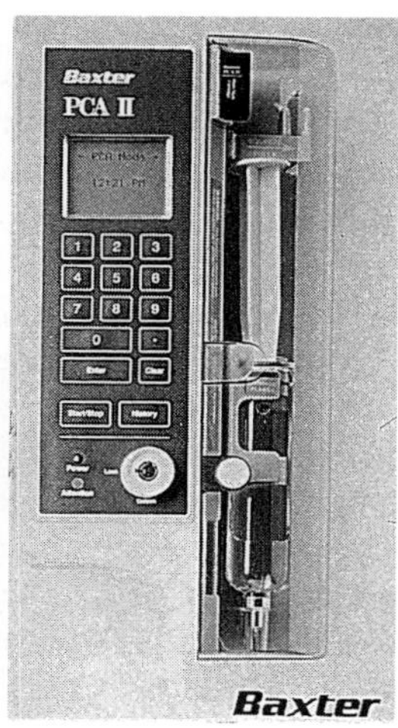

Figure 14-10 Examples of continuous infusion pumps. **A**, Portable wrist model. **B**, Patient-controlled analgesia (PCA) pump is designed for patient- or clinician-activated medication delivery. (Courtesy Baxter Healthcare Corporation, Deerfield, Ill.).

cation. Because it is lightweight (about 15 oz) and easily worn, ambulation by mobile clients is not impaired.

The client's current pain treatment requirements and degree of pain control determine the initial infusion rate. Infusion rate adjustments thereafter are based on objective and subjective evidence of pain relief and side effects. The client should be monitored for potential respiratory depression every hour for the first 4 hours and routinely thereafter. If the client's respiratory rate falls below the established limit, the nurse should reduce the rate of flow, notify the prescriber, and have naloxone, an opioid antagonist, ready to administer. Mechanical ventilation may be preferred to naloxone to relieve the respiratory depression, since naloxone will also diminish the client's pain relief.

Duramorph, a morphine sulfate solution that is preservative free, is commonly prescribed for intravenous, epidural, or intrathecal use. Morphine's relatively poor lipid solubility delays the onset of analgesia when morphine is administered by epidural or injection (see Table 14-4). Thereafter additional "breakthrough" analgesics may be prescribed. The risk of inducing respiratory depression is reportedly greater by the intrathecal route than by epidural administration (*USP DI*, 1996). Although nurses do not usually directly administer drugs intraspinally, the filling of a drug reservoir of an implanted intraspinal delivery system may be required. Special training of the nurse is required, and the manufacturer's directions should be followed closely.

The nurse should be aware of the potential side effects of the opioids, such as nausea, vomiting, sedation, and respiratory depression. With epidural administration, pruritus is common as well.

Nursing Management

Opioid Therapy

Assessment. A thorough assessment of the client's pain regarding location, severity, quality, and intensity needs to be accomplished to establish a baseline for management of the client's condition. It is necessary to individualize the drug dose and its frequency based on the potency and duration of action of the specific drug used, severity of pain, use of a pain scale, condition of the client, other medications that the client is receiving concurrently, and the client's response to the analgesic regimen (see the previous discussion of assessment in the nursing management of pain therapy section).

The client should be assessed for preexisting conditions for which the use of opioids would be contraindicated, such as hypersensitivity to the prescribed drug, acute respiratory depression, or diarrhea associated with pseudomembranous colitis caused by cephalosporins, lincomycins, or penicillins,

! MANAGEMENT OF DRUG OVERDOSE

Opioids

- If an oral opioid overdose occurs, emesis or gastric lavage is employed to empty the stomach. If respiratory depression or any other life-threatening adverse effect is present, the treatment for these effects would take precedence.
- For respiratory depression establish a patent airway and controlled respiration. Administer naloxone (Narcan) to reverse the opioid-induced respiratory depression and sedation by displacing the opioids at the receptor site. In opioid-dependent individuals, it can also induce acute drug withdrawal. The intravenous route of administration is the preferred method of administering naloxone. Its effects are seen within 2 minutes. It can also be given intramuscularly or subcutaneously, but the onset of action is then seen within 2 to 5 minutes. Naloxone is shorter acting than most opioids; therefore, to prevent the recurrence of respiratory depression, it must be administered by a continuous infusion or by repeated injections (intramuscularly or subcutaneously). See the drug monograph on naloxone, p. 256, for additional information.

or caused by poisoning because all of these conditions may be worsened. For epidural or intrathecal administration, the contraindications would include coagulation defects, which might result in uncontrollable CNS hemorrhage, or infection at or near the site of administration, which might spread the infection into the CNS. Opioids should be used with extreme caution in conditions such as acute bronchial asthma or any respiratory impairment or chronic disease, increased intracranial pressure (may increase), or severe inflammatory bowel disease (risk of toxic megacolon). See the Pregnancy Safety box below for FDA pregnancy safety classifications.

The client's concurrent drug therapy should be assessed for significant drug interactions. When morphine is given with:

Drug	Possible effect and management
alcohol or other CNS depressants	May result in enhanced CNS depression, respiratory depression, and hypotension. Reduce dosage of one or both drugs and monitor closely for decreased respiratory rate and blood pressure, slowed reflexes, and drowsiness.
buprenorphine (Buprenex)	**May result in additive effect of respiratory depression if given concurrently with low doses of mu receptor agonists or with kappa-receptor agonist. Avoid concurrent usage. Buprenorphine has partial agonist effects on the mu receptor. If given before or after an opioid agonist, it may reduce the analgesic effects of the opioid.**
carbamazepine (Tegretol)	**Concurrent use with propoxyphene may result in decreased metabolism and increased carbamazepine serum concentration, thus increasing the potential for toxicity. Avoid concurrent drug administration.**
monamine oxidase (MAO) inhibitors (furazolidone [Furoxone], procarbazine [Matulane])	**Test dose with one fourth of the dose of morphine (or any prescribed opioid analgesics) to ascertain compatibility of the medications. The possibility of inducing excitability, hypertension, or hypotension; increased sweating; convulsions; respiratory depression; fever; and cardiac dysfunctions exists. Therefore it is usually recommended that caution be taken and reduced dosages of opioids be prescribed for clients receiving MAO inhibitors. Concurrent administration with meperidine has resulted in very severe, and at times, fatal reactions. The effects include sudden excitation, increased sweating, rigidity, very severe hypertension (or hypotension in some persons), coma, seizures, hyperpyrexia, and collapse. The use of meperidine is contraindicated in any clients receiving or having received an MAO inhibitor within 2 to 3 weeks (USP DI, 1996).**
naltrexone (Narcan)	Will produce withdrawal symptoms in clients dependent on opioid medications. Avoid concurrent administration in clients receiving opioids therapeutically.
rifampin (Rifadine)	May increase methadone metabolism and so may precipitate withdrawal symptoms in clients being treated for opioid dependence. Methadone dosage adjustment may be required.
zidovudine (AZT)	**Morphine may decrease clearance of zidovudine. Concurrent use should be avoided as toxicity of one or both drugs may occur.**

Pregnancy Safety

Category	Drug
B	diclofenac, flurbiprofen, ketoprofen, naloxone, naproxen
C	auranofin, aurothioglucose, buprenorphine, codeine, dezocine, diflunisal, etodolac, fentanyl, hydrocodone, hydromorphone, ketorolac, morphine, nabumetone, naltrexone, opium, oxaprozin, pentazocine, tolmetin, mefenamic acid
Unclassified	butorphanol, fenoprofen, indomethacin, levorphanol, meclofenamate, meperidine, methadone, nalbuphine, oxycodone, oxymorphone, penicillamine, piroxicam, propoxyphene, sulindac, tiaprofenic acid

Nursing diagnosis. In many instances, the effects described below may be overcome by appropriate nursing care (see Nursing Care Plan on p. 246).

Implementation

Monitoring. The nurse should observe the client's response to the analgesic and record the degree and duration of pain relief and any adverse effects that may occur. Vital signs, particularly the respiratory rate, should be taken and recorded before morphine sulfate is given. Morphine can cause respiratory depression; if the client's respiratory rate is less than 12/min, the dose may need to be withheld or decreased. In addition, the nurse should monitor the client's orientation, reflexes, bilateral grip strength, level of consciousness, pupil size, bowel sounds, urinary output, and liver and kidney function tests. The nurse's assessment is important information required by the prescriber to determine the possibility of adverse drug effects on the client. Signs of opioid overdose are cold and clammy skin, drowsiness, dizziness, restlessness and mental confusion, miosis (pinpoint pupils), and decreasing pulse rate and blood pressure. Oral and injectable opioid analgesics produce unacceptable or undesirable effects such as nausea and vomiting, constipation, urinary retention, cough reflex suppression, and CNS effects.

Tolerance is another undesirable effect of narcotic analgesics. An increase in analgesic dosage may be needed to provide for the same degree of analgesic effectiveness. Lack of reliable data has led to many misconceptions about tolerance. Tolerance, for example, does not always occur. It is sporadic and unpredictable. One client may take the same

Nursing Care Plan

Selected Nursing Diagnoses Related to Opioid Therapy

Nursing diagnosis	Outcome criteria	Nursing interventions
Ineffective airway clearance related to cough reflex suppression	Evidence of good pulmonary ventilation Absence of rhonchi	Reposition the immobile client frequently. Teach turning, coughing, and deep breathing.
Ineffective breathing pattern: hypoventilation related to CNS depressant effects of drug	Respiratory rate 16-20/min Absence of cyanosis	Assess respiratory rate before administering each dose; if below 12/min, hold dose. Administer oxygen. Elevate head of bed. Have narcotic antagonist and respiratory support systems nearby during IV administration.
Risk for fluid volume excess related to nausea and/or vomiting	Absence of and/or decrease in nausea and/or vomiting	Administer prescribed antiemetics. Administer oral analgesics with food. Reduce noxious environmental stimuli. Apply cool cloth to the face. Provide small, frequent meals.
Constipation	Evidence of client's normal bowel patterns	Assess client's bowel status. Increase fluid consumption. Instruct in high-fiber diet. Encourage ambulation. Obtain an order for a stool softener and/or a bulk-forming laxative. Provide relaxed environment for elimination.
Urinary retention	Evidence of urinary status without urgency and/or retention	Increase fluid intake to about 2500 ml daily, unless contraindicated. Administer sitz bath. Provide relaxed environment for elimination. Suggest a dose reduction or switch to alternative therapy.
Risk for injury related to sensory/perceptual alterations	Absence of injury	Assist to ambulate. Caution against driving and other hazardous activities. Caution against taking alcohol and other CNS depressants concurrently.

dosage of the same opioid for years and never need an increase, whereas other clients with similar pain problems may require periodic increases. In the majority of clients with genuine pain who are receiving opioids in therapeutic doses, the dependence liability is relatively uncommon; most do not report euphoria or psychologic dependence. Tolerance in clients needing pain relief (not tolerance in clients who take drugs for pleasure) is managed by gradually decreasing the dose when analgesic effect is achieved. Once pain is controlled (e.g., removal of a tumor that is causing the pain), a lower dose will maintain analgesic effects. The need for an increase in the analgesic dosage will usually be a result of the disease process or progression. The nurse should assess for pupillary constriction. As the drug is eliminated from the body, the pupils return to normal. Continued constriction of the pupils with early return of the symptoms for which the medication was administered may indicate a developing tolerance because the drug has not yet been eliminated from the body but has diminished effectiveness. **Abstinence syndrome**, a collection of symptoms such as restlessness, chills and hot flashes, piloerection, rhinorrhea, drowsiness, lacrimation, mydriasis, sneezing, yawning, generalized anxiety, abdominal cramps, lower back pain, lower extremity cramps, vomiting and diarrhea, anorexia, diaphoresis, muscular twitching, and a craving for the drug, may occur on withdrawal of opioid analgesics after prolonged use and physical dependence. Gradually decreasing the dosage of the medication as the severity of the pain decreases may diminish the development of withdrawal symptoms.

Intervention. Preventive pain treatment with analgesics involves the frequent administration of analgesics on a regular fixed-time interval in anticipation of pain. Analgesics are to be given before the client's anticipation of the recurrence of pain or before it reaches an intensity that makes the client feel a loss of control. The client should actively participate in the pain treatment process with trust and confidence and be able to assist in planning a schedule of pain medication based on lifestyle. This fixed-schedule method of administration decreases suffering until the next scheduled dose because a blood level of the analgesic has been reached that controls the client's pain. If the fixed-time schedule is inappropriate, it is the nurse's responsibility to teach the client to request

BOX 14-2

Epidural Analgesia

Epidural analgesia is a therapeutic modality that offers an alternative to traditional methods of pain control. It can be administered as an intermittent injection or continuous infusion of opiate into the epidural space. The nursing management of clients receiving epidural analgesia to manage postoperative pain is an essential one for client comfort and safety. Generally, the client should understand the purpose and the benefits of epidural analgesia and provide consent to the modality before surgery.

With the client in a side-lying position, the epidural catheter is inserted most commonly at L2 level by the anesthesiologist. Once it is tested for placement, it is stabilized with an occlusive dressing. It should be taped in such a manner that the tubing will not pull or kink. If the catheter becomes dislodged or the dressing becomes loose or wet, the anesthesiologist should be notified. The catheter may be connected to a continuous infusion or capped. It should be carefully labeled "for epidural use only." Because some preservatives might be toxic to neural tissue, medications for epidural use must not contain preservatives.

Although rare, respiratory depression can occur with the administration of spinal opiates. The respiratory status of the client receiving intermittent epidural analgesia should be monitored once each hour for the first 12 hours or until the respiratory rate exceeds 12/min, then every 2 hours for 12 hours, and then every 4 hours. With continuous infusion of the analgesic agent, monitor the client every hour for the first 24 hours or until the respiratory rate is greater than 12/min, then once every 4 hours. Clients with low respiratory rates should be monitored as necessary. Naloxone is usually kept in the immediate client environment according to agency policy. The anesthesiologist is called immediately if respiratory depression occurs. Naloxone 0.4 mg IV is usually ordered, but remember this dose may reverse the analgesic effect of the opiate and the client will experience pain.

Pruritus is experienced by about one third of all clients receiving spinal opioids. Although the mechanism is unclear, it is felt that this pruritus is the result of the epidural opiates producing sensory sensations that are interpreted by the sensory cortex as itching. Low doses of naloxone are administered to relieve the pruritus without concomitant reversal of analgesia. Nausea and vomiting may also be an issue with some clients. Fluid balance monitoring and assessment of bladder distention should be maintained while the client is receiving epidural analgesia to detect any urinary retention that may occur.

The client's level of comfort should be assessed every 2-4 hours for the first 24 hours after surgery using a pain scale. Supplemental parenteral analgesics may be required for "breakthrough" pain. Assess the level of consciousness every 2 hours for the first 24 hours and then every 4 hours for the duration of therapy. In addition, some agencies require a motor and sensory assessment at least every 8 hours and before ambulation. Blood pressure and pulse should be determined before ambulating the client for the first time.

Instruct the client to notify the nurse if pain is experienced and if increased drowsiness and/or leg numbness and weakness occur. Epidural analgesia is not usually continued past the fifth postoperative day.

From Keeney (1993).

medication before the pain becomes severe. Often clients are unaware that they need to ask for pain medication, since none of their other medications may be on a demand schedule.

The nurse should encourage client and family willingness and belief to participate in the reinforcement of the pain-treatment process. Combinations of optimal doses of NSAIDs and opioid agonists indicated for pain may permit lower doses of the opioid agonist. A stepped-care or flow chart approach (see Figure 14-9) is the optimal plan to follow because it uses nonopioid analgesics progressing to other stronger analgesics to manage the client's pain with the most effective dosage.

After administering the medication, the nurse should provide comfort measures to allow the best effect: reduction of environmental stimuli, assisting the client to a comfortable position, and back massage. Nonpharmacologic measures for pain such as these and others (relaxation techniques and cutaneous stimulation) may be used concurrently, as well as considered as substitutes for pharmacologic interventions with some clients. Provide for the client's safety (such as with assisted ambulation) if CNS effects occur.

Injection sites should be rotated to prevent induration and abscess. If analgesic medication is required for more than 2 weeks, oral, intravenous, or other routes of administration should be considered. For prolonged pain relief, epidural or intrathecal administration may be considered (Boxes 14-2 and 14-3). When a narcotic is administered by the epidural, intrathecal, or intravenous route, naloxone must be on hand because the risk of respiratory distress is significantly in-

BOX 14-3

Intraspinal Analgesic Infusion

Another type of analgesic therapy—continuous intraspinal morphine infusion—reduces the client's pain without diminishing CNS functioning. An implantable infusion device is connected to an implantable catheter placed in the epidural and intrathecal space. The system, which is refilled by injection through a septum into a central chamber of the device, administers the medication continuously. In the home setting, the client and family are taught how to care for the device and how to evaluate the response to the therapy. The device is usually refilled every 2 weeks by a home health care nurse. Study is continuing with this unique method of pain control, which promises relief for clients with intractable pain while increasing the quality of life.

BOX 14-4

Analgesic Equivalency Chart

All analgesics are compared with 10 mg (IM) morphine to determine an analgesic dosage equivalent. Such information is very useful for health care professionals assessing potency and considering drug alternatives.

Analgesic	IM dose (mg)	Oral dose (mg)
morphine	10	20-60*
hydromorphone	1.5	7.5
oxycodone	not available	30
levorphanol	2	4
methadone	10	20
meperidine	75	300

Suppository dosage form

Hydromorphone, 3 mg, is approximately equivalent to 1.5 mg IM dosage.

Morphine, 10-30 mg, is considered equivalent to the oral dosage. Individualize dosage according to client response.

Oxymorphone, 5-10 mg, is approximately equivalent to 1 mg of IM oxymorphone.

*For a single dose or intermittent use. Chronic administration may decrease oral dose to 20 or 30 mg equivalent.

creased with these routes of administration. Repeated intramuscular or subcutaneous administration of opioids to clients in shock, who may have impaired tissue perfusion, may result in an overdose when the client's circulation is restored.

Morphine sulfate intensified oral solution (Roxanol, 20 mg/ml) comes with a specific calibrated dropper; no other dropper should be used for dosing. The medication is diluted in 30 ml or more of fluid or semisolid food. The nurse or client should make sure the entire dose is removed from the dropper.

When the prescriber is changing the client's medication from one route of administration to another, the nurse should check the dosage against the Analgesic Equivalency Chart (Box 14-4).

Other side effect/adverse reactions of opioid therapy can be managed by nursing actions as discussed in the Nursing Care Plan on p. 246.

Education. Since orthostatic hypotension (a form of low blood pressure that occurs when a person stands) can occur in ambulatory clients, caution the client about rising quickly from a supine position. Opioids can impair the client's mental and physical abilities, so caution should be exercised when the drug is prescribed for ambulatory clients or for anyone who will be driving a car or operating any type of machinery. Clients should be instructed to call for assistance if they wish to ambulate. A client taking opioids needs to be reminded that the combination of ethanol and the normal dosage of the drug can render them incapable of normal functioning.

Roxanol is the most convenient method for receiving oral morphine but requires careful instruction of the client. Because it is a controlled substance, the client should be instructed to prevent theft by drug-dependent individuals.

The dose may be altered by a prescriber if a client is receiving other opioid analgesics, CNS depressants, cyclic antidepressants, neuroleptics, anxiolytics, ethanol, or sedative-hypnotics, since the combination of any of these can produce CNS depression.

Evaluation. Because opioid analgesics are frequently used inappropriately, the nurse should be aware and report any instances of suspected abuse. Since some health professionals are not well versed in pain control, nurses should take the initiative in reversing the undertreatment of clients in pain. Educating others within the clinical setting is important to promote comfort for the client. The client should report relief from pain after administration of the drug, the respiratory status should be within the normal limits, and other adverse responses to the drug such as CNS depression, urinary retention, and constipation should not occur.

Opium Preparations

Opium contains several alkaloids that include morphine and small amounts of codeine and papaverine. The effects of opium result from the presence of morphine in the preparations. The mechanism of action and pharmacokinetics are the same as or similar to morphine.

Opium tincture contains 10 mg morphine/ml and is used as an antidiarrheal agent and, when diluted, for the treatment of neonatal opioid dependence.

Camphorated tincture of opium (paregoric) contains 2 mg morphine/5 ml. It is an antidiarrheal agent. In some instances, it has been used to treat neonatal opioid dependence, but this use is controversial. Paregoric contains camphor, which can cause serious toxicity including seizures and respiratory depression, and benzoic acid, which can displace bilirubin from albumin. Both substances may enhance the typical problems seen in such infants (such as convulsions and hyperbilirubinemia); therefore many prescribers seem to prefer the use of diluted opium tincture to paregoric.

Opium alkaloid hydrochloride injection (Pantopon) contains 10 mg morphine/ml. This product is only available in Canada. Opium and belladonna suppositories (B & O Supprettes, No. 15A) contain 30 mg powdered opium (10% morphine and other alkaloids) and 16.2 mg powdered belladonna alkaloid (principle belladonna alkaloids are atropine and scopolamine). Number 16A contains 60 mg powdered opium and 16.2 mg belladonna extract. The preparations are used to relieve moderate to severe pain reported with ureteral spasms and have also been prescribed for breakthrough pain between injections of opioids. For side effects/adverse reactions and significant drug interactions see the discussion on morphine.

Adult dosage for opium tincture is 0.3 to 1 ml PO four times daily; maximum 6 ml daily. Camphorated tincture of opium (paregoric) is 5 to 10 ml PO one to four times daily; maximum 10 ml four times daily. Pediatric paregoric dose for 2 years and older is 0.25 to 0.5 ml/kg body weight 1 to 4 times daily.

■ Nursing Management
Opium Preparation Therapy

In addition to the nursing management discussed within the section on opioid therapy, opium tincture may be diluted with water for administration; the solution will become milky. Other liquid forms of opioids may be given with fruit juice to increase their palatability. If opium tincture is given as an antidiarrheal, monitor its effectiveness by checking the frequency and character of stools. If rectal suppositories are being used to administer opioids, the rectum should be emptied first to enhance absorption of the drug.

codeine [koe' deen] (Paveral)

Codeine is available in sulfate and phosphate salts and marketed as oral tablets, oral solution, and injectable dosage forms. Codeine is absorbed well after either oral or parenteral administration and is excreted by the kidneys. Oral administration is used for analgesic, antitussive, and antidiarrheal effects. Codeine may also be injected for treatment of mild to moderate pain. See Tables 14-4 and 14-6 for pharmacokinetic overview and dosing data for opioid analgesics.

■ Nursing Management
Codeine Therapy

In addition to the nursing management discussed within the morphine section, oral codeine should be administered with milk or food to reduce any gastrointestinal distress. Codeine has been added to cough elixirs because it acts as a cough suppressant. The nurse should encourage fluid hydration, which will help to liquify sputum and reduce the constipating effects of codeine.

hydrocodone bitartrate [hye droe koe' doen] (Vicodin, Hycodan)

Hydrocodone is marketed in combination with homatropine in the United States. But in Canada, Hycodan is hydrocodone bitartrate only. Although the product name is similar in both countries, the formulation is not identical. Hydrocodone bitartrate is used as an analgesic and antitussive. See Tables 14-4 and 14-6 for additional information.

hydromorphone [hye droe mor' fone] (Dilaudid, Dilaudid HP)

Hydromorphone is a semisynthetic opioid that has a faster onset of action but a shorter duration of action than morphine. It is prescribed for its analgesic and antitussive effects. See Tables 14-4 and 14-6 for additional information.

meperidine [me per' i deen] (Demerol, Pethidine)

Meperidine is an effective analgesic for short-term use but is considered "the least potent of the common opioid analgesics, and is administered in the largest doses" (Mather & Denson, 1992, p 81). A commonly prescribed opioid, it has a pharmacologic profile similar to morphine, with the following noted differences:

1. Meperidine is less apt to release histamine or to increase biliary tract pressure than morphine; thus is often prescribed for clients with acute asthma, biliary colic, and pancreatitis (Sinatra & Savarese, 1992).
2. Its duration of action is shorter than morphine, thus a more frequent dosing schedule is necessary (see Table 14-4).
3. Meperidine has poor oral bioavailability. To achieve an approximate analgesic equivalency to a 75 mg intramuscular dose requires an oral dose of 300 mg (*USP DI*, 1996). Because the largest oral form of meperidine marketed is a 100 mg tablet, this preparation is often prescribed in dosages that are less effective than the injectable dosage form. See Table 14-6 for dosing data.
4. Meperidine is metabolized in the liver to normeperidine, a CNS neurotoxic metabolite. Normeperidine has a half-life between 15 and 20 hours in persons with normal renal function. Prolonged administration or use of high doses of meperidine, or use in older adults or in clients with impaired renal or hepatic function, has resulted in normeperidine-induced CNS toxicity. This neurotoxicity may produce significant mood changes such as sadness, anger, restlessness and apprehension, increased irritability, nervousness, tremors, agitation, quivering, convulsions, and myoclonus (*AHFS*, 1996; Jacox et al, 1994). Neurotoxicity has also been reported in clients with sickle cell anemia, burn injuries, or cancer who had normal renal and hepatic function but were receiving repeated large doses of meperidine (*AHFS*, 1996).

   Although the use of meperidine for only a few days may generally result in mild and tolerable problems, meperidine should be avoided in clients requiring prolonged usage or high-dose therapy and when renal or liver dysfunction is present. (The

TABLE 14-6 Dosing data for opioid analgesics

Drug	Approximate equianalgesic oral dose	Approximate equianalgesic parenteral dose	Recommended starting dose (adults more than 50 kg body weight)		Recommended starting dose (children and adults less than 50 kg body weight)*	
			Oral	Parenteral	Oral	Parenteral
Opioid agonist						
morphine†	30 mg q3-4h (around-the-clock dosing) 60 mg q3-4h (single dose or intermittent dosing)	10 mg q3-4h	30 mg q3-4h	10 mg q3-4h	0.3 mg/kg q3-4h	0.1 mg/kg q3-4h
codeine‡	130 mg q3-4h	75 mg q3-4h	60 mg q3-4h	60 mg q2h (intramuscular/subcutaneous)	1 mg/kg q3-4h§	Not recommended
hydromophone† (Dilaudid)	7.5 mg q3-4h	1.5 mg q3-4h	6 mg q3-4h	1.5 mg q3-4h	0.06 mg/kg q3-4h	0.015 mg/kg q3-4h
hydrocodone (in Lorcet, Lortab, Vicodin, others)	30 mg q3-4h	Not available	10 mg q3-4h	Not available	0.2 mg/kg q3-4h§	Not available
levorphanol (Levo-Dromoran)	4 mg q6-8h	2 mg q6-8h	4 mg q6-8h	2 mg q6-8h	0.04 mg/kg q6-8h	0.02 mg/kg q6-8h
meperidine (Demerol)	300 mg q2-3h	100 mg q3h	Not recommended	100 mg q3h	Not recommended	0.75 mg/kg q2-3h

methadone (Dolophine, others)	20 mg q6-8h	10 mg q6-8h	20 mg q6-8h	10 mg q6-8h	0.2 mg/kg q6-8h	0.1 mg/kg q6-8h
oxycodone (Roxicodone, also in Percocet, Percodan, Tylox, others)	30 mg q3-4h	Not available	10 mg q3-4h	Not available	0.2 mg/kg q3-4h§	Not available
oxymorphone† (Numorphan)	Not available	1 mg q3-4h	Not available	1 mg q3-4h	Not recommended	Not recommended
Opioid agonist-antagonist and partial agonist						
buprenorphine (Buprenex)	Not available	0.3-0.4 mg q6-8h	Not available	0.4 mg q6-8h	Not available	0.004 mg/kg q6-8h
butorphanol (Stadol)	Not available	2 mg q3-4h	Not available	2 mg q3-4h	Not available	Not recommended
nalbuphine (Nubain)	Not available	10 mg q3-4h	Not available	10 mg q3-4h	Not available	0.1 mg/kg q3-4h
pentazocine (Talwin, others)	150 mg q3-4h	60 mg q3-4h	50 mg q4-6h	Not recommended	Not recommended	Not recommended

From Carr DB, Jacox AK, Chapman CR et al: *Acute pain management: operative or medical procedures and trauma. Clinical practice guideline,* AHCPR Pub No 92-0032, Rockville, Md, 1992, Agency for Health Care Policy and Research, USDHSS, PHS.

Note: Published tables vary in the suggested doses that are equianalgesic to morphine. Clinical response is the criterion that must be applied for each patient; titration to clinical response is necessary. Because there is not complete cross tolerance among these drugs, it is usually necessary to use a lower than equianalgesic dose when changing drugs and to retitrate to response.

Caution: Recommended doses do not apply to patients with renal or hepatic insufficiency or other conditions affecting drug metabolism and kinetics.

**Caution:* Doses listed for patients with body weight less than 50 kg cannot be used as initial starting doses in babies less than 6 months of age. Consult the *Acute Pain Management: Operative or Medical Procedures and Trauma. Clinical Practice Guideline* section on management of pain in neonates for recommendations.

†For morphine, hydromorphone, and oxymorphone, rectal administration is an alternate route for patients unable to take oral medications, but equianalgesic doses may differ from oral and parenteral doses because of pharmacokinetic differences.

‡*Caution:* Codeine doses above 65 mg often are not appropriate due to diminishing incremental analgesia with increasing doses but continually increasing constipation and other side effects.

§*Caution:* Doses of aspirin and acetaminophen in combination opioid-NSAID preparations must also be adjusted to the patient's body weight.

Nursing Research

Postoperative use of meperidine

Administration of narcotic analgesic is an integral part of nursing care for postoperative clients. Yet moderate to severe pain remains the norm for most hospitalized clients. Undertreatment of pain appears to be the most common explanation for the frequency and severity of pain experienced by postoperative clients. The purpose of this study was to describe the types and amounts of narcotic analgesics administered postoperatively to clients by nurses.

The postoperative administration of narcotic analgesics was examined with 180 uncomplicated adult appendectomy clients. Narcotic analgesia doses were transcribed from the hospital records of these clients for the entire postoperative period. Equianalgesic doses were calculated so that all medications were comparable with meperidine. Eighty-three percent (n=150) of the clients received meperidine. Patients who received meperidine were given significantly more narcotic analgesics than those who received morphine sulfate. The amount of narcotic analgesics received by clients was significantly related to their length of stay. Meperidine and Tylenol #3 (acetaminophen with codeine phosphate) comprised the significantly associated analgesics. These findings suggest a need to reexamine the current use of meperidine in postoperative analgesia.

Critical thinking questions

- What is specific about meperidine's pharmacokinetics that might have contributed to this finding?
- Within the data of this research was a finding that eight people received no narcotic analgesic at all. How might this result occur?
- What other factors might result in the association between meperidine and extended length of hospital stay for clients?

From McDonald DD (1993). Postoperative narcotic analgesic administration. *Applied Nursing Research* 6(3):106.

Nursing Research box above discusses research on the postoperative use of meperidine.) The nurse should be aware that naloxone (opioid antagonist) will antagonize meperidine but not normeperidine and may in some instances cause further CNS excitation and seizures. Management for normeperidine toxicity includes stopping meperidine and substituting an alternate opioid, such as morphine. If seizures occur, an anticonvulsant may be used.

5. Meperidine produces a vagolytic effect, resulting in significant tachycardia; therefore its use should probably be avoided or closely monitored in clients with dysrhythmias or myocardial infarction.
6. Review the drug interaction section, especially for concurrent use of MAO inhibitors with meperidine. Very severe, unpredictable life-threatening reactions may result.

■ Nursing Management

Meperidine Therapy

Assessment. The administration of meperidine is contraindicated with clients with severe dysfunction of the liver because the drug is inactivated in the liver; certain conditions involving the gallbladder and the bile ducts because it causes biliary spasm; head injury and increased intracranial pressure because it may mask neurologic parameters; and chronic obstructive pulmonary disease because it may result in respiratory depression and shock. Respiratory depression occurs as with morphine but is of shorter duration. Meperidine causes CNS excitation ranging from irritability to seizures. When administered with a phenothiazine such as promethazine, which also lowers the seizure threshold, the client is at higher risk for seizures. Meperidine should be used with caution in clients who have atrial flutter or other supraventricular tachycardia, since meperidine may increase ventricular response through vagolytic action. Meperidine is not administered for chronic pain, because of its short duration of action. It may be given orally but is more effective intramuscularly.

A thorough assessment of the client's pain regarding location, severity, and quality needs to be done as for the nursing management of the previously discussed opioid therapy.

Nursing diagnosis. In addition to the nursing diagnoses considered within the nursing management of opioid therapy, clients are at risk for impaired tissue integrity (fibrotic areas) related to intramuscular administration and sensory/perceptual alterations related to CNS stimulation.

Implementation

Monitoring. Vital signs should be monitored and recorded before and after administration of meperidine. It can cause tachycardia and hypotension. Observation of behavioral changes are indicated. Observations of the client are the same as discussed for morphine.

Intervention. Before mixing meperidine in solution with another medication, consult a specific reference, because it tends to be physically and chemically incompatible with a wide range of substances.

Tissue irritation is common with the administration of intramuscular meperidine. Clients frequently experience muscle damage, poor absorption, and pain during injection. Rotation of injection sites is essential.

Meperidine is diluted for IV administration; however, it is not the recommended route of administration. It needs to be titrated for the client's response because of its respiratory depressant effects.

Meperidine dosage should be gradually tapered because abstinence symptoms, such as nausea, vomiting, and diarrhea, can occur. Such symptoms should be reported to the prescriber so that the dosage may be adjusted.

Education. Client teaching is the same as for the client education discussed in the section on morphine, p. 248. (See also the case study at right.)

Case Study

Pain Management

Daniel Watkins is a 53-year-old man who was admitted to the hospital for severe abdominal pain. A bowel resection was done to relieve an obstruction. By his fourth postoperative day he is ambulating and tolerating oral intake. He has been taking both injections and oral medication for pain. The following medications are currently ordered:

meperidine, 50-75 mg IM q4h prn for pain
Tylox, one or two capsules PO q4h prn for pain
Tylenol, 650 mg PO q4h prn for headache and fever

Mr. Watkins is complaining of pain around his incision after a dressing change and removal of surgical drains. He is very anxious and upset. He is requesting pain medication. He had his last dose of meperidine 6 hours ago. He took one capsule of Tylox 2 hours ago for mild pain after ambulating.

1. What assessment data does the nurse need in order to decide how to intervene at this time?
2. The nurse decides to administer meperidine 50 mg IM. What assessment should be done to monitor for adverse reactions to the meperidine?
3. What should the nurse document in the client's chart about the pain management?
4. Mr. Watkins complains that the drugs do not always help when he has severe pain. What is the nurse's appropriate action for this situation?
5. What measures can the nurse teach Mr. Watkins to promote more effective pain management?
6. When Mr. Watkins complains of a headache, what medication would be most appropriate for the nurse to administer?

methadone [meth' a done] (Dolophine, Methadose)
Methadone is an effective analgesic with properties similar to morphine, with the exception of its extended half-life. The duration of action for methadone is usually listed at 4 to 6 hours, but with repeated oral dosing, the half-life may extend from 22 to 48 hours (perhaps even longer in the elderly and clients with renal dysfunction). This extended half-life is *not* related to its analgesic effect. To control pain methadone is administered every 6 to 8 hours, based on the individual's response. See Table 14-6 for dosing information.

Because of its extended half-life, methadone is approved by the FDA for use in state approved detoxification and maintenance treatment programs. In Canada, it is available through specially authorized physicians. Oral administration is preferred for detoxification and required for maintenance programs. Methadone dependence is substituted in individuals who are physiologically dependent on heroin, opium, or other opioids. See Chapter 9 for information on methadone treatment programs. The mechanism of action of methadone is similar to that of morphine, as are the pharmacokinetics (see Table 14-4). Side/adverse reactions are also similar to those for morphine, although methadone's miotic and respiratory depressant effects may be present for more than 24 hours. Excessive sedation is reported in some clients following a regular dosing schedule.

■ Nursing Management

Methadone Therapy

See also the nursing management discussion on opioid therapy, p. 244.

Assessment. When the client is receiving methadone for treatment of heroin abuse, the nurse should be aware of possible outside sources of OTC drugs (liquid cough preparations with alcohol) and alcohol (such as alcohol or alcohol beverages brought in by friends and family), which may potentiate the action of methadone.

Implementation

Monitoring. Although most adverse effects dissipate in the initial 3 weeks of therapy, constipation and diaphoresis may persist.

Intervention. Overdosage of this drug can cause extreme respiratory depression. Naloxone should be readily available for intravenous administration. The antagonist action is only 1 to 3 hours, and the action of methadone is 36 to 48 hours or more; thus repeated doses of naloxone for up to 8 to 24 hours may be required to treat respiratory depression.

When methadone is used for detoxification and maintenance therapy, it is administered as an oral liquid. If dispersable tablets are used, they are dissolved in 120 ml of water or citrus-flavored solution, such as Tang, Kool-Aid, or fruit juice. Dissolution takes a minute or so and may be enhanced by using cold and/or acidic solvents. If the concentrated oral solution is used, it should be diluted in at least 90 ml of solution to enable the complete dosage to be received. It has also been used for the treatment of the terminally ill.

Education. Since methadone is commonly given on an outpatient basis for withdrawal from heroin or morphine-like drugs, the client should be cautioned about operating a car or other potentially dangerous equipment because mental and physical abilities may be impaired. Orthostatic hypotension is a common side effect, which can last for several weeks. Clients should be instructed to rise slowly from a recumbent position and to sit or lie down in the event of dizziness or faintness.

Evaluation. If methadone is administered for detoxification, the client should demonstrate effective management of the therapeutic regimen by remaining free of the abused substance and by participating in the psychiatric, social, and vocational rehabilitation programs.

levorphanol [lee vor' fa nole] (Levo-Dromoran)
Levorphanol is an opioid analgesic used for moderate-to-severe pain. See Tables 14-4 and 14-6 for additional information.

For nursing management of levorphanol therapy, review the discussion of opioid therapy. The actions of levorphanol are identical to morphine, but the effective dose is one fourth to one fifth that of morphine. Note, too, that the duration of action is 6 to 8 hours and if administered with the frequency of other opioids, it will accumulate in the body and place the client at risk for respiratory depression.

oxycodone [ox i koe' done] (Percodan, Tylox, Percocet)
Oxycodone is approximately 10 times more potent than codeine. It is available alone, in combination with aspirin (Percodan) or acetaminophen (Tylox, Percocet) and in an extended-action dosage form (OxyContin). (See Tables 14-4 and 14-6 for additional information.) The suppository dosage form is not available in the United States but is available in Canada. Review the nursing management of opioid therapy.

oxymorphone [ox i mor' fone] (Numorphan)
Oxymorphone is pharmacologically similar to morphine with the following exceptions: in equianalgesic dosages, oxymorphone usually causes more nausea, vomiting, and psychic effects (euphoria) than morphine; and it may also be less constipating and cause less suppression of the cough reflex than morphine. Oxymorphone is a potent analgesic used for moderate-to-severe pain, preoperative medication, obstetric analgesia, and as adjunct therapy for the treatment of anxiety caused by dyspnea resulting from pulmonary edema associated with left ventricular failure. See Tables 14-4 and 14-6 for additional information.

■ Nursing Management
Oxymorphone Therapy

Oxymorphone should be given with milk or meals to decrease the incidence of gastrointestinal distress. It tends to cause more nausea and vomiting than **equianalgesic** (producing approximately the same degree of analgesia) doses of morphine sulfate. Oxymorphone suppositories need to be stored in the refrigerator but protected from freezing.

fentanyl [fen' ta nil]
Fentanyl is an opioid analgesic available in a preservative-free solution (Sublimaze), in combination with droperidol (Innovar), and as a topical transdermal patch (Duragesic). Fentanyl solution and fentanyl with droperidol are used parenterally (IV) for analgesia as a premedication, as an adjunct to anesthesia, and in the immediate postoperative period. Parenteral administration of fentanyl should be restricted to those experienced with this product and with the management of fentanyl-induced respiratory depression. Fentanyl and the fentanyl derivative sufentanil (Sufenta), if given rapidly in large doses, may cause chest wall muscle rigidity, which then requires supportive respiratory ventilation and perhaps a rapid-acting muscle relaxant. This depression is dose related (*USP DI*, 1996).

Fentanyl is metabolized in the liver and excreted in urine. Drug interactions and side effect/adverse reactions are similar to the other opioids. The patch system is available in 25, 50, 75, and 100 μg/hr dosage forms. The manufacturer publishes an equianalgesic potency chart and a morphine to fentanyl conversion chart that should be utilized to determine the fentanyl dose.

■ Nursing Management
Fentanyl Transdermal System

In addition to the nursing management discussed with opioid therapy:

Assessment. In opioid-naive clients (persons not taking any opioid medication), in elderly clients (60 years and older), and in cachectic or debilitated clients, the starting dose should not be higher than 25 μg/hr. This product is used in the management of chronic pain as an alternative to the other opioids, especially for clients who have difficulty swallowing or complying with a schedule of oral medications.

Implementation

Monitoring. Monitor respiratory status and keep naloxone and resuscitative equipment available.

Intervention. Remove the transdermal system from the package immediately before applying. Use water to clean the skin area before application. Do not use soap, oils, lotions, alcohol, or other products because they may alter the absorption of this product. Apply it to a dry, flat (hairless) area of the upper torso, front or back. Do not apply to skin that is burned, cut, irritated, very oily, or recently shaved. If the skin area is hairy, cut the hair with a scissors. Hold the patch in place 10 to 20 seconds to be sure it is securely fastened to the client. Then check the patch to make certain skin contact is complete and the edges of the system adhere to the skin. Wash hands after application of the patch. Use large amounts of water in washing, especially if the gel accidentally came in contact with your skin. Avoid use of soap, alcohol, or any other solvent. The patch releases fentanyl continuously by absorption through the skin, which aids in controlling pain around the clock for 72 hours.

After application fentanyl is absorbed and concentrated in the upper layers of skin. Serum levels increase slowly, usually reaching a plateau between 12 and 24 hours. It is recommended that during the initial application of the patch a short-acting analgesic be prescribed for the first 20 to 24 hours, since peak serum levels of fentanyl usually occur between 24 and 72 hours. Thereafter the person should have an order for a short-acting opioid for breakthrough pain.

Average half-life of fentanyl is 17 hours (range is 13 to 22 hours). Because it may take as long as 6 days to reach steady-state levels of a new dose, dosage adjustments after the initial 72-hour change should be instituted on an every 6-day schedule.

If another system is required after 72 hours, apply to a new site. Withdraw the drug gradually. Because the serum level of fentanyl decreases slowly, give half the equianalgesic dose of the new analgesic 12 to 18 hours after removal.

Education. Instruct the client to dispose of the system by folding the adhesive sides together and then flushing the system down the toilet.

Evaluation. The client will experience pain relief without breakthrough pain or any adverse effects of the drug.

propoxyphene [proe pox' i feen] (Darvon) propoxyphene napsylate combinations (Darvocet-N)

Propoxyphene is a synthetic analgesic structurally related to methadone that is indicated for the treatment of mild to moderate pain. Controlled studies have reported that propoxyphene 65 mg is equivalent to or less effective than acetaminophen 650 mg, aspirin 650 mg, codeine 32 mg, pentazocine (Talwin) 30 mg, or meperidine (Demerol) 50 mg (McCaffery & Beebe, 1989). When combined with aspirin or acetaminophen, propoxyphene combinations usually provide analgesia greater than either medication alone.

Propoxyphene binds to opioid receptors and produces an analgesic effect similar to codeine and the opioids. The hydrochloride dosage form is more rapidly absorbed than the water-insoluble napsylate formulation, although peak serum levels are approximately equivalent. The bioavailability of propoxyphene hydrochloride 65 mg is equivalent to that of propoxyphene napsylate 100 mg. The duration of action of propoxyphene is 4 to 6 hours. Propoxyphene crosses into the CNS and is believed to cross the placenta. Metabolism occurs mainly in the liver where approximately one fourth of the dose is metabolized to norpropoxyphene, a toxic metabolite with a half-life of 30 to 36 hours (*USP DI,* 1996). Propoxyphene is also more apt to cause convulsions than most of the other opioid analgesics. See Table 14-4 for pharmacokinetic information.

The usual adult dose for propoxyphene and propoxyphene napsylate is one every 4 hours when needed. The pediatric dose is not established.

■ Nursing Management
Propoxyphene Therapy

Propoxyphene should be used with caution with clients who have a history of excessive alcohol intake, and it is contraindicated in those who are suicidal or addiction prone. Preparations containing propoxyphene taken in excessive doses or in combination with alcohol or other CNS depressants are a major cause of drug-related deaths. Ambulatory clients should be cautioned about driving a car or operating dangerous machinery, since their judgment may be impaired.

OPIOID ANTAGONISTS

Naloxone and naltrexone are opioid antagonists; they competitively displace the opioid analgesics from their receptor sites, thus reversing their effects. The major difference is that naloxone must be administered parenterally, whereas naltrexone is available as an oral dosage formulation.

Antagonists block the subjective and objective opioid effects and can precipitate withdrawal symptoms in individuals physically dependent on opioids. Naloxone and naltrexone are used to reverse the adverse or overdose effects of opioids (codeine, diphenoxylate, fentanyl, heroin, hydromorphone, levorphanol, meperidine, methadone, morphine, oxymorphone, opium derivatives, and propoxyphene) and of the partial agonists (agonist-antagonist drugs such as butorphanol, nalbuphine, and pentazocine). Respiratory depression induced by nonopioids (barbiturates, etc.), CNS depression, or a disease progression will usually not respond to antagonist drug therapy.

In an opioid analgesic overdosage, naloxone and naltrexone will reverse the respiratory depression, sedation, pupillary miosis (constriction), and euphoric effects; they may also reverse the psychotomimetic effects of the agonist-antagonists analgesics (pentazocine and others). Both drugs

BOX 14-5

tramadol (Ultram)

Tramadol is indicated for the treatment of moderate to moderately severe pain. In animal studies, tramadol appears to act centrally to inhibit reuptake of norepinephrine and serotonin, and it also binds to mu-opioid receptors. An early release stated this drug was not chemically related to the opiates, had less potential for causing respiratory depression, and while it could cause dependence, there was little proof of drug abuse in countries where the drug was used (News, 1995). It was promoted as being comparable to Tylenol (acetaminophen) with codeine #3 in both safety and efficacy.

In 1996, the manufacturer sent a letter to health care professionals to warn them of potential seizures, anaphylactoid reactions, and drug abuse associated with tramadol (FDA News and Product Notes, 1996). Therefore, this product is not recommended for use in persons with a history of opioid allergy, dependence, or a past or present history of addiction.

Tramadol is well absorbed orally with an onset of action within 60 minutes, peak effect in 2 hours, and a half-life of 6 to 7 hours. It is metabolized in the liver and primarily excreted in urine. Side/adverse effects include abdominal distress, anorexia, increased anxiety, weakness, constipation, confusion, dizziness, insomnia, sweating, visual disturbances, and urinary retention and frequency.

Usual adult dose is 50 to 100 mg every 6 hours. Maximum daily dose is 400 mg.

FDA News and Product Notes (1996). *Ultram Formulary,* 31:450.
News (1995). New Oral Analgesic, Tramadol, Gains Marketing Approval. *American Journal Health-System Pharmacy,* 52:1153-4.

TABLE 14-7 Naloxone and naltrexone: side effects/adverse reactions

Drugs	Side effects*	Adverse reactions†
naloxone	Nausea, vomiting, tremors, increased sweating, nervousness	Tachycardia, hypertension
naltrexone	Insomnia, nervousness; nausea, vomiting, abdominal distress; headaches, tiredness, generalized joint and muscle pain; chills; constipation, anorexia, diarrhea	Hallucinations, paranoia, confusion, severe depression; rash; stomach pain; earache; increased temperature; tinnitus; edema and phlebitis

*If side effects continue, increase, or disturb the client, inform the prescriber.
†If adverse reactions occur, contact prescriber because medical intervention may be necessary.

are believed to work at all three receptor sites, but their greatest activity is for mu receptors.

naloxone hydrochloride [na lox' one] (Narcan)
Naloxone is inactivated orally, but is very effective parenterally. Its onset of action is 1 to 2 minutes (IV) and 2 to 5 minutes (IM or SC). Half-life is between 60 and 100 minutes. Duration of action depends on the dose administered and the route of administration. Usually the IM dose results in a prolonged effect. Naloxone is widely distributed throughout the body and also crosses the placenta. It is metabolized in the liver and excreted via the kidneys. Naloxone adult dose is 0.4 to 2 mg as single dose or 0.1 to 0.2 mg for postoperative opioid depression. For continuous infusion, 2 mg of naloxone may be diluted in 500 ml of normal saline or 5% dextrose injection. Because naloxone is shorter acting than most opioids, repeated naloxone injections or a continuous infusion is necessary to prevent the recurrence of respiratory depression. See Table 14-7 for side/adverse effects.

naltrexone [nal trex' one] (ReVia)
This drug is indicated for adjuvant treatment in the detoxified opioid-dependent person. Absorption is rapid, but it undergoes an extensive first-pass metabolism in the liver to the major metabolite 6-beta-naltrexol, which also has opioid antagonist effects. Peak serum concentration is reached in 1 hour; elimination half-life for naltrexone is 4 hours, metabolite in approximately 13 hours. Duration of action is dose dependent. Excretion is via the kidneys. Table 14-7 lists side/adverse effects. Treatment with naltrexone is started cautiously; usually 25 mg orally with close monitoring for withdrawal signs and symptoms for approximately 1 hour. If no withdrawal effects occur, the balance of the daily dosage is given. Maintenance is usually 50 mg orally daily.

Nursing Management

Opioid Antagonist Therapy

Nurses administer opioid antagonists in the emergency treatment of opioid overdose, as well as in maintenance therapy of former opioid addicted individuals. The nurse must have an understanding of opioid analgesics and opioid antagonists to provide nursing care to these clients.

Assessment. Clients should be observed carefully; opioid antagonists should either not be administered or administered with extreme caution if the client is known or suspected to be physically dependent on opioids (including newborns of dependent mothers) because abrupt and complete reversal of opioid effects will produce an acute abstinence syndrome in the physically dependent client. Naloxone should be used with caution in clients with preexisting ventricular irritability because ventricular tachycardia and fibrillation may occur. Naltrexone is contraindicated in clients with acute hepatitis or hepatic failure because there is an increased risk of hepatotoxicity.

A baseline assessment should include hepatic function studies for naltrexone, as well as the status of the symptoms for which the opioid antagonist is being administered.

Nursing diagnosis. The client being administered naloxone is at risk for the nursing diagnosis of altered comfort related to withdrawal symptoms (anxiety, irritability, body aches, diarrhea, tachycardia, runny nose, sweating, yawning, anorexia, nausea, vomiting, trembling, shivering) and the potential complication of decreased cardiac output related to the cardiovascular effects (tachycardia, hypotension, hypertension) of the drug.

In addition to these symptoms, the neonate may also experience convulsions with naloxone. With naltrexone, altered comfort may be a concern as described above, with additional symptoms (abdominal cramping, headache, joint and muscle pain), but also the client may experience impaired skin integrity (rash occurs in 1% to 10% of clients); constipation (up to 10%); and sexual dysfunction in men (up to 10%). Although the symptoms of body aches, abdominal discomfort, nausea and vomiting, lethargy, and anxiety may be the same as for withdrawal symptoms, these symptoms may disappear with continued use.

Implementation

Monitoring. Continued nursing observation is necessary for the client who has responded to naloxone; doses should be repeated as necessary, since the duration of action of some opioids exceeds the duration of action of naloxone. Monitor closely for airway obstruction and maintain suction equipment at the bedside until the client is recovered. Monitor vital signs, particularly respirations, minimally every 5 minutes until the client is stable. The respiratory rate should increase within 1 to 2 minutes of the first dose. The intravenous infusion rate of administration should be titrated according to the client's response. An intensive care unit is probably the most appropriate place for this client until the effects of the drug have completely abated. Clients should be observed for a day or longer regardless of the apparent recovery.

With naltrexone, monitor hepatic studies monthly for the first 6 months and then periodically after that. Naltrexone should be discontinued if significant hepatic abnormalities occur.

Intervention. In addition to opioid toxicity, one of the major indications for naltrexone is the treatment of opioid dependency and addiction, and it should be used as an adjunctive measure to a comprehensive drug rehabilitation program involving counseling and psychotherapy. Naltrexone therapy should not be instituted until the client has been completely detoxified as evidenced by being opioid free for 7 to 10 days, by absence of withdrawal symptoms, and by abstinence verification via a negative urinalysis for opioids or naloxone challenge test. If, in an emergency situation, an opioid analgesic is required for a client receiving naltrexone therapy, its administration should be accomplished in a hospital setting where careful monitoring is available. Because high doses of the analgesic will be required to overcome the effects of naltrexone, the client will be at risk for prolonged respiratory depression and circulatory collapse. Naltrexone does not cause physical or psychologic dependence.

To verify abstinence from opioids, as is frequently done before naltrexone therapy, a naloxone challenge test may be done. This test should not be done in the presence of withdrawal symptoms (body aches, diarrhea, gooseflesh, sneezing and runny nose, irritability, diaphoresis, trembling and weakness, abdominal cramping, tachycardia, nausea and vomiting) or opioids in the urine. If administered intravenously, an initial dose of 0.2 mg is given and the client is observed for 30 seconds for symptoms of withdrawal. If no symptoms occur, an additional 0.6 mg may be administered and the client is observed for 20 minutes. If administered subcutaneously, 0.8 mg is given, and the client is observed for 45 minutes. If withdrawal symptoms occur, the test should be repeated at an appropriate interval. It should be remembered that naloxone has no effect on respiratory depression caused by nonopiate drugs. If the client has taken multiple drugs, the naloxone will reverse only the opioids.

It is recommended that naloxone not be mixed with other agents because it becomes unstable. After dilution, any unused solution should be discarded after 24 hours. Additional resuscitative measures, such as oxygen and mechanical ventilation, should be available when necessary to counteract opioid overdosage.

Education. When opioid antagonists are used in emergency treatment, client education should be focused on assisting the client to cope with the immediate situation. Instructions should be given to keep the client informed of what is to occur and to help the client cooperate with treatment procedures, even when the client appears unresponsive. Discussion of the dangers of drug abuse or dependence may be appropriate at some time after emergency treatment. Compliance with long-term naltrexone therapy is improved if someone other than the client (health care provider or family member) administers the naltrexone.

With naltrexone, stress the importance of regular visits to the prescriber for hepatic function studies to detect hepatotoxicity, the need to maintain other parts of the rehabilitation program (counseling sessions, support group meetings, etc.), notifying other health care providers of naltrexone use, and carrying an identification indicating the use of this drug. Alert the client not to take opioid medications for pain relief, diarrhea, or cough because they will not be effective. Warn the client not to take large doses of opioids to overcome the effects of the drug because that may result in coma and death. The drug should not be shared with others, including those dependent on opioids.

Evaluation. After administration of antagonists, evaluation takes place to help identify the development of opioid withdrawal syndrome in the possible opioid-dependent client. When naltrexone is used for maintenance of the opioid-free state in former opioid-addicted individuals, follow-up evaluations are needed to reinforce and ensure compliance.

In the reversal of opioid toxicity, the respiratory rate and volume will increase and the blood pressure will return to normal if it has been depressed.

OPIOID AGONIST-ANTAGONIST AGENTS

Although the exact mechanism of action of the **opioid agonist-antagonist agents** is unknown, these agents have both agonist and antagonist effects on the opioid receptors. For example, buprenorphine (Buprenex) is a partial agonist at the mu receptors while butorphanol (Stadol), nalbuphine (Nubain), and pentazocine (Talwin) produce agonist effects at the kappa and sigma receptors and may displace agonists (opioids) from their mu receptor sites, thus inhibiting their effects and perhaps inducing a drug withdrawal reaction in clients physically dependent on agonist opioids. Dezocine (Dalgan) is a partial agonist at the mu receptor with some effect at the sigma receptors after high doses. Generally, these drugs are less potent analgesics and have a lower dependency potential than opioids, and withdrawal symptoms are not as severe as those reported with the opioid agonist medications.

The opioid agonist-antagonist agents have pharmacokinetics, adverse effects, and significant drug interactions similar to morphine. Table 14-8 lists agonist-antagonist pharmacokinetics, equivalency, and dosing.

butorphanol tartrate (byoo tor' fa nole) (Stadol)
Butorphanol tartrate is indicated for treatment of moderate-to-severe pain and as an anesthetic adjunct. It is administered parenterally (IM or IV).

TABLE 14-8 Agonist-antagonist: pharmacokinetics, equivalency, and dosing

Drug	Equivalent dose* (mg)	Onset (min)	Peak (min)	Duration (hrs)	Half-life (hrs)	Usual dose
buprenorphine (Buprenex)						
IV	0.3	<15	<60	6	2-3	0.3 mg q6h
IM	0.3	15	60	6	2-3	
butorphanol (Stadol)						
IV	2	2-3	30	2-4	2-4	0.5-2 mg q3-4h
IM	2	10-30	30-60	3-4	2-4	
dezocine (Dalgan)						
IV	10	<15	—	2-4†	2	2.5-10 mg q2-4h
IM	10	<30	1-2	2-4†	2	
nalbuphine (Nubain)						
IV	10	2-3	30	3-6	5	10 mg q3-6h
IM	10	<15	60	3-6	5	
SC	10	<15	—	3-6	5	
pentazocine (Talwin)						
PO	180	15-30	60-90	3	2-3	50 mg PO or 30 mg parenteral q3-4h
IM	60	15-20	30-60	2-3	2-3	
IV	60	2-3	15-30	2-3	2-3	
SC	60	15-20	30-60	2-3	2-3	

min, minutes.
*Equivalent to 10 mg morphine IM dose.
†Dose dependent.

■ Nursing Management

Butorphanol Therapy

In addition to the nursing management discussed within opioid therapy:

Assessment. Use with caution as a preoperative medication with hypertensive clients because butorphanol may increase the blood pressure. It should not be administered to clients with acute myocardial infarction because the cardiovascular effects tend to increase the workload on the heart. However, butorphanol may be used with clients with gallbladder disease or gallstones because biliary spasm has not been reported.

If the client is suspected of being physically dependent on narcotics, butorphanol should not be given until the person is detoxified. Since butorphanol is a narcotic agonist-antagonist, it would only counteract the effects of the original narcotic, set up a need for an increase in the dosage, and precipitate an abstinence syndrome.

Butorphanol may elevate CSF pressure; therefore it should be used with caution in clients with head injuries or preexisting increased CSF pressure. Because butorphanol is metabolized in the liver, it should be given with caution to clients with compromised or impaired renal or hepatic function. Because of decreased metabolism of the drug in the liver, side effects and greater activity may result.

The safety of the use of butorphanol in pregnancy before the labor period has not been established, but the safety to the mother and fetus after the administration of butorphanol during labor has been established. Clients receiving butorphanol during labor have experienced no adverse effects other than those observed with commonly employed analgesics; however, this drug should be used with caution in women delivering premature infants.

The client receiving butorphanol therapy should be assessed for significant drug interactions. When butorphanol is given concurrently with:

Drug	Possible effect and management
alcohol or CNS depressants	May increase the potential for CNS depression, respiratory depression, and hypotension. Monitor closely for adverse effects because one or both drugs may need to be reduced.
buprenorphine (Buprenex)	**May reduce the therapeutic effects of butorphanol, nalbuphine, or pentazocine at the kappa receptors. Increased respiratory depressant effects may occur when buprenor-phine is given with low doses of other mu receptor agonists or kappa receptor agonists. Avoid concurrent administration.**
monoamine oxidase (MAO) inhibitors	Use opioid analgesics (other than meperidine) cautiously in reduced dosages. For safety's safe, one fourth of the usual anal gesic dose should be given to determine client's response to this combination.

Drug	Possible effect and management
naltrexone (Narcan)	Use of naltrexone will precipitate withdrawal symptoms in the butorphanol-dependent client. It will also negate any therapeutic use of the drug.

Nursing diagnosis. The client receiving butorphanol therapy is at risk for injury related to the CNS effects of the drug and altered comfort related to the underlying condition and the ineffectiveness of the drug.

Implementation

Monitoring. Monitor for pain relief. Butorphanol tartrate can cause respiratory depression if the dose exceeds 4 mg as a single dose. If the usual intramuscular dose of 2 mg is insufficient to relieve the client's pain, the dose can be increased by 1 to 4 mg every 3 to 4 hours. It is important for the nurse to assess the client's response to this medication and to be aware of any signs of respiratory depression. These could be changes in rate, depth, or regularity of respiratory rate. Monitor for adverse CNS reactions, such as confusion and vertigo, fluctuations in blood pressure, and bowel function for constipation.

Intervention. SC route is not recommended; do not administer rapid IV. Ensure that naloxone and resuscitative equipment are in the immediate environment. Provide for the client's safety.

Education. Instruct the client to change positions slowly and to avoid activities that require concentration and alertness. Instruct in measures to prevent constipation such as high fiber diet and adequate hydration, although butorphanol is not as constipating as other opioids. It also has a lower risk of dependence and the withdrawal symptoms are not as severe as opioid agonists.

Evaluation. The client will have relief from pain without any adverse effects from the drug.

dezocine [dez' oh seen] (Dalgan)

Dezocine, a potent parenteral opioid agonist-antagonist comparable to morphine in analgesic potency, onset, and duration of action, is indicated for the treatment of pain. It is administered parenterally, IM or IV.

When dezocine is used concurrently with other CNS depressants, an additive CNS depressant effect may occur. It is suggested that the dose of either or both drugs be reduced.

More frequent side effects reported include nausea, vomiting, drowsiness, and injection site reactions. Less frequent include dizziness, increased sweating, chills, hypotension or hypertension, chest pain, dry mouth, constipation, muscle pain or cramps, increased anxiety, crying spells, and headaches. Adverse reactions include respiratory depression, urinary retention, and delirium. See also Nursing Management: Opioid Therapy.

▲ **pentazocine** [pen taz' oh seen] (Talwin)

The analgesic pentazocine is not indicated for pain caused from an acute myocardial infarction because of its effects on cardiac function. It increases cardiac workload by increasing systemic and pulmonary arterial pressure, systemic vascular resistance, and left ventricular end-diastolic pressure. It also has a higher incidence of psychotomimetic side effects than the majority of other analgesics, thus limiting its usefulness, especially in terminally ill clients or those who are already anxious or fearful.

Pentazocine tablets are combined with naloxone (Narcan) in the United States because of the high incidence of pentazocine abuse. Naloxone taken orally is not pharmacologically active, but if this combination is dissolved and injected, naloxone will block the effects of pentazocine. Significant drug interactions are the same as those for butorphanol. SC administration is to be avoided because of tissue damage at the injection sites; IM sites should be routinely rotated for the same reason. See Nursing Management: Opioid Therapy.

nalbuphine [nal' byoo feen] (Nubain)

Nalbuphine an analgesic for moderate-to-severe pain, is also used preoperatively as an adjunct to anesthesia and for obstetric analgesia. Drug interactions are similar to pentazocine. See Nursing Management: Opioid Therapy for nursing considerations.

buprenorphine [byoo pre nor' feen] (Buprenex)

Buprenorphine dissociates very slowly from the mu receptor; thus it will reduce or block the effect of concurrent or subsequent dosing with opioid agonist drugs. It can precipitate withdrawal symptoms if administered to persons physically dependent on opioids. Buprenorphine induced respiratory depression and other adverse effects are often difficult to reverse because naloxone is not very effective in treating buprenorphine-induced adverse effects. When naloxone is ineffective, the respiratory stimulant doxapram is recommended (*USP DI*, 1996).

Significant drug interactions. When buprenorphine is given with:

Drug	Possible effect and management
other CNS depressants or MAO inhibitors	May result in increased CNS depressant effect, respiratory depression, and hypotension. Monitor closely since one or both drugs may need to be decreased by the prescriber.
opioid analgesics	**The therapeutic effects of the opioid may be reduced. In physically opioid-dependent clients, withdrawal symptoms may be precipitated by coadministration of buprenorphine. Avoid this combination.**

See Nursing Management: Opioid Therapy for nursing management of buprenorphine.

NONOPIOID ANALGESICS

The nonopioid analgesics are effective for mild to moderate pain and are often combined with opioid analgesics to enhance pain control in cases of severe pain. They correspond, in combination with a weak opioid, to step 2 in Figure 14-9. The major drugs in this classification include acetaminophen, aspirin, nonsteroidal antiinflammatory drugs

MANAGEMENT OF DRUG OVERDOSE

Acetaminophen

- Early symptoms: sweating, anorexia, nausea or vomiting, abdominal pain or cramping and/or diarrhea; usually occur in 6 to 14 hours after ingestion, lasting for approximately 24 hours
- Late symptoms: abdominal area may exhibit swelling, tenderness, or pain in 2 to 4 days after ingestion (hepatotoxicity)
- Treatment: gastric lavage or emesis. Start acetylcysteine administration as soon as possible. Determine acetaminophen serum levels at 4 hours or more, after ingestion. Hepatotoxicity is possible if serum acetaminophen is over 150 µg/ml at 4 hours; 100 µg/ml at 6 hours, 70 µg/ml at 8 hours, 50 mcg/ml at 10 hours or 3.5 µg/ml at 24 hours. Administer acetylcysteine orally as soon as possible, within 24 hours of ingestion. See *USP DI* for dosage instructions.
- Perform liver, renal, and cardiac function tests. Institute supportive measures as indicated.

MANAGEMENT OF DRUG OVERDOSE

Aspirin

- The treatment of an aspirin overdose may include gastric lavage or emesis followed by the administration of activated charcoal. Close monitoring is necessary to institute appropriate nursing or medical interventions such as correcting hyperthermia, fluid and electrolyte imbalance, acid-base imbalances, hyperglycemia, or hypoglycemia (especially in children).
- Serum salicylate levels are monitored until the concentration is lowered to a nontoxic level. For example, if large amounts of aspirin have been consumed and the salicylate concentration 2 hours after ingestion is 500 µg/ml (50 mg/dl), it would indicate a serious toxicity, whereas a serum level of 800 µg/ml (80 mg/dl) is potentially fatal. Prolonged monitoring of salicylate serum levels is indicated in massive salicylate overdose situations.
- The nurse should be aware that serum levels are not reliable for measuring degree of toxicity after consumption of large amounts of the delayed release formulations.
- Exchange transfusion, hemodialysis, peritoneal dialysis, or hemoperfusion may be necessary in severe salicylate overdoses.

(NSAIDs), and the adjunct analgesics. These agents are used for the treatment of mild to moderate pain, fever, inflammation caused by rheumatoid arthritis, osteoarthritis and various other acute and chronic musculoskeletal and soft tissue inflammations. The NSAIDs are also used to treat metastatic bone pain, usually in combination with an opioid analgesic (Twycross, 1994). Information about the over-the-counter (OTC) dosage forms of these preparations are discussed in Chapter 11.

Aspirin (acetylsalicylic acid) may also be prescribed to reduce the risk of transient ischemic attacks (TIAs), myocardial infarcts, and stroke.

Mechanism of action. Aspirin and the NSAIDs peripherally inhibit the synthesis and release of prostaglandins. This effect on inflamed tissue is believed to be responsible for their analgesic and antiinflammatory action. Salicylates also block the generation of pain impulses and may have a central analgesic action in the hypothalamus. The NSAIDs also inhibit leukocyte migration and the release of the lysosomal enzymes, which contributes to their antiinflammatory effect.

Aspirin also inhibits the formation of platelet aggregation in the blood vessels by inhibiting prostacyclin. Prostacyclin is a platelet aggregation (reversible) inhibitor in blood vessels. Both effects may be dose dependent. Prescription salicylates include controlled release aspirin, 800 mg (Zorprin), salsalate (Disalcid and others), Trilisate, and magnesium salicylate (Magan). Salsalate is converted to salicylate during absorption from the GI tract and in the liver. It (and Trilisate) have the advantage of producing little, if any, adverse gastrointestinal effects, and does not affect platelet aggregation. Salsalate's analgesic effects are equivalent to aspirin. The magnesium from magnesium salicylate may be absorbed, which may result in systemic toxicity in clients with renal impairment.

Acetaminophen appears to produce its analgesic effect by inhibition of prostaglandin synthesis in the CNS (predominant effect) and peripherally. Although exact mechanisms of action are unknown, antiinflammatory effects are minimal. The antipyretic effect for these agents is mediated centrally, via the hypothalamus. See the Management of Drug Overdose boxes above.

NONSTEROIDAL ANTIINFLAMMATORY DRUGS

Approximately 20 different nonsteroidal antiinflammatory drugs (NSAIDs) are now available in the United States. Although aspirin is also an NSAID, this term most commonly refers to the newer aspirin substitutes on the market. Aspirin and the OTC NSAIDs are reviewed in Chapter 11. The NSAIDs have analgesic, antipyretic, and antiinflammatory effects, although the indications for the individual NSAID may vary according to specific testing and clinical data submitted to the FDA for approval.

The NSAIDs inhibit cyclooxygenase and prevent the synthesis of prostaglandins and thromboxane, which are responsible for the therapeutic effects and some of the adverse reactions of this drug classification (Figure 14-11). The nurse should be aware, however, that the inflammatory process has a purpose in the body; it attempts to neutralize, destroy, or

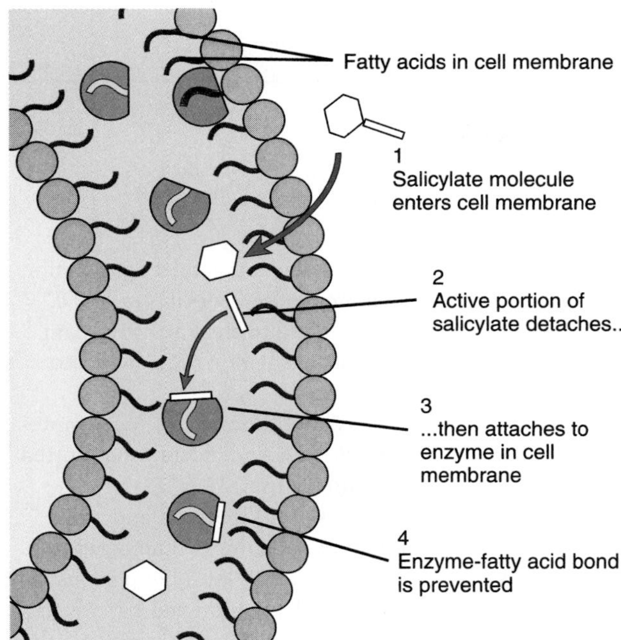

Figure 14-11 Inhibition of prostaglandin production. Inflammatory diseases and local injuries often lead to an increased production of prostaglandins. Nonsteroidal antiinflammatory drugs (NSAIDs) act peripherally by entering the cell membrane (*1*), the active portion (salicylate) detaches (2), and attaches to the enzyme (cyclooxygenase) in the cell membrane (3). This new complex (*4*) cannot react with fatty acids to induce prostaglandin synthesis, thus reducing inflammation and pain in the affected area.

prevent the dissemination of the toxic or foreign substances. The cardinal signs of inflammation that result include swelling, pain, redness, and heat at the site. By interfering with prostaglandin synthesis, the NSAIDs tend to reduce the inflammatory process and ultimately provide pain relief. It is quite possible that other actions (currently unknown) may also contribute to the therapeutic effects of these medications.

The NSAIDs are indicated for the treatment of acute or chronic rheumatoid arthritis, osteoarthritis, ankylosing spondylitis, and other rheumatic diseases; mild to moderate pain, especially when the antiinflammatory effect is also desirable (such as after dental procedures, obstetric and orthopedic surgery, and soft tissue athletic injuries); gouty arthritis, fever, nonrheumatic inflammation, and dysmenorrhea. Refer to a current package insert or *USP DI* for a listing of approved and investigational NSAIDs use. The primary NSAIDs include:

Acetic acids:

diclofenac [dye kloe' fen ak] (Voltaren, Voltaren-XR)
etodolac [eh toe' doe lak] (Lodine)
indomethacin [in doe meth' a sin] (Indocin)
ketorolac [kee' toe role ak] (Toradol)
nabumetone [na byoo' me tone] (Relafen)
sulindac [sul in' dak] (Clinoril)
tolmetin [tole' met in] (Tolectin)

Fenamates:

meclofenamate [me kloe fen am' ate] (Meclomen)
mefenamic [me fe nam' ik] (Ponstel)

Oxicams:

piroxicam [peer ox' i kam] (Feldene)

Propionic acids:

fenoprofen [fen oe proe' fen] (Nalfon)
flurbiprofen [flure bi' proe fen] (Ansaid)
ibuprofen [eye byoo proe' fen] (Motrin, Advil)
ketoprofen [kee toe proe' fen] (Orudis)
naproxen [na prox' en] (Naprosyn)
oxaprozin [ox a pro' zin] (Daypro)

Salicylates (which would also include aspirin, salsalate, etc):

diflunisal [dye floo' ni sal] (Dolobid)

The following are general pharmacokinetics; for specific pharmacokinetics, usual adult dose, and comments see Table 14-9.

Oral absorption of these drugs is very good. Food may delay absorption but it has not been proven to significantly change the total amount absorbed. Protein binding is high (greater than 90%). Sulindac is an inactive substance (prodrug) that is converted by the liver to an active sulfide metabolite. Most of the agents are metabolized by the liver and excreted by the kidneys. Table 14-9 lists dosing recommendations and comments.

Nursing Management

NSAID Therapy

Assessment. The nurse should establish the client's allergies before administering these drugs. In individuals with a documented history of allergy or hypersensitivity to aspirin, the anaphylactoid reaction is life threatening. Clients with the triad of aspirin allergy, nasal polyps, and bronchospastic disease experience may bronchospasm, leading to respiratory failure with the use of the NSAIDs. Clients sensitive to one NSAID may be sensitive to any of the other NSAIDs. The NSAIDs are contraindicated in individuals when the drugs have caused asthmatic symptoms, rhinitis, urticaria, nasal polyps, angioedema, or bronchospastic events. In addition, diclofenac is contraindicated for clients with a history of or active blood dyscrasias or bone marrow depression because these conditions will be precipitated or worsen. In addition to all of the above contraindications, phenylbutazone may cause sodium and water retention and so places clients at risk for fluid volume excess, such as those with cardiac disease, cardiac failure, or cardiopulmonary disease. The potential for increased phenylbutazone blood concentration and possible toxicity exists for clients with renal and hepatic impairment; clients with active ulcer disease risk perforation and bleeding.

NSAIDs are to be used with caution in elderly clients, who are more prone to upper gastrointestinal, hepatic, or

TABLE 14-9 Nonsteroidal antiinflammatory drugs: pharmacokinetics, dosing, and comments

NSAID	Onset of action (hr)	Half-life (hr)	Usual adult dosage (mg/day)	Comments*
Acetic acids				
diclofenac (Voltaren)	0.5	1.2-2	50 mg tid or qid	Has less effect on platelet aggregation that most other NSAIDs (*USP DI*, 1996). Used to treat arthritis, pain, primary dysmenorrhea, and acute gout attacks.
etodolac (Lodine)	0.5	6-7	200, 300, or 400 mg tid or qid	Also has uricosuric effects. Gastrointestinal distress and ulceration reported less often (Insel, 1996).
indomethacin (Indocin)	0.5	4-6	25 or 50 mg bid to qid	Higher risk for GI effects and renal function impairment than other agents. Use cautiously in persons with epilepsy, depression and Parkinson's disease because it may aggravate these conditions.
ketorolac (Toradol)	IM-10 min (dose dependent)	PO-4 IM-6	30 mg IM/IV q6h, then 10 mg PO q4-6h	Should not be given by any route for longer than 5 days. Risk of GI bleeding and other severe effects increase with duration of treatment. Do not give preoperatively or intraoperatively if bleeding control is necessary. Severe allergic reactions or anaphylaxis may occur with first dose.
nabumetone (Relafen)	—	22	500, 750, or 1000 mg daily (hs) or in two divided doses	Pro-drug (inactive), converted to active metabolite (6-MNA) in liver. Absorption increased by food and milk. Has lower reports of GI ulceration and bleeding than other NSAIDs.
sulindac (Clinoril)	—	8	150-200 mg bid	Renal calculi and biliary obstruction containing sulindac metabolites reported although it is less likely than most NSAIDs to cause renal toxicity.
tolmetin (Tolectin)	—	5	400 mg tid	High evidence of anaphylactic reactions and may also cause serum sickness or flu-like syndrome (*USP DI*, 1996).
Fenamates				
meclofenamate (Meclomen)	1	2-3	50 mg tid or qid	Less effect on platelet aggregation than most other NSAIDs. Use cautiously in persons on sodium-restricted diet (*USP DI*, 1996).
mefenamic acid (Ponstel)	—	2	250 mg q6h	Less effect on platelet aggregation but can prolong prothrombin time. Used for short-term treatment of pain and dysmenorrhea; also for acute gouty attacks and vascular headaches.

CAP, Capsule; *ERC*, extended-release capsules; *ERT*, extended-release tablets.
*All oral NSAIDs should be taken with 8 oz of water with person remaining upright for at least 15 to 30 minutes afterward (*USP DI*, 1996).

TABLE 14-9 Nonsteroidal antiinflammatory drugs: pharmacokinetics, dosing, and comments—cont'd

NSAID	Onset of action (hrs)	Half-life (hrs)	Usual adult dosage (mg/day)	Comments
Oxicams				
piroxicam (Feldene)	2-4	24	20 mg daily or 10 mg bid	Contraindicated in renal impairment. May cause flu-like syndrome. May accumulate in elderly women (*USP DI,* 1996).
Propionic acids				
fenoprofen (Nalfon)	—	3	300 to 600 mg tid or qid	Contraindicated in persons with renal impairment. Food decreases absorption and peak serum levels therefore administer 30 minutes before or 2 hr after meals unless GI distress occurs, then administer with milk.
flurbiprofen (Ansaid)	—	5.7	100 mg daily bid or tid	Similar to other agents in this category. Currently under study in transdermal patch, to treat soft tissue lesions (Insel, 1996).
ibuprofen (Motrin, Advil)	0.5	2	300 to 800 mg tid or qid	Available in tablets, liquid, and OTC. May decrease blood glucose levels (*USP DI,* 1996). Incidence of GI side effects less than with aspirin (Insel, 1996).
ketoprofen (Orudis)		CAP-1.6 ERC-5.4 ERT-3-4	25 to 75 mg tid or qid	Can cause fluid retention and increase in creatinine levels, especially in persons receiving diuretics and the elderly. Monitor renal function closely (Insel, 1996).
naproxen (Naprosyn)	1	13	250, 375, or 500 mg bid	Available in liquid, tablet, and extended-release tablets. Use tablets and liquid with caution in persons on sodium-restricted diet (*USP DI,* 1996).
oxaprozin (Daypro)		21-25	600 mg daily or bid	Has a long half-life that accumulates with chronic dosing. Half-life may be 40 to 60 hrs or more, which increases with age (Insel, 1996). Discontinue oxaprozin at least 1 to 2 weeks before elective surgery because it has greater tendency to cause perisurgical bleeding (*USP DI,* 1996).
Salicylates				
diflunisal (Dolobid)	1	8-12	250-500 mg bid	Higher risk of causing renal impairment but less apt to cause antiplatelet effect than other NSAIDs (*USP DI,* 1996). Does not have any antipyretic effects (Insel, 1996).

Geriatric Implications

NSAIDs

The incidence of perforated peptic ulcers and/or bleeding is more common in the elderly taking an NSAID than in younger adults. Serious consequences more often occur in this age group.

Clients with renal impairment may be at increased risk for NSAID-induced liver or renal toxicity and often require a dosage reduction to prevent drug accumulation.

Clinicians have recommended that clients 70 years or older be started at one-half the usual adult dose with close monitoring and careful dosage increases. Dosage increase should be based on the client's therapeutic response and lack of signs and symptoms of toxicity. Specific drug warnings include:

1. Flurbiprofen (Ansaid) may result in elevated peak serum levels in females between 74 and 94 years old. This serum level has not been documented in elderly male clients (*USP DI,* 1996). Therefore elderly females may need a lower dose to produce a therapeutic response.
2. Indomethacin (Indocin) is responsible for a higher incidence of CNS side effects, especially confusion in the elderly.
3. Naproxen (Naprosyn) administration in the elderly results in a higher proportion of unbound (free) naproxen, which may not be reflected by the total serum level. The steady state concentration of unbound naproxen may be nearly double that of a younger adult, which may result in an increase in side/adverse/toxic effects, even with a normal serum level range. The nurse should be aware of this potential because the prescriber may need to be notified about the possible need for a dosage reduction (*USP DI,* 1996).

---

renal effects of these agents. Dosages of indomethacin may start with less than half the adult dose with elderly clients. See the Geriatric Implications box above.

These drugs should be used cautiously in individuals with preexisting hepatic impairment. Prudent long-term management for clients should include liver enzyme monitoring and determinations of the baseline level. Cautious use in individuals with impaired renal function is required; creatinine clearance should be closely monitored in these clients. A reduced dosage should be employed in clients with diminished renal function to prevent drug accumulation. Cautious use is also required with clients with inflammatory or ulcerative disease of the small or large bowel; hemophilia or other bleeding problems (increased risk of bleeding as a result of platelet aggregation inhibition); or stomatitis (may mask the symptoms of blood dyscrasias). In addition, indomethacin is to be used cautiously with clients with mental depression and other psychiatric problems because they may be aggravated. Sulindac may cause renal calculi in clients with a history of kidney stones; adequate hydration and cautious use is necessary. For all rectal forms of NSAIDs, clients with a history or active case of anal or rectal bleeding, hemorrhoids, inflammatory lesions of the anus or rectum, or proctitis may have the condition reactivated or exacerbated.

Obtain a baseline assessment of the client's pain before initiating therapy. Hematologic determinations should occur before beginning phenylbutazone therapy.

Review the client's current medication regimen for the risk of significant drug interactions, such as those that may occur when NSAIDs are given concurrently with the drugs listed below.

Drug	Possible effect and management
anticoagulants, oral (coumarin or indanedione, heparin, or thrombolytic agents)	May increase the risk of gastrointestinal ulcers or hemorrhage. Monitor closely for signs of these effects. Coumarin or indanedione anticoagulants may be displaced from protein-binding sites, resulting in an increased risk of bleeding episodes. Monitor closely with laboratory coagulation testing. **Platelet inhibition may be dangerous for individuals receiving anticoagulant or thrombolytic agents. Avoid concurrent drug administration if possible.** If an NSAID is necessary, the usual dosages of diclofenac, diflunisal, meclofenamate, and mefenamic acid reportedly are less likely to significantly affect platelets (*USP DI,* 1996). With concurrent therapies, monitor closely for potential serious side effects.
antihypertensives, diuretics (especially triamterene [Dyrenium])	Flurbiprofen, indomethacin, ibuprofen, naproxen, oxaprozin, and piroxicam may reduce the effectiveness of antihypertensive agents. Monitor antihypertensive effect closely whenever an NSAID is used concurrently. Concurrent use of an NSAID and a diuretic may result in a decrease in diuretic, natriuretic, and antihypertensive diuretic effect. Diflunisal has not been reported to decrease furosemide's effectiveness, although diflunisal is reported to increase the serum level of hydrochlorothiazide and decrease the hyperuricemic response to hydrochlorothiazide or furosemide. May increase the risk of inducing renal failure in some clients. **Triamterene and indomethacin reportedly caused acute renal failure or renal function impairment; therefore this drug combination should be avoided.**
Administration of two NSAIDs concurrently, especially diflunisal (Dolobid) and indomethacin (Indocin) or aspirin	**May increase the risk of gastrointestinal side effects, such as duodenal ulcers or hemorrhage. These combinations should be avoided.**

Drug	Possible effect and management
cefamandole, (Mandol), cefoperazone (Cefobid), cefotetan (Cefotan), plicamycin (Mithracin), or valproic acid (Depakene)	**These drugs may cause a decrease in prothrombin blood levels and an inhibition of platelet aggregation. Concurrent administration with an NSAID may increase the risk for bleeding episodes, gastrointestinal ulceration, and hemorrhage. Avoid concurrent administration if possible.**
cyclosporine, gold compounds, nephrotoxic drugs	Concurrent use with NSAIDs may result in increased serum levels of cyclosporine and possibly gold compounds, resulting in an increased potential for nephrotoxicity. Concurrent use of nephrotoxic drugs and NSAIDs may also increase the risk for nephrotoxicity. Monitor closely during concurrent drug use.
lithium (Lithane)	Diclofenac, ibuprofen, indomethacin, naproxen and piroxicam may decrease excretion of lithium, which may result in an increased lithium serum level and toxicity. Thus the possibility of inducing this effect with the other NSAIDs exists. Monitor lithium serum levels and for clinical symptoms of lithium toxicity during concurrent therapy and after the NSAID is discontinued.
methotrexate (Mexate)	**Concurrent use of methotrexate with low to moderate doses of an NSAID may result in methotrexate toxicity. Adjust methotrexate as necessary according to methotrexate serum levels and the client's renal function. This reaction can be severe and even fatal; therefore close monitoring is necessary.**
probenecid (Benemid)	May result in an increase in serum levels of the NSAIDs and an increased risk of toxicity. Concurrent use with ketoprofen is not recommended. If probenecid is given with an NSAID, monitor closely, since a decrease in NSAID dosage may be indicated.
zidovudine (AZT)	**When given concurrently with indomethacin, a decrease in the metabolism of zidovudine may result, leading to increased serum levels and toxicity. It is also possible that an increase in indomethacin serum levels and toxicity may occur. Avoid concurrent use of these medications.**

A baseline assessment should include blood pressure, temperature, pulse, respirations, adventitious lung sounds, orientation, CBC, clotting times, renal and hepatitic function tests, stool guaiac, and a detailed description of the client's discomfort.

Nursing diagnosis. Clients receiving NSAID therapy have the potential for the following nursing diagnoses: altered bowel elimination pattern (constipation or diarrhea); altered comfort related to ineffective dosage of the NSAID, gas, mild stomach distress, or skin rash; sensory-perceptual alterations evidenced by visual changes, tinnitus, or dizziness; fluid volume excess (periorbital edema, peripheral edema, respiratory rales); altered protection related to hy-

Nursing Care Plan

Selected Nursing Diagnoses Related to Administration of Nonsteroidal Antiinflammatory Analgesics

Nursing diagnosis	Outcome criteria	Nursing interventions
Risk for alteration in comfort related to CNS, GI, dermatologic effects	Absence of dizziness and changes in sensorium	Institute safety measures if CNS symptoms develop
	Absence of GI symptoms; nausea, and vomiting, abdominal pain or cramps, indigestion	Administer with food or after meals. Provide small, frequent meals. Caution against alcohol ingestion
	Absence of rash, hives, pruritus, and SLE-type syndrome	Provide comfort measures to reduce pain, inflammation, and other dermatologic effects Report adverse symptoms to the prescriber Institute emergency procedures if severe adverse symptoms occur
Risk for injury related to CNS, GI, and sensitivity effects	No symptoms of injury occur	Assist to ambulate Caution against driving and other hazardous activities. Advise against alcohol ingestion. Report sore throat, fever, rash, itching, sudden weight gain, edema of ankles and fingers, changes in vision, and black tarry stools
Knowledge deficit related to drug therapy	Self-administers drug with accuracy and safety Relates signs and symptoms of side/adverse effects and those to report to prescriber	Instruct client in name and dosage of drug and its relationship to client's own condition. Avoid concurrent use of OTC medications and steroids. Teach signs and symptoms of side/adverse effects and how to prevent/minimize as in interventions above

poprothrombinemia; and altered health maintenance related to insufficient knowledge of contraindications, potential hazards, or signs and symptoms of bleeding. The potential complications of convulsions, acute renal failure, hemorrhage, and gastrointestinal ulcers and perforation exist with the administration of NSAIDs. See the Nursing Care Plan on p. 265 for selected nursing diagnoses related to administration of nonsteroidal antiinflammatory analgesics.

Implementation

Monitoring. The client's pain and mobility of affected areas should be monitored periodically.

Clients require close monitoring of their prothrombin time if they are receiving concomitant anticoagulant therapy or if they have other intrinsic hemostatic coagulation defects. Clients taking other NSAIDs should have hematologic determinations only if symptoms of blood dyscrasias occur.

Precipitation of acute renal failure may occur in clients with preexisting diminished sodium excretion, congestive heart failure, cirrhosis, hypertension, or renal disease.

The surfacing of eye problems during therapy should be handled by an ophthalmologic examination, and the drug therapy should be discontinued until evaluation has ruled out the drug therapy as a causal agent.

Monitor fluid intake and output and other symptoms of fluid volume excess (weight gain, edema, increase in blood pressure) with the administration of diclofenac, fenoprofen, flurbiprofen, indomethacin, ketoprofen, nabumetone, naproxen, phenylbutazone, and tolmetin. In addition, clients taking indomethacin need to be monitored periodically for confusion, mood changes, and hallucinations.

Intervention. The doses may be taken 30 to 60 minutes before meals or 2 hours postprandially to reach a blood level more readily. Administer with a full glass of water and have the client remain in an upright position for 15 to 30 minutes to minimize the risk of tablets becoming lodged in the esophagus, which may cause esophageal irritation. Administration with a meal followed by a full glass of water will also aid in preventing gastric upset. Indomethacin may be taken with antacids to prevent gastric irritation, however, it shouldn't be mixed with antacids or other medications.

Indomethacin suppositories need to remain in the rectum to be effective. Administer IV indomethacin over 5 to 10 seconds; avoid extravasation because it is irritating to the tissues. Usually fluids are restricted with IV administration.

Ketorolac is the first injectable analgesic NSAID that is stated to be comparable to morphine and meperidine in efficacy without the undesirable side effects/adverse reactions. It has no respiratory depression effects and produces far fewer CNS side effects compared with the opioids. It currently is reported to have little or no potential for abuse or addiction, so it has no special handling procedures required by the federal government. Ketorolac is indicated for the short-term management of pain but should not be used as an obstetrical preoperative medication or for obstetrical analgesia.

The nurse should be aware that headache and drowsiness occur in about 15% of individuals taking fenoprofen.

Mefenamic acid is not administered for more than 7 days.

Education. When clients are self-managing their NSAID therapy, they should be made aware of the need for periodic determinations of WBCs, hemoglobin, and/or hematocrit.

The woman who is pregnant or intends to become pregnant while using an NSAID should notify her health care provider, since these drugs may interfere with maternal and infant blood clotting and prolong the duration of pregnancy and parturition. There is an increase in the incidence of stillbirths and neonatal deaths in humans. If the mother intends to breastfeed, she should be made aware of the fact that salicylates are detected in the breast milk and are cleared from the body more slowly by infants. See the Pregnancy Safety box on p. 245 for the FDA classification of the various NSAIDs.

The client with a clinical problem such as erosive gastritis, ulcers, bleeding disorders, mild diabetes, or gout or those individuals receiving anticoagulant drugs should be warned to discuss this new change with their prescriber before commencing therapy again with an NSAID. Large doses of salicylates are to be avoided in clients with carditis. The effect of edema caused by these agents should be considered in individuals with diseases such as congestive heart failure and hypertension.

The client who omits a scheduled dose should not double the next dose but resume the usual dosing interval. The analgesia provided by NSAIDs is subject to a ceiling effect; higher than recommended dosages may not provide more therapeutic effect in the treatment of pain not associated with inflammation.

Alcoholic beverages produce a synergistic effect with NSAIDs in causing gastrointestinal bleeding.

The nurse should discuss with the client the most common side effects and adverse reactions, which, however, are not always an indication of excessive dosage and should be reported to the prescriber. Clients should be told that if a skin rash, itching, visual disturbances, edema, persistent headache, or dark stools occur, they should immediately notify their prescriber. A therapeutic alternative may be evaluated.

Some individuals have drowsiness and dizziness and should be cautioned about performing tasks with which the drug would interfere. The problem of morning stiffness in affected joints may be overcome by taking the last dose as late as possible in the evening.

The client should be cautioned not to use any OTC analgesics concurrently with the NSAID unless the prescriber specifically recommends them. Compliance may be an issue for some NSAIDs because the time until effectiveness is lengthy, such as 2 weeks with indomethacin.

Because photosensitivity occurs with diflunisal and ibuprofen, advise the client to avoid the use of sun lamps and prolonged exposure to the sunlight.

Ibuprofen is available without prescription in the 200 mg strength for self-medication. Clients using ibuprofen as an OTC medication should be instructed to report to their health care provider if their symptoms do not improve, if fever persists for more than 3 days, or if swelling or redness occurs in the painful area.

Case Study
The Client Taking NSAIDs

Rita Amherst is a 35-year-old woman who has had vague aches and pains along with malaise for the past 8 months. In recent months, she has noticed that her finger joints have been somewhat swollen and painful. Several weeks ago, her left knee also began to stiffen, which she attributed to a recent fall. She went to her local physician, who examined her and referred her to a rheumatologist. He had a diagnostic workup done on an outpatient basis. Rita has no history of serious medical illness.

Rita is placed on a regimen of aspirin 0.9 g PO qid with the dose to be increased until antiinflammatory effects are seen. She is also placed on diflunisal to reduce the acute inflammatory process.

1. What two actions of NSAIDs seem to be most responsible for their therapeutic effects?
2. For what interaction should Rita be monitored while taking aspirin concurrently with diflunisal?
3. What are some of the most frequently observed side effects of diflunisal?
4. Why is it important for Rita to contact her prescriber if she suspects she is pregnant?

Evaluation. The client reports increased comfort and increased range of motion and ability to perform activities of daily living. There is decreased or absence of joint swelling, redness, and warmth. If administered as an antipyretic, the client's temperature will be within normal limits. The client will not experience any untoward effects of NSAID therapy.

THROMBOXANE (TXA_2)

Thromboxane A_2 is a potent vasoconstrictor that stimulates additional platelet aggregation, therefore inhibiting thromboxane A_2 formation, which decreases platelet aggregation. Aspirin inhibits thromboxane synthetase, thereby preventing prostaglandin formation. Aspirin irreversibly blocks prostaglandin synthetase, whereas the other NSAIDs are primarily reversible inhibitors (*USP DI*, 1996).

OTHER DRUGS

Other products, such as the antimalarial agents (Chapter 61), gold salts, and penicillamine, are also used to treat inflammation in clients who have not responded to or cannot tolerate salicylates or NSAIDs. In addition, adjuvant analgesic medications are added to opioid medications to enhance analgesia.

Although in use for over 50 years in the treatment of rheumatoid arthritis, gold compounds are generally much slower acting and more toxic than the other products. Therefore they are reserved for individuals who demonstrate continued or increased disease activity while receiving conservative therapy.

auranofin [au rane' oh fin] (Ridaura)
aurothioglucose suspension [aur oh thee oh gloo' kose] (Solganal)
gold sodium thiomalate injection (Myochrysine)

While the exact antiinflammatory mechanism of action is unknown, these drugs appear to suppress the synovitis of the acute stage of rheumatoid disease. Proposed mechanisms of action include inhibition of sulfhydryl systems, various enzyme systems, suppression of phagocytic action of macrophages and leukocytes, and alteration of immune response.

Gold products are indicated for the treatment of rheumatoid arthritis; aurothioglucose and gold sodium thiomalate are also used to treat juvenile arthritis. The onset of action after oral administration is in 3 to 4 months, while parenterally it is in 6 to 8 weeks. Half-life of oral gold is 21 to 31 days in blood, 42 to 128 days in body tissues. Auranofin is rapidly metabolized, but the metabolism of aurothioglucose and gold sodium thiomalate is unknown. Excretion is primarily by the kidneys.

Most frequent side effects that are more common with auranofin include abdominal distress or pain, gas, diarrhea, nausea, and vomiting. These effects are rare in the other gold products. Most frequent adverse effects include sore, irritated tongue or gums (less with auranofin), allergic skin reaction, and mouth ulcers or fungus.

The adult dosage for auranofin is 6 mg daily, maximum daily dose is 9 mg/day. Pediatric dosage has not been determined. The adult dosage for aurothioglucose suspension and gold sodium thiomalate injection is 10 mg IM the first week, increasing weekly according to manufacturer's schedule until a total dose of 800 mg to 1 g has been reached. Maintenance dosage is 25 to 50 mg IM every 2 to 4 weeks, according to manufacturer's schedule. In children 6 to 12 years old, the dosage is 2.5 mg IM the first week and increased weekly according to schedule until the total dose of 200 to 250 mg has been reached. Maintenance dosage is 6.25 to 12.5 mg IM every 3 to 4 weeks.

The gold sodium thiomalate pediatric dosage is 10 mg IM the first week, then 1 mg/kg (up to 50 mg/dose) following the adult recommendations for weekly intervals.

■ Nursing Management
Gold Therapy

Assessment. Clients should be assessed for a sensitivity to gold and other heavy metals, since they may also be intolerant to gold salts. In addition, clients with a history of bone marrow dysplasia, exfoliative dermatitis, necrotizing enterocolitis, or pulmonary fibrosis may have the condition recur. Gold therapy is used with caution with clients with renal dysfunction, severe debilitation, Sjogren's syndrome in rheumatoid arthritis (an immunologic disorder characterized by deficient moisture production of the lacrimal, salivary, and other glands), inadequate cerebral or cardiovascular circulation, systemic lupus erythematosus, urticaria, eczema, colitis (especially for auranofin), or blood dyscrasias.

A baseline assessment should include the extent of joint involvement, discomfort and mobility, and hepatic and renal function values, WBC, platelet count, and urinalysis.

When gold compounds are given concurrently with penicillamine, the risk for very serious kidney or blood adverse reactions is increased. Avoid administration of this combination.

Nursing diagnosis. Assessment of the client receiving gold compounds should include consideration of the following nursing diagnoses: impaired skin integrity related to pruritus (auranofin, 17%), rash (auranofin, 24%), and exfoliative dermatitis; altered protection related to leukopenia, thrombocytopenia, and anemia; altered comfort evidenced by numbness and tingling of the hands and feet (peripheral neuritis), abdominal cramps (auranofin, 14%), metallic taste, and conjunctivitis (auranofin); fluid volume deficit related to anorexia, nausea, and vomiting (auranofin, 10%); altered oral mucous membranes evidenced by glossitis, gingivitis, or stomatitis (auranofin, 13%); altered thought processes related to CNS effects evidenced by confusion and hallucinations; diarrhea (auranofin, 47%); visual alterations related to iritis or corneal ulcers; and the potential complications of allergic reaction, hepatitis, and renal toxicity.

Implementation

Monitoring. Platelet counts, WBCs, and urinalyses should be completed periodically during therapy (urinalysis before every injection and platelets and WBCs before every second injection). All three should be accomplished monthly with auranofin therapy. Also with auranofin therapy, renal and hepatic function studies are required before and periodically during the course of therapy.

Glossitis, gingivitis, and stomatitis may result from gold compound therapy. Since these conditions may cause a lack of appetite, monitor the client's nutritional status.

Skin symptoms such as itching and rash are quite common with auranofin. Gastrointestinal symptoms such as abdominal cramps and diarrhea are quite common. Both should be reported promptly to the prescriber.

Intervention. Therapy is often begun with the concurrent administration of NSAIDs during the first few months of gold therapy, until it becomes effective. If the client experiences mild adverse symptoms, gold therapy is discontinued until the symptoms have resolved, then reinstituted at a lower dosage. Adverse responses such as anaphylaxis, angioedema, and syncope may result after an injection. Have emergency equipment available. If the client experiences a severe reaction, gold therapy is discontinued and not restarted.

To administer the intramuscular injection, the nurse must first shake the vial vigorously and warm it to body temperature to ease drawing the suspension into the syringe. An 18-gauge, 1½-inch needle should be used to deposit the gold deep into the muscular tissue of the upper quadrant of the gluteal region. A 2-inch needle may be used for obese clients.

Education. Advise clients that dental work should not be undertaken if the administration of gold compounds has had a leukopenic or thrombocytopenic effect. In addition, instruction should be provided by the nurse regarding appropriate oral hygiene, including gentle toothbrushing and flossing and the avoidance of the use of toothpicks.

Caution the client that exposure to sunlight may aggravate gold-induced dermatitis or cause a rash.

Encourage effective self-management of the therapeutic regimen; relief from symptoms may not occur for 3 to 6 months. Regular visits to the health care provider are necessary to monitor progress.

With parenteral forms of the medication, there is the possibility of a nitritoid reaction (hypotension, flushing, lightheadness, and fainting) after the injection and joint pain for 1 to 2 days after an injection.

Alert the client that side effects may occur even after the discontinuation of gold compounds.

Evaluation. After 2 to 6 months, the client reports increased comfort and increased range of motion and ability to perform activities of daily living. There is a decrease in or absence of joint swelling, redness, and warmth. The client will not experience any untoward effects of gold therapy.

penicillamine [pen i sill' a meen] (Cuprimine, Depen)
Penicillamine is a *chelating agent* for heavy metals, such as mercury, lead, copper, and iron. The metals are made more soluble so that they can be readily excreted by the kidneys. The mechanism of action as an antirheumatic agent is unknown, although lymphocyte function is improved and IgM rheumatoid factor and immune complexes located in the serum and synovial fluids are reduced. The relationship of these effects to rheumatoid arthritis is unknown.

Penicillamine is indicated for the prophylaxis and treatment of Wilson's disease; treatment of rheumatoid arthritis (especially for individuals with severe arthritis who have not responded to other therapies); and in the treatment of cystinuria. Most common side effects include anorexia, diarrhea, loss of taste senses, nausea, vomiting, and abdominal pain. Adverse reactions reported include allergic reactions and stomatitis.

The adult dosage of penicillamine as a chelating agent is 250 mg PO, four times daily. As an antirheumatic agent, 125 or 250 mg PO daily and increased if necessary at 2 to 3 month intervals, up to a maximum of 1.5 g/day. The dosage as an antiurolithic agent is 500 mg orally 4 times daily. For infants over 6 months and young children, the chelating dosage is 250 mg daily, administered in fruit juice while the antirheumatic agent has not been determined.

■ Nursing Management

Penicillamine Therapy

In addition to the following discussion, see the section on general nursing management for NSAIDs on p. 261.

Assessment. Because penicillamine is chemically related to penicillin, determine the client's allergy to penicillin before the first dose. Use with caution in clients with hepatic or renal dysfunctions.

Implementation

Monitoring. If penicillamine is given as an antirheumatic, monitor the client's joint involvement, pain, and mobility.

Twenty-four-hour urinary copper analyses are recommended for clients with Wilson's disease to determine optimum penicillamine dosages. For clients developing moderate proteinuria, 24-hour urinary protein determinations are recommended at 1- to 2-week intervals. Take urinalyses and complete blood and platelet counts and hemoglobin determinations twice a month for the first 6 months and each month thereafter to monitor for toxicity.

Hepatic function studies should be completed every 6 months for the first 18 months of therapy to monitor for toxic hepatitis.

For clients with cystinuria, x-ray examinations for renal calculi should be done on an annual basis.

Intervention. Administer the drug on an empty stomach at least 1 hour apart from any other drug, food, antacid, or milk. If the course of therapy is interrupted, it needs to be restarted at a low dosage and gradually increased to the appropriate dosage. Penicillamine dosage should be reduced to 250 mg if the client is going to have surgery because of the drug's effects on collagen and elastin, which results in increased skin friability. Return to the usual dosage should be delayed until wound healing is complete.

If penicillanine is administered for cystinuria, the client should be on high fluid intake, especially at night when the urine is more acidic and concentrated; 500 ml at bedtime and 500 ml once in the middle of the night is adequate. The greater the fluid intake, the lower the therapeutic dose of penicillamine.

For clients with impaired nutrition, pyridoxine 250 mg daily is recommended because penicillamine increases the requirement of this vitamin. If therapy is interrupted for any reason, it should be reinstituted at lower dosages to prevent adverse reactions.

Education. The client should be encouraged to comply with the medication regimen, since an interruption in the medication for even a few days may cause a sensitivity reaction when it is restarted.

Long-term compliance may be especially difficult for clients with rheumatoid arthritis because an improvement in the status of their illness may require 2 to 3 months of therapy.

If administered for Wilson's disease, the dosage is calculated on the basis of the urinary copper excretion; the objective is to maintain a negative copper balance. The client should be advised that a low copper diet may be necessary. This means omitting mushrooms, chocolate, dried fruit, nuts, shellfish, liver, molasses, and broccoli. Suggest the use of distilled water, since most tap water flows through copper pipes.

Alert the client that taste may be impaired. The ability to taste may be enhanced by administering 5 to 10 mg of copper daily, except for individuals with Wilson's disease, in whom copper intake is restricted.

Evaluation. The client with Wright's disease will experience increased urinary copper excretion on 24-hour urine specimen, hepatic and renal function studies within normal limits, and a reduction or absence of neurologic symptoms. If penicillamine is administered as an antiurolithic, the client will not evidence any cystine calculi.

Adjuvant Medications

Adjuvant (coanalgesic) medications are used in combination with other analgesics to enhance pain relief or to treat symptoms that exacerbate pain, or in some instances they are used alone to treat specifically identified pain. The nonsteroidal antiinflammatory drugs (NSAIDs) are often listed with the adjuvant analgesics, but with this exception, the primary indications for adjuvant medications are not for the treatment of pain. Nevertheless, these agents have been reported to have an analgesic effect in some pain conditions.

Adjuvant analgesic medications include a variety of medications such as anticonvulsants, antidepressants, antihistamines, corticosteroids, local anesthetics, antiarrhythmics, psychostimulants, clonidine, and capsaicin.

Anticonvulsants, antidepressants, anesthetics, and antiarrhythmics are often prescribed for the treatment of neuropathic pain. They are frequently used in combination with opioids for cancer-associated nerve pain (Jacox et al, 1994; Salerno, 1996).

Corticosteroids are beneficial for cancer pain that originates in a fairly restricted area, such as intracranially, alongside a nerve root; or in pelvic, neck, or hepatic areas. Dexamethasone is prescribed for an increase in intracranial pressure and for relief of pain caused by pressure on a nerve. Corticosteroids may also relieve pain by suppressing the release of prostaglandins and thus inhibiting the inflammatory process.

The antihistamine hydroxyzine (Vistaril) is reported to have some analgesic properties (Haddox, 1992). It also has anxiolytic and sedative effects that may be useful in some clients. Psychostimulants, such as methylphenidate (Ritalin) and dextroamphetamine (Dexedrine), potentiate opioid analgesia and also help to increase alertness or reduce persistent, opioid-induced sedation in some clients. The analgesic effects are postulated to occur centrally and in the descending spinal inhibitory pathways. Opioid-induced cognitive impairment in cancer and AIDS clients has improved with administration of a psychostimulant drug (Bruera & Watanabe, 1994).

The usual approach to opioid-induced persistent sedation is to reduce the opioid dose and increase daily drug frequency. If the client does not appropriately respond to this method, the opioid should be switched. If the sedation problem persists with these alternative strategies, a psychostimulant may be added to the opioid regime (Jacox et al, 1994).

Additional useful adjuvant analgesics include clonidine (Catapres) and capsaicin. Clonidine is a centrally acting, $alpha_2$ adrenergic agonist that has been used for the treatment of pain associated with reflex sympathetic dystrophy (Rauck et al, 1993), diabetic neuropathy, postherpetic neuralgia, spinal cord injury, phantom pain, and pain in cancer patients who were opioid tolerant (Portenoy, 1993).

BOX 14-6

Bladder Pain

Pentosan polysulfate sodium (Elmiron) is a semi-synthetic heparin-like derivative used to treat bladder pain or discomfort from interstitial cystitis. This product is a weak anticoagulant and fibrinolytic but its analgesic mechanism of action is unknown. It has been postulated that pentosan adheres to the bladder wall mucosa to prevent irritating substances in the urine from reaching bladder cells.

Pharmacokinetically, pentosan is administered orally, has an elimination half-life of approximately 5 hours, is metabolized primarily in the liver and spleen, and is excreted in urine. Side/adverse effects include urinary frequency, alopecia, diarrhea, nausea, headache, dyspepsia, and stomach distress. Recommended dose is 100 mg three times a day, an hour before or two hours after meals (Elmiron, 1996).

Elmiron (1996). Package Insert, Baker Norton Pharmaceuticals, #1001218, Rev 960B.

Capsaicin, an alkaloid found in chili peppers, is formulated into a topical cream (Zostrix) that is indicated for the treatment of neuralgia and arthritic pain. On application it causes an initial release and then a depletion of substance P from nerve fibers, which results in a decrease in pain transmission (Salerno, 1996). See references for additional information on adjuvant medications.

SUMMARY

Pain continues to be a worldwide health problem. It disables and distresses more people than any other symptom and is probably the most common reason a person seeks health care. Few things that a nurse does are more important than alleviating pain. The delicate task of balancing the therapeutic relief of analgesics against their toxicity continues to be a challenge for nurses. Attitudes, fears, and biases of clients, families, and caregivers contribute to the unnecessary undertreatment of pain. It requires skill and knowledge on the part of the nurse to assess accurately and intervene effectively for the relief of the pain of the clients in his or her care.

Morphine and other opioid angonists, the earliest substances to be used for pain relief, are still among the more effective. The nurse, however, needs to be alert to the toxic symptoms of inappropriate use of these analgesics. Naloxone and natrexone are opioid antagonists used for the reversal of opioid toxicity. Opioid agonist-antagonists are also used for pain relief.

Nonsteroidal antiinflammatory drugs (NSAIDs) are used to treat the signs and symptoms of inflammation, fever, and pain. Since the mid-1970s, these aspirin substitutes have become quite popular for the treatment of mild to moderate pain and for the antiinflammatory treatment of arthritis. Although widely available, these agents are not without adverse gastrointestinal, hepatic, and renal effects. Gold compounds, also used in the treatment of arthritis, are much slower acting and much more toxic than the NSAIDs.

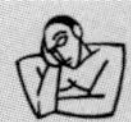

Critical Thinking

1. Tyrone Scali, age 42, has come to the emergency department after a fall while playing tennis. The health care provider diagnoses a sprained ankle, wraps his ankle with an elastic bandage, and advises him to elevate the ankle and keep it at rest. Aspirin 650 mg PO every 4 hours prn for pain is prescribed. Before instructing Mr. Scali regarding his aspirin therapy, you review his health history. What data would you be looking for which might contraindicate the use of aspirin for Mr. Scali?
2. Sarah Smith, age 53, has just returned to the general surgical unit from the postanesthesia recovery unit after having had a thyroidectomy. Her physician has prescribed morphine 10 mg IM q4h prn for postoperative pain. She is requesting pain medication for "a stabbing pain in her throat." What assessments will be critical before an analgesic is administered?
3. Robert Staysa, age 85, has osteoarthritis, which causes pain in his back, hips, and knees. His physician prescribes ibuprofen 400 mg PO qid. Why would the physician prescribe ibuprofen rather than a low-dose opioid analgesic? Given his age, what adverse reaction of NSAID therapy is Mr. Staysa most at risk for?
4. Jessie Holstein, age 72, is receiving auranofin for her rheumatoid arthritis. Why would gold salts be used rather than NSAIDs for clients with arthritis? While you are reviewing Mrs. Holstein's blood work, you notice that her platelet count is 155,000/mm^3. What action would you take?

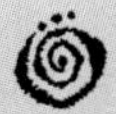

Collaborative Learning Activities

1. Across the top of the board write two headings: "Acute pain" and "Chronic pain." Down the left side of the board list the following descriptors: characteristics, sign/symptoms, therapeutic goals, drug, administration timing, dose, route. Have two teams of students, one for each type of pain, take 10 minutes to reach a consensus on the factors without using their books.
2. A student team will present assessment of the client receiving opioid therapy and discuss the treatment of an overdose.
3. A pair of students will prepare a demonstration on appropriate administration and related nursing implementation for the administration of the fentanyl transdermal system.
4. Create a large side effects/adverse reactions chart, listing each down the left side of the board. Relate nursing diagnoses and nursing intervention appropriate to the listed reactions.

BIBLIOGRAPHY

American Hospital Formulary Service (1996). *AHFS: Drug information '95.* Bethesda, MD: American Society of Hospital Pharmacists.

Anderson KN, et al. (Eds.) (1994). *Mosby's medical, nursing, and allied health dictionary* (4th ed.). St. Louis: Mosby.

Beers MH, Ouslander JG, Fingold SF, et al. (1992). Inappropriate medication prescribing in skilled-nursing facilities, *Ann Intern Med* 117(8):680-684.

Bobak IM, Lowdermilk DL, & Jensen MD (1995). *Essentials of maternity nursing* (4th ed.). St Louis: Mosby.

Bruera E & Watanabe S (1994). Psychostimulants as adjuvant analgesics. *J Pain & Sympt Manag* 9(6):412-415.

Carr DB, Jacox AK, Chapman CR, et al. (1992). *Clinical practice guideline. Acute pain management: Operative or medical procedures and trauma.* AHCPR Pub No. 92-0032. Rockville, MD: Agency for Health Care Policy and Research, Public Health Service, US Department of Health and Human Services.

Cleeland CS, Gonin R, Hatfield AK, et al. (1994). Pain and its treatment in outpatients with metastatic cancer, *New Engl J Med* 330:592-6.

Cohen FL (1980). Postsurgical pain relief: Patients' status and nurses' medication choices, *Pain* 9:265.

Covington TR (Ed.) (1996). *Handbook of nonprescription drugs* (11th ed.). Washington, DC: American Pharmaceutical Association.

Cushing M (1992). Pain management on trial, *Amer J Nurs* 92(2):21-2.

Foley KM (1991). The relationship of pain and symptom management to patient requests for physician-assisted suicide, *J Pain & Sympt Manag* 6(5):289-97.

Gossel TA & Wuest JR (1993). Control of chronic cancer pain, *Fla Pharm Today* 57(4):21.

Gu X & Belgrade MJ (1993). Pain in hospitalized patients with medical illnesses, *J Pain & Sympt Manag* 8(1):17-21.

Haddox JD (1992). Neuropsychiatric drug use in pain management. In Raj PP (Ed.). *Practical management of pain* (2nd ed.) St Louis: Mosby.

Hammack JE & Loprinzi CL (1994). Use of orally administered opioids for cancer-related pain, *Mayo Clin Proc* 69:384-390.

Insel PA (1996) Analgesic-antipyretic and antiinflammatory agents and drugs employed in the treatment of gout. In Hardman JG & Limbird LE (Eds.). *Goodman & Gilman's the pharmacological basis of therapeutics* (9th ed.). New York: McGraw-Hill.

Jacox A, Carr DB, Payne R, et al (1994). *Management of cancer pain: Clinical practice guideline no. 9.* AMCPR Publication No 94-0592. Rockville, MD: Agency for Health Care Policy and Research, U.S. Dept. of Health and Human Services, Public Health Service.

Keeney SA (1993). Nursing care of the postoperative patient receiving epidural analgesia, *MEDSURG Nurs* 2(3):191-6.

Kenyon J (Ed.) (1993). Fear of adverse effects should not hinder opioid use, *Drugs Therapy Perspect* 1(6):13.

Kinzbrunner B & Salerno E (1994). *Vistas pain management formulary.* Miami: Vistas Healthcare Corp.

Lipman AG (1993). The argument against therapeutic use of heroin in pain management, *Amer J Hosp Pharm* 50(5):996.

Mather LE & Denson DD (1992). Pharmacokinetics of systemic opioids for the management of pain. In Sinatra RS, Hord AH, Ginsberg B, & Preble LM (Eds.). *Acute pain* (pp 78-92). St Louis: Mosby.

McCaffery M & Beebe A (1989). *Pain: Clinical manual for nursing practice.* St Louis: Mosby.

McCaffery M & Ferrell B (1992). Pain control decisions, *Nursing* 22(8):48.

McCarthy RL & Montagne M (1993). The argument for therapeutic use of heroin in pain management, *Amer J Hosp Pharm* 50(5):992.

McGrath PA (1990). *Pain in children: Nature, assessment, and treatment.* New York: Guilford Press.

Melzack R & Wall PD (1965). Pain mechanisms: A new theory, *Science* 150:971-9.

Olin BR (Ed.) (1996). *Facts and comparisons.* Philadelphia: JB Lippincott.

Patt RB (1993). Classification of cancer pain and cancer pain syndromes. In Patt RB. *Cancer pain.* Philadelphia: JB Lippincott.

Patt RB (1996). Using controlled-release oxycodone for the management of chronic cancer and noncancer pain, *Amer Pain Soc Bull* 6(4):1-6.

Peat S (1995). Providing pain relief for the surgical patient, *Care Crit Ill* 11(1):16-9.

PDR (1996). *Physicians' desk reference.* Oradell, NJ: Medical Economics Co.

Portenoy RK (1993). Adjuvant analgesics in pain management. In Doyle D, Hanks GWC, & Macdonald N (Eds.). *Oxford textbook of palliative medicine.* New York: Oxford University Press.

Porter J & Jick H (1980). Addiction rare in patients treated with narcotics, *New Engl J Med* 302:123.

Rauck RL, Eisennach JC, Jackson K, et al (1993). Epidural clonidine treatment for refractory reflex sympathetic dystrophy, *Anesthesiology* 79(6):1163-9.

Salerno E (1996). Pharmacologic approaches. In Salerno E & Willens JS. *Pain management handbook.* St Louis: Mosby.

Salerno E & Willens JS (1996). *Pain management handbook.* St Louis: Mosby.

Sinatra RS & Savarese A (1992). Parenteral analgesic therapy and patient-controlled analgesia for pediatric pain management. In Sinatra RS, Hord AH, Ginsberg B, & Preble LM (Eds.). *Acute pain.* St Louis: Mosby.

Twycross R (1994). *Pain relief in advanced cancer.* Edinburgh: Churchill Livingstone.

United States Pharmacopeial Convention (1996). *USP DI: Drug information for the health care professional* (16th ed.). Rockville, MD: The Convention.

Wallace M (1994). Assessment and management of pain in the elderly, *MEDSURG Nurs* 3(4):293-298.

Warfield CA (Ed.) (1993). *Principles and practice of pain management.* New York: McGraw-Hill Inc.

Waters L (1992). Pharmacologic strategies for managing pain in children, *Ortho Nurs* 11(1):34.

Watt-Watson JH & Donovan MI (1992). *Pain management: Nursing perspective.* St Louis: Mosby.

Weissman DE & Haddox JD (1989). Opioid pseudoaddiction—an iatrogenic syndrome, *Pain* 36(3):363-6.

Welk TA (1991). An educational model for explaining hospice services, *Amer J Hospice Palliat Care* 8(5):14-17.

Willcox SM, Himmelstein DU, & Woolhandler S (1994). Inappropriate drug prescribing for the community-dwelling elderly, *JAMA* 272(4):292-296.

Willens JS (1996). Introduction to Pain Management. In Salerno E & Willens JS. *Pain management handbook.* St Louis, Mosby.

World Health Organization (1989). *Freedom from pain cancer pain: Educational lecture for health care professionals.* Geneva: WHO.

Zhukovsky DS, Gorowski E, Hausdorff J, et al. (1995). Unmet analgesic needs in cancer patients, *J Pain & Sympt Manag* 10(2):113-119.

Chapter 15

Anesthetics

Chapter Focus

The advances of modern surgical technique would not be possible without the developments that have occurred in anesthesia. Anesthetic agents prevent the pain that would otherwise be experienced during surgery. These agents protect the client from the trauma of surgical pain and provide the surgeon the time and exposure to the surgical field necessary to accomplish sophisticated procedures. Nursing during the perioperative period involves three distinct phases: preoperative, intraoperative, and postoperative. Although the care the nurse provides in each of these phases varies in its approach, the ultimate goal is the safety and well-being of the client. The following objectives and key terms are important for a good understanding of this chapter.

Key Terms

balanced anesthesia (p. 274)
caudal anesthesia (p. 293)
conduction anesthesia (p. 293)
dissociative anesthesia (p. 285)
general anesthesia (p. 274)
infiltration anesthesia (p. 293)
local anesthesia (p. 288)
neurolepsis (p. 285)
neuroleptanesthesia (p. 283)
regional anesthesia (p. 288)
saddle block (p. 293)
spinal anesthesia (p. 293)

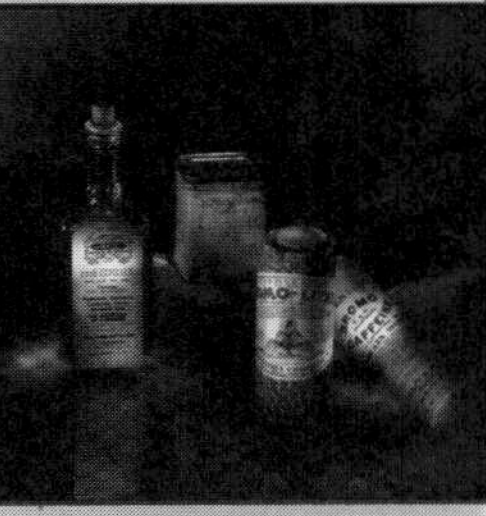

Key Drug [▲]

halothane

Objectives

1. Describe common general anesthetic agents.
2. Identify the significant physiologic changes observable in the client at each stage of anesthesia.
3. List common drugs that interact with anesthetic agents and the possible result of concomitant use.
4. Identify disease and risk factors that can alter the response to anesthesia.
5. Discuss nursing measures to prevent or treat common postoperative complications.
6. Discuss the use and side effects of local anesthetics.
7. Apply the nursing process to the client receiving general or local anesthetic agents.

Anesthetic drugs are central nervous system (CNS) depressants used to induce a loss of sensation, especially the sensation of pain. There are two major categories of anesthesia: general and regional (local). General anesthesia induces a state of unconsciousness and varying amounts of analgesia, amnesia, muscle relaxation, and loss of reflexes (sensory and autonomic). This state is achieved by intravenous or inhalation routes of drug administration. Regional or local anesthesia blocks pain sensations in specific areas of the body without loss of consciousness. Generally the effect of application of regional anesthesia is related to the target nerve and its distribution in the body, whereas local anesthesia is a blockade of the nerves in the infiltrated tissues. Local anesthesia may be achieved topically or by setting up a field block in an area that encircles the operative field (infiltration anesthesia). Spinal, epidural, caudal, and nerve block anesthesia have been referred to as both regional and local anesthesia.

GENERAL ANESTHESIA

General anesthesia is the absence of sensation and consciousness, induced generally by inhalation or intravenous injection of various anesthetic agents. The CNS alters to produce varying degrees of analgesia, depression of consciousness, skeletal muscle relaxation, and reflex reduction. It is an important mode of therapy, especially for surgical procedures.

MECHANISM OF ACTION

At concentrations that produce anesthesia, general anesthetics affect all excitable tissues of the body. They vary widely in their individual effects and in the concentration necessary for each to produce a given state of anesthesia. Although many theories of anesthesia have been proposed, none satisfactorily explains the basic mechanisms of action. Indeed, different anesthetics may have different modes of action, and no single theory may suffice.

The pattern of depression is similar for all general anesthetics—irregular and descending. The medullary centers are depressed last. Fortunately, the medulla is spared temporarily, since it contains the vital centers concerned with heart action, blood pressure, and respiration. Initially, anesthesia produces a loss of the perception of sight, touch, taste, smell, awareness, and hearing. Usually unconsciousness is produced. The two classes of general anesthetics are inhalation anesthetics (gases or volatile liquids) and intravenous agents.

Balanced anesthesia. A combination of drugs is necessary to produce all the desired effects sought with anesthesia. Analgesia, muscle relaxation, unconsciousness, and amnesic effects are not produced safely by a single anesthetic. The induction of anesthesia by using a combination of drugs, each for its specific effect, rather than by using a single drug with multiple effects, is termed **balanced anesthesia**. For example, anesthesia may be induced by premedicating with a short-acting barbiturate or a benzodiazepine and then an opioid analgesic and a skeletal muscle relaxant, followed by an anesthetic gas administered by the anesthetist. The specific drugs and dosages will depend on the procedure to be done, the physical condition of the client, and the client's response to the medications. The advantage of balanced anesthesia is a lower reported incidence of postoperative nausea, vomiting, and pain.

STAGES OF GENERAL ANESTHESIA

General anesthesia generally consists of four stages. The stages of anesthesia vary with the choice of anesthetic, speed of induction, and skill of the anesthetist. The current practice of inducing general anesthesia with an intravenously administered anesthetic before inhalation anesthesia promotes rapid transition from consciousness to surgical anesthesia, and the early stages of anesthesia are not seen. If the drug is given slowly enough, however, usually all stages can be observed. They are most easily seen when an anesthetic gas is used as the only anesthetic. Not all stages occur with all anesthetics.

Stage 1: analgesia. This stage begins with the onset of anesthetic administration and lasts until loss of consciousness. Smell and pain are abolished before consciousness is lost. Vivid dreams and auditory or visual hallucinations may be experienced. Speech becomes difficult and indistinct. Numbness spreads gradually over the body. The body feels stiff and unmanageable. Hearing is the last sense lost.

The nurse should maintain a quiet and tranquil environment for the client because even low voices and equipment sounds may be interpreted as excessively loud and may be counterproductive to the anesthetic. Before anesthesia is begun, restraining straps are placed on the client, and the client, is covered for warmth and modesty.

Stage 2: excitement. This stage varies greatly with individuals. Reflexes are still present and may be exaggerated, particularly with sensory stimulation such as noise. The client may struggle, shout, laugh, swear, or sing. Autonomic activity, muscle tone, eye movement, and rapid and irregular breathing increase. Irregular respiration may cause uneven absorption of anesthetic; a period of apnea followed by a few deep breaths may produce a high concentration of anesthetic in the blood. Vomiting and incontinence sometimes occur in this stage.

The variability in this stage results from (1) the amount and type of premedication, (2) the anesthetic agent used, and (3) the degree of external sensory stimuli. Since the advent of balanced anesthesia, the signs and duration of this stage have been reduced.

Except to restrain for safety reasons, the client should not be touched during this stage.

Stages 1 and 2 constitute the *stage of induction.*

Stage 3: surgical anesthesia. The third stage is divided into four planes of increasing depth of anesthesia. Which plane a client is in is determined by the character of the respirations, eyeball movement, and pupil size, and the degree to which reflexes are present. Most operations are done in plane two or in the upper part of plane three. As the client moves into plane one, the respiratory irregularities of the second stage usually have disappeared and respiration becomes full and regular. As anesthesia deepens, respiration becomes more shallow and more rapid. Paralysis of the intercostal muscles is followed by increased abdominal breathing; finally, only the diaphragm is active. A loss of reflexes occurs in a cephalocaudal direction, from the head downward. The eyelid reflex is lost and the eyeballs, which exhibit a rolling movement at first, gradually move less and then cease to move. Normally, if the pupils were reflexively dilated in the second stage, they now constrict to about their size in natural sleep. The reaction to light becomes sluggish. The pupils dilate as plane 4 is approached.

The client's face is calm and expressionless and may be flushed or even cyanotic. The musculature becomes increasingly relaxed as reflexes are progressively abolished. Most abdominal surgery cannot be performed until the abdominal reflexes are absent and the abdominal wall is soft. The body temperature is lowered as the anesthetic state continues. The pulse remains full and strong. Blood pressure may be elevated slightly, but in plane four the blood pressure drops and the pulse weakens. The skin, which was warm, now becomes cold, wet, and pale.

Because each phase of anesthesia is closely monitored by the anesthetist, he or she will give approval to begin the procedure. Obtain this approval before preparing the skin, surgically draping the client, and proceeding with surgery.

Stage 4: medullary paralysis (toxic stage). Respiratory arrest and vasomotor collapse characterizes the fourth stage. Respiration ceases before the heart action, so by lightening the anesthetic state by reducing the gaseous agent, this stage may be reversed.

The nurse is part of the surgical team in providing resuscitative measures; the necessary drugs, equipment, supplies; and other assistance as necessary.

SIGNIFICANT DRUG INTERACTIONS

Among the dangers facing a surgical client is an unexpected drug interaction occurring in preparation or during anesthesia. Anesthetists must always be familiar with the interactions between anesthetics and the maintenance drug therapies used in a wide range of illnesses. A serious drug interaction may be underway before surgery, and the surgical anesthesia may complicate the interaction. A critical analysis of the surgical candidate's drug regimen (prescribed, OTC, and alternative/complementary medications) should be done in relation to the anesthetic drugs and preanesthetic drugs to be used.

Although it is the anesthetist's responsibility to obtain the preoperative drug history, the nurse should also be aware of all the medications the client consumed in the 2- to 3-week preoperative period. Various pharmacologic classes of medication may result in adverse reactions in clients anesthetized for surgery. For example, *anticoagulants* such as heparin and coumarin are usually discontinued 48 hours before surgery to reduce the increased risk of hemorrhage, while *CNS depressants* such as opioids and hypnotics may increase the risk of enhanced CNS-depressant effects.

Antidysrhythmics such as propranolol hydrochloride may induce a decreased cardiac output, decreased heart rate, and bronchospasm. Quinidine, procainamide, and lidocaine may reduce cardiac conduction, increase peripheral vasodilation, and potentiate neuromuscular blocking agents, such as tubocurarine.

Combining local anesthetic agents with *sympathomimetic or vasoconstrictive agents* (such as epinephrine, phenylephrine, or methoxamine) can cause ischemia, leading to sloughing of tissue or gangrene in fingers, toes, or areas that have end arteries. If combined with local anesthetics, these agents should be carefully dosed and closely monitored.

Selected *antihypertensive agents* such as guanethidine (Ismelin) and methyldopa (Aldomet) deplete the synthesis or storage of norepinephrine in the sympathetic (adrenergic) nerve endings and may result in severe hypotension when combined with anesthetics and analgesics. Prescribers may consider reducing or stopping such medications before surgery.

When used as long-term therapy, *corticosteroids* usually produce adrenal gland suppression, which may result in hypotension during surgery. Since the stress of anesthesia and surgery usually increases the need for and release of endogenous corticosteroids, it is recommended that corticosteroid dosages be increased in the perioperative period.

Cholinesterase inhibitors such as echothiophate iodide (Phospholine Iodide) and demecarium bromide (Humorsol), and exposure to organophosphate insecticides may prolong succinylcholine blockade. Extended apnea and death have been reported with this combination. It is generally recommended that the cholinergic eyedrops be stopped approximately 2 weeks before elective surgery.

Antibiotics—particularly aminoglycoside antibiotics (e.g., amikacin and gentamicin), clindamycin, tetracyclines, and polymyxin antibiotics—may potentiate the neuromuscular blocking agent or cause neuromuscular blockade. A reduction in the dose of the neuromuscular blocking agent may be necessary, along with careful titration or careful dosing of the drug for the client, to response. Clients with myasthenia gravis, Parkinson's disease, or other neuromuscular disorders must be monitored carefully.

Many other drugs have the potential for inducing an unwanted effect intraoperatively or postoperatively. Concurrent administration of various drugs with anesthetic agents requires close supervision and monitoring of the surgical client. As a general guideline, if a drug is needed for treatment preoperatively, it should be continued through surgery. Unnecessary drugs are discontinued for a period at least five times the half-life of the drug before surgery. Drugs having significant interactions with anesthetic agents are replaced, when possible, with an alternative medication before surgery.

SPECIAL ANESTHESIA CONSIDERATIONS

Many disease states and risk factors can alter the individual's response to anesthesia. The preoperative assessment of the client's health status by the nurse includes, among other factors, acute and chronic medical conditions.

Alcoholism. The alcoholic client may have a variety of associated disease states, including liver dysfunction, pancreatitis, gastritis, and esophageal varices. The anesthetic requirements for such a client may be increased because of the increase in liver-metabolizing enzymes and the development of cross-tolerance. The alcoholic client is monitored closely during the postanesthetic period for alcohol withdrawal syndrome, since its onset may be delayed because of the administration of medications for pain relief. Pharmacologic intervention with diazepam or other agents may be required to prevent the occurrence of withdrawal symptoms.

Obesity. Overweight or obese clients may have cardiac insufficiency, respiratory problems, atherosclerosis, hypertension, or an increased incidence of diabetes, liver disease, or thrombophlebitis. In such clients, obtaining the desired depth of anesthesia and muscle relaxation may be a problem. Generally, fat-soluble anesthetics, especially those with toxic metabolites such as methoxyflurane (Penthrane), should be avoided.

Smoking. Individuals who smoke usually have an increasingly rigid arterial vascular system, adrenal gland stimulation, and perhaps lung disease (bronchitis, emphysema, carcinoma, etc.). Therefore postoperative complications are six times more common in smokers than in nonsmokers. Smoking also increases the client's sensitivity to muscle relaxants.

Pregnancy. See the Pregnancy Safety box above for the FDA rating of anesthetic drug safety during pregnancy. Before any drug is used, the expected drug benefits should be considered against the possible risk to the fetus. Box 15-1 describes risks to health care providers.

Young age. The physical characteristics of a neonate may predispose the infant to upper airway obstruction or laryngospasm during anesthesia or resuscitation. A small mandible and neck, a narrow cricoid ring, and a large body water compartment with a high extracellular water turnover rate, immaturely functioning liver and kidneys, and a rapid metabolic rate all contribute to the need for careful consideration of the infant or pediatric client. Drug dosages and administered fluids must be carefully calculated using the body weight or the surface area of the child. Halothane and nitrous oxide are commonly used in pediatrics because the incidence of hepatitis in children is considered rare after halothane usage. Neonates are usually more sensitive to the nondepolarizing muscle-relaxing agents (see Chapter 23).

Advanced age. Aging results in a generalized decline in organ function (approximately 1% per year after age 30), the existence of chronic disease processes, or both. As the number and complexity of illnesses increase with age, the complexity of drug treatment also increases, which results in greater potential for drug interactions and side effects. Generally, an increased and prolonged drug effect is seen in the elderly. Mortality rates for the aged client undergoing major surgery may be 4 to 8 times higher than for younger clients.

Pregnancy Safety

Category	Drug
B	etidocaine, lidocaine, prilocaine, methohexital, enflurane, propofol
C	alfentanil, bupivacaine, chloroprocaine, dibucaine, etomidate, fentanyl, mepivacaine, methoxyflurane, sufentanil, tetracaine, thiopental
Unclassified	droperidol, halothane, ketamine, isoflurane, procaine, sevoflurane

BOX 15-1

Waste Anesthetic Gases as Occupational Health Hazard

Chronic exposure of health care providers in the operating room to waste anesthetic gases may present a significant occupational health hazard. Studies have demonstrated an increased incidence of spontaneous abortions among women exposed to nitrous oxide, as well as among wives of men who are exposed. In addition, neurologic, hepatic, and renal disorders have been seen in the chronically exposed. Health care providers should protect themselves by avoiding the area within a foot of the client's mouth and nose when the breath contains exhaled anesthetic agents. Health care providers should be active in establishing exposure monitoring programs to detect unsafe levels caused by faulty equipment and unsafe practices.

■ Nursing Management

General Anesthetics

Nursing during the perioperative period encompasses three distinct phases: preoperative, intraoperative, and postoperative. While these phases are a continuum, nursing care during each phase differs in its approach to the client and nursing care goals.

Preoperative

One of the major responsibilities of the nurse in the client's preoperative period is to accomplish a focus assessment, the acquisition of selected or specific data as determined by the nurse and the client or as directed by the client's condition (Carpenito, 1995). Although general health data are gathered upon admission of the client to the health care agency, it is important to focus on those factors that will influence the client's experience with anesthetic agents to achieve optimal anesthesia without adverse effect.

One of these factors is the client's underlying acute and chronic conditions and the medications the client has recently or is currently taking. Disease states and risk factors that can alter the individual response have been discussed previously.

The nurse must also assess the client's experience with previous surgeries to allay anxiety and to identify risk factors to prevent adverse reactions, particularly malignant hyperthermia. Malignant hyperthermia is a condition characterized by often fatal hyperthermia. It is important to ask if the client or a family member has had problems with anesthesia, because it is associated with an autosomal dominant trait.

The night before surgery, sedatives or hypnotics may be administered to ensure a sound and restful sleep. The time of the administration of this medication provides an opportunity to assess the client's emotional state regarding the anticipated operative procedure. Many clients have anxieties regarding the experience of anesthesia, such as fear of not waking up, having pain during surgery, talking while they are anesthetized, or having nausea and vomiting after surgery. These anxieties can be minimized if the client and family are well prepared about the anesthetic agents to be used.

Questions about the rationale for a particular agent or method can best be answered by the surgeon or the anesthesiologist. Although very few clients talk while anesthetized, and those who do are generally unintelligible, clients do have other concerns that are valid regarding anesthesia and that need to be discussed to ensure that there is informed consent for the anesthesia. Clients can be reassured that they will have close surveillance throughout the surgical procedure and in the immediate postoperative period. Clients who persist in their fears regarding the anesthesia or the surgery need consultation with the surgeon and/or the anesthesiologist before final preparation for surgery. Severe anxiety or fear, unless allayed, affects both the autonomic and central nervous systems and may cause reactions that are detrimental physiologically and psychologically. Anxious clients may resist relaxation and fight the anesthetic. A greater amount of anesthetic therefore would be required, and toxic levels of drugs might be administered inadvertently. Preoperative teaching and counseling by the nurse help in allaying the client's anxiety. This preoperative counseling may be managed, particularly with day or short stay surgeries by a case manager or by preoperative visits to the hospital.

Besides the preanesthetic medications, all of the preparation for surgical procedures should be carefully explained to clients. Most clients are not familiar with the procedures related to the perioperative experience. The necessity for postoperative coughing, deep breathing, frequent turning, and use of spirometers should be taught to the client preoperatively. These activities help to prevent the postoperative complications of general anesthetics, such as hypostatic pneumonia and atelectasis. The preoperative teaching promotes cooperation when the client is asked to do these activities that often cause discomfort after a surgical procedure.

Food is usually withheld after the evening meal, and standard procedure is to give the client nothing to eat or drink after midnight. This procedure helps prevent aspiration if vomiting occurs as a response to anesthesia.

Attention should be given to the client's drug history in preoperative preparation. Withholding maintenance medications while the client is NPO for surgery will have the physiologic effect of abrupt withdrawal. Specific orders should be obtained from the primary prescriber regarding rescheduling the time of administration, a change in the route of administration of the client's standing medications, or both. When a parenteral form of medication is not available, permission may sometimes be given for the client to take oral medications with a small amount of water (30 to 60 ml) while the client is NPO before surgery.

In addition, as previously discussed, some medications may remain in the client's system and interact to cause serious problems such as arterial hypotension and circulatory collapse or respiratory depression.

Using premedication is less common now than in the past. Drug choice considers the client's age, weight, physical condition, and level of anxiety, the anesthetic method selected, and the duration and type of surgery. Not including drugs in the preoperative preparation of some clients may be appropriate, while others may need aggressive pharmacologic intervention to produce the desired preoperative state. When drugs are prescribed, a combination of drugs, such as morphine or meperidine (Demerol), hydroxyzine (Atarax), and atropine, is generally used for the immediate preoperative preparation of the client for major surgery. In this instance, atropine is used to block the action of acetylcholine at parasympathetic nerve endings, to overcome vagal effects of anesthesia, and to dry secretions.

Opioid analgesics, barbiturates, or benzodiazepines (the anxiolytics most commonly used) may be administered before the client is taken to surgery to promote serenity and amnesia, smooth induction, and decrease the amount of anesthetic agent required to produce anesthesia. It is important that the nurse administer the preoperative medications at the exact time ordered. If they are given too close to the time of administration of the general anesthetic, they may achieve full effect during anesthesia and cause severe respiratory depression or hypotension.

The time it takes to complete specific surgical procedures is variable, so it becomes impossible for many preoperative medications, other than for the first cases of the day, to be ordered for a specific time. For other than the first cases of the day, the preoperative medication is ordered "on call" from the operating room.

All the physical tasks involved with the client's preparation for surgery (i.e., signing surgical permits, final voiding before surgery, taking vital signs) should be accomplished before the preoperative medication is administered. Once the medication is administered, the client should be placed on bed rest with the side rails up and the call light within reach. This decreases stimulation and favors the action of the medication. In addition, the consent for anesthesia, surgery, or both is not considered valid if the client has received sedation before signing.

Intraoperative

The nurse has a highly specialized role within the operating room. The nursing responsibilities entail the maintenance of safety, physiologic monitoring, and psychologic support for the client, but the nurse's role in relation to the administration of anesthetic agents is that of a supportive one to the anesthesiologist, or the nurse anesthetist, administering the anesthetic. The operating room nurse should monitor for factors that may result in hypotension, nerve injury, or malignant hyperthermia.

Hypotension may result from an excess of nonvolatile drugs that depress the vasomotor center. When opioids are given, the client's pain must be assessed thoroughly and vital signs recorded. Avoid these drugs because they may increase hypotension. However, severe pain can also cause hypotension. In these cases an opioid may both alleviate pain and increase blood pressure.

A second complication that the operating room nurse must be on the alert for is nerve injury, which may follow spinal anesthesia or malpositioning during general anesthesia. Brachial, radial, ulnar, and perineal nerves are the most likely to be injured. The operating room nurse is responsible for ensuring that the client is positioned properly to prevent injury from nerve damage. A knowledge of proper positioning for the particular surgical procedure is essential.

A rare but very dangerous adverse effect of inhaled, fat-soluble anesthetics is *malignant hyperthermia*. This is an emergency in which the client's temperature suddenly escalates; if it is not treated appropriately and promptly, the client may die. Individuals susceptible to malignant hyperthermia have an underlying muscle disorder, an autosomal dominant trait. The use of neuromuscular blocking agents has also been associated with this adverse effect, especially when they are used with the inhalation anesthetics. With concurrent use of succinylcholine, the onset may be more abrupt. The body temperature may increase as much as 1° C (1.8° F) every 5 minutes, reaching reported highs of 43° C (109.4° F). Although the condition is relatively rare, 1 in 50,000 surgical clients, it is a life-threatening condition with a mortality rate of 30% to 40%. The operating room personnel, with whom the nurse has a key role, should have a preplanned course of action, including the availability of dantrolene sodium (discussed more fully in Chapter 23), a complete change of anesthesia circuit, hyperventilation with 100% oxygen, methods to lower body temperature rapidly, and other symptomatic treatment. Dantrolene sodium has been used prophylactically and in the treatment of this disorder.

The clinical role of the nurse anesthetist, who assumes the direct responsibility for the administration of anesthetics, requires a formal certification program for advanced practice of that specialty.

Postoperative

The major objective of the immediate postoperative period is to help the client in recovering from the effects of the anesthesia and the surgery safely, comfortably, and as quickly as possible.

Assessment. A general postoperative assessment should include:

- Airway and breathing—the adequacy of the airway and airway reflexes (gag, cough, swallow); type of airway in place; rate and quality of respiration; breath sounds; ability to cough and deep breathe; amount and method of oxygen administered and the time it was initiated.
- Circulation—pulse rate, peripheral pulses; blood pressure readings; cardiac monitor pattern (if applicable); skin color and temperature.
- Metabolic—skin integrity and turgor; temperature; urine output; type and rate of IV fluids administered.
- General—location, condition, and output from drains and catheters; muscle strength and response; bowel sounds; status of the surgical incision; position of client; pain; level of consciousness and ability to communicate (Beare & Myers, 1994).

Nursing diagnosis. The client receiving a general anesthetic may experience the following nursing diagnoses: ineffective airway clearance related to inadequate cough and tenacious secretions; ineffective breathing pattern related to excess or cumulative effects of drugs administered during anesthesia; risk for aspiration related to nausea and vomiting, because of gastrointestinal distention, medication and anesthesia, stimulation of the vomiting center or chemoreceptor trigger zone, or anoxia during anesthesia; pain; hypothermia; sensory/perceptual alterations; and the potential complications of urinary retention, abdominal distention or paralytic ileus, and shock.

Implementation

Monitoring. At frequent intervals depending on the client's condition, evaluate the client's status as in the initial assessment.

Intervention. Neuromuscular blocking agents such as curare, succinylcholine, and *d*-tubocurarine can cause hypoventilation. Maintaining a patent airway until the client has fully responded is important in the postoperative period. Nursing measures include encouraging clients to deep breathe and cough frequently. Change of position to prevent pooling of pulmonary secretions also can help to improve ventilation and prevent atelectasis. Most clients receiving general anesthesia will be administered supplemental oxygen until they are fully recovered from the anesthesia. Mobilization and alternating contraction and relaxation of muscles promote circulation.

Postoperatively the nurse can administer a prescribed antiemetic and position the client on his or her side to prevent aspiration. Maintain the client without any oral sustenance until peristalsis returns. Normal bowel sounds and progression to an appropriate diet are the client outcomes sought.

Early detection of impending shock and institution of proper therapy may prevent or at least modify its severity. Rate, volume, and rhythm of the pulse should be noted, as well as the client's color and skin temperature. A rapid, thready, weak pulse; cyanosis or extreme pallor; cold, clammy skin; and low blood pressure are characteristic signs of shock. Checking for bleeding at the operative site is important; if the client continues to lose blood postoperatively, hemorrhagic shock may occur. Postoperative shock also may result from extensive surgical trauma, prolonged operating time, prolonged deep anesthesia, or even inadequate anesthesia.

Education. With increasing numbers of surgeries being done at ambulatory surgical centers, the nurse should be concerned with client-family teaching for the client who is returning home, to help him or her recover more fully from the anesthesia and the surgery. In addition to specifics regarding the client's operative procedure and its relevant postoperative care, the nurse should prepare the client for some psychomotor impairment and sensory/perceptual alterations during the first 24 hours following anesthesia. Caution the client against attempting tasks that require alertness and coordination, such as driving. The client should be instructed to avoid using alcohol or other CNS depressants within the first 24 hours unless they are prescribed by the health care provider.

Evaluation. The client will effectively maintain his or her own airway, have an effective cough, have normal respiratory rate and depth, and have normal breath sounds. The temperature, blood pressure, and pulse will be within normal limits. The client will experience no postoperative pain or an acceptable level of postoperative discomfort. The client's urinary output will be more than 30 to 50 ml/hr without complaints of urgency or bladder fullness. The client is oriented to person, time, and place.

TYPES OF GENERAL ANESTHETICS

General anesthetics are usually divided into two groups: (1) the inhalation anesthetics, which include gases and volatile liquids, and (2) intravenous anesthetics, which include barbiturates and nonbarbiturates.

Inhalation Anesthetics

Inhalation, or *volatile*, anesthetics are gases or liquids that can be administered by inhalation when mixed with oxygen. These can effect a concentration in the blood and brain to depress the CNS and cause anesthesia. They have the following characteristics:

- They are complete anesthetics and thus can abolish superficial and deep reflexes.
- They provide for controllable anesthesia, since depth of anesthesia is easily varied by changing the inhaled concentration.
- Allergic reactions to these agents are uncommon.
- Rapid recovery can occur as soon as administration ceases, since the anesthetic is excreted in expired air.

■ Nursing Management

Inhalation Anesthetic Agents

The actual administration of general anesthesia is conducted by a physician or nurse who has specialized training in anesthetic management, which is beyond the scope of this textbook. General nursing measures discussed herein are focused on the care of the client after surgery has been completed and are in addition to the previous discussion of the nursing management of general anesthetics.

Implementation

Monitoring. Monitor the client's temperature, blood pressure, pulse, and respiratory rate closely during the immediate postoperative period. The recovery phase for volatile anesthetic agents is generally short, and they leave no analgesia residue; thus the postoperative analgesia phase will be short. Thoroughly assess the client for postoperative pain. Shivering and tremors may be observed postoperatively.

Intervention. Use caution when changing the client's position during the recovery phase. Besides the vasodilation, compensatory vasoconstriction mechanisms are depressed, which may result in a significant drop in blood pressure with position changes (postural hypotension). Oxygen is administered during the immediate recovery period to compensate for the respiratory depression from the anesthetic agents as well as the increased oxygen needs of the body from shivering. Pain relief medications will provide relief for immediate postoperative pain. However, *the nurse should remember that any sedative or analgesic probably will need to be decreased by one half to one fourth for the first dose after surgery,* because of the combined effects of the CNS depressants, e.g., residual anesthetic agents and analgesics. Measures to avoid heat loss from vasodilation include using warm blankets, covering the head with a blanket, and using a hyperthermic automatic blanket.

Education. To allay fears, explain preoperatively to these clients that they will receive oxygen during the recovery period and be closely monitored until the anesthetic effects have completely worn off.

Evaluation. The client should demonstrate normal breath sounds and an effective cough and gag reflex. Vital signs should be within normal limits, and the client should be able to respond to verbal commands.

Inhalation Anesthetics

While ether and chloroform as volatile liquids, and cyclopropane and nitrous oxide as gases, were commonly used over the years, only nitrous oxide is clinically still in use today. Chloroform is hepatotoxic, and ether and cyclopropane are highly flammable; thus these agents have been replaced by safer anesthetics. In 1956, halothane (Fluothane), a nonflammable agent, largely replaced the older volatile liquids. Halothane, though, has been associated with hepatic dysfunction and failure. Since then, newer less toxic volatile liquids have been developed: desflurane (Suprane), enflurane (Ethrane), isoflurane (Forane), methoxyflurane (Penthrane), and sevoflurane (Ultane).

Gases

nitrous oxide [nye' trus ox' ide]
Nitrous oxide, an anesthetic gas, is the most commonly used agent for dental surgery, minor surgery, and obstetric analgesia. It is often combined with other anesthetics to enhance its effects, so it is also used extensively in major surgery. It is excreted 100% unchanged through the lungs. Its few side effects primarily consist of postoperative nausea, vomiting, or delirium, and it has no known significant drug interactions.

For general anesthesia, the recommended dosage is 70% with 30% oxygen inhalation for induction, 30% to 70% with oxygen for maintenance.

At the termination of nitrous oxide anesthesia, the rapid movement of large amounts of nitrous oxide from the circulation into the lungs may dilute the oxygen in the lungs. This dilution may result in a phenomenon known as diffusion hypoxia. To prevent this, the anesthesiologist or anesthetist usually administers 100% oxygen to clear the nitrous oxide from the lungs. During recovery the client should be administered humidified oxygen by mask, and encouraged to breathe deeply to promote ventilation.

Volatile Liquid Anesthetics

▲ **halothane** [ha' loe thayn] (Fluothane, Somnothane♣)
Halothane is used primarily as a general anesthetic. Pharmacokinetics are detailed in Table 15-1. A list of the drug's side effects/adverse reactions also appears in Table 15-1. Postoperative nausea and vomiting may occur in many clients and may be more frequent if nitrous oxide is used to supplement other anesthetics. A rare complication of halothane is liver damage, or *halothane hepatitis,* although this view is controversial. While the mechanism is not known, some experts believe the liver damage to be caused by a hypersensitivity-type reaction to a metabolite of halothane. The diagnosis is made on the clinical findings of unexplained fever, eosinophilia, rashes, and abnormal liver function tests within 2 weeks of exposure, especially after a repeat exposure. The syndrome is more common in older or obese clients and is not seen in children.

Significant drug interactions. Halothane sensitizes the myocardium to the effects of catecholamines (epinephrine, norepinephrine, or dopamine) or sympathomimetic agents (e.g., ephedrine, metaraminol). These agents may produce serious cardiac dysrhythmias in the presence of halothane. Levodopa, which pharmacologically increases the quantity of dopamine in the CNS, should be discontinued at least 6 to 8 hours before halothane is administered. Halothane is the only volatile anesthetic agent that sensitizes the myocardium.

Systemic aminoglycosides, lincomycins, polymyxins, and capreomycin, when given concurrently with any of the volatile anesthetics, may result in skeletal muscle weakness, respiratory depression, or apnea (absence of respiration). Clients usually require mechanical ventilation. If these medications are used, the dosage of the nondepolarizing neuromuscular blocking drugs should be decreased to one third or one half of the usually prescribed dosage.

Dosage and administration. See Table 15-1.

desflurane [des floo' rayn] (Suprane)
Released in late 1992, desflurane is an alternative to halothane and isoflurane. It produces a more rapid induction and emergence from anesthesia than the following agents. The use of desflurane has been associated with a moderately high incidence of airway irritation, coughing, and laryngospasm. For this reason it is not indicated for anesthesia induction in pediatric clients, although it is approved for anesthesia maintenance in infants and young children.

enflurane [en floo' rayn] (Ethrane)
Enflurane is indicated for induction and maintenance of general anesthesia. It is only slightly metabolized in the body. Its clinical effects are similar to those of halothane, but it is less potent. Enflurane may cause seizures when given at high concentrations; therefore, it is not recommended for use with clients who are seizure-prone, such as those with epilepsy or head injuries.

isoflurane [eye soe floo' rayn] (Forane)
Isoflurane is indicated for induction and maintenance of general anesthesia. It undergoes an extremely low degree of metabolism. Until the release of desflurane, it was promoted as having a more rapid action than the other inhalation agents and causing less cardiovascular depression. Nephrotoxicity is minimal with the use of isoflurane.

methoxyflurane [me thox' i floo rayn] (Penthrane)
Methoxyflurane is used for anesthesia and analgesic effects. It is a potent anesthetic agent used for obstetric analgesia. It is given in concentrations of 0.3% to 0.8%. Methoxyflurane is highly metabolized, and a by-product of its metabolism is free fluoride, which is toxic to the kidney (nephrotoxic). Because of methoxyflurane's potential for nephrotoxicity, its use is limited to minor surgical procedures and obstetrics.

sevoflurane [sev oe floo' rayn] (Ultane)
Sevoflurane is an inhalation general anesthetic indicated for induction and maintenance during surgery. While the induction dose is individualized, the usual adult inhalation dose is between 0.5% to 3% alone or combined with nitrous oxide (*USP DI Update,* 1995). Sevoflurane was released in 1995 and it has a faster uptake, distribution, and rate of elimination

TABLE 15-1 Volatile liquid anesthetic agents

Agent	Pharmacokinetics: Absorption	Pharmacokinetics: Metabolism	Pharmacokinetics: Excretion	MAC (%)*	Toxicity	Side effects/adverse reactions
halothane (Fluothane, Somnothane✤)	By lungs	Up to 20% by liver	60%-80% unchanged by the lungs; remainder excreted or metabolized through kidneys	0.75	May cause "halothane hepatitis" (see p. 280)	Hypotension, cardiovascular depression, lowered body temperature, respiratory depression, malignant hyperthermia Emergence delirium—shivering and trembling, confusion, hallucinations, nervousness, increased excitability
desflurane (Suprane)	By lungs	<0.2% by liver	Primarily lungs	7.3	Airway irritation, severe laryngospasm, coughing	See halothane
enflurane (Ethrane)	By lungs	About 2.5% by liver	80% unchanged by lungs; remainder excreted as metabolites through kidneys	1.68		See halothane
isoflurane (Forane)	By lungs	Less than 1% by liver	Almost all through lungs: less than 1% as metabolites through kidneys	1.15		See halothane
methoxyflurane (Penthrane)	By lungs	About 50% by liver	35% unchanged by lungs; remainder excreted as metabolites through kidneys	0.16	Dose-related nephrotoxicity (renal tube damage) from fluoride metabolite	See halothane
sevoflurane (Ultane)	By lungs	—	Primarily lungs	2.1	Cardiac depressant (bradycardia)	See halothane

**MAC*, Minimum alveolar concentration (percent in oxygen) that prevents movement in 50% of patients exposed to painful stimuli. May need higher concentrations in some patients; generally, highest in very young children, lowest with increasing age, pregnancy, hypotension, or concurrent CNS depressant use.

than isoflurane and halothane. When compared with desflurane, it has a slower uptake and distribution but the rate of elimination is similar to desflurane (Olin, 1995).

Intravenous Anesthetics

Intravenous anesthetic agents are used for induction or maintenance of general anesthesia, to induce amnesia, and as an adjunct to inhalation-type anesthetics. The major groups include ultrashort-acting barbiturates, nonbarbiturates, dissociative anesthetics, and neuroleptanesthesia. Intravenous anesthetics are valuable to allay emotional distress, since many clients dread having a tight mask placed over the face while they are fully conscious. These anesthetics reduce the amount of inhalation anesthetic required. Box 15-2 lists advantages and disadvantages of intravenous anesthetics.

The intravenous anesthetics most commonly used are the ultrashort-acting barbiturates. These drugs are rapidly taken up by brain tissue because of their high solubility. For example, equilibrium between brain and blood occurs within 1 minute after injection of thiopental. Shortness of action results from the drug being quickly redistributed into the fat depots of the body. The amount of body fat affects drug action; the greater the amount of body fat, the briefer the effect of a single intravenous dose. With prolonged administration or large doses, however, prolonged drug action results in delayed recovery. This is caused by saturation of fat depots and the slow rate of drug release (10% to 15% per hour).

■ Nursing Management
Intravenous Anesthetic Agents

In this text the nurse's role in intravenous general anesthetics does not include the administration of the anesthetic. The focus of the role does include, however, client care during the recovery period that follows the anesthesia.

BOX 15-2

Advantages and Disadvantages of Intravenous Anesthetics

Disadvantages. Swelling, pain, ulceration, tissue sloughing, and necrosis if drug infiltrates into tissue; thrombosis and gangrene if arterial injection occurs; and hypotension, laryngospasm, and respiratory failure from overdosage or prolonged administration. Muscle relaxation and analgesic effects are minimal.

Advantages. Rapidity with which unconsciousness is induced, amnesic effects, prompt recovery with minimal doses, and simplicity of administration. Intravenous anesthetics are nonirritating to mucous membranes, and use is not accompanied by the hazard of fire or explosion.

Assessment. The nurse should note that intravenous anesthetics are seldom used alone for anesthesia, except for short procedures such as electroconvulsive therapy, cast application or removal, and hypnosis. *The nurse should remember that the dose of any postoperative sedative or analgesic probably will need to be decreased by one third to one fourth for the first dose after surgery;* after that the dose of the analgesic will be titrated according to the client's needs. The nurse must assess the client's response to the analgesic and relay the information to ensure adequate medication dosage.

Nursing diagnosis. Nursing diagnoses related to the administration of intravenous anesthesia may include but are not limited to: ineffective airway clearance; ineffective breathing pattern; impaired gas exchange; risk for aspiration; and the potential complications of thrombophlebitis at the infusion site and decreased cardiac output.

Implementation

Monitoring. Assessment of the client's cardiovascular and respiratory status should be done at frequent intervals, as well as assessment of the client's behavioral response to intravenous anesthetic agents. Monitor the IV site for color, temperature, swelling, pain, and patency.

Intervention. When intravenous anesthetic agents are administered, resuscitative equipment should be within the immediate environment.

Education. Generally there is some impairment of psychomotor skills for 24 hours after the administration of these drugs. Instruct the client not to engage in any activities requiring alertness and coordination, such as driving. Caution the client to avoid alcohol and CNS depressants for the first 24 hours after taking these drugs, except as prescribed.

Evaluation. The client should demonstrate normal breath sounds and an effective cough. Vital signs should be within normal limits, and there should be no evidence of a thromboembolic event.

Ultrashort-Acting Barbiturates

Ultrashort-acting barbiturates include thiopental sodium (Pentothal) and methohexital sodium (Brevital Sodium). These ultrashort-acting barbiturates are CNS depressants that produce hypnosis and anesthesia without analgesia. They frequently are combined with other drugs for muscle relaxation and analgesia in balanced anesthesia. Their exact mechanism of action for anesthesia, anticonvulsant effects, or the reduction of intracranial pressure (an indication for thiopental) is unknown, although a variety of theories have been proposed. General anesthesia with ultrashort-acting barbiturates is believed to result from suppression of the reticular activating system.

The onset of action for these barbiturates is generally rapid—20 to 60 seconds—with an extremely short duration. They are distributed rapidly throughout the body with accumulation in the fatty tissues, followed by redistribution from brain to lean body mass in emergence. These drugs are metabolized in the liver and excreted through the kidneys.

The most common side effects during the recovery period are shivering and trembling. Less frequently reported are nausea, vomiting, prolonged somnolence, and headache. Serious adverse reactions include emergence delirium (increased excitability, confusion, and hallucinations); cardiac dysrhythmias (tachycardia, bradycardia, or myocardial depression); allergic response (bronchospasm, rash, hives, edema of eyelids, lips, or face, and hypotension); respiratory depression; and thrombophlebitis.

Careful assessment and close monitoring are required when the intravenous barbiturates are used in combination with other CNS depressants, which may result in enhanced depression effects, as well as diuretics, antihypertensive agents, and calcium-blocking drugs, since hypotension may occur.

Dosages for induction of general anesthesia and resultant duration of action vary. Methohexital requires 1 to 2 mg/kg for induction, with a duration of action of 5 to 7 minutes. Thiopental is individually dosed according to the client's response.

■ Nursing Management

Ultrashort-Acting Barbiturates

Intravenous barbiturates must be administered by personnel trained in their use and in management of possible complications. Continuous monitoring is essential while these barbiturates are being administered. Barbiturates cause depression of respiratory and cardiovascular functions. Resuscitation equipment, a laryngoscope, an endotracheal tube, suction, and oxygen must be on hand when ultrashort-acting barbiturates are administered for anesthesia.

In addition to the nursing management described for intravenous anesthetic agents, the injection site should be monitored closely. Ultrashort-acting barbiturates are very alkaline and therefore irritating to the tissues. Take care to avoid extravasation of the drug into the tissues during intravenous injection; pain, swelling, ulceration, and necrosis may occur. Intraarterial injection may result in tissue necrosis and gangrene.

Intravenous barbiturates are incompatible with a wide range of solutions, including bacteriostatic diluents and lactated Ringer's solution. The nurse should consult the drug insert or a specialized reference before mixing substances, and they should not be administered if they are cloudy or there is a precipitate. Thiopental solutions should be freshly prepared and used within 24 hours.

Nonbarbiturates

Nonbarbiturate intravenous anesthetic agents include the benzodiazepines midazolam, diazepam, and lorazepam; the short-acting hypnotics etomidate and propofol; the opioids fentanyl, sufentanil, and alfentanil; and ketamine, a dissociative anesthetic. Several drugs also may be combined to produce **neuroleptanesthesia**, a general anesthesia produced by the administration of a neuroleptic agent, a narcotic analgesic, and nitrous oxide in oxygen.

midazolam [mid' a zoe lam] (Versed)
diazepam [dye az' e pam] (Valium)
lorazepam [lor az' e pam] (Ativan)

Benzodiazepines are given intravenously as premedication or for induction of anesthesia. Diazepam and lorazepam are not water soluble; thus their nonaqueous solutions may cause local irritation. Midazolam is water soluble and thus less irritating locally. In the body midazolam becomes more lipid soluble; therefore it can readily cross the blood-brain barrier. These agents generally have a slower onset of CNS effects than the barbiturates and a more prolonged post-anesthetic recovery period, and they often produce an amnesic effect.

Midazolam also causes a decrease in cerebrospinal fluid pressure and thus may be selected for anesthesia induction in clients with intracranial lesions. Intravenously, midazolam has a rapid onset of action (1 to 3 minutes) and a short elimination half-life of approximately 2.5 hours. It is metabolized in the liver and excreted by the kidneys.

Concurrent use of benzodiazepines with alcohol or CNS depressing drugs may result in hypotension, respiratory depression, and possibly respiratory and cardiac arrest. A reduction in drug dosage and close monitoring are indicated if such drugs are used concurrently. Debilitated clients and those 55 years and older require a smaller than normal midazolam dose administered at a slower rate (Wangaman & Foster, 1991). Check a current reference for dosing recommendations. If concurrent CNS depressant drugs are used, the midazolam dose should be reduced by at least 50% and diazepam by 33%.

etomidate [eh toe' mid date] (Amidate)

Etomidate is a short-acting, nonbarbiturate hypnotic used for the induction of general anesthesia. Etomidate is reported to decrease the activity of the reticular formation in the brainstem (in animals). Its cardiac and respiratory effects are minimal, so this product may be advantageous for the client with impaired cardiac functions, respiratory functions, or both. Etomidate is used intravenously in induction of general anesthesia and in concomitant anesthesia for supplementation of a subpotent anesthetic agent (nitrous oxide in oxygen).

Etomidate (Amidate) induces hypnosis within 1 minute, with a duration of action between 3 and 5 minutes. To reduce recovery time in adults, a 0.1-mg IV dose of fentanyl is administered 1 or 2 minutes before anesthesia induction, thus reducing the amount of etomidate needed. Etomidate is metabolized in the liver and excreted by the kidneys.

The side effects most commonly reported during the recovery period are nausea and vomiting; less often reported are hypotension, hypertension, dysrhythmias, and breathing difficulties. Involuntary muscle movements have been reported, especially when fentanyl is not given before induction with etomidate. Pain at the injection site is also reported. SPECIAL WARNING: Etomidate can suppress the adrenal gland production of steroid hormones (cortisol, etc.), which can result in a temporary gland failure. Electrolyte imbalance, hypotension, and shock may result. Seriously ill or postoperative patients may need adrenal cortex supplementation.

Significant drug interactions. When etomidate is given with other CNS depressants, the client should be monitored for enhanced CNS depression. For less significant but potential drug interactions, see the listing under IV barbiturates.

Dosage and administration. See Table 15-2.

For the nursing management of clients receiving etomidate, see the nursing management for intravenous anesthetic agents in general. The client should be monitored for enhanced CNS depression if other CNS depressing drugs are administered. For less significant but potential drug interactions, see the listing under IV barbiturates.

propofol [pro poe' foal] (Diprivan)
Propofol is a rapidly acting, nonbarbiturate hypnotic used for the induction and maintenance of general anesthesia. It has a rapid onset of action of within 40 seconds and the duration of effect is only from 3 to 5 minutes. Its redistribution from the brain to other body tissues explains the short effect. This agent's elimination half-life is 3 to 12 hours.

TABLE 15-2 Nonbarbiturates: dosage and administration

Agent	Adults	Children
alfentanil (Alfenta)		
Adjunct to general anesthesia	8-20 μg (0.008-0.02 mg)/kg body weight IV initially. Additional dosages of 3-5 μg/kg as needed for short duration (up to 30 min). For induction anesthesia, may use initial dose of 130-245 μg (0.130-0.245 mg)/kg body weight.	Adjunct to anesthesia: IV 30-50 μg (0.03-0.05 mg)/kg body weight initially, then 0.5-1.5 μg/kg body weight by continuous infusion
etomidate (Amidate)		
Anesthesia induction	0.2-0.6 mg/kg body weight administered over 30-60 seconds	Children over 10 yr, 0.2-0.6 mg/kg body weight
fentanyl (Sublimaze)		
Adjunct to general anesthesia		
Minor surgery	2 μg (0.002 mg)/kg body weight IV	Children less than 2 yr, no established dosage
Major surgery	2-20 μg (0.002-0.02 mg)/kg body weight IV. High doses are used for open-heart surgery, complicated neurosurgery, or orthopedic procedures, i.e., 20-50 μg (0.02-0.05 mg)/kg body weight IV	
Primary agent in major surgery	50-100 μg (0.05-0.1 mg)/kg body weight IV given with oxygen, nitrous oxide, or both and neuromuscular blocking agent	Children 2-12 yr, 2-3 μg (0.002-0.003 mg)/kg body weight IV
Presurgical or postoperative use	0.07-1.4 μg (0.0007-0.0014 mg)/kg body weight IM	
sufentanil (Sufenta)		
Adjunct to general anesthesia	Low dosages, 0.5-1 μg (0.0005-0.001 mg)/kg body weight IV initially. Additional dosages of 10-25 μg may be given as needed. Moderate dosages, 2-8 μg/kg body weight IV initially. Additional dosages of 10-50 μg may be given as needed	
Primary agent in major surgery	8-30 μg/kg body weight IV initially with oxygen. Additional dosages of 25-50 μg may be given as needed	Cardiovascular surgery: initially, 10-25 μg/kg body weight IV given with 100% oxygen. Maintenance, up to 25-50 μg IV

From *USP DI* (1996).

This agent is a respiratory depressant and may produce apnea and cardiac depression depending on the dose, rate of administration, and concurrent drugs administered. Bradycardia and hypotension may also occur frequently. Nausea, vomiting, and involuntary muscle movement are commonly reported.

The nursing management of the client receiving propofol is as for other IV anesthetics.

fentanyl [fen' ta nil] (Sublimaze)
sufentanil [soo fen' ta nil] (Sufenta)
alfentanil [al fen' ta nil] (Alfenta)

Adjunct medications for anesthesia include fentanyl (Sublimaze), sufentanil (Sufenta), and alfentanil (Alfenta). These agents have been theorized to produce their effects at the mu receptor. All three are opioid analgesics used for balanced anesthesia (see earlier section) and in combination with oxygen, nitrous oxide, or both for the induction and maintenance of anesthesia. When combined with an agent such as droperidol that produces **neurolepsis** (an altered state of consciousness characterized by quiescence, reduced motor activity and anxiety, and indifference to surroundings) then fentanyl, sufentanil, and alfentanil may be used for neuroleptsis or neuroleptanesthesia (see p. 286).

The most commonly reported side effects/adverse reactions are drowsiness, hypotension, bradycardia, and respiratory depression (allergic reaction). Less frequent are chills, nausea, vomiting, increased weakness, dizziness, constipation, depression, pruritus, muscle spasms, and increased excitability (paradoxical reaction). Convulsions are reported with fentanyl; dysrhythmias are reported with sufentanil.

Concurrent use of these drugs with CNS depressants may result in an enhanced CNS depressant effect, hypotension, and respiratory depression. Dosage adjustment and careful monitoring are required. When other opioid agonist analgesics are used during the recovery phase from fentanyl or sufentanil anesthesia, the dosage should be one fourth to one third the usually recommended dosage. Naltrexone blocks the effects of opioid analgesics. If an opioid is necessary for elective surgery, naltrexone should be stopped for several days before the scheduled operation.

Information on dosage and administration of these drugs appears in Table 15-2.

Fentanyl (Sublimaze), sufentanil (Sufenta), and alfentanil (Alfenta) all cross the blood-brain barrier and are rapidly distributed to various tissues. They are highly protein bound, with a triphasic half-life—that is, distributive phase, redistributive phase, and elimination.

Fentanyl produces an analgesic effect in 7 to 15 minutes when given intramuscularly or 1 to 2 minutes when given intravenously. The rate of the loss of consciousness depends on the dose and the rate of administration (usually 4 to 5 minutes at the rate of 0.4 mg/min IV). Its peak effect occurs at 3 to 5 minutes when given IV, and at 20 to 30 minutes when given IM. The duration of effect is 0.5 to 1 hour IV, 1 to 2 hours IM.

Sufentanil has an immediate analgesic effect, with the time until loss of consciousness depending on dose and rate of administration (usually 1 to 1.6 minutes at the rate of 0.3 mg/min). The duration of action is less than 1 hour.

Alfentanil has an immediate analgesic effect, producing a peak effect in 1 to 2 minutes. The duration of action is dose dependent but is usually less than 10 to 15 minutes.

All three drugs are metabolized in the liver, although sufentanil may also have some intestinal metabolism. They are excreted by the kidneys.

■ Nursing Management
Fentanyl, Sufentanil, Alfentanil

Nurses should carefully monitor all clients receiving fentanyl during surgery, since respiratory depression is a side effect, and all precautions need to be taken; an oral airway and oxygen should be readily available. CNS depressants can potentiate the respiratory and sedative effects of fentanyl, so the dosage of any sedative or analgesic should be reduced by one third to one fourth. The client should be made to lie down if he or she is experiencing nausea, vomiting, dizziness, or syncope. See also Nursing Management for Opioid Analgesics, Chapter 14.

Dissociative Anesthetic

ketamine hydrochloride [keet' a meen] (Ketalar)

Ketamine is a rapid-acting, nonbarbiturate, intravenous anesthetic. It is a derivative of the psychotomimetic drug of abuse phencyclidine. Ketamine acts on the midbrain within the reticular formation, as do the barbiturates. It produces analgesia and amnesia but not muscular relaxation. The mechanism of action is not fully known. Ketamine blocks afferent transmission of impulses associated with the affective-emotional aspect of pain perception. It may also suppress spinal cord activity. Ketamine produces a **dissociative anesthesia**; an anesthesia characterized by analgesia and amnesia without loss of respiratory function or pharyngeal and laryngeal reflexes. It produces a cataleptic state in which the client appears to be awake but detached from his or her environment and unresponsive to pain. The client's eyelids usually do not close, nystagmus (rapid, involuntary oscillation of the eyeballs) is common, and slight involuntary and purposeless movements may occur.

Ketamine increases secretions of salivary and bronchial glands; therefore the administration of an anticholinergic agent (such as atropine) may be necessary. Ketamine may increase blood pressure, muscle tone, and heart rate. Respiration is usually not depressed. After recovery, the client has no recall of events while under the influence of ketamine.

Ketamine is best suited for short diagnostic or surgical procedures not requiring skeletal muscle relaxation. It is also used to induce anesthesia before administration of general anesthetics and as an adjunct to low-potency anesthetics, such as nitrous oxide.

When ketamine is given intravenously, the onset of anesthesia occurs within 30 seconds. When it is administered intramuscularly, the onset of action occurs within 3 to 4 minutes. The duration of action is 5 to 10 minutes for an IV dose of 2 mg/kg body weight or 12 to 25 minutes for an IM dose of 10 mg/kg.

Ketamine is metabolized in the liver. Termination of anesthetic action occurs with redistribution from the central nervous system and liver biotransformation. Ninety percent is excreted in the kidneys.

The most commonly reported side effects/adverse reactions of ketamine include hypertension and increased pulse rate and an emergence reaction, such as distortion in body image, delirium, explicit dreams, illusions, and dissociative-type experiences. In some clients, flashbacks of vivid dreams with or without illusions may occur weeks later. Less commonly reported side effects include hypotension, bradycardia, respiratory depression, and vomiting. No significant drug interactions have been reported.

The recommended adult dosage for anesthesia induction is 1 to 2 mg/kg body weight IV or 5 to 10 mg/kg body weight IM. The recommended rate for maintenance is 10 to 50 µg/kg body weight by infusion at a rate of 1 to 2 µg/min. As with any anesthetic, the dosage needs to be carefully assessed and individualized.

▪ Nursing Management

Ketamine Hydrochloride

Assessment. Obtain a baseline assessment of the client's vital signs and mental status before ketamine administration. Ketamine is contraindicated in clients with hypertension, increased intracranial pressure, intracranial lesions, intracranial surgery, or a history of psychiatric problems or alcoholism.

Nursing diagnosis. The following nursing diagnoses may be identified with a client receiving ketamine: risk for injury related to the drug's dissociative reaction; ineffective breathing pattern related to the drug's respiratory depressive effects; risk for aspiration; and sensory/perceptual alterations (visual and auditory).

Implementation

Monitoring. Ketamine produces a dissociative state; the client may not appear to be asleep but is dissociated from the environment. Observe ketamine-anesthetized clients for blood pressure elevation, tachycardia, bradycardia, dreaming, delirium, hallucinations, euphoria, and increased muscle tone. Monitor cardiac status and observe for respiratory depression.

Intervention. When clients are given ketamine, protect them from visual, tactile, and auditory stimuli during emergence to decrease the possibility of psychic effects. Up to 50% of unpremedicated clients report dreams and hallucinations as the medication wears off. If they are disturbing, these responses may be alleviated with diazepam. These dreams and hallucinations can occur up to 24 hours after administration of ketamine. Keep environmental stimulation to a minimum during recovery to reduce the risk of an emergent reaction. Do not arouse these clients until they awake on their own.

Education. Caution the client against driving, other hazardous activities, and alcohol ingestion for at least 24 hours after recovery from ketamine, because of psychomotor impairment.

Evaluation. The expected outcomes are that the client experiences effective anesthesia and the safety of the client is maintained. The airway is patent, and adequate ventilatory status is maintained. Sensory/perceptual alterations are minimized or absent.

Neuroleptanesthesia

Neuroleptanesthesia is a general anesthesia produced by a combination of a neuroleptic (antipsychotic) such as droperidol (Inapsine), diazepam (Valium), or ketamine (Ketalar) and a narcotic analgesic, most commonly fentanyl but sometimes meperidine (Demerol), morphine, or pentazocine (Talwin). It is used primarily for procedures that require the client's cooperation.

An example of this classification is droperidol and fentanyl (Innovar injection). Innovar consists of 1 part fentanyl to 50 parts droperidol.

droperidol [droe per'i dole] and fentanyl [fen'ta nil] (Innovar injection)

Droperidol is used to produce neuroleptic anesthesia. Droperidol is a neuroleptic drug with prolonged action. This combination produces a state in which clients are neither asleep nor awake but in a state of profound analgesia and psychomotor sedation. This state permits the client to undergo short procedures requiring consciousness and cooperation, such as bronchoscopy and cystoscopy, without pain. Droperidol is also used as a premedication for anesthesia and as an adjunct for induction and maintenance of anesthesia. Droperidol has lost some of its earlier popularity, since clinical investigation has demonstrated that the depression of respiratory rate and alveolar ventilation may persist longer than the analgesic effect.

The onset of action for droperidol, when given either intravenously or intramuscularly, is between 3 and 10 minutes, with peak effect at 30 minutes. The duration of action is 2 to 4 hours. Alteration of consciousness may persist up to 12 hours. Droperidol is metabolized in the liver and excreted in the kidneys.

The most commonly reported side effects/adverse reactions are hypotension, hypertension, dystonia, increased hyperexcitability, anxiety, and sweating. Less frequently reported effects include bronchospasm, emergence delirium (hallucinations), chills, shivering, depression, and nightmares. Respiratory depression has been reported when the drug is used in combination with an opioid analgesic; this can lead to respiratory arrest. Concurrent use should be avoided, but if it is necessary, the dosage of the opioid should be reduced to one fourth to one third of the usual dosage. Concurrent use of other CNS depressants may result in enhanced CNS depressant effects. Table 15-3 lists dosage and administration recommendations.

TABLE 15-3 Droperidol and fentanyl (Innovar): dosage and administration

Use	Adults	Children
Premedication for general anesthesia	0.5 to 2 ml IM given ½-1 hr before surgery	Over 2 years old, 0.25 ml per 20 pounds body weight
General anesthesia adjunct		
Induction	1 ml per 20 to 25 pounds body weight administered slowly IV. Individualize dosage, since smaller dosages have been found adequate depending on client's response	
Without general anesthesia for diagnostic procedures	0.5 to 2 ml IM approximately ½-1 hr before procedure	

From *PDR* (1995).

■ Nursing Management

Droperidol

Assessment. Droperidol produces neuroleptic anesthesia. The client is usually free of pain, not necessarily asleep, easily aroused, able to cooperate, but psychologically indifferent to the environment, which is beneficial when the client must participate in the procedure. Obtain a baseline assessment of the vital signs and general physical status before drug administration. Droperidol should be used with caution in clients with renal, respiratory, cardiovascular, or hepatic impairment.

Nursing diagnosis. The client receiving droperidol may have the following nursing diagnoses: ineffective breathing pattern related to the drug's respiratory depressive effects; risk for injury related to sedation; risk for aspiration; sensory/perceptual alterations (visual and auditory); and the potential complication of decreased cardiac output related to drug-induced hypotension.

Implementation

Monitoring. Assess the client frequently for any signs of respiratory depression, because increased rigidity of the respiratory muscles may result in insufficient breathing. Since droperidol has hypotensive effects, monitor blood pressure until the drug effects have dissipated completely. Orthostatic hypotension is possible. Postoperatively, the client may not complain of pain because droperidol alters *perception* of pain. In these clients pain may manifest itself as restlessness, agitation, or any number of other nonspecific complaints.

Intervention. If the postoperative client who has received droperidol does experience pain, the normal dosage of analgesic may be decreased to one third or one fourth of the usual dosage. Droperidol potentiates the actions of barbiturates and narcotics, so the analgesic dosage will be decreased until all the droperidol is eliminated. Some alteration of consciousness may last for 12 hours after the last dose.

If the drug is given preoperatively, the client should be assisted if ambulation is necessary. Move and position the client slowly during anesthesia to prevent hypotension. If the hypotension is caused by hypovolemia, several approaches may need to be taken. Fluids may be ordered to treat hypotension, the client may be repositioned to improve venous return (supine with feet elevated), and a vasopressor may be given. Resuscitative equipment and a narcotic antagonist should be available in the immediate environment.

Evaluation. The expected outcomes for the client are: respiratory status and blood pressure remain within normal limits and sedation is achieved, and the recovery from Innovar is without adverse occurrence.

PREANESTHETIC AGENTS/ANESTHETIC ADJUNCTIVE AGENTS

Various medications are used as preanesthetic agents, or as adjuncts to anesthesia, to reduce undesirable effects produced by apprehension or by induction and maintenance of anesthesia. Table 15-4 reviews some of the common agents. Narcotic analgesics not only reduce anxiety and provide analgesia but also allow for a reduction in the dosage of anesthetic administered, because of their additive effects. See Box 15-3 for a rapid-acting opioid used during anesthesia. The administration of muscle relaxants provides surgeons easier access and increased visualization of the abdominal cavity during abdominal surgery or in cases in which controlled mechanical ventilation is required. Many nondepolarizing neuromuscular blocking agents are available, including atracurium (Tracrium), cisatracurium (Nimbex), doxacurium (Nuromax), mivacurium (Mivacron), pipecuronium (Arduan), rocuronium (Zemuron), and vecuronium (Norcuron) (Olin, 1997).

TABLE 15-4 Preanesthetic agents

Drug classification	Agents most frequently used	Desired effect
Narcotic analgesics	morphine meperidine (Demerol)	Sedation to decrease tension and anxiety; provide analgesia, and decrease amount of anesthetic used
Barbiturates	pentobarbital (Nembutal) secobarbital (Seconal)	Decreased apprehension Sedation Rapid induction
Phenothiazines	promethazine (Phenergan)	Sedation Antihistaminic Antiemetic Decreased motor activity
Anticholinergics	glycopyrrolate (Robinol) atropine scopolamine	Inhibition of secretions, vomiting, and laryngospasms, plus sedation (with scopolamine)
Skeletal muscle relaxants	succinylcholine (depolarizing) (Anectine, Quelicin, Sucostrin) *d*-tubocurarine (nondepolarizing) (Sux-cert)	Promotion of muscular relaxation

BOX 15-3

Rapid-Acting Opioid for Use during General Anesthesia

Remifentanil (Ultiva) is a short-acting analgesic used during induction and maintenance of general anesthesia and also for the immediate postoperative period. This drug should only be administered under the direct supervision of an anesthesiologist or nurse anesthetist.

A mu-receptor agonist, remifentanil has a rapid onset of action, is metabolized by nonspecific esterases in blood and tissues, and lasts between 5 to 10 minutes after the drug is discontinued. To control postoperative pain, adequate analgesia should be instituted before discontinuation of remifentanil (New Ultiva, 1996). Side/adverse effects include hypoxia, apnea, respiratory depression, and muscle rigidity. See current reference or package insert for additional information.

New Ultiva (1996). Letter from Glaxo Wellcome, Glaxo Wellcome Inc, #ULT037RO.

LOCAL ANESTHESIA

Local anesthesia refers to the direct administration of an anesthetic agent to tissues to induce the absence of sensation in a portion of the body. Unlike general anesthesia, consciousness is not depressed with local anesthesia. Local anesthetic agents may be applied to an area or injected into tissues, where they produce their effect in the immediate area only; hence the term *local anesthesia*. Local anesthetic drugs may also be injected around a nerve or nerve trunk (spinal, epidural) to produce anesthesia in a large region of the body. This is referred to as **regional anesthesia**.

SURFACE OR TOPICAL ANESTHESIA

The use of surface, or topical, anesthesia is restricted to mucous membranes, damaged skin surfaces, wounds, and burns. The anesthetic is applied in the form of a solution, ointment, gel, cream, or powder to produce loss of sensation by paralyzing afferent nerve endings. Topical anesthetics do not penetrate unbroken skin. Topical anesthesia is used to relieve pain and itching and to anesthetize mucous membranes of the eye, nose, throat, or urethra for minor surgical procedures. Cocaine in a 4% to 10% solution continues to be one of the most widely used agents for topical anesthesia.

Local anesthesia may also be achieved by freezing. Low temperatures in living tissues produce diminished sensation. This form of anesthesia is sometimes employed for minor operative procedures. A caution is that tissues that are frozen too intensely for too long may be destroyed. Ethyl chloride is a local anesthetic that can be used to produce this effect, although it is not employed extensively.

LOCAL ANESTHETICS

Local anesthetics are drugs used to abolish pain sensation in a particular part of the body (Tables 15-5 and 15-6). The basic mechanism of action of these drugs is unknown, but most act by stabilizing or elevating the threshold of excitation of the nerve cell membrane without affecting resting potential (blockage of sodium channels). This action is a result of re-

TABLE 15-5 Local anesthetics: administration and use

Method	Tissue affected	Preparation used	Examples of drugs used	Therapeutic use
Topical	Sensory nerve endings in mucous membranes and dermis	Solution Ointment Cream Powder	cocaine benzocaine ethyl aminobenzoate lidocaine tetracaine bupivacaine	Relief of pain or itching Examination of conjunctiva
Infiltration	Sensory nerve endings in subcutaneous tissues or dermis	Injection	etidocaine procaine prilocaine lidocaine chloroprocaine mepivicaine	Minor surgery
Block	Nerve trunk	Injection	etidocaine procaine prilocaine lidocaine chloroprocaine mepivacaine	Dental and limb surgery Sympathetic block
Spinal (subarachnoid block)	Spinal roots	Injection	procaine tetracaine lidocaine	Abdominal surgery Surgery of the lower extremities Muscle relaxation

duction of membrane permeability to all ions; thus depolarization and transmission of nerve impulses are prevented.

Table 15-6 presents some commonly used local anesthetics and their properties. Benzyl alcohol, an aromatic alcohol of low potency, is used topically with procaine to extend procaine's duration of action. The choice of a local anesthetic for a particular procedure depends on the duration of drug action desired. Table 15-7 lists short, intermediate, and long-acting local anesthetic drugs. Vasoconstrictors, such as epinephrine and norepinephrine, are used with the local anesthetic to decrease systemic absorption and prolong the anesthetic's duration of action. They are not used for nerve blocks in areas where there are end arteries (fingers, toes, ears, nose, penis) because ischemia may develop, resulting in gangrene.

A number of local anesthetic agents cannot be injected. However, because they are absorbed slowly, they can be used safely on open wounds, ulcers, and mucous membranes. They occasionally cause dermatitis and allergic sensitization, which necessitate their discontinuance. The ester-type local anesthetics (cocaine, procaine, tetracaine, benzocaine) are metabolized to *p*-aminobenzoic acid (PABA) metabolites, which are mainly responsible for allergic reactions in some clients. The amide anesthetics (lidocaine, mepivacaine, bupivacaine, etidocaine, prilocaine) are not metabolized to PABA derivatives; thus allergic reactions induced by these anesthetics are very rare (Katzung, 1992).

Topical anesthetics for skin disorders are used primarily to relieve pruritus, discomfort, pain, and soreness; indications for mucous membranes are similar. The anesthetics are poorly absorbed through the intact skin, but from mucous membranes and skin breaks and sores (e.g., abrasions, trauma, and ulcers) absorption is increased, leading to the possibility of systemic involvement. When they are employed in the oral cavity (mouth and pharynx), interference with swallowing may occur and the client is at risk for aspiration. The client is assessed for a returning gag reflex by gentle touching of the back of the pharynx with a tongue blade. All food and fluid are withheld until the reflex returns.

Local anesthetics are capable of abolishing all sensation, but pain fibers are affected first, probably because they are thinner, unmyelinated, and more easily penetrated by these drugs. Loss of pain is followed in sequence by loss of response to cold, warmth, touch, and pressure. Most motor fibers also can be anesthetized when an adequate concentration of the drug is present over sufficient time.

The parenteral local anesthetics have complete systemic absorption, which is decreased by the addition of a vasoconstrictor such as epinephrine. The half-lives of selected anesthetics are as follows: bupivacaine, 3½ hours; etidocaine, 2¾ hours; lidocaine, 1½ hours; and mepivacaine, 2 hours. Onset of action is a function of the anesthetic technique employed, the type of block desired, dosage, and the pK_a (negative logarithm of ionization constant) of each anesthetic.

TABLE 15-6 Properties of commonly used local anesthetics

	Procaine	Cocaine	Benzocaine
Trade names	Novocain	—	Americaine Hurricaine
Potency	—	2-3 times that of procaine	Very low
Onset of action	2-5 min	1 min	Immediate
Duration	½-1 hr	½-1 hr	15-20 min
Dose	0.25%-2%, depending on method of administration 10% for spinal anesthesia Not used topically	1%-4% topically	Variable 5%-20% ointment topically
Toxicity	Least toxic of all local anesthetics	More toxic than procaine when injected subcutaneously	Relatively nontoxic
Precautions	Overdose of rapid injection may cause CNS stimulation	Not recommended for infiltration, nerve block, or spinal anesthesia Repeated use causes psychologic dependence	Suitable for topical use only Sensitization may develop

The time it takes for a drug to reach a peak concentration depends on the type of block but ranges from 10 to 30 minutes.

Reactions to Local Anesthetics

Local anesthetics produce vasodilation by direct action on blood vessels and by anesthetizing sympathetic vasoconstrictor fibers. This action can cause rapid absorption of the drug; when the rate of absorption exceeds the rate of elimination, toxic effects can occur. To decrease rate of absorption and incidence of toxic effects by allowing more time for metabolic degradation and to prolong local anesthetic effects, epinephrine or other vasoconstrictor drugs are used. The dosages of vasoconstrictors must be carefully determined to prevent ischemic necrosis at the injection site. Since local anesthetics are potentially toxic drugs, a client's age, weight, physical condition, and liver function must be taken into account in determining drug dosage. Most reactions to local anesthetics result from overdosage, rapid absorption into systemic circulation, or individual hypersensitivity or allergic response.

Central nervous system. At first the CNS may be stimulated and cause anxiety, restlessness, confusion, dizziness, tremors, and even convulsions. Then depression may occur, and unconsciousness and death may ensue.

Cardiovascular system. Myocardial depression, bradycardia, and hypotension can occur because of smooth muscle relaxation and inhibition of neuromuscular conduction. The client suddenly becomes pale, feels faint, and has a drop in blood pressure. Cardiac arrest can be the result of a cardiovascular reaction.

Anesthetics containing a vasoconstrictor are employed with caution in clients receiving drugs that may change blood pressure, such as monoamine oxidase inhibitors, phenothiazines, and tricyclic antidepressants. The combination may produce severe hypotension or hypertension. Cardiac dysrhythmias occur when catecholamine vasoconstrictors (e.g., epinephrine) are used in clients receiving cyclopropane, halothane, or trichloroethylene.

Allergic reaction. True allergic reactions are said to be uncommon. Sometimes a reaction is thought to be allergic when it is really caused by overdosage. However, allergic reactions can occur. They may be relatively mild (hives, itching, skin rash), or they may be acutely anaphylactic.

The allergic reactions are characteristically manifested by cutaneous lesions, urticaria, or edema. They may result from various factors, such as hypersensitivity, idiosyncrasy, or diminished tolerance. These rare allergic reactions are usually limited to the ester type of anesthetics. The most important risk of local anesthetics is a dose-related CNS toxicity, which may progress from sleepiness to convulsion.

Small test doses are frequently given to gauge the extent of the client's sensitivity to the anesthetic agent. The anesthetic agent chosen, its concentration, the rate of injection, and physical and emotional factors in the client all influence reactions to local anesthetics.

■ Nursing Management

Local Anesthetics

Unlike general anesthetics, nurses often administer topical local anesthetic agents. Therefore the nurse has a much broader role in relating to these agents.

Assessment. Assess the client for previous response to local anesthetics and the existence of preexisting diseases or drug allergies.

Nursing diagnosis. The following nursing diagnoses may be identified with the client receiving a local anesthetic agent: pain related to an inadequate block, risk for injury related to the loss of sensation, and decreased cardiac output related to adverse response to drug. The potential complication of allergic reaction exists.

Lidocaine	Tetracaine	Mepivacaine
Xylocaine	Pontocaine	Carbocaine
2 times that of procaine 2-5 min 1-3 hr 0.5%-4% for injection 2% and 5% topically	10 times that of procaine 3-10 min 1->3 hr 1% topically 0.15%-0.25% for injection	2 times that of procaine Less rapid than procaine 1-3 hr 1%-2% solution
See procaine When administered rapidly or in large doses, may cause convulsions and hypotension	More toxic than procaine, but toxic effects rare because of low dosage used Drug interaction with cholinesterase inhibitors and sulfonamides	2 times that of procaine; less than lidocaine Combined with vasoconstrictor to delay drug absorption and prolong duration Avoid in pregnancy—may cause constriction of uterine artery

TABLE 15-7 Selected injected local anesthetic drugs: pharmacokinetic overview

Name	Metabolism	Use	Dosage and administration
Short-acting (½-1 hr)			
procaine (Novocain)	Ester compound—same as chloroprocaine	Infiltration, nerve block, spinal anesthesia, epidural block	Usual adult dosage for infiltration: 350-600 mg as 0.25%-0.5% solution Peripheral nerve block: 500 mg as 0.5%, 1%, or 2% solution Spinal and epidural dosage, vary with individual client, procedure, and degree of anesthesia desired Pediatric dosage: not available
chloroprocaine (Nesacaine, Nesacaine-MPF)	Ester compound—metabolized by cholinesterases in plasma and liver to a PABA compound. Excretion: kidneys	Nesacaine—infiltration and regional anesthesia Nesacaine-CE—for caudal and epidural anesthesia	Usual adult dosage for infiltration nerve blocks: 30-800 mg as 1% or 2% solutions, depending on site and length of surgical procedure Caudal and epidural: 40-500 mg as 2% or 3% solution, without epinephrine Usual pediatric dosage for infiltration nerve blocks: up to 20 mg/kg body weight
Intermediate duration (1-3 hr)			
lidocaine (Xylocaine, Xylocard♣)	Amide compound Metabolism: liver to active and toxic metabolites Excretion: kidneys	Infiltration, nerve block, spinal epidural	Usual adult dosage depends on site and length of surgical procedure Pediatric dosage: same as adult Lidocaine is available with and without epinephrine
mepivacaine (Carbocaine)	Amide compound—see above	Infiltration, nerve blocks, caudal, epidural	Available alone and with levonordefrin (vasoconstrictor). Dosage depends on site and length of surgical procedure Adult maximum dosage: Dental, up to 6.6 mg/kg body weight (300 mg maximum per appointment). Other usages, up to 7 mg/kg body weight. Pediatric, up to 5 or 6 mg/kg body weight

Continued

TABLE 15-7 Selected injected local anesthetic drugs: pharmacokinetic overview—cont'd

Name	Metabolism	Use	Dosage and administration
Intermediate duration (1-3 hr)—cont'd			
prilocaine (Citanest, Citanest Forte)	Amide compound—see above	Infiltration, peripheral nerve blocks, caudal, epidural	Available alone or with epinephrine (vasoconstrictor). Although dosages vary with site and length of procedure, the adult maximum dosages are as follows: Dental, up to 400 mg as a 4% solution in 2-hr period. Other procedures, individualize. Pediatric maximum: Dental, children up to 10 yr, 40 mg (4% solution) maximum. Other procedures, individualize
Long duration (3-10 hr)			
bupivacaine (Marcaine, Sensorcaine)	Amide type—see above	Infiltration, caudal, epidural, peripheral nerve blocks	Available alone or with dextrose (Marcaine spinal) or with epinephrine. Dosages vary with site, additional drugs, and length of procedure
etidocaine (Duranest)	Amide type—see above	Infiltration; peripheral nerve blocks, caudal and epidural nerve blocks	Available alone and with epinephrine. Dosages vary with site and length of procedure
tetracaine (Pontocaine)	Ester compound—see above	Saddle block (low spinal), up to costal margin, spinal anesthesia	Available alone and with dextrose. Dosages vary with site and length of procedure

Implementation

Monitoring. During and after administration of a local anesthetic, monitor the client for signs of pain, allergy, or other adverse reactions. Minimal monitoring parameters for clients receiving local anesthesia should include blood pressure, heart rate and rhythm, respiratory rate, oxygen saturation, skin condition, and mental status. It is especially important to monitor hypertension and cardiac status for dysrhythmias when a local anesthetic containing a vasoconstrictor such as epinephrine is administered.

Intervention. Do not use the local anesthetic solution if it is cloudy, discolored, or if it contains crystals. Solutions that do not contain preservatives should be discarded after the vial has been opened. Most commercial preparations of local anesthetic agents are acidic solutions. Some surgeons may adjust the pH of the solution by mixing it with sodium bicarbonate to decrease pain upon infiltration. This increase in pH is also reported to make the onset more rapid and increase the duration of sensory analgesia (Watson, 1991).

Resuscitative equipment must be available in case the client has an anaphylactic reaction.

If local anesthetics are used as ointments or creams, thoroughly cleanse and dry the area before applying. When the suppository form of the agent is used, chill in the refrigerator 30 minutes, remove wrapper, and moisten with water or lubricant to insert.

Note that when local anesthetics are used topically in the nose or throat, they may cause paralysis of the upper respiratory tract, leading to possible aspiration. Measure the preparation accurately. Apply it with a cotton swab; swishing should be used for mouth and gums and gargling for application to the throat. Do not allow the local anesthetic to be swallowed unless specifically cleared with the prescriber. After local anesthesia of the nasopharyngeal area, test for the adequacy of the client's gag reflex by touching the back of the throat with a tongue depressor or swab. Food or drink should be withheld until this reflex returns, to prevent aspiration.

The client who has regional anesthesia needs to be protected from trauma to the anesthetized portion of the body, since the perception of pain and pressure, the body's normal protective mechanism, has been diminished or obliterated. Pressure from side rails and other objects normally perceived and avoided by the client may cause injury.

After the use of spinal anesthetics, the client should be well hydrated and remain lying down for up to 12 hours to minimize the risk of spinal headache.

Education (for local anesthetics that may be self-administered by the client). Instruct the client to use the preparation exactly as prescribed—not to use more, or more often, or for a longer period of time. Caution the client not to inhale while using the topical aerosol or spray dosage forms. Instruct the client in the use of the provided applicator for rectal aerosol foam preparation. Avoid using if bleeding hemorrhoids are present.

If local anesthetic preparations are used topically in the nose or throat, instruct the client not to eat for 1 hour after administration, since this may lead to aspiration. Because of the variability in response, each client must be able to swallow before food is offered. Advise the client not to chew gum while the anesthetic is in effect, since there is the risk of biting the tongue or buccal mucosa.

Evaluation. The expected outcome is that the client experiences an effective sensory block without any adverse response to the drug.

ANESTHESIA BY INJECTION

Anesthesia by injection is accomplished by infiltration or by conduction (spinal, caudal, or saddle block).

Infiltration anesthesia is produced by injecting dilute solutions (0.1%) of the agent into the skin and then subcutaneously into the region to be anesthetized. Epinephrine often is added to the solution to intensify the anesthesia in a limited region and to prevent excessive bleeding and systemic effects. Repeated injection will prolong the anesthesia as long as needed. The sensory nerve endings are anesthetized. This method of administration is used for minor surgery such as incision and drainage or excision of a cyst (see Table 15-7).

Conduction (block) **anesthesia** means a loss of sensation, especially pain, in a region of the body, produced by injecting a local anesthetic into the vicinity of a nerve trunk and thus inhibiting the conduction of impulses to and from the area supplied by that nerve, the region of the operative site. The injection may be made at some distance from the surgical site. A single nerve may be blocked, or the anesthetic may be injected where several nerve trunks emerge from the spinal cord (paravertebral block). A more concentrated solution is required because of the thickness of nerve trunk fibers. This method of anesthesia is often used for foot and hand surgery.

Spinal anesthesia is a type of extensive nerve block sometimes called a subarachnoid block. The anesthetic solution is injected into the subarachnoid space and affects the lower part of the spinal cord and nerve roots.

For low spinal anesthesia, the client is placed in a flat or Fowler's position. A solution with a specific gravity greater than that of cerebrospinal fluid is used, since it tends to diffuse downward. For high spinal anesthesia, Trendelenburg's position with the head sharply flexed is used, along with an anesthetic solution of lower specific gravity than that of cerebrospinal fluid (which tends to diffuse upward) or a solution with the same specific gravity as cerebrospinal fluid (which may diffuse upward or downward, depending on position used). Solutions with the same specific gravity as cerebrospinal fluid act primarily at the site of injection.

The onset of anesthesia usually occurs within 1 to 2 minutes after injection. The duration of anesthesia is 1 to 3 hours, depending on the anesthetic used. Spinal anesthesia is used for surgical procedures on the lower abdomen, inguinal area, or lower extremities. It may be the method of choice for clients with severe respiratory problems or with liver, kidney, or metabolic disease. Marked hypotension, decreased cardiac output, and respiratory inadequacy tend to occur during anesthesia and are considered to be disadvantages of this method of anesthesia.

Postoperatively, headache is the most common complaint; this may be accompanied by difficulty in hearing or seeing. Headache may be postural and occur only in the head-up or sitting or standing position. This symptom is the result of the opening in the dura made by the large spinal needle, which may persist for days or weeks, permitting loss of cerebrospinal fluid.

Headache and auditory and visual problems after lumbar puncture result from decreased intracranial pressure. These symptoms usually are alleviated when cerebrospinal fluid pressure returns to normal. Paresthesias such as numbness and tingling may occur after spinal anesthesia; they are usually limited to the lumbar or sacral areas and disappear within a relatively short time. The success and safety of spinal anesthesia depend primarily on the anesthetist's skill and knowledge.

Caudal anesthesia is produced by injecting an anesthetic solution into the caudal canal, the sacral part of the vertebral canal containing the cauda equina, or the bundle of spinal nerves that innervates the pelvic viscera. It is used in obstetrics and for pelvic or genital surgery. Its advantage over spinal anesthesia is that the anesthetic does not have direct access to the spinal cord and medullary centers. Thus the respiratory muscles and blood pressure are not directly affected, and undesirable effects are less likely to occur.

Saddle block is sometimes used in obstetrics and for surgery involving the perineum, rectum, genitalia, and upper parts of the thighs. The client sits upright while the anesthetic is injected after a lumbar puncture. The client remains upright for a short time, until the anesthetic has taken effect. The body parts that contact a saddle when riding become anesthetized; hence the name.

Injectable Local Anesthetics

The injectable local anesthetics are listed in Table 15-7. Generally the onset of action for an anesthetic is the result of drug concentration and the targeted nerve-tissue area. Potency and duration of anesthetic action increase with a drug's lipid solubility. For more information on metabolism, indications, and pharmacokinetics, see Table 15-7.

Side effects/adverse reactions. The adverse reactions of injected local anesthetics generally require medical intervention.

Cyanosis caused by methemoglobinemia is one of the most common adverse reactions reported with an epidural block or high spinal injection. It has been reported with all local anesthetics but is most prevalent with prilocaine (Citanest). Symptoms may include weakness, breathing difficulties, increased heart rate, dizziness, or collapse.

Other reactions reported with an epidural block or high spinal injection include diaphoresis, hypotension, bradycardia or irregular heart rate, pale skin color (cardiovascular depression), diplopia, seizures, tinnitus, increased excitability, shivering, involuntary shaking (caused by stimulation of CNS), nausea, and vomiting.

Effects most commonly reported with ester compounds include skin rash and an allergic reaction manifested by edema of face, lip, mouth, or throat. Anaphylaxis and severe hypotension are reported rarely.

With central nerve block anesthesia, the most common adverse reactions are in the form of neuropathies or neurologic effects, including headaches. Other adverse reactions include paresthesia or paralysis of lower legs, breathing difficulties, severe hypotension, bradycardia, and backache. Some clients report a reduction or loss of sexual functions, bladder control, or bowel movements.

Meningitis-type effects are most often reported with spinal anesthesia. These include headaches, nausea, vomiting, and stiff or sore neck.

Allergic effects manifested by dental anesthesia are numbing or tingling of lips and mouth, as well as edema of lips or mouth, while sympathomimetic or adrenergic effects are reported with epinephrine or other vasoconstrictors. These most commonly include hypertension, shaking, increased anxiety or nervousness, tachycardia, headache, and chest pain.

Significant drug interactions. The significant drug interactions are limited, but this does not preclude a variety of unexpected responses, thus indicating the need for close observation.

Prior or concurrent administration of CNS depressant drugs may result in additive CNS depression effects. Adjust dosages and monitor closely.

Vasoconstrictor agents, such as epinephrine, norepinephrine, or phenylephrine, in combination with local anesthetics may cause impaired circulation of the area, resulting in sloughing of tissue. If vasoconstrictor agents are used for end arteries, such as toes or fingers, ischemia resulting in gangrene may develop. Extreme caution is advised.

Dosage and administration. See Table 15-7.

SUMMARY

Anesthetic agents are invaluable in the limiting of pain and suffering. By either altering consciousness or interfering with the conduction of impulses to the pain centers of the central nervous system, these agents allow surgical procedures and other painful therapies to be performed.

There are two major categories of anesthesia: general and regional or local. General anesthesia may be achieved either intravenously or by inhalation. Regional anesthesia is obtained by injecting an anesthetic drug near a nerve trunk or into a specific site. Local anesthesia may be accomplished by topical application or by infiltration of the operative area. Because no anesthetic agent produces analgesia, muscle relaxation, unconsciousness, and amnesic effects with perfect safety, generally a combination of agents is used, each for its specific effect; this technique is called balanced anesthesia.

Although nurses do not administer general anesthetics unless they are certified nurse anesthetists, they may be called upon to assist the physician to a degree depending on the clinical setting. And it is necessary for the nurse to have an understanding of the effects of anesthetic agents in order to provide appropriate nursing care in the perioperative period. In the preoperative period, the emphasis of the nurse is on the thorough assessment and preparation of the client to alleviate anxiety and to minimize the potential for physiologic injury intraoperatively and in the postoperative period. Immediately after surgery, the need is to help the client to recover from the effects of the anesthetic safely, comfortably, and as quickly as possible. Common postoperative complications for which the nurse should be alert are hypotension, nausea and vomiting, hypoventilation, oliguria, nerve injury, paralytic ileus, thrombosis, shock, atelectasis, hypothermia/hyperthermia, and malignant hyperthermia.

Inhalation therapy can be administered by gases or volatile liquids. Because these agents are primarily exhaled and excreted through the lungs, their anesthetic effect can be rapidly reversed if respiration is maintained satisfactorily.

Intravenous anesthetic agents are used to induce amnesia, for induction and maintenance of general anesthesia, and as adjuncts to inhalation anesthetics. Because of the risk of respiratory and cardiovascular depression, the client's vital signs need to be closely monitored and resuscitation equipment must be at hand in the clinical setting where these agents are administered.

Neuroleptanesthesia is a type of general anesthesia that results from the combined use of a neuroleptic agent and a narcotic analgesic; it is used for procedures in which the client's cooperation is desired. Although easily aroused, the client remains psychologically indifferent to events; however, hypotension and respiratory depression may still occur.

With local anesthesia consciousness is not depressed, but a portion of the body is rendered insensitive to pain. Because the perception of pain and pressure is a protective mechanism of the body, the observations of the nurse are important to ensure that the client does not aspirate (if topical anesthesia has been used in the nose and throat) or that tissue damage does not occur through trauma to anesthetized parts of the body.

The role of the nurse in the administration of anesthetics is generally not a direct one, but one in which assessment and the protection of the client take priority.

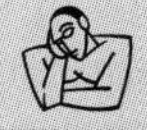

Critical Thinking

1. Mrs. Clarke, age 42, has been admitted to the hospital for an abdominal hysterectomy. On the night before surgery, as you are reviewing the preoperative routine with her, she asks why she should get an injection before she goes to the operating room. How do you respond?
2. Differentiate between the different regional block anesthesias—caudal, saddle, and spinal. Under what circumstances would each be the regional block of choice?
3. What would be the additional nursing observations required if the client received a local anesthetic with epinephrine rather than one without epinephrine?

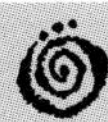

Collaborative Learning Activities

1. Analyze an actual anesthesia record from a clinical record, identifying the type of anesthesia used, route of administration, fluctuation in client's vital signs throughout the course of anesthesia, fluids administered compared with fluids lost, any other data provided, and any problems or complications encountered during anesthesia administration.
2. Students will develop a postoperative plan of care for the client whose anesthesia record was examined based on this client's specific anesthesia experience.

BIBLIOGRAPHY

American Hospital Formulary Service (1996). *AHFS drug information '96*. Bethesda, MD: American Society of Hospital Pharmacists.

Anderson KN, et al. (Eds.) (1994). *Mosby's medical, nursing, & allied health dictionary* (4th ed.). St Louis: Mosby.

Beare PG & Myers JL (1998). *Principles and practice of adult health nursing* (3rd ed.). St Louis: Mosby.

Carpenito LJ (1995). *Nursing diagnosis: Application to clinical practice* (6th ed.). Philadelphia: JB Lippincott.

Katzung BG (1992). *Basic and clinical pharmacology* (5th ed.). Norwalk, CT: Appleton & Lange.

Kendall F (1993). Documenting local anesthesia patient care, *AORN J* 58(4):715.

Meyer C (1993). New drugs: A faster exit from recovery, *Amer J Nurs* 93(9):50.

Olin BR (Ed.) (1995). *Facts and comparisons*. St. Louis: Facts and Comparisons.

Olin BR (Ed.) (1997). *Facts and comparisons*. St. Louis: Facts and Comparisons.

Parnass SM (1993). Ambulatory surgical patient priorities, *Nurs Clin North Amer* 28(3):531-45.

Phillips M (1994). Into the land of Nod: Drugs used during anesthesia in day surgery, *Canad Oper Room Nurs J* 12(4):5-9.

Physician's desk reference (1995). (49th ed.). Montvale, NJ: Medical Economics.

Riley TN & DeRuiter J (1993). New drugs 1992, *US Pharmacist* 18(3):35.

Smith CJ (1994). *Preparing nurses to monitor patients receiving local anesthesia: Using the decision-making process*, *AORN J* 59(5):1036-41.

United States Pharmacopeia Convention (1996). *USP DI: Drug information for the health care provider* (16th ed.). Rockville, MD: The Convention.

United States Pharmacopeia Convention (1995). *USP DI: Volumes I and II update*. (November). Rockville, MD: The Convention.

Wangaman WR & Foster SD (1991). New advances in anesthesia, *Nurs Clin North Amer* 26(2):451.

Watson DS (1991). Safe nursing practices involving the patient receiving local anesthesia, *AORN J* 53(4):1055.

Chapter 16

Antianxiety, Sedative, and Hypnotic Drugs

Chapter Focus

Anxiety and sleep disorders are common health problems across the life span. Anxiety with apprehension, tension, or uneasiness related to anticipated danger is often a normal and beneficial response to a situation. However, excessive anxiety can interfere with daily functioning. As a group, the anxiety disorders affect about 15% of the population. During the course of a year 35% of adults report episodes of insomnia, making it by far the most common sleep disorder. The antianxiety, sedative, and hypnotic drugs discussed in this chapter, along with supportive nursing care, should enable clients to increase their psychologic and physiologic comfort. The following objectives and key terms are important for a good understanding of this chapter.

Key Terms

amnesic effect (p. 303)
antianxiety or anxiolytic agent (p. 297)
anxiety (p. 297)
hypnotic (p. 297)
insomnia (p. 300)
non-REM sleep (p. 297)
REM sleep (p. 297)
sedative (p. 297)

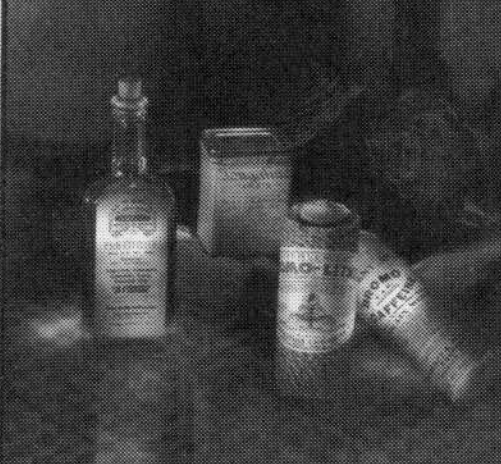

Key Drug [▲]

diazepam

Objectives

1. Describe the physiology and stages of sleep.
2. Differentiate between antianxiety, sedative, and hypnotic drug effects.
3. Discuss specific nursing interventions for the use of antianxiety, sedative, and hypnotic agents in pediatric and geriatric clients.
4. Identify the characteristics of commonly used benzodiazepines and barbiturates.
5. Formulate an appropriate plan of care for a specific client who requires the administration of an antianxiety, sedative, or hypnotic agent.

The **antianxiety** or **anxiolytic agents** reduce feelings of excessive anxiety, such as apprehension, fear, nervousness, worry or panic. **Anxiety** is a state or feeling of apprehension, uneasiness, agitation, uncertainty, and fear resulting from the anticipation of some threat or danger, usually of intrapsychic origin, whose source is generally unknown or unrecognized. It is usually a normal psychologic and physiologic response to a personally threatening situation, such as a threat to one's health, body, loved ones, job, or lifestyle. Generally this anxiety stimulates the person to take a purposeful or deliberate action to counteract or offset the anxiety-producing state. When a person is unable to cope with a persistently stressful situation because excessive anxiety interferes with daily functioning, help is necessary. Although many nonpharmacologic modalities are available, antianxiety agents are commonly prescribed for the treatment of anxiety. For proposed site of action for the benzodiazepines, see the section on the limbic system in Chapter 13, Overview of the Central Nervous System.

Sedatives are CNS depressant drugs that were commonly prescribed before the advent of the benzodiazepine family. Their general use today has declined. Sedatives are chemical substances that reduce nervousness, excitability, or irritability by producing a calming or soothing effect. **Hypnotics** are drugs used to induce sleep. The major difference between a sedative and a hypnotic is the degree of CNS depression induced. A small dose may be used for a sedative effect, whereas larger dosages may be used for hypnotic effects. Barbiturates have been used extensively as sedative-hypnotic agents, but because of their low degree of selectivity and safety, they have been largely replaced by the safer benzodiazepines.

PHYSIOLOGY OF SLEEP

Sleep is a recurrent, normal condition of inertia and unresponsiveness during which an individual's overt and covert responses to stimuli are markedly reduced. During sleep a person is no longer in sensory contact with the immediate environment and stimuli that have bombarded the senses of sight, hearing, touch, smell, and taste during waking hours. Such factors no longer attract attention or exert a controlling influence over voluntary and involuntary movements or functions. It is not difficult to understand that everyone needs to escape from constant stimuli.

Research has shown that sleep is not one level of unconsciousness; it consists of two basic stages that occur cyclically:

1. Non-rapid eye movement (non-REM)
2. Rapid eye movement (REM)

During sleep the individual moves through the four stages of **non-REM sleep** (the first four stages of sleep characterized on an electroencephalogram (EEG) by alpha waves, slow and of low amplitude), with stage 4 considered the deepest level of non-REM sleep, and then through **REM sleep**, the fifth stage of sleep, characterized by rapid eye movement, dreaming, and by delta waves on EEG (Figure 16-1). Alternating periods of REM and non-REM sleep occur throughout the night (McCance & Huether, 1994). It should be kept in mind that REM sleep is not synonymous with light sleep. It takes a more powerful stimulus to arouse a person from REM sleep than from synchronous slow-wave sleep.

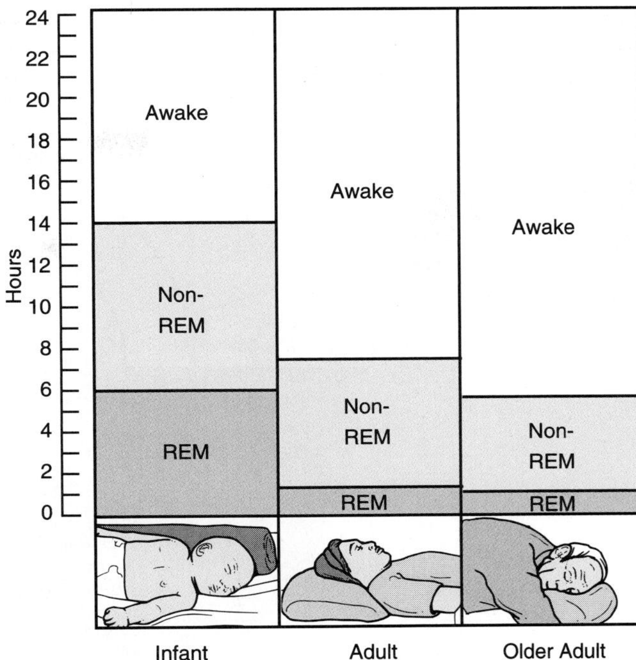

Figure 16-1 Sleep-wake cycles across the life span. Infants: approximately 40% of total sleep time is REM. Adults: 20% of total sleep time is REM. Older adults: total sleep time is slightly reduced; REM remains 20% of total. (From Beare PB & Myers JL (1994). Principles and practice of adult health nursing [2nd ed.]. St. Louis: Mosby.)

The stages of sleep are based on electrical activity that can be observed in the brain by means of an electroencephalogram (EEG). The EEG provides graphic illustrations of brain waves, which are an indication of the electrical activity occurring in the brain (Figure 16-2).

Sleep research indicates that there are psychologic and physiologic reasons for the body to maintain an equilibrium between the various stages of sleep. The physiologic functions of the body tend to be depressed during nondreaming sleep. For example, it is known that:

1. Blood pressure falls (10 to 30 mm Hg)
2. Pulse rate is slowed
3. Metabolic rate is decreased
4. Gastrointestinal tract activity is slowed
5. Urine formation slows
6. Oxygen consumption and carbon dioxide production are lowered
7. Body temperature decreases slightly
8. Respirations are slower and more shallow
9. Body movement is minimal

Dreaming sleep tends to increase most of these parameters. Body movements are more noticeable—turning, jerking, moving of the arms and legs, talking, crying, or laughing and,

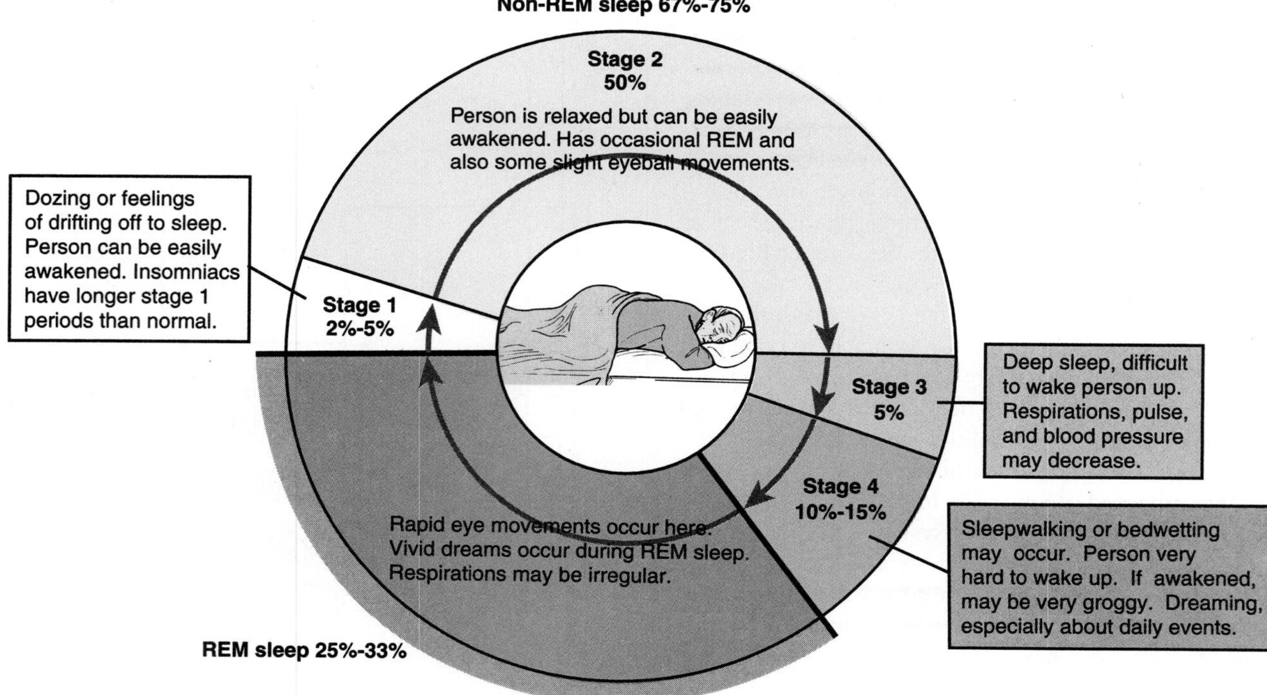

Figure 16-2 Stages of sleep.

of course, eye movements show under the closed lids. The dynamic physiologic equilibrium of the body continues to be maintained even during sleep. Depression of physiologic functions occurs during deep sleep, and an increase in functions occurs during dreaming. Studies have shown that when individuals are deprived of deep sleep, they become physically uncomfortable, tend to withdraw from their friends and society, are less aggressive and outgoing, and manifest concern over vague physical complaints and changes in bodily feelings. The overall impression made by persons deprived of deep sleep is that of a depressive and hypochondriac reaction.

Dream sleep is also important as studies indicate that individuals deprived of dreaming sleep (every time the subjects attempted to dream, as evidenced by rapid eye movements, they were awakened and not permitted to dream), had a variety of undesirable effects afterward. During waking hours the individuals became less integrated and less effective and exhibited signs of confusion, suspicion, and withdrawal. They appeared anxious, insecure, and irritable; they had greater difficulty concentrating; they had a marked increase in appetite with a definite weight gain; and they were introspective and unable to derive support from other people.

Many psychologists and psychiatrists believe that wish fulfillment finds expression in dreams, and potentially harmful thoughts, feelings, and impulses are released through dreams so that there is no interference with the functioning of the personality during waking hours.

It is also known from dream deprivation studies that the longer dream deprivation continues, the greater the increase in attempts to dream, until the individual begins to dream almost on falling asleep. When subjects are finally allowed to dream, a marked increase in dreaming is noted for the entire night, and as much as 75% of the night may be spent in dreaming. This amount diminishes for each succeeding recovery night until the individual has again established his or her normal sleep pattern.

Research has shown that deep sleep takes priority over dreaming sleep when there has been prolonged sleep deprivation. In other words, deep sleep needs will be met first, after which dreaming sleep needs will be met. The body then attempts to reestablish the normal equilibrium between the sleep stages.

Each individual establishes his or her own normal sleep pattern, which may vary from night to night and which is influenced by the individual's emotional and physical state. For most individuals, any alteration in sleeping habits will cause problems in falling asleep, staying asleep, or both. Because drugs affect physical and emotional states, they also influence an individual's sleep pattern. Box 16-1 lists selected drugs that may cause insomnia.

PEDIATRIC DRUG USE

The use of antianxiety, sedative, or hypnotic agents in children is limited. Because young children are much more sensitive to the CNS-depressant effects of this classification of drugs, counseling and psychotherapy are usually tried first. Paradoxical reactions, or reactions contrary to the expected reaction, have been reported with the use of barbiturates in both children and geriatric clients. These reactions include increased excitability, hostility, confusion, hallucinations,

BOX 16-1

Drugs Associated with Inducing Insomnia

alcohol
beta-adrenergic blocking agents (Inderal, etc.)
captropril (Capoten)
CNS stimulants (caffeine, Ritalin, etc.)
enalapril (Vasotec)
fluoroquinolones (Cipro, Floxin, Maxaquin, Noroxin, Penetrex)
gemfibrozil (Lopid)
levodopa (Larodopa, etc.)
levothyroxine (Synthroid, etc.)
maprotiline (Ludiomil, etc.)
methyldopa (Aldomet, etc.)
metoclopramide (Reglan, etc.)
metronidazole (Flagyl, etc.)
nicotine
nicotine gum (Nicorette)
oxybutynin (Ditropan, etc.)
protriptyline (Vivactil)
pentoxifylline (Trental)
phenylpropanolamine combinations (Contac, Dimetapp, Triaminic, etc.)
pseudoephedrine combinations (Seldane-D, Sudafed, etc.)
quinapril (Accupril)
theophylline (Slo-Bid, Theo-24, Theobid, etc.)
thyroid

Withdrawal from CNS depressants
alcohol
barbiturates
tricyclic antidepressants, such as amitriptyline, imipramine, doxepin, and trimipramine
triazolam (Halcion)
hypnotic drugs

Miscellaneous drugs with potential for inducing insomnia
contraceptives, oral
phenytoin
corticosteroids
MAO inhibitors

and perhaps an acute elevation of body temperature. However, sedation may be indicated for particular situations if the drug and dosage are carefully selected for the individual child (e.g., the treatment of severe anxiety associated with an acute attack of asthma, as an adjunct preanesthetic agent, or in the treatment of convulsive disorders). Close monitoring and assessment by the health care providers is required (see the Pediatric Implications box at right).

GERIATRIC DRUG USE

Although they make up approximately 12% of our population, geriatric Americans consume between 35% and 40% of all sedative hypnotics prescribed. The elderly have more fragmented sleeping patterns, they go to bed earlier and wake up earlier and may take multiple daytime naps. This in part may be due to the changes in the stages of sleep pattern reported in this age group, such as a progressive decline in REM sleep (Gottlieb, 1990).

The Federal guidelines for use of hypnotics in long-term care residents specify that: (a) short-acting benzodiazepines should be tried before the long-acting agents are used; (b) hypnotic agents should not be used for more than 10 consecutive days in any 30-day period; and (c) no benzodiazepine should be used longer than 3 to 4 months for treatment of anxiety (Regimen, 1995).

Careful drug selection and dosage are necessary to avoid producing excessive CNS depression in the elderly. The aging process may also be associated with physiologic alter-

Pediatric Implications

Antianxiety agents and sedatives

Young children are more susceptible to the CNS-depressant effects of the benzodiazepines. In neonates, profound CNS depression may result because of the lower rate of drug metabolism by the immature liver.

Chronic use of clonazepam may result in impaired physical or mental functions in the developing child, which may not become apparent until years later.

Buspirone use has not been studied in persons under 18 years; therefore it is not recommended for use in this age group.

Although diazepam (Valium) may be used in infants 6 months and over, this drug and other benzodiazepines should not be used to treat a hyperactive or psychotic child.

To reduce or minimize potential adverse CNS-depressant effects, carefully follow the manufacturer's dosage instructions and, whenever possible, avoid concurrent administration of other CNS-depressant types of drugs.

Monitor child for excessive sedation, lethargy, and lack of coordination; if any of these effects are present, dosage adjustments may be necessary.

Paradoxical reactions have been reported in both children and the elderly with the use of barbiturates. (See description under Pediatric Drug Use, p. 298)

ations, including a decline in metabolism and in many organ functions, especially liver and kidney functions. Because drug half-lives may be extended, agents with shorter half-lives and no active metabolites may be safer for the geriatric client. Monitor the elderly client for paradoxical reactions (i.e., increased excitability, rage, hostility, confusion, and hallucinations), which have been reported with the barbiturates and, in rare instances, the benzodiazepines. The appearance of such adverse reactions requires immediate discontinuance of the medication and consultation with the prescriber. See Chapter 8 for additional information on inappropriate drug use in the elderly.

The short-acting benzodiazepines are much safer than the barbiturates, which are less effective anxiolytic and hypnotic agents. Oxazepam, lorazepam, temazepam, alprazolam, and triazolam have short to intermediate half-lives, and they are usually recommended for an elderly client who requires a benzodiazepine. Barbiturates should be avoided in the elderly because enhanced CNS depression, confusion, ataxia, and paradoxical reactions are commonly reported.

One of the most frequent concerns of the elderly is **insomnia,** difficulty falling asleep, staying asleep, or early morning awaking. See the Geriatric Implications box below for discussion. Age-related physiologic changes may also contribute to the changes in sleep patterns reported. Many other factors may also result in sleep disturbances, such as retirement, death of a close friend or spouse, social isolation, increased use of medications, and many other issues.

A study of 430 geriatric persons reported that the most common sleep-related problem was staying asleep (Dopheide, 1995). The three most common reasons for not being able to maintain sleep were respiratory difficulties, pain, and muscle or leg cramps. Appropriate therapy for insomnia should be limited to identification of the cause and treatment of the specific problem.

Gottlieb (1990) indicates that older women report more difficulties with their sleeping patterns than men, are more apt to take hypnotic medications than men, and that sleep deprivation in women is more likely to result in mood alterations.

Chloral hydrate and benzodiazepines are usually the agents of choice for treating insomnia in the elderly. When possible, prescribers often suggest that the elderly limit their hypnotic intake to three or four times a week, allowing clients to select the nights on which they need to take their medication. This schedule usually results in enhanced effectiveness, less daytime drowsiness or sedation, and a decreased potential for inducing tolerance to the medication. Regular and careful assessment, monitoring, and reevaluation of the need for hypnotics are highly recommended.

It has been reported that many anxiolytic benzodiazepines may also be very effective hypnotic agents. Clients receiving a daytime benzodiazepine (such as alprazolam [Xanax], diazepam [Valium] or lorazepam [Ativan]) who also require temporary use of a hypnotic drug may be prescribed an equivalent hypnotic dose of the anxiolytic agents. For example, 0.5 mg alprazolam, 5 mg diazepam, and 1 mg of lorazepam are considered equivalent to 15 mg flurazepam (Dalmane), 15 mg temazepam (Restoril), or 0.25 mg triazolam (Halcion) (Crismon, 1992).

Geriatric Implications

Insomnia and hypnotics

Sleep latency increases while REM and stage 4 sleep may be absent in the geriatric client. Sleep disturbance is one of the most frequent concerns of the elderly.

Evaluate the individual for preexisting health conditions, since various illnesses such as arthritic pain, hyperthyroidism, cardiac dysrhythmia, and paroxysmal nocturnal dyspnea may alter sleep patterns.

Hypnotics should be reserved to treat acute insomnia and, when prescribed, limited to short-term or intermittent use to avoid the development of tolerance and dependency.

A hypnotic with a short duration of action is preferred. When longer-acting hypnotics are given, daytime sedation, ataxia, and memory deficits may result.

Encourage the older client to use nonpharmacologic approaches to promote sleep.

Be aware that the elderly, children, and persons with CNS dysfunction may experience a paradoxical reaction (CNS stimulation) to hypnotics and antihistamines.

Common side effects with the antihistamine sleeping aids (which may be prescribed but are also usually in OTC drugs) include dizziness, tinnitus, blurred or altered vision, gastrointestinal disturbance, and dry mouth.

■ Nursing Management

Sedative-Hypnotic Therapy

The following nursing management is common to drugs prescribed for sedative-hypnotic therapy. Nursing issues unique to specific sedatives/hypnotics will be described as that drug is discussed.

Assessment. The nurse should find out what the client's sleep habits are and how a good night's sleep is ensured at home. A thorough sleep history is required before a regimen of medications is begun. Such a history includes the following information:

- What does the client do about environmental control, which includes ventilation, lighting, and noise?
- What does the client do about physical care? Does he or she shower or bathe before retiring or go for a walk?
- What does the client do about food? Does he or she snack before retiring?
- Does the client have quiet recreation, such as reading, before sleep?

Various problems may cause the client to have insomnia (see Box 16-1). These include circadian rhythm irregularities, sleep apnea, restless leg syndrome, intake of alcohol or caffeine, various medications, and poor sleep hygiene, which is characterized by irregular bedtimes, daytime napping, and strenuous exercise or heavy eating just before bedtime.

If the client's disturbed sleep pattern is due to discomfort or pain at night, an opioid or an increased opioid dose at bedtime may be indicated. Joint pain or stiffness that results in insomnia will usually respond to a nonsteroidal antiinflammatory drug (NSAID) such as ibuprofen (Motrin) or naproxen (Naprosyn).

When a client is admitted, a thorough drug history should be taken, including the use of both prescription and over-the-counter sleep preparations. All sleep medication brought from home should be removed for the client's safety. Concern for drug interactions for sedatives and hypnotics in general would be with alcohol and other CNS depressants.

The general health status of the client should be determined because the elderly and children are more sensitive to the effects of these drugs. Clients with hepatic and renal function dysfunctions will require smaller doses or less frequent ones. The use of these drugs should be avoided in pregnant and breastfeeding clients. See the box below for FDA pregnancy safety classifications.

Nursing diagnosis. With the administration of sedatives/hypnotics to clients, the following nursing diagnoses/collaborative problems may be identified: sleep pattern disturbance related to the client's underlying problem; sensory/perceptual alterations (blurred vision, diplopia); altered thought processes (confusion); risk for injury related to the drugs' CNS effects (daytime sedation, dizziness, incoordination, ataxia, withdrawal syndrome); knowledge deficit related to sedative/hypnotic therapy; and the potential complication of paradoxical stimulation (increased irritability, hyperactivity).

Pregnancy Safety

Category	Drug
B	buspirone
C	chloral hydrate, ethchlorvynol, paraldehyde
D	alprazolam, barbiturates, halazepam, lorazepam (parenteral), midazolam (parenteral)
X	temazepam, triazolam quazepam
Unclassified	other benzodiazepines meprobamate, hydroxyzine estazolam

Implementation

Monitoring. Evaluation of effectiveness may be facilitated by use of a written "sleep diary." Among the information recorded in the diary are activities and eating before sleep, bedtimes, waking times, naps, and medication administration. Review of the diary will help identify the success of therapy or areas of poor sleep hygiene. Monitor for symptoms of overdosage, such as inappropriate sleepiness, slurred speech, confusion, and respiratory depression; and tolerance, such as continuing and increasing anxiety and insomnia.

Intervention. Because nurses are in a strategic position to influence the client's sleep, it cannot be stressed enough that caution must be exercised when decisions are made about giving or repeating an hs or prn order for a sleeping medication. Immediately administering a sleeping medication when a client complains of being unable to sleep may be doing the client more harm than good. An assessment of the client and alternative methods of relaxing the client must be considered. The nurse should try using supportive nursing measures (e.g., a back rub, reduction of environmental stimuli, relaxation therapy, or a warm drink) either alone, before a hypnotic is given, or together with the drug.

If the client is depressed or has a history of attempted suicide, precautions should be taken to prevent hoarding of sedatives/hypnotics. Ensure that the client has swallowed each dose.

Every effort should be made not to disrupt the sleeping client. If at all possible, other medications are scheduled before sedatives/hypnotics are given. Take the vital signs before the client falls asleep. Many interruptions for various aspects of care can do nothing but further alter the client's sleep pattern.

Because clients can become physically and psychologically dependent on these sedative/hypnotic drugs, gradually taper off the medications to avoid an abstinence syndrome reaction. Although not recommended, some hypnotics are used on a long-term basis. To reduce or avoid the development of tolerance, intermittent nightly use of the drug is suggested; for example, if the client has one or two nights of "good" sleep (as defined by the client), it may be possible to omit the drug the next night.

Education. Caution the client against driving a car, operating machinery, or participating in any activity that may be dangerous while taking these drugs until the drug's effects are known. Although the client may deny feeling sleepy the next day, activity performance may show definable impairment because serum levels of some of these drugs are retained. Alert the client to call for assistance in ambulating if required.

Clients and their families need to be taught ways to promote restful sleep without resorting to OTC sleep aids such as Sominex, NyTol, Sleep-eze, or Unisom. Instruct the client that nonpharmacologic approaches to promote sleep will enhance the effectiveness of any agent prescribed (Box 16-2).

Explain to the client that sedative or hypnotic drugs taken in combination with alcohol, antihistamines, antianxiety agents, antidepressants, or antipsychotic agents will produce

BOX 16-2

Nonpharmacologic Approaches to the Promotion of Sleep

1. Restrict use of caffeinated beverages or any caffeine-containing product within 8 hours of bedtime. Read labels because many OTC drugs also contain caffeine.
2. Establish set times for retiring and arising from bed. Avoid daytime napping whenever possible. Try to make the bedroom quiet and dark.
3. Avoid alcohol consumption and smoking cigarettes within 8 hours of bedtime or during the night.
4. Avoid heavy meals several hours before bedtime.
5. Avoid strenuous exercise before bedtime. Exercising during the day is recommended if physical condition permits it.
6. Relax in the evening before retiring by reading, utilizing relaxation techniques, taking a warm bath, listening to relaxing music, or going for a pleasant walk.
7. Try not to worry if unable to sleep because anxiety will add to or cause insomnia. If you cannot sleep, get out of bed and go to another room until sleepy.
8. Do not use the bedroom for wake-time activities, such as eating or watching television.
9. If recurrent and disturbing thoughts interfere with sleep, it may help to write them down and consider a plan of action to solve the problem.
10. Drink warm, noncaffeinated drinks, such as warm milk with honey, before bedtime. Home remedies that help induce sleep include eating a snack high in carbohydrate and low in protein or a few crackers or cookies with a glass of warm malted milk.

an enhanced CNS-depressant effect. This combination should be avoided.

Evaluation. The client will report feeling rested and wakeful without residual drowsiness or "drug hangover" during the daytime.

BENZODIAZEPINES

The benzodiazepines are among the most widely prescribed drugs in clinical medicine, primarily because of their advantages over the older agents (such as the barbiturates, meprobamate, and alcohol). Their popularity probably results from their anxiolytic and hypnotic dose-related effects, which have the following advantages: (a) lower fatality rates with acute toxicity and overdose, (b) lower potential for abuse, (c) more favorable side/adverse effect profiles, and (d) fewer potentially serious drug interactions reported when administered with other medications.

Mechanism of action. Benzodiazepines do not exert a general CNS-depressant effect. Instead a wide range of selectivity is seen with the various members of this class. Some general pharmacologic properties of this class include muscle relaxant, antianxiety, anticonvulsant, and hypnotic effects.

At least two benzodiazepine receptors have been identified, BZ_1 and BZ_2. The BZ_1 receptors are primarily located in the cerebellum and are believed to mediate the antianxiety and sedative effects. BZ_2 receptors are found in the basal ganglia and hippocampus, and so are associated with muscle relaxation and cognitive effects (memory and sensory functions). Both benzodiazepines and barbiturates potentiate the effects of gamma-aminobutyric acid (GABA), the inhibitory neurotransmitter. Benzodiazepines bind to specific benzodiazepine receptors in the brain and spinal cord, which increases the effect of GABA on chloride influx. This results in hyperpolarization of cell membrane and nerve inhibition.

Barbiturates increase GABA binding to receptors sites, and in high concentrations may directly depress calcium-dependent action potentials and increase chloride flux without GABA. Therefore barbiturates result in a broader effect than the benzodiazepines because they also depress excitatory transmitters and nonsynaptic membranes, resulting in a more pronounced CNS depressant effect.

The limbic system, associated with the regulation of emotional behavior, contains a highly dense area of benzodiazepine receptors in the amygdala that appear to correspond to specific antianxiety effects of certain drugs. These proposed benzodiazepine receptors may share some sites of action with other drugs (alcohol, meprobamate, barbiturates) and may further explain cross-tolerance to these drugs.

Indications. The most common indications for benzodiazepines include anxiety disorders, alcohol withdrawal, preoperative medication, insomnia, seizure disorders, and neuromuscular disease. They are also used to induce amnesia during cardioversion and endoscopic procedures.

Anxiety disorders. Alprazolam (Xanax), bromazepam (Lectopam♣), chlordiazepoxide (Librium), chlorazepate (Klonopin), diazepam (Valium), halazepam (Paxipam), ketazolam (Loftran), lorazepam (Ativan), oxazepam (Serax), and prazepam (Centrax) are the benzodiazepines used as antianxiety agents. In addition, alprazolam (Xanax), lorazepam (Ativan)(oral), and oxazepam (Serax) are used as adjunct medications to treat anxiety associated with depression.

Alcohol withdrawal. The benzodiazepines most often used for treatment of alcohol withdrawal syndrome are chlordiazepoxide (Librium), clorazepate (Tranxene), diazepam (Valium), and oxazepam (Serax). These drugs are very useful for the acute agitation, tremors, and other symptoms of acute alcohol withdrawal.

Preoperative medication. Parenteral chlordiazepoxide (Librium), diazepam (Valium), lorazepam (Ativan), and midazolam (Versed) are used preoperatively to reduce anxiety and to help induce general anesthesia; the last three drugs may also decrease the client's memory of the procedure. These three drugs are also used for endoscopic procedures to decrease anxiety and tension and to produce an anterograde **amnesic effect**, a loss of memory about the procedure.

Sleep disorders. Flurazepam (Dalmane), quazepam (Doral), temazepam (Restoril), and triazolam (Halcion) are usually prescribed for sleep disorders such as insomnia. Generally these drugs are indicated for short-term treatment of insomnia only.

Seizure disorders. Clonazepam (Klonopin) is available orally as an anticonvulsant (see Chapter 17). Parenteral diazepam (Valium) is indicated for intractable, repetitive seizures, such as status epilepticus. Oral diazepam may be used for short-term adjunct therapy (1 to 2 weeks) with other anticonvulsants for the treatment of convulsions.

Neuromuscular disease. Benzodiazepines, especially diazepam (Valium), may be useful as adjunct medications for the treatment of skeletal muscle spasms caused by muscle or joint inflammation or spasticity resulting from upper motor neuron dysfunction, such as cerebral palsy and paraplegia.

Pharmacokinetics. Oral benzodiazepines are readily absorbed from the GI tract. Clorazepate (Tranxene) and diazepam (Valium) are the most rapidly absorbed drugs in this class. Usually the more rapidly absorbed benzodiazepines produce a more prompt and intense onset of action.

The more lipid soluble (lipophilic) benzodiazepines, such as diazepam (Valium), are widely distributed in the body and brain and are also highly protein bound. After multiple doses benzodiazepines accumulate in the body's fluids and tissues. This saturation of storage sites allows for greater blood concentration and longer action. Accumulation in storage sites also accounts for the prolonged action of benzodiazepines after they have been discontinued.

The GI tract and the liver are the sites of metabolism for either the active drug or metabolite dosage forms of the inactive metabolites. The acid environment of the stomach is the site of conversion of clorazepate (Tranxene) to its active form, desmethyldiazepam. Prazepam (Centrax) also undergoes metabolism in the stomach and liver to the active metabolite desmethyldiazepam. Chlordiazepoxide (Librium), chlorazepate (Tranxene), diazepam (Valium), flurazepam (Dalmane), halazepam (Paxipam), ketazolam (Loftran♣) and prazepam (Centrax) are converted to active metabolites, notably desmethyldiazepam, a long-acting metabolite (30 to 100 hours) (*USP DI*, 1996). Therefore, long-acting benzodiazepines and their active metabolites are more apt to accumulate, especially in the elderly, resulting in increased risk for falls and hip fractures (*USP DI*, 1996).

These drugs are highly protein bound and lipid soluble and are excreted by the kidney. Protein binding is reduced in newborns, alcoholic clients, and those with cirrhosis or renal insufficiency. Oxazepam (Serax) and lorazepam (Ativan) are metabolized to inactive metabolites; thus they may be preferred agents in elderly clients and persons with liver disease.

The injectable benzodiazepines include chlordiazepoxide (Librium), diazepam (Valium), and lorazepam (Ativan). The onset of anticonvulsant, antianxiety, and muscle relaxant effects of these agents after intravenous administration is approximately 1 to 5 minutes. After intramuscular injection, the onset of action is approximately 15 to 30 minutes. Table 16-1 gives a pharmacokinetic overview of selected benzodiazepine drugs.

Side effects/adverse reactions. The most frequent side effects of benzodiazepines include drowsiness, hiccups (especially with midazolam [Versed]), lassitude, and loss of dexterity. Less frequent side effects include dry mouth, nausea, vomiting, headaches, constipation, abdominal cramping, unsteadiness, dizziness, and blurred vision. If side effects continue, increase, or disturb the client, inform the prescriber. Adverse reactions include increased behavioral problems, which are seen mostly with children (anger, decreased ability to concentrate). Neurologic reactions include insomnia, increased excitability, hallucinations, and apprehension (paradoxical reaction). In addition, the client may experience pruritus, skin rash, sore throat, elevated temperature, increased bruising or bleeding episodes, mental depression, hepatitis, confusion, mouth or throat sores, and muscle weakness. Finally, clients using midazolam (Versed) have reported muscle tremors, tachycardia, shortness of breath, or breathing difficulties. If adverse reactions occur, contact prescriber because medical intervention may be necessary. See the box below for the treatment of benzodiazepine overdose.

Significant drug interactions. Significant drug interactions, such as enhanced CNS depressant effects, may occur when benzodiazepines are used in combination with alcohol and CNS depressants, opioid analgesics, anesthetics, or tricyclic antidepressants. Close monitoring is necessary because the dosage of one or both drugs may need to be adjusted. Concurrent administration of benzodiazepines with zidovudine (AZT), an antiviral drug, may inhibit zidovudine metabolism, leading to an increased potential for its accumu-

! MANAGEMENT OF DRUG OVERDOSE

Benzodiazepine

In conscious clients, administer an emetic followed by activated charcoal to adsorb the benzodiazepine. For unconscious clients a gastric lavage with a cuffed endotracheal tube may be used.

Ensure maintenance of an adequate airway, closely monitor vital signs, administer oxygen for depressed respirations, and promote diuresis by the administration of intravenous fluids.

Medications that may be used include IV administration of flumazenil (Romazicon) as a benzodiazepine antagonist and vasopressors such as norepinephrine, metaraminol, or dopamine to treat hypotension. Do not use barbiturates to treat excitation effects as they may exacerbate the condition.

Dialysis is of limited value in treating a benzodiazepine overdose.

TABLE 16-1 Pharmacokinetic overview: benzodiazepines

Name	Duration of action*	Time to peak plasma concentration (hr) (oral)	Half-life (hr)*	Active metabolites (half-life in hr)
alprazolam (Xanax)	S-I	1-2	11-16	None
chlordiazepoxide (Librium, Libritab Medi-lium♣)	L	0.5-4	5-30	desmethylchlordiazepoxide (18) demoxepam (14-95) desmethyldiazepam (30-100) oxazepam (5-15)
clonazepam (Klonopin, Rivotril♣)	S-I	1-2 (some patients from 4-8 hr)	18-50	None
clorazepate (Tranxene, Novoclopate♣)	L	0.5-2	Parent drug not active	desmethyldiazepam (30-100) oxazepam (5-15)
diazepam (Valium, Apo-Diazepam♣)	L	0.5-2	20-70	desmethyldiazepam (30-100) temazepam (9.5-12.4) oxazepam (5-15)
estazolam (Prosom)	S-I	2	10-24	None
flurazepam (Dalmane, Apo-Flurazepam♣)	L	0.5-1	2.3	desalkylflurazepam (30-100) N-1-hydroxyethylflurazepam (2-4)
halazepam (Paxipam)	L	1-3	14	desmethyldiazepam (30-100)
ketazolam (Loftran♣)	L	3	2	desmethyldiazepam (30-100) N-methylketazolam (34-52) diazepam (20-70)
lorazepam (Ativan, Apo-Lorazepam♣)	S-I	1-6	10-20	None
midazolam HCl (Versed)	S	0.25-1	2.5	1-hydroxymethyl and 4-hydroxy midazolam
oxazepam (Serax, Ox-pam♣)	S-I	1-4	5-15	None
prazepam (Centrax)	L	2.5-6 hr for metabolite desmethyldiazepam (single dose)	Parent drug not active	desmethyldiazepam (30-100) oxazepam (5-15)
quazepam (Doral)	L	2	39	desalkylflurazepam (30-100) 2-oxoquazepam (39)
temazepam (Restoril)	S-I	1-2	8-15	None
triazolam (Halcion)	S-I	within 2	1.5-5.5	None

From *USP DI*, 1996. *S*, Short; *S-I*, short to intermediate acting; *L*, long acting.
*Elimination half-life.

lation and toxicity. If used concurrently, monitor closely for adverse effects.

In 1996 the manufactures of Halcion and Xanax issued warnings that these benzodiazepines are contraindicated for use in persons receiving ketoconazole and itraconazole. Caution and close monitoring is suggested whenever these drugs are administered in combination with other medications (Drug Product Update, 1996).

Dosage and administration. Table 16-2 lists dosage and administration information.

Nursing Management

Benzodiazepine Therapy

Concern about the overuse or overprescribing of benzodiazepines leading to tolerance, dependency, and withdrawal problems is discussed in Chapter 9. Several general guidelines are offered to reduce the potential for drug abuse with this drug classification.

First, benzodiazepines are antianxiety agents (i.e., they are used to control the symptoms of anxiety but are not curative agents).

Second, benzodiazepines are indicated for short-term therapy or on an as-needed basis. The dosage should be the minimum necessary to produce the desired effect. The client should be reevaluated every 2 weeks to detect the effectiveness of the medication, the need for continued therapy, or both.

Third, when a benzodiazepine is being discontinued, the dosage should be tapered over 2 weeks. In clients receiving the short-acting benzodiazepines (lorazepam [Ativan], alprazolam [Xanax]), severe withdrawal symptoms have been reported if the medications have been abruptly stopped. Switching for a few weeks to a benzodiazepine that has a

TABLE 16-2 Benzodiazines: FDA approved indications, dosage, and administration

Drug	FDA approved indications*	Dosage and administration
alprazolam (Xanax, generic)	anxiety, panic	*Adults:* antianxiety, 0.25-4 mg/day in divided doses. Antipanic, up to 10 mg/day. *Children up to 18 yrs old:* not recommended.
chlordiazepoxide (Librium, generic)	anxiety, sedative-hypnotic (alcohol withdrawal)	*Adults:* antianxiety, 5-25 mg po 3 or 4 times a day. Alcohol withdrawal, 50-100 mg PO initially, repeat as needed up to 400 mg/day. Parenteral, 50-100 mg IM or IV 3 or 4 times/day. Preoperative, 50-100 mg IM 1 hr before surgery. *Children:* 6 yrs and older, 5-10 mg PO 2 to 3 times a day. Parenteral up to 12 yrs, not established; 12 and over, 25-50 mg IM or IV.
clonazepam (Klonopin)	seizures, panic	See Chapter 17 for information.
clorazepate (Tranxene, generic)	anxiety, seizures, sedative-hypnotic (alcohol withdrawal)	*Adults:*antianxiety, 7.5-15 mg PO 2 to 4 times a day. Alcohol withdrawal, 30 mg initially, then 15 mg 2 to 4 times eventually reduced to 3.75 mg (see current reference for dosing guidelines). Anticonvulsant, 7.5-30 mg 3 times a day per recommended schedule (see current reference for dosing guidelines).
diazepam (Valium, generic)	anxiety, sedative-hypnotic, seizures, skeletal muscle relaxant	*Adults:* antianxiety, 2-10 mg PO 2 to 4 times a day. Sedative-hypnotic (alcohol withdrawal), 5-10 mg 3 or 4 times a day. Anticonvulsant or skeletal muscle relaxant (adjunct), 2-10 mg 3 or 4 times a day. Parenteral, IM or IV, individualized dose (usually 5 up to 20 mg depending on procedure). See current guidelines.
estazolam (Prosom)	sedative-hypnotic	*Adults:* 1-2 mg PO. *Children up to 18 yrs old:* not recommended.
flurazepam (Dalmane, generic)	sedative-hypnotic	*Adults:* 15-30 mg PO. *Children up to 15 yrs old:* not recommended.
halazepam (Paxipam)	anxiety	*Adults:* 20-40 mg 3 or 4 times a day. *Children up to 18 yrs old:* not recommended.
lorazepam (Ativan, generic)	anxiety, sedative-hypnotic	*Adults:* antianxiety, 1-3 mg 2 or 3 times a day. Sedative-hypnotic, 2-4 mg at bedtime. Parenteral, 0.5 mg/kg IM up to maximum of 4 mg or 0.044 mg/kg or total dose of 2 mg IV (whichever is less). *Children up to 12 yrs old:* PO not recommended. Parenteral not recommended for children up to 18 yrs old.
midazolam (Versed)	preoperative sedation and amnesia, conscious sedation	*Doses are individualized, generally adults:* 70-80 µg/kg ½ to 1 hr before surgery. Also see Chapter 15.
oxazepam (Serax, generic)	anxiety, sedative-hypnotic	*Adults:* antianxiety, 10-30 mg 3 or 4 times a day. Sedative-hypnotic (alcohol withdrawal), 15 or 30 mg 3 or 4 times a day. *Children up to 12 yrs old:* dosage not established.
prazepam (Centrax, generic)	anxiety	*Adults:* 10-20 mg PO 3 times a day or 20-40 mg at bedtime. *Children up to 18 yrs old:* dosage not established.
quazepam (Doral)	sedative-hypnotic	*Adults:* 7.5-15 mg at bedtime. *Children up to 18 yrs old:* dosage not established.
temazepam (Restoril, generic)	sedative-hypnotic	*Adults:* 7.5-15 mg at bedtime. *Children up to 18 yrs old:* dosage not established.
triazolam (Halcion)	sedative-hypnotic	*Adults:* 125-250 µg at bedtime. *Children up to 18 yrs old:* dosage not established.

**USP DI*, 1996

longer half-life before starting the tapering procedure has helped to reduce the more serious withdrawal symptoms, such as tonic-clonic seizures.

Finally, concurrent consumption of two or more benzodiazepine agents, even for daytime anxiety and bedtime insomnia, is considered inappropriate therapy. Using one benzodiazepine to accomplish both purposes is preferred because (1) effectiveness is usually equivalent, (2) the drug will be better tolerated and controlled by the client, and (3) the therapy will be less expensive.

In addition to the general nursing management of sedative-hypnotic therapy previously discussed, benzodiazepine therapy involves the following nursing management (see also the case study below).

Assessment. Initially it should be determined if the client has a hypersensitivity to any of the benzodiazepines, since there may be a cross-sensitivity to other benzodiazepines. Pregnant women usually should avoid using benzodiazepines because their use is associated with increased risk of congenital anomalies. Female clients of childbearing age should be advised that if they should become pregnant or intend to become pregnant during anxiolytic therapy, they should immediately notify the prescriber. Then a decision about discontinuing the drug must be made.

Nursing mothers should not be given benzodiazepines. Because of their molecular size, the benzodiazepines and their metabolites probably are excreted in breast milk.

For elderly or debilitated clients the initial dose should be small and increments added gradually, based on the response of each client, to preclude ataxia or excessive sedation. Doses of benzodiazepines sufficient to control anxiety cause unwanted drowsiness less frequently than equivalent doses of barbiturates or meprobamate. The benzodiazepines have high therapeutic effectiveness and low addiction potential and lethality. They are generally desirable agents for anxious elderly clients. These drugs occasionally cause paradoxical reactions such as agitation and confusion, but these occur to a lesser degree than with barbiturates.

The nurse should remember that elderly clients are more vulnerable to the adverse effects of benzodiazepines. Excretion is delayed in this population, and thus the half-life increases. This response may allow the client to attain therapeutic blood levels with a single dose rather than two or three doses per day. Daytime sedation can be reduced if the single daily dose is administered at bedtime. If the elderly client is continent, ambulatory, and alert, excessive doses of the benzodiazepines may result in incontinence, loss of the ability to ambulate, or confusion. Careful titration to individual needs is essential in elderly clients.

When depression accompanies the client's anxiety, the incidence of suicidal tendencies is significant. This may require further protective measures to avoid self-destructive acts such as multidrug overdosage. As small an amount of the drug as possible should be available to such a client at any

Case Study

The Client Taking Antianxiety Agents

Anna Smith is a 45-year-old mother of four children. She is an attractive and intelligent woman of medium build. She describes herself as being somewhat of a perfectionist and a very sensitive person. In the last few months, she has become increasingly concerned with various family problems. Her 19-year-old son has dropped out of college and has developed new friends she is concerned about. She suspects that his behavior changes are related to drugs.

Lately she has been feeling very fatigued during the day, yet is unable to sleep at night because of "worrying" over problems. She doesn't feel that she can talk to her husband, because he has been working long hours at his executive job and falls right to sleep as soon as he goes to bed. She tried an over-the-counter medication (Vivarin) to get some pep, but found it just made her feel jittery and nervous, and made it even more difficult to get to sleep.

She went to her family doctor, who initially prescribed diazepam (Valium) 5 mg PO tid and pentobarbital (Nembutal) 100 mg PO at bedtime. After 2 weeks' time, she found that she still had the same difficulty in sleeping and had become more depressed and irritable. She found that she could not manage to keep the house clean because she just did not have the energy, and would have crying spells late each afternoon when no one else was home except her 4-year-old son. Her physician then ordered some blood tests, and after ascertaining that they were normal, he advised Anna to see a psychiatrist. The psychiatrist prescribed alprazolam (Xanax) 0.025 mg PO tid for her anxiety and the same drug 0.025 mg, 1 or 2 tablets prn at bed time. Over the next 4 weeks her anxiety began to decrease and she was able to sleep through the night.

1. How would benzodiazepines affect Anna's anxiety levels?
2. For what side effects/adverse reactions should Anna be monitored?
3. What are some of the important points to stress to Anna while she is on Xanax?
4. While Anna was taking Xanax, she was to attend an obligatory cocktail party given by her husband's business associates. How would you advise her when she asks you, "Would it hurt if I have a cocktail or two?"

one time. This requires accurate medical office data about prescriptions and their refill dates and ensures greater control by the prescriber/case manager.

Because of their anticholinergic effects, benzodiazepines should be used with caution in clients with glaucoma. Their use may also result in respiratory failure in clients with severe chronic obstructive pulmonary disease.

A baseline assessment of the client should include a description of the client's underlying condition and CNS and mental status, and also a complete blood count and liver function tests. Also the usual precautions in treating clients with impaired renal or hepatic function should be observed. In animal studies hepatomegaly and cholestasis were observed.

Dosages should be carefully determined for clients with renal impairment, especially when chlordiazepoxide (Librium) and diazepam (Valium) are administered, since active metabolites may accumulate and produce toxicity. Flurazepam hydrochloride (Dalmane) should be avoided, whereas other agents, such as clonazepam (Klonopin), lorazepam (Ativan), oxazepam (Serax), and temazepam (Restoril), seem to pose no risk of toxicity for clients who have renal impairment.

Clients frequently experience a number of physical and psychiatric problems at the same time and may require treatment with several drugs. This multiple drug therapy is sometimes called "polypharmacy." Many clients may benefit diagnostically and therapeutically from a health evaluation made during a drug-free period of time. However, some clients abruptly withdrawn from high doses or therapeutic doses of benzodiazepines taken over prolonged periods exhibit symptoms of withdrawal. These symptoms may resemble those of anxiety for which the drug was originally prescribed. A mild withdrawal syndrome is characterized by feelings of tension or anxiety, anorexia, GI symptoms such as diarrhea, weakness, lethargy, light-headedness, tremor, and mild numbness. Clients who exhibit moderately severe symptoms report anxiety, apprehension, restlessness, insomnia, increased frequency of dreaming, anorexia-induced weight loss, dysphoric moods, and palpitations. Rarely, clients exhibit seizures and delirium. Symptoms usually begin 24 to 72 hours after withdrawal. When the client is withdrawn from a short-acting benzodiazepine, symptoms peak in about 5 to 7 days and subside after 7 to 10 days. The withdrawal syndrome of the long-acting benzodiazepines peaks at about 5 days but may last 2 to 4 weeks. Withdrawal symptoms can be relieved by administering a dose of the anxiolytic agent. The withdrawal syndrome can be avoided by gradually tapering the dose of the anxiolytic agent and supporting the client during this period with other anxiety-relieving techniques.

Nursing diagnosis. Because of the CNS effects of benzodiazepine therapy, clients are at risk for injury related to dizziness, incoordination, and ataxia; alteration in sensory-perceptual function (blurred vision, diplopia); altered thought processes (anterograde amnesia, memory impairment, and vivid dreams); impaired communication (slurred speech); and a disturbance in sleep pattern (daytime sedation and hangover). There may occasionally also be an alteration in bowel function (constipation) and alteration in urinary pattern (urinary retention). Rarely there is drug-related depression.

Implementation

Monitoring. Reassessment of the medication's effectiveness as an antianxiety agent or as a sedative-hypnotic should be done periodically over the course of therapy. Clients receiving benzodiazepines for prolonged periods should have periodic blood counts to monitor for neutropenia, as well as liver function tests. Monitoring of mental status, and of CNS, bowel, and urinary functioning should occur.

Intervention. Avoid intramuscular administration because the benzodiazepines are highly alkaline and irritating to tissues. Absorption is also erratic by this route of administration. Administer intravenous preparations slowly because apnea, hypotension, bradycardia, and cardiac arrest have been associated with rapid administration. Arteriospasm, with resultant gangrene, results from accidental intraarterial, rather than intravenous, administration. After receiving a parenteral dose of a benzodiazepine, the client needs close observation for at least 3 hours, preferably at bed rest.

Education. Nonpharmacologic interventions for the reduction of anxiety related to the stress of everyday life should be encouraged because the benzodiazepines are not indicated for the long-term management of this anxiety. Stress-reduction techniques such as self-coaching, thought stopping, guided imagery, and progressive relaxation exercises may be used as adjuncts to the benzodiazepines.

Instruct the client to avoid alcoholic beverages, sleep-inducing OTC medications, and other CNS depressants while taking benzodiazepines. Caution the client not to take more than the prescribed dosage if the medication seems less effective, and to consult the prescriber. If on a scheduled dosing regimen (such as use as an anticonvulsant rather than as a prn medication), the client should take a missed dose within 1 to 2 hours of when it should have been taken. If it is remembered much later, the client should not double the next dose but should skip the missed dose and continue the regimen.

Evaluation. If a drug is being used for its antianxiety properties, the client should report an increase in psychologic and physiologic comfort and should appear to have relaxed facial expressions and body movements. Clients using a benzodiazepine for nighttime sedation should relate an increase in the amount and quality of sleep and daytime wakefulness if the agent is effective.

Benzodiazepines

alprazolam [al pray' zoe lam] (Xanax)

Alprazolam is used as an antianxiety and antipanic agent. Accumulation is minimal after multiple doses and elimination rapidly follows termination of therapy. Reports of violent and aggressive behavior have been associated with alpra-

Cultural Aspects — Racial Differences in Response to Alprazolam

Awareness of the potential for unusually high plasma concentrations of some drugs in Asian clients may help nurses detect and prevent adverse drug effects. Results from a study by Lin et al (1988) of blood plasma levels of alprazolam (Xanax), a widely prescribed benzodiazepine, in 42 healthy men (14 American-born Asians, 14 foreign-born Asians, and 14 Caucasians) indicate that Asian clients require smaller doses to achieve the same blood plasma levels as Caucasian subjects. In both Asian groups the drug remained in the blood longer. Body heights and weights were not a factor (Kudzma, 1992).

zolam use (Glod, 1992). However, in some clients rapid decreases in dosage or abrupt discontinuation of therapy has resulted in seizures, delirium, and withdrawal reactions. The risk of seizures is greatest within 1 to 3 days after alprazolam is abruptly discontinued. To reduce or avoid the potential for these adverse effects alprazolam should be gradually tapered, at 3- to 5-day intervals until discontinued. See the Cultural Aspects box above for racial differences in response to alprazolam.

chlordiazepoxide [klor dye az e pox' ide] (Librium, Libritab)
Besides its use as an antianxiety agent, chlordiazepoxide is also used as a sedative-hypnotic, an antitremor drug, an antipanic agent (parenteral), and for relief of acute alcohol withdrawal symptoms. It has also been used to treat tension headaches.

Parenterally IV administration is preferred to IM injection because intramuscular absorption is slow and erratic. Intravenous administration should be slow, over a period of at least 1 minute. The nurse should be careful *not* to use the intramuscular diluent when preparing solution for intravenous administration, since it tends to form air bubbles.

When preparing a chlordiazepoxide solution for intramuscular administration, use only the manufacturer's diluent and administer the drug deeply into the muscle. Mixing the drug with sodium chloride or sterile water for injection will cause pain on injection. Solutions should be used immediately after reconstitution, and any unused solution should be discarded.

After receiving the drug parenterally the client should rest in bed and be monitored carefully for up to 3 hours for decreases in respiratory rate, heart rate, and blood pressure. Because of the long-acting metabolites that remain in the bloodstream for several days, the client should be monitored for accumulative effects of the drug.

clonazepam [kloe na' ze pam] (Klonopin, Rivotril♣)
Clonazepam is used as an anticonvulsant and for the treatment of panic disorders. When used as an anticonvulsant, clients receiving long-term therapy should avoid abrupt withdrawal because this may result in seizures.

Clonazepam administered concurrently with carbamazepine may result in a decrease in the serum levels and half-life of clonazepam. Monitor the client closely whenever the client receives combination anticonvulsant therapies.

clorazepate [klor az' e pate] (Tranxene, Novoclopate♣)
Clorazepate is used as an antianxiety agent, sedative-hypnotic, anticonvulsant, and for relief of acute alcohol withdrawal symptoms. When given orally, it is one of the most rapidly absorbed benzodiazepines.

▲ **diazepam** [dye az' e pam] (Valium, Apo-Diazepam♣)
Diazepam is used as an antianxiety agent, sedative/hypnotic, anticonvulsant, skeletal muscle relaxant, antitremor, and antipanic agent. It is also indicated for treatment in acute alcohol withdrawal, status epilepticus, tension headache, temporomandibular joint disorders, and as a preoperative medication. The parenteral diazepam also has an amnesic indication.

Intravenous administration should be accomplished slowly, at least 1 minute for each 5 mg of the drug, to prevent apnea, hypotension, bradycardia, or cardiac arrest. The client should be observed at bed rest for at least 3 hours after parenteral administration. Intravenous injection should be made into a large vein, not small veins such as found on the back of the hand and wrist.

Diazepam is not compatible with aqueous solutions. Continuous intravenous infusion is not recommended, since diazepam may precipitate in the infusion bag and the medication may be absorbed by the plastic infusion bags and tubing. If direct intravenous injection is not possible, the drug should be slowly injected through an infusion port as close to the point of needle or cannula insertion in the client as possible.

When diazepam is administered parenterally for peroral endoscopy, the use of a topical anesthetic for the insertion of the endoscope is recommended. Increased coughing, decreased respirations, dyspnea, hyperventilation, and laryngospasm have been known to occur; resuscitation measures to assist with respirations should be available.

See Chapter 17 for nursing management of diazepam as an anticonvulsant therapy.

estazolam [es tay' zoe lam] (ProSom)
Estazolam is similar to the other hypnotic benzodiazepines. It is indicated for the short-term treatment of insomnia. It is widely distributed in the body and easily crosses the blood-brain barrier. Having an intermediate to long half-life, estazolam is less likely to cause rebound insomnia after drug withdrawal.

flurazepam [flure az' e pam] (Dalmane, Apo-Flurazepam♣)
Flurazepam is indicated only for use as a sedative/hypnotic. Although the sleep pattern will improve the first night, the client should be instructed that 2 to 3 nights may be required

before flurazepam becomes fully effective. Elimination is slow, since metabolites remain in the body several days. This may produce unwanted daytime carry-over effects that result in poor coordination and drowsiness. The carry-over effects may be overcome by using lower doses and administering medication every other evening. The client must be warned of the sustained effect of the active metabolites.

halazepam [hal az' e pam] (Paxipam)
Halazepam is indicated for use only as an antianxiety agent. It has a long half-life and active metabolites, which may be significant when multiple doses are administered. Elimination may take several days or even weeks.

lorazepam [lor a' ze pam] (Ativan, Novolorazem♣)
Lorazepam is indicated for use as an antianxiety agent, sedative-hypnotic, amnestic, antitremor, adjunct skeletal muscle relaxant, anticonvulsant (parenteral only), antiemetic in cancer chemotherapy (parenteral only), and for the treatment of acute alcohol withdrawal symptoms and tension headaches.

Lorazepam must be mixed with an equal amount of a compatible diluent immediately before intravenous use. It may be infused directly into a vein or through intravenous tubing. Infusion rates are not to exceed 2 mg/min. Intraarterial injection may cause arteriospasm and possible gangrene, so avoid using the drug intraarterially. Intramuscular lorazepam is injected undiluted into deep muscle mass.

After receiving a parenteral dose of lorazepam, the client should be observed at bed rest for at least 1 hour for decreases in respiratory rate, heart rate, and blood pressure.

The tablet dosage form may be administered orally or sublingually.

midazolam [mid' ay zoe lam] (Versed)
Midazolam is used preoperatively for sedation and amnesic effects, and as an adjunct to general anesthesia. Midazolam is only used in parenteral form. Unlike diazepam (Valium), it does not cause thrombophlebitis and irritation on injection.

Dosages should be individualized according to the health status of the client. The range between therapeutic dosage and unconsciousness or disorientation is narrow, necessitating close monitoring of the client.

Instruct the client not to engage in tasks requiring alertness, such as driving, until the effects of midazolam have abated or until the day after administration, whichever is longer.

Intravenous midazolam has been associated with severe respiratory depression and arrest, especially when given concurrently with an opioid analgesic or when administered too rapidly. A warning has been issued for the intravenous use of this drug: it should be administered only in a hospital or ambulatory care setting that has continuous respiratory and cardiac monitoring and resuscitative drugs and equipment available.

As with diazepam (Valium), when midazolam (Versed) is used for peroral endoscopic procedures, a topical anesthetic agent should also be used for the insertion of the endoscopy tube. Measures to support respiration (oxygen, suction airway) should be available.

oxazepam [ox a' ze pam] (Serax, Ox-pam)
Oxazepam is indicated for anxiety associated with mental depression and for the treatment of acute alcohol withdrawal symptoms. Drug accumulation is minimal during multiple-dose therapy and the drug is rapidly eliminated when discontinued.

prazepam [pra' ze pam] (Centrax)
Prazepam is indicated only as an antianxiety agent. It is one of the most slowly absorbed benzodiazepines after oral administration, and accumulation of active metabolites may be significant in long-term therapy. Lethargy and increased fatigue are more often reported with prazepam than with most other benzodiazepines.

quazepam [kway' ze pam] (Doral)
Quazepam, a benzodiazepine hypnotic, has a greater affinity for the BZ_1 receptors than any of the other hypnotic benzodiazepines. Because of its extended drug half-life and active metabolites, steady state serum levels occur between 7 to 13 days. Daytime drowsiness is more common with quazepam than with most of the other benzodiazepines, but its prolonged half-life makes rebound insomnia less likely to occur after drug withdrawal.

temazepam [te maz' e pam] (Restoril)
Temazepam is indicated as a sedative-hypnotic. Only minimal accumulation occurs during multiple doses, and elimination is rapid when therapy is discontinued. Temazepam's slow absorption pattern means it usually takes 1 to 2 hours to reach effective blood levels. Its effectiveness for inducing sleep can be enhanced by proper scheduling of its administration, 1 to 1½ hours before bedtime.

triazolam [try az' oh lam] (Halcion)
Triazolam is indicated only as a sedative-hypnotic. Although anterograde amnesia may occur with any benzodiazepine, triazolam ". . . may be associated with more frequent psychiatric disturbances than other agents in this class . . . " (McCue et al, 1993). In several European countries the 0.5 mg dose of triazolam was taken off the market because of the frequency of reports of amnesia and other adverse reactions. In the United States the FDA has required stronger product labeling and client information. It appears that triazolam reduces the amount of REM sleep, which may contribute to the development or exacerbation of a mental or behavior-type disorder (Jellin, 1991). Effects reported include memory impairment, confusion, depersonalization, and severe anxiety.

Paradoxical rage reactions have also been reported with the benzodiazepines. This reaction is more commonly reported with triazolam according to foreign and domestic studies (Crismon, 1992). The symptoms include depersonalization, increased anxiety and restlessness, agitation, paranoid behavior, rage, panic reactions, and hallucinations. This response may be dose related, since dosages in excess of 0.5 mg/day were recorded in the majority of individuals (Crismon, 1992).

The benzodiazepines have been associated with changes in cognitive function and an increased risk for falls and injuries in the elderly. Altered pharmacokinetics in the geriatric client may increase the risk for benzodiazepine adverse effects; thus close professional supervision along with clear guidelines for benzodiazepine use is necessary. The package insert information cautions the client not to take the medication for more than 7 to 10 days without prescriber consultation, to report any unusual thoughts or behavior during treatment to the prescriber, and to avoid the use of alcohol and other drugs including OTC medications unless prescriber approval has been obtained (*USP DI*, 1996). Avoid the use of this product when a full night's sleep is not possible, such as airline flights of less than 7 or 8 hours. Amnestic episodes caused by lack of drug elimination from the body have been reported in such situations. Although many people have taken triazolam (Halcion) without reports of the adverse effects, it may be prudent to avoid the use of this product in the elderly because they generally have an increase in susceptibility to memory loss and other adverse drug reactions (Sherman, 1991).

New Benzodiazepines Not Available in the United States

Several benzodiazepines currently unavailable in the United States include clobazam (Frisium), an anticonvulsant and anxiolytic similar to diazepam; and nitrazepam (Mogadon), a hypnotic used in Europe and Canada for many years. Both products have long half-lives, which increases the potential for drug accumulation and side effects. They are similar to drugs already marketed in the United States (Olin, 1995). Abecarnil, a partial benzodiazepine-receptor agonist, may have a number of advantages over the currently marketed benzodiazepines. This product initially appears to have less potential for inducing sedation, drug tolerance, ataxia, amnesia, drug dependence, and abuse (Edmonds, 1995). Further studies are necessary to clinically validate such claims.

Benzodiazepine Antidote

Flumazenil (Romazicon), a benzodiazepine-receptor antagonist, is indicated for the treatment of a benzodiazepine overdose or to reverse the sedative effects of benzodiazepines following surgical or diagnostic procedures. This drug will not reverse the effects of opioids or other nonbenzodiazepine drugs. Although it can reverse the sedative effects of benzodiazepines, a reversal of the benzodiazepine-induced respiratory depression has not been demonstrated (Abramowicz, 1992). Therefore hypoventilation must include the establishment of an airway, assisting ventilation and interventions to support circulation (*USP DI*, 1996).

Kirkwood (1991) has suggested using flumazenil to differentiate between accumulation of benzodiazepines or their metabolites in the elderly and physical deterioration from other causes in suspected benzodiazepine overdose situations.

The mechanism of action for flumazenil is that it competes with the benzodiazepine at the receptor sites in the CNS. It is administered intravenously with antagonistic effects occurring within 1 to 2 minutes, peak effect in 6 to 10 minutes, and duration of action of approximately 1 to 3 hours, depending on the dose of benzodiazepine consumed. Because most benzodiazepines have a longer half-life than 1 hour, repeated injections of flumazenil are necessary. Flumazenil is metabolized in the liver and excreted by the kidneys.

Side effects reported with this drug include headache, visual disturbance, excess sweating, increased anxiety, nausea, and lightheadedness. Pain at the injection site can be significantly decreased by infusing the drug through a freely running IV solution into a large vein. Flumazenil may cause convulsions in clients taking benzodiazepines to control epilepsy. Seizures have also been reported in clients who consumed an overdose of a tricyclic antidepressant and a benzodiazepine. Cardiac arrhythmias have also been reported with the use of flumazenil. Caution is advised when giving flumazenil to clients who are known to use benzodiazepines chronically because moderate to severe withdrawal symptoms may be precipitated in such individuals.

Flumazenil dosage to reverse sedation is an initial intravenous dose of 0.2 mg injected over 15 seconds. This dose may be repeated at 1-minute intervals up to a maximum of 1 mg. For a benzodiazepine overdose the same initial dose is given, usually over 30 seconds, and then additional doses of 0.3 and 0.5 mg may be given at 1-minute intervals up to a maximum of 3 mg of flumazenil. See current package insert for additional dosing information.

BARBITURATES

The barbiturates were once the most commonly prescribed class of medications for hypnotic and sedative effects. With only a few exceptions, they have been largely replaced by the benzodiazepines. Phenobarbital is generally considered the prototype drug for this classification.

Classification. The barbiturates are classified according to the duration of their action as long-, intermediate-, short-, and ultrashort-acting drugs. The short-acting drugs produce an effect (onset) in a relatively short time (10 to 15 minutes) and peak over a relatively short period (3 to 4 hours). Short-acting barbiturates are used for treating insomnia, for preanesthetic sedation, and in combination with other drugs for psychosomatic disorders.

Long-acting barbiturates require more than 60 minutes for onset and peak over a period of 10 to 12 hours. Long-acting barbiturates are used for treating epilepsy, other chronic neurologic disorders, and for sedation in clients with high anxiety.

Ultrashort-acting barbiturates are used as IV anesthetics. Thiopental sodium, which belongs to the ultrashort-acting group of barbiturates, acts rapidly and can produce a state of anesthesia in a few seconds.

Intermediate-acting barbiturates have an onset of 45 to 60 minutes and peak in 6 to 8 hours.

Mechanism of action. The mechanism of action for barbiturates is nonselective depression of the central nervous system. High doses of the barbiturates may induce anesthesia. Barbiturates similar to the benzodiazepines appear to enhance systems that use gamma-aminobutyric acid (GABA) as an inhibitory transmitter. In addition, barbiturates may also decrease excitatory neurotransmitter effects. The ascending reticular formation receives stimuli from all parts of the body and relays impulses to the cortex (thus promoting wakefulness and alertness); barbiturate depression of the ascending reticular formation decreases cortical stimuli, reducing the need for wakefulness and alertness.

The extent of barbiturate effect varies from mild sedation to deep anesthesia, depending on the drug selected, method of administration, dosage, and the reaction of the individual's nervous system. The barbiturates are not regarded as analgesics and cannot be depended on to produce restful sleep when insomnia is caused by pain. However, when a barbiturate is combined with an analgesic, the sedative action seems to reinforce the action of the analgesic and to alter the client's emotional reaction to pain.

When used in large doses, all barbiturates depress the motor cortex of the brain, but phenobarbital, mephobarbital (Mebaral), and metharbital (Gemonil) exert a selective action on the motor cortex, even in small doses. This explains their use as anticonvulsants.

Therapeutic doses have little or no effect on medullary centers, but large doses, especially when administered intravenously, depress the respiratory and vasomotor centers.

Indications. The most common indications for the use of barbiturates include as adjuncts to anesthesia, treatment of seizure disorders, and several are indicated for treatment of insomnia. However, these agents have generally been replaced by the benzodiazepine family of drugs. Barbiturates are only indicated for short-term use in insomnia because they tend to lose their effectiveness in 14 days or less.

Barbiturates have been used for sedative effects in treating anxiety and nervousness. But for daytime use the benzodiazepines have largely replaced the barbiturates, primarily because they produce less drowsiness or ataxia.

Short-acting barbiturate anesthetics, such as thiopental and methohexital, are used for selected surgical procedures, especially for surgery of short duration. These barbiturates are discussed more fully in Chapter 15. The short-acting barbiturates, such as pentobarbital (Nembutal), may be used for their preanesthetic effect, to reduce anxiety and facilitate anesthesia induction. Diazepam (Valium) and other benzodiazepines are often used today for this purpose—as a preanesthetic agent to help with anesthesia induction, to reduce anxiety, and to induce an amnesic effect.

Anticonvulsant. Barbiturates are also used to prevent or control convulsive seizures associated with tetanus, strychnine poisoning, meningitis, eclampsia, and epilepsy. They may be prescribed alone or in conjunction with other anticonvulsant drugs. Phenobarbital is used in the treatment of epilepsy (generalized tonic-clonic) and for seizures induced by fever, whereas mephobarbital (Mebaral) and metharbital (Gemonil) may be alternative agents for phenobarbital.

Narcoanalysis. Intravenous amobarbital may be used in narcoanalysis, a form of psychotherapy that helps a client to talk about suppressed feelings and events.

Hyperbilirubinemia. Although not approved for treatment of hyperbilirubinemia, phenobarbital (oral and injectable) is often used to prevent or treat this condition in neonates and in clients with congenital nonhemolytic unconjugated hyperbilirubinemia.

Pharmacokinetics. Barbiturates are readily absorbed after oral, rectal, and parenteral administration. The soluble sodium salts are absorbed faster than the free acids. Most of the barbiturates undergo change in the liver before they are excreted by the kidney. The longer-acting barbiturates are metabolized more slowly than the rapidly acting barbiturates. The slower a barbiturate is altered or excreted, the more prolonged is its action. If excretion is slow and administration prolonged, cumulative effects will result.

Side effects/adverse reactions. The more frequent side effects of barbiturates include ataxia, drowsiness, dizziness, and hangover effect. Less frequent side effects are nausea, vomiting, insomnia, constipation, restlessness, faintness, headache, and night terrors. If side effects continue, increase, or disturb the client, inform the prescriber. The most common adverse reactions to these drugs include a hypersensitivity reaction such as skin rash, exfoliative dermatitis, sore throat, fever, edema, serum sickness, apnea, bronchospasms, urticaria, and Stevens-Johnson syndrome. Stevens-Johnson syndrome is a severe, occasionally fatal inflammatory disease of children and young adults, characterized by fever, bullae of the skin, and ulcers of the mucous membranes of mouth, nose, eyes, and genitalia.

Clients of any age, but especially elderly or debilitated clients, may exhibit confusion, disorientation, and mental depression. In children and elderly or debilitated clients, a paradoxical reaction (increased excitability) may occur. Long-term barbiturate use may result in osteomalacia and rickets (bone pain or aching, anorexia, myalgia, loss of weight). Finally, toxic signs include very severe confusion and persistent irritability. Acute toxic effects may include bradycardia, confusion, respiratory problems (apnea, laryngospasm), ataxia, extreme weakness, and visual disturbances.

Dosage and administration. See Table 16-3.

TABLE 16-3 Selected barbiturates: pharmacokinetics, indications, and dosage

Name	Onset of action (min)	Duration of action (hr)	Indications/dosage*
Short-acting			
pentobarbital (Nembutal)	10-15	3-4	*Adults:* hypnotic, 100 mg PO/IV, 150 to 200 mg IM, or 120 to 200 mg rectally at bedtime. Daytime sedative, 20 mg PO or 30 mg rectally 2 to 4 times a day. Preoperative, 100 mg PO or 150 or 200 mg IM. Anticonvulsant, 100 to 500 mg IV. *Children:* sedative-preoperative, 2-6 mg/kg or maximum 100 mg/dose.
secobarbital (Seconal)	10-15	3-4	*Adults:* hypnotic 100 mg PO, 100 to 200 mg IM, or 50 to 250 mg IV at bedtime. Daytime sedative, 30-50 mg 3-4 times daily. *Children:* daytime sedative, 2 mg/kg; preoperative, 2-6 mg/kg or maximum 100 mg/dose given 1-2 hr before surgery.
Intermediate-acting			
butabarbital (Butisol)	45-60	6-8	*Adults:* hypnotic and preoperative, 50-100 mg; daytime sedative, 15-30 mg 3-4 times daily. *Children:* sedative-preoperative, 2-6 mg/kg to maximum of 100 mg/dose.
Long-acting			
amobarbital (Amytal)	60+	10-12	*Adults:* hypnotic, 65 to 200 mg PO, IM, or IV at bedtime. Daytime sedative, 50-300 mg PO in divided doses or 30 to 50 mg IM or IV 2 or 3 times daily. Anticonvulsant, 65 to 500 mg IV. *Children:* sedative, 2 mg/kg PO 3 times daily; preoperative (6 yr and over), 3-5 mg/kg.
phenobarbital	60+	10-12	*Adults:* hypnotic, 100-320 mg PO or IV hs; daytime sedative, 30-120 mg PO/IM/IV in 2-3 divided doses daily; anticonvulsant, 60-250 mg PO daily or 100 to 320 mg IV. *Children:* anticonvulsant, 1-6 mg/kg/day.

*Barbiturates have generally been replaced by benzodiazepines for daytime sedation and hypnotic effects. See current references for additional information (*USP DI*, 1996).

■ Nursing Management

Barbiturate Therapy

Because of the potential for barbiturate dependence, tolerance, abuse, or misuse, the role of the nurse is essential in providing safe and effective drug therapy. In addition to the general nursing management of sedative/hypnotic therapy previously discussed, the following nursing activities should be considered.

Assessment. The nurse should assess and note the sleeping pattern of the client. This observation can influence the prescriber's decision about the type of barbiturate to prescribe.

Avoid giving barbiturates to clients who are hypersensitive to them or have respiratory conditions (involving dyspnea or obstruction), previous dependency on barbiturates, or renal or hepatic impairment, and to elderly persons and children with a history of paradoxical reactions. Acute intermittent porphyria may be aggravated through barbiturate inducement of the enzyme necessary for porphyrin (molecular components of hemoglobin, myoglobin, and various enzymes) synthesis.

Client assessment must include the concurrent drug regimen. The following effects may occur when barbiturates are given with the drugs listed below:

Drug	Possible effect and management
alcohol and CNS depressants	Enhanced CNS-depressant effects may result. Monitor closely for respiratory pattern changes, and perhaps decrease the dosage of one or both drugs to reduce the possibility of inducing the effect.
anticoagulants warfarin (Coumadin)	Decrease in anticoagulant effects caused by enhanced metabolism. Prothrombin time tests may be necessary to monitor therapeutic response to anticoagulant and to determine dosage changes of the anticoagulant.
anticonvulsants carbamazepine (Tegretol)	Monitor serum levels closely whenever carbamazepine or a succinimide is added or discontinued from a drug regimen. Increased metabolism of the anticonvulsant may occur, leading to decreased serum levels and therapeutic effects.

Drug	Possible effect and management
anticonvulsants divalproex sodium (Depakote) or valproic acid (Depakene)	Monitor barbiturate serum levels closely because the metabolism of barbiturates may decrease, leading to elevated levels and an increase in CNS depression and neurologic dysfunction. The half-life of valproic acid may also be reduced, which would also require monitoring of blood levels and dosage adjustments. Phenobarbital may also increase valproic acid hepatotoxicity; monitor closely for jaundice, hepatomegaly, anorexia, abdominal discomfort, clay-colored stools, and dark urine.
contraceptives, oral	Enhanced metabolism of estrogen (particularly oral estrogen) may result in a decrease in contraceptive effects. The prescriber may need to consider a nonhormonal birth control method or progestin-only oral contraceptive.
corticosteroids	When given with barbiturates (especially phenobarbital), corticosteroids may enhance metabolism and have decreased therapeutic effects. Dosage adjustments may be necessary. Monitor closely for a lack of therapeutic response to corticosteroid.

A baseline assessment of the client should include a description of the client's underlying condition, mental status, blood pressure determination, and CBC and liver function studies.

Nursing diagnosis. Because of the CNS effects of barbiturate therapy, clients are at risk for injury (drowsiness), altered thought processes (confusion, depression), and a disturbance in sleep pattern (daytime drowsiness, hangover). There may also be an alteration in bowel pattern (constipation) as a result of the drug's gastrointestinal effects. There is risk for impaired tissue integrity (redness, swelling, pain at injection site—thrombophlebitis) if the drug is administered intravenously. Respiratory problems may present as ineffective airway clearance or hypoventilation because of the respiratory depressant effects of barbiturates. The following potential complications exist: Stevens-Johnson syndrome (a serious inflammatory disease characterized by the sudden onset of fever, bullae of the skin, and ulcers on the mucous membranes of the lips, eyes, mouth, nasal passage, and genitalia); drug-induced hepatitis (jaundice); paradoxical reaction (unusual excitement); agranulocytosis (sore throat, fever); megaloblastic anemia (lethargy, weakness); thrombocytopenia (unusual bleeding or bruising); and allergic reaction (urticaria, wheezing, or tightness in chest).

Implementation

Monitoring. Continuous assessment of the client is focused on detection of adverse reactions or side effects, monitoring compliance, and monitoring effectiveness of the therapy. Indicators of effectiveness include sleep time, daytime wakefulness, and client reports about feelings of rest and wakefulness. Tolerance develops to all barbiturates during long-term therapy, but it develops at unpredictable rates. The development of tolerance, as well as possible dependence, should be closely evaluated. Monitoring for paradoxical reactions, allergic reactions, or drug interactions is also essential. The nurse should function as a client advocate when evaluation suggests that a change in drug therapy is needed.

Intervention. The nurse should be aware that long- and short-acting barbiturates may be combined in the same capsule so that the medication can be used to advantage for the client who has difficulty both in falling asleep and in remaining asleep for the desired number of hours.

To hasten the onset of sleep with oral administration, the rate of absorption may be increased by administering barbiturates well diluted or on an empty stomach.

With the exception of anesthesia and control of status epilepticus, barbiturates are infrequently prescribed to be administered by the intravenous route. If the intravenous barbiturates have been prescribed, dilute according to the package insert directions and administer slowly. If the barbiturate is to be infused in an intravenous solution, use an infusion control device and monitor the infusion rate closely, since rapid injection can be dangerous. The airway should be patent and emergency resuscitative equipment should be available when the medication is given intravenously.

For intravenous injection, use the larger veins to decrease the risk of irritation. The intravenous site should be assessed for any signs of thrombophlebitis or extravasation.

Barbiturates may be administered rectally with a retention enema if the oral or parenteral route is undesirable.

Clients who become disoriented or confused by a barbiturate should not be restrained. Rather, the client should be reoriented and a calm environment promoted.

Education. Instruct the client to use the barbiturate only as directed. The client should not alter the dosage or take the drug more often or for a longer period than ordered. Barbiturates may impair mental and physical functioning. The client should avoid dangerous activities if affected by barbiturates in this manner.

Barbiturates may affect the developing fetus. If a client is pregnant or may become pregnant during therapy, she should discuss barbiturate use with her nurse-midwife, nurse practitioner, or physician. Barbiturates will also pass into breast milk and may affect the nursing infant.

Barbiturates may cause mental or physical dependence or tolerance. Clients should consult their prescriber if they experience the signs or symptoms of dependence or no longer receive the full effect of the drug.

If the client is following a scheduled dosing regimen (as when a barbiturate is used as an anticonvulsant) and a dose is missed, it should be taken immediately if remembered within 1 to 2 hours of the scheduled time; otherwise, the client should skip the dose and continue with the regimen.

Abrupt withdrawal may precipitate seizures in the epileptic client. Abstinence syndrome (see Chapter 9) may be seen after abrupt withdrawal in any client after long-term therapy. Barbiturates interact with many other drugs and alcohol. Inform the client not to take any additional medications while taking a barbiturate unless they have been approved by the prescriber or pharmacist. Dangerous interactions may occur.

Evaluation. If the barbiturate has been administered for sedation, the client will report feeling relaxed or having slept well. If the indication for barbiturate use was seizures, the client will demonstrate a marked decrease or absence of seizures.

MISCELLANEOUS SEDATIVES AND HYPNOTICS

A number of antianxiety agents/sedatives and hypnotics do not fall into the previously discussed drug classes, but they will be discussed here because they are available for client use with prescription.

Antianxiety Agents/Sedatives

buspirone [byoo spye' rone] (BuSpar)

Buspirone is not related pharmacologically to other medications discussed in this chapter. It is indicated for the treatment of anxiety disorders and is considered to be equivalent in efficacy to the benzodiazepines usually with less sedation. The exact mechanism of action is unknown, but the drug has a high affinity for serotonin receptors and a moderate affinity for brain D_2-dopamine receptors in the CNS. It does not affect GABA, nor does it have any significant affinity to the benzodiazepine receptors.

Absorption of the drug is very good, but it undergoes extensive first-pass metabolism in the liver. Protein binding is high (95%) and the onset of effect may take 1 to 2 weeks. The drug does not cause muscle relaxation or sedation, so clients may not notice any effects from the medication during this time. The half-life (elimination) is between 2 and 3 hours after a single 10- to 40-mg dose. Buspirone is metabolized in the liver; one of the metabolites is active. It is eliminated through the kidneys and feces.

The most common side effects include headache, nausea, increased nervousness, and faintness. Less frequent side effects include tinnitus, abdominal distress, insomnia, nightmares, increased weakness, dry mouth, blurred vision, muscle pain or spasms, and decreased ability to concentrate. Rarely are adverse reactions reported. They include chest pain, tachycardia, muscle weakness, paresthesia, sore throat, elevated temperature, depression, and confusion.

The recommended dosage for adults is 5 mg orally 3 times daily, increased by 5 mg per day, every 2 to 3 days, until the desired response is achieved. Maximum dose is 60 mg per day. No dosage has been established for persons under 18 years old.

■ Nursing Management

Buspirone Hydrochloride Therapy

Assessment. Contraindications to the use of buspirone therapy would be hepatic or renal impairment, since the drug is metabolized in the liver and excreted by the kidneys. It should be used with caution for clients who are also receiving digoxin therapy, since it displaces digoxin from the plasma protein binding sites and so increases the effects of the digoxin. Avoid concurrent administration with MAO inhibitors, since severe hypertension may occur.

The baseline assessment of the client should include the underlying condition for which buspirone is prescribed as well as the client's CNS status.

Nursing diagnosis. Clients receiving buspirone are at risk for the following nursing diagnoses/collaborative problems: anxiety related to the client's underlying problem and the ineffectiveness of the drug; altered thought processes (depression, confusion); risk for injury related to drug-induced CNS response (dizziness, lightheadedness); and altered comfort (headache, nausea).

Implementation

Monitoring. Continuous assessment should include the client's level of anxiety, mental status, neuromuscular coordination, and vital signs.

Intervention. Administer with food to prevent gastrointestinal distress.

Education. In addition to the general discussion under the nursing management of sedatives and hypnotics, instruct clients to use ice chips or sugarless candies to manage the side effect of dry mouth if it occurs. Inform clients that 1 or 2 weeks of therapy may be necessary before the effects of buspirone therapy are evidenced. Chest pain, alterations in thought processes, palpitations, sensory or motor changes in the hands and feet, or fever or sore throat should be reported to the prescriber.

Evaluation. The expected outcome is that clients will state that they are less anxious and will not experience any adverse effects from the buspirone.

hydroxyzine [hye drox' i zeen] (Atarax, Vistaril)

Hydroxyzine, a piperazine antihistamine, is an antianxiety agent, sedative-hypnotic, antihistamine, and antiemetic. The antianxiety effect may be due to hydroxyzine's suppression of activity in selected subcortical areas of the CNS although its full mechanism of action is unknown. Its antihistamine and sedative effects may be due to competition with histamine at H_1 receptor sites. Hydoxyzine's antiemetic, antimotion sickness and anti-vertigo effects may be the result of central anticholinergic activity and decreased vestibular stimulation and labyrinthine function. Hydroxyzine may also have an effect on the chemoreceptive trigger zone.

Absorption of hydroxyzine is good. Onset of action occurs within 15 to 30 minutes after an oral dose. Duration of effect is 4 to 6 hours when the drug is given orally; half-life is 20 to 25 hours. Hydroxyzine is metabolized in the liver and excreted by the kidneys.

The most common side effects include sedation, which usually disappears after a few days of therapy or when the dose is reduced. Less frequent and usually reported with high drug doses are anticholinergic side effects, such as dry mouth. Adverse reactions, rarely reported, include skin rash and trembling or seizures (in doses higher than recommended).

The recommended adult dose of hydroxyzine is 25 to 100 mg orally, 3 to 4 times daily as necessary. When the drug is administered to children as an antianxiety agent or sedative-hypnotic, the dosage is 0.6 mg/kg body weight orally. For antihistamine or antiemetic effects, administer 0.5 mg/kg body weight orally every 6 hours when necessary. Parenterally the adult dosage is 25 to 100 mg IM every 4 to 6 hours if necessary. When used in children as an antiemetic or adjunct to narcotic medication, hydroxyzine should be administered 1 mg/kg body weight IM.

■ Nursing Management

Hydroxyzine Therapy

In addition to the nursing management of sedative and hypnotic therapy discussed in the previous section, the following nursing measures need to be considered for the administration of hydroxyzine.

Assessment. The nurse needs to be aware that because of its antiemetic effects, hydroxyzine may mask symptoms of serious conditions that might be evidenced by nausea and vomiting, such as brain lesions, appendicitis, and other gastrointestinal disorders.

When hydroxyzine is given concurrently with alcohol or CNS depressants, the CNS-depressant effects may be enhanced. A dosage reduction may be necessary.

Nursing diagnosis. In addition to the anxiety related to the client's underlying condition and the ineffectiveness of the drug, the client may be at risk of altered mucous membranes related to drug-induced dry mouth. The potential complication of seizures exists.

Implementation

Monitoring. The client's level of anxiety, vital signs, and neuromuscular functioning should be monitored.

Intervention. The drug is not to be administered subcutaneously, intravenously, or intraarterially because significant tissue damage may occur. Hydroxyzine needs to be administered by deep intramuscular injection; the Z-track injection is preferred.

Education. Clients may be instructed to use ice chips and sugarless candy or gum to manage any symptoms of dry mouth that occur. Involuntary motor activity, such as trembling and shaking, should be reported to the prescriber; a change in medication dosage may be indicated.

Evaluation. The expected outcome is that clients state that they are less anxious and do not experience any adverse effects.

Hypnotics

chloral hydrate [klor al hye' drate] (Noctec, Novochlorhydrate🍁)

The CNS-depressant effects produced are believed to be caused by the drug's active metabolite, trichloroethanol, although its exact mechanism of action is unknown. Chloral hydrate is indicated as a sedative and as a hypnotic. Oral and rectal forms are rapidly absorbed. Chloral hydrate is metabolized in the liver and erythrocytes to its active metabolite, trichloroethanol; further liver metabolism is to inactive metabolites. Onset of action of a hypnotic dose occurs within 30 minutes; half-life is approximately 7 to 10 hours. The drug is excreted by the kidneys. Side/adverse effects include nausea, abdominal distress, ataxia, dizziness, drowsiness, confusion, excitability (paradoxical reaction), hallucinations, and skin rash.

Adult hypnotic dose is 0.5 to 1 g PO or rectally 15 to 30 minutes before bedtime. Daytime sedative dose is 250 mg 3 times daily, after meals. Use extreme caution with administration of chloral hydrate to children as pediatric deaths have occurred with the use of this drug. If administered, the child should be in a health care facility that can provide continuous monitoring (*USP DI*, 1996).

■ Nursing Management

Chloral Hydrate Therapy

In addition to the nursing management discussed in the previous section on sedatives and hypnotics, the following nursing measures need to be considered for the administration of chloral hydrate.

Assessment. The client should be assessed for medical conditions in which chloral hydrate might need to be administered with caution, such as esophagitis, gastritis, or gastric or duodenal ulcers, because these may be exacerbated with the oral forms of the drug. Consider, too, hepatic impairment since choral hydrate is metabolized in the liver, and renal impairment, since the drug is excreted by the kidneys.

The concurrent medication regimen of the client needs to be considered because the following effects may occur when chloral hydrate is given with the drugs listed below:

Drug	Possible effect and management
alcohol or other CNS depressants	Enhanced CNS depression effects may result. Monitor closely for respiratory depression and/or lethargy, since the dosage of one or both drugs may need to be reduced.
anticoagulants (coumarin, indanedione)	Especially within the first few days or weeks, the anticoagulant may be displaced from its protein binding, leading to an enhanced hypoprothrombinemic effect. Monitor closely for bleeding tendencies.

Nursing diagnosis. The client receiving chloral hydrate has the potential for the following nursing diagnoses/collaborative problems: sleep pattern disturbance related to the client's underlying problem and the ineffectiveness of the drug; altered thought processes (confusion); altered comfort (nausea); sleep pattern disturbance (daytime drowsiness, hangover); risk for injury related to the adverse CNS reactions to the drug (dizziness, lightheadedness); and the potential complications of allergic reaction, paradoxical reaction, and convulsions.

Implementation

Monitoring. The client's sleep pattern and CNS responses to the drug should be monitored.

Intervention. The unpleasant taste and odor of the elixir make it difficult for clients, particularly children, to take. To make the elixir more palatable, mix it with fruit juice or some type of chilled fluid (such as ginger ale). If the client is being given the elixir as a preoperative medication, when only a small amount of liquid should be ingested, a flavored extract (e.g., peppermint extract, banana extract) should be added to make it more palatable.

Because the drug can cause gastric irritation, administer it after meals with 8 oz of fluid, unless it is being administered as a preoperative medication.

Client safety is essential. If the client shows signs of somnambulism, confusion, or dizziness, he or she should be assisted with ambulation. In addition, the prescriber should be consulted for a dosage reduction or a change in medication for nighttime sedation.

Education. Because chloral hydrate may interfere with urine glucose testing in diabetics, instruct clients in the use of home blood glucose monitoring methods.

Evaluation. As with other sedative-hypnotics, the client should report the drug effective in inducing nighttime sleep and daytime wakefulness without adverse effects. Client safety is maintained.

ethchlorvynol [eth klor vi' nole] (Placidyl)

The CNS depressant effects are similar to those of chloral hydrate and barbiturates, although the exact mechanism of action is unknown. Ethchlorvynol is indicated for use as a sedative-hypnotic.

Absorption is good from the gastrointestinal tract. The drug's distribution is highly localized in lipid or fat tissues; the drug has also been located in cerebrospinal fluid, brain, bile, liver, kidneys, and spleen. This drug has a half-life of approximately 10 to 20 hours; onset of action within 15 to 60 minutes and a duration of action of approximately 5 hours. Ethchlorvynol is metabolized in the liver and excreted by the kidneys.

Side/adverse effects include visual disturbances, nausea, vomiting, abdominal distress, increased weakness, facial numbness, unpleasant aftertaste, allergic reactions, paradoxical (increased excitability or nervousness) reaction and thrombocytopenia. Significant drug interactions are the same as those for chloral hydrate, discussed on p. 315.

When ethchlorvynol is administered to adults as a sedative-hypnotic, the recommended dose is 500 to 1000 mg orally at bedtime. The elderly may require lower doses because they are more sensitive to the drug. This drug is not available for use with children.

■ Nursing Management

Ethchlorvynol Therapy

The drug may produce transient giddiness and ataxia in some clients because it is absorbed rapidly. The symptoms can be minimized by administering the drug with milk or food. If the client awakens in the early morning hours after a bedtime dose of ethchlorvynol, a single additional dose of 100 to 200 mg may be administered. The nurse should check to see that the dosage for elderly, debilitated clients is reduced to the smallest effective amount. The client should be instructed to report any yellowing of the skin or eyes (which might be signs of cholestatic jaundice), rash, or excessive bruising (which might indicate thrombocytopenia). See also nursing management for sedative-hypnotic therapy.

meprobamate [me proe ba' mate] (Equanil, Miltown)

Meprobamate functions as a CNS depressant with an unknown mechanism of action. It is indicated for use as an antianxiety agent. Absorption is good; the drug has a half-life of approximately 10 hours. It is metabolized in the liver and excreted by the kidneys.

Side/adverse effects include ataxia, drowsiness, visual disturbances, nightmares, muscle twitching, euphoria, headache and allergic reactions. Clients taking meprobamate concomitantly with alcohol or CNS depressants may experience increased alcohol and CNS-depressant effects.

The recommended adult dosage is 400 mg orally 3 or 4 times daily or 600 mg twice daily, up to a maximum of 2.4 g/day. Elderly clients may be more sensitive to this drug; their dosage should be lowered and/or they should be monitored closely. Meprobamate is not recommended for children under 6 years old. For children 6 to 12 years old, the dose is 100 to 200 mg orally 2 or 3 times daily. The effectiveness of meprobamate beyond 4 months of therapy has not been studied.

For the nursing management of the client receiving meprobamate, consult the general nursing management for antianxiety, sedative, and hypnotic agents.

paraldehyde [par al' de hyde] (Paral)

Paraldehyde's CNS-depressant effects, while similar to those of alcohol, barbiturates, and chloral hydrate, has an unknown mechanism of action. It depresses various levels of the CNS, including the ascending reticular activating system. Paraldehyde is indicated as an anticonvulsant and in the past has been used as a sedative-hypnotic. The latter is no longer an approved indication as safer and more effective agents are available.

Absorption is good from the gastrointestinal tract and intramuscular sites; the drug reaches peak serum levels in ½ to 1 hour after oral administration or in 2½ hours after rectal administration. It has a half-life of 3 to 10 hours, is metabolized in the liver (70% to 90%) with trace amounts excreted by the kidneys. The unmetabolized paraldehyde is excreted via exhalation.

Side/adverse effects include unpleasant taste, drowsiness, abdominal distress, nausea, vomiting, skin rash, muscle cramps, trembling, and confusion.

The recommended anticonvulsant adult dose is up to 12 ml (diluted to a 10% solution) via gastric tube as needed orally every 4 hours. The rectal dose is 10 to 20 ml. The pediatric anticonvulsant dose is 0.3 ml/kg orally or rectally.

■ Nursing Management

Paraldehyde Therapy

Assessment. Because paraldehyde is excreted partly through the lungs and increases respiratory secretions, its administration is contraindicated in clients with bronchopulmonary disease. Oral administration would be of concern in clients with gastroenteritis, since paraldehyde is a GI irritant.

Significant drug interactions are seen when paraldehyde is used in combination with alcohol and CNS depressants (see data on chloral hydrate). The drug also interacts with disulfiram; disulfiram (Antabuse) decreases paraldehyde metabolism, which may lead to increased blood levels of paraldehyde and acetaldehyde. Do not give disulfiram to clients receiving paraldehyde.

Nursing diagnosis. In addition to the other potential nursing diagnoses/collaborative problems for sedatives and hypnotics, clients receiving paraldehyde parenterally may be at risk for an alteration in comfort (pain) related to the injection, and for impaired gas exchange related to its effects on pulmonary capillaries.

Implementation

Monitoring. Monitor the client's mental status and level of consciousness. Vital signs and breath sounds should be assessed periodically in keeping with the client's status. Liver function studies should be monitored.

Intervention. When giving the drug orally, dilute paraldehyde well in flavored syrup, iced fruit juice, or milk; the fluid should be chilled to minimize its odor and taste. Dilution also decreases gastric irritation. Administer in a glass container, since paraldehyde reacts with plastic. When given by the intramuscular or intravenous route, a glass syringe should be used. Paraldehyde will react with plastic syringes and cause the plastic to decompose into toxic compounds.

When giving this drug by a parenteral route (rarely done), the nurse should have resuscitative equipment available in the event of a cardiorespiratory arrest. The client should be kept in the side-lying position to prevent aspiration of bronchial secretions, which are increased after administration of the drug.

Because the drug cannot be used if the container has been open for more than 24 hours, label the container with the date and time it was opened. Do not use the drug if it is colored or has the odor of acetic acid.

When giving this drug by the intramuscular route, administer no more than 5 ml per injection site and rotate the sites. Subcutaneous administration should be avoided because paraldehyde irritates the tissues. Ensure the client is in a well-ventilated room, since the exhaled drug can be very pungent.

For rectal doses paraldehyde should be diluted with 1 to 2 parts of olive oil, cottonseed oil, or normal saline solution to prevent rectal tissue irritation.

Because the solution is extremely volatile, avoid contact with eyes, skin, and clothing. The solution and its fumes should be kept away from a heat source, open flame, or spark.

Education. The nurse should prepare the client and family or caregiver for the strong unpleasant breath odor that results from administration of the drug and should instruct the client in oral hygiene. The client will need to be instructed to report symptoms that might result from the paraldehyde, such as yellowing of the skin or eyes, which might indicate hepatitis, and/or bloody stools, which might result from the irritation of the intestinal mucosa.

Evaluation. When paraldehyde is given as an anticonvulsant, the client will have a marked decrease or absence of seizure activity.

zolpidem tartrate (Ambien)

Zolpidem tartrate is the first of a new class, nonbenzodiazepine hypnotic approved for short-term treatment of insomnia. It is more selective in its binding to the GABA receptor than the benzodiazepines are; thus it has some pharmacologic properties that are similar to those of benzodiazepines. The benzodiazepines bind to $omega_1$, $omega_2$, and $omega_3$ GABA receptors whereas zolpidem only binds to $omega_1$ receptors. Being more selective, it lacks the anticonvulsant, muscle relaxant, and anti-anxiety properties associated with the benzodiazepines.

The adult dosage is 10 mg at bedtime. A 5 mg initial dose is recommended for geriatric, debilitated clients and persons with hepatic insufficiency. No dosage has been established for children under 18 years old.

The client should be advised to avoid concurrent intake of alcohol and CNS depressants. It is also recommended to take this medication on an empty stomach because food decreases its absorption. The most commonly reported side effects are headaches, drowsiness, and myalgia. See the general discussion of nursing management for sedatives and hypnotics.

SUMMARY

When a client is unable to cope with a persistently stressful situation because excessive anxiety interferes with daily functioning, an antianxiety agent may be prescribed. Benzodiazepines are the most commonly used drugs in this group. Before their advent, sedatives were used to reduce nervousness or irritability by producing a soothing effect. Hypnotics are used to induce sleep. Sedatives and hypnotics differ only in the degree of CNS depression.

Benzodiazepines do not exert a general CNS-depressant effect, and their wide range of selectivity of action allows their use for a variety of conditions—as anticonvulsants, hypnotics, muscular relaxants, and antianxiety agents. Barbiturates, on the other hand, are used for mild sedation to deep anesthesia. Although a barbiturate is not an analgesic, when administered with an analgesic it reinforces analgesic effects and alters the client's emotional response to pain.

Sleep is important for humans, and both REM sleep and non-REM sleep are essential for good mental health. Antianxiety, sedative, and hypnotic drugs may be prescribed to assist sleep. Both pediatric clients and geriatric clients are much more sensitive to the CNS-depressant effects of these drugs. Children usually respond better to counseling and psychotherapy than to antianxiety agents; the elderly, because of a decline in organ function, are more effectively treated with shorter-acting benzodiazepines. Both groups of clients are at greater risk for paradoxical reactions than the general population.

The nurse's role in sedative-hypnotic therapy is to assess the extent of the client's sleep pattern disturbance, its cause, and the client's previous ways in coping with it. Nonpharmacologic nursing interventions to induce sleep should be used in place of or as adjuncts to medicating the client with a sedative-hypnotic agent. Client education should focus on safe self-administration, emphasizing that performance may be impaired because blood levels of some of these drugs are retained. Effectiveness will be indicated by the client reporting feelings of rest without residual drowsiness during the day.

Benzodiazepines are among the most frequently prescribed drugs today for a variety of disorders: anxiety disorders, alcohol withdrawal, preoperative medication, neuromuscular disease, and sleep and seizure disorders. Barbiturates, previously more widely used, have been largely replaced by the benzodiazepines. However, barbiturates are still indicated as hypnotic, antianxiety, anesthetic, preanesthetic, anticonvulsant, antihyperbilirubinemic, and narcoanalytic agents.

Although antianxiety, sedative, and hypnotic drugs create many of the same responses within the client, the nurse must be knowledgeable about the specific agents used. Because these agents exert CNS effects, the nurse needs to be aware that the client may be at risk for injury, alteration in sensory/perceptual function, alteration in self-concept, and a further disturbance of sleep pattern. The gastrointestinal effects of many of these agents may result in constipation. As with all agents, clients and their families may also experience a knowledge deficit related to their drug therapy.

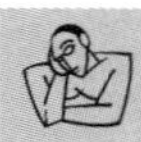

Critical Thinking

1. What factors would need to be included in an education plan for a client taking benzodiazepines? if the client were a young married woman? an elderly client? an Asian client? a child?
2. What nonpharmacologic nursing measures should accompany the administration of a sleep medication?
3. What actions might a nurse take if a client had altered comfort at night as well as insomnia?

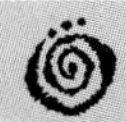

Collaborative Learning Activities

1. Assign student teams each of the components of the first critical thinking question above. Have the teams present their responses to the questions in the class with the rationale for their answer.

BIBLIOGRAPHY

Abramowicz M (Ed.) (1992). Flumazenil, *Med Lett* 34(874):66.

American Hospital Formulary Service (1996). *AHFS drug information '95*. Bethesda, MD: American Society of Hospital Pharmacists.

American Medical Association (1995). *Drug evaluations annual 1995*. Chicago: The Association.

Anderson KN, et al. (Eds.) (1994). *Mosby's medical, nursing, & allied health dictionary* (4th ed.). St Louis: Mosby.

Crismon ML (1992). Insomnia. In Koda-Kimble MA & Young LY. *Applied therapeutics* (5th ed.). Vancouver: Applied Therapeutics.

DiPiro JT, et al. (Eds.) (1993). *Pharmacotherapy* (2nd ed.). Norwalk, CT: Appleton & Lange.

Dopheide JA (1995). Sleep disorders. In Young LY & Koda-Kimble MA. *Applied therapeutics: The clinical use of drugs* (6th ed.). Vancouver, WA: Applied Therapeutics.

Drug Product Update (1996). Halcion, Xanax Changes, *ASHP Newsletter* 29(10):5.

Edmonds S, et al. (Eds.) (1995). Abecarnil shows promise in generalized anxiety disorder, *Drugs & Ther Perspect* 5(12):7-8.

Glod CA (1992). Xanax: Pros and cons, *J Psychosoc Nurs Ment Health Serv* 30(6):36-7.

Gottlieb GL (1990). Sleep disorders and their management—special considerations in the elderly, *Am J Med* 88(suppl 3A):29S.

Grimsley SR (1995). Anxiety disorders. In Young LY and Koda-Kimble MA. *Applied therapeutics: The clinical use of drugs* (6th ed.). Vancouver, WA: Applied Therapeutics.

Hartmann PM (1995). Drug treatment of insomnia: Indications and newer agents, *Amer Family Phys* 51(1):191-4.

Hoehns JD & Perry PJ (1993). Zolpidem: A nonbenzodiazepine hypnotic for treatment of insomnia, *Clin Pharmacy* 12(11):814-828.

Jellin JM (Ed.) (1991). Neurology/psychiatry, *Pharm Lett* 7(11):61.

Kirkwood CF (1991). Flumazenil—a benzodiazepine receptor antagonist, *P & T* 16(3)243.

Kudzma EC (1992). Drug responses: All bodies are not created equal, *Amer J Nurs* 92(12):48-50.

Lammon CA & Adams AH (1993). Recognizing benzodiazepine overdose, *Nursing* 23(1):33.

Lin DM, et al. (1988). Comparison of alprazolam plasma levels in normal Asian and Caucasian volunteers, *Psychopharmacol Bull* 96:365.

McCance KL & Huether SE (1994). *Pathophysiology: The biologic basis for disease in adults and children* (2nd ed.). St Louis: Mosby.

McCue JD, et al. (1993). *Geriatric drug handbook for long-term care.* Baltimore: Williams & Wilkins.

Mejo SL (1992). Anterograde amnesia linked to benzodiazepines, *Nurse Pract* 17(10):44.

Melmon KL, et al. (1992). *Clinical pharmacology* (3rd ed.). New York: McGraw-Hill.

Morton MR (1992). Managing anxiety disorders in the older adult, *Clin Consult* 11(4):7.

News Capsules (1993). P & T update: New approvals and dosage forms, *Hosp Formul* 28(3):207.

Olin BR (Ed.) (1995). *Facts and comparisons.* St. Louis: Facts and Comparisons.

Pagel JF (1994). Treatment of insomnia, *Amer Family Phys* 49(6): 1417-21.

PDR (1995). *Physicians' desk reference* (49th ed.). Montvale, NJ: Medical Economics.

Regimen: An update on long-term care drug therapy (1995). Monitoring psychoactive drug use in nursing home patients, *NARD* *118*(3):1-4.

Sherman D (1991). Evaluation and treatment of sleep disorders, *Contemp Long Term Care* *14*(12):70.

Silcox MM (1992). Flumazenil useful in reversing effects of benzodiazepines, *J Emerg Nurs* *18*(4):301.

United States Pharmacopeia Convention (1996). *Drug information for the health care professional* (16th ed.). Rockville, MD: The Convention.

Wong DL (1995). *Whaley & Wong's nursing care of infants and children* (5th ed.). St Louis: Mosby.

Chapter 17

Anticonvulsants

Chapter Focus

Epilepsy is the second most common neurologic disease in North America (after stroke); it affects 1 out of 50 children and 1 out of 100 adults. As in other chronic disorders, nurses play a key role in assisting clients to effectively manage their epilepsy. This chapter will provide you with information about anticonvulsant medications as a basis for that role. The following objectives and key terms are important for a good understanding of this chapter.

erms

epilepsy (p. 321)
focal seizure (p. 321)
primary (idiopathic) epilepsy (p. 321)
secondary epilepsy (p. 321)
serum half-life (p. 324)
status epilepticus (p. 322)
tonic-clonic generalized (grand mal) epilepsy (p. 321)
toxemia of pregnancy (p. 339)

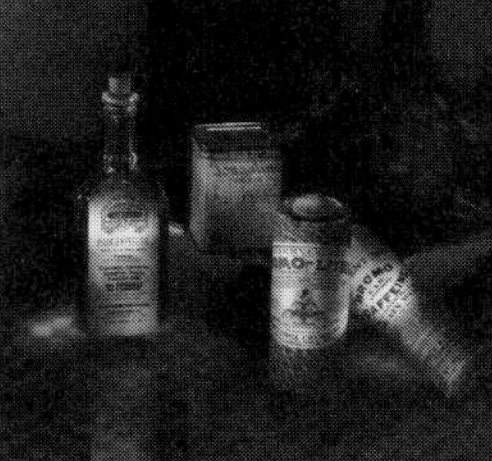

Key Drugs [▲]

phenobarbital
phenytoin

Objectives

1. Describe the international classification of epileptic seizures.
2. Identify observations to be made about a client having a seizure.
3. Discuss the nursing management for anticonvulsant therapy.
4. Identify the major anticonvulsant drug classifications including examples of drugs and their primary methods of seizure-control activity.
5. List the common side effects/adverse reactions of anticonvulsants.
6. Implement an appropriate plan of care for a client receiving an anticonvulsant drug or drugs.

Epilepsy is a group of chronic neurologic disorders characterized by sporadic recurrent episodes of convulsive seizures, sensory disturbances, abnormal behavior, loss of consciousness, or all of these symptoms resulting from a brain dysfunction or an abnormal discharge of cerebral neurons. Although nearly 70% of seizures do not have an identifiable cause (**primary or idiopathic epilepsy**), approximately 30% have an underlying cause (**secondary epilepsy**) that is treatable (e.g., head injury, cerebrovascular infarct or hemorrhage, infection, brain tumor, drug toxicity, or a metabolic imbalance).

CLASSIFICATION OF SEIZURES

The choice of an appropriate anticonvulsant drug for treatment of an individual client depends on accurate diagnosis and classification of the seizure type. A complete medical history, laboratory tests, a neurologic exam, and an electroencephalogram (EEG) are necessary for classification. Computerized tomography (CT) and magnetic resonance imaging (MRI) may also be used to detect anatomic defects or to locate small focal brain lesions. Identifying specific seizure types is critical to the development of a treatment plan.

The terminology currently used with epileptic seizures is illustrated in Box 17-1 on the international classification of seizures. In practice, however, many health care providers still use the common terms—grand mal, Jacksonian, psychomotor, and petit mal—therefore the student should be familiar with both seizure classifications. This text will use both classifications.

BOX 17-1

International Classification of Seizures

Partial seizures

Simple (no impairment of consciousness)
- Motor symptoms (formerly called Jacksonian)
- Sensory (hallucinations of sight, hearing, or taste); somatosensory (tingling)
- Autonomic—autonomic nervous system responses
- Psychic (personality changes)

Complex (impaired consciousness)
- Cognitive (memory impairment, confusion)
- Affective (bizarre behavioral effects)
- Psychosensory (automatisms—repetition, purposeless behaviors)
- Psychomotor (complex symptoms that may include an aura, automatism [i.e., chewing, swallowing movements], unreal feelings, bizarre behaviors, and motor seizures)
- Compound (tonic, clonic, or tonic-clonic seizures)

Partial seizures, secondarily generalized
- Unilateral seizures
- Predominantly unilateral seizures

Generalized seizures (convulsive or nonconvulsive)
Widespread involvement of both cerebral hemispheres
- Tonic-clonic seizures (formerly called grand mal)
- Tonic (sustained contractions of large muscle groups)
- Clonic (various dysrhythmic contractions in the body)
- Myoclonic (unaltered consciousness, isolated clonic contractions)
- Absence (formerly called petit mal—brief loss of consciousness for a few seconds, no confusion, EEG demonstrates 3/sec spike wave patterns.
- Atonic (head drop or falling down symptoms)

Unclassified seizures
Available data incomplete, inadequate, or lacks classification status (such as neonatal seizures)

TYPES OF EPILEPSY

Partial simple motor (Jacksonian) epilepsy is described by some as a type of **focal seizure**; it is associated with irritation of a specific part of the brain. A single body part, such as a finger or an extremity, may jerk and such movements may end spontaneously or spread over the whole musculature. Consciousness may not be lost unless the seizure develops into a generalized convulsion.

Partial complex (psychomotor) seizures are characterized by brief alterations in consciousness, unusual stereotyped movements (such as chewing or swallowing movements) repeated over and over, changes in temperament, confusion, and feelings of unreality. These seizures are often associated with grand mal seizures and are likely to be resistant to therapy with drugs.

Generalized absence, simple or complex (petit mal), seizures are most often seen in childhood and consist of temporary lapses in consciousness that last for a few seconds. Clients appear to stare into space or daydream, are inattentive, and may exhibit a few rhythmic movements of the eyes (slight blinking), head, or hands. They do not convulse. They may have many attacks in a single day. The EEG records a 3/sec spike wave pattern. Sometimes an attack of generalized absence seizures is followed by a generalized tonic-clonic type of seizure. When the child reaches adulthood, other types of seizures may occur.

Tonic-clonic generalized (grand mal) epilepsy is the type most commonly seen. Such attacks may be characterized by an aura, a sudden loss of consciousness and motor control. The aura is specific to the individual; it may consist of numbness, visual disturbance, or a particular form of dizziness that warns the client of an approaching seizure. The client falls forcefully and has a series of tonic (stiffening, increased muscle tone) and clonic (rapid, synchronous jerking) muscular contractions. The eyes roll upward, the arms flex, and the legs extend. The force of the muscular contractions causes air to be forced out of the lungs, which accounts for the cry that the client may make on falling. Respiration is suspended temporarily, the skin becomes diaphoretic and cyanotic, perspiration and saliva flow, and the client may froth at the mouth and bite the tongue if it gets caught between the teeth. Incontinence may occur. When the seizure subsides, the client regains partial consciousness, may complain of aching, and then tends to fall into a deep sleep.

Status epilepticus is a clinical emergency. It is the state of recurrent seizures of more than 30 minutes without an intervening stay of consciousness. A 10% to 20% mortality rate results from anoxia in this state. *The major cause of status epilepticus is noncompliance with the drug regimen*; other causes include cerebral infarction, CNS tumor or infection, trauma, or low blood concentration of calcium or glucose.

Mixed seizures are seen in some clients who have more than one type of seizure disorder. This is significant because different types of seizures respond specifically to certain anticonvulsant drugs. The aim of therapy is to find the drug or drugs that will effectively control the seizures with a minimum of undesirable side effects and restore physiologic homeostasis to arrest convulsive activity.

RELATIONSHIP OF AGE TO SEIZURES

A relationship of age to onset of an epileptic seizure state exists. Most clients diagnosed as having epilepsy have their initial seizure before the age of 20; however, seizures may have an onset at any age in life. Idiopathic (undefined, unascertainable, or genetic in origin or cause) seizures are often diagnosed between the ages of 5 and 20. Onset before or after this age period is often from nonidiopathic (identifiable, ascertainable) causes and is termed *symptomatic* (acquired, organic) epilepsy.

Neonates. Neonatal seizures occur in newborn children less than 1 month old. Among the more common causes of neonatal seizures in this age group are congenital defects or malformation of the brain, abnormality or infections (meningitis, encephalitis, abscess) within the CNS, hypoxia (in utero or during delivery), premature birth, and defects in metabolism. These epileptic seizures are also referred to as *organic, symptomatic,* or *acquired* because they may be caused by an identifiable preceding condition or cause.

Infants. In infants less than 2 years of age, the seizure types most frequently diagnosed include generalized tonic-clonic seizures and partial seizures. The atonic epileptic seizure seen in later development (ages 2 to 5 years) may be preceded by infantile spasms in those less than 2 years. The infantile spasm is not classified as a type of epileptic seizure itself. Among the more common causes of infant seizures are those reported in the neonatal state and, additionally, injury in the perinatal period, infection, exposure to toxins (in utero caused by maternal exposure or drug use, misuse, or abuse), maternal exposure to x-rays, and postnatal trauma.

Children. In children 2 to 5 years old, the seizure types that are frequently diagnosed include generalized tonic-clonic seizures and atonic seizures. The causes are similar to those mentioned in newborns and infants with the addition of chronic diseases involving the CNS. The parents of the child may wrongly believe the child has a behavioral disorder rather than a treatable seizure disorder.

In children aged 6 years and older, brain tumors and vascular disease may cause seizures. Sometimes the convulsive seizure is associated with a brain infection, head trauma, fever, growth of scar tissue, cerebrovascular disease, the presence of a toxin or a poison, or drug withdrawal.

In children 5 to 16 years old, the seizure types that emerge in diagnosis are absence seizures and generalized tonic-clonic seizures, which may be idiopathic in origin. Seizure types such as partial, myoclonic, and less commonly generalized tonic-clonic seizures may be caused by neurologic diseases, infection, postnatal trauma, or head trauma (accident or sport).

Young adults. Within the age group 16 to 25 years, generalized seizures may be idiopathic in origin. The partial seizure and less commonly seen generalized seizures may result from the use of alcohol, social/recreational drug use, drug abuse or misuse, or head injury.

Adults. In clients over 20 years of age the seizures emerging often are of the generalized type, which may be idiopathic. Also seen are partial seizures and less commonly generalized seizures, which may have been precipitated by trauma to the head or a tumor of the brain.

Elderly. Persons over the age of 60 are at greater risk from seizure episodes. In this population osteoporosis and cerebrovascular disease are common, and therefore seizures may lead to fractures, intracranial bleeding, neurologic deficit, cognitive impairment, and severe limitation in daily functioning. Common causes of seizures in the elderly include trauma, brain tumors, vascular disease, embolic stroke, and Alzheimer's disease (Rowan, 1995).

ANTICONVULSANT THERAPY

Although secondary seizures usually respond to correction of the underlying condition and perhaps short-term use of anticonvulsants, primary recurrent seizures require long-term anticonvulsant drug therapy. The primary goal of drug therapy is to control or prevent the recurrence of the seizure disorder. Although there is no ideal anticonvulsant drug, if there were, the following characteristics would be highly desirable:

- The drug should be highly effective but exhibit a low incidence of toxicity.
- The drug should be effective against more than one type of seizure and for mixed seizures.
- The drug should be long-acting and nonsedating so that the client is not inconvenienced with the need for multiple daily drug dosing or excessive drowsiness.
- The drug should be well tolerated by the client and inexpensive, since the client may have to take it for years or for the rest of his or her life.
- Tolerance to the therapeutic effects of the drug should not develop.
- The drug should control seizures and permit the client to function effectively in any environment.

The major drugs used in the treatment of partial seizures and generalized tonic-clonic seizures are phenytoin (Dilantin), carbamazepine (Tegretol), and the barbiturates.

TABLE 17-1 Pharmacokinetic overview of selected anticonvulsant drugs

Name	Fate	Therapeutic plasma levels in adults (μg/ml)	Serum half-life (hr)
carbamazepine (Tegretol)	Absorption: slow and variable Metabolism: liver Excretion: urine, feces	4-12	1 dose: 25-65 Multidose: Adults 12-17
clonazepam (Klonopin, Rivotril ♣)	Absorption: good Metabolism: liver Excretion: urine	0.02-0.08	18-50
divalproex (Depakote, Epival ♣)	Absorption: 1-4 hr Metabolism: liver Excretion: urine, small amount from feces and lungs	50-100	6-16
ethosuximide (Zarontin)	Absorption: good Metabolism: liver Excretion: urine	40-100	Adults: 56-60 Children: 30-36
felbamate (Felbatol)	Absorption: good Metabolism: liver Excretion: urine and feces	Not determined	13-23
methsuximide (Celontin)	Absorption: good Metabolism: liver Excretion: urine	10-40	1-3 Active metabolite: 36-45
phenobarbital (Luminal and others)	Absorption: good Metabolism: liver Excretion: urine	10-40	Adults 53-118 Children: 40-70
phenytoin (Dilantin)	Absorption: orally, slow; poor in neonates Metabolism: liver Excretion: urine and feces	10-20	Adults: 22 (range 7-42)
primidone (Mysoline, Sertan ♣)	Absorption: good Metabolism: liver Excretion: urine	5-12	primidone: 3-24 and metabolites phenobarbital: 75-126 PEMA: 10-25
valproic acid (Depakene)	Absorption: complete and rapid Metabolism: kidney Excretion: urine, small amount from lungs and feces	50-100	Adults: 6-16

Phenytoin is the oldest nonsedating anticonvulsant drug in clinical use and is the most commonly prescribed anticonvulsant in North America. Several more recently released anticonvulsants include felbamate (Felbatol) and gabapentin (Neurontin).

Although the exact mode and site of action of these drugs are complex and incompletely understood, a major mechanism of action appears to relate to stabilization of the cell membrane by altering cation transport, especially sodium, potassium, and calcium. For example, phenytoin (hydantoins) decreases abnormal seizure discharge by blocking sodium channels and perhaps calcium influx. Thus phenytoin suppresses seizures by stabilizing cell membrane excitability, and reducing the spread of seizure discharge. Carbamazepine also enhances inactivation of the sodium channel, which alters neuronal excitability (decreases synaptic transmission). Thus the two main pharmacologic effects are:

- To increase motor cortex threshold to reduce its response to incoming electric or chemical stimulation
- To depress or reduce the spread of a seizure discharge from its focus or origin by depressing synaptic transport or decreasing nerve conduction.

Anticonvulsants fall into five major classifications: hydantoins, barbiturates, succinimides, benzodiazepines, and a miscellaneous group. The miscellaneous anticonvulsants include carbamazepine (Tegretol), valproic acid (Depakene), primidone (Mysoline), acetazolamide (Diamox), magnesium sulfate, felbamate (Felbatol) and gabapentin (Neurontin), drugs that are not chemically similar to one another (Table 17-1 and Box 17-2).

BOX 17-2

Anticonvulsant Agents for Seizure Disorders

The agents considered most effective with the least toxicity in treatment of seizure disorders are as follows:*

Generalized tonic-clonic (grand mal)	Absence seizures (petit mal)	Simple or complex partial	Myoclonic
valproic acid	ethosuximide	carbamazepine	valproic acid
phenytoin	valproic acid	phenytoin	clonazepam
carbamazepine		valproic acid	

*Listed in order of preference (Lott, 1995).

■ Nursing Management

Anticonvulsant Therapy

A client for whom anticonvulsants have been prescribed is treated most effectively with a holistic approach. This client has many special problems, including the fear of sudden loss of physical and emotional control and the stigma of seizures. In recent years, emphasis has been placed on public education on epilepsy to dispel the myths associated with it. This individual needs information about the seizure condition and its management, along with psychosocial support from the nurse. The client should understand that the condition can be controlled or modified with medication. The goal is to attain maximum seizure control with minimal medication side effects. The anticonvulsant or combination of such drugs prescribed depends on the type of seizure, whether the client is having more than one type of seizure, or whether the seizures are difficult to control. Finding the appropriate regimen for each client takes time.

The clinical effectiveness of anticonvulsant therapy varies with the drug's pharmacokinetics, mechanism of action, and serum levels achieved with scheduled drug dosing. The nurse should be aware that anticonvulsants may exhibit varying blood levels in different clients after each client has received the same dose. This variation results from a complex of interrelated factors including individual absorption, metabolism, distribution, and excretion, which may be caused by genetic and/or environmental factors; concomitant ailments, such as renal or hepatic dysfunctions; concurrent medication; diet; individual client compliance; and physical status. The dosage of certain drugs needs to be adjusted in order to obtain optimal therapeutic effects, and this dosage may have wide client variation.

Therapeutic dosage ranges are intended to serve merely as rough guides to therapy; they are not inflexible limits. The ranges provide a point from which the dosage of a drug may be individualized to account for the extremes in variation to response and adverse effects. The client beginning anticonvulsant therapy should have serum levels measured to establish individual level/dose ratio. This level tends to be a constant measure for an individual, although it varies considerably among clients. The time required to reach a steady serum level is generally about four to five times the elimination half-life of a drug. A convenient time for serum level measurement is 1 month after initiating therapy, since levels measured much earlier may be lower than the steady-state level finally achieved.

Pregnancy Safety

Category	Drug
C	acetazolamide, carbamazepine, ethotoin, lamotrigine, phenytoin
D	barbiturates, paramethadione, valproic acid, divalproex, felbamate, gabapentin
Unclassified	succinimides, primidone, diazepam, clonazepam, clorazepate, mephenytoin

The **serum half-life** of a drug (the time required for the drug serum level to drop 50% of its initial value when no additional drug is administered) is a measure of its rate of excretion and depends on the client's age. As discussed in Chapter 3, the pharmacokinetics of a drug are affected by age. For example, drug metabolism is relatively slow in the neonate, but in infants and young children it is higher on a milligram per kilogram of body weight basis than it is for an adult. Usually the elderly, whose metabolism is decreased, require a lower dosage schedule (see Chapter 8).

Epilepsy may worsen during pregnancy, and status epilepticus increases in frequency during gestation and labor. (See the above box for Pregnancy Safety of Anticonvulsants.) Some anticonvulsants appear in breast milk. Emotional stress (psychologic, occupational, physiologic, marital, economic) may influence seizure frequency.

Assessment. Along with a general assessment and drug history, assessment of the client with a convulsive disorder includes data specific to the seizures. These data include the number of seizures within a specific time; precipitating events or activities; presence of sensations or perceptions that the client experiences before a seizure, called an *aura*; and the character of seizures.

The nurse should assess the presence or absence of an aura and its nature. It may also be helpful to evaluate the ability of the client to describe it (somatic, visceral, psychic). It can also be useful to note the presence or absence of a cry. The onset of seizure should be assessed for site of initial body movements, deviation of head and eyes, chewing and salivation, posture of body, and sensory changes.

After onset of seizure it is important to note characteristics of the tonic and clonic phases. Characteristics include movements of body as the seizure progresses; skin color; airway clearance; pupillary changes; incontinence; and duration of each phase.

After the tonic and clonic phases, the nurse should try to assess duration of and behavior during the relaxation (sleep) phase. During the postictal phase, not only the duration should be noted but also general behavior; ability to remember anything about the seizure; orientation; pupillary changes; headache; and, finally, any injuries present. Finally, as accurate a picture as possible should be assessed of the duration of the entire seizure, level of consciousness, and length of unconsciousness if present. Often the nurse will not be present when a seizure has occurred. In this situation family, friends, or other witnesses may provide valuable information about the seizure.

In addition, the nurse should assess the client's understanding and management of the anticonvulsant medication regimen. One of the most common causes of seizure exacerbations is the mismanagement of the medications by the client. Up to 50% of clients do not take their medications regularly (Legion, 1991). Many do not understand the concepts of steady blood levels and half-life. Some clients use the drugs as they would aspirin, taking extra doses when they are afraid they might have a seizure. Some are afraid of the harm they think that their medications could cause, whereas others are concerned about becoming addicted to the drugs. The nurse should understand clients' use of medications as an attempt to gain control and provide information to allow them to manage the therapeutic regimen effectively.

Nursing diagnosis. In addition to the selected nursing diagnoses presented in the Nursing Care Plan below, the client receiving anticonvulsant therapy should be assessed

Nursing Care Plan

Selected Nursing Diagnoses for the Client on Anticonvulsant Medications

Nursing diagnosis	Outcome criteria	Nursing interventions
Knowledge deficit related to newly prescribed or altered anticonvulsant drug therapy	The client will describe: the seizure condition; how the drug therapy relates to the condition; how and when to take the medications; common drug interactions; safety precautions; common side effects and which of these warrant reporting; storage requirements of the drugs. The client will: demonstrate less anxiety related to fear of the unknown, loss of control, and misconceptions	Assess learning needs and learning readiness Plan with the client and family for the achievement of realistic goals Provide information to meet outcome criteria
Ineffective management of therapeutic medication regimen	The client will: self-administer medications safely and accurately	Determine the client's reasons for inaccuracies of dosing and take appropriate teaching/counseling interventions Provide needed drug information concerning rationale for the specific client's seizure status Discuss the increased possibility of seizures with ineffective management of the regimen
Risk for injury related to effects of anticonvulsant drug therapy	The client will: maintain anticonvulsant drug therapy without untoward side effects, adverse reactions, and toxicity	Administer drug safely and accurately Observe client for drowsiness, ataxia, behavioral changes, slurred speech, mental confusion, vertigo, and excessive sedation (see drug monographs for drug-specific side effects/adverse reactions) Instruct client about symptoms to be reported Explain the importance of Medic Alert card/tag Discourage self-altering of medication regimen Caution against activities requiring coordination and alertness until responses to drugs are known

for the following nursing diagnoses: activity intolerance related to anticonvulsant-induced weakness; altered bowel elimination (constipation or diarrhea) related to GI effects; altered comfort related to headache, nausea and vomiting, or dermatologic effects; altered protection related to drug-induced hematologic dysfunction; altered thought processes related to adverse CNS effects of drug; body image disturbance related to hydantoin-induced enlargement of the facial features, hirsutism, alopecia, or gynecomastia (in males); fluid volume excess related to carbamazepine-induced water intoxication; risk for injury related to client's underlying seizure activity, the ineffectiveness of anticonvulsant drug coverage and the CNS, visual, or hypotensive effects of the drug; impaired home maintenance management related to drug-imposed restrictions on driving and other activities; impaired skin integrity related to drug-induced rash; and altered respiratory pattern (hypoventilation) related to respiratory depressant effects of phenobarbital. The potential collaborative problems are: gingival hyperplasia (hydantoin), cognitive impairment, allergic reaction, blood dyscrasias, and hepatotoxicity.

Implementation

Monitoring. Therapeutic alternatives are selected (monotherapy or polytherapy) that best control the client's seizure. Many anticonvulsants have known blood levels of an optimal therapeutic range, the level of medication needed to control seizures. Therapeutic drug monitoring includes interpreting results of serum concentrations with the client's clinical response. This monitoring has reduced the need of polydrug anticonvulsant therapy and added greater efficiency in drug selection for each client.

Increased anticonvulsant serum levels may signal impending toxic effects. Generally, adverse effects are more serious at higher serum levels. Maintaining a serum level within the therapeutic range is a challenge for some clients (see the Pediatric and Geriatric Implications boxes below). The challenge surfaces when other drugs are added or deleted from the client's regimen, a client mismanages the medication regimen, there is an organ system dysfunction as seen in the hepatorenal systems, or undesirable drug effects cause the client to withdraw from drug therapy. Fully informing clients about the drug therapy and the need for serum concentrations within the therapeutic range may reduce therapeutic failures caused by adverse effects or the client's ineffective management of the medication regimen.

The most common medical test to evaluate seizure activity is the electroencephalogram (EEG), a recording of electrical activity generated by the brain made by placing electrodes on the scalp. Monitoring the results of EEGs will

Pediatric Implications

Anticonvulsants

Chewable phenytoin tablets are not indicated for once-daily administration.

If skin rash develops with use of phenytoin, discontinue drug immediately and notify prescriber.

Avoid intramuscular phenytoin injections.

Be aware that neonates whose mothers received hydantoin drugs during pregnancy may require vitamin K to treat hypoprothrombinemia.

The young client (under age 23) is more susceptible to gingival hyperplasia, especially with phenytoin or mephenytoin therapy. Gingivitis or gum inflammation usually starts during the first 6 months of drug therapy, although severe hyperplasia is unlikely in dosages under 500 mg/day. A dental program of teeth cleaning and plaque control started within 7 to 10 days of initiating drug therapy helps to reduce the rate and severity of this condition.

Coarse facial features and excessive body hair growth are more frequently reported in young clients.

Impaired school performance is reported with long-term, high-dose, hydantoin therapy (especially at high or toxic serum levels).

Whenever possible, other anticonvulsants should be considered first because they are less apt to cause the adverse effects induced by the hydantoins.

Children receiving valproic acid, especially those up to 2 years old or those receiving multiple anticonvulsant drugs, are at a greater risk for developing serious hepatotoxicity. This risk decreases with advancing age.

From *USP DI* (1996).

Geriatric Implications

Anticonvulsants

If skin rash develops with the use of phenytoin, discontinue drug immediately and notify the prescriber.

Debilitated clients or persons with renal or liver disease have a greater risk of developing toxicity with the anticonvulsant agents. Lower doses of the anticonvulsants will help to avoid adverse reactions.

The elderly tend to metabolize anticonvulsants more slowly; thus drug accumulation and toxicity may occur. Monitor closely because dosage adjustments (lower doses) may be necessary.

Serum albumin levels may be lower in geriatric clients, thus resulting in decreased protein binding of bound drugs, such as phenytoin and valproic acid. Monitor closely because lower drug doses may be necessary.

Administer intravenous doses at a rate slower than the recommended rate for an adult. Elderly rate of administration for phenytoin should be 5 to 10 mg/minute up to a maximum of 25 mg/minute.

From *USP DI* (1996).

indicate the client's progress by decreased seizure activity of the brain.

Subjective data to be obtained include the client's understanding and reaction to the convulsive disorder and drug therapy.

In addition, baseline vital signs and liver function and blood studies should be accomplished.

Intervention. One of the characteristics of the anticonvulsant drugs is that either the parent drug or the active metabolite has a long serum half-life, so the exact daily medication schedule is seldom critical. Administration of these drugs may be one to three times daily.

The first serum concentration after the first intravenous dose is half the peak value attained during long-term administration. Therefore the client can attain steady-state serum concentration quickly if the first intravenous dose is twice the maintenance dose. In adults, for example, a loading (intravenous) dose of phenytoin (1000 mg or 13 to 14 mg/kg, which is more than twice the usual maintenance dose of 300 mg/half-life of about 24 hours) will produce a therapeutic serum concentration of 10 to 20 μg/ml. The intravenous route is necessary because phenytoin is absorbed very slowly and erratically by the intramuscular route because the water solubility of the drug decreases and phenytoin crystals precipitate in the muscle. A high degree of local irritation has also been reported with intramuscular injection.

Although anticonvulsant agents are usually given orally, there are a few parenteral forms. These are reserved for occasions when the parenteral form is the best choice of therapy. Table 17-2 lists these conditions or situations and the parenteral drugs indicated for the treatment of each. Anticonvulsant drugs should be administered intravenously in emergency situations (such as status epilepticus) because of the slow absorption from the intramuscular injection site and the low peak serum levels achieved.

Anticonvulsant drugs should be administered using as long an interval between doses as possible, depending on their half-life. The anticonvulsant drugs that have an elimination half-life of 24 hours or more generally need to be administered only once a day to maintain a therapeutic serum concentration. The daily dose may be administered at bedtime to overcome the sedation seen with peak levels of anticonvulsant drugs.

In a nonemergency situation it is best to make changes in drug therapy with one drug at a time. The nurse and the client must be aware that each time a new anticonvulsant drug is started or the dose of a drug is increased or decreased, it takes four to five elimination half-life intervals (so the concentration of the drug has dropped by 95%) to reach the new steady-state serum concentration and to achieve the total therapeutic effect of the new drug regimen.

When serum levels of anticonvulsants are ordered, they should be scheduled for a time greater than 8 hours since the last dose of medication was given.

Several studies have shown that after 2 to 5 years of seizure control, medication can be stopped without recurrence of the seizures (at least for several years) in about 50% to 60% of all clients, and better in children (Dichter, 1992). Clients with the best chance of remaining seizure-free are those who have had no seizures for 2 to 5 years preceding the discontinuance of medication, who had relatively few seizures before control was attained, who required a single drug for control, who have a normal neurologic examination, and whose EEG is normal. The withdrawal procedure should be initiated with close medical supervision. More than 90% of recurrences will occur within the first year of withdrawal, and most will occur during the withdrawal period or shortly thereafter (Dichter, 1992). However, seizures may occur even after long periods that were seizure free. Fewer seizures occur when the withdrawal is planned or gradual or when the dose is reduced to minimal maintenance therapy.

TABLE 17-2 Indications for parenteral use of anticonvulsants

Parenteral drug	Use
barbiturates, especially phenobarbital, also amobarbital, pentobarbital sodium, and secobarbital sodium	Eclampsia, status epilepticus, severe recurrent seizures, tetanus, convulsant drug toxicity, other convulsive states
phenytoin	Status epilepticus, seizure during neurosurgery
magnesium sulfate	Severe toxemias of pregnancy (preeclampsia and eclampsia)
benzodiazepines: diazepam, lorazepam	Status epilepticus, severe, recurrent seizures

Education. The client should be encouraged to adopt a moderate lifestyle, follow an appropriate diet, and get sufficient rest and exercise. Stressful situations should be avoided; if this is not possible, the prescriber should be notified for dosage adjustment in ongoing stressful conditions. Drinking alcohol and taking OTC medications should be cautioned against (see specific drugs for interactions or effects). The client should understand that anticonvulsants take days or weeks to reach an effective level in the body. A missed dose may result in a seizure in a few days, and taking an extra dose will not prevent an impending seizure.

Although the client may be seizure free for some time and may perceive that a "cure" has occurred, the medication dose should not be decreased or stopped without consultation with the prescriber.

During initiation or change of therapy, the client should avoid activities that require coordination and alertness, such as driving, or situations that might be hazardous, such as swimming or ladder climbing, until response to the drug therapy has been determined.

Medications should be stored at home away from light and heat and out of the reach of children, since overdosage is especially dangerous in children. Outdated and discontinued medications should be flushed down the toilet.

TABLE 17-3 Central nervous system effects of selected anticonvulsants

Drug	Behavioral alterations	Cognitive effects
Barbiturates, especially phenobarbital	May see paradoxical effect, especially in elderly, children, or compromised clients (e.g., increased activity or excitement, irritability, altered sleep patterns, increased tiredness)	Impaired judgment, short-term memory impairment, decreased attention span
carbmazepine	Increased irritability, insomnia, behavioral changes, especially in children, depression	Less than phenytoin, phenobarbital, or primidone
phenytoin	Fatigue, increased clumsiness, confusion, mood alterations	Decreased attention span, decreased ability to problem solve

The nurse should suggest that the family keep a daily record of the number and type of seizures that occur during drug therapy. This is one measure of the efficacy of the medication(s) and will help the prescriber determine if increased dosage or an additional agent is needed.

Instruct the client and family in seizure precautions, and the importance of wearing a Medic Alert tag/card (obtainable at local pharmacy) should be explained. A valuable resource for both the nurse and the client is the Epilepsy Foundation of America (located at 4351 Garden City Drive, Landover, MD 20785; phone (301) 459-3700).

Evaluation. Evaluation of the client's progress on anticonvulsant therapy should be assessed in terms of achievement of the outcome criteria and the response to nursing interventions for the specific client. The client will experience a decrease in or absence of seizure activity and maintain therapeutic blood levels of the drug without experiencing any adverse effects of the drug. Some of the behavioral and cognitive effects reported with the anticonvulsants are listed in Table 17-3. And as with all drugs, the client will administer the drug safely and accurately when managing his or her own medication regimen.

HYDANTOINS

The prototype hydantoin is phenytoin (Dilantin, Diphenylan), which was developed from a search for an anticonvulsant that would cause less sedation than the barbiturates. Phenytoin is a drug for the treatment of all types of epilepsy except absence seizures. Two other hydantoin drugs are used for their anticonvulsant effects, ethotoin (Peganone) and mephenytoin (Mesantoin). Ethotoin and mephenytoin are usually prescribed only for those clients whose symptoms cannot be controlled with other drugs or those who had significant adverse effects from other anticonvulsants. In addition, both drugs are only available in the oral form, which limits their usefulness when a rapid response or parenteral route is needed.

Mechanism of action. See the previous section for a complete explanation of the mechanism of action. In addition, the hydantoins as a group act to reduce the maximal activity of brainstem centers responsible for the tonic phase of grand mal seizures.

▲ **phenytoin** [fen' i toyn] (Dilantin, Infatabs, various)
phenytoin sodium extended (Dilantin)

Phenytoin is more effective for grand mal than petit mal seizures. It is also frequently prescribed in combination with phenobarbital, and it may be prescribed for clients after surgery on the brain, after head trauma, and for status epilepticus to prevent seizures. See Table 17-1 for the drug's pharmacokinetics.

Side/adverse effects include hirsutism, constipation, nausea, vomiting, drowsiness, dizziness, and gingival hyperplasia (bleeding, sensitive gum tissue or overgrowth of gum tissue). The usual adult dosage is 100 mg PO 3 times a day. When proper dose is established, only the extended phenytoin capsules may be given once a day, depending on the individual's tolerance. For status epilepticus, the dose is 15 to 20 mg/kg IV at a rate of up to 50 mg/min (or in the elderly, 5 to 25 mg/min). The pediatric dose is 5 mg/kg PO in divided doses initially, then for maintenance dosing 4 to 8 mg/kg PO in two or three doses daily. For status epilepticus, 15-20 mg/kg administered IV at a rate of 1 mg/kg/min. Do not exceed 50 mg/min (*USP DI,* 1996).

■ Nursing Management
Hydantoin Therapy

Assessment. The client's history should be reviewed for conditions that contraindicate the use of phenytoin, such as a known sensitivity to the drug and impaired cardiac function, because parenteral administration of the drug may affect ventricular automaticity and cause ventricular arrhythmias. The review should also include conditions that require the cautious use of phenytoin. There is an elevated incidence of birth defects in children born to mothers taking phenytoin, although most deliver normal infants. The drug is excreted in breast milk. Pediatric clients are at higher risk for gingival hyperplasia and coarsening of the facial features and excessive body hair growth. Because of decreased serum albumin and low protein binding of the drug, elderly clients have an increased possibility of toxic effects of the drug. Clients with a history of blood dyscrasias will be at greater risk for serious infection and those with porphyria may experience an exacerbation. Toxic serum concentrations of phenytoin may occur with clients with impaired hepatic and renal function caused by altered protein binding.

The client's medications should be assessed for likely drug interactions. There exists a serious interaction between phenytoin and alcohol with the development of cross-tolerance to phenytoin in clients with epilepsy who are also heavy drinkers. Chronic alcohol use speeds up the metabolism of the drug apparently by enzyme induction and makes normal doses inadequate. The following effects may occur when hydantoins are given with the drugs listed below:

Drug	Possible effect and management
antacids	Concurrent use may decrease the bioavailability of phenytoin, administer 2-3 hr apart.
anticoagulants warfarin (Coumadin)	A decrease in metabolism may cause an increased serum level and hydantoin toxicity. Anticoagulant effect may be initially increased but will decrease with continuous combined use. Monitor closely for symptoms of thromboembolism.
adrenocorticoids, corticosteroids, estrogens, or oral contraceptives	An increase in metabolism of these drugs may result from hydantoin's induction of hepatic microsomal enzymes, which may decrease the therapeutic effects of these medications; monitor closely because a dosage adjustment may be necessary. Breakthrough bleeding and an increased risk of conception may occur with estrogen-containing contraceptives.
carbamazepine (Tegretol)	A decrease in therapeutic effect may occur with one or both drugs. Serum drug levels should be closely monitored.
chloramphenicol (Chloromycetin), cimetidine (Tagamet), disulfiram (Antabuse), isoniazid (INH), amiodarone (Cardarone), oral anticoagulants, or sulfonamides	A decrease in metabolism may cause an increased serum level and toxicity of hydantoins. Dosage adjustment may be required.
alcohol, CNS depressants	May result in enhanced CNS depression. Monitor closely for respiratory depression and drowsiness.
calcium	Calcium supplements or calcium sulfate may decrease phenytoin absorption by approximately 20%. Space medications 1 to 3 hours apart.
diazoxide, oral (Proglycem)	**May decrease phenytoin effects and decrease the hyperglycemic action of diazoxide. Avoid or a potentially serious drug interaction may occur.**
fluconazole (Diflucan)	May decrease phenytoin metabolism, resulting in increased plasma levels of phenytoin and toxicity. Monitor phenytoin serum levels.
folic acid	Hydantoins deplete folate from the body. Increased folic acid intake may lower the serum hydantoin levels, leading to a possible loss of seizure control.
lidocaine, propranolol (Inderal), and possible other beta-blocking agents	If given with IV phenytoin, additive cardiac depressant effects may occur. Hydantoins may also increase the metabolism of lidocaine.
methadone	Methadone metabolism may be increased by chronic dosing of phenytoin, which may precipitate an acute withdrawal reaction in clients being treated for narcotic dependence. Methadone dosages may need to be adjusted whenever phenytoin is started or discontinued.
phenacemide (Phenurone)	Increased risk of toxicity when both drugs are used concurrently.
streptozocin (Zanosar)	**Phenytoin is reported to protect pancreatic beta cells from streptozocin therapeutic effects. Avoid or a potentially serious drug interaction may occur.**
sucralfate (Carafate)	Concurrent use may decrease absorption of hydantoin anticonvulsants. Space medications at least 2 hours apart.
valproic acid (Depakene)	Monitor serum levels of phenytoin (preferably unbound phenytoin) closely, since variable responses have been reported. Adjustments of dosage may be necessary according to client's clinical response.
xanthines	Monitor serum concentrations of both drugs. If phenytoin plasma levels are in the therapeutic range, an increase in metabolism of xanthines (except for dyphylline) will occur. Also, if given with xanthines, a decrease in phenytoin absorption may result; monitor closely.

Nursing diagnosis. The following nursing diagnoses/collaborative problems may be identified in a client receiving phenytoin: risk for injury related to the client's underlying seizure activity and ineffectiveness of anticonvulsant therapy; body image disturbance related to the coarsening of facial features, hirsutism, alopecia, and in males, gynecomastia; powerlessness related to chronicity of seizure disorder therapy; and the potential complications of cognitive impairment, blood dyscrasias, hepatotoxicity, and gingival hyperplasia.

Implementation

Monitoring. Monitor the effectiveness of therapy by documenting seizure activity and signs and symptoms of adverse responses to phenytoin. The nurse should monitor closely for documented drug interactions that may alter the client's response to medications. Because some drugs can impair or enhance the effects of phenytoin, monitoring of drug serum levels will be important for accurate dosage administration and as a mechanism of determining compliance.

When clients are taking phenytoin, serum levels should be monitored. It takes approximately 7 to 10 days before recommended serum levels are achieved although peak plasma levels are usually reached in 8 to 12 hours. It is particularly important that serum levels be monitored closely in clients with renal and hepatic impairment. Clients with impaired liver function, the elderly, or those who are very ill may demonstrate early signs of toxicity. A small percentage of persons metabolize the drug slowly because of limited enzyme availability that may be genetically determined. The metabolism of phenytoin is dose dependent at therapeutic doses. Liver function tests and blood counts should be monitored periodically.

Intervention

Enteral administration. When using the suspension form of the medication, shake the container vigorously before measuring out the dose in a graduated or exact measuring device (oral syringe). Clients with enteral tube feedings and pediatric clients have been undermedicated and later overmedicated from the same container because of improper shaking of the container.

Oral preparations should be given with meals to decrease gastric distress. The appearance of side effects or adverse reactions may require nursing intervention ranging from basic nursing skills to urgent consultation with the prescriber. Note that the 100-mg capsule of phenytoin sodium contains only 92% phenytoin and so is not equivalent to two 50-mg phenytoin chewable tablets that contain 100% phenytoin.

Nasogastric tube administration. Administration of phenytoin suspension without dilution, or follow-up irrigation of the nasogastric tube after the phenytoin is given prevents adequate absorption and leads to a significant decrease in plasma phenytoin concentrations. Until further research is performed, it is recommended that phenytoin suspension be diluted before administration and that the nasogastric tube be irrigated with 20 ml of fluid (D_5W, normal saline) before and after administration. When phenytoin is administered to clients receiving enteral feedings, a significant decrease in absorption of oral phenytoin may occur. If the client is receiving an enteral feeding, the phenytoin should be administered intravenously; if this is not feasible, serum concentrations of phenytoin should be monitored frequently. Abrupt withdrawal may precipitate status epilepticus.

Parenteral administration. If the state of the client is such that immobilization of an extremity is impossible because of convulsions or inaccessible veins, then the intramuscular route may be useful. If the administration does not terminate the seizure, the nurse must consult with the prescriber to consider other anticonvulsants, intravenous barbiturates, general anesthesia, or other measures. The intramuscular route is not recommended for the treatment of status epilepticus, since the plasma levels of phenytoin in the therapeutic range cannot be readily achieved. Because muscle tissue is more acidic than the phenytoin solution, phenytoin crystallizes when given intramuscularly. The absorption of these crystals is slow and erratic, and pain and necrosis may occur at the injection site.

The manufacturer supplies a special diluent for parenteral use. Because the preparation dissolves slowly, warming the vial in warm water after the diluent has been added is recommended to hasten dissolution. Only a clear solution is to be administered.

Because intravenous phenytoin is an irritant to the veins (and is incompatible with many solutions and medications), it is recommended that the intravenous line be flushed with normal saline (0.9% sodium chloride injection) before and after this drug is administered.

Some clients complain of burning and pain at the intravenous injection site. Because phenytoin is a highly alkaline solution (pH 11.4), burning and pain raise suspicion that there may be a poorly seated needle, extravasation, or a fluid load that is being infused too quickly into a small vein. The nurse should restart the infusion into a large vein, using a larger-gauge needle. Subcutaneous injection may cause inflammation and necrosis and should not be done.

The addition of phenytoin solution to an intravenous infusion is not recommended because of its lack of solubility (the solution is made with propylene glycol 40%, alcohol 10%, water 50%, and pH adjusted with sodium hydroxide to 12) and the resultant precipitation.

The manufacturer does not recommend adding parenteral phenytoin sodium to intravenous solutions or mixing it with any other medications, since precipitation (even microcrystals) may occur. Since a number of physicians prescribe intermittent infusions of phenytoin, the *USP DI* (1996) has recommended that all the following criteria must be met in such situations:

- Parenteral phenytoin sodium is mixed with 50 ml of sodium chloride 0.9% injection (normal saline). The mixture is made immediately before administration of the infusion. The concentration of phenytoin in solution is between 1 and 10 mg/ml.
- A 0.22 to 0.45 μ filter must be used in the administration of this solution and the infusion should be finished within 1 hour. The IV tubing should be flushed with 0.9% sodium chloride injection before and after the infusion. Carefully observe the admixture for crystals, cloudiness, or precipitation.
- The administration rate for the infusion should be a maximum of 50 mg/min. Reduce to 25 mg/min in clients who might develop hypotension, have cardiovascular disease, or are receiving sympathomimetic adjuvant medications. ECG monitoring is recommended during the infusion for these clients. Elderly, seriously ill, or debilitated clients or clients with liver function impairment should generally receive a lower dose at a much slower rate of administration.
- Monitor blood pressure and cardiac function closely.

The nurse can readily determine that the rate and time for dilantinization are a function of the client's clinical situation. The dose-related side effects increase with the rapidity at which the client is dilantinized to the therapeutic range. Proceeding cautiously and slowly is clinically prudent. Nystagmus (bilateral and vertical) develops at levels of 10 to 20 μg/ml; ataxia, drowsiness, and diplopia are seen at levels about 30 μg/ml; and lethargy is seen at 40 μg/ml.

Monitor closely for side effects/adverse reactions. Signs of overdose or toxicity include blurred or double vision, nausea, vomiting, slurred speech, clumsiness, unsteadiness or staggering gait, dizziness, fatigue, confusion, and hallucinations. In addition, the diverse signs of toxicity seen with intravenous phenytoin are cardiovascular collapse, CNS depression, and hypotension (seen with rapid intravenous administration resulting from propylene glycol solvent). The rate of administration (not to exceed 50 mg over 1 minute) is important, since severe cardiotoxic reactions and fatal outcomes are reported in the elderly or gravely ill.

Education. One of the side effects of hydantoins is gum hyperplasia; it is therefore important that oral hygiene be emphasized. Clients should be encouraged to brush frequently, floss, and massage their gums. Because the tissue overgrowth is usually greater and more apparent anteriorly than posteriorly, the client, particularly the adolescent, may have body image concerns. A program of professional dental prophylaxis and an aggressive program of plaque control by the client will minimize hyperplasia. Clients should be instructed to inform their dentists that they are taking hydantoins, so that the dentist can observe and monitor for periodontal problems.

Clients who have diabetes should be instructed to report any changes in blood or urine sugar concentrations. Hydantoins may affect blood sugar levels.

The client should be advised of possible skin changes. An erythematous-type rash with or without fever should be reported immediately to the prescriber. Hirsutism or excessive body and facial hair growth is reported in some clients. This side effect is particularly troublesome in young women. This alteration in body image will require supportive nursing care.

The client should be cautioned against changing brands of the drug, since the bioavailability of phenytoin may vary. Generic phenytoin and Dilantin from Parke-Davis are not the same. Dilantin capsules are the only form of extended phenytoin sodium available; all the rest are prompt-acting and are not intended for once-a-day dosage. Generic phenytoin capsules are a prompt-acting form of the drug as are the chewable tablets from Parke-Davis. The extended form can be used for once-a-day dosing and for clients who are stabilized on a 300-mg divided dosage. It is important that this information be explained clearly to the client and family.

When discussing the appropriate means of administration of the suspension dosage form, the nurse should stress that very vigorous shaking of the container is mandatory before measuring out the dose in a graduated or exact measuring device (oral syringe). Clients should be cautioned against unsupervised self-administration of other drugs while taking any of the hydantoins, since they interact with a variety of drugs.

Any client with epilepsy should carry an identification card or wear a Medic-Alert bracelet that indicates the anticonvulsant being taken.

Evaluation. The client will experience less or no seizure activity; maintain a serum level of phenytoin within the therapeutic range of 10 to 20 μg/ml; demonstrate no adverse effects to phenytoin; and administer the drug safely and accurately when self-managing the medication regimen.

fosphenytoin [foss fen' i toy in] (Cerebyx)

Fosphenytoin, a prodrug of phenytoin sodium (Dilantin), was formulated to avoid the problems associated with intravenous administration of phenytoin, i.e., pain and burning at site of administration. The product is rapidly converted to phenytoin in the body and may be administered by intramuscular and intravenous injection (Drug Updates, 1996). Phenytoin derived from fosphenytoin has the same pharmacologic profile as phenytoin sodium.

Fosphenytoin 150 mg is equivalent to 100 mg phenytoin sodium, although it may be administered at a faster rate than phenytoin, (150 mg/min) (Cloyd, 1996; Olin 1996).

mephenytoin [me fen' i toyn] [Mesantoin]

Mephenytoin is chemically similar in structure, activity, and pharmacokinetics to phenytoin, but it is less potent as an anticonvulsant. It produces more sedation than phenytoin, but this side effect is dose related. It also has a greater potential for producing blood dyscrasias and dermatologic effects than the other hydantoins. This product is usually reserved for clients whose seizures are not controlled with safer anticonvulsants.

The usual adult dose is 50 to 100 mg orally daily, increased weekly as necessary up to a 1.2 g/day maximum; for children the dose is 25 to 50 mg daily.

ethotoin [eth' oh toyn] (Peganone)

Ethotoin is similar to phenytoin but less effective and offers little advantage over phenytoin. Side effects of ataxia, hirsutism, and gum hyperplasia are rare, and ethotoin may be substituted for phenytoin to reduce these side effects. Ethotoin is available only for oral administration, with dosage individualized according to response. Maintenance dosage (usually divided into four to six doses) of less than 2 g is usually not effective.

BARBITURATES

Barbiturates, especially phenobarbital, have been used for many years for the treatment of generalized tonic-clonic and partial seizures. This class of medications is relatively inexpensive, efficacious, and has a low incidence of side effects. The most commonly prescribed barbiturate is phenobarbital.

Mephobarbital (Mebaral) is converted by the liver metabolizing enzymes to phenobarbital, whereas metharbital (Gemonil) is metabolized to barbital in the liver. All three barbiturates are long-acting compounds, but there is little or no advantage in using the latter two instead of phenobarbital, the most commonly prescribed barbiturate.

The parenteral dosage forms of amobarbital, phenobarbital, and secobarbital have been used in emergency treatment of seizures (see Table 17-2). The oral dosage forms are generally not indicated for the treatment of seizure disorders because of their potent sedative-hypnotic effects. See Table 17-1 for a pharmacokinetic overview of selected anticonvulsant agents.

The adverse effects of apnea, bronchospasm, and respiratory depression may occur after rapidly administered intravenous injections of barbiturates. Severe symptoms of withdrawal may occur in individuals who have a barbiturate dependency from prolonged use at high dosages. Anxiety, trembling, nausea, vomiting, insomnia, orthostatic hypotension, seizures, hallucinations, and even death may result if the drug is withdrawn abruptly. Gradual withdrawal in a controlled setting is usually recommended for the treatment of dependence.

▲ **phenobarbital** [fee noe bar' bi tal] (Barbita, Luminal)
Phenobarbital is the prototype barbiturate to treat epilepsy. There are many dosage forms (tablets, elixirs, solutions, and parenteral) and strengths available. The nurse must exercise special caution to ensure that the proper dose is given as prescribed.

Several weeks of phenobarbital therapy may be necessary to achieve the maximum anticonvulsant effects. When administered intravenously, 15 to 30 minutes is required to reach the maximum anticonvulsant effect. To avoid excessive barbiturate-induced depression it is important to wait for the anticonvulsant effect to develop before administering additional doses. When administered intravenously, phenobarbital should be administered slowly to avoid respiratory depression; a rate of 60 mg/min should not be exceeded. Resuscitative equipment should be readily available.

The optimal blood concentration of phenobarbital should be determined by seizure control and absence of toxic effects. A serum concentration of 10 to 40 μg/ml is usually desired. Dosage and administration of phenobarbital are addressed in Table 16-3.

amobarbital [am oh bar' bi tal] (Amytal)
Amobarbital is indicated for use as a sedative-hypnotic and anticonvulsant. Only the parenteral form is used as an anticonvulsant. Amobarbital should be administered deep intramuscularly to reduce the possibility of sterile abscesses and sloughing of tissue. When administered intravenously to an adult, the rate of injection should not exceed 100 mg/min. Parenteral solutions should be clear and without precipitate when reconstituted. The solution should be used within 30 minutes of reconstitution, since it hydrolyses easily.

mephobarbital [me foe bar' bi tal] (Mebaral)
Mephobarbital is a barbiturate indicated for use only as an anticonvulsant. Therapy is usually begun with small doses and increased over a period of 4 to 5 days until the optimal dosage has been established. Because mephobarbital is metabolized to phenobarbital, serum levels of phenobarbital may be monitored. Mephobarbital is available in oral dosage forms only.

metharbital [meth ar' bi tal] (Gemonil)
Metharbital is used only as an anticonvulsant. It is metabolized to barbital, and serum barbital concentrations may be monitored. Metharbital is available in oral dosage forms only.

Nursing Management
Barbiturate Therapy

Assessment. Combination of these drugs with alcohol, antihistamines, antianxiety agents, antidepressants, or antipsychotic agents should be avoided because they may result in an enhanced CNS-depressant effect.

Pediatric and geriatric clients may be more sensitive to barbiturates and may respond to lower doses or may have reactions such as depression, confusion, or even excitement. These drugs should be used very cautiously in pregnant women because they can cause neonatal hemorrhage and an increased incidence of teratogenic effects. If given throughout the third trimester, physical drug dependence and withdrawal reactions have been reported in the neonate from birth to approximately 2 weeks.

Barbiturates are to be used with caution if any of the following conditions are present: hypersensitivity to barbiturates; history of drug abuse, because the client is predisposed to dependence; hepatic impairment, which would interfere with barbiturate metabolism; respiratory disease, because of the risk of ventilatory depression; or pain, because symptoms of an underlying condition may be masked. Barbiturates are contraindicated for clients with porphyria or a history of the disease, because they may increase symptoms by stimulating enzymes for porphyrin synthesis.

The client's concurrent drug regimen should be reviewed to detect any significant drug interactions. The following effects may occur when barbiturates, especially phenobarbital, are given with the drugs listed below:

Drug	Possible effect and management
adrenocorticoids or corticosteroids (prednisone, etc.)	The effects of these drugs may be decreased because of enhanced metabolism caused by barbiturates. Dosage adjustment may be necessary.
alcohol, anesthetics, CNS depressants (sedatives, hypnotics, narcotics)	Enhanced CNS depressant effects, respiratory depression; use extreme caution in combining such medications. Usually the dosage of one or both drugs should be reduced.
anticoagulants warfarin (Coumadin)	Effects may be decreased because of enhanced metabolism produced by barbiturates. Closely monitor prothrombin time. Dosage adjustment of anticoagulants may be necessary.
carbamazepine (Tegretol)	Concurrent drug administration may result in a decrease in the serum level and half-life of carbamazepine. Monitor serum levels whenever carbamazepine is prescribed or discontinued from combination drug therapy.
hydantoin anticonvulsants	Unpredictable effects on hydantoin metabolism may occur. Serum levels should be closely monitored when drugs are given concurrently.

Drug	Possible effect and management
divalproex sodium (Depakote) or valproic acid (Depakene)	Two effects may result from this combination: (1) valproic acid half-life may be decreased, which would require a dosage ad justment to maintain control; or (2) metabolism of barbiturates may be decreased, which can result in elevated barbiturate serum levels and toxicity. Monitor barbiturate levels, since a dosage adjustment may be necessary. Phenobarbital may also increase the potential for valproic acid hepatotoxicity—monitor liver function study results closely.

Nursing diagnosis. The client receiving anticonvulsant therapy with barbiturates should be assessed for the following nursing diagnoses/collaborative problems: sleep pattern disturbance (daytime sedation, hangover); risk for injury related to dizziness; altered thought processes (confusion); and the potential complications of Stevens-Johnson syndrome, blood dyscrasias, and paradoxical excitement.

Implementation

Monitoring. In addition to the evaluation needed for anticonvulsant therapy in general, during prolonged barbiturate therapy, liver and renal function will be monitored (usually through blood and urine testing) at periodic intervals determined by the client's prescriber.

Determination of serum drug levels may be performed to monitor drug levels. The optimal blood levels are determined by response to seizure control and appearance of toxic effects.

Intervention. If barbiturates are administered intravenously, ensure that the airway is patent and resuscitative equipment is readily available.

When drug therapy is initiated, the client may have some drowsiness and dizziness. Safety precautions should be taken when the client is ambulatory until the response to the medication has been ascertained.

Because the drug dosage schedule initially will vary until the correct dosage maintenance level is achieved, it is important that the nurse follow the dosage schedule accurately. The appearance of side effects or adverse reactions may require basic nursing measures such as reassurance, safety, or comfort, or it may indicate the need for further consultation.

If barbiturates are used during pregnancy, the nurse should consult with the client's prescriber to see if the client is to receive vitamin K in the last month of pregnancy to prevent hemorrhagic complications of delivery and in the newborn.

Education. Clients should be instructed to return to their prescriber routinely for CBC, blood chemistry studies, and drug blood level tests.

The client should be cautioned to avoid driving a car or operating potentially hazardous machinery until the response to drug therapy has been determined.

Self-alteration of prescribed medications or consumption of OTC drugs without consultation with the prescriber should be discouraged. OTC drugs may interfere with or enhance the drug's effectiveness. If used in combination with alcohol, CNS depression may occur. Abrupt withdrawal of the drug is contraindicated and could result in severe abstinence syndrome. Dosage should be tapered under medical supervision.

Clients taking oral estrogen-containing contraceptives should be aware that concurrent use of barbiturates may result in decreased contraceptive reliability, and they may wish to use a nonhormonal method of birth control or consult with their prescriber about a progestin-only oral contraceptive.

Case Study

The Client on Anticonvulsant Therapy

Carla Blomquist, a 25-year-old school teacher, was admitted 1 week ago to the hospital for a work-up to determine the cause of grand mal seizures that began suddenly 2 weeks previously. Carla has no history of head trauma or recent infection. She takes no medications, and her health has been very good, with no major illnesses or hospitalizations.

Carla's blood pressure is within normal limits. All tests for space-occupying lesions and infections have proved negative. Electroencephalographic (EEG) changes are not diagnostic. No cause for the seizures has been determined. However, she is concerned about the effects her seizures may have on her job and family life. Her physician has prescribed the following medications:

Phenytoin (Dilantin) 100 mg PO qid
Phenobarbital (Luminal) 30 mg PO tid

Her activity level has not been restricted, but she has been directed not to drive for a month. When a month has passed, she is to return to the clinic for evaluation of the medication therapy. Carla has had no seizures since the medications were begun.

1. What is the major action of phenytoin? Why is phenobarbital also used?
2. What are some of the CNS effects that Carla might have in relation of taking phenytoin and phenobarbital?
3. You are discharging Carla; what instructions will enhance her ability to effectively manage her therapeutic regimen?

Women using this drug therapy should be instructed to inform their prescriber if they become pregnant. Barbiturates have been shown to cause an increase in fetal abnormalities. Barbiturates are excreted in breast milk and can cause CNS depression in the nursing infant.

Evaluation. The client will experience fewer seizures or remain seizure free, maintain a phenobarbital plasma concentration of 15 to 40 µg/ml, and be free of adverse reactions to the drug.

SUCCINIMIDES

The succinimides include ethosuximide (Zarontin), methsuximide (Celontin), and phensuximide (Milontin). These agents produce a variety of effects, such as increasing the seizure threshold and reducing the EEG spike-and-wave pattern of absence seizures by decreasing nerve impulses and transmission in the motor cortex.

Ethosuximide and phensuximide are indicated for the treatment of absence seizures, whereas methsuximide is reserved for absence seizures that are nonresponsive to other medications. Pharmacokinetics are discussed in Table 17-1.

Side/adverse effects include headache, epigastric pain, anorexia, hiccups, nausea, vomiting, rash, pruritus (possibly Stevens-Johnson syndrome), mood changes, and agranulocytosis. Dosage and administration issues are presented in Table 17-4.

■ Nursing Management
Succinimide Therapy

Assessment. In addition to the baseline assessment of the client's seizure activity, the nurse should determine if the client has any preexisting health problems for which the succinimides would be contraindicated. Primarily these are the blood dyscrasias (because of the drugs' adverse hematologic effects) and hepatic and renal dysfunction (because changes may occur in these organs with succinimide therapy). It should also be determined if there are significant drug interactions with the client's concurrent drug regimen. The following effects may occur when succinimides are given in combination with the drugs listed below:

Drug	Possible effect and management
carbamazepine (Tegretol), phenobarbital, or phenytoin ((Dilantin)	Results in increased metabolism of succinimide anticonvulsants and decreased serum levels. Monitor serum levels especially when either drug is added, increased, decreased, or deleted from the drug regimen.
haloperidol (Haldol)	May change the pattern or frequency of seizures. Dosage of the anticonvulsant may need to be adjusted. Serum levels of haloperidol may be reduced, which may result in decreased effectiveness.
phenothiazines, thioxanthenes, antidepressants, loxapine (Loxitane), maprotiline (Ludiomil), or CNS depressants	May decrease the effectiveness of the anticonvulsant, enhance CNS depression, and lower the seizure threshold. Monitor closely for respiratory depression and drowsiness because dosage modifications may be necessary.

Nursing diagnosis. In addition to the nursing diagnoses/collaborative problems discussed previously for anticonvulsant therapy, the client receiving succinimide therapy has the potential for the following: altered protection related to the development of blood dyscrasias; and the potential complications of Stevens-Johnson syndrome (fever, bulla on the skin, ulcers of the mucous membranes of lips, eyes, mouth, and genitalia), blood dyscrasias (agranulocytosis, thrombocytopenia), and systemic lupus erythematosus (muscle ache, swollen glands, sore throat, fever, skin rash).

Implementation

Monitoring. In addition to monitoring the client's seizure activity, liver, renal, and hematologic studies should be evaluated periodically because of the drug's possible effects on these systems. Report any signs of liver, kidney, or hematologic disorders to the prescriber.

TABLE 17-4 Succinimides: dosage and administration

Drug	Adults	Children
ethosuximide (Zarontin)	Orally: initially 250 mg twice a day, in increased as necessary at 4- to 7-day intervals; maximum total daily dose is 1.5 g.	Orally: children 6 yr old and older, follow adult schedule. For children up to 6 yr, initial dose is 250 mg/day, increased by 250 mg at 4- to 7-day intervals. Maximum total daily dose is 1 g.
methsuximide (Celontin)	Orally: initial dose is 300 mg daily, increased as necessary by 300-mg increments at 1-wk intervals until seizures controlled or maximum daily dose of 1.2 g reached.	Dosage is individualized. 150-mg capsules available for pediatric dosage adjustments.
phensuximide (Milontin)	Orally: initial dose is 500 mg two or three times a day, increase by 500-mg increments at 1-wk intervals until seizures controlled or maximum daily dose of 3 g reached.	Pediatric dose similar to adult schedule.

Intervention. To decrease stomach distress, the succinimides may be taken with milk, food, or antacids.

Education. Although their incidence is rare with the succinimides, the blood dyscrasia effects may result in gingival bleeding, delayed healing, and an increase in the number of infections for the client when they do occur. Dental work should be deferred until blood counts are within the normal range. Clients may have to modify their dental hygiene with cautious use of toothbrushes and dental floss. The client should alert other health care providers about the succinimide regimen if surgery, dental work, or emergency medical care is required.

The nurse should caution the client about drowsiness and other possible CNS disturbances. When dosage adjustments are made or medications added, serum drug levels may be ordered. The nurse should explain the importance of serum blood levels to the client who needs to have serum levels drawn frequently. The client should be cautioned that withdrawal of the succinimides may precipitate absence seizures. Adverse personality changes can occur while the client is taking this medication; the nurse should stress the importance of reporting any behavioral changes to the prescriber.

If the client is taking phensuximide, the nurse should caution him or her that the drug may change the color of the urine to pink, red, or red-brown; this is harmless.

Evaluation. The client should have diminished seizures or remain free of seizures without any untoward effects of the drug.

BENZODIAZEPINES

The benzodiazepines include clonazepam (Klonopin), diazepam (Valium), clorazepate (Tranxene), and parenteral lorazepam (Ativan). These drugs appear to suppress the propagation of seizure activity produced by foci in the cortex, thalamus, and limbic areas.

Clonazepam (Klonopin) is a long-acting drug used to treat absence seizures and myoclonic seizure disorders. It has been used alone, but more often it is prescribed as an adjunct to other anticonvulsants to establish seizure control. Diazepam (Valium) may be used parenterally for status epilepticus and in severe recurrent convulsive seizures, but the oral dosage form is not effective for maintenance control. The oral form of diazepam has been used as an adjunctive medication for short-term treatment in convulsive disorders. Diazepam is not effective alone and use beyond 4 months has not been clinically evaluated (*PDR*, 1996).

Clorazepate (Tranxene) has been prescribed as an adjunct medication for the treatment of simple partial seizures. Parenteral lorazepam (Ativan) is also used for the treatment of status epilepticus (*USP DI*, 1996).

See Table 17-1 and Chapter 16 for the pharmacokinetics and side/adverse effects of these drugs.

Dosage and administration (Table 17-5.) Dosage is usually individualized for each client and is increased with caution to avoid adverse effects. In elderly or debilitated persons and those taking other CNS-depressant-type medications, a lower dose with a slow increase is prudent.

■ Nursing Management

Benzodiazepine Therapy

Assessment. See Chapter 16 for the detailed client assessment required before benzodiazepine therapy may be initiated.

Nursing diagnosis. See Chapter 16 for nursing diagnoses/collaborative problems associated with benzodiazepine therapy.

TABLE 17-5 Benzodiazepine anticonvulsants: dosage and administration

Drug	Adults	Children
clonazepam (Klonopin)	Orally: initially 0.5 mg three times daily with increases of 0.5-1 mg every third day until seizures are controlled, side effects occur, or the maximum of 20 mg/day is reached.	Orally (less than 10 years old or 30 kg), initial 0.01-0.03/kg in divided doses (three times a day); if necessary, increase by 0.25-0.5 mg every 3 days until seizures are controlled, side effects occur, or the maximum maintenance dose of 0.1-0.2 mg/kg is reached.
diazepam (Valium)	5-10 mg IV initially; repeat at 10-15 min intervals if necessary to a maximum of 30 mg; inject slowly—at least 1 minute for each 5-mg dose administered intravenously. Orally, 2-10 mg three to four times daily.	1 mo to 5 yr of age, 0.2-0.5 mg by slow IV every 2-5 min to a maximum of 5 mg; this regimen may be repeated if necessary, in 2-4 hr. 5 yr or older 1 mg every 2-5 min by slow IV to a maximum of 10 mg; this regimen may be repeated if necessary, in 2-4 hr.
clorazepate (Tranxene)	Orally, initially up to 7.5 mg three times daily; increase if necessary by 7.5 mg/wk to a maximum of 90 mg/day.	9-12 yr old, orally, up to 7.5 mg twice daily; increase if necessary by 7.5 mg/wk to a maximum of 60 mg daily.

USP DI, 1996.

Implementation. Discussion here will be limited to the use of benzodiazepines for urgent seizure control. Consult Chapter 16 for general nursing management of the client receiving benzodiazepines.

Monitoring. Baseline vital signs should be taken before parenteral forms of diazepam (Valium) or lorazepam (Ativan) are given, and then the client should be observed at bed rest after administration (for at least 3 hours for diazepam and 8 hours for lorazepam) for decreases in respiratory rate, heart rate, and blood pressure.

Intervention. Diazepam (Valium) is insoluble in water; therefore each milliliter of the parenteral form contains 40% propylene glycol, 10% ethyl alcohol, 5% sodium benzoate, and benzoic acid as buffers, and 1.5% benzyl alcohol as a preservative. If this ratio is altered, the diazepam is insoluble. If direct intravenous injection is not possible, diazepam may be injected through the infusion tubing as close to the insertion point as possible. Inject slowly, at least 1 minute for each 5 mg.

Lorazepam (Ativan) must be diluted with a compatible diluent immediately before intravenous use. It may be infused directly into a vein or through intravenous tubing. Infusion rates should not exceed 2 mg/min.

Because of the short-lived effect of intravenous benzodiazepine administration, seizures, although brought under prompt control, may recur. The nurse should be ready to readminister the drug.

Benzodiazepines are not for maintenance; once seizure control is achieved, agents useful in long-term seizure control should be considered. Tonic status epilepticus has been precipitated in some clients treated with intravenous diazepam for petit mal status or petit mal variant status. The nurse must exercise extreme care (monitor respirations every 5 to 15 minutes and before each intravenous dose) in administering benzodiazepines (especially by the intravenous route) to elderly or very ill clients or those with compromised pulmonary reserve because of the possibility of apnea and cardiac arrest.

Resuscitative equipment should be available because of the possible occurrence of hypotension, tachycardia, and respiratory depression.

In the neonate (age 30 days or less) the efficacy and safety of parenteral diazepam are not established. Prolonged CNS depression has been reported in the neonate, probably resulting from the inability to biotransform diazepam into the inactive metabolites.

The benzoate in the injectable form has been reported to displace other drugs and bilirubin from the plasma protein binding sites, causing jaundice.

To minimize the occurrence of thrombophlebitis after intravenous injection of diazepam, the vein can be flushed with 1 ml of saline per milligram of diazepam.

If benzodiazepines are intended to be given along with a narcotic, the dose of the narcotic should be reduced. Diazepam is a drug that may be subject to abuse by medical and nursing professionals and clients. This is a controlled drug; therefore the nurse is responsible for proper documentation of the drug's distribution and use.

Education. When benzodiazepines are given for treating convulsive disorders, an abrupt withdrawal of the medication can cause an increase in frequency or severity of seizures. Clients should be instructed to take their medication as directed.

Diazepam does cross the placental barrier and has been associated with causing cleft lip in the infant. The risk-to-benefit ratio should be carefully considered in the client during pregnancy.

It is not advisable that alcohol or other CNS depressants be combined with benzodiazepines. Severe drowsiness, respiratory depression, and apnea may occur.

Evaluation. The client will experience a decrease in the severity and frequency of seizures without any adverse effects of the drug.

Miscellaneous Anticonvulsants

acetazolamide [a set a zole' a mide] (Diamox)
Acetazolamide is a carbonic anhydrase inhibitor usually prescribed for the treatment of open-angle glaucoma. It is used in combination with other anticonvulsant agents for the treatment of absence seizures, generalized tonic-clonic seizures, mixed seizures, and myoclonic seizure patterns. Acetazolamide's mechanism of action is unknown. It has been theorized that inhibiting carbonic anhydrase in the CNS may result in an increase in carbon dioxide that retards neuronal activity. Systemic metabolic acidosis may also play a part in its action. See Chapter 34 for pharmacokinetics and side effects/adverse reactions.

Dosage and administration. Adult and pediatric: anticonvulsant therapy, oral 4 to 30 mg/kg/day (initial dose is usually 10 mg/kg/day) in four divided doses (usually 375 to 1000 mg/day).

For the nursing management of acetazolamide therapy, consult the previous discussion of the nursing management of anticonvulsant therapy and Chapter 34, Diuretics, for the drug monograph.

carbamazepine [kar ba maz' e peen] (Tegretol)
The exact mechanism of action is unknown, although this drug's effects are somewhat similar to those of phenytoin. Carbamazepine is indicated in the treatment of partial seizures with complex symptomatology, for generalized tonic-clonic seizures, for psychomotor seizures, and for mixed seizure patterns. This drug is also indicated in the treatment of pain associated with true trigeminal neuralgia.

See Table 17-1 for a pharmacokinetic overview. Autoinduction of metabolism occurs, and half-life decreases with repeated doses. Side/adverse effects include vertigo, drowsiness, nausea, vomiting, dizziness, blurred or other visual disturbances, ataxia, confusion, muscle aches or cramps, allergic reaction, Stevens-Johnson syndrome, systemic lupus erythematosus–type syndrome and the syndrome of increased release of antidiuretic hormone (SIADH).

Dosage and administration. In adults, carbamazepine should be given initially at 200 mg twice daily, increased by 200 mg/day weekly in divided doses until response is noted;

maximum dose is 1200 mg/day, with a maintenance range of 800 to 1200 mg/day in divided doses. For children up to 6 years, the initial dose is 10 to 20 mg/kg/day in divided doses; increase weekly if necessary to 100 mg/day. Maintenance usually requires between 250 and 300 mg daily to maintain therapeutic serum level. The dose for children 6 to 12 years is initially 100 mg twice a day; increase by 100 mg/day weekly until desired response is obtained. Maintenance is usually between 400 and 800 mg/day in divided dosages.

■ Nursing Management

Carbamazepine Therapy

Assessment. Carbamazepine therapy is contraindicated with clients with absence, atonic, or myoclonic seizures because of the possibility of the seizures becoming more generalized with use of the drug. There is also risk of exacerbation of AV heart block, blood disorders, and bone marrow depression for clients with a history of these preexisting conditions. The risk/benefit of carbamazepine should be considered for the client with the following health conditions: active alcoholism (potentiates CNS depression); behavioral disorders (may activate latent psychosis); cardiac damage or coronary artery disease; and renal or hepatic impairment.

The client's concurrent medication regimen should be reviewed to detect any significant drug interactions. The following effects may occur when carbamazepine is given with the following drugs:

Drug	Possible effect and management
anticoagulants, oral warfarin (Coumadin)	Monitor for a decreased anticoagulant effect. Increased hepatic microsomal enzyme activity may increase anticoagulant metabolism, resulting in a decreased half-life and therapeutic effect. Dosage adjustments of anticoagulant may be necessary during and after treatment with carbamazepine.
anticonvulsants (hydantoin or succinimide); barbiturates; benzodiazepines metabolized by hepatic enzymes, especially clonazepam (Klonopin), primidone (Mysolinc), or valproic acid (Depakene)	Concurrent drug administration may result in increased drug metabolism and decreased serum levels and therapeutic effectiveness of these medications. Monitor blood levels whenever any of these medications is added to or discontinued in clients receiving carbamazepine, since dosage adjustment may be necessary. Valproic acid, however, may prolong the half-life of carbamazepine.
clarithromycin (Biaxin)	Concurrent use may result in elevated carbamazepine levels. Monitor serum levels closely.
cimetidine (Tagamet), diltiazem (Cardizem), or verapamil (Calan)	May increase plasma levels of carbamazepine, which can result in toxicity. Monitor closely.
corticosteroids	Concurrent administration may decrease steroidal effect because of increase in hepatic metabolism. Monitor closely for lack of response to corticosteroid therapy; dosage adjustment may be necessary.
erythromycin	Concurrent use may reduce carbamazepine metabolism, resulting in increased serum levels and toxicity. Avoid this combination and use a different antibiotic with clients taking carbamazepine.
estrogen-containing contraceptives	Decrease in contraceptive reliability; clients should be advised to use a nonhormonal birth control method or to discuss the possibility of an oral progestin product with their prescriber.
isoniazid (INH)	Carbamazepine may increase liver metabolism of isoniazid releasing an intermediate metabolite that can lead to hepatotoxicity. Also isoniazid may increase serum concentrations of carbamazepine, which may result in toxicity.
loxapine, (Loxitane), maprotiline (Ludiomil), thioxanthenes, or tricyclic antidepressants	May reduce the convulsive threshold and enhance CNS depressant effects; dosage adjustment may be necessary to control seizures and reduce side effects. Monitor closely for seizure activity.
monoamine oxidase (MAO) inhibitors	**Hypertensive crisis, elevated temperatures, severe convulsions, and even death have been reported with this combination. When switching from one therapy to another (MAO inhibitors to carbamazepine or vice versa), a drug-free interval of at least 14 days is recommended. Avoid or a potentially serious drug interaction may occur.**
quinidine	Because of increased metabolism, concurrent use may decrease quinidine's therapeutic effects. Monitor closely for cardiac arrhythmias; dosage adjustment may be necessary.
propoxyphene (Darvon, others)	May result in increased carbamazepine serum levels and toxicity. If an analgesic is necessary, it is recommended that another analgesic be selected.

Blood studies (CBC, liver function studies, BUN), urinalysis, physical examination, ophthalmic examinations, and ECG should be done before beginning carbamazepine therapy.

Nursing diagnosis. The client receiving carbamazepine therapy should be evaluated for the following nursing diagnoses/collaborative problems: risk for injury related to CNS toxicity (blurred or double vision, nystagmus); excess fluid volume related to water intoxication; altered mucous membranes (dry mouth); altered thought processes (confusion); altered bowel elimination (diarrhea); and altered comfort (headache, nausea and vomiting, aching joints and muscles); and the potential complications of Stevens-Johnson syndrome, systemic lupus erythematous–like syndrome, and blood dyscrasias.

Implementation

Monitoring. The level of seizure activity of the client should be monitored as well as the plasma carbamazepine concentrations. Weigh daily and monitor the client's intake and output to determine fluid retention. The client should be observed for any symptoms of adverse reactions to the drug.

Blood studies should be done every 2 weeks during the second and third months and then every month while the client is taking this medication.

Intervention. Carbamazepine should be administered with meals to reduce gastrointestinal irritation. The importance of compliance with drug therapy should be stressed with all clients taking this drug; abrupt withdrawal of the drug (in clients with epilepsy) can precipitate a seizure.

Education. Clients should report to the prescriber if they have any signs of hematologic dysfunction such as easy bruising, bleeding, sore throat or mouth, or malaise. It is not uncommon for the client to be drowsy during the initial therapy; clients should be cautioned about this so that they can avoid driving a car or operating hazardous equipment.

This drug is also used specifically for the pain of trigeminal neuralgia. It should not be used as a routine analgesic.

Carbamazepine can cause breakthrough bleeding in women taking oral contraceptives. Women should be told that it may interfere with the effectiveness of the contraceptive, so other birth control measures may need to be used. Carbamazepine is excreted in breast milk, so it may not be recommended in nursing mothers.

In middle-aged or elderly clients carbamazepine may decrease salivary flow and contribute to the development of caries, periodontal disease, or discomfort. Ice chips, chewing gum, and sugarless candies may ease the discomfort caused by the dry mouth.

Evaluation. The client will: have decreased severity and frequency of seizures; have plasma carbamazepine concentrations of 6 to 12 μg/ml; and be without adverse reactions to the drug.

felbamate [fel' bah mate] (Felbatol)

Felbamate is an antiepileptic used for the treatment of partial and secondary generalized seizures. It is also used as adjunct therapy for partial and generalized seizures associated with Lennox-Gastaut syndrome in children. Its mechanism of action is unknown although it has some properties in common with the other anticonvulsants; it may increase seizure threshold, have an inhibitory effect on GABA receptor binding, and reduce the spread or progression of a seizure.

See Table 17-1 for pharmacokinetic profile. Side/adverse effects include gastric distress, nausea, vomiting, taste alterations, anorexia, constipation, headache, insomnia, dizziness, fever, abnormal gait, and red-purple skin spots.

The usual adult (14 years old and over) dose is 1200 mg/day in divided doses. Children, 2 to 14 years old, receive 45 mg/kg/day or 3600 mg/day, whichever is less, in divided doses.

■ Nursing Management

Felbamate Therapy

In addition to the general nursing management for anticonvulsant drug therapy, consider the following:

Assessment. Felbamate is contraindicated, unless absolutely necessary, for use with clients with, or having a history of, blood disorders, bone marrow depression, or hepatic impairment because conditions may be exacerbated.

The baseline assessment of the client should include status of the underlying condition, mental status, vital signs, liver function studies, and CBC.

Nursing diagnosis. The client receiving felbamate should be assessed for the following nursing diagnoses/collaborative problems: sleep pattern disturbance (daytime sedation); activity intolerance related to malaise and flu-like symptoms; altered thought processes (agitation, aggressive reactions); altered nutrition, less than required related to anorexia, nausea, and vomiting; altered bowel pattern (constipation); and the potential complications of blood dyscrasias, hepatic dysfunction, and Stevens-Johnson syndrome.

Implementation

Monitoring. Although the value of routine monitoring of felbamate blood levels has not been established, it may be necessary to monitor the blood levels of the client's other anticonvulsant medications, because of the drug's impact upon them. Monitor for signs and symptoms of side/adverse effects.

Intervention. Shake the oral suspension thoroughly before administering.

Education. Take as prescribed and consult with prescriber before taking any other medications, including OTCs.

Evaluation. The client will experience a decrease in the frequency and severity of seizures without adverse effects of the drug.

gabapentin (ga ba pen' ten) (Neurontin)

Gabapentin is an antiepileptic for the treatment of adult partial seizures with or without secondary generalization. It was tested in refractory partial seizure clients and was reported to significantly reduce seizure frequency. The mechanism for its anticonvulsant action is unknown.

Gabapentin is absorbed orally, distributed unbound in the circulation and excreted by the kidneys unchanged. Side/adverse effects include drowsiness, dizziness, tiredness, ataxia and nystagmus.

The recommended adult dose is 300 to 600 mg three times a day.

■ Nursing Management

Gabapentin Therapy

In addition to the general nursing management for anticonvulsant drug therapy, consider the following:

Assessment. Gabapentin seems to be well tolerated with its adverse effects mild to moderate in severity and self-limiting.

Nursing diagnosis. The client receiving gabapentin should be assessed for the following nursing diagnoses/collaborative problems: altered sleep patterns (daytime somnolence, 19% of clients); risk of injury (dizziness, ataxia, 12.5%-17%); and fatigue (11%).

Implementation

Monitoring. The addition of gabapentin does not appreciably alter the serum levels of other anticonvulsant medications, so monitoring of serum levels is not necessary for the adjustment of concurrent anticonvulsant medications when gabapentin is added. The value of monitoring gabapentin serum levels has not been established.

Intervention. When administered with antacids, the absorption of gabapentin is reduced. Therefore, it is recommended that gabapentin be administered 2 hours after antacids. When switching to another anticonvulsant or stopping gabapentin, it is recommended that gabapentin be tapered down, over a minimum of 7 days (Olin, 1996).

Education. Advise clients not to drive or operate dangerous machinery until the effects of gabapentin on the individual can be determined.

Evaluation. With the addition of gabapentin to the client's anticonvulsant regimen, seizures should decrease in frequency and severity.

lamotrigine [la moe trih' jeen] (Lamictal)

Lamotrigine is an anticonvulsant whose mechanism of action is unknown. It is believed that lamotrigine stabilizes seizures by blocking sodium channels and thus inhibiting the release of excitatory neurotransmitters (glutamate, aspartate). These substances are believed to have a role in development and spread of epileptic seizures (*AHFS*, 1996). It is indicated as adjunct therapy for the treatment of partial seizures in adults (16 years and older) with epilepsy.

This drug is well absorbed orally, reaches peak serum levels in 1.4 to 4.8 hours, and has a half-life of 10 to 25 hours if taken with no other medications. If lamotrigine is administered with an enzyme-inducing anticonvulsant, half-life is 8 to 20 hours; with valproic acid only, half-life is 59 hours; with both enzyme-inducing and valproic acid anticonvulsants, half-life is 28 hours. It is metabolized in the liver and excreted primarily by the kidneys.

Side/adverse effects include headache, dizziness, drowsiness, abdominal distress, ataxia, rash, and visual disturbances. The usual adult dose if given with enzyme-inducing anticonvulsants is 50 mg daily for 2 weeks, then 50 mg twice a day for 2 weeks. Dose is adjusted according to response. If lamotrigine is administered with enzyme-inducing and valproic acid anticonvulsants, the dose is 25 mg every other day for 2 weeks, then 25 mg daily for 2 weeks. After 2 weeks, the dose is adjusted according to client response.

For nursing management of lamotrigine therapy, see the general nursing management for anticonvulsant therapy.

primidone [pri' mi done] (Mysoline)

Primidone and its metabolites, phenobarbital and phenylethylmalonamide (PEMA), contribute to anticonvulsant activity. The mechanism of action is unknown, but primidone and its metabolites all appear to have active anticonvulsant effects. Primidone is used for control of generalized tonic-clonic (grand mal) and complex seizures. For a pharmacokinetics overview, see Table 17-1.

Side/adverse effects include drowsiness, ataxia, dizziness, allergic reaction, and possibly paradoxical reactions in children and the elderly.

Dosage and administration. Adults, 100 to 125 mg at bedtime for 3 days, increased by 100 or 125 mg twice a day for the fourth through the sixth day, then increased by 100 to 125 mg 3 times a day until the ninth day. On day 10, the dose of 250 mg three times a day is established and may be altered according to the needs of the client to a maximum of 2 g/day.

For children up to 8 years, the initial dose is 50 mg orally at bedtime for 3 days, increased to 50 mg twice a day through day 6, then increased to 100 mg twice daily through day 9. On day 10, a maintenance dose of 125 or 250 mg 3 times a day, adjusted according to client response.

For the nursing management of primidone therapy, see barbiturate discussion in this chapter except for the following differences. Clients with reported reactions to barbiturates may be intolerant of primidone. If administered concurrently, monoamine oxidase (MAO) inhibitors may prolong the effects of primidone; dosage adjustments may be necessary. Monitor closely. The nurse should shake the oral suspension well for consistent dosing.

magnesium sulfate [mag nee' zhum]

Magnesium sulfate has a depressant effect on the CNS, which reduces striated muscle contractions. In addition, magnesium sulfate blocks peripheral neuromuscular transmission by reducing acetylcholine release at the myoneural junction, reducing the sensitivity of the motor endplate and lowering the excitability of the motor membrane.

The drug has three major indications. As an anticonvulsant, it is used in the prevention and control of seizures related to acute nephritis in children and seizures related to toxemias of pregnancy (Box 17-3). As a uterine relaxant, it is used in the treatment of uterine tetany and to inhibit con-

BOX 17-3

Toxemia of Pregnancy (Preeclampsia and Eclampsia)

Toxemia of pregnancy is a syndrome of elevated blood pressure, edema, and proteinurea, which occurs in about 5% of all pregnancies in North America. The syndrome is described in clinical terms because its cause is unknown. Preeclampsia is another term for the syndrome. Depending on the severity of symptoms, preeclampsia may be classified as mild, which may be treated at home, or severe, which requires hospitalization for monitoring and treatment. If the disease progresses, convulsions will occur and the syndrome is classified as eclampsia, which is derived from a Greek word used to described convulsions. Sensory changes that occur in severe preeclampsia and eclampsia include headache, epigastric pain, blurred vision, and hyperreflexia. Therapeutic goals for the treatment of toxemia of pregnancy are control of blood pressure, prevention of convulsions, maintenance of renal function, and provision of optimal conditions for the fetus. Treatment is symptomatic because the only "cure" for toxemia is delivery of the baby. Convulsions may still occur up to 48 hours after delivery, necessitating continued therapy in the immediate postpartum period.

tractions of premature labor. Finally, it is used as replacement therapy for magnesium deficiency.

About one third of dietary ingested magnesium is absorbed from the GI tract. With intravenous administration, onset of action is immediate, with approximately 30 minutes duration of action; with intramuscular administration, onset is about 1 hour, with a 3- to 4-hour duration of action. Magnesium undergoes no metabolism and is excreted by the kidneys. See the box at right for Management of Magnesium Sulfate Overdose.

Dosage and administration. For seizures caused by toxemia in pregnancy: administer 4 to 5 g (32-40 mEq) IV in 250 ml of D_5W or NS, administered over ½ hour. In addition, administer IM doses of up to 10 g (maximum 5 g in each buttock).

Pregnancy safety. Magnesium sulfate is administered in the treatment of toxemias of pregnancy. The drug crosses the placenta, with fetal blood levels approximately equal to maternal blood levels, and produces similar effects in the neonate as in the mother. Decreased reflexes, muscle tone, blood pressure, and respiratory depression may be seen if the mother received magnesium shortly before delivery. It is recommended that magnesium sulfate *not* be administered during the 2 hours before delivery, if possible.

■ Nursing Management

Magnesium Sulfate Therapy

Assessment. Magnesium sulfate should not be used in the presence of heart block, significant heart damage, or renal failure (creatinine clearance <20 ml/min). Caution must be exercised in the presence of severe renal function impairment because of the risk of hypermagnesemia and magnesium toxicity.

The client's current drug regimen should be reviewed to detect significant drug interactions.

Drug	Possible effect and management
CNS depressants	Dosage of barbiturates, opiates, general anesthetics, or other CNS depressants should be adjusted to avoid additive CNS depressant effects.
neuromuscular blocking agents	Excessive neuromuscular blockade has occurred when these drugs are administered with magnesium sulfate.

A baseline assessment should include blood pressure and respiratory rate determination, deep tendon reflexes, ECG for cardiac function, renal function determinations (especially urine output), and serum magnesium levels.

Nursing diagnosis. The client on magnesium sulfate therapy should be assessed for the following nursing diagnoses/collaborative problems: risk for injury related to hypotension and electrolyte imbalances; activity intolerance related to hypotonia; and the potential complication of cardiac dysrhythmias and respiratory paralysis.

Implementation

Monitoring. Monitor seizure activity. Take vital signs every 15 minutes while the drug is administered IV. Respirations should minimally be 16/min before each parenteral dose. Monitor intake and output; urinary output should be at least 100 ml in the 4 hours before each dose. The client must be closely monitored for the possible development of magnesium toxicity. ECG should be monitored continuously during intravenous administration. Serum magnesium determinations may be obtained as clinically indicated. Normal average serum magnesium concentrations are 1.6 to 2.6 mEq/L. Approximate serum concentrations (mEq/L) indicative of hypermagnesemia are as follows:

- 4 to 6: therapeutic range, mild depression of deep tendon reflexes
- 5 to 10: depression of deep tendon reflexes; prolonged PQ interval or widened QRS interval on ECG
- 10: loss of deep tendon reflexes
- 12 to 15: respiratory paralysis; complete heart block
- 25: cardiac arrest

The patellar reflex or knee jerk is an indication of CNS depression from magnesium. The patellar reflex should be checked before beginning therapy and before each dose. The disappearance of the reflex indicates excessive serum levels of magnesium.

Intervention. Extreme care must be taken to avoid overdosage and toxic serum concentrations. Intravenous infusions should be administered with a regulating or controlling device. A calcium salt that can be administered IV (calcium gluconate, calcium gluceptate, or calcium chloride) should be available when parenteral magnesium is administered.

Education. Alert the client as to the adverse actions of the drug so that the client may report them as soon as they are experienced.

Evaluation. The client will be seizure free without any adverse effects of the drug.

> **! MANAGEMENT OF DRUG OVERDOSE**
>
> **Magnesium sulfate**
>
> Signs of hypermagnesemia, which may begin at a serum concentration at or above 5 mEq/L, include flushing, hypotension, sweating, depressed reflexes, reduced respiratory rate, hypothermia, flaccid paralysis, circulatory collapse, slowed heart rate, and CNS depression.
>
> Treatment includes artificial respiration, calcium gluconate IV (5 to 10 mEq of calcium) injected slowly to reverse respiratory depression and heart block. In reduced renal function, dialysis may be necessary.

phenacemide [fen nass' e mide] (Phenurone)
Phenacemide is used for clients with severe epilepsy, especially partial seizures with complex symptoms that are refractory to other medications. This drug is extremely toxic and should be reserved for use *after* all available anticonvulsants have been proven ineffective. It may cause liver, blood, and psychologic problems (such as personality changes);

bone marrow depression; and hepatitis. Deaths have been reported with its use, so some prescribers believe it is too toxic for routine use.

■ Nursing Management
Phenacemide Therapy

In addition to the nursing considerations of anticonvulsant drug therapy discussed earlier:

Assessment. Determine if the client has any preexisting medical conditions, since the administration of phenacemide might have significant clinical risk, such as: sensitivity to phenacemide or other anticonvulsant drugs; history of blood dyscrasias (drug-induced aplastic anemia deaths have occurred); history of renal impairment (may be aggravated); history of hepatic impairment (drug-induced liver damage deaths have occurred); and history of personality disorders (suicide attempts and psychoses requiring hospitalization have occurred). Concurrent administration of other anticonvulsants, especially ethotoin, significantly increases the risk of additive toxicity, and causes paranoia.

A baseline assessment should include the client's mental status, blood cell counts, and hepatic and renal function studies.

Nursing diagnosis. While receiving phenacemide therapy, the client is at risk for the nursing diagnosis of altered thought processes (suicidal ideation, paranoid delusions, psychosis); and the potential complications of allergic reaction (skin rash), blood dyscrasias (leukopenia, neutropenia, aplastic anemia), hepatitis, and nephritis.

Implementation

Monitoring. Observe client for sore throat, fever, fatigue, and any unusual bleeding or bruising that might be indicative of blood dyscrasias. Report also any behavioral changes, such as decreased interest in surroundings, depression, or aggressiveness. Monitor blood cell counts and hepatic and renal function studies.

Intervention. Because of its potential for toxicity, minimal dosages should be prescribed for seizure coverage. Any withdrawal or change to or from other anticonvulsant drugs should be made gradually.

Education. Instruct client to avoid alcoholic beverages and not to take other drugs without consultation with the prescriber. Caution against activities requiring alertness, such as driving because of the possibility of drowsiness.

Evaluation. The client will experience a decrease in the frequency and severity of seizures without any adverse effects of phenacemide.

valproic acid [val proe' ik] (Depakene)
divalproex sodium [dye val' proe ex] (Depakote)

The mechanism by which valproic acid exerts its anticonvulsant effects has not been fully established. It has been proposed that its activity is related to directly or indirectly increasing or enhancing brain levels of the inhibitory neurotransmitter GABA. By competitive inhibition it may prevent the reuptake of GABA by glial cells and axonal terminals.

Valproic acid and divalproex sodium are indicated for use as sole and adjunctive therapy in the treatment of absence seizures, including petit mal, and as adjunctive therapy in clients with multiple seizure types, including absence seizures. See Table 17-1 for a pharmacokinetic overview. Chemically, valproate sodium is converted in the stomach to valproic acid, which is rapidly absorbed from the gastrointestinal tract. Divalproex sodium is a prodrug, a combination of valproic acid and valproate sodium, in an enteric-coated tablet. Divalproex dissociates into valproate, which is then absorbed in the small intestine.

Side effects/adverse effects include tremors, mild gastric distress, diarrhea, weight gain, irregular menses, and hepatotoxicity. The adult and pediatric dose is initially 15 mg/kg/day, increased at weekly intervals as needed. Maximum daily dose is 60 mg/kg/day (*PDR,* 1996).

■ Nursing Management
Valproic Acid Therapy

Assessment. Hepatic disease in the client would contraindicate the use of valproic acid therapy because there have been some instances of fatal hepatotoxicity with use of the drug. It is also recommended that caution be used with valproic acid therapy in clients with blood dyscrasias, organic brain disease, hypoalbuminemia, and renal function impairment. The drug is excreted in breast milk and can cause CNS depression in the nursing infant. Birth defects (spina bifida) have occurred when this drug was taken during the first trimester of pregnancy. Clients taking this drug who are considering pregnancy may need to be given another anticonvulsant that has no documented risk of causing birth defects.

The client's concurrent medication regimen should be reviewed for significant drug interactions. The following effects may occur when valproic acid and divalproex sodium (a drug that contains 50% valproic acid and sodium valproate) are given with the drugs listed below:

Drug	Possible effect and management
alcohol, anesthetics (general), CNS-depressant type drugs	May result in potentiated CNS-depressant effects.
anticoagulants, warfarin (Coumadin), heparin, or thrombolytic agents	Increased risk of bleeding and hemorrhage; monitor closely for early signs if given in combination.
aspirin, dipyridamole, (Persantine), or sulfinpyrazone (Anturane)	Increased risk of bleeding and hemorrhage; monitor closely; the prescriber might consider alternative therapeutic agents.
barbiturates or primidone (Mysoline)	Phenobarbital and primidone serum levels may increase, resulting in increased depression and toxicity. Monitor closely because the prescriber may need to adjust dosage.

Continued

Drug	Possible effect and management
carbamazepine (Tegretol) and phenytoin (Dilantin)	Breakthrough seizures may occur because of decreased serum levels of carbamazepine or valproic acid. Phenytoin protein binding may be affected when combined with valproic acid; therefore monitor closely, using serum levels as a guide, perhaps, for dosing adjustments by the prescriber.
mefloquine (Lariam)	Concurrent use may result in lower valproic acid serum levels and loss of seizure control. Monitor valproic acid levels; dosage adjustments during and after mefloquine therapy may be necessary.

Nursing diagnosis. The client receiving valproic acid therapy has the potential for the following nursing diagnoses/collaborative problems: risk of injury related to visual effects (double vision, nystagmus); altered nutrition, less than required related to anorexia, indigestion, and nausea and vomiting; altered bowel pattern (diarrhea); and the potential complications of hepatotoxicity, adverse ophthalmologic effects, pancreatitis (abdominal pain, nausea and vomiting), cognitive impairment, and thrombocytopenia (unusual bruising or bleeding).

Implementation

Monitoring. In addition to monitoring the client's seizure activity and serum valproate concentrations, the nurse should observe for early signs of the drug's adverse effects. Baseline and periodic evaluations of bleeding time, blood cell counts, and renal and hepatic function studies are recommended.

Intervention. The drug should be administered with or after meals to avoid gastric irritation. The client should avoid chewing or crushing the tablets and capsules; the nurse should avoid giving the tablet form with milk because of possible early dissolution and local irritation to the mouth and throat. The drug is available in syrup form for clients unable to swallow tablets or capsules. Divalproex sodium is prescribed for clients unable to tolerate the gastrointestinal irritation produced by valproic acid. When other anticonvulsant drugs are used in combination, the dosage of valproic acid and/or the other anticonvulsants may need to be adjusted to maintain serum levels and seizure control.

Education. The client should be instructed not to chew the tablet or capsule, since it will irritate the mouth and throat. Combining this drug with alcohol or other CNS depressants can cause a potentiation of sedation.

This drug can cause a false-positive urine ketone test in clients with diabetes mellitus; these clients should be instructed to consult their prescriber about using some other diagnostic tool for ketones. The client should be instructed to be aware of signs of decreasing mental alertness, which can occur when valproic acid is given alone or in combination with other anticonvulsants.

The client should be told to report to the prescriber if any of the following side effects occur: visual disturbances, rash, and diarrhea. Valproic acid has been shown to cause liver dysfunction; therefore the client should be instructed to report signs of liver dysfunction, such as spontaneous bleeding and bruising, light-colored stools, jaundice, and protracted vomiting to the prescriber immediately. The client should have liver function studies done at least every month during the first 6 months of therapy when hepatotoxicity is most likely to occur.

Evaluation. The outcome criteria being sought are that the client will experience a decrease in the frequency and severity of seizures with a predose serum valproate concentration of at least 50 μg/ml without adverse effects of the drug.

SUMMARY

Epilepsy, a symptom of a disorder of the brain rather than a disease itself, occurs in only a small percentage of the population. Epileptic seizures have various causes and so are classified by symptoms. The nurse needs to be particularly observant in the assessment and documentation of seizures. The drugs used for the treatment of seizures are also varied: barbiturates, hydantoins, succinimides, oxazolidinediones, benzodiazepines, and others. Each client's therapy is individualized by taking into account a complex of interrelated factors, such as the pharmacokinetics of the drug in an individual, concurrent ailments and medications, diet, physical status, and the client's compliance with the regimen. The nurse must use a holistic approach, not only to manage the client's physical symptoms but also to provide psychosocial support. Moderation is the key for these clients, in rest, exercise, diet, and avoidance of stress. The most common nursing diagnoses for clients receiving anticonvulsant therapy are knowledge deficit and ineffective management of the therapeutic regimen and risk for injury related to the side effects/adverse reactions of these drugs. An important evaluation factor is the effectiveness of the regimen in controlling and minimizing seizures.

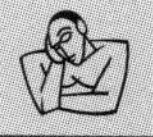

Critical Thinking

1. Why is the assessment essential in determining a therapeutic anticonvulsant medication regimen for a client? What part does the client's age play?
2. Mrs. Curtis, a 24-year-old, and her husband, have decided to start a family. She has been on phenytoin since childhood for a seizure disorder and would prefer to discontinue the medication before getting pregnant. What criteria will be involved in the decision to wean Mrs. C. from her medication?

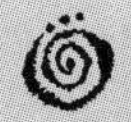

Collaborative Learning Activities

1. Because the nurse plays a crucial role in the treatment management of a client on anticonvulsant therapy, four student groups will prepare a 10 minute presentation on one of the following aspects of nursing management: assessment, nursing diagnosis, implementation, and evaluation.

BIBLIOGRAPHY

American Hospital Formulary Service (1996). *AHFS drug information '96*. Bethesda, MD: American Society of Hospital Pharmacists.

Anderson KN, et al. (Eds.) (1994). *Mosby's medical, nursing, & allied health dictionary* (4th ed.). St. Louis: Mosby.

Carpenito LJ (1995). *Nursing diagnosis: Application to clinical practice* (6th ed.). Philadelphia: JB Lippincott.

Carter JR (1994). *The use of new antiepileptic medications in pediatric patients with epilepsy, J Pediatr Health Care* 8(6):277-82.

Chipps EM, Clanin NJ, & Campbell VG (1992). *Neurologic disorders*. St Louis: Mosby.

Cloyd J (1996). Pharmacologic considerations of fosphenytoin therapy. *P & T Supplement* 21(55):13s-20s.

Dichter MA (1992). Deciding to discontinue antiepileptic medication, *Hosp Pract* 27(20):16.

Drug Update (1996). Pharmacy News, *J Am Pharm Assoc NS* 36(10):566.

Hardman JG & Limbird LE (Eds.) (1996). *Goodman & Gilman's the pharmacological basis of therapeutics* (9th ed.). New York: Macmillan.

Killam P (1992). Childhood epilepsy: Myth vs. reality, *Am J Nurs* 92(3):77.

Legion V (1991). Health education for self-management by people with epilepsy, *J Neuroscien Nurs* 23(5):300.

Lott RS (1995). Seizure Disorders. In Young LY & Koda-Kimble MA (Eds.). *Applied therapeutics: The clinical use of drugs*. Vancouver, WA: Applied Therapeutics.

Olin BR (Ed.) (1996). *Facts and comparisons*. St. Louis: Facts and Comparisons.

PDR (1996). *Physicians' desk reference* (50th ed.). Montvale, NJ: Medical Economics.

Rowan AJ (1995). Recognition and assessment of seizure disorders in the elderly: Epidemiology, pathophysiology, and differentiation, *Consult Pharmacist* 10(suppl A):4-8.

Steiner JF (1994). Pharmacologic treatment of epilepsy, *J Amer Acad Physic Asst* 7(7):508-16.

United States Pharmacopeial Convention (1996). *USP DI: Drug information for the health care professional* (15th ed.). Rockville, MD: The Convention.

US Gabapentin Study Group (1994). The long-term safety and efficacy of gabapentin (Neurontin) as add-on therapy in drug-resistant partial epilepsy, *Epilepsy Res* 18:67-73.

Wertz EM (1995). Understanding AEDs . . . anti-epileptic drugs, *Emergency* 27(1):18,23-5.

Chapter 18

Central Nervous System Stimulants

Chapter Focus

The CNS stimulants may produce dramatic effects, but their therapeutic usefulness is limited because of their multiple actions and side effects. Continuous use and misuse of these drugs (especially amphetamines) have resulted in the development of drug tolerance, drug dependence, and drug abuse. Large doses of the CNS stimulants may precipitate convulsive seizures, coma, and exhaustion. Although the number of drugs that stimulate the central nervous system is large, only a few of these are actually used for this purpose. The nurse needs to be knowledgeable about the therapeutic uses of CNS stimulants as well as the nontherapeutic effects of these drugs that are commonly abused in our society. The following objectives and key terms are important for a good understanding of this chapter.

Key Terms

amphetamines (p. 346)
analeptics (p. 346)
anorexiants (p. 346)
attention deficit disorder (p. 346)
cataplexy (p. 346)
narcolepsy (p. 346)

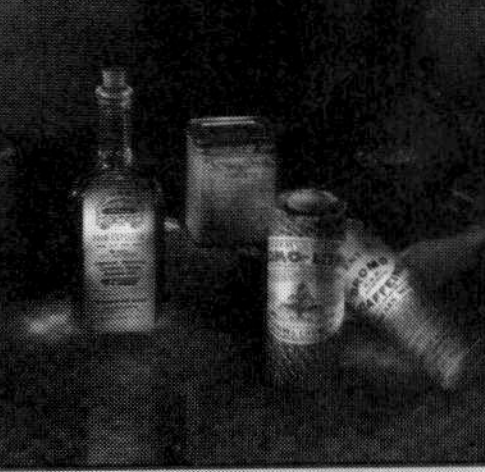

Key Drugs [▲]

amphetamine
methylphenidate
caffeine

Objectives

1. Discuss attention deficit disorder (ADD) with hyperactivity and the drug treatment for ADD.
2. Define the terms *analeptic* and *anorexiant drugs.*
3. Describe common CNS-stimulant drugs and the indications for their use.
4. Identify common physical and psychic changes attributable to CNS stimulants.
5. List caffeine-containing food and beverages, along with their approximate caffeine content.
6. Implement an appropriate plan of care for the client receiving CNS-stimulant drugs.

The classification of stimulants depends on where in the nervous system they exert their major effects—on the cerebrum, the medulla and brainstem, or the hypothalamic limbic regions. **Amphetamines** are mainly stimulants of the cerebral cortex; **analeptics** primarily affect the centers in the medulla and the brainstem; and **anorexiants** suppress the appetite, perhaps by a direct stimulant effect on the satiety center in the hypothalamic and limbic regions. Central nervous system stimulants act by increasing the neuronal discharge or by blocking an inhibitory neurotransmitter. These drugs may also affect other parts of the nervous system.

Cerebral stimulants were commonly prescribed in the past for obesity and to counteract CNS-depressant overdosage, but such use today is considered obsolete. Although the CNS stimulants suppress appetite, tolerance develops to the anorexic effect usually before the weight reduction goal is reached. Treatment of severe CNS depression with stimulants is also discouraged, since close monitoring and supportive measures have been found to be quite successful without the production of undesirable adverse reactions. With their narrow therapeutic index between effectiveness and toxicity, CNS stimulants may induce cardiac dysrhythmias, hypertension, convulsions, and violent behavior. Thus the CNS stimulants have limited use in practice today; they are primarily used for the treatment of **attention deficit disorder** (ADD) with hyperactivity and narcolepsy.

ADD with hyperactivity is a syndrome characterized by distractibility, a short attention span, impulsive behavior, hyperactivity, and learning and behavior disabilities. Improper functioning of the neurotransmitter systems (noradrenergic, dopaminergic, and serotonergic) have been implicated in this syndrome (Sakled & Curtis, 1995). Stimulant medications tend to decrease the distractibility and hyperactivity, resulting in an increased attention span.

The onset of ADD with hyperactivity usually occurs between the ages of 3 and 7 years, with boys affected more often than girls by a 10:1 ratio (Bolinger et al, 1992). Usually professional intervention is unnecessary until the child enters the school setting. Attention deficit hyperactivity disorder (ADHD) may persist into adulthood. In one report, 31% of young adults that had ADHD in childhood still had the full syndrome. Adults with ADHD may have a higher incidence of substance abuse, antisocial personality disorders, anxiety, and depression when compared with a control group. Children treated with stimulants, however, were reported to have a better outcome as adults (Saklad & Curtis, 1995). Management of this disorder requires a behavioral modification program with use of pharmacologic therapy as an adjunct if necessary.

Approximately 15% to 20% of children do not respond or their symptoms actually increase with the stimulant drugs. Antidepressant therapy (imipramine [Tofranil], desipramine [Norapramin]) should be considered for these individuals, especially if they present with ADHD with anxiety or depression symptoms. Clonidine (Klonopin) has been used, especially for persons that have both ADHD and Tourette's syndrome, but this product should not be used for children with ADHD and depression, since it can worsen the condition (Saklad & Curtis, 1995).

Although stimulant medications are available in short-acting (4-hour) and long-acting (8-10 hour) forms, it is general practice to establish a daily schedule using the short-acting form. The dosage required will be learned from empiric experience. For this reason the prescriber needs to work closely with the child, the parents, and school personnel in evaluating results and planning dosages.

The child's distractibility and hyperactivity must be managed during school hours. But it may be equally important to contain these symptoms at other times of the day to promote the child's psychosocial development by participating in clubs, religious activities, or social events. Rather than having a continuous approach to dosing, it is more helpful to consider the child's life in 4-hour units and to provide a dose appropriate to the needs of that time block. For example, the child might take 10 mg of a short-acting stimulant at 8 AM and again at noon on a school day but add another dose at 4 PM if a music lesson is planned for that evening.

Narcolepsy is a condition characterized by excessive drowsiness and uncontrollable sleep attacks during the daytime. In addition, the client may exhibit a sleep paralysis (inability to move that occurs immediately on falling asleep or on awakening), **cataplexy** (stress-induced generalized muscle weakness), and hypnagogic illusions or hallucinations (vivid auditory or visual dreams occurring at onset of sleep). CNS stimulants are useful in controlling the daytime drowsiness and excessive sleep patterns, whereas tricyclic antidepressants are being tested in conjunction with the stimulants for cataplexy and sleep paralysis.

The mechanism of action for the cerebral stimulants (amphetamines) includes the release of norepinephrine from storage and also a direct stimulating effect on alpha and beta receptor sites. While the central nervous system effects are unknown, the primary action centrally appears to be in the cerebral cortex and possibly the reticular activating system. Stimulation results in an increase in motor function and mental alertness, decreased sense of fatigue, and usually a euphoric effect (AHFS, 1996).

Animal studies indicate amphetamine blocks reuptake of dopamine and norepinephrine from the synapse, inhibits monoamine oxidase (MAO) action and also increases the release of catecholamines (*USP DI*, 1996).

ANOREXIANT DRUGS

Anorexiant or appetite-suppressant drugs include a variety of medications that are used to treat exogenous obesity (Table 18-1). The anorexiant drugs are lipid soluble and cross the blood-brain barrier.

Phendimetrazine affects norepinephrine and, like amphetamine, produces marked euphoria, stimulation, and abuse potential. Phentermine and diethylpropion affect norepinephrine and produce mild euphoria and mild to moderate stimulation with minimal abuse potential.

TABLE 18-1 Anorexiant medications

Drug	Recommended dosages
benzphetamine (Didrex)	Adults, 25-50 mg orally, daily, Not recommended in children less than 12 yr old.
diethylpropion	
Tablets (Tenuate)	Adults, 25 mg 3 times daily, 1 hr before meals. Not recommended in children less than 12 yr old.
Extended-release tablets (Tenuate Dospan, Tepanil Ten-tab)	Adults, 75 mg orally daily at mid-morning. Not recommended in children less than 12 yr old.
fenfluramine	
Tablets (Pondimin, Ponderal🍁)	Adults, 20 mg initially orally, 3 times daily, ½-1 hr before meals. May increase by 20 mg daily at weekly intervals up to 40 mg 3 times a day. Not recommended in children less than 12 yr old.
Extended-release capsules (Ponderal Pacaps🍁)	Adults, 60 mg orally, initially, daily. May be increased to 120 mg daily if necessary. Not recommended in children less than 12 yr old.
mazindol (Mazanor, Sanorex)	Adults, 1 mg initially orally once a day before breakfast. Increase to 1 mg 3 times daily, an hour before meals or 2 mg daily, an hour before lunch. Not recommended in children less than 12 yr old.
phendimetrazine	
Tablets (Adphen, Bontril PDM, and others)	Adults, 17.5-35 mg orally, 2 or 3 times daily, an hour before meals. Not recommended in children less than 12 yr old.
Capsules (Obalan)	Adults, 35 mg 2 or 3 times a day, 1 hour before meals.
Extended-release capsules (Adipost, Bontril Slow Release)	Adults, 105 mg orally daily, ½-1 hour before breakfast. Not recommended in children less than 12 yr old.
phentermine	
Tablets (Phentride)	Adults, 15-37.5 mg daily before breakfast. Not recommended in children less than 12 yr old.
Capsules (Fastin)	Adults, capsules same as above.
Resin capsules (Ionamin)	Adults, 15 or 30 mg orally daily before breakfast. Not recommended in children less than 12 yr old.

Mazindol affects dopamine and adrenergic receptors and has the same CNS effects as diethylpropion, with minimal abuse potential. Fenfluramine increases serotonin, which depresses the CNS while suppressing the appetite. It also increases glucose use and has minimal abuse potential. Fenfluramine may be the drug of choice for anxious individuals or for clients who should avoid the use of CNS-stimulant drugs (such as those with hyperthyroidism, agitation, and advanced arteriosclerosis).

Anorexiants have a number of limitations, so careful selection of the clinical choices is necessary to minimize the unwanted effects. As appetite suppressants they are recommended as an adjunct to other regimens, such as physical exercise, behavior modification, and restriction of caloric intake, and are prescribed for a short time, since tolerance to the anorectic effect may occur within a few weeks (*USP DI*, 1996).

Side effects/adverse reactions. Most frequently reported side effects include euphoria, increased irritability, nervousness, and insomnia with all except fenfluramine. Other less frequent side effects are visual disturbance, diarrhea or constipation, dry mouth, difficulty on urination, tachycardia, impotence, headaches, sweating, and nausea and vomiting. Fenfluramine side effects include ataxia, nightmares, increased weakness, and difficulty in talking.

Adverse reactions include hypertension with all stimulant drugs except fenfluramine. Less frequently reported is CNS depression and confusion, allergic rashes or hives, and psychosis. Pulmonary hypertension has been reported with fenfluramine. See the box on p. 348 for Management of Anorexiant Overdose.

■ Nursing Management

Anorexiant Therapy

Assessment. Anorexiant drugs are used to treat altered nutrition: more than body requirements. The nurse should work with the client to determine the causative factors for the obesity that results from the ingestion of calories in excess of metabolic need: sedentary lifestyle, lack of nutritional knowledge, or increased food intake related to stress, low self-esteem, or boredom. Nursing interventions can then be planned based on the specific etiologic factor to which the anorexiant drug therapy serves as a short-term adjunct. A realistic goal for weight loss should be 1 to 2 pounds a week, although obese clients will tend to have a greater weight loss than this, at least initially.

MANAGEMENT OF DRUG OVERDOSE

Anorexiant

There is no specific antidote for an overdose of anorexiant drugs. Institute symptomatic and supportive measures according to the individual client's requirement.

Generally, emesis and/or use of gastric lavage is indicated, followed by administration of activated charcoal to adsorb any remaining drug in the GI tract. Do not use this measure for fenfluramine because an overdose of this drug usually induces unconsciousness.

Excessive stimulation may be counteracted with barbiturates, chlorpromazine, or haloperidol (to decrease anticholinergic effects). Seizures may be controlled with diazepam or phenobarbital.

Monitor vital signs and respiratory functions frequently. Closely monitor cardiac and respiratory functions. Medications usually utilized are: for hypertension, IV phentolamine or nitrites; for hypotension, IV fluids; for arrhythmias, lidocaine IV; and for tachycardia, a beta-adrenergic blocking agent.

Urine acidification and forced diuresis is also recommended.

Anorexiants are, in general, contraindicated for clients with agitated states; arteriosclerotic disease; cardiovascular disease, particularly those with dysrhythmias; cerebral ischemia; glaucoma; moderate to severe hypertension; hyperthyroidism; and psychosis, since anorexiant therapy may worsen their condition. Dependence on anorexiants may develop with clients with a history of drug abuse or dependence. Uremia may alter excretion of the drug.

The use of fenfluramine is contraindicated in clients with alcoholism because depression and psychosis have occurred. It is also contraindicated in clients with a history of depression, since they become depressed or more depressed following withdrawal of the drug. This is because fenfluramine is a CNS depressant, whereas the other anorexiants are CNS stimulants.

The client's concurrent medication regimen needs to be assessed to determine if there would be significant drug interactions with anorexiant therapy. Concurrent use or use within 14 days of monamine oxidase (MAO) inhibitors with anorexiants should be avoided, since potentiated sympathomimetic effects, including hypertensive crisis, may result. Avoid administration of concurrent CNS-depressant drugs, including alcohol, with fenfluramine because enhanced CNS depression may result. Anorexiants with thyroid medications may increase CNS stimulant effects and side effects. These drugs should be administered with caution to clients with diabetes, since the need for insulin may be decreased as a result of the concomitant dietary regimen. Blood and urine glucose levels should be monitored closely. General anesthetics should be administered with caution. Sensitivity to the specific drug and other sympathomimetics should be determined.

A baseline assessment should include height and weight, vital signs, lifestyle issues related to obesity, knowledge level, and mental status.

Nursing diagnosis. Once the client is started on anorexiant therapy, the nurse should be alert for the following nursing diagnoses: disturbance in sleep pattern and altered thought processes (depression) related to CNS effects; altered comfort related to dry mouth, rash, headache, or gastrointestinal or urinary effects; disturbance of self-concept related to changes in sexual desire or decreased sexual ability; and the potential complication of altered cardiac output related to cardiovascular effects.

Implementation

Monitoring. The client's weight needs to be monitored on an ongoing basis. Adverse effects of these drugs, except for fenfluramine, usually relate to overstimulation, such as nervousness, restlessness, insomnia, and anxiety. Blood pressure and pulse should be monitored to assess whether the client is responding adversely to the drug. Tolerance is a frequent occurrence with anorexiants, and the client should be assessed for the possibility of habituation and addiction.

Fenfluramine is different from the other anorexiants because its adverse effects are drowsiness and depression. Diarrhea may be significant enough to decrease the dosage or end the course of fenfluramine.

Intervention. Because these drugs are to be used only for a short term, emphasis is on a total weight reduction program that includes a suitable diet, appropriate exercise regimen, and behavior modification related to the cause of the overeating.

Preparations administered daily should be administered in the morning to decrease insomnia. Avoid administering anorexiant drugs within 4 to 6 hours, or 10 to 14 hours for extended release or long acting dosage forms, of anticipated sleep times.

After prolonged high dosages, the drug should be discontinued gradually to avoid a rebound increase in appetite and withdrawal symptoms.

Education. Clients should be instructed to consult the prescriber if the drug seems to be less effective than desired; they should not self-regulate the dosage. Instruct the client to avoid caffeine-containing beverages, which increase the effects of the stimulant anorexiant drugs. Caution the client that these drugs may impair the client's ability to perform tasks requiring physical coordination and alertness. Clients should be instructed about ways to minimize unpleasant taste and dryness of mouth with mouth rinses, ice chips, chewing gum, and sugarless candies.

In addition, the client should receive appropriate education regarding lifestyle changes, such as nutrition and exercise, to support weight loss.

Evaluation. The expected outcomes for the client should include: decreased appetite with accompanying weight loss.

BOX 18-1

dexfenfluramin (Redux)

Dexfenfluramine is a serotonin reuptake inhibitor and releasing agent approved for the management of obesity. It is used to induce and maintain weight loss in individuals who are also on a reduced-calorie diet. Dexfenfluramine is chemically similar to fenfluramine (dextrorotary isomer) and amphetamines, but it differs in that it is a pure serotonin agonist and does not produce CNS stimulation (*AHFS Suppl A,* 1996).

This drug is metabolized to an active metabolite d-norfenfluramine that also has similar effects on serotonin. It is well absorbed orally, reaches peak serum level in 1½ to 8 hours, and has a half-life of 17 to 20 hours. It is metabolized in the liver and excreted primarily in urine.

Dexfenfluramine is contraindicated for use in clients with pulmonary hypertension and in persons receiving monoamine oxidase inhibitor (MAOI) drugs. Serious and fatal reactions may occur in persons that were also receiving an MAOI drug concurrently or within the previous 2 weeks of starting dexfenfluramine. An additional recommendation is that 3 weeks should elapse after the discontinuation of dexfenfluramine before starting an MAOI medication. If the anti-migraine medications sumtriptan (Imitrex) and dihydroergot-amine (DHE 45) are taken concurrently with dexfenfluramine, a serotonin syndrome may result. This syndrome includes confusion, ataxia, hypothermia, shivers, vomiting, tachycardia, excitation, disorientation, and other effects (Olin, 1966).

The most common side/adverse effects include headache, diarrhea, insomnia, dry mouth, and sedation. Dexfenfluramine can also cause a false-positive urine test for amphetamines for up to a day after taking a 30-mg dose (*AHFS Suppl A,* 1996). The usual adult dose is 15 mg twice daily with meals, which may be continued for up to 1 year. If the individual has not lost at least 4 pounds in the first month of therapy, the prescriber is advised to reevaluate the need to continue this drug. The safety and effectiveness of this drug beyond a year has not been established. Pregnancy safety is FDA category C (Olin, 1966).

The client should also be able to sleep without difficulty and not experience any other adverse effects of the drug.

AMPHETAMINES

The mechanism of action was previously reviewed in this chapter. Amphetamines used over long periods can produce psychologic and physical dependence. Prolonged use of amphetamines leads to the development of tolerance. Because of their potential for abuse, amphetamines are not recommended for use as appetite suppressants; instead they are indicated for the treatment of ADD with hyperactivity and in the treatment of narcolepsy.

Amphetamines are well absorbed and are distributed to body tissues, with especially high concentrations in the brain and cerebrospinal fluid. The half-life depends on urinary pH. Generally they are as follows: amphetamine, 10 to 30 hours; dextroamphetamine, 10 to 12 hours for adults and 6 to 8 hours in children; methamphetamine, 4 to 5 hours. These drugs are metabolized in the liver and excreted by the kidneys. Excretion is pH dependent; it is increased in an acidic urine and decreased in a more alkaline urine.

The nurse should be aware that long-term amphetamine abuse can lead to chorea, a condition characterized by involuntary, purposeless, rapid motions, which is mediated by alterations in the physiology of the basal ganglia; chorea is also seen with the administration of cocaine, which reduces dopamine levels.

The most frequently reported side effects with amphetamine use includes euphoria, increased irritability, nervousness, insomnia, and restlessness. Less frequently reported are visual disturbance, excessive sweating, dry mouth, abdominal cramps, impotence, alterations in sexual desire, diarrhea or constipation, dizziness, anorexia, nausea or vomiting, and weight loss. The most frequently reported adverse reactions include tachycardia or irregular heart rate. Less frequent are allergic reactions including urticaria, hives, angina or chest pain, tremors, hyperreactive reflexes, dyskinesia, and Tourette's syndrome. With high dosage or prolonged consumption, CNS mood changes including depression, increased agitation, and psychosis may occur. Drug dependency and tolerance may also develop.

Dosage and administration. See Table 18-2.

Treatment of amphetamine overdose. In addition to symptomatic and supportive care as outlined in the management of an anorexiant overdose, if the client has taken the long-acting dosage forms, a saline cathartic is indicated. Monitor vital signs and respiratory functions closely.

■ Nursing Management

Amphetamine Therapy

In addition to the nursing management of anorexiant therapy, the nursing activities that are presented next should be considered with amphetamine therapy.

Assessment. The nurse should be aware that amphetamines, like other CNS stimulants, should be avoided by persons with hypertension and cardiovascular disease and by those who are unduly restless, anxious, agitated, and excited. Amphetamines should be used with caution in elderly and debilitated clients or those with a history of homicidal or suicidal tendencies.

Individuals with bronchial asthma who are sensitive to tartrazine dye should not use the dosage forms that contain the dye.

The client's concurrent drug regimen should be reviewed to identify any potential significant drug interactions. The

TABLE 18-2 Amphetamines: dosage and administration

Drug	Adults	Children
amphetamine tablets		
Narcolepsy	5-20 mg 1-3 times daily	Children to 6 yr, dosage not determined; 6-12 yr, 2.5 mg orally twice daily; increase by 5 mg/day at 1-wk intervals until therapeutic effect or adult dosage achieved. Children 12 yr and older, 5 mg twice daily orally, increasing dose by 10 mg/day at weekly intervals until therapeutic effect or adult dosage achieved.
Attention deficit disorder	Not applicable	Children up to 3 yr, not recommended. 3-6 yr, 2.5 mg orally; increased by 2.5 mg/day at weekly intervals until therapeutic response achieved. 6 yr and older, 5 mg orally 1 or 2 times/day; increase by 5 mg/day at weekly intervals until therapeutic response achieved.
dextroamphetamine tablets		
Narcolepsy	5-60 mg orally 1-3 times daily	Children up to 6 yr, dosage not determined. 6-12 yr, 5 mg daily; increase by 5 mg/day at weekly intervals until therapeutic effect or adult dosage achieved. 12 yr and older, 10 mg daily; increase by 10 mg/day at weekly intervals until therapeutic effect or adult dosage achieved.
Attention deficit disorder	Not applicable	Children up to 3 yr, not recommended. 3-6 yr, 2.5 mg orally daily; increase by 2.5 mg/day at weekly intervals until therapeutic response achieved. 6 yr and older, 5 mg orally once or twice/day; increase dosage by 5 mg daily at weekly intervals until therapeutic response achieved. Dextroamphetamine extended-release capsules may be used after therapeutic dosage per day is established.
methamphetamine tablets (Desoxym), methamphetamine extended-release tablets (Desoxyn)		
Attention deficit disorder	Not applicable	Children up to 6 yr, not recommended. 6 yr and older, 5 mg orally 1 or 2 times daily; increase by 5 mg/day at weekly intervals until therapeutic effect achieved (usually 20-25 mg/day).

following effects may occur when amphetamines are given with the drugs listed below.

Drug	Possible effect and management
antidepressants, tricyclic	**May result in adverse cardiovascular effects, such as arrhythmias, tachycardia, or severe hypertension. Monitor the pulse and blood pressure closely; dosage adjustments may be necessary. Avoid or a potenially serious drug interaction may occur.**
beta-adrenergic blocking drugs (systemic and ophthalmic)	**May cause unopposed alpha-adrenergic effects resulting in hypertension, bradycardia, and possible heart block. If necessary to use both classifications, labetalol, a beta-blocking agent that also has alpha-blocking effects, may reduce the risk of producing the above effects. Monitor closely for dysrhythmias. Avoid or a potenially serious drug interaction may occur.**
CNS stimulants such as appetite suppressants, caffeine, methylphenidate, pemoline, sympathomimetics, theophylline, amantadine	**May result in an increase in adverse cardiovascular effects, nervousness, insomnia, and convulsions. Avoid or a potentially serious drug interaction may occur.**
digitalis glycosides	**May result in an increase in cardiac dysrhythmias. Avoid usage or, if necessary, monitor apical pulse very closely. Concurrent use not recommended or contraindicated because of possible serious outcome.**

Drug	Possible effect and management
meperidine (Demerol)	**Although some investigators believe the analgesic effect of meperidine might be enhanced, concurrent use should be avoided because it may result in severe respiratory depression, seizures, hyperpyrexia, severe hypotension, cardiovascular collapse, and death in some clients. Avoid or a potentially serious drug interaction may occur.**
monoamine oxidase (MAO) inhibitors	**Avoid concurrent usage because increased release of catecholamines, headaches, dysrhythmias, vomiting, sudden severe hypertension, and possibly hyperpyretic crisis may result. Avoid or a potentially serious drug interaction may occur. Do not administer during or for 2 weeks after the discontinuance of an MAO inhibitor.**
thyroid hormones	**May result in enhanced effects of thyroid or amphetamines. If client has coronary artery disease, the potential for inducing coronary insufficiency is increased. Avoid or a potentially serious drug interaction may occur.**

Nursing diagnosis. Amphetamine therapy may put the client at risk for the following nursing diagnoses: ineffective coping related to the client's underlying disorder or development of abuse problem; altered nutrition: more than body requirements related to the ineffectiveness of amphetamine therapy; altered nutrition: less than body requirements (particularly for children receiving amphetamine therapy for ADD); sleep pattern disturbance related to drug-induced insomnia; altered thought processes related to the CNS effects of the drug; and altered oral mucous membranes related to dry mouth.

Implementation

Monitoring. Nurses should assess pulse and blood pressure of clients receiving amphetamines to monitor for adverse cardiovascular effects of the drug. Caution should be used and the possibility of psychologic dependence and addiction should be considered in clients with a history of addiction to alcohol or other drugs. The nurse should evaluate for potential dependence in all clients receiving the drug. The client's weight and dietary intake, sleep patterns, compliance with therapy, and mental status should be monitored on an ongoing basis.

Children receiving amphetamines for a prolonged period should have their growth carefully monitored because these drugs are thought to mildly inhibit growth. Growth usually catches up during drug-free periods. Amphetamines should be discontinued periodically in children with ADD to reevaluate the need for therapy; they should be reinstituted only if behavioral symptoms return.

Intervention. The last dose of the day should be administered not later than 6 hours before the client's bedtime; if a sustained-release product is used, the last daily dose should be administered not less than 10 to 14 hours before bedtime to avoid insomnia. If before-meals dosing is prescribed, the dose should be given 30 to 60 minutes before the client's meal. Modification of diet and behavior is essential if the drug is to be successful as an anorexiant. If weight loss is not desired, administer the drug with or after meals. Help client overcome a dry mouth with sugarless candy, gum, or ice chips.

The dosage should be gradually tapered before discontinuing the drug after prolonged high dosage to avoid withdrawal manifestations such as psychotic symptoms and lethargy. Because fatigue occurs as the drug effects diminish, the nurse should be aware that the client will need more rest and sleep.

Education. The client should be instructed not to self-regulate the dose; the habit-forming potential should be stressed. If the effect of the drug seems to decrease, the nurse should caution the client not to increase the dosage but to consult the prescriber. The sustained-release tablet should be swallowed whole; it should not be broken, chewed, or crushed. The nurse should inform the client of the CNS and cardiovascular side effects of the drug that need to be reported.

Clients should be cautioned that amphetamines may impair their functioning in the performance of tasks requiring mental alertness and physical coordination. These drugs are frequently abused by athletes, students, and drivers for the purpose of increasing alertness but may result in an impaired ability to function. The nurse should caution the client to store the drug securely to avoid unintended use by another person.

Evaluation. The expected outcome will be the client demonstrating clinical improvement—the child will have an increased attention span and decreased restlessness, be able to sleep without difficulty, and show no evidence of adverse effects.

OTHER CENTRAL NERVOUS SYSTEM STIMULANTS

doxapram [dox' a pram] (Dopram)

At low dosages doxapram stimulates respiration by acting on the peripheral carotid chemoreceptors; at higher dosages the medullary respiratory center is stimulated. This drug is used for the treatment of respiratory depression induced by a drug overdose, chronic obstructive pulmonary disease, or postanesthetic effects.

Doxapram is a parenteral drug administered intravenously. It has an onset of effect at 20 to 40 seconds and a peak effect at 1 to 2 minutes. Doxapram's duration of action is 5 to 12 minutes. It is excreted primarily in the feces.

Infrequent side effects include urinary retention or incontinence, headache, diarrhea, dizziness, cough, hiccups, confusion, warm or burning feeling, nausea or vomiting, and sweating. Infrequent or rare adverse reactions include chest pains, tachycardia, extrasystoles, hemolysis, thrombophlebitis, dyspnea, and tachypnea. Signs of overdosage are hypertension, convulsions, trembling, tachycardia, and increased deep tendon reflexes.

TABLE 18-3 Doxapram: dosage and administration

Indication	Adults	Children
postanesthesia respiratory depression	Administer IV 0.5-1 mg/kg body weight; do not exceed 1.5 mg/kg as single dose. If needed, dose may be repeated every 5 minutes up to maximum total dose of 2 mg/kg body weight.	Not recommended in children less than 12 yr old.
acute respiratory insufficiency in chronic obstructive pulmonary disease (COPD)	IV infusion, administer 1-2 mg/min; if necessary, administration rate may be increased to 3 mg/min. Maximum time for infusion with no additional infusions recommended is 2 hours.	

Administration of doxapram with monoamine oxidase (MAO) inhibitors or vasopressors may result in an increase in blood pressure or a hypertensive crisis. Monitor the vital signs closely.

Dosage and administration. (Table 18-3).

▪ Nursing Management

Doxapram Therapy

Assessment. The client's assessment should include a determination of other conditions for which the doxapram may be contraindicated, such as head trauma or seizure disorders (because of the risk of drug-induced seizures) and cardiovascular disorders (because of the drug's vasopressor effects). Doxapram is also contraindicated if the client is experiencing incompetence of ventilatory mechanism as a result of airway obstruction, pneumothorax, or flail chest and other respiratory diseases because the condition may be worsened. Cautious use is recommended with cardiac dysrhythmias because of the risk of hypoxia and aggravation of the dysrhythmic disorder, increased intracranial pressure or cerebral edema, pheochromocytoma, or hyperthyroidism because of the drug's vasopressor effects.

The nurse should obtain a baseline pulse, blood pressure, and deep tendon reflexes and then monitor those indicators frequently to avoid overdosage; and the rate of the infusion should be adjusted on the basis of these assessments. Arterial blood gases should be analyzed before initiation of therapy as a baseline and every 30 minutes during the 2-hour period of infusion to avoid the possibility of respiratory acidosis when doxapram is administered to clients with chronic obstructive pulmonary disease.

Nursing diagnosis. When doxapram is administered, the client is at risk for the following nursing diagnoses: ineffective breathing pattern related to anesthesia-induced respiratory depression (for which the doxapram is ordered); risk for aspiration; risk for injury related to the drug's vasopressor effects; and the potential complication of drug-induced seizures.

Implementation

Monitoring. Doxapram hydrochloride has a narrow margin of safety. The nurse should observe for early signs of toxicity, such as increased blood pressure and pulse rate, dysrhythmias, dyspnea, and increased skeletal response with increased deep tendon reflexes and spasticity. Because narcosis may recur, close monitoring of the client is necessary until full alertness has been maintained for 1 hour.

Intervention. Before administering the drug to clients with respiratory depression, a patent airway should be established and an adequate oxygen supply ensured in an attempt to prevent aspiration. Because intravenous administration tends to cause hemolysis, only diluted solutions should be administered at a slow rate of infusion. To decrease local tissue reaction and thrombophlebitis, various injection sites should be used to avoid extravasation. Doxapram is a *temporary* measure to correct acute respiratory insufficiency. Mechanical assistance with ventilation is safer, more reliable, and effective for long-term (more than 2 hours) therapy.

Evaluation. The expected outcomes will be that the client's respirations are within normal limits compared with baseline and the return of the cough and gag reflex. The arterial CO_2 of the client with chronic obstructive pulmonary disease will be within normal limits as compared with baseline.

▲ methylphenidate hydrochloride

[meth ill fen' i date] (Ritalin)

The mechanism of central action is unknown. Pharmacologic actions are similar to those of amphetamines, with CNS and respiratory stimulation; sympathomimetic activity is also reported. Sites of action are the cerebral cortex and subcortical areas.

Methylphenidate also appears to block the reuptake of dopamine into the dopaminergic neurons. In ADD with hyperactivity, methylphenidate decreases motor activity and increases the attention span. In narcolepsy it appears to stim-

TABLE 18-4 Methylphenidate: dosage and administration

Drug	Adults	Children
methylphenidate tablets (Ritalin)	5-20 mg 2 or 3 times daily with or after meals.	ADHD: Children up to 6 yr, dosage not established; 6 yr and older, 5 mg twice daily (after breakfast and lunch), increase if needed by 5 to 10 mg weekly up to maximum of 60 mg/day. If no improvement after dosage increases over 30 days, stop medication.
methylphenidate extended-release (Ritalin-SR)	20 mg 1 to 3 times daily every 8 hours.	Children up to 6 yr, dosage not established; 6 and older, see adult dosing recommendations.

ulate the cortex and subcortex, including the thalamic area, to increase alertness, lift the spirits, and increase motor activity. The drug is indicated for treatment of ADD and narcolepsy.

Methylphenidate is well absorbed. Peak serum concentration of tablets is 1.9 hours in children; the extended-release tablets reach peak serum concentration in 4.7 hours in children. This drug is metabolized in the liver and excreted by the kidneys.

The more frequently reported side effects of methylphenidate include anorexia, increased nervousness, and insomnia (usually more frequent in children). Less frequent side effects are headache, nausea, abdominal pain, drowsiness, and dizziness. The more frequent adverse reactions include hypertension and tachycardia. Less frequent are chest pain, trembling or uncontrolled movement of body, rash, fever of unknown origin, and increased bruising. Signs of overdosage may include confusion, delirium, dry mouth, euphoria, increased fever and sweating, severe headaches, hypertension, tremors, muscle twitching, irregular heartbeats, vomiting, convulsions, and possibly coma.

There is no specific treatment for an overdose of methylphenidate; treatment is symptomatic and supportive. Emesis or gastric lavage is implemented initially in treatment. The client should be in quiet surroundings and, if necessary, a short-acting barbiturate might be used in severe overdose situations. Monitor and maintain cardiovascular and respiratory functions carefully.

Dosage and administration. (Table 18-4).

■ Nursing Management

Methylphenidate Therapy Assessment

Assessment. Methylphenidate must be used cautiously in clients with epilepsy because the drug can lower the convulsive threshold. The drug is usually contraindicated for use in clients with glaucoma, motor tics other than Tourette's disorder, anxiety, and depression because it may worsen the condition. It also should be used with caution in clients with hypertension. Some clients with Tourette's syndrome may benefit with cautious use.

Use of methylphenidate in pregnant or lactating women is not recommended and is also contraindicated in clients with glaucoma, agitation, depression, or fatigue.

The client's concurrent medication regimen should be reviewed to identify any significant drug interactions. The following effects may occur when methylphenidate hydrochloride is given with the drugs listed below:

Drug	Possible effect and management
other CNS stimulants	May result in additive CNS stimulation effects causing increased nervousness, irritability, insomnia, dysrhythmias, and convulsions. Monitor apical pulse, mental status, and behaviors closely.
Monoamine oxidase (MAO) inhibitors	**May result in hypertensive crisis. Do not give drugs concurrently or within 14 days of administration of an MAO inhibitor. Avoid or a potentially serious drug interaction may occur.**
pimozide (Orap)	Should not be administered together. Withdraw client from methylphenidate before starting pimozide therapy. Concurrent use may mask reason for tic development because methylphenidate may also induce tics. Pimozide is indicated for the treatment of tics in clients with Tourette's syndrome.

A baseline assessment should include an evaluation of the child's growth and development status, complete blood counts, and blood pressure determination.

Nursing diagnosis. Once methylphenidate therapy has begun the client should be assessed for the following nursing diagnoses: sleep pattern disturbance; altered thought processes (confusion, depression); altered nutrition, less than required (children especially); risk for injury related to its CNS effects; and altered nutrition related to its anorexiant effects; and the potential complication of altered cardiac output (hypertension, tachycardia) related to the drug's cardiovascular effects.

Implementation

Monitoring. Clients should be monitored for weight loss from appetite suppression. Children, in particular, should be assessed on a regular basis for physical growth, since there may be suppression of normal weight gain.

Methylphenidate must be used cautiously in emotionally unstable persons and in those with a history of drug dependence or alcoholism. Drug abusers have used it as a substitute for amphetamines. The drug should be discontinued periodically to reassess therapeutic need as indicated by the return of symptoms. Long-term therapy should be accompanied by repeated medical examinations and tests for complete blood and platelet counts.

Intervention. Dosage should be calculated for each client based on the response to the drug. Extended-release forms of the drug should be used only after the initial therapy has established the appropriate dosage for the client. The nurse should administer the last daily dose of the non–extended-release form several hours before bedtime to avoid insomnia.

Sole dependence on methylphenidate for treatment of ADD is discouraged. Other therapies (psychologic, educational, social) should be used in conjunction with the drug therapy. When symptoms of ADD improve, interruption of drug therapy during times of low stress may be possible. The client may be given medication-free weekends, holidays, or vacations.

Education. The client should be instructed to take the medication on an empty stomach 30 to 45 minutes before eating. Extended-release forms should be swallowed whole, not crushed, broken, or chewed.

Do not increase the dose if the medication seems less effective. Regular visits with the client's prescriber are needed to monitor progress of the drug therapy. If the client takes large doses over an extended period, withdrawal must be gradual. Caution the clients that they should *not* stop taking the medication without checking with the prescriber, because of the risk of depression on withdrawal. Careful supervision is required during withdrawal for that reason. Tolerance and psychologic dependence have occurred with long-term use, and abnormal behavior and psychotic episodes have been observed.

Evaluation. The expected outcomes will be that the client demonstrates clinical improvement, that the child will have an increased attention span with a decreased restlessness and be able to sleep without difficulty and not evidence adverse effects.

pemoline [pem' oh leen] (Cylert)

The mechanism of central action is unknown. Pemoline may act by means of dopaminergic mechanisms. It is indicated for treatment of ADD with hyperactivity. Pemoline has good absorption and a half-life of 12 hours. Peak serum concentration occurs in 2 to 4 hours with peak effect reached in 3 to 4 weeks (*USP DI,* 1996). Pemoline is partially metabolized in the liver and is excreted by the kidneys.

More frequent side effects include anorexia, insomnia, and weight loss. Less frequent are dizziness, daytime sedation, irritability, depression, nausea, rash, and abdominal pain. A rare adverse reaction is jaundice.

Signs of overdosage include increased agitation, confusion, euphoria, hallucinations, severe headaches, hypertension, elevated temperatures, increased sweating, convulsions, tachycardia, dilated pupils, vomiting, and uncontrollable muscle movements of eyes.

No significant drug interactions have been reported. Dosage is as follows: children younger than 6 years, not established; 6 years or older, 37.5 mg orally each morning. Dosage may be increased by 18.75 mg daily on a weekly basis until therapeutic response is noted or a maximum of 112.5 mg/day is reached.

■ Nursing Management

Pemoline Therapy

See the discussion of the nursing management of methylphenidate therapy. Pemoline must be used cautiously in emotionally labile clients and in clients with a history of drug dependence or alcoholism. The drug should be discontinued periodically to reassess the need for its administration as indicated by a return of symptoms. The nurse should caution the client that the most common side effects are insomnia and anorexia. These are dose related and may be decreased by a dosage adjustment by the prescriber.

The client should be prepared for an initial weight loss with a return to normal weight curve in 3 to 6 months. Parents should be counseled that the beneficial effect of the medication may not be apparent for 3 to 4 weeks, but that it is important to the success of the regimen that the drug be administered as prescribed.

▲ caffeine [kaf feen']

Caffeine is a stimulant found in many beverages, foods, OTC drugs, and prescription drugs (Box 18-2). It is probably the most commonly used stimulant worldwide. It has been estimated that 7 million kilograms of caffeine are consumed annually in the United States. Many persons do not consider caffeine to be a drug, but this product can produce many therapeutic and adverse effects. For example, a large daily intake of caffeine-containing products may increase alertness but may also induce insomnia and heart arrhythmias in some persons, especially the elderly. A withdrawal syndrome of increased irritability, headache, and increased weakness has been reported when users of more than 600 mg/day of caffeine, or approximately 6 cups of coffee, decrease or eliminate this intake. Caffeine has also been implicated in many adverse health effects, such as cancer, fibrocystic breast disease, and birth defects. See Box 18-3 for caffeine-free OTC analgesic medications.

Short- and long-term effects. The mechanisms of action for caffeine were previously postulated to be an increase in cyclic adenosine monophosphate (cAMP) levels by blocking the enzyme phosphodiesterase. Recent studies though indicate caffeine's effects are primarily due to antagonism of the central adenosine receptors (adenosine is a neurotransmitter that is structurally similar to caffeine). Because caffeine has an effect on many body functions, both its short-term and possible long-term effects are of concern. Discussion of these effects, as they involve each body system, follows.

CNS. Although all levels of the CNS may be affected, regular doses of caffeine (100 to 150 mg) will stimulate the

BOX 18-2

Caffeine Content in Selected Products

	Caffeine per tablet/capsule
Analgesics*	
OTC medications	
Anacin	32 mg
Cope	32 mg
Excedrin Extra Strength	65 mg
Vanquish Caplets	33 mg
Prescription medications	
Cafergot	100 mg
Fiorinal	40 mg
Wigraine	100 mg
Menstrual medications*	
Midol Maximum	60 mg
Beverages	
Brewed coffee, automatic drip	60-180 mg/5 oz
Brewed coffee, percolator	40-170 mg/5 oz
Brewed tea, U.S.	20-90 mg/5 oz
Instant coffee	30-120 mg/5 oz
Instant tea	25-50 mg/5 oz
Brewed decaffeinated coffee	2-5 mg/5 oz
Chocolate milk	2-7 mg/8 oz
Soft drinks*	
Mountain Dew	54 mg/12 oz
Coca-Cola	45 mg/12 oz
Diet Coke	45 mg/12 oz
Pepsi-Cola	38 mg/12 oz
Diet Pepsi	36 mg/12 oz
Ginger Ale	0
7-Up	0
Sunkist Orange	0

Modified from *Nonprescription products: formulations & features '97-'98* (1997). Washington, DC: American Pharmaceutical Association.

BOX 18-3

Caffeine-free OTC Analgesic Medications

Aleve	Midol Menstrual
Aspergum	Motrin IB
Bayer Aspirin	Tempra 1, 2, or
Bromo-Seltzer	Tylenol Infants
Bufferin Extra Strength	Tylenol Regular Strength
Bufferin Arthritis Strength	Tylenol Extra Strength
Liquiprin for children	

Modified from *Nonprescription products: formulations & features '97-'98* (1997). Washington, DC: American Pharmaceutical Association.

cortex to produce increased alertness and decreased motor reaction time to both visual and auditory events. Drowsiness and fatigue generally disappear. Larger doses may affect the medullary, vagus, vasomotor, and respiratory centers, resulting in slowing of the heart rate, vasoconstriction, and increased respiratory rate. Studies attribute such effects to competitive blockade of adenosine receptors. Thus caffeine is still under investigation for the treatment of neonatal apnea, generally as an adjunct to nondrug measures and as an alternative to theophylline.

Analgesic adjunct, vascular effect. Caffeine constricts cerebral blood vessels, resulting in decreased cerebral blood flow and oxygen tension in the brain. Thus caffeine is used in analgesic products and in combination with ergotamine to enhance pain relief and, perhaps, to hasten the onset of action. When caffeine is given with ergotamine, the enhanced effect is believed to be a result of better absorption of the ergotamine in the presence of caffeine.

Respiratory stimulant. Although the mechanism of action is not clearly defined, caffeine appears to stimulate the medullary respiratory center. Thus it may be useful for the treatment of apnea in preterm infants and for Cheyne-Stokes respiration in adults.

Cardiovascular. Caffeine stimulates the myocardium, increasing both the heart rate and the cardiac output. This effect is antagonistic to that produced on the vagus center; consequently, a slight slowing of the heart may be observed in some individuals and an increased rate in others. The latter effect usually predominates after large doses. Overstimulation may cause tachycardia and cardiac irregularities.

Depending on the dose, caffeine may cause an increase in systemic vascular resistance. This can cause an increase in blood pressure. This effect may be secondary to stimulation of the sympathetic nervous systems and by blocking adenosine-induced, vasodilation.

Skeletal muscles. Caffeine affects voluntary skeletal muscles to increase the contractual force and decrease muscle fatigue.

Gastrointestinal. Caffeine increases secretion of pepsin and hydrochloric acid from the parietal cells. This is why coffee is restricted in clients who have a gastric or duodenal ulcer.

Renal. Caffeine produces a mild diuretic effect by increasing renal blood flow and glomerular filtration rate and by decreasing the reabsorption of sodium and water in the proximal tubules.

Additional effects. Caffeine also increases metabolic activity, inhibits uterine contractions, transiently increases glucose levels by stimulating glycolysis, and increases catecholamine levels in plasma and urine.

Indications and pharmacokinetics. Caffeine is used in the treatment of fatigue or drowsiness and as an adjunct to analgesics to enhance relief of pain. Its absorption is good, and it is distributed to all body compartments; it will cross the blood-brain barrier and enter the CNS and readily through the placenta. Caffeine is metabolized in the liver.

! MANAGEMENT OF DRUG OVERDOSE

Caffeine

Institute symptomatic and supportive measures according to the individual client's requirement.

If treatment is started within 4 hours of overdose, induce emesis with ipecac syrup and/or gastric lavage followed by activated charcoal. A magnesium sulfate (Epsom salts) laxative should also be considered.

Maintain fluid and electrolyte balance, ventilation, and oxygenation.

For hemorrhagic gastritis, administer antacids and iced saline lavage; for seizures, IV diazepam, phenobarbital or phenytoin.

Pregnancy Safety

Category	Drug
B	diethylpropion, doxapram, pemoline
C	amphetamines, caffeine, fenfluramine
X	benzphetamine
Unclassified	mazindol, methylphenidate, phendimetrazine, phentermine

In adults caffeine is metabolized to theophylline and theobromine, whereas in the neonate only a small portion is metabolized to theophylline. Caffeine's half-life is 3 to 7 hours in adults and 65 to 130 hours in neonates. Peak plasma level is achieved within 50 to 75 minutes, with therapeutic plasma levels at 5 to 25 μg/ml. In adults, caffeine is excreted by the kidneys, with only 1% to 2% excreted unchanged; in neonates it is excreted by the kidneys, with approximately 85% excreted unchanged.

Side effects/adverse reactions. More frequent side effects include increased nervousness or jittery feelings and irritation of GI tract resulting in nausea. More frequent adverse reactions in neonates include abdominal swelling or distension, vomiting, body tremors, tachycardia, jitters, or nervousness.

Signs of overdose are increased temperature, headache, increased irritability and sensitivity to pain or touch, increased urination, confusion, dehydration, abdominal pain, agitation, muscle twitching, nausea and vomiting, tinnitus, insomnia, and convulsions. See the box above for Management of Caffeine Overdose.

The adult dose is 100 to 200 mg orally, repeated in 3 to 4 hours if necessary to a maximum of 1000 mg daily. Extended-release dosage form (200 to 250 mg) has the same recommendations as the tablets. Caffeine is not recommended for use in children up to 12 years old (*USP DI,* 1996).

▪ Nursing Management

Caffeine Assessment

Assessment. Assessment of caffeine intake should be a routine part of the nursing drug history. This includes caffeine intake from foods and beverages as well as from medications.

Caffeine may exacerbate gastric ulceration in peptic ulcer disease and so should be used cautiously in clients with a history of peptic ulcers. Because of its suspected potential for causing dysrhythmias, it is recommended that clients with symptomatic cardiac dysrhythmias or palpitations and clients in the recovery phase of acute myocardial infarctions avoid using caffeine.

The FDA has warned women to avoid or to decrease caffeine consumption during pregnancy. Studies in humans have shown that heavy caffeine use by pregnant women may increase the risk of spontaneous abortion and intrauterine growth retardation (*USP DI,* 1996). Nurses in various settings should instruct pregnant and childbearing-age women to avoid drugs and sodas containing caffeine. Women who continue to drink coffee during their pregnancy should be encouraged to drink decaffeinated or instant coffee and to limit their coffee intake to 2 to 3 cups a day. Those who drink tea should decrease the brewing time or select a decaffeinated brand or herb tea. The best solution would be to substitute fruit and vegetable juices or water for beverages that contain caffeine.

The client's concurrent medications should be reviewed to identify significant drug interactions that might occur with caffeine ingestion. The following effects may occur when caffeine is taken with the drugs listed below:

Drug	Possible effect and management
other CNS-stimulating drugs, other caffeine-containing medications or drinks	May result in increased CNS stimulation and undesirable side effects, such as increased nervousness, irritability, insomnia, dysrhythmias, and seizures. Monitor client's apical pulse and behaviors closely.
monoamine oxidase (MAO) inhibitors	**Concurrent use with caffeine may result in severe hypertension or dangerous dysrhythmias. Small amount of caffeine may induce increased heart rate. Avoid or a potentially serious drug interaction may occur.**

A baseline assessment of the infant's cardiovascular and respiratory status should be accomplished before caffeine therapy is initiated.

Nursing diagnosis. The client taking caffeine may be at risk for the following nursing diagnoses: sleep pattern disturbance; altered thought processes (confusion, irritability);

altered comfort (GI distress, headache); and ineffective management of therapeutic regimen (if the client is on caffeine restrictions).

Implementation

Monitoring. When caffeine is administered for neonatal apnea, monitor serum caffeine levels 24 hours after loading dose and then 1 to 2 times a week, or every 2 weeks after the infant is stabilized, to ensure therapeutic levels.

Education. A client who is or may become pregnant should be advised to avoid or limit her consumption of caffeine-containing foods (e.g., coffee, tea, cola drinks, cocoa, and milk chocolate) and drugs (e.g., OTC stimulants, analgesic combinations, and cold preparations).

Caffeine passes into breast milk and may accumulate in nursing infants. Research suggests that when nursing mothers consume large amounts of caffeine, their babies may appear jittery and have trouble sleeping. Breastfeeding mothers should be advised to limit their intake of caffeine-containing beverages to 1 to 2 a day.

When taken close to bedtime, caffeine-containing medications and beverages may interfere with sleep. Caffeine is not intended to replace sleep and should not be used for that purpose. Clients with a hypersensitivity to caffeine should be alerted to its combination with analgesics (acetaminophen, aspirin, and phenacetin) for the treatment of headache. Because the adverse CNS effects for the drug are increased in children, these same combination preparations should not be given to children.

The question is sometimes raised whether or not caffeine causes physical and psychologic dependence. Many persons note that if they do not have their usual cup or two of coffee in the morning, they feel irritable and nervous and develop a headache. This probably indicates psychologic and physical dependence. Such clients should be instructed to decrease their caffeine intake by gradually reducing the number of servings of coffee, cola, and tea or by mixing the amounts with decaffeinated preparations and gradually decreasing the proportion of the caffeinated form.

Evaluation. The expected outcome for the infant receiving caffeine for sleep apnea is that the respiratory status will be within the normal limits related to the baseline. If the client is taking caffeine for other reasons, the client will experience a restful sleeping pattern and not evidence any adverse effects of caffeine.

SUMMARY

The CNS stimulants have limited use in practice today. Although used in the past for the treatment of obesity, their narrow therapeutic index and the rapid development of tolerance before significant weight reduction occurs have discouraged this use. Their prime indications are for attention deficit disorder and narcolepsy. When used for their anorexiant effect, they are an adjunct to a regimen of diet and exercise. Because stimulation of the CNS occurs, clients may experience sleep pattern disturbance, altered thought processes, sexual dysfunction, and altered comfort related to side effects such as dry mouth, headache, rash, and gastrointestinal or urinary effects. Caffeine, although not often thought of as a drug, is also a CNS stimulant, and the nurse should take an active role in educating clients on the effects of its ingestion.

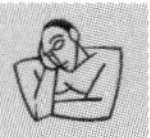

Critical Thinking

1. Herbert Poulin, a client with insulin-dependent diabetes, has been prescribed amphetamine sulfate for short-term treatment of exogenous obesity. He asks why he has to be on a total weight reduction program in addition to anorexiant therapy. What would you tell him? What would be included in such a program? Will the amphetamine affect his management of his diabetic regimen? What other information should be provided for this client?
2. The instructor of your health education class has given you the topic of caffeine habituation to present to the student group. What would you consider to be the most relevant information for your college-aged group? How would you present this topic?

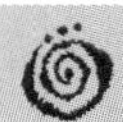

Collaborative Learning Activities

1. Two students will role play a nurse-client interaction in which the client has just indicated to the nurse, "I'm glad the doctor gave me a prescription for that appetite suppressant because now I don't have to worry about what I eat!"
2. List dietary sources of caffeine on the board. Without looking in the text, students should rank the preparations from the highest to the lowest caffeine content. Then add the mg caffeine content to the preparations listed on the board. Have the students calculate their caffeine intake for the last 24 hours.

BIBLIOGRAPHY

AHFS Supplement A (1996). Dexfenfluramine hydrochloride, *AHFS drug information '96*. Bethesda, MD: American Society of Hospital Pharmacists.

American Hospital Formulary Service (1996). *AHFS drug information '96*. Bethesda, MD: American Society of Hospital Pharmacists.

Anderson KN, et al. (Eds.) (1994). *Mosby's medical, nursing, & allied health dictionary* (4th ed.). St Louis: Mosby.

Bolinger AM, et al. (1992). General pediatric therapy. In Koda-Kimble MA & Young LY (Eds.). *Applied therapeutics: The clinical uses of drugs* (5th ed.).Vancouver: Applied Therapeutics.

Bray GA (1993). Use and abuse of appetite-suppressant drugs in the treatment of obesity, *Annual Intern Med 119*(7)707-12.

Covington TR (Ed.) (1996). *Handbook of nonprescription drugs* (11th ed.). Washington, DC: American Pharmaceutical Association.

Klein RG & Mannuzza S (1988). Hyperactive boys almost grown up: Methylphenidate effects on ultimate height, *Arch Gen Psychiatry 45*(12):1131-4.

Leung AKC, et al. (1994). Attention-deficit hyperactivity disorder: Getting control of impulse behavior, *Post grad Med 95*(2):153-60.

Newcomb P (1991). Tricyclic antidepressants and children, *Amer J Primary Health Care 16*(5):26.

Olin BR (Ed.) (1996). *Facts and comparisons*. St. Louis: Facts and Comparisons.

Saklad JJ & Curtis JL (1995). Psychiatric disorders in children, adolescents, and people with developmental disabilities. In Young LY & Koda-Kimble MA (Eds.). *Applied therapeutics: The clinical uses of drugs* (6th ed.). Vancouver: Applied Therapeutics.

Theesen KA & Stimmel GL (1993). Psychiatric disorders. In DiPiro JT, et al. *Pharmacotherapy* (2nd ed.) Norwalk, CT: Appleton & Lange.

United States Pharmacopeial Convention (1996). *USP DI: Drug information for the health care professional* (16th ed.). Rockville, MD: The Convention.

Chapter 19
Psychotherapeutic Drugs

Chapter Focus

Providing nursing care for clients receiving psychotherapeutic agents can be challenging. Nursing responsibilities include not only planning, implementing, and evaluating drug therapy, but doing so via a meaningful therapeutic relationship with the client. Whether the setting is an acute psychiatric facility, a nursing home, or a community environment, the nurse's knowledge base of psychotherapeutic drugs provides for direct care, as well as for teaching and counseling of the client and caregivers for safe and accurate self-administration of these agents. The following objectives and key terms are important for a good understanding of this chapter.

Key Terms

affective disorder (p. 378)
endogenous depression (p. 379)
exogenous depression (p. 379)
mania (p. 388)
tardive dyskinesia (TD) (p. 373)
tranquilizer (p. 364)

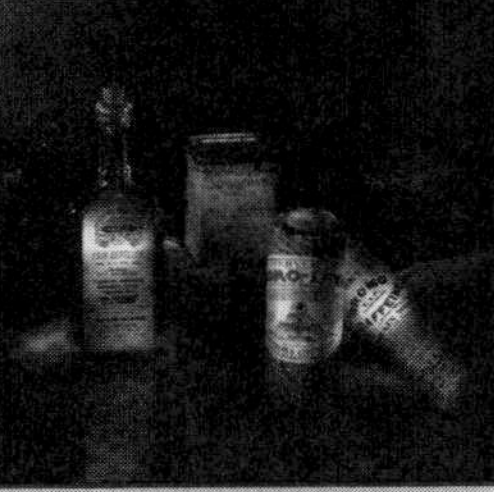

Key Drugs [▲]

chlorpromazine
haloperidol
imipramine
risperidone

Objectives

1. Discuss the use of drug therapy in psychiatry.
2. Identify the common psychotropic drugs.
3. Differentiate between phenothiazine derivatives, tricyclics, monoamine oxidase (MAO) inhibitors, and lithium.
4. Discuss nursing management of the common side effects/adverse reactions of psychotherapeutic agents.
5. Identify common tyramine-containing substances and their interactions with MAO inhibitor drugs.
6. Implement an appropriate plan of care for clients who require the administration of psychotherapeutic agents.

Medications used to treat psychoses and affective disorders, especially schizophrenia (antipsychotic agents), depression (antidepressants), and mania (lithium and others) are reviewed in this chapter. Refer to Chapter 13 for a review of the physiology and functions of the various components of the central nervous system (CNS). It is necessary to review the CNS functional systems (i.e., reticular activating system [Figure 19-1], limbic and extrapyramidal systems, plus acetylcholine and catecholamines) to enhance understanding of this chapter.

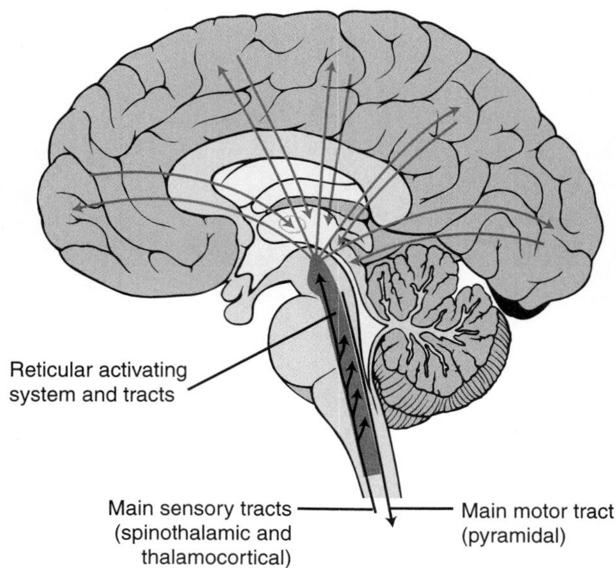

Figure 19-1 Reticular activating system.

CENTRAL NERVOUS SYSTEM AND EMOTIONS

A holistic view of human beings and their experience no longer allows the health care practitioner to separate the functions of the mind from the body. The CNS is responsible for consciousness, behavior, memory, recognition, learning, and the more highly developed attributes such as imagination, abstract reasoning, and creative thought. In addition, it serves to coordinate such vital regulatory functions as blood pressure, heart rate, respiration, salivary and gastric secretions, muscular activity, and body temperature.

The interrelationships among the various circuits in the brain produce patterns of behavior that can be modified by external situations or by internal autonomic adjustments. This allows the individual to adapt to changes in both the external and the internal environments.

Autonomic Regulation

The functions of the sympathetic and parasympathetic visceral nervous systems are discussed in Chapter 20. These systems play an important role in the production of behavior. An understanding of these mechanisms is the basis for learning the actions and side effects of the drugs that affect mood and behavior.

Biochemical Mechanisms

The functions of the CNS depend on the actions of certain neurohormonal agents located in the brain and peripheral tissues. These neurohormones are stored in inactive forms and at the right moment, nerve impulses release their free forms to stimulate transmission of appropriate reactions. The neurotransmitter exerts its action by interacting with the receptor (a specialized protein), located on the outermost part of the postsynaptic cell, which produces both electric and biochemical changes within the postsynaptic cell.

Acetylcholine, norepinephrine, and serotonin have been found in the CNS. Tyrosine and dopamine are normal constituents of the brain and known precursors of norepinephrine synthesis. High concentrations of norepinephrine are found in the hypothalamus, medulla, limbic system, and cranial nerve nuclei. Dopamine is found in high concentrations in the striatum and caudate nucleus. It is believed that both norepinephrine and dopamine function as transmitters. They have widespread inhibitory and excitatory effects on a wide variety of centrally mediated functions, such as sleep and arousal, affect, and memory. Thus some central synapses are adrenergic.

Areas rich in serotonin include the hypothalamus, pineal gland, midbrain, and spinal cord. Alteration of serotonin levels in the nervous system is associated with changes in behavior. Many drugs mimic or block the action of serotonin on peripheral tissues and produce changes in mood and behavior, which suggests that they interfere with the action of serotonin and norepinephrine in the brain.

The relationship of dopamine to the major psychoses has received much attention. There are a variety of dopamine receptors in the brain especially the basal ganglia and limbic areas, but D_1 and D_2 are the primary ones involved with the antipsychotic agents. While both receptors are involved with movement disorders in the basal ganglia, blockade of the D_2 receptors (causing supersensitivity) in animals has resulted in tardive dyskinesia. Thus further research in this area may result in the development of more specific treatment agents that have less adverse effects (Ereshefsky & Richards, 1992). Antipsychotic agents with a low affinity for D_2 receptors, such as clozapine, are less apt to cause extrapyramidal side/adverse effect (Hardman & Limbird, 1996).

ROLE OF DRUG THERAPY IN PSYCHIATRY

Drugs play an important role in contemporary approaches of psychiatric care. Drug therapy reduces or alleviates symptoms and allows the client an opportunity to participate more easily in other forms of treatment. Drugs temporarily modify behavior, whereas other therapies, such as psychotherapy, can shape behavior and produce a permanent change. However, any enduring effects on behavior are more likely to result from the individual's concurrent interaction with the environment. Because incoming information must be translated into biochemical changes before it can affect nervous system function, environmental transactions, as with drugs, may affect similar pathways before influencing behavior. The effects of drugs can be additive, potentiating, or antagonistic, depending on their nature and direction. The milieu may potentiate the effectiveness of the drug or may detract from it.

Generally prescribers select psychotherapeutic agents on the basis of the diagnostic category—schizophrenia, manic-depressive syndrome, or psychoneurosis. The prescriber will try to match a particular drug's therapeutic advantages to the client's symptoms, assuming the person's diagnosis warrants the use of an antipsychotic agent. Since their introduction the antipsychotic and other psychotropic agents have been widely prescribed and, in many instances in the elderly, inappropriately used. Inappropriate prescriptions expose the older person to an increased risk of adverse or serious drug reaction that is often detrimental to the client's cognitive and functional health status. Such studies have resulted in regulations governing Medicare and Medicaid recipients in long-term care facilities.

In 1992 the OBRA Long Term Care Requirements Act for long-term care facilities was implemented. Although this act applies to all the drugs a client receives, the Health Care Financing Administration's (HCFA) surveyors initially focused their attention on the major CNS drug categories: antipsychotics, antianxiety, sedatives, hypnotics, and benzodiazepines. The purpose of this law was to review the indication, dosage (including duplicate-type drug orders), duration, and monitoring parameters, to determine if the drugs were given in the presence of side/adverse effects. The surveyors may cite a facility for deficiencies in these areas (Carley, 1992).

For a nursing home resident to be prescribed antipsychotic drugs, an appropriate specific condition must be documented, such as schizophrenia, schizo-affective disorder, delusional disorder, psychotic mood disorder, acute psychotic episode, brief reactive psychosis, schizophreniform disorder, atypical psychosis, Tourette's disorder, or Huntington's disease, all of which are organic mental syndromes that have associated psychotic or agitation features. The latter features are defined as (1) specific behaviors that can be quantitatively and objectively documented (biting, kicking, scratching, etc.) and that cause the client to present a danger to himself or others and actually interfere with the nursing staff's ability to provide care to the client; or (2) the presence of psychotic symptoms (delusions, hallucinations, or paranoid behavior) that are not a result of a previously mentioned disorder but cause the resident extreme distress (Box 19-1). To treat the symptoms of hiccups, nausea, vomiting, or pruritus, short-term therapy of 1 week is permissible.

The purpose of the regulations was to eliminate or reduce the inappropriate prescribing of such potent medications for behaviors that may be controlled by nonpharmacologic approaches. For example, insomnia, pacing, wandering, restlessness, crying spells or screaming episodes, deficient memory, uncooperativeness, nervousness, or depression would not alone warrant the use of an antipsychotic agent. Such symptoms would have to be associated with an appropriate diagnosis as mentioned previously to be indicated.

BOX 19-1

Positive and Negative Symptoms in Schizophrenia

Clients with schizophrenia present with a wide variety of symptoms that range from the most responsive (or positive) to less responsive (or negative) to the antipsychotic agents. Most antipsychotic agents produce an effect on the following positive symptoms: agitation, anxiety, hallucinations, poor hygiene and dress, hyperactivity, delusions, paranoia, and hostility, while the negative symptoms of flat affect, social inadequacy, diminished speech patterns, judgment, insight, and others are usually less responsive to drug therapy.

The target symptoms are used as monitoring parameters to evaluate the individual's response to the medication. The atypical antipsychotic drugs such as clozapine and risperidone appear to be more effective than other neuroleptic agents against negative symptoms (Marken & Stanislav, 1995).

Drug Selection

When the prescriber establishes the need for drug therapy, it must be decided what agent or combination of agents is best suited for the client's total health needs. This requires an intimate knowledge of the behavioral actions, pharmacologic effects, and potential adverse reactions of the agents used, as well as an awareness of the many individual and environmental factors present (see the Nursing Research box on p. 362 and the Cultural Aspects box on p. 363).

The additional effects or side effects profile of a drug is a useful tool in helping the prescriber select an appropriate antipsychotic agent (Table 19-1). If a drug with a strong sedation property is desired, chlorpromazine (Thorazine) or thioridazine (Mellaril) might be prescribed. If extrapyramidal side effects are troublesome, thioridazine, with the greatest anticholinergic effect, has less potential for inducing extrapyramidal side effects.

If anticholinergic side effects such as dry mouth, blurred vision, constipation, and urinary retention continue and are disturbing to the client, the prescriber could select an agent with less potential for inducing such effects, such as fluphenazine (Prolixin, Permitil), thiothixene (Navane), or haloperidol (Haldol). Therefore, continuous nursing and medical evaluations based on observation of the client for the drug's effects, therapeutic and adverse, are necessary.

Nurses play an important role in the evaluation and assessment of a client's response to drug therapy. They should

Text continued on p. 364

Nursing Research

Gender differences in pharmacokinetics and pharmacodynamics of psychotropic medication

There are theoretical reasons to suggest gender-related drug effects, but there are limited clinical data to support such hypotheses for different psychopharmacologic agents. The issue discussed in the Yonkers et al (1992) article is particularly important because Phase I studies, which determine therapeutic doses, have been conducted on male subjects, but women seek treatment and receive psychotropic medication more frequently than men. The authors concluded that there are potential sex differences in pharmacokinetics related to absorption and bioavailability, distribution, metabolism, and menstrual cycle effects, which require empirical studies of specific drugs. The reader may consult Yonkers' article for the specific citations of the research reviewed.

The literature analyzing the pharmacokinetics, pharmacodynamics, and side effects of psychotropic drugs is most substantial for antipsychotic drugs. Women have been found to have higher blood levels for fluphenazine and fluspipirilene than men of similar weight and age with comparable dosing. Women have had greater improvement than men after treatment with pimozide and chlorpromazine. It has been hypothesized that this greater efficacy in young women is due to the presumed antidopaminergic effect of estrogen. This same protective effect for premenopausal women may hold true for antipsychotic-induced side effects, in that there is a higher prevalence of severe dyskinesias in young men and the severity of tardive dyskinesia is far greater in women over 67. Although estrogen has not been directly tested as an antipsychotic agent in humans, age needs to be considered when looking at gender differences because of the critical interactions between gender and age.

The preponderance of evidence suggests that benzodiazepines that are conjugatively metabolized have slower elimination rates in women than in men. Oral contraceptives have been found to decrease the clearance of benzodiazepines, so that cognitive and psychomotor tasks were more impaired during the week off hormones in women taking oral contraceptives because benzodiazepines peaked more quickly. This suggests that a change in absorption rates for the week off hormones leads to a dose of benzodiazepines that suddenly becomes intoxicating. More studies are needed to test the physiologic response throughout the menstrual cycle.

Given the literature citing the higher prevalance of depressive disorders in women, the paucity of studies addressing sex-specific medication effects is surprising. In evaluating the efficacy of tricyclic antidepressants (TCAs) and MAOIs by gender in three types of atypical depression, it was found that depressed women with panic attacks had a more favorable response to MAOIs than to TCAs, whereas men who were more depressed and had panic attacks responded more favorably to TCAs. When the studies were controlled for the use of oral contraceptives, no significant gender differences were found in plasma levels of amitriptyline and nortriptyline.

Lithium carbonate has been the subject of several case reports suggesting menstrual cycle effects on serum levels. Because some women do show a phasic difference, it may be helpful to correlate lithium levels to symptoms throughout the menstrual cycle. Adverse reactions to lithium may occur with more frequency in women, particularly lithium-induced hypothyrodism.

In the Yonkers et al (1992) article, despite the limitations of the studies reviewed, the authors conclude that there is evidence suggesting gender-related variations. These findings include: (1) the potential for women to have higher plasma levels of psychotropic drugs (especially when given with oral contraceptives) and (2) greater efficacy of antipsychotic agents and a greater likelihood of adverse reactions, such as hypothyroidism and, in older women, tardive dyskinesia. These suggested sex-related differences clearly require further investigation.

Critical thinking questions

- In what ways could this research influence your nursing practice in the administration of psychotropic medications?
- What instructions would you provide to Nora Parton, a 27-year-old female client who has been prescribed benzodiazepines while she is on oral contraceptives?

From Yonkers KA et al (1992).

Cultural Aspects — Culture as a Variable in Drug Therapy

To deal with cultural issues in psychiatric care, attempts are usually made to promote recognition and appreciation of cultural influences in the hope that a more sensitive and therapeutic approach might result. Keltner and Folks (1992) believe that while relatively little research on the topic of culture and psychopharmacology exists, the work that has been published is of significance to nurses administering psychotropic agents.

Do individuals from varying cultural, ethnic, and racial backgrounds respond to psychotropic drugs differently?

Asians reportedly require lower doses than do Caucasians for drugs such as neuroleptics, tricyclic antidepressants (TCAs), and lithium. There are fewer studies of Hispanics and African-Americans. It has been reported that Hispanic clients require lower doses of antidepressant medication than non-Hispanics and that Afro-Americans generally improve more rapidly with the use of neuroleptics, TCAs, and anxiolytics than their white counterparts. Lithium has a significantly longer half-life in African-Americans than in Caucasians or Asians.

How can these differences in dosage of psychotropics be explained?

Cultural, ethnic, and racial differences in drug response and metabolism have been appreciated by pharmacologists for some time. Differences in pharmacokinetics may be genetic or caused by environmental influences. Only about 9% of African-Americans and Caucasians are considered to be slow metabolizers as compared to as many as 32% of Asians. Individuals who metabolize drugs more slowly will experience a greater drug effect. There is also evidence of variability in protein binding based on ethnicity. Habits such as smoking and drinking alcohol are known to speed drug metabolism, whereas a low-protein, high-carbohydrate diet is known to slow metabolism. The fact that Caucasians and African-Americans drink significantly more alcohol than Asians and eat differently may provide an environmental explanation for the greater drug response by Asians.

Do individuals of various cultural backgrounds experience side effects differently?

Asians are more sensitive to neuroleptics than Caucasians are. In one study, Asian clients began experiencing extrapyramidal effects (EPS) at dosages that were about half of those for Caucasians. At equivalent doses, 95% of Asians experienced EPS whereas only 67% of Caucasians and African-Americans experienced those side effects (Lin, 1986). Hispanic clients taking TCAs are reported to experience side effects at half the dosages observed in white non-Hispanics (Marcos & Cancro, 1982). African-Americans apparently are far more susceptible to TCA delirium than are Caucasians. However, one study determined that there was no observed difference in the frequency and severity of tardive dyskinesia among Caucasian, African-American, and Hispanic clients (Sramek et al, 1991).

Undoubtedly, individuals from all cultural, ethnic, and racial backgrounds are helped by psychotropic drugs. However, there is growing evidence that differences influence the course and outcome of psychopharmacologic therapy.

How would this research influence your nursing practice in administering psychotropic agents?

From Keltner NL & Folks DG (1992).

TABLE 19-1 Selected antipsychotic agents, potency, and major side effects

Chemical, generic name (trade name)	Equivalent* PO dose (mg)	Frequency of selected effects & side effects†				
		Antiemetic	Sedation	Hypotension‡	Anticholinergic	EPS§
Phenothiazines						
aliphatic						
chlorpromazine (Thorazine)	100	3	3	3	2	2
piperidine						
thioridazine (Mellaril)	100	1	3	3	3	1
mesoridazine (Serentil)	50	1	3	3	3	1
piperazine						
fluphenazine (Permitil)	2	1	1	1	1	3
perphenazine (Trilafon)	10	3	1	1	1	3
prochlorperazine (Compazine)	15	3	2	1	1	3
trifluoperazine (Stelazine)	5	3	1	1	1	3

From Olin (1996); *USP DI*, (1996).
*Equivalent dosages are from low potency (50 to 100 mg) to intermediate potency (10 to 49 mg) to high potency (1 to 9 mg).
†Grading: 1, low; 2, moderate; 3, high.
‡Orthostatic hypotension.
§*EPS*, extrapyramidal side effects include akathisia, dystonia, parkinsonism, and tardive dyskinesia.

Continued

TABLE 19-1 Selected antipsychotic agents, potency, and major side effects—cont'd

Chemical, generic name (trade name)	Equivalent* PO dose (mg)	Frequency of selected effects & side effects†				
		Antiemetic	Sedation	Hypotension‡	Anticholinergic	EPS§
Thioxanthenes						
thiothixene (Navane)	4	—	1	1	1	3
Other compounds						
butyrophenone						
haloperidol (Haldol)	2	2	1	1	1	3
dihydroindolone						
molindone (Moban)	10	—	1	1	1	3
dibenzoxapine						
loxapine (Loxitane)	15	—	2	2	1	3
atypical agents						
clozapine (Clozaril)	50	1	3	3	3	1
risperidone (Risperdal)	—	—	1	1	1	0/1

—Undocumented or unknown

be aware of the criteria the prescriber uses in selecting psychotherapeutic drugs and of the expected effects so they can observe and report on the client's progress. This progress is evaluated by monitoring the client's behavioral and affective responses to the medications; the client's knowledge of the drug therapy; the presence and extent of expected side effects and adverse reactions and their response to dosage adjustment and supportive nursing interventions; and the potential for, or existence of, drug or food interactions. Knowledge of the action of drugs also assists health care professionals in understanding the interpersonal responses that occur in the therapeutic relationship with the client.

ANTIPSYCHOTIC OR NEUROLEPTIC AGENTS

Historical Background

Between 1900 and 1950 the population of the United States doubled while the population in public mental hospitals quadrupled. During this time the average length of confinement was usually years, and the trend was definitely toward an increase in clients admitted to such institutions yearly. Also, client and employee injuries caused by combative or abusive clients led to the common use of physical restraints and client isolation.

Before the antipsychotic agents the treatment of mentally disturbed clients consisted of isolation (i.e., hidden in cellars or attics in their homes), or if they came to the attention of local authorities, they were transferred to jails or homes for the insane. Actual therapies used before the advent to the antipsychotic agents were water or ice pack therapies, strait-jackets or other physical restraints, shock therapy with insulin or electricity, lobotomy, and the use of a few drugs such as paraldehyde, chloral hydrate, and the barbiturates.

The first antipsychotic agent that is also the prototype phenothiazine was chlorpromazine (Thorazine). This was the first **tranquilizer** (a drug prescribed to calm an agitated or anxious individual) released in the early 1950s. However, the term *tranquilizer* had been used approximately 200 years ago by Dr. Benjamin Rush. Dr. Rush, an early pioneer in the mental health field and a signer of the Declaration of Independence, invented a restraining chair named the "tranquilizer chair" (Lyons & Petrucelli, 1978). This chair was modified by the addition of a pulley system, so that the extremely agitated client would be seated and restrained in the chair and the chair was raised off the ground and rocked back and forth until the person was quieted (Figure 19-2).

The student should be aware that neither the tranquilizer chair nor the tranquilizing (antipsychotic) agents cure mental illness. They have been and are used to control the symptoms associated with this disease state; the chair provided physical and eventually physiologic restraints, whereas the antipsychotic and tranquilizing agents constitute a chemical control of the symptoms.

The use of the antipsychotic drugs proved to be a revolutionary force in the psychiatric field. The duration of institutionalization decreased from years to months for many clients, and others live at home and are treated at community mental health centers. The reported incidence of injuries

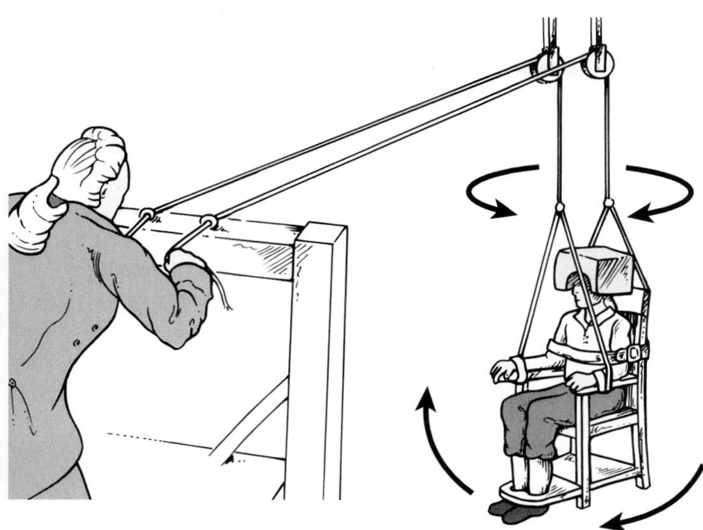

Figure 19-2 Tranquilizer or restraining chair used in the eighteenth century to "tranquilize" the agitated patient.

declined along with the closing of many large public mental health facilities.

This chapter will review the antipsychotic agents, antidepressant therapy, and antimanic medications.

ANTIPSYCHOTIC AGENTS

The discussion of antipsychotic medications will be divided into phenothiazines, thioxanthenes, and other compounds.

Phenothiazine Derivatives

The first phenothiazine, ▲ chlorpromazine (Thorazine), was widely accepted for the treatment of mental illness. Since then, many other drug products have been developed so that phenothiazines now comprise the largest group of psychotropic agents. Phenothiazines are divided chemically into the following three subgroups: (1) the aliphatic compounds (e.g., chlorpromazine), (2) the piperidine compounds (e.g., thioridazine), and (3) the piperazine compounds (e.g., fluphenazine).

Aliphatic phenothiazine derivatives include chlorpromazine (Thorazine and others), methotrimeprazine (Levoprome, Nozinan 🍁), promazine (Sparine), and triflupromazine (Vesprin).

Piperidine phenothiazine derivatives include mesoridazine (Serentil), and thioridazine (Mellaril, Apo-Thioridazine 🍁).

Piperazine phenothiazine derivatives consist of fluphenazine (Prolixin, Permitil), perphenazine (Trilafon, Apo-Perphenazine, prochlorperazine (Compazine, Stemetil 🍁), and trifluoperazine (Stelazine, Novo-Flurazine 🍁) (see Table 19-3 for phenothiazine dosing).

Classification. Antipsychotic medications have been classified as low-potency, intermediate-potency, and high-potency drugs. The basis for the classification is the quantity of medication necessary to produce an equivalent effect when compared with other agents in the same category. For example, 100 mg of chlorpromazine (Thorazine) is considered to be approximately equivalent to 50 mg of mesoridazine (Serentil) or 2 mg haloperidol (Haldol). Thus chlorpromazine is a low-potency agent, mesoridazine an intermediate-potency agent, and haloperidol is a high-potency drug (see Table 19-1 for antipsychotic equivalency dosages). The student is cautioned not to confuse potency with effectiveness; potency refers to the quantity of a drug necessary to produce an equivalent effect as compared with another drug in the same classification. Effectiveness measures the therapeutic response to various agents, and this may range from less effective, to equivalent in effectiveness, or to more effective, depending on the individual drugs being studied.

Although the exact mechanism of action for the antipsychotic effects is unknown, the major therapeutic effects and side/adverse effects are the result of dopamine blockade in specific areas of the CNS. Phenothiazines also produce an alpha-blocking effect (hypotension), inhibit or block dopamine at the chemoreceptor trigger zone (CTZ), and peripherally inhibit the vagus nerve in the gastrointestinal tract (antiemetic effect). They also produce an antianxiety effect by depression of the brainstem reticular system. Most phenothiazines and haloperidol increase prolactin release, which infrequently results in swelling of the breast and milk secretion. Methotrimeprazine (Levoprome) is a phenothiazine with primarily analgesic and sedative effects. It is not used as an antipsychotic drug in the United States.

Indications. Various phenothiazine derivatives are used in the treatment of psychosis, nausea and vomiting, pain, sedation, and as adjuncts to the treatment of tetanus, acute intermittent porphyria, and intractable hiccups.

Pharmacokinetics. Phenothiazines are well absorbed orally with an onset of action between ½ and 1 hour; IM onset of action is within 30 minutes with the exception of the long-acting parenteral forms. The onset of antipsychotic effect is achieved gradually, usually requiring several weeks, while peak therapeutic effect is between 6 weeks to 6 months. Duration of action for these products ranges from 6 to 24 hours or more, depending on dosage and frequency of drug administration. Phenothiazines are metabolized in the liver and excreted primarily by the kidneys. Table 19-2 lists side effects/adverse reactions.

Dosage of antipsychotic agents varies according to the individual, the reason for treatment, and the client's response to the medication. It is best to titrate from a low dose, increasing when necessary to produce a therapeutic response, which usually occurs within days to a couple of months. Continue at this dosage for 14 days and then gradually decrease dosage to the lowest amount that produces a therapeutic response.

When stopping antipsychotic therapy, gradually reduce the dosage over 2 or 3 weeks. When antipsychotic agents

TABLE 19-2 Antipsychotic medications: side effects/adverse reactions

Side effects*	Adverse reactions†
More frequent: sleepiness, dizziness, dry mouth, constipation, and nasal congestion reported with aliphatic and piperidine phenothiazines and thioxanthenes. Incidence is less with the piperazine phenothiazines, with the exception of perphenazine.	Visual changes, hypotensive episodes (more common with aliphatic and piperidine phenothiazines, thioxanthenes, and possibly, molindone)
thioxanthenes: skin sensitivity to the sun	Dystonia and/or parkinson-type effects including shuffle in walk, arm or leg stiffness, tremors, masklike facial expression, dysphagia, imbalance, muscle spasms or unusual twisting effects of face, neck, or back (more common with aliphatic and piperazine phenothiazines, thioxanthines, loxapine, molindone, resperidone, and haloperidol)
loxapine: most often seen are blurred vision, confusion, dizziness, dry mouth, and increase in body weight	Akathisia (abnormal restlessness and agitation), increased pacing, and insomnia (more often reported with haloperidol, loxapine, thioxanthene)
haloperidol: usually blurred vision, constipation, dry mouth, and increase in body weight	Tardive dyskinesia, a very serious adverse reacton; although rare, neuroleptic malignant syndrome (NMS) may occur
molindone: usually sedation, blurred vision, dry mouth, and constipation	Clozapine can cause agranulocytosis, hypotension, tachycardia, and seizures
clozapine: may cause sedation, dizziness, constipation, insomnia, headaches, tremor, and nausea	Hyperkinesia, agitation, aggressive behavior
risperidone: nausea, dizziness, sedation, insomnia, headache	

*If side effects continue, increase or disturb the client, inform the prescriber.
†If adverse reactions occur, contact the prescriber, since medical intervention may be necessary.

have been given to clients in high doses or for a long time and are suddenly discontinued, nausea, vomiting, dizziness, tremors, and dyskinesia have been reported. Table 19-3 describes dosage and administration.

Acetophenazine (Tindal), promazine (Sparine), and triflupromazine (Vesprin) are available on the market but are not commonly used today.

Thioxanthenes

chlorprothixene [klor proe thix' een] (Taractan)
flupenthixol [floo pent ' ole] (Fluanxol ♣, Fluanxol Depot ♣)
thiothixene [thye oh thix' een] (Navane)

Thioxanthenes resemble the piperazine phenothiazines in their antipsychotic effects, including the high incidence of extrapyramidal adverse effects (see Table 19-2). Their antipsychotic indication, side effects, precautions, and drug interactions are similar as those for the phenothiazines. Table 19-4 lists dosage and administration guidelines. See the general nursing management for antipsychotic drugs.

Other Antipsychotic Compounds

Butyrophenone Derivatives

▲ **haloperidol** [ha loe per' i dole] (Haldol)

The butyrophenones, while structurally different from the other antipsychotic agents, have similar properties in terms of antipsychotic efficacy. Haloperidol appears to have a selective CNS effect; it competitively blocks D_2 receptors in the mesolimbic system and also causes an increased turnover of brain dopamine to produce its antipsychotic effect. It has less effect on the norepinephrine and epinephrine receptors and is associated with a significant degree of extrapyramidal effects. The drug has both antiemetic and antipsychotic effects.

Haloperidol is used to treat psychotic disorders, severe behavioral problems in children and Tourette's syndrome, a rare central nervous system disorder that results in involuntary, rapid, and repetitive motor movements of muscle groups that are usually accompanied by involuntary vocalizations. This syndrome is more common in males, usually appearing before the age of 14, and may present initially as tics (facial grimaces and blinking). Other symptoms include vocal tics or noises, such as grunting, barking, shouting, sniffing, compulsive swearing (coprolalia), and movement disorders (involuntary, purposeless movements). The individual's intellectual functions are normal. The symptoms may peak and wane throughout the person's life. Although there is no cure for Tourette's syndrome, haloperidol (Haldol) and pimozide (Orap) have produced dramatic improvement in some clients.

For dosage and administration, see Table 19-4.

Very low doses of haloperidol have also been found to be useful for the treatment of severe agitation, combativeness, and psychosis in the demented patient. Generally, divided doses of 0.5 mg to 2 mg/day are sufficient for the elderly client.

TABLE 19-3 Phenothiazine indications and dosage*

Chemical classification generic (Trade Name)	Indication	Starting dose: Adults	Starting dose: Children
Phenothiazines			
aliphatic			
chlorpromazine (Thorazine)	antipsychotic	PO 10-25 mg 2-4 times times daily IM 25-50 mg, repeat in 1 hr if needed, then q3-12h prn	6 mo & older, PO 0.55 mg/kg q4-6h IM 0.55 mg/kg q 6-8 h
	antiemetic	PO 10-25 mg q4h IM 25-50 mg q3-4h Supp 50-100 mg rectally q6-8h	Same as above Supp 1 mg/kg q6-8h
	hiccups or porphyria	PO 25-50 mg 3-4 times daily IM hiccups, 25-50 mg 3-4 times daily Porphyria, 25 mg q6-8h until oral therapy can be started	—
	tetanus	IM 25-50 mg 3 or 4 times daily	IM 0.55 mg/kg q6-8h
piperidine			
thioridazine (Mellaril)	antipsychotic	PO 25-100 mg 3 times daily	PO 2-12 yr; 0.25-3 mg/kg 4 times daily
mesoridazine (Serentil)	antipsychotic	15-50 mg 2-3 times daily	No established dose for up to 12 yr old; 12 yr & older, see adult dosage
piperazine			
fluphenazine (Prolixin)	antipsychotic	PO 2.5-10 mg in divided doses 6-8h IM 1.25-2.5 mg q6-8h Decanoate: 12.5-25 mg, repeat q1-3wk	PO 0.25-0.75 mg 1-4 times daily IM not established Under 12 yr, not established; 12 or older, see adult dosing
perphenazine (Trilafon)	antipsychotic antiemetic	PO 4-16 mg 2-4 times daily PO 8-16 mg daily in divided doses IM 5-10 mg q 6 hr	PO/IM not established under 12; 12 or older, see adult dosing
prochlorperazine (Compazine)	antipsychotic	PO 5-10 mg 3 or 4 times daily IM 10-20 mg q 2-4 hr IV 2.5-10 mg slowly injected Supp 10 mg 3-4 times/day	PO 2-12 yr old, 2.5 mg 2-3 times/day. Over 12, see adult dosing IM 2-12 yr, 0.132 mg/kg
	antiemetic	PO 5-10 mg 3-4 times/day IM 5-10 mg q3-4h Supp 25 mg rectally twice daily	PO/supp is dosed according to weight; see current package insert
trifluoperazine (Stelazine)	antipsychotic	PO 2-5 mg twice daily IM 1-2 mg q4-6h	PO 6 yr & older, 1 mg 1-2 times/day IM 6 yr & older, 1 mg 1-2 times/day

*Doses are titrated as needed and tolerated by the individual.

TABLE 19-4 Thioxanthene and other compounds, indications and dosing*

Chemical classification generic (Trade Name)	Indication	Starting dose: Adults	Starting dose: Children
Thioxanthene			
thiothixene (Navane)	antipsychotic	PO 2 mg tid IM 4 mg 2-4 times/day	Oral dose is not established for up to 12 yr old; 12 yr and older, see adult dosage IM same as above
Other compounds			
butyrophenone			
haloperidol (Haldol)	antipsychotic	PO 0.5-5 mg 2-3 times/day IM 2-5 mg q2-4h initially, then q4-8h afterward	PO/IM not established
dihydroindolone			
molindone (Moban)	antipsychotic	PO 50-75 mg in 3 or 4 divided doses	Oral dose not established
dibenzoxapine			
loxapine (Loxitane)	antipsychotic	PO 10 mg bid	Oral dose not established
Atypical agents			
clozapine (Clozaril)	antipsychotic	PO 25 mg 1-2 times/day	Oral dose not established
risperidone (Risperdal)	antipsychotic	PO 1 mg twice/day	Oral dose not established

*Doses are titrated as needed and tolerated.

Dihydroindolone Derivative

molindone [moe lin' done] (Moban)

Molindone is an antipsychotic agent representing a new chemical class. In theory, molindone blocks dopamine receptors in the reticular activating and limbic systems, with activity similar to major tranquilizers such as phenothiazines. Similar to haloperidol, molindone causes little sedation and few anticholinergic and cardiovascular adverse effects but it reportedly has a high incidence of causing extrapyramidal symptoms.

Molindone is administered orally. In adults, the initial dose is 50 to 75 mg daily in divided doses. Dosages may increase to 100 mg daily in 3 or 4 days. Dosage must be individualized to a maximum daily dose of usually 225 mg/day. Dosage for the elderly client is lower than the adult dosage and is increased as necessary according to response or development of side effects. Molindone is not recommended for children younger than 12 years of age.

Dibenzoxapine Derivative

loxapine succinate [lox' a peen] (Loxitane, Loxapac ♣)

Loxapine, while structurally similar to the phenothiazines, is a member of a distinct chemical class of antipsychotic drugs, the dibenzoxapines. It causes a moderate degree of sedation and orthostatic hypotension, has few anticholinergic effects, and has a high incidence of causing extrapyramidal symptoms.

Loxapine adult oral dose (liquid or capsule) is 10 mg twice daily, increased slowly during the first 7 to 10 days as necessary. Maintenance dose is 15 to 25 mg orally 2 to 4 times daily. Maximum dosage is 250 mg/day. Dosage for the elderly is 3 to 5 mg twice daily initially. Dosage for children younger than 16 years old has not been established. Injectable loxapine is administered to adults at 12.5 to 50 mg IM every 4 to 6 hours as necessary, up to a maximum of 250 mg/day.

Nursing Management

Antipsychotic Agent Therapy

Assessment. Before starting antipsychotic drug therapy, the client should have a complete history and physical assessment completed. Of particular importance is a neurologic examination and documentation of orientation, affect, and cognition as a baseline assessment.

The client should also be assessed for health conditions that contraindicate the use of a particular agent or ones that would require cautious use and special monitoring interventions.

Antipsychotic agents may cause a number of cardiovascular effects, including hypotension (caused by alpha-adrenergic blockade), tachycardia (anticholinergic effect), myocardial depressant effects, and electrocardiographic alterations affecting ST, T wave, and widening of QRS interval. The most cardiotoxic agents are chlorpromazine (Thorazine) and thioridazine (Mellaril). A high-potency antipsychotic, such as haloperidol (Haldol) has fewer cardiotoxic effects so it may be the preferred agent with clients with cardiovascular disease.

These drugs are contraindicated in clients with severe cardiovascular disease, severe CNS depression, or who are comatose. They are administered with caution to clients with active alcoholism because these drugs may potentiate

Pediatric Implications

Psychotherapeutic agents

Children are at a greater risk of developing neuromuscular or extrapyramidal side effects, especially dystonias. Monitor closely if antipsychotic agents are administered.

Pediatric clients with chickenpox, CNS infections, measles, dehydration, gastroenteritis, or other acute illnesses will be at special risk of developing adverse reactions and possibly Reye's syndrome. Avoid use of phenothiazine antiemetic therapy in such clients.

The tricyclic antidepressants are usually not recommended for the treatment of depression in children under 12 years old. Some agents, though, such as amitriptyline (Elavil), desipramine (Norpramin), and imipramine (Tofranil) have been used in children over the age of 6 for major depressions. Several of these agents are also used in the treatment of enuresis and attention deficit disorder. Be aware that children are very sensitive to an acute overdose, which should always be considered very serious and potentially fatal. Adolescents often require a decreased dose because of their sensitivity to this drug category.

Adverse effects reported in children receiving the tricyclic antidepressants include changes in electrocardiogram patterns, increased nervousness, sleep disorders, complaints of tiredness, hypertension, and mild stomach distress.

Lithium may decrease the bone density or bone formation in children. If necessary to use, monitor closely serum levels and for signs of toxicity.

From *USP DI* (1996).

Pregnancy Safety

Category	Drugs
B	bupropion, clozapine, fluoxetine, maprotiline, sertraline
C	amitriptyline, amoxapine, haloperidol, loxapine, nefazodone, pimozide, phenelzine, risperidone, trimipramine, trazodone, venlafaxine
D	lithium
Unclassified	desipramine, doxepin, imipramine, isocarboxazid, molindone, nortriptyline, phenothiazines, (although not recommended during pregnancy), protriptyline, thiothixene, tranylcypromine

CNS depression, liver impairment, and place the client at higher risk of heat stroke. With decreased metabolism by the liver, there may be increased sensitivity to CNS effects and Reye's syndrome in children and adolescents (see Pediatric Implications box above). Clients with the following disorders may find their symptoms increased: blood dyscrasias, cardiovascular disease, glaucoma, Parkinson's disease, peptic ulcer, urinary retention, and chronic respiratory disorders. The thioxanthenes in particular are contraindicated in clients with blood dyscrasias and bone marrow depression. Antipsychotic drugs should be used cautiously in clients with a history of convulsive disorders because of their action in reducing the convulsive threshold. Adequate anticonvulsant therapy needs to be maintained. The risk of administering these drugs to pregnant women should be weighed against the expected therapeutic outcome (see Pregnancy Safety box above for FDA rating).

An ophthalmologic exam is recommended before the onset of antipsychotic agent therapy, to include measurement of visual acuity with and without refraction, a color vision test, and a slit lamp study of the fundus and exam of the visual fields.

Before beginning antipsychotic therapy, a drug history of the client (especially of the geriatric client) should be taken. The elderly may experience unusual adverse drug reactions as compared with younger persons (See Geriatric Implications box 370). Confusion, depression, and hallucinations have been reported with a wide variety of drugs in the elderly; thus the possibility of a drug-induced effect must be addressed (Abrams & Berkow, 1990).

The client's current drug regimen should be reviewed to determine if there are any significant drug interactions. The following effects may occur when antipsychotic agents are given with the drugs listed below:

Drug	Possible effect and management
alcohol, CNS depressants	**May result in enhanced CNS depression, respiratory depression, and increased hypotensive effects. The drug dosage should be reduced to one fourth to one half the usual dose. Titrate according to client response.** **Concurrent alcohol use may increase the risk of inducing a heat stroke. Avoid or a potentially serious drug interaction may occur.** Barbiturates may decrease chlorpromazine serum levels through an increase in the metabolizing enzymes in the liver. Thioridazine (Mellaril) may decrease serum phenobarbital serum levels. Monitor closely for loss of therapeutic effect of barbiturates, since a dosage adjustment may be necessary.

Continued

Drug	Possible effect and management
anticholinergics	Concurrent drug use may result in an increase in anticholinergic side effects.
antihypertensive agents	Concurrent drug use with the phenothiazines may result in an increase in hypotensive side effects.
antithyroid medications	Increase the risk for agranulocytosis when phenothiazines are given concurrently.
epinephrine	**Antipsychotic agents block alpha-adrenergic receptors, thus administration of epinephrine to treat phenothiazine-induced hypotension may result in severe hypotension. With the alpha receptors blocked, epinephrine stimulates beta receptors, which can result in severe lowering of blood pressure and in tachycardia. Avoid or a potentially serious drug interaction may occur.**
extrapyramidal-inducing medications (such as amoxapine (Asendin), metoclopramide (Reglan), reserpine (Serpalan, etc.)	May result in increased frequency and severe extrapyramidal effects.
guanadrel (Hylorel) or guanethidine (Ismelin)	Concurrent use with antipsychotic agents, especially loxapine and thiothixenes, may reverse the hypotensive drug effectiveness. Closely monitor BP of all clients receiving this drug combination.
levodopa (L-dopa)	Concurrent use with the antipsychotic agents may render levodopa ineffective in controlling Parkinson's disease.
lithium (Eskalith)	(1) May decrease GI absorption of chlorpromazine (Thorazine) by as much as 40%; (2) phenothiazines may increase the rate of lithium excretion in the kidneys; (3) may result in an increase in extrapyramidal symptoms; (4) may increase the risk of seizures, confusional states, neuroleptic malignant syndrome, and dyskinesia; and (5) phenothiazines and molindone may mask nausea and vomiting, which are early signs of lithium toxicity. Haloperidol (Haldol) may also increase extrapyramidal side effects. Although controversial, there are reports of irreversible neurologic and brain damage when both drugs are given for longer periods than several weeks. If both drugs are given concurrently, monitor clients closely for neurologic changes, since dosage reductions may be necessary.
metrizamide (Amipaque)	When given concurrently with phenothiazines, may lower the seizure threshold. Discontinue phenothiazines at least 2 days before and also for 1 day after a myelogram.
quinidine	**When given concurrently with the thioxanthenes (chlorprothixene, thiothixene), an increase in cardiac effects may occur. Avoid or a potentially serious drug interaction may occur.**
tricyclic antidepressants, inhibitors, and procarbazine (Matulane)	**Concurrent use may increase the MAO duration and intensify the sedative and anticholinergic side effects of these medications. Metabolism of the phenothiazines and the antidepressants may be inhibited.**
tricyclic antidepressants, inhibitors, and procarbazine (Matulane)	May enhance the risk of inducing neuroleptic malignant syndrome (NMS)—hyperthermia, dehydration, cardiovascular instability, hypoxemia, and muscular rigidity. Avoid or a potentially serious drug interaction may occur.

Geriatric Implications

Psychotherapeutic agents

The elderly tend to have higher serum levels of the antipsychotic and antidepressant drugs because of changes in drug distribution resulting from a decrease in lean body mass, less total body water, less serum albumin, and usually an increase in body fat. Therefore, these clients require a lower drug dose and a more gradual drug dose titration than the younger adult client.

Geriatric clients are more prone to have orthostatic hypotension, anticholinergic side effects, extrapyramidal side effects, and sedation. They should be carefully evaluated before starting such potent medications, and if the antipsychotic agents are necessary, close supervision and the prescribing of the lowest dose possible is recommended.

The elderly client generally should receive half the recommended adult dose. The client with organic brain syndrome should only receive 33% to 50% of the usual adult dose with increases in dosage at 7- to 10-day periods. When clinical improvement is noted, attempts at tapering and discontinuing the drug should be instituted.

The tricyclic antidepressants may cause increased anxiety in the geriatric client. If the client has cardiovascular disease, the use of the tricyclic antidepressants increases the risk of inducing arrhythmias, tachycardia, stroke, congestive heart failure, and myocardial infarction.

Lithium is more toxic in the geriatric client; therefore, lower lithium dosages, a lower lithium serum level, and very close monitoring is critical in this age group. The elderly are more prone to develop CNS toxicity, lithium-induced goiter, and clinical hypothyroidism than the average adult. Generally, excessive thirst and elimination of large volumes of urine may be early side effects of lithium toxicity frequently seen in the elderly.

From *USP DI* (1996).

Nursing diagnosis. Once a client has started antipsychotic therapy, the nurse needs to assess for potential problems that may occur as the result of the drug's side effects and adverse reactions. The Nursing Care Plan at right describes selected more common nursing diagnoses. In addition, the client may experience: urinary retention related to the anticholinergic effects; impaired skin integrity (rash); altered protection related to bone marrow depression; and the potential complications of allergic reaction, heat stroke, hepatotoxicity, Reye's syndrome, neuroleptic malignant syndrome (NMS), persistent tardive dyskinesia, and priaprism.

Nursing Care Plan

Selected Nursing Diagnoses Related to Antipsychotic Medication Administration

Nursing diagnosis	Outcome criteria	Nursing interventions
Alteration in bowel elimination: constipation related to drug's anticholinergic effects	The client will maintain his or her usual bowel elimination pattern; select foods high in fiber from the daily menu; maintain a fluid intake of 2500 ml daily; increase activity as allowed	Assess client's usual bowel elimination pattern; monitor and record bowel movements Instruct client to establish a routine for bowel elimination; select foods high in fiber; maintain fluid intake of 2500 ml/day and perform isometric abdomminal strengthening exercises, unless contraindicated; increase activity as allowed
Altered comfort related to dry mouth	The client will maintain a healthy oral cavity as evidenced by pink, moist, intact mucosa	Provide ice chips, sugarless candies, and frequent mouth hygiene if dry mouth occurs
Risk for injury related to increased sensitivity to the sun, visual effects, and the development of dizziness, hypotension, akathisia, parkinsonian, extrapyramidal effects, and tardive dyskinesia	The client will not experience sunburn, falls, symptoms of tardive dyskinesia	Monitor blood pressure at appropriate intervals; keep client in recumbent position for 30 minutes after injection; provide assistance with ambulation if sedation, dizziness, orthostatic hypotension, or visual changes occur Instruct client to change position from recumbent to upright slowly Alert client to hypersensitivity to sun and the use of sunscreens and sunglasses Monitor for and instruct client in the early signs of tardive dyskinesia (facial tics, grimacing, blinking, lip smacking, tongue protrusion, writhing motions of the arms, hands, and fingers). Report immediately
Knowledge deficit related to newly prescribed or altered psychotherapeutic agents	The client will describe his condition; how the drug therapy relates to the condition; how and when to take the medications; common drug interactions; common side effects and which of these warrant reporting; storage requirements of the drug; demonstrate less anxiety related to fear of the unknown, loss of control, and misconceptions	Assess learning needs and learning readiness Plan with the client and family for the achievement of realistic goals Provide information to meet outcome criteria
Ineffective management of therapeutic regimen	The client will self-administer medications safely and accurately	Determine the client's reasons for ineffective management of therapeutic regimen and take appropriate teaching/counseling interventions Discuss the increased possibility of the return of symptoms with ineffective management of therapeutic regimen

Implementation

Monitoring. In the past, many clients said to be resistant to drug therapy were found to be noncompliant with the prescribed therapy. Many psychotic clients deny their illness or associate the consumption of medications with dependence or weakness. Clients refractory to antipsychotic medications should be reviewed for:

- **Compliance.** The prescriber may order a plasma serum level of the medication, if such a test is available, to determine the client's reliability, or the drug order may be switched to a liquid formulation to be administered in a supervised setting.
- **Inadequate dosage.** The prescriber should adjust the dosage according to the individual needs of the client. Inadequate dosage or the development of drug tolerance may result in an inadequate response to the medication.

BOX 19-2

Neuroleptic Extrapyramidal Adverse Effects

Akathisia

Description:

Motor restlessness; person unable to sit or stand still, feels urgent need to move, pace, rock, or tap foot.

May also present as apprehension, irritability, and general uneasiness and may be mistaken for agitation.

More common in females than males; usually occurs in 5 to 30 days (up to 90 days) of starting drug therapy.

Treatment: lower dose of neuroleptic agent, switch to a different drug, or administer an antiparkinson drug, such as benztropine (Cogentin).

Dystonia

Description:

Acute reaction requiring immediate intervention. Client exhibits muscle spasms of face, tongue, neck, jaw, and/or back. Hyperextension of neck and trunk and arching of back.

Tongue may protrude; facial grimaces; exaggerated posturing of head, neck, or jaw; difficulty swallowing and/or talking. Person may have a fixed upward gaze and/or eye muscle spasms. May be accompanied by excessive salivation.

Commonly occurs after large doses of neuroleptics, usually within an hour up to a week of drug therapy. Occurs more often in males than females.

Treatment: depending on the severity of reaction, one or more of the following may be necessary; lower neuroleptic dose, administer benztropine (Cogentin) IM or IV, or diphenhydramine (Benadryl) IM.

Drug-induced parkinsonism

Description:

Symptoms similar to Parkinson's disease; shuffling gait, drooling, tremors, increased rigidity (cogwheel). Bradykinesia (slow movements) and akinesia (immobility) also reported.

Treatment:

Add antiparkinson drug, such as benztropine (Cogentin) diphenhydramine (Benadryl), etc.

Physician may switch to a neuroleptic less likely to induce this effect, such as thioridazine (Mellaril).

Tardive Dyskinesia

Description:

Oral/facial dyskinesias, i.e. abnormal involuntary muscle movements around the mouth, lip smacking, tongue darting, constant chewing movements, tics, etc.

Person may also have involuntary movements of arms or legs. More common in older women but has been reported in younger persons.

Treatment:

Prevention is vital, may be irreversible. No effective treatment.

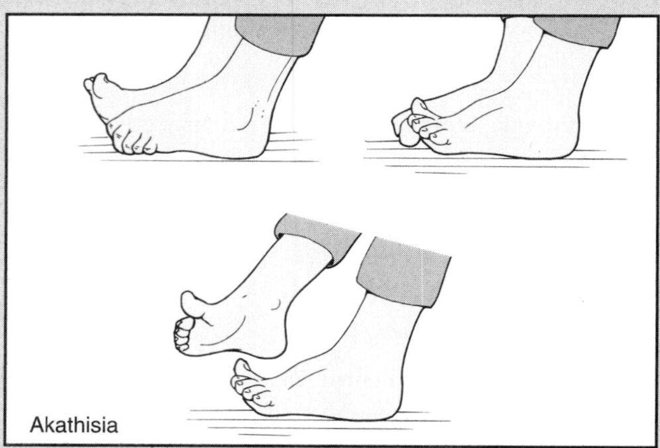
Akathisia

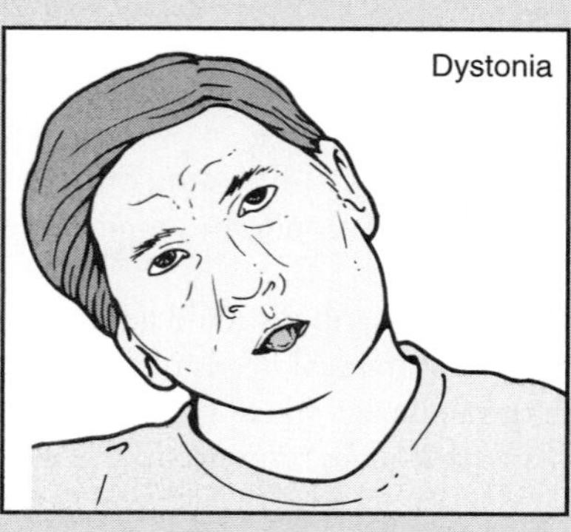
Dystonia

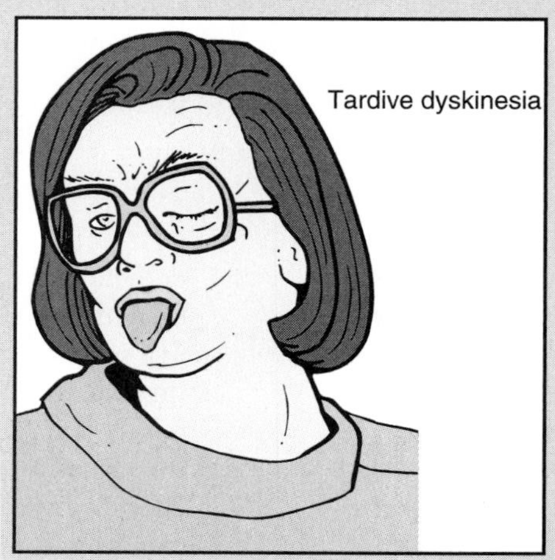
Tardive dyskinesia

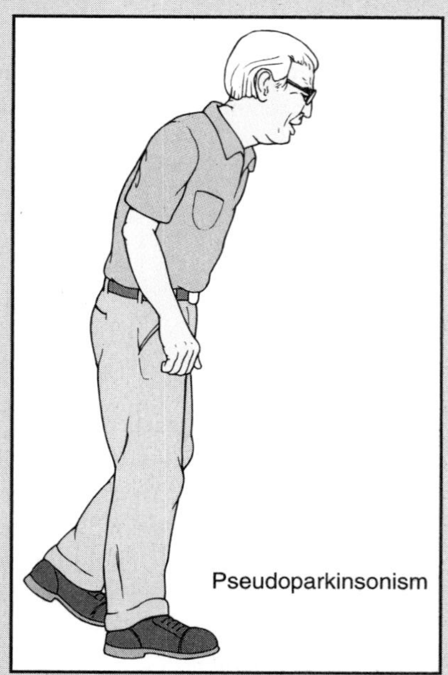
Pseudoparkinsonism

- **Questionable oral bioavailability.** Although this is not known to be a common possibility, it is a variable to be considered. The prescriber may switch from an oral solid dosage form to a liquid formulation and also adjust the dosage as necessary, based on the individual's response or development of side effects. Switching to another antipsychotic agent may also be considered.

Observe the client for orthostatic hypotension, especially after parenteral administration; monitor BP before and after injections. If orthostatic (postural) hypotension occurs and causes severe difficulties or serious hazards, the nurse should alert the prescriber, who may institute one of the following remedial measures: (1) a change of medication to one of the phenothiazine derivatives that does not produce this side effect with such frequency, (2) reduction of dosage, or (3) discontinuation of medication for 24 hours with a gradual buildup of dosage as tolerated. If hypotension necessitating drug intervention occurs, norepinephrine or phenylephrine (Neo-Synephrine) may be administered. Because phenothiazines tend to reverse epinephrine's vasopressor effects, epinephrine may not be effective in reversing hypotension.

The nurse should be alert to signs of agranulocytosis such as sore throat, fever, or weakness in clients taking these drugs; this usually occurs between weeks 4 and 10. When these symptoms appear, the drug is usually discontinued; the nurse should hold the dose and notify the prescriber as soon as possible. White blood cell and differential counts are required periodically.

Because of possible ocular changes, including particle deposition in the cornea and lens and pigmentary retinopathy (decreased vision, brownish coloring of vision, impaired night vision, and pigment deposits on the fundus), contact the prescriber. These changes may be related to dosage levels or therapy duration. The client on a long-term regimen or on moderate-to-high dose therapy should have periodic ophthalmologic examinations.

Observe the client for neuroleptic extrapyramidal adverse effects (Box 19-2). The nurse should particularly monitor the client closely for early signs of tardive dyskinesia, usually small, wormlike motions of the tongue. Since there is no known effective treatment for tardive dyskinesia, the drug should be discontinued immediately and the prescriber notified (Box 19-3).

The nurse should monitor the client for neuroleptic malignant syndrome (NMS) (hyperthermia, dehydration, cardiovascular instability, hypoxemia, and muscular rigidity). Therapy is essentially symptomatic and supportive with the drug being discontinued immediately.

An ECG should be performed periodically and with every adjustment in loxapine (Loxitane) dosage because the drug may potentiate cardiac dysrhythmias.

The client should be monitored for signs and symptoms of urinary hesitancy or retention, prostatic hypertrophy, narrow-angle glaucoma, or respiratory problems (e.g., intake and output for urinary retention and constipation) because of the anticholinergic effects of the drugs.

Hepatic function tests and urine tests for bilirubin and bile should be done weekly during the first month of therapy to assist in the detection of cholestatic jaundice, which is more likely to occur between the second and fourth week. Clinically, the client should be observed for yellow skin, nausea, flulike symptoms, and rash. The drug should be discontinued immediately.

Depression, especially if the client is not closely supervised, may account for the greater incidence of suicide in psychiatric clients undergoing drug therapy than in those receiving only institutional care.

The client's emotional status should be assessed carefully because there may be a rapid mood swing from mania to depression when haloperidol (Haldol) is administered to the client with a bipolar disorder.

Observe the client and note if the mental status has changed from the baseline assessment to demonstrate the efficacy or inefficacy of the drug.

BOX 19-3

Tardive Dyskinesia

Tardive dyskinesia (TD) is a potentially irreversible neurologic disorder that primarily involves the buccolingual and masticatory muscles. This adverse effect to the antipsychotic agents may occur within a few months or years of treatment or after these agents have been discontinued. The risk of inducing TD increases with total dosage of the drug given and the length of the treatment period.

Incidence: Although 0.5% to 65% of the treated population may develop this syndrome, recent reports place the percentage of clients at risk as 10% to 20%.

Presenting features:
- Facial: grimacing or scowl expression, facial tics, arching of the eyebrows
- Ocular: blinking, eyelid spasms (blepharospasm)
- Oral/buccal: lip smacking, lower lip thrusting, sucking, puffing of cheeks, chewing of the cheeks (the inside of the mouth should be checked for this)
- Lingual/masticatory: lateral jaw movements, tongue protrusion or thrusting such as "fly catching movements," tongue in lip or cheek resulting in an observable bulge in the specific area
- Systemic effects: foot tapping; rocking from side to side; arms, hands, and fingers may display a jerking and/or a writhing motion (choreoathetoid motion); pelvic thrusting motions.

Treatment: Prevention only. Early assessment and diagnosis is crucial in preventing the development of an irreversible disorder. Decreasing or discontinuing the antipsychotic agent if possible is the recommended procedure. At present, there is no known effective treatment for TD.

Data from Kalachnik (1983); *USP DI* (1996).

Intervention. Rapid neuroleptization or high-dose therapy is appropriate in certain cases. For instance, aggressive treatment is used in clients with acute psychosis who may exhibit dangerous and/or destructive behaviors. Usually intramuscular therapy with a high-potency antipsychotic agent (such as haloperidol [Haldol] or thiothixene [Mellaril]) is given, often on an hourly schedule, until the desired effects are achieved. If a client will take oral medication, high-dose oral therapy may be substituted. Because of the half-life of the intramuscular doses, the first oral dose should be given 12 to 24 hours after the last intramuscular dose.

Once a client is stabilized on antipsychotic medications, the entire daily dosage may be prescribed to be given at bedtime. The long duration of action of these drugs makes a single bedtime dosage feasible. This dosage schedule has increased client compliance, lowered medication costs, decreased side effects, and decreased or eliminated the need for simultaneous hypnotic medication. This dosage schedule would require both careful drug selection and client assessment before implementation. Using a drug with a high anticholinergic potential in an elderly client or an individual with cardiovascular disease may result in an increased potential for cardiotoxic effects. In such cases, smaller, multiple (two or three times daily) daily doses are indicated.

Long-acting injections are frequently useful in antipsychotic therapy. Depot fluphenazine enanthate (Prolixin Enanthate), fluphenazine decanoate (Prolixin Deconate), and haloperidol decanoate (Haldol Deconate) are available for clients who are persistently noncompliant, do not understand the need for taking medications, or have a high frequency of relapses (psychotic episodes). Fluphenazine decanoate is often a better choice than the enanthate because its duration of action is approximately 2 weeks longer.

Clients receiving fluphenazine decanoate may also exhibit a slight decrease in extrapyramidal side effects as compared with clients taking the enanthate formulation. The enanthate formulation results in a more variable fluphenazine plasma level and the effect is not as prolonged as the decanoate formulation. Converting from an oral antipsychotic agent to fluphenazine decanoate is complicated, therefore the reader is referred to Ereshefsky and Richards (1992) for more information.

Clients being considered for haloperidol decanoate therapy should first receive oral haloperidol. Dosage and dosing interval adjustments should be carefully chosen and closely monitored. In some persons the effects of haloperidol decanoate may last up to 6 weeks.

Dosages of phenothiazines and other antipsychotic agents are individualized according to client response so that the lowest effective dose may be used. Dosages are increased more slowly and in smaller increments with elderly or debilitated clients.

Note that in most cases concurrent treatment with more than one neuroleptic agent is not indicated. If the client does not respond to a particular drug, usually the dose of that drug should be increased or a different drug prescribed. Occasionally a client may respond best to a combination of two drugs from different classes. However, the potentiation and lowered margin of safety of such combinations require greater precautions for client safety.

Because administration of large doses over a prolonged time may lead to anticholinergic psychoses or tardive dyskinesia, adverse reactions may be prevented by providing periodic "drug-free holidays" during which the client does not receive phenothiazines. Because of the long elimination half-life of these drugs, "holidays" should last several weeks. Maintenance dosage should be periodically evaluated for a possible reduction in the dosage or cessation of drug therapy. Clients with preexisting renal or hepatic disease may require reduced dosage.

The oral route of administration is preferred unless the client is unable to take an oral dose. Oral forms of phenothiazines should be administered with at least 120 ml of fruit juice or other liquids or semisoft foods to decrease gastric irritation and to make the drug more palatable. However, the client should be informed that the medication is in the substance. Phenothiazines should not be administered concurrently with antacids or antidiarrheals; times of administration should be altered to allow 2 hours between doses of these medications. Administration of the maintenance dosage at bedtime facilitates sleep and decreases drowsiness during the daytime.

The fluphenazine hydrochloride (Prolixin) and perphenazine (Trilafon) oral concentrate solutions should not be mixed with fluids containing caffeine (coffee, tea, cola), tannic acid (tea), or pectinates (apple juice) because a physical incompatibility may occur. Instead, dilute with at least 60 ml of lemon-lime carbonated beverage or pineapple, orange, tomato, or grapefruit juice for each 5 ml of concentrate.

A special dropper should be used for oral liquid haloperidol (Haldol) administration; if diluted with tea or coffee, a precipitate will form. Haloperidol may be administered from a premeasured oral syringe without diluting if desired. If dilution is desired, use at least 60 ml of diluent and mix just before administration to prevent precipitation.

The nurse should administer the loxapine succinate (Loxitane) oral concentrate with the calibrated dropper, which has 1 ml equal to 25 mg only. The drug should be mixed with orange or grapefruit juice shortly before administration.

When preparing phenothiazines, the nurse should be aware that the injectable forms tend to be physically and/or chemically incompatible with a wide range of solutions. The nurse should check the package insert for compatibility information about the specific drugs being prepared. Avoid freezing phenothiazine solutions. Discolored solutions, slightly yellowed, may be used. However, if marked discoloration or a precipitate is apparent, the solution should not be used. Skin and eye contact with phenothiazine solutions should be avoided because it may cause contact dermatitis and irritation. Exposed areas should be washed immediately to minimize the effect.

When given intramuscularly, antipsychotic drugs should be injected deeply and slowly in divided doses of not more than 1 ml per injection site into large muscle mass, such as the ventrogluteal or dorsogluteal site. Rotate and document the rotation of injection sites. Irritation of the subcutaneous tissues can be reduced by diluting the drug with 0.9% sodium chloride injection and/or the addition of 2% procaine, injecting the drug by the "Z track" technique (see Figure 5-8). Massaging the injection site helps reduce local irritation.

Decanoate and enthanthate, the long-acting forms of fluphenazine (Prolixin), are oil preparations. They may be given intramuscularly or subcutaneously using a 21-gauge or larger needle.

Some clients have been known to develop abscesses at the injection site, which are believed to result from large doses of drug being administered in one area. Use of the intramuscular route when administering antipsychotic drug is usually indicated when the client refuses the tablet or concentrate form or when the most immediate effect of the drug is desired. If the client is severely agitated, combative, or struggling, the nurse should take care to follow safe administration technique. This technique usually requires enough well-trained personnel to restrain the client adequately while the medication is being given.

Loxapine hydrochloride (Loxitane) is to be administered only intramuscularly and usually only in acute-care settings where clients may be closely monitored. Because of the drug's orthostatic hypotensive effects, the client should remain lying down for 30 minutes after an injection.

Intravenous administration of undiluted chlorpromazine (Thorazine) should be avoided. If used for direct intravenous administration, it should be diluted to at least 1 mg/ml and administered at a rate of 1 mg/min for adults and 0.5 mg/min for children. For intravenous infusion the drug should be added to 500 to 1000 ml of 0.9% sodium chloride solution and administered slowly. In both instances the client should be kept recumbent to minimize hypotension.

Intravenous administration of perphenazine (Trilafon) is limited to recumbent hospitalized adult clients and requires the availability of resuscitative equipment and drugs for the treatment of severe hypotensive episodes or extrapyramidal responses in the client. If administered by fractional intravenous injection, the solution should be diluted to 0.5 mg/ml of 0.9% sodium chloride and administered slowly, 1 mg per injection at intervals of at least 1 to 2 minutes. Blood pressure and pulse should be assessed continuously during intravenous administration.

Gradual reduction of the antipsychotic dosage over several weeks for clients on high or long-term dosages will help prevent withdrawal symptoms of nausea, vomiting, irritability, trembling, and transient dyskinetic signs. The only rationale for abrupt withdrawal is the occurrence of severe side effects/adverse reactions.

Education. The client who complains of dizziness, light-headedness, or palpitation may be experiencing orthostatic hypotension. This can easily be confirmed when the client's blood pressure is compared in the prone and standing positions. The client should be instructed to rise slowly from the recumbent position and to sit on the edge of the bed for a few minutes before attempting to stand. Support and reassurance may be necessary to allay the client's anxiety. Explaining orthostatic hypotension also may help him or her understand this experience and reduce anxiety. Clients should be encouraged to remain in a recumbent position for 1 hour after initial doses, parenterally administered doses, or large oral doses (rarely) of the phenothiazines to minimize hypotensive episodes.

The nurse should caution clients against driving, operating dangerous machinery, or performing tasks that require absolute precision, motor coordination, and mental alertness. Tolerance to drowsiness develops as therapy continues. The client should be told that the antipsychotic medication may take several weeks to treat the disorder effectively.

To prevent photosensitivity, the nurse should advise the client to stay out of the sun, use sunscreen lotion, or wear protective clothing to prevent solar erythema, or the nurse should assist clients by providing the necessary protective measures. A dark, purplish-brown skin pigmentation induced by light (photosensitivity) has been reported in hospitalized psychiatric clients who were given large doses of phenothiazines for 3 to 10 years. Exposure to light also increases the possibility of ocular changes; therefore, the client should be instructed to wear sunglasses.

The nurse should caution the client that dry mouth can be a bothersome adverse effect and contribute to the development of caries, gum disease, and oral candidiasis. The client should be instructed in the use of proper oral hygiene. Xerostomia may affect the fitting of full dentures; referral should be made for dental care for this and other dental problems.

Long-term therapy with phenothiazines necessitates dietary increases in riboflavin. Good dietary sources of vitamin B_2 are muscle meats, organ meats, milk, eggs, leafy and yellow vegetables, and enriched cereals and breads. However, if the client has altered nutrition, it may be beneficial to use a vitamin supplement until adequate nutrition is assured.

Phenothiazines also affect regulation of body temperature; clients should be cautioned to avoid extremes of environmental temperature (i.e., swimming in cold water or walking in hot, humid weather), which could lead to hypothermia and respiratory distress or hyperthermia and heat prostration, respectively.

The client should be instructed to avoid alcohol and other CNS depressants, since they increase the CNS depressant effects of the antipsychotic agents. Using these drugs concurrently with extrapyramidal reaction-causing medications will increase the frequency and severity of extrapyramidal effects.

The tablet form of molindone (Moban) contains calcium sulfate, which may impair the absorption of tetracyclines and phenytoin (Dilantin). The client should be informed about this interaction.

With the extended-action injectable form of these drugs, the effects may last up to 6 weeks; therefore, clients should be counseled that precautions and other side effects information will apply during this time.

Evaluation. With successful antipsychotic therapy the client will be able to perform activities of daily living independently without adverse effects of the drugs. The client will also safely and accurately self-administer the medication.

Atypical Antipsychotic Agents

clozapine [kloe' za peen] (Clozaril)

Clozapine is considered an "atypical" antipsychotic agent. It differs from the other neuroleptics by being active at the limbic dopamine receptors, affecting both receptors but with less affinity for D_2, thus it is less apt to induce extrapyramidal side effects. It binds more to serotonin (5-HT_2), $alpha_1$ and histamine (H_1) receptors than dopamine receptors. Because it has the potential for causing agranulocytosis, a potentially life-threatening effect, this drug is reserved for treatment-resistant schizophrenia or for when the adverse effects of other drugs preclude their continued use. Treatment resistance has been defined as the client not responding to an appropriate course of standard antipsychotic agents after trying at least two antipsychotic medications (*USP DI*, 1996).

Treatment with clozapine is closely monitored, with the manufacturer recommending dispensing of only weekly supplies and the performance of weekly WBC testing. The adult dose is 25 mg once or twice daily increased by 25 to 50 mg/day until 300 to 450 mg/day is reached by the end of the second week of therapy. Thereafter, increases should not exceed 100 mg once or twice a week. The maximum daily dose is 900 mg. Clients should be closely monitored because high doses may result in an increase in adverse effects, such as seizures (*USP DI*, 1996).

■ Nursing Management

Clozapine Therapy

In addition to the general nursing management for antipsychotic therapy, the following should be noted:

Assessment. Clozapine is contraindicated in cases of severe CNS depression, blood dyscrasias, or a history of bone marrow depression because these conditions will be potentiated. Because of this drug's effect on myeloproliferation, it is essential that the client's white cell count be determined at the start of therapy, at weekly intervals, and for 4 weeks after the last dose. Therapy should not be initiated if the WBC is less than 3500/mm^3, and should be discontinued at any time there is a substantial decline from the client's baseline WBC or if it falls below 3000/mm^3. Consideration of the risk-benefit should also be given if the client has narrow-angle glaucoma, prostatic hypertrophy, or seizure disorders because these conditions may be worsened.

Review the client's drug regimen. The concurrent administration of alcohol or CNS depressant drugs may enhance the CNS depressant effects of clozapine; concurrent administration of a bone marrow depressant may potentiate the myelosuppressive adverse effect, and concurrent use with lithium increases the risk of inducing seizures, confusion, neuroleptic malignant syndrome, and dyskinesias. Whenever possible, avoid concurrent administration of these agents.

Implementation

Monitoring. The client should be assessed for flu-like symptoms or infection. Cardiovascular effects may occur, such as tachycardia and hypotension, but these may be minimized if the client is started on low doses with gradual increments. White blood cell count (WBC) and differential counts are done at weekly intervals and for 4 weeks after clozapine therapy ends. Therapy is discontinued if the WBC is less than 3000/mm^3 or the granulocyte count less than 1500 per mm^3.

Education. Safety precautions related to hypotension should be reviewed with the client. In addition, there is reported to be clozapine dose-related seizure activity with seizures occurring in 1% to 2% of clients receiving low doses (<300 mg/day), 3% to 4% of clients receiving moderate doses (300 to 599 mg/day), and 5% of clients receiving high doses (>600 mg/day). Clients with a history of seizures are at higher risk. Appropriate teaching and safety precautions should be taken.

▲ **risperidone** [ris peer' i dohn] (Risperdal)

Risperidone is the first benzisoxazole from a new chemical class of antipsychotic drugs that blocks both serotonin and dopamine receptors. It is indicated for the treatment of psychotic disorders and improves both the positive and negative symptoms of schizophrenia.

This drug is orally well absorbed. Peak serum level is within 1 to 2 hours, and it is metabolized in the liver to 9-hydroxyrisperidone, an active metabolite that is therapeutically active. Elimination half-life is 20 to 24 hours with excretion primarily via the kidneys.

Most common side effects include fatigue, cough, constipation or diarrhea, dry mouth, increase in dreaming, nausea, and weight gain. Adverse effects that should be reported to the prescriber include insomnia, visual changes, sexual dysfunction, agitation, increased anxiety, and extrapyramidal reactions.

The usual adult dose is 1 mg twice daily, increasing by 1 mg twice daily on the second and third day if tolerated. Thereafter, dosage increases may be instituted at weekly intervals. In the elderly, dosage is 0.5 mg twice daily, titrated according to response. Safety in children up to 18 years old is not established.

■ Nursing Management

Risperidone Therapy

In addition to the nursing management cited in the section on the nursing management of antipsychotic drugs, consider the following:

Assessment. Risk/benefit should be considered if the client has cardiovascular disease or renal or hepatic function impairment. Risperidone is contraindicated in pregnancy and lactation. Hypotensive clients will have their symptoms aggravated.

Drug interactions to be concerned with in the drug history include increased CNS depression effects with alcohol and other CNS depressing medications; enhanced hypotensive effects with antihypertensive agents; reduced levodopa effects when given with bromocriptine (Parlodel), levodopa

(L-dopa) or pergolide (Permax); increased clearance from the body when administered with carbamazepine (Tegretol) and decreased clearance if administered with clozapine (Clozaril).

A baseline assessment includes blood pressure, temperature, pulse, respirations, adventitious lung sounds; mental status, reflexes, liver and liver function studies, CBC, urinalysis, and ECG.

Nursing diagnosis. The client on risperidone therapy may experience the following nursing diagnoses: anxiety; sleep pattern disturbance (insomnia); altered comfort (headache, agitation, nausea, vomiting); constipation; and the potential complications of neuroleptic malignant syndrome and tardive dyskinesias.

Implementation

Monitoring. If client has difficulty with dizziness and light-headedness, take sitting and standing blood pressures to assess orthostatic hypotension. Monitor body temperature. If client's temperature is elevated without signs of infection, notify prescriber. WBCs and ECGs are done periodically.

Intervention. Dosage is increased gradually to the most effective dosage and the client should be weaned from the drug gradually. Risperidone is not to be discontinued suddenly.

Education. Alert client to change positions slowly to prevent orthostatic hypotension; safety instructions about driving and operating hazardous equipment; and photosensitivity precautions. Women should practice contraception and contact the prescriber if they suspect they are pregnant or if they wish to become pregnant. Clients should report to their prescriber any symptoms of fatigue, weakness, palpitations, mouth ulcers, sore throat, or fever.

Evaluation. The client should experience a decrease of psychotic symptoms without any adverse effects of the drug and be able to self-administer risperidone safely and accurately.

pimozide [pi' moe zide] (Orap)

Pimozide is indicated for the treatment of severe motor and vocal tics in persons with Tourette's syndrome that have failed to respond to haloperidol (Haldol). Although the mechanism of action is unknown, pimozide blocks dopamine in the central nervous system. Pimozide is administered orally, is metabolized in the liver to two major metabolites, produces peak effect in 6 to 8 hours, has a half-life of 29 hours, and within a week about 50% is primarily excreted by the kidneys.

The most frequent side effects include dry mouth, orthostatic hypotension, skin rash, pruritus, visual disturbances, constipation, sedation, breast soreness, and perhaps milk secretion. The most frequent adverse effects reported are akathisia, behavioral alterations, ventricular arrhythmias, and drug-induced parkinsonian and extrapyramidal effects. With the exception of mood or behavioral changes, the other adverse effects occur most commonly during the first few days of therapy. Less frequent reactions include intense, irregular muscle spasms (dystonia), tardive dyskinesia, jaundice, neuroleptic malignant syndrome, and blood dyscrasias.

Dosage and administration. In adults and children 12 and older, administer 1 to 2 mg orally in divided doses. Increase dosage gradually every other day as necessary. For children under 12 the dosage has not been established. Maximum daily dosage is 20 mg in divided doses.

Nursing Management

Pimozide Therapy

Assessment. It should be determined that the client does not have an underlying condition such as cardiac arrhythmias or severe CNS depression for which pimozide is contraindicated; pimozide potentiates these conditions. The risks of cardiovascular and extrapyramidal effects are such that pimozide should not be used to treat tics other than those of Tourette's syndrome. Women with a history of breast cancer need to consider the risk-to-benefit ratio of the drug because the disease may be aggravated by increased serum prolactin concentrations as a result of pimozide therapy. Pimozide should not be administered in the presence of hypokalemia because of the heightened risk for ventricular arrhythmias.

The client's concurrent drug therapy should be reviewed to exclude the occurrence of significant drug interactions. The following effects may occur when pimozide is given with the drugs listed below:

Drug	Possible effect and management
alcohol, CNS depressants	May enhance CNS depressant effects. Monitor closely.
amphetamines, methylphenidate (Ritalin), pemoline (Cylert)	These drugs may cause tics, therefore they should be discontinued before pimozide therapy is begun.
anticholinergic drugs	May result in enhanced anticholinergic side effects, such as dry mouth, constipation, blurred vision, and excitability.
antidepressants, tricyclic; disopyramide (Norpace), maprotiline (Ludiomil), phenothiazines, procainamide (Pronestyl), or quinidine	**May enhance or potentiate cardiac arrhythmias. Avoid or a potentially serious drug interaction may occur.**
extrapyramidal-causing medications, including phenothiazines	May result in an increase in the extrapyramidal side effects of both medications. May also increase the anticholinergic and CNS depressant effects.

A baseline assessment of the client's behaviors, including the character and frequency of symptoms, should be recorded to enable the evaluation of client progress, the therapeutic usefulness of the pimozide therapy, and the occurrence of any adverse effects. A baseline ECG is essential to monitor the cardiac effects of the drugs.

BOX 19-4

New Antipsychotic Agent

Olanzapine (Zyprexa), the first agent from the thienobenzodiazepine class, was approved in 1996 for the treatment of schizophrenia. It is a monoaminergic antagonist that binds with adrenergic alpha$_1$, dopamine, histamine, serotonin, and muscarinic receptors in the body. While its mechanism of action is unknown, its effectiveness has been proposed to be due to its dopamine and serotonin type 2 blocking action. Action at the other receptors may account for some of olanzapine's other effects and side effects. This product appears to control both positive and negative symptoms with usually, a low incidence of adverse reports (Stat/Gram, 1996).

Pharmacokinetically, olanzapine is well absorbed orally, reaching peak serum levels in 6 hours. Its half-life is between 21 to 54 hours. It is metabolized and excreted in urine and feces. Side/adverse effects include headache, agitation, constipation, orthostatic hypotension, sedation, weight gain, and somnolence.

Usual dose is 5 to 10 mg once daily, titrating weekly as necessary. Antipsychotic efficacy was reported at dose ranges between 10 to 15 mg/day (Zyprexa, 1996).

Nursing diagnosis. The client receiving pimozide therapy is at risk for the following nursing diagnoses: social isolation and low self-esteem related to the symptoms of the Tourette's syndrome and the ineffectiveness of the drug; decreased cardiac output related to prolonged QT interval (fast or irregular pulse); risk for injury related to blurred vision and orthostatic hypotension; altered bowel elimination (constipation or diarrhea); altered mucous membranes (dry mouth); altered comfort (nausea and vomiting, sore breasts, headache); altered thought processes (depression); the potential complications of extrapyramidal (parkinsonian and dystonic) effects, and the development of tardive dyskinesia, neuroleptic malignant syndrome, obstructive jaundice, and blood dyscrasias.

Implementation

Monitoring. The client's vital signs should be monitored for hypotension and arrhythmias. Serial ECGs will be taken over the course of therapy. The client's symptoms should be recorded.

Intervention. Periodic attempts should be made to decrease the dosage of pimozide to evaluate the status of the tic behaviors.

Education. Alert the client to avoid alcoholic beverages and other CNS depressants during pimozide therapy. Precautions should be taken regarding the use of hazardous equipment until the client's response to the medication has been determined. Caution the client to rise slowly from a sitting or lying position because of the hypotensive effect of the drug. Sugarless gums and candies or ice chips may be used to relieve the symptom of dry mouth if this is of concern to the client. Advise the client to wear or carry a medical identification so that other health care providers will be aware that the client is receiving pimozide therapy. Symptoms of the adverse effects of pimozide should be reviewed with the client to enable him or her to know which should be reported to the prescriber.

Evaluation. The client's tics will be diminished or absent without the client experiencing any ill effects of the drug.

See Box 19-4 for a new antipsychotic agent.

ANTIDEPRESSANT THERAPY

Affective Disorders

Affective disorders, or mood disturbances, include depression, which is the most common affective disorder, and mania or elation. Mania is discussed later in this chapter.

Etiology of Affective Disorders

No single factor has been identified as the cause of affective disorders. Psychiatrists who believe in psychosocial therapies will probe to identify stressful events or mental conflicts that preceded the onset of depression, while others adhering to the biologic theory tend to explain affective disorders by the monoamine theory (i.e., catecholamine [norepinephrine, dopamine, epinephrine] and indolamine [serotonin] levels in the CNS). Many practitioners today believe that both psychosocial and biologic factors lead to a common pathway that results in an affective disorder.

Many factors are involved with affective disorders; some of these are genetics, psychosocial events (divorce, death of a mate), physiologic stress (illness, infection, childbirth), and personality traits. Any combination of these factors may also affect the CNS's biochemical mechanisms, lending weight again to the theory that affective disorders have a common pathway.

Monoamine Theory in Affective Disorders

Centrally acting monoamines, especially norepinephrine and serotonin, have been theorized to be the cause of depression and mania. A deficiency in central norepinephrine has been associated with depression, whereas an excess of norepinephrine is believed to be related to mania.

The tricyclic antidepressants may block the reuptake of one or both monoamines into the adrenergic neuron. This blockade will lead to elevated levels of norepinephrine and serotonin in the synapse areas. Monoamine oxidase (MAO), an enzyme found in the mitochondria of nerve cells, is responsible for metabolizing norepinephrine within the nerve. Monoamine oxidase inhibitors (MAOIs) block this enzyme, leading to increased levels of norepinephrine available for release to the synapse area.

Although the mechanism of action of many antidepressants is inhibition of the reuptake of norepinephrine or sero-

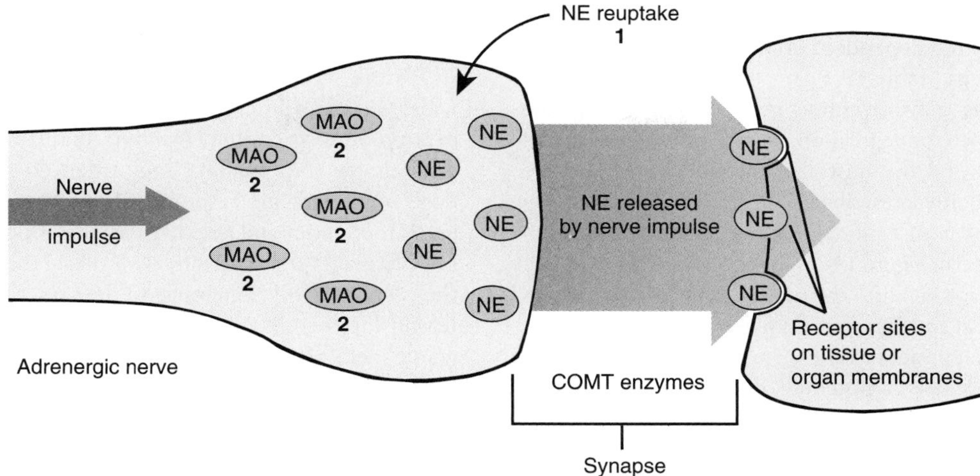

Figure 19-3 Proposed action of antidepressant drug therapy. Normally norepinephrine (NE) is released from storage sites within the adrenergic nerve by the arrival of a nerve impulse. The released NE may be metabolized within the nerve by MAO enzyme or after the activity of NE at the receptor sites, by catechol-O-methyltransferase (COMT) enzymes located in the synaptic cleft. Most NE is taken back into the nerve and stored by way of the reuptake mechanism. Antidepressant drug therapy: (1) tricyclic antidepressants block the reuptake of released NE and prevent it from reentering the adrenergic nerve. (2) MAO inhibitors block MAO located on surface of the cell mitochondria. The result is more NE available for release or available in the synapse area.

tonin, or inhibition of the MAO enzyme system, not all antidepressants have this effect. Therefore it is believed that the full range of the antidepressant central activity of these medications is probably unknown (Figure 19-3).

Depression

Over the years many classifications of depression have been used, such as the time during life that depression occurred (childhood, adolescent, or senile depression), or the reason for the depression, such as **exogenous** (reactive) **depression** or endogenous depression. Reactive or secondary depressions are often a person's response to a loss (loss of pleasure or interest in activities and everyday living caused perhaps by the loss of a loved one or the presence of a debilitating illness) or disappointment (from not meeting one's expectations or loss of a job, pet, friend, etc.). This is usually referred to as "the blues" or normal depression, which generally remits in several months without the use of antidepressant medications. The mobilization of support systems and, if necessary, psychotherapy are useful adjuncts in exogenous depression.

Unipolar or **endogenous depression** is characterized by the absence of external causes for depression. This type of depression may be caused by genetic determination and biochemical alterations (Katzung, 1992). Antidepressant medications are very useful in the treatment of this type of depression.

The current classification of depressive disorders has eliminated the use of the above terminology. Instead, major affective disorders are defined as bipolar disorders (mixed type and manic) and major depression as unipolar (single episode or recurrent episodes), along with atypical affective disorders, which include depression. Psychiatrists have debated over whether the new classification is an improvement over the previous types of classification, since it is important for the clinician to have a diagnostic framework from which to work.

Criteria for major depression include the presence of mood changes (sadness, despondency, anxiety, crying spells, guilt feelings, self-pity, pessimism, loss of interest in life and social activities), psychologic symptoms (low self-esteem, poor concentration, hopeless or helpless feelings, suicidal tendencies or increased focus on death), physiologic manifestations (sleep disturbances that may range from insomnia to hypersomnia, decreased interest in sex, complaints of fatigue, loss of energy, menstrual dysfunction, headaches, palpitations, constipation, loss of appetite, and weight loss or weight gain), and thinking alterations (a decrease in concentration or attention span, complaints of poor memory, confusion, delusions relating to health, persecution, or religion, and hallucinations if the client is also psychotic). Mood variations are usually diurnal and often worse in the morning.

Measures to treat depression include electroshock therapy, psychotherapy, reduction of environmental stressors, and milieu therapy. In a number of cases, antidepressant drug therapy in combination with one or more adjunct measures is more effective than drug therapy alone.

Selection of an Antidepressant

The primary antidepressants available include the tricyclic antidepressants (TCAs), heterocyclics, selective serotonin reuptake inhibitors (SSRIs), monoamine oxidase inhibitors (MAOIs), and other miscellaneous antidepressants. The therapeutic response rate is similar with all antidepressants; thus selection is often dependent on the side effect profile of the individual drugs (Table 19-5).

In the past, the tricyclic antidepressants were usually the first drugs prescribed for depression. Today, second-generation drugs, the SSRIs, and the miscellaneous antidepressants are often more commonly prescribed. The mechanism of action for the tricyclic and MAO antidepressants was discussed previously and illustrated in Figure 19-3. The SSRIs selectively block the reuptake of serotonin into the nerve terminal while the actions of the atypical antidepressants are less well defined.

Selection of an antidepressant is empiric, taking into consideration the side effect potential of each antidepressant compared with the medical problems of the individual client. For example, prescribers might select a sedating antidepressant (amitriptyline [Elavil], doxepin [Sinequan], or fluoxetine [Prozac]) for the agitated depressed person or the potent blockers of norepinephrine reuptake (desipramine [Norpramin], nortriptyline [Aventyl]) for a withdrawn depressive client. The Agency for Health Care Policy and Research (Depression Guideline Panel, 1993) issued tables on the selection and side effect profiles of antidepressant medications (Box 19-5 and Table19-6).

Plasma levels of the tricyclic antidepressants can vary widely between different individuals and, with the possible exception of nortriptyline (Aventyl), imipramine (Tofranil) and desipramine (Norpramin), they often do not correlate with dose or therapeutic response. Prescribers may order serum levels to monitor and help identify the noncompliant client. A low plasma level should initially indicate the need to interview the client to verify adherence to the prescribed schedule. The reason for the client's ineffective management of the therapeutic medication regimen (side effects that are intolerable to client, misunderstanding of directions, potential drug interaction, lack of finances to purchase medications) can then be identified and perhaps resolved (Laird & Benefield, 1995).

If compliance is verified and serum levels still remain low, dosage adjustments may be necessary or the prescriber might consider switching to a different antidepressant. If the client is nonresponsive to a predominantly norepinephrine-potentiating medication, a serotonin-potentiating agent might be indicated (see Table 19-5) as the individual may have bio-

TABLE 19-5 Pharmacology of antidepressant medications

Drug	Therapeutic dosage range (mg/day)	Average (range) of elimination half-lives (hr)*	Potentially fatal drug interactions
Tricyclics			
amitriptyline (Elavil, Endep)	75-300	24 (16-46)	Antiarrhythmics, MAOIs
clomipramine (Anafranil)	75-300	24 (20-40)	Antiarrhythmics, MAOIs
desipramine (Norpramin, Pertofrane)	75-300	18 (12-50)	Antiarrhythmics, MAOIs
doxepin (Adapin, Sinequan)	75-300	17 (10-47)	Antiarrhythmics, MAOIs
imipramine (Janimine, Tofranil)	75-300	22 (12-34)	Antiarrhythmics, MAOIs
nortriptyline (Aventyl, Pamelor)	40-200	26 (18-88)	Antiarrhythmics, MAOIs
protriptyline (Vivactil)	20-60	76 (54-124)	Antiarrhythmics, MAOIs
trimipramine (Surmontil)	75-300	12 (8-30)	Antiarrhythmics, MAOIs
Heterocyclics			
amoxapine (Asendin)	100-600	10 (8-14)	MAOIs
bupropion (Wellbutrin)	225-450	14 (8-24)	MAOIs (possibly)
maprotiline (Ludiomil)	100-225	43 (27-58)	MAOIs
trazodone (Desyrel)	150-600	8 (4-14)	—
Selected serotonin reuptake inhibitors (SSRIs)			
fluoxetine (Prozac)	10-40	168 (72-360)†	MAOIs
paroxetine (Paxil)	20-50	24 (3-65)	MAOIs‡
sertraline (Zoloft)	50-150	24 (10-30)	MAOIs‡
Monoamine oxidase inhibitors (MAOIs)§			For all 3 MAOIs:
isocarboxazid (Marplan)	30-50	Unknown	Vasoconstrictors‖, decongestants,‖
phenelzine (Nardil)	45-90	2 (1.5-4)	meperidine, and possibly
tranylcypromine (Parnate)	20-60	2 (1.5-3)	other narcotics

Adapted from Depression Guideline Panel. Depression in Primary Care: Volume 2. *Treatment of Major Depression*. Clinical Practice Guideline, Number 5. Rockville, MD: U.S. Department of Health and Human Services, Public Health Service, Agency for Health Care Policy and Research. AHCPR Pub. No. 93-0551. April, 1993.

*Half-lives are affected by age, sex, race, concurrent medications, and length of drug exposure.

†Includes both fluoxetine and norfluoxetine.

‡By extrapolation from fluoxetine data.

§MAO inhibition lasts longer (7 days) than drug half-life.

‖Including pseudoephedrine, phenylephrine, phenylpropanolamine, epinephrine, norepinephrine, and others.

chemical differences that would indicate a trial with the opposite reuptake blocking agent.

The elderly often have reduced liver drug metabolizing enzymes, and thus higher serum drug levels and a greater potential for side effects exist. Many prescribers start geriatric clients at one third to one half the usual adult dosage, adjusting as necessary according to therapeutic response or presence of undesirable side effects.

Tricyclic Antidepressants

Tricyclic antidepressants are indicated for the treatment of depression, enuresis (imipramine), and obsessive-compulsive disorder (clomipramine). They are well absorbed when given orally. The onset of antidepressant effect occurs within 2 to 3 weeks, and they are metabolized primarily in the liver and excreted by the kidneys. Active metabolites produced in the liver have in some instances, resulted in the marketing of new antidepressants, which are noted in parentheses.

generic (Brandname): active metabolite (Brandname if marketed)

amitriptyline (Elavil): nortriptyline (Aventyl, Pamelor)
amoxapine (Asendin): 7- and 8-hydroxyamoxapine
desipramine (Norpramin): 2 hydroxydesipramine
doxepin (Sinequan): desmethyldoxepin
imipramine (Tofranil): desipramine (Norpramin)
fluoxetine (Prozac): norfluoxetine

For half-life and additional information, see Table 19-5; side effects/adverse reactions, see Table 19-6.

clomipramine [kloe mi' pra meen] (Anafranil)
Clomipramine an analogue of imipramine, is a potent inhibitor of serotonin reuptake, and its active metabolite inhibits norepinephrine reuptake. It is indicated for the treatment of obsessive-compulsive disorders.

It is well absorbed orally, reaching the peak plasma level within 2 to 4 hours. It has a half-life of 19 to 37 hours and reaches steady-state levels in 1 to 2 weeks. Metabolism is via the liver, and excretion is in the urine.

Side effects/adverse reactions and drug interactions are similar to the other tricyclic agents. The initial adult dose is 25 mg daily gradually increased as necessary and tolerated, to 100 mg during the first 14 days. Administer in divided doses to reduce the gastrointestinal side effects. After 2 weeks the dose may be increased over several more weeks if necessary, to a maximum dose of 250 mg/day. After the dose is established, the total daily dose may be given at bedtime to reduce daytime sedation effects. In children and adolescents the initial dose is 25 mg/day; increased as necessary during the first 14 days, to a daily maximum of 3 mg/kg or 100 mg (whichever is the smaller dose). The dose may later be increased to 3 mg/kg or 200 mg (whichever is smaller) as

BOX 19-5

Selecting Among Antidepressant Medications for Depressed Outpatients

I. First- and second-line choices
   A. Secondary amine tricyclics (e.g., nortriptyline, desipramine)*
   B. Bupropion
   C. Fluoxetine
   D. Paroxetine
   E. Sertraline
   F. Trazodone
II. Alternative agents for patients with special presentations or needs
   A. Tertiary amine tricyclics (e.g., amitriptyline, imipramine)
      Special considerations:
      Absence of serious medical illnesses, including cardiac disease, that preclude use
      Need for rapid sedation
   B. Monoamine oxidase inhibitors (MAOIs)
      Special considerations:
      Nonresponse or intolerance to at least one tricyclic and one heterocyclic
      Family or personal history of MAOI response
      Atypical symptom features
   C. Selected anxiolytic medications†
      Special considerations:
      Medical contraindications to FDA-approved antidepressant medications
      No adverse cardiovascular effects
      Low side-effect profile
      Substantial withdrawal with long-term use
      Limited exposure time expected (<3 months)
      Patient has no history of substance abuse
      Quick action needed

Adapted from Depression Guideline Panel. Depression in Primary Care: Volume 2. *Treatment of Major Depression.* Clinical Practice Guideline, Number 5. Rockville, MD: U.S. Department of Health and Human Services, Public Health Service, Agency for Health Care Policy and Research. AHCPR Pub. No. 93-0551. April, 1993.
*Other first- and second-line choices are recommended for patients with arrhythmias, cardiac conduction defects, ischemic heart disease, cardiomyopathy, or cardiac valve disease.
†Evidence is clearest for alprazolam. Not recommended in severe depressions because studies reveal reduced efficacy. Not recommended for prolonged care because no studies longer than 12 weeks are available. Not recommended when FDA-approved antidepressant medications can be used safely. For buspirone, efficacy is suggested in those with primary anxiety disorders and mild associated depressive symptoms.
Note: Evidence for efficacy with severely depressed inpatients is more abundant for the standard tricyclics than for newer agents.

TABLE 19-6 Side-effect profiles of antidepressant medications

	Side effect						
		Central nervous system		Cardiovascular			Other
Drug	Anticholinergic	Drowsiness	Insomnia/agitation	Orthostatic-hypotension	Cardiac arrhythmia	Gastrointestinal distress	Weight gain (over 6 kg)
Amitriptyline	4+	4+	0	4+	3+	0	4+
Desipramine	1+	1+	1+	2+	2+	0	1+
Doxepin	3+	4+	0	2+	2+	0	3+
▲Imipiramine	3+	3+	1+	4+	3+	1+	3+
Nortriptyline	1+	1+	0	2+	2+	0	1+
Protriptyline	2+	1+	1+	2+	2+	0	0
Trimipramine	1+	4+	0	2+	2+	0	3+
Amoxapine	2+	2+	2+	2+	3+	0	1+
Maprotiline	2+	4+	0	0	1+	0	2+
Trazodone	0	4+	0	1+	1+	1+	1+
Bupropion	0	0	2+	0	1+	1+	0
Fluoxetine	0	0	2+	0	0	3+	0
Paroxetine	0	0	2+	0	0	3+	0
Sertraline	0	0	2+	0	0	3+	0
Monoamine oxidase inhibitors (MAOIs)	1	1+	2+	2+	0	1+	2+

Adapted from Depression Guideline Panel. Depression in Primary Care: Volume 2. *Treatment of Major Depression.* Clinical Practice Guideline, Number 5. Rockville, MD: U.S. Department of Health and Human Services, Public Health Service, Agency for Health Care Policy and Research. AHCPR Pub. No. 93-0551. April, 1993.

*0 = absent or rare
1+
2+ = in between
3+
4+ = relatively common
†Dry mouth, blurred vision, urinary hesitancy, constipation

necessary. Once the titrated dose is established, the entire daily dose may be administered at bedtime.

■ Nursing Management

Tricyclic Antidepressant Therapy

Assessment. Tricyclic antidepressants should not be administered to clients in the acute recovery phase of a myocardial infarction. The benefits of this drug therapy versus the risks must be considered for clients with increased intraocular pressure, prostatic hypertrophy, history of urinary retention, or history of narrow-angle glaucoma, because tricyclic antidepressants possess significant anticholinergic properties; for clients with hyperthyroid conditions or those taking thyroid medication, because of the possibility of cardiovascular toxicity; and for individuals with a past history of seizure disorders, because this class of drugs has been demonstrated to lower the seizure threshold. Conditions that may be aggravated by the administration of tricyclic antidepressants are asthma, blood disorders, GI disorders (risk of paralytic ileus), and cardiovascular disorders (risk of arrhythmias, congestive heart failure, heart block, or stroke). Clients with active alcoholism may potentiate any CNS depressant effects of the antidepressants. Those with hepatic and renal dysfunction may experience accumulation of the drug because of impairment of the drug's metabolism and excretion. In addition, clients with schizophrenia may have their condition activated, and those with bipolar disorders may have their swings from mania and depression and back accelerated. When tricyclic antidepressants are administered to pregnant clients, the potential benefits should be weighed against the potential risks to the fetus.

A thorough drug history is required to ensure that the client does not have any drug allergies to tricyclic antidepressants, carbamazepine (Tegretol), maprotiline (Ludiomil), or trazodone (Desyrel) for which the drug would be contraindicated, or that the concurrent drug regimen does not have any significant drug interactions. The following effects may occur when tricyclic antidepressants are given with the drugs listed below:

Drug	Possible effect and management
alcohol or CNS depressants	May result in enhanced CNS depressant effects; avoid concurrent use if possible, or reduce dosage of one or both drugs and monitor closely.
antithyroid drugs	**May increase risk of inducing agranulocytosis. Avoid or a potentially serious drug interaction may occur.**

Drug	Possible effect and management
cimetidine (Tagamet)	May inhibit metabolism of tricyclic agent, leading to increased serum levels and toxicity; lower tricyclic dosage by 20% to 30% and monitor closely.
clonidine (Catapres), guanadrel (Hylorel), or guanethidine (Ismelin)	May decrease the antihypertensive effects of these drugs; monitor BP closely because dosage changes or alternate antihypertensive agents may be necessary. Clonidine and tricyclic antidepressants may increase risk of CNS depression; monitor closely for lethargy, confusion, and respiratory depression.
contraceptives, oral	May increase or decrease tricyclic serum levels; monitor closely for decreased therapeutic response or drug toxicity; dosage adjustments may be necessary.
extrapyramidal-inducing medications; amoxapine (Asendin), phenothiazines, haloperidol (Haldol), metoclopramide (Reglan), reserpine (Serpalan), thioxanthenes	May increase risk and severity of extrapyramidal adverse effects. With phenothiazines, sedative and anticholinergic side effects may be enhanced; monitor closely.
metrizamide intrathecal (Amipaque)	Concurrent use of tricyclic antidepressants increases risk of inducing seizures because of a lowered seizure threshold. Discontinue tricyclic agents at least 2 days before and 1 day after a myelogram.
MAO inhibitors	Should be contraindicated in outpatient settings; hypertensive crises, severely elevated temperatures, convulsions, and death have been reported with concurrent administration of MAO inhibitors and tricyclic antidepressants. Before switching from one classification to the other, at least a 2-week drug-free period from either category should be instituted. If concurrent use is prescribed in an inpatient setting, it would require strict supervision and close monitoring because of the potentially serious adverse effects. See current *USP DI* for dosing recommendations.
sympathomimetics	**May increase possibility of potentiating cardiovascular toxicities (severe hypertension, dysrhythmias, tachycardia) or severely elevated body temperatures. Avoid or a potentially serious drug interaction may occur.**

Clients must be closely assessed at the start of therapy and monitored closely throughout therapy for suicide potential. The risk of suicide increases as therapy improves the client's depressed state and energy levels increase.

Nursing diagnosis. Clients receiving tricyclic antidepressants may experience the following nursing diagnoses: altered thought processes related to the ineffectiveness of the drugs; risk for injury related to the drug's adverse CNS effects (blurred vision, confusion, tremors, hypotension, drowsiness); altered mucous membranes (dry mouth); altered nutrition: more than required related to appetite stimulating effects of the drug; altered comfort (nausea, headache); and the potential complications related to the drug's anticholinergic properties (confusion, hallucinations, blurred vision, urinary retention, constipation).

Implementation

Monitoring. The client's blood pressure and pulse should be monitored at appropriate intervals. Note that the possibility of suicide is inherent in any severely depressed client and persists until a significant remission occurs. The suicidal risks of tricyclic antidepressants are especially high, and suicide attempts with tricyclic antidepressants are frequently seen in many emergency departments. When a client has a serious overt suicidal potential and is not hospitalized, the quantity of the tricyclic antidepressant should not exceed 1 week's supply. See the box on p. 384 for management of tricyclic antidepressant overdose.

In clients with schizophrenia, activation of the psychosis may occur, requiring reduction of the dosage or the addition of a major tranquilizer to the therapeutic regimen. Manic or hypomanic episodes may occur in individuals with the cyclic type of disorders. If this occurs, the tricyclic antidepressant should be discontinued until the episode is relieved and then may be reinstituted at a lowered dosage if still needed in the therapy.

Use extreme caution (ECG, BP and pulse monitoring, nursing observations) when the tricyclic antidepressants are administered to clients who have any evidence of cardiovascular disease because of the possibility of conduction defects, dysrhythmias, myocardial infarction, cerebrovascular accidents, and tachycardia. The quinidine-like cardiac effects are well documented in the literature. With amoxapine (Asendin), monitor closely for early symptoms of tardive dyskinesia.

Intervention. Initial dosages in adolescent, elderly, and debilitated clients should be lower and increased gradually. The medication should not be withdrawn abruptly. In resistant cases of depression in adults, a dose of 2.5 mg/kg body weight/day or higher may have to be exceeded in the hospital. If such a dose or higher is necessary, maintain ECG monitoring during the initiation of therapy and at appropriate intervals during stabilization of the dose.

If the client is to be evaluated by plasma tricyclic determination because of a failure to respond to treatment, increased side effects, or questionable compliance, blood samples should be taken immediately before the first morning dose or at least 8 hours after a dose.

Education. During initiation or change of therapy the client should avoid activities that require coordination and alertness until psychomotor response to the tricyclic antidepressant therapy has been determined.

Alert the client to report anticholinergic effects of the drugs, such as blurred vision, altered thought processes, constipation, difficulty starting urinary stream, and eye pain, which may be indicative of glaucoma. The client

⚠ MANAGEMENT OF DRUG OVERDOSE

Tricyclic antidepressant

Tricyclic antidepressant (TCA) overdose can be life-threatening, resulting in serious adverse reactions such as heart block, cardiac arrhythmias, hypotension, seizures, coma, and in some instances fatalities. In the United States, the third most common drug-induced death is due to TCA overdoses (Montano, 1994).

Montano (1994, p 32) also states that "70% to 80% of people who take overdoses of TCAs do not reach the hospital alive." It is therefore critically important that health care professionals know how to deal with a tricyclic overdose.

Signs and symptoms

The signs and symptoms of a TCA overdose may vary in severity, depending on numerous factors including the amount ingested and absorbed, the age of the individual, and the interval between ingestion and initiation of a treatment modality. Any acute overdose or unwarranted ingestion of a TCA in children or adults must be considered serious and potentially fatal.

CNS abnormalities include agitation, ataxia, choreoathetoid movements, drowsiness, hyperactive reflexes, muscle rigidity, restlessness, stupor, seizures, and coma. Cardiac abnormalities may include dysrhythmia, ECG evidence of impaired conduction, signs of congestive heart failure, and tachycardia. Quinidine-like adverse effects are common in poisonings with tricyclic antidepressants.

Treatment

Symptomatic and supportive measures are instituted according to the individual client's requirement. They may include:

- emesis and/or use of gastric lavage to empty stomach followed by administration of activated charcoal to absorb any remaining drug in the GI tract.
- close monitoring of cardiovascular functioning for at least 5 days. Cardiac dysrhythmias have occurred up to 6 days after massive TCA doses, which may require treatment with lidocaine or phenytoin.
- maintainance of body temperature and respiratory and cardiac functions.
- for all tricyclics except amoxapine, physostigmine salicylate may need to be administered. The use of this product is directed at persons with life-threatening signs such as coma with respiratory depression, very serious cardiac arrhythmias, severe hypertension, or uncontrollable convulsions. Physostigmine salicylate is not administered for amoxapine overdoses because it has the potential of increasing seizure activity.
- administration of anticonvulsants such as diazepam (Valium), phenytoin (Dilantin), paraldehyde, or an inhalation anesthetic to control seizures.

Be aware that hemodialysis, peritoneal dialysis, forced diuresis, and exchange transfusions are not successful in treating a TCA overdose (*USP DI*, 1996).

should be advised to schedule regular appointments with the health care professional for periodic blood cell counts, glaucoma tests, and hepatic and renal function studies. Because dry mouth is a common side effect, the client should be taught appropriate oral hygiene to prevent caries and other dental problems. In addition, breath mints may be reassuring to the client in social situations. Ice chips and sugarless candies are also helpful in promoting comfort.

Self-alteration of the prescribed medications or consumption of other medication, including over-the-counter medications, should not be done without the prescriber's approval. Clients should be specifically instructed to avoid alcoholic beverages during the tricyclic antidepressant regimen because CNS depression may be heightened.

Orthostatic hypotension may occur. The nurse should instruct the client to come to a standing position slowly and carefully to avoid feeling faint.

The nurse should caution the client that therapeutic response to tricyclic antidepressants is not immediate. It may be 10 to 14 days before there is demonstrated effect and 30 days for full effect.

Note that an emerging public health problem is tricyclic antidepressant poisoning or overdose in children. Doses in excess of 10 mg/kg body weight are potentially dangerous. The incidents are characterized as accidental because most occur when the drug is given to a household member for depression or to an enuretic child. Alert the adult family member to the possibility of accidental overdose and the need for security and administrative responsibility over the medication.

Evaluation. If tricyclic antidepressant therapy is successful, the client will report an improvement of depression. Clinically the client will participate in more activities, initiate social interaction, and take more of an interest in his or her own appearance. Vital signs, ECG, and bowel elimination will be normal and the client will not experience any adverse CNS effects of the tricyclic antidepressants.

Heterocyclic Antidepressants

The heterocyclic or second-generation antidepressants include amoxapine (Asendin), bupropion (Wellbutrin), maprotiline (Ludiomil), mirtazapine (Remeron), and trazodone (Desyrel). Generally, these agents have fewer long-term side effects (such as weight gain) than the tricyclic antidepressants, plus they have other advantages and disadvantages that need to be considered.

Amoxapine (Asendin), an active metabolite of loxapine (an antipsychotic agent), inhibits the reuptake of norepinephrine and is a potent dopamine-blocking agent. The latter effect may result in extrapyramidal side effects and neuroleptic malignant syndrome (Olin, 1996). With therapeutic doses, amoxapine and maprotiline have fewer cardiovascular side effects than the tricyclic agents (Laird & Benefield, 1995). An amoxapine overdose, though, may result in seizures and status epilepticus within 12 hours of ingestion. Renal failure has also been reported with an amoxapine overdose.

Bupropion's (Wellbutrin) mechanism of action is unknown although it weakly blocks the reuptake of dopamine, serotonin and norepinephrine. This drug and the newer agents are used for persons who are nonresponsive to other antidepressants. Bupropion has fewer anticholinergic effects, rarely produces hypotension or sexual dysfunction but is reported to cause agitation, insomnia, tremors and dose-related seizures (Abramowicz, 1994).

Maprotiline (Ludiomil) is similar to the tricyclic antidepressants except it is associated with an increased risk of skin rash (redness, swelling, pruritus) and seizures. Seizures have been reported with therapeutic daily doses of maprotiline in persons without any history of seizures (Wells, 1994). Therefore this product is contraindicated in anyone with a history of seizures.

Trazodone (Desyrel) is chemically different from the other antidepressants. It blocks serotonin reuptake and also produces changes in the binding at serotonin receptors. Trazodone has few if any anticholinergic effects and thus has minimal effects on cardiac conduction. The prescriber should still use caution in using this drug with persons with a history of cardiac disease because several cases of ventricular arrhythmia have been reported with its use. However, in the United States trazodone overdoses alone have not resulted in severe cardiac abnormalities and death (Brown & Bryant, 1992).

Monoamine Oxidase (MAO) Inhibitor Antidepressants

Monoamine oxidase inhibitors (MAOIs) are indicated as second- or third-line antidepressants for the treatment of depression that does not respond to other, safer antidepressants (Depression Guideline Panel, 1993). These agents have numerous drug interactions with prescription and OTC medications, caffeine, and tyramine-containing foods and beverages. The major adverse reaction with these agents is the occurrence of a sudden and possibly very severe hypertension that if untreated can progress to vascular collapse and fatality.

Monoamine oxidase, an enzyme found in nerve terminals, the liver, and the brain, is necessary to the inactivation and degradation of tyramine, catecholamines, serotonin, and various medications. The MAOIs interfere with this inactivation, which may result in a potentiation of vasopressor effects and serious adverse effects.

Two types of MAO enzymes have been identified and named—MAO-A and MAO-B. MAO-A appears to have a preference for serotonin and is located throughout the body, with high concentrations located in the human placenta. MAO-B is mainly contained in human platelets, but approximately equal amounts of both types are found in the liver and brain. The MAO inhibitor drugs in current use are nonselective.

The MAOIs are capable of blocking or diminishing the activity of MAO, resulting in a net increase in brain amine levels. Current research indicates that the MAOIs produce desensitization of the $alpha_2$ or beta and serotonin receptors (down-regulation). During early clinical trials of MAOIs as antidepressants, orthostatic hypotension was encountered as a common but inconsistent side effect, thus many MAOIs were produced and studied specifically as antidepressant and antihypertensive agents.

The MAOIs discussed in this section are those used as antidepressants: the hydrazines—isocarboxazid (Marplan) and phenelzine (Nardil)—and the nonhydrazine, tranylcypromine sulfate (Parnate). The MAOIs are indicated primarily in resistant depression and anxious and hostile depression, especially those also involving panic attacks or phobic symptoms.

MAOIs can increase the concentration of all central amines, although different effects on the individual amines are possible. For example, some of the MAOIs may increase dopamine or norepinephrine concentrations to a more extensive degree than serotonin concentrations, whereas other MAOIs may raise the level of serotonins to a greater degree than those of norepinephrine and dopamine. The increase in amine concentration is associated with behavioral hyperactivity (amphetamine-like psychomotor stimulation with large doses) produced by the MAOIs and, in some cases, with the exacerbation of psychotic symptoms. In lower doses antiphobic and antidepressant activities are seen. In general these compounds are most effective in reversing the dysphoric state and its attendant vegetative disturbances in clients with depressive syndromes.

The therapeutic doses of the MAOIs take from days to weeks to attain a maximal therapeutic effect. MAOIs produce an irreversible inactivation of MAO by forming a stable complex with the enzyme; recovery from the effect of MAOIs thus depends on enzyme regeneration, which may occur over several weeks. Inhibition occurs only in very high doses and may be responsible for some of the toxic effects of MAOIs. The mechanism of action of MAOIs was discussed in the previous section. The MAOIs are well absorbed orally; onset of action in some individuals occurs from 7 to 10 days while full effect usually takes from 4 to 8 weeks of therapy. These agents irreversibly bind MAO activity; recovery may take 10 days to 2 weeks. MAOIs are metabolized in the liver and excreted primarily by the kidneys. Side effects/adverse reactions are discussed in Table 19-6.

Dosage and administration. See Table 19-5. See box on p. 369 for pregnancy safety ratings.

■ Nursing Management

MAO Inhibitor Therapy

Assessment. MAOIs should not be administered to clients with active alcoholism, congestive heart failure, pheochromocytoma (because the tumors secrete pressor substances), severe hepatic impairment (may precipitate hepatic precoma), or renal function impairment (drug may accumulate). Clients with the following conditions should consider the risk-benefits of taking MAOIs: cardiac arrhythmias, cardiovascular or cerebrovascular disease (ischemia and conduction disturbances may occur); headaches (may mask hypertensive reaction); or hypotension or history of sympathectomy (hypotension may be potentiated). Hypertensive clients may experience a hypertensive crisis from dietary lapses. MAOIs may aggravate psychosis in clients with schizophrenia. The nurse should be aware that overactive, overstimulated, or agitated clients usually do not respond well to MAO inhibitors since the drugs may cause stimulation. These drugs are also contraindicated in many other conditions.

Because MAO inhibitors interact with numerous drugs, often with severe consequences, it is important for the nurse to complete a thorough drug history to determine any significant drug interactions. This should include the month prior to the administration as well as the concurrent therapy. The following effects may occur when MAO inhibitors are given with the drugs listed below:

Drug	Possible effect and management
alcohol or CNS depressants	May enhance CNS depressive effects. If alcohol contains tyramine, may result in severe hypertensive reaction. Avoid or a potentially serious drug interaction may occur.
local anesthetics containing epinephrine or cocaine	May result in very severe hypertensive reaction. Cocaine should not be administered during or within 2 weeks after an MAO inhibitor. Avoid or a potentially serious drug interaction may occur.
antidepressants, tricyclics, carbamazepine (Tegretol), maprotiline (Ludiomil), other MAO inhibitors, furazolidone, (Furoxone), selegiline (Eldepryl) or procarbazine (Matulane)	May result in severely elevated temperatures, hypertensive crises, severe seizures, and death. Avoid or a potentially serious drug interaction may occur. Before switching from one of these medications to an MAO inhibitor or vice versa, a 2-week drug-free period should be instituted. Several studies have used tri-cyclic antidepressants with an MAO inhibitor for refractory depression. See current USP DI for explicit instructions on proper dosing and monitoring of this combination.
antidiabetic agents (oral or insulin)	Enhanced hypoglycemic effects reported. Reduction in oral hypoglycemic agent may be required during or even after concurrent drug therapy.
bupropion (Wellbutrin)	Concurrent use increases the risk of bupropion toxicity. A 2 week interval is recommended from the discontinuance of MAOIs and the start of bupropion therapy.
buspirone (BuSpar)	May cause hypertension. Avoid or a serious drug interaction may occur.
caffeine (e.g., drug products, coffee, tea, chocolate, cola) carbamazepine (Tegretol), cyclobenzaprine (Flexeril), maprotiline (Ludiomil), or other MAO inhibitors	May result in severe cardiac dysrhythmias or hypertension. Avoid or a serious drug interaction may occur. May result in severe hypertensive crises, convulsions, and death. At least a 2-week drug-free interval is recommended to avoid this reaction.
dextromethorphan (Benylin DM, Robitussin DM)	May result in increased excitability, hyperpyrexia, and hypertension. Avoid or a serious drug interaction may occur.
doxapram (Dopram)	Enhanced and severe hypertensive effects may result. Avoid or a potentially serious drug interaction may occur.
fluoxetine (Prozac)	May result in agitation, restlessness, gastrointestinal distress, or seizures and hypertensive crises. Avoid or a potentially serious drug interaction may occur. For client safety, a minimum of a 2-week drug-free period should be instituted when switching from an MAO inhibitor to fluoxetine. When switching from fluoxetine to an MAO inhibitor, a 5-week drug-free period should be implemented.
guanadrel (Hylorel), guanethidine (Ismelin), or rauwolfia alkaloids	May result in severe hypertension. Withdraw MAOI at least 7 days before starting therapy with these agents. Rauwolfia alkaloid: if an MAOI is added to a medication schedule already containing a rauwolfia alkaloid, serious CNS depression may result. If a rauwolfia alkaloid is added to a medication schedule that already includes an MAOI, hypertension and increased excitability may result. Avoid or a potentially serious drug interaction may occur.
levodopa (L-dopa)	*Avoid this combination.* Severe and sudden hypertensive crisis reported. Before starting levodopa therapy, the client should be withdrawn from MAOIs with at least a 2 to 4 week drug-free period.
meperidine (Demerol) and perhaps other opioid narcotics	Severe hypertension, increased excitability, sweating, and rigidity reported with concurrent use. Also in some individuals, hypotension, seizures, elevated temperature, respiratory depression, cardiovascular collapse, coma, and death reported, which may be caused by serotonin accumulation from the MAOI. Avoid or a potentially serious drug interaction may occur. Do not use meperidine for at least 14 to 21 days after an MAOI is stopped. Morphine and other narcotics are not reported as causing such a severe reaction, but it is recommended that the opioid dosage be reduced to one-fourth (test dose) the usual dosage. Monitor closely whenever opioids or anesthesia adjuncts (fentanyl [Sublimaze], sufentanil [Sufenta]) are given to clients who have received MAOIs in the previous 2 or 3 weeks.
methyldopa (Aldomet)	Severe headache, hypertension, hallucinations, and increased excitability have been reported. Avoid or a serious drug interaction may occur.
methylphenidate (Ritalin)	Concurrent use may result in a hypertensive crisis. Avoid or a serious drug interaction may occur. At least a 2-week drug-free period should be allowed before instituting methylphenidate therapy.
sympathomimetics, systemic	Direct-acting (dopamine, mephentermine, metaraminol, dobutamine, methoxamine, and phenylephrine) or indirect-acting (amphetamines, phenylpropanolamine, and pseudoephedrine) or combination effects (ephedrine) should not be given during or within 2 weeks of an MAOI. Severe hypertensive crisis, elevated temperatures, cardiac dysrhythmias,

Drug	Possible effect and management
sympathomim—cont'd	**headaches, and vomiting have been reported. Avoid or a serious drug interaction may occur.**
tryptophan, especially tranylcypromine (Parnate)	May result in hyperventilation, increased temperature, shivering, disorientation, mania, or hypomania. If necessary to use both drugs, start tryptophan in low doses and increase dose slowly. Monitor mental status and blood pressure closely.
tyramine or high pressor-containing foods and beverages (see Box 19-6)	**Sudden, severe hypertensive crisis has been reported. Avoid or a potentially serious drug interaction may occur. Client teaching is crucial for individuals receiving MAOI drugs. MAO inhibitors and tyramine or high pressor amine-containing foods or beverages must be avoided during therapy and for a minimum of 2 weeks after therapy is discontinued.**

A baseline assessment should include a documentation of the client's symptoms of depression, blood pressure, and renal and hepatic function studies.

Nursing diagnosis. The client receiving MAO inhibitor therapy has the potential for the following selected nursing diagnoses: sleep pattern disturbance related to CNS stimulation; activity intolerance (weakness); altered comfort (headache, increased perspiration); diarrhea; risk for injury related to blurred vision, orthostatic hypotension, or weakness; fluid volume excess (edema); altered nutrition: more than required, related to carbohydrate craving; sexual dysfunction (anorgasmia, ejaculatory disorders, impotence); and the potential complications of CNS stimulation (restlessness, twitching, agitation), hypertensive crises, hepatitis, leucopenia, and the anticholinergic effects of MAOIs (blurred vision, dry mouth, urinary retention, constipation).

Implementation

Monitoring. The client's statements and behaviors related to depression should be documented. Blood pressure should be monitored regularly to detect evidence of dangerous fluctuations in pressure during therapy, such as pressor amine response and orthostatic hypotension. Monitor ECG for changes. Weigh biweekly and maintain intake and output. Periodic liver function tests (bilirubin, alkaline phosphatase, or transaminase) should be performed, and darkened urine and jaundice as signs of drug-induced hepatitis should be reported to the prescriber.

It should be noted that the suicidal tendencies present with the client's condition may compound the nursing care issues because of the delayed effect of these drugs in relieving suicidal tendencies. This effect presents an additional risk to the client during initial phases of drug therapy. The nurse should be alert to the possibility of any impulsive ingestion of these substances.

Because the risk of suicide is frequently higher near the end of the depressive cycle, attention should be given to the possibility of suicidal attempts during this period. Overt client behavior may indicate a remission of depressive symptoms; however, this may be caused by drug action and not by alleviation of pathologic processes. Antidepressants should generally be continued for several months after the remission of symptoms and should never be discontinued abruptly, since a relapse may occur.

Intervention. During hospitalization the nurse should note that the depressed client's anorexia may prompt well-meaning family members or friends to bring supplementary foods to the client or a little wine to stimulate the appetite. Careful nursing observation during visiting hours and instruction of the family regarding restrictions on tyramine or high pressor-containing foods and beverages can avoid serious consequences. Communication with the hospital dietitian may also prevent these foods from appearing on the client's hospital menu. The drug should be discontinued immediately when any adverse signs and symptoms occur. Fever should be managed by external cooling. To control severe hypertension reactions, phentolamine mesylate (Regitine) should be on hand (5 mg to be administered slowly intravenously to avoid hypotensive effect).

Because these drugs usually cause some agitation and insomnia, they are not administered late in the evening.

Education. Because of the possible food-drug interactions, the nurse should teach the client and family which foods

BOX 19-6

Tyramine-Containing Substances

Tyramine content of foods varies according to the references reviewed. This variation may result from different conditions or preparation of the foods, different food samples, or different producers or manufacturers. The major goal should be to advise the client to avoid foods and drinks with reported moderate- to high-tyramine content as follows:

Cheese: aged (blue, boursault, natural brick, brie, camembert, cheddar, emmenthaler, gruyere, mozzarella, parmesan, romano, roquefort, stilton)

Meat and fish: beef and chicken liver, unrefrigerated, fermented; caviar, fish, unrefrigerated, fermented; fish, dried; herring, dried, salted, and pickled; fermented sausages (bologna, pepperoni, salami, summer sausage) and any other unrefrigerated, fermented meats

Vegetables: overripe avocado and overripe fava beans

Fruit: overripe figs, bananas, and raisins

Alcoholic beverages: red wines, especially Chianti; sherry; beer; liquors

Other foods may contain tyramine or high-pressor amines but when eaten in moderation and only when fresh, they are said to be less apt to cause a serious reaction (*USP DI*, 1996). Such foods include yogurt, sour cream, cream cheese, cottage cheese, chocolate, and soy sauce.

may cause a severe reaction (Box 19-6). Tyramine-containing foods and beverages should not be ingested for at least 2 to 3 weeks after discontinuance of drug therapy. As the client's depression lifts or if electroshock therapy is used concomitantly with drug therapy, reinstruction of the client may be necessary.

The nurse should teach the client and family to recognize the adverse effects of this drug, to know the dietary precautions, and to understand drug reactions that precipitate adverse reactions. This knowledge may avert the cardiovascular effects. Because orthostatic hypotension is a common side effect, the nurse should instruct the client to come to a sitting or lying position slowly to avoid syncope.

Drowsiness occurs during initiation or change of therapy, so the client should be instructed to avoid activities requiring coordination and alertness until the response to therapy has been determined.

The client should be alerted to the signs and symptoms of hypertensive crisis: severe headache or chest pain, increased photosensitivity, nausea and vomiting, bradycardia or tachycardia, and diaphoresis. The client should check with a physician or hospital emergency department immediately. The client should wear a medical identification band that indicates MAOI therapy and should be instructed to alert health care providers to the MAOI regimen if dental or emergency care is required.

The nurse should advise the client to observe all the rules of caution involved in MAOI therapy for at least 14 days after medication is discontinued.

Evaluation. The client's behavior and communication indicate an improvement of depression without the client experiencing adverse CNS or cardiovascular symptoms.

SSRIs

Selective serotonin reuptake inhibitors (SSRIs) are safer and as effective as the other antidepressants. Fluoxetine (Prozac), the first SSRI released in this category, was followed by fluvoxamine (Luvox), paroxetine (Paxil) and sertraline (Zoloft). All but fluvoxamine are used to treat depression while fluoxetine and fluvoxamine are used to treat obsessive-compulsive disorders. Unlike the tricyclic agents that often cause weight gain, the SSRIs, with the exception of paroxetine, may cause anorexia and weight loss (Olin, 1996).

See Table 19-5 for pharmacology and dosing information.

Fluoxetine and paroxetine are well absorbed, sertraline absorption is slow but fairly consistent; onset of action is 1 to 4 weeks; metabolism in the liver with excretion via the kidneys and feces. See Table 19-6 for side effects.

Other Miscellaneous Antidepressants

The other miscellaneous antidepressants include nefazodone (Serzone) and venlafaxine (Effexor). While the mechanism of action for nefazodone is unknown, it does inhibit serotonin and norepinephrine reuptake and also is a serotonin receptor antagonist. The greatest effect of venlafaxine and its active metabolite is interference with the reuptake of serotonin. To a lesser degree it also interferes with reuptake of norepinephrine and dopamine.

Both products are well absorbed orally; half-life of nefazodone is 2 to 4 hours while venlafaxine and its active metabolite is 3 to 5 hours and 9 to 11 hours, respectively. With both drugs, the onset of antidepressant effects is several weeks. They are metabolized in the body and liver and excreted primarily by the kidneys.

Reported nefazodone (Serzone) side effects include nightmares, constipation or diarrhea, sedation, dry mouth, agitation, increase in appetite and cough, insomnia, nausea, vomiting, paresthesia, peripheral edema, and tremors. Adverse effects include ataxia, blurred vision or visual disturbances, lightheadedness, skin rash, pruritus, and tinnitus.

Venlafaxine (Effexor) side effects include nightmares, anorexia and weight loss, weakness, chills, constipation or diarrhea, lightheadedness, dry mouth, dyspepsia, sweating, insomnia, nausea, vomiting, abdominal gas or pain, taste alterations, tremors and rhinitis; adverse effects include sexual dysfunction, visual disturbances, and headaches. Some of these effects such as sexual dysfunction, nausea, vomiting, anorexia, tremors, and chills, may be dose-related.

The usual adult dose for nefazodone is 100 mg bid; for venlafaxine 25 mg tid with food. Doses may be increased according to the individual's response and tolerance for the product. See the box on p. 369 for pregnancy safety.

ANTIMANIC THERAPY

Mania is characterized by the presence of speech and motor hyperactivity, reduced sleep requirements, flight of ideas, grandiosity, elation, poor judgment, aggressiveness, and possibly hostility. The manic state is seen with recurrent manic symptoms with little or no depression, whereas bipolar affective disorders have both an acute manic phase and a hypomanic state or alternating periods of mania and depression. Counseling, psychotherapy, and drug therapy are useful for the treatment of bipolar disorders. While lithium is considered the drug of choice for this disorder, carbamazepine (Tegretol) and valproic acid (Depakene) have been used investigationally for persons that are not responsive or unable to take lithium (*USP DI*, 1996; Love & Grothe, 1995). These agents are approved as anticonvulsants and are reviewed in Chapter 17. The following is a list of lithium products:

lithium carbonate capsules [lith' ee um] (Eskalith, Carbolith ♣)
lithium carbonate tablets (Eskalith, Lithane)
lithium carbonate extended-release tablets (Lithobid, Eskalith CR)
lithium citrate syrup (Cibalith-S)

Lithium's mechanism of action has not been established. It is theorized that lithium accelerates the presynaptic destruction of catecholamines (serotonin, dopamine, and norepinephrine), inhibits transmitter release at the synapse, and decreases postsynaptic receptor sensitivity with the result that the presumed overactive catecholamine systems in mania are corrected.

Sodium in the cells has been reported to increase as much as 200% in manic clients. Lithium and sodium are both actively transported across cell membranes, but lithium cannot be as effectively pumped out of the cell as sodium. Thus lithium may stabilize cell membranes.

The third mechanism is lithium blockade of the inositol tri- and diphosphate system in the CNS, that is, its effects on the second messengers necessary for alpha-adrenergic and muscarinic transmission. At the current time, the latter is the most accepted theory (Katzung, 1992).

The drug is indicated in the treatment of manic-depressive illness, although it is being investigated for other uses. With the exception of the slow-release dosage form, lithium is completely absorbed in 6 to 8 hours and has a half-life in adults of 24 hours, in adolescents of 18 hours, and in geriatric clients of up to 36 hours. Time to peak serum levels is for syrup, 30 minutes; capsules/tablets, 1 to 3 hours; and extended-release tablets, 4 hours. Therapeutic serum levels for the treatment of bipolar disorder is: acute, 0.8 to 1.2 mEq/L and maintenance, 0.5 to 1 mEq/L. Clinical response is usually reported in 1 to 3 weeks. Lithium is not metabolized and is primarily excreted by the kidneys unchanged.

The most frequent side effects include tremors of hands (slight), thirst, nausea, increased urination, and diarrhea. Less frequent adverse reactions include tachycardia, increased weakness, weight gain, respiratory difficulties (on exertion), fainting, and irregular pulse rate. Early signs of toxicity include diarrhea, anorexia, muscle weakness, nausea, vomiting, tremors, slurred speech, and drowsiness. Later signs are blurred vision, convulsions, severe trembling, confusion, ataxia, and increased production of urine.

The usual adult dose for acute mania for lithium is 300 to 600 mg 3 times daily, adjusted according to client's response and tolerance up to a maximum dose of 2.4 g/day. Maintenance dose is 300 mg 3 or 4 times a day. Geriatric clients usually require a lower dosage. The dose for children up to 12 years old is 15-20 mg/kg in 2 or 3 divided doses, adjusted according to response.

■ Nursing Management

Lithium Therapy

Assessment. Lithium is contraindicated in clients with a history of leukemia, since it may be reactivated with its administration. In addition, lithium may exacerbate cardiovascular disease; CNS conditions, such as epilepsy and parkinsonism; and psoriasis. If the client has a severe infection with prolonged sweating, diarrhea, or vomiting, it may necessitate a reduction in the lithium dosage to prevent toxicity caused by dehydration. When lithium excretion is delayed by renal insufficiency, it may also lead to toxicity.

Lithium should not be administered to pregnant women during the first trimester unless the potential benefits outweigh the risks to the fetus. Lithium is excreted in the breast milk of lactating mothers in quantities sufficient to cause lithium toxicity in the child; this prohibits its use in breast-feeding mothers.

The client's concurrent medication regimen should be reviewed to detect any significant drug interactions. The following effects may occur when lithium is given with the drugs listed below:

Drug	Possible effect and management
antithyroid drugs, calcium iodide, potassium iodide, or iodinated glycerol	May enhance the hypothyroid goitrogenic effects of lithium or these medications; monitor closely for lethargy, intolerance to cold, etc.
antiinflammatory analgesics, nonsteroidal	May decrease excretion of lithium leading to increased lithium levels and toxicity; monitor closely for blurred vision, confusion, and dizziness.
chlorpromazine (Thorazine), possibly other phenothiazines	Concurrent use has reduced absorption of chlorpromazine (and possibly other phenothiazines) up to 40%. Reduced serum levels may lead to treatment failure. Also, an increased rate of lithium excretion has been reported. Adverse effects, especially neurotoxic and extrapyramidal ones, and delirium are reportedly increased in the elderly. Nausea, vomiting, and other signs of lithium toxicity may be masked by the phenothiazines. Monitor physical symptoms and drug serum levels closely.
diuretics	Decreased lithium excretion resulting in an increased lithium level and toxicity. A reduction in lithium dosage may be indicated. Monitor closely (see Box 19-7 for other factors affecting lithium serum levels).
fluoxetine (Prozac)	Lithium serum levels may be altered. Monitor serum lithium levels.
haloperidol (Haldol)	Concurrent use in early therapy has been associated with irreversible neurologic toxicity and brain damage in some cases. The clients usually had organic brain syndrome or another CNS impairment. However, this interaction is controversial within the professions. Be aware that extrapyramidal signs and symptoms may be increased with this combination and clients should be closely monitored whenever this combination is used.
molindone (Moban)	Concurrent use may result in neurotoxicity, as evidenced by confusion, convulsions, delirium, or abnormal EEG changes. Avoid concurrent administration.

BOX 19-7

Factors Affecting Lithium Serum Levels

	Excretion:
Increased by:	
Diarrhea	Decreased
Diuretics or dehydration	Decreased
Low-salt diets	Decreased
High fevers or strenuous exercise	Decreased
Decreased by:	
High salt intake	Increased
High intake of sodium bicarbonate	Increased
Pregnancy	Increased

A baseline assessment should include documentation of the client's symptoms, weight, BP, ECG, electrolyte and renal function determinations, and WBC and differential count.

Implementation

Monitoring. The nurse should assess the history of manic episodes, occurrence, and degree of severity, along with the cyclic appearance of pattern. Family intervention for treatment when manic-depressive symptoms appear is essential.

Serum lithium determinations are recommended once or twice weekly during the client's manic phase and until the client is stabilized; testing is done every 2 to 3 months while the client is in remission. Test samples are to be drawn just before the morning dose of lithium when there is maximum stabilization of the serum concentrations. Serum lithium levels above 1.5 mEq/L produce toxic reactions to the drug.

Monitor the client's WBC and energy level for tiredness because of possible leukemia. Monitor ECG for changes and the BP for hypotension. Weigh client daily and check for indicators of edema. Monitor electrolytes (hyponatremia, hypercalcemia, and hypophosphatemia) and renal and thyroid (hypothyroidism) studies.

Intervention. Administer after meals to prevent laxative action and to decrease gastric upset, tremors, or weakness by prolonging the absorption rate. Dilute the syrup in juice before administration and do not mix with or administer at the same time as any other medication that contains a basic form. Ensure that the client has an adequate fluid intake of 2.5 to 3 L daily and sufficient sodium intake.

Education. Client compliance, cooperation, and commitment to adhere strictly to all therapy are essential. The family should be advised in language they can understand of all ramifications of therapy, including effects related to serum level. The nurse should discuss the overt clinical signs of lithium toxicity with the client, family, or closest companion. Some of these symptoms are diarrhea, vomiting, tremors, mild ataxia, lack of coordination, drowsiness, and muscular weakness. If any of these signs appear, the client is to discontinue therapy and notify the prescriber promptly. Advise the client of facilities where prompt and accurate serum lithium determinations may be obtained.

Discuss with the client and family the importance of a normal diet because lithium decreases sodium reabsorption by the renal tubules, which may produce sodium depletion. An intake of 2500 to 3000 ml of liquid daily during the initial stabilization period is essential. The client should be cautioned to avoid fluid depletion; coffee, tea, and cola intake should be limited because of the diuretic effect and exercise, saunas, and exposure to hot weather should be avoided. The client should be advised to seek the assistance of a health care provider for illnesses that cause diaphoresis, vomiting, or diarrhea.

The nurse should advise the client that it is necessary to take the medication consistently—initially because it takes 1 to 3 weeks for improvement of the condition and thereafter even though the symptoms may abate. The nurse should assess carefully for compliance to the regimen, particularly if the client has had an increase in weight. Weight gain is a major cause of noncompliance, especially in female clients. The importance of regular visits to the prescriber for the monitoring of serum lithium levels should be stressed with the client.

Impairment of alertness may occur, so the client should be instructed to avoid activities that require coordination and close attention until the response to therapy has been determined.

Evaluation. The client will demonstrate improved mental status behaviors without adverse effects of the drug.

SUMMARY

Emotions, and therefore behaviors, are the result of a final, unified effect of the central nervous system, autonomic regulation, and biochemical mechanisms. As a result of their ability to modify these processes, drugs are important adjuncts to the treatment of psychiatric disorders. However, it is essential that antipsychotic drugs be prescribed only for appropriate, specific disorders to assist the client to cope more effectively with the environment and better use nonpharmacologic therapies. Use of these drugs as a substitute for a therapeutic milieu constitutes misuse.

Since the advent of tranquilizers in the early 1950s, institutionalization for psychiatric disorders has decreased, not only in duration for the individual client, but also as the sole alternative as a setting for psychiatric care. Many clients are now treated at community mental health centers as a result of the administration of psychotherapeutic agents.

Phenothiazine derivatives constitute two thirds of all antipsychotic drugs. They are divided into three subgroups: the aliphatic, piperidine, and piperazine compounds. Although the exact mechanism of their antipsychotic effect is not known, a primary effect is dopamine blockade in specific areas of the CNS. A major role for nursing with the phenothiazine derivatives is the assessment of the client for the development of side effects and adverse reactions, since many of them are debilitating and irreversible. Because many clients are treated in the community, it is essential that health teaching for the safe and accurate self-administration of these medications be accomplished.

Antidepressant therapy is used for the treatment of affective disorders, or mood disturbances, with tricyclic antidepressants being used for major depressions and the MAO inhibitors for atypical depressions. Lithium is considered the drug of choice for bipolar affective disorders. There is no ideal psychotherapeutic agent, since all of them produce undesirable side or adverse effects. Therefore the nurse's teaching role is important for the safe and accurate self-administration of these agents and the assessment of the untoward effects of the drugs.

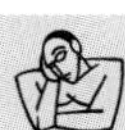

Critical Thinking

1. Mrs. Thomas, age 84, has been admitted to an extended-care facility. Over the first 3 days she has become increasingly combative. One of the nursing assistants has indicated that she does not want to be assigned to care for Mrs. Thomas because she is afraid of her. As the nurse on the unit you must decide whether Mrs. Thomas meets the necessary criteria that must be met before an antipsychotic can be prescribed to a resident in an extended-care facility. What will you do?
2. Barbara Walton has a manic-depressive disorder for which she has been prescribed lithium 300 mg PO bid. On a recent visit to the clinic her lithium blood level was 1.7 mEq/L. What action should you take?
3. Mr. Shapiro has had his depression treated unsuccessfully with tricyclic antidepressants. The prescriber is going to try to treat him with MAO inhibitors. During the drug history, Mr. Shapiro lists the following dietary intake for yesterday: breakfast—black coffee, bran cereal with skim milk and sliced banana on top; lunch—diet soda, bologna sandwich, and potato chips from the local lunch wagon; and dinner—salad, spaghetti with a little red wine, and garlic bread. He also stopped on the way home from work and had a "couple of beers with the guys." What instruction will you provide to assist Mr. Shapiro to manage his therapeutic regimen on MAOIs effectively?

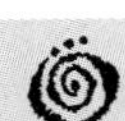

Collaborative Learning Activities

1. Before class the students will write what conditions and features of organic mental syndromes must be present before an antipsychotic agent may be prescribed. Discuss how these symptoms might be managed nonpharmacologically in a nursing home setting. Discuss the legal requirement for the use of antipsychotic agents in this setting.
2. Teams of students will present an analysis of the types of extrapyramidal reactions and symptoms associated with drug-induced parkinsonian effects, akathisia, dystonia, and tardive dyskinesia.

BIBLIOGRAPHY

Abrams WB & Berkow AB (Eds.) (1990). *The Merck manual of pediatrics.* Rahway, NJ: Merck Sharp & Dohme Research Laboratories.

Abramowicz M (Ed.) (1994). Drugs for psychiatric disorders, *Med Lett 36*(933):89-96.

American Hospital Formulary Service (1996). *AHFS drug information '96.* Bethesda, MD: American Society of Hospital Pharmacists.

Anderson KN, et al. (Eds.) (1994). *Mosby's medical, nursing, and allied health dictionary* (4th ed.). St Louis: Mosby.

Bond WS.(1991). Ethnicity and psychotropic drugs, *Clin Pharm 10*:467-70.

Brown CS & Bryant SG (1992). Major depressive disorders. In Koda-Kimble MA & Young LY (Eds.). *Applied therapeutics* (5th ed.). Vancouver: Applied Therapeutics.

Carley M (1992). Unnecessary drug requirements, *Contemp Long Term Care 15*(12):68.

Depression Guideline Panel (1993). *Depression in primary care: Volume 2. Treatment of major depression. Clinical practice guideline, #5.* Rockville, MD: U.S. Department of Health and Human Services, Public Health Service, Agency for Health Care Policy and Research.

Ereshefsky L & Richards AL (1992). Psychoses. In Koda-Kimble MA & Young LY (Eds.). *Applied therapeutics* (5th ed.). Vancouver: Applied Therapeutics.

Hardman JG & Limbird LE (Eds.) (1996). *Goodman and Gilman's the pharmacological basis of therapeutics* (9th ed.). New York. Macmillan.

Harrington C et al. (1992). Psychotropic drug use in long-term care facilities: A review of the literature, *Geront 32*(6):822-7.

Kalachnik JE (1983). Tardive dyskinesia, *Minn Pharmacist 37*(4):14.

Katzung BG (1992). *Basic and clinical pharmacology* (5th ed.). Norwalk, CT: Appleton & Lange.

Keltner NL & Folks DG (1993). *Psychotropic drugs.* St Louis: Mosby.

Keltner NL & Folks DG (1992). Culture as a variable in drug therapy, *Persp Psychiatr Care 28*(1):33-6.

Laird LK & Benefield WH (1995). Mood disorders I: Major depressive disorders. In Young LY & Koda-Kimble MA. *Applied therapeutics* (6th ed.). Vancouver, WA: Applied Therapeutics.

Lin T (1986). Multiculturalism and Canadian psychiatry: opportunities and challenges, *Canad J Psychiatr 31*(7):681.

Love RC & Grothe DR (1995). Mood Disorders II: Bipolar affective disorders. In Young LY & Koda-Kimble MA. *Applied therapeutics* (6th ed.). Vancouver, WA: Applied Therapeutics.

Lyons AS & Petrucelli RJ (1978). *Medicine: An illustrated history.* New York: Harry N Abrams.

Marcos L & Cancro R (1982). Pharmacotherapy of Hispanic depressed patients: Clinical observations, *Amer J Psychother 36*:505.

Marken PA & Stanislav SW (1995). Schizophrenia. In Young LY & Koda-Kimble MA. *Applied therapeutics* (6th ed.). Vancouver, WA: Applied Therapeutics.

Maxmen JS & Ward NG (1995). *Psychotropic drugs: Fast facts* (2nd ed.). New York: WW Norton.

Medicare and Medicaid (1989). *OBRA requirements for long-term care facilities.* Section 483.60 Level A Requirement: Pharmacy services; Section 483.10 Level A Requirement: Resident rights; Section 483.20 Level A Requirement: Resident assessment; Section 482.25 Level A Requirement: Quality of Care and Interpretive Guidelines. Washington, DC: Health Care Financing Administration (HCFA).

Montano CB (1994). Recognition and treatment of depression in a primary care setting, *J Clin Psychiat 55*(12 suppl):18-34.

Olin BR (Ed.) (1996). *Facts and comparisons.* St. Louis: Facts and Comparisons.

PDR (1996). *Physician's desk reference* (50th ed.). Oradell, NJ: Medical Economics.

Stat/Gram (1996). Letter from Eli Lilly and Company, OL-0077.

Stramek R, et al. (1991). Prevalence of tardive dyskinesia among three ethnic groups of chronic psychiatric patients, *Hosp Commun Psychiat 42*:590.

Tieaskie L (1992). NMS: Rare and dangerous drug reaction, *Amer J Nurs 92*(2):67-70.

United States Pharmacopeial Convention (1996). *USP DI: Drug information for the health care professional* (16th ed.). Rockville, MD: The Convention.

Wells BG (Ed.) (1994). *Therapeutic options in the treatment of depression: A special report.* Washington, DC: American Pharmaceutical Association.

Yonkers KA, et al. (1992). Gender differences in pharmacokinetics and pharmacodynamics of psychotropic medication, *Amer J Psychiat 149*(5):587-95.

Zal HM (1994). Depression in the elderly: Differing presentations, wide choice of therapies, *Consultant 34*(3):354-6, 358, 361.

Zyprexa (1996). Package insert. Eli Lilly Industries, Inc, #PV2960.

Chapter 20

Overview of the Autonomic Nervous System

Chapter Focus

Because the autonomic nervous system (ANS) regulates the functions of internal viscera such as the heart, blood vessels, digestive organs, and reproductive organs, a functional knowledge of the ANS is essential. An understanding of this chapter will allow the nurse to predict general responses to a variety of stimuli, explain responses to changes in the environment, understand symptoms that result from ANS dysfunction, and know how drugs affect the ANS. The following objectives and key terms are important for a good understanding of this chapter.

Key Terms

adrenergic (p. 401)
autonomic nervous system (ANS) (p. 394)
catecholamine (p. 399)
cholinergic (p. 401)
conduction (p. 395)
feedback control mechanism (p. 394)
muscarinic (M) receptors (p. 399)
neuroeffector junction (p. 395)
neurohumoral transmission (p. 395)
nicotinic (N) receptors (p. 399)
reflex arc (p. 394)
somatic nervous system (p. 394)
synaptic junction (p. 395)

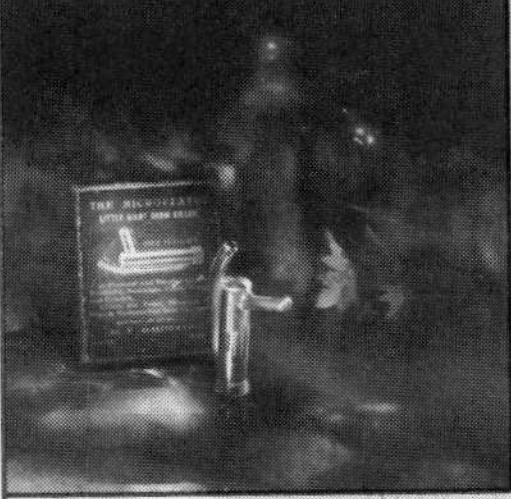

Objectives

1. Describe the reflex control system.
2. Explain the major differences between the parasympathetic and sympathetic divisions of the autonomic nervous system.
3. Name the primary neurotransmitters for each system.
4. Relate the primary disposition of the neurotransmitters following release from their respective nerves.
5. Identify the three basic characteristics of the autonomic nervous system.

The **autonomic nervous system** (ANS) functions primarily as a regulatory or self-governing system for maintaining the internal environment of the body at an optimal level (homeostasis). This system automatically controls the function of smooth muscle, cardiac muscle, and glandular secretions, which interact in many vital physiologic tasks. Digestion of a meal, maintenance of the pressure of circulating blood, and many other processes are internally regulated by the ANS.

REFLEX CONTROL SYSTEM

The nervous system is the important control and communication system within the body. It collects information about conditions inside and outside of the body. The simplest means by which the nervous system responds to environmental change is through the action of the reflex arc. The reflex arc is the automatic motor response to sensory stimuli. In any reflex a nerve fiber conducts a nerve impulse; these impulses are the basis of communication of information through the nervous system.

The reflex act consists of two major functional processes: the sensory input and the motor output. The first component of the reflex arc is the receptor, which detects environmental changes such as temperature, pressure in blood vessels, and distention in the viscera. These changes are responsible for producing a stimulus in the receptor. Information from the sensitized receptor is then transmitted as a nerve impulse along the afferent neuron to the central nervous system (CNS), the site of integration. The CNS then issues instructions as an altered motor nerve impulse along the efferent neuron to the effector, which produces the appropriate movements of muscles and glands.

The information carried *to* the central nervous system (sensory input) and instructions sent *from* the central nervous system (motor output) constitute a **feedback control mechanism**. Information fed back to the central nervous system from a receptor is modulated so that nerve impulses may vary in frequency and pattern according to the degree of activity required of the effector. The control of visceral function is involuntary, so the feedback mechanism must include all the components of a control system essential for performing the reflex act. Therefore reflex action functions as a feedback mechanism, operating from a receptor to an effector. Its purpose is to prevent extreme changes in function that may create a disturbance in the internal environment.

A good example of feedback control is the blood pressure-regulating reflex. Again, the sequence of events follows the pattern of the reflex arc. The carotid sinus in the carotid artery and the aortic sinus in the aortic arch serve as pressure receptors (baroreceptors) that are highly sensitive to stretch, and the degree of wall stretching is determined by the amount of pressure within these vessels. Thus any increase in blood pressure stimulates the baroreceptors, and this information is conveyed as nerve impulses along the afferent neuron to the vasomotor center in the medulla.

The medulla is the central nervous system site for integration of blood pressure. After the appropriate neuronal connections, a decrease in sympathetic discharge is conducted along the efferent neuron to the effectors, which produces relaxation of arteriolar smooth muscles. This relaxation causes dilation of the arteries and a reduction in blood pressure. This is only a partial explanation of blood pressure regulation, since a decrease in arterial pressure produces the opposite response in the same neuronal pathway. In addition, this control mechanism operates in coordination with cardiac function.

NERVOUS SYSTEM CLASSIFICATION

The nervous system is classified on the basis of the reflex arc. The two main divisions are the central nervous system and the peripheral nervous system. The central nervous system consists of the brain and spinal cord and performs the important integrative functions from the peripheral sources. The peripheral system has two divisions: the **somatic nervous system**, which innervates voluntary or skeletal muscles, and the autonomic nervous system, which influences the involuntary activities of smooth muscles, cardiac muscles, and glands. The afferent fibers of both systems are the first link in the reflex arc by carrying sensory information to the central nervous system. After integration at various levels in the brain, the outflow from the central nervous system is conducted along either the somatic efferent system or the autonomic efferent system. Both of these systems constitute the final link in the reflex arc (Figure 20-1).

Several centers in the central nervous system integrate all autonomic nervous system activities. There is evidence

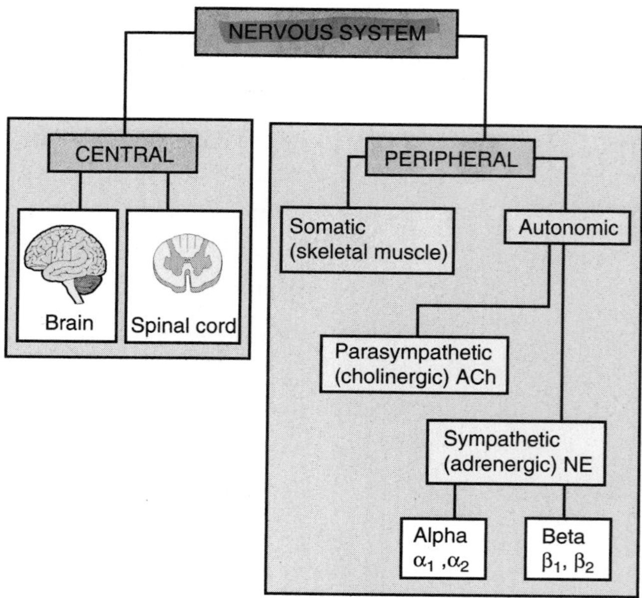

Figure 20-1 Divisions of the nervous system.

that the hypothalamus, in particular, performs such integrating activities. It contains centers that regulate body temperature, water balance, and carbohydrate and fat metabolism. It also integrates mechanisms concerned with emotional behavior, the waking state, and sleep. The medulla oblongata integrates the control of blood pressure, respiration, and cardiac function. A series of "vital centers," including the vasomotor center, respiratory center, and cardiac center, respectively, coordinate these activities. The midbrain, limbic system, cerebellum, and cerebral cortex, are all involved in the control of and in physiologic functions regulated by the autonomic nervous system.

DIFFERENCES BETWEEN THE PARASYMPATHETIC AND SYMPATHETIC SYSTEMS

The autonomic nervous system is organized into two subdivisions: (1) the parasympathetic system and (2) the sympathetic system (Box 20-1). The anatomic arrangement of each system consists of two motor nerves, a preganglionic nerve and a postganglionic nerve, with a ganglion (group of nerve cell bodies) connecting the two neurons (Figure 20-2).

Physiologic differences. Since the parasympathetic system and the sympathetic system simultaneously innervate many of the same organs, the opposing actions of the two systems balance one another. The parasympathetic system functions mainly to conserve energy and restore body resources of the organism, otherwise known as the system of rest and digestion. These include cardiac deceleration, a rise in gastrointestinal activity associated with increased digestion and absorption, and an increase in excretion. In contrast, the sympathetic system mobilizes the organism during emergency and stress situations, and so it is called the "fight or flight" system. These functions involve expenditure of energy and increases in the blood sugar concentration, heart activity, and blood pressure (Table 20-1).

Anatomic and pharmacologic differences. The parasympathetic or cholinergic system's preganglionic fibers emerge with the cranial nerves III, VII, IX, and X and at the sacral spinal levels from about S3 through S4. The tenth cranial nerve or vagus nerve has extensive branches that supply fibers to the heart, lungs, and almost all the abdominal organs.

The sympathetic (adrenergic) system is also called the thoracolumbar system because its preganglionic fibers originate in the spinal cord from the thoracic segment T1 to the lumbar segment at L2 level (Figure 20-3 and Table 20-2).

BOX 20-1

ANS Terminology

Over the years, various terminology has been used to describe the division of the autonomic nervous system. The anatomic names are sympathetic and parasympathetic, and the corresponding functional terms, which relate to the primary neurotransmitters for each system, are adrenergic and cholinergic, respectively. Generally, the terms are used interchangeably—that is, sympathetic or adrenergic and parasympathetic or cholinergic nervous systems. It is important to understand the terms parasympatho*mimetic* and sympatho*mimetic*, which means to mimic or produce an effect similar to activation of either system. Parasympatho*lytic* or sympatho*lytic* implies blocking the normal effects seen with activation of either system. Anticholinergic is synonymous with parasympatholytic.

Anatomic	*Functional*	*Primary neurotransmitter*
Sympathetic	Adrenergic	norepinephrine (NE)
Parasympathetic	Cholinergic	acetylcholine (ACh)

NEUROHUMORAL TRANSMISSION

There is general agreement that information in the nervous system is transmitted both electrically and chemically. This phenomenon occurs because nerve cells have two special characteristics: (1) They can conduct electrical signals. The passage of a nerve impulse or an action potential along a nerve fiber or a muscle fiber is called **conduction.** (2) They have intercellular connections with other nerve cells and with innervated tissues such as muscles and glands. The presence of a specific chemical at these connections determines the type of information a neuron can receive and the range of responses it can yield in return. The passage of a nerve impulse across a synaptic or neuroeffector junction with the use of a chemical is called **neurohumoral transmission.**

Although each nerve fiber may conduct an impulse along the neuron, it is solely the chemical substance called the neurotransmitter or neurohormone that permits the action potential of a neuron to cross (1) the **synaptic junction** from one neuron to another neuron, or (2) the **neuroeffector junction** from a neuron to an effector organ. In this mechanism the arrival of an action potential at a nerve terminal starts the release of the neurotransmitter. The hormone or mediator then acts as a messenger by which nerve cells communicate information to the structures they innervate. The neurotransmitter exerts its influence primarily at the junctional spaces (synaptic junction or neuroeffector junction) to facilitate the transmission of impulses to their final destination. Many drugs may also act selectively at these junctions.

Types of Neurohumoral Transmission

The neurohormones acetylcholine and norepinephrine are responsible for neurohumoral transmission. Nerves that contain acetylcholine are called *cholinergic neurons,* and they are involved in cholinergic transmission. Nerves that contain norepinephrine or epinephrine (from adrenal medulla) are known as *adrenergic neurons,* and they are associated with adrenergic transmission.

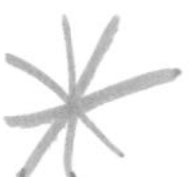

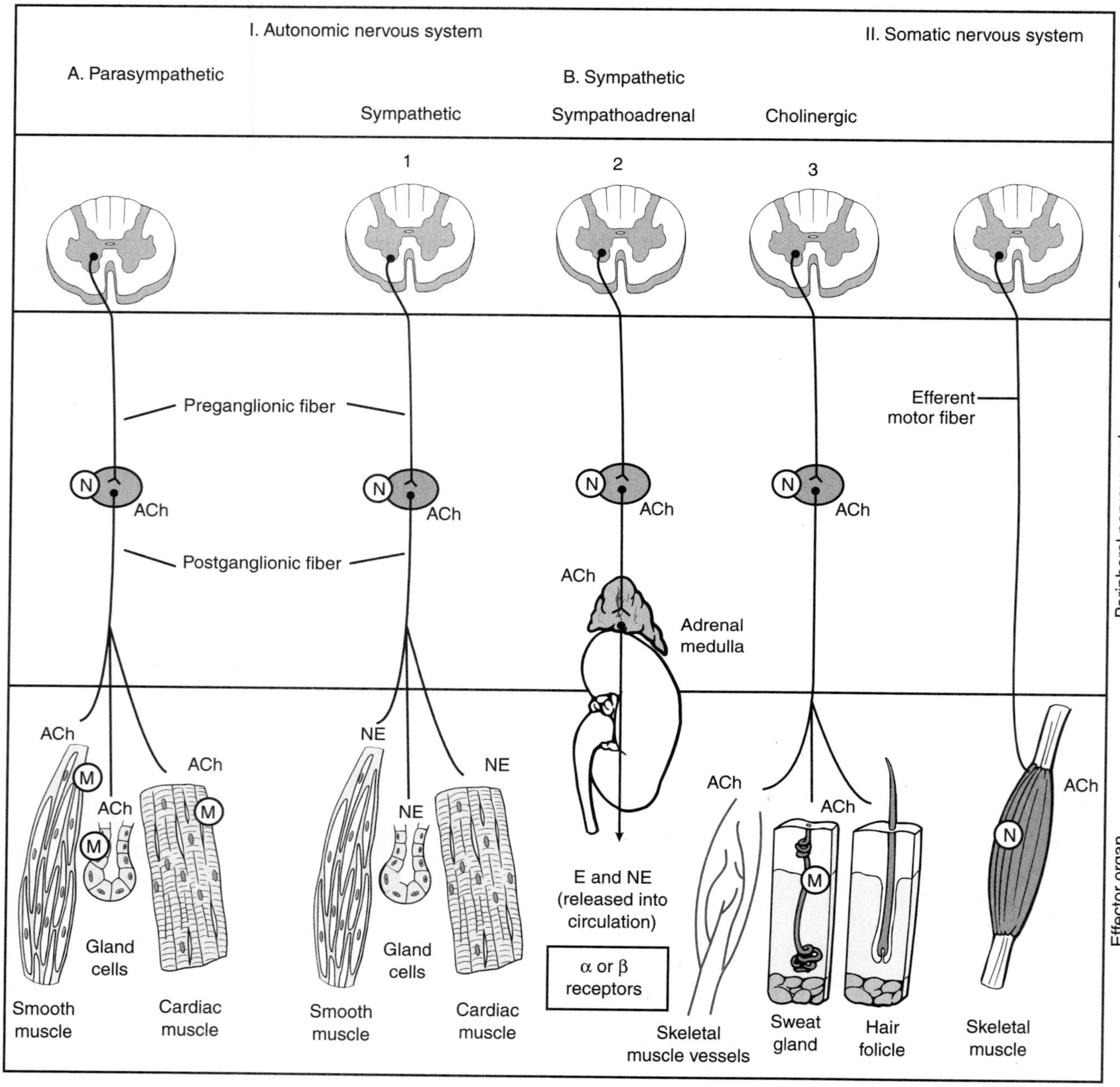

Figure 20-2 Schema of receptor sites for neurohumoral transmission. **I**, Autonomic nervous system, where preganglionic fibers of both parasympathetic and sympathetic nerves synapse in the ganglia. **II**, Somatic motor nervous system. *N*, Nicotinic sites; *M*, muscarinic sites; *ACh*, acetylcholine; *E*, epinephrine; *NE*, norepinephrine.

TABLE 20-1 Classification of the effector organ responses to autonomic nerve impulses

Effector organs	Responses to parasympathetic (cholinergic) impulses	Response to sympathetic (adrenergic) impulses: Receptor	Response to sympathetic (adrenergic) impulses: Response
Cardiovascular system			
Heart			
Sinoatrial node	Decreased heart rate	$Beta_1$	Increased heart rate
Atrioventricular node	Decreased conduction velocity	$Beta_1$	Increased automaticity and conduction velocity
Ventricles	No innervation	$Beta_1$	Increased force of contraction and conduction velocity
Arterioles (smooth muscle)			
Coronary	Dilation	Alpha, $beta_2$, dopaminergic	Constriction and dilation
Skin and mucosa	Dilation	Alpha	Constriction
Skeletal muscle	No innervation	Cholinergic	Dilation
Cerebral	Dilation	Alpha	Slight constriction
Mesenteric	None	Alpha, $beta_2$, dopaminergic	Constriction and dilation
Renal	None	Alpha, $beta_2$, dopaminergic	Constriction and dilation
Veins	None	Alpha, $beta_2$	Constriction and dilation
Lung			
Bronchial muscle	Bronchoconstriction	$Beta_2$	Relaxation (bronchodilation)
Bronchial glands	Stimulation		Inhibition
Gastrointestinal tract			
Motility	Increased motility	Alpha, $beta_2$	Relaxation (decreased motility)
Sphincters	Relaxation	Alpha	Contraction
Exocrine glands	Increased secretion	?	Decreased secretion
Salivary glands	Dilation: copious, watery secretion	Alpha	Constriction: thick, viscous secretion
Gallbladder and ducts	Contraction		Relaxation
Kidney	None	$Beta_2$	Renin secretion
Urinary bladder			
Detrusor muscle	Contraction	$Beta_2$	Relaxation
Sphincter	Relaxation	Alpha	Contraction
Eye			
Radial muscle Iris	Contraction of sphincter muscle (miosis, pupillary constriction)	Alpha	Contraction of radial muscle (mydriasis)
Ciliary muscle	Contracted for near vision		Relaxed for far vision
Liver	Glycogen synthesis	Beta	Glycogenolysis, gluconeogenesis
Pancreas	Secretion	Alpha	Decreased secretion
Skin	None	$Beta_2$	Increased secretion
Sweat glands	No innervation	Cholinergic	Increased sweating
Pilomotor muscle	No innervation		Contraction (gooseflesh)
Lacrimal glands	Increased secretion		No innervation
Nasopharyngeal glands	Increased secretion		No innervation
Male sex glands	Erection		Ejaculation

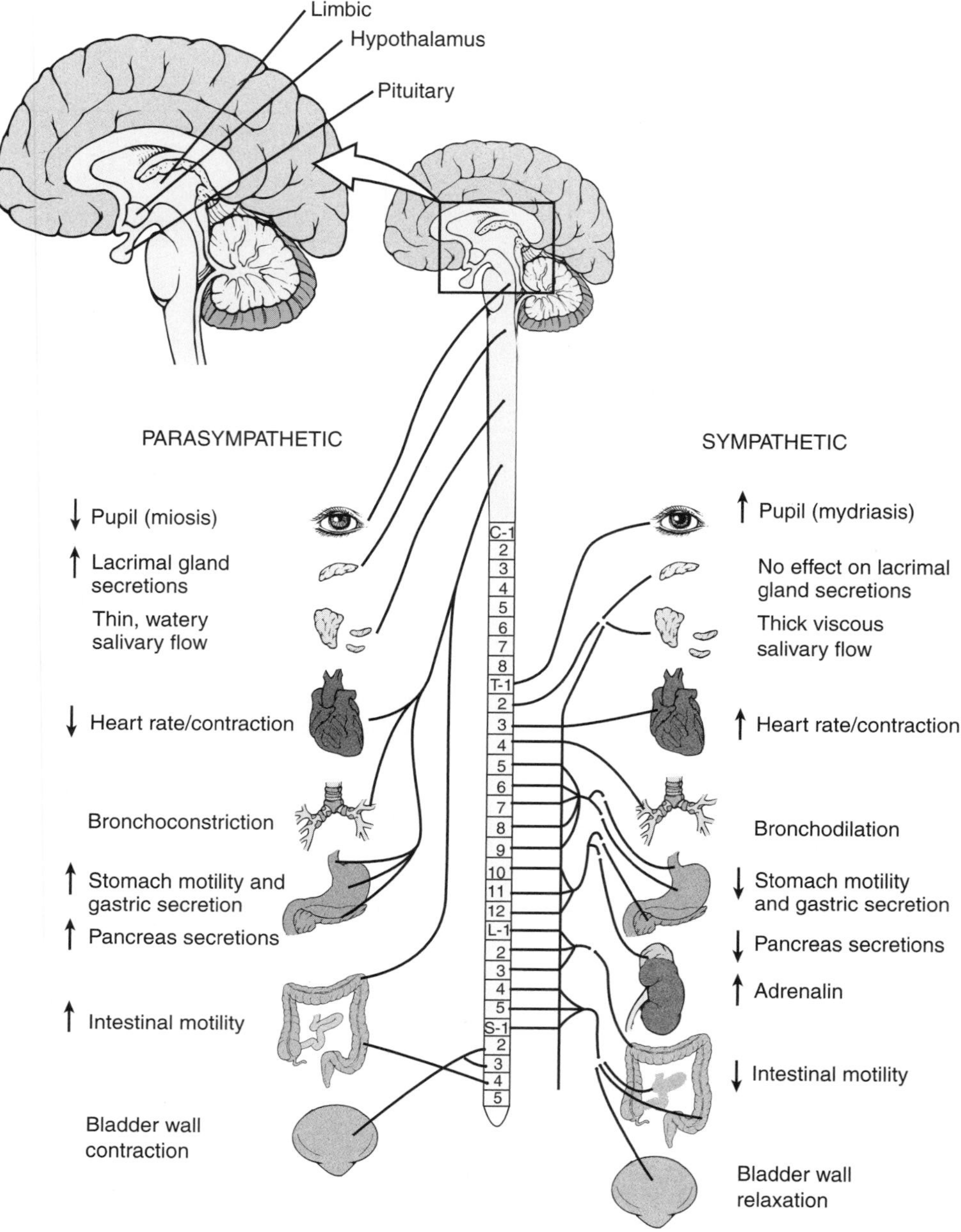

Figure 20-3 Diagram of the autonomic nervous system.

In neurohumoral transmission the sequence of events includes (1) biosynthesis, (2) storage, (3) release, (4) action, and (5) inactivation of the mediator (Figures 20-4 and 20-5). Many autonomic drugs affect one of these individual events, so it is essential to understand the basic mechanisms involved in this complicated process. These drugs have been useful in treating many persons afflicted with autonomic disorders.

Cholinergic Transmission

Synthesis and storage. Acetylcholine is synthesized in the cytoplasm of the nerve terminal. Once synthesized, the acetylcholine is stored in packets called synaptic vesicles or granules, which are located in the nerve terminal (see Figure 20-4, *A*-2).

Release and action. The arrival of an action potential at the nerve ending causes the vesicle to approach the membrane and release the acetylcholine molecules into the synaptic cleft or space. Calcium ions must be present for an efficient release. Once free, the acetylcholine diffuses across the synaptic or junctional cleft and attaches itself to specialized receptors (postjunctional sites) on the membrane of the next neuron or neuroeffector. The binding of acetylcholine to the receptor increases the permeability of the membrane to sodium and potassium ions; thus a depolarizing action

TABLE 20-2 Differentiating characteristics between the parasympathetic and sympathetic nervous systems

Characteristic	Parasympathetic nervous system	Sympathetic nervous system
Origin	Craniosacral	Thoracolumbar
Structure innervation	Cardiac muscle Smooth muscle Glands Viscera	Cardiac muscle Smooth muscle Glands Viscera
Ganglia	Near the effector (vagus, atria of heart)	Near central nervous system
Length of fibers	Preganglionics (long) Postganglionics (short)	Preganglionics (short) Postganglionics (long)
Ratio of preganglionics to postganglionics	Branching is minimal (1:2), very discrete, fine responses	High degree of nerve branching (1:11, 1:17)
Response	Discrete	Diffuse
Ganglion transmitter	Acetylcholine	Acetylcholine
Transmitter substance (postganglionic nerve endings)	Acetylcholine	Norepinephrine (most cases); epinephrine and norepinephrine (adrenal medulla) Acetylcholine for sweat glands and blood vessels of skeletal muscles
Blocking drugs (postganglionic nerve endings)	Cholinergic blocking agents (atropine)	Adrenergic blocking agents Alpha: phentolamine Beta: propranolol

finally results in excitation or inhibition of neural, muscular, or glandular activity (see Figure 20-4, *A-3*).

Cholinergic receptors. The cholinergic receptor sites that are stimulated by acetylcholine are either nicotinic or muscarinic. **Nicotinic** (N) **receptors** appear in the ganglia of both the parasympathetic and sympathetic fibers, the adrenal medulla, and the skeletal (striated) muscle that is supplied by the somatic motor system. **Muscarinic** (M) **receptors** (postganglionic sites) are located in the smooth muscle, cardiac muscle, and glands of the parasympathetic fibers and the effector organs of the cholinergic sympathetic fibers. The N and M receptors are shown in Figure 20-2.

Inactivation. Once acetylcholine has exerted its effect on the postjunctional sites, the excess amount is inactivated rapidly by the enzyme acetylcholinesterase. The metabolites formed in this reaction are chemically inactive and are the same compounds from which acetylcholine is formed. Inactivation of this neurohormone is shown as a reverse action in the preceding formula (see Figure 20-4, *A-5*).

Adrenergic Transmission

The term **catecholamine** refers to a group of chemically related compounds: norepinephrine (noradrenalin), epinephrine (adrenaline), and dopamine. They are all involved in some aspect of adrenergic transmission.

Synthesis and storage. The catecholamines produced by the sympathetic nervous system include norepinephrine and epinephrine. The complex pathway for synthesis of these neurotransmitters is mediated by different enzymes located in the postganglionic nerve terminals and in the chromaffin cells of the adrenal medullary glands.

The formation of norepinephrine is initiated by tyrosine, which is an amino acid derived from proteins in the diet. When tyrosine enters the cytoplasm of the nerve terminal, it is converted into dopa, which in turn is decarboxylated to dopamine. Dopamine is then taken up into the storage vesicles, or granules, where it is transformed into the neurotransmitter norepinephrine by the enzyme dopamine ß–hydroxylase. Figure 20-5 shows the steps of the synthetic process.

In the adrenal medullary gland, the enzyme methyl transferase converts norepinephrine to epinephrine. On stimulation, both epinephrine (E) and norepinephrine (NE) are released from the adrenal medulla and carried by the circulation to all parts of the body.

Release. The arrival of an action potential at the nerve terminal of the postganglionic fibers causes the vesicles to fuse with the cell membrane and release the stored supply of norepinephrine into the junctional cleft. Calcium ions must be present to enhance the release of norepinephrine from the vesicles. The free form of norepinephrine then diffuses across the cleft to the receptor sites on the postjunctional membrane of neuroeffector cells (smooth muscle, cardiac muscle, or glands) (see Figure 20-5).

Action. Once the norepinephrine combines with either the alpha or beta receptor sites on the membrane of the neuroeffector cells, a series of chemical and electrical events produces either an excitatory or an inhibitory effect. The alpha receptor activation is primarily responsible for excitatory

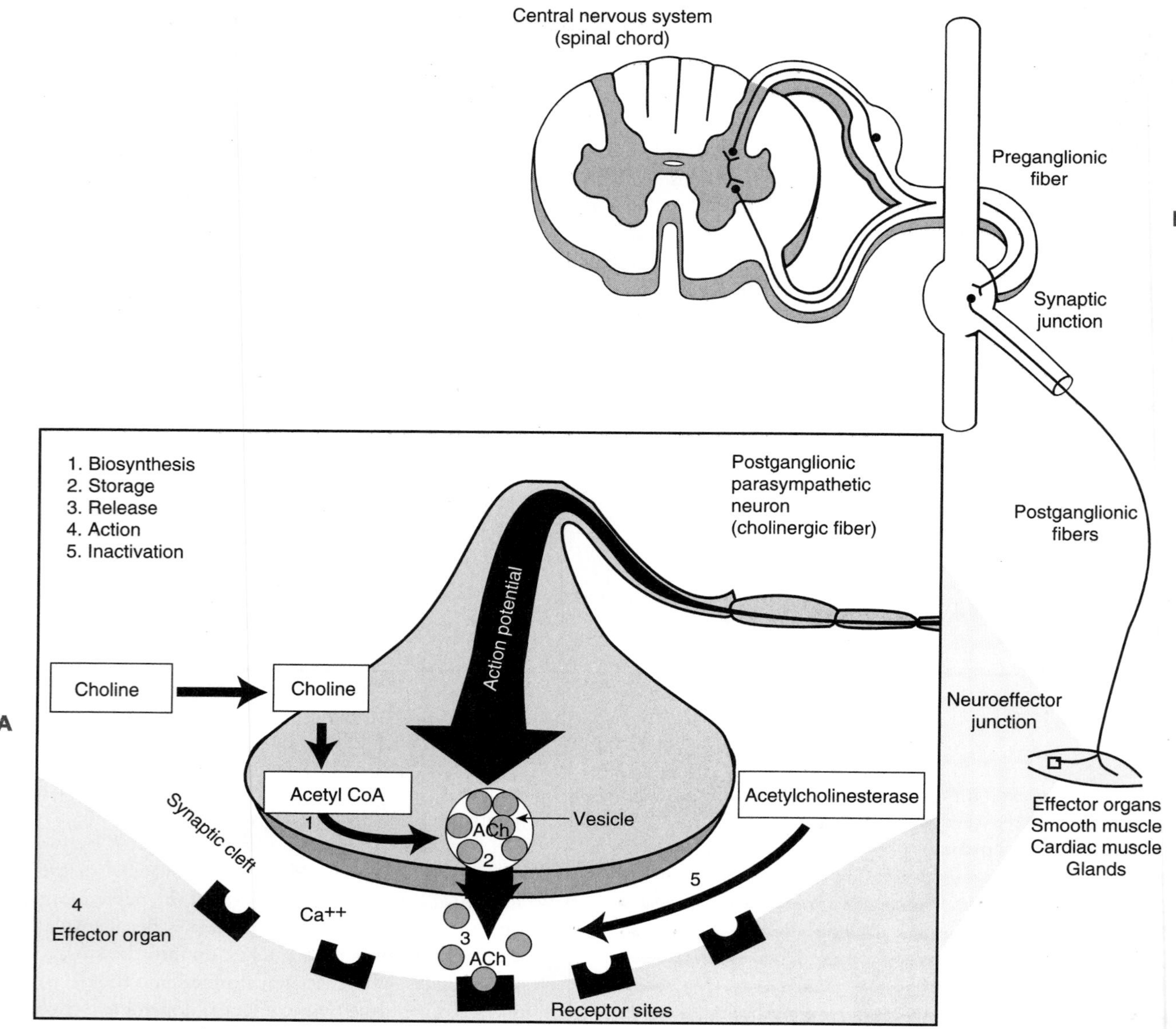

Figure 20-4 **A,** Cholinergic transmission. Schematic diagram of parasympathetic postganglionic neuron, showing steps in cholinergic transmission at the neuroeffector junction. *1, Biosynthesis* of acetylcholine (ACh): Choline is taken up by the nerve terminal, and it interacts with acetyl coenzyme A to synthesize ACh. *2, Storage:* Following synthesis, ACh is stored in the vesicle until the arrival of a nerve impulse. *3, Release:* An action potential of the nerve terminal causes the vesicle to attach itself to the membrane and release ACh. The neurohormone then diffuses across the synaptic cleft and combines with the receptors on the effector cell. *4, Action:* The interaction of ACh with the receptor sites results in a motor response. *5, Inactivation of ACh:* At the synaptic cleft, ACh is hydrolyzed by the enzyme acetylcholinesterase. **B,** Schematic representation to show the relationship between a neuron in the central nervous system, a neuron in a peripheral ganglion, and an effector organ supplied by the parasympathetic nerve.

response, although it results in intestinal relaxation. By contrast, beta receptor activation is usually inhibitory except in the myocardial cells, where norepinephrine produces an excitatory effect.

Adrenergic receptors. The adrenergic receptor sites that are stimulated by the endogenous catecholamines—norepinephrine, epinephrine, and dopamine—are classified as alpha and beta receptors. Both classes have two subtypes. The alpha receptors are identified by neuronal location: (1) $alpha_1$ sites are located on the postsynaptic effector cells, and (2) $alpha_2$ sites appear on the presynaptic nerve terminals, controlling the amount of norepinephrine release that operates through a negative feedback mechanism. By contrast, the beta receptors are designated by organ location:

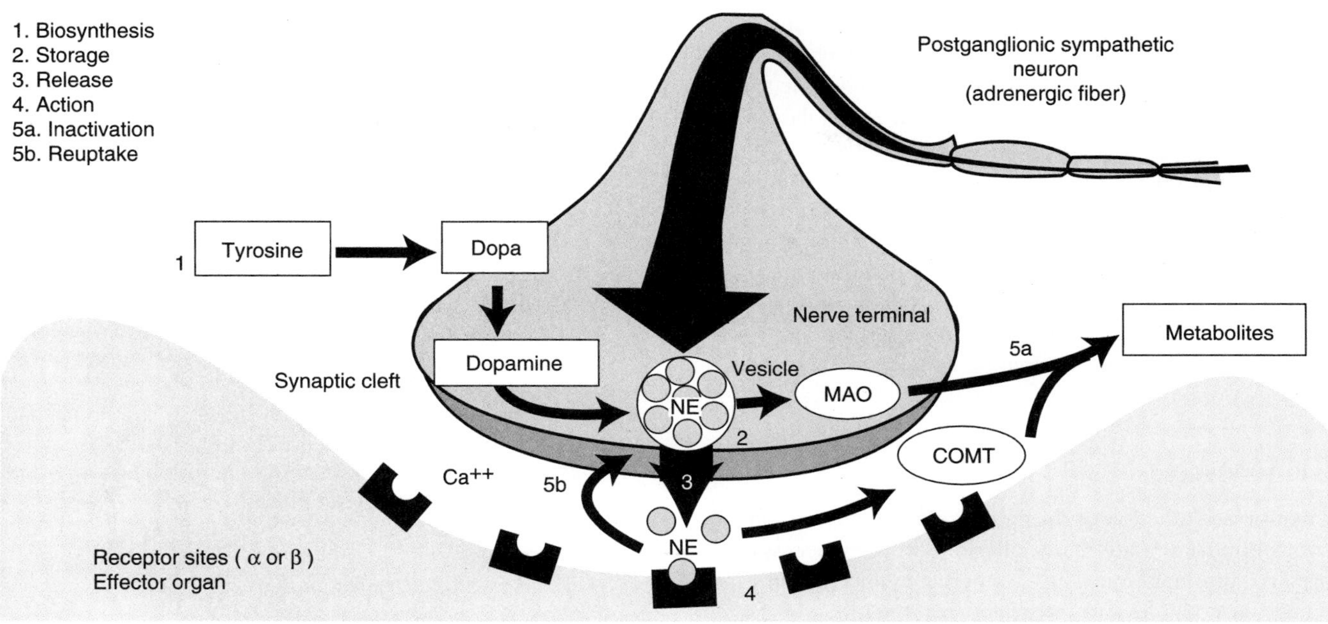

Figure 20-5 Adrenergic transmission at the neuroeffector junction.

(1) beta$_1$ receptors are located primarily in the heart, and (2) beta$_2$ receptors appear in the smooth muscle of the bronchioles, arterioles, and various other visceral organs in the body. At least five types of dopamine receptors have been identified in the CNS. D_1 and D_2 receptors are associated with the antipsychotic medications and movement disorders, such as Parkinson's disease. Stimulation of D_2 receptors is primarily responsible for antiparkinson drug activity, and the D_1 receptors may play a similar although smaller role in this area.

Inactivation. Once norepinephrine has performed its adrenergic function, its action must be rapidly stopped to prevent prolongation of its effects, which could lead to a loss of regulatory control of visceral function. The inactivation of norepinephrine occurs by (1) enzymatic transformation, (2) reuptake of the norepinephrine into nerve terminals, and (3) diffusion.

Catecholamines are metabolized by two enzymes, monoamine oxidase (MAO) and catechol-o-methyltransferase (COMT). Free norepinephrine *within* the cytoplasm of the nerve terminal is metabolized by MAO, which is stored in the mitochondria of sympathetic neurons. COMT, which is located *outside* the neuron or at the synaptic cleft, participates in the inactivation or metabolism of norepinephrine outside the neuron.

The mechanism of norepinephrine reuptake plays a more significant role than enzymatic transformation in catecholamine inactivation. In the reuptake process, norepinephrine is removed by the active transport ("amine pump") from the junctional sites (synaptic and neuroeffector junctions) and is returned to the sympathetic nerve terminal and storage vesicles. In this way, an adequate supply of norepinephrine is provided by reuptake, as well as by the process of synthesis.

Finally, a small portion of norepinephrine released at the synaptic cleft may be picked up by the circulation and metabolized elsewhere in the body. This is known as the diffusion process. Figure 20-5 portrays the steps in adrenergic transmission.

General Actions of Autonomic Transmitters

In 1933 Dale and co-workers determined the chemical differences between fibers that release acetylcholine (**cholinergic** fibers) and those that release norepinephrine and epinephrine (**adrenergic** fibers). In the autonomic nervous system, all the preganglionic fibers originate in the central nervous system and synapse with the ganglia of the postganglionic fibers. The terminals of all the preganglionic fibers release acetylcholine and interact with nicotinic receptors in the membrane of the postganglionic fibers or the adrenal medulla.

In the parasympathetic system the terminals of the postganglionic fibers also release acetylcholine and interact with muscarinic receptors in the membrane of the smooth muscle, cardiac muscle, and glands.

In the sympathetic nervous system there are three different kinds of postganglionic neurons: (1) The sympathetic neuron, the major type, releases norepinephrine and activates either alpha or beta receptors in the membrane of the smooth muscle, cardiac muscle, and glands. (2) The sympathoadrenal neuron, in which the preganglionic fiber synapses with a modified sympathetic ganglion, the adrenal medulla, releases mostly epinephrine and a small amount of norepinephrine, which are secreted into the circulation and carried to all parts of the body. (3) The cholinergic sympathetic neuron releases acetylcholine and stimulates muscarinic receptor sites on the sweat glands to produce sweating and on the blood vessels in skeletal muscle to increase vasodilation and enhance blood flow.

In the somatic (sensory) nervous system a single neuron, the efferent (motor) fiber, releases acetylcholine and interacts with the nicotinic sites on the skeletal muscle membrane. The autonomic drugs play an important role by enhancing or inhibiting physiologic activity at these sites of neurohumoral transmission (see Figure 20-2 and Table 20-2).

SUMMARY

The primary function of the autonomic nervous system is to control and integrate many physiologic tasks necessary to preserve internal homeostasis, emergency mechanisms, and repair. Its activities are integrated by a number of centers within the central nervous system: the hypothalamus, medulla oblongata, midbrain, limbic system, cerebellum, and cerebral cortex. The autonomic nervous system innervates the smooth muscles, cardiac muscles, and glands. It is composed of two divisions, the parasympathetic and the sympathetic; their actions oppose and balance each other.

1. Although both systems are present in the body, only one will be predominate at any given time.
2. If an autonomic nervous system function is blocked, the opposite effect will take precedence.
3. Drugs are available to stimulate or block either system.

Functions stimulated by the parasympathetic system are chiefly those concerned with digestion, excretion, near vision, cardiac deceleration, and anabolism. Functions stimulated by the sympathetic system are primarily those concerned with the expenditure of energy and are called into play by physical or emotional stress.

Nerve impulse transmission is caused by the activity of chemical substances called neurotransmitters: acetylcholine and the catecholamines. Nerve fibers that synthesize and liberate acetylcholine are known as cholinergic fibers; those that synthesize and secrete norepinephrine and epinephrine are called adrenergic fibers.

For the nurse to achieve an understanding of the pharmacology of autonomic drugs, a basic knowledge of the anatomy and physiology of the autonomic nervous system is essential. This information helps to predict the effects of drugs that stimulate or block autonomic function.

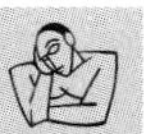

Critical Thinking

1. Your client's blood pressure has suddenly dropped. How would sympathetic reflexes that control blood vessels respond (1) to a sudden decrease in blood pressure or (2) to a sudden increase in blood pressure?
2. Clients with diabetes mellitus may develop autonomic neuropathy, that is, degeneration of the ANS nerves. Which parts of the ANS are involved with the following symptoms:
   a. Lack of pain with a heart attack
   b. Constipation
   c. Impotence
   d. Decreased pupillary response to light

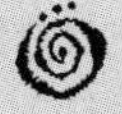

Collaborative Learning Activities

1. One pair of students will compare and contrast the parasympathetic and sympathetic systems for the rest of the class.
2. Another pair of students will present the characteristics of nerve cells in neurohumoral transmission, types of transmission, and the sequence of events involved.

BIBLIOGRAPHY

Anderson KN, et al. (Eds.) (1994). *Mosby's medical, nursing, & allied health dictionary* (4th ed.). St Louis: Mosby.

Guyton AC (1990). *Textbook of medical physiology* (8th ed.). Philadelphia: WB Saunders.

Hardman JG & Limbird LE (Eds.) (1996). *Goodman and Gilman's the pharmacological basis of therapeutics* (9th ed.). New York: McGraw Hill.

McCance KL & Huether SE (1990). *Pathophysiology: The biological basis for disease in adults and children*. St Louis: Mosby.

Seeley RR, et al. (1996). *Anatomy and physiology* (2nd ed.). St Louis: Mosby.

Thibodeau GA & Patton KT (1996). *Anatomy and physiology* (3rd ed.). St Louis: Mosby.

VanWynsberghe D, Norback CR, & Carola R (1995). *Human anatomy and physiology* (3rd ed.). New York: McGraw-Hill.

Vinik AI & Vinik E (1992). The diabetes complication no one talks about, *Diabet Forecast* 45(7):70.

Chapter 21

Drugs Affecting the Parasympathetic Nervous System

Chapter Focus

The parasympathetic component of the autonomic nervous system (ANS) innervates various organs and acts on the heart, gastrointestinal tract, urinary bladder, and respiratory tract. In conjunction with its counterpart, the sympathetic component of the autonomic nervous system (ANS), it works to control body functions that occur without conscious thought. Drug therapy associated with this system can influence autonomic processes by mimicking acetylcholine at receptor sites, or it can inhibit the breakdown of acetylcholine at these same sites, prolonging its action. In either case, the nurse needs to be knowledgeable about the drugs related to the parasympathetic nervous system because they are used across a wide variety of human conditions. The following objectives and key terms are necessary for a good understanding of this chapter.

Key Terms

adrenergic (p. 404)
adrenergic blocking (p. 404)
anticholinergic (p. 408)
antimuscarinic (p. 408)
cholinergic (p. 404)
cholinergic blocking (p. 408)
direct-acting cholinergic drug (p. 404)
indirect-acting cholinergic drug (p. 406)
muscarinic effect (p. 404)
parasympatholytic (anticholinergic) (p. 408)
parasympathomimetic (p. 404)
sympatholytic (p. 404)
sympathomimetic (p. 404)

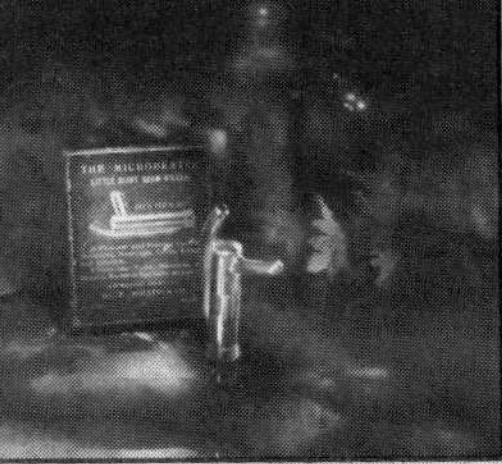

Key Drugs [▲]

atropine
bethanechol
nicotine

Objectives

1. Explain the difference between the muscarinic and nicotinic actions of acetylcholine.
2. Describe the side effects/adverse reactions of cholinergic, cholinergic blocking, and synthetic antispasmodic agents.
3. Describe the physiologic effects of the belladonna alkaloids.
4. List the physiologic effects of nicotine.
5. Describe the use of ganglionic blocking drugs.
6. Implement the nursing management of the care of clients receiving agents affecting the parasympathetic nervous system.

AUTONOMIC DRUGS

Autonomic drugs may mimic, intensify, or block the effects of the parasympathetic and sympathetic divisions of the autonomic nervous system. They are divided into the following groups:

1. **Cholinergic (parasympathomimetic)** drugs (e.g., bethanechol) act like mediators of the parasympathetic nervous system
2. **Cholinergic blocking (parasympatholytic or anticholinergic)** drugs (e.g., atropine) block the action of the parasympathetic nervous system
3. **Adrenergic (sympathomimetic)** drugs (e.g., norepinephrine) act like mediators of the sympathetic nervous system
4. **Adrenergic blocking (sympatholytic)** drugs (e.g., propranolol, a beta blocking agent) block the action of the sympathetic nervous system

CHOLINERGIC DRUGS

As discussed in Chapter 20, acetylcholine plays an important role in transmission of nerve impulses in both the parasympathetic and sympathetic divisions of the autonomic nervous system.

Acetylcholine has two major actions on the nervous system: (1) it has stimulant effects on the ganglia, adrenal medulla, and skeletal muscle, and (2) it has stimulant effects at postganglionic nerve endings in cardiac muscle, smooth muscle, and glands. The first action resembles the effects of nicotine, such as tachycardia, elevated blood pressure, and peripheral vasoconstriction, and is referred to as the "nicotine effect" of acetylcholine. The second action of acetylcholine at the postganglionic nerve endings is like that of muscarine (an alkaloid obtained from the toadstool *Amanita muscaria*) and is referred to as the **muscarinic effect** or cholinergic effect of acetylcholine. (Table 21-1; see Figure 20-2 on p. 396 to review nicotine [N] and muscarinic [M] sites.)

Cholinergic drugs are agents that bring about effects in the body similar to those produced by acetylcholine. These agents are also called parasympathomimetics because they mimic the action produced by stimulation of the parasympathetic nervous system.

Cholinergic fibers are widespread: they are present in heart, spleen, uterus, vas deferens, colon, and the vessels of the skin and muscles. Cholinergic fibers probably are present in many more tissues of the body. In the gastrointestinal tract parasympathetic innervation predominates: it stimulates both motor and secretory action.

Although acetylcholine is important physiologically, it has no therapeutic value because (1) its actions are very brief owing to rapid hydrolysis by acetylcholinesterase, and (2) no selective purpose can be achieved through its use, since it has several sites of action.

Cholinergic drugs may be obtained from natural (plant) or synthetic sources. The synthetic drugs are more stable and have a more selective action on particular organs. The two groups of cholinergic drugs available are (1) *direct-acting* and (2) *indirect-acting*. **Direct-acting cholinergic** drugs combine directly with the cholinergic receptors in postsynaptic membranes innervated by parasympathetic neurons and evoke effects similar to those produced by acetylcholine. By contrast, instead of a direct effect on receptors, **indirect-acting cholinergic** drugs act primarily on the enzyme inhibiting the action of cholinesterase (acetylcholinesterase) that normally de-

TABLE 21-1 Acetylcholine: sites for muscarinic and nicotinic actions

Site	Muscarinic action*	Nicotinic actions
Cardiovascular		
Blood vessels	Dilation	Constriction } With large doses after atropine
Heart rate	Slowed	Increased } With large doses after atropine
Blood pressure	Decreased	Increased } With large doses after atropine
Gastrointestinal		
Tone	Increased	Increased
Motility	Increased	Increased
Sphincters	Relaxed	—
Glandular secretions	Increased salivary, lacrimal, intestinal, and sweat secretion	Initial stimulation, then inhibition of salivary and bronchial secretions
Skeletal muscle	—	Stimulated
Autonomic ganglia	—	Stimulated
Eye	Pupil constriction Decreased accommodation	—
Blocking agent	Atropine	Tubocurarine
Remarks	Above effects increase as dosage increases	Increased dosage inhibits effects and causes receptor blockade

*Usual sites for therapeutic effects.

grades acetylcholine. This results in an accumulation of acetylcholine at all the sites where it is liberated (see Figure 20-4, A-5, p. 400). By rendering the enzymatic action ineffective, the anticholinesterase drugs cause a prolonged and intensified cholinergic response at the various effector sites.

Cholinergic drugs may be used:

1. To stimulate the intestine and bladder postoperatively thus increasing peristalsis and urination
2. To lower intraocular pressure in clients with glaucoma
3. To promote salivation and sweating
4. To terminate curarization (neuromuscular blockade used as an adjunct to general anesthesia)
5. To treat myasthenia gravis symptomatically*

The therapeutic effectiveness of cholinergic drugs depends primarily on their muscarinic action, but some of them also possess nicotinic action. This nicotinic action usually requires doses much larger than those used therapeutically. However, some drugs may exhibit more nicotinic than muscarinic effects (see Table 21-1).

The ideal cholinergic or anticholinesterase drug would:

1. Mimic or inhibit the effect of acetylcholine on a particular structure or organ
2. Be effective when administered orally
3. Be more stable and less easily inactivated than the drugs now available
4. Produce a therapeutic effect with minimal side effects

Although these ideal drugs are not yet available, progress is being made in this direction.

*Cholinergic, but not parasympathomimetic, action involves the somatic nervous system, innervating skeletal muscle.

Cholinergic drugs used primarily to lower intraocular pressure are discussed in Chapter 43, Ophthalmic Drugs. These include pilocarpine and carbachol. Table 21-2 lists the prominent cholinergic and anticholinesterase drugs.

Direct-Acting Cholinergic Drugs (Choline Esters)

Drugs that are chemically similar to the neurotransmitter acetylcholine include bethanechol, carbachol, and methacholine. All compounds in this group are quaternary amines so they are poorly absorbed orally. Their actions are comparable although longer acting then the physiologic mediator acetylcholine. The side effects of these drugs are a consequence of parasympathetic stimulation which includes bradycardia, hypotension, sweating, salivation, vomiting, diarrhea, and intestinal cramps.

▲ **bethanechol chloride** [be than' e kole] (Urecholine, Duvoid ♣)

Bethanechol is a synthetic choline ester with actions similar to those of acetylcholine. It produces the effects of stimulation of the parasympathetic nervous system. It has predominant muscarinic action with particular selectivity on the detrusor muscle of the urinary bladder and smooth muscle of the gastrointestinal tract. Hence contraction of the smooth muscle of the bladder is sufficiently strong to initiate micturition and empty the urinary bladder. In the gastrointestinal tract, the drug stimulates gastric motility, increases gastric tone, and often restores impaired peristaltic activity of the esophagus, stomach, and intestine. It also promotes defecation. Unlike acetylcholine, bethanechol is not de-

TABLE 21-2 Cholinergic agents: direct acting and indirect acting (anticholinesterase) agents

Generic name	Usual adult dose (24 hrs)	Usual route of administration
ambenonium (I) (Mytelase)	5 mg tid to qid	Oral
bethanechol (D) (Urecholine)	10-50 mg tid to qid 5 mg tid or qid	Oral Subcutaneous
isoflurophate (I) (Floropryl)	Thin strip (0.5 cm) of 0.025%, variable instructions	Topical (eye) ointment
neostigmine bromide (I) (Prostigmin)	15 mg q3-4h	Oral
neostigmine methylsulfate (I) (Prostigmin)	0.5 mg dose variable	Intramuscular or subcutaneous
physostigmine (I) (Eserine)	1 drop, 0.25%-0.5% solution bid or tid	Topical (eye)
physostigmine (I) (Antilirium)	0.5 mg-2 mg (maximum)	IM or IV
pilocarpine (D)	1 drop, 0.5%-4% qid	Topical (eye)
pyridostigmine (I) (Mestinon)	Highly variable	Oral

D, direct acting; *I*, indirect acting.

stroyed by cholinesterase, and therefore its effects are more prolonged than that of the natural neurotransmitter. Therapeutic test doses in normal human subjects have little effect on heart rate, blood pressure, or peripheral circulation.

Bethanechol (Urecholine) has generally been replaced by more effective drugs, but it is approved in the United States for the treatment of postoperative and postpartum nonobstructive urinary retention and for neurogenic atony of the urinary bladder associated with retention. Although not indicated on its U.S. product labeling, it has also been used to relieve postoperative abdominal distention and gastric atony or stasis and reflux esophagitis associated with decreased pressure of lower esophageal sphincter.

Despite being poorly absorbed from the gastrointestinal tract, bethanechol chloride is effective orally. It is widely distributed to organs innervated by the parasympathetic nervous system. Onset of action is within 30 to 90 minutes after oral administration, peak effect within 1 hour, and duration of action up to 6 hours, depending on the dose administered. If administered subcutaneously, the onset of action is within 5 to 15 minutes, peak effect within 15 to 30 minutes, and duration of action approximately 2 hours. Route of excretion is currently unknown. Table 21-3 lists side effects/adverse reactions.

Dosage and administration. Oral dosage for adults, 10-50 mg orally, 3 to 4 times daily; for children, 0.6 mg/kg body weight in 3 or 4 divided doses per day. Parenteral dosage for adults, 5 mg *subcutaneously*, 3 or 4 times/day when needed; and for children, *subcutaneous use only*, 0.2 mg/kg body weight in 3 or 4 divided doses per day.

▪ Nursing Management

Bethanechol Therapy

Assessment. Bethanechol should not be used after gastrointestinal anastomosis or bladder surgery until healing has occurred. Its risk-benefit should be considered when peptic ulcer (increase in gastric acid secretion may aggravate ulcer) or peritonitis, gastrointestinal or urinary obstruction, or an inflammatory disease of the gastrointestinal tract is present when increased muscular activity might be harmful. It is also used with caution during pregnancy or in clients with coronary disease and hyperthyroidism (increased risk of atrial fibrillation), hypotension (may decrease BP), bradycardia (may slow heart rate), or asthma (may cause bronchospasm).

The nurse should be aware of the following possibilities when bethanechol is given with the drugs listed below:

Drug	Possible effect and management
other cholinergic or anticholinesterase medications	**Enhanced cholinergic effects and perhaps toxicity. Monitor closely for adverse effects or, if possible, avoid this combination of medications (see Table 21-3).**
ganglionic blocking agents	**May result in severe abdominal distress followed by a precipitous fall in blood pressure. Avoid or a potentially serious drug interaction may occur.**
procainamide or quinidine	Cholinergic effects may be antagonized. Monitor closely for dry mouth, urinary retention, blurred vision, confusion, and ataxia.

The client's vital signs, as well as a description of the symptoms for which it is being prescribed, should be taken as a baseline assessment before bethanechol therapy is initiated.

Nursing diagnosis. The client receiving bethanechol should be assessed for the following nursing diagnoses: altered comfort related to belching or parasympathetic stimulation (headache, increased salivation or sweating, nausea or vomiting, nervousness, flushing of the skin, and abdominal discomfort); altered bowel elimination pattern (diarrhea); altered urinary pattern, (frequency related to effects of drug or retention related to the ineffectiveness of the drug); risk of injury related to blurred vision, change in near or distant vision, or orthostatic hypotension; and the potential complications of bronchoconstriction (shortness of breath, wheezing, tightness in chest) and seizures.

Implementation

Monitoring. Observe the client closely for side effects or adverse reactions, particularly with subcutaneous administration. Monitor vital signs and carefully check respiration for 30 to 60 minutes after injection. Keep available 0.6 mg atropine in a syringe to counteract severe side effects. Evaluate the effectiveness of the drug by monitoring intake and output, or residual urine volumes if applicable, when administering bethanechol for postoperative urinary retention. If the bladder sphincter fails to relax as the urinary bladder contracts in response to bethanechol administration, urine may be forced up the ureter into the kidney. If the client has bacteriuria, this reflux of urine into the kidney may cause a kidney infection. Intake and output must be carefully monitored in these clients. Box 21-1 describes the use of bethanechol in rehabilitation settings with clients having neurogenic bladder.

Intervention. Administer bethanechol on an empty stomach to minimize the possibility of nausea and vomiting. Bethanechol is to be parenterally administered only subcutaneously. Do not administer intramuscularly or intravenously because severe symptoms of cholinergic overstimulation (flushing of the skin, headache, severe hypotension, hypothermia, bradycardia, nausea and vomiting, abdominal cramps, bloody diarrhea, shock, or cardiac arrest) may occur.

Education. Instruct the client to move slowly from a lying to a sitting or standing position because orthostatic hypotension is a common effect of bethanechol.

Evaluation. Without experiencing any adverse effects of the drug, the client should be able to urinate without experiencing retention.

Indirect-Acting Cholinergic Drugs

The **indirect-acting cholinergic drugs** are anticholinesterases or cholinesterase inhibitors because they inhibit the action of the enzyme cholinesterase, thereby prolonging the effect of acetylcholine. Anticholinesterase agents (e.g., neostigmine, physostigmine) exert their influence on both muscarinic and nicotinic sites. They are used in the treatment of myasthenia gravis and glaucoma (see Chapters 23 and 43, respectively). Physostigmine salicylate is used for overdosage

TABLE 21-3 Drugs affecting the parasympathetic nervous system: side effects/adverse reactions

Drug(s)	Side effects*	Adverse reactions†
Cholinergic		
bethanechol chloride (Urecholine, Duvoid♣)	More frequent with high dosages, unsteadiness; faintness; nausea or vomiting; headache; flushed skin; abdominal pains or upset; increased salivation and sweating Less frequent: diarrhea; increased urination; blurred or disturbed vision; gas complaints	Rare and usually reported with subcutaneous injection: difficulty in breathing, shortness of breath, feeling of pressure in the chest In overdosage or in persons hypersensitive to drug: hypotension; profuse and bloody diarrhea; shock; possibly sudden cardiac arrest
Cholinergic blocking (parasympatholytic)		
atropine	More frequent: inhibition of sweating; constipation; complaints of dry mouth, throat, and skin Less frequent: abdominal distention; blurred vision; inhibition of lactation; urinary retention or dysuria; sedation; headache; photophobia; drowsiness; weakness; nausea or vomiting	Less frequent or rare: urticaria; dermatitis; eye pain from increased intraocular pressure Overdosage/toxicity: blurred vision; ataxia; confusion; disorientation; severe dryness of mouth, throat, and nose area; hyperpyrexia; hallucinations; restlessness; delirium; tachycardia; difficulty in breathing
scopolamine (Transderm-Scop)	Same as atropine, plus euphoria; amnesia, insomnia or increased drowsiness reported more often with scopolamine	Dilated and fixed pupil on side where disk was applied have been reported with use of transdermal disk behind the ear. To avoid extensive neurologic exams, unconscious individuals appearing with above symptoms should be checked first for the use of a disk behind the ear. If the disk is removed, this syndrome usually abates within 2 weeks. To avoid misdiagnosis, drops of 1% pilocarpine solution may be instilled in the eye; this will reverse the nonneurogenic dilated pupil
Synthetic antispasmodics		
dicyclomine (Bentyl, Antispas)	More frequent: abdominal distention, headache, dizziness Less frequent: nausea, vomiting, sedation, nervousness, decreased sexual ability, blurred or disturbed vision, confusion (especially in older clients) Rare: inhibition of sweating, tachycardia, dry mouth	More frequent: usually constipation (especially in older cllients) Less frequent: dysuria Rare: dermatitis
glycopyrrolate (Robinul)	More frequent: dry mouth, nose, throat, and skin Less frequent/rare: the following may occur more often if high doses are given: abdominal distention, blurred vision, constipation, decreased lactation, inhibition of sweating, dysuria, sedation, headache, amnesia (especially in older clients), photophobia, nausea, vomiting, insomnia, weakness, decrease in sexual ability	Rarely reported: faintness, hypotension, dizziness, eye pain, dermatitis Overdosage: respiratory difficulties; severe muscle weakness; extreme tiredness; drowsiness or a paradoxical effect of increased excitability; nervousness, restlessness; tachycardia; warm, dry, and red flushing of skin

*If side effects continue, increase, or disturb the client, the physician should be informed.
†If adverse reactions occur, the prescriber should be contacted because medical intervention may be necessary.

Continued

TABLE 21-3 Drugs affecting the parasympathetic nervous system: side effects/adverse reactions—cont'd

Drug(s)	Side effects*	Adverse reactions[†]
Synthetic antispasmodics—cont'd		
clidinium (Quarzan)	More frequent: dry mouth, nose, throat and skin Less frequent: abdominal distention, blurred vision, constipation, decreased lactation, insomnia, nausea, vomiting, increased weakness, headache, drowsiness, dysuria (especially in elderly men), inhibition of sweating, decrease in sexual ability	Rare: faintness, hypotension (especially in older clients); dermatitis Overdosage: same as glycopyrrolate
Ganglionic blocking drugs		
trimethaphan camsylate (Arfonad)	Side effects are dose related: loss of appetite, nausea, vomiting, constipation, dilated pupil, dry mouth, impotency, pruritis, hives, hypotension, increased heart rate, urinary retention, and use may precipitate angina attack	Overdosage: severe hypotension, respiratory arrest

BOX 21-1

Use of Bethanechol with Clients Having Neurogenic Bladder

Bethanechol is used as an adjunct therapy in clients with chronic neurogenic bladder. After several baseline measurements of residual urine volume, the adult client is administered 5 mg of bethanechol chloride subcutaneously every 4 hours. Twelve hours after the first dose of bethanechol, the client is asked to void, and a residual urine volume is measured. If the amount of residual urine is less than the baseline volume, the drug is continued for another 24 hours. At that time the drug's effectiveness is again evaluated by another residual urine volume measurement. If this too is below the baseline volume, the drug is continued for another 24 to 48 hours on the "every 4 hours" schedule. After that period, the dosage should be decreased to 2.5-5 mg every 4 hours. When the residual urine is less than 50 mL, the dosage is changed to an oral form, 50 mg every 4 hours. According to the client's response, the dosage interval may be gradually increased and the dosage decreased.

and anticholinergic substance toxicity. (See the discussion about tricyclic antidepressant overdosage treatment in Chapter 19.)

Drugs Used to Treat Myasthenia Gravis

Myasthenia gravis is a condition characterized by weakness of the skeletal muscles innervated by the somatic efferent fibers. Since the disease affects cholinergic transmission, the anticholinesterase drugs are used because they elevate the concentration of acetylcholine at the myoneural junctions. The prolonged activity of the neurohormone at these sites results in a dramatic increase in muscle strength and function. There is a more extensive discussion of myasthenia gravis and its treatment in Chapter 23. (See also Figure 20-2, p. 396, for site of action.)

CHOLINERGIC BLOCKING DRUGS

Muscarinic Blocking Drugs

The **cholinergic blocking**, or **parasympatholytic**, drugs have many important uses in medicine. More specifically, these agents are called **antimuscarinic** or **anticholinergic** drugs because they block the muscarinic effects of acetylcholine. When the nerve fiber is stimulated, the acetylcholine liberated from the terminal is unable to bind to the receptor site and fails to produce a cholinergic effect. Thus these agents also are referred to as anticholinergic drugs. (See Figure 20-2, p. 396, for muscarinic [M] sites.)

Belladonna Alkaloids

The best known muscarinic or cholinergic blocking drugs are the belladonna alkaloids. The major drugs in this class are atropine, hyoscyamine, and scopolamine (Table 21-4). A number of plants belonging to the potato family (*Solanaceae*) contain similar alkaloids. *Atropa belladonna* (deadly nightshade), *Hyoscyamus niger* (henbane), *Datura stramonium* (jimson weed or thorn apple), and several species of *Scopolia* also contain belladonna alkaloids. The principal alkaloids of these plants are atropine, scopolamine (hyoscine), and hyoscyamine. Atropine is the prototype of the antimuscarinic drugs. It has been in use for over half a century and

TABLE 21-4 Selected anticholinergic agents containing specific alkaloids*

Alkaloid formation†	Trade name
hyoscyamine	Anaspaz
	Cystospaz
	Cystospaz-M
	Levsin
hyoscyamine and scopolamine	Bellafoline
scopolamine	Buscopan ♣
	Transderm-Scop
	Transderm-V
atropine, hyoscyamine, scopolamine, and phenobarbital	Barbidonna
	Barophen
	Donnatal
	Donnatal Extentabs
	Kinesed
atropine and phenobarbital	Antrocol
belladonna and butabarbital	Butibel
belladonna and phenobarbital	Chardonna-2
hyoscyamine and phenobarbital	Levsin-PB

*Specific alkaloids include the active alkaloids of belladonna, such as hyoscyamine, atropine, and scopolamine.
†The alkaloid formulation lists the active ingredients as marketed under the various trade names. Individual salts, strengths, and dosing intervals may vary according to the manufacturer's instructions.

continues to be a popular drug because of its therapeutic effectiveness.

▲ **atropine sulfate** [a' troe peen] (Atropine, Isopto Atropine)

Mechanism of action. As a competitive antagonist, atropine acts by occupying the muscarinic (M) receptor sites, thereby preventing or reducing the muscarinic response of acetylcholine (see Figure 20-2, p. 396). The drug-receptor complex is formed at the neuroeffector junctions of smooth muscle, cardiac muscle, and exocrine glands.

Atropine has very little effect on the actions of acetylcholine at nicotinic receptor sites. So at autonomic ganglia, where transmission normally involves the action of acetylcholine, relatively high doses of atropine are required to produce even a partial block. At the neuromuscular junctions of the somatic nervous system, where the receptors are exclusively nicotinic, extremely high doses of atropine are required to produce any degree of block. See Figure 20-2 (p. 396) for nicotinic (N) sites on the ganglia or parasympathetic and sympathetic nerve divisions, and for N sites on effector organ (skeletal muscle) of the somatic motor system.

Atropine can produce a wide range of pharmacologic effects because a vast distribution of parasympathetic cholinergic nerves normally exists in the body. Furthermore, drug activity is dose-dependent. Small doses depress salivary and bronchial secretions and sweating. Large doses dilate the pupils, inhibit accommodation of the eyes, and increase heart rate by blocking vagal effects of the heart. Larger doses inhibit micturition and decrease the tone and motility of the gut by inhibiting parasympathetic control of both the urinary bladder and the gastrointestinal tract. In addition, still larger doses are required to inhibit gastric secretion and motility.

Pharmacologic properties

Eye. The pupil is dilated (mydriasis), and the ciliary muscle (muscle of accommodation) is relaxed (cycloplegia). The sphincter muscle of the iris and the ciliary muscle are both innervated by cholinergic nerve fibers and therefore are affected by atropine. Since the sphincter muscle is unable to contract normally, the radial muscle of the iris causes the pupil to dilate.

Pupil dilation may reduce outflow of aqueous humor, causing a rise in intraocular pressure. This is a hazardous situation for clients with glaucoma (angle closure). These effects in the eye are brought about by both local and systemic administration of atropine, although the usual single therapeutic dose of atropine given orally or parenterally has little effect on the eye. After the pupil is dilated, photophobia occurs, and when the drug has reached its full effect, the usual reflexes to light and accommodation disappear.

Systemic absorption of ophthalmic medications resulting in undesirable side effects or adverse reactions have been reported with atropine and a number of other eye preparations. Therefore ophthalmic preparations should be included in the review of the client's current medications because an ophthalmic preparation may be an offending agent (*USP DI*, 1996).

Skin and mucous membranes. Since the sweat glands of the skin are supplied by sympathetic cholinergic nerves, atropine decreases or abolishes their activity. This causes the skin to become hot and dry. Further, since the flow of secretions from glands lining the respiratory tract is reduced, drying of the mucous membranes of the mouth, nose, pharynx, and bronchi occurs. Clients who have been given atropine, particularly for preoperative preparation, often complain of a dry mouth and thirst.

Respiratory system. Secretions of the nose, pharynx, and bronchial tubes are decreased. The muscles of the bronchial tubes relax, and the airway widens to ease breathing. Atropine and scopolamine are less effective than epinephrine as bronchodilators and are seldom used for asthma.

Cardiovascular system. When low doses are given or an intravenous dose is administered slowly, the cardiac rate is temporarily and slightly slowed because of the central action of the drug on the cardiac center in the medulla (paradoxical bradycardia). Larger intravenous doses given rapidly will block the vagal effect on the SA node and AV junction and cause an increased heart rate.

In therapeutic doses atropine has little or no effect on blood pressure. This is expected because most vascular beds lack significant cholinergic innervation. However, large (and sometimes ordinary) doses cause vasodilation of vessels in the skin of the face and neck. This may result from a direct dilator action or from histamine release. Reddening of the face and neck is seen, especially after large or toxic doses.

Gastrointestinal tract. It appears that the amount and character of the gastric secretion are little affected by atropine given in ordinary therapeutic doses. The secretion of acid in the stomach is presumably less under vagal control than under hormonal or chemical control. The effect of atropine on the secretion of the pancreas and intestinal glands is not therapeutically significant. Atropine and other belladonna alkaloids decrease tone and peristalsis in the stomach and small and large intestines. Atropine does not affect the secretion of bile, but it exerts a mildly antispasmodic effect in the gallbladder and bile ducts.

Urinary tract. The drug relaxes the ureter, especially when it has been in a state of spasm. Therapeutic doses decrease the tone of the fundus of the urinary bladder. When the detrusor muscle is hypertonic, it is relaxed by atropine. It also causes constriction of the internal sphincter, which can produce urinary retention.

Central nervous system. Atropine has prominent effects on the central nervous system and in large doses causes excitement and maniacal behavior. These behavioral effects suggest the existence of important cholinergic pathways and receptors within the central nervous system.

Small or moderate doses of atropine have little or no cerebral effect. Large or toxic doses cause the patient to become restless, wakeful, and talkative. This condition may develop into delirium and finally stupor and coma. The exalted, excited stage has sometimes been called a "belladonna jag." A rise in temperature is sometimes seen, especially in infants and young children. This is probably the result of suppression of sweating rather than action on the heat-regulating center.

Atropine has been used to diminish tremor in Parkinson's disease. It probably reduces cholinergic synaptic transmission. Therapeutic doses of atropine stimulate the respiratory center and make breathing faster and sometimes deeper. When respiration is seriously depressed, atropine is not always reliable as a stimulant; in fact, it may deepen the depression. Large doses stimulate respiration, but they can also cause respiratory failure and death.

Small doses stimulate the vagus center in the medulla, causing primary slowing of the heart. The vasoconstrictor center is stimulated briefly and then depressed. Because depression follows soon after stimulation, atropine has been called a borderline stimulant of the central nervous system.

Topical effects. There is a slight amount of absorption when atropine or belladonna is applied to the skin, especially if it is an alcoholic preparation or in the form of a transdermal patch.

Indications. Atropine is indicated for the treatment of irritable bowel syndrome, spastic biliary tract disorders, and genitourinary disorders; and as an antidote for cholinergic toxicity from excessive amounts of cholinesterase inhibitors, muscarinics, or organophosphate pesticide poisoning. Atropine is also used to treat sinus bradycardia and Parkinson's disease, to prevent excessive salivation and respiratory tract secretions as a preanesthetic agent, and as an adjunctive medication for peptic ulcers and for gastrointestinal radiography.

Pharmacokinetics. Atropine is readily absorbed from oral and parenteral administration; it is also absorbed from mucous membranes.

After oral administration, the maximum effect is reached within 1 hour; duration of action is 4 to 6 hours. It is widely distributed in fluids of the body and easily passes the placental barrier to the blood of the fetus and the blood-brain barrier. Atropine is metabolized primarily in the liver, approximately 30% to 50% of atropine is excreted unchanged in the urine. For side effects/adverse reactions, see Table 21-3.

Dosage and administration. The oral anticholinergic adult dose for atropine sulfate for an adult is 0.3 to 1.2 mg PO, every 4 to 6 hours. The pediatric dose is 0.01 mg/kg, not exceeding 0.4 mg, every 4 to 6 hours. The adult oral dose to prevent excessive salivation and respiratory tract secretions during anesthesia is 0.4 to 0.6 mg. The dose should be titrated as necessary to client's response or to the appearance of side effects. The adult parenteral anticholinergic dose is 0.4 to 0.6 mg IM, IV, or SC every 4 to 6 hours. The pediatric anticholinergic dose is 0.01 mg/kg IM, IV, or SC, not exceeding 0.4 mg. The dose may be repeated every 4 to 6 hours if necessary. The adult parenteral dose to treat bradycardia (dysrhythmia) is 0.4 to 1 mg IV, every 1 to 2 hours, up to a maximum of 2 mg; the pediatric dysrhythmic dose is 0.01 to 0.03 mg/kg.

■ Nursing Management

Atropine Therapy

See also Nursing Management: Anticholinergic Therapy (Chapter 23, p. 455).

Assessment. Use atropine with caution in elderly clients and children under 6 years of age because they are more susceptible to adverse reactions, such as excitement, sleepiness, or confusion. Toxicity may occur in the elderly even when the drug is prescribed within the normal adult dosage range. Sensitivity to the drug should be determined.

Anticholinergics should be used with caution in individuals over 40 years of age because of the risk of precipitating undiagnosed glaucoma. The use of atropine (or belladonna alkaloids) should be avoided in clients with a medical history of severe cardiac disease (increases heart rate), reflux esophagitis (decreased GI motility promotes gastric retention), GI tract obstructive disease states or intestinal atony (decreased motility may result in obstruction), urinary retention (aggravates symptoms), prostatic hypertrophy (aggravates symptoms), or myasthenia gravis (aggravates condition by inhibition of acetylcholine). Do not use in clients with open-angle glaucoma (mydriatic effect increases intraocular pressure), ulcerative colitis, or renal or hepatic disease (increases effects of drug). Administer systemic forms carefully to clients with chronic pulmonary disease because bronchial secretions may be sufficiently decreased to result in bronchial plugs. Use with caution in infants, blondes, clients with Down's syndrome, and pediatric clients with spastic paralysis and brain damage because they tend to be more sensitive to the drug's effects.

Assess the client's concurrent medication regimen for significant drug interactions. The following effects may occur when atropine (and other belladonna alkaloids) are given with the drugs listed below:

Drug	Possible effect and management
antacids or antidiarrheal agents	May reduce absorption and therapeutic effectiveness of atropine. Space medications at least 2 to 3 hours apart.
other anticholinergics	Increase in anticholinergic effects reported. Monitor for such symptoms as decreased perspiration, dry mouth, blurred vision, and confusion, because dosage adjustment may be necessary.
ketoconazole (Nizoral)	Increase in gastrointestinal pH by atropine may result in reduced absorption of ketoconazole. Atropine should be administered preferably 2 hours after ketoconazole.
potassium chloride, especially wax matrix formulations	Increased contact with gastrointestinal tract may result in mucosal irritation and lesions. Liquid formulations of potassium should be considered a replacement for the wax matrix formulation in this situation.

Obtain a baseline assessment of the client's vital signs and urinary and bowel status. For geriatric and debilitated clients, a mental status assessment will be helpful to determine if the client is having any drowsiness or CNS stimulation as a result of the drug. If the drug is used as an antiarrhythmic, a baseline ECG is required. For clients on long term therapy, a baseline intraocular pressure determination is indicated.

Nursing diagnosis. The client receiving atropine therapy is at risk for the following nursing diagnoses: hyperthermia related to the suppression of sweat gland activity; risk for injury related to blurred vision, dizziness or lightheadedness; impaired tissue integrity (irritation at injection site); altered thought processes (confusion, agitation); altered comfort related to dry mouth or increased sensitivity of eyes to light; urinary retention related to the drug's anticholinergic effects; altered bowel elimination pattern (constipation) related to decreased motility of the gastrointestinal tract; and the potential complication of allergic reaction and decreased cardiac output related to the drug's ineffectiveness.

Implementation

Monitoring. Monitor pulse, which is a sensitive indicator of client's response to atropine. Also be alert to any change in blood pressure, temperature, and respiration, particularly after intravenous administration. ECG recordings are monitored when atropine is used for arrhythmias. Monitor client for urinary output and bowel regularity. Notify prescriber of any significant changes. Observe elderly clients for excitement, agitation, and delirium. Assess for constipation, dryness of mouth, and, in the elderly male client, urinary retention. Because of the mydriatic effects of atropine, intraocular pressure determinations should be done at regular intervals for clients having extended atropine therapy.

Intervention. Administer oral preparations 30 to 60 minutes before meals. Administer antacids or antidiarrheal medications at least 1 hour after the administration of atropine. Have physostigmine on hand to treat atropine overdose.

Education. Inform client of possible side effects. Advise the client about the use of sugarless gum and candy, ice, or saliva substitutes to relieve dry mouth. Instruct the client to avoid alcohol and other CNS depressants while taking atropine.

Counsel the client involved in long-term use to follow a consistent dental hygiene program, including semiannual visits to the dentist because the decreased salivary flow promotes caries, buccal candidiasis, and periodontal disease.

Instruct the client to avoid exposure to high environmental temperatures, exercise in warm, humid weather, or prolonged hot baths. These activities may lead to heat prostration. The client should report any fever to the prescriber because the medication may have to be discontinued.

Inform the client using an ophthalmic preparation that his or her vision will be impaired for a few days. The client should protect his or her eyes by wearing dark glasses. The client's ability to judge distance will also be impaired; therefore the client should avoid driving a car or operating machinery. The drug should be discontinued if signs of local irritation or follicular conjunctivitis occur. This may happen after prolonged periods of ophthalmic therapy.

Evaluation. The client's ECG indicates the underlying arrhythmia has been corrected without any tachycardia. The client does not experience any adverse effects of the atropine, such as constipation or urinary retention. If the drug is taken for an ophthalmic condition, the client will experience therapeutic mydriasis without systemic adrenergic-like effects.

For additional atropine preparations see Chapters 41 and 43.

scopolamine [skoe pol' a meen] (Transderm-Scop, Transderm-V)
scopolamine hydrobromide

See the preceding discussion of atropine for mechanism of action. Scopolamine's peripheral effects are similar to atropine, but it differs in its effects on the central nervous system. At therapeutic doses, it depresses the CNS and causes drowsiness, euphoria, memory loss, relaxation, sleep, and relief of fear. It does not increase blood pressure or respiration.

It is used in the treatment of irritable bowel syndrome; renal and ureteral colic; and for dysrhythmias induced during surgery owing to increased vagal stimulation. Because of its depressant action on vestibular function, it is used for motion sickness to prevent nausea and vomiting. It is used as an adjunct medication with general anesthesia to check secretions, to prevent laryngospasm, and for its sedative (twilight sleep) and amnesic effects.

Scopolamine's pharmacokinetics are the same as atropine. The transdermal dosage form produces its antiemetic effects for up to 72 hours. For side effects/adverse reactions, see Table 21-3.

An oral dosage form is not available in the United States. The parenteral dose in adults for use as an anticholinergic and an antiemetic is 0.3 to 0.6 mg as a single dose. Used as an adjunct to anesthesia or for sedation-hypnosis, administer 0.6 mg IM, IV, or SC, 3 or 4 times daily. For amnesia give 0.32 to 0.6 mg IM, IV, or SC. The elderly are more sensitive to scopolamine. If used, lower doses than the adult ones are recommended. In children, when used as an antiemetic, give 6 μg (0.006 mg)/kg IM, IV, or SC as a single dose. To reduce excess salivation during anesthesia, various IM doses are recommended according to age; see current reference. When administering scopolamine transdermally as an adult antiemetic or antivertigo, apply patch (0.5 mg) behind ear for a period of 3 days. For antiemetic effect, apply 4 hours before desired effect is required. The elderly are more sensitive to this drug at adult dosage; monitor closely for hyperpyrexia, confusion, blurred vision, and ataxia. The drug is not recommended for children.

■ Nursing Management
Scopolamine Therapy

See the previous discussion of atropine sulfate. In addition, concurrent use of scopolamine with alcohol and other CNS depressants may result in increased CNS depression effects. Clients should be monitored closely for drowsiness and altered thought processes.

For the transdermal application of scopolamine, instruct the client to wash and dry hands before and after application of the patch. It is to be applied to the hairless skin area behind the ear. It is not to be applied over abrasions or rashes. Alert the client that drowsiness and dilated pupils (photophobia and blurred vision) may occur, and if they occur, tasks such as driving or mowing the lawn may be hazardous.

If scopolamine has been administered as part of a preoperative medication for a day stay or ambulatory procedure, caution the client before discharge about the effects on memory and motor tasks. These effects may persist for a few hours.

Synthetic Substitutes for Atropine

The usefulness of atropine is limited by the fact that it is a complex drug that produces effects in a number of organs or tissues simultaneously. When it is administered for its antispasmodic effects, it also produces prolonged effects in the eye, causing dilated pupils and blurred vision. It also causes dry mouth and possibly rapid heart rate. When the antispasmodic effect is desired, other effects become side effects, which may be distinctly undesirable.

A large number of drugs have been synthesized in an effort to capture the antispasmodic effect of atropine without its other effects. Drugs of this type are frequently used to relieve hypertonicity and hypersecretion in the stomach.

Many products are marketed as antispasmodic and anticholinergic agents, but their formulations are either modifications of a belladonna alkaloid or include one or more of the natural alkaloids as their active ingredients. The pharmacologic properties are therefore similar to the previously reviewed substances and will not be repeated here (see Table 21-4). The more commonly used or newer systemic agents—dicyclomine (Bentyl), glycopyrrolate (Robinul), and clidinium bromide (Quarzan)—will be discussed.

dicyclomine [dye sye' kloe meen] (Bentyl, Bentylol ♣, and others)

Dicyclomine produces both a direct effect on smooth muscle, resulting in a decreased tone, and motility of the gastrointestinal, biliary, and urinary tracts. It only appears to produce the typical anticholinergic (antimuscarinic) effect when administered in large doses. Dicyclomine is indicated for the treatment of the irritable bowel syndrome.

Little has been determined about the pharmacokinetics of this product. It is rapidly absorbed after oral or parenteral administration, and about 50% of the dose is excreted by the kidneys and the other 50% in the feces. Half-life is 1.8 hours initially and 9 to 10 hours for the second phase.

For side effects/adverse reactions, see Table 21-3.

Dosage and administration. The adult oral dose is 10 to 20 mg 3 or 4 times daily. Dosage may be adjusted according to response, up to a maximum of 160 mg/day. For children: less than 6 months old, it is not recommended; 6 months to 2 years old, 5 to 10 mg orally (syrup available, 5 mg/tsp) 3 or 4 times daily, adjust as necessary; and 2 years old and older, 10 mg orally 3 or 4 times daily, adjust as necessary. Parenterally: Adults, 20 mg IM every 4 to 6 hours. *Do not administer intravenously.* For children, the dosage is not established.

■ Nursing Management
Dicyclomine Therapy

See the discussion of nursing management of atropine sulfate therapy. The significant drug interactions with antacids and antidiarrheal agents, other anticholinergics, ketoconazole (Nizoral), and potassium chloride are the same as for atropine. Dicyclomine injections should only be given intramuscularly. Administer oral preparations with food or milk to minimize gastric distress. The syrup form may be diluted with equal parts of water to make administration easier. When administering the parenteral form, ensure that the client is lying or sitting down because some temporary lightheadedness could be experienced. Alert the client that blurred vision may occur and should be reported to the prescriber. When prescribed as adjunctive therapy for peptic ulcers and other GI disorders, the client should experience relief from GI pain.

glycopyrrolate [glue koe pye' roe late] (Robinul, Robinul Forte)

This is a synthetic anticholinergic product with effects similar to atropine. Unlike atropine, it is unable to easily cross lipid membranes (such as blood-brain barrier) and therefore has minimal central nervous system side effects. It also appears to be less likely to produce pupillary or ocular eye effects.

Glycopyrrolate is indicated as an anticholinergic (antimuscarinic) to prevent or reduce hypersecretion or reduce arrhythmias induced during anesthesia; and to prevent or reduce toxicities induced by cholinesterase inhibitors (neostigmine or pyridostigmine). It is administered orally, IV, IM, or SC. The onset of action of intravenous dose occurs within 1 minute. For IM or SC routes, onset of action is 15 to 30 minutes. Vagal blocking action lasts from 2 to 3 hours, while the antisialagogue effect, the inhibition of the flow of saliva, may last up to 7 hours. Glycopyrrolate is excreted by the kidneys. For side effects/adverse reactions, see Table 21-3.

The significant drug interactions are the same as dicyclomine (see previous section). In addition, administering cyclopropane with glycopyrrolate IV may result in ventricular arrhythmias. To reduce this possibility, give smaller dosages of glycopyrrolate IV (0.1 mg or less) and monitor client closely.

Dosage and administration. For adults in the treatment of peptic ulcer, 1 to 2 mg orally 2 or 3 times daily and when necessary, 2 mg at bedtime; then reduce to 1 mg twice daily or adjust dosage according to client's response and tolerance. The elderly may be more sensitive to this glycopyrrolate dosage, so a lower dosage schedule should be considered. For children the dosage is not established.

Parenterally for adults as an anticholinergic for the treatment of peptic ulcer, administer glycopyrrolate 0.1 to 0.2 mg IM or IV every 4 hours if necessary, up to a maximum of 4 doses per 24 hours. To prevent or reduce excessive salivation and respiratory tract secretions or gastric hypersecretory situations during anesthesia, 4.4 μg/kg of body weight is given parenterally, 30 to 60 minutes before anesthesia. For dysrhythmias during anesthesia or in surgery, 0.1 mg IV is given at 2 to 3 minute intervals as necessary. As a cholinergic adjunctive medication, glycopyrrolate 0.2 mg IV is given for each 1 mg of neostigmine or 5 mg of pyridostigmine and may be administered in the same syringe.

Parenteral dosages for children with peptic ulcer have not been determined. To prevent or reduce excessive salivation and respiratory tract secretions or gastric hypersecretory situations during pediatric anesthesia, 4.4 to 8.8 μg/kg body weight IM is given 30 to 60 minutes before anesthesia. For children with dysrhythmias during anesthesia or in surgery, 4.4 μg/kg of body weight IV given every 2 or 3 minutes, as necessary. As a cholinergic adjunctive medication with children, glycopyrrolate 0.2 mg IV is given for each 1 mg of neostigmine or 5 mg of pyridostigmine and may be administered in the same syringe.

■ Nursing Management

Glycopyrrolate Therapy

Alert the client to have ophthalmic examinations for intraocular pressure periodically. Intraocular pressure may become elevated because of the mydriasis produced by the drug. If blurred vision occurs, it should be reported to the prescriber. When contemplating mixing glycopyrrolate in a syringe with other drugs, consult the package insert, because the drug is unstable at a pH higher than 6 and will form a precipitate when combined with some other agents. See atropine sulfate discussion for additional nursing management.

clidinium [kli di' nee um] (Quarzan)

Clidinium is a synthetic product related to the belladonna alkaloids, especially atropine. It competitively antagonizes acetylcholine at the postganglionic parasympathetic receptor sites in both smooth muscles and the secretory glands, thus reducing GI motility and gastric acid secretion. Ganglionic blockade may be produced if high doses of clidinium are given. Unlike atropine, it produces few, if any, CNS side effects or alterations on the eye.

Clidinium is indicated as an adjunctive treatment for peptic ulcers. Following oral absorption the onset of action occurs within 1 hour; duration of action lasts up to 3 hours. Clidinium is metabolized in the liver and excreted primarily by the kidneys. For side effects/adverse reactions, see Table 21-3.

The oral dose of clidinium for adults is 2.5 to 5 mg 3 or 4 times daily, before meals and at bedtime. Adjust dosage according to individual response. Dosage for elderly is 2.5 mg orally 3 times a day, before meals. Pediatric dosage has not been determined.

■ Nursing Management

Clidinium Therapy

The significant drug interactions are the same as for atropine. Administer ½ hour to 1 hour before meals to enhance absorption. The client should have intraocular pressure determinations done periodically, since intraocular pressure increases because of the drug's mydriatic effect. Blurred vision may occur and should be reported to the prescriber.

For further nursing management, see atropine sulfate discussion.

GANGLIONIC DRUGS

The major neurotransmitter of all autonomic ganglia is acetylcholine. This includes ganglionic synapses of both the parasympathetic and sympathetic nervous system. Acetylcholine activates the nicotinic receptor at the ganglionic sites, which is unlike that of the nicotinic receptors on the effector organ, the skeletal muscle. Thus stimulation of the preganglionic neuron results in the release of acetylcholine from its terminal.

Acetylcholine then activates the nicotinic receptors on the ganglia of the postganglionic parasympathetic or sympathetic neurons, or adrenal medulla.

This interaction ultimately generates a nerve impulse down the postganglionic fibers to produce specific effects on smooth muscle, cardiac muscle, and glands (see Figure 20-2). Ganglionic stimulation influences nerve impulse transmission to the entire autonomic nervous system, and because of such pervasive activity ganglionic drugs have limited therapeutic value.

The drugs that affect nicotinic or cholinergic receptor sites on autonomic ganglia are (1) ganglionic stimulating drugs and (2) ganglionic blocking drugs.

GANGLIONIC STIMULATING DRUGS

Nicotine

Nicotine is a liquid alkaloid, freely soluble in water. It turns brown on exposure to air and is the chief alkaloid in tobacco. Nicotine has no therapeutic use but is of great pharmacologic interest and toxicologic importance. Its use in experiments performed on animals has helped to increase understanding of the autonomic nervous system. Nicotine is readily absorbed from the gastrointestinal tract, respiratory mucous membrane, and skin.

Pharmacologic Effects

Nicotine may produce a variety of complex and often unpredictable effects in the body. Many actions are dose related, with generally small doses inducing activation or stimulation and larger doses producing a decreased or depressed response. Because nicotine acts on multiple systems within the body, the ultimate response may be the sum of the different stimulation and depressant actions of this chemical.

At the autonomic ganglia, nicotine temporarily stimulates all sympathetic and parasympathetic ganglia. This is followed by depression, which tends to last longer than the period of stimulation. Its effects on skeletal muscle are similar to its effects on the ganglia; a depressant phase follows stimulation. During the depressant phase nicotine exerts a curare-like action on skeletal muscle.

Nicotine stimulates the central nervous system, especially the medullary centers (respiratory, emetic, and vasomotor). Large doses may cause tremor and convulsions. Stimulation is followed by depression. Death may result from respiratory failure, although it may be caused more by the curare-like action of nicotine on nerve endings in the diaphragm, rather than by action on the respiratory center.

The actions and effects of nicotine on the cardiovascular system are complex. Heart rate is frequently slowed at first but later may be accelerated above normal. Various disturbances in rhythm have been observed. The small blood vessels in peripheral parts of the body constrict but later may dilate, and the blood pressure will fall; this occurs in nicotine poisoning. Nicotine also has an antidiuretic action. Repeated administration of nicotine causes development of tolerance to some of its effects.

Toxicity

Nicotine has both short- and long-term toxic effects that are extremely important to the health care professional. Nicotine toxicity has resulted from misuse of insecticides containing nicotine, which at times has led to the death of farmworkers. And because nicotine is a major ingredient in tobacco products, both acute toxicity (with ingestion of such products by small children) and chronic toxicity are well documented (Box 21-2).

BOX 21-2

Acute Symptoms of Nicotine Toxicity

Increased flow of saliva
Nausea and vomiting
Abdominal cramps
Diarrhea
Confusion
Cold sweat
Headache
Fainting
Hypotension
Tachycardia
Prostration and collapse
Convulsions may occur
Death results from respiratory failure

Tobacco Smoking and Nicotine

Burning of tobacco can generate approximately 4000 compounds in a gaseous and a particulate or particle phase. Gas phase substances include carbon monoxide, carbon dioxide, hydrogen cyanide, ammonia, volatile nitrosamines, and many other substances. The particulate phase contains mainly nicotine, water, and tar. Known carcinogens have been identified as etiologic factors in a variety of neoplastic diseases, such as cancer of the bladder, lung, buccal cavity, esophagus, and pancreas. Other smoking-related illnesses include pulmonary emphysema, chronic bronchitis, coronary heart disease, and myocardial infarction. Chronic dyspepsia may develop in heavy smokers, and clients with gastric ulcer are usually advised to avoid smoking. Of considerable importance is the fact that smokers absorb sufficient nicotine to exert a variety of effects on the autonomic nervous system. See Box 21-3 for a discussion of nurses and smoking.

In individuals with peripheral vascular disease such as thromboangiitis obliterans (Buerger's disease), nicotine is generally believed to be a contributing factor in the disease. It may cause spasms of the peripheral blood vessels thus reducing the blood flow through the affected vessels. Vasospasm in the retinal blood vessels of the eye, associated with smoking of tobacco, is thought to cause serious disturbance of vision.

Passive smoking, the inhalation of cigarette smoke by nonsmokers, also has harmful effects. The fetus of a smoking mother may have a low birth weight and increased congenital abnormalities. Children of parents who smoke have an increased incidence of sudden infant death syndrome, an increased incidence of respiratory infections and allergic reactions, and an increased likelihood of becoming smokers. Special effort should be made to assist women to stop smoking, particularly during the childbearing years. Smoking by women is still prevalent and may be higher and even increasing within some cultural groups (see the Cultural Aspects box at right).

BOX 21-3

Nurses and Smoking

Nurses, besides having the most prolonged contact with clients and their families, have the knowledge and skills to teach them about the hazards of smoking. Unfortunately, nurses continue to smoke at a frequency higher than other health professionals. In the United States, although 64% of physicians and 61% of dentists who have smoked in the past have stopped smoking, only 36% of nurses have stopped. This is particularly important because Dalton (1986) found that currently smoking nurses were likely to agree that smoking was a major cause of cancer and other health problems and to counsel clients about those hazards. Nurses need to be role models and this should decrease their smoking habits if they are to contribute to a change in the public's smoking behaviors.

An effective program of smoking cessation should incorporate acceptance, support, specific information, and regular opportunities for monitoring progress. Stretcher (1985) found that even a minimal-contact smoking cessation program, including a brief practitioner consultation with self-help manuals conducted in health care settings, produced significant reductions in cigarette smoking.

Besides educating and counseling clients and their families about the benefits of smoking cessation, nurses can participate in community antismoking activities. Such activities include supporting clean indoor air acts and teaching health education courses in schools.

Cultural Aspects: Prevalence of Cigarette Smoking in Hispanic Women of Childbearing Age

Because of the relationship between maternal smoking and poor perinatal outcome, the prevalence of cigarette smoking in women of childbearing age is of importance. A secondary analysis of Hispanic Health and Nutrition Examination Survey data was conducted to determine the prevalence and degree of cigarette smoking among large probability samples of Cuban-American, Mexican-American, and Puerto Rican women of childbearing age. Percentages, means, and 95% confidence intervals were used to determine age-adjusted and age-specific rates for each Hispanic group. Age-adjusted smoking prevalence rates were 23.2%, 22.6%, and 33.5% for Mexican-Americans, Cuban-Americans, and Puerto Ricans, respectively. Age-specific rates indicated that all Puerto Rican women under the age of 40, Mexican-American women in their forties, and Cuban-American women in their thirties had smoking prevalence higher than the national average for women. The high fertility rates for Hispanic women and the high prevalence rates for subgroups of Hispanic women support the need for smoking behavior interventions. Puerto Rican women in their twenties are of particular concern because of their high smoking prevalence (42.2%) in conjunction with the high fertility (61% of births to all Hispanics) of Hispanic women in their twenties. Although most Hispanic women were relatively light smokers, prevention and cessation interventions need to be developed for Puerto Rican women of childbearing age who demonstrated high smoking prevalence. Because of the diversity among Hispanics, campaigns and interventions need to include strategies that are sensitive to the social, educational, economic, and cultural situations of Hispanic peoples.

Critical thinking questions

- What are some considerations related to cigarette smoking and concepts of behavior change that might be relevant for young Hispanic women?
- What factors would be useful in planning and implementing smoking cessation interventions for Hispanic women of childbearing age?

From Pletsch PK (1991). Prevalence of cigarette smoking in Hispanic women of childbearing age, *Nurs Research* 40(2):103.

Nonsmoking adults exposed to smokers have increased symptoms as in those with chronic heart or lung disease also. Higher rates of cancer have also been reported in nonsmoking spouses.

The addictive component of tobacco is nicotine. Many drugs are reported to interact with nicotine. See the discussion below for drug interactions requiring an adjustment in dosage to produce their therapeutic effect for clients who smoke and those for whom nicotine replacement has been prescribed as part of a smoking cessation program.

nicotine gum [nik' oe teen] (Nicorette)
nicotine transdermal systems (Habitrol, Nicoderm, Nicotrol, Prostep),
nicotine nasal spray (Nicotrol NS)

Nicotine is available in a gum (resin), transdermal systems (patches), and nasal spray for use in smoking cessation programs. The nicotine resin is in the form of chewing gum and provides a source of nicotine for the nicotine-dependent client who is undergoing acute cigarette withdrawal. When the client has a strong urge to smoke, a stick of gum is chewed instead, which relieves the physical symptoms of nicotine withdrawal. The number of pieces of gum chewed is gradually reduced over a 2 to 3 month period. For mechanism of action, see the discussion of pharmacologic effects of nicotine.

Nicotine gum is indicated for adjunct treatment of nicotine dependence. It is absorbed through buccal mucosa, slower than if inhaled while smoking. It is metabolized primarily by the hepatic route, with smaller amounts metabolized in the kidney and lung. Half-life is 1 to 2 hours. Elimination is primarily renal with 10% excreted unchanged and the remainder as metabolites; the drug is excreted in breast milk.

Nicotine transdermal systems (patches) are also available to aid the client in withdrawing from smoking. The Nursing Research box on p. 416 discusses current research related to the use of nicotine patches. Three of the patches (Habitrol, Nicoderm, and Prostep) are worn for 24 hours whereas Nicotrol was formulated to be worn for 16 hours a day. The latter patch was designed to mimic the individual's natural smoking pattern, which usually has higher nicotine serum

Nursing Research

Efficacy of transdermal patches for smoking cessation

Nicotine replacement is effective for reducing withdrawal symptoms during smoking cessation. In double-blind clinical trials, transdermal nicotine therapy has been more effective than placebos in reducing nicotine craving and tobacco withdrawal symptoms, such as headache, poor concentration, and irritability. Short-term smoking cessation rates were higher in those using the patch. In placebo-controlled studies involving individuals who had smoked a pack of cigarettes per day, using a 30 mg patch produced higher cessation rates at 6 weeks, 71% with the nicotine patch, 34% with the placebo patch; in another with a 14 mg patch at 4 weeks, the rates were 39% with the nicotine patch and 13.5% with the placebo patch.

The data on long-term smoking cessation rates are less encouraging. In the previous study mentioned, the cessation rates declined at 6 months to 22% with the nicotine patch and 8% with placebo. In a 16-week study using another nicotine patch, 53% succeeded in not smoking after 6 weeks and only 17% of those on placebo. Only 12% of the treated clients, however, continued to abstain from smoking 2 years later. Another trial used a patch for up to 18 weeks; cessation rates at 6 weeks were 77% with the nicotine patch and 39% with the placebo. One year later, only 29% of those treated with the nicotine patch had succeeded in stopping smoking.

Studies show that using the transdermal nicotine patches in conjunction with behavioral-modification programs achieves better smoking-cessation results than using the patch alone. One placebo-controlled trial divided 131 smokers into three groups: behavioral modification only, behavioral training with a nicotine patch, or behavioral training without a nicotine patch. After 9 weeks of therapy, the cessation rate for behavioral-modification group was 44.4%, whereas the rate for the nicotine patch with behavioral modification was 69%. Those clients given the placebo patch with behavioral modification had a cessation rate of 51%.

Critical thinking questions

- Given this research, do you believe transdermal nicotine delivery systems are beneficial to the client? Why?
- If so, how would you recommend that transfermal nicotine delivery system be used?

*From Holdcroft (1992).

levels during the day with lower nicotine levels overnight. Thus a decrease in nicotine serum levels will theoretically not affect the client's sleeping patterns. A potential disadvantage is the drug-free period may result in early morning craving for a cigarette. (Box 21-4 lists products and dosage forms.) To achieve long-term smoking abstinence, all four products should be used in conjunction with a behavioral modification program (Abramowicz, 1992).

Nicotine nasal spray administers 1 mg of nicotine per two sprays to the nasal membrane. The spray is comparable in efficacy to the gum and patches but it has a faster onset of action. The client should be instructed to stop smoking before using the spray and to not use any other nicotine products while using this product. The FDA recommends the spray be used for at least 3 months but not longer than 6 months because it is possible to become dependent on the spray (New Drugs/Drug News, 1996).

More frequent side effects include belching, fast heart beat, mild headache, increased appetite, increased watering of mouth, and sore mouth or throat. Less frequently encountered are constipation, coughing, dizziness, or lightheadedness, dry mouth, hiccups, hoarseness, laxative effect, loss of appetite, irritability, indigestion, and difficulty in sleeping. Transdermal patches may cause pruritus and/or erythema under the patch, a generalized rash, nausea, dizziness, myalgias, coughing, difficulty in sleeping, and nightmares.

More frequently encountered adverse reactions of nicotine gum include injury to mouth, teeth, or dental work. A rare adverse reaction is irregular heartbeat. Early signs of overdose are nausea and vomiting, severe increased watering of the mouth, severe abdominal pain, diarrhea, cold sweat, severe headache, severe dizziness, disturbed hearing and vision, confusion, and severe weakness. Advanced signs of overdose are fainting, hypotension, difficulty breathing, fast, weak, or irregular pulse, and convulsions.

Dosage and administration. Oral: 2 mg as a chewing gum, repeated as needed to curb the client's urge to smoke, up to 30 pieces of gum per day maximum. The gum should be chewed intermittently and very slowly when the client has the urge to smoke. Most clients require about 10 pieces of gum per day during the first month of treatment. Transdermal systems: patches are reapplied every 24 hours except in the case of Nicotrol, which is worn for 16 hours each day.

■ Nursing Management

Nicotine Replacement Smoking Cessation Therapy

Assessment. A baseline assessment of smoking history should be done and cardiovascular status should be assessed before the initiation of therapy. It should be determined before the initiation of therapy with nicotine that the client does not have severe angina pectoris, severe cardiac arrhythmias, or a myocardial infarction, because these will be worsened by the catecholamine action on the heart (increased heart rate and blood pressure), or temporomandibular joint disorder, which might be aggravated by the chewing of nicotine gum. Other disorders that would require the cautious use of the gum would be insulin-dependent diabetes mellitus (increases serum concentrations of insulin); hypertension, hyperthyroidism, or vasospastic dis-

BOX 21-4

Nicotine Transdermal Systems

Brand name	Dosage per patch	Recommended duration of use
Habitrol	21 mg/24 hr	4-8 wk
	14 mg/24 hr	2-4 wk
	7 mg/24 hr	2-4 wk
Nicotrol	15 mg/16 hr	4-12 wk
	10 mg/16 hr	2-4 wk
	5 mg/16 hr	2-4 wk
Nicoderm	21 mg/24 hr	6 wk
	14 mg/24 hr	2-4 wk
	7 mg/24 hr	2-4 wk
Prostep	22 mg/24 hr	4-8 wk
	11 mg/24 hr	2-4 wk

eases (increased heart rate and blood pressure); dental problems; or esophagitis, inflammation of the mouth, or peptic ulcer, which may be exacerbated. Nicotine smoking cessation therapy is contraindicated in pregnant women because it may cause fetal harm. Sensitivity to nicotine should also be determined.

The client's medication regimen needs to be assessed for significant drug interactions. The following effects may occur when nicotine is taken with the drugs listed below:

Drug	Possible effect and management
acetaminophen, caffeine, oxazepam [Serax], pentazocine (Talwin), propranolol (Inderal), propoxyphene (Darvon), and theophylline	Smoking increases drug metabolism, which may result in lower blood levels of these medications. Thus some clients may require higher or more frequent drug dosing. Smoking cessation will generally reverse this effect.
adrenergic agonists or blocking agents, catecholamines, and cortisol	Smoking and nicotine increase cortisol and catecholamine levels; therefore therapy with the adrenergic agonists or blocking agents may require dosage adjustment based on the individual's response.
furosemide (Lasix)	When used in combination with nicotine (smoking), a decrease in diuretic effect and cardiac output has been reported. These effects may be reversed if the client stops smoking.
insulin	Smoking cessation may result in an increased insulin effect; dosage reduction may be necessary. Monitor closely for symptoms of hypoglycemia.

Nursing diagnosis. The client participating in nicotine replacement smoking cessation therapy is at risk for the following nursing diagnoses: injury to mouth, teeth, or dental work related to viscosity of the gum; altered comfort related to headache, increased watering of the mouth, jaw muscle-ache, fast heartbeat, sore throat or mouth; altered health maintenance related to negative health habits; impaired skin integrity related to localized reaction to transdermal patch altered sleep pattern (insomnia); and altered thought processes (unusual irritability).

Implementation

Monitoring. Assess client's tolerance of smoking cessation. Observe client for symptoms of nicotine toxicity (see Box 21-2).

Intervention. Over the course of therapy, the dosage delivered by the transdermal system may be adjusted approximately every 2 weeks.

Education

Gum. The client is instructed that when the urge to smoke occurs, one piece of nicotine gum is chewed slowly for about 30 minutes. At that point, most of the nicotine will have been released. The amount of nicotine released depends on the rate of chewing and amount of time the saliva is in contact with the gum. Instruct the client not to chew more than 30 pieces in a day. The number of pieces of gum should be reduced each day over a 2 to 3 month period. The gum should be carried at all times during therapy. The use of the gum for more than 3 months is not advised and may indicate its use as a substitute for the maintenance of nicotine dependency. At 6 months of use a gradual withdrawal program should be instituted.

Because its viscosity is greater than regular gum, it may cause damage to dentures, inlays, fillings, and natural teeth. Excessive chewing may lead to some temporomandibular joint discomfort. Have the client use sugarless hard candies between doses of gum to meet the need for oral stimulation and relieve oral discomfort. Instruct the client to discontinue use and consult with physician or dentist if gum sticks to dental work. The client should *not* smoke while being treated with nicotine gum.

Nicotine gum should be combined with a supervised program for smoking cessation including education, counseling, and psychological support. Nicotine replacement products should not be used during pregnancy.

Because an overdose of nicotine can be fatal, particularly in small children, the gum should be kept out of the reach of children. If many pieces are chewed at once or in rapid succession, an overdose may occur in an adult; however, the consequences of overdose may be mitigated by the early nausea and vomiting that generally occur with excessive nicotine intake.

Transdermal system. The client should be instructed to select a nonhairy, clean, dry, and intact area of the front or the back of the torso or the outer aspect of the upper arm for the placement of the patch. The patch should only be removed from its sealed pouch just before application or it will lose efficacy. Remove the protective liner from the sticky side of the patch, and touching this side of the patch as little as possible, apply the patch to the selected skin site. Press the patch to the skin with the palm of the hand for about 10 seconds to ensure it sticks well, especially around the edges. Fold the previous used patch in half with the sticky side together and place in the newly opened pouch of the replacement patch. Throw the pouch away in the trash away from children and pets. Nicotine can be very toxic and the patches contain enough nicotine to poison children and pets. If a child plays with a patch, take it away from the child and contact a poison control center or health center immediately. Washing hands immediately after patch application is essential because the nicotine on the hands could get into the eyes and cause irritation. The client should change patches every 24 hours, about the same time each day, selecting a different site. Water will not harm the patch and the client may swim, shower, or use a hot tub while wearing a patch. If it should come off, a new patch is to be applied to a new site, but the patch may be changed to be in keeping with the client's usual 24-hour schedule or the time of application may be changed to 24 hours after the replacement patch was applied. Clients should be alerted that the skin under the patch may be reddened, but it should not stay red for more than a day after the patch is removed. If the patch site becomes swollen or very red, patches should be discontinued and the prescriber should be consulted.

Women of childbearing age should be advised to use effective birth control to avoid pregnancy because of nicotine's link with low birth weight infants and a decrease in fetal breathing movements, possibly the result of decreased placental perfusion.

Evaluation. Evaluation of the client's progress toward smoking cessation should occur at least monthly and determination of the efficacy of the gum or the transdermal systems in the therapy program made. If the client is still smoking after 6 months of gum therapy, or 4 weeks of transdermal patch therapy, treatment should be discontinued because the client is unlikely to quit on this attempt. The expected outcome would be that the client is no longer smoking and denies any adverse drug effects.

GANGLIONIC BLOCKING DRUGS

Ganglionic blocking drugs block transmission of both sympathetic and parasympathetic nerve impulses at the nicotinic receptors on the ganglia. In 1950 the methonium derivatives were introduced, and hexamethonium chloride became the drug of choice in managing severe and malignant hypertension.

Despite the difficulties in managing individuals receiving hexamethonium because of its erratic absorption and action and severe side effects, its use demonstrated that severe hypertension could be controlled. Since 1961 the ganglionic blocking agents have been rarely used. Newer antihypertensive drugs that have more selective action and fewer severe side effects are preferred.

However, the student should be aware of these products because some prescribers may select trimethaphan as an alternative for clients resistant to the effects of sodium nitroprusside. Other prescribers may use a ganglionic blocking agent such as trimethaphan for the treatment of a hypertensive crisis in individuals with an acute dissecting aortic aneurysm. The two ganglionic blocking agents available are mecamylamine hydrochloride (Inversine tablets) and trimethaphan camsylate (Arfonad injection). Since mecamylamine has many side effects and is not considered a first line drug in the treatment of hypertension, the nurse is referred to the package insert or current *USP DI* for additional information on this product.

trimethaphan camsylate [trye meth' a fan] (Arfonad) Ganglionic blocking agents lower arterial pressure by blocking the action of acetylcholine on the ganglion cells. This results in reduced transmission of impulses from preganglionic to postganglionic fibers in both sympathetic and parasympathetic nerves. Blocking transmission of impulses through the sympathetic ganglia abolishes vasoconstrictor tone; the blood vessels dilate and arterial pressure falls.

Trimethaphan camsylate is used in the treatment of hypertension and is administered by intravenous infusion. It is also used to produce controlled hypotension during surgery. Onset of action is immediate, and duration of effect is 10 to 15 minutes. Metabolism is probably by pseudocholinesterase. The drug is excreted mostly unchanged by the kidneys.

For side effects/adverse reactions, see Table 21-3.

Dosage and administration. Adults: for hypertensive emergency, initially, 0.5 mg to 1 mg/min by intravenous infusion. Adjust dosage is according to client response. Maintenance dosage is 1 to 5 mg/min by intravenous infusion. To control blood pressure during surgery: initially, 3 to 4 mg/min, adjusted as necessary. Maintenance dose is 0.2 to 6 mg/min by intravenous infusion.

The elderly may be more sensitive to trimethaphan so a lower dosage with close monitoring of the blood pressure is indicated. With children, the dosage is initially 0.05 to 0.15 mg/min, adjusted according to individual response, administered by intravenous infusion.

■ Nursing Management

Trimethaphan Camsylate Therapy

For a detailed discussion of the nursing care of the client receiving antihypertensive agents, see Chapter 27, Antihypertensives.

Assessment. Use trimethaphan with caution for children and elderly clients, who tend to be more sensitive to its hypotensive effects. The risk benefit of its use should be determined for clients with Addison's disease, anemia and hypovolemic shock (may increase hypoxia), diabetes, hepatic disease (may decrease hepatic perfusion and worsen condition), renal disease (may increase effects of drug),respiratory insufficiency (hypoxemia may be aggravated), cardiovascular or cerebrovascular insufficiency (ischemia may be aggravated by hypotension), and for clients taking other antihypotensive or steroid medications. The client's baseline blood pressure should be assessed.

The client's concurrent medication regimen should be assessed for significant drug interactions. The following effects may occur when trimethaphan is given with the drugs listed below:

Drug	Possible effect and management
ambenonium (Mytelase), neostigmine (Prostigmin), or pyridostigmine (Mestinon)	**The antimyasthenic effects of these drugs will be blocked, which may result in increased weakness and inability to swallow. Avoid or a potentially serious drug interaction may occur.**

Nursing diagnosis. The client receiving trimethaphan camsylate therapy should be assessed for the following nursing diagnoses: altered comfort related to nausea and vomiting, dry mouth, itching, and anginal pain; altered bowel elimination pattern (constipation); risk for injury related to blurred vision, weakness, and orthostatic hypertension; and the potential complications of hypoventilation (respiratory depression), paralytic ileus (with IV use over 48 hours), and urinary retention.

Implementation

Monitoring. Clients receiving trimethaphan camsylate should be in an intensive care setting for appropriate monitoring. Emergency equipment should be available in the event of respiratory arrest. Monitor the client's blood pressure and respiratory function frequently. Monitor intake and output because renal blood flow may be reduced or urinary retention may occur.

Intervention. The solution should be diluted with dextrose 5% injection only and administered by infusion pump or micro-drip regulator to ensure a precise regulation of the flow rate. The prepared intravenous solution is stable at room temperature for 24 hours. Oral antihypertensive therapy should be started as soon as possible because a pseudotolerance to the drug may occur in some individuals.

The client should be in a supine position to avoid cerebral anoxia. Oxygen therapy should be instituted while the client is receiving trimethaphan. Assist the client with activities of daily living if trimethaphan-induced weakness is an issue. Antiemetics may be used to mitigate nausea caused by the drug. If used for controlled hypertension during surgery, the drug should be discontinued before the wound is closed to allow the client's blood pressure to return to normal.

Education. Alert the client to change positions cautiously because orthostatic hypotension is possible. Ice chips and sugarless candies can be used to alleviate dry mouth.

Evaluation. The client's blood pressure is within normal limits without the client experiencing adverse effects of the drug.

SUMMARY

Drugs that mimic, intensify, or inhibit the effects of the parasympathetic and sympathetic divisions of the autonomic nervous system are known as the autonomic drugs. They are grouped as cholinergic, cholinergic blocking, adrenergic, and adrenergic blocking drugs. The cholinergic (parasympathomimetic) drugs have nicotinic effects that stimulate the ganglia, adrenal medulla, and skeletal muscle, and muscarinic effects that stimulate the postganglionic nerve endings in glands, and in cardiac and smooth muscle. They are used primarily to stimulate the intestine and bladder postoperatively, to terminate curarization, to lower intraocular pressure, to promote salivation and sweating, to dilate peripheral blood vessels, and to treat myasthenia gravis symptomatically. Anticholinergic (parasympatholytic) drugs block the muscarinic effects of acetylcholine, which can produce a wide range of pharmacologic effects. They are used to treat illnesses in which spasm is a component, such as irritable bowel syndrome, spastic biliary disorders, and urinary disorders. Because anticholinergics decrease respiratory secretions, they are administered as a preanesthetic drug and to control the excessive salivation of some disorders, such as Parkinson's disease. The ganglionic drugs are either ganglionic stimulating or ganglionic blocking drugs. Nicotine is a ganglionic stimulating drug. It has, however, no therapeutic use, but the nurse should be knowledgeable about its effects for health teaching purposes. In the 1950s, ganglionic blocking drugs were used for the management of severe and malignant hypertension, but since the 1960s the advent of more selective effective antihypertensive drugs has limited their use.

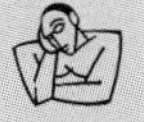

Critical Thinking

1. Nurses in schools and other community agencies are well placed to serve as consultants and counselors to students and be advocates for smoking cessation. As children relate better to the present rather than the future consequences of their activities, what would you share with a class of fourth graders about the immediate physiologic consequences of smoking?
2. Harry Johnson is receiving atropine 0.4 mg PO q4h as part of his treatment for irritable bowel syndrome. He complains of intolerance to heat, dry mouth, and constipation. How will you explain these symptoms to him? What instruction will you provide to assist him to effectively manage his therapeutic regimen?

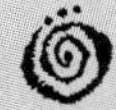

Collaborative Learning Activities

1. Two teams of students will provide a brief smoking cessation presentation to the class; one as in critical thinking question #1, with an audience of fourth graders, and the other, a college age audience. Considering the life span developmental issues of the two groups, differ the style and content of the programs.

BIBLIOGRAPHY

Abramowicz M (Ed.) (1992). Nicotine patches, *Med Lett* 34(868):37.

American Hospital Formulary Service (1996). *AHFS drug information '96*. Bethesda, MD: American Society of Hospital Pharmacists.

American Medical Association (1995). *AMA drug evaluations 1995*. Chicago: The Association.

Anderson KN, et al. (Eds.) (1994). *Mosby's Medical, nursing, & allied health dictionary* (4th ed.). St Louis: Mosby.

Dalton JA & Swenson I (1986). Nurses and smoking: Role modeling and counseling behaviors. *Oncol Nurs Forum* 13(2):45.

Geiger-Bronsky MJ (1995). Anticholinergic therapy in the critically ill patient with bronchospasm, *AACN Clin Issues Adv Pract Acute Crit Care* 6(2):287-96.

Hardman JG & Limbird LE (Eds.) (1996). *Goodman and Gilman's the pharmacological basis of therapeutics* (9th ed.). New York: McGraw Hill.

New Drugs/Drug News (1996). nasal spray smoke cessation approved, *P&T* 21(6):303.

Holdcroft C (1992). Efficacy of transdermal patches for nicotine replacement and smoking cessation, *Nurs Pract* 17(7):46.

Strecher WJ, et al. (1985). Evaluation of a minimal contact smoking cessation program in a health care setting, *Patient Educ Couns* 7 (4):395.

United States Pharmacopeia Convention (1996). *Drug information for the health care professional* (16th ed.). Bethesda, MD: The Convention.

Chapter 22

Drugs Affecting the Sympathetic (Adrenergic) Nervous System

Chapter Focus

Adrenergic receptors regulate cardiac, arteriolar, bronchial, and gastrointestinal smooth muscle. Pharmacologic intervention related to these receptors is commonplace and varied. Management of clients receiving drugs that affect the sympathetic, or adrenergic, nervous system challenges nurses daily. The following objectives and key terms are important for a good understanding of this chapter.

Key Terms

alpha-adrenergic blocking agents (p. 441)
beta-adrenergic blocking agents (p. 447)
calorigenic effect (p. 425)
chronotropic effect (p. 424)
dromotropic effect (p. 424)
inotropic effect (p. 424)
sympathomimetic drugs (p. 422)

Key Drugs [▲]

dopamine
epinephrine
norepinephrine
propranolol

Objectives

1. Discuss the three types of adrenergic drugs.
2. Differentiate between alpha$_1$, alpha$_2$, beta$_1$, and beta$_2$ adrenergic effects.
3. Describe the effects of the three naturally occurring catecholamines on the body.
4. List common adrenergic drugs and blocking agents, their effects, and side effects/adverse reactions.
5. Implement nursing management of the care of clients receiving adrenergic and adrenergic-blocking drugs.

ADRENERGIC DRUGS

Sympathomimetic drugs are medications that enhance or mimic the effects of sympathetic nerve stimulation. These drugs are designed to produce actions similar to those of the neurotransmitters. The sympathomimetic drugs are also called adrenergic drugs and there are three types of adrenergic drugs: (1) direct-acting, (2) indirect-acting, and (3) dual-acting (direct and indirect) agents.

Direct-Acting Adrenergic Drugs

Catecholamines

The three naturally occurring catecholamines in the body—dopamine, norepinephrine, and epinephrine—are synthesized by the sympathetic nervous system. While dopamine is a precursor of norepinephrine and epinephrine, it also has a transmitter role of its own, in certain portions of the central nervous system. (For information on adrenergic transmission see Figure 20-5 and the discussion in Chapter 20.)

Epinephrine is primarily an emergency hormone while norepinephrine is an important transmitter of nerve impulses. The latter is also an intermediary in epinephrine biosynthesis. Catecholamines that depend on their ability to interact *directly* with adrenergic receptors (alpha and beta) are called *direct-acting* drugs. Thus the response of these agents is mediated by directly stimulating the adrenergic receptors. In the sympathetic nervous system the adrenergic effector cells contain two distinct receptors, the alpha (α) and beta (β) receptors.

There is evidence that the alpha receptors appear on two primary locations. The $alpha_2$ receptors are found on the presynaptic nerve terminals, platelets and smooth muscle and thus are called presynaptic (prejunctional) receptor sites. It has been suggested that the function of the presynaptic receptor is associated with the control of the *amount* of transmitter released per nerve impulse. The rate of transmitter synthesized can be regulated by a feedback mechanism. Thus when the concentration of transmitter released from the nerve terminal into the synaptic cleft reaches a high level, it stimulates the presynaptic receptors and prevents further release of the transmitter. This kind of feedback prevents excessive and prolonged stimulation of the postsynaptic cell. The postsynaptic receptors, which are located on the effector organs, are known as $alpha_1$ receptors.

The beta receptors are subdivided on the basis of their responses to drugs. $Beta_1$ receptors are located mainly in the heart, whereas $beta_2$ receptors mediate the actions of catecholamines on smooth muscle, especially bronchioles and arterial smooth muscle.

Norepinephrine acts mainly on alpha receptors causing vasoconstriction. Epinephrine acts on both alpha and beta receptors producing a mixture of vasodilation and vasoconstriction. Isoproterenol, a synthetic catecholamine, acts only on beta receptors. For a discussion of receptor sensitivity, see Box 22-1.

The most important alpha-adrenergic activities in humans are these: (1) vasoconstriction of arterioles in the skin and splanchnic area, resulting in a rise in blood pressure, (2) pupil dilation; and (3) relaxation of the gut. Beta-adrenergic activity includes (1) cardiac acceleration and increased contractility, (2) vasodilation of arterioles supplying skeletal muscles, (3) bronchial relaxation, and (4) uterine relaxation. The effects of both alpha and beta stimulation result from a summation of action where they are interrelated. That is, a change in blood pressure will depend on the degree of vasoconstriction

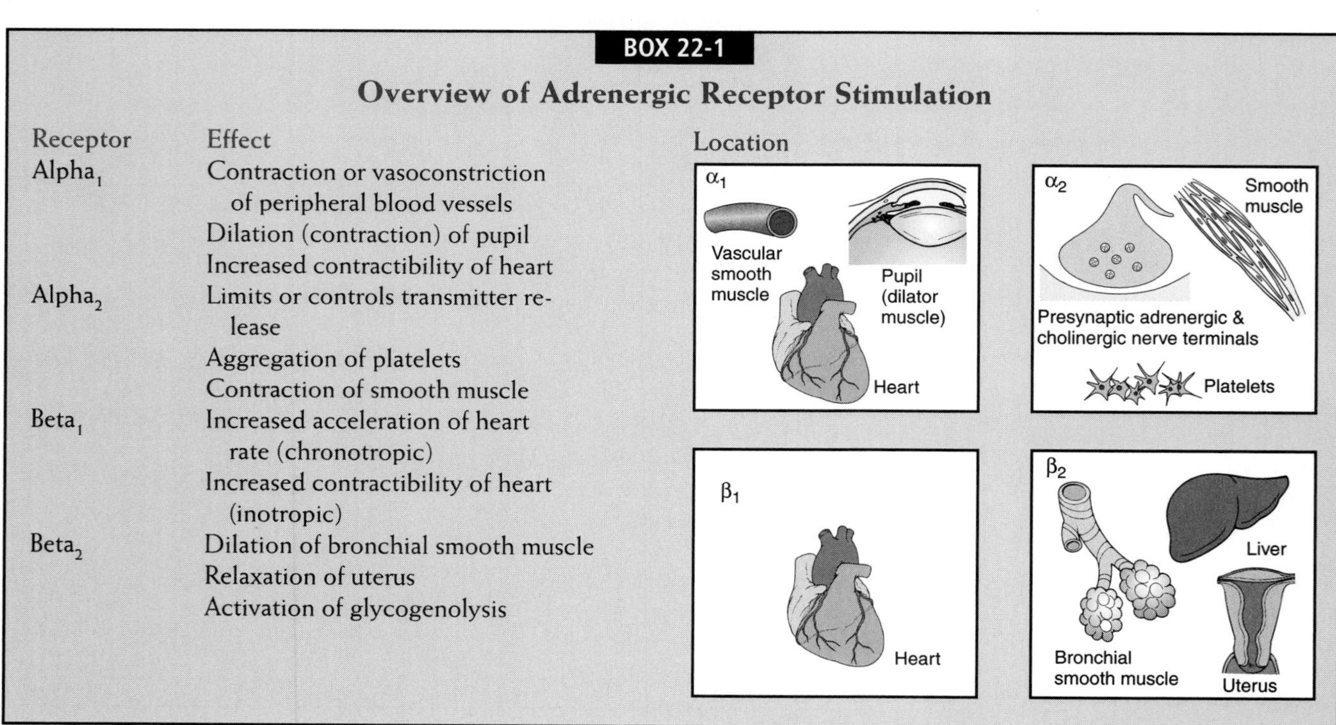

BOX 22-1

Overview of Adrenergic Receptor Stimulation

Receptor	Effect
$Alpha_1$	Contraction or vasoconstriction of peripheral blood vessels Dilation (contraction) of pupil Increased contractibility of heart
$Alpha_2$	Limits or controls transmitter release Aggregation of platelets Contraction of smooth muscle
$Beta_1$	Increased acceleration of heart rate (chronotropic) Increased contractibility of heart (inotropic)
$Beta_2$	Dilation of bronchial smooth muscle Relaxation of uterus Activation of glycogenolysis

in the skin and splanchnic area *and* the extent of vasodilation in skeletal muscles, along with changes in heart rate. Large arteries and veins contain both alpha and beta receptors; the heart contains only beta receptors (Table 22-1).

Specific drugs are available that stimulate or block alpha and beta receptors. These agents work at peripheral autonomic sites, which distinguishes them from ganglionic blocking agents that act at the ganglia.

As catecholamines, norepinephrine and epinephrine are important neurohormones in neural and endocrine integration. They are always present in arterial blood, although the amount varies widely during any one day. Certain physiologic stimuli such as stress and exercise significantly increase blood levels of catecholamine. Studies indicate that the major sources of circulating norepinephrine are stimulated sympathetic nerve endings. Organs such as the heart

TABLE 22-1 Adrenergic receptor stimulation

Effector organs	Receptor type	Adrenergic response
Heart		
Cardiac muscle (atria, ventricles)	β_1	Increased force of contraction (inotropic action)
Sinoatrial node	β_1	Increased heart rate (chronotropic action)
Atrioventricular node	β_1	Increased automaticity and conduction velocity; shortened refractory period (chronotropic action)
Blood vessels		
Arterioles		
Coronary	α_1, β_2, dopaminergic	Constriction, dilation*
Cerebral	α_1	Constriction
Pulmonary	α_1, β_2	Constriction,* dilation
Mesenteric visceral	α_1, β_2	Constriction,* dilation
Renal	α_1, β_2, dopaminergic	Constriction,* dilation
Skin, mucosa	α_1, α_2	Constriction
Skeletal muscle	α, β_2	Constriction, dilation
Veins	α_1, β_2	Constriction, dilation
Lung		
Bronchial smooth muscle	β_2	Bronchodilation
Bronchial glands	α_1, β_2	Inhibition
Gastrointestinal tract		
Smooth muscle (motility, tone)	α_1, α_2, β_2	Decreased
Sphincter	α_1	Contraction
Secretion	?	Inhibition
Gallbladder and ducts	—	Relaxation
Liver	β_2	Glycogenolysis
Spleen capsule	α_1, β_2	Contraction,* relaxation
Pancreas: insulin secretion	α_2	Decreased
Adipose tissue	β_1	Lipolysis
Urinary bladder		
Detrusor muscle	β_2	Relaxation
Sphincter	α_1	Contraction
Kidney ureter	α_1	Contraction
Kidney secretion (renin)	β_1	Increased
Uterus		
Pregnant	α_1	Contraction
Nonpregnant	β_2	Relaxation
Sex organs, male	α_1	Ejaculation
Skin		
Pilomotor muscles	α_1	Contraction
Sweat glands	α_1, cholinergic	Increased secretion
Eye		
Radial muscle, iris (pupil size)	α_1	Contraction—pupil dilation (mydriasis)
Ciliary muscle	β_2	Relaxation for far vision

*Predominant response.

and blood vessels receive a large fraction of blood and possess large numbers of sympathetic nerve endings, thus they contain the greatest amount of catecholamines. The number of sympathetic nerve endings or adrenergic nerves to various organs determines the magnitude of response of these organs to increased levels or injections of catecholamines.

Pharmacologic Effects

Catecholamines produce a variety of physiologic responses.

Cardiac. Epinephrine and norepinephrine produce almost the same cardiac responses when injected. A significant increase in myocardial contraction (positive **inotropic effect**) is the result of increased influx of calcium into cardiac fibers. The strong myocardial contractions result in more complete emptying of the ventricles and an increase in cardiac work and oxygen consumption. Strong contractions brought about by isoproterenol and epinephrine also increase cardiac output, or volume. Norepinephrine, on the other hand, may not alter cardiac output and may even decrease it slightly.

This effect of norepinephrine is believed to result from its potent vasoconstriction action, which increases resistance to ejection of blood from the heart. The increased work of the heart to move the blood against increased pressure is "pressure work" rather than "volume work."

It has been shown experimentally and clinically that 0.5 mg of epinephrine injected into arterial or venous blood and circulated by cardiac compression or massage may stimulate spontaneous and vigorous cardiac contractions. Even though the heart is in ventricular fibrillation, epinephrine increases fibrillation vigor and frequently promotes successful electric defibrillation of the individual. In these situations the drug may be injected repeatedly. However, epinephrine cannot be used repeatedly to improve the function of a failing heart (congestive heart failure), since it increases oxygen consumption by cardiac muscle. It can also cause anginal pain in clients with angina pectoris because it increases cardiac oxygen demand. Therefore, although it increases coronary blood flow, its use is contraindicated for clients with angina. The production of strong contractions provides the rationale for the use of epinephrine in cardiac arrest.

A significant increase in cardiac rate (positive **chronotropic effect**) is the result of the increased rate of membrane depolarization in the pacemaker cells in the sinus node during diastole. Action potential threshold is reached sooner, pacemaker cells fire more often, and heart rate increases.

Norepinephrine, with its predominantly alpha adrenergic activity, may not produce as severe a tachycardia as epinephrine. The increased vasoconstriction and increased blood pressure may cause a reflex bradycardia. Isoproterenol usually produces a tachycardia, since its direct and reflex effects act in the same direction. Dosage and client variables affect these responses.

An increase in atrioventricular conduction (positive **dromotropic effect**) is another physiologic response. Because epinephrine increases atrioventricular conduction, some cardiologists use it in the treatment of heart block.

Catecholamines may also produce spontaneous firing of Purkinje fibers, which may cause them to exhibit pacemaker activity. This effect may cause ventricular extrasystoles and increase the susceptibility of ventricular muscle to fibrillation. These effects are more likely to occur with epinephrine than norepinephrine.

Vascular. Vascular effects of the catecholamines depend on the dose and the vascular bed affected. Low doses of epinephrine may decrease total peripheral vascular resistance and decrease blood pressure. In large doses epinephrine activates alpha receptors in the greater peripheral vascular system, which increases resistance and increases blood pressure. Norepinephrine elevates blood pressure by increasing peripheral resistance and decreasing blood flow through skeletal muscles.

Norepinephrine, a vasoconstrictor, increases total peripheral resistance. Isoproterenol is not a vasoconstrictor but a pure vasodilator; epinephrine is both a vasoconstrictor and vasodilator, with vasodilation being greater in its overall net effects. For example, during great stress the release of epinephrine from the adrenal medulla constricts blood vessels in the skin and splanchnic areas but dilates those of skeletal muscles, thus shunting blood to the areas needed for "fight or flight" responses.

Renal artery constriction and resistance is greater with epinephrine than with norepinephrine. In large doses epinephrine may actually stop blood flow through some nephrons and stimulate release of antidiuretic hormone (ADH), thereby reducing urinary excretion.

Central nervous system. Epinephrine and isoproterenol in sufficient amounts can lead to alertness, tremulousness, respiratory stimulation, and anxiety. Norepinephrine is less likely to cause anxiety and tremulousness. Beneficial cerebral effects from epinephrine and norepinephrine in cases of hypotension are thought to be the result of increased systemic pressure with a resultant improvement in cerebral blood flow.

Smooth muscle. Generally the catecholamines relax nonvascular smooth muscles and when smooth muscle of the gastrointestinal (GI) tract is relaxed, amplitude and tone of intestinal peristalsis are reduced. Theoretically this may retard propulsion of food and gastrointestinal emptying; however, this effect is rare in humans with therapeutic doses of catecholamines.

In some situations smooth muscle of some organs react like vascular smooth muscle and contract. For example, radial and sphincter muscles of the iris contract, and the smooth muscle of the lids may contract, giving rise to the widened, staring eyes seen in sympathetically stimulated individuals.

In the urinary bladder epinephrine causes trigone and sphincter constriction and detrusor relaxation with a delay in the desire to void.

Respiratory. Catecholamines dilate bronchial smooth muscle. Isoproterenol is a more active bronchodilator than epinephrine, while epinephrine is a stronger bronchodilator than norepinephrine.

Glandular. Epinephrine may increase the amount of viscid saliva excreted, but, as a rule, sympathomimetics decrease secretion and produce a dry mouth. Catecholamines may produce local sweating on the palms of the hands and in the axillary and genital areas. The exact mechanism for these effects is not clear.

Metabolic. Epinephrine inhibits insulin secretion. Catecholamines have antagonistic effects on gluconeogenesis, and they decrease liver and skeletal muscle glycogen and increase lipolysis in adipose tissue. The result of these effects is a rise in blood sugar and an increase in free fatty acids. Thus in response to stress ("fight or flight" response) there can be an abundant supply of fuel and energy (Figure 22-1).

Catecholamines also have a **calorigenic effect** (capable of generating heat, which increases oxygen consumption) resulting from the sum of the preceding effects. Norepinephrine's action in relation to these effects is weaker than that of epinephrine or isoproterenol.

▲ **epinephrine** [ep i nef' rin] (Adrenalin)

Epinephrine is available in solutions for inhalation and nebulization, parenteral and ophthalmic administration. Many bronchodilator aerosols are available over the counter in solutions containing up to 1% of the epinephrine base. For example:

- epinephrine inhalation aerosol (Bronkaid Mist, Bronkaid Mistometer ♣)
- epinephrine bitartrate inhalation aerosol (Asthma-Haler, Medihaler-Epi)
- racepinephrine inhalation solution (AsthmaNefrin, Vaponefrin)

Parenteral dosage forms and ophthalmic solutions include:

- epinephrine injection (Adrenalin, EpiPen Auto-Injector)
- sterile epinephrine suspension (Sus-Phrine)
- Ophthalmic epinephrine is discussed in Chapter 43.

Mechanism of action. Epinephrine is a direct-acting catecholamine that is naturally released from the adrenal medulla in response to sympathoadrenal stimulation. It also is prepared synthetically. Epinephrine stimulates alpha and beta receptors. Its primary action is on the beta receptors of the heart, the smooth muscle of the bronchi, and the blood vessels. The $beta_1$ action stimulates the heart by increasing heart rate, force of myocardial contraction, and cardiac output. The $beta_2$ action on the smooth muscle of the bronchioles produces bronchodilation, thereby increasing tidal volume and vital capacity of the lung. Stimulation of alpha receptors constricts arterioles of the bronchioles and inhibits histamine release, thus reducing nasal congestion and edema. In contrast, $beta_2$ adrenergic activity of the smooth muscle of arterioles causes vasodilation.

Another effect of epinephrine is alpha activity, which results in contraction of the radial muscle in the iris ($alpha_1$), causing dilation of the pupil (mydriasis). Constriction of the blood vessels in the skin also is activated by alpha activity. The detrusor muscle in the urinary bladder contains beta receptors and is relaxed by epinephrine (see Table 22-1).

Indications

1. Used for symptomatic treatment of bronchial asthma and other obstructive pulmonary diseases, such as chronic bronchitis and emphysema, that cause bronchospasm.
2. Used for symptomatic relief of acute hypersensitivity reactions. Indicated in the emergency treatment of acute anaphylactic shock and severe acute reactions to drugs, animal serums, insect stings, and other allergens

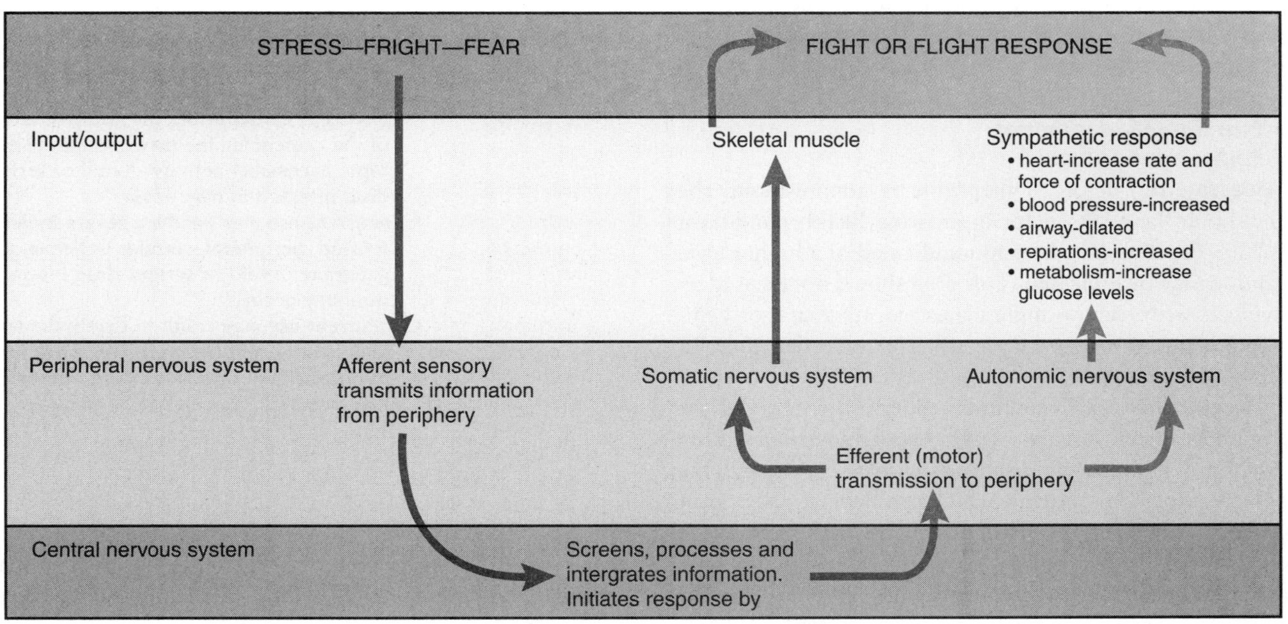

Figure 22-1 Nervous system response to severe fright or stress.

to relieve bronchospasm, urticaria, hives, angioneurotic edema, and swelling of nasal mucosa. Pulmonary congestion is also alleviated by constriction of mucosal blood vessels.

3. Used as an adjunct with local anesthetics. Concurrent administration of epinephrine with local anesthetics reduces circulation to the site, which results in a slowing of vascular absorption. This promotes a local effect of the anesthetic and also prolongs its duration of action, thus reducing the risk of anesthetic toxicity.
4. Administered as a hemostatic agent to control superficial bleeding from arterioles and capillaries in the skin, mucous membranes, or other tissues.
5. Used in ocular surgery to control bleeding, induce mydriasis and conjunctival decongestion, and decrease intraocular pressure.
6. Used to treat cardiac arrest or cardiac standstill. On occasion it may be given by intracardiac injection in acute attacks of ventricular standstill, after physical measures and electrical defibrillation have failed.

Pharmacokinetics. Epinephrine should not be given orally because it is rapidly metabolized in the mucosa of the GI tract and liver, so serum levels achieved would be inadequate. It is well absorbed after IM or SC injection.

Epinephrine has a rapid onset of action, from 3 to 5 minutes by inhalation or between 6 and 15 minutes after SC injection. The duration of action of epinephrine is 1 to 3 hours by inhalation, and from 1 to 4 hours after IM or SC injection. In severe anaphylaxis, asthma, or cardiac arrest, epinephrine doses may need to be repeated every 5 to 20 minutes, depending on dosage used and client's response. Epinephrine is metabolized in the liver and excreted in the kidneys.

Side/adverse effects include increased nervousness, restlessness, insomnia, tachycardia, tremors, sweating, increased blood pressure, nausea, vomiting, pallor and weakness; and with inhalation devices, bronchial irritation and coughing (with high doses), dry mouth and throat, headaches, and flushing of face and skin.

Dosage and administration. See Table 22-2.

■ Nursing Management

Epinephrine Therapy

Assessment. Before epinephrine is administered, the client should be assessed for preexisting health conditions for which the drug may be contraindicated or a higher level of caution may be indicated. This drug should not be used by individuals with narrow-angle glaucoma, traumatic or hemorrhagic shock (increases myocardial oxygen demand), or organic brain damage.

Use epinephrine with caution in elderly clients and those with cardiovascular disease, hypertension, hyperthyroidism, or psychosis because the drug may worsen the underlying condition. Pulmonary edema, which can be fatal, may occur because of peripheral constriction. Use with caution in clients with bronchial asthma or emphysema who also have degenerative heart disease. Clients with coronary insufficiency may develop anginal pain. Clients with diabetes mellitus may require increased insulin dosage because of a epinephrine-induced hyperglycemia.

Epinephrine should be administered to the pregnant client with great caution. It is known to cross the placenta, and although appropriate studies have not been conducted in humans to demonstrate the teratogenic effects seen in rat studies, it may cause anoxia in the fetus. If administered during labor, it may delay the second stage because of the relaxation of uterine muscles. When epinephrine is given parenterally to maintain maternal blood pressure during delivery, it can cause acceleration of the fetal heart rate. It is contraindicated if the maternal blood pressure is greater than 130/80.

A review of the client's current medication regimen is necessary to detect possible significant drug interactions. The following interactions may occur when epinephrine is given with the drugs listed below.

Drug	Possible effect and management
anesthetics, such as cyclopropane, halothane (Fluothane), enflurane (Ethrane), isoflurane (Forane), trichloroethylene, etc.	May sensitize the heart, increasing risk of severe dysrhythmias. Monitor closely because a reduction in epinephrine (sympathomimetics) is usually necessary.
local parenteral anesthetics	When used in end artery areas, such as fingers, toes, or penis, the reduced blood supply to the area may result in ischemia and gangrene. Use very cautiously in such areas and monitor closely.
beta-adrenergic receptor blocking agents, including ophthalmics	**Therapeutic effects of both agents may be inhibited. With bronchodilators having both alpha and beta stimulating effects (epinephrine), with beta receptor blockade, stimulation of alpha receptors may result in hypertension, severe bradycardia with possibly heart block. Avoid or serious drug interaction may occur.**
digitalis glycosides	**Digitalis sensitizes the myocardium to the effects of epinephrine; the additive effect of the catecholamine may precipitate ectopic pacemaker activity. Avoid or serious drug interaction may occur.**
ergotamine or ergoloid mesylates (Hydergine)	**Concurrent use may produce severe hypertension, peripheral vascular ischemia, and gangrene. Avoid or serious drug interaction may occur.**
maprotiline (Ludiomil), tricyclic antidepressants, MAO inhibitor antidepressants, or cocaine	**Concurrent use may result in dysrhythmias, tachycardia, and hypertension, or hyperpyrexia. Avoid or serious drug interaction may occur.**

A baseline assessment of the client's cardiopulmonary status should be obtained by ECG, blood pressure, and auscultation of the heart and lung sounds.

TABLE 22-2 Epinephrine: dosage and administration

Indication	Adults	Children
Parenteral		
Bronchodilator	SC 0.2-0.5 mg every 20 min up to 4 hr as needed, with dosage increase to max. 1 mg/dose if needed.	SC 0.01 mg/kg every 15 min for 2 doses, then every 4 hr if needed. Max. dose 0.5 mg/dose.
Anaphylaxis	IM/SC 0.2-0.5 mg repeated every 10-15 min as needed, with dosage increase to max. of 1 mg/dose if needed.	SC 0.01 mg/kg repeated every 15 min for 2 doses, then every 4 hr as needed; severe cases: dosage may increase to 0.5 mg/dose.
Cardiac stimulant	IV or intracardiac injection 0.1-1 mg (base) diluted to 10 ml with sodium chloride injection given to restore myocardial contractility. After intracardiac administration, external cardiac massage should be applied to enhance drug entry into coronary circulation. May repeat every 5 min if needed. Endotracheal tube instillation dosage is 1 mg (base) for cardiac resuscitation.	IV or intracardiac, 0.005-0.01 mg/kg; repeat every 5 min or follow with IV infusion at initial rate of 0.001 mg/kg/min. May be increased in increments of 0.0001 mg/kg/min if necessary to max. of 0.0015 mg/kg/min.
Anesthetic (local) adjunct	Intraspinal 0.2-0.4 mg added to anesthetic spinal mixture. With local anesthetic: 0.1 to 0.2 mg in a 1:200,000 to 1:20,000 solution.	See adult dosing.
Auto-injection		
Auto-injector for emergency self-treatment of anaphylaxis (EpiPen Auto-Injector)	Available in 0.5 mg/ml and 1 mg/ml.	
Suspension (Sus-phrine)		
Bronchodilator	SC 0.5 mg initially, followed by 0.5-1.5 mg every 6 hr as necessary.	SC 0.025 mg/kg. May be repeated in 6 hr. If child weighs 30 kg, max. single dose is 0.75 mg.
Inhalation		
Bronchodilator 1:100 (1%) solution	Proper dose automatically dispensed by metered nebulizer. Allow 1-5 min between inhalations. Use fewest possible inhalations.	
Topical		
Nasal decongestant	1-2 drops (0.1% solution) every 4-6 hr.	
Antihemorrhagic	0.002%-0.1% (1:50,000 to 1:1000) solution of epinephrine applied locally.	

Nursing diagnosis. Because of the CNS effects of dizziness or lightheadedness, nervousness or restlessness, trembling, and insomnia, the client with epinephrine therapy should be evaluated for the nursing diagnoses of altered comfort, sleep pattern disturbance, anxiety, altered thought processes, and risk for injury. There also may be altered comfort because of the drug's gastrointestinal, respiratory, and local effects. Evaluate for ineffective airway clearance related to the client's preexisting health status to determine the drug's effectiveness. The cardiovascular effects—headache, hypertension, palpitations, tachycardia, flushing of the face—may indicate the complication of altered cardiac output.

Implementation

Monitoring. Assess the client's vital signs and auscultate the heart and lungs periodically. During intravenous administration of epinephrine, monitor vital signs and observe electrocardiogram (ECG) results continuously until stabilized. Monitor for signs of excess fluid volume such as peripheral edema, sudden weight gain, and distended neck veins. Since epinephrine increases blood glucose levels, observe individuals with diabetes for loss of diabetic control.

Intervention. Avoid epinephrine overdosage, particularly inadvertent intravenous administration of the usual SC dosages, which may cause extreme hypertension. Cerebrovascular hemorrhage may result, particularly in the elderly client. Read labels very carefully; epinephrine ophthalmic, nasal, and topical solutions must not be injected.

Store medication in tight, light-resistant container at a temperature between 15° and 30° C (59° and 86° F). Do not use if solution is pink or brown in color or contains a precipitate. This color change is caused by oxidation of the drug; multiple-use vials in which air is injected to withdraw the solution are more prone to this change.

Parenteral administration. Carefully recheck solution strength, dosage, expiration date, and route of administration of drug. Avoid medication errors by not confusing the 1:100 solution with the 1:1000 solution. Overdosage has resulted in fatalities. Use a small syringe (tuberculin syringe) to assure accuracy in measurement of parenteral injection. Aspirate syringe before parenteral injection (subcutaneous and intramuscular) to prevent intravenous injection that can result in sudden hypertension. Intraarterial injection is contraindicated because the marked vasoconstriction that results may cause gangrene. Injection sites need to be rotated because repeated local injections may result in necrosis secondary to the vasoconstricting effects of the drug. Massage of the injection site will promote absorption of the drug. For the same reasons, epinephrine should not be administered intramuscularly into the buttocks. The presence of the anaerobic organism *Clostridium welchii* and reduced oxygen tension within the tissues as a result of the administration of epinephrine creates the potential for gas gangrene.

The use of sterile epinephrine in a suspension allows for the frequency of parenteral injection to be effective to up to 10 hours; however, when administering the suspension, inject it promptly after it is withdrawn from the vial to prevent the solution from settling. A 1:1000 solution must be diluted with a 10 ml sodium chloride injection before intravenous or intracardiac administration.

In emergency situations epinephrine may be administered intracardially, in which case it should be done by team members with experience in this technique. If the client is intubated, the drug can be injected directly into the bronchial tree via the endotracheal tube at the same dosage as for intravenous administration.

Inhalation. Epinephrine and other beta-adrenergic agents may be used interchangeably; however, allow 4 hours between doses when changing from one to another. Do not administer concurrently.

Nasal administration. To prevent drug from entering the throat, instill nose drops with head low in lateral position. Rinse nose dropper with hot water to prevent contamination of medication.

Education. Instruct the client to take the medication exactly as prescribed and, if required, take it around the clock. Caution the client against the repeated or prolonged use of epinephrine, which can cause *tolerance* or "epinephrine fastness." If the drug is withheld 12 hours to several days, its effectiveness usually returns. The client should avoid self-medicating with any OTC preparations without prescriber consultation. Contact the prescriber if experiencing tachycardia, shortness of breath, or chest pain.

Emergency autoinjection. Remind the client that the medication requires a prescription. Instruct the client to consult the prescriber or pharmacist before taking any OTC drug concurrently with epinephrine. Review with the client in detail the operation of the EpiPen autoinjector. The package insert *must* be read carefully. Remind the client that the autoinjector contains the drug that the client injects intramuscularly in the anterolateral region of the thigh or the deltoid part of the arm. Instruct the client *not* to inject the drug into buttock because of the increased risk of infection owing to fecal contaminants on the skin.

Emphasize the importance of keeping the drug on hand in case of emergency and that the drug should be stored in a dark, cool place to prevent deterioration. Supplies should also be rotated so that the client uses the oldest supplies first. Caution the client to check the auto-injector to make sure the solution is neither brown in color nor contains a precipitate. If so, the drug must be discarded.

Inhalation. Teach the client how to use the metered dose nebulizer. (See the box in Chapter 38 on p. 660.) Instruct the client to take pulse rate before inhalation therapy. Allow 2 minutes between doses, and do not administer more frequently than required to relieve symptoms. Excessive repeated use may cause paradoxical bronchospasm. To prevent drug tolerance, caution the client not to overuse the drug. Instruct the client to notify the prescriber if the symptoms are not relieved with the usual dosage, since this may be an indication of worsening of the bronchospasm requiring reassessment of therapy. The prescriber should also be notified if the pulse rate increases more than 20 to 30 beats/min. The client may expect that the symptoms should be relieved in 20 minutes. Instruct the client to rinse his or her mouth with water to prevent mucosal absorption of drug. Teach clients with a history of allergic reaction or bronchial asthma how to self-inject epinephrine subcutaneously in case of emergency.

Nasal administration. Inform the client that this route of application may produce a stinging sensation. Forewarn the client that rebound congestion may occur with prolonged use, which may cause rhinitis. Nose drops should not be used for more than 3 to 5 days.

Ophthalmic administration. Alert the client that lightheadedness, increased perspiration and heart rate, trembling, and pallor are signs of systemic absorption. These symptoms may be avoided by limiting the amount of medication that enters the systemic circulation by proper instillation of eye drops. Instruct the client to create a pocket for the solution by gently pinching the skin below the lower eyelid and pulling it away from the eye. Place a drop of the solution into the pocket and hold it open for 1 or 2 seconds to allow the solution to settle. Have the client look down and then gently release the lower eyelid. Press just under the inner corner of the eye for 1 minute. This obstructs the nasolacrimal duct and minimizes the absorption of the drug into the bloodstream.

Administer drug at bedtime or following a miotic to minimize discomfort, blurred vision, and sensitivity to light caused by mydriasis.

Instruct the client to discontinue drug and notify the prescriber if signs of allergy develop (itching, edema of lids, discharge from lids). Advise the client that after initial administration, stinging of the eyes and headache may occur, but with continued drug use these symptoms disappear. Notify the prescriber if these symptoms, which may be controlled by lower dosage, persist. Recommend to the client that intraocular pressure determinations should be scheduled periodically.

The client should be alerted that after long-term use of epinephrine, brownish pigment deposits caused by oxidation of the drug may occur in the eyelids and conjunctiva or as large dark casts in the lacrimal sac or nasolacrimal duct. These may be mistaken as foreign objects in the eye. The casts may be removed by irrigation. Instruct clients who wear soft contact lenses to consult with the prescriber regarding concurrent use of ophthalmic epinephrine instillation because the medication may discolor lens.

Evaluation. The client's symptoms are relieved and vital signs are within the normal range without adverse effects of the drug.

isoproterenol hydrochloride [eye soe proe ter' e nole] (Isuprel)
isoproterenol sulfate (Medihaler-Iso)

Isoproterenol, a synthetic catecholamine, is a nonselective beta adrenergic drug; it stimulates $beta_1$ and $beta_2$ adrenergic receptors. The $beta_1$ receptor activity produces an increase in force of myocardial contraction and heart rate. The $beta_2$ receptor response of the smooth muscle of the bronchi, skeletal muscle, gastrointestinal tract, and blood vessels of the splanchnic bed causes a relaxation of these organs. More important, isoproterenol can greatly relax the smaller bronchi and may even dilate the trachea and main bronchi. This drug also stimulates insulin secretion and releases free fatty acid.

Hemodynamically, the $beta_1$ activity of the heart increases cardiac output and venous return to the heart. Moreover, peripheral vascular resistance is reduced and in normal individuals it may cause a significant drop in blood pressure with excessive dosage.

Isoproterenol is used as a cardiac stimulant in cardiac arrest, Adams-Stokes syndrome, atrioventricular (AV) block, and carotid sinus hypersensitivity. It also may be used as adjunct therapy in treatment of cardiogenic shock, and it relieves bronchospasm associated with bronchial asthma, pulmonary emphysema, and bronchitis.

Isoproterenol is readily absorbed when given parenterally or by inhalation. Absorption of sublingual isoproterenol is erratic and unreliable. Its duration of action is usually up to 2 hours after oral inhalation or subcutaneous administration, less than 1 hour after IV administration. Isoproterenol is metabolized in the GI tract, liver, and lungs and is excreted in the urine.

The side/adverse effects of isoproterenol are similar to epinephrine with the following exceptions: inhalation and sublingual dosage forms may induce a pink to red discoloration of saliva, which is an expected alteration.

Dosage and administration

Cardiac standstill and dysrhythmias. Adult isoproterenol IV dose is 0.02 to 0.06 mg initially, then 0.01 to 0.2 mg if necessary. When administering IM, 0.2 mg initially, then 0.02 to 1 mg if necessary. For IV infusion, intracardiac and subcutaneous dosing, see current drug reference. Dosage in children has not been determined and is individualized by prescriber.

Bronchodilator. Sublingual dose for adults is 10 to 15 mg 3 to 4 times/day; for children it is 5 to 10 mg 3 times/day.

Inhaler. Follow individual manufacturer's instructions carefully when administering isoproterenol by inhalation. Generally, with a metered-dose nebulizer, 1 inhalation is administered, which may be repeated in 1 to 5 minutes if necessary, 4 to 6 times daily. In bronchospasm of chronic obstructive pulmonary disease (COPD), the second dose should be given 3 to 4 hours after the initial dose. When treating acute asthma in children, give oral inhalation of a 0.5% nebulized solution (5 to 15 deep inhalations). If necessary, repeat in 5 to 10 minutes. Dosage may be repeated up to 5 times daily.

■ Nursing Management

Isoproterenol Therapy

Assessment. Use with great caution in clients with cardiovascular disorders such as arrhythmias, coronary insufficiency and hypertension (condition may be worsened); hyperthyroidism (adverse effect more apt to occur); pheochromocytoma; diabetes (drug-induced hyperglycemia may occur); or sensitivity to sympathomimetic amines. Excessive use may decrease effectiveness.

A review of the client's current medication regimen will detect any possible drug interactions. With the exception of the local-parenteral anesthetic interactions, the drug interactions with isoproterenol are similar to those listed under epinephrine. In addition, avoid concurrent administration of epinephrine and isoproterenol because of the possibility of increased additive effects and cardiotoxicity. When the action of one medication is considered complete (usually 4 hours), a second one may be administered.

Baseline assessments of the client's health status to be obtained are the same as for epinephrine.

Nursing diagnosis. Because of the CNS effects of dizziness or lightheadedness, nervousness or restlessness, trembling, and insomnia, the client should be evaluated for the nursing diagnoses of altered comfort, sleep pattern disturbance, anxiety, altered thought processes, and risk for injury. There also may be altered comfort because of the drug's gastrointestinal, respiratory, and local effects. Evaluate for ineffective airway clearance related to the client's preexisting health status to determine the drug's effectiveness. The potential complication of altered cardiac output may be evidenced by headache, hypertension, palpitations, tachycardia, and flushing of the face.

Implementation

Monitoring. With intravenous administration, record baseline blood pressure and pulse before starting isoproterenol therapy. During infusion, check blood pressure every 2 minutes until stabilized, then every 5 minutes during drug administration. Adjust the flow rate to maintain blood pressure, usually at systolic 80 to 100 mm Hg or in hypertensive clients, 30 to 40 mm Hg below preexisting blood pressure. Monitor ECG pattern and central venous pressure, as well as urine volume and blood gases for clients in shock. Follow prescriber's guidelines for titrating flow in relation to heart rate, central venous pressure, blood pressure, ECG changes, and volume of urine flow. If precordial pain occurs, stop drug. If heart rate exceeds 110 beats/minute, a slower infusion rate or temporarily discontinuance of the drug will be prescribed. With doses that cause a heart rate of 130 beats/minute, anticipate the development of ventricular dysrhythmias. Intravenous isoproterenol frequently causes dysrhythmias in clients with heart disease. Monitor respiratory pattern and lung sounds during administration.

For sublingual use, assess the effectiveness of the sublingual dosage forms carefully because absorption of the drug may be erratic and unpredictable. Discontinue medication if severe paradoxical airway resistance develops; institute alternative therapy.

Isoproterenol may increase blood glucose levels. Observe individuals with diabetes for loss of diabetic control. The dosage of insulin or oral hypoglycemic agents may need to be increased. Evaluate the client's extremities for paresthesias, color changes, and coldness. The client receiving isoproterenol may also experience altered comfort related to dryness of the mouth.

Intervention. Read labels carefully; solution for oral inhalation must not be administered intravenously.

Before intravenous therapy, hypovolemia should be corrected if possible. Plan nursing care so that the client is constantly attended while receiving the drug. Never leave the client unattended during the infusion. Use a two-bottle setup so that an intravenous infusion can be kept running if this drug is discontinued. Use an infusion pump to precisely regulate infusion rate. Have oxygen and other resuscitative equipment available. Barbiturates may be used for adjunct sedative therapy to manage the side effects of CNS stimulation.

Education. For sublingual administration, instruct the client to allow sublingual tablet to dissolve under tongue without swallowing saliva until tablet is completely dissolved. Swallowing the drug with saliva causes epigastric pain. Instruct the client to rinse mouth thoroughly with water between sublingual doses. Prolonged use can cause tooth decay. Instruct the client to swallow sustained-release tablets whole and not to chew them.

With oral inhalation, instruct the client to use oral inhalation correctly. (See box in Chapter 38 on p. 660.) The instructions for the metered powder nebulizer are the same as for metered dose nebulizer except that deep inhalation is not necessary. The client should allow 1 to 5 minutes between first and second inhalations. Advise the client that there should be no more than six inhalations in an hour in any 24 hour period. If the client needs more than three aerosol treatments within a 24 hour period, the prescriber should be contacted. If the client has 3 to 5 treatments in a 6 to 12 hour period with minimal or no relief, the therapeutic regimen needs to include other medications in addition to the aerosol.

Advise the client that the drug may turn sputum and saliva pink. Caution against overuse since tolerance can develop and sudden deaths have been reported. Instruct the client to notify the prescriber if prescribed doses are not producing desired relief or if there are adverse effects.

Store drug in tight light-resistant container. Do not use if precipitate or discoloration is present (solutions become pink or brownish pink on exposure to light, air, heat, or on contact with metal or alkali).

Evaluation. The client will demonstrate relief from respiratory distress with vital signs within the normal range without experiencing any adverse effects of the drug.

▲ **norepinephrine bitartrate** [nor ep i nef' rin] (Levophed)

Norepinephrine is a direct-acting sympathomimetic amine identical to the body catecholamine synthesized in the postganglionic nerve ending of the sympathetic nervous system. This agent has a high affinity for the alpha receptors. Since the blood vessels of the skin and mucous membrane contain only alpha receptors, norepinephrine produces a powerful constriction in these tissues. In addition, the blood vessels (both arteriolar and venous beds) in the visceral organs, including the kidneys, contain predominantly alpha receptors. Consequently, norepinephrine causes vasoconstriction and a reduced blood flow through the kidneys and other visceral organs. This agent also activates $beta_1$ receptors in the heart and exerts an increase in the force of myocardial contraction, resulting in an increase in cardiac output.

The main therapeutic effect of norepinephrine results from peripheral arteriolar vasoconstriction in all vascular beds. Both systolic and diastolic pressures are elevated, causing an increase in mean arterial pressure. Of importance during shock is constriction of the venous capacitance vessels, which reduces splanchnic and renal blood flow. This is brought about by severe restriction of tissue perfusion in these regions. In persistent hypotension after blood volume deficit has been corrected, norepinephrine helps to raise the blood pressure to an optimal level and establishes a more adequate circulation.

Norepinephrine is selectively employed for restoring blood pressure in certain acute hypotensive states such as sympathectomy, myocardial infarction, pheochromocytomectomy, and blood transfusion reaction. When used to treat hypotension associated with an acute myocardial infarction, an increase in cardiac output and oxygen demand plus the possibility of inducing dysrhythmias may offset the benefits of using the drug to increase blood pressure. This would have to be carefully considered when selecting norepinephrine for use in such conditions.

Norepinephrine is also used as adjunct therapy in cardiac arrest and profound hypotension. Since the advent of dopamine, the use of norepinephrine to treat shock has declined significantly. It is usually prescribed for clients whose shock produces severe hypotension and vasodilation of the peripheral blood vessels.

Norepinephrine is administered only by intravenous infusion because oral norepinephrine is destroyed in the GI tract and subcutaneous norepinephrine is poorly absorbed. Onset of action is immediate or rapid by intravenous infusion and distribution mainly concentrates in sympathetic tissues; duration of action is approximately 1 to 2 minutes after an intravenous infusion is discontinued. The drug is metabolized in the liver and other tissues, and by reuptake into the sympathetic nerves and is excreted in the kidneys.

The side/adverse effects of norepinephrine include anxiety, dizziness, pallor, tremors, insomnia, headache, pounding heart rate, and perhaps swelling of thyroid gland in neck.

Stimulation of alpha and $beta_1$ receptors with norepinephrine is dose-related. At low doses (<2 μg/minute), $beta_1$ receptors are stimulated thus producing an inotropic and chronotropic response. Doses higher than 4 μg/minute result in stimulation of the alpha receptors or increase total peripheral resistance.

When norepinephrine is used in the treatment of hypotension in adults, an IV infusion of 0.5 to 1 μg/minute; the dosage is adjusted as necessary to raise and maintain the desired pressure. The maintenance dose ranges from 2 to 12 μg/minute with dosage adjustment as necessary to raise and maintain the desired pressure.

■ Nursing Management

Norepinephrine Therapy

Assessment. Review the client's health status for preexisting conditions that may preclude the use of norepinephrine or cause it to be used with particular caution. It is not to be used in clients who are in hypovolemic states except as an emergency measure to maintain cerebral and coronary artery blood flow. Hypovolemia should be corrected before the administration of norepinephrine.

Norepinephrine is contraindicated in pheochromocytoma because hypertension may be worsened. It may also increase the ischemia of myocardial infarction. Do not give to clients with mesenteric or peripheral vascular thrombosis because of the risk of increasing ischemia and extending the thrombosis. Because of its vasoconstricting effects, norepinephrine should be used with caution for clients with occlusive vascular diseases, such as Buerger's disease or arteriosclerosis. It is also contraindicated in profound hypoxia or hypercapnia and pregnancy. Determine if the client is intolerant of sulfites, because the injection dosage form of norepinephrine contains sodium bisulfite as a preservative (Box 22-2).

Assess the client's current drug regimen for possible drug interactions. Norepinephrine's drug interactions with hydrocarbon inhalation anesthetics (such as halothane), beta-adrenergic blocking agents, digitalis glycosides, maprotiline (Ludiomil), cocaine, ergotamine, and ergoloid mesylates are the same as with epinephrine. In addition, when given concurrently with doxapram (Dopram), an increase in central nervous system stimulation and blood pressure may occur. Monitor closely because dosage adjustments may be required. Also, when given concurrently with methyldopa (Aldomet), the hypotensive effect of methyldopa is decreased while the hypertensive action of norepinephrine may be enhanced. If norepinephrine is given to individuals receiving methyldopa, initiate with very small doses with close monitoring.

Use with extreme caution in clients receiving MAO inhibitors and tricyclic antidepressants because prolonged hypertension may result. The nurse should be aware that norepinephrine solutions are incompatible with iron salts, alkalies (sodium bicarbonate), and oxidizing agents.

Nursing diagnosis. The client receiving norepinephrine therapy should be assessed for the following selected nursing diagnoses: risk for injury related to dizziness, impaired integrity of the skin related to extravasation (sloughing of skin), altered comfort (headache), disturbed sleep pattern (insomnia), and the potential complications of sulfite allergy (rash, hives, swelling of the face, difficulty breathing) and altered cardiac output (arrhythmias and hypertension).

BOX 22-2

Sulfite Sensitivity

Sulfite is contained in the commercially available formulations of:

- amrinone (Inocor)
- dobutamine (Dobutrex)
- dopamine (Intropin)
- epinephrine (Adrenalin)
- metaraminol (Aramine)
- methoxamine (Vasoxyl)
- norepinephrine (Levophed)
- phenylephrine (Neo-Synephrine)

They should not be administered to individuals with a known sensitivity to sulfite agents (sulfur dioxide, potassium or sodium bisulfite, potassium or sodium metasulfite, sodium sulfite).

Symptoms of sulfite sensitivity include:

Skin: clamminess, flushed, pruritus, urticaria, cyanosis
Respiratory: bronchospasm, shortness of breath, wheezing, laryngeal edema, respiratory arrest
Cardiovascular: hypotension, syncope
CNS: severe dizziness, loss of consciousness
Other: anaphylaxis, death

Implementation

Monitoring. During infusion, adjust dosage according to prescriber's guidelines. This includes the client's response, with particular attention to urinary output, respiration, blood pressure, pulse, and observation of extremities for color and temperature (for peripheral ischemia). These parameters must be accurately recorded to attain precise titration of drug. It is advised that the blood pressure be taken every 2 to 3 minutes during norepinephrine administration until the desired blood pressure is reached; then it should be measured every 5 minutes until the drug is discontinued. If the client was previously hypotensive, the desired systolic blood pressure range is 80 to 100 mm Hg; however, for those previously hypertensive, it should be maintained at 30 to 40 mm Hg below their preexisting systolic values. Monitor by ECG; reduce or discontinue medication if cardiac dysrhythmia occurs.

Inspect the infusion site for extravasation every 10 to 15 minutes. If extravasation occurs, notify the prescriber immediately. Observe the client for blanching along route of infused vein and for cold, hard swelling around injection site.

Observe the client for mentation (cerebral circulation), temperature of extremities, and color of earlobes, lips, and nail beds; also monitor for paresthesia.

Monitor intake and output. After prolonged use of the drug a decrease in urinary output may indicate necrosis of the kidney.

Intervention. Be aware of the importance of maintaining adequate blood volume before administering norepinephrine. Blood should be administered separately. This is to prevent tissue ischemia that can result from the vasoconstrictive effect of the drug. Administer norepinephrine only intravenously; its vasoconstrictor effect prohibits IM or SC administration.

Anticipate that infusion will be administered through a plastic catheter deep into a large vein to minimize risk of extravasation. The veins of the leg are not recommended because of poor circulation, which can result in occlusive vascular disease.

If extravasation occurs, the area should be quickly infiltrated with 5 to 10 mg of phentolamine (Regitine) in 10 to 15 ml of sodium chloride with a fine-gauge needle to dilate blood vessels. Have phentolamine ready. To prevent sloughing of the skin secondary to extravasation, 5 to 10 mg of phentolamine may be added to every liter of norepinephrine solution.

Norepinephrine should be diluted with 5% dextrose in distilled water or 5% dextrose in sodium chloride solution because the dextrose prevents a significant loss of potency by oxidation. Anticipate the addition of heparin to infusion solution to prevent thrombosis of infused vein in clients with severe hypotension after myocardial infarction.

Never leave the client unattended during infusion. An intravenous pump flow regulator should be used for accuracy of the flow rate in drops per minute. Discontinue therapy gradually by slowing infusion rate, and continue to monitor client and vital signs to ensure circulatory adequacy.

Store medication by protecting it from light. The solution deteriorates after 24 hours; discard it after that time. Do not use solution if it is discolored or if precipitate is present.

Education. Alert the client to report any difficulty in breathing, discomfort at the infusion site, or headache immediately.

Evaluation. The client on norepinephrine therapy will demonstrate an improvement of blood pressure and coronary artery blood flow by having a blood pressure >90 to 100 mm Hg systolic and an absence of the clinical signs of shock (urinary output <30 ml/hour, weak thready pulse, restlessness, confusion).

Drugs Used for Circulatory Shock

In any instance of shock, treatment must be directed to the cause. A main concern is the need to improve circulation so that enough oxygen is available for tissue perfusion. Hypoxia that denotes impaired tissue perfusion may result from inadequate pumping action of the heart, decreased blood volume, decreased peripheral resistance of arterial vessels, or increased size of the venous bed.

During circulatory shock the autonomic nervous system plays an essential compensatory role in an attempt to restore normal circulation. Therefore many sympathomimetic drugs are used to manage this condition. Although there are other agents, the five drugs that are widely used for circulatory shock are dopamine, epinephrine, and norepinephrine, which are all vasopressors, and dobutamine and isoproterenol, which possess cardiogenic activity. Amrinone (Inocor), which has positive inotropic and vasodilator effects, can also be used for clients with congestive heart failure who are not responsive to standard therapy. Milrinone (Primacor), an analogue of amrinone, is also available for short-term use in congestive heart failure. (See Chapter 25, "Cardiac Glycosides.")

Vasopressors have strong alpha activity, and dopamine produces less vasoconstriction than epinephrine and norepinephrine. Dobutamine and isoproterenol are important for improving cardiac output because of their capability to stimulate beta1 receptors in the heart. Most of the agents are nonselective beta acting drugs, but norepinephrine lacks $beta_2$ activity. Also, with the exception of isoproterenol and amrinone, all of these agents stimulate alpha receptors (Table 22-3).

dobutamine hydrochloride [doe byoo' ta meen] (Dobutrex)

Dobutamine is a synthetic catecholamine that acts directly on the heart muscle to increase the force of myocardial contraction. This response is attributed to the direct stimulation of the $beta_1$-adrenergic receptors of the heart. At the same time dobutamine produces comparatively little increase in heart rate or peripheral vascular resistance. By enhancing stroke volume, this agent is an effective positive inotropic drug. Because of its minimal influence on heart rate and blood pressure (both major determinants of myocardial oxygen demand), it is valuable for use in individuals with low cardiac output syndrome.

Dobutamine is administered intravenously in the *short-term* management of clients requiring inotropic support, as in congestive heart failure or after cardiac surgery. It is used to strengthen the decompensated heart in individuals with the low cardiac output syndrome. Its beneficial effects include a

TABLE 22-3 Vasopressor effects in shock

Drug	Receptor site effects*			Organ response†		
	β_1	β_2	α_1	Kidneys	Cardiac	BP
epinephrine	+++	+/++	+++	D	I	D
dobutamine	+++	+	0/+	0	I	
dopamine	+++	0/+	++	I		0/I
isoproterenol	+++	+++	0	I/D	I	#
norepinephrine	++	0	+++	D	0/D	I

*Receptor site effects: β_1, intropic effects; blood vessel effects; β_2, vasodilation; α_1, vasoconstriction.
†Organ response kidneys—renal perfusion; cardiac—cardiac output; BP—blood pressure.
+, minimal effect; ++, moderate effect; +++, greatest effect; 0, no effect; *I*, increased; *D*, decreased; # usual doses maintain or increase systolic pressure.

progressive increase in cardiac output and a decrease in pulmonary capillary wedge pressure, thereby improving ventricular contraction.

In clients with congestive heart failure or after an acute myocardial infarction, the concomitant use of sodium nitroprusside and dobutamine is sometimes beneficial. It results in a higher cardiac output and a lower pulmonary capillary wedge pressure than when either drug is used alone. Because of the vasodilating effect of nitroprusside, the decrease in peripheral resistance lessens the workload on the heart.

Dobutamine is administered by intravenous infusion with an onset of action within 1 to 2 minutes; plasma half-life is 2 minutes as it is rapidly metabolized by the liver and is excreted in the urine.

The side/adverse effects of dobutamine (less frequently reported) include nausea, headache, angina, respiratory distress, palpitation, increased heart rate and blood pressure, and perhaps premature ventricular beats.

Adult dosage is by intravenous infusion, 2.5 to 15 μg/kg/minute. For children, the dosage ranges between 5 to 20 μg/kg/minute.

■ Nursing Management

Dobutamine Therapy

Assessment. Use cautiously in clients with tachycardia and increased blood pressure because the drug may intensify both of these conditions. Safe use of this drug after myocardial infarction is not established. There is concern that a drug that increases the force of myocardial contraction and heart rate may intensify the ischemia by increasing oxygen demand. Note that dobutamine is contraindicated in idiopathic hypertrophic subaortic stenosis (obstruction may increase). Use dobutamine cautiously in individuals with occlusive vascular disease such as Buerger's or Raynaud's disease, atherosclerosis, diabetic endarteritis, or arterial embolism, or with arrhythmias such as tachydysrhythmias and ventricular fibrillation. Note that dobutamine is contraindicated in pheochromocytoma. If the client is hypovolemic, this state should be corrected before dobutamine therapy is begun. Adequate fluid balance is required for the course of therapy. Clients with pheochromocytoma may experience severe hypertension.

The nurse should be aware of potential drug interactions with hydrocarbon inhalation anesthetics (such as halothane, may increase risk of ventricular arrhythmias), beta-adrenergic blocking agents (may cancel the beta_1 adrenergic effects of the drug), digitalis glycosides, maprotiline (Ludiomil), cocaine, ergotamine, and ergoloid mesylates are the same as with norepinephrine. In addition, when given concurrently with doxapram (Dopram), an increase in central nervous system stimulation and blood pressure may occur. Monitor closely because dosage adjustments may be required. Also, when given concurrently with methyldopa, the hypotensive effect of methyldopa (Aldomet) is decreased while the hypertensive action of dobutamine may be enhanced; initiate with very small doses with close monitoring.

Use with extreme caution in clients receiving MAO inhibitors. The coadministration of an MAO inhibitor may result in severe headaches, cardiac dysfunction, or a hypertensive and/or hyperpyretic crisis. Clients receiving an MAO inhibitor within several weeks of dopamine should have the initial dose of dopamine reduced to 10% of the usual adult dose. Monitor closely because dosage adjustments may be necessary.

Nursing diagnosis. The client receiving dobutamine therapy should be monitored for the following: altered comfort (nausea, chest pain, palpitations, headache, nervousness); impaired tissue perfusion related to peripheral vasoconstriction (changes in color, tingling or numbness in fingers or toes); decreased cardiac output (hypotension, hypertension, tachycardia); and the potential complication of hypokalemia, angina, and dysrhythmias.

Implementation

Monitoring. During therapy, the electrocardiogram and blood pressure should be continuously monitored to ascertain any alteration in cardiac output. If possible, the pulmonary capillary wedge pressure and cardiac output also should be monitored to ensure safe infusion and precise titration of the drug. If the client responds by an increase in the heart rate (30 beats/min or more) and an increase in systolic blood pressure (50 mm Hg or greater) during the course of treatment, a reduction of dosage usually reverses these adverse effects because the drug is rapidly metabolized. Monitor extremities for color and temperature for peripheral ischemia.

Monitor intake and output. Increased urinary output indicates improved cardiac output and urinary perfusion. NOTE: Clients with atrial fibrillation and rapid ventricular response should be treated with a digitalis preparation before dobutamine therapy.

If a significant decrease in pulse pressure (disproportionate rise in diastolic pressure) is observed, decrease the infusion rate. Continue to observe the client for further evidence of vasoconstrictor activity. Decrease medication or stop temporarily and notify the prescriber if the following occurs: reduced urinary output without hypotension, increasing tachycardia, dysrhythmia, and marked decrease in pulse pressure. When appropriate, decrease the dosage gradually to prevent severe hypotension. Monitor for sulfite sensitivity (see Box 22-2).

Continue to observe client carefully after drug therapy is discontinued. The duration of action of the drug is brief, and the beneficial effects of the drug may be quickly terminated.

Intervention. Administer using an infusion pump or other device to control the rate of flow and avoid bolus dosing. Adjust dosage based on the clinical response of the client as for norepinephrine and isoproterenol. (See nursing management for intravenous administration of isoproterenol.) The concentration of dobutamine solution for administration should not exceed 5 mg/ml of dobutamine.

For precautions and care regarding extravasation, see norepinephrine nursing management. Have available a syringe with phentolamine mesylate (Regitine), 5 mg in 10 ml saline for use by the physician if extravasation occurs.

Intravenous solution remains stable for 24 hours. A color change during this period indicates some oxidation, but there is no loss of potency during the first 24 hours. Dobutamine is incompatible with alkaline solutions and should not be mixed with products such as 5% sodium bicarbonate injection. Check for drug incompatibilities when considering administration through an intravenous line with other drugs.

Education. Alert the client to report any difficulty breathing, headache, or chest pain immediately.

Evaluation. The client with dobutamine therapy will demonstrate an improvement in cardiovascular status with vital signs within normal limits, improved hemodynamic monitor measurements (central venous pressure and pulmonary wedge pressures), urinary output >30 ml/hr, absence of adventitious lung sounds, and improved pulmonary wedge pressures.

▲ **dopamine hydrochloride** [doe' pa meen] (Intropin) Dopamine is a catecholamine that occurs as an immediate precursor of norepinephrine (see Figure 20-5). It acts both directly and indirectly by releasing norepinephrine. It stimulates dopaminergic receptors, $beta_1$ receptors, and in high doses, alpha receptors. Actually, receptor activity is dose dependent, it depends on the amount of drug administered.

Unlike norepinephrine, in low doses (0.5 to 2 μg/kg/min), dopamine is unique because it acts mainly on dopaminergic receptors to cause vasodilation of the renal and mesenteric arteries. Renal vasodilation increases renal blood flow with usually a greater amount of urine and sodium excretion. This prevents kidney failure secondary to shock.

In low to moderate doses (usually 2 to 10 μg/kg/min), dopamine acts directly on the $beta_1$ receptors on the myocardium and indirectly by releasing norepinephrine from its neuronal storage sites in the sympathetic neuron.

These actions increase myocardial contractility and stroke volume, thereby increasing cardiac output. Systolic blood pressure and pulse pressure may increase with either no effect or a slight elevation in diastolic blood pressure. Nevertheless, total peripheral resistance is usually unchanged. Coronary blood flow and myocardial oxygen consumption increase. However, heart rate increases only slightly at low doses.

In higher doses of dopamine (10 μg/kg/min or more), alpha adrenergic receptors are stimulated, increasing peripheral resistance. Because of a rise in cardiac output, blood pressure increases. As a consequence, a high dose level may reduce urinary output, eliminating the benefit of vasodilation because the renal artery becomes constricted. From the therapeutic standpoint, it is important to note that dopamine in low to moderate doses causes vasodilation in the renal, mesenteric, coronary, and cerebral blood vessels. These vasodilator properties suggest the presence of specific dopamine receptors.

Therefore, unlike norepinephrine, dopamine helps alleviate inadequate tissue perfusion through the vital splanchnic organ systems. The combination of cardiac and circulatory effects has led to dopamine's successful use in the treatment of circulatory shock and refractory heart failure. Dopamine is used to correct hemodynamic imbalances associated with shock syndrome caused by myocardial infarction, trauma, endotoxin septicemia, open heart surgery, renal failure, and chronic cardiac decompensation (as in congestive heart failure).

Administration of dopamine must be by intravenous infusion. The drug has rapid onset of action (2 to 5 minutes) and a short duration of action (5 to 10 minutes), is widely distributed by the body but does not cross the blood-brain barrier. Dopamine is rapidly metabolized by the liver, kidney, and plasma to inactive substances. The drug is excreted in the urine.

The side/adverse effects of dopamine include headaches, nausea, vomiting, angina, respiratory difficulties, decreased blood pressure or less frequently, hypertension, irregular or ectopic heart beats, tachycardia, and palpitations.

For vasopressor effects, adult dose ranges by effect desired (see previous section). Pediatric IV infusion rate ranges between 5 to 20 μg/kg/minute.

For nursing management of dopamine therapy, see the discussion of dobutamine.

Indirect- and Dual-Acting Adrenergic Drugs

The direct-acting adrenergic (catecholamines) drugs, act directly on alpha and beta receptors to stimulate adrenergic response. The indirect-acting adrenergic drugs act indirectly on receptors by first triggering the release of the catecholamines, norepinephrine and epinephrine, from their storage sites; these neurotransmitters then activate the alpha and beta receptors.

Finally, the *dual-acting* adrenergic drugs have both indirect and direct effects. These drugs have many and varied uses in medicine.

ephedrine [e fed' rin] (Ephed II)
Ephedrine has both a direct and an indirect sympathomimetic action. It acts indirectly by stimulating release of norepinephrine from presynaptic nerve terminals and also acts directly on both alpha and beta receptors. Like epinephrine and norepinephrine, ephedrine has positive inotropic (myocardial stimulation) and chronotropic (increased heart rate) activities, but it is a less effective vasoconstrictor. However, it does raise the blood pressure and is used for this purpose during spinal anesthesia and to treat orthostatic hypotension.

Parenteral ephedrine has been used in hypotensive clients who do not respond to fluid replacement, position changes, and specific antidotes in the case of drug overdosage. Be aware though, if severe peripheral vasoconstriction is present, ephedrine may be ineffective and may actually worsen the situation (Table 22-4).

Ephedrine has been used to produce bronchodilation in the treatment of milder forms of bronchial asthma but generally more beta$_2$-selective drugs are preferred, such as albuterol, metaproterenol, and terbutaline. It is also used to relieve nasal mucosal congestion.

Ephedrine is also used as a pressor agent in hypotensive states during spinal anesthesia or after sympathectomy. Absorption of the drug is rapid after oral, IM, or SC administration. Onset of action for bronchodilation occurs within 15 to 60 minutes with oral dosage form, and within 10 to 20 minutes with intramuscular dosage form. Duration of action is 3 to 5 hours after oral dosage form, and 30 to 60 minutes after IM or SC injections of 25 to 50 mg doses. The pressor effects and cardiac responses after parenteral administration of ephedrine usually occur within 60 minutes. The drug is metabolized in the liver and excreted in the kidneys.

The side/adverse effects of ephedrine are similar to epinephrine although it is not available in aerosol so coughing and local irritation are not reported. In addition, ephedrine may cause mood changes and hallucinations.

Dosage and administration. For vasopressor effects, the adult ephedrine dose, IM or SC, is 25 to 50 mg, repeated if necessary. If a faster effect is desired, it may be administered IV. For bronchodilator or decongestant effect, the dose is 25 to 50 mg orally or 12.5 to 25 mg SC, IM or slow IV every 3 or 4 hours as needed. For decongestion, several drops of a 0.5% to 1% ephedrine solution may be applied topically and repeated every 4 hours if necessary.

■ Nursing Management

Ephedrine Therapy

Assessment. The client's health status needs to be reviewed for conditions for which ephedrine may be contraindicated or used with additional caution. Use ephedrine with caution in clients with hypertension, hyperthyroidism, prostatic hypertrophy, and diabetes mellitus. Use with caution in children under 6 years and with elderly clients. Do not use in clients with severe hypertension, narrow-angle glaucoma, or history of hypersensitivity to sympathomimetic drugs or with those receiving digitalis or MAO inhibitor therapy.

Ephedrine's significant drug interactions with anesthetics, antidepressants (tricyclic and MAO inhibitors), beta-blocking agents, cocaine, digitalis glycosides, ergoloid mesylates, and ergotamine are the same as reported with epinephrine.

A baseline assessment of the client's cardiovascular and respiratory status is required.

Nursing diagnosis. The client receiving ephedrine therapy should be assessed for the following selected nursing diagnoses: disturbed sleep pattern (insomnia); anxiety; altered comfort (headache); and risk for sensitivity (rash, facial edema, wheezing). Altered urinary output pattern may occur evidenced by sphincter spasm and retention caused by ephedrine's effects. There is the potential complication of decreased cardiac output (tachycardia, arrhythmias).

Implementation

Monitoring. During intravenous administration, closely monitor blood pressure repeatedly during first 5 minutes, then check every 3 to 5 minutes until it is stable. Never leave client unattended during intravenous administration.

If administered parenterally to maintain blood pressure in conjunction with spinal anesthesia during delivery, ephedrine may cause the fetal heart rate to accelerate and it should be discontinued when the maternal blood pressure reaches 130/80.

Monitor intake and output, and advise the client to report any difficulty in urinating (particularly older male patients).

Intervention. Administer only if the solution is clear; discard any unused portion. If used within a cough and cold remedy, administer a few hours before bedtime and avoid administering at night to help prevent insomnia, an altered sleep pattern.

Education. If self-administered for respiratory symptoms, advise client not to take OTC drugs unless the prescriber is consulted first. Caution client not to overuse drug because tolerance may develop. It may be necessary to withhold medication for several days to restore effectiveness. Instruct client to follow correct dosage and report any side effects or adverse reactions immediately to the prescriber. Also, advise client not to swallow nose drops so as to avoid systemic effects.

Evaluation. The client on ephedrine therapy will demonstrate an improvement in cardiovascular status with vital signs within normal limits, urinary output >30 ml/hr, absence of confusion and restlessness, and improved hemodynamic monitor measurements (central venous pressure and pulmonary wedge pressures). If administered for respiratory congestion, the client will demonstrate easier breathing without wheezing and rhinitis.

TABLE 22-4 Indirect- and dual-acting adrenergic drug effects

Receptors, action sites	Ephedrine	Phenylephrine	Mephentermine	Metaraminol	Methoxamine
Trade names	Ephedrine Sulfate	Neo-Synephrine	Wyamine	Aramine	Vasoxyl
Mode of action					
Alpha receptors	Stimulates	Stimulates	Stimulates	Stimulates	Stimulates
Beta receptors	Stimulates More prolonged but less intense action than epinephrine	N.S.*			
Effects					
Cardiovascular					
Myocardium	Variable	N.S. Bradycardia may occur reflexively	Increases contractility and rate May cause bradycardia	Some increase in contractility Bradycardia may occur	— Reflex bradycardia may occur
Pacemaker cells	N.S.	N.S.	N.S.	—	—
Coronary vessels	Dilates—increases blood flow	Dilates—increases blood flow	Dilates—increases blood flow	—	—
Blood pressure	Increases	Increases	Increases	Increases	Increases
Bronchi	Dilates	Dilates but less than epinephrine	Dilates but less than epinephrine	N.S.	—
Cerebral effects	Stimulating action	N.S.	N.S.	—	—
Blood vessels					
Skeletal muscle	N.S.	—†	N.S.	N.S.	Decreases blood flow
Kidney	Constricts	Constricts	Constricts but less than ephedrine	Constricts—decreases blood flow	
Gastrointestinal tract	Decreases peristalsis	Decreases motility	Relaxes smooth muscle—inhibits	Some inhibition	Inhibits
Metabolic	Increases metabolic rate	Some increase in metabolic rate	N.S.	N.S.	N.S.
Remarks	Serious dysrhythmias may occur if used with digitalis Can be given orally			Prolonged duration of action cumulative effects may occur—give drug slowly May cause tissue sloughing—do not give subcutaneously	
Uses	Vasopressor Allergic states Nasal decongestant Enuresis Myasthenia gravis	Nasal decongestant Vasopressor Paroxysmal atrial tachycardia Mydriatic	Vasopressor	Vasopressor	Vasopressor Paroxysmal atrial tachycardia

*N.S., Not significant.
†Effect is slight, nonexistent, or unknown in humans.

phenylephrine systemic [fen ill ef' rin] (Neo-Synephrine injection)

phenylephrine nasal (Neo-Synephrine, Alconefrin)

Phenylephrine is primarily a direct-acting agent, its main effects are stimulation of the alpha receptors, resulting in vasoconstriction, and an increase in both diastolic and systolic blood pressures. The drug has little effect on the $beta_1$ receptors of the heart. Its vasoconstricting action is more prolonged than that of norepinephrine thus it may be used for acute hypotension that occurs from spinal anesthesia. It is not effective in shock caused by loss of blood volume. Phenylephrine is also contained in many combination cough-cold, antihistamine and decongestant, and ophthalmic preparations.

It is a synthetic adrenergic drug chemically related to epinephrine, norepinephrine, and ephedrine. Phenylephrine exhibits fewer side effects than epinephrine and has longer-lasting therapeutic effects. It has little or no effect on the central nervous system.

When applied topically to mucous membranes, phenylephrine reduces swelling and congestion by constricting the small blood vessels. It is useful in the treatment of sinusitis, vasomotor rhinitis, and hay fever. It is sometimes combined with local anesthetics to retard their systemic absorption and to prolong their action.

Phenylephrine is used as a mydriatic for certain conditions in which dilation of the pupil is desired without cycloplegia paralysis of the ciliary muscle) and may be applied intranasally for congestion caused by colds, hay fever, sinusitis, or allergies.

Administered IV, phenylephrine produces an immediate effect with a duration of action of 5 to 20 minutes. The drug is metabolized partially in gastrointestinal tract tissues and in the liver by the enzyme monoamine oxidase. The route of excretion is not identified.

The side/adverse effects of phenylephrine while uncommon include anxiety, restlessness, dizziness, tremors, difficult breathing, pallor, increased weakness, angina and allergic reactions with the preparations that contain sulfites (see Box 22-2). For dosage and administration, see Table 22-5.

■ Nursing Management

Phenylephrine Therapy

Assessment. Before administering phenylephrine, it should be assessed as to whether the client has a preexisting health problem for which the drug would be contraindicated or used only with extreme caution. Risk-benefit should be considered if phenylephrine is used in clients with narrow-angle glaucoma (ophthalmic preparations), severe coronary disease, severe hypertension, or ventricular tachycardia. Use with caution in individuals with hyperthyroidism, hypertension, diabetes mellitus, ischemic cardiac disease, or cerebral arteriosclerosis.

The client's current medication regimen should be reviewed for significant drug interactions. The following interactions

TABLE 22-5 Phenylephrine: dosage and administration

Dose/indication	Adults	Children
Hypotension	IM or SC: initially, 2-5 mg of 1% solution. If necessary, may repeat every 10-15 min. IV: 0.2 mg, repeat in 15 min if necessary. IV infusion: Initial, 100-180 µg/min until blood pressure stabilizes. (Solution contains 10 mg phenylephrine to 500 ml 5% dextrose injection or 0.9% sodium chloride injection.) When client is stabilized, give 40-60 µg/min.	For hypotension during spinal anesthesia, IM or SC, 0.5 mg - 1 mg/25 lbs body weight.
To prolong spinal anesthesia	Add 2-5 mg to anesthetic solution.	
Nasal congestion		
Nasal solution or spray (0.25% - 0.5%)	2 or 3 drops or 1 or 2 sprays in each nostril every 3 - 4 hr as necessary.	Children 6 to 12 yr (0.25%): 2 or 3 drops every 3-4 hr as necessary. Spray (0.25%): 1 or 2 sprays every 3-4 hr as necessary. Less than 6 yr (0.125%): 2 or 3 drops every 3-4 hr as necessary.
Nasal decongestant	Oral, 10 mg every 3-4 hr as necessary.	
Ophthalmic preparations		
Ophthalmoscopy, 2.5% solution	1 drop to conjunctiva, 15-30 min before examination.	See adult dose.
Mydriasis and vasoconstriction	1 drop topically to conjunctiva of a 2.5% to 10% solution. If necessary, may repeat in 1 hr.	1 drop of a 2.5% solution topically to conjunctiva. If necessary, may repeat in 1 hr.

may occur when phenylephrine is given with the drugs listed below:

Drug	Possible effect and management
alpha receptor-blocking agents	May reduce or block the vasopressor effect of phenylephrine, resulting in hypotension.
anesthetics, inhalation of hydrocarbons such as chloroform, enflurane, halothane, and others, plus digitalis glycosides	**Increases risk of inducing serious cardiac dysrhythmias. If necessary to use concurrently, monitor closely with ECG read ings because therapeutic interventions may be necessary. Avoid or serious drug interaction may occur.**
beta-blocking agents	Therapeutic effects of both drugs may be inhibited. This can occur with both oral and ophthalmic beta-adrenergic blocking drugs. Avoid concurrent use.
ergotamine and ergoloid mesylates	**Increases vasoconstriction; severe hypertension and peripheral vascular ischemia and gangrene may occur. This combined use is not recommended. Avoid or serious drug interaction may occur.**
doxapram (Dopram)	The vasopressor effects of either or both drugs may increase. Monitor blood pressure closely since dosage adjustments may be necessary.
cocaine, maprotiline (Ludiomil), or tricyclic antidepressants	May potentiate cardiovascular effects of phenylephrine, such as dysrhythmias, increase heart rate, and cause severe hypertension and elevated body temperature. Monitor client's vital signs closely.
monoamine oxidase (MAO) inhibitors	**May cause increased release of accumulated neurotransmitters into the synapse area, causing severe headaches, dysrhythmias, vomiting, severe hypertension, and/or high fevers. Avoid or serious drug interaction may occur. Phenylephrine should not be given during or within 2 weeks after the administration of an MAO inhibitor.**

Obtain a baseline assessment of the client's underlying condition for which the phenylephrine is being prescribed.

Nursing diagnosis. The client's risk of altered comfort is related to phenylephrine's cardiovascular (chest pain) and neurologic effects (restlessness, trembling), as well as the local effects of topical preparations (stinging). Altered cardiac output should be considered as a potential complication with the administration of phenylephrine related to its cardiovascular effects (hypertension, arrhythmias).

Implementation

Monitoring. The blood pressure of clients with hypertension should be monitored carefully while they are receiving phenylephrine, even nasal or ophthalmic preparations. Any signs of angina should be reported to the prescriber immediately. Monitor the infusion site for extravasation. Monitor intake and output. Observe client for rebound miosis (pupil constriction) after ophthalmic administration.

Monitor for sulfite sensitivity (see Box 22-2). Pediatric clients are more likely to be sensitive to the vasopressor effects. Elderly clients may demonstrate confusion, sedation, hypotension, dryness of mouth, and urinary retention.

Intervention. After each use, wash nasal droppers with hot water to prevent contamination of solution; eye droppers should not touch the eye or any other surface. Solutions lose potency with exposure to air, strong light, or heat. Keep container tightly sealed and away from light. Discard if solution is dark brown or contains a precipitate.

If nasal or ophthalmic phenylephrine preparations are administered to clients with hypertension, timing of the doses should not be at the end of dosing periods of the antihypertensive drugs when therapeutic levels of antihypertensive medications are low.

Nasal preparations. Before administration of drug, instruct client to blow nose to clear nasal passages. Instill drops by having client tilt head back and remain in position a few minutes to permit medication to spread through nose. When administering a spray, have head upright, and squeeze bottle firmly and quickly to produce spray into each nostril; after 3 to 5 minutes blow nose and repeat.

IV administration. See nursing management under norepinephrine for intravenous administration. Have phentolamine (Regitine) available to treat hypertensive emergencies.

Ophthalmic preparations. Instruct client to apply pressure to lacrimal sac during administration of phenylephrine eye drops and for 1 or 2 minutes after instillation. The client with contact lenses should consult the physician for specific instructions.

Education. For intravenous administration, alert the client to report discomfort at the infusion site, headache, or chest pain immediately. With nasal applications, instruct client not to swallow the solutions, in order to avoid systemic effects. Instruct the client to swallow the extended-release capsules whole.

Emphasize to client the importance of adhering to drug regimen. Consult prescriber about any modification—dose, time interval, and others. Alert client to the risk for injury, because dizziness and drowsiness are common side effects of the phenylephrine; activities should be modified to consider those effects. Advise client to avoid the ingestion of alcohol and other CNS depressants that would increase the severity of these effects. Notify the prescriber if insomnia, dizziness, or tremors occur.

Tell the client that phenylephrine inhibits salivation, and long-term use promotes caries, gum disease, and oral candidiasis. Regular dental checkups are advised.

Caution client about burning and stinging sensation after instillation of eye drops. Inform client that after instillation of drops, pupils will be dilated and may be sensitive to light. Notify prescriber if sensitivity persists beyond 12 hours after discontinuation of drug.

Evaluation. For hypotensive conditions, the client on phenylephrine therapy will demonstrate a blood pressure >90 to 100 mm Hg systolic, urinary output >30 ml/hour and an absence of symptoms of shock (weak thready pulse, restlessness, confusion). For nasal congestion, the client will demonstrate easier breathing and report less nasal discharge and congestion. For pupillary dilation, the client will demonstrate dilated pupils and decreased intraocular pressure by tonometry.

mephentermine sulfate [me fen' ter meen] (Wyamine)

Mephentermine's effects are similar to ephedrine, but it produces more cerebral stimulation. Mephentermine is a dual-acting (primarily) sympathomimetic. It releases catecholamines from storage sites in the heart and other tissues (indirect action). Therefore it tends to bring about both alpha and beta stimulating effects, including inotropic and chronotropic effects on the heart. Since mephentermine improves cardiac contraction and mobilizes blood from venous pools, thereby increasing cardiac output, it acts as a peripheral vasoconstrictor (see Table 22-4).

The drug is used as a pressor agent in the treatment of hypotension secondary to spinal anesthesia and as adjunct therapy for hypotension secondary to hemorrhage, medications, and shock due to brain tumor or trauma.

Administered IM, the drug's onset of action occurs within 5 to 15 minutes; duration of action is 1 to 4 hours. Administered IV, mephentermine is nearly immediate in action; duration of action is 15 to 30 minutes. The drug is metabolized in the liver and excreted in the kidneys.

The side/adverse effects of mephentermine (less frequent) include anxiety, nervousness, restlessness and tachycardia.

For hypotension: Adult mephentermine dosage is 30 to 45 mg IV in a single injection. Repeat doses of 30 mg as needed to maintain blood pressure. Dosage for children has not been established.

■ Nursing Management

Mephentermine Therapy

Assessment. The client's health status should be evaluated to ensure the client does not have a condition for which mephentermine would be contraindicated or require extreme caution. Use cautiously in individuals with arteriosclerosis, hypertension, cardiovascular disease, hyperthyroidism, and chronically ill clients. Clients having hypoxia should have the condition corrected before the administration of mephentermine or the response to the drug may be decreased or the risk of adverse effects may be increased.

Drugs may cause uterine contraction; therefore it should not be administered to pregnant women.

The client's current medication regimen should be reviewed to detect significant drug interactions. See phenylephrine drug interactions for potential drug interactions that may also occur with mephentermine.

Obtain a baseline assessment of the client's underlying condition for which the mephentermine is being prescribed.

Nursing diagnosis. The client receiving mephentermine therapy is at risk for the following selected nursing diagnoses: altered comfort (restlessness, headache) and anxiety; and the complication of altered cardiac output (arrhythmias, hypertension).

Implementation

Monitoring. Monitor closely blood pressure, pulse, ECG, central venous pressure, and urinary output. The blood pressure and pulse should be checked every 2 minutes until stabilized, then every 5 to 15 minutes thereafter during therapy. The blood pressure should be maintained at slightly less than the client's normal blood pressure. In clients with hypertension, maintain at 30 to 40 mm Hg below usual blood pressure.

Observe client for possible development of tolerance if repeated injections are administered. Note that blood volume replacement must be instituted as soon as possible in treatment of secondary shock.

Intervention. Administer mephentermine using an infusion device to precisely regulate dosage according to the response of the client. Do not use if the solution is discolored or a precipitate has formed.

Education. Alert the client to report headache and anxiety as early symptoms of overdose.

Evaluation. The client on mephentermine therapy will demonstrate a blood pressure >90 to 100 mm Hg systolic, urinary output >30 ml/ hr, and an absence of symptoms of shock (weak thready pulse, restlessness, confusion).

metaraminol [met a ram' i nole] (Aramine)

Metaraminol is a vasopressor agent with both direct (primarily) and indirect effects on the sympathetic system. It acts indirectly by releasing norepinephrine from tissues and storage sites and directly on alpha receptors, as a neurohormone.

Metaraminol has positive inotropic effects. Since it constricts blood vessels, increases peripheral resistance, elevates both systolic and diastolic blood pressure, and improves cardiac contractility and cerebral, coronary, and renal blood flow, the drug is used for the treatment of shock.

Since metaraminol exhibits beta- and alpha-adrenergic activity, it is often effective in raising blood pressure when alpha adrenergic agents are ineffective. This may be because of its ability to bring about more effective venous flow. It does not appear to cause dysrhythmias. It generally lacks CNS stimulatory effects and its side effects are rare and often related to rapid drug administration. Although similar to norepinephrine in action, it is generally considered a less potent drug.

Metaraminol is used for acute hypotensive states occurring with spinal anesthesia. It is also administered for the prevention and treatment of acute hypotension associated with surgery, drug-induced reactions, and shock.

The drug is administered parenterally only. When given IV, onset is within 1 to 2 minutes; SC or IM, the onset of action is within 10 minutes. Duration of action is between 20 to 60 minutes and it is metabolized in the liver and excreted in the bile and kidneys.

The metaraminol adult dose given SC or IM is 2 to 10 mg to prevent acute hypotension. To avoid cumulative effects, wait 10 minutes before giving additional doses. When given via IV infusion, administer 15 to 100 mg in 500 ml of sodium chloride injection (0.9%) or 5% dextrose in water at rate determined by the prescriber to maintain the desired blood pressure response. The drug is given by direct IV injection for severe shock, 0.5 to 5 mg followed by the infusion described above. Pediatric dosage has not been established.

▪ Nursing Management

Metaraminol Therapy

Assessment. The client's health status should be reviewed for contraindications before the initiation of metaraminol therapy. The drug is to be used with caution in individuals with acidosis, hypertension, heart disease, peripheral vascular disease, thyroid disease, diabetes mellitus, or cirrhosis of liver. Clients with hypoxia should have this condition corrected before or concurrently with the administration of metaraminol, or its effectiveness may be reduced or the risk of adverse effects may be increased. Do not use in individuals sensitive to metaraminol.

Review client's current medication regimen for significant drug interactions. See phenylephrine drug interactions for potential drug interactions that may also occur with metaraminol.

Obtain a baseline assessment of the client's underlying condition for which the metaraminol is being prescribed.

Nursing diagnosis. The client with metaraminol therapy may experience the nursing diagnosis of impaired tissue integrity related to extravasation of IV fluid (sloughing at infusion site); and the potential complications of allergic reaction to sulfites (rash, facial edema, wheezing) and altered cardiac output (hypertension, arrhythmias, hypotension when the drug is discontinued).

Implementation

Monitoring. Closely monitor blood pressure every 2 to 5 minutes during infusion (client must be constantly attended). Since the drug has a prolonged effect, adjust flow rate carefully to avoid a cumulative response. Before terminating infusion, reduce flow rate gradually to avoid abrupt withdrawal of drug, which otherwise might result in severe hypotension. If possible, correct plasma volume before starting therapy. Continue to monitor blood pressure closely after the drug has been discontinued. If severe hypotension occurs, the drug should be resumed quickly.

Monitor for cardiac arrhythmias. Monitor intake and output; also monitor sodium and potassium loss because clients with cirrhosis of liver may suffer from diuresis. Monitor for sulfite sensitivity (see Box 22-2).

Monitor infusion site frequently for extravasation because it will result in sloughing of the skin.

Intervention. Subcutaneous injection is rarely given since it causes tissue necrosis. Moreover, avoid extravasation during intravenous infusion. The use of larger veins may be helpful during infusion. Veins of the ankle and back of the hand should be avoided, particularly in clients with peripheral vascular disease and diabetes mellitus. Have on hand phentolamine (decreases pressor effect) and atropine (for bradycardia). Metaraminol must be diluted before administration. Once diluted, it should be used within 24 hours. Because metaraminol is incompatible with many drugs, it should not be administered in a solution containing other medications.

Education. Alert the client to report discomfort at the infusion site.

Evaluation. The client on metaraminol therapy will demonstrate a blood pressure >90 to 100 mm Hg systolic, urinary output >30 ml/ hr, and an absence of symptoms of shock (weak thready pulse, restlessness, confusion).

methoxamine hydrochloride [meth ox' a meen] (Vasoxyl)

Methoxamine is an alpha-adrenergic stimulator devoid of beta receptor activity, except in high doses. The direct-acting sympathomimetic agent is pharmacologically related to phenylephrine. Since it has no stimulating effect on the heart, the rise in blood pressure causes a reflex bradycardia. This effect makes it useful in treating paroxysmal supraventricular tachycardia and in restoring or maintaining blood pressure during anesthesia. (See Table 22-4.)

Parenterally administered, with IV administration, the effects of methoxamine are immediate; duration of action as a vasopressor is 5 to 15 minutes. Following IM administration the effects are seen within 15 to 20 minutes, with duration of effects between 60 and 90 minutes. Metabolism and excretion routes are unknown.

The side/adverse effects of methoxamine are infrequent and include sweating, severe headaches, hypertension, vomiting and urinary urgency with high doses.

The adult vasopressor dose is 10 to 15 mg IM or 3 to 5 mg given slowly by direct IV. Dose for children is not established.

▪ Nursing Management

Methoxamine Therapy

Assessment. Use methoxamine cautiously in clients with acidosis, hyperthyroidism, pheochromocytoma, cardiovascular disease, or hypertension and also following parenteral injection of ergot alkaloids. Clients with hypoxia should have this condition corrected before or concurrently with the administration of methoxamine, or its effectiveness may be reduced or the risk of adverse effects may be increased.

Review the client's current medications for significant drug interactions. See drug interactions for phenylephrine.

Obtain a baseline assessment of the client's underlying condition for which the methoxamine is prescribed.

Nursing diagnosis. In addition to altered cardiac output, the client with methoxamine therapy may also experience altered comfort related to methoxamine's effects of headache, increased perspiration, and the sensation of urinary urgency.

Implementation

Monitoring. Monitor the blood pressure and pulse continuously during therapy and titrate the dose accordingly. The BP should be maintained at slightly less than the client's normal blood pressure. In clients with hypertension, maintain at 30 to 40 mm Hg below usual BP. Observe client for severe bradycardia with ECG rhythm strips.

Monitor intake and output because output increases when normal blood pressure levels occur (if the client is not hypovolemic). Observe client for sudden changes of blood pressure after the drug is terminated. Monitor for sulfite sensitivity (see Box 22-2).

BOX 22-3

Midodrine (ProAmatin)

Midodrine (ProAmatine) is indicated for the treatment of symptomatic orthostatic hypotension. It is a prodrug that is converted to an active metabolite desglymidodrine, and $alpha_1$ agonist that activates arteriolar and venous receptors to increase blood pressure. It can raise systolic blood pressure by 15 to 30 mm Hg in 1 hour after a 10 mg dose.

Pharmacokinetics

Midodrine metabolite peaks in 1 to 2 hours; half-life is 3 to 4 hours with metabolism in many tissues including the liver. It is excreted renally.

Side/adverse effects include paresthesia, pruritus, dysuria, and supine hypertension. Adult dose is 10 mg PO three times daily during daytime hours (every 4 hours but not later than 6 PM). Because of the risk of supine hypertension, do not give midodrine after evening meal or less than 4 hours before retiring (Olin, 1997).

Intervention. Intramuscular doses may need to be repeated. If so, allow sufficient time for previous injection to have taken effect before considering administering another. Administer IV slowly if the systolic pressure falls below 60 or in another emergency. Have atropine available if bradycardia occurs.

Evaluation. The client with methoxamine therapy will demonstrate a blood pressure >90 to 100 mm Hg systolic, urinary output >30 ml/hr, and an absence of symptoms of shock (weak thready pulse, restlessness, confusion).

See Box 22-3 for midodrine (ProAmatin).

ADRENERGIC BLOCKING DRUGS

Alpha-Adrenergic Blocking Drugs

Most **alpha-adrenergic blocking agents** are competitive blockers; they compete with the catecholamines at receptor sites and inhibit adrenergic sympathetic stimulation. They are more effective against the action of circulating catecholamines than against catecholamines released from storage sites in the neurons. These drugs may be obtained from natural sources, such as ergot and its derivatives, or they may be synthesized.

The alpha-adrenergic blocking agents fall into three categories:

1. Noncompetitive, long-acting antagonists (e.g., phenoxybenzamine [Dibenzyline]): action persists for several days or weeks because a stable bond is formed between a specific component of the drug and the alpha receptor site.
2. Competitive, short-acting antagonists (e.g., phentolamine [Regitine], tolazoline [Priscoline]): the blocking action is reversible and competitive at the alpha receptor site and the effects last only several hours.
3. Ergot alkaloids: usually act as partial alpha-adrenergic antagonists. However, the drugs produce primarily a spasmogenic effect on smooth muscle of blood vessels, thereby causing vasoconstriction.

Noncompetitive, Long-Acting Antagonists

phenoxybenzamine [fen ox ee ben' za meen] (Dibenzyline)

Phenoxybenzamine is a long-acting, irreversible alpha-adrenergic blocking agent that abolishes or decreases the receptiveness of alpha receptors to adrenergic stimuli. Since phenoxybenzamine competes with the catecholamines, it is also useful in decreasing the blood pressure of clients with pheochromocytoma. It does not block sympathetic impulses on the heart and therefore does not directly impair cardiac output.

All $alpha_1$ blockers are also used to relieve symptoms of benign prostatic hyperplasia, although this indication is not included in the U.S. product labeling. By noncompetitively blocking alpha adrenergic receptors of the bladder neck and proximal urethra, the internal sphincter is relaxed improving voiding efficiency in clients with functional outlet obstruction.

Phenoxybenzamine is used in the management of pheochromocytoma: preoperative preparation of client for surgery, chronic treatment of individuals with malignant pheochromocytoma, and individuals for whom surgery of pheochromocytoma is contraindicated. However, because a 2 year study in rats employing large doses of phenoxybenzamine demonstrated basal cell growth in the stomach, the manufacturer recommends its use only for emergency, short term use, such as preoperative management of pheochromocytoma (AMA, 1995).

Oral absorption of the drug is variable. Onset of action occurs in 2 hours. The drug can persist for 3 or 4 days since it forms a stable bond with the receptor. The half-life is about 24 hours with metabolism in the liver and excretion in the kidney and bile.

The side/adverse effects of phenoxybenzamine include dizziness (postural hypotension), miosis, tachycardia, nasal congestion, confusion, dry mouth, headache and inhibition of ejaculation.

The initial adult dose is 10 mg twice daily orally; dosage may be increased by 10 mg every other day until the desired effect is noted. Maintenance dose is 20 to 40 mg two or three times daily. Initial pediatric dose is 0.2 mg/kg PO up to a maximum of 10 mg, administered once daily. Dosage may be increased every 4 days until the desired effect is noted. Maintenance dose is 0.4 mg to 1.2 mg/kg body weight, given in 3 or 4 divided doses.

■ Nursing Management

Phenoxybenzamine Therapy

Assessment. Use phenoxybenzamine with caution in clients with renal insufficiency, and upper respiratory infection (may aggravate nasal congestion). Do not use in clients with compensated congestive failure or coronary artery disease because it will cause angina and congestive heart failure, or in conditions when a decrease in blood pressure might be dangerous, such as cerebrovascular insufficiency. Sensitivity to the drug should be determined.

A review of the client's current medication regimen should be accomplished to detect significant drug interactions. When phenoxybenzamine is given with other sympathomimetics, such as epinephrine, metaraminol, methoxamine, and phenylephrine, the results may be as follows:

1. Blocking of the alpha-adrenergic receptor effects of epinephrine (Adrenalin), which may result in severe hypotension and tachycardia.
2. Decrease in the vasopressor effects of metaraminol (Aramine).
3. Blocking of the vasopressor effect of methoxamine (Vasoxyl), resulting in severe hypotension.
4. Decrease in the vasopressor effect to phenylephrine (Neo-Synephrine). Avoid concurrent drug administration if at all possible.

Obtain a baseline assessment of the client's blood pressure and cardiovascular status.

Nursing diagnosis. The client receiving phenoxybenzamine is at risk for the following nursing diagnoses: altered comfort (headache, dry mouth); activity intolerance related to weakness and lethargy; sexual dysfunction related to alpha-adrenergic blockade (inability to ejaculate); and risk for injury related to miosis, postural hypotension and confusion.

Implementation

Monitoring. Monitor blood pressure and pulse rate both in recumbent and standing positions during period of dosage adjustment, particularly when dosage is increased. Observe client for signs of hypotension and tachycardia. Inform client that these signs usually disappear with continued therapy. However, with the vasodilation associated with exercise, drinking alcohol, or eating a large meal, these signs may recur. Urinary catecholamines determinations during initial treatment help to determine appropriate dosage.

Intervention. Administer the oral drug with milk to reduce gastric irritation. The dosage should be adjusted according to the clinical response and level of urinary catecholamines. Dosage increases will be gradual from the lowest therapeutic dose, but the increments should be no more frequent than every 4 days. Treat overdosage by intravenous infusion of norepinephrine. Do not use epinephrine since it will cause a further drop in blood pressure.

Education. Advise client to make position changes slowly (from recumbent to upright posture) to prevent orthostatic hypotension. Instruct client to dangle legs and exercise feet for a few minutes at the bedside before standing. If faintness or weakness occurs, a head-low position should be assumed or the person must lie down immediately. Elastic support stockings help to prevent orthostatic hypotension. Because of the risk of injury related to orthostatic hypotension, instruct the client not to drink alcohol, to avoid standing for long periods, and not to exercise during hot weather because the possibility of this effect would be increased. Advise the client to modify activities if dizziness and/or drowsiness occur, because of the risk for injury.

Advise the client that because the drug inhibits salivary flow and thus promotes the development of caries, periodontal disease, and buccal candidiasis, regular dental checkups are required. Dryness of the mouth can be relieved and the comfort of the client promoted by ice chips and sugarless gum. Warn client against using any other drug, particularly OTC sympathomimetics (such as cough, cold, or allergy preparations) without consulting the prescriber.

An effect of this drug can be inhibition of ejaculation, which should be reported to the prescriber.

Evaluation. Clients with pheochromocytoma will note decreases in blood pressure, pulse, and sweating that are signs of therapeutic effectiveness. The client's blood pressure will be within normal limits.

Competitive, Short-Acting Antagonists

phentolamine mesylate [fen tole' a meen] (Regitine, Rogitine ♣)

Phentolamine is an alpha adrenergic blocking agent that competitively blocks $alpha_2$ (presynaptic) and $alpha_1$ (postsynaptic) receptors. The action occurs at both arterial and venous vessels. This direct relaxation of vascular smooth muscle lowers total peripheral resistance. Accordingly, hypertension is inhibited when there are excessive levels of epinephrine and norepinephrine. It also decreases pulmonary vascular resistance.

The drug is used to prevent or control hypertensive episodes in the individual with pheochromocytoma. It is also used to reverse the vasoconstrictive action of an overdose or excessive response to IV administration or extravasation of norepinephrine (Levophed) or dopamine. The subcutaneous injection of phentolamine (Regitine) following extravasation of intravenous norepinephrine or dopamine will prevent tissue necrosis if prompt action is taken.

Parenteral phentolamine is administered IV, half-life is approximately 19 minutes. Metabolism and excretion sources are unknown; because only 13% (approximately) of the drug is found in urine after parenteral administration.

The side/adverse effects of phentolamine include diarrhea, dizziness (postural hypotension), nausea, vomiting, abdominal pain and tachycardia.

When phentolamine is used preoperatively, 5 mg IV is administered 1 to 2 hours before surgery, dosage may be repeated if necessary during surgery. As an antiadrenergic preoperative in children, 1 mg (IM or IV) is administered 1 to 2 hours before surgery, repeated if necessary.

■ Nursing Management

Phentolamine Therapy

Assessment. Use phentolamine with caution in clients with coronary artery disease and myocardial infarction because reflex tachycardia as a result of the drug may precipitate congestive heart failure. Gastritis and peptic ulcer may be aggravated by phentolamine. Do not use in clients with hypersensitivity to phentolamine.

Significant drug interactions are the same as for phenoxybenzamine.

The client's blood pressure and cardiovascular status are essential for a baseline assessment.

Nursing diagnosis. Clients receiving phentolamine should be evaluated for risk for injury related to the drug's cardiovascular effects (orthostatic hypotension, reflex tachycardia). Diarrhea and altered comfort (abdominal cramping, nasal stuffiness, facial flushing, nausea and vomiting) may also be an issue. If administered in a norepinephrine IV infusion or for extravasation, observe client for impaired tissue integrity at the infusion site. With parenteral administration, the potential complications of cerebrovascular spasm (confusion, sudden loss of coordination or slurring of speech) and myocardial infarction (chest pain) may occur.

Implementation

Monitoring. Monitor blood pressure and pulse every 2 minutes until stabilized. Observe extravasation site for tissue necrosis.

Intervention. When administered intravenously as an antiadrenergic, the client should be in a supine position because the drug may cause severe and prolonged hypotension with fainting, tachycardia, and cardiac arrhythmias.

When phentolamine is used to prevent sloughing of tissue with administration of norepinephrine, 10 mg may be added to every liter of intravenous fluids containing norepinephrine without affecting its vasopressor effect. If extravasation has already occurred, 5 to 10 mg of phentolamine in 10 ml of 0.9% sodium chloride injection should be immediately infiltrated into the affected area. However, this treatment is ineffective if 12 or more hours have passed since the extravasation.

Education. After therapy, advise the client to rise slowly from bed and remain in sitting position for a few minutes before standing upright, to prevent orthostatic hypotension.

Evaluation. The client's blood pressure will be within normal limits. There will be an absence of tissue necrosis at the IV infusion site.

tolazoline [toe laz' a leen] (Priscoline)

Like phentolamine, tolazoline produces a moderately effective competitive alpha-adrenergic blocking action although tolazoline is considerably less potent. It acts as a vasodilator by a direct relaxant effect on vascular smooth muscle. It usually reduces pulmonary arterial pressure and peripheral vascular resistance.

The drug is used to treat persistent pulmonary hypertension in the newborn when systemic arterial levels of oxygen cannot be maintained by oxygen supplementation and/or mechanical ventilation machines.

Parenterally, the onset of action is within 1/2 hour of initial dose. Half-life in neonates is 3 to 10 hours. Tolazoline is excreted in the kidneys, mainly unchanged.

The side/adverse effects of tolazoline include GI bleeding, systemic alkalosis, hypotension, thrombocytopenia and oliguria or acute renal failure.

The parenteral dose for children is 1 to 2 mg/kg (IV) initially via a scalp vein over a 5 to 10 minute period. The maintenance dose is 0.2 mg/kg for each 1 mg/kg loading dose, by IV infusion. When arterial blood gases appear to be remaining stable, the drug may be gradually withdrawn.

■ Nursing Management

Tolazoline Therapy

Assessment. Tolazoline should not be used when systemic hypotension (systolic blood pressure less than 40 mm Hg) exists. Caution must be used when administering in the presence of acidosis (may increase pulmonary vasoconstriction) or mitral stenosis (drug may increase or decrease pulmonary artery pressure and total pulmonary resistance). Determine sensitivity to tolazoline.

If epinephrine or norepinephrine are used to treat a tolazoline overdose, a paradoxical hypotension effect followed by an exaggerated hypertensive response may occur. Avoid using epinephrine or norepinephrine with large amounts of tolazoline.

A baseline assessment should include the client's blood pressure, pulse, ECG, CBC, electrolytes, and blood gases. If long-term therapy is considered, renal function studies should be obtained.

Nursing diagnosis. Evaluate the client for the risk for injury related to the tolazoline's cardiovascular (systemic hypotension) and gastrointestinal (hemorrhage) effects. Altered comfort may occur due to the drug's adverse effects of nausea and vomiting, goose flesh, and flushing of the skin. Altered bowel elimination (diarrhea) may occur. The potential complications of acute renal failure, tachycardia and thrombocytopenia may occur.

Implementation

Monitoring. Monitor the client's response to the drug through ECG, blood gases, blood pressure, and pulse rates. Also observe CBCs, serum electrolyte levels, particularly sodium and potassium levels. Renal function studies are to be done periodically.

To monitor for gastrointestinal bleeding, perform a hematest of gastric aspirates. Monitor for pain in upper abdominal area, increased pulse, and coffee-ground emesis.

Intervention. This drug is administered only in pediatric or neonatal intensive care units where respiratory support is immediately available. Use an infusion pump or micro-drip regulator for administration to allow for precise flow regulation. Do not mix in a syringe or solution with other drugs. Pretreating the client with antacids may be necessary to prevent stress ulcers secondary to the increase in gastric secretion caused by the drug. Provide a warm environment for the infant to enhance the efficacy of the drug. Check the diluent carefully, use of diluents containing benzyl alcohol is not recommended for neonates and may lead to fatal toxic syndrome.

Evaluation. The client's arterial blood gases will be within the normal limits.

Ergot Alkaloids

Ergot is a fungus that grows on rye, and when it is hydrolyzed, many of its derivatives dissociate to yield lysergic acid diethylamide (LSD). These alkaloids have diverse and somewhat contradictory effects. Ergot alkaloids are partial agonists or antagonists at alpha-adrenergic receptors. The primary effect of the ergot alkaloids used to treat or prevent migraine and other vascular headaches is alpha-adrenergic blockade. Only ergoloid mesylates is not used to treat headaches; it is indicated as adjunct therapy to treat dementia symptoms (*USP DI*, 1996). Mechanism of action is reviewed later in this section. The following are examples of ergot preparations.

dihydroergotamine mesylate [dye hye droe er got' a meen] (D.H.E. 45)
ergoloid mesylates [er' goe loid mess' i lates] (Hydergine)
ergotamine tartrate [er got' a meen] (Ergomar, Gynergen ♣)
ergotamine tartrate and caffeine (Cafergot)
ergotamine tartrate inhalation (Medihaler Ergotamine)
ergotamine, belladonna alkaloids, and phenobarbital (Bellergal-S, Bellergal ♣)
methysergide maleate [meth i ser' jide] (Sansert)

The exact mechanism of action of ergoloid mesylates is unknown, but it may increase nerve cell metabolism which can result in improved oxygen uptake and cerebral metabolism. Thus lowered neurotransmitter levels may increase to normal. The other ergot alkaloids stimulate smooth muscle, especially of the blood vessels and the uterus, so they decrease the cerebral blood supply.

The early phase of a migraine attack is associated with constriction of the cranial blood vessels. It is characterized by visual symptoms and malaise and appears as a warning or "aura" of an oncoming attack. This is followed by the painful phase of a migraine headache that results in cranial vasodilation. The increase in blood flow in the vessels produces pulsations that appear to be the source of the pain. The ergot alkaloids act as alpha-adrenergic blocking agents and depress the central vasomotor center. They cause direct vasoconstriction of cranial blood vessels during the vasodilation phase, thereby reducing the pulsation thought to be responsible for the headache. These drugs also possess antiserotonin activity.

Abnormalities in serotonin metabolism may play a role in the migraine syndrome. Evidence exists that the drugs that act favorably in alleviating migraine influence on serotonin metabolism. Methysergide is a serotonin inhibitor and also acts as a potent vasoconstrictor. (See Chapter 39 for serotonin activity.) Ergotamine tartrate inhalation is used to abort or reduce a migraine attack, whereas ergotamine, belladonna alkaloids, and phenobarbital are used in combination to prevent vascular headaches. Some of these drugs are used for treatment of vascular headaches, such as migraine and cluster headaches. The drug (dihydroergotamine mesylate or ergotamine tartrate) must be given early in the attack; it does not prevent migraine attacks.

Dihydroergotamine is administered parenterally. The ergoloid mesylates and ergotamine tartrate (and its combinations without caffeine) are slowly and erratically absorbed from the GI tract. Caffeine is said to aid oral absorption. The aerosol dosage form, like methysergide, is well absorbed. Rectal suppositories of ergotamine tartrate (available in combination products) produce higher plasma concentrations than oral and may be used if other routes are ineffective.

The onset of action for dihydroergotamine mesylate IM/SC/IV is fairly rapid, 15 to 30 minutes after IM, within minutes after IV; half life is 1.4 to 15 hours; duration of action for IM dose is 3 to 4 hours; and is mainly excreted in the bile. Ergotamine tartrate and its combinations have onset of action within 1 to 2 hours; and half-life of about 2 hours. Methysergide maleate has an onset of action and duration of 24 to 48 hours; the half-life of ergoloid mesylates is 3.5 hours.

The ergot alkaloids are metabolized in the liver. Dihydroergotamine mesylate and methysergide maleate are both excreted in the kidney.

The side/adverse effects of ergot alkaloids include dizziness, nausea, vomiting, headache, diarrhea, pruritus, edema of lower extremities, and peripheral vasoconstriction or vasospasms (dose-related) which may result in cold hands or feet, leg weakness, pain in arms, legs, or lower back.

For information on dosage and administration, see Table 22-6.

■ Nursing Management

Ergot Alkaloids

Assessment. Do not use with clients with severe hypertension because it may be aggravated or those with unstable angina or recent myocardial infarction (drug-induced vasospasm may precipitate a recurrence). Clients with a history of CVA or transient ischemic attack (TIA) may be prone to recurrence as a result of increased blood pressure. Caution should also be used if the client has vascular surgery, cardiovascular or peripheral vascular disease (may increase ischemia), sepsis (more sensitive to effects of ergonovine), or hepatic (may result in ergot overdose) or renal disease. Elderly clients are also more at risk from the drug's vasospastic and hypothermic effects. Ergotamine is not recommended for use during pregnancy because of its oxytocic effects. It is contraindicated in clients who are breastfeeding because it inhibits lactation and may cause peripheral ischemia or nausea and vomiting in the infant.

When ergot alkaloids are given with other ergot alkaloids, vasopressors, or vasoconstrictors, the combination may result in increased vasoconstriction, ischemia, and possibly gangrene. Avoid this drug combination. Vasospasms have been reported when oral contraceptives (estrogen and progestin) were given concurrently with ergotamine tartrate and dihydroergotamine. With chronic use of the latter product, breakthrough bleeding and a decrease in contraceptive effectiveness have also been reported.

TABLE 22-6 Ergot alkaloids: dosage and administration

Alkaloid	Adult	Children
dihydroergotamine mesylate	IM: 1 mg at start of attack; repeat in an hr if necessary up to 3 mg maximum per day; 6 mg per week.	6 yrs and older, IM 0.5 mg at beginning of attack repeated in 1 hr if necessary.
	IV: 0.5 mg at beginning of attack given with an antiemetic. May repeat once in 1 hr if needed.	IV: 0.25 mg initially may repeat once in 1 hr if needed.
ergoloid mesylates	1-2 mg orally or sublingually, three times daily.	Not established.
ergotamine tartrate	Oral: 1-2 mg initially, repeat in ½ hr if needed. Maximum 6 mg/day; no more than twice a week that is at least 5 days apart.	Not established.
	Sublingual: 2 mg initially, repeat instructions as above (oral).	
	Aerosol: one inhalation at beginning of attack, repeat every 5 min if necessary, to maximum of 6 sprays/day.	
ergotamine tartrate and caffeine	Oral: 1-2 tablets at beginning of attack, repeat in 30/min intervals as needed, to maximum of 6 tablets/day. Limit to twice a week, at least 5 days apart.	6-12 yrs old-Oral: 1 tablet initially, repeat once or twice if necessary.
	Suppositories: one-fourth to one rectally initially; if necessary, a second may be inserted in 1 hr. Maximum: 2 suppositories per migraine attack, or 5 suppositories/1 week.	Not established.
methysergide	Oral: 4-6 mg daily in divided doses. Take with milk or after meals.	Not established.

Obtain a baseline assessment of the client's headaches; precipitating factors, aura, frequency, severity, and past efforts and success of relief.

A baseline assessment of blood pressure and ECG is essential. The examination of the extremities and palpation of peripheral pulses provides a baseline for older clients.

Nursing diagnosis. The client receiving ergot alkaloid therapy may experience the following selected nursing diagnoses: altered comfort related to the underlying vascular headache because of ineffectiveness of the drug or a developing tolerance to the drug, dizziness, or nausea; and risk for injury related to a decrease in peripheral sensation because of vasoconstriction (paleness, coolness, numbness, or tingling of fingers and toes). Fluid volume excess (edema) may occur. The potential complications of CNS toxicity, cardiovascular effects, and pleural or retroperitoneal fibrosis may also occur.

Implementation

Monitoring. Discuss with client the frequency and severity of headaches. Examine extremities and palpate peripheral pulses at monthly intervals to detect ischemia and edema as early as possible. Blood pressure and ECG monitoring is necessary with multiple dosing.

Intervention. Nonpharmacologic interventions for pain relief of migraine should be used to supplement the medication, such as a quiet environment, relaxation therapy, and other measures specific to the client. Because nausea and vomiting may be increased by the administration of ergotamine before relief of the headache occurs, phenothiazine antiemetics may be required to promote the comfort of the client. Safety measures should be taken to prevent injury to the client's extremities and they should be monitored for the ischemic effects of the drug.

Education. Tell client to take initial dose of drug during early part of migraine attack, during "aura" (visual field defects, scintillating scotomas, paresthesia, and nausea). The client then should lie down in a quiet, dark room for several hours. Assure the client that the quality of relief is related to the promptness with which the medication is started after the onset of symptoms.

Warn client to take drug exactly as prescribed. Prolonged use or overdose can cause circulatory impairment (ergot poisoning): numbness, tingling sensation, weakness, intermittent claudication, cyanosis of extremities, muscle pain, and coldness of extremities. Report symptoms immediately to prescriber. If not corrected, gangrene may develop. Severe peripheral vasoconstriction may be treated by administering intravenous sodium nitroprusside. Discontinuing the drug for 2 to 3 days may relieve these symptoms.

Instruct the client to avoid alcohol ingestion because it aggravates the headache. Counseling should be provided for smoking cessation since nicotine increases the peripheral vasoconstriction effects of the drug. For the same reason, clients should be instructed to avoid exposure to cold. Alert the client to the signs and symptoms of infection with the caution to report these to the prescriber as infection increases the sensitivity to the drug.

Instruct client how to monitor for fluid volume excess by checking for edema, taking daily weights, and maintaining low salt intake. Inform client of possible occurrence of hypotension. Position changes from recumbent to upright should be made slowly to avoid dizziness or fainting. Alert the client to the possible need to modify activities if dizziness and drowsiness occur as side effects.

Warn female clients of childbearing age not to use ergot alkaloids because of potential oxytocic effects during pregnancy. Clients with migraine may require assistance to identify physical and emotional stresses that cause migraine attack. Relaxation techniques, adequate rest, and avoidance of stressful situations may alleviate the severity or frequency of attacks.

Instruct the client in the proper method of taking sublingual tablets, including the avoidance of eating, drinking, and smoking until the tablet is completely dissolved. Correct use of inhaler should be advised. If suppositories are to be used and only half a dose required, instruct client to cut them in half lengthwise after refrigeration.

Evaluation. The client on ergot alkaloid therapy will experience diminished headaches, or will not experience headaches.

methysergide maleate [meth i ser' jide] (Sansert)
Although methysergide is not as potent a vasoconstrictor as ergotamine, the preceding nursing measures should be observed. Administer the oral dosage of methysergide with food to minimize gastrointestinal irritation.

Methysergide is not administered continuously for more than 6 months; a drug-free period of 3 to 4 weeks must occur before the drug is restarted. Advise client to withdraw drug gradually over 2 to 3 week period to prevent "headache rebound" resulting from abrupt drug withdrawal. If the drug does not provide a therapeutic response after a 3 week trial period, it is unlikely that longer administration will be of benefit.

Because there is a potential for serious side effects with methysergide, the client should be advised to report dyspnea and chest or abdominal pain and to keep clinical appointments so that blood count, sedimentation rate, renal function, pulmonary function, and cardiac status may be assessed. Regular examination must be performed by prescriber for possible development of fibrotic (formation of tissue) and vascular complications. Retroperitoneal fibrosis, as well as cardiac fibrosis, have been noted in a small number of individuals. Often these conditions regress when the drug is discontinued.

For further nursing management of methysergide, refer to ergot alkaloids.

sumatriptan [soo ma trip' tan] (Imitrex)
Sumatriptan is an antimigraine product that is believed to produce its effects at serotonin receptor subtype (5-HT_{1d}) selectively, which results in a binding and stimulation of these receptors located on cranial blood vessels. The receptors' response is constriction of blood vessels, and perhaps, cerebral blood vessel constriction that results in the reduction of pulsation associated with pain from vascular headaches (*USP DI,* 1996). Sumatriptan may also decrease mediators of inflammation that are somehow involved with serotonergic mechanisms. This product has no effect on other receptors in the body.

Pharmacokinetics. Sumatriptan is available in oral and parenteral dosage forms. Orally it is rapidly, although incompletely absorbed; has onset of action within ½ hour; reaches peak effect in 2 hours (in 50% to 75% of clients); is metabolized in liver and excreted renally. Parenterally, it is administered subcutaneously with an onset of action (relief of headache pain) within 10 minutes; reaches peak serum level within 1 hour; is metabolized in liver and excreted via the kidneys.

The side/adverse effects of sumatriptan include nausea, vomiting, dizziness, weakness, drowsiness and fatigue. As these symptoms also occur during and/or after a migraine headache, it is difficult to determine sumatriptan's contribution to these effects. Chest pain, difficulty swallowing, tightness in chest and/or neck may also occur. Several deaths have resulted 3 hours or more after its administration (strokes, cerebral hemorrhage) and it is not certain if they were due to underlying disease or directly related to sumatriptan. Individuals with migraines are at increased risk for cerebrovascular accidents or a transient ischemic attack and it has been postulated that maybe, a cerebrovascular attack rather than a migraine caused the symptoms that resulted in the administration of sumatriptan (*USP DI,* 1996).

The adult antimigraine oral dose is 100 mg. If the client responds to this dose, it may be repeated if the headache pain returns or increases in intensity. The maximum dosage is a 100 mg dose, 3 times in 24 hours. Parenterally, 6 mg SC is injected in outer thigh or outer upper arm. If the client responds to this dose in 1 to 2 hours, an additional dose may be given if the headache pain returns or increases.

▪ Nursing Management
Sumatriptan Therapy

Assessment. The client should be assessed for conditions for which sumatriptan would be contraindicated, such as sensitivity to the drug, and ischemic heart disease, Prinzmetal's angina, or uncontrolled hypertension (may worsen the condition). Sumatriptan is used cautiously in clients with a history of cardiovascular disease and potential for childbearing. The drug's safety has not been established for use during pregnancy, lactating clients, or children.

A baseline assessment should include a description of the aura, location, severity, duration, and any associated symptoms (nausea and vomiting, photophobia) that the client experiences during a migraine episode.

Nursing diagnosis. The client with sumatriptan therapy may experience the following nursing diagnoses/collaborative problems: pain related to migraine and the ineffectiveness of the drug; risk for injury related to dizziness and vertigo; fatigue; anxiety; impaired tissue integrity (site of injection); sensory/perceptual alterations (warm or cold sensations, tingling, burning, numbness); and the potential complications of coronary vasospasm, angina, and myocardial infarction (chest pain/pressure).

Implementation

Monitoring. If the client is receiving sumatriptan for the first time, monitor blood pressure before and for one hour following dose. If chest pain occurs, monitor with ECG for ischemic changes.

Intervention. Administer initial SC injection under observation in a health agency.

Education. Instruct the client on SC administration of the drug. Advise the client that any injection site redness or tenderness usually lasts an hour.

Instruct client that sumatriptan should only be used during a migraine episode; it will not prevent or reduce the number of migraines. It should be administered as soon as an migraine attack begins, but may be used at any time during an attack. A second injection may be used after an hour, if the first was ineffective, but no more than 2 injections may be used in a 24 hour period.

Sumatriptan tablets have a special coating to disguise an unpleasant taste; swallow them whole, do not break, crush, or chew them.

Advise the client that resting in a darkened room after taking the medication will also help to relieve the migraine. To prevent injury secondary to dizziness, caution the client against hazardous activities until the response to the drug has been determined. Advise female clients on contraception methods while they are on sumatriptan therapy.

If the client experiences chest pain or tightness with use, notify the prescriber before using sumatriptan again. If the pain is severe, notify the prescriber or other health care provider immediately. If the usual dose fails to relieve three consecutive headaches, notify the prescriber, and alternative therapy will be sought.

Evaluation. With sumatriptan, the client should experience relief from the migraine attack.

Beta-Adrenergic Blocking Agents

Beta blocking agents inhibit beta receptors by competing with the catecholamines at the receptor site. Beta-adrenergic blocking agents are differentiated into two subclasses: $beta_1$ and $beta_2$ blockers. Drugs that selectively inhibit only one type of receptor—$beta_1$ or $beta_2$—are called selective. $Beta_1$ selective blocking agents are frequently referred to as cardioselective blockers because these agents block the $beta_1$ receptors in the heart. Drugs that inhibit both types of receptors, $beta_1$ and $beta_2$ are referred to as nonselective beta-adrenergic blocking agents.

A further differentiation often identifies beta-adrenergic blocking agents that have intrinsic sympathomimetic activity (ISA). The ISA property was initially believed to be advantageous when compared with agents that only possess beta blocking effects. It was projected that fewer serious side effects would occur with such agents, but clinically, the significance of this property has not been proven. Intrinsic sympathomimetic activity causes partial stimulation of the beta-receptor although this effect is less than a pure agonist. For example, if the client has a slow heart rate at rest, the partial agonists may help to increase the heart rate by their partial agonist property. But if the person has a rapid heart rate or tachycardia from exercise, these agents may help to slow down the heart rate secondary to the predominate beta-blocking effect. It is believed the only role for the ISA property might be to treat clients that experience severe bradycardia from the non-ISA medications (Carter, Furmaga & Murphy, 1995). These drugs should also not be used to prevent myocardial infarction, because of their partial agonist properties.

Examples of adrenergic blocking drugs by classification include (Carter et al, 1995; Olin, 1996):

$Beta_1$ antagonist effects

1. Selective $beta_1$-adrenergic blocking agents (cardioselective) include atenolol (Tenormin), betaxolol (Kerlone), bisoprolol (Zebeta), esmolol (Brevibloc), and metoprolol (Lopressor).
2. Selective $beta_1$-adrenergic blocking agents with ISA effects include acebutolol (Sectral).

$Beta_1$ and $beta_2$ antagonist effects

3. Nonselective beta-adrenergic blocking agents include labetalol* (Normodyne), nadolol (Corgard), propranolol (Inderal), sotalol (Betapace) and timolol (Blocadren).
4. Nonselective beta-adrenergic blocking agents with ISA effects include carteolol (Cartrol), carvedilol* (Coreg), penbutolol (Levatol), and pindolol (Visken).

The prototype beta-adrenergic blocking drug is ▲ propranolol.

Mechanism of action. Beta-adrenergic blocking agents compete with beta-adrenergic agonists (e.g., catecholamines) for available beta receptor sites located on the membrane of cardiac muscle, smooth muscle of bronchi, and smooth muscle of blood vessels. Cardiac muscle contains $beta_1$ receptors while the smooth muscle sites contain primarily $beta_2$ receptors. Pharmacologically, the $beta_1$ adrenergic blocking action in the heart decreases heart rate, conduction velocity, myocardial contractility, and cardiac output.

The antiangina effects produced by the beta blockers are primarily caused by their ability to lower the myocardial oxygen requirements. Their antihypertensive actions are not specifically identified, but these effects may result from a decrease in cardiac output, a diminished sympathetic outflow from the vasomotor center in the brain to the peripheral blood vessels, and an inhibition of renin release by the

*Carvedilol also is an $alpha_1$ antagonist.

kidney. The result is a decrease in peripheral vascular resistance that lowers blood pressure.

To prevent a recurrence of a myocardial infarction, beta blockers (without ISA properties) are used for their antidysrhythmic effect plus their ability to decrease the myocardial oxygen demands on the heart. The latter effect may reduce the progression of ischemia and its severity on the heart.

Various mechanisms may be involved in the prevention of vascular headaches, such as, prevention of arterial vasodilation, inhibition of platelet aggregation, and increased oxygen release to tissues.

Indications. Used to treat chronic angina pectoris, hypertension, hypertrophic cardiomyopathy, tremors and anxiety; prevent and/or treat cardiac dysrhythmias, a second myocardial infarction and vascular headaches; as an adjunct to thyrotoxicosis and pheochromocytoma therapy and to treat mitral valve prolapse syndrome. Esmolol (Brevibloc) is a parenteral agent indicated for treatment of supraventricular tachycardia and noncompensatory sinus tachycardia.

For the pharmacokinetics and usual adult dose of the beta-adrenergic blocking agents, see Table 22-7. Propranolol, metoprolol, and penbutolol are highly lipid soluble, therefore they have a larger volume of distribution in the body, a greater first-pass liver metabolism, and also, a wider range of effective doses (individual variability) than the other agents. For example, the range for propranolol is 10 to 640 mg/day (see Table 22-7) as compared to a drug with a less-lipophilic (more water soluble) profile, such as atenolol (50 to 100 mg), betaxolol (10 to 20 mg), and others. The less-lipophilic agents are not as affected by liver metabolism and are excreted more unchanged by the kidneys, therefore requiring dosage adjustments in persons with renal impairment (Carter et al, 1995).

The side/adverse effects of beta-adrenergic drugs include drowsiness, weakness, trouble sleeping, anxiety, nasal congestion, abdominal distress, dizziness, bradycardia, nausea, vomiting, depression, cold hands and feet, and difficulty breathing (bronchospasm).

TABLE 22-7 Beta-adrenergic blocking agents: pharmacokinetics and adult dosing

Drug	Time to peak effect (hr)	Half-life (hr)	Metabolism/ excretion (%)*	Usual adult dose (range)
acebutolol (Sectral)	2.5-3.5	3-8	liver/renal (30-40) bile/feces	200 mg twice daily (600-1200 mg/day)
atenolol (Tenormin)	2-4	6-7	renal (85-100)	50 mg daily (50-100 mg/day)
betaxolol (Kerlone)	3-4	14-22	liver/renal (>80)	10 mg daily (10-20 mg/day)
bisoprolol (Zebeta)	N/A	9-12	liver/renal (50)	5 mg daily (2.5-20 mg/day)
carteolol (Cartrol)	1-3	6	liver/renal (60-70)	2.5 mg daily (2.5-10 mg/day)
carvedilol (Coreg)	N/A	7-10	liver renal (2) bile/feces	6.25 mg twice daily (6.25-50 mg/day)
labetalol (Normodyne)	PO: 2-4 IV: 5 min	6-8 5.5	liver/renal (55-60)	PO: 100 mg twice a day (400-1200 mg/day) IV: 20 mg intravenously
metoprolol (Lopressor)	PO: 1-2	3-7	liver/renal (3-10)	100 mg daily (50-450 mg/day)
nadolol (Corgard)	4	20-24	renal (70)	40 mg daily (40-240 mg/day)
penbutolol (Levatol)	1.5-3	5	liver/renal (90)	20 mg daily (10-40 mg/day)
pindolol (Visken)	1-2	3-4	liver/renal (40)	5 mg twice daily (5-45 mg/day in Canada; 60 mg/day in US)
propranolol (Inderal)	1-1.5	3-5	liver/renal (<1)	40 mg twice daily (10-640 mg/day)
sotalol (Betapace)	2-3	7-18	liver/renal (75)	80 mg twice daily (80-320 mg/day)
timolol (Blocadren)	1-2	4	liver/renal (20)	10 mg twice daily (10-60 mg/day)

*Percent excreted unchanged. Olin (1996); *USP DI* (1996).

Nursing Management

Beta-Adrenergic Blocking Drug Therapy

Assessment. The client's health status should be reviewed for preexisting health problems that might contraindicate the use of beta-adrenergic blocking agents or indicate a need for special precautions with the client. For pregnancy safety, see the box below.

The risk of decreasing myocardial contraction, thus increasing the risk of heart failure, must be considered when selecting a beta blocking agent. So such agents are contraindicated with clients with cardiac failure, cardiogenic shock, second or third degree heart block, and sinus bradycardia (<45 beats/min). Long-term use of beta-adrenergic blockers may aggravate congestive heart failure because of decreased cardiac output. If a beta blocking agent is necessary for a client with stabilized congestive heart failure, labetalol or drugs with ISA activity, such as pindolol, at low dosages may be the agents of choice.

Blockade of the $beta_2$ receptors of the bronchial smooth muscle leads to bronchoconstriction. This effect is particularly hazardous for individuals with a history of allergy, or asthma, bronchitis, and emphysema. There is less risk of inducing bronchospasm in these clients when a cardioselective beta blocker ($beta_1$ blocker) is used.

$Beta_2$-adrenergic blockade prevents the appearance of the warning signs and symptoms (sweating, increased heart rate, and anxiety) of acute hypoglycemia. Because these agents mask the appearance of the warning signs of hypoglycemia, they should be used with caution in individuals with diabetes mellitus who take insulin or hypoglycemic drugs. Labetalol and other selective $beta_1$-adrenergic blockers generally, do not potentiate insulin-induced hypoglycemia.

Pregnancy Safety

Category	Drug
B	acebutolol, pindolol
C	amrinone, betaxolol, bisoprolol, carteolol, dopamine, ephedrine, epinephrine, isoproterenol, labetalol, mephentermine, metaraminol, metoprolol, nadolol, norepinephrine, penbutolol, phenoxybenzamine, phenylephrine, propanolol, timolol, tolazoline
X	ergotamine tartrate
Unclassified	dihydroergotamine,* dobutamine, ergoloid mesylates, methysergide, phentolamine

*Not recommended.

Because these drugs may mask clinical signs of hyperthyroidism (e.g., tachycardia), they give a false impression of improvement of hyperthyroidism. Abrupt withdrawal of the drug will exacerbate symptoms of hyperthyroidism, and therefore therapy should be discontinued gradually.

Exacerbation of depression has been reported in clients with depression or with a history of depression; they should be closely monitored if taking a beta blocking agent.

The client's current medication regimen is to be reviewed for significant drug interactions. The following interactions are possible when beta-adrenergic blocking agents are given with the drugs listed below:

Drug	Possible effect and management
allergen immunotherapy or allergic extracts for skin testing	**Use of these agents place client at risk for serious systemic reaction; another drug should be substituted for the beta-adrenergic blocking agent. Avoid or a potentially serious drug interaction may occur.**
antidiabetic agents, oral hypoglycemic agents or insulin	May cause hyperglycemia or hypoglycemia. Symptoms of hypoglycemia, such as increased heart rate and decreased blood pressure, may be blocked, thus making it difficult to monitor. Monitoring of blood glucose levels and dosage adjustments of the hypoglycemic agent may be necessary.
calcium channel blocking agents, clonidine (Catapres), or guanabenz (Wytensin)	May result in potentiated antihypertensive effects; monitor BP closely. If therapy with a beta-adrenergic blocking agent, clonidine, or guanabenz is to be discontinued, taper the dose of the beta blocker gradually over several days. When it is discontinued, the clonidine or guanabenz may then be tapered and discontinued also over several days. Closely monitor blood pressure throughout this procedure. Use caution when high doses of calcium blocking agents are given concurrently with a beta-adrenergic blocking agent. Nifedipine (Procardia, Adalat) may, in some instances, result in excessive hypotension in clients receiving concurrent therapy.
cocaine	May reduce or cancel the effects of the beta-adrenergic blocking agents. Also, while beta blocking agents are used to treat symptoms induced by cocaine (i.e., increased heart rate, cardiac arrhythmias, etc.), an increased risk of inducing hypertension, severe bradycardia, and heart block can occur. If a beta blocker is necessary, labetalol may present less risk than the other beta-adrenergic blocking agents (because of its alpha-adrenergic blocking effect).
monoamine oxidase (MAO) inhibitors	**This combination is not to be used; severe hypertension may result, even up to 14 days after the MAO inhibitor is discontinued. Avoid or a potentially serious drug interaction may occur.**

Continued

Drug	Possible effect and management
monoamine oxidase (MAO) inhibitors—cont'd	**The effects of both drugs may be reduced or blocked (sympathomimetics with beta activity). In sympathomimetics with both alpha and beta activity, beta blockade may result in increased alpha effects; i.e., hypertension, severe bradycardia, and possibly heart block. Avoid or a potentially serious drug interaction may occur.**
sympathomimetics	Labetalol may be used if combination therapy is necessary because it has alpha blocking effects. In sympathomimetic drugs with beta-adrenergic activity, the beta blocking agent may cancel the $beta_1$ cardiac activity of dopamine or dobutamine; or the $beta_2$ bronchodilating effects of isoproterenol, metaproterenol.
xanthines (aminophylline or theophylline)	Therapeutic response of both drugs may be reduced or blocked. May also result in theophylline accumulation in the body. Monitor vital signs closely when this drug combination is prescribed.

Obtain a baseline assessment of the client's underlying condition for which the beta-adrenergic blocking agent is being prescribed. This may include pulse, blood pressure, ECG, and other cardiac functioning determinations.

Nursing diagnosis. The client receiving beta-adrenergic blocking agents may experience the following nursing diagnoses: altered thought processes (depression); sexual dysfunction (decreased sexual ability); risk for injury related to dizziness; ineffective airway clearance (bronchospasm); disturbed sleep pattern (insomnia, drowsiness); activity intolerance related to lethargy and weakness; and the potential complication of altered cardiac output (bradycardia, arrhythmias, congestive heart failure).

Implementation

Monitoring. Always check the apical pulse rate before administering the drug. If it is slower than 60 beats/minute or rate is irregular, hold drug and call prescriber immediately. Also check and report significant variations in blood pressure. Low parameters indicate overdosage.

Because of the potential for altered cardiac output and ineffective airway clearance related to the blockade of cardiac and bronchial beta-adrenergic receptors, when these agents are administered intravenously, monitor ECG, blood pressure, and pulmonary wedge pressure. Have available atropine (for bradycardia), vasopressors (for hypotension), and bronchodilators (for bronchoconstriction). Institute oral therapy as soon as tolerated to reduce the risk of decreased cardiac output. Report to the prescriber a considerable slowing of the pulse rate however the drug is administered. Beta blocking action can result in cardiac standstill.

Monitor closely hypertensive individuals who have congestive heart failure that is controlled by digitalis and diuretics. The effects of digitalis and beta blockers are additive in depressing AV conduction. Discontinue therapy if cardiac failure continues with digitalis administration. Cardiac failure may be precipitated because of drug-depressed myocardial contractility. Evaluate the effectiveness of drug therapy by assessing the frequency of anginal attacks and activity tolerance. When the drug is used as an antihypertensive, a reduction in blood pressure will indicate effectiveness.

To monitor for potential/actual fluid volume excess, measure intake and output and weigh client daily. Fluid retention may cause dyspnea, orthopnea, nocturnal cough, pulmonary rales, distended neck veins, and edema, which are all signs of impending heart failure. Report weight gain and other such symptoms to the prescriber.

Observe client for possible signs of thyrotoxicosis, since the drug may mask clinical signs of hyperthyroidism. In individuals with renal and hepatic impairment, monitor for signs of excessive drug accumulation.

Monitor for adherence to the therapeutic regimen; noncompliance may be an issue related to sexual dysfunction, fatigue, and/or depression.

Intervention. To minimize variations in absorption, be consistent in administering oral beta blocking agents with regard to taking them with food or on an empty stomach. Although the manufacturer recommends giving the drug before meals and at bedtime, there is disagreement about whether food enhances or delays bioavailability.

Notify anesthesiologist if client is scheduled for surgery and is receiving a beta blocker; because caution should be used if a hydrocarbon anesthetic, such as halothane, is to be administered. Note that the drug must be withdrawn slowly (see Box 22-4). Otherwise the client will suffer from abrupt withdrawal syndrome: tremors, sweating, severe headache, malaise, palpitation, rebound hypertension, life-threatening dysrhythmias, myocardial infarction (in clients with cardiac problems and angina pectoris), and hyperthyroidism in clients with thyrotoxicosis. If drug is to be discontinued, reduce dosage over a 1 to 2 week period. It may be recommended that the drug be withdrawn well before surgery. In individuals with pheochromocytoma, the drug is usually not discontinued before surgery.

For administration of labetalol, the client should be in a supine position during injection and for 3 hours afterward. Increase client's activity and move client to an upright position gradually.

BOX 22-4

Withdrawal of a Beta Blocking Agent

Withdraw beta-adrenergic blocking agents slowly by tapering or lowering the dose over approximately 14 days.

Advise client to avoid vigorous physical exercises or activity during this time to decrease the risk of a reinfarction or cardiac dysrhythmia.

If withdrawal signs occur (angina or chest pain, sweating, tachycardia, respiratory distress), temporarily reinstitute the beta blocking agent to stabilize the client; then slowly lower the dose with close supervision.

Education. Instruct the client to take his or her own pulse rate before each dose; also, withhold medication and inform the prescriber if pulse rate drops below 60 beats/min.

Counsel client not to alter the drug regimen established by prescriber. The drug controls hypertension, but does not cure, so lifetime compliance is necessary. Medication should be taken even if the client feels well, and the client should always have an adequate supply of drug available so that strict compliance is observed. Advise the client of the hazards of untreated hypertension. Emphasize the importance of keeping appointments for periodic laboratory tests.

Advise the client to carry medical identification to alert health professionals in an emergency situation that a beta blocker is being taken.

Caution the client not to take OTC medications, especially decongestants and cough and cold medications, but to consult with the health care provider.

While the drug is being withdrawn, advise the client to avoid physical exertion to reduce the risk of myocardial infarction and/or dysrhythmias. Instruct client to restrict sodium intake to prevent unnecessary fluid retention. Caution client to avoid cold temperatures because there is an increased sensitivity to cold. Painful, cold, and tender hands and feet are a sign of impaired circulation. Take peripheral pulse to monitor decrease in peripheral circulation.

Advise hypertensive clients to make position changes slowly to prevent lightheadedness and dizziness. Alcohol ingestion, standing still for long periods, exercise, and hot weather enhance the orthostatic hypotensive effects of the drug. If the problem continues to exist, notify prescriber. Drowsiness and dizziness are common side effects, so caution client about operating a car or hazardous equipment.

In angina pectoris, exercise tolerance should increase and pain should be reduced with the drug. Caution client to avoid overexertion because he or she has less pain. Instruct client to inform prescriber if adequate relief is not obtained from the drug.

Instruct client to monitor weight and to report to prescriber the possible signs of congestive heart failure: weight gain of 3 to 4 pounds a day, dyspnea, cough, fatigue, rapid pulse, and anxiety. (Weight gain of 1 pound represents approximately 500 ml of retained fluid; 4 pounds of weight gain represents about a half gallon of retained fluids.)

Alert clients with diabetes that these drugs mask the signs and symptoms of hypoglycemia, may prolong hypoglycemia, or may cause increased levels of blood glucose.

Evaluation. The client will experience an absence of signs and symptoms of the underlying condition without adverse effects of the drug. If the drug is given for hypertension, the blood pressure will be within normal limits; for arrhythmias, there will be a normal sinus rhythm on the ECG.

SUMMARY

Because of the sympathetic nervous system's ability to produce generalized physiologic responses, drugs that act on the system may affect a wide range of body functions. These agents are described as either adrenergic (sympathomimetic) drugs—those that mimic the effects of sympathetic nerve stimulation—or adrenergic blocking (sympatholytic) drugs—those that compete with the catecholamines at receptor sites and inhibit adrenergic sympathetic stimulation. The adrenergic drugs may be direct-acting, indirect-acting, or dual-acting (direct and indirect) agents. Knowledge of these agents is essential, since many of them are used to rectify life-threatening situations when the nurse must act quickly to provide the necessary pharmacologic intervention. Other drugs that act on the sympathetic nervous system are used quite commonly in practice for a wide range of clients.

The adrenergic direct-acting drugs, catecholamines, interact with and stimulate adrenergic effector cells, which are alpha and beta receptors. Alpha-adrenergic activity includes vasoconstriction of arterioles in the skin and splanchnic area, which increases blood pressure, pupil dilation, and relaxation of the gut. Beta-adrenergic activity includes cardiac acceleration and increased contractility; vasodilation of arterioles of skeletal muscles; bronchial relaxation; and uterine relaxation. Beta receptors can be either beta$_1$ receptors, located mainly in the heart, or beta$_2$ receptors within the bronchioles and arterial smooth muscle. Understanding the placement of these receptor cells assists the nurse in conceptualizing the activities of the various drugs that affect the sympathetic nervous system.

Epinephrine is a direct-acting catecholamine that stimulates alpha, beta$_1$, and beta$_2$ receptors. It is considered to be the classic or standard drug of this classification because of its long history of use for symptomatic treatment of asthma, emergency treatment of anaphylactic shock and cardiac arrest, local hemostasis, and management of simple open-angle glaucoma. Isoproterenol is a nonselective beta-adrenergic drug.

Norepinephrine, on the other hand, has a high affinity for alpha receptors. Dobutamine is valuable for individuals with low cardiac output because it directly stimulates the beta$_1$-adrenergic receptors of the heart. Dopamine acts mainly to cause vasodilation of the renal and mesenteric arteries. All of these drugs are used for the treatment of circulatory shock.

The indirect-acting adrenergic agents act indirectly on receptors by triggering the release of epinephrine and norepinephrine from their storage sites, which then stimulate alpha and beta receptors. Dual-acting adrenergic agents have both indirect and direct effects. Ephedrine has both a direct and an indirect sympathomimetic action and is used more commonly for bronchodilation for milder forms of asthma and as a nasal decongestant. Phenylephrine is also commonly found in many combination cough-cold, antihistamine and decongestant, and ophthalmic preparations. Mephentermine sulfate and metaraminol, as dual-acting adrenergic agents, are used primarily for their vasopressor effects with hypotensive clients.

The adrenergic blocking, or sympatholytic, drugs are also classified by alpha and beta receptors, and by their ability to inhibit adrenergic sympathetic nervous stimulation at these sites. There are noncompetitive, long-acting antagonists, such as phenoxybenzamine, which is used mainly for vasodilation and inhibition of vasospasm; competitive, short-acting antagonists, such as phentolamine, used locally to reverse the action of an extravasation of vasoconstricting drugs, and tolazoline, which is indicated for pulmonary hypertension in the newborn; and the ergot alkaloids, which are used for the management of vascular headaches.

The beta-adrenergic blocking agents are differentiated into selective $beta_1$-adrenergic blocking agents, such as atenolol and metoprolol, which decrease heart rate, conduction velocity, myocardial contractility, and cardiac output; and the nonselective beta-adrenergic blocking agents such as carteolol, penbutolol, pindolol, propranolol, and timolol. The nonselective beta-adrenergic blocking agents affect cardiac muscle and smooth muscle of the bronchi and blood vessels but are used primarily to treat chronic angina, hypertension, and cardiac dysrhythmias and to prevent a second myocardial infarction, vascular headaches, and cardiac dysrhythmias.

Being knowledgeable about drugs affecting the sympathetic nervous system is essential for all areas of nursing practice.

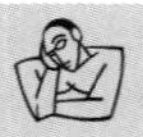

Critical Thinking

1. Sean Murphy is admitted to the emergency department with a massive myocardial infarction. His blood pressure has dropped to 80/40 mm Hg, his pulse has increased to 128/min, and his skin is cool and moist. The physician indicates that Mr. Murphy is in cardiogenic shock and orders an infusion of dopamine, 10 μg/kg/min. How will this dose affect adrenergic receptors? What would you expect to occur as the result of Mr. Murphy receiving this infusion? What monitoring by the nurse should take place? What action should the nurse take if the infusion infiltrates?
2. Mrs. Melanie Freedman is 43 years old and has a history of migraine headaches. She has tried a number of therapies without success. Ergotamine tartrate (Ergomar) has now been prescribed for her. Mrs. Freedman calls the clinic and indicates that she has vomited each time she has taken the drug. How should the nurse respond to Mrs. Freedman's comment?
3. Dr. Harry Lewis, a 56-year-old university professor, has been admitted to the hospital with atrial tachycardia. He has been started on propranolol (Inderal), 30 mg qid. What nursing interventions will you take because Dr. Lewis also has diabetes mellitus?

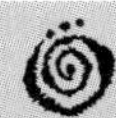

Collaborative Learning Activities

1. Two teams of students will design a teaching plan for a client with a newly prescribed epinephrine inhaler and a client prescribed a beta-adrenergic blocking agent. The teams will role play an instructional session with the client.

BIBLIOGRAPHY

American Hospital Formulary Service (1996). *AHFS drug information '96*. Betheseda, MD: American Society of Hospital Pharmacists.

American Medical Association (1995). *Drug evaluations: Annual 1995*. Chicago: The Association.

Anderson KN, et al. (Eds.) (1994). *Mosby's medical, nursing & allied health dictionary* (4th ed.). St Louis: Mosby.

Brown KK (1993). Boosting the failing heart with inotropic drugs, *Nursing* 23 (4):34.

Carter BL, Furmaga EM, & Murphy CH (1995). Essential hypertension. In Young LY & Koda-Kimble MA (Eds.). *Applied therapeutics* (6th ed.). Vancouver, WA: Applied Therapeutics.

Clark BK (1992). Beta-adrenergic blocking agents: Their current status, *AACN* 3(2):447.

Clements JV (1992). Sympathomimetics, inotropics, and vasodilators, *AACN* 3(2):393.

Fitzgerald M (1995). Pharmacologic highlights: The beta-2 agonists, *J Amer Acad Nurse Pract* 7(6):304-7.

Hardman JG & Limbird LE (Eds.) (1996). *Goodman and Gilman's the pharmacological basis of therapeutics* (9th ed.). New York: McGraw Hill.

Jackson G (1993). The management of stable angina, *Hosp Pract* 28(1):59.

Katzung BG (1992). *Basic and clinical pharmacology* (5th ed.). Norwalk: Appleton & Lange.

Long K, et al. (1994). Treating benign prostatic hyperplasia with medications, *Nurse Pract Forum* 5(3):126-7.

Olin BR (Ed.) (1996-1997). *Facts and comparisons*. St Louis: Facts and Comparisons.

Sterling LP (1995). Beta adrenergic agonists, *AACN Clin Issues Adv Pract Acute Crit Care* 6(2): 271-8.

United States Pharmacopeial Convention (1996). *Drug information for the health care professional* (16th ed.). Rockville, MD: The Convention.

Chapter 23

Drugs for Specific CNS-Peripheral Dysfunctions

Chapter Focus

Parkinson's disease, myasthenia gravis, dementia, Alzheimer's disease, and skeletal muscle relaxants are discussed in this chapter. CNS-peripheral dysfunctions are often progressive and incapacitating. Therefore appropriate assessment, intervention, and evaluation are important measures for nursing. The following objectives and key terms are important for a good understanding of this chapter.

Key Terms

akinesia (p. 455)
Alzheimer's disease (p. 468)
anticholinergic drug (p. 455)
anticholinesterase agent (p. 464)
dementia (p. 468)
designer drugs (p. 454)
dystonia (p. 470)
myasthenia gravis (p. 464)
on-off syndrome (p. 459)
Parkinson's disease (p. 454)
spasms (p. 470)
spasticity (p. 470)

Key Drugs [▲]

baclofen
benztropine
levodopa
selegiline
tacrine

Objectives

1. Explain the neurotransmitter balance theory in Parkinson's disease.
2. Name the two neurotransmitters that centrally affect motor function and balance.
3. Discuss medications used to treat Parkinson's disease, myasthenia gravis, dementia, Alzheimer's disease, and muscle spasm/spasticity.
4. Describe the physiology of muscle movement and motor nerve response.
5. Compare the manifestations of the two primary types of muscle spasticity.
6. Compare the action of central-acting and direct-acting skeletal muscle relaxants.
7. Summarize the drug interactions associated with skeletal muscle relaxants.
8. Implement nursing management of drug therapy prescribed for the treatment of Parkinson's disease, myasthenia gravis, dementia, Alzheimer's disease, and muscle spasm/spasticity.

The personal tragedy of the progressive nature of Parkinson's disease, myasthenia gravis, dementia, and Alzheimer's disease, the emotional distress of the family members, and the increasing cost of care to society all challenge health care providers to develop and manage rational pharmacologic treatments. Because there are no "cures" at present, drug therapy attempts to minimize the symptoms of these conditions.

Skeletal muscle spasticity can also be debilitating, but these muscles are affected by many pharmacologic substances. Their effects may be at the neuromuscular junction or at different levels in the central nervous system, i.e., at the brain or the spinal cord. These agents are also discussed in this chapter.

PARKINSON'S DISEASE

Parkinson's disease is a progressively debilitating disorder of the CNS characterized by resting tremor, forward flexion of the trunk, and muscle rigidity and weakness. It occurs usually between the ages of 50 to 80, affecting both sexes equally. Approximately 1% of the American population or 1 million persons currently have Parkinson's disease (Flaherty & Gidal, 1995). While the cause is unknown, genetic factors, viral influences, and environmental contaminants have been suspected. The disease is caused by a disorder of the extrapyramidal system in the brain, especially the basal ganglia area. Degeneration of the dopamine-producing neurons in this area produces a dopamine/acetylcholine imbalance, a progressive loss of dopamine (inhibitory neurotransmitter), and an increase in acetylcholine (excitatory neurotransmitter). It has also been induced by designer drugs (Box 23-1). The correct balance of dopamine and acetylcholine is important in regulating posture, muscle tone, and voluntary movement (Figure 23-1). Other neurotransmitters such as norepinephrine and serotonin are also decreased in the brain of a person with Parkinson's disease.

The central nervous system has two major types of dopamine receptors, D_1 and D_2 receptors. The D_1 receptor role is not currently known but D_2 and especially D_{2A} receptors are involved with the effects of levodopa and the other dopamine agonists (Flaherty & Gidal, 1995). The use of drug therapy is aimed at correcting this dopamine/acetylcholine imbalance by increasing dopamine levels and blocking acetylcholine levels. The classes of drugs used in treatment are: (1) drugs with central anticholinergic activity (anticholinergics and antihistamines) and (2) drugs that affect brain dopamine levels to enhance dopaminergic mechanisms.

BOX 23-1

Parkinson's Disease Induced by Designer Drugs

Designer drugs, or chemical variations of illegal or controlled substances, are an ever-increasing problem in North America. Such products are usually not illegal but generally are produced to induce the psychoactive effects of selected illegal products. Often the user consumes an unknown substance that may or may not be the desired product. Reports indicate that MPTP, a chemical produced as an analog of meperidine in clandestine laboratories, has been sold on the streets as heroin, cocaine, or a contaminant of other products.

MPTP has reportedly induced a degenerative CNS disorder characterized by tremors and muscle paralysis similar to the symptoms of Parkinson's disease. In a number of cases the paralysis reported has been permanent.

Drugs with Central Anticholinergic Activity

Symptoms of Parkinson's disease caused by an excess of cholinergic activity are muscle rigidity and muscle tremor. The muscle rigidity or increased tone appears as "ratchet resistance," or "cogwheel rigidity," wherein the affected muscle moves easily, then meets resistance or remains fixed in the new position. The muscle tremors appear to have a "to-and-fro" movement caused by the sequence of contractions of agonistic and antagonistic muscles involved. The tremors are usually worse at rest and are commonly manifested as a "pill-rolling" motion of the hands and a bobbing of the head. Anticholinergics are more

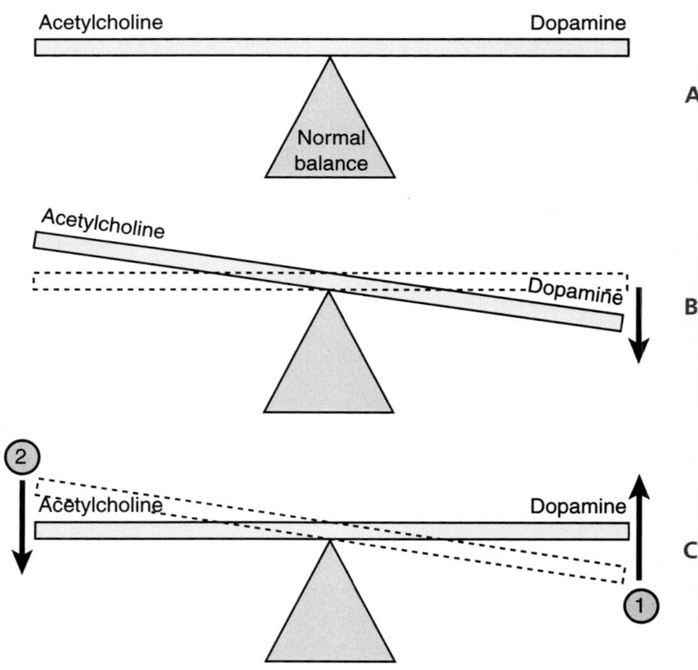

Figure 23-1 Central acetylcholine/dopamine balance. **A,** Normal "balance" of acetylcholine and dopamine. **B,** In Parkinson's disease, a *decrease* in dopamine results in an acetylcholine/dopamine imbalance. **C,** Drug therapy in Parkinson's disease aims at increasing the dopamine level, which restores the acetylcholine/dopamine balance toward normal by (1) increasing the supply of dopamine or (2) blocking or lowering acetylcholine levels.

useful early in the course of this disease because the dopamine depletion side effects are not prominent at this stage.

Various drugs with central anticholinergic activity are used to treat Parkinson's disease, such as benztropine (Cogentin), trihexyphenidyl (Artane), and diphenhydramine (Benadryl). These agents are used in the treatment of mild Parkinson's disease and as an adjunct to dopamine replacement.

Anticholinergic Agents

Drugs that inhibit or block the effects of acetylcholine are referred to as **anticholinergic drugs**. The belladonna alkaloids, atropine and scopolamine, were the first centrally active (i.e., crossing the blood-brain barrier) anticholinergic agents used to treat Parkinsonism and for many years were the only drugs available for such treatment. These drugs have been supplanted by synthetic anticholinergics, which were developed in an effort to produce drugs as effective as the belladonna drugs but with fewer side effects.

The anticholinergics that readily cross the blood-brain barrier can produce some improvement in functional capacity. The usefulness of these drugs is limited because of their side effects and their tendency to be less effective with continued use. Some anticholinergics are also used to control extrapyramidal reactions, such as rigidity, **akinesia** (difficulty in or lack of ability to initiate muscle movement), tremor, and akathisia, which are caused by antipsychotic drugs such as the phenothiazines.

Anticholinergic drugs block central cholinergic excitatory pathways, returning the dopamine/acetylcholine balance in the brain (especially in the basal ganglia) to normal. The effects of the anticholinergic agents include decreased salivation and relaxation of smooth muscle with a decrease in tremors. Decreased rigidity and akinesia (in nearly 50% of the clients) are also reported.

Anticholinergic agents are indicated for use as antidyskinetics, for treatment of Parkinson's disease, and for treatment of drug-induced extrapyramidal reactions. These drugs are very well absorbed and the onset of action for specific drugs is as follows: benztropine oral, 1 to 2 hours; benztropine IM/IV within minutes; biperiden IM within 10 to 30 minutes, IV within minutes; and trihexyphenidyl oral, 1 hour. For onset of action for diphenhydramine, see the section on antihistamines in Chapter 38. Duration of effect for specific agents is as follows: benztropine (Cogentin) oral, IM, or IV, 24 hours; biperiden (Akineton) IV, 1 to 8 hours; procyclidine (Kemadrin, Procyclid) oral, 4 hours; and trihexyphenidyl (Artane) oral, 6 to 12 hours. Metabolism of the anticholinergics is undetermined. They are most likely excreted by the kidneys.

The side/adverse effects of anticholinergic drugs include blurred vision, mydriasis, constipation, dry skin, anhidrosis, urinary hesitancy, pain on urination, nausea, vomiting, photophobia, drowsiness, xerostomia, and dysphagia. Table 23-1 lists dosage and administration information.

■ Nursing Management

Anticholinergic Therapy

Assessment. The nurse should note that clients who display an intolerance for one belladonna alkaloid or derivative may also respond similarly to other belladonna alkaloids or derivatives. Anticholinergics are contraindicated in breastfeeding clients because they inhibit lactation, and also in children younger than 3 years because they are very susceptible to the toxic effects of these drugs (see Pediatric Implications box on p. 456). Elderly clients are also at risk for the development of health problems, such as dryness of the mouth, constipation, and urinary retention, particularly in males, caused by the anticholinergic effects of these agents (see Geriatric Implications box on p. 456).

TABLE 23-1 Anticholinergic drugs: dosage and administration

Drug	Adults*	Children
▲ benztropine (Apo-benztropine ♣, Cogentin)	PD: 1-2 mg PO, IM, or IV daily, adjusted as necessary. DIE: 1-4 mg PO, IM, or IV once or twice daily, maximum 6 mg/day.	Less than 3 yr, not recommended 3 yr and older, individualize dose
biperiden (Akineton)	PD: 2 mg PO 3-4 times/day; or 2 mg IM or slow IV, which may be repeated at ½ hr intervals to maximum of 4 doses/day.	Not established DIE: 0.4 mg/kg IM
procyclidine (Kemadrin, Procyclid ♣)	PD or DIE: 2.5 mg PO 3 times daily after meals, increased gradually as needed.	Not established
trihexyphenidyl (Artane),	PD: 1-2 mg PO day 1, increased by 2 mg at 3-5 day intervals as necessary. Usual dose is 6-10 mg in divided doses. Extended release capsules are available, 5 mg after breakfast, adjusted as necessary. DIE: 1 mg PO initially daily, increased as necessary. Usual dose is 5-15 mg.	Not established

PD, Parkinson's disease; *DIE*, drug-induced extrapyramidal reactions.
*Elderly clients usually require lower dosages as they are more sensitive to these medications.

Pediatric Implications

Anticholinergics

Infants and young children are very susceptible to anticholinergic side/adverse effects.

Closely monitor pediatric clients with spastic paralysis or brain damage, since they generally have an increased reaction to these agents, thus requiring a dosage reduction.

Anticholinergics, especially high doses, may cause a paradoxical type reaction of increased nervousness, confusion, and hyperexcitability.

Children receiving these agents where hot weather prevails or environmental temperatures are high have an increased risk of developing a rapid body temperature increase (anticholinergic drugs suppress sweat gland activity).

Dosage adjustments are often necessary for infants, clients with Down's syndrome, and blonds since they generally have an increased response to this drug category. Flushing, increased temperature, irritability, and increased pulse and respiratory rate may occur.

Start with low doses and increase gradually, as needed and tolerated.

Geriatric Implications

Anticholinergics

The elderly are highly susceptible to anticholinergic side effects especially constipation, dry mouth, and urinary retention (usually in males).

Avoid use of these agents in clients with narrow-angle glaucoma or a history of urinary retention.

Memory impairment has been reported with continuous administration of these agents, especially in older clients.

When usual adult doses are administered, some elderly may have a paradoxical reaction: hyperexcitability, agitation, confusion, and sedation.

Chronic use decreases or inhibits the flow of saliva, which may contribute to oral discomfort, periodontal disease, and candidiasis.

Overheating resulting in heat stroke has been reported in persons receiving anticholinergic drugs during vigorous exercise or periods of hot weather.

Blurred vision and/or increased sensitivity to light may occur.

Anticholinergic dosing in the elderly should begin at the lowest dose with gradual increases until maximum improvement is noted or intolerable side effects occur.

Geriatric clients may respond to usual doses with agitation, sleepiness, and altered thought processes. Because the anticholinergics block the actions of acetylcholine, which supports many functions of the brain including memory, elderly clients, particularly those with existing memory problems, may become more impaired with continued use of anticholinergics. Caution should be exercised with the use of anticholinergics in individuals over the age of 40 because of the possibility of precipitating undiagnosed glaucoma.

The anticholinergic activity that decreases tone and motility of the gastrointestinal tract necessitates caution in the use of these drugs in instances of reflux esophagitis, hiatal hernia, intestinal atony, paralytic ileus, pyloric obstruction, or ulcerative colitis. In addition, clients with or who have a predisposition to prostatic hypertrophy, urinary retention, or other obstructive uropathy may find the condition precipitated or exacerbated. Because the heart rate may be increased, it should be carefully considered before anticholinergics are administered to clients with preexisting tachycardia or other cardiac conditions such as arrhythmias, congestive heart failure, coronary heart disease, and mitral stenosis, in whom such an increase would be undesirable. The mydriatic effect of these drugs increases intraocular pressure, which may precipitate an acute episode of angle-closure glaucoma or necessitate an adjustment in the therapy of clients with open-angle glaucoma.

The client's current medication regimen should be reviewed to detect any significant drug interactions. The following effects may occur when anticholinergics are given with the drugs listed below:

Drug	Possible effect and management
alcohol and CNS depressant	May result in enhanced CNS depressant effects. Monitor closely for hypoventilation, sedation, confusion, and ataxia.
antacids	Concurrent administration may reduce absorption and therapeutic effects of anticholinergic agents. Separate administration of antacids and anticholinergics by at least 1 to 2 hours.
anticholinergic or other antimuscarinic* medications	May result in enhanced anticholinergic effects. Monitor for constipation because bowel impaction and/or paralytic ileus may be produced. Increased fluid intake, exercise, stool softeners, and/or laxatives may be necessary.
ketoconazole (Nizoral)	Anticholinergics may increase GI pH resulting in a marked reduction in the absorption of ketoconazole. Clients should be advised to take the drugs 2 hours apart.

*Drugs that block cholinergic receptors at postganglionic parasympathetic synapses and a small number of postganglionic sympathetic synapses (atropine, scopolamine) (see Chapter 21).

A baseline assessment should include the client's mobility status and other symptoms related to the underlying disease for which the anticholinergic agent is being prescribed. Intraocular pressure should be measured for those clients at risk for glaucoma.

Nursing diagnosis. Once the client begins anticholinergic therapy, assessment should relate to the potential development of a number of nursing diagnoses/collaborative problems related to the drug. There may be sensory-perceptual alterations related to the drug's effects on vision and somatosensory function, especially in the elderly. Geriatric clients are also more at risk for altered thought processes (confusion) and are at risk for injury related to the CNS effects. There may be alteration in elimination patterns: bowel function (constipation), because of the GI effects, and altered patterns of urinary elimination, primarily resulting from urinary retention. Comfort may be altered related to xerostomia, blurred vision, rash, and the GI and GU effects of anticholinergics. Potential complications might be decreased cardiac output (dysrhythmias), paralytic ileus, and increased intraocular pressure.

Implementation

Monitoring. The vital signs should be monitored and changes in the cardiac status should be observed and reported. Dysrhythmias have been noted as a result of these drugs, but they are dose related.

In clients with bladder neck obstruction, urinary retention may occur. Male clients, in particular, should be monitored for difficulty in starting their urinary stream. The nurse should observe the client for symptoms of paralytic ileus and report symptoms of abdominal pain, distention, and constipation to the prescriber. Increasing dyspepsia in clients with hiatal hernias may indicate an aggravation of esophageal reflux because of gastric retention.

Because of the decrease in peristalsis, gastrointestinal transit is prolonged and the absorption of other drugs may be impaired. For this reason, these drugs are also contraindicated in clients with diarrhea. If the cause is infectious, the diarrheal symptoms will be prolonged by retention of bowel contents.

Caution should be taken with clients with chronic pulmonary disease because the resultant decrease in bronchial secretions may lead to bronchial mucus plugs.

Elderly clients are more sensitive to these drugs and require less than the usual adult dose. Monitor closely for agitation, sleepiness, and altered thought processes.

The nurse should observe the client for xerostomia, a reduction in the volume of saliva. This symptom is important and should be reported, not only because the extreme dryness of the mouth usually is a discomfort to the client but also because the severity of xerostomia limits the amount of drug that can be administered. From this symptom, the progression of adverse effects is interference with visual accommodation and difficulty in urination.

Intervention. With beginning therapy, the dosages are low, increasing every 5 to 6 days until a therapeutic level can be obtained. When the drug is to be withdrawn, it is done so in the same fashion—gradually. Sudden withdrawal may cause vomiting, lassitude, and excessive sweating and salivation. Tolerance may develop if the therapy is prolonged, which may require an increase in dosage. If another antiparkinsonism agent is to be substituted for the initial drug, the dosage of the first drug should be gradually decreased while the substitute is gradually increased.

Oral dosage forms of anticholinergics should be administered 30 minutes to 1 hour before meals to maximize absorption. If the client has gastrointestinal distress, it can be minimized by administering the drug with meals; however, absorption will be delayed. Antacids and antidiarrheal agents should not be administered within 1 hour of taking oral anticholinergics. With the parenteral administration of anticholinergics, the client may experience a temporary sensation of lightheadedness and the nurse should take precautions to meet the client's safety needs by having him or her rest in a sitting or preferably prone position for about 20 minutes. Local irritation may also occur with parenteral administration.

Education. The nurse should arrange for the client to check with a pharmacist, physician, or other prescriber for drug interactions before taking any other drugs, including OTC drugs. The client should be instructed to avoid CNS depressants such as alcohol, barbiturates, and narcotics while taking the drugs.

The client should be cautioned that anticholinergics impair physical and mental functioning (i.e., they cause drowsiness and blurred vision) and that care should be taken when driving or operating machinery. The nurse should alert the client to the dangers of heat exhaustion and inform him or her to avoid exercise during warm weather because of the decreased ability to perspire. This caution should also be of concern to clients with fever because hyperthermia may result. The client should also be instructed to change position slowly if orthostatic hypotension is a problem.

The nurse should advise the client to use sugarless hard candy, gum, mouthwash, or bits of ice to relieve dryness of the mouth.

The client should be counseled to have yearly ophthalmic examinations. Intraocular pressure determinations are of particular importance because increased ocular tension may occur with these anticholinergic agents.

Evaluation. The client on anticholinergic therapy for parkinsonism will demonstrate improved mobility with a reduction in muscular rigidity and tremor without any ill effects of the drug.

Drugs Affecting Brain Dopamine

Three classifications of drugs affect brain dopamine: those that release dopamine, those that increase brain levels of dopamine, and dopaminergic agonists. The drugs of choice in the treatment of Parkinson's disease are those that increase the brain levels of dopamine. The other two classifications are used as adjuncts or when therapy normally used is contraindicated.

The drugs affecting brain dopamine have their major effect on the akinesia seen in Parkinson's disease. Akinesia is the difficulty in or the lack of ability to initiate muscle movement caused in Parkinson's disease by decreased levels of brain dopamine. The client with akinesia exhibits a masklike facial expression, impairment of postural reflexes, and eventually an inability for self-care. Drugs affecting brain dopamine increase the level of brain dopamine, thus creating a balance between dopamine and acetylcholine in the brain, especially in the basal ganglia area.

Drugs That Increase Brain Levels of Dopamine

▲ **levodopa** [lee voe doe' pa] (L-Dopa, Dopar, Larodopa) A small percentage of levodopa crosses the blood-brain barrier intact. It is decarboxylated to dopamine, stimulates dopamine receptors, and helps to balance the dopamine/acetylcholine concentrations. Levodopa is indicated for treatment of Parkinson's disease (idiopathic, postencephalitic, symptomatic, or parkinsonism associated with cerebral atherosclerosis).

Levodopa is absorbed by active transport; approximately 30% to 50% reaches systemic circulation. The drug is distributed to most body tissues; the CNS receives less than 1% of the dose because of peripheral metabolism. The enzyme decarboxylase converts levodopa (95%) to dopamine in the stomach, intestines, and also the liver. Levodopa has a half-life of 1 to 3 hours.

Usually improvement is seen within 2 to 3 weeks (although other clients may require levodopa for up to 6 months to obtain a therapeutic effect). Peak concentration is achieved in 1 to 3 hours. Duration of action is up to 5 hours per dose. The drug is excreted by the kidneys.

The side/adverse effects of levodopa include anxiety, nervousness, confusion (especially in the elderly), constipation, nightmares, difficult urination, depression, orthostatic hypotension, mood changes, increased aggressiveness, irregular heart rate, severe nausea or vomiting, and choreiform and involuntary movements of the body (face, arms, hands, tongue, head, and upper body).

Levodopa (Dopar, Larodopa) dose for children 12 years and older and adults is 250 mg orally 2 to 4 times daily, increased by 100 to 750 mg/day at 3 to 7 day intervals until therapeutic response is achieved. The maximum dose is 8 g/day. Elderly and postencephalitic clients may require lower doses because they are more sensitive to this medication. Dosage for children younger than 12 years has not been established.

■ Nursing Management

Levodopa Therapy

Assessment. The client's health status should be assessed for any preexisting conditions for which the administration of levodopa would place the client at higher risk of injury or would require it to be administered with a greater degree of caution. Levodopa is not recommended for children younger than 12 years old, pregnant women, or clients with undiagnosed skin lesions or a history of melanoma because these lesions may be activated. For pregnancy safety ratings, see the box above. Levodopa may inhibit lactation in nursing mothers. Levodopa should be administered with great caution to clients with severe cardiovascular, renal, hepatic, or endocrine disease; peptic ulcer (increases risk of GI bleeding); diabetes; or psychiatric disturbances (increases risk of depression). Levodopa may increase dysrhythmias in predisposed clients. It may aggravate pulmonary conditions. Intraocular pressure may increase and precipitate an acute attack of glaucoma. The administration of levodopa may precipitate or aggravate urinary retention, particularly in male clients.

In addition, the client's current drug regimen should be reviewed for significant drug interactions. The following effects may occur when levodopa is given with the drugs listed below:

Drug	Possible effect and management
anesthetics, hydrocarbon inhalation	May result in dysrhythmias. Discontinue levodopa 6 to 8 hours before hydrocarbon anesthetics, especially halothane.
anticonvulsants, haloperidol (Haldol), or phenothiazines	May result in decreased levodopa effects because hydantoin anticonvulsants increase levodopa metabolism and haloperidol and phenothiazines block dopamine receptors in the brain. When hydantoin and levodopa are given concurrently, monitor closely; increased doses of levodopa may be necessary. If at all possible, avoid the combination of haloperidol or phenothiazines with levodopa.
cocaine	May result in increased risk of arrhythmias. If medically necessary to give both drugs concurrently, reduce doses and monitor closely with ECG monitoring.
monoamine oxidase (MAO) inhibitors	**This combination may result in a hypertensive crisis. Avoid or a potentially serious drug interaction may occur. MAO inhibitors should be discontinued 2 to 4 weeks before starting levodopa therapy.**
pyridoxine (vitamin B_6)	Dosages of 10 mg or more may reverse the antiparkinsonian effect of levodopa. Monitor closely.
selegiline (Eldepryl)	Although this combination may be used, it may result in increased levodopamine-induced nausea, dyskinesias, confusion, hypotension, and hallucinations. If this combination is used, the dose of levodopa should be reduced within several days of starting the selegiline.

Pregnancy Safety

Category	Drug
B	pergolide
C	amantadine, biperiden, carbidopa/levodopa, edrophonium, neostigmine, selegiline
Unclassified	ambenonium, benztropine, bromocriptine, levodopa, procyclidine, pyridostigmine, trihexyphenidyl

The nurse should obtain a baseline assessment of the client's parkinsonian symptoms. This should include self-care deficits and the amount of assistance required for the client to accomplish activities of daily living as well as the client's physical and emotional adaptation to the illness.

Nursing diagnosis. After beginning levodopa therapy, the client should be assessed for the following nursing diagnoses: impaired physical mobility related to the underlying Parkinson's disease and dose-related side effects of choreiform movements (50% to 80% of clients); altered thought processes (anxiety, confusion, nervousness, depression) related to adverse CNS effects of the drug; disturbed sleep pattern (nightmares, insomnia); risk for injury related to orthostatic hypotension (30% of clients in early therapy); altered bowel elimination (constipation); altered comfort (headache, nausea and vomiting); and the potential complications of hypertension, duodenal ulcer, hemolytic anemia, and dysrhythmias.

Implementation

Monitoring. The client's vital signs should be monitored during periods of dosage regulation for indications of hypotension and dysrhythmias. Monitor the client's progress by observing body movements for signs of improvement. Periodic evaluations need to be done for hepatic, cardiovascular, and renal functioning, including hemoglobin determinations and complete blood count. Ophthalmologic testing for glaucoma is especially important with the administration of levodopa.

Nightmares and mood changes, such as agitation, anxiety, and confusion, are symptoms for which the client should be observed in addition to the side effects previously mentioned.

Intervention. Levodopa should be administered before meals because food impedes the drug's action. Nausea and vomiting occur in 80% of the clients early in levodopa therapy. However, tolerance develops with continued use of the drug. For geriatric clients and individuals receiving other medications, the dosage of levodopa should be titrated to reach the client's therapeutic level with minimal side effects.

Education. The client should be instructed to change to the upright position slowly if orthostatic hypotension is a problem. Hypotension can be minimized with the use of elastic stockings. In addition, elderly clients who respond to levodopa therapy, particularly those with osteoporosis, should be cautioned to resume higher activity levels gradually to minimize the risk of fractures. Because levodopa has mydriatic effects, clients should be encouraged to have their intraocular pressure checked periodically for the detection of glaucoma.

The client should be instructed to call the prescriber if symptoms of overdosage develop (involuntary muscle twitching and involuntary winking). The nurse should caution the client receiving prolonged high-dose therapy that "on-off" syndrome may occur (Box 23-2). The client should be advised that involuntary movement of the face, mouth, tongue, and head often develop with prolonged therapy and that the prescriber should be notified of these symptoms so that drug dosage can be adjusted.

BOX 23-2

Levodopa On-Off Syndrome

On-off syndrome refers to a complication following prolonged levodopa therapy (2 years or more). The client fluctuates from being symptom free ("on") to demonstrating full-blown Parkinson's symptoms ("off") during therapy. These effects may last from minutes to hours and may be due to a decrease in delivery of dopamine centrally; an alteration in sensitivity of the dopamine receptors; variation in amount and rate of drug absorption; a dopamine metabolite interference; or a combination of effects.

Treatment may require more frequent administration of levodopa or levodopa-carbidopa and perhaps, the addition of a direct-acting dopamine agonist, bromocriptine. Following a drug holiday (drug withdrawal) of several days to a week, some persons may demonstrate an improved response to the drug therapy. This may be because of the reestablishment of dopamine receptor sensitivity to levodopa, which is usually only temporary. Because many individuals worsen during the drug-free period, this approach should be instituted in a hospital setting (Flaherty & Gidal, 1995).

Clients need to be alerted that the response to levodopa may not occur until several weeks after the treatment has begun. Urine and perspiration may be darker, but this is of no significance. Clients with diabetes need to be aware that levodopa may interfere with urine tests for sugar and ketones. Alert clients to the necessity for compliance as full withdrawal of the drug may worsen parkinsonian symptoms, depression, immobility, and increase the risk of thromboembolic disease.

Dietary counseling should be provided regarding protein and pyridoxine (B_6) ingestion. Proteins are metabolized into the amino acids, which may compete with levodopa for transport to the brain, making the response to levodopa unpredictable. Rather than restrict the client's protein intake, it should be divided in equal parts to be taken over the entire day. Vitamin compounds and foods high in pyridoxine, such as pork, beef, liver, ham, egg yolks, avocado, beans, sweet potato, dry skim milk, and oatmeal may decrease the effects of levodopa and should be avoided. Dietary teaching should include the necessity of a high fiber and fluid intake to minimize the side effect of constipation with the drug, along with gradual increases in activity and the establishment of an elimination routine.

Evaluation. The client on levodopa therapy will demonstrate an improvement in mobility with a decrease in muscular rigidity and tremor.

levodopa-carbidopa [lee voe doe' pa/kar bi doe' pa] (Sinemet)

Sinemet and Sinemet CR (control or extended release) are combinations of levodopa with the dopa decarboxylase inhibitor, carbidopa. Carbidopa competes for the enzyme dopa decarboxylase, thus retarding the peripheral breakdown of levodopa. Carbidopa does not cross the blood-brain barrier like levodopa, and therefore it does not interfere with the intracerebral transformation of levodopa to dopamine. Because carbidopa prevents much of the peripheral conversion of levodopa to dopamine, the incidence of systemic side effects of levodopa, such as nausea, vomiting, and cardiac dysrhythmias, is decreased. The CNS effects of levodopa are a greater risk with this combination because more levodopa is reaching the brain to be converted to dopamine.

The addition of carbidopa to levodopa reduces the required dose of levodopa to approximately 20% to 25% of the original levodopa dosage. The available levodopa-carbidopa combination dosage forms include 10/100 (10 mg of carbidopa and 100 mg of levodopa), 25/100 (25 mg of carbidopa and 100 mg levodopa), and 25/250 (25 mg of carbidopa and 250 mg of levodopa). To obtain the peripheral inhibitor effect of carbidopa, a minimum of 75 mg (range, 75 to 100 mg) per day is necessary. Saturating peripheral dopa decarboxylase requires between 75 to 100 mg/day of carbidopa (Flaherty & Gidal, 1995). Nausea and vomiting are reported in clients receiving dosages lower than 75 mg/day of carbidopa. Therefore three combination dosage forms are available to permit greater flexibility in prescribing sufficient amounts of both levodopa and carbidopa for the client. The manufacturer recommends that not more than 200 mg/day of carbidopa be prescribed. As with levodopa alone, the decarboxylation to dopamine replaces the missing brain dopamine and restores a balance to dopamine/acetylcholine concentrations.

Levodopa/carbidopa is indicated for the treatment of idiopathic, postencephalitic, and symptomatic Parkinson's disease. For levodopa's pharmacokinetics, see the previous section. Between 40% and 70% of an oral dose of carbidopa is absorbed. The drug is distributed widely to many body tissues with the exception of the CNS. The drug's metabolism is insignificant. It is excreted by the kidneys.

Side effects/adverse reactions are similar to those for levodopa. Eyelid spasms or closing may be an early sign of drug overdose. Mental or mood changes may also occur earlier and may be dose related.

Drug interactions are the same as for levodopa, with the exception of the pyridoxine interaction. The interaction between levodopa and pyridoxine does not occur in the presence of carbidopa.

For clients not previously on levodopa therapy, start oral dosage at 10/100 or 25/100 3 times daily. Increase dose as needed every 1 or 2 days until the desired response is obtained. For clients previously on levodopa therapy, discontinue levodopa at least 8 hours before instituting combination therapy. If the client is receiving less than 1.5 g levodopa daily, start with 10/100 or 25/100 of carbidopa/levodopa 3 or 4 times daily; increase at 1- or 2-day intervals until the desired response is obtained. If the client is receiving more than 1.5 g of levodopa daily, administer 25/250 carbidopa/levodopa orally 3 or 4 times daily, increasing if necessary at 1- or 2-day intervals until the desired response is obtained.

Be aware that conversion from levodopa to combination levodopa-carbidopa requires only 25% of the original dosage of levodopa initially, with a maximum of up to 200 mg carbidopa and 2 g levodopa daily. If additional levodopa is necessary, give as a single agent. See the case study at right for further study.

Geriatric and postencephalitic clients may require a lower dose because they are more sensitive to this combination. Dosage for children under the age of 18 years has not been established. See nursing management for levodopa.

Dopamine-Releasing Drug

amantadine [a man' ta deen] (Symmetrel)

Amantadine is a synthetic antiviral compound. While its exact mechanism of its action is not completely known, it is postulated that amantadine releases dopamine and other catecholamines from neuronal storage sites. It also blocks the uptake of dopamine into presynaptic neurons, thus permitting peripheral and central accumulation of dopamine. Amantadine may also give the client a sense of well-being and elevation of mood. It is less effective than levodopa but produces more rapid clinical improvement and causes fewer untoward reactions.

Amantadine is indicated for use as an antidyskinetic (treatment of Parkinson's disease) and as an antiviral (systemic agent). Amantadine is well absorbed; it is not metabolized. The drug has a half-life of 11 to 15 hours. Peak serum levels are reached within 2 to 4 hours, with onset of antidyskinetic action within 48 hours. Steady-state is reached within 2 to 3 days with daily drug administration; drug serum level is 0.2 to 0.9 μg/ml. Levels above 1 μg/ml are considered toxic. Amantadine is excreted by the kidneys.

The side/adverse effects of amantadine include impaired concentration, dizziness, increased irritability, anorexia, nausea, nervousness, purple-red skin spots (livedo reticularis, usually seen with chronic therapy), confusion, hallucinations, mental or mood variations, orthostatic hypotension, and difficult urination. Symptoms of overdose include severe confusion, insomnia, nightmares, and seizures.

Adult antidyskinetic dose is 100 mg orally once or twice daily. Maximum dosage is 400 mg/day. The elderly are dosed at 100 mg daily to start, titrating to 2 or 3 times a day as necessary.

■ Nursing Management

Amantadine Therapy

Assessment. Before the initiation of amantadine therapy the client should be assessed for preexisting peripheral edema, congestive heart failure, and epilepsy because these conditions may be exacerbated by the drug. In addition, because amantadine is not metabolized and is excreted by the kidneys, clients who have renal function impairment are at risk for drug toxicity and will require a reduced dosage.

Case Study

Parkinson's Disease

Mr. Edwards is a 64-year-old man who has been diagnosed with Parkinson's disease. He is to begin taking levodopa-carbidopa (Sinemet) 10/100 tid. After 3 days his dosage is increased by one tablet a day. His final dosage is now one tablet of Sinemet, 25/100 qid.

1. How does levodopa contribute to the improved function of the client with Parkinson's disease?
2. Explain the rationale for giving carbidopa with the levodopa.
3. What points should the nurse include in teaching Mr. Edwards about his drug therapy?

After 2 years of therapy, Mr. Edwards' symptoms have improved, with adverse effects limited to occasional nausea, dry mouth, and anorexia. However, periodically he has increases in his disease symptoms even though he continues to take his medication. The prescriber has decided to add amantadine (Symmetrel) 100 mg daily to the drug treatment.

4. Why did Mr. Edwards experience an increase in his symptoms?
5. Symmetrel is pharmacologically classified as an antiviral agent. Explain its role in the treatment of Parkinson's disease.

Six months later Mr. Edwards comes to the clinic reporting that he has begun having episodes of confusion, insomnia, nightmares, and hallucinations. He has waited several months before discussing these episodes and expresses concern that he is "losing his mind." In addition the nurse notices while talking with him that he has developed some involuntary movements of his tongue and face.

6. How should the nurse respond to Mr. Edwards' concerns?
7. What is the significance of the involuntary movements noted in the nurse's assessment of the client?

After reviewing Mr. Edwards' case, the prescriber decides to discontinue the Symmetrel. Within 6 weeks Mr. Edwards reports that the nightmares and insomnia have stopped. He no longer experiences the hallucinations, and the confusion is minimal. The involuntary movements have decreased significantly.

A baseline assessment of the client's vital signs and parkinsonian movements should be documented.

The client's concurrent medication regimen should be reviewed for significant drug interactions. The following effects may occur when amantadine is given with the drugs listed below:

Drug	Possible effect and management
alcohol	**Increased CNS side effects, such as confusion, lightheadedness, orthostatic hypotension, and fainting spells reported. Avoid or a potentially serious drug interaction may occur.**
anticholinergics	May enhance anticholinergic side effects, such as confusion, hallucinations, frightening dreams, etc. Dosage adjustments may be necessary. Also monitor for paralytic ileus.
CNS stimulants	Additive CNS stimulation reported; side effects include increased nervousness, irritability, difficulty sleeping, and at times seizures and cardiac dysrhythmias. Closely monitor clients receiving concurrent stimulant therapy.

Nursing diagnosis. The client receiving amantadine should be assessed for the following nursing diagnoses: altered thought processes (confusion, mental or mood variations); altered sleep patterns (insomnia); risk for injury related to blurred vision, dizziness and orthostatic hypotension; altered nutrition; altered comfort related to rash, headache, xerostomia, anorexia and nausea; altered elimination patterns: urinary (retention) and bowel (constipation); and the potential complications of CNS toxicity (seizures, depression), congestive heart failure, corneal deposits (impaired vision) and livedo reticularis (red blotchy spots on skin).

Implementation

Monitoring. The client's mobility status should be monitored for muscular rigidity, tremor, and the ability to accomplish activities of daily living. The side effects of nausea, dizziness, insomnia, nervousness, and impaired concentration are common with this drug. For clients receiving doses greater than 200 mg/day, there is a higher risk of CNS toxicity; these clients should be monitored carefully. Vital signs should be monitored 4 times a day when dosages are increased. Clients with epilepsy are at greater risk for seizures and so should be monitored accordingly. In long-term therapy, monitor for congestive heart failure, with symptoms such as increased edema of feet and lower legs, difficulty in breathing, and rapid increase of body weight.

Intervention. Changing the client's medication schedule from a once-a-day to a twice-a-day schedule may decrease some of the unpleasant side effects such as lightheadedness, insomnia, and nausea, but be aware that increasing the number of doses of a drug increases the risk of ineffective management of the medication regimen by the client. Therapy should be discontinued gradually. Abrupt cessation of the drug may cause exacerbations of symptoms of parkinsonism within 24 hours and onset of parkinsonian crisis within 3 days.

Education. The client should be informed that a reduction in benefits occurs after 4 to 12 weeks of therapy. Increasing the dose or taking a brief holiday from the drug will restore its benefits. Compliance with a full course of therapy is necessary.

The nurse should instruct the client not to drink alcohol while taking this drug because it may result in dizziness, fainting, and confusion. See also the general discussion of nursing management of anticholinergic therapy.

Evaluation. The client will demonstrate improved mobility with decreased muscular rigidity and tremor without adverse effects of the drug.

Dopaminergic Agonists

bromocriptine [broe moe krip' teen] (Parlodel)

Bromocriptine is an ergot alkaloid derivative marketed as the first agonist of dopamine receptor activity. It activates postsynaptic dopamine receptors, stimulating the production of dopamine and correcting the brain dopamine/acetylcholine imbalance. The drug is indicated as an antidyskinetic, growth hormone suppressant, antihyperprolactinemic, and prophylactic for lactation after second or third trimester pregnancy loss. Approximately 28% of a dose is absorbed, but only 6% reaches systemic circulation.

Bromocriptine's half-life is biphasic: alpha, 4 to 4½ hours; beta, 15 hours. Onset of activity from a single dose used for antiparkinsonism is 30 to 90 minutes, reaching a peak concentration at 2 hours. The drug is metabolized in the liver. Metabolites of bromocriptine are excreted primarily in bile.

The side/adverse effects of bromocriptine include drowsiness, headache, nausea, hypotension, and, less frequently, confusion, hallucinations, and uncontrolled movements of body, face, tongue, arms, hands, and head.

The adult oral antidyskinetic dose is 1.25 to 2.5 mg orally daily, titrated as necessary. Maintenance dosage may range from 2.5 to 100 mg daily in divided doses. Dosage for children younger than 15 years has not been established.

■ Nursing Management

Bromocriptine Therapy

Assessment. Bromocriptine should not be administered to mothers expecting to breastfeed, because the drug inhibits lactation. In addition, bromocriptine is contraindicated for clients with a history of hypertension or pregnancy-induced hypertension because it may be aggravated. Use with caution in clients with hepatic dysfunction, because metabolism of the drug may be reduced. Clients with psychiatric disorders may have a worsening of symptoms with the administration of bromocriptine.

Bromocriptine has an additive effect with other antiparkinsonism drugs. Clients with an intolerance of ergot derivatives may also be intolerant of bromocriptine. When bromocriptine is given with estrogens, progestins, or oral contraceptives, the hormones may cause amenorrhea and possibly galactorrhea, which counteracts the effects of bromocriptine. Do not administer concurrently.

A baseline assessment of the client's health status should include blood pressure determination as well as a description of the client's motor status. If the drug is being administered for hyperprolactinemia, a baseline serum prolactin should be obtained. To rule out a pituitary tumor causing the hyperprolactinemia, a CT scan or an MRI of the sella turcica is recommended.

Nursing diagnosis. Clients receiving bromocriptine therapy have the potential for the following nursing diagnoses: risk for injury related to hypotension and CNS effects (confusion, hallucinations); altered comfort (headache, nausea, dry mouth, stuffy nose, leg cramps); altered bowel function (constipation, diarrhea); depression; and the potential complications of myocardial infarction (chest pain, shortness of breath, sweating, weakness), seizure or stroke (headache, vision changes, sudden weakness), peptic ulcer (stomach pain, black tarry stools), Raynaud's phenomenon (tingling or pain of fingers and toes when exposed to cold), and retroperitoneal fibrosis (abdominal pain, anorexia, nausea, and vomiting).

Implementation

Monitoring. Blood pressure should be monitored; 1% to 5% of the clients have symptomatic hypotension. Other common effects include constipation, nausea, nasal congestion, and tingling or pain in the fingers and toes when exposed to the cold. These effects occur in 30% to 60% of the clients being treated for Parkinson's disease with this medication. The most common side effects occur when the client first begins therapy and most of them are dose related, seldom occurring with doses less than 20 mg daily.

If bromocriptine is administered for female infertility, periodic serum prolactin levels and ovulation evaluations are recommended. If used for the treatment of acromegaly, growth hormone serum levels aid in determining dosages.

Intervention. The nurse should administer bromocriptine with meals or milk to decrease the adverse effect of nausea. Bedtime administration may minimize the effects of dizziness and nausea for the client. Give the first dose at bedtime or with the client lying down, because the hypotensive effects of the drug are more likely to occur after the initial dose. The dosage is initiated at a low level and gradually increased to the minimum effective dosage.

Education. The nurse should caution clients with infertility not taking the drug for that indication to use a contraceptive measure because this drug may result in a restoration of fertility. A mechanical barrier device, such as a diaphragm or condom, should be suggested rather than oral contraceptives, because oral estrogen contraceptives increase the risk of stimulating prolactin-secreting cells. Pregnancy tests should be performed every 4 weeks during therapy, along with the use of contraceptive measures. A positive result of a pregnancy test should be reported to the prescriber immediately.

The nurse should caution clients bromocriptine may impair physical and mental functioning and that they should take care when driving or operating machinery. The client should be instructed to limit alcohol consumption because it increases CNS side effects. Also, taking this drug with alcohol may result in a disulfiram-type reaction, tachycardia, pounding heart rate, facial flushing, sweating, nausea, vomiting, headache, blurred vision, chest pain, and lethargy.

The client should be taught to prevent or minimize constipation by increasing dietary fiber, increasing fluid intake to 3000 ml daily, performing moderate exercise daily, and establishing a regular time of day for bowel elimination. The nurse should advise the client to limit exposure to the cold or to wear protective clothing to prevent discomfort of the fingers and toes.

The client should be cautioned to get up slowly from a sitting or supine position because of bromocriptine's hypotensive effects. Regular dental examinations are advised because bromocriptine inhibits salivation and thereby increases the client's risk of discomfort, caries, and peridontal disorders. See also the general discussion of nursing management related to anticholinergic therapy.

Evaluation. The client will demonstrate an increase in physical mobility with a decrease in muscular rigidity and tremor without any adverse effects of the drug. If bromocriptine is administered for infertility, conception will occur.

pergolide [per' go lide] (Permax)

Pergolide is a dopamine agonist, usually used in conjunction with levodopa or levodopa-carbidopa to treat the signs and symptoms of Parkinson's disease. It is more potent and longer acting than bromocriptine and directly stimulates both D_1 and D_2 receptors (Flaherty & Gidal, 1995). In combination the dose of levodopa or levodopa-carbidopa is often reduced. According to Flaherty and Gidal, up to 75% of non–levodopa-responding clients improved with the addition of pergolide to levodopa. Also, clinical fluctuations reported in clients receiving levodopa-carbidopa may be reduced; that is, the "on" period was prolonged while the "off" period was decreased in most of the clients studied.

Pergolide stimulates dopamine receptors in the nigrostriatal area but, unlike bromocriptine, its action is independent of dopamine synthesis or dopamine storage sites. It also inhibits prolactin secretion. Pergolide is indicated as an adjunct treatment for Parkinson's disease. It is well absorbed; serum protein binding is high (about 90%); the drug is excreted in the kidneys.

The side/adverse effects of pergolide include stomach distress/pain, constipation, lightheadedness, sedation, hypotension, cold-type symptoms, nausea, lower back pain, confusion, dyskinesias such as uncontrollable body movements, and hallucinations.

The recommended dose for adults and elderly clients is 0.05 mg PO daily for 2 days, increased by 0.1 to 0.15 mg every 3 days over the next 12 days. The dose may then be increased by 0.25 mg every 3 days until maximum therapeutic effect is reached. Doses should be divided and given 3 times daily. The maximum dose is 5 mg/day. Pediatric dosage has not been established.

■ Nursing Management

Pergolide Therapy

Assessment. Individuals with a previous allergic experience with ergot alkaloids should not be administered pergolide. Clients with altered thought processes such as confusion or hallucinations may experience a worsening of these symptoms. The increased risk of atrial premature contractions and sinus tachycardia should be considered before pergolide is administered to clients with cardiac arrhythmias. The drug is contraindicated in mothers who anticipate breastfeeding, since it inhibits lactation.

No significant drug interactions are reported to date, but the nurse should be aware that dopamine antagonists, such as the phenothiazines and haloperidol (Haldol), may decrease the effects of the pergolide. Medications that produce hypotension may have an additive hypotensive effect.

A baseline assessment of the client's mobility status, including previous "on-off" fluctuations as well as a blood pressure determination, is essential to monitoring the effectiveness of pergolide therapy.

Nursing diagnosis. The client receiving pergolide therapy should be assessed for the following nursing diagnoses: altered thought processes (confusion, hallucinations); risk for injury related to CNS toxicity (dyskinesias), urinary tract infection (burning on urination), and hypotension; altered comfort (dry mouth, rhinitis, nausea); altered bowel elimination (constipation); and the potential complications of myocardial infarction (chest pain, shortness of breath, tachycardia, weakness), and cerebrovascular hemorrhage (severe headache, vision changes, seizures, sudden weakness).

Implementation

Monitoring. The client's blood pressure should be monitored on a regular basis because changes in blood pressure occur. Hypotension is more common than hypertension. Fluctuations in blood pressure are more apt to occur in periods of dosage adjustment. Monitor the client's comfort level, mental status, mobility status, and bowel elimination pattern.

Intervention. The dosage of pergolide should be titrated so the client obtains the maximum therapeutic benefits and side effects are minimized. Administer pergolide with meals to minimize nausea and vomiting, although these effects usually subside with continued therapy. Nausea and dizziness are not uncommon with the first dose. These effects can be mitigated by administering the first dose at bedtime or while the client is lying down. Careful oral hygiene is required because of the reduced salivary flow.

Education. Encourage the client to seek regular appointments with the prescriber so that the client's progress may be monitored. Alert the client that possible sleepiness or dizziness may make it unsafe for him or her to drive or perform other tasks that require alertness. The client should be taught to come slowly to an upright position from a sitting or prone position because of the drug's hypotensive effects. Advise the client that sugarless candies or gum, ice chips, and saliva substitute may be used to minimize the possible dryness of the mouth.

Evaluation. The client will demonstrate increased mobility with decreased muscular rigidity and tremor, and longer "on" periods and shorter "off" periods without adverse effects of the drug.

Monoamine Oxidase Inhibitor

▲ **selegiline** [sel ee' jell een] or deprenyl (Eldepryl)
Selegiline is used in combination with levodopa or levodopa and carbidopa to treat Parkinson's disease. There are two types of monoamine oxidase in the body: monoamine oxidase A is necessary to metabolize norepinephrine and serotonin; monoamine oxidase B metabolizes dopamine. Selegiline irreversibly inhibits monoamine oxidase B, thus preventing the breakdown of dopamine. As a result it will enhance or prolong levodopa's antiparkinson's effect, which may result in a lowering of the daily dose of levodopa.

Selegiline is well absorbed orally, reaches peak serum level in ½ to 2 hours, and has three active metabolites (with half-lives of 2 to 20 hours). It readily crosses the blood-brain barrier and is excreted slowly via the kidneys.

The side/adverse effects of selegiline include dry mouth, nausea, vomiting, insomnia, dizziness, stomach distress or pain, dyskinesias, and mood alterations.

The usual adult dose of selegiline is 5 mg at breakfast and lunch.

■ Nursing Management

Selegiline Therapy

The nursing management of the client on selegiline therapy is essentially the same as for pergolide except for its significant drug interactions. The following effects may occur when selegiline is given with the drugs listed below:

Drug	Possible effect and management
fluoxetine (Prozac)	**Concurrent use may result in mania and a reaction similar to the serotonin syndrome (confusion, restlessness, hyperreflexia, sweating, shivering, tremors, diarrhea, ataxia, and fever). Avoid or a potentially serious drug interaction may occur. Fluoxetine should not be initiated until at least 2 weeks after selegiline is discontinued. Selegiline should not be initiated in persons taking fluoxetine until at least 5 weeks after fluoxetine has been discontinued (*USP DI*, 1996).**
levodopa (L-dopa)	Although it is indicated to be given concurrently with levodopa, the nurse should be aware that this combination may increase levodopa-induced side effects, such as dyskinesias, nausea, hypotension, confusion, and hallucinations. To reduce this potential, the dose of levodopa should be lowered within 2 to 3 days after selegiline therapy is initiated.
meperidine (Demerol)	**Concurrent drug administration may result in severe adverse reactions, such as severe hypertension, respiratory depression, sweating, excitation, rigidity, seizures, hyperpyrexia, vascular collapse, coma, and death. Avoid or a potentially serious drug interaction may occur. Avoid administration of meperidine for at least 2 to 3 weeks after use of an MAO-inhibiting (MAOI) drug. Although the use of other opioids, such as morphine, is not as likely to result in such a severe reaction, they should also be used very cautiously in lowered doses in any person receiving an MAOI.**
tyramine	**The use of tyramine or foods and beverages that contain tyramine or high pressor amines should be avoided, or if consumed in very small quantities, should be very carefully monitored. This combination may result in an immediate, severe hypertensive episode requiring medical attention. Avoid or a potentially serious drug interaction may occur. It is recommended that dietary restrictions must continue for at least 2 to 3 weeks after the discontinuance of an MAOI.**

MYASTHENIA GRAVIS

Myasthenia gravis is a progressive, incurable disease characterized by the loss of or decrease in acetylcholine receptors caused by an autoimmune process resulting in skeletal muscle weakness and fatigue. Because of its involvement with the production of antibodies, the thymus gland is believed to have a role in the causation of myasthenia gravis. Nearly 15% of all myasthenia gravis clients have a thymoma, or tumor of the thymus gland.

Symptoms of myasthenia gravis usually become worse with exertion and are less noticeable with rest. Stress, infection, menses, surgery, and other factors may also increase the symptoms. The most common early reported symptoms are ptosis and diplopia. Dysarthria, dysphagia, and limb weakness, especially of the upper extremities, also occur in the advanced stages. The client may complain of shoulder fatigue after shaving or combing the hair, or of hand weakness, finding it difficult to open doors or kitchen jars or to perform repetitive tasks, such as lawn work or playing the piano (Figure 23-2).

The most serious effects of myasthenia gravis are dysphagia and respiratory muscle weakness, since these may result in aspiration pneumonia or respiratory failure. Treatment of this disease state may include thymectomy, cholinesterase inhibitors, plasmapheresis, and, at times, corticosteroids. The mainstay, though, is cholinesterase-inhibitor drugs, such as anticholinesterase drugs.

Anticholinesterase Agents

The **anticholinesterase agents**, or antimyasthenics, are drugs that enhance cholinergic action by blocking the effect of cholinesterase. These drugs act by inactivating or inhibiting cholinesterase at the sites of acetylcholine transmission, permitting the accumulation of acetylcholine. Because of their ability to increase the amount of acetylcholine at the

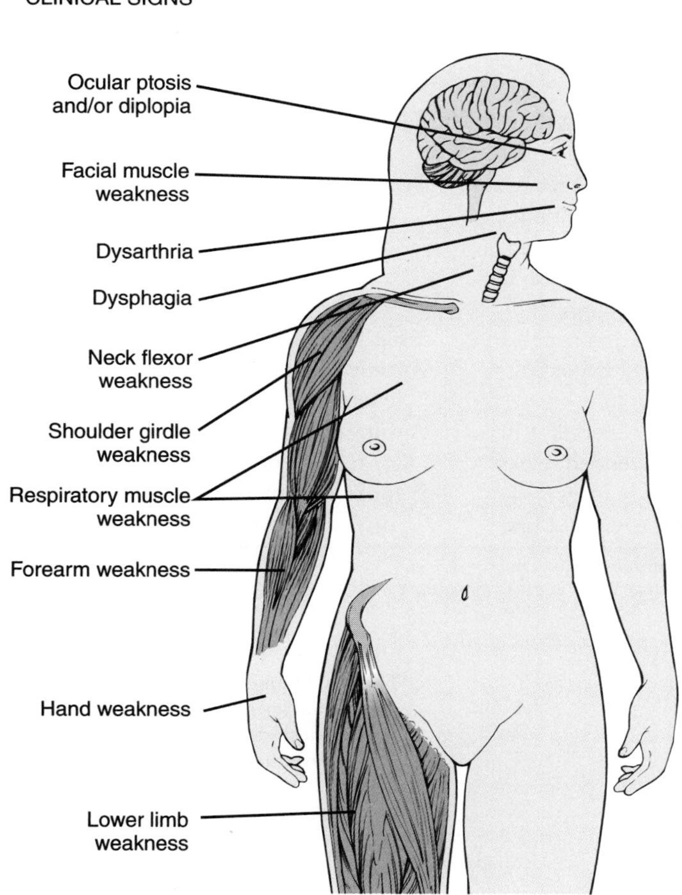

SYMPTOMS

- Drooping of upper eyelids
- Double vision
- Diminished expression
- Slurred speech
- Difficulty swallowing
- Shoulder tiredness
- Exhaustion, decrease in respirations
- Arm fatigue and/or weakness

IMPLICATIONS

- Symptoms become worse with exertion but will improve with rest.
- Stress, menses, infections, surgery, and vigorous physical exercise may worsen symptoms.
- Symptom severity may fluctuate from morning to night and from day to day.
- Muscle weakness common; sensory loss and coordination difficulties not reported in myasthenia gravis clients.

Figure 23-2 Signs, symptoms, and implications of myasthenia gravis.

myoneural junction, the cholinesterase inhibitors are primarily used for the diagnosis and treatment of myasthenia gravis and for their local effects in the eye (see Chapter 43). These drugs are used also for urinary retention and paralytic ileus and as an antidote for the curariform effects of the nondepolarizing skeletal muscle relaxants, such as tubocurarine (Tubarine) and pancuronium (Pavulon).

Orally, all are poorly absorbed from the gastrointestinal tract. Onset of action of these drugs is as follows: ambenonium (Mytelase), within 30 minutes; edrophonium (Tensilon), IM within 2 to 10 minutes and IV within 30 to 60 seconds; neostigmine (Prostigmin), orally within 45 to 75 minutes, IM within 30 minutes, and IV within 4 to 8 minutes; and pyridostigmine (Mestinon) oral tablet or syrup within 30 to 45 minutes, extended-release tablet, 30 to 60 minutes, IM within 15 minutes, and IV within 2 to 5 minutes.

Duration of effect of each is as follows: ambenonium, 3 to 8 hours; edrophonium IM within 5 to 30 minutes and IV approximately 10 minutes; neostigmine oral and parenteral, 2 to 6 hours; and pyridostigmine oral syrup or tablets, 3 to 6 hours; extended-release tablet, 6 to 12 hours; and parenteral, 2 to 4 hours. Neostigmine and pyridostigmine are metabolized mainly in the liver and are excreted in the kidneys.

The side/adverse effects of anticholinesterase agents include nausea, vomiting, diarrhea, abdominal cramps, increased sweating, drooling, increased urge to urinate, pinpoint pupils, eye watering, and increased bronchial secretions. Overdose effects include blurred vision, severe diarrhea, increased salivation, increase in bronchial secretions, severe nausea or vomiting, respiratory difficulties, severe abdominal pain, bradycardia, increased weakness, ataxia, confusion, slurred speech, and muscle weakness.

Ambenonium (Mytelase) is a slowly reversible cholinesterase inhibitor; therefore it may accumulate at cholinergic synapses and produce increased, prolonged effects. Because of the narrow margin between first appearance of side effects and serious toxicity, ambenonium is usually reserved for clients who have not responded adequately to neostigmine or pyridostigmine or for clients who are hypersensitive to the bromide component in both drugs.

Edrophonium chloride injection (Tensilon) is used to diagnose myasthenia gravis. Because of its short duration of

TABLE 23-2 Cholinesterase inhibitors: dosage and administration

Drug	Adults	Children
ambenonium (Mytelase)	Antimyasthenic dose: 5 mg PO 3 or 4 times daily, adjusted as necessary.	0.3 mg/kg divided in 3 or 4 doses, adjusted as necessary, every 1-2 days.
edrophonium (Tensilon)	Diagnostic: 10 mg IM, if cholinergic reaction results, repeat test in ½ hr using a 2 mg dose to rule out possible false-negative effect. IV, 2 mg given every 15-30 sec; if no response after 45 sec give 8 mg.*	See current reference for dosing recommendations.
neostigmine (Prostigmin)	15 mg PO every 3-4 hr, adjusted as necessary. Antimyasthenic dose: 0.5 mg IM or SC, adjusted as necessary.	2 mg/kg divided into 6 or 8 doses. Antimyasthenic: 0.01-0.04 mg/kg IM or SC every 2-3 hr†
pyridostigmine (Mestinon)	Antimyasthenic: 30-60 mg PO every 3-4 hr, adjusted as necessary; or extended release tablets 180-540 mg 1-2 times daily. Parenteral: 2 mg IM or IV every 2-3 hrs.	Antimyasthenic: 7 mg/kg PO divided in 5 or 6 doses daily. Neonates of myasthenic mothers: 0.05-0.15 mg/kg IM every 4 to 6 hr.

*If a cholinergic effect results after a 2 mg dose, discontinue test and give atropine IV (0.4 mg).
†Dose of 0.01 mg/kg of atropine may be given with each dose or with alternate doses to offset muscarinic side effects.

action, it is not indicated for the treatment of myasthenia gravis (Table 23-2).

■ Nursing Management

Anticholinesterase Therapy

Assessment. Caution should be used in clients with asthma, pneumonia, or atelectasis. An increase in bronchial secretions may aggravate these conditions. Antimyasthenics may cause an increase in cardiac dysrhythmias. Clients who have a hypersensitivity to bromides, usually demonstrated by a rash, may also be sensitive to the bromide ion of neostigmine or pyridostigmine. Note that these drugs are contraindicated in clients with urinary tract infection or obstruction, because an increase in bladder muscle tone may aggravate symptoms. They should be avoided in clients with decreased gastrointestinal motility because the drug may accumulate and cause toxicity when gastrointestinal motility is restored.

Anticholinesterase agents need to be considered carefully before they are administered during pregnancy. Muscular weakness has been demonstrated in some newborns whose mothers received these agents during pregnancy. In addition, anticholinesterase agents promote uterine irritability and may induce early labor in pregnant women who are near term.

The client's current medication regimen should be reviewed for any significant drug interactions. The following effects may occur when cholinesterase inhibitors are given with the drugs listed below:

Drug	Possible effect and management
other cholinesterase inhibitors such as demecarium (Humorsol), echothiophate (Phospholine), and isoflurophate (Floropryl)	**This combination of drugs is not recommended. Avoid or a potentially serious drug interaction may occur.**
guanadrel (Hylorel), guanethidine (Ismelin), mecamylamine (Inversine), or trimethaphan (Arfonad)	**These are ganglionic blocking agents that may antagonize the action of the cholinesterase-inhibitor drugs, resulting in increased muscle weakness, respiratory muscle weakness, and difficulty in swallowing. Avoid or a potentially serious drug interaction may occur.**
procainamide (Pronestyl) or quinidine	The neuromuscular blocking action and possibly antimuscarinic effect of procainamide may antagonize the action of the cholinesterase inhibitor drugs. If used concurrently, monitor client closely.

Assess neuromuscular status (ptosis, diplopia, speed, ability to swallow, respiratory function, extremity strength) before administration of the drug. A baseline assessment should include the client's neuromuscular and respiratory status.

Nursing diagnosis. Once the client begins antimyasthenic therapy the nurse's assessment should focus on the potential development of nursing diagnoses/collaborative problems related to the effects of the drugs. There may be alterations in the client's patterns of elimination related to the parasympathomimetic effects (diarrhea); risk for injury related to the visual and CNS effects exists, especially in the elderly client; and altered urinary patterns of urinary frequency, urgency, and incontinence are possible. The increase in bronchial secretions may result in ineffective airway clearance. The client's comfort may also be altered because of rash, GI effects, and muscle weakness.

Implementation

Monitoring. When treatment is initiated, the client should be observed closely for signs of toxic effects. Atropine sulfate and equipment for respiratory support should be on hand. Observation for cholinergic effect should be ongoing when these drugs are used. The time of onset of weakness indicates whether the weakness is caused by overdosage or underdosage. If the weakness begins about 1 hour after administration of the drug, overdosage is a possibility. If it occurs after 3 or more hours, the weakness is usually caused by underdosage.

The nurse should observe for subtle changes in the client's speech and facial expression. Ptosis increases and the ability to swallow decreases early, since weakness increases with an increase in the nicotinic effects.

Blood pressure, pulse, respirations, movement of the respiratory muscles, respiratory rate, tidal volume, and inspiratory force should be monitored.

The nurse should check vital capacity by asking the client to take a deep breath and count as high as possible without taking another breath; most people can count as high as 40 or 50. All these observations are important because symptoms usually seen in respiratory distress, such as nasal flaring and intercostal or suprasternal retractions, may not occur because of muscle weakness. Arterial blood gases should also be monitored. Dosage, route of administration, and frequency of the medication depend on the client's clinical response, the remissions and exacerbations of the disease, and the stresses experienced by the client.

CNS effects are evidenced by altered thought processes (confusion, irritability), increasing unsteadiness, slurred speech, dyspnea, and seizures. Blurred vision, bradycardia, increasing bronchial secretions and salivation, severe vomiting, and diarrhea result from the muscarinic effects.

Intervention. These drugs are initiated at a dosage less than that required to produce the client's maximum strength, and the dosage is gradually increased at intervals of 48 hours or more according to the severity of the disease and the response of the client. Oral dosage forms may take several days to produce any change. If the last dosage increment does not produce a corresponding increase in the client's muscle strength, the dose will need to be reduced to its previous level. Because it is essential that the smallest dose for maximum result be used, the nurse's assessment and documentation of the client's health status are crucial.

The drugs administered for myasthenia gravis are best given with food or milk to decrease adverse muscarinic effects, such as abdominal cramping, nausea, and vomiting. However, if dysphagia is a problem, the medication should be administered 30 to 45 minutes before meals and a rest period from the time of medication until meal time should be provided to allow for peak muscle strength for eating. This may be enhanced by serving frequent, regular, soft foods and encouraging the client to take small bites of food with frequent rest intervals. The main meal should be served at the time of day when the client has the most strength.

The nurse should be prepared for crisis intervention with medications, (edrophonium and neostigmine) for myasthenic crisis and (atropine) for cholinergic crisis. Basic resuscitative equipment should be available: suction catheters, AMBU bag, oxygen, and intubation tray.

The drugs should be administered on time because they are rapidly metabolized. A delay of 15 to 20 minutes in administration may cause beginning impairment of the muscles involved in swallowing and respiration.

The nurse must be especially alert to the route of administration because the oral dosage is 30 times greater than parenteral doses.

It should be noted that atropine sulfate, 0.06 to 1.2 mg, may be administered before or concurrently with these drugs to prevent adverse effects such as excessive secretions or bradycardia.

When using these agents to counteract the neuromuscular blocking agents (e.g., tubocurarine), the nurse should administer them along with artificial ventilation and oxygen therapy. They should be used only when some definite sign of voluntary respiration can be observed.

The nurse should administer intravenous pyridostigmine bromide (Mestinon) very slowly to prevent thrombophlebitis. The syrup dosage form of pyridostigmine may be more easily tolerated by clients with impaired swallowing or when the client's condition warrants frequent fractional doses, less than 60 mg. Although there is an extended-release form of pyridostigmine, it is usually not recommended because it increases the risk of cholinergic crisis, may need to be supplemented temporarily with other oral dosage forms to control symptoms, or may pass intact through the GI tract if the client has increased intestinal activity or diarrhea.

A client who has had prolonged drug therapy may become refractory to the drug. By decreasing the dosage or withdrawing the drug for a few days under medical supervision, responsiveness may be restored.

Education. The client with myasthenia gravis should be instructed to take the medication as ordered, using an alarm clock for precise timing of doses if necessary. An adequate supply of medications should be kept on hand. The family should also be instructed about timing of doses.

The client and family should maintain a log of symptoms. This will assist them to be aware of what events, such as emotional stress, menstruation, or infection, worsen the symptoms and how the client responds to medication. The client should be taught to observe for therapeutic effects of the drug: a decrease or absence of ptosis; improved chewing, swallowing, and speech; increased skeletal muscle strength; and less fatigue. Activities should be planned to take advantage of the drug's peak effectiveness.

When stabilized, the client can be taught to recognize muscarinic effects (diaphoresis, salivation, slowed heart rate, and decreased blood pressure) and modify the medication dosage or take atropine if needed. The greater the control the client has over the therapeutic regimen, the less the client's feeling of powerlessness in the face of a devastating and debilitating disease.

The client should be cautioned to avoid alcoholic beverages for 1 hour after medications because they hasten drug absorption. Tonic water should be avoided because it may contain quinine, which increases weakness.

Evaluation. The client will demonstrate greater muscle strength and an increased ability to swallow, chew, and speak without adverse effects of the drug.

DEMENTIA

Dementia, a progressive mental disorder characterized by chronic personality disintegration, confusion, and deterioration of intellectual capacity and impulse control, affects 3% to 16% of Americans over the age of 65. Alzheimer's disease accounts for approximately 50% to 60% of dementia while vascular dementia (including multi-infarct dementia, formerly known as cerebrovascular arteriosclerosis), Pick's disease, Parkinson's disease dementia, and other forms comprise the balance (Williams, 1995). It has been estimated that irreversible dementias occur in about 90% of persons with dementia (Bravyak & Schechter, 1992).

Reversible dementias may be caused by drugs, emotion, metabolic or endocrine alterations, nutrition, trauma, infection, alcoholism, and systemic illness. The medications most associated with this type of dementia include anticholinergic agents, cardiac drugs, selected antihypertensives and psychotropics. Box 23-3 lists selected potentially reversible causes of dementia.

BOX 23-3

Potentially Reversible Causes of Dementia

Drugs, chemicals, or toxins
- a. Bromides
- b. Mercury
- c. Drugs such as butyrophenones, phenothiazines, diuretics, sedatives

Emotional problems
- a. Depression
- b. Chronic alcoholism

Metabolic disorders
- a. Hyperglycemia
- b. Hypothyroidism
- c. Hypopituitarism

Eye/ear deprivation
- a. Blindness
- b. Deafness

Nutritional deficits
- a. Vitamin B_{12} deficiency
- b. Folic acid deficiency
- c. Niacin deficiency

Tumors/trauma, acute
- a. Subdural hematoma
- b. Brain metastasis
- c. Brain tumors

Infections and/or fever
- a. Viral infections
- b. Bacterial (tuberculosis)
- c. Bacterial (endocarditis)

Arteriosclerotic events
- a. Vascular occlusion
- b. Stroke

Modified from Lamay PP (1980). *Prescribing for the elderly*. Littleton, CO: PSG Publishing.

The syndrome of dementia usually develops slowly. Early signs include depression, loss of ability to concentrate, and increased anxiety, irritability, and agitation. Intellectual ability is usually the first to decline; then recent memory (such as names of acquaintances or recent events); followed by the loss of orientation to time, place, and person. Personal habits will change. The person may become loud or obscene, or some personality characteristics that were present might become magnified.

Helplessness, total dependency, and loss of manual skills may occur next. In the final stages, the person may be bedridden with loss of sphincter control and eventually will die, usually of bronchopneumonia.

The prescriber should rule out all the possible reversible causes of dementia first. Then treatment should be instituted to try to prevent or reduce the ongoing damage and to support the client and family in managing this disease process. Drug treatment is only indicated for symptom control, that is, the use of low-dose antipsychotic agents for treating severe agitation, delusions, and hallucinations, or antidepressants for severe depression. Supportive care should include proper nutrition, moderate exercise if permitted, vitamins if indicated, and the use of environmental aids in a consistent fashion, such as night lights and daily calendar reminders.

ALZHEIMER'S DISEASE

Alzheimer's disease is a presenile dementia characterized by confusion, memory failure, disorientation, restlessness, speech disturbances, and hallucinosis, and is tragically incurable. It affects approximately 4 million Americans with about 250,000 new cases diagnosed annually (Lamy, 1992). It has been estimated to be the major underlying reason for over 50% of all nursing home admissions (Miller, 1995). It has been estimated that approximately 3% of Americans over the age of 65 have Alzheimer's disease, which increases with age to 19% in persons between 75 and 84 years old and 47% in elders 85 years and older (Miller, 1995).

Clinically, a progressive decline in intellectual functions is noted, such as memory loss, loss of logical thinking or judgment, time and space disorientation, and an increased tendency to wander as a result of progressive disorientation. As the disease progresses, profound memory loss, personality changes, hyperactivity, hostility, and paranoia may present. This middle phase in Alzheimer's disease is also characterized by the presence of aphasia (loss of speech or ability to express oneself), apraxia (loss of complex or intentional movements), and anomia (loss of ability to remember names of persons and objects). In the terminal phase, nearly all higher mental functioning is lost and the person needs assistance with activities of daily living; thus the person requires continuous nursing care.

In this final period clients may be unable to speak intelligibly, walk, sit up in bed, eat or groom themselves, smile, or recognize simple objects or familiar persons. Table 23-3 explains the Staging of Cognitive Decline.

In the terminal or last phase, the client wants to touch or examine all objects with the mouth (hyperorality), exhibits a decrease or loss in emotions, may be bulimic, and may also have a compulsion to touch everything in sight. Insomnia, nighttime wandering, and restlessness have also been reported. The progressive deterioration of brain cells may lead to increased dependency for all needs, decreased mobility to the point of being bedridden, and eventually death.

While researchers are still searching for the cause of Alzheimer's disease, many theories have been proposed. Currently the theories under study include: (1) a deficiency in acetylcholine, a major neurotransmitter, and perhaps other neurotransmitters in the brain; (2) a slow virus or infection that attacks selected brain cells; (3) genetic predisposition; (4) autoimmune theory—that the body fails to recognize host tissue and attacks itself; and (5) beta-amyloid protein accumulation in the CNS (Williams, 1995). A primary hypothesis is that Alzheimer's disease results from the loss of related cholinergic nerves in the CNS (Miller, 1995).

Current pharmacotherapy is directed toward improving cognitive functioning or limiting disease progression and symptom control.

Unfortunately, no known current medication cures, retards, or prevents Alzheimer's disease. Two medications, the ergoloid mesylates (Hydergine) and tacrine (Cognex), have been approved by the Food and Drug Administration (FDA) to treat memory deficits. The ergoloid mesylates have been used to treat early dementia but its use is controversial in Alzheimer's disease. One study reported no improvement with its use and instead, some worsening of cognitive ability and behaviors (*USP DI*, 1996).

▲ **Tacrine** (Cognex), a centrally acting cholinesterase inhibitor, has a longer duration of action than physostigmine. This product appears to improve cognitive function in a limited number of persons with mild to moderate Alzheimer's disease. Side effects include nausea, vomiting, diarrhea, headache, ataxia, and muscle aches. Hepatic alterations such as hepatocellular necrosis, jaundice, and increases in serum alanine aminotransferase have been reported. Weekly monitoring of serum alanine aminotransferase for the first 18 weeks of therapy is recommended. Afterward the testing may be reduced to every 3 months. The oral adult dose is 10 mg four times daily, increased at 6-week intervals as necessary. The maximum daily dose is 160 mg (Williams, 1995). The benefits from tacrine have been limited, and therefore many other drugs are under investigation. These agents include the nonsteroidal antiinflammatory agents (piracetam [Nootropil], oxiracetam and indomethacin [Indocin]); velnacrine maleate (Mentane), a centrally acting cholinesterase inhibitor; nimodipine (Nimotop) a calcium antagonist; and selegiline (Eldepryl), an MAO-B inhibitor that may have antioxidant effects and also increases serotonin and norepinephrine concentrations (Eggert & Crismon, 1994; Bravyak & Schechter, 1992). It has also been reported that postmenopausal women treated with estrogen were less likely to get Alzheimer's than those that were untreated (Williams, 1995). Serotonin antagonists and angiotensin-converting enzyme (ACE) inhibitors are also under investigation. To date the etiology and effective treatment for Alzheimer's disease are still unknown.

TABLE 23-3 Staging of cognitive decline

Stage	Clinical phase	Symptoms
1	Normal	No change in cognition
2	Very mild	Forgets object location, some deficit in word finding
3	Mild (early confusion)	Early cognitive decline in one or more areas; memory loss, decreased ability to function in work situation, name-finding deficit, some decrease in social functioning, recall difficulties, anxiety
4	Moderate	Unable to perform complex tasks such as managing personal finances, planning a dinner party, concentration, and knowledge of current events
5	Moderately severe (early dementia)	Usually needs assistance for survival; reminders to bathe, help in selecting clothes, and other daily functions; may be disoriented as to time and recent events although this can fluctuate; may become tearful
6	Severe (dementia)	Needs assistance with dressing, bathing, and toilet functions (flushing, etc.); may forget spouse, family, and caregivers names, details of their personal life, and generally be unaware of their surroundings; incontinence of urine and feces may occur in this stage; increase in CNS disturbances such as agitation, delusions, paranoia, obsessive anxiety and increase potential for violent behavior
7	Very severe (late dementia)	Unable to speak (speech limited to 5 words or less), person may scream or make other sounds; unable to ambulate, sit up, smile, or feed themselves; unable to hold head erect, will ultimately slip into stupor or coma

BOX 23-4

Donepezil (Aricept)

Donepezil is the second drug approved by the Food and Drug Administration for symptomatic treatment of Alzheimer's disease. This product inhibits the enzyme acetylcholinesterase, which permits an increased accumulation of acetylcholine in the brain. It is indicated for mild to moderate Alzheimer's disease.

Side/adverse effects include nausea, diarrhea, vomiting, muscle cramps, dizziness, and insomnia. The usual dose is 5 mg or 10 mg daily (Olin, 1997).

See Box 23-4 for donepezil, the second drug released for the treatment of Alzheimer's disease.

Symptom management includes small dosages of antipsychotic agents such as haloperidol (Haldol), 0.5 to 5 mg/day, for delusions and hallucinations. Two precautions exist however: first, start with a low dosage and only gradually increase it if necessary. Monitor the client closely for side effects. Second, be aware that antipsychotic agents or any medications with a high anticholinergic potential could worsen the cognitive functioning of the client.

For depression, antidepressants with a low anticholinergic profile, such as desipramine (Norpramin) or trazodone (Desyrel, Trazon), have been used. Start at one third to one half the usual adult dose for clients with Alzheimer's disease and increase slowly as necessary. The antianxiety agents, especially those with a short-to-intermediate half-life, such as lorazepam (Ativan), oxazepam (Serax), or alprazolam (Xanax), are generally selected for clients who exhibit severe anxiety. Be aware that if such agents are used to treat agitation in clients with dementia (or specifically, Alzheimer's disease), the potential for inducing a paradoxical reaction is present. Such clients may respond with an increase in activity, restlessness, and agitation. So it is important for the prescriber to differentiate between agitation and anxiety. If the benzodiazepine antianxiety agents are used, they should be closely monitored because symptoms change with time. Short-term use or reevaluation at least every 3 to 6 months is necessary.

Nursing Management

Drug Therapy for Alzheimer's Disease

In the pharmacologic management of clients with Alzheimer's disease, care needs to be taken to provide for their safety and comfort. The nurse should understand that the elderly excrete and metabolize most of the medications prescribed for the treatment of Alzheimer's disease less efficiently. Smaller dosages are required to produce the desired effect. The nurse's assessment and documentation of subtle changes in the client's health status will allow prescribers to individualize medication dosages more closely. Drugs that have the side effects of depression, confusion, and alteration of sleep patterns, or those that compromise respiratory function should be avoided.

Alzheimer's disease remains, in many ways, a perplexing illness. Besides providing appropriate care, the nurse should keep abreast of medical and nursing research findings, be committed to conducting nursing studies on the care of clients with Alzheimer's disease, and share ideas about effective nursing interventions with colleagues.

SKELETAL MUSCLE RELAXANTS

Most muscle strains and spasms are self-limited and respond to rest and physical therapy and short-term skeletal muscle relaxants. However, **spasticity** (a form of muscular hypertonicity with increased resistance to stretch) as the result of stroke, closed head injuries, cerebral palsy, multiple sclerosis, spinal cord trauma, and other neurologic disorders requiring long-term use of these agents will challenge the nurse's rehabilitative skills and knowledge. In both short- and long-term care, the nurse's role, in addition to medication administration, is to provide comfort and rehabilitative measures in collaboration with physical therapists and other members of the health care team.

Neuromuscular Junction

Skeletal muscles are striated (striped) muscles attached to the skeleton. They are usually under voluntary control. These muscles produce body movements, maintain body position against the force of gravity, and counteract environmental stressors such as wind. A muscle is made of numerous muscle cells or muscle fibers. Each muscle cell is connected to only one motor nerve fiber, but each of the nerve fibers is connected to several muscle cells. Therefore stimulation of one nerve fiber will cause stimulation and activation of a group of muscle cells. The region where a motor nerve fiber makes functional contact with a skeletal muscle fiber (synaptic contact) is known as the neuromuscular junction.

Skeletal Muscle Spasm and Spasticity

Skeletal muscle **spasms** result when there is an involuntary contraction of a muscle or group of muscles that is accompanied by pain or limited function. Most skeletal muscle spasms are caused by local injuries, but some may result from low calcium levels or epileptic myoclonic seizures. Each type of spasm is treated according to its cause.

Skeletal muscle injuries are usually self-limiting and can be treated with rest; physical therapy; immobility by use of casts, neck collars, crutches, or arm slings; or whirlpool baths. With tissue damage and edema, however, antiinflammatory drugs may be used.

Central skeletal muscle relaxants are used mainly for conditions in which muscle spasms do not quickly respond to other forms of therapy. Such conditions include musculoskeletal strains and sprains, trauma, and cervical or lumbar radiculopathy as a result of degenerative osteoarthritis, herniated disk, spondylosis, or laminectomy. Unlike diazepam (Valium), the centrally acting drug, baclofen (Lioresal), which is used for skeletal muscle spasticity, has not been found useful in the treatment of muscle spasms.

Skeletal muscle spasticity, characterized by skeletal muscle hyperactivity, occurs when gamma motor neurons (which tonically control muscle spindle contractile activity) become hyperactive. There are two primary types of muscle spasticity: spinal and cerebral. Spinal spasticity can be identified by a marked loss of inhibitory influences with hyperactive tendon stretch reflexes, clonus (alternate contraction and relaxation of muscles), primitive flexion withdrawal reflexes, and a flexed posture. Varying degrees of spasticity of the bladder and bowel can also be seen. Cerebral spasticity has less reflex excitability, increased muscle tone, and no primitive flexion withdrawal reflexes or flexed posture. **Dystonia,** an impairment of muscle tone, may also be present in individuals with cerebral spasticity.

Muscle spasticity is most commonly seen in clients with central nervous system injuries and strokes. Moderate to severe spasticity can be seen in two thirds of clients with multiple sclerosis. Individuals with cerebral palsy and rare neurologic disorders can also have muscle spasticity, but it is seen less frequently in these instances.

Central-acting and direct-acting skeletal muscle relaxants are the drugs of choice in the treatment of muscle spasticity. These drugs include baclofen (Lioresal), diazepam (Valium), and dantrolene (Dantrium). They are more effective in the treatment of spinal spasticity than cerebral spasticity. However, optimal therapy cannot be achieved in the treatment of either unless physical therapy is given concurrently.

CENTRAL-ACTING SKELETAL MUSCLE RELAXANTS

The exact mechanism of action of the central skeletal muscle relaxants is not known. Action results from CNS depression in the brain (brainstem, thalamus, and basal ganglia) and spinal cord that results in relaxation of striated muscle spasm. Removal of the central nervous depressive action from the skeletal muscle relaxation action of the central-acting skeletal muscle relaxants is not possible currently. As a result, these drugs create the side effects of drowsiness, blurred vision, lightheadedness, headache, and feelings of weakness, lassitude, and lethargy that make their long-term use undesirable. The drugs used primarily as antispastic agents are baclofen, diazepam, and dantrolene. Dantrolene, a direct-acting skeletal muscle relaxant (peripheral action) is discussed later in this chapter.

■ Nursing Management

Central-Acting Skeletal Muscle Relaxant Therapy

Assessment. The client should be assessed for a history of allergic reaction to the specific agent. Central nervous system depression may be exacerbated with the administration of central-acting muscle relaxants, so caution should be taken with these clients. The drugs should also be used cautiously in the presence of hepatic or renal dysfunction and in pregnant women. The FDA disapproves of prolonged administration of these drugs and discourages their use for periods longer than 3 weeks.

Obtain a baseline assessment of the client's spasticity: frequency, location, severity, and factors that exacerbate and ameliorate the spasm.

Nursing diagnosis. Once the client begins taking a central-acting skeletal muscle relaxant, the nurse's assessment should consider the potential development of a number of nursing diagnoses/collaborative problems related to the effects of the drug. Because of the CNS effects of the drug, the client may experience altered thought processes (confusion), activity intolerance related to weakness, and a risk for injury related to ataxia, drowsiness, dizziness, or syncope. Elimination patterns may be altered, such as with constipation and urinary frequency. Altered comfort may evidence as muscle weakness, nausea, headache, stomach discomfort, hiccough, and rash.

Sensory-perceptual alterations (visual and auditory hallucinations) may also occur. With overdosage, the potential complications of seizures and respiratory depression exist.

Implementation

Monitoring. Document the progress of the client's muscle spasticity. Assess for the nursing diagnoses/collaborative problems above.

Intervention. For ease of administration, the tablets may be crushed and mixed with fluid, jelly, or other food. The drugs should be administered with meals or milk to prevent the side effects of nausea, vomiting, heartburn, and abdominal distress associated with large doses.

Education. Inform individuals taking these agents to avoid activities that require mental alertness, judgment, and physical coordination, such as operating dangerous machinery or driving an automobile. Instruct the client that alcohol and other CNS depressants will increase the CNS effects of these drugs. Because many clients have postural hypotension with these medications, clients should be cautioned about standing suddenly and instructed to rise slowly, in keeping with individual physical limitations.

Evaluation. The client will demonstrate increased comfort, decreased involuntary movement and muscle tonicity, and increased range of motion without adverse effects of the drug.

▲ **baclofen** [bak' loe fen] (Lioresal)

Baclofen, a GABA inhibitory neurotransmitter, inhibits transmission of monosynaptic and polysynaptic reflexes. Although its exact mechanism of action is unknown it is a spasmolytic agent at the spinal level, where it inhibits transmission. It is used in the treatment of spasticity resulting from multiple sclerosis or from injuries to the spinal cord. Baclofen may reduce pain in spastic patients by inhibiting substance P release in the spinal cord (Katzung, 1992).

Absorption is generally good but may vary with different individuals. Time to peak concentration is 2 to 3 hours. Onset of action is variable and may occur in hours or up to weeks. Baclofen has a half-life of 2.5 to 4 hours and a therapeutic serum level of 80 to 400 ng/ml. Baclofen is metabolized in the liver and excreted in the kidneys.

The side/adverse effects of baclofen include transient drowsiness, vertigo, confusion, sleepiness, weakness, and nausea. Adult dose is 5 mg orally three times daily, increased by 5 mg per dose every 3 days until desired response is

Case Study
The Client Receiving Skeletal Muscle Relaxants

Jimmy Culver is a 17-year-old male high school student who sustained a T3–T4 spinal cord injury a year ago as a result of being in a car accident. He has been hospitalized for a recurrent urinary tract infection and (R) ischial decubitus ulcer. Additionally, he has severe muscle spasms in his lower extremities. The prescriber has ordered baclofen (Lioresal) 10 mg PO bid and diazepam (Valium) 10 mg PO bid for his muscle spasms.

1. What should a baseline assessment of Jimmy include before the administration of baclofen and diazepam is begun?
2. Jimmy tells you that he is still having the muscle spasms, even after he has been taking baclofen for a week. What should you tell him?
3. What side effects of baclofen should Jimmy or his parents be looking for?
4. If for some reason Jimmy stops taking baclofen, what adverse reactions should be looked for?
5. Jimmy tells you that sometimes he experiences severe nausea and abdominal distress after taking tablets between classes. How can you help alleviate his discomfort?

achieved, not to exceed 80 mg/day. Dosage for children has not been determined.

■ Nursing Management
Baclofen Therapy

In addition to the nursing management discussed as appropriate to central-acting skeletal muscle relaxant therapy in general, baclofen requires the following management. (See also the case study above.)

Assessment. The combination of baclofen and alcohol or other CNS depressants may result in enhanced CNS depressant effects and hypotension. Monitor closely because reduction in dosage of one or both drugs may be necessary.

Nursing diagnosis. Some clients receiving baclofen, particularly by intrathecal administration, may experience activity intolerance related to decreased extensor tone as an effect of the drug. Risk of injury related to drowsiness (up to 63%), dizziness (up to 15%), confusion (up to 11%) is a significant nursing diagnosis with the administration of baclofen. Others to be considered are: constipation (2% to 6%), altered thought processes (paranoia), sexual dysfunction in males, altered urinary pattern (2% to 6%), and altered comfort (nausea, nervousness).

Implementation

Monitoring. Administration of baclofen may increase the diabetic client's blood glucose levels, thus requiring an adjustment of the insulin dosage during therapy and when baclofen therapy is stopped. Geriatric clients are at risk for adverse CNS reactions. They should be assessed for the development of altered thought processes, such as hallucinations, depression, confusion, and excessive sedation. Observe for increased seizure activity in clients with epilepsy because the seizure threshold may be lowered. Monitor the client's clinical state and EEG results during therapy.

Intervention. The dosage should be increased gradually to therapeutic levels to decrease the incidence of adverse effects. A gradual reduction in dosage over a period of 2 weeks is recommended, since abrupt withdrawal may cause hallucinations, paranoia, nightmares, confusion, and rebound spasticity.

Education. Tell the client that the maximum benefit of the medication may not be reached for 1 to 2 months.

If abrupt withdrawal is required, instruct the client that hallucinations and rebound spasticity may occur. Alert the client to possible side effects such as dermatitis, CNS effects, and syncope. If orthostatic hypotension is a concern, instruct the client to come to an upright position slowly and stay seated until the lightheadedness dissipates.

Evaluation. The client will experience increased comfort and demonstrate decreased involuntary movement and muscle tonicity and increase range of motion without adverse effects of the drug.

diazepam [dye az' e pam] (Valium, Apo-Diazepam ♣)

While the mechanism of action for diazepam is unknown, it appears to act primarily by inhibiting afferent spinal polysynaptic (and possibly monosynaptic) pathways. It may also directly suppress muscle function at the neuromuscular synapse. Diazepam is used in the treatment of skeletal muscle spasm caused by reflex spasm to local pathologic conditions, such as inflammation of muscle and joints or secondary to trauma. It is also used to treat spasticity caused by upper motor neuron disorders (cerebral palsy and paraplegia), athetosis, tetanus, and stiff-man syndrome (to overcome the widespread chronic muscular rigidity, pain, and skeletal muscle spasms). See Chapter 16 for more information on diazepam.

■ Nursing Management
Diazepam Therapy

In addition to the nursing management discussed as appropriate to central-acting muscle relaxant therapy in general, greater detail relating to diazepam may be found in Chapter 16. Some unique nursing management of diazepam muscle relaxant therapy follows:

Assessment. Baseline vital signs should be assessed before diazepam is given and then frequently after the injection.

Implementation

Monitoring. Observe clients, particularly the elderly, for oversedation and impairment of coordination. Clients

TABLE 23-4 Other central-acting skeletal muscle relaxants: pharmacokinetics

Drug	Onset of action	Time to peak concentration (hr)*	Peak serum concentration*	Duration of action (hr)	Half-life (hr)	Metabolism/ excretion
carisoprodol	30 min	4 (350 mg)	4-7 μg/ml	4-6	8	liver/kidneys
chlorphenesin	N/A	1 to 3	3.8-17 μg/ml (800 mg)	N/A	2.5-5	liver/kidneys
chlorzoxazone	within 60 min	1 to 2	10-30 μg/ml (750 mg)	3-4	1-2	liver/kidneys
cyclobenzaprine	within 60 min	3 to 8	15-25 ng/ml (10 mg)	12-24	24-72	GI tract and liver/kidneys
metaxalone	60 min	2 (800 mg)	295 μg/ml (800 mg)	N/A	2-3	liver/kidneys
methocarbamol	PO, within 30 minutes	2 (2 g)	16 μg/ml (2 g)	N/A	0.9-2.2	may be liver/ kidneys and feces
	IV, immediate	nearly immediate	19 μg/ml (1 g)	N/A		
orphenadrine						
extended release	within 60 min	6 to 8 (100 mg)	60-120 ng/ml (100 mg)	12	14†	liver/kidneys and feces
IM	5 min	½ (60 mg)				
IV	immediate	immediate				
orphenadrine HCl	within 60 min	3 (50 mg)	110-210 ng/ml (100 mg)	8	14†	liver/kidneys and feces

N/A, not available.
*Single dose.
†Parent drug half-life. Metabolites may range between 2 and 25 hours.

undergoing long-term therapy can become physically dependent on the drug and show signs and symptoms of withdrawal when the drug is discontinued.

Intervention. Diazepam is insoluble in water, and so the parenteral form is prepared in a specific solvent. Do not mix or dilute parenteral dosages with other fluids or add to intravenous fluids. Administer intramuscular injections slowly and deeply into a large muscle to diminish local irritation.

Administer intravenous diazepam slowly, at least 1 minute for each 5 mg of the drug, to prevent apnea, hypotension, bradycardia, or cardiac arrest. After receiving a parenteral dosage, the client should be observed and should stay in bed for at least 3 hours. Resuscitative equipment should be available. To avoid phlebitis and venous thrombosis, small veins on the back of the hand and wrist should not be used for intravenous administration. To minimize the occurrence of thrombophlebitis after intravenous administration of diazepam, flush the vein with 1 ml of saline per 1 mg of diazepam.

Continuous intravenous infusion is not recommended because diazepam may precipitate in the infusion bag and the medication may be adsorbed to the plastic of infusion bags and tubing. If the drug cannot be administered by direct intravenous infusion, it may be injected through the intravenous tubing, but the injection should be as close as possible to the insertion point.

Education. The client should be alerted to the risk for injury related to the drug's CNS effects of drowsiness, dizziness, and confusion.

Evaluation. The client will report feeling relaxed and demonstrate decreased involuntary movement and muscle tonicity and increased range of motion without adverse effects of the drug.

Other Central-Acting Skeletal Muscle Relaxants

carisoprodol [kar eye soe proe' dole] (Soma)
chlorphenesin carbamate [klor fen' e sin] (Maolate)
chlorzoxazone [klor zox' a zone] (Paraflex)
cyclobenzaprine [sye kloe ben' za preen] (Flexeril)
metaxalone [met ax' ah lone] (Skelaxin)
methocarbamol [meth oh kar' ba mole] (Robaxin, Marbaxin)
orphenadrine [or fen' a dreen] (Disipal)
orphenadrine extended-release (Norflex)

Muscle spasms are treated with central-acting skeletal muscle relaxants that are analogs to various antianxiety medications. The exact mechanism of action of these drugs has not been determined, but it is believed the muscle relaxant effects of many of these drugs may be related to this CNS-depressant activity. Carisoprodol interferes with nerve transmission in the descending reticular formation and spinal cord while chlorzoxazone produces its effects in the spinal cord and subcortical brain areas. In addition to skeletal muscle relaxant effects, orphenadrine is also an analgesic.

These drugs are used in adjunct treatment for skeletal muscle spasms along with rest and physical therapy. For information on their pharmacokinetics, see Table 23-4. The side/adverse effects of these central-acting skeletal muscle re-

TABLE 23-5 Central-acting muscle relaxants: dosage and administration

Drug	Adults	Children
carisoprodol (Soma)	350 mg PO 4 times daily	Under 5 yr, not recommended; 5-12 yr 6.25 mg/kg 4 times daily.
chlorphenesin (Maolate)	800 mg PO 3 times daily initially; later decreased to 400 mg 4 times daily	Not determined
chlorzoxazone (Paraflex)	250-750 mg PO 3-4 times daily, adjusted as necessary	20 mg/kg in 3 or 4 divided doses daily
cyclobenzaprine (Flexeril)	20-40 mg daily in divided doses	Not determined
metaxalone (Skelaxin]	800 mg PO 3-4 times daily	Not determined
methocarbamol (Robaxin)	1.5 g PO 4 times daily for 2-3 days, increased if necessary; parenteral: 1-3 g IM or IV daily for 3 days	Not determined
orphenadrine (Disipal, Norflex)	50 mg PO 3 times daily or 100 mg twice daily for extended-release dosage; parenteral: 60 mg IM or IV every 12 hr	Not determined

laxants include drowsiness, dizziness, dry mouth, and abdominal distress. In addition, metaxalone (Skelaxin) may cause nausea, vomiting, increased excitability and restlessness while methocarbamol (Robaxin) and orphenadrine (Disipal) may cause visual disturbances.

When a skeletal muscle relaxant is given with alcohol, CNS depressants, or opioid analgesics, enhanced CNS depressant effects may occur. Monitor closely because the dosage of one or both drugs should be reduced. For the dosage and administration for these agents, see Table 23-5.

■ Nursing Management

Other Central-Acting Skeletal Muscle Relaxants

For all of the following drugs, see also the general discussion of the nursing management of central-acting skeletal muscle relaxant therapy.

Carisoprodol (Soma). Carisoprodol is found in the milk of lactating mothers at levels two to four times the maternal plasma concentration, causing sedation and gastrointestinal distress in the infant. Risk and benefit should be considered before using this drug for a pregnant or lactating client. Carisoprodol is contraindicated in clients with acute intermittent porphyria. On occasion, an idiosyncratic reaction to carisoprodol has occurred within minutes or hours of the first dose. Symptoms may include disorientation, agitation, vision disturbances, impaired verbal communication, and extreme weakness. The symptoms are temporary, but supportive therapy may be needed and may require hospitalization. There have been rare reports of psychologic dependence and abuse. Drowsiness is more frequent with carisoprodol than with most other muscle relaxants.

Chlorphenesin (Maolate). Watch for sensitivity reactions. Hold the dose and notify the prescriber if unusual reactions occur. Observe for unusual bleeding and indications of blood dyscrasia. Safety when used for longer than 8 weeks has not been determined.

Chlorzoxazone (Paraflex). Chlorzoxazone is contraindicated in individuals with hepatic disease. Liver function studies should be monitored closely during therapy because hepatotoxicity is a possible side effect. Tell the client that the drug may discolor the urine orange or purple-red. Drowsiness and/or dizziness is more common with chlorzoxazone than with most other muscle relaxants.

Metaxalone (Skelaxin). Metaxalone is contraindicated in individuals with renal and hepatic disease. Monitor liver function studies. Monitor blood studies because hemolytic anemia may occur. Clinitest and Benedict's solution may give a false-positive reading in urine tests of clients taking metaxalone. Use Clinistix, Diastix, or Testape instead. Caution the client to notify the prescriber if skin rash or yellowish discoloration of skin or eyes occurs (signs of liver-related jaundice). Gastrointestinal irritation with nausea, vomiting, and abdominal cramps is more common with metaxalone than with other muscle relaxants.

Methocarbamol (Robaxin, Marbaxin). Be aware that methocarbamol is not recommended for individuals receiving anticholinesterase agents or for those who have epilepsy or for those who are in renal failure (because this may increase preexisting acidosis and urea retention). Have epinephrine, injectable steroids, and/or injectable antihistamines available for IV injection to treat syncope should it occur. Anaphylactic reaction has occurred after IM and IV administration. Have the client recumbent during IV infusion and remain recumbent 10 to 15 minutes after infusion to decrease the incidence of adverse effects such as syncope, hypotension, and bradycardia.

Do not give subcutaneously. Administer deep (IM) injection to decrease local irritation. Avoid IV extravasation; thrombophlebitis, pain, and tissue sloughing may result. The IV infusion should not be refrigerated. In addition, its compatibility with other solutions is limited; see a specialized reference before mixing. It may be diluted in normal saline or 5% dextrose in water, but do not dilute to more than 10 ml (1 g) in 250 ml. If administering intravenously undiluted, inject at a rate not greater than 3 ml/min. Note that tablets may

TABLE 23-6 Dantrolene: dosage and administration

Adults	Children
Antispastic	
25 mg PO daily initially, increased by 25 mg as necessary every 4-7 days until adequate response or 100 mg 4 times a day is reached.	0.5 mg/kg PO twice daily, increased by 0.5 mg/kg/day as necessary every 4-7 days until adequate response or a 3 mg/kg four times a day until dosage is reached. Do not exceed 400 mg/day.
Prophylaxis for malignant hyperthermic crisis	
4-8 mg/kg PO in 3 or 4 divided doses daily for 24-48 hr before surgery. Last dose is given 3-4 hr before surgery, with minimum water. IV infusion: 2.5 mg/kg over 1 hr before anesthesia.	Not available
Acute malignant hyperthermic reaction	
IV push of minimum of 1 mg/kg; continue this dose until symptoms abate or maximum cumulative dose of 10 mg/kg is reached. After IV therapy, 4-8 mg/kg PO in four divided doses daily is given for 1-3 days.	See adult dose

Pregnancy Safety

Category	Drug
B	cyclobenzaprine
Unclassified	baclofen, diazepam,* carisoprodol, chlorphenesin, chlorzoxazone, metaxalone, methocarbamol, orphenadrine, dantrolene

*To be avoided during pregnancy, especially during the first trimester.

be crushed and suspended in water or saline for administration via a nasogastric tube.

Advise client to notify the prescriber if skin rash, itching, fever, or nasal congestion occurs. Tell the client that urine, if it is left standing, may darken to green, black, or brown.

Orphenadrine (Disipal). Use with caution in individuals with cardiac decompensation, coronary insufficiency, cardiac dysrhythmias, or tachycardia. Note that orphenadrine is contraindicated in clients with glaucoma, prostatic hypertrophy, obstruction of the neck of the bladder, and myasthenia gravis. Periodic blood, urine, and liver function studies should be done with prolonged therapy. Discuss side effects with the client.

See the Pregnancy Safety box above for FDA classification of the skeletal muscle relaxants.

Direct-Acting Skeletal Muscle Relaxant

dantrolene [dan' troe leen] (Dantrium)

Dantrolene is used in the prophylaxis and treatment of malignant hyperthermia (see Chapter 15) and spasticity, especially upper motor neuron disorders, such as multiple sclerosis, cerebral palsy, spinal cord insults, and cerebrovascular accident (CVA). Dantrolene acts directly on skeletal muscles to produce skeletal muscle relaxation by inhibiting the release of calcium from the sarcoplasmic reticulum to the myoplasm. This results in a decreased muscle response to the action potential and decreased muscle contraction. As an antispastic agent, dantrolene's direct effect on skeletal muscle dissociates the excitation-contraction coupling. This effect is probably induced by the interference with calcium ion release from the sarcoplasmic reticulum. Dantrolene reduces both monosynaptic- and polysynaptic-induced muscle contractions.

Dantrolene is available orally and parenterally. The drug's oral absorption is fair; onset of action when dantrolene is used to treat the spasticity of upper motor neurons is 1 week or more. The drug has a half-life (orally) of 8.7 hours (100-mg dose); the IV half-life is 4 to 8 hours. Time to peak concentration is 5 hours (oral dose). It is metabolized in the liver and excreted in the kidneys.

The side effects of dantrolene include diarrhea, dizziness, sleepiness, uncomfortable feelings, unusual fatigue, muscle weakness, nausea, and vomiting. Less frequently reported adverse effects include severe diarrhea, respiratory difficulty and respiratory depression. For dosage and administration, see Table 23-6.

■ Nursing Management

Dantrolene Therapy

Assessment. Dantrolene should not be administered to clients with active hepatic disease because of the increased risk for hepatotoxicity. Use caution in clients with impaired cardiac, hepatic, or pulmonary function. These precautions do not apply to the short-term intravenous use of dantrolene to treat malignant hyperthermia. Women over 35 are also at higher risk for hepatotoxicity. Lactose intolerant clients may also react adversely to dantrolene capsules, which contain lactose. Determine if there is sensitivity to dantrolene.

Careful assessment of the client is particularly important when dantrolene has been prescribed for spasticity. Because there is no way of knowing if a client will benefit without a clinical trial, the observations of the relief of spasticity are critical. The decision for long-term use of dantrolene depends on the balance between the drug-induced weakness and other adverse effects and the beneficial effects of the drug. Paraplegic clients may not consider the adverse effect of weakness as detrimental as spasticity. Ambulatory clients who use spasticity to remain upright or balance are not candidates for dantrolene therapy.

The client's current medications should be reviewed to detect significant drug interactions. The following effects may occur when dantrolene is given with the drugs listed below.

1. When given for short-term use (1 to 3 days) or chronic use with alcohol or CNS depressants: enhanced CNS depression may occur. Dosage of one or both drugs may need to be decreased. Monitor closely.
2. When given for chronic use only with hepatotoxic drugs: the risk of inducing liver toxicity increases. Women over 35 years of age taking estrogen products are at particular risk for this toxicity.
3. When given intravenously for malignant hyperthermia only, with the calcium channel-blocking agent, verapamil): avoid this combination while attempting management of a malignant hyperthermic emergency. There is some evidence to suggest these drugs may interact to produce cardiovascular collapse.

A baseline assessment of the client's involuntary movement, muscle tonicity, and range of motion should be determined. Because of the risk of hepatotoxicity, hepatic functions studies should be done before the start of chronic dantrolene therapy.

Nursing diagnosis. The client receiving dantrolene therapy is at risk for the following selected nursing diagnoses/collaborative problems: impaired physical mobility related to muscle spasm related to the ineffectiveness of the drug; impaired gas exchange related to respiratory depression; altered bowel elimination (diarrhea, constipation); altered urinary pattern (frequency); risk for injury related to dizziness, or weakness; altered comfort (headache, nausea); impaired skin integrity (acne-like rash); fatigue; or altered thought processes (depression) and the potential complication of pleural effusion with pericarditis, convulsions, hepatotoxicity, and thrombophlebitis.

Implementation

Monitoring. When dantrolene has been administered to prevent malignant hyperthermia, carefully monitor the client postoperatively for possible delayed effects of the drug. The client receiving long-term therapy should be monitored for blood cell counts and hepatic and renal functioning. The risk of hepatotoxicity is greater in clients with previous liver disease, those taking 800 mg daily in the short-term therapy or 200 mg daily for longer than 2 months, and women over 35 concurrently receiving estrogen therapy. Hepatitis most frequently occurs between 3 and 12 months into therapy and is generally preceded by gastrointestinal symptoms such as anorexia, nausea, and vomiting. Side effects may be minimized by starting with low dosages and increasing them gradually. With short-term use, diarrhea may be a concern and may be severe enough to discontinue therapy. In chronic use, constipation may occur and health teaching should focus on its prevention.

The client's spasticity should be assessed periodically early in therapy, but effects may not be seen for a week. If no improvement is noted after 45 days, therapy should be discontinued.

Intervention. The contents of the capsule may be mixed with fruit juice for oral administration to a client unable to swallow capsules. Administer immediately after mixing. When intravenous dantrolene is used to treat malignant hyperthermia, use of all anesthetic agents is discontinued, oxygen is administered, metabolic acidosis and fluid and electrolyte imbalances are corrected, and the client is cooled. Reconstitute intravenous dantrolene with 60 ml of sterile water for injection without a bacteriostatic agent and shake the mixture until it is clear. Use within 6 hours of preparation. Dantrolene is incompatible with acidic solutions, including 5% dextrose injection and 0.9% sodium chloride injection. Oral dantrolene may be given after the intravenous dose to prevent recurrence of symptoms. Avoid extravasation of intravenous dantrolene. It is painful and irritating to the tissue because of the high pH of the solution.

Dantrolene may be given, orally or IV, for malignant hyperthermic crisis prophylaxis: IV, administered over a 1 hour period before anesthesia; and orally, 1 to 2 days before surgery with the last dose 3 to 4 hours before scheduled surgery with a minimum of water.

Education. Caution clients that photosensitivity is possible with dantrolene, so they should avoid exposure to the sun. However, improvement should be seen within 45 days or the drug should be discontinued. Regular visits to the prescriber should be encouraged for assessment of progress and to monitor for side effects with blood studies. For other nursing considerations, see the nursing management of central-acting skeletal muscle relaxant therapy.

Evaluation. The client will demonstrate increased comfort and decreased involuntary movement and muscle tonicity and increased range of motion without adverse effects of the drug. If the drug is administered for malignant hyperthermia, the client will not demonstrate fever, cardiac arrhythmias, or muscle rigidity.

SUMMARY

The major CNS-neuromuscular disorders discussed in this chapter—Parkinson's disease, myasthenia gravis, dementia, Alzheimer's disease, and muscle spasticity—are progressive and often incapacitating syndromes. Pharmacologic therapy is essential for symptom control, which allows the client to function as independently as possible for as long as possible.

Clients with Parkinson's disease require correction of the disorder's imbalance of dopamine/acetylcholine. For that reason, the client is treated with drugs that have central anticholinergic activity, anticholinergics and antihistamines, and drugs that affect dopamine levels to enhance dopaminergic mechanisms. Because the condition is debilitating and long term, clients and caregivers require support and education to maintain compliance with the medication regimen.

Myasthenia gravis, characterized by skeletal muscle weakness and fatigue, is also progressive and incurable. Central to the treatment of this disorder are the anticholinesterase drugs.

For dementia and Alzheimer's disease the drug therapy is not as specific. Low doses of antipsychotic drugs are used in both disorders to control severe agitation, delusions, and hallucinations.

Pharmacologic agents administered as skeletal muscle relaxants affect skeletal muscle at the neuromuscular junction or at different levels in the central nervous system, such as the spinal cord or the brain. With central-acting skeletal muscle relaxants, the drugs' effects result from CNS depression in the brain and spinal cord. Direct-acting skeletal muscle relaxants affect striated muscle to dissociate the excitation-contraction coupling and so reduce monosynaptic- and polysynaptic-induced muscle contractions. Although most skeletal muscle spasm is the result of local injury, other instances may be of a more systemic nature; but the treatment of each type of spasm is related to its cause.

An essential part of the nurse's role is to identify the subtle changes in the client's health status in any of the discussed conditions, which enables the prescriber to individualize the medication regimen and sustain the highest quality of life for the client.

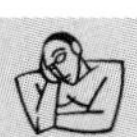

Critical Thinking

1. Mrs. Ross has been diagnosed with myasthenia gravis, for which she has been prescribed pyridostigmine syrup. Her most distressing symptom is a mild dysphagia. How could the nurse best manage Mrs. Ross's drug therapy?
2. Mrs. Kelly brings her 72-year-old husband to the clinic for a periodic assessment of his Alzheimer's disease and the effectiveness of his drug therapy. Formulate a line of inquiry to elicit from Mrs. Kelly information that will assist you to determine the effectiveness of his drug therapy.
3. To evaluate the effectiveness of skeletal muscle relaxant therapy for a client with spasticity, what would constitute an appropriate assessment of the client's status?
4. What would be essential to be included in a teaching plan for a client who would be self-administering muscle relaxant therapy?

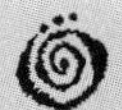

Collaborative Learning Activities

1. Three student teams will present the case study on the client with Parkinson's disease. The first team will cover the first questions related to Mr. Edwards' initial therapy. Team two will focus on his course of therapy after the first 2 years, and team three will discuss his response to the addition of amantadine to his therapy.

BIBLIOGRAPHY

American Hospital Formulary Service (1996). *AHFS drug information '96*. Bethesda, MD: American Society of Hospital Pharmacists.

American Medical Association (1995). *Drug evaluations: Annual 1995*. Chicago: The Association.

Anderson KN, et al. (Eds.) (1994). *Mosby's medical, nursing, & allied health dictionary* (4th ed.). St Louis: Mosby.

Bravyak JAT & Schechter BR (1992). *Alzheimer's disease management*. Philadelphia: Philadelphia College of Pharmacy and Science.

Cutson TM, et al. (1995). Pharmacological and nonpharmacological interventions in the treatment of Parkinson's disease, *Phys Ther* 75(5):363-73.

Eggert A & Crismon ML (1994). Current concepts in understanding Alzheimer's disease, *Clin Pharm Newswatch* 1(1):1-8.

Flaherty JF & Gidal BE (1995). Parkinson's Disease. In Young LY & Koda-Kimble MA (Eds.). *Applied therapeutics: The clinical use of drugs* (6th ed.). Vancouver: Applied Therapeutics.

Katzung BG (1992). *Basic and clinical pharmacology* (5th ed.). Norwalk, CT: Appleton & Lange.

Kernick CA, et al. (1995). Myasthenia gravis: Pathophysiology, diagnosis and collaborative care, *J Neurosci Nurs* 27(4):207-18.

Kimble MA (1996) *Applied therapeutics: The clinical use of drugs* (6th ed.). Vancouver, WA: Applied Therapeutics.

Lamy PP (1992). Alzheimer's disease: 1906-1991, *Elder Care News* 8(4):27-37.

Lopate G & Pestronk A (1993). Autoimmune myasthenia gravis, *Hosp Pract* 28(1):109.

Miller S (1995). Management strategies for the Alzheimer's disease patient, *Clin Consult* 14(1):1-9.

Schneider LS, et al. (1994). Emerging drugs for Alzheimer's disease: Mechanisms of action and prospects for cognitive enhancing medications, *Med Clin North Am* 78(4):911-34.

Segatore M, et al. (1995). The pharmacotherapy of spinal spasticity: A decade of progress. II. Therapeutics, *Sci Nurs* 12(1):2-7.

United States Pharmacopeial Convention(1996). *USP DI: Drug information for the health care professional* (16th ed.). Rockville, MD: The Convention.

Waldman HJ (1994). Centrally acting skeletal muscle relaxants and associated drugs, *J Pain Symptom Manage* 9(7):434-41.

Whitehouse PJ, et al. (1994). Pharmacotherapy for Alzheimer's disease, *Clin Geriatr Med* 10(2):339-50.

Williams BR (1995). Geriatric Dementias. In Young LY & Koda-Kimble MA. *Applied therapeutics: The clinical use of drugs* (6th ed.). Vancouver, WA: Applied Therapeutics.

Chapter 24
Overview of the Cardiovascular System

Chapter Focus

While progress has been made in increasing the public's awareness about lifestyle changes necessary to promote good cardiovascular health, more than 75 million people in North America have some type of cardiovascular disorder. Because one-third of all female deaths annually is due to heart disease, cardiovascular disease is the leading cause of death in American women (Sifton, 1994). "Heart disease kills more women each year than cancer, accidents, and diabetes combined" (Sifton, 1994, p. 127). As longevity increases, it can be expected that more people will be living with chronic cardiovascular conditions and coping with the results of acute ones. As a result, nurses will be providing care within acute facilities, as well as assisting clients to effectively manage their therapeutic cardiovascular regimens in a variety of community and home settings. A thorough knowledge of anatomy and physiology is essential for assessment of the client, interpretation of diagnostic examinations, provision of care, and client teaching. The following objectives and key terms are important for a good understanding of this chapter.

Key Terms

action potential (p. 481)
atria (p. 479)
automaticity (p. 483)
AV junction (p. 483)
cardiac output (p. 479)
conduction system (p. 483)
conductivity (p. 484)
depolarization (p. 481)
diastole (p. 482)
electrocardiogram (ECG) (p. 484)
electrophysiologic properties (p. 483)
myocardium (p. 479)
refractoriness (p. 484)
repolarization (p. 481)
rhythmicity (p. 483)
sarcomere (p. 479)
stroke volume (p. 483)
systole (p. 482)
ventricles (p. 479)

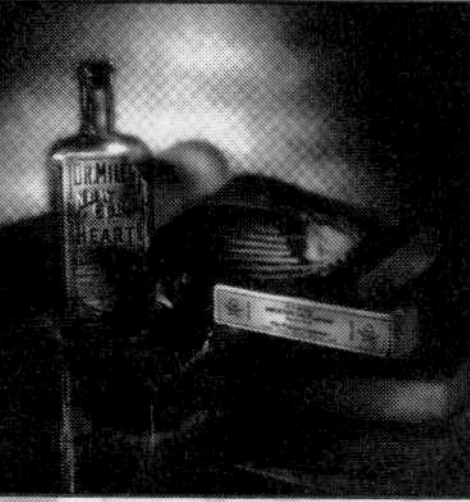

Objectives

1. Describe the anatomy and physiology of the heart.
2. Name the three major tissues of the heart.
3. Describe the role of electrical excitation in myocardial contraction.
4. Explain ion exchange during depolarization and repolarization of the myocardial cell.
5. Describe the events occurring in the cardiac cycles, systole and diastole.
6. Describe the vagus nerve's effect on the heart.
7. Describe the energy balance between expenditure and restoration maintained by the coronary blood vessels.

Rapidly developing science and technology have resulted in new knowledge and a greater understanding of cardiac activity. The resulting anatomic, electrophysiologic, and pharmacologic information has permitted greater precision in diagnosing and treating cardiac disease, particularly the dysrhythmias. Along with these advances has come the increased use of electrocardiographic monitoring of acutely ill clients and those with known or suspected cardiovascular disorders. In addition, the nurse's clinical role has expanded and now includes care of clients on many other types of monitoring equipment as well. This requires the nurse to recognize and understand abnormal electrocardiographic patterns and in some cases to begin therapy, including pharmacologic therapy, to prevent serious complications and unnecessary deaths. Therefore nurses must understand the electrical and physiologic properties of the heart and the effects drugs have on cardiac activity to keep their knowledge current and their nursing care therapeutically effective.

Microelectrode techniques have grown increasingly sophisticated and helped provide greater understanding of the electrical properties of cardiac fibers and the causes of various cardiac disorders. Fortunately, these advances have led to the discovery of new drugs that are useful in treating cardiac conditions.

Cardiac drugs largely affect three major tissues of the heart: cardiac muscle (myocardium), conduction system, and coronary vessels. In this chapter the normal function of these structures is discussed. The physiologic properties of these structures and the drug groups used therapeutically are summarized in Table 24-1.

THE HEART

The heart is a hollow muscular organ that consists of two main pumping chambers: the right ventricle, which is linked with the pulmonary circulation, and the left ventricle, which is connected to the systemic circulation. The cardiac muscle or myocardium is the largest and most important structure of the heart. As a contractile muscle, under normal conditions it can adapt its performance by adjusting the **cardiac output** according to the body's needs. Cardiac output is the volume of blood expelled by the ventricles of the heart, equal to the amount of blood ejected at each beat multiplied by the number of beats in the time used in computation. However, when the heart cannot produce a variable output, the therapeutic use of digitalis or cardiac glycosides (i.e., the digitalis drugs) produces changes at the cellular level. The following description of myocardial ultrastructure and the contractile process facilitates an understanding of the basic mechanisms in cardiac glycoside action.

Cardiac Muscle

The pumping action of the heart depends on the ability of the cardiac muscle to contract. The **myocardium,** a thick, contractile, middle layer of the heart, is composed of many interconnected branching fibers or cells that form the walls of the two **atria,** the upper chambers of the heart, and two **ventricles,** the two lower chambers of the heart. Each individual myocardial fiber contains a nucleus in the middle and a plasma membrane (cell membrane), the sarcolemma (Figure 24-1, 2 and 3). By joining end to end, the cells form a long fiber, with each cell separated from the other by a plasma membrane called the intercalated disk. This disk is believed to provide sites of low electrical resistance to permit the spread of exciting impulses throughout the cardiac muscle.

Each individual muscle fiber (cell) comprises a group of multiple parallel myofibrils, and each myofibril is arranged end to end in a series of repeating units called the **sarcomere,** (Figure 24-1, 4). By light microscope examination, the muscle fiber reveals its most characteristic feature, alternating light and dark bands. These bands result from crossing of the multiple parallel myofibrils, which are aligned in register with one another (Figure 24-1, 3). At the level known as the Z line, the sarcolemma of the muscle fiber interlocks (invaginates) at its end with the sarcomere to form the transverse sarcotubule or T system, which penetrates deeply into the cell. Furthermore, internal membranes form an extensive network called

TABLE 24-1 Effect of cardiac drug groups on cardiac tissues

Cardiac tissue	Physiologic property	Drug group	Pharmacologic action
Cardiac muscle (myocardium)	Force of myocardial contraction (Frank-Starling's law)	Cardiac glycosides	Positive inotropic effect—increases cardiac output
Sarcomere (functional unit)	Contractility and conductivity		
Cardiac conduction system	Automatically (rhythm and rate)	Antidysrhythmic drugs	Converts to normal sinus rhythm or abolishes dysrhythmia
	Conductivity	Calcium channel blockers	
Coronary arteries	Nutritional blood flow to myocardium and other cardiac structures	Antianginal drug Calcium channel blockers	Coronary vasodilation or lessens work of the heart

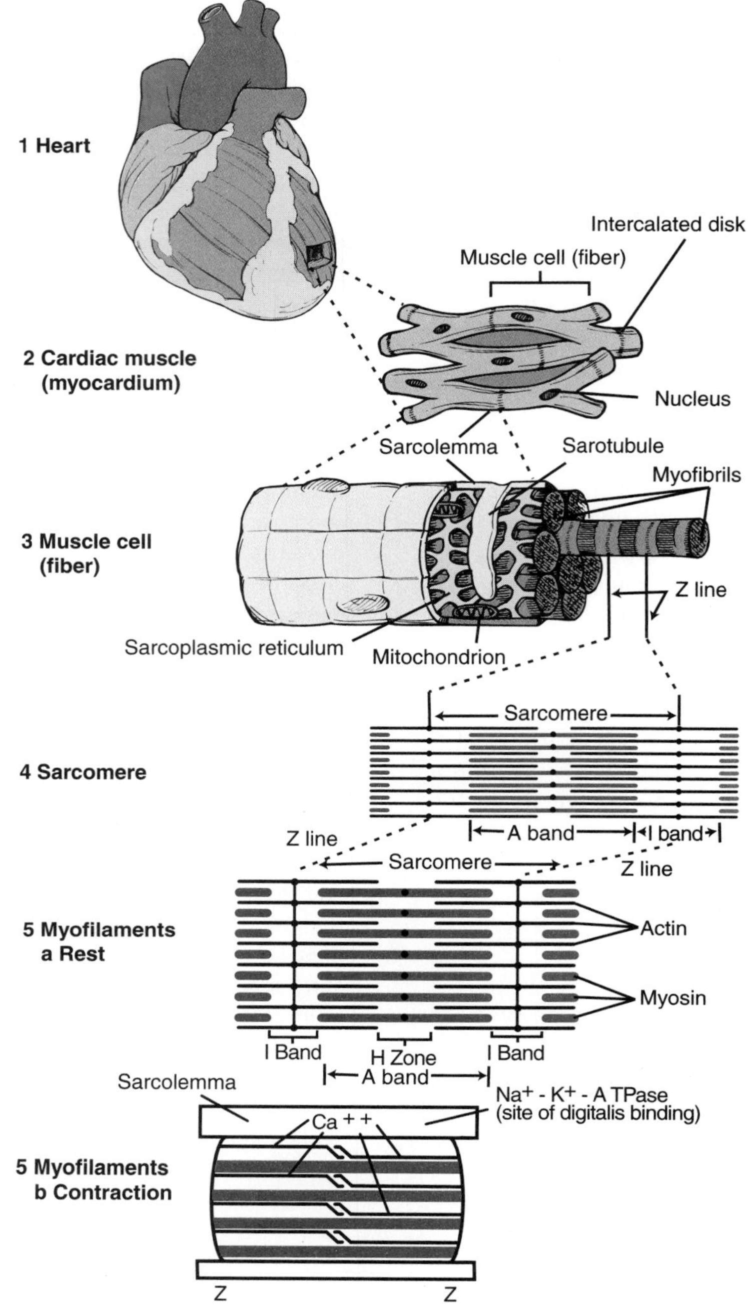

Figure 24-1 Structure of heart and cardiac muscle cell fibers. The heart (*1*) is mainly a muscular organ. The enlargement of the square illustrates a portion of the cardiac muscle (myocardium) (*2*), which is composed of myocardial cells. Each cell contains a centrally located nucleus and a limiting plasma membrane (sarcolemma), which forms the intercalated disk at the termination of each cell. An individual muscle cell (fiber) (*3*) consists of multiple parallel myofibrils. Each myofibril is arranged longitudinally in a series of light and dark repeating units, and the content of a unit is called a sarcomere. At the Z line, the sarcolemma invaginates to form the transverse sarcotubules or T system. An extensive network, called the sarcoplasmic reticulum, encircles groups of myofibrils and makes contact with the sarcotubules. The sarcoplasmic reticulum contains a high concentration of calcium ions. The mitochondria appear in long chains between the myofibrils. The sarcomere (*4*) is the unit of muscle contraction. It is composed of two types of bands, the A band and the I band. The latter is divided by the Z line. Myofilaments (*5*) of the sarcomere include the thin filament, actin, and the thick filament, myosin. The dark appearance of the A band is caused by the myosin and the lighter appearance of the I band by the actin. Here, the sarcomere is at rest (*a*). On contraction (*b*) the sarcomere shortens so that the thick filaments approach the Z line and the width of the H zone narrows between the thin filaments. Calcium ions are needed for systolic contractions.

the sarcoplasmic reticulum. This structure encircles groups of myofibrils and makes contact with the sarcotubules. The tremendous energy requirements for cardiac muscle contraction may be seen by the great numbers of mitochondria lined up in long chains between the myofibrils (Figure 24-1, *3*). Figure 24-1, *4*, shows the sarcomere, which is the basic unit of contraction in the heart. It lies between two successive Z lines and in part of the myofibril. The sarcomere consists of dark bands called A bands and lighter I bands. The end unit of the myofibril is the myofilament. The darkness of the A band results from the thicker myosin filaments, and the lightness of the I bands reflects the thinner actin filaments. Crossbridges, which are small projections that extend from the sides of the myosin filament, appear along the entire length of the thick filament. The interaction between these crossbridges of myosin and the active sites of actin produces contraction. In the sarcomere, the H zone represents the middle, less dense portion of the A band, and the myosin filament runs the entire length of this band. The I band, on the other hand, is divided by the Z line. The actin filament runs through the whole I band and terminates at the H zone. This arrangement is shown in Figure 24-1, *5*.

Myocardial Contraction

During the past decade our understanding of the fundamental mechanisms governing contraction of cardiac muscle in both normal and pathologic states has increased tremendously. Yet some aspects of this complicated process are still unknown. Cardiac muscle contraction begins with a rapid change in the cell membrane's electrical charge. This electrical current spreads to the interior of the cell where it causes release of calcium ions from the sarcoplasmic reticulum. The calcium ions then initiate the chemical events of contraction. The overall process for controlling cardiac muscle contraction, called excitation-contraction coupling, involves electrical excitation, mechanical activation, and contractile mechanisms.

Electrical excitation. Cardiac muscle contraction begins with electrical excitation or stimulus of the myocardial fiber. The source of electricity in the heart is found in the charges of ion concentration—mainly sodium, potassium, and calcium ions—across the cardiac cell membrane of the sarcolemma. The **action potential**, the difference in electrical charge, which produces the rapid ion changes, occurs in the membrane of the myocardial cell and results in a self-propagating series of polarization and depolarization. The *resting state* of an inactive muscle cell in the ventricle is created by the difference in electrical charge across the sarcolemma. In this case the inside of the cell is negative with respect to the cell's outside, which is positively charged. Because the sarcolemma separates these opposite charges, the membrane in effect is polarized. At rest, the extracellular environment is rich in sodium ions (Na^+) and the intracellular environment in potassium ions (K^+), with calcium ion (Ca^{++}) concentration in the region of the sarcolemma and where it invaginates on the sarcotubule (Figure 24-2, *B*).

The cardiac action potential is divided into two stages: **depolarization** (the stage in which an electrical impulse results in contraction of the ventricular muscle represented by the QRS interval on ECG), and **repolarization** (the recovery phase after muscle contraction represented by the T wave). These stages are subdivided into five phases of ionic changes. The resting potential of an inactive myocardial cell is called phase 4; in this phase the membrane is polarized with a charge of approximately −90 millivolts (mv). At this voltage the interior of the cell is negative with respect to the cell's exterior. During this time the membrane cannot be penetrated by ions. However, any stimulus that changes the resting membrane potential to a critical value, called the threshold, can generate an action potential. (Follow Figure 24-2, *A*, for steps of the action potential.)

Threshold may be reached by normal pacemaker activity or by propagation of an electrical impulse from a nearby cell, which opens the sodium channels. The fast inward current of sodium ions (fast channel), results in a membrane that is positively charged to +20 mv. This difference in membrane potential results in depolarization and is designated as phase 0 of the action potential. Phase 0 in the ventricular muscle is the contraction phase and is represented by QRS on the surface electrocardiogram. Soon after, the repolarization period occurs in three phases. The beginning of phase 1 is the overshoot, and it makes a brief change toward repolarization. Phase 2 is a slow period that forms a plateau with a slow inward current of calcium ions (slow channel) and outward flow of potassium ions. Calcium ion entry into the cell is essential for the excitation-contraction coupling mechanism, which will be explained later. Phase 3 is accomplished by rapid potassium ion efflux from the cell. After repolarization, phase 4 recovery or resting period ensues represented by the T wave, whereby the cell membrane actively transports sodium ions outside and potassium ions inside, returning the cell membrane to a state of rest or polarization. These cation exchanges during recovery require the energy-utilizing transport mechanism of the Na^+-K^+ pump, or Na^+-K^+ ATPase. The adenosine triphosphatase (ATPase), which is powered by oxygen, is an enzyme that is located in the cell membrane or sarcolemma; it furnishes the energy needed for active transport to return sodium ions and potassium ions to their original resting positions at the membrane. Digitalis plays a key role at this site. By binding to the sarcolemma Na^+-K^+-ATPase, digitalis inhibits the return of sodium ions and potassium ions to their resting positions. Consequently, digitalis allows more sodium ions and calcium ions to enter the cell to strengthen myocardial contraction. However, it is also thought that if an excessive amount of these ions appears intracellularly, digitalis toxicity may occur.

Mechanical activation. As previously stated, the unit that contracts is the sarcomere. It consists of two contractile proteins, actin and myosin. Myosin, the thicker filament, contains the ATPase enzyme system that is needed to hydrolyze ATP. Hydrolysis is required to provide the energy for contraction. ATP is synthesized in the mitochondria, which are normally abundant in cardiac muscle. Actin, the thin filament, is involved with calcium ion activity. These two filaments combine to help effect cardiac contraction.

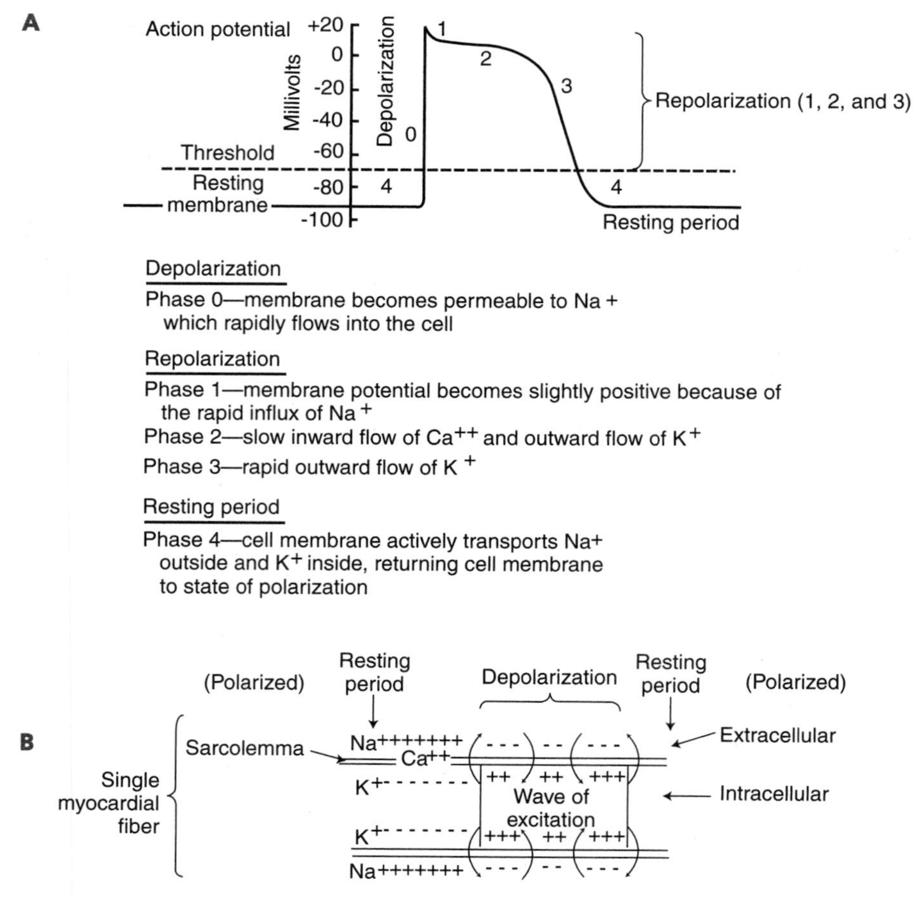

Figure 24-2 A, Action potential of a single myocardial fiber (cell). B, Ionic exchanges that occur across the cell membrane of a single myocardial fiber during an action potential.

Contraction is initiated when the nerve impulse reaches the myocardial cell and travels along the sarcolemma of the muscle fiber. As the depolarization wave spreads along the sarcotubules, it arrives at the sarcoplasmic reticulum, causing the release of its large quantities of calcium ions. These ions then bind to special receptors on the actin filaments. Hence the plateau, which is phase 2 of the action potential, is reached through the slow inward calcium current flow (slow channel). *Calcium ion movement is the chief component that links or couples electrical excitation of the sarcolemma with muscle activation of the myofilaments in the sarcomere.* Thus *mechanical activation* finally is accomplished when calcium ions bind to troponin, a regulator protein located on the actin filaments. This in turn mediates the interaction of actin and myosin.

Contractile mechanism. As soon as the actin filaments are activated by the calcium ions, the myosin filaments become attracted to the active sites of the actin filament. This interaction pulls the actin along the immobile myosin filaments toward the center of the A band, thus shortening the sarcomere and producing muscle contraction. In this process the lengths of individual filaments remain unchanged. The I band narrows as the thick filaments approach the Z line, and the H zone narrows between the ends of the thin filaments when they meet at the center of the sarcomere (Figure 24-1, *5a* and *5b*). The greater the quantity of calcium ions delivered to troponin, the faster the rate and numbers of interactions between actin and myosin. As a result of this response, the development of tension and contractility is increased.

When magnesium is present, ATP is cleaved by myosin ATPase. This reaction releases the energy needed to perform work. *The conversion of chemical energy to mechanical energy by ATP plays an essential role in energizing muscle shortening.* In other words, it provides the energy so the actin-myosin filaments move and produce muscle contraction. Although this is a somewhat simplified explanation of the contractile mechanism, it illustrates the important events pertinent to understanding cardiotonic drug action.

Finally, muscle relaxation depends on removing calcium ions from the sarcomere. The calcium ATPase (located in the walls of the sarcoplasmic reticulum) actively returns calcium ions to the sarcoplasmic reticulum and the sarcolemma, thereby allowing the actin-myosin filaments of the sarcomere to return to their resting positions.

In the normal heart, the Frank-Starling relationship holds true. This relationship means that the longer the muscle fibers are at the end of **diastole** (period of heart relaxation), the more forceful the contraction will be during **systole** (the period of contraction). This mechanism applies only when

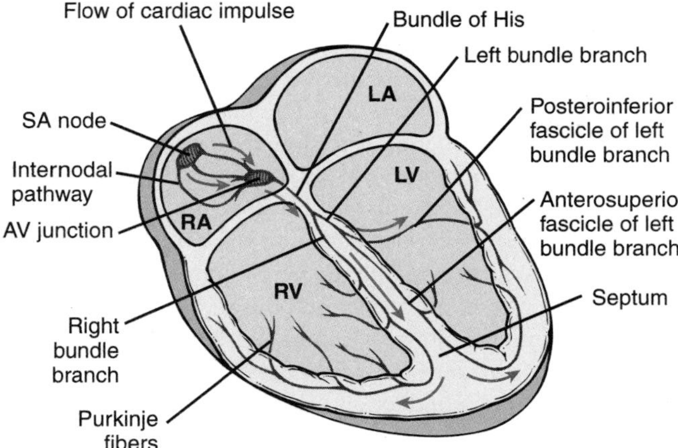

Figure 24-3 Conduction system of the heart. The cardiac impulse is initiated at the SA node and is transmitted through the internodal pathways to the two atria, resulting in atrial contraction. At the AV node, the electrical impulse is delayed. Conduction then speeds up at the bundle of His, with the impulse traveling through the right bundle branch and the left bundle branch and continuing through the posteroinferior fascicle and anterosuperior fascicle of the latter bundle branch. Finally, the arrival of impulses at the Purkinje fibers results in their distribution to all parts of both ventricles, where, upon excitation, ventricular contraction is produced. *RA,* Right atrium; *RV,* right ventricle; *LA,* left atrium; *LV,* left ventricle.

the muscle fiber is lengthened within physiologic limits. If a diseased heart is dilated and the fibers are stretched to a critical point beyond their limits of extensibility, the forces of contraction and cardiac output are both diminished and ineffective. Thus the functional significance of the Frank-Starling relationship is that effective cardiac output can be brought about only by adequate relaxation and refilling of cardiac chambers after each myocardial contraction.

Cardiac Conduction System

The effective pumping action of the heart depends on the regularity of events occurring in the cardiac cycle. Each cycle consists of a period of relaxation, diastole, followed by a period of contraction, systole. The rhythm and rate of the cardiac cycle are regulated by the **conduction system,** specialized tissue that has the ability to initiate and transmit the electrical impulses needed to stimulate contraction of the cardiac muscle.

The conduction system is made up of the following structures: (1) sinoatrial (SA) node, (2) internodal pathways, (3) atrioventricular (AV) node, (4) bundle of His, (5) right and left bundle branches, and (6) Purkinje fibers. The Purkinje fibers penetrate the endocardium and end in the myocardial cells. The AV node and the His area form the **AV junction,** which extends from the atrial fibers through the AV node to the bifurcation of the bundle of His. When referring to this region, the term *AV junction* is considered to be more accurate than *AV node* (Figure 24-3).

In the normal heart the SA node initiates the heartbeat. The impulses generated here are then conducted through the internodal pathways to the "working" fibers of the atrial myocardium, producing atrial contraction. When the impulses move through the AV junction, electrical conduction is delayed. However, at the bundle of His, conduction speeds up and the impulses travel through the right bundle branch and the left bundle branch, then through the posteroinferior and anterosuperior fascicles of the left bundle branch. The transmission of impulses at the Purkinje fibers, which consist of tiny fibrils that spread around the ventricles and connect directly with the myocardial cells, is very rapid. Finally, the simultaneous depolarization of both ventricles produces ventricular contraction, resulting in **stroke volume,** the volume of blood being propelled through the pulmonary artery and aorta by the ventricles.

Electrophysiologic Properties

The coordinated pumping action of the heart is initiated and regulated by the specialized fibers of the conduction system. The individual fibers of this system possess three basic **electrophysiologic properties:** (1) automaticity, (2) conductivity, and (3) refractoriness.

Automaticity. The specialized fibers of the conduction system have the inherent ability to spontaneously initiate an electrical impulse without any external stimuli. This is the most fundamental mechanism of impulse formation, and the cells that possess this property of **automaticity,** the ability to initiate an impulse, are called pacemaker cells. They are found in specialized conducting tissues such as the SA node, the AV junction, and the His-Purkinje system. Normally, the impulse of the heart is spontaneously and regularly initiated at the pacemaker cells of the SA node. During resting potential (phase 4), the membrane of the cell depolarizes itself—spontaneously and gradually—until it reaches threshold and an action potential occurs. The slow depolarization of the membrane in the resting state is called spontaneous diastolic depolarization, or phase 4 depolarization, and defines automaticity. Thus the membrane of pacemaker cells is never at rest, and this property is attributed to the continuous influx of sodium ions into the interior of the cells, which readily drives the membrane to threshold. The resting potential of automatic pacemaker cells differs from that of the nonautomatic myocardial cells. After full repolarization, the membrane of myocardial cells maintains a steady resting potential until an external stimulus causes it to achieve threshold. To summarize, automaticity is a property of fibers of the conduction system that normally controls heart rhythm; it is not a feature of "working" muscle—atria and ventricles. However, under pathologic conditions, myocardial cells do have the potential to exhibit spontaneous depolarization.

The spontaneous excitation of pacemaker cells establishes the normal rhythm of the heart. The regularity of such pacemaking activity is termed **rhythmicity.** Under normal circumstances, only one functional pacemaker, the SA node, predominates because it has the highest frequency of depolarization. The normal rate of impulse formation is about 72 beats/min. If the SA node decreases its rate of impulse formation to a level below the AV junction (40 to 60 beats/min), then the AV junction becomes the primary pacemaker of the heart and will drive the heart at about 40 beats/min.

Conductivity. **Conductivity** refers to the ability to transmit an action potential or nerve impulse from cell to cell. The property of conductivity therefore exists not only in the cells of the conduction system but also in the cardiac musculature. The speed of impulse conduction varies as it passes from one tissue to another in the heart. It is slowest in the AV junction and fastest in the Purkinje fibers. The significant delay of conduction at the AV junction allows more time for ventricular filling. On the other hand, the rapid depolarization of Purkinje fibers creates an instantaneous spread of impulses from the terminals to the ventricular muscles. Simultaneous activation of the musculature is essential for producing powerful ventricular contraction.

Velocity of conduction. The speed with which electrical activity is spread within the sinus node is quite slow, about 0.05 m/sec. The impulse then spreads out rapidly over the atrial musculature at a rate of about 1 m/sec. When the impulse reaches the AV node, a delay of about 0.05 m/sec occurs and atrial systole takes place. The impulse then spreads rapidly, 2 to 4 m/sec, along the right and left bundle branches and Purkinje fibers. Studies indicate that no more than 22 m/sec may elapse during this time. This rapid activation of contractile elements evokes a synchronous contraction of the ventricles.

The velocity of conduction is determined by the size of the resting potential of the cell membrane and the rate of rise of phase 0 of the action potential. This defines membrane responsiveness. Antidysrhythmic drugs may affect conduction by slowing phase 0 depolarization rate, thereby decreasing membrane responsiveness.

Refractoriness. Cardiac tissue is nonresponsive to stimulation during the initial phase of systole (contraction). This is known as **refractoriness** and it determines how closely together two action potentials can occur. Throughout most of repolarization, the cell cannot respond to a stimulus. The effective refractory period represents that period in the cardiac cycle during which a stimulus, no matter how strong, fails to produce an action potential. Antidysrhythmic drugs can lengthen or shorten the refractory period of cardiac tissues by influencing the level of responsiveness of the cell membrane. After the effective refractory period and as repolarization nears completion, a relative refractory period occurs. This is defined as that period during which a propagated action potential can be elicited, provided the stimulus is stronger than normally required in diastole. When this happens, the fiber is stimulated to contract prematurely.

Autonomic Nervous System Control

Although the conduction system possesses the inherent ability for spontaneous, rhythmic initiation of the cardiac impulse, the autonomic nervous system has an important role in the regulation of the rate, rhythm, and force of myocardial contraction of the heart. The heart is innervated by both the parasympathetic and sympathetic nerves. Vagal nerve fibers of the parasympathetic branch are found primarily in the SA node, atrial muscles, and AV junction, whereas the sympathetic fibers innervate the SA node, AV junction, and the atrial and ventricular muscles.

Vagal stimulation to the heart is mediated by the release of the acetylcholine, a neurohormone that acts on the muscarinic receptors to decrease heart rate and is also believed to decrease ventricular contraction. The main effect of acetylcholine on the AV junction is to slow the rate of conduction and lengthen the refractory period. By contrast, sympathetic fiber stimulation is mediated by the release of norepinephrine, which acts specifically on the $beta_1$ receptors in the cardiac tissue. Circulating epinephrine from the adrenal medulla may also elicit cardiac responses. By acting on the beta adrenergic receptors, norepinephrine and epinephrine increase both heart rate and force of myocardial contraction. They also increase conduction velocity and shorten the refractory period of the AV junction. Epinephrine has a very potent effect on the heart. In large doses its direct effect on the electrophysiologic properties of cardiac tissue can create cardiac dysrhythmias (Box 24-1). Normally the heartbeat is under the continuous influence of both parasympathetic and sympathetic control, so that the resting heart rate is the result of their opposing influences.

Electrocardiograms

Electrocardiograms are graphic representations of electrical currents produced by the heart. Nurses caring for clients on monitoring equipment should be able to detect and interpret

BOX 24-1

Common Cardiac Dysrhythmias

Heart block—impaired impulse conduction through the heart; usually the impaired conduction occurs between atria and ventricles

First-degree heart block—conduction time is prolonged but all impulses are conducted from atria to ventricles

Second-degree heart block—some but not all atrial impulses are conducted to ventricles

Third-degree heart block—no atrial impulses are conducted to ventricles

Ectopic beats—a contraction of the heart that originates some place other than the sinoatrial node

Extrasystole "premature beat"—a premature contraction of the heart that arises independent of the normal rhythm

Tachycardia—unusually rapid heart rate (usually over 100 beats/min in adult)

Bradycardia—unusually slow heart rate (usually less than 60 beats/min in adult)

Atrial flutter—extremely rapid rate of atrial contraction; may be 200 to 350 beats/min

Atrial fibrillation—rapid and incoordinated contraction of the atria

Ventricular fibrillation—rapid and incoordinated contraction of the ventricles; because of the incoordination of contractions, there is little or no effective pumping of blood; death will result if not immediately treated

changes in the cardiac rate or rhythm or in the conduction of the wave of electric activity or excitation. The electrocardiogram (ECG) is a useful tool in determining the therapeutic effectiveness of certain drugs. Drugs used to treat cardiovascular disease may alter the electric activity of the heart. The ECG may provide the earliest objective evidence of a drug's effectiveness or its toxic manifestations. A knowledgeable and observant nurse can use the information obtained from the ECG to assess the effectiveness of drug therapy for cardiac dysrhythmias.

Electrical activity always precedes mechanical contraction. Immediately after a wave of electrical activity moves through atrial muscle, the muscle contracts and blood flows from the atria into the ventricles. (Figure 24-4 shows an illustration of the normal ECG.) The P wave is produced by a wave of excitation through the atria (atrial depolarization). The onset of the P wave follows the firing of the SA node. After the P wave, a short pause or interval (PR interval) occurs while the electrical activity is transmitted to the AV junction, conduction tissue, and ventricles. Repolarization, or recovery, of the ventricles is indicated by the T wave. Atrial recovery or repolarization does not show on the ECG because it is hidden in the QRS complex.

Physiology of Fast and Slow Channels of Cardiovascular Fibers

To understand the clinical application of calcium channel blockers, one must review the normal physiology of the fast and slow channels that exist in the membrane of the cardiovascular fibers. The cell membrane is composed of two types of channels that are controlled by "gates." When opened, they allow the movement of an inward current of (1) sodium ions through the fast channels and (2) calcium ions through the slow channels into the cell, depending on the type of fibers involved. These channels appear in the cell membrane of three types of cardiovascular fibers. The heart contains two types: (1) fast-channel fibers, which appear in the myocardial cells of the atria and ventricles and the Purkinje fibers, and (2) slow-channel fibers, which occur in the SA node and the AV junction. Last, the third type, slow fibers, are present in the smooth muscle of the coronary and peripheral arterial vessels.

In this mechanism, the role of calcium ions is essential in affecting three physiologic processes:

1. Increasing the strength of myocardial contraction (fast fibers)

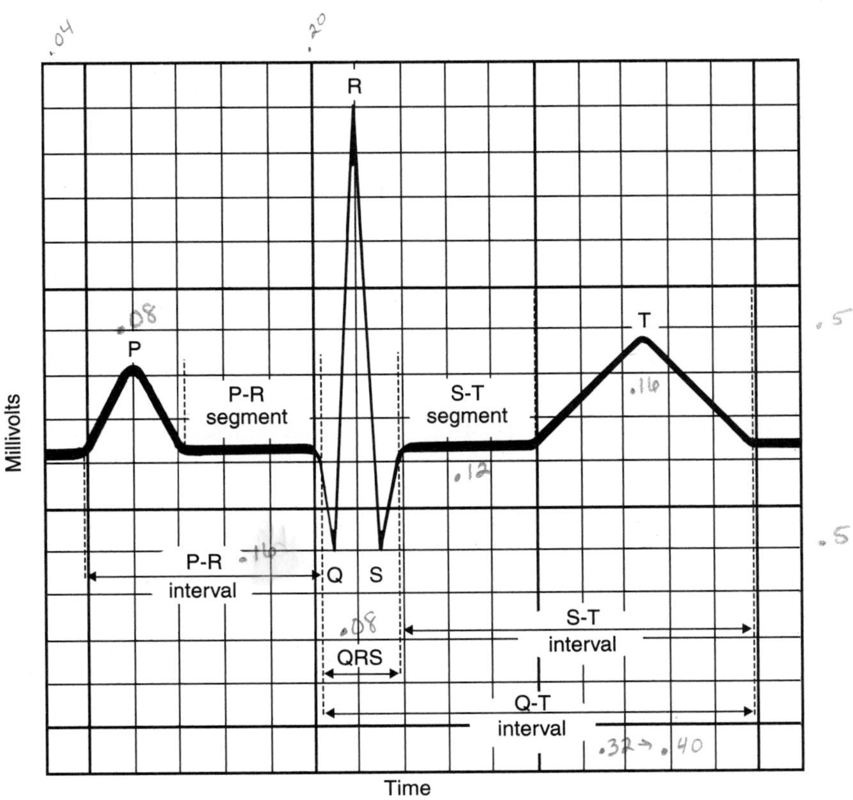

Figure 24-4 Graphic representation of the normal electrocardiogram. Vertical lines represent time, each square represents 0.04 second, and every five squares (set off by heavy black lines) represents 0.20 second. The normal P-R interval is less than 0.20 second; the average is 0.16 second. The average P wave lasts 0.08 second; the QRS complex is 0.08 second; the S-T segment is 0.12 second; the T wave is 0.16 second; and the Q-T interval is 0.32 to 0.40 second if heart rate is 65 to 95 beats/min. Each horizontal line represents voltage; every five squares equals 0.5 millivolt.

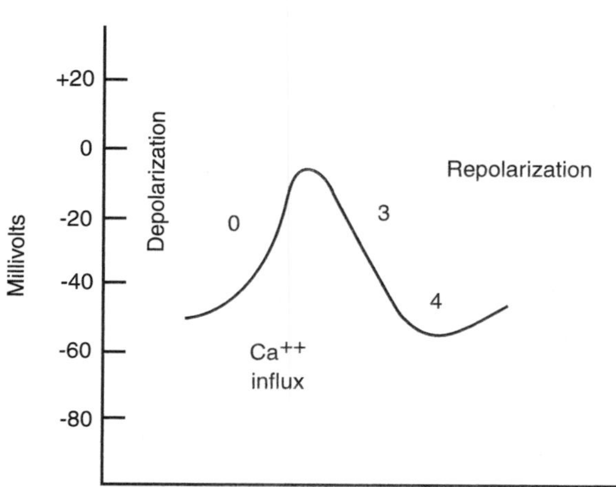

Figure 24-5 Action potential of slow channel fiber, the SA node. It consists of three phases. Unlike the fast fibers of myocardial cells, depolarization (phase 0) is attributed primarily to Ca^{++} inflow through slow channels of the cell membrane. Repolarization involves only phase 3, which is followed by phase 4.

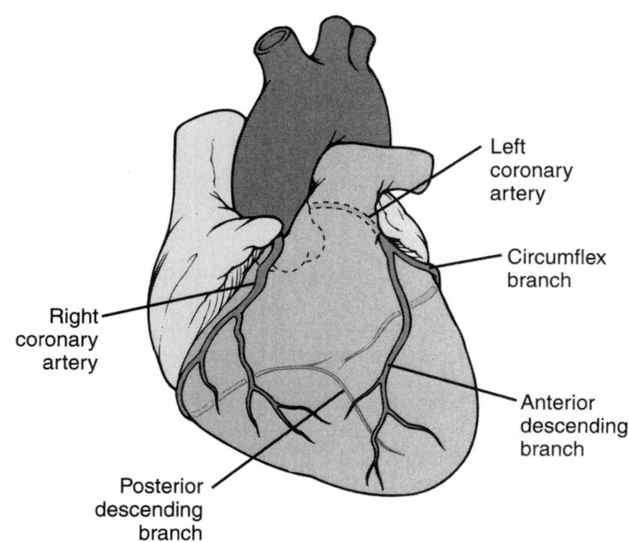

Figure 24-6 Coronary blood supply to the heart. Dark shaded vessels are those located on the external surface of the ventricles; light shaded vessels show penetration of arterial branches toward the endocardial surface.

2. Enhancing automaticity and conduction speed (slow fibers)
3. Vasoconstriction of coronary arteries and peripheral arterioles (slow fibers)

As previously described, the action potential that generates excitation-contraction coupling in the fast fibers consists of five phases. Depolarization (phase 0) results from an electrical stimulus that produces a fast inward current of sodium ion (fast channel). This is then followed by repolarization, which begins with a short phase 1; but, more importantly, phase 2, the plateau phase, produces a slow inward current of calcium ions into the cell (slow channel). The influx of calcium ions is responsible for linking electrical excitation to myocardial contraction (excitation-contraction coupling) required to promote the sliding of actin and myosin filaments for myocardial contraction (positive inotropic effect). Rapid repolarization occurs during phase 3; and, finally, phase 4 reestablishes the resting state. (See configuration of action potential in Figure 24-2, *A*.) In the slow fibers of the SA and AV nodes, the action potential consists of only three phases. The principal distinguishing feature of the pacemaker fiber resides in phase 4. A slow spontaneous depolarization occurs that requires no external stimulus and is termed *diastolic depolarization*. This is responsible for automaticity. Also, unlike the fast fibers of the myocardium, depolarization (or phase 0) is achieved by the slower current carried by both calcium ions and sodium ions through the slow channels of nodal cells. Thus phase 0 results in a slower conduction velocity in nodal cells than in myocardial cells. Calcium channel blockers inhibit these slow channels. Repolarization is more gradual and involves only phase 3. The membrane then finally returns to phase 4 (Figure 24-5). The smooth muscle of blood vessels depends primarily on the presence of calcium ions to initiate and sustain contraction. The main source of calcium ions in cardiac muscle cells is the sarcoplasmic reticulum. In the action potential for smooth muscle, it is believed that the onset of depolarization (phase 0) is caused mainly by calcium ions rather than by sodium ions. Calcium ions enter the smooth muscle cell through slow channels, and it is the rise in free calcium ion concentration that is considered to be the primary event in excitation-contraction coupling that is responsible for increasing muscle tone and vasoconstriction. In addition, activation of smooth muscle can reduce the caliber of small vessels markedly, as is apparent from the "spasm" that may occur in coronary vessels. The calcium channel blockers (specifically verapamil, nefidipine, and diltiazem) are capable of blocking the slow calcium ion influx in smooth muscle of blood vessels, thereby producing relaxation.

CORONARY VASCULAR SUPPLY OF THE HEART

The entire blood supply to the myocardium is provided by the right and left coronary arteries, which arise from the base of the aorta (Figure 24-6). The right atrium and ventricle are supplied with blood from the right coronary artery. The left coronary artery divides into the anterior (descending) branch and the circumflex branch and supplies blood to the left atrium and ventricle. These main coronary vessels continue to divide, forming numerous branches. The result is a profuse network of coronary vessels. The major arterial vessels are located on the external surface of the ventricles. Arterial branches penetrate the myocardium toward the endocardial surface.

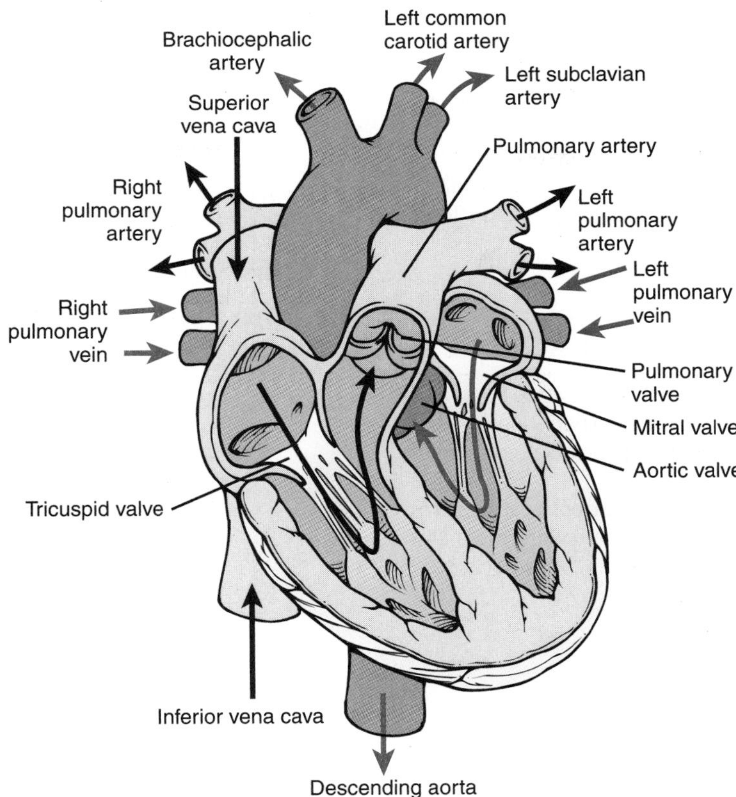

Figure 24-7 Overview of heart, blood flow, and valves.

Increased oxygen delivery to the myocardium is supported almost exclusively by increased coronary blood flow. When the demand for oxygen and nutrients by body tissues is increased, the heart must increase its output. At the same time, the heart muscle itself must be supplied with enough oxygen and nutrients to replace the energy expended. In other words, a balance must be maintained between energy expenditure and energy restoration. During systole the myocardial contraction compresses the coronary vascular bed. This restricts coronary inflow but increases coronary outflow. Coronary inflow in the left ventricle occurs primarily during diastole when the ventricles have relaxed and the coronary vessels are no longer compressed. Blood is driven through the coronary arteries by aortic pressure perfusing the myocardium.

A change in heart rate is accomplished by shortening or lengthening diastole. With tachycardia the increased number of systolic contractions per minute reduces the time available for diastole and coronary inflow. An increase also occurs in the metabolic needs of the rapidly beating heart. Normally, coronary dilation occurs in an attempt to meet increased metabolic demand and to overcome restricted blood inflow. With bradycardia, the decreased number of systolic contractions per minute prolongs the diastolic period. Resistance to coronary flow and metabolic requirements of the myocardium are reduced.

Whenever the delivery of oxygen to the myocardium is inadequate to meet the heart's oxygen consumption needs, myocardial ischemia occurs. One of the major causes of ischemia is coronary artery disease. Figure 24-7 gives an overview of heart, blood flow, and valves.

SUMMARY

Understanding the electrical and physiologic properties of the heart and the effects of drugs on cardiac activity is essential knowledge for nurses. The drugs used therapeutically effect the myocardium, the conduction system, and coronary vessels. The action of the myocardium to adjust cardiac output according to the body's needs is based on electrical excitation, mechanical activation, and the contractile mechanism of myocardial fiber. However, effective cardiac output can be achieved only with adequate relaxation and refilling of the cardiac chambers after each contraction. The cardiac conduction system initiates and transmits electrical impulses required for the contraction of the myocardium. Automaticity, conductivity, and refractoriness are the essential properties of the fibers of the conduction system. The sequence of cardiac excitation is graphically represented by electrocardiography. The ECG is a useful tool for monitoring cardiac activity to assist nurses to evaluate the effectiveness of a number of drugs used to treat cardiovascular disease.

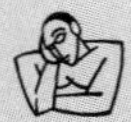

Critical Thinking

1. What is the role of systole and diastole in the cardiac conduction system?
2. What are the effects of acetylcholine, norepinephrine, and epinephrine on vagal stimulation of the heart, sympathetic fiber stimulation, heart rate, myocardial contraction force, and conduction velocity?

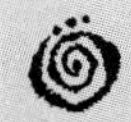

Collaborative Learning Activities

1. Three teams of students will present to the class the effects of acetylcholine, norepinephrine, and epinephrine on vagal stimulation of the heart, heart rate, myocardial contraction force, and conduction velocity.
2. Distribute copies of normal and abnormal electrocardiograms. Small groups of students will compare these with Figure 24-4 and determine abnormalities and describe the dysfunction.

BIBLIOGRAPHY

Anderson KN, et al. (Eds.) (1994). *Mosby's medical, nursing, & allied health dictionary* (4th ed.). St Louis: Mosby.

Gilman AG, et al. (Eds.) (1990). *Goodman & Gilman's the pharmacological basis of therapeutics.* (8th ed.). New York: Macmillan.

Guyton AC (1987). *Human physiology and the mechanism of disease.* (4th ed.). Philadelphia: WB Saunders.

Martini F, et al. (1992). *Fundamentals of anatomy and physiology* (2nd ed.). Englewood Cliffs, NJ: Prentice Hall.

Seeley RR, Stephens TD, & Tate P (1996). *Anatomy & physiology* (2nd ed.). St Louis: Mosby.

Sifton DW (1994). *The PDR family guide to women's health and prescription drugs.* Montvale, NJ: Medical Economics.

Thibodeau GA & Patton K (1996). *Anatomy and physiology* (3rd ed.). St Louis: Mosby.

Van Wynsberghe D, Noback CR, & Carola R (1995). *Human anatomy and physiology* (3rd ed.). New York: McGraw-Hill.

Chapter 25 Cardiac Glycosides

Chapter Focus

Cardiac glycosides have been used since the first century A.D. and are still frequently prescribed for the treatment of specific cardiac disorders. However, there is a very narrow therapeutic range and toxicity is life-threatening. Nurses must be knowledgeable about the administration of these drugs and be able to recognize the toxicities that commonly occur with them. The following objectives and key terms are important for a good understanding of this chapter.

Key Terms

chronotropic (p. 490)
congestive heart failure (p. 490)
digitalization (p. 495)
dromotropic (p. 490)
inotropic (p. 490)

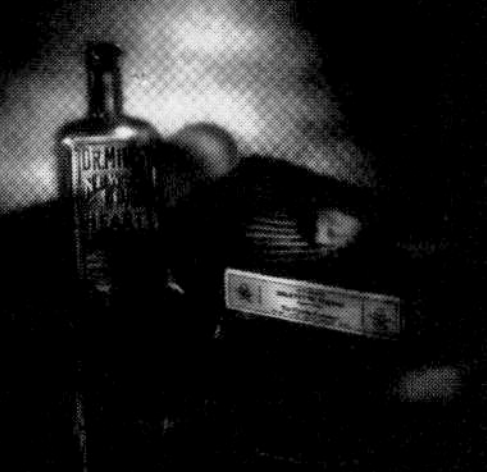

Key Drug [▲]

digoxin

Objectives

1. Describe right- and left-sided heart failure, including at least three major signs and symptoms.
2. Name the two primary mechanisms of action for digitalis glycosides.
3. Describe the first symptoms of digitalis toxicity and the different arrhythmias usually seen in young children and in adults.
4. Name at least three drugs that interact with digitalis glycosides, and describe possible effects and management of any interaction.
5. Describe both the fast (rapid) and slow method of digitalization.
6. Discuss factors predisposing a client to digitalis toxicity.
7. Implement the nursing management of the care for clients who are receiving cardiac glycosides.

Various medications may change the force of myocardial contraction and the rate and rhythm of the heart. Pharmacologic terms that have specific meaning for the actions of drugs on the cardiovascular system include the following: "inotropic," "chronotropic," and "dromotropic" effects.

Drugs with an **inotropic** (Gr. *inos*, fiber; *tropikos*, a turning or influence) effect influence myocardial contractility. Drugs with a positive inotropic effect, strengthen or increase the force of myocardial contraction (e.g., digitalis, dobutamine, dopamine, epinephrine, and isoproterenol) while drugs with a negative inotropic effect weaken or decrease the force of myocardial contraction (e.g., lidocaine, quinidine, and propranolol).

Drugs with **chronotropic** (Gr. *chronos*, time) action affect heart rate. A positive chronotropic effect is produced if the drug accelerates the heart rate by increasing the rate of impulse formation in the sinoatrial (SA) node (e.g., norepinephrine). A negative chronotropic drug has the opposite effect and slows the heart rate by decreasing impulse formation (e.g., acetylcholine).

Dromotropic (Gr. *dromos*, a course) effect refers to drugs that affect conduction velocity through specialized conducting tissues. A drug having a positive dromotropic action speeds conduction (e.g., phenytoin) while a negative dromotropic action drug delays conduction (e.g., verapamil).

Drugs in the digitalis group are among the oldest drugs known as therapeutic agents for treatment of heart failure. The effects of digitalis glycosides are twofold. They increase the strength of contraction (positive inotrope) and alter the electrophysiologic properties of the heart by slowing the heart rate (negative chronotrope) and slowing conduction velocity (negative dromotrope). Other agents may produce varying effects with the same objective of treating heart failure. To better understand the beneficial and toxic effects of the digitalis glycosides and other agents, the mechanisms of heart failure will first be described.

HEART FAILURE

Congestive heart failure (CHF) occurs in 2 to 4 million Americans annually, nearly twice as often in males as in females. After 50 years old, prevalence increases every decade of life until approximately 9% of the over 80 population is affected (Kradjan, 1995). Because CHF adversely affects quality of life and has a high mortality rate, an understanding of its etiology and appropriate interventions is important.

Congestive heart failure or pump failure is a pathologic state in which the weakened myocardium is unable to pump sufficient blood from the ventricles (i.e., cardiac output) to sustain normal circulation required to meet the metabolic demands of the body organs. The etiologic factors of heart failure are listed in Table 25-1. Despite the etiologic factors, depressed myocardial contractility is primarily the underlying cause of heart failure. Therefore, in heart failure, it is important to identify and remove the cause and correct the problem whenever possible, and then treat the heart failure state, as follows:

1. Remove excess water and salt in the body. Sodium restrictions, reduction of physical activity, and initiation of diuretic and/or digitalis glycoside therapy are the usual measures taken.
2. Enhance myocardial contraction. The positive inotropic effect of digitalis has been related to excitation contraction coupling. (See Chapter 24 for an explanation of this phenomenon.)

The nurse should be aware that drugs may exacerbate or precipitate congestive heart failure (Box 25-1). Also, many drugs contain sodium; the avoidance of their use must be considered with a salt-restricted diet (Table 25-2).

Heart failure appears to be associated with a defect in the excitation-contraction coupling, and in some individuals dysfunction of *contractile proteins* may occur as an additional abnormality. Ineffective calcium pumping by the sarcoplasmic

TABLE 25-1 Etiology of heart failure

Organic heart disorders	Other causes
cardiac dysrhythmia	alcoholism
hypertension	anemia
infective endocarditis	hyperthyroidism
valvular disorders (mitral valve stenosis, regurgitation, etc.)	liver disease
myocardial infarction	nutritional deficiency
pulmonary embolism	renal disease

BOX 25-1

Drugs That May Precipitate or Exacerbate Heart Failure

1. Drugs that cause sodium and water retention or expand intravascular volume:
   albumin
   androgens
   corticosteroids (cortisone, hydrocortisone, fludrocortisone [Florinef], etc.)
   diazoxide (Proglycem, Hyperstat)
   estrogens
   guanethidine (Ismelin)
   mannitol
   methyldopa (Aldomet)
   minoxidil (Loniten)
   NSAIDs
   urea
2. Drugs that inhibit myocardial contractility (negative inotropic or cardiotoxic agents):
   beta-blocking agents
   calcium channel blockers (especially verapamil)
   disopyramide (Norpace)
   doxorubicin (Adriamycin)
   quinidine

reticulum may alter the normal relaxation process. Furthermore, the mitochondria—*not* the sarcoplasmic reticulum—may act as the dominant calcium uptake storage site. If so, less calcium is available for release from the sarcoplasmic reticulum to activate contraction. Thus the amount of coupling is reduced, and depressed myocardial contractility ensues.

With regard to dysfunction of contractile proteins in heart failure, attention has been focused on abnormal energy utilization. Some researchers have shown that the activity of myosin adenosine triphosphatase (ATPase) is decreased. When the activity of this enzyme is reduced in heart failure, the interaction between actin-myosin filaments is reduced in intensity, and thus the force of contractility is lowered.

An important consequence of inadequate performance of the myocardium is hemodynamic alterations. Compensatory mechanisms are activated, and incomplete emptying of the heart during ventricular systole eventually allows blood to accumulate inside the heart chambers, causing dilation or enlargement of the heart and is referred to as low output, systolic dysfunction. During this process, blood backs up into the atria.

In the left atrium, this can lead to pulmonary congestion; in the right atrium, systemic congestion, including ascites, may occur. During the interim, the heart attempts to pump the blood forward in the circulation, but instead the increased fluid in the left ventricle produces stretching of the myocardial fibers and dilation of the ventricles.

Athletes commonly have cardiac hypertrophy, which is an enlargement of cardiac muscle and of the ventricular chambers. Thus the overall effectiveness of the heart as a pump is increased. Frank-Starling's law states that an increase in the length of the heart's muscle fibers results in increased contraction and cardiac output. This stretching of cardiac muscle results from increased preload, an increased amount of blood returned to the heart and entering the heart chambers. Therefore the more the cardiac muscles are stretched during diastole, the greater the contraction in systole.

Congestive heart failure is a myocardial dysfunction resulting in a decreased cardiac output. Regardless of the primary cause, the result is that preload can increase until a massive overload results. The ventricles are unable to meet the needs for contraction or pumping. Mechanisms to compensate, involving sympathoadrenergic stimulation, may occur as the body attempts to maintain an adequate cardiac output. But the increased heart rate and peripheral vascular resistance also elevate the heart's demand for oxygen, thus further contributing to myocardial dysfunction. The inability to obtain adequate cardiac output is referred to as myocardial insufficiency or cardiac decompensation. Furthermore, chronic progressive ventricular failure generally leads to congestive heart failure, which means that the heart's ability to contract decreases to the extent that the heart pumps out less blood than it receives. Subsequently, myocardial infarction produces circulatory failure.

A decrease in cardiac output means less blood is in the blood vessels, and the body's various organs are receiving less blood. The kidneys respond by retaining more water and

TABLE 25-2 Sodium content of selected prescription and over-the-counter medications

Medications	Sodium/unit	Sodium/maximum daily dose (adult)
Antibiotics		
carbenicillin disodium (Geopen, Pyopen)	108-150 mg/g	4.5 to 6 g/40 g
ticarcillin injection (Ticar)	120-150 mg/g	2.9 to 3.6 g/24 g
ampicillin sodium (Polycillin-N, Omnipen-N, and others)	62-78 mg/g	1 to 1.2 g/16 g
cephalosporins		
cefamandole naftate (Mandol)	77 mg/g	0.9 g/12 g
ceftriaxone sodium (Rocephin)	83 mg/g	0.33 g/4 g
cephradine injection (Velosef)	136 mg/g	1 g/8 g
Over-the-counter medications		
Alka-Seltzer Effervescent Pain Reliever and Antacid Tablets	0.5 g/tablet	
Alka-Seltzer, Lemon-Lime	506 mg	
Alka-Seltzer, Original	567 mg	
Bellans	144 mg	
Bromo-Seltzer powder	0.76 g/capful	
Eno Powder	0.8 g/tsp	
Rolaids	53 mg/tablet	
Soda Mint Tablets	90 mg/tablet	
Food supplements		
Ensure	844/L	
Meritene	880-1078 mg/L	
Osmolite	549/L	
Sustacal	924-940/L	

electrolytes, producing fluid retention and electrolyte disturbances. This is called right-sided heart failure; the clinical signs include jugular vein distention, hepatomegaly, ascites, and peripheral edema. On the other hand, left-sided heart failure leads to fluid accumulation in the lungs—pulmonary edema—producing dyspnea, as well as interference with oxygen and carbon dioxide exchange. Failure of one side of the heart is usually followed by failure of the other side, which produces total heart failure (Figure 25-1).

In summary, the failing heart may show increases in both preload (increased blood volume return to the heart chambers) and afterload (the increased pressure in the aorta that the ventricle muscles must overcome to open the aortic valve and push blood through). The decrease in renal perfusion just described may activate the renin-angiotensin-aldosterone (RAA) feedback mechanism. Then sodium and water are retained and intravascular volume and blood flow back to the heart increase. In less serious situations, this is usually enough to maintain arterial blood pressure, thus turning off the RAA system. But in individuals who have conditions bordering on heart failure, this can produce a frank decompensation or acute heart failure. The increase in circulatory blood volume increases the demands on the heart, which may result in acute pulmonary edema. Thus cardiotonic drugs such as digitalis glycosides (to increase contractility); diuretics (to reduce increased blood volume and edema); vasodilators (nitrates that pool blood in the extremities, thus reducing blood return or preload, and arterial vasodilators that decrease arterial resistance, reducing afterload); and angiotensin converting enzyme (ACE) inhibitors (to decrease peripheral vascular resistance [afterload], pulmonary capillary wedge pressure [preload], pulmonary vascular resistance and secretion of aldosterone) are all important drugs in the treatment of heart failure. Usually ACE inhibitors such as captopril, enalapril, and lisinopril are used with digitalis and diuretics to treat CHF unresponsive to other therapies. In this chapter, the discussion focuses on digitalis glycosides, digoxin immune fab (Digibind), amrinone (Inocor), and milrinone lactate (Primacor).

DIGITALIS GLYCOSIDES

The story of the origin of digitalis is interesting in that it demonstrates an herbal remedy that was used for hundreds of years by common people (called "housewife's recipe") and it was prepared by farmers and housewives for dropsy (fluid accumulation). More than 400 years ago Dr. Leonhard Fuchs recommended that physicians use it "to scatter the dropsy, to relieve swelling of the liver, and even to bring on menstrual flow" (Silverman, 1942). Dr. Fuchs was a botanist-physician, and at that time, the medical profession paid little attention to a "mere flower picker."

In the mid-1700s, a female patient shared an old family recipe for curing dropsy with Dr. William Withering, which

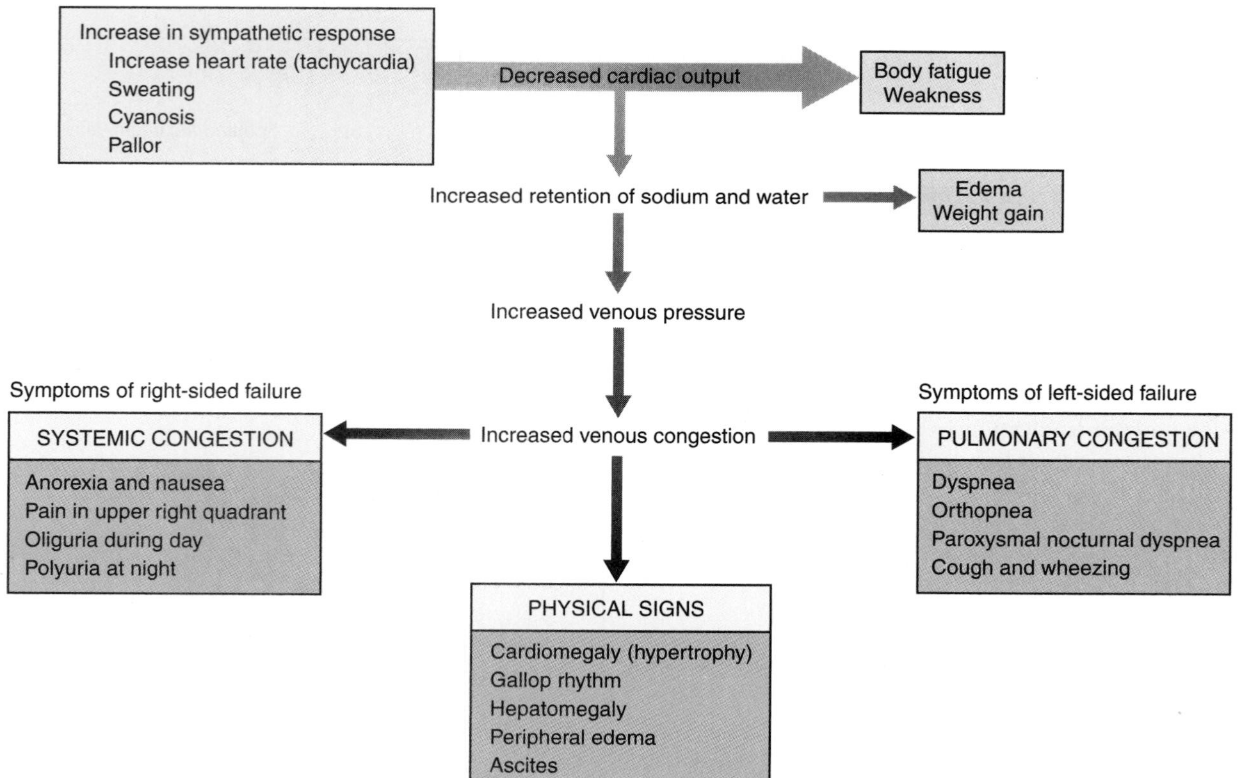

Figure 25-1 Signs and symptoms of heart failure.

he used for his dropsy patients, and after spending 10 years studying digitalis, he published his conclusions in *An Account of the Foxglove.* This remarkable publication stressed instructions that are still valid today—the necessity of individualizing dosage according to the client's response. Digitalis was finally admitted to the London Pharmacopeia in 1722.

The digitalis glycosides belong to many different botanical families. The action of each is fundamentally the same, so that the description for digitalis, with minor differences, applies to all. The principal forms are discussed here.

digitoxin [di ji tox' in] (Crystodigin)
▲ **digoxin** [di jox' in] (Lanoxin, Lanoxicaps)

Digoxin is the most commonly used digitalis glycoside and is generally considered the prototype drug in this classification. Digitalis affects cardiac function through two important mechanisms:

1. Positive inotropic action.
2. Negative chronotropic and negative dromotropic actions.

Positive inotropic action. The main function of digitalis is inotropic. The increased myocardial contractility is associated with more efficient use of available energy. If the failing heart is enlarged, the positive inotropic action of digitalis can cause the myocardium to beat more forcefully, thereby increasing cardiac output and decreasing oxygen use. Thus the improved pumping action of the heart in individuals with congestive heart failure may reach levels that approach normal because the net effect is not only reduced heart size but also decreased venous pressure to relieve edema. The positive inotropic mechanism is not precisely known. However, one theory asserts that digitalis is bound to sites on the myocardial cell membrane (sarcolemma), where it inhibits the action of membrane-bound Na^+-K^+-ATPase enzyme. Normally, this enzyme hydrolyses ATP to provide the energy for the Na^+-K^+ pump needed to release Na^+ and transport K^+ into the cardiac cell during repolarization. By binding specifically to Na^+-K^+-ATPase, digitalis inhibits the active transport of Na^+ and K^+ (Figure 24-1, *5b*). Then intracellular Na^+ accumulates, which stimulates the release of large quantities of free calcium ion from the sarcoplasmic reticulum. The free calcium ion is essential for linking the electrical excitation of the cell membrane to the mechanical contraction of the myocardial cell, a mechanism known as excitation-contraction coupling.

Thus, more free calcium ion produces a greater degree of coupling of actin and myosin to form actinomyosin, which results in more forceful myocardial contraction with a concomitant increase in cardiac output. Inhibition of Na^+-K^+-ATPase activity is projected to be the mechanism by which the cardiac glycosides increase myocardial contraction without causing increased oxygen consumption. (See Myocardial Contraction in the Cardiac Muscle section in Chapter 24.)

Negative chronotropic and negative dromotropic actions. Digitalis has negative chronotropic (decreased heart rate) and negative dromotropic (slowed conduction velocity) effects because it can alter three electrophysiologic properties of cardiac tissues:

1. *Automaticity.* Cardiac tissue has the inherent ability to initiate and propagate an impulse without external stimulation. This property affects the rate and rhythm of the heart. Low to moderate doses of digitalis slow the heart rate because the SA node depolarizes less frequently. On the other hand, toxic concentrations of digitalis can directly increase automaticity. This increases the rate of both action potentials and spontaneous depolarization. This is one of the mechanisms responsible for digitalis-induced ectopic pacemakers. Toxic doses of digitalis may significantly increase impulse formation in latent or potential pacemaker tissue, causing dysrhythmia.
2. *Conduction velocity.* All concentrations of digitalis decrease conduction velocity. The AV conduction velocity is slowed both by the direct action of digitalis and by increased vagal action. The ECG shows a prolonged P-R interval, and in toxic doses the drug can lead to increased heart block (Figure 25-2).
3. *The refractory period* effects of digitalis vary in different parts of the heart. If the refractory period in the ventricles is reduced, nearly toxic amounts of digitalis are required. A prolonged refractory period occurs in the AV conduction system, which is very sensitive to digitalis action. This action is partly direct and partly caused by increased vagal tone. Toxic doses of digitalis may prolong the refractory period and depress conduction in the AV conduction system until complete heart block may occur.

Congestive heart failure. A heart in failure is no longer capable of supplying body tissue with adequate oxygen and nutrients or of removing metabolic waste products. The positive inotropic effect of digitalis that results in increased myocardial contractility benefits the client with a failing heart.

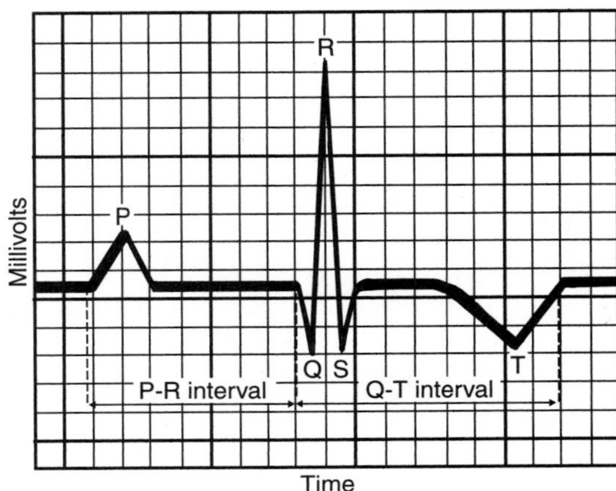

Figure 25-2 Representation of typical effects of digitalization on the electric activity of the heart as shown on the electrocardiogram. Note the prolonged P-R interval, the shortened Q-T interval, and the T wave inversion.

The increased force of systolic contraction causes the ventricles to empty more completely. Also, a slower heart rate permits more complete filling, which results in the following:

1. Venous pressure falls, and the pulmonary and systemic congestion and their accompanying signs and symptoms are either diminished or completely abolished.
2. Coronary circulation is enhanced, myocardial oxygen demand is reduced, and the supply of oxygen and nutrients to the myocardium is improved.
3. Heart size is often decreased toward normal.

Some cardiac glycosides have a true but mild diuretic effect. However, marked diuresis in the edematous client primarily results from improved heart action, improved circulation to all body tissues, and improved tissue and organ function including renal function. When digitalis is effective, the client is noticeably improved and has an increased sense of well-being.

Atrial fibrillation. During atrial fibrillation several hundred impulses originate from the atria, but only a fraction of them are transmitted through the AV junction. (Figure 25-3 shows the electrocardiographic pattern of atrial fibrillation.) Digitalis is ideal for slowing the ventricular rate because it increases the refractory period of the AV junction and also slows conduction at this site. It is important to know that the purpose of using digitalis in atrial fibrillation is to slow the ventricular rate to reduce the possibility of inducing ventricular tachycardia. It also may prevent or eliminate cardiac failure. Digitalis does not convert the fibrillating atria into normally contracting ones.

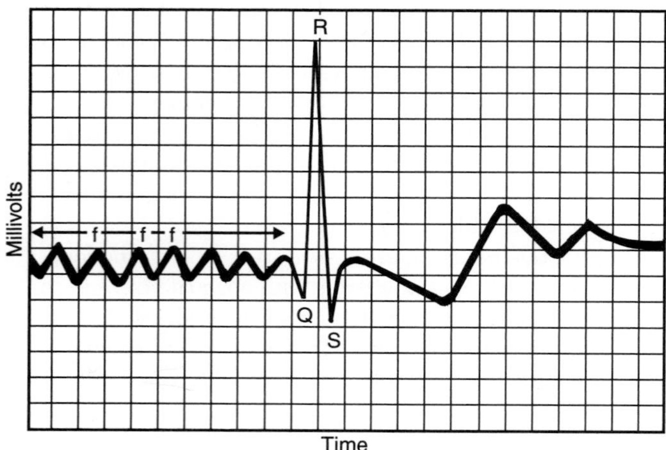

Figure 25-3 Graphic representation of atrial fibrillation as seen on the electrocardiographic monitor or tracing paper. No true P waves are noted; but f (fibrillation) waves consisting of rapid, small, and irregular waves are noted. The QRS complex is normal in configuration and duration but occurs irregularly.

Indications. These drugs are used in the treatment of congestive heart failure and in the treatment or prevention of cardiac arrhythmias, especially atrial fibrillation, atrial flutter, and paroxysmal atrial tachycardia. They are also used in the treatment of cardiogenic shock associated with pulmonary edema.

Pharmacokinetics. Digoxin's bioavailability is approximately 60% to 80% with tablets, 70% to 85% with the elixir, and 90% to 100% with the capsule dosage form. Digitoxin is very lipophilic, so it is almost completely absorbed orally.

The cardiac glycosides can be categorized into two main groups: rapid-acting agents and long-acting agents. Table 25-3 lists specific pharmacokinetic information.

The side/adverse effects of the digitalis glycosides include anorexia, nausea, bradycardia, stomach pain and dysrhythmias.

Although glycoside serum levels are of limited value in establishing therapeutic serum levels, they are sometimes helpful as an indicator of toxicity. For example, the elderly population may have age-related, renal, or hepatic impairment and a decreased volume of distribution for digitalis; thus lower doses are necessary to avoid digitalis toxicity.

Dosage and administration (Table 25-4). The nurse should also be aware of the following issues related to cardiac glycosides:

Bioavailability. Bioavailability (discussed in more detail in Chapter 3) refers to the amount of the administered drug that is usable in the target tissue. Bioavailability must be considered when a client is transferred from one dosage form to another; a dosage adjustment may be required to compensate for the pharmacokinetic differences of the dosage form. A 100 µg (0.1 mg) dose of the injection or of the digoxin-solution capsule is bioequivalent to a 125-µg (0.125-mg) dose of the tablet or elixir. When clients are switched from capsules to tablets, or vise versa, this difference in bioavailability must be kept in mind.

TABLE 25-3 Cardiac glycosides: pharmacokinetic parameters

Drug	Route	Onset of action	Peak effect (hr)	Plasma half-life	Duration of action	Therapeutic plasma level (ng/ml)	Metabolism	Excretion
Rapid acting								
digoxin (Lanoxin)	IV	5-30 min	1-4	36-48 hr	6 days	0.5-2	Liver	Kidney (50%-70% unchanged)
	Oral	½-2 hr	2-6	36-48 hr	6 days	0.5-2	Liver	Same as above
Long acting								
digitoxin (Crystodigin)	Oral	1-4 hr	8-14	5-9 days	14 days	13-25	Liver	Kidney (metabolites)

Digitalization. **Digitalization** is the saturation of body tissues with enough digitalis glycoside to cause the signs and symptoms of heart failure to disappear. Although nomograms and formula calculations are available to estimate digoxin dosage based on lean body weight and renal function, most prescribers still prescribe digoxin according to body weight of the client. (See dosage chart, Table 25-4.) However, digitalis glycosides have a very narrow therapeutic index; in other words, the therapeutic dose is very close to the toxic dose. Many clients experience digitalis toxicity, so it is vital for the nurse to monitor, and to teach the client to watch for, signs and symptoms of improvement and of drug toxicity. Drug serum levels should also be monitored. There are essentially two methods of digitalization: the rapid (fast) method, which requires hospitalization of the client, and the slow method, which is usually prescribed in an ambulatory setting.

The rapid digitalization (loading) method is reserved for the client in acute distress from heart failure. If the client has not previously received any digitalis glycoside, then intravenous digoxin is given in divided doses in a 24-hour period. The goal of treatment is to obtain the maximum therapeutic effect of the glycoside as rapidly as possible. With this method, the drug toxicities will quickly become evident, while the client is in the controlled environment of the hospital unit. An advantage is that the toxicities can be easily correlated to a specific drug concentration. For example, the prescriber decides to intravenously administer to an individual a total dose of 1 mg digoxin. Digoxin may be prescribed as 0.5 mg IV now and 0.25 mg IV every 6 hours for two doses for a total of 1 mg. The nurse is expected to observe the client for signs of improvement. If the client demonstrates digitalis toxicity after the 1 mg dose, the

TABLE 25-4 Cardiac glycosides: dosage and administration

		Dosage range	
Drug	**Route**	**Digitalizing (loading)**	**Maintenance**
digitoxin (Crystodigin, Digitaline 🍁)	oral	*Adults:* RAPID: 0.6 mg initially, followed in 4-6 hr by 0.4 mg and then 0.2 mg every 4-6 hr SLOW: 0.2 mg 2 times a day for 4 days *Children:* Not recommended	0.05-0.3 mg/day
digoxin (Lanoxicaps, Lanoxin)	IV	*Adults:* 0.4-0.6 mg initially then 0.1-0.3 mg every 6-8 hr as needed	0.125-0.5 mg daily as a single dose or in divided doses daily
	IV	*Children:* give in following divided doses: ½ dose at once, remainder in fractional doses at 4-8 hr intervals: Premature infant, rapid: 15-25 μg/kg	 20%-30% of loading dose daily in divided doses
		Full-term infant, rapid: 20-30 μg/kg	20%-35% of loading dose daily in divided doses
		Infant (1-24 months), rapid: 30-50 μg/kg	25%-35% of loading dose daily
	IV	*Children:* 2 to 5 yr—25-35 μg/kg 5 to 10 yr—15-30 μg/kg Over 10 yr—8-12 μg/kg	25%-35% of loading dose in divided doses 2 or 3 times a day 25%-35% of loading dose once a day
	tablet	*Adults:* RAPID: 0.75-1.25 mg divided into 2 or more doses, each administered at 6-8 hr intervals SLOW: 0.125-0.5 mg once a day for 7 days	0.125-0.5 mg once a day
		Children: 2 to 10 yr: 0.03-0.04 mg/kg in divided doses every 6-8 hr	20%-30% of digitalizing dose daily
	capsule	*Adults:* RAPID: 0.4-0.6 mg followed by 0.1-0.3 mg every 6-8 hr as necessary SLOW: 0.05-0.35 mg daily in 2 divided doses; repeat dosage for 1-3 weeks to reach steady state serum levels *Children:* See current literature because dosages vary according to age	0.05-0.35 mg orally once or twice daily, as necessary

prescriber would know that this person was not able to tolerate a 1 mg total dose and in the future would avoid any dosage regimen that might reach this level.

The slow method of digitalization is generally used in less acute situations in the ambulatory setting. The length of time before an individual has reached full digitalization is much longer than with the rapid method. An oral maintenance dose of digitalis daily may be prescribed, and the client would not reach full digitalization until approximately the fifth half-life of the drug. Digoxin, which has a 36 hour half-life, would take approximately 7 days for digitalization, whereas digitoxin (with a half-life of 7½ days) would require more than a month. The advantages of the slow method include these: (1) the individual may be treated on an outpatient basis, (2) it is a safer method, (3) close monitoring is not required, and (4) the doses may be taken orally. The disadvantages are these: (1) the extended length of time before the individual is digitalized and (2) the difficulty of determining when digitalis toxicity occurs, since the onset of symptoms may be very gradual.

Geriatric Implications

Cardiac glycosides

Digoxin, one of the most commonly prescribed drugs in the world, must be closely monitored as the treatment dose is approximately 60% of the toxic dose (Long & Rybacki, 1995). Elderly clients often have a reduced tolerance for the cardiac glycosides and thus lower doses may be necessary to reduce the potential for drug toxicity.

Early toxic signs often include anorexia, nausea, and vomiting; difficulty with reading, which may appear as visual alterations such as green and yellow vision, double vision, or seeing spots or halos; headaches; dizziness; fatigue; weakness; confusion; depression; increased nervousness; and diarrhea. Decreased libido and impotency have been reported in approximately 35% of males as a result of digoxin's estrogen-type effects. Also, male breast enlargement and breast tenderness have been reported (Long & Rybacki, 1995).

Be aware that exercise reduces serum digoxin levels because of increased uptake in skeletal muscles. The nurse must be cognizant of the physical activity of their clients taking digoxin (Semla, Beinzer & Higbee, 1993).

Research indicates that bisacodyl (Dulcolax, Fleet Laxative) may reduce absorption of Lanoxin (digoxin) (Graedon & Graedon, 1995). Do not administer these drugs concurrently.

Nursing Management

Cardiac Glycoside Therapy

Assessment. The client's health status should be assessed for underlying conditions (e.g., ventricular fibrillation or a toxic effect from a previous administration of the drug) for which digitalis glycosides might be contraindicated. Digitalis glycosides are to be used cautiously when the following conditions are noted:

- Dysrhythmias. They may be caused by underlying heart disease or reflect digitalis intoxication; the drug should be withheld if the latter occurs.
- Progression of AV block. Incomplete AV block may progress to advanced or complete heart block in digitalizing clients; this means that heart failure may need to be managed by other measures.
- Elderly clients. Because of their small body mass (i.e., lean body weight) and frequent renal impairments, elderly clients must be given digoxin cautiously. Digitoxin is less affected by renal function impairment (see the Geriatric Implications box above).
- Clients with electronic cardiac pacemakers. These clients require careful titration of their dosage because they may demonstrate symptoms of toxicity at dosages usually tolerated by other individuals.
- Electrolyte imbalances. Hypokalemia and hypomagnesemia increase the risk of digitalis toxicity. Also exercise great caution in giving the drug to clients with hypercalcemia and hyperkalemia to avoid digitalis-induced dysrhythmia, principally heart block. Hypocalcemia may decrease the effectiveness of digitalis glycosides; calcium supplementation may be necessary.
- Ventricular dysrhythmias. Clients with premature ventricular contractions or ventricular tachycardia are at risk for exacerbation with the administration of digitalis glycosides.
- Myocardial pathology. Clients with acute myocarditis or myocardial infarction or ischemic heart disease are at higher risk for digitalis-induced arrhythmias because of the increased sensitivity of the effects of the drug.
- Conduction disorders. The condition of clients with Wolff-Parkinson-White or sick sinus syndrome may worsen.
- Renal dysfunction. Clients with renal impairment (digoxin only) and those with acute glomerulonephritis may have reduced excretion and so greater risk of toxicity.
- Myxedema, severe pulmonary disease, or carotid sinus hypersensitivity predispose the client to the toxic effect of digitalis glycosides.

The client's current medication regimen should be reviewed for significant drug interactions. The following interactions may occur when digitalis glycosides are given with the drugs listed below:

Drug	Possible effect and management
amiodarone (Cordarone)	May increase digoxin serum levels (possibly other digitalis glycosides also) to toxic levels. Reduce dosage of digitalis preparation and monitor serum digoxin levels closely.

Drug	Possible effect and management
antacids (especially aluminum and magnesium types)	May decrease digitalis glycoside absorption 25% to 35%. Space medications apart, preferably giving digitalis glycoside 1 to 2 hours before antacids.
antidysrhythmic agents, injectable calcium salts, succinylcholine, or sympathomimetics	**Concurrent administration may enhance risk of cardiac dysrhythmias. Avoid or a potentially serious drug interaction may occur.**
antidiarrheal adsorbents (kaolin, pectin, etc.), cholestyramine (Questran), colestipol (Colestid), or large quantities of dietary fiber (bran)	May reduce absorption of digitalis glycosides, resulting in a decreased therapeutic response. Administer digitalis products 1 to 2 hours before these agents, then monitor closely for digitalis effectiveness.
calcium channel blocking agents (verapamil [Calan, Isoptin], diltiazem [Cardizem])	Concurrent use may require reduced digitalis glycoside dosages. Monitor closely for digitalis-related dysrhythmias.
indomethacin (Indocin)	Renal excretion of digitalis glycosides is reduced, leading to increased serum levels and possibly toxicity. Reduce digitalis glycoside dosage by 50% when indomethacin is started. Monitor closely for both therapeutic and toxic effects and make dosage adjustments accordingly.
magnesium sulfate injection	**Use with extreme caution in individuals receiving digitalis. Alterations in cardiac conduction and heart block may result. Avoid or a potentially serious drug interaction may occur.**
potassium-depleting drugs, such as amphotericin B (parenteral), corticosteroids, or potassium-depleting diuretics	The potential for inducing hypokalemia with these medications may, if used concurrently with digitalis preparations, increase the possibility of digitalis toxicity. Monitor potassium levels closely and the client for signs and symptoms of hypokalemia.
potassium salts	Although potassium salts are commonly prescribed to treat hypokalemia, especially when clients are also taking a digitalis glycoside, potassium salts are not indicated in clients with severe heart block who are receiving digitalis. Hyperkalemia may be very dangerous in such individuals.
propafenone (Rhythmol)	Concurrent use may increase digoxin levels by 25% to 85%, resulting in digitalis toxicity. Careful monitoring of serum digoxin levels and dosage adjustments may be necessary.
quinidine	May result in an increased serum level of digoxin and digitoxin. Monitor serum levels and client's response closely; dosage reductions may be necessary.
spironolactone (Aldactone)	Concurrent administration may increase half-life of digoxin. Monitor closely; dosage reduction may be needed.
sucralfate (Carafate)	Concurrent use decreases absorption of digoxin; space apart by at least 2 hours.

A baseline assessment of the client with congestive heart failure should include the following: weight; blood pressure, pulse pressure, and any postural change in blood pressure; apical pulse rate and rhythm; apical-radial pulse deficit; heart sounds; jugular vein distention; edema; lung sounds; capillary refill time; skin color and temperature; urinary output; determination of presence of chest discomfort (pain or pressure), shortness of breath, syncope, fatigue, nausea, and perception of heart rate ("skipping beats"); level of consciousness and anxiety; cardiac enzymes; serum electrolyte levels, blood urea nitrogen, and creatinine levels; and ECG.

Nursing diagnosis. The client receiving cardiac glycosides is at risk for the following selected nursing diagnoses/collaborative problems: altered comfort (headache, nausea, vomiting); altered visual perceptions (halos of green-yellow light around objects); altered bowel elimination (diarrhea); altered thought processes (confusion, depression); risk for injury (electrolyte imbalance, drowsiness); and the potential complications of allergic reaction, decreased cardiac output, and dysrhythmias.

Implementation

Monitoring. Because altered cardiac output may occur related to the drug's positive inotropic effects, take the adult client's apical pulse for 1 minute before drug administration. Note rate, rhythm, and quality of pulse. If the pulse is 60 or below or a dysrhythmia that had not previously occurred is noted, withhold the drug and report immediately to the prescriber. In children, also take the apical pulse 1 minute before administering the drug. Consult with the prescriber to determine the apical rate at which the drug should be withheld. The pediatric baseline rate usually is higher than adults (see the Pediatric Implications box on p. 498).

Take apical and radial pulse for 1 minute to monitor for atrial fibrillation. In clients with atrial fibrillation, determine pulse deficit (apical pulse minus radial pulse).

Check the following parameters during digitalization: Observe the client for a positive response to digitalization. An increase in cardiac output reflects a more effective cardiac function, which includes improvement in rate and rhythm of heartbeat and in respiration, diuresis, reduction in weight (e.g., decrease in edema), and feeling of well-being.

Know therapeutic digitalis serum levels and normal potassium, calcium, and magnesium ion serum levels. A fall in potassium serum level enhances digitalis effect and the risk of digitalis toxicity. Clients taking digitalis often receive potassium-depleting diuretics, which promote renal potassium excretion and lower serum potassium levels. Monitor serum potassium levels closely. Observe client for symptoms of hypokalemia, such as drowsiness, hypoperistalsis, mental depression, paresthesia, muscle weakness, anorexia, depressed

Pediatric Implications

Cardiac glycosides

A fall in serum potassium levels enhances digitalis effect and increases the risk of digitalis toxicity. Monitor serum potassium levels closely.

Early signs of CHF include tachycardia (especially during rest and minimum activity), increased fatigue and irritability, a sudden weight gain, respiratory distress and profuse scalp sweating especially noted in infants.

Individualize dosing with very close monitoring, especially in infants. Be extremely careful in calculating digitalis dosages; one decimal point placement error can increase the dose tenfold. Double check all calculations with another health care professional (nurse, pharmacist, or physician).

Common signs of digoxin toxicity in children include nausea, vomiting, anorexia, bradycardia, and dysrhythmias.

Give digoxin on a regular time schedule, either 1 hour before or 2 hours after feedings.

From Wong (1995).

BOX 25-2

Serum Digoxin Concentration Determinations

The therapeutic serum digoxin concentration is 0.5 to 2 ng/ml. But be aware that serum levels do not clearly delineate toxic from nontoxic clients. It has been reported that 38% of actual toxic individuals had a digoxin serum level below 2 µg/ml. Some clients with hypokalemia had digoxin toxicity with serum levels of 1.5 ng/ml (Kradjan, 1995). Therefore use serum levels only as a guide; clinical impressions or evaluations are best in measuring therapeutic outcome.

Criteria for use of serum digoxin levels:

1. Suspected toxicity
2. Client's compliance is questionable or unreliable
3. Client not responding appropriately to therapy
4. Presence of impaired renal function
5. Use of drugs with documented interference (quinidine, calcium channel blocking agents, etc.)
6. Confirm an unusual or seriously abnormal digoxin serum level

The time a blood sample is drawn for a digoxin serum level is critical. It is recommended that serum levels obtained 6 to 8 hours after the last oral dose, 2 hours after an intravenous dose, or just before a dose is scheduled are the most reliable.

reflexes, orthostatic hypotension, and polyuria (Cooke, 1992). Provide client taking potassium-depleting diuretics with foods that contain a high potassium content, such as bananas and orange juice if tolerated.

Also monitor serum blood urea nitrogen (BUN) and creatinine levels as evidence of renal function, especially in the elderly.

Observe the rhythm strip for digitalis-induced dysrhythmias if the client is on an ECG monitor. Dysrhythmias that might indicate digoxin toxicity are atrial tachycardia with AV block, progressing AV blocks, accelerated junctional rhythms, and ventricular dysrhythmias, including ventricular bigeminy and ventricular tachycardia (Kelso, 1992). Discontinue the drug if drug intoxication occurs. Serum digitalis level is ordered by prescriber if toxicity is suspected (Box 25-2). Be aware that the range of the therapeutic index of digitalis is extremely narrow. Note that digitoxin has the greatest potential for toxicity because its slow elimination can produce cumulative effects in the body, but may be preferred if the prescriber wants to ensure that body stores will not be rapidly depleted if the client misses a dose. Digoxin may be preferred in individuals with impaired liver function because the drug does not require extensive hepatic metabolism, whereas digitoxin is slowly eliminated from the body by the liver, not the kidneys, which may make it the drug of choice for clients with renal disease.

Observe the client's food intake. Anorexia is almost always the first sign of toxicity; nausea and vomiting, sometimes with abdominal discomfort and increased salivation, usually occur 1 to 2 days after the anorexia.

Monitor intake and output. Delayed or diminished renal excretion of the drug can lead to toxicity. Weigh the client daily, preferably before breakfast, to monitor for an alteration in fluid balance. A sudden weight gain is an early sign of fluid retention. Monitor the client for signs and symptoms of excess fluid volume such as dependent edema (pedal or sacral), basilar crackles in the lungs, and jugular distention.

Intervention. Rapid-acting digoxin is the most commonly prescribed form of a digitalis glycoside used in the coronary care unit (CCU). It may be given intravenously, intramuscularly, or orally. Administer intravenously as an undiluted digoxin (0.25 mg/ml) slowly at 0.25 mg/min. Avoid rapid administration to prevent pulmonary edema. The drug may be administered in diluted form. Administer intravenously with caution to clients with hypertension since it temporarily causes an increase in blood pressure. Avoid intramuscular injections of digoxin because it is painful and the bioavailability of the IM injected drug is low, with unpredictable absorption, especially in clients with severe heart failure, edema, and poor tissue perfusion (Marcus, 1991).

Case Study

The Client with Cardiovascular Disease

Grace Markham is a 63-year-old widow who lives alone. She has a history of rheumatic heart disease manifested by moderate mitral valve stenosis with slight mitral insufficiency. She has been maintained on digoxin, 0.125 mg PO, daily for several years with few adverse effects. Compliance with therapy has generally been excellent. She understands the drug therapy and her 2-g sodium diet.

She was admitted to the hospital complaining of dyspnea on exertion, ankle edema, mild chest pain on exertion, and fatigue. The ECG shows no signs of infarction but does show atrial fibrillation with a ventricular response of 124 beats per minute. Her serum digoxin level was 0.9 ng/ml. A repeat cardiac catheterization showed no changes in the mitral valve but did indicate some early coronary artery narrowing. While she was in the hospital the following medications were ordered for Ms. Markham:

digoxin, 0.25 mg PO, daily
Lasix, 20 mg PO, twice a day
K-Dur, 20 mEq PO, daily
verapamil SR, 240 mg PO, daily
Isordil, 10 mg PO, three times a day

1. Describe the relationship between digoxin, Lasix, and K-Dur in the management of Ms. Markham's symptoms.
2. What additional data should be included in the assessment of the client related to the use of these three medications?
3. What is the significance of the serum digoxin level of 0.9 ng/ml?
4. How will the use of digoxin affect Ms. Markham's atrial fibrillation?

Several weeks later Ms. Markham comes to the clinic complaining of nausea, vomiting, and diarrhea. She reports having had these symptoms for several days. She has continued to take her medications except for the K-Dur, which she found increased the nausea.

5. What additional assessment data (subjective, objective, laboratory) do you want to gather related to these new symptoms?
6. A serum digoxin level for Ms. Markham was 2.5 ng/ml. Explain the significance of this change in relationship to the symptoms she was having.

However, if ordered IM, give digoxin deep into large muscle mass and follow with massage.

The maintenance dose may be given orally if the client can tolerate food; otherwise intravenous injections are required. *Do not administer oral preparation with meals having a high fiber content.* Studies with digoxin show that the drug binds with the fiber, thereby reducing the amount of medication available for absorption from the gut. Advise the client to take drug 1 hour before or 2 hours after meals.

Be aware that digitoxin, though infrequently used, can be given undiluted intravenously (slowly) or orally to avoid pulmonary edema. Oral administration is more consistently absorbed and is safer for individuals with renal disease because the metabolites excreted in the urine are inactive and do not affect the half-life of a digitalis glycoside.

Education. Instruct the client to take digitalis at the same time each day, precisely as prescribed. Do not skip or double a dose if missed. Also, do not change the brand of drug when prescription is refilled because of the difference in the bioavailability in generic forms and Lanoxin. Inform the client that digoxin and Lanoxin are essentially the same drug; in some cases, clients were prescribed both, each by a different prescriber. If using an elixir form of the drug, the dose should be determined using the special dropper that comes with the preparation. Caution client not to take other medications without prior approval of prescriber.

Instruct the client to restrict sodium intake to 2 g daily. Advise clients who are not hospitalized to report weight gain of 1 to 2 pounds a day. Caution clients to avoid licorice because it can induce sodium and water retention.

Advise the client to carry medical identification and to alert health professionals unfamiliar with his or her drug regimen that the drug is being taken.

Teach the client how to take his or her pulse and recommend taking the pulse before each dose of the medication. The dose should be withheld and the prescriber notified if the pulse is below 60 or above 110 and/or is erratic or if the client suffers from anorexia, diarrhea, nausea, vomiting, sudden weight gain, or apparent edema (see the case study above). Visual disturbances, such as blurred vision or green or yellow halos around objects, should also be reported to the prescriber.

Evaluation. The client will demonstrate a normal sinus rhythm on ECG and clinical improvement, e.g., absence of S_3 and basilar crackles and dependent edema, improved activity tolerance, decreased cardiomegaly on x-ray, increased sense of well-being.

Antidote for Digitalis Glycosides

digoxin immune Fab (ovine) (Digibind)

This drug is an antidote for severe digitalis glycoside toxicity. Digoxin immune Fab (ovine) binds and makes complex molecules with digoxin or digitoxin in the serum. These molecules are then excreted by the kidneys. As more tissue

BOX 25-3

Digitalis Toxicity

Almost every type of dysrhythmia can be produced by digitalis toxicity. The type of dysrhythmia produced varies with the age of the client and other factors. Premature ventricular contractions and bigeminal rhythm (two beats and a pause) are common signs of digitalis toxicity in adults, whereas children tend to develop ectopic nodal or atrial beats. Digitalis-induced dysrhythmias are caused by depression of the SA and AV nodes of the heart. This results in various conduction disturbances (first- or second-degree heart block or complete heart block). Digitalis may also cause increased myocardial automaticity, producing extrasystoles or tachycardias.

Nurses must be aware of the predisposing factors to digitalis toxicity. The presence of any of these factors in clients indicates the need for close observation for signs and symptoms of digitalis intoxication:

1. Potassium loss. Hypokalemia (low potassium levels) can increase digitalis cardiotoxicity. Since potassium inhibits the excitability of the heart, a depletion of body or myocardial potassium increases cardiac excitability. Low extracellular potassium is synergistic with digitalis and enhances ectopic pacemaker activity (dysrhythmias). The following are causes of potassium loss:
   a. Hypokalemia occurs if large amounts of body fluids are lost as a result of vomiting, diarrhea, and gastric suctioning.
   b. The use of various diuretic agents (carbonic-anhydrase inhibitors, ammonium chloride, furosemide and thiazide preparations) induces potassium diuresis along with sodium and water diuresis.
   c. Poor dietary intake or severe dietary restrictions decreasing electrolyte intake can cause loss of potassium.
   d. Adrenal steroids cause potassium loss and sodium retention.
   e. Surgical procedures associated with severe electrolyte disturbances such as abdominoperineal resection, colostomy, ileostomy, colectomy, and ureterosigmoidostomy can cause loss of potassium.
   f. Use of potassium-free intravenous fluids can cause hypokalemia.
2. Hypercalcemia. Excess calcium in the presence of digitalis may cause sinus bradycardia, atrioventricular conduction block, and ectopic dysrhythmia.
3. Pathologic conditions. Kidney, liver, and severe heart disease are major factors in digitalis toxicity. Approximately 80% of digoxin is excreted by the kidneys, whereas approximately 90% of digitoxin is first metabolized by the liver. Therefore, in a clinical setting, the physician may choose digitoxin as the drug of choice for a client in renal failure, because of its mode of excretion, i.e., liver metabolism. For a client with liver impairment, the physician may select digoxin as the drug of choice, mainly because it does not rely on the liver for metabolism before excretion. The long half-life of digitoxin is a disadvantage in treatment. If the client should develop digitalis toxicity, the half-life of digoxin may increase from 36 hours to 120 hours, whereas the half-life of digitoxin increases from 120 to 210 hours.

digoxin is released into the serum to maintain an equilibrium, it will be bound and removed by this product, which results in lower levels of digoxin in serum and body tissues.

The drug is indicated for treatment of life-threatening digoxin or digitoxin overdose (Box 25-3).

Onset of action takes place in less than 1 minute, with a half-life of 15 to 20 hours. Initial signs of improvement in digitalis toxicity can be seen in 15 to 30 minutes after administration but can take up to several hours. Arrhythmias and hyperkalemia are usually reversed first, whereas inotropic effect reversal may take several hours. The drug is excreted in the kidneys.

Side/adverse effects. Close monitoring is necessary since withdrawal of digitalis may result in a decrease in cardiac output, congestive heart failure, and hypokalemia. An increase in ventricular rate may be seen in persons with atrial fibrillation. No significant drug interactions have been reported.

Dosage in adults may be calculated on the amount of digoxin or digitoxin consumed or it may be based on steady-state serum levels. Usually a 38-mg dose of digoxin immune Fab (ovine) for injection will bind approximately 0.5 mg of digoxin or digitoxin. The formulas in Box 25-4 may be applied to determine the dose of the antidote.

Miscellaneous Agents

amrinone (Inocor)

The mechanism of action of amrinone has not been fully identified. Amrinone increases force and velocity of myocardial tissues, resulting in a positive inotropic effect. Experiments indicate that amrinone inhibits phosphodiesterase

BOX 25-4

Formulas for Digoxin Immune Fab (ovine)

For digoxin tablets, oral solution, or IM injection:

$$\text{Dose (mg)} = \frac{\text{dose ingested (mg)} \times 0.8}{0.5} \times 38$$

For digitoxin tablets, digoxin capsules, or IV digoxin:

$$\text{Dose (mg)} = \frac{\text{dose ingested (mg)}}{0.5} \times 38$$

When the amount of digitalis ingestion is unknown and the steady-state serum level is also not available, then 760 mg of digoxin immune Fab (ovine) is usually administered because it is reportedly sufficient to treat most life-threatening ingestions.

activity, which in turn increases cellular cAMP concentration and cardiac contractility. Amrinone appears to produce a direct relaxant effect on the vascular smooth muscle (vasodilation) and reduced preload and afterload. It is used to treat congestive heart failure in individuals who do not respond to standard therapies, such as digitalis glycosides, diuretics, and vasodilators.

Administered intravenously, time to peak action is within 10 minutes. Duration of effect is dose-related. If 0.75 mg/kg is administered, duration of action is approximately 30 minutes. If 3 mg/kg is administered, duration is approximately 120 minutes. The half-life when administered in CHF is between 5 to 8.3 hours. The drug is metabolized in the liver and excreted primarily via the kidneys.

The side/adverse effects of amrinone, although infrequent, include nausea, vomiting, abdominal pain, fever, taste alterations, hypotension, arrhythmias, chest pain, and thrombocytopenia. Inotropic effects are additive to those of digitalis. Adult dose is 0.75 mg/kg IV slowly over 2 to 3 minutes; if necessary, repeat in 30 minutes. The maintenance dose by intravenous infusion is 5 to 10 μg/kg/min, individualized according to response. Maximum dosage is 10 mg/kg/day, but in several reports, dosages up to 18 mg/kg/day were given for short time periods.

For neonates and infants, the initial dose is 3 to 4 mg/kg, in divided doses; maintenance dose is 3 to 5 μg/kg/minute for neonates and 10 μg/kg/minute for infants. For FDA category, see the Pregnancy Safety box above.

■ Nursing Management

Amrinone Therapy

Assessment. The nurse should ascertain the status of the client's sensitivity to sulfites since amrinone lactate injection contains sodium metabisulfite to which the client may be intolerant. Amrinone is not to be used with clients with severe aortic or pulmonic valvular disease. It is to be used with caution in clients with impaired hepatic or renal

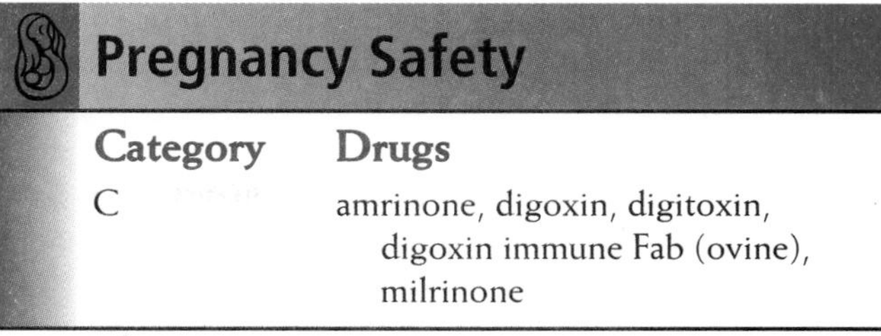

Pregnancy Safety

Category	Drugs
C	amrinone, digoxin, digitoxin, digoxin immune Fab (ovine), milrinone

function; a dosage adjustment may be required because the elimination of the drug will be impaired. Amrinone may aggravate outflow tract obstruction in hypertrophic cardiomyopathy; use with caution.

Nursing diagnosis. The client receiving amrinone is at risk for the following nursing diagnoses/collaborative problems: altered comfort (burning at infusion site, chest pain, nausea, vomiting, abdominal pain); risk for injury related to hypotension (dizziness); hyperpyrexia; and the potential complications of decreased cardiac output, dysrhythmias, dose-dependent thrombocytopenia, hepatotoxicity, and hypersensitivity reactions.

Implementation

Monitoring. Blood pressure and pulse should be monitored to assess hypotensive and dysrhythmic effects of the drug. The infusion rate should be slowed or stopped if the client becomes hypotensive. The appropriate range for blood pressure readings should be prescribed. In addition, assess cardiac index and pulmonary wedge pressure if warranted. Assess electrolytes, central venous pressure, urine output, body weight, and the status of any orthopnea, dyspnea, and fatigue to evaluate the drug's effectiveness and the client's progress.

Assess platelet counts before and frequently during therapy. Observe for unusual bleeding and bruising, which are clinical signs of thrombocytopenia. The drug may be discontinued if the platelet count falls below 150,000/mm^3.

Because of the possibility of hepatotoxicity, liver function studies are usually done and the client is monitored for clinical signs of jaundice. These signs include yellowish skin or sclera, dark urine, and pruritus. Report nausea and vomiting to the prescriber. It may be severe enough to require that the drug be discontinued.

If the drug is monitored through plasma concentrations, the therapeutic range is 0.5 to 7 μg/ml but optimal level is about 3 μg/ml. Monitor for sulfite sensitivity (see Box 22-2). Monitor, too, for tachyphylaxis to the effects of amrinone, a common occurrence, usually taking place within the first 72 hours of therapy.

Intervention. Examine the solution for color changes and/or precipitation. Amrinone is incompatible with dextrose because it loses its potency. However, it may be diluted in saline and administered as a bolus through a line containing freely running D_5W. Do not mix with furosemide (Lasix) or inject it into the same tubing because it precipitates.

For direct intravenous administration, it may be administered by direct injection over 2 to 3 minutes or diluted in 0.45% or 0.9% saline solution to a concentration of 1 to 3 mg/ml and given by continuous infusion. Use prepared solution within 24 hours. Administer slowly intravenously, over 2 to 3 minutes, to minimize pain and burning at the injection site. Avoid extravasation. Change infusion sites every 48 hours; administer with an infusion pump.

Education. Instruct the client to move slowly from a sitting or lying position to a more upright position because of the drug's hypotensive effects.

Evaluation. The client will demonstrate a normal sinus rhythm on ECG and clinical improvement, e.g., absence of S_3 and basilar crackles, dependent edema; improved activity tolerance; decreased cardiomegaly on x-ray; and increased sense of well-being.

milrinone injection (Primacor IV)

Milrinone is indicated for the short-term treatment of congestive heart failure. It is a selective inhibitor of cAMP isozymes in cardiac and vascular muscle; thus it improves cardiac function, contractility and vasodilation, without increasing myocardial oxygen consumption and heart rate. It is a positive inotrope and vasodilator with very little chronotropic activity.

After IV (loading dose) administration, hemodynamic improvement has been reported within 5 to 15 minutes, lasting up to 2 days after a 50 µg/kg dose (Sanofi Winthrop Letter, 1992). Significant drug interactions have not been reported, but its administration with other hypotension-producing drugs may have an additive effect.

A chemical interaction (precipitate) has been reported when furosemide (Lasix) was administered via an IV line containing a milrinone infusion. This procedure should be avoided.

Significant side effects/adverse reactions include headaches, hypotension, and ventricular arrhythmias; and rarely, angina and thrombocytopenia. See current guidelines for dosing recommendations.

The nursing management is the same as for amrinone.

SUMMARY

Cardiac glycosides increase the strength of cardiac contraction and alter the electrophysiologic properties of the heart by slowing conduction velocity, which accounts for their therapeutic properties for the treatment of heart failure. Clients may be hospitalized for rapid digitalization—which is the saturation of the body tissues with enough digitalis glycoside to cause the signs and symptoms of heart failure to disappear—or they may receive digitalization at a slower rate prescribed in an ambulatory setting. In either case, because the therapeutic index of the drug is so narrow, the nurse has the responsibility to closely monitor the client for signs of toxicity and to also teach the client about the drug's therapeutic and nontherapeutic effects. The nurse must be aware of the predisposing factors to digitalis toxicity and assist the client in also recognizing some of them. Potassium loss is the most common risk factor for digitalis toxicity. Digoxin immune Fab (ovine) for injection is used as an antidote for severe digitalis glycoside toxicity.

The nurse has a major assessment and educational role with clients using cardiac glycosides, since many clients take these drugs on a long-term basis. It is important not only that they take them accurately, but also that they are knowledgeable about the drugs to minimize the risk for injury inherent in their administration.

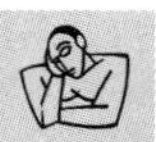

Critical Thinking

1. What electrolyte imbalances affect the development of digitalis glycoside toxicity? In what way?
2. Mrs. Stacy, a 74-year-old client with chronic congestive heart failure, is leaving the hospital with a medication regimen that includes digoxin, furosemide, and potassium supplements. What instructions would be essential to include in a teaching plan for Mrs. Stacy to enable her to safely and accurately self-administer her medications?

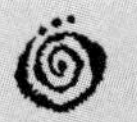

Collaborative Learning Activities

1. Three teams of students will present the case study of the client with cardiovascular disease. The first team should answer question one of the case and develop a plan of care related to her medications using only the three nursing diagnoses of highest priority. The second team is to answer the rest of the questions related to her present hospitalization. Team three is to discuss the rest of the questions and develop a plan of care for following Mrs. Markham at home.

BIBLIOGRAPHY

American Hospital Formulary Service (1996). *AHFS drug information '96.* Bethesda, MD: American Society of Hospital Pharmacists.

American Medical Association (1995). *Drug evaluations: Annual 1995.* Chicago: The Association.

Anderson KN, et al. (Eds.) (1994). *Mosby's Medical, nursing, & allied health dictionary* (4th ed.). St Louis: Mosby.

Cawley M (1994). The role of digoxin in the treatment of atrial fibrillation, *J Cardiopulm Rehab 14*(6):373-5.

Cooke DM (1992). Shielding your patient from digitalis toxicity, *Nursing 22*(7):44-7.

Cooke DM (1991). Current perspectives on intravenous administration of digoxin, *J Intraven Nurs 15*(6):310-4.

Covington TR (1995). *Handbook of nonprescription drugs: Product updates* (10th ed.). Washington, DC: American Pharmaceutical Association.

Graedon J & Graedon T (1995). *The people's guide to deadly drug interactions.* New York: St. Martin's Press.

Kelso LA (1992). Dysrhythmias associated with digoxin toxicity, *AACN 3*(1):220-5.

Kradjan WA (1995). Congestive heart failure. In Young LY & Koda-Kimble MA. *Applied therapeutics: The clinical use of drugs* (6th ed.). Vancouver: Applied Therapeutics.

Long JW & Rybacki JJ (1995). *The essential guide to prescription drugs.* New York: HarperCollins.

Marcus FI (1991). Digitalis: How well are you using it?, *Patient Care 25*(17):21.

Meisser JE & Gever LN (1993). Reducing the risks of digitalis toxicity, *Nursing* 23(7):47-51.

New Medicines (1995). 107 medicines in testing for two leading causes of death in Americans, *PhRMA*. Pharmaceutical Manufacturers Association.

Olin BR (Ed.) (1995). *Facts and comparisons: Drug information*. St Louis: Facts and Comparisons.

Sanofi Winthrop Pharmaceutical Priority Letter (1992). *Primacor IV*. (J Coelho, Senior Associate Medical Director). 60-225580.

Semla TP, Beizer JL, & Higbee MD (1993). *Geriatric dosage handbook*. Hudson, OH: Lexi-Comp.

Silverman M (1942). *Magic in a bottle*. New York: Macmillan.

United States Pharmacopeial Convention (1996). *USP DI: Drug information for the health care professional* (16th ed.). Rockville, MD: The Convention.

Wong DL (1995). Whaley & Wong's *Nursing care of infants and children* (5th ed.). St Louis: Mosby.

Wright JM (1995). Pharmacologic management of congestive heart failure, *Crit Care Nurse Q* 18(1):32-44.

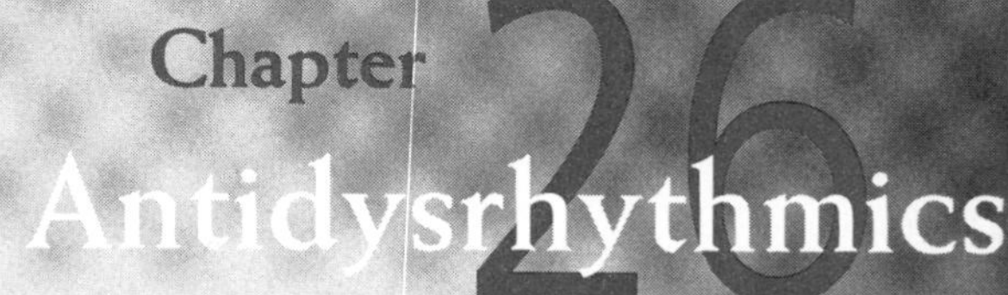

Chapter 26
Antidysrhythmics

Chapter Focus

While during the last decade the use of antidysrhythmic drugs has increased tremendously, the nurse should be aware that they are as life saving as they can be life threatening (Stier, 1992). The benefit versus the risk requires evaluation with each client. The quality of client care is enhanced by the nurse's role in client teaching and knowledge of antidysrhythmic therapy. The following objectives and key terms are important for a good understanding of this chapter.

Key Terms

Adams-Stokes syndrome (p. 513)
automaticity (p. 505)
conductivity (p. 505)
dysrhythmia (arrhythmia) (p. 505)
sinus bradycardia (p. 505)
sinus tachycardia (p. 505)
Wolff-Parkinson-White syndrome (p. 513)

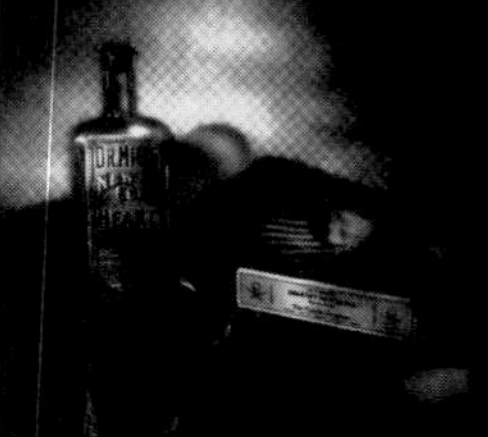

Key Drugs [▲]

lidocaine
procainamide
quinidine

Objectives

1. Identify the medications most commonly used as antidysrhythmic agents.
2. Describe the primary electrophysiologic effects and ECG effects of the major antidysrhythmic agents.
3. Relate at least three nursing evaluation strategies to monitor client response to antidysrhythmic therapy.
4. List the most common adverse reactions experienced by the elderly client receiving specific antidysrhythmic therapy.
5. Implement nursing management of the care for individual clients who require the administration of an antidysrhythmic agent.

A cardiac **dysrhythmia** may be defined as any deviation from the normal rhythm of the heartbeat. Dysrhythmia is caused by some disorder that modifies the electrophysiologic properties of the cells of the conduction system or cardiac muscle cells. For a review of the electrophysiologic events of a normal action potential, see Chapter 24, Overview of the Cardiovascular System.

Antidysrhythmic drugs are used for the treatment and prevention of disorders of cardiac rhythm. Dysrhythmias often develop in individuals about 4 to 72 hours after myocardial infarction ("heart attack"). In addition, abnormal rhythm may occur in those recovering from cardiac surgery, in clients with coronary artery disease, and in individuals with extracardiac disorders, such as pheochromocytoma, electrolyte imbalance, or thyroid disease.

DISORDERS IN CARDIAC ELECTROPHYSIOLOGY

Disorders of cardiac rhythm arise as a result of (1) abnormality in spontaneous initiation of an impulse, or **automaticity**, or (2) abnormality in impulse conduction, or **conductivity.** In some conditions, a combination of both processes may occur.

Abnormality in automaticity. A disturbance in automaticity may alter the heart's rate, rhythm, or site of origin of impulse formation. When the rate of pacemaker activity is affected, a decrease in automaticity of the SA node produces **sinus bradycardia** (an abnormal condition in which the myocardium contracts steadily but at a rate less than 60 contractions per minute) whereas an increase in automaticity of the SA node results in **sinus tachycardia** (an abnormal condition in which the myocardium contracts regularly but at a rate greater than 100 beats per minute). On the other hand, a shift in the site of origin of impulse formation can generate an abnormal pacemaker or an ectopic focus, resulting in activation of some part of the heart other than the SA node. This is called an ectopic pacemaker, and it may discharge at either a regular or an irregular rhythm. It occurs because the cardiac fibers depolarize more frequently than the SA node. Consequently, abnormal automaticity may develop in cells that usually do not initiate impulses, for example, atrial or ventricular cells. Clinical disorders such as hypoxia or ischemia can activate sympathetic receptors that in turn become centers to initiate impulses. In addition, ischemic sites can cause impulse disturbances in automaticity and also in conductivity, and both manifestations are responsible for ectopic beats. The ectopic beats are classified as escape beats, premature beats or extrasystoles, and ectopic tachydysrhythmia.

Abnormality in conductivity. Altered conduction of the cardiac impulse probably accounts for more dysrhythmias than a change in automaticity. A disturbance in conductivity may be caused by (1) delay or block of impulse conduction or (2) the reentry phenomenon.

Delay or block of impulse conduction. Normally, the SA node and AV junction are poor conductors of impulse transmission. Under abnormal circumstances, conduction of an atrial impulse to the ventricles may be delayed or blocked in the AV junction or structures beyond this region in the conduction pathway. However, impaired impulse transmission generally appears in the AV junction and occurs in varying degrees of block. In the first-degree AV block the impulses from the SA node pass through to the ventricles very slowly, and this is noted by a prolonged P-R interval on the ECG. In the second-degree block some atrial beats fail to pass into the ventricles through the AV junction. Finally, in the third-degree block or complete heart block, no impulses reach the ventricle, in which case the Purkinje fibers initiate their own spontaneous depolarization at a very slow rate. This results in independent ventricular and atrial rhythms referred to as ventricular "escape."

Reentry phenomenon. Reentry phenomenon is the mechanism responsible for initiating ectopic beats. A necessary condition for reentry is unidirectional block. Normally, when an impulse travels down the Purkinje fiber, it spreads along two branches and when it enters the connecting branch, impulses are extinguished at the point of collision in the center (Figure 26-1, *A*). At the same time, other impulses that begin laterally from the Purkinje fibers activate ventricular muscle tissue. In an abnormal situation the impulse descending from the central Purkinje fiber travels down the right branch normally but encounters a block in the left branch as a result of ischemia or injury (Figure 26-1, *B*). This is a unidirectional block, because the impulse is capable of passing in one direction but not in the other. As a result, in the left branch, where the impulse is blocked in the forward direction at the site of injury, a retrograde or reverse impulse from the ventricular tissue penetrates or reenters the depressed region from the other direction, provided that the pathway proximal to the block is no longer refractory. When the effective refractory period of the blocked area is over, reentry of the impulse from the ventricular muscle into this site causes the impulse to circulate or recycle repetitively through the loop, resulting in a circus-type movement that produces dysrhythmia.

As shown in Figure 26-1, *C*, reentry is abolished by certain drug groups, which are explained later in this chapter. *Drugs that decrease or slow conduction velocity can convert unidirectional block to a two-way or bidirectional block.* As the impulses traveling in the antegrade or forward direction and those appearing in a retrograde or reverse direction are blocked at the injured site, the reentry pathway is interrupted, thereby abolishing the ectopic beats. In Figure 26-1, *D*, the conditions required for preventing reentry by another mechanism are also illustrated. *The Group I-B drugs have no effect on conduction velocity, thus they eliminate reentry by stopping unidirectional block entirely.* Consequently, the normal impulse conduction along the right and left branches of the Purkinje fibers is again restored.

■ ■ ■

In recent years an increasing number of antidysrhythmic drugs have required classification into categories based on their fundamental mode of action on cardiac muscle. Such a

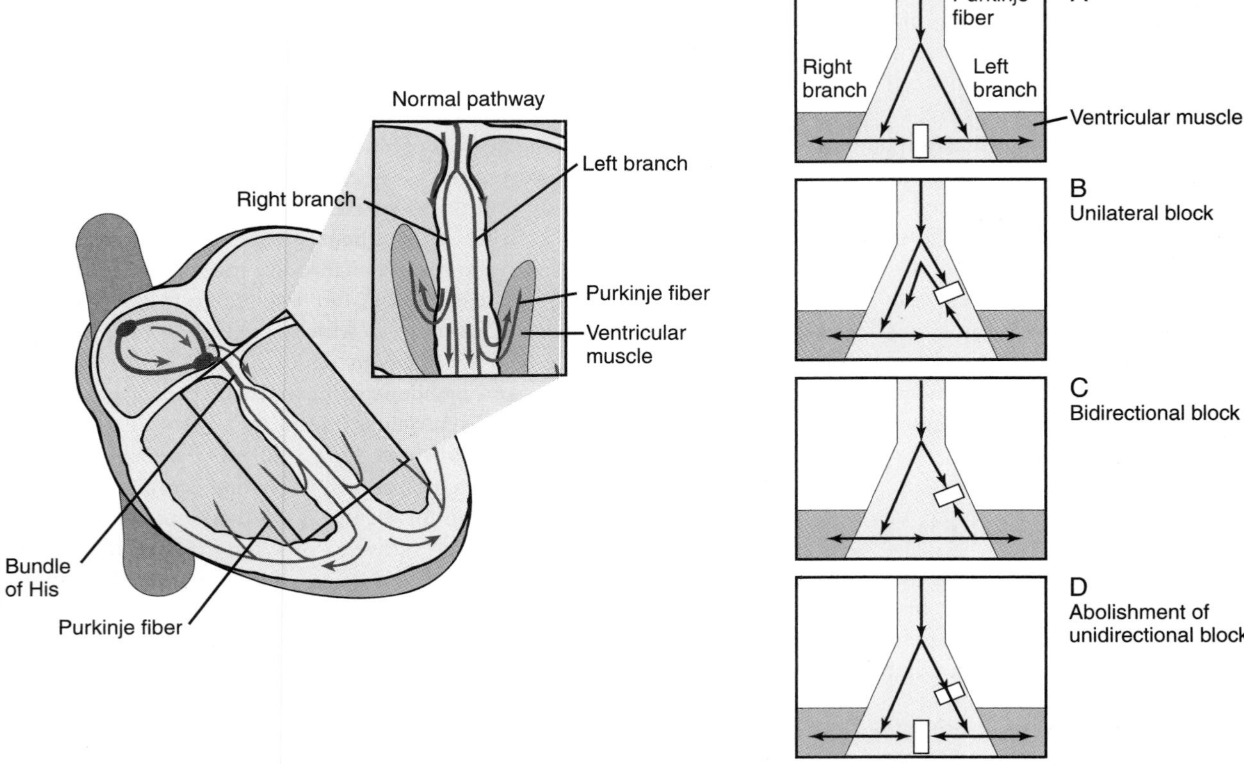

Figure 26-1 Reentry phenomenon. Illustration of a branched Punkinje fiber that activates ventricular muscle.

grouping of antidysrhythmic mechanisms should prove of value in predicting the drug's therapeutic efficacy. Although all drugs belonging to a particular class do not necessarily possess totally identical actions. In some cases a given agent may have subsidiary properties (extracardiac effects) that alter the basic electrophysiologic actions on the cardiac muscle. The currently available antidysrhythmic drugs are classified into four categories according to their mechanisms of action (Box 26-1). However, these drugs have one major electrophysiologic property in common: they all have the ability to suppress automaticity.

Group I compounds are subdivided into groups I-A, I-B, or I-C to reflect the similar electrophysiologic effects of each subgroup. The only exception to the sub-category division is moricizine. Moricizine (Ethmozine) is listed under Group I as it has characteristics of all three groups, 1A, 1B, and 1C (Olin, 1996). Class 1 drugs bind to sodium channels interfering with sodium influx during phase 0 of the action potential, thus depressing conduction velocity. Group I-A drugs include disopyramide (Norpace), procainamide (Pronestyl), and quinidine (Cin-Quin); Group I-B are lidocaine, mexiletine (Mexitil), phenytoin (Dilantin), and tocainide (Tonocard) while Group I-C includes flecainide (Tambocor), and propafenone (Rhythmol). Group 1-C drugs, because of their prodysrhythmic effects, should be carefully selected and closely monitored when prescribed.

BOX 26-1

Antidysrhythmic Classifications

Group I drugs—fast sodium channel blockade in cardiac muscle, resulting in an increased refractory period

(Subclasses I-A, I-B, and I-C further define the differences between the drugs).

Group II drugs—beta-adrenergic blocking agents that reduce adrenergic stimulation on the heart

Group III drugs—generally do not affect depolarization but work by prolonging cardiac repolarization

Group IV drugs—block the slow calcium channel, resulting in depression of myocardial and smooth muscle contraction, decreased automaticity, and, perhaps, decreased conduction velocity

Propranolol (Inderal), acebutolol (Sectral), and esmolol (Brevibloc) are considered Group II drugs because of their beta-adrenergic blocking action.

Group III drugs include bretylium (Bretylol), amiodarone (Cardarone), ibutilide (Corvert), and sotalol (Betapace). The principal action of bretylium is antiadrenergic; it also has a positive inotropic action and prolongs repolarization. Amiodarone increases the refractory period and increases the P-R interval, QRS complex, and Q-T interval, contrary to the typical effects of bretylium.

The last category, which is identified as Group IV agents, is characterized by a selective calcium antagonistic action. For this reason, verapamil is classified independently of other conventional compounds and is discussed in Chapter 28. Adenosine is listed under the unclassified antiarrhythmic agents.

■ Nursing Management

Antidysrhythmic Therapy

Assessment. Careful evaluation is necessary to determine the effect of a dysrhythmia for a specific client. Depending on the individual's health status and the degree of dysrhythmia, the effect may range from benign to life threatening. A thorough history, physical assessment, and an interpretation of the dysrhythmia on ECG are essential for formulating the possible nursing diagnoses.

A baseline assessment of the client with dysrhythmias should include: blood pressure, pulse pressure, and any postural change; apical pulse rate and rhythm; apical-radial pulse deficit; heart sounds; jugular vein distention; edema; capillary refill time; urinary output; determination of presence of chest discomfort (pain or pressure), shortness of breath, syncope, fatigue, nausea, and perception of heart rate ("skipping beats"); level of consciousness and anxiety; serum electrolyte levels; and ECG.

Nursing diagnosis. Possible nursing diagnoses/collaborative problems that the client receiving an antidysrhythmic agent might experience may include but are not limited to the following: altered comfort (nausea); risk for injury related to hypotension and dizziness; activity intolerance; knowledge deficit; anxiety; and the potential complications of altered cerebral and peripheral tissue perfusion and decreased cardiac output. The nurse will need to consider these issues in the care and education of clients taking antidysrhythmic agents.

Implementation

Monitoring. To determine the effectiveness of the therapy, the nurse should continue to assess the indicators of the baseline assessment. The client should be questioned as to episodes of lightheadedness, dizziness, or confusion. The ECG is monitored for changes.

Intervention. Although some clients with cardiac dysrhythmias may require an artificial pacemaker to control their dysrhythmia, most are treated with antidysrhythmic agents sometime in the course of their illness.

Education. Instruction of the client receiving antidysrhythmic agents provides the opportunity for the client to self-administer the medications safely and accurately. Much anxiety can be allayed through instruction regarding the dysrhythmia and its management. This is essential because medications may have to be taken for a lifetime. The client should be able to take and assess pulse rate and rhythm accurately, counting for 1 full minute. He or she should be able to describe the medication regimen, including dosage scheduling, rationale, and side effects/adverse reactions of the prescribed medications. Coffee, tea, and cola drinks may need to be limited since caffeine can cause an increase in abnormal heart rhythm. The client should be able to state signs and symptoms to report to the prescriber, including chest pain, dizziness, low blood pressure, gastrointestinal distress, blurred vision, a change in respiratory status or pulse rate or rhythm, swollen feet or ankles, or a sudden weight gain. He or she should be able to state the need for ongoing care and the importance of adherence to the prescribed treatment regimen.

Evaluation. The administration of antidysrhythmic agents has the expected outcomes of having the client maintain cardiac output, evidenced by blood pressure, pulse, and capillary refill within normal limits; increase activity tolerance, as evidenced by less fatigue and less dyspnea; have less chest pain, palpitations, and associated symptoms; and demonstrate no dysrhythmias on ECG tracings. The efficacy of these medications for a particular client is determined by the achievement of these goals. Modification of the nursing care plan may be necessary for the client to achieve the goals for management of the dysrhythmia.

GROUP I-A DRUGS

The pharmacologic effects of procainamide, quinidine, and disopyramide are similar: they bind to sodium channels and interfere with sodium influx during phase 0 of the action potential. The result is depression of conduction velocity. EKG effects of these drugs include widening of the QRS and a prolonged QT. Of these agents quinidine has been most widely used and serves as the key drug for this group.

▲ **quinidine gluconate** [kwin' i deen] (Duraquin, Quinaglute)
▲ **quinidine polygalacturonate** (Cardioquin)
▲ **quinidine sulfate** (Cin-Quin)

Quinidine stabilizes the cell membrane by preventing ready movement of sodium and potassium across this cellular barrier. This inhibition of cation exchange results in a decrease in the rate of diastolic depolarization from resting potential during phase 4 and an increase in the threshold potential (the voltage shifts toward 0 mv). Therefore quinidine decreases impulse conduction and delays repolarization in the atria, ventricles, and Purkinje fibers. By decreasing impulse generation at ectopic sites, quinidine suppresses or abolishes dysrhythmias. Fortunately, abnormal or ectopic pacemaker tissue appears to be more sensitive to quinidine than normal pacemaker tissue (SA node), thus permitting the SA node to reestablish control over impulse formation in the heart.

Widening of the QRS complex indicates a decrease in intraventricular conduction, and lengthening of the P-R interval represents slower conduction through the AV junction, which are changes observed on the ECG when quinidine is used. Thus caution must be used when the drug is given to individuals with intraventricular conduction disorders.

Perhaps the most significant action of quinidine is its ability to prolong the effective refractory period of atrial and ventricular fibers. A delay in completion of repolarization probably exerts an important antifibrillatory action. The tissue remains refractory for a period of time after full restoration of the resting membrane potential. This property is believed to influence the conversion of unidirectional block to bidirectional block, thereby abolishing the reentry type of dysrhythmia (see Figure 26-1, C).

The indirect anticholinergic effect of quinidine inhibits vagal action on the SA node and AV junction. This atropine-like effect permits the sinus node to accelerate and often may provoke a dangerous sinus tachycardia. Therefore digoxin, a beta blocker, or verapamil are usually administered before quinidine to prevent ventricular acceleration, when one is attempting to convert atrial fibrillation to normal sinus rhythm. Finally, the chief noncardiac action of quinidine is peripheral vasodilation, which results from quinidine's alpha-adrenergic blocking effect on vascular smooth muscle. The combined effect of a decrease in peripheral vascular resistance and a reduced cardiac output caused by depressed myocardial contractility contributes to the development of hypotension, a condition that may reach serious proportions during quinidine therapy.

Quinidine is used in the management of ventricular and supraventricular arrhythmias. Pharmacokinetics are detailed in Table 26-1. The side/adverse effects of quinidine include anorexia, diarrhea, bitter taste, nausea, vomiting, abdominal distress, flushing, rash, tinnitus, confusion, and visual changes.

Quinidine salts contain different percentages of active drug: quinidine gluconate, 62%; quinidine polygalacturonate, 80%; quinidine sulfate, 83%, therefore they are not interchangeable without an appropriate dosage adjustment. Quinidine sulfate 200 mg is considered equivalent to 275 mg of quinidine gluconate or of quinidine polygalacturonate. The usual quinidine sulfate adult dose is 200 to 300 mg PO 3 to 4 times daily; the pediatric dose is 6 mg/kg body weight in 5 divided doses.

■ Nursing Management

Quinidine Therapy

In addition to the general nursing management for antidysrhythmic therapy:

Assessment. The client's health status should be assessed to determine whether he or she has a medical condition for which the administration of quinidine might be contraindicated or incur some risk. Do not use in clients with complete atrioventricular (AV) block or AV or intraventricular conduction defects, because of additional cardiac depression. If quinidine is administered to clients with myasthenia gravis, it may increase muscle weakness because of its weak curare-like action. Quinidine should be used with caution with clients with a history of thrombocytopenia. Clients with hepatic or renal function impairment may require decreased dosages to avoid accumulation of the drug. With incomplete AV block and digitalis toxicity, the additive effects of quinidine will increase conduction inhibition and result in more cardiac depression. Clients sensitive to quinine may also be sensitive to quinidine.

The nurse should review the client's current medication regimen for significant drug interactions. The following significant drug interactions may occur when quinidine is given with the drugs listed below.

Drug	Possible effect and management
antidysrhythmic agents	May result in enhanced cardiac response. Monitor ECG tracings closely.
anticoagulants, such as warfarin (Coumadin)	Monitor for signs of additional anticoagulant effects, such as excessive bruising, bleeding gums, black stools, hematuria, hematemesis. It may be necessary to adjust anticoagulant dosage both during therapy and after quinidine therapy is discontinued.
neuromuscular blocking agents	Monitor for increased or enhanced blocking effects, especially in the postsurgical client.
pimozide (Orap)	May potentiate cardiac dysrhythmias. Monitor closely, preferably with an ECG, since intervention may be necessary.
urinary alkalizers, such as carbonic anhydrase inhibitors, citrus fruit juices in large amounts, antacids	May result in increased reabsorption of quinidine and elevated serum levels; dosage adjustments may be necessary.

Nursing diagnosis. With the administration of quinidine, the client may experience the following nursing diagnoses/collaborative problems: altered comfort (skin flushing, bitter taste, anorexia, nausea and vomiting, and abdominal cramping); risk for injury related to cinchonism (blurred vision, dizziness, headache, altered hearing), hypotension (syncope), and anemia (tiredness, weakness); altered nutrition related to gastrointestinal effects; and altered thought processes (confusion), and the potential complications of allergic reaction (fever, rash, wheezing, dyspnea); thrombocytopenia (unusual bruising or bleeding); and further dysrhythmias.

Implementation

Monitoring. Use caution during intravenous administration of quinidine because of possible vasodilation, depressed cardiac contraction, and cardiovascular collapse, which may lead to profound shock. NOTE: The intravenous (IV) route is seldom used. Continuously monitor both the ECG and the systemic arterial blood pressure during and immediately after parenteral administration. Toxic effects include widening of QRS complex in excess of 25%, abolition of P waves, and ventricular extrasystoles. Notify the prescriber immediately when such effects occur.

Monitor intake and output, blood counts, serum electrolyte determinations, and kidney and liver function tests during prolonged therapy. The effect of quinidine is reduced if hypokalemia is present.

Use quinidine with caution in clients with atrial fibrillation or flutter. The vagal blocking effect of the drug may increase the number of atrial beats conducted across the AV junction, resulting in sudden acceleration in ventricular rate.

TABLE 26-1 Selected antidysrhythmics: pharmacokinetics

Drug	Time to peak level or effect (hr)	Duration of action* (hr)	Therapeutic serum level‡ (μ/ml)
Group I-A drugs			
disopyramide	0.5-3	1.5-8.5	3-6
procainamide	1-1.5	3	4-10
quinidine	1-4	6-8	3-6
Group I-B drugs			
lidocaine	IV: 1 min	10-20 min	1.5-5
	IM: 3-15 min	60-90 min	
tocainide	½-2	8	6-15
mexiletine	2-3	—	0.5-2
Group I-C drugs			
flecainide	3	—	0.4-1
encainide	0.5-1.5	—	—
propafenone	1-3.5	—	0.2-1.5 (trough)
Group I (A, B, C)			
moricizine	0.5-2 level 6-14 effect	10-24	—
Group II drugs			
propranolol	1-1.5	3-5	—
Group III drugs			
bretylium	IV: 5-10 min†		
	IM: 1†	6-24	0.5-2.5
amiodarone	3-7	Variable	—
sotalol	2-3	7-18	—
Group IV drugs			
Calcium antagonists—see Chapter 28			

(Olin, 1996; *USP DI*, 1996; Chow & Kertland, 1995.)
*Metabolism/excretion is primarily via the liver/kidneys with the exception of amiodarone, which is mainly excreted via bile.
†To treat ventricular fibrillation.
‡Steady state plasma level.

Prior administration of digitalis slows AV conduction and reduces the hazard of ventricular tachycardia. Monitor ECG and blood serum levels of the two drugs to avoid toxicity. Reduction in digoxin dosage is suggested when quinidine is given simultaneously. Check plasma quinidine levels carefully. Be aware that concomitant administration with digitalis (digoxin) readily induces toxicity because the two drugs lead to an excessively high plasma concentration of digoxin (less digoxin is excreted by the kidney).

Be alert to premature ventricular contractions not noted before drug administration (appears as an ectopic foci by reentry phenomenon) because they may lead to ventricular tachycardia or fibrillation and subsequently to cardiac standstill (asystole). Note that another form of ventricular disorder can cause "quinidine syncope." It produces ventricular tachycardia or fibrillation, causing a decrease in cardiac output and thereby diminishing blood flow to the brain. The symptoms are a feeling of faintness, loss of consciousness, and ultimately sudden death.

Intervention. To determine if the client may have an idiosyncratic response or hypersensitivity to quinidine, give a test dose of 200 mg orally a few hours before the initiation of therapy. A parenteral dose of 200 mg is also administered before intramuscular (IM) or intravenous (IV) therapy if time permits. Observe the client for fever, acute asthma, angioedema, and anaphylactic shock. Cinchonism may also be manifested by headache, dizziness, fever, tinnitus, nausea, tremor, and visual disturbances. Administer oral preparation on an empty stomach 1 to 2 hours after meals with a full glass of water to promote absorption. However, quinidine may be given with food to decrease gastric distress if it occurs.

Education. Instruct the client to report any symptoms of rash, ringing in the ears, or visual disturbances. Caution client to immediately report feeling faint (see Quinidine Syncope in a subsequent nursing management section). Also, examine buccal mucosa for petechial hemorrhage. If bleeding occurs, report immediately. The drug will be discontinued because of possible thrombocytopenic purpura.

Advise the client to have regular dental checkups and to practice good dental hygiene since the antimuscarinic effects of the drug inhibit salivary flow and so contribute to caries and gum disease, particularly in the elderly. Recommend that the client carry medical identification. Caution the client to alert health professionals, including dentists, that quinidine is being taken.

Evaluation. The client's ECG will demonstrate an absence of atrial and ventricular ectopy.

disopyramide [dye soe peer' a mide] (Norpace)

Disopyramide effects are similar to quinidine with the exception that its anticholinergic effects are more prominent. This is the reason a drug that slows AV conduction is administered with disopyramide when it is used in the treatment of atrial flutter or atrial fibrillation. Reentrant dysrhythmias are abolished by converting a unidirectional block into a bidirectional block (see Figure 26-1).

Disopyramide is indicated to treat ventricular dysrhythmias. For pharmacokinetics see Table 26-1. The side/adverse effects of disopyramide are similar to quinidine with exception of tinnitus, visual changes and rash. In addition, disopyramide may cause dry mouth and throat, difficulty in urination, weight gain, and sexual impotency.

Dosage is individualized according to response and tolerance. The usual adult loading dose is 300 mg for clients 50 kg or greater; maintenance dose is 150 mg every 6 hours. Elderly clients usually require a reduction in dosage, since they are more sensitive to the effects produced by the usual adult dosage. Pediatric dose varies by age; check a current reference for specific dosing recommendations.

■ Nursing Management

Disopyramide Therapy

In addition to the general nursing management of antidysrhythmic therapy previously discussed, the following should be considered:

Assessment. Despite the fact that little effect has been shown on the AV junction conduction time, do not use this drug in clients with greater than first-degree block. Drug should be discontinued if second- or third-degree block occurs during therapy; the P-R interval will be prolonged. Do not use in clients with cardiogenic shock or known hypersensitivity to the drug.

Disopyramide may cause hypoglycemia in clients with diabetes mellitus. Administer disopyramide phosphate cautiously in pregnant clients because it has been reported to produce uterine contractions in such clients.

The drug's anticholinergic properties may cause urinary retention in clients with prostatic enlargement or bladder neck obstruction or a myasthenic crisis if the client has myasthenia gravis. This anticholinergic activity of the drug may also precipitate an acute condition in clients with a history of closed-angle glaucoma. If administered to clients with either renal or hepatic function impairment, an accumulation of disopyramide may result; dosage reductions may be required. Administration to clients with cardiac conditions such as cardiac conduction abnormalities resulting in decreased conduction, congestive heart failure, and cardiomyopathies is not recommended because of its cardiac depressive effects. The client's serum potassium level must be within the normal range; if it is too high, then serious dysrhythmias may occur; if it is too low, the drug may not be effective.

The nurse should review the client's current medication regimen for significant drug interactions. The following interactions may occur when disopyramide is given with the drugs listed below:

Drug	Possible effect and management
Other antiarrhythmic agents, such as diltiazem (Cardizem), flecainide (Tambocor), lidocaine, procainamide (Pronestyl), beta-adrenergic blocking agents, quinidine, tocainide (Tonocard), or verapamil (Calan)	**Monitor closely for prolonged electrophysiologic conduction and decreased cardiac output. Beta-adrenergic blocking agents may exacerbate heart failure, especially in individuals with compromised ventricular function. Avoid or a potentially serious drug interaction may occur. Do not administer disopyramide concurrently or within 48 hours before or 24 hours after verapamil, since fatalities have been reported.**
pimozide (Orap)	Concurrent therapy may prolong the QT interval, which may result in cardiac arrhythmias. If used concurrently, monitor closely.

In addition to the assessment indicators discussed within the general nursing management of antidysrhythmic therapy, a baseline assessment of the client receiving disopyramide should include blood glucose determination, intraocular pressure, complete blood cell counts, and hepatic and renal function.

Nursing diagnosis. With the administration of disopyramide, the client has the potential for development of the following nursing diagnoses/collaborative problems: urinary retention related to the drug's anticholinergic effects (10% to 20%); altered comfort related to chest pain (1% to 10%), dry mouth (40%); altered thought processes (confusion [1% to 10%], depression [<1%]); excess fluid volume (1% to 10%) (swelling of the feet and lower legs, rapid weight gain, shortness of breath); risk for injury related to dizziness, syncope, and weakness of hypotension (1% to 10%), blurred vision, and hypoglycemia (<1%); altered bowel elimination (constipation) related to the anticholinergic effects(1% to 10%); altered self-concept related to decreased sexual ability (1% to 10%) and the potential complications of decreased cardiac output (1% to 10%) and agranulocytosis (<1%) (sore throat and fever).

Implementation

Monitoring. Monitor blood pressure carefully; disopyramide should be discontinued if hypotension, bradycardia, or congestive heart failure becomes worse. The symptoms of congestive heart failure are difficulty in breathing, shortness of breath, weight gain, distended neck veins, and pulmonary rales.

Monitor ECG intervals carefully to avoid cardiac toxicity. The following signs are indications to collaborate with the prescriber in planning for drug withdrawal:

- If QRS complex widens more than 25%
- If Q-T interval is prolonged more than 25% (dose monitoring required and consideration of discontinuing the drug)

ECG monitoring is essential for clients with severe cardiac disease, hypertension, or renal or hepatic impairment.

Monitor serum potassium level; it should be normal to achieve optimal effect. Toxic reactions are enhanced by excessive potassium levels. Measure intake and output, particularly in clients with impaired renal function or prostatic hypertrophy. Urinary retention may require stopping the use of disopyramide. Monitor blood glucose concentrations for those clients at risk for hypoglycemia.

Intervention. Clients with preexisting closed-angle glaucoma should receive disopyramide only if cholinergic eye drops are also administered to control the ocular anticholinergic effects of the drug. If the client receives a loading dose of disopyramide, monitor for hypotension and congestive heart failure closely. Clients stabilized on other antidysrhythmic agents may be changed to disopyramide: 6 to 12 hours after the last dose of quinidine sulfate, and 3 to 6 hours after the last dose of procainamide. Those clients with atrial flutter and fibrillation should be digitalized before disopyramide therapy begins to ensure the enhanced AV conduction does not increase the ventricular rate to inappropriate levels.

Education. Instruct client to make position changes slowly from recumbent posture if hypotension should occur. Advise client about possibility of dry mouth, which can be relieved by sugarless hard candy, gum, or frequent clear water rinses. Recommend regular dental checkups for the prevention of caries and periodontal disease. Also, avoid alcoholic beverages because of potential hypotensive effects.

Emphasize the importance of not skipping or stopping medication without consulting the prescriber since adverse cardiac effects may occur upon sudden withdrawal.

Instruct client to weigh daily to monitor fluid retention. Report to the prescriber a weight gain of 2 or more pounds within a 24-hour period. Observe for edema.

Caution the client about driving or other hazardous activities, since blurred vision and dizziness may occur. Alert clients about the hypoglycemic effects of the drug, particularly clients with diabetes. Teach signs and symptoms of hypoglycemia; if they occur, instruct the client to take a form of sugar and notify the prescriber. Caution the client that heat intolerance and reduced perspiration will occur and to avoid exertion and hot weather. Constipation may result from the anticholinergic effects of the drug. Instruct clients about high-fiber diet, increased fluid intake, moderate exercise, and regular bowel patterning.

Evaluation. The client on disopyramide therapy will have regular palpable pulses and demonstrate on ECG the absence of or a decrease in ventricular ectopy.

▲ **procainamide** [proe kane' a mide] (Pronestyl, Procanbid) Procainamide's electrophysiologic effects are similar to quinidine with the following exceptions:

1. Procainamide appears to be less effective in controlling abnormal ectopic pacemaker activity.
2. Procainamide has fewer anticholinergic effects than quinidine.
3. Procainamide has more potent negative inotropic effects than quinidine.

The result is the direct depressant effect of procainamide on the SA node and AV junction may not be as effectively balanced by vagal blockade as it is with quinidine. In clients with a preexisting ventricular dysfunction, procainamide may also cause severe congestive heart failure.

The primary indications for procainamide are to treat atrial and ventricular arrhythmias, such as premature ventricular contractions, ventricular tachycardia, atrial fibrillation, and paroxysmal atrial tachycardia. It is also used to treat cardiac dysrhythmias associated with anesthesia and surgery. For pharmacokinetics see Table 26-1. The side/adverse effects of procainamide are similar to quinidine with the exception of tinnitus and visual changes. In addition an SLE-type reaction may occur, that is, fever, chills, painful joints and rash.

Adult antiarrhythmic dose is 50 mg/kg PO or IM in 8 divided doses daily. Pediatric oral dose is 12.5 mg/kg four times daily. Procanbid is an extended release tablet that is dosed twice daily.

■ Nursing Management

Procainamide Therapy

In addition to the general management for antidysrhythmic therapy previously discussed, the following should be considered:

Assessment. Procainamide is contraindicated for use in second- or third-degree or complete AV block unless the client has an electrical pacemaker because of its additive cardiac depressive effects. Clients with torsades de pointes (a type of ventricular tachycardia) may have their condition aggravated. Use with caution in atrial fibrillation or flutter because the ventricular rate may increase suddenly since the atrial rate is slowed. Embolization may result from dislodgement of mural thrombi caused by forceful contraction of the atrium with conversion to sinus rhythm. There is a risk with AV block, bundle branch block, or digitalis toxicity of increased cardiac depression. Congestive heart failure, hepatic and renal impairment may cause drug accumulation, leading to toxicity. For those clients with a history of lupus erythematosus, procainamide may precipitate an active episode. The drug may also increase muscle weakness in clients with myasthenia gravis.

The nurse should review the client's current medication regimen for significant drug interactions. The following interactions may occur when procainamide is given with the drugs listed below.

Drug	Possible effect and management
other antiarrhythmic agents	Monitor for enhanced or additive cardiac effects.
antihypertensives	Increased hypotension has been reported, especially when parenteral (intravenous) procainamide is given with antihypertensive agents. Monitor closely, since dosage adjustments may be necessary.
antimyasthenia agents	The effect of antimyasthenic agents on skeletal muscle may be blocked by the antimuscarinic effects of procainamide. Monitor closely, since dosage adjustments of the antimyasthenic agent may be required.

Continued

Drug	Possible effect and management
neuromuscular blocking agents	Concurrent use may result in enhanced neuromuscular blockade. Monitor closely since reversal of blockade may be prolonged.
pimozide (Orap)	Prolonged Q-T intervals and cardiac dysrhythmias may be reported with concurrent use. Monitor closely, preferably with an ECG, since intervention may be necessary.

In addition to the indicators for a baseline assessment of the client receiving antidysrhythmic therapy, the baseline assessment for the administration of procainamide should also include complete blood cell counts.

Nursing diagnosis. With the administration of procainamide, the client may experience the following nursing diagnoses/collaborative problems: altered thought processes related to CNS effects (confusion, hallucinations, depression); risk for injury related to dizziness; risk for infection related to leukopenia and agranulocytosis (fever, sore mouth, gums, and throat); altered bowel elimination, diarrhea; and the potential complications of allergic reaction, systemic lupus erythematosus-like syndrome (30%)(fever, chills, skin rash, arthralgia), hemolytic anemia, and thrombocytopenia (unusual bleeding and bruising).

Implementation

Monitoring. Continue to monitor general cardiovascular status. Monitor intravenous administration constantly, and observe the following:

- Infusion pump: maintain desired flow rate. Keep client in supine position. Avoid rapid administration to prevent "speed shock" (irregular pulse, tight feeling in chest, flushed face, headache, loss of consciousness, shock, cardiac arrest).
- ECG monitoring: discontinue therapy if QRS complex is widened greater than 50% and P-R interval is prolonged.
- Arterial blood pressure: during loading dose take BP every 5 minutes; if blood pressure drops more than 15 mm Hg, discontinue infusion. Have pressor solutions available: dopamine or norepinephrine to treat hypotension. Elderly clients are more apt to exhibit hypotension.

Monitor serum electrolytes as hypokalemia predisposes the client to arrhythmias.

With oral dosages, BP, ECG, serum potassium levels, and complete blood cell counts should be monitored.

Intervention. To initiate intravenous therapy, the drug should be diluted in 5% dextrose to facilitate control of the dosage range; the dose should be administered at a rate not greater than 50 mg/min by direct intravenous administration or infusion. Also, intravenous therapy is limited to use in hospitals where monitoring facilities are available. Once prepared, the solution is stable for 24 hours at room temperature or 7 days if refrigerated. Procainamide is physically incompatible with many substances; check specific references when considering mixing with other drugs. The first oral dose should be administered at least 3 to 4 hours after the last intravenous dose.

Education. Urge the client on long-term therapy to keep appointments for periodic laboratory work: antinuclear antibody (ANA) titers, blood counts, and plasma procainamide and N-acetylprocainamide (NAPA) determinations. This is particularly important in clients with congestive heart failure, those with hepatic or renal function impairment, or those changing from regular oral to extended-release preparation of the drug. Symptoms of systemic lupus erythematosus (polyarthralgia, cough, fever, and pleuritic pain) and steady increases in ANA titers should be reported to the prescriber so that the drug can be discontinued.

Counsel clients to report symptoms such as unusual bleeding and/or bruising; sore mouth, gums, or throat; fever; rash; or symptoms of an upper respiratory tract infection to the prescriber. These symptoms are more apt to occur with the extended-release dosage form.

Some clients, particularly elderly clients, may be prone to dizziness. Alert them that driving and operating other mechanical equipment might be hazardous. Instruct the client in gradual positional changes to avoid postural hypotension.

Advise the client to continue to take the medication even though he or she is feeling well. Instruct the client that if a regular oral preparation dose is missed but remembered within 2 hours, to take it (within 4 hours for extended-release form), if a missed dose is remembered after this time *it should not be taken.* Instruct the client not to double up on doses. Alert the client not to discontinue the medication without consulting the prescriber, since a gradual withdrawal may be necessary to prevent worsening the condition.

Recommend that the client carry medical identification. The client should be instructed to alert health professionals, including dentists, that he or she is taking procainamide. The secondary anticholinergic effects of the drug decrease salivary flow and may contribute to caries and periodontal disease; recommend that the client maintain regular dental appointments. The oral forms of procainamide are hygroscopic (they will absorb moisture). Advise the client to keep them tightly closed in their original container and not to transfer them to other less tightly sealed containers or to leave them exposed to air.

Caution the client receiving the extended-release form of the medication that the dose is contained in a wax matrix that may be detected in the stools. This has no effect on the drug's absorption.

Evaluation. The client on procainamide therapy should demonstrate a regular palpable pulse and an absence of or decrease in atrial and ventricular ectopy on ECG.

GROUP I-B DRUGS

The Group I-B drugs (e.g., lidocaine [Xylocaine], phenytoin [Dilantin], tocainide [Tonocard], and mexiletine [Mexitil]) differ from Group I-A drugs in that they either increase or have no effect on conduction velocity. While not approved by the FDA, phenytoin is used in the therapy of digitalis-induced dysrhythmias. Lidocaine, tocainide, and mexiletine are related therapeutically and are particularly useful for acute ventricular dysrhythmias. Mexiletine's high incidence of side effects/adverse reactions has limited its use. Tocainide can cause the serious adverse reaction of agranulocytosis, therefore it is usually reserved for clients who have not responded to other drug therapies.

lidocaine [lye' doe kane] (Xylocaine, Xylocard ♣) Lidocaine, an agent used extensively as a local and topical anesthetic agent, is also an antidysrhythmic agent, especially for ventricular dysrhythmias seen after cardiac surgery or an acute myocardial infarction. Lidocaine appears to act primarily on the sodium channel, blocking both the activated and inactivated sodium channels, although its greater effect is in depolarized or ischemic tissues. These effects are indicative of the efficacy of lidocaine for suppressing arrhythmias associated with depolarization (such as ischemia, digitalis-induced toxicity) and its lack of effectiveness in arrhythmias that occur in normal polarized tissues (atrial fibrillation, atrial flutter). Lidocaine has few electrophysiologic effects in normal cardiac tissue.

Unlike quinidine and procainamide, lidocaine has no vagolytic properties nor does it influence cardiac output and arterial pressure. Also, it does not depress myocardial contractility and thereby provides no potential for the development of congestive heart failure. Since it exerts a limited effect, if any on the SA node and atrial myocardium, the drug has no use in the treatment of supraventricular tachycardias. Because electric activities are primarily limited to the ventricular cells, the major use of lidocaine is in abolishing ventricular dysrhythmias (see Figure 26-1, *D*) (See Table 26-1 for pharmacokinetics).

The side/adverse effects of lidocaine include dizziness, anorexia, nausea, vomiting, chest pain, and breathing difficulties.

Lidocaine adult dose is by IV bolus, 1 mg/kg at a rate of 25 to 50 mg/min, which may be repeated in 5 minutes if necessary (maximum dose per hour is 300 mg). Children receive the same 1 mg/kg dose initially, but repeat dosages in 5 minutes should not exceed a total dose of 3 mg/kg. By IV infusion, the dose is usually 20 to 50 μg/kg/min given at a rate of 1 to 4 mg/min for both adults and children.

■ Nursing Management

Lidocaine Therapy

In addition to the general nursing management for antidysrhythmic therapy, the following should be considered:

Assessment. Do not administer lidocaine to clients with severe degrees of sinoatrial, atrioventricular, or intraventricular block, or **Adams-Stokes syndrome** (sudden recurring episodes of loss of consciousness, caused by transient interruption of cardiac output by incomplete or complete heart block), because it may worsen the heart block. Risk/benefit should be considered with clients with a known history of hypersensitivity to amide type of local anesthetics. Use with caution in individuals with hypovolemia, shock, all forms of heart block, sinus bradycardia, and **Wolff-Parkinson-White syndrome** (a supraventricular tachycardia), because these conditions may be aggravated. Use with caution and in lower doses in individuals with congestive heart failure or reduced cardiac output and in the elderly. To prevent toxicity in clients with impaired renal and hepatic function, employ caution with prolonged use since the drug is metabolized mainly in the liver and excreted by the kidney.

Its use during human pregnancy is not established by adequate studies. Administer only when potential benefits outweigh potential hazards to the fetus because lidocaine may constrict uterine arteries, resulting in fetal hypoxia. It is not recommended for pediatric usage.

A significant drug interaction may occur when lidocaine is administered with phenytoin (hydantoin anticonvulsant), which may result in enhanced cardiac depressant effects. Also, the anticonvulsant may reduce lidocaine serum concentration by increasing the liver metabolism of lidocaine.

The client's baseline assessment should include the indicators described within the discussion of the general nursing management of antidysrhythmics.

Nursing diagnosis. With the administration of lidocaine, the client should be assessed for the following selected nursing diagnoses/collaborative problems: altered comfort related to the use of parenteral dosage forms (pain at the site of injection) and related to specific serum levels of the drug (nervousness, dizziness, drowsiness, and feelings of numbness, cold, and heat); risk for injury related to drug toxicity (blurred vision, nausea, vomiting, tinnitus, tremors, dizziness, seizures, bradycardia); and the potential complications of allergic reaction (skin rash, urticaria, and dyspnea) and decreased cardiac output related to cardiac conduction disturbances (hypotension, arrhythmias, heart block, and cardiac arrest).

Implementation

Monitoring. Constant ECG monitoring is essential for IV administration and recommended during intramuscular administration to observe for signs of toxicity. Monitor ECG and blood pressure to avoid potential overdosage and toxicity. If excessive cardiac depression occurs, such as prolongation of PR interval, QRS complex, or aggravation of dysrhythmias, stop infusion immediately. Serum electrolyte levels should be determined periodically during prolonged lidocaine infusions to correct imbalances. Observe the client for adverse effects of lidocaine (Box 26-2). Monitor serum lidocaine levels to minimize the chance of toxicity if high-dose infusions are used or if the client is receiving other drugs that might affect lidocaine clearance.

If the intravenous administration should run for more than 24 hours, observe for local thrombophlebitis and assess the client for the risk of accumulation.

Intervention. Recheck drug label; only lidocaine hydrochloride *without preservatives or epinephrine,* which specifically reads "IV use for cardiac dysrhythmias," should be administered. Preparations intended for use as an anesthetic contain epinephrine and *should not* be used for treating dysrhythmias. Intravenous infusions of lidocaine are usually prepared by adding 1 g of lidocaine to 1 L of 5% dextrose solution for a 1 mg/ml solution. The solution is stable for 24 hours. Do not add to blood transfusions. For IV route, use a precision IV volume control set for continuous infusion.

Usually a bolus dose is given to rapidly attain therapeutic serum concentrations. If the loading dose does not provide the desired therapeutic effect within 5 minutes, a second dose may be administered, one half to one third of the initial dose. However, give no more than 200 to 300 mg in a 1-hour period. Monitor the prescribed IV rate of flow, usually at no more than

BOX 26-2

Adverse Effects Related to Serum Concentrations of Lidocaine

1.5-6 μg/ml	6-8 μg/ml	>8 μg/ml
Anxiety, nervousness, drowsiness, dizziness, sensations of cold, heat, or numbness	Tremors, twitching, blurred or double vision, nausea, vomiting, tinnitus	Dyspnea, severe dizziness, fainting, bradycardia, convulsions

4 mg/min. Terminate IV infusion as soon as cardiac rhythm is stable or signs of toxicity develop. Have resuscitative equipment and drugs available to treat adverse reactions involving the cardiovascular system, respiratory system, and CNS.

Note that IV infusions are rarely continued beyond 24 hours. The client is then given an oral antidysrhythmic agent for maintenance therapy. Intramuscular administration is only for instances in which ECG is not available and the risk/benefit ratio has been considered by the prescriber. In such an emergency, the deltoid muscle is used for the intramuscular site because therapeutic blood levels are reached faster than in gluteus or lateral thigh muscles. Aspirate during the process of injection to ensure that intravascular injection will be avoided. Intramuscular use may increase creatinine phosphokinase levels and interfere with diagnostic enzyme tests for myocardial infarction.

After initial use, discard partially used solutions of lidocaine that contain no preservatives.

In clients over 65 or in those with congestive heart failure or renal or hepatic function impairment, the dose and rate of infusion is generally reduced by one half and then adjusted in response to the client's condition.

Education. Instruct the client on the procedure for self-injection and have the client state and demonstrate the procedure. The client should ensure that the medication is always readily available and that it is not out of date. If symptoms of heart attack occur, instruct the client to contact the prescriber immediately. The client should not administer the medication unless instructed to do so by the prescriber. To administer, the client should remove the safety cap, place the black end of the cylinder on thickest part of thigh, and press hard; the client should feel a needle stick. The needle is held in place for a slow count of 10 and then area is massaged for a slow count of 10. Instruct the client not to drive after administering the drug unless there is no other alternative. The client should seek medical attention immediately.

Evaluation. The client will have regular palpable pulses and the absence of or a decrease in ventricular ectopy on ECG.

mexiletine [mex il' e teen] (Mexitil)
tocainide [toe kay' nide] (Tonocard)

Mexiletine and tocainide are chemically and therapeutically related to lidocaine. Because they resist first pass liver metabolism, they may be administered orally. Arrhythmias that respond to parenteral lidocaine are usually responsive to these drugs. They are indicated for the treatment and/or prevention of ventricular arrhythmias. See Table 26-1 for pharmacokinetics. .

Side/adverse effects are similar to lidocaine. In addition, paresthesia of fingers and toes, rash, tremors, and with tocainide primarily, pneumonitis and sweating are reported.

The mexiletine adult dose is usually 200 mg PO every 8 hours, titrated as necessary. The tocainide adult dose is 400 mg PO every 8 hours. Geriatric clients should receive smaller doses because they may be more sensitive to these drugs. Pediatric dosages are not established.

■ Nursing Management

Tocainide Therapy

In addition to the general nursing management for antidysrhythmic therapy, the following should be considered:

Assessment. Determine that the client is not sensitive to amide-type anesthetics and has no AV block preexisting second- or third-degree without an electrical pacemaker. Note whether the client has renal or hepatic function impairment, since tocainide must be used cautiously, with intensive monitoring, because of reduced elimination and biotransformation of the drug. Clients with congestive heart failure may have their condition worsen because of the drug's small negative inotropic effect. Caution should be used with clients with atrial flutter or fibrillation because acceleration of ventricular rate may infrequently occur. A baseline health assessment specific to this drug should include an ECG, chest x-ray examination, and blood counts. No significant drug interactions are reported to date.

Nursing diagnosis. With the administration of tocainide, the client should be assessed for the development of the following nursing diagnoses: altered comfort related to CNS effects (dizziness, headache, blurred vision, trembling, numbness or tingling of the fingers and toes), and gastrointestinal effects (anorexia, nausea, vomiting); altered thought processes (confusion); risk for infection related to the development of leukopenia or agranulocytosis (fever, chills); and impaired skin integrity related to skin reactions (peeling, scaling, and blisters of skin), and the potential complications of thrombocytopenia (unusual bruising or bleeding), pneumonia, pulmonary fibrosis or edema (cough, dyspnea), and decreased cardiac output related to further cardiac arrhythmias.

Implementation

Monitoring. Take blood counts at periodic intervals to detect bone marrow suppression and monitor ECG tracings for medication effectiveness. Chest x-ray examinations are required at the first sign of pulmonary complications, such as pneumonia, pulmonary edema, or pulmonary fibrosis. If the client evidences tremor, it may be an indication that the highest tolerable dose has been reached.

Intervention. Administer with food or milk to reduce gastric distress. If the client has adverse reactions shortly after taking a dose of tocainide, each individual dose may be decreased but administered with greater frequency. If the dysrhythmia returns before the next scheduled dose, a higher dosage or more frequent dosing should be considered.

Education. Instruct the client to take medication even though he or she is feeling better. Doses should not be missed and should be evenly spaced. If a forgotten dose is remembered within 4 hours, it should be taken. If a longer interval has passed, the dose is not to be taken until the next scheduled time. Advise the client to maintain regular visits to the prescriber to monitor progress. Recommend that a medical identification card be carried or a bracelet worn.

Alert the client that dizziness may occur and that caution should be taken when driving or operating other mechanical equipment. The elderly client has an increased risk of falling. Instruct the client to report signs and symptoms of leukopenia and thrombocytopenia (evidence of infection, delayed healing, fever, chills, sore throat, unusual bleeding, and bruising). If these symptoms occur, the client should postpone dental work and should be instructed to use toothbrushes, dental floss, and toothpicks cautiously.

Evaluation. The client will have regular palpable pulses and the absence of or a decrease in ventricular ectopy on ECG.

■ Nursing Management
Mexiletine Therapy

The nursing management of the client receiving mexiletine is much the same as for tocainide, except these clients may also experience altered bowel elimination related to the gastrointestinal effects of the drug, either constipation or diarrhea; the risk for impaired skin integrity related to skin reactions is not quite so severe. Refer to the earlier discussion for tocainide for more detail.

GROUP I-C DRUGS

The Group I-C drugs include flecainide (Tambocor) and propafenone (Rhythmol), which are used to treat and/or prevent supraventricular tachydysrhythmias. These agents can cause sinus arrest, AV block, and life-threatening ventricular arrhythmias. This prodysrhythmic effect is of special concern especially in clients with poor left ventricular function or sustained ventricular arrhythmias. The Group I-C drugs can also aggravate congestive heart failure.

flecainide [fle kay' nide] (Tambocor)

Flecainide is a sodium channel blocking agent used to treat ventricular arrhythmias; it has minimal effects on repolarization and no anticholinergic properties. It suppresses premature ventricular contractions and in high doses may exacerbate arrhythmias in clients with a preexisting ventricular tachydysrhythmia or in persons with a previous myocardial infarction. It is indicated for the treatment of ventricular arrhythmias and as prophylaxis of supraventricular arrhythmias, such as AV junction reentrant tachycardia. See Table 26-1 for pharmacokinetics.

The side/adverse effects of flecainide include blurred vision, dizziness, headaches, constipation, nausea, weakness, chest pain, irregular heartbeats and arrhythmias. Flecainide, if administered with other antidysrhythmic agents, may result in enhanced adverse cardiac effects. In persons with hypotensive ventricular tachycardia, irreversible ventricular tachycardia or ventricular fibrillation has been reported. Avoid concurrent usage.

Flecainide adult dose is 50 to 100 mg PO every 12 hours, titrated every 4 days as necessary.

■ Nursing Management
Flecainide Therapy

The nursing management is essentially the same as for tocainide, except pulmonary symptoms such as pneumonia and pulmonary fibrosis are not a concern with flecainide.

propafenone [proe pa feen' one] (Rhythmol)

Propafenone is similar to flecainide in action and therapeutic uses. It also has some beta blocking and weak calcium channel blocking activity. It prevents the passage of sodium ions into the fast sodium channels (phase 0), resulting in a decrease in depolarization rate. It also prolongs the refractory period in cardiac tissues. It is indicated for the treatment of life-threatening ventricular arrhythmias. For pharmacokinetics, see Table 26-1.

The side/adverse effects of propafenone include dizziness, nausea, headaches, constipation, weakness, chest pain, irregular heartbeats, and arrhythmias.

The usual adult dose is 150 mg PO every 8 hours, with dosage adjustments at 3 to 4 day intervals as necessary. Pediatric dosage is unknown.

■ Nursing Management
Propafenone Therapy

In addition to the general nursing management of antidysrhythmic therapy, consider the following:

Assessment. The client's blood pressure and pulse should be known before propafenone is administered since it is contraindicated in marked hypotension and bradycardia. The drug is also contraindicated in preexisting second or third degree AV block or right bundle branch block associated with left hemiblock without an electric pacemaker because of the risk of complete heart block. Its use should be carefully considered in clients with congestive heart failure because of its negative inotropic effects and with cardiogenic shock or sinus bradycardia because further myocardial depression may result. With sick sinus syndrome, sinus node recovery may be prolonged resulting in sinus bradycardia, sinus pause, or sinus arrest. The effective dose for the elderly client may be lower because of impaired hepatic or renal function in this age group. As with the other antidysrhythmic agents, an ECG should be obtained before beginning therapy. Any electrolyte imbalances should also be corrected because the effects of propafenone will be altered if such a state exists.

A potentially significant drug interaction with digoxin has been reported; digoxin serum levels may increase from 35% to 85% depending on the dose of propafenone consumed, which increases the potential for digitalis toxicity.

The digoxin dose should be reduced when propafenone is started. Warfarin plasma concentrations also increase with concurrent administration, which may lead to an increase in prothrombin times (25% increase). Monitor closely because warfarin dosage adjustments are usually necessary.

Nursing diagnosis. Once propafenone has been administered to the client, the nurse should assess the client for the following nursing diagnoses/collaborative problems resulting from the effects of the drug: altered comfort (chest pain, headache, nausea and vomiting, rash, and dizziness); sensory-perceptual alterations related to CNS effects (trembling, shaking, blurred vision); altered bowel elimination (diarrhea or constipation); risk for infection related to hematologic effects (agranulocytosis); and the potential complication of decreased cardiac output related to further dysrhythmias and the development of hypotension, bradycardia, ventricular tachycardia, and/or congestive heart failure.

Implementation

Monitoring. Continuous ECG monitoring is recommended during the initiation of therapy. Periodic monitoring of CBC is recommended. If the client is also receiving digoxin, serum digoxin levels should be monitored.

Intervention. The therapeutic response to the drug should be carefully recorded because the dosage of propafenone is titrated by the prescriber on the basis of the client's response and tolerance (see the case study below).

Evaluation. An expected outcome of propafenone therapy is that the client's ventricular dysrhythmia will be suppressed or will diminish in severity.

GROUP I DRUGS (A, B, C)

moricizine [mor' i siz een] (Ethmozine)

Moricizine (Ethmozine) has properties of all three classes (A,B,C) and does not belong to one individual classification. It is a fairly potent sodium channel blocking agent that does not prolong the action potential duration. It has local anesthetic action and a membrane stabilizing effect; thus it decreases AV junction and His-Purkinje conduction. It is indicated for the treatment of life-threatening ventricular arrhythmias. See Table 26-1 for the drug's pharmacokinetics.

The side/adverse effects of moricizine include lightheadedness, dry mouth, blurred vision, nausea, vomiting, weakness, chest pain, heart failure, and ventricular tachyarrhythmias. The *USP DI* (1996) does not list any significant drug interactions.

Adult dose is 200 to 300 mg PO 3 times daily, every 8 hours, titrated as necessary at 3 day intervals. Maximum daily dose is 900 mg.

■ Nursing Management

Moricizine Therapy

The nursing management is essentially the same as for propafenone.

GROUP II DRUGS

propranolol [proe pran' oh lole] (Inderal)
acebutolol [a se byoo' toe lole] (Sectral)
esmolol [ess' moe lol] (Brevibloc)

All three drugs are beta-adrenergic blocking agents used to control cardiac dysrhythmias caused by excessive sympathetic nerve activity. Dysrhythmias caused by increased sympathetic discharge (hyperthyroidism) are effectively blocked by the beta-adrenergic blocking action of propranolol. Acebutolol is used to treat ventricular arrhythmias, such as ventricular premature beats, whereas esmolol is indicated for short-term treatment of supraventricular tachycardia induced by atrial fibrillation or atrial flutter (see drug monographs in Chapter 22).

GROUP III DRUGS

The electrophysiologic properties of drugs in this group differ markedly from the drugs previously discussed. Drugs in this group prolong the effective refractory period by prolonging the action potential (delay repolarization).

Case Study

The Client Taking Antidysrhythmics

James Cameron is a 62-year-old manager of a fast-food restaurant who had rheumatic heart disease as a child and who has a long family history of heart disease. He has been having chest pain for the past 3 months, which can usually be relieved by rest. This time, however, the pain was more severe than usual and not relieved by rest, so he came to the emergency room, His ECG shows elevated ST segments: the chest pain persists; and his vital signs are BP 184/90, pulse 114 and irregular, respirations 24. The physician finds that he has developed ventricular arrhythmias that are not only difficult to control with the usual medications—verapamil and lidocaine—but are becoming life-threatening to him. The physician prescribed propafenone hydrochloride (Rhythmol). Mr. Cameron is receiving 150 mg PO q8h.

1. What nursing diagnoses should be monitored with propafenone administration?
2. What side effects should the nurse be alert to?
3. What drug interactions are possible in coadministration of propafenone?

bretylium tosylate [bre til' ee um] (Bretylol, Bretylate ♣)
Unlike the other antiarrhythmics, bretylium does not suppress automaticity and has no effect on conduction velocity. The direct electrophysiologic action on the heart appears to be prolongation of the action potential and lengthening of the effective refractory period. It is believed this mechanism helps to terminate dysrhythmias caused by the reentry phenomenon. Bretylium is also taken up and concentrated in the adrenergic nerve terminals where, after an initial release of norepinephrine, it prevents any further release. This sympatholytic action significantly increases the threshold, producing an antifibrillatory response in the ventricles. Bretylium produces a positive inotropic effect, increasing myocardial contractility. With long-term treatment, the drug shows increased responsiveness to circulating epinephrine and norepinephrine, which may account for the increased myocardial contractility. For pharmacokinetics, see Table 26-1.

The side/adverse effects of bretylium include anorexia, headaches, nausea, vomiting, bitter taste, impotency, dizziness, cough, breathing difficulties, fever, paresthesia of fingers or toes, hand tremors, and weakness.

The usual adult dose is for life-threatening ventricular fibrillation is 5 mg/kg IV of undiluted solution, followed by 10 mg/kg every 15 to 30 minutes if needed, to a total of 30 mg/kg in 24 hours. For dosage recommendations for other ventricular arrhythmias, see a current reference.

■ **Nursing Management**
Bretylium Therapy

In addition to the general nursing management of antidysrhythmic therapy, consider the following:

Assessment. Bretylium should be administered with caution to clients with conditions involving reduced cardiac output, such as aortic stenosis and pulmonary hypertension, because severe hypotension may occur as a result of reduced peripheral resistance without an increase in cardiac output. Clients with renal function impairment require increased dosage intervals because elimination of the drug is reduced.

Do not administer digitalis glycosides to clients receiving bretylium. The initial release of norepinephrine produced by bretylium may increase digitalis toxicity.

Nursing diagnosis. With the administration of bretylium, the client may be assessed for the following nursing diagnoses: altered comfort related to rapid IV administration (nausea and vomiting); ineffective breathing pattern related to possible neuromuscular block (<0.1%)(dyspnea, respiratory depression); risk for injury related to postural hypotension (dizziness, syncope); and the potential complications of angina (chest pain) and decreased cardiac output.

Implementation

Monitoring. Continuously monitor ECG and blood pressure.

Intervention. Administer bretylium to clients in an area that is adequately staffed by qualified personnel and equipped with appropriate facilities for constant ECG monitoring and use of emergency equipment. Anticipate the possible development of transient hypertension and dysrhythmias during the early stage of therapy. This is caused by the initial release of norepinephrine from adrenergic nerve terminals.

Bretylium is always diluted for intermittent or continuous intravenous administration, unless it is a situation of life-threatening ventricular fibrillation. In this case, it is administered undiluted and as quickly as possible. But in general, administer intravenous doses slowly to prevent nausea and vomiting.

Rotate IM injection site. Do not administer more than 5 ml at one site. Necrosis, muscle atrophy, or fibrosis may occur if injection is repeatedly given at the same site. Note that IM injection is rarely used.

Bretylium is generally discontinued in 3 to 5 days and an alternate antidysrhythmic agent may be substituted if indicated.

Education. Instruct the client to remain in a supine position during therapy until tolerance to the hypotensive effect of the drug occurs.

Evaluation. The client on bretylium therapy will have regular palpable pulses and will evidence an absence of ventricular tachycardia or fibrillation on ECG.

amiodarone [a mee' oh da rone] (Cordarone)
Amiodarone increases the refractory period in all cardiac tissues by a direct effect on the tissues. It decreases automaticity, prolongs AV conduction, and decreases the automaticity of fibers in the Purkinje system. It may block potassium, sodium and calcium channels, and beta receptors. It has the potential of causing a variety of complex effects on the heart and has serious adverse effects. Therefore, it is usually reserved for the prevention and treatment of life-threatening ventricular dysrhythmias in persons not responding to or tolerating other drug therapies. For pharmacokinetics, see Table 26-1.

The side/adverse effects of amiodarone are similar to bretylium. In addition, constipation, flushing, and ataxia are reported.

Usual adult dose for ventricular dysrhythmias is 800 mg to 1.6 g PO daily for 1 to 3 weeks until a therapeutic response is noted or side effects appear. The dose is then reduced to 600 to 800 mg daily for 1 month, eventually decreasing to the lowest effective dose. See the box on p. 518 for FDA pregnancy safety guidelines.

The pediatric dose is 10 mg/kg/day for 10 days or until a therapeutic response is noted or side effects appear. Dose is then decreased and tapered to lowest effective dose as outlined in package insert.

■ **Nursing Management**
Amiodarone Therapy

In addition to the general nursing management for antidysrhythmic therapy, consider the following:

Assessment. Determine that the client does not have, AV block preexisting second- or third-degree without a pacemaker because of the risk of complete heart block, or syncope as a result of severe bradycardia or sinus node function impairment unless controlled by a pacemaker because of the risk of atropine-resistant sinus bradycardia. Use caution if the client

Pregnancy Safety

Category	Drug
B	lidocaine, moricizine
C	adenosine, bretylium, disopyramide, flecainide, mexiletine, procainamide, propafenone, quinidine, tocainide
D	amiodarone
Unclassified	sotalol

has congestive heart failure or impaired hepatic or thyroid function. Hypokalemia should be corrected before the initiation of amiodarone therapy to ensure the drug's effectiveness.

The nurse should review the client's medication regimen for significant drug interactions. The following drug interactions may occur when amiodarone is given with the drugs listed below.

Drug	Possible effect and management
other antidysrhythmic agents	May increase cardiac effects and the risk of inducing tachyarrhythmias. It also increases serum levels of quinidine, procainamide, flecainide, and phenytoin. If amiodarone must be given with Group I antidysrhythmic agents, reduce the dose of the Group I antidysrhythmic drug by 30% to 50% several days after starting amiodarone and gradually withdraw the Group I drug. If additional treatment with amiodarone is necessary, start therapy at half the usual recommended dosage.
anticoagulants, warfarin (Coumadin)	May increase anticoagulant effect. Dose of anticoagulant should be reduced by one third to one half of the dose when adding amiodarone to the client's drug regimen. Prothrombin times should also be closely monitored.
digitalis glycosides	May increase the serum level of digoxin and other digitalis glycosides, resulting in toxicity. Digitalis glycosides should be stopped or the dose reduced to 50% whenever amiodarone is given. Monitor serum levels closely. May also see additive effects of both drugs on the SA node and AV junction.
phenytoin (Dilantin)	May result in increased serum levels of phenytoin, possibly resulting in toxicity. Monitor serum levels of phenytoin.

Nursing diagnosis. With the administration of amiodarone, the client should be assessed for the development of the following nursing diagnoses/collaborative problems: altered comfort (dizziness, bitter taste, headache, flushing, nausea, and vomiting); altered self-concept related to decreased libido, blue-gray coloring of the skin of the face, hands, and arms; altered bowel elimination, 25% (constipation); altered nutrition, less than required related to anorexia, 25% (severe weight loss); and the potential complications of neurotoxicity, which occurs in 20% to 40% of clients (ataxia, tremors of the hands, numbness and tingling of fingers and toes, weakness of the arms and legs); photosensitivity; pulmonary fibrosis or pneumonitis, 10% to 15% (cough, dyspnea, fever); hyperthyroidism, 2% (weight loss, insomnia, nervousness, sensitivity to heat); hypothyroidism, 10% (weight gain, tiredness, sensitivity to cold, dry skin); ocular toxicity (blurred vision, corneal deposits [10%]); allergic reaction (rash); hepatitis (yellow skin and eyes); decreased cardiac output related to new dysrhythmias, sinus bradycardia, congestive heart failure (pulmonary edema, edema of feet and lower legs); and noninfectious epididymitis (pain and swelling of the scrotum).

Implementation

Monitoring. Perform ECG, thyroid function studies, liver function studies ALT (SGPT), AST (SGOT), and serum alkaline phosphatase), chest x-ray examinations, and pulmonary studies before the initiation of therapy and periodically thereafter. Vital signs and fluid balance monitoring should occur with these clients. Ophthalmologic examinations should be done initially and if eye symptoms occur. Pulmonary fibrosis may occur in 10% to 30% of the clients receiving long-term amiodarone therapy. Because this is usually reversible if detected early enough, chest x-ray examinations every 3 months are recommended. Thyroid function studies are to be done at periodic intervals.

Intervention. Begin the loading dose phase at the beginning of amiodarone therapy in the hospital, because of the difficulty in adjusting dosage and the potential for adverse effects, such as neurotoxicity and ocular, pulmonary, and thyroid toxicity. Since gastrointestinal disturbances occur in 25% of clients during loading, take care to minimize these as much as possible. Provide the client a high-fiber diet and increased fluid intake, unless contraindicated, to prevent constipation. Administer with food or milk to decrease nausea. Make efforts to stimulate appetite to counteract anorexia.

Education. Instruct the client to continue the medication even if he or she is feeling well. If a dose is missed, the client should be advised not to take it at all, to avoid doubling up on doses. If two or three doses are missed, instruct the client to contact the prescriber.

Instruct the client to maintain regular contact with the prescriber to monitor drug use. Advise the client to carry medical identification at all times. Instruct the client to alert health professionals unfamiliar with the medication regimen to the amiodarone administration.

Photosensitivity is a potential adverse effect with this drug. Caution client to avoid exposure to the sun and to wear sun-protective clothing and dark glasses. Sun-screen agents are not effective because they do not block UVB light, so barrier sun blocks are needed, such as zinc or titanium oxide. In addition, a blue-gray coloration of the skin occurs with long-term use (more than 1 year) and affects sun-exposed parts of the body, such as face, neck, and arms, and those with fair skin.

Alert clients to report any of the following signs and symptoms to the prescriber: cough, dyspnea, fever (pulmonary toxicity); ataxia, numbness, tingling, weakness, or spasm of extremities (neurotoxicity); blurred vision or increased sensitivity of the eyes to light (ocular toxicity); unusual weight gain or loss, increased sensitivity to heat or cold (thyroid toxicity); pain and swelling of the scrotum; jaundice (hepatic toxicity); or swelling of the feet and lower legs (congestive heart failure).

Evaluation. The client on amiodarone therapy will have regular palpable pulses and will evidence an absence of or decrease in atrial and ventricular ectopy on ECG.

ibutilide [eye byoo' ti lide] (Corvert)

Ibutilide has class III effects; it prolongs the action potential and increases atrial and ventricular refractory period. It produces its effect mainly at the sodium channels. It is indicated for the treatment of atrial fibrillation or atrial flutter.

Administered intravenously, ibutilide has an average 6 hour elimination half-life with excretion mainly in the urine. Significant side/adverse effects include ventricular extrasystoles, headaches, tachycardia, hypotension, and other potentially serious cardiac arrhythmias.

Adult dose for persons weighing less than 60 kg is 1 mg diluted in dextrose 5% 50 ml. If necessary, a second dose may be administered 10 minutes later (Olin, 1996).

■ Nursing Management

Ibutilide Therapy

In addition to the general nursing management for antidysrhythmic agent therapy, the following should be considered:

Assessment. Ascertain that the client is hypersensitive to ibutilide or any of the other product components. Ibutilide can induce or worsen ventricular arrhythmias. Avoid its use in clients with prolongation of the QT interval.

Review the client's medication regimen to determine any significant drug interactions that might occur with the concurrent administration of ibutilide. Concomitant antiarrhythmics, such as the Class IA drugs, disopyramide, quinidine, and procainamide, and other Class III drugs, such as amiodarone and sotalol, should not be administered concurrently or within 4 hours after infusion because of their potential to prolong refractoriness. Avoid any other drugs that might prolong the QT interval, such as phenothiazines, tricyclic and tetracyclic antidepressants, and some antihistamine agents (H_1 receptor antagonists). Ibutilide-induced supraventricular arrhythmias may mask the cardiotoxicity associated with excessive digoxin levels.

Nursing diagnosis. The client receiving ibutilide is at risk for the following nursing diagnoses/collaborative problems: risk for injury related to postural hypotension (2%) and the potential complications of ventricular arrhythmias and congestive heart failure.

Implementation

Monitoring. The client requires continuous ECG monitoring in an environment with personnel trained in the identification and management of acute ventricular arrhythmias, including intracardiac pacing facilities, a cardioverter/defibrillator, and medication for the treatment of sustained VT. Observe ECG monitoring for at least 4 hours after the ibutilide infusion or until QT has returned to baseline.

Intervention. If the client has had atrial fibrillation of more than 2 to 3 days duration, he or she should be anticoagulated at least 2 weeks before ibutilide therapy is initiated. If the arrhythmia does not end within 10 minutes after the infusion, a second infusion of equal strength may be administered 10 minutes after the end of the first infusion. Correction of any electrolyte imbalances is necessary before therapy is begun.

Education. Explain the procedure and equipment to client.

Evaluation. The client will not experience atrial flutter/fibrillation or any adverse effects of ibutilide.

sotalol [soe' ta lole] (Betapace)

Sotalol is a beta adrenergic blocking agent that prolongs the action potential duration, increasing the effective refractory period in atrial, ventricular, and AV junction. It is indicated for life-threatening ventricular arrhythmias. See Chapter 22 for additional information.

■ Nursing Management

Sotalol Therapy

In addition to the following, see the discussion of general nursing management of beta-adrenergic agents in Chapter 22 and of antidysrhythmic therapy in this chapter.

Assessment. The client should be assessed for health conditions for which the use of sotalol is contraindicated, such as bronchial asthma, sinus bradycardia, second- and third-degree AV block, congenital or acquired long Q-T syndrome, cardiogenic shock, uncontrolled CHF, and hypersensitivity to sotalol. Determination should also be made of conditions for which there are precautions to sotalol use, such as reduced renal function and nonallergic bronchospasm. Sotalol may mask signs of hypoglycemia in clients with diabetes mellitus and tachycardic symptoms of hyperthyroidism. Hypotension may occur in clients receiving anesthesia. Further dysrhythmias may be provoked in clients with conduction disturbances, proarrhythmias, CHF, hypokalemia, acute myocardial infarction, and sick sinus syndrome (Dunnington, 1993).

An assessment should include the client's current medication regimen to detect significant drug interactions as for other beta-adrenergic agents (see Chapter 22, p. 449).

A baseline assessment is the same as for other antidysrhythmic agents.

Nursing diagnosis. The client receiving sotalol therapy is at risk for the following nursing diagnoses/collaborative problems: fatigue; altered sexuality pattern related to decreased libido and/or impotence; altered comfort (headache); altered thought processes (depression); ineffective airway clearance related to bronchospasm; and the potential complications of heart failure, hypoglycemia in diabetic clients, and exacerbation of peripheral vascular disease.

Implementation

Monitoring. Monitor the client's cardiovascular status as for other antidysrhythmic therapies.

Intervention. Absorption may be reduced by food, especially milk and milk products, due to an interaction with calcium; administer 1 hour before food or 2 hours afterward.

Education. Instruct the client on how to monitor pulse and other pertinent indicators. Advise clients with ischemic heart disease not to abruptly discontinue the medication because it may result in angina.

Evaluation. The client will demonstrate an improvement in the underlying symptoms and a diminished dysrhythmia.

GROUP IV: MISCELLANEOUS DRUG GROUP

Calcium antagonists are selective antiarrhythmic agents that are reviewed in Chapter 28.

UNCLASSIFIED ANTIARRHYTHMIC AGENT

adenosine (a den'o sin)

Adenosine is a natural constituent of muscle tissue, is used to slow AV node conduction, and thus is indicated for the conversion of paroxysmal supraventricular tachycardia (PSVT) to normal sinus rhythm.

Administered by intravenous bolus, it is nearly immediately taken up by red blood cells and vascular endothelial cells and metabolized to inosine and adenosine monophosphate (AMP) in the body. The side/adverse effects include dyspnea, flushing, nausea, headache, and chest pain/pressure.

Usual dose is 6 mg administered rapidly IV bolus over 1 to 2 seconds. If the arrhythmia is still present in 1 to 2 minutes after the injection, then a 12 mg dose may be administered.

■ Nursing Management

Adenosine Therapy

In addition to the nursing management of antidysrhythmic therapy discussed previously, the following should be considered:

Assessment. The client should be assessed to determine that there is no AV block or preexisting second- or third-degree block without a pacemaker, because there is the risk of complete heart block if the drug is administered in such circumstances. In the client with sick sinus syndrome, the administration of adenosine may result in sinus node recovery time being prolonged and sinus bradycardia or sinus arrest may occur.

Review the client's medications, since adenosine's effects are potentiated by coadministration of carbamazepine (Tegretol) and dipyridamole (Persantin), and caffeine and theophylline reduce or antagonize adenosine's effects. If possible, avoid concurrent drug administration.

A baseline assessment of the client's blood pressure, pulse, and respiration, and an ECG should be obtained to confirm the efficacy of adenosine.

Nursing diagnosis. The client receiving adenosine may experience the following nursing diagnoses/collaborative problems: altered comfort (flushing of the face, headache, nausea, or numbness or tingling in the arms) and ineffective airway clearance related to transient bronchoconstriction. The potential complications of new arrhythmias and heart block exist.

Implementation

Monitoring. The client should be on a cardiac monitor, or the heart rate and blood pressure should be monitored every 15 to 30 seconds for several minutes.

Intervention. Adenosine is administered by IV rapidly, 6 mg over 1 to 2 seconds. It is administered rapidly to achieve the desired negative dromotropic and chronotropic effect. Give directly into the vein or if given by IV line, inject as proximal as possible and follow with a rapid saline flush. If the first dose is not effective within 1 to 2 minutes, a second one of 12 mg may be given in the same fashion and repeated if necessary. If a high level block occurs after the dose, do not repeat the dose. Resuscitation equipment and drugs should be available during adenosine therapy. The solution may crystallize if refrigerated; warm to room temperature. Ensure the solution is clear before administering. Discard any unused solution as it contains no preservatives.

Education. Alert the client that flushing of the face may occur and to report any symptoms of cough, dizziness, headache, nausea, or numbness or tingling of the arms.

Evaluation. The dysrhythmia for which the adenosine was administered will resolve without the client experiencing any adverse reactions to the drug.

SUMMARY

Antidysrhythmic agents are used for the treatment and prevention of disorders of cardiac rhythm that result from some abnormality in the electrophysiologic properties of the cells of the cardiac conduction system or cardiac muscle cells. Although all drugs in this grouping have the ability to suppress automaticity, they are subdivided into groups I-A, I-B, and I-C to reflect the similar electrophysiologic properties of each subgroup. Group I-A includes disopyramide, procainamide, and quinidine, all of which decrease conduction velocity and prolong the action potential. Group I-B drugs, lidocaine, phenytoin, tocainide, and mexiletine, either increase or have no effect on conduction velocity. Group I-C drugs, flecainide and propafenone, are used to treat or prevent supraventricular tachydysrhythmias; however, they have prodysrhythmic effects that are of concern and require careful monitoring of the client. Group II drugs have beta-adrenergic blocking action and are discussed in Chapter 22. The Group III agents, bretylium and amiodarone, are antiadrenergic. Group IV consists of miscellaneous agents; some have selective calcium antagonistic action, such as verapamil, which is discussed in Chapter 28.

Nursing management of cardiac dysrhythmias with the administration of antidysrhythmic agents should have the expected outcomes of having the client maintain cardiac output within normal limits, increase activity tolerance, experience less chest discomfort and associated symptoms, and evidence decreased or no dysrhythmias on ECG tracings. Client education is focused on the development of the client's knowledge of health status and medications, skill at pulse taking, and ability to recognize changes in health status that are reportable to enable the client to self-administer antidysrhythmic agents safely and accurately.

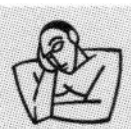

Critical Thinking

1. How would the differences in the groupings of antidysrhythmic agents affect nursing management of the client's care?
2. What concerns do you perceive a client who is receiving antidysrhythmic therapy might have?

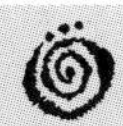

Collaborative Learning Activities

1. Six teams of students will represent the antidysrhythmic classes: I-A, I-B, I-C, II, III, and IV. The students will contrast the indications, assessment, monitoring, intervention, client education, and evaluation for each of these classes. The teams will select the nursing diagnoses of highest priority that would apply to all of the classes as a total group and each team will select one that would be unique to their class of antidysrhythmic agents.

BIBLIOGRAPHY

Abramowicz M (Ed.) (1994). Drugs for cardiac arrhythmias, *Med Lett* 36(937):111-4.

American Hospital Formulary Service (1996). *AHFS drug information '96*. Bethesda, MD: American Society of Hospital Pharmacists.

Anderson KN, et al. (Eds.) (1994). *Mosby's medical, nursing, & allied health dictionary* (4th ed.). St Louis: Mosby.

Benz MR (1991). Pharmacologic management of ventricular arrhythmias, *Crit Care Nurs Q* 14(3):8-15.

Brzozxowski LA (1993). Antiarrhythmic propafenone: Improving patient outcomes, *Dimens Crit Care Nurs* 12(3):116-22.

Chow MSS & Kertland & HR (1995). Cardiac arrythmias. In Young LX & Koda-Kimble MA. *Applied therapeutics* (6th ed.). Vancouver: Applied Therapeutics.

Dreifus LS, Longano J, & Phibbs BP (1992). Symptomatic arrhythmias, *Patient Care* 26(18):176-8, 183, 187, 190, 193, 196, 198-208, 213-20.

Dunnington CS (1993). Sotalol hydrochloride (Betapace): A new antiarrhythmic drug, *Amer J Crit Care* 2(5):397-406.

Formulary Drug Review (1990). A review of propafenone, *Hosp Pharmacy* 25(2):177.

Hanisch DG & Perron L (1992). Complex dysrhythmias in infants and children, *AACN* 3(1):255-67.

Olin BR (Ed.) (1996). *Facts and comparisons: Drug information.* St Louis: Facts and Comparisons.

Paul SC (1993). New pharmacologic agents for emergency management of supraventricular tachydysrhythmias, *Crit Care Nurs Q* 16(2):35-45.

Porterfield LM, Porterfield JG, & Collins SW (1993). The cutting edge in arrhythmias, *Crit Care Nurse* (June supplement):8-9.

Stier F (1992). Antidysrhythmic agents, *AACN* 3(2):483.

United States Pharmacopeial Convention (1996). *USP DI: Drug information for the health professional* (16th ed.). Rockville, MD: The Convention.

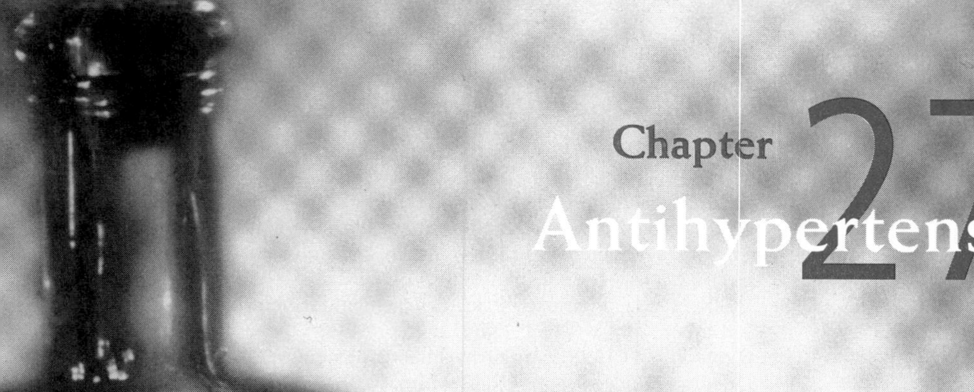

Chapter 27 Antihypertensives

Chapter Focus

Hypertension (sustained, elevated blood pressure) is a chronic circulatory disease that affects millions of Americans. It has been estimated that approximately 50 million Americans have hypertension or systolic and/or diastolic blood pressures higher than 140/90 (Oates, 1996). Untreated hypertension or subtherapeutic treatment of hypertension increases the risk of stroke, cerebral hemorrhage, congestive heart failure, coronary heart disease, and renal failure. Risk factors for essential hypertension include family history, race (most common in African Americans), stress, obesity, a high dietary intake of saturated fats or sodium, use of tobacco or oral contraceptives, sedentary lifestyle, and aging. The role of nursing is important, not only in the direct care of the hypertensive client but even more so in the prevention and management of the condition through client education. The following objectives and key terms are important for a good understanding of this chapter.

Key Terms

adrenergic inhibitors (p. 529)
baroreceptor reflex (p. 524)
diuretics (p. 529)
hypertension (p. 523)
potassium-sparing diuretic agents (p. 529)
primary (idiopathic or essential) hypertension (p. 524)
rebound hypertension (p. 529)
renin-angiotensin-aldosterone mechanism (p. 524)
secondary hypertension (p. 524)
stepped treatment approach (p. 526)
thiazides (p. 529)
vasodilators (p. 542)

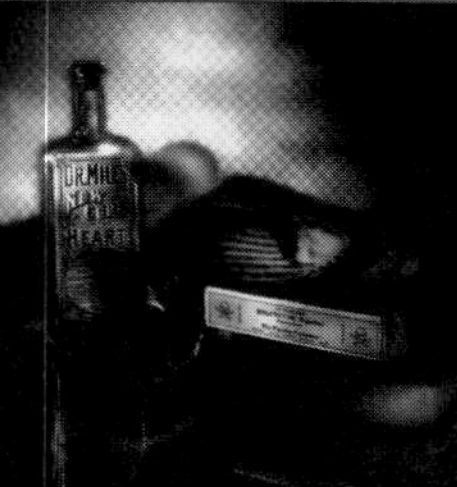

Key Drugs [▲]

captopril
clonidine
nitroprusside
prazosin

Objectives

1. Describe the physiologic control of blood pressure.
2. Define hypertension on the basis of the criteria established by the Joint National Committee on Detection, Evaluation, and Treatment of High Blood Pressure.
3. Describe the stepped-care approach used in drug therapy for hypertension.
4. Discuss the special considerations for antihypertensive drug therapy: sexual dysfunction, concerns with the pediatric, geriatric, pregnant, or surgical client.
5. Define the five major categories of antihypertensive drugs: diuretics, adrenergic inhibitors, vasodilators, angiotensin-converting enzyme (ACE) inhibitors, and calcium antagonists.
6. Identify commonly used antihypertensive drugs as to mechanism of action, pharmacokinetics, side effects and adverse reactions, interactions, and dosages.
7. Implement nursing management of the care of individual clients with antihypertensive drug regimens.

Since 1972, the mortality rate from coronary heart disease has decreased by 50% and the mortality rate from stroke has declined by 57%. According to the Joint National Committee on Detection, Evaluation, and Treatment of High Blood Pressure (JNC V) (1992), the early detection, treatment, and control of hypertension are believed to have significantly contributed to these declines. Despite this improvement, though, cardiovascular disease is still the number one cause of death in North America.

DEFINITION OF HYPERTENSION

Hypertension is defined as an elevated systolic blood pressure, diastolic blood pressure, or both. The classification for adult hypertension was defined by JNC V (1992) as follows:

Hypertension	Systolic (mm Hg)	Diastolic (mm Hg)
Normal	<130	<85
Stage 1 (mild)	140-159	90-99
Stage 2 (moderate)	160-179	100-109
Stage 3 (severe)	180-209	110-119
Stage 4 (very severe)	210 and over	120 and over

The prevalence of hypertension increases with age, is higher in African Americans than in Caucasians, and in both races is more common in the lower socioeconomic groups. In youth to early middle age, high blood pressure is greater in men than women. This tends to reverse later in life (JNC V, 1992). The nurse should be aware that clients with elevated blood pressure are frequently asymptomatic. Because there is a potential for a steady progression of secondary organ damage that may become fatal, untreated hypertension is known as the "silent killer" (see the Nursing Research box below).

Two or more diastolic or systolic blood pressures, taken on two or more occasions after an initial screening, are necessary to diagnose an individual as hypertensive. Persons with a blood pressure equivalent to or greater than 140/90 should be treated (nonpharmacologically and/or pharmacologically) to reduce the risk of premature death and disability. Uncontrolled high blood pressure has resulted in increased risks of morbidity, disability, and mortality; thus the development of a classification based on risk to the individual at specific blood pressure ranges was developed.

Obtaining a careful and detailed drug history before diagnosis is also important, since many over-the-counter (OTC) and prescription medications may increase blood pressure or interfere with the effectiveness of an antihypertensive agent. Oral contraceptives (estrogen-containing agents), corticosteroids, nonsteroidal antiinflammatory agents, antidepressants, nasal decongestants, and appetite-suppressing agents are typical examples of interfering substances. Figure 27-1 illustrates sites of drug effects that can induce or exacerbate hypertension.

Clients who are at high risk for developing cardiovascular disease or who are 50 years or older with mild hypertension should receive antihypertensive agents, since studies indicate a decrease in cardiovascular mortality and morbidity in this age group when medicated.

Nursing Research

Hypertension as a silent killer

Not only is hypertension "silent" in its symptoms, but it is also silent in that as prevalent as it is, there is little public knowledge about the condition. Few lay people understand that it may begin in childhood and become evident in adulthood, certainly not the children themselves. Desmond et al (1992) examined knowledge level and perceptions of hypertension in high school students. Using a closed-format Health Belief Model questionnaire, this study assessed 448 low socioeconomic-level African American and white, male and female, junior and senior high school students' knowledge and perceptions regarding hypertension. Approximately two thirds of the students stated that they had a family member with high blood pressure. However, the students had a mediocre knowledge of hypertension and did not perceive themselves as susceptible to hypertension. The knowledge level was low despite the fact that many students had family members with hypertension. There was no significant difference in the scores of black and white students. Socioeconomic status, not ethnic group, may be responsible for differences in risk factors. Further controlled studies are needed to evaluate the effectiveness of health education in homes and schools in promoting students' health in adulthood.

Critical thinking questions

- How could socioeconomic status contribute to differences in risk factors? How could socioeconomic status contribute to differences in knowledge about risk factors?
- Given the results of the study, how would you increase the awareness of the risks of hypertension in this student population?

From Kirkpatrick MK (1992). Review NAACOG's *Women's Health Nursing Scan* 6(5):9.

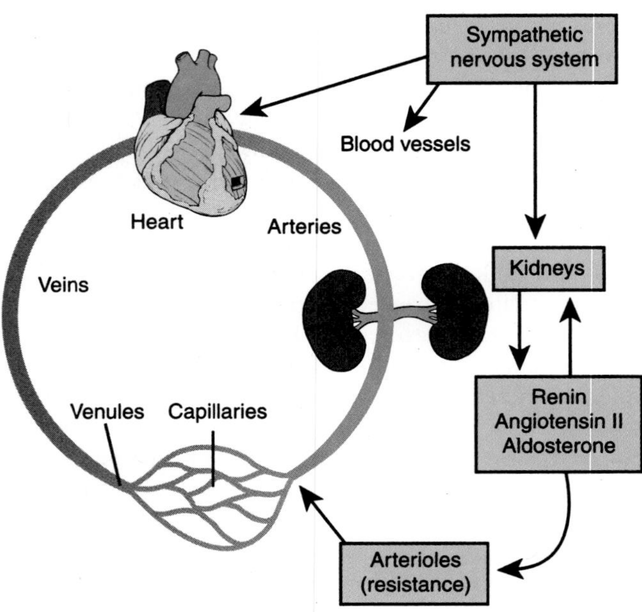

Figure 27-1 Sites of drug effects that can induce or exacerbate hypertension. Many drugs can do either. The sympathetic nervous system is affected by many drugs that can increase blood pressure by their action on the heart and blood vessels (i.e., sympathomimetics): cocaine, amphetamine, ergotamine, estrogen, MAO inhibitors, and NSAIDs. The kidneys are affected by NSAIDs, estrogens, corticosteroids, cocaine, and amphetamine. The renin-angiotensin II-aldosterone system is affected by estrogens, alcohol, and glycyrrhizic acid (licorice). Arterioles are affected by alcohol, sympathomimetics, cocaine, amphetamine, and ergotamine.

CLASSIFICATION OF HYPERTENSION

In **essential,** or **idiopathic,** or **primary hypertension** the specific cause of the hypertension is unknown. This group accounts for approximately 90% of cases. **Secondary hypertension,** representing approximately 10% of cases, may be a symptom of pheochromocytoma, toxemia of pregnancy, or renal artery disease or may result from use of specific medications. If the cause of secondary hypertension is corrected, the blood pressure will usually return to normal.

PHYSIOLOGIC CONTROL OF BLOOD PRESSURE

Control of blood pressure involves a complex interaction between the nervous, hormonal, and renal systems, since all play a part in regulating arterial blood pressure (Figure 27-2). The body has two primary mechanisms to control blood pressure:

1. Adrenergic nervous system or baroreceptor reflex—a rapid-acting system
2. Renin-angiotensin-aldosterone mechanism—a long-acting system

Adrenergic Nervous System

The adrenergic or sympathetic nervous system uses a reflex mechanism, the **baroreceptor reflex,** to maintain blood pressure. The baroreceptors are nerve endings located in the walls of the internal carotid arteries and the aortic arch. These sensory receptors rapidly respond to changes in blood pressure. Any elevation in pressure stretches the receptors causing an impulse to be transmitted along the afferent neuron (vagus nerve) to the vasomotor center in the brainstem. The vasomotor center responds to the impulse by causing (1) a decrease in heart rate and force of myocardial contraction, which lowers cardiac output, and (2) vasodilation of peripheral vessels, which decreases total peripheral resistance. The subsequent reduction in blood pressure is attributed to the reflex activity of the baroreceptor reflex.

When blood pressure is low, this information is projected to the vasomotor center that then activates sympathetic nerves. The sympathetic nervous system is mediated by two hormones: norepinephrine and epinephrine. Norepinephrine acts mainly on alpha-adrenergic receptors, located in the arterioles, while epinephrine acts on both alpha- and beta-adrenergic receptors. The affinity of norepinephrine for these receptors produces vasoconstriction, with a resultant increase in blood pressure. The $beta_1$-adrenergic receptors prevalent in the heart are also activated by norepinephrine. This response increases both the heart rate and the force of myocardial contraction, thereby indirectly causing an elevation in blood pressure.

Because it produces dilation of skeletal muscle blood vessels, epinephrine does not cause any increase in peripheral resistance. However, epinephrine does produce a considerable increase in heart rate and force of myocardial contraction, so the elevation in cardiac output indirectly raises the blood pressure (Box 27-1).

This reflex functions as a rapidly acting system for short-term control of pressure, both low and high blood pressure. It has been demonstrated that over a prolonged period the rate of firing of the baroreceptors diminishes even if the blood pressure remains elevated. Therefore in hypertension it has been speculated that these receptors are "reset" to maintain a higher level of blood pressure.

Renin-Angiotensin-Aldosterone Mechanism

The **renin-angiotensin-aldosterone mechanism** regulates blood pressure by increasing or decreasing the blood volume through kidney function (Figure 27-3). The initiating factor is renin, an enzyme secreted from the juxtaglomerular cells located in the afferent arteriolar walls of the nephron. When blood flow through the kidneys is reduced, renal arterial pressure is reduced, which causes release of renin into the circulation. Here, renin catalyzes the cleavage of a plasma protein to form angiotensin I, a weak vasoconstrictor. Subsequently, in the small vessels of the lung, angiotensin I is converted by angiotensin-converting enzyme (ACE) to angiotensin II.

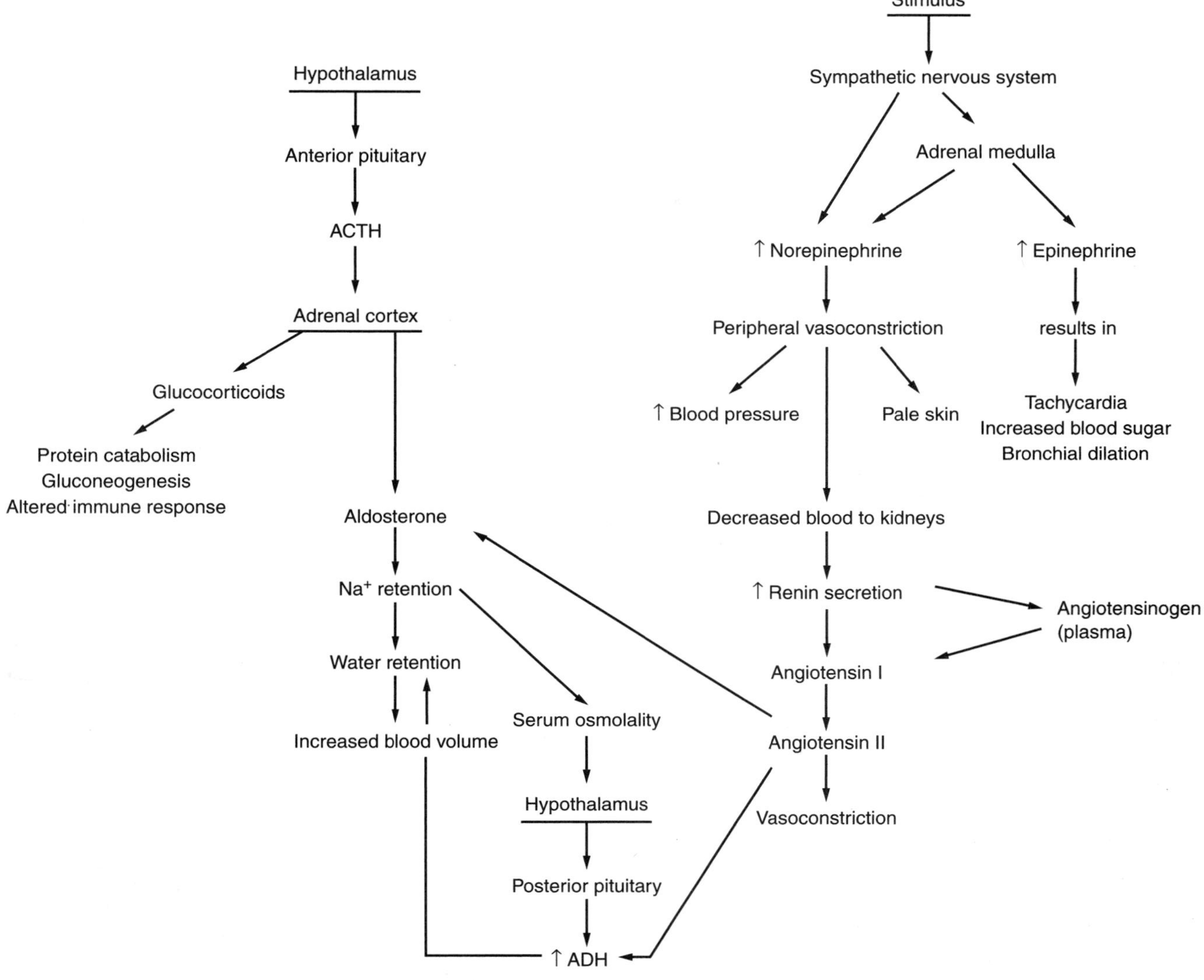

Figure 27-2 Physiologic control of blood pressure. Activation of the sympathetic nervous system results in an increased release of norepinephrine, resulting in peripheral vasoconstriction and increased blood pressure. An increased release of epinephrine increases heart rate and the force of myocardial contractions, also resulting in elevation of blood pressure. Vasoconstriction results in increased blood pressure plus decreased blood supply to the kidneys, which activates the angiotensin system. Ultimately, the release of angiotensin II (a potent vasoconstrictor) results in an increase in aldosterone release from the adrenal cortex, an increase in release of ADH, and increased blood volume. See the text for a description of mechanisms.

Angiotensin II is one of the most potent vasoconstrictors known. It is particularly effective in constricting arterioles, which increases peripheral resistance and raises blood pressure. In addition, angiotensin II acts on the adrenal cortex to stimulate the secretion of aldosterone, a hormone that promotes reabsorption of sodium by the kidneys. The increased sodium elevates the osmotic pressure in the plasma, causing a release of antidiuretic hormone from the hypothalamus. Angiotensin II acts on the kidney tubules to promote reabsorption of water.

Excessive fluid retention is controlled by the negative-feedback mechanism operating within this system so that fluid balance is restored to a normal level. Thus the renin-angiotensin-aldosterone system involves slow adjustments to changes in fluid volume. The kidneys are by far the most important organs in the body for long-term regulation of blood pressure. When the operation of the urinary system fails, increased peripheral resistance and retention of fluid volume produce a combination of hypertensive effects, which keep blood pressure constantly elevated.

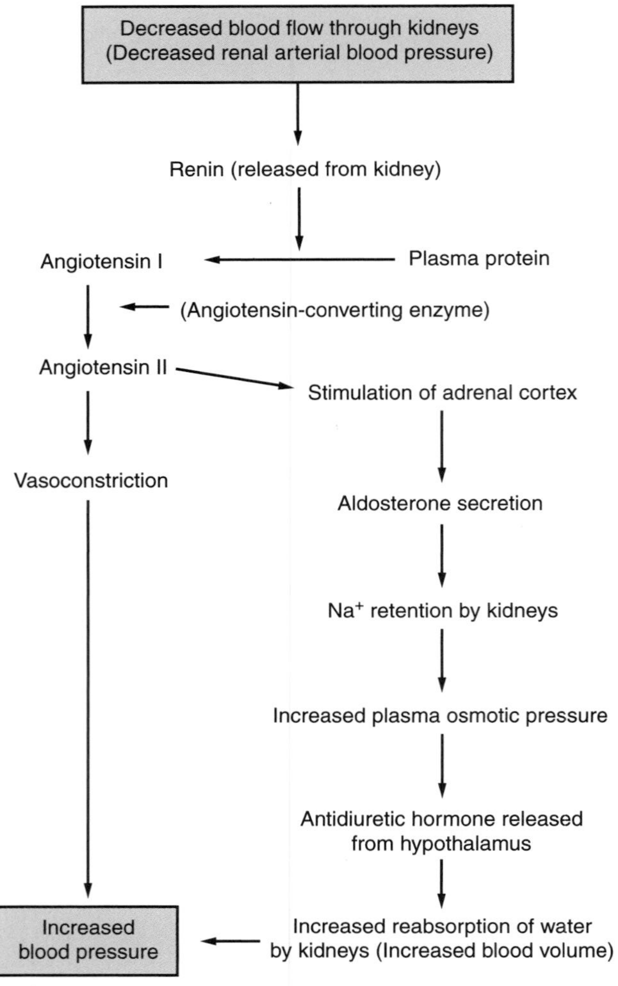

Figure 27-3 The renin-angiotensin-aldosterone system.

BOX 27-1

Basic Blood Pressure Equations

Blood pressure (mean arterial pressure) = cardiac output × peripheral resistance

Cardiac output = stroke volume × heart rate

Thus knowledge of the normal mechanisms for blood pressure control has led to the development of the pharmacologic agents. For example, the beta-blocking agents suppress renin release while the ACE inhibitors prevent the conversion of angiotensin I to angiotensin II. The mechanism of action for the antihypertensive agents is reviewed in this chapter.

ANTIHYPERTENSIVE THERAPY

Client participation in antihypertensive therapy is essential for control of blood pressure. The client needs to understand that hypertension is usually asymptomatic and that therapy does not cure but only controls hypertension. Long-term therapy is necessary to prevent the morbidity and mortality that result from primary hypertension. Compliance with an individualized antihypertensive regimen is associated with a good prognosis and healthy lifestyle.

Nonpharmacologic approaches are legitimate interventions. These measures include weight control if the client is overweight, sodium restriction (Box 27-2), elimination of tobacco, limited consumption of alcohol, reduction in dietary saturated fats, a regular exercise program, and behavior modification to promote relaxation. They may be used independently in mild hypertension and always as an adjunct to drug therapy for clients with moderate to severe hypertension. Adherence by the client to a prescribed nonpharmacologic regimen may allow reduction in medication dosage and subsequent side effects.

BOX 27-2

Fruits and Vegetables Low in Sodium and Calories and High in Potassium

artichokes	cantaloupe	peaches
bananas	carrots	potatoes
broccoli	honeydew melon	strawberries
brussels sprouts	oranges	tomatoes
	orange juice	

Careful use of antihypertensive drugs can effectively control the blood pressure in a majority of hypertensive individuals, with less risk of serious complications and intolerable side effects. The JNC V (1992) report proposes a new pharmacologic treatment approach for hypertension. Figure 27-4 explains the **stepped treatment approach** for hypertension, an antihypertensive therapy program that becomes more aggressive with each level of treatment.

If over a 3 to 6 month period the blood pressure remains at or above 140/90 mm Hg and the client has followed the recommended lifestyle modifications plus has target organ disease (retinopathy, transient ischemic attack (TIA), stroke, left ventricular hypertrophy, etc.) and/or any other known risk factors for cardiovascular disease, then antihypertensive medications should be started. In stages 1 and 2, monotherapy with a diuretic or a beta-blocking agent is indicated. Currently, these are the only drug classifications that have been reported to reduce cardiovascular morbidity and mortality in controlled clinical trials. While the alternative medications—ACE inhibitors, calcium antagonists, alpha$_1$-blocking agents, and the alpha-beta blockers—are as effective in reducing blood pressure although results from long-term studies are not currently available. Thus evidence indicating their effectiveness in reducing morbidity and mortality is lacking. In the step approach, these agents may be utilized as additional drugs in stage 3 or 4.

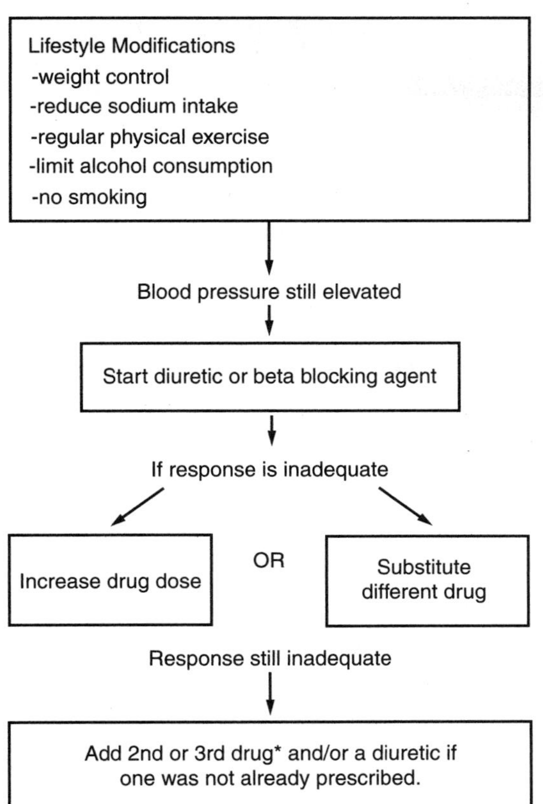

Figure 27-4 Stepped treatment approach for hypertension. *ACE inhibitors, calcium antagonists, alpha-blocking agents, or beta-blocking agents.

Special Concerns

Demographics. African Americans generally respond better to diuretics and calcium antagonists than to ACE inhibitors or beta blocking agents. See the Cultural Aspects box below for additional clinical responses to antihypertensive agents among racial and ethnic groups.

Gender differences in blood pressure response to antihypertensive agents have not been identified. Hypertension has been reported to be 2 to 3 times more common in women who have used oral contraceptive agents for 5 years or longer as compared with those not taking any oral contraceptives. This risk increases with age, smoking, and higher doses of estrogen and progesterone. If hypertension occurs, the usual treatment is to discontinue the oral contraceptive, and usually blood pressure normalizes in 3 to 6 months. If the blood pressure does not return to normal, lifestyle modifications and antihypertensive drugs should be instituted.

Age differences also affect blood pressure. A significant proportion of persons over 65 years of age have elevated systolic or diastolic blood pressure or both, which increases their risk of cardiovascular morbidity and mortality. Nonpharmacologic means of blood pressure reduction (weight reduction if necessary, dietary sodium restriction, etc.) are indicated. Antihypertensive drugs should be started with smaller than usual doses, increased by smaller than usual amounts, and scheduled at less frequent intervals with the elderly, since they are more sensitive to volume depletion and sympathetic inhibition than younger clients. They commonly have impaired cardiovascular reflexes, which make them more susceptible to hypotension.

In elderly clients with isolated systolic hypertension who are treated with antihypertensive drugs, the systolic pressure should be cautiously decreased to 140 to 160 mm Hg. Only if this medication level is tolerated without side effects should consideration be given to further lowering the systolic value. This population's response to both nonpharmacologic and pharmacologic therapies should be monitored closely.

The goal of therapy for hypertensive children and adolescents is to reduce the blood pressure without adverse effects that limit compliance or interfere with normal growth and development. The type of intervention will be determined by the causative factors, the presence of complications, and the degree of hypertension. Nonpharmacologic measures (weight control, reduction of dietary sodium, exercise, avoidance of smoking and alcohol, and reduction of saturated fat) are strongly recommended. If children do not respond to nonpharmacologic measures or if their blood pressures place them at risk for organ damage, then pharmacologic therapy should be considered.

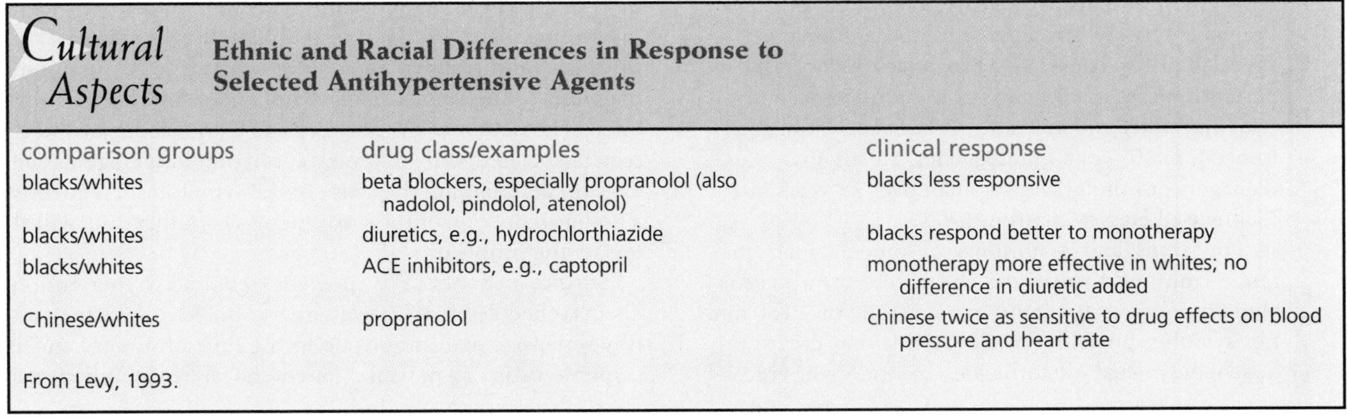

Cultural Aspects — Ethnic and Racial Differences in Response to Selected Antihypertensive Agents

comparison groups	drug class/examples	clinical response
blacks/whites	beta blockers, especially propranolol (also nadolol, pindolol, atenolol)	blacks less responsive
blacks/whites	diuretics, e.g., hydrochlorthiazide	blacks respond better to monotherapy
blacks/whites	ACE inhibitors, e.g., captopril	monotherapy more effective in whites; no difference in diuretic added
Chinese/whites	propranolol	chinese twice as sensitive to drug effects on blood pressure and heart rate

From Levy, 1993.

Pharmacologic interventions for children also follow the stepped approach. Continued assessment of the child and family is necessary to ensure satisfactory blood pressure control and compliance with the therapeutic program, whether pharmacologic or nonpharmacologic.

Concomitant disease states. Beta-blocking agents may aggravate asthma, diabetes, and peripheral ischemia. In such instances, a diuretic may be the preferred agent. Beta-adrenergic blocking agents can cause bronchospasm and therefore should be avoided in clients with a history of bronchial asthma or chronic obstructive pulmonary disease. The beta-blocking agents may also reduce the client's control of diabetes mellitus by interfering with the individual's normal response to hypoglycemia. This may lead to prolonged hypoglycemia and severe hypertension. Although the beta blockers are not contraindicated for use in diabetic clients, individuals receiving such drugs should be educated about this potential problem and taught alternate methods for self-monitoring.

Several antihypertensive agents, such as the thiazide and loop diuretics and beta blockers, may increase serum lipid levels in some clients. Beta blockers with an intrinsic sympathomimetic effect and labetalol do not appear to have this effect on lipids. The ACE inhibitors and calcium antagonists also have no reported adverse effect on serum lipid levels. Therefore, it is apparent that careful selection and monitoring of antihypertensive agents are necessary, especially in clients with coexisting chronic illnesses.

Alternatively, beta blockers may improve angina pectoris and migraine headaches and may extend life after a myocardial infarction (*USP DI,* 1996). Beta-adrenergic blocking agents may provide initial therapy for the younger person with tachycardia and marked lability of blood pressure.

Pregnancy. Hypertension during pregnancy is a serious condition that requires early detection and treatment. Two major diagnostic categories and treatment are:

1. Chronic hypertension—hypertension present before pregnancy or diagnosed before the twentieth week of gestation. Diuretics, methyldopa (Aldomet), or other antihypertensive medications may be utilized, with the exception of ACE inhibitors. ACE inhibitors are to be avoided; serious neonatal problems, including renal failure and death, have been reported. See the Pregnancy Safety box above for more information.
2. Preeclampsia-eclampsia—a pregnancy-induced hypertension that is a primary factor in maternal and fetal morbidity and mortality. It has been estimated to occur in 10% of all pregnancies, mostly in teenagers or primigravida woman over 35 years old (Sagraves, Letassy & Barton, 1995).

   The signs and symptoms of preeclampsia may range from mild to severe; the severe form may include blood pressure ≥110 mm diastolic or ≥160 mm Hg systolic; proteinuria, elevated serum creatinine, headache, visual disturbance, gastric pain, retinal damage (hemorrhage, exudate, etc), pulmonary edema, decreased platelet count (<100,000/mm^3), and/or eclampsia or convulsions or seizures in a woman with preeclampsia.

Pregnancy Safety

Category	Drug
B	methyldopa, guanadrel, guanfacine
C	clonidine, diazoxide, doxazosin, hydralazine, prazosin, guanabenz, guanethidine, reserpine, minoxidil, nitroprusside, terazosin, all ACE inhibitors in first trimester
D	All ACE inhibitors in second and third trimesters, trimethaphan

Therapy includes bed rest, hospitalization (controversial today), and, if the fetus is mature, a timely delivery. Use of antihypertensive agents is based on maternal safety, and most clinicians initiate treatment when the diastolic blood pressure is ≥100 mm Hg. If delivery is not planned for within 24 hours, an oral agent such as methyldopa (Aldomet) is the drug of choice, although labetalol (Normodyne), magnesium sulfate, parenteral hydralazine, calcium blocking agents, and various beta-adrenergic agents have also been utilized. Published studies are suggesting the use of low-dose aspirin (60 mg) to prevent preeclampsia in high-risk clients. Aspirin reverses the imbalance between prostacyclin and thromboxane that may be responsible for preeclampsia. The ACE inhibitors are not recommended for use during pregnancy as mentioned previously (Sagraves, et al, 1995).

Mothers receiving continuous antihypertensive therapy should be advised not to breastfeed, since most of the agents are transferred to breast milk.

Sexual dysfunction. Sexual dysfunction is a common complication of antihypertensive medications and may be manifested in males as decreased libido, impotence, impaired or retrograde ejaculation, and gynecomastia. In females it may be manifested as decreased libido, decreased vaginal lubrication, and inability to achieve orgasm. Such symptoms may lead to the client's poor compliance with the drug regimen. The nature of the disorder and a knowledge of the effects associated with different antihypertensive agents will assist in determining the cause of the symptoms. Frequently, a dosage reduction or the substitution of another drug will alleviate the problem.

Surgical clients. To prevent rebound hypertension, clients scheduled for elective surgery should receive their antihypertensive medications up to the time of surgery and as soon afterward as possible. Parenteral diuretics, adrenergic

BOX 27-3

Rebound Hypertension and Hypertensive Crisis

The abrupt withdrawal or discontinuation of antihypertensive medications may result in rebound hypertension and possibly a hypertensive crisis. **Rebound hypertension** refers to the sudden increase of blood pressure to the pretreatment level or above. Hypertensive crisis or hypertensive emergency is the elevation of diastolic blood pressure above 120 to 130 mm Hg (Hawkins et al, 1993).

Symptoms of rebound hypertension depend on the elevation of the blood pressure. Usually the symptoms involve sympathetic system hyperactivity, such as sweating, anxiety, tachycardia, insomnia, muscle cramps, chest pain, headache, and nausea. In a hypertensive emergency or crisis, the extremely elevated rise in blood pressure may cause target organ damage, such as to the eyes (retinal), heart, kidneys, or neurologic system.

In both instances, therapy is instituted to reduce blood pressure as soon as possible (Hawkins et al, 1993).

inhibitors, and vasodilators, plus sublingual nifedipine or transdermal clonidine, are available for clients who are unable to take oral medications. Clients taking an adrenergic inhibitor before surgery are more at risk for rebound hypertension (Box 27-3).

The client's electrolyte status should be carefully checked before surgery. If hypokalemia is detected, it should be corrected before the scheduled operation. The anesthesiologist should always be completely informed about the client's medication regimen; this is vital information that may alter the medications or the monitoring methods used.

■ ■ ■

The antihypertensive drugs currently used to reduce blood pressure are classified into five major categories: diuretics, adrenergic inhibitors (central and peripheral), angiotensin-converting enzyme (ACE) inhibitors, calcium antagonists, and vasodilators. The use of diuretics or the beta-blocking agents in hypertension have resulted in a reduction in morbidity and mortality.

DIURETIC DRUGS

Diuretic drugs play a vital role in lowering blood pressure. The use of **diuretics**, agents that promote the formation and excretion of urine, results in a loss of excess salt and water from the body by renal excretion. The decrease in plasma and extracellular fluid volume subsequently depresses vascular reactivity to sympathetic stimulation. Thus volume depletion, plus a direct diuretic effect on the arterioles that produces vasodilation, results in lowering of the blood pressure. This response causes an initial decline in cardiac output, followed by a decrease in peripheral resistance and a lowering of blood pressure (Figure 27-5).

The **thiazides** and related sulfonamide diuretics, such as chlorthalidone and metolazone, when used in maximum therapeutic doses, are moderately effective in decreasing blood pressure. Therefore these mild diuretics can be used alone for individuals with early stages of hypertension. By contrast, many of the other types of antihypertensive agents, when used alone on a long-term basis, cause a gradual retention of sodium and water, expansion of plasma fluid volume. Thus a low dose diuretic is often given in combination with ACE inhibitors, alpha blocking agents, vasodilators, or adrenergic inhibitors to prevent fluid retention.

The **potassium-sparing agents,** such as spironolactone and triamterene, are useful in counteracting potassium loss induced by other diuretics. They promote sodium and water loss without accompanying loss of potassium. These drugs are indicated for management of hyperaldosteronism and renal vascular hypertension when the client's condition is resistant to other diuretics. See Chapter 34 for monographs on diuretic drugs.

ADRENERGIC INHIBITING (SYMPATHOLYTIC) AGENTS

Adrenergic inhibitors, the most effective antihypertensive drugs, inhibit the activity of the sympathetic nervous system. The heart, blood vessels, and kidneys influence arterial pressure through various reflex mechanisms. Sympathetic stimulation increases heart rate and force of myocardial contraction, constricts arterioles (resistance vessels) and venules (capacitance vessels), and releases renin from the kidneys. Adrenergic inhibiting agents then are effective in reducing blood pressure and preventing serious cardiovascular complications. The sites at which these drugs modify sympathetic nervous system activity vary widely and usually involve complex mechanisms.

Beta-Adrenergic Blocking Agents

The beta-blocking agents decrease cardiac output and inhibit renin secretion, which results in a lowering of blood pressure. By competing with epinephrine for available beta receptor sites, they inhibit typical organ or tissue response to

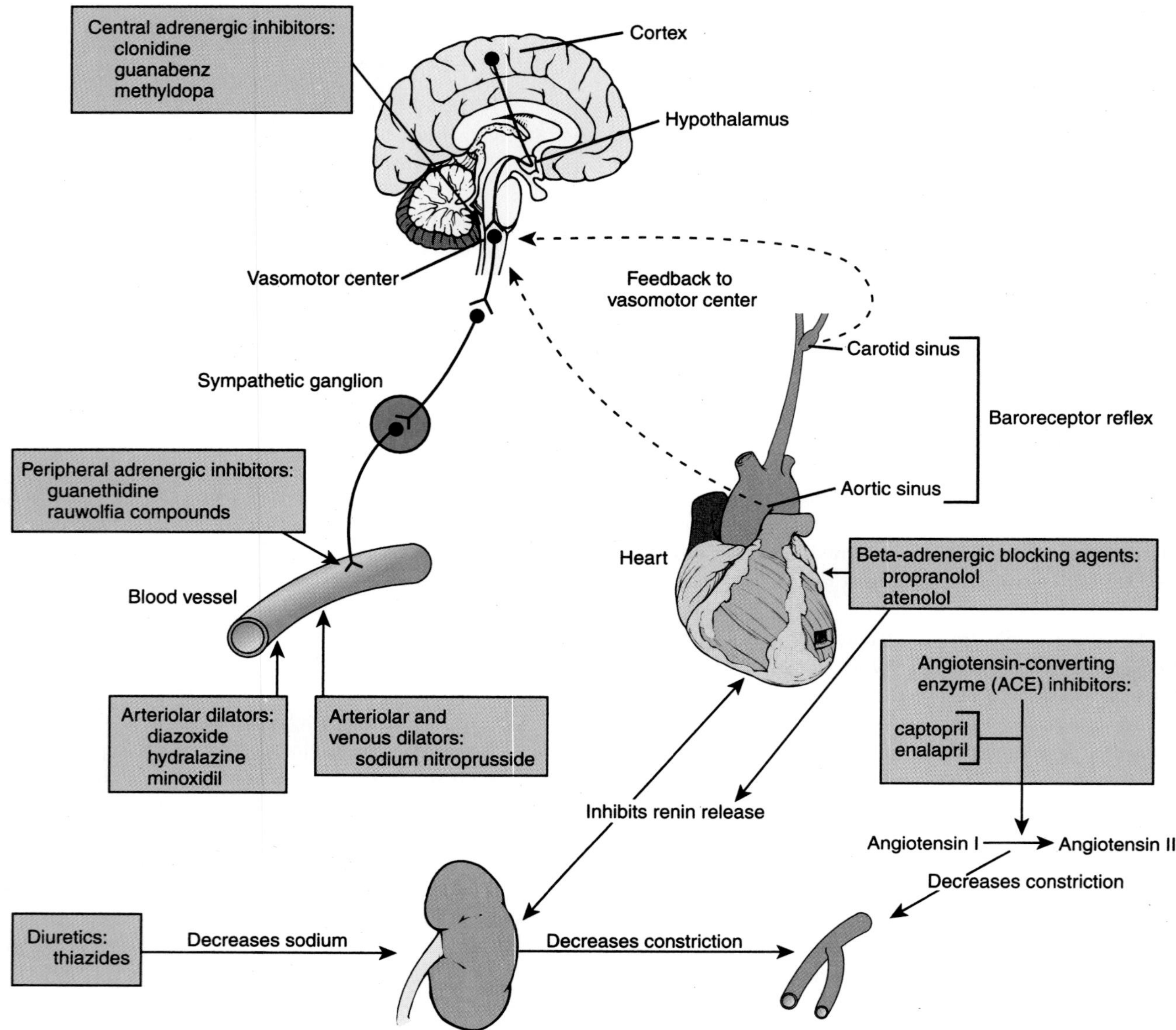

Figure 27-5 Site and method of action for various antihypertensive drugs, based on reported clinical and experimental evidence.

beta stimulation. For additional information about this drug category, see Chapter 22.

The other adrenergic inhibitors are also effective in lowering blood pressure and generally have multiple sites of action or may have unknown mechanisms of action. For clarification, the drugs are characterized by their primary proposed site of action.

Centrally Acting Adrenergic Inhibitors

The centrally acting agents clonidine (Catapres), methyldopa (Aldomet), guanfacine (Tenex), and guanabenz (Wytensin) are effective antihypertensives, especially when combined with a diuretic. When given as a single agent, clonidine and methyldopa (guanfacine and guanabenz to a lesser extent) usually produce sodium and water retention.

▲ **clonidine hydrochloride** [kloe' ni deen] (Catapres, Catapres-TTS)

Clonidine reduces systolic and diastolic blood pressure by stimulation of central $alpha_2$ receptors, which decreases sympathetic outflow of norepinephrine from the brain to the blood vessels and heart. Blood pressure is lowered by decreasing cardiac output, heart rate, and peripheral vascular resistance. The depressed cardiac output is the result of a reduction in both heart rate and stroke volume. Consequently, this action can cause bradycardia.

While not approved indications in the United States, clonidine is also used in the diagnosis of pheochromocytoma;

prophylaxis of migraine or vascular headaches; treatment of dysmenorrhea, menopause, and Gilles de la Tourette's syndrome; and nicotine and opioid withdrawal (*USP DI,* 1996).

The decreased sympathetic outflow to the kidneys reduces renal vascular resistance and thus preserves renal blood flow. In some clients, renin activity may be suppressed (Hoffman & Lefkowitz, 1996). With continued clonidine use, a diuretic is prescribed to correct fluid retention.

Oral clonidine has an onset of action within ½ to 1 hour; peak effect in 2 to 4 hours; and duration of action up to 8 hours. The serum half-life is between 12 and 16 hours; metabolized in the liver and primarily excreted by the kidneys. Clonidine transdermal is best absorbed from the chest and upper arm. Onset of action and time to peak effect are 2 to 3 days, while duration of action is approximately a week if the drug is in continuous contact with the body (about 8 hours if removed from the body). Metabolism and excretion are the same as for oral clonidine.

The side/adverse effects of clonidine include dry mouth, headaches, constipation, weakness, postural hypotension, impotency or decreased sexual drive, insomnia, anxiety, anorexia, nausea, vomiting, and pruritus.

The adult dose is 0.1 mg twice daily initially; increased every 2 to 4 days by 0.1 or 0.2 mg as necessary to control blood pressure. For maintenance, the dose is 0.2 to 0.6 mg daily in divided doses. The dosage for children has not been established.

Catapres-TTS (clonidine transdermal system). Clonidine transdermal is available in various strengths (0.1, 0.2, or 0.3 mg) programmed to deliver the specified strength daily for 1 week. The system is composed of four layers: a film that contains a drug reservoir of clonidine, a membrane that controls the rate of drug delivery, an adhesive layer that also contains clonidine to initially saturate the skin site, and a top backing or cover layer. The system was formulated for the drug to flow from a higher concentration to the lower concentration in the body, which is limited by the rate-controlling membrane layer. It takes approximately 2 to 3 days to reach a therapeutic clonidine serum level on initial application; replacing the system weekly at a new body site will maintain the therapeutic serum level.

■ Nursing Management

Clonidine Therapy

Assessment. Use clonidine therapy cautiously with clients who have coronary insufficiency, recent myocardial infarction, or cerebrovascular disease as a decrease in blood pressure may decrease tissue perfusion and so increase ischemia. Chronic renal failure will decrease elimination and the drug and so increase the risk of toxicity. Those with thromboangiitis, Raynaud's disease, or a history of mental depression may have their condition worsen. Clients with sinus or atrioventricular node dysfunction may experience further impairment. Elderly clients, too, are more sensitive to clonidine's hypotensive effects and are at risk of injury related to orthostatic hypotension. Dosage adjustments may be necessitated by age-related renal function impairment.

If the transdermal dosage form of clonidine is to be applied, the client's skin should be assessed for any irritation or abrasion so that they can be avoided since absorption may be increased if the drug is applied to these areas. On the other hand, areas of skin involvement with disorders such as systemic lupus erythematosus or scleroderma might decrease drug absorption if the drug were applied to them, so avoid these areas.

A baseline assessment of the client's blood pressure, health status, and lifestyle should be done before clonidine therapy is started.

The client's current medication regimen should be reviewed for significant drug interactions, such as the ones that may occur if clonidine is given with the drugs listed below:

Drug	Possible effect and management
beta-adrenergic blocking agents	Concurrent administration with clonidine may lead to loss of blood pressure control. Additive bradycardia effects may also occur. Monitor pulse rate closely. If the prescriber wants to discontinue both drugs, the beta blocking agent should be stopped first. Discontinuing clonidine first may increase the risk of inducing a withdrawal hypertensive crisis.
tricyclic antidepressants	The antihypertensive effectiveness of clonidine may be reduced. This usually occurs in the first or second week of therapy. Monitor closely, since dosage adjustments and/or alternative hypotensive agents may need to be considered by the prescriber.

Nursing diagnosis. The client receiving clonidine therapy has the potential for the following nursing diagnoses: risk for injury related to orthostatic hypotension, rebound hypertension, or the ineffectiveness of clonidine therapy; impaired skin integrity related to allergic reaction to transdermal system (itching, redness of skin); excess fluid volume related to sodium and water retention (edema); altered thought processes (mental depression); altered bowel elimination (constipation) (10%); altered sleep patterns (drowsiness) (33% with oral use); altered mucous membranes (dry mouth) (40% with oral use); fatigue (10%); sexual dysfunction (impotence, loss of libido); and the collaborative problem of overdose (dyspnea, syncope, pinpoint pupils, bradycardia, fatigue). See the Nursing Care Plan on p. 532 for other selected nursing diagnoses related to antihypertensive therapy.

Implementation

Monitoring. Closely monitor blood pressure and pulse during initiation of therapy, and continue to observe these parameters until dosage is properly titrated. Blood pressure should decrease within 30 to 60 minutes after administration, and the decrease may persist for 8 hours. Regularly monitor the blood pressure and pulse rate on a long-term basis to determine clonidine effectiveness.

Observe the client for drug tolerance evidenced by rising blood pressure levels. The prescriber may increase the dosage or add a diuretic to obtain the required antihypertensive response.

Nursing Care Plan

Selected Nursing Diagnoses Related to Antihypertensive Therapy

Nursing diagnosis	Outcome criteria	Nursing interventions
Knowledge deficit related to newly prescribed or altered antihypertensive drug therapy	Client will describe hypertension; how drug therapy relates to condition; how and when to take medications; common drug interactions, particularly with OTC drugs; safety precautions; common side effects and which are reportable; storage requirements of drugs; and will monitor effectiveness of drug therapy with sequential blood pressure readings.	Assess learning needs and learning readiness. Plan with client and family for achievement of realistic goals. Provide information to meet outcome criteria.
Ineffective management of the therapeutic regimen	Client will self-administer medications safely and accurately.	Check refill frequency to determine adherence to the medication regimen. Explore with client reasons for nonadherence and take appropriate teaching/counseling interventions. Provide needed drug information concerning rationales for specific client's hypertensive status. Emphasize that drug therapy does not cure but controls hypertension and possible need for life-long therapy. Discuss possibility of rebound hypertension with nonadherence to the medication regimen.
Sexual dysfunction related to antihypertensive drug therapy	Client will describe nature of dysfunction, consult with prescriber for dosage reduction or drug substitution, and resume sexual activity.	Assess for causative factors. Encourage client to share concerns. Provide health teaching and referral when needed. Encourage return to sexual activity.

Weigh the client daily for 3 to 4 days after initiation of therapy, since fluid volume excess may occur because of sodium retention and edema. Monitor intake and output; check the client for dependent edema. If fluid retention does not disappear, it may be necessary to add a diuretic to the regimen.

Monitor for the anticholinergic effects of dry mouth, constipation, and urine retention.

Closely monitor a client with a history of mental depression because the drug may intensify this condition. Altered self-concept related to impotence may also occur.

Intervention. When applying clonidine using the transdermal system, select a hairless intact area of the client's upper arm or torso. Do not trim the patch, since doing so would alter the dosage. Reapply once every 7 days on a different skin site. If the system loosens, cover it with an adhesive overlay from the drug package to ensure good adhesion. The patch should remain in place during bathing or showering. Replace the patch if it falls off or becomes very loose. Discard used patches by folding them in half with adhesive sides together. If local skin irritation occurs before the patch has been in place for 7 days, it may be removed and a new one applied to a different skin area. A change from transdermal therapy may be required if skin irritation persists.

Prescribed dose reductions are done over 2 to 4 days or preferably longer (1 to 2 week period) to prevent rebound hypertension, a potentially serious adverse syndrome.

With clients who cannot effectively manage the therapeutic regimen, consultation with the prescriber may result in a change from oral doses to the transdermal therapeutic system or another antihypertensive drug because of the risk of rebound hypertension. When a client is being switched from an oral dosage form of clonidine to the transdermal form, the oral dose needs to be reduced over 2 to 3 days to avoid a withdrawal response because the transdermal dosage form's onset will take 2 to 3 days.

Education. Emphasize the importance of periodic follow-up visits so that the clonidine level and blood pressure are closely monitored. Be explicit in instructions concerning the serious consequences of rebound hypertension caused by missing drug doses or by abrupt cessation of the drug. Clients with serious side effects should immediately report the problem to the prescriber so that the dosage may be adjusted or the drug may be withdrawn gradually over a period of 2 to 4 days. Abrupt withdrawal, including omission of sequential doses, can result in hypertensive crisis within 8 to 24 hours. The symptoms of hypertensive crisis are anxiety, sweating, tachycardia, insomnia, salivation, abdominal and muscle cramps, headache, and chest pain. The client and caregivers should be taught to perform blood pressure monitoring at home and record the results and then to report the results at regular visits to the health care provider.

Instruct the client to keep an adequate supply of the drug at all times, particularly during travel. Instruct the client to take the last dose before bedtime to ensure continuous blood pressure control during the night and reduce daytime drowsiness, which occurs in about 33% of clients using oral dosage forms. Instruct the client to make position changes slowly. The client should move slowly from the recumbent to the upright position and dangle the feet from the edge of the bed to prevent dizziness and fainting. The client needs to be cautioned to avoid alcohol ingestion, prolonged standing and strenuous exercising, and exercising during hot weather, because the potential for orthostatic hypotension is greatly increased.

Altered comfort related to dry mouth may occur in 40% of the clients using oral dosage forms. Encourage the client to use sugarless candy or gum or ice to obtain relief. A saliva substitute such as Orex or Oralube may also be used. If dry mouth persists longer than 2 weeks, the prescriber or dentist needs to be consulted because of the increased risk of caries and oral candidiasis.

Altered bowel function occurs as constipation in about 10% of clients. Instruction should be provided concerning adequate fluid and fiber intake, regular exercise, and establishing a regular bowel pattern to prevent or minimize constipation.

Advise the client on long-term therapy to have a periodic eye examination (every 6 to 12 months) to identify possible retinal degeneration; this has occurred in rats to which clonidine has been administered. Instruct the client to carry a medical identification card or Medic Alert bracelet or pendant. Warn the client not to take OTC medication without consulting the health care provider. Caution the client about the increased sedative effects of alcohol, barbiturates, and other CNS depressants during clonidine therapy, particularly if the individual is operating a car or machinery.

Instruct the client on how to apply the patch and place the patch at a different site each week.

Advise the client in nonpharmacologic management of hypertension, which includes sodium restriction, weight reduction, regular exercise, smoking cessation, moderate consumption of alcohol, reduction in dietary saturated fats, behavior modification to promote relaxation, and adequate dietary intake of potassium, calcium, and magnesium.

Evaluation. The client's blood pressure will remain within normal limits. The client and family will state an understanding of effective self-management of the therapeutic clonidine regimen.

methyldopa [meth ill doe' pa] (Aldomet)
methyldopate injection [meth ill doe'pate] (Parenteral Aldomet)

Although the exact hypotensive mechanism is unknown, the theory is that a metabolite of methyldopa (alpha methylnorepinephrine) stimulates the central alpha$_2$ receptors, which results in a reduction in norepinephrine (sympathetic) outflow to the heart, kidneys, and peripheral vasculature. It lowers blood pressure in a similar way to clonidine.

Methyldopate is hydrolyzed to methyldopa in the body, which then must undergo the previous theoretical process to produce the hypotensive effect. The antihypertensive effect produced by the parenteral dosage form begins in approximately 4 to 6 hours, so it should not be used as the primary single drug in a hypertensive emergency.

Methyldopa's peak effect is 4 to 6 hours after a single dose or 48 to 72 hours with multiple dosing. The duration of action is 12 to 24 hours (after oral single dose), 1 to 2 days (after multiple oral doses), or 10 to 16 hours (after IV administration). Methyldopa is metabolized centrally to alpha methylnorepinephrine. Excretion is primarily by the kidneys.

Side/adverse effects include drowsiness, dry mouth, headaches, edema of feet and legs, postural hypotension, impotency, insomnia, depression, anxiety, and nightmares.

The initial adult oral dose is 250 mg two to three times daily for 2 days, adjusted according to the individual client's response. Maintenance dose is 500 to 2000 mg/day, divided into 2 to 4 individual doses (maximum daily dosage is 3 g/day). Children's dose is initially 10 mg/kg PO initially in 2 to 4 divided doses, increased at 2-day intervals according to the child's response, up to 65 mg/kg or 3 g/day, whichever is less.

In the administration of parenteral methyldopa, the adult dose is 250 to 500 mg in dextrose 5% injection (100 ml) administered over ½ to 1 hour every 6 hours as needed. The maximum dose is 1 g every 6 to 12 hours. The pediatric IV infusion dose is 20 to 40 mg/kg in dextrose 5% injection over ½ to 1 hour administered every 6 hours as needed up to 65 mg/kg or 3 g/day, whichever is less.

■ Nursing Management
Methyldopa Therapy

Assessment. Do not use methyldopa in clients with active hepatic disease, such as hepatitis or cirrhosis, or hypersensitivity to methyldopa. Use with caution in clients with a history of autoimmune hemolytic anemia, pheochromocytoma (interference with catecholamines), or previous liver disease in association with the administration of methyldopa. Risks and benefits must be considered in childbearing and lactating women.

A baseline assessment should be obtained of the client's blood pressure, and a complete blood cell count and a direct Coombs test should be performed.

The client's current medication regimen should be reviewed for significant drug interactions. The following interactions may occur when methyldopa is given with the drugs listed below:

Drug	Possible effect and management
monoamine oxidase (MAO) inhibitors	**Hyperexcitability, hallucinations, headache, and hypertension have been reported with this combination. Avoid or a serious drug interaction may occur.**
sympathomimetics (cocaine, norepinephrine, phenylephrine, and others)	**A decrease in methyldopa's antihypertensive effect is reported. Avoid or a serious drug interaction may occur. If it is necessary to use sympathomimetics, the prescriber should prescribe very small doses of the sympathomimetic agent. Monitor closely.**

Nursing diagnosis. The client receiving methyldopa therapy has the potential for the following nursing diagnoses: risk for injury related to orthostatic hypotension or the ineffectiveness of methyldopa therapy; altered protection related to leukopenia or thrombocytopenia; excess fluid volume related to sodium and water retention (edema); altered thought processes (mental depression); anxiety; altered bowel elimination (diarrhea); altered sleep patterns (drowsiness, [>5%]); altered mucous membranes (dry mouth, [>5%]); altered comfort (headache, [>5%]); activity intolerance related to hemolytic anemia; sexual dysfunction (decreased libido, ejaculation failure); and the collaborative problems of drug fever (fever within the first 3 months of therapy), myocarditis (fever, chills, tachycardia), pancreatitis (abdominal pain with nausea and vomiting), systemic lupus erythematosus (weakness, joint pain, rash); cholestasis or hepatitis (dark urine, pale stools, jaundice).

Implementation

Monitoring. Take blood pressure and pulse as prescribed during initiation of therapy, and continue until the drug dosage is properly titrated. Take blood pressure at regular intervals, with the client in lying, sitting, and standing positions, to determine methyldopa effectiveness.

Observe the client for drug tolerance within the second or third month of therapy, evidenced by rising blood pressure levels. The prescriber may increase the dosage or add a diuretic to obtain the required antihypertensive response. Observe the client for drug-induced depression and report any symptoms to the prescriber. Observe the client for side effects, especially unexplained fever or jaundice, and immediately report any to the prescriber.

If unexplained fever or rash occurs, obtain liver function studies (e.g., AST [SGOT], bilirubin), especially during the first 2 or 3 months of therapy. If jaundice is present, the drug is discontinued to avoid drug-induced hepatitis.

Monitor for fluid volume excess by measuring intake and output, weighing the client daily, and checking for dependent edema. Report fluid retention to the prescriber. If fluid retention occurs, it may be necessary to add a diuretic to the regimen.

Hemolytic anemia may occur in 4% of clients, with possible fatal complications. A complete blood count and a direct Coombs test should be done periodically during treatment. A positive Coombs test may or may not indicate hemolytic anemia. With prolonged use of methyldopa, 10% to 20% of patients develop a positive direct Coombs test; this is not a contraindication to further use of the drug. If a positive Coombs test leads to a diagnosis of hemolytic anemia, the prescriber will discontinue therapy. Positive Coombs test results produced by methyldopa therapy may interfere with the crossmatching of blood. If thrombocytopenia or reversible leukopenia occurs, drug therapy should be discontinued.

The refill frequency may be checked to determine the effectiveness of the client's management of the therapeutic regimen.

Intervention. Dosage increases should be initiated with the evening dose to minimize the effects of sedation.

Intramuscular or subcutaneous administration is not recommended because of unreliable absorption. Administer an intravenous infusion slowly over 30 to 60 minutes. When changing a client from the intravenous to the oral form once the blood pressure has stabilized, the same dosage is used.

Education. Emphasize to the client the importance of keeping clinical laboratory visits for blood cell counts and hepatic function studies. Methyldopa hepatotoxicity (reversible) may occasionally develop 2 to 4 weeks after initiation of therapy. The client should report any flu-like symptoms of chills, fever, headache, anorexia, fatigue, arthralgia, or pruritus. If the results of the liver function tests are positive, therapy will be discontinued. Instruct the client to follow the same precautions as for oral clonidine.

Evaluation. The client's blood pressure will be within normal limits without the client experiencing adverse effects from methyldopa therapy. The client and/or caregivers will effectively manage the methyldopa regimen.

guanabenz acetate [gwahn' a benz] (Wytensin)

The mechanism of action of guanabenz acetate is believed to be the same as for clonidine; it is a centrally acting alpha$_2$ agonist. Cardiac output remains unchanged and the antihypertensive effect occurs without major changes in peripheral resistance. Nevertheless, peripheral resistance does eventually decrease with continued therapy.

Guanabenz has an onset of action within 1 hour (for a single dose), the peak effect occurs in 2 to 4 hours, and the duration of action is 12 hours. The serum half-life is 6 hours. The drug is metabolized in the liver, and excretion is via the kidneys and feces. The side/adverse effects of guanabenz include drowsiness, headaches, nausea, and impotency or decreased sexual drive.

Initial adult dose is 4 mg given PO twice daily, increased if necessary every 1 to 2 weeks by increments of 4 to 8 mg/day up to a maximum of 32 mg/day. The dosage for children is not established.

■ Nursing Management

Guanabenz Therapy

Assessment. Guanabenz is used during pregnancy only if the benefits outweigh the potential risk of adverse effects to the fetus. In animal studies an increase in skeletal abnormalities has been observed, along with increased fetal loss and diminished body weight of the neonate. Always inquire whether a female client is pregnant or plans to become pregnant. Do not use in clients who are hypersensitive to guanabenz. The drug should be used with caution for clients with cerebrovascular or cardiovascular disease or renal or hepatic impairment. A baseline assessment of the client's blood pressure should be obtained.

Giving guanabenz concurrently with a beta-adrenergic blocking agent or other hypotensive agents may result in additive hypotensive effects. Monitor blood pressure closely because dosage adjustments may be necessary. When discontinuing both drugs in a client—for example, a beta-blocking drug and guanabenz—taper the beta blocker first to prevent a withdrawal hypertensive reaction.

Nursing diagnosis. As with other antihypertensive agents, the administration of guanabenz might be an indication for the following nursing diagnoses: risk for injury related to the syncope or ineffectiveness of guanabenz therapy (hypertension); altered comfort (headache or nausea); altered mucous membranes (dry mouth); fatigue; altered sleep pattern (drowsiness); sexual dysfunction; and the collaborative problem of sympathetic overactivity (anxiety, chest pain, tachycardia, nausea, insomnia, headache, increased salivation, and sweating).

Implementation

Monitoring. Closely monitor blood pressure and pulse during the initiation of therapy and until the dosage is properly titrated. Closely observe clients with severe hepatic or renal failure, severe coronary insufficiency, recent myocardial infarction, or cerebrovascular disease, and elderly clients, who are particularly sensitive to the drug's hypotensive effects. The client's blood pressure should be monitored on a long-term basis.

Intervention. The last dose of each day should be taken at bedtime to ensure overnight control of blood pressure and reduce daytime drowsiness.

Guanabenz is usually not discontinued before surgery; however, the anesthesiologist must be aware that the client is receiving the drug.

Education. Emphasize the importance of periodic follow-up visits so that the guanabenz dosage and blood pressure are monitored. Some clients may be instructed to take their own blood pressure and report the readings at regular visits to the prescriber.

Caution the client against abrupt withdrawal of the drug. There is the possibility of withdrawal symptoms, although rebound hypertension does not generally occur.

Inform the client of the possible side effects, particularly dry mouth, and about the increased sedative effects if taken with alcohol, barbiturates, or other central nervous system depressants; caution in operating a car or other machinery is indicated. Caution the client not to take OTC medications without consulting with the prescriber. Instruct the client to take the last dose before bedtime to ensure continuous blood pressure control during the night. Instruct the client to carry a medical identification card or a Medic Alert bracelet or pendant.

Advise the client not to discontinue the drug even if he or she is experiencing unpleasant side effects, since withdrawal symptoms may occur. Instead the prescriber should be consulted for recommendations as to how to proceed.

Instruct the client in nonpharmacologic management of hypertension; see Figure 27-4.

Evaluation. The client will maintain a blood pressure within normal limits without experiencing any adverse effects of guanabenz.

guanfacine [gwahn' fa seen] (Tenex)

Guanfacine (Tenex) is a centrally acting alpha$_2$-adrenergic agonist antihypertensive similar to clonidine. Thus peripheral vascular resistance, heart rate, and blood pressure are lowered.

Guanfacine is well absorbed orally, with peak effect in 8 to 12 hours (single dose) or 1 to 3 months (long-term dosing). The onset of action occurs within 7 days of chronic dosing. The duration of effect is 1 day (single dose). Metabolism occurs in the liver with excretion by the kidneys. The side/adverse effects of guanfacine include constipation, dry mouth, sedation, lightheadedness, headache, nausea, vomiting, insomnia, impotency, dry or itching eyes, weakness, and depression.

Adult dose is 1 mg orally daily at bedtime, increased if needed in 3 to 4 weeks (to 2 mg/day). If necessary, a third increase may be instituted in another 3 to 4 weeks. The pediatric dose has not been determined.

■ Nursing Management

Guanfacine Therapy

Except for the precaution regarding the use of guanabenz during pregnancy, the nursing management for guanfacine is the same as for guanabenz. There is also the added concern that the client may experience depression with the use of guanfacine. The client and family/caregiver should report any symptoms of depression, which include: appetite disturbance (anorexia or overeating); significant weight gain or loss; sleep disturbance (insomnia or hypersomnia); fatigue; agitation; loss of interest or pleasure in activities; feelings of guilt or worthlessness; difficulty in concentration or decision making; or suicidal thoughts.

Peripheral Adrenergic Inhibitors

The peripherally active, adrenergic inhibitors include guanethidine (Ismelin) guanadrel (Hylorel) and reserpine (Serpalan).

guanethidine sulfate [gwahn eth' i deen] (Ismelin)

Guanethidine sulfate is a powerful antihypertensive drug that acts as a postganglionic adrenergic neuron blocking agent. Guanethidine enters the storage vesicles of the adrenergic nerve terminal, where it gradually displaces the stored norepinephrine. The subsequent depletion of norepinephrine inhibits transmission of nerve impulses at the neuroeffector junction. Although there is no significant change in peripheral resistance, the drug reduces blood pressure by decreasing vascular tone, primarily at the venous side and secondarily at the arterial side of the circulatory system.

A lower venous return reduces cardiac output, which consequently decreases cerebral, splanchnic, and renal blood flow. The venous pooling of blood is responsible for the severe orthostatic hypotension that is reported with this drug. This is a limiting factor for the use of this product. The reduction in blood pressure is noticeably greater with the client in the standing position than in the recumbent position.

The adrenergic blocking action of guanethidine increases gastrointestinal motility, frequently causing diarrhea. The drug does not affect the catecholamines in the adrenal medulla. It is contraindicated for use in pheochromocytoma because it may cause the release of catecholamines, thus producing a hypertensive crisis.

Guanethidine has a variable absorption orally (3% to 30% absorbed) with long-term dosing. Peak effect is within 8 hours (single dose) or 1 to 3 weeks (with long-term dosing). It has a biphasic half-life; that is, alpha is 1 to 2 days, beta is between 4 and 8 days. When the drug is stopped (with long-term dosing), there is a gradual blood pressure increase to pretreatment levels within 1 to 3 weeks. Guanethidine is metabolized in the liver and excreted by the kidneys.

The side/adverse effects of guanethidine include orthostatic hypotension, weakness, impaired ejaculation, diarrhea, bradycardia, stuffy nose, alopecia, blurred vision, ptosis of eyelids, nausea, vomiting, muscle pain or tremors, dry mouth, headache, edema, and chest pain (angina).

Dosage and administration. For adult ambulatory clients the dose is 10 or 12.5 mg PO daily initially, increased by 10 or 12.5 mg increments at 5 to 7 day intervals as necessary. The maintenance dose is 25 to 50 mg daily. For hospitalized clients, the initial dose is 25 to 50 mg PO daily, increased by 25 to 50 mg increments at daily or every-other-day intervals as necessary.

The pediatric dose is 0.2 mg/kg PO daily, increased at 7 to 10 day intervals as necessary for blood pressure control.

■ Nursing Management

Guanethidine Therapy

Assessment. Do not use in clients who are hypersensitive to guanethidine. The risk-benefit ratio should be considered carefully with clients with pheochromocytoma as the release of catecholamines may exacerbate symptoms, or with frank congestive heart failure not caused by hypertension, which may be worsened by fluid retention.

Anticipate that hospitalized clients will receive a higher initial dosage than ambulatory clients because they can be watched more carefully. Baseline measurement of the client's blood pressure is necessary.

Review the client's current medication regimen for significant drug interactions, such as those that may occur when guanethidine is given with the drugs listed below:

Drug	Possible effect and management
oral antidiabetic medications or insulin	May result in an increased hypoglycemic effect. Monitor blood glucose levels closely and communicate with prescriber, since dosage adjustments may be necessary.
minoxidil (Loniten) or hypotension-producing medications	**Concurrent use with guanethidine is not recommended, since antihypertensive effects may be potentiated.**
monoamine oxidase (MAO) inhibitors	**Severe hypertension may result. Avoid or a serious drug interaction may occur. It is recommended that MAO inhibitors be discontinued for a minimum of 1 week before starting guanethidine.**
metaraminol (Aramine), and possibly other sympathomimetics	**The antihypertensive effectiveness of guanethidine may be reduced. Concurrent use of metaraminol and guanethidine may result in cardiac arrhythmias, severe prolonged hypertension, or a hypertensive crisis. Avoid or a serious drug interaction may occur.**
tricyclic antidepressants, loxapine (Loxitane), thioxanthenies, and possibly other psychotropic medications	May reduce the antihypertensive effect of guanethidine by blocking its access to the adrenergic nerve site. Monitor closely, since dosage adjustments or alternate antidepressant medications on a trial basis may be ordered by the prescriber.

Nursing diagnosis. With the administration of guanethidine, the client may experience the following nursing diagnoses: altered tissue perfusion (renal, cerebral, and/or cardiopulmonary) related to the drug's ineffectiveness with the underlying condition or the drug's ischemic effects secondary to hypotension; fluid volume excess (dependent edema); sexual dysfunction evidenced by ejaculation difficulties; altered comfort related to headache or chest pain (angina); altered mucous membranes (dry mouth, stuffy nose); altered bowel elimination (diarrhea); fatigue; and risk for injury related to the orthostatic hypotensive effects of the drug. The potential complications of bradycardia may also occur.

Implementation

Monitoring. The most frequent problem with guanethidine is orthostatic hypotension. As a baseline for comparison, take blood pressure readings before initiation of drug therapy; during therapy, continue to keep a record of blood pressures while the client is supine and standing. The hypotensive effect of the drug is greater with the client in the standing position than in the supine position. Therefore dosage adjustment of guanethidine is determined by blood pressure taken first while the client is in the supine position, then again after the client has been standing for 10 minutes or performing mild exercise. If there is *no decrease* from the previous levels, an increase in dosage is indicated. Dosage should be reduced when the client has normal supine blood pressure, excessive fall in orthostatic pressure, or severe diarrhea.

Monitor intake and output, observing for reduced urine volume, particularly in clients with limited cardiac or renal function. Weigh the client daily, and watch for signs of edema or fluid retention. Report increased weight (2 pounds or more in 24 hours) to the prescriber. Carefully monitor the client's pulse rate. If bradycardia occurs, report readings to the prescriber. Closely monitor a client receiving long-term therapy, because the effects of guanethidine are cumulative.

Monitor the blood glucose levels of clients who are receiving antidiabetic medication, since guanethidine may produce additive hypoglycemic effects.

Intervention. Note that guanethidine has a long duration of action as well as a prolonged half-life. Also, the full therapeutic benefits may not be noticed for 1 to 3 weeks. This means that dosage increases, when needed, are made at intervals of 5 to 7 days.

Education. Forewarn the client that orthostatic hypotension (dizziness, lightheadedness, or syncope) occurs frequently and is prominent when one is rising from sleep or making rapid position changes. Instruct the client to change position gradually. Venous return to the heart can be increased by flexing arms and legs slowly before sitting or standing. Recommend that the client don elastic stockings before getting out of bed.

During dosage adjustment, the hospitalized client should receive help when getting out of bed. Inform the client that orthostatic hypotension is aggravated by hot showers or baths, hot weather, prolonged standing, physical exercise, and alcohol ingestion. During an episode of orthostatic hypotension, caution the client to sit or lie down at the first sign of dizziness or weakness.

Instruct the client to report any signs of diarrhea. If it persists, the prescriber may order an anticholinergic agent (atropine), paregoric, or a kaolin-pectin preparation. Guanethidine may be discontinued or the dosage may be reduced. Note the state of hydration of the client, and check the level of electrolyte balance during this episode.

Alert the client to inform surgeons, anesthesiologists, and dentists that he or she is taking guanethidine before any invasive procedures are considered. Instruct the client to carry a medical identification card or a Medic Alert bracelet or pendant.

Emphasize the importance of drug compliance. Report side effects so that the prescriber can modify the drug regimen without discontinuing medication. Also, advise the client to avoid emotional encounters or any other form of stress; instruction on stress management techniques should be offered. Instruct the client not to take any other medication or over-the-counter drugs, which may contain sympathomimetic agents, without consulting the prescriber. Stress the importance of keeping follow-up appointments with the prescriber.

As with guanabenz and other antihypertensive agents, instruct the client in the nonpharmacologic measures to take for blood pressure reduction.

Evaluation. The client will maintain a blood pressure within normal limits without experiencing any adverse effects of guanethidine.

guanadrel [gwahn' a drel] (Hylorel)

The mechanism of action for guanadrel is the same as guanethidine. Guanadrel has an onset of action within 2 hours and peak effect between 4 and 6 hours (after single dose). The half-life is variable, but generally it is about 10 hours. The duration of effect is about 9 hours. The drug is metabolized by the liver and excreted by the kidneys.

The side/adverse effects of guanadrel include hypotension, weakness, impaired ejaculation, increased urination at night, muscle pain or tremors, dry mouth, headache, edema, and chest pain.

Metaraminol (Aramine) and other sympathomimetics, monoamine oxidase inhibitors (MAOI), tricyclic antidepressants, loxapine (Loxitane) thioxanthenes, and psychotropic agents (especially chlorpromazine [Thorazine]) may cause drug interactions; see under guanethidine. In addition, trimeprazine (Arfonad) may reduce the antihypertensive effect of guanadrel by displacement and blocking guanadrel's access to the adrenergic neuron. Monitor blood pressures closely.

The initial adult oral dose is 5 mg twice daily, which may be increased at daily, weekly, or monthly intervals as necessary for blood pressure control. The maintenance dosage is 20 to 75 mg per day in two to four divided doses. Pediatric doses have not been established.

For nursing management, see the discussion of guanethidine on p. •••.

Rauwolfia Derivatives

reserpine [re ser' peen] (Serpalan)

Rauwolfia derivatives are alkaloids obtained primarily from *Rauwolfia serpentina*, a shrub endemic to India and various tropical areas of the world. Reserpine, a rauwolfia alkaloid, lowers blood pressure by depleting the storage sites of norepinephrine in the peripheral postganglionic adrenergic neuron. Without adequate norepinephrine available for release, discharges of nerve impulses from the peripheral sympathetic neurons, which supply the smooth muscle of arterioles, produce little or no effect on these blood vessels. The resultant vascular relaxation decreases peripheral resistance, thereby reducing blood pressure. These compounds also decrease heart rate and thus lower cardiac output. Reserpine also depletes stores of serotonin.

Reserpine has an onset of antihypertensive action of days to 3 weeks with multiple dosing, and a peak antihypertensive effect within 3 to 6 weeks. The half-life is initially 4.5 hours, but with long-term dosing it is extended to 45 to 168 hours. Reserpine is metabolized in the liver and excreted primarily fecally.

The side/adverse effects of reserpine include nausea, vomiting, anorexia, diarrhea, dizziness, dry mouth, stuffy nose, lightheadedness, fluid retention, sexual dysfunction, chest pain, bradycardia, and bronchospasms.

The adult dose is 0.1 to 0.25 mg PO daily.

■ Nursing Management

Reserpine Therapy

Assessment. Determine if the client has a history of mental depression, in which case the drug is used cautiously. Reserpine therapy is discontinued at the first sign of despondency; otherwise continued therapy could result in suicide. Use reserpine cautiously in clients with a history of gallstones to prevent biliary colic, or with a history of renal insufficiency (diuretic is usually required) to avoid the decreased renal tissue perfusion that may result from lower blood pressure levels. Use cautiously in clients with epilepsy, cardiac arrhythmias, respiratory problems, parkinsonism, or pheochromocytoma. Clients with ulcerative colitis or acute peptic ulcer disease may experience increased gastrointestinal motility; use reserpine with caution. Do not use reserpine with clients who are hypersensitive to *Rauwolfia* derivatives.

A baseline assessment should be obtained of the client's blood pressure. Review the client's current medication regimen for significant drug interactions, such as the following, which may occur when reserpine is given with the drugs listed below:

Drug	Possible effect and management
CNS depressants and/or alcohol	Enhanced CNS depressant effects. Monitor vital signs, level of consciousness, and mental status closely.
MAO inhibitors	**May result in hyperpyrexia and hypertension (moderate, severe, or even crisis level). Concurrent administration is not recommended. Clients receiving MAO inhibitors should be taken off this medication for at least 1 week before a *Rauwolfia* alkaloid is started.**

Nursing diagnosis. With the administration of reserpine, the client may experience the following nursing diagnoses: altered tissue perfusion related to the client's underlying condition; risk for injury related to cardiovascular and CNS effects (lightheadedness, dizziness, orthostatic hypotension); altered thought processes (depression); sexual dysfunction (impotence or decreased sexual interest); altered bowel elimination (diarrhea); altered mucous membranes (dry mouth, stuffy nose); altered sleep pattern (nightmares, early morning insomnia); altered protection (thrombocytopenia); altered comfort (abdominal cramps, headache, chest pain); anxiety; and the collaborative problems related to GI effects (tarry stools, hematemesis, peptic ulcer) or arrhythmias.

Implementation

Monitoring. Monitor the client's blood pressure and pulse rate frequently and compare with baseline readings, particularly before parenteral administration. A decrease in blood pressure may be a result of bradycardia. Weigh the client daily. Excessive weight gain indicates fluid retention, which should be reported to the health care provider.

Intervention. Administer oral medication with meals or with milk or other food to minimize gastric irritation, since the drug increases gastric secretions.

Note that the *Rauwolfia* derivatives have a slow onset of action and a long duration of action, so therapeutic benefits may take about 2 weeks to develop. This means that dosage adjustments should be made no more frequently than every 7 to 14 days so that the full effect of the previous dosage can be evaluated. Action may persist for approximately 1 month after discontinuation of therapy. If a client requires general anesthesia, including dental surgery, reserpine no longer needs to be withdrawn; however, the anesthesiologist must be aware of the therapy. It is recommended that reserpine be withdrawn 2 weeks before electroconvulsive therapy is instituted.

Education. Although orthostatic hypotension does not usually occur, advise the client to make position changes slowly to avoid potential dizziness and fainting. Alert the client that the drug may cause drowsiness and to take precautions about driving and other hazardous activities until the CNS effects are known. Advise the client not to take alcohol or other CNS depressants, which will increase the sedative effects of reserpine.

Teach the client or caregiver the possible side effects that may occur and that should be reported to the prescriber, such as nightmares, weight gain, nasal stuffiness, or a significant change in blood pressure. Mental depression (anorexia, self-depreciation, detached attitude, and powerlessness) may lead to suicide. This usually occurs in clients who receive high dosages.

If nasal stuffiness occurs, nasal decongestants or other OTC preparations containing sympathomimetics should not be used without first consulting the prescriber. Dry mouth may be relieved by rinsing with warm water, OTC saliva substitutes (Xero-Lube), sugarless gum, or sour hard candy.

Emphasize the importance of drug compliance even if the client is feeling well. Instruct the client not to discontinue the drug suddenly but to report unpleasant side effects to the prescriber. Also stress the need for medical follow-up visits. Instruct the client to carry a medical identification card or a Medic Alert bracelet or pendant.

As with other antihypertensive agents, instruct the client in the nonpharmacologic measures to take for blood pressure reduction.

Evaluation. The client will maintain a blood pressure within normal limits without experiencing any adverse effects of reserpine.

Alpha-Adrenergic Blocking Drugs

The alpha-adrenergic blocking agents used in the management of hypertension include phenoxybenzamine (Dibenzyline), phentolamine (Regitine) doxazosin (Cardura) prazosin (Minipress), and terazosin (Hytrin). Phenoxybenzamine and phentolamine are alpha blockers that are relatively nonselective because they antagonize responses mediated by both $alpha_1$ and $alpha_2$ receptors. Hence, they lower blood pressure by preventing norepinephrine from activating alpha$_1$ receptors on vascular smooth muscle to produce vasoconstriction. See Chapter 22 for monographs of phenoxybenzamine and phentolamine. Doxazosin, prazosin, and terazosin are more selective in activity and are classed as alpha$_1$-adrenergic blocking agents.

doxazosin [dox ay' zoe sin] (Cardura)
▲ **prazosin hydrochloride** [pra' zoe sin] (Minipress)
terazosin [ter ay' zoe sin] (Hytrin)

Doxazosin, prazosin, and terazosin are selective alpha$_1$-adrenergic blocking agents that dilate both arterioles and veins. This action results in a decrease in peripheral vascular resistance and lowered blood pressure. With prazosin and terazosin, the lowering of blood pressure is not associated with reflex tachycardia, while doxazosin may cause a small increase in heart rate. Prazosin has been used as adjunct therapy to digoxin and diuretics, in the treatment of congestive heart failure. This combination, though, has not resulted in improved survival (*USP DI*, 1996). While all three drugs have been used to treat benign prostatic hyperplasia to improve urinary flow and the symptoms of BPH, only doxazosin and terazosin are FDA approved for this indication (*USP DI*, 1996). (Doxazosin may be used in normotensive clients with BPH since it does not appear to significantly lower blood pressure. In individuals with both hypertension and BPH, it is effective in treating both conditions.)

The onset of action for doxazosin is 1 to 2 hours, peak effect in 5 to 6 hours, and the duration of action is 1 day. Prazosin has an onset of action within 0.5 to 1.5 hours; reaches peak effect within 2 to 4 hours (in congestive heart failure, peak effect is in 1 hour); duration of effect in clients with hypertension is 7 to 10 hours (single drug dose), whereas with congestive heart failure it is 6 hours. Terazosin is rapidly absorbed orally with onset of action within 15 minutes; peak effect in 2-3 hours; duration of action is approximately 1 day. Metabolism for all three drugs (active and inactive metabolites) is in the liver with excretion primarily in feces.

The side/adverse effects of alpha-adrenergic blocking drugs include weakness, nausea, vomiting, stuffy nose, orthostatic hypotension, angina, edema of lower extremities, headaches, syncope, and shortness of breath. There are no known major drug interactions with these drugs to date.

The initial doxazosin adult dose is 1 mg PO daily at bedtime, increased if necessary, every 2 weeks. Maximum daily dose is 16 mg. A pediatric dosage has not been established. Prazosin adult dose is 0.5 mg PO 2 or 3 times daily for at least 3 days. If tolerated, the dose may be increased if necessary, according to individual response. The pediatric dose is 0.05 to 0.4 mg/kg/day, administered in 2 or 3 divided doses. Terazosin adult oral dose is 1 mg PO daily at bedtime. The maintenance dose is between 1 and 5 mg daily, as needed to control blood pressure. The maximum daily dose is 20 mg. A pediatric dosage has not been established.

■ Nursing Management

Alpha-Adrenergic Blocking Agent Therapy

Assessment. Do not administer if the client has a sensitivity to the drug. Clients with impaired renal function may require lower doses of these drugs. With the administration of alpha-adrenergic blocking agents, elderly clients may be more sensitive to the effects of the drug. For prazosin, use caution in clients who have angina pectoris or severe cardiac disease. Document a baseline blood pressure.

Nursing diagnosis. Nursing diagnoses to be considered with these agents might be the following: risk for injury related to the cardiovascular and CNS effects (drowsiness, dizziness, and orthostatic hypotension); fluid volume excess (dependent edema, shortness of breath, and weight gain); fatigue; altered mucous membranes (dry mouth); altered comfort (nasal stuffiness, headache, chest pain, joint pain, nausea, and vomiting); altered cardiac output (tachycardia, palpitations); and the collaborative problem of "first-dose orthostatic hypotensive reaction." With prazosin, the client may also experience altered urinary elimination (urinary incontinence) and sexual dysfunction (priapism).

Implementation

Monitoring. Monitor blood pressure and pulse rate frequently, and observe for any sudden drop in blood pressure and for tachycardia.

Intervention. "First-dose hypotensive reaction", a syncope along with dizziness, lightheadedness, or sudden loss of consciousness, may occur, generally within ½ to 2 hours after an initial dose or a rapid dose increase of the drug. These symptoms may also appear when other antihypertensive agents are added to the regimen. Occasionally, the syncopal episode is preceded by severe tachycardia (heart rate of 120 to 160 beats/min). To minimize this reaction, limit the initial dose of these drugs to 1 mg; then increase the dosage slowly. When adding a diuretic or other antihypertensive agent, reduce the drug to 1 or 2 mg and then increase the dosage as needed. It is recommended that the initial dose be administered at bedtime to minimize the "first-dose hypotensive reaction."

Education. Inform the client of "first-dose hypotensive reaction." Instruct the client to avoid rapid postural changes, particularly from recumbent to upright positions. Also, if dizziness occurs, the client should be instructed to lie down. Reassure the client that this effect tends to disappear with continued use of the drug or dosage reduction. Instruct the client not to drive or operate hazardous machinery during the early period of adjustment to drug therapy. Note that the full effect of the drug may not be achieved for 4 to 6 weeks.

Teach the client to weigh daily and report any significant increase (over 1 kg a day) to the prescriber. Because these agents tend to increase fluid retention, instruct the client to minimize sodium intake.

Emphasize the importance of drug compliance and keeping appointments with the prescriber. If tolerance develops, ineffectiveness usually occurs within several months and the prescriber will need to alter the drug regimen.

Instruct the client not to take any other drugs without first consulting the prescriber. This includes OTC medications that contain sympathomimetic agents used for a cold, cough, or allergic condition.

As with other antihypertensive agents, instruct the client in nonpharmacologic measures to be taken to reduce hypertension (see Figure 27-4).

Evaluation. The client will maintain a blood pressure within normal limits and not experience any untoward effects of the alpha-adrenergic blocking agent.

ANGIOTENSIN-CONVERTING ENZYME INHIBITORS

Angiotensin-converting enzyme (ACE) inhibitors competitively block the angiotensin I converting enzyme necessary for the conversion to angiotensin II. Angiotensin II is a powerful vasoconstrictor that raises blood pressure and also causes aldosterone release, resulting in sodium and water retention. Thus the inhibition of ACE has the following results: (1) a decrease in vascular tone, thereby directly lowering blood pressure; (2) inhibition of aldosterone release, reducing sodium and water reabsorption; the resultant excretion of fluid is thought to cause only a secondary reduction in blood pressure (decrease in aldosterone secretion does lead to a slight elevation in serum potassium); and (3) an increase in plasma renin activity, caused by a loss of negative feedback on renin release. See Figures 27-2 and 27-3 for physiologic blood pressure control and the renin-angiotensin-aldosterone system.

Other indications for the ACE inhibitors include the following:

Captopril, enalapril, and lisinopril are also used in combination with digoxin and diuretics for the treatment of congestive heart failure not responsive to standard therapies.

Captopril has been utilized to treat diabetic nephropathy and also left ventricular dysfunction after a myocardial infarction. It has been reported to increase survival and the incidence of heart failure in such persons (*USP DI*, 1996).

It is apparent that a disturbance of the basic function of the renin-angiotensin-aldosterone system can cause increased vascular resistance or hypertension (Hawkins et al, 1993). Furthermore, a damaged kidney that cannot regulate its renin release through normal feedback mechanisms may easily cause an elevation in blood pressure in certain individuals. This evidence has led to the development of the angiotensin II inhibitors. Benazepril (Lotensin), captopril (Capoten), enalapril (Vasotec), fosinopril (Monopril), lisinopril (Prinivil, Zestril), moexipril (Univasc), quinapril (Accupril), ramipril (Altace), and trandolapril (Mavik) are angiotensin-converting enzyme inhibitors. Also, benazepril and the calcium blocking agent amlodipine are combined and marketed as Lotrel in the United States.

Blood pressure is lowered to about the same extent in clients in supine and upright positions. Although orthostatic hypotension and tachycardia are uncommon, they have been reported in volume-depleted individuals. For pharmacokinetics and adult dosage, see Table 27-1.

The side/adverse effects of ACE inhibitors include dry cough, headaches, diarrhea, loss of taste, weakness, nausea, dizziness, hypotension, rash, fever and joint pain. The Management of Drug Overdose box below describes treatment of ACE inhibitor overdosage.

MANAGEMENT OF DRUG OVERDOSE

ACE Inhibitor

- For hypotension, institute fluid volume expansion.
- If angioedema of face, mucous membranes of mouth, lips, and extremities occurs, an antihistamine may be useful. If the angioedema affects the tongue, glottis, or larynx, then withdraw the ACE inhibitor and hospitalize the client. Epinephrine SC, IV diphenhydramine, and IV hydrocortisone may be necessary.
- Hemodialysis will remove captopril, enalaprilat, and lisinopril.

TABLE 27-1 ACE inhibitors: pharmacokinetics and dosing

Drug	Onset of action (hr)	Duration of effect (hr)	Active metabolite	Usual adult dosage (mg/day)*
benazepril (Lotensin)	within 1	24	benazeprilat	5-40
▲ captopril (Capoten)	0.25-1	6-12	—	25-100
enalapril (Vasotec)	1	24	enalaprilat	5-40
fosinopril (Monopril)	within 1	24	fosinprilat	10-40
lisinopril (Prinivil, Zestril)	1	24	—	10-40
moexipril (Univasc)	1	24	moexiprilat	7.5-30
quinapril (Accupril)	within 1	up to 24	quinaprilat	10-80
ramipril (Altace)	1-2	24	ramiprilat	2.5-20

*Oral doses titrated as needed and tolerated (Olin, 1996; *USP DI*, 1996).

Nursing Management

ACE Inhibitor Therapy

Assessment. ACE inhibitors may cause fetal and neonatal morbidity and mortality when administered to pregnant women; discontinue when pregnancy is suspected. Clients with a history of angioedema will be at risk of ACE inhibitor–related angioedema. Because of the risk of hyperkalemia, clients with reduced renal function may require lower or less frequent doses of ACE inhibitor drugs. The risk should be considered for clients who have hyperkalemia, hyponatremia, volume depletion, diabetes mellitus, or a sensitivity to the drug. Clients with cerebrovascular insufficiency or coronary insufficiency may have their ischemia aggravated by the reduced blood pressure, resulting in cerebrovascular accident or myocardial infarction.

Before the beginning of therapy, a baseline assessment of the client's blood pressure, a complete white cell count, and a proteinuria determination are necessary.

Review the client's current medication regimen for significant drug interactions, such as may occur when ACE inhibitors are given with the following drugs:

Drug	Possible effect and management
alcohol or diuretics	**Concurrent administration with an ACE inhibitor may result in a sudden, very severe hypotensive episode. Avoid or a potentially serious drug interaction may occur. To reduce this reaction, either discontinue the diuretic for approximately a week before starting ACE inhibitor therapy, or increase the salt intake of the client for 1 week before, or start the ACE inhibitor at low dosages. Generally, this reaction does not recur with continued dosing, and the diuretic may be given later, if necessary.**
potassium-sparing diuretics, low-salt milk, potassium supplements, or potassium-containing medications and salt substitutes (see also the case study below)	Closely monitor serum electrolytes, especially potassium because of the high risk for hyperkalemia.

Nursing diagnosis. With the administration of ACE inhibitors, clients may experience the following nursing diagnoses: altered nutrition, less than body requirements, related to taste impairment; risk for injury related to hypotension; altered protection related to neutropenia and agranulocytosis; impaired skin integrity (rash); altered comfort (nausea, headache, dry cough, joint pain, or chest pain); and the collaborative problems of anaphylaxis, pancreatitis, and hyperkalemia (confusion, weakness, cardiac arrhythmias).

Case Study

The Client with Hypertension

Ronald Sanford, age 37 years, is diagnosed with essential hypertension. His blood pressure has been ranging between 148 and 176 systolic and 90 and 110 diastolic. His average blood pressure is 150/94. There is a strong family history of hypertension and stroke on both sides of the family. Mr. Sanford is married with two school-aged children. He works full-time as a loading dock supervisor for a long-distance trucking company. His elevated blood pressure was found during a routine physical examination. He reports no other manifestations. At this time there is no evidence of renal insufficiency or retinopathy.

Mr. Sanford is to begin taking atenolol, 50 mg daily, and hydrochlorothiazide, 50 mg daily.

1. Atenolol is a beta-adrenergic blocking agent. How will this drug contribute to the control of Mr. Sanford's blood pressure?
2. Describe the antihypertensive action of the hydrochlorothiazide.
3. What will Mr. Sanford need to know about taking his medications and avoiding adverse reactions?
4. In addition to drug therapy, what nonpharmacologic measures will you teach Mr. Sanford to help lower his blood pressure?
5. After 6 months on this drug therapy, Mr. Sanford's blood pressure is maintained at 124 to 138 systolic and 78 to 88 diastolic. However, he complains that he doesn't seem to have the energy he used to have and that he is having some decrease in sexual activity. What will you tell Mr. Sanford about these concerns and their relationship to the drug therapy?

Over the next 2 years, Mr. Sanford experiences a gradual increase in his blood pressure. Dosage adjustments in the atenolol and hydrochlorothiazide fail to effectively lower his blood pressure. Captopril, 25 mg three times a day, is added to his treatment program.

6. How does captopril lower blood pressure?
7. What does Mr. Sanford need to know about taking the captopril in order to achieve maximum therapeutic benefit?

Implementation

Monitoring. Obtain white blood cell and differential counts every month for the first 3 to 6 months of therapy and periodically thereafter. Instruct the client to report any sign of infection (e.g., sore throat, fever), which indicates possible neutropenia.

Proteinuria associated with nephrotic syndrome may occur, particularly in clients with previous renal disease. Perform urinary protein determinations periodically. If proteinuria is greater than 1 g/day, the drug should be reevaluated. Have the client report any edema or weight gain that may occur.

An elevation in potassium level may occur because of depressed aldosterone levels. Monitor the serum potassium level. Serum sodium levels should also be monitored.

Monitor blood pressure closely because a precipitous fall can occur in 1 to 3 hours, particularly in clients who have been receiving salt-restricted diets, diuretics, or dialysis. Vomiting, diarrhea, and dehydration can intensify hypotension. The client is to be instructed to discontinue the salt-restricted diet. The hypotensive effect is the same in both standing and supine positions. Monitor the pulse rate. If bradycardia occurs, document and report readings to the prescriber.

Intervention. Whenever possible, before initiating therapy the current antihypertensive regimen should have been discontinued for at least 1 week. All other medications need prescriber approval. Captopril, moexipril, quinapril, and ramipril will have reduced absorption if given with meals. The absorption of the other ACE inhibitors is not affected by food (Olin, 1996).

Clients with renal disease, particularly those with renal artery stenosis, may have an increase in BUN and serum creatinine levels. Reduce the dosage of the ACE inhibitor or discontinue diuretic therapy if necessary.

During the first 4 weeks of therapy, skin rash occurs in approximately 10% of clients. Dosage reduction or cessation or administration of an antihistamine usually causes the rash to disappear.

Education. Inform the client that the full therapeutic benefits of the drug will not be noticed until after several weeks of therapy. Therefore emphasize the importance of drug compliance. Report side effects so that the prescriber can modify the drug regimen without discontinuing medication. Advise the client against suddenly discontinuing the drug. Also, advise the client to avoid emotional encounters or any forms of stress.

Advise the client that signs of infection (e.g., sore throat or fever) and easy bruising or bleeding (possible agranulocytosis) should be reported to the prescriber. If taste impairment (dysgeusia) occurs, it generally disappears in 2 or 3 months, but it may cause weight loss. Provide the client with nutritional guidance.

Instruct the client not to use potassium supplements or substances containing large amounts of potassium (i.e., salt substitutes or low-sodium milk, which may contain up to 60 mEq potassium/L) without prescriber approval. Caution clients with heart failure to increase their physical activity slowly in response to decreased chest pain.

As with other antihypertensive agents, instruct the client in the nonpharmacologic measures to be taken to reduce hypertension; see Figure 27-4.

Evaluation. The client will maintain a blood pressure within the normal limits without adverse effects of the ACE inhibitor agents.

See Box 27-4 for a new angiotensin II antagonist.

CALCIUM ANTAGONISTS

Calcium channel blocking agents are used for the treatment of hypertension, angina pectoris, supraventricular tachycardia, and vascular headaches. See Chapter 28 for additional information.

VASODILATORS

Vasodilators exhibit a direct action on the smooth muscle walls of the arterioles and veins, thereby lowering peripheral resistance and blood pressure. Although various theories have been proposed, the mechanism of action, at least in part, involves the direct relaxation of vascular smooth muscle by stimulation of the calcium-binding process. The drop in blood pressure stimulates the sympathetic nervous system and activates the baroreceptor reflexes, increasing heart rate and cardiac output. This also increases renin release. Therefore combined therapy is recommended. To inhibit sympathetic reflex response, use of a beta-adrenergic blocker such as propranolol (Inderal) has been advocated, along with a diuretic to alleviate the sodium and water retention that occurs during vasodilator therapy.

There are two types of vasodilators: (1) arteriolar dilators, such as diazoxide (Hyperstat IV), hydralazine (Apresoline), and minoxidil (Loniten), which exert a selective effect on arterioles, and (2) arteriolar and venous dilator, such as sodium nitroprusside (Nipride, Nitropress), which lowers blood pressure by acting on both arteriolar resistance vessels and venous capacitance vessels.

BOX 27-4

Angiotensin II Antagonist

Losartan (Cozaar) is the first in a new class of antihypertensives, that is, it blocks angiotensin II (AT_1) at its receptor site. Both losarten and its active metabolite antagonize or block AT_1 receptors. Losartin is available alone and in combination with hydrochlorothiazide (Hyzaar).

Side/adverse effects include dizziness, diarrhea, cough, insomnia, muscle cramps, nasal congestion, and sinusitis. Usual oral dose is 50 mg daily (25 mg in individuals treated with diuretics or those with hepatic impairment) (Olin, 1996).

Arteriolar Dilator Drugs

diazoxide [dye az ox' ide] (Hyperstat IV)

The antihypertensive action results from direct relaxation of smooth muscles in the peripheral arterioles, which causes a decrease in peripheral resistance. As blood pressure is reduced, a reflex increase in heart rate and cardiac output occurs, with resultant maintenance of coronary and cerebral blood flow. This cardiovascular reflex mechanism also inhibits the development of orthostatic hypotension.

When administered intravenously, diazoxide is a potent antihypertensive agent. However, the oral form (Proglycem) produces only a slight decrease in blood pressure. Its main action is to stimulate hyperglycemia and decrease plasma insulin levels by suppressing insulin release (see Chapter 50).

Diazoxide is administered intravenously to reduce blood pressure promptly in *hypertensive emergencies* such as malignant hypertension and hypertensive crisis. Intravenous diazoxide is ineffective in reducing elevated blood pressure in clients with MAO-induced hypertension or pheochromocytoma. Because of its adverse effects, the drug is not used for treatment of chronic hypertension.

Administered by IV push, the onset of action is 1 minute; peak effect occurs within 2 to 5 minutes; half-life is approximately 28 hours; duration of effect is 2 to 12 hours. Diazoxide is metabolized in the liver and excreted by the kidneys.

The side/adverse effects of diazoxide include nausea, vomiting, tachycardia, anorexia, headache, constipation, abdominal cramps, changes in taste perception, and edema.

The adult dose is up to 150 mg IV administered within 10 to 30 seconds, repeated in 5 to 15 minutes if necessary, up to a maximum of 1.2 g/day. After the emergency period, give diazoxide for several days, until an oral hypertensive agent is effective. Pediatric dosage is 1 to 3 mg/kg IV, repeated if necessary in 5 to 15 minutes.

■ Nursing Management

Diazoxide Therapy

Assessment. Clients who are unable to tolerate thiazide diuretics or sulfonamide-type medications may also show intolerance to diazoxide. Do not use intravenous injection of diazoxide in the treatment of compensatory hypertension, such as in aortic coarctation or arteriovenous shunt. Use with caution in clients with impaired cerebral or cardiac circulation since an abrupt drop in blood pressure may seriously reduce blood flow to these organs. Risk-benefit should be considered with clients with inadequate cardiac reserve, such as uncompensated congestive heart failure. Use cautiously with clients with hypokalemia, history of gout, or hepatic or renal function impairment.

A baseline assessment of the client should include blood pressure and urine ketones and blood glucose determinations.

Review the client's current medication regimen since diazoxide given concurrently with other antihypertensive medications or peripheral vasodilators may result in a severe hypotensive reaction. If concurrent use is necessary, smaller doses may be indicated. A concurrent use of hydantoin anticonvulsants and diazoxide may result in the diminished efficacy of both drugs. The client should be monitored closely for several hours for hypotension. Simultaneous use of anticoagulants with diazoxide may require reduction in dosage of anticoagulants because diazoxide potentiates their action.

Nursing diagnosis. With the administration of diazoxide, the client may be assessed for the following nursing diagnoses: risk for injury related to hypotension; altered protection related to thrombocytopenia; altered tissue integrity related to extravasation of intravenous preparation of diazoxide; altered comfort (anorexia, nausea, vomiting, or abdominal distention); altered bowel elimination (constipation); excess fluid volume related to sodium and water retention, evidenced by edema of the lower extremities and pulmonary edema; altered self-concept related to excessive hairiness with long-term use of the drug; and the collaborative problems of angina, myocardial infarction, extrapyramidal effects, hyperglycemia (drowsiness, fruity breath odor, polyuria), and allergic reaction.

Implementation

Monitoring. With IV administration, monitor blood pressure every 5 minutes until it is stable, then every hour during the duration of drug action. Before ending surveillance, take blood pressure with the client standing. Take the pulse before and during therapy. If tachycardia occurs with intravenous administration, report it immediately to the prescriber. For oral administration, monitor blood pressure on a regular basis.

Because of sodium and water retention, weigh the client daily. Measure intake and output, and report any weight gain to the prescriber because a diuretic may be indicated. After repeated injections, observe the client closely for signs of congestive heart failure (edema, dyspnea, cough, pulmonary rales, distended neck veins, and fatigue).

During IV diazoxide treatment, monitor blood and urinary glucose levels, serum electrolytes, and complete blood counts. (Hypokalemia potentiates hyperglycemia.) Overdosage of diazoxide requires that the client with hyperglycemia be observed up to 7 days, until the blood sugar level is stabilized. Hyperglycemia occurs in most clients, especially when injections are repeated; closely monitor blood glucose levels, particularly in individuals with diabetes mellitus. In some instances insulin may be indicated. Monitor the infusion site for extravasation.

Intervention. Intravenous diazoxide should be administered only in a peripheral vein through an established IV line to avoid cardiac dysrhythmias. Avoid extravasation, because the solution is alkaline and will cause pain and cellulitis of the tissue. If extravasation occurs, treat with cold packs.

Place the client in recumbent position during therapy and keep him or her in the same position for at least 30 minutes after injection. If a diuretic such as furosemide (Lasix) is administered, the diuretic generally is given ½ to 1 hour before diazoxide. Have the client remain supine for 8 to 10 hours because of additive hypotensive effect. The entire dose should be given by rapid intravenous injection (in less than 30 seconds). Slower administration may result in reduced effect or decreased duration of effect. Notify the prescriber if symptoms of abdominal distention, absence of bowel sounds, or constipation occur.

Education. With the oral forms of diazoxide, instruct the client to monitor blood pressure, test urine for sugar and ketones, and take weight daily. The client should report any significant changes to the prescriber.

Alert the client not to take other medications without consulting the prescriber and to maintain regular appointments for surveillance. As with other antihypertensive medications, instruct the client in nonpharmacologic therapies to reduce blood pressure (see Figure 27-4).

Evaluation. The client will maintain a blood pressure within normal limits without any adverse effects of diazoxide.

hydralazine [hye dral' a zeen] (Apresoline)

Hydralazine hydrochloride is believed to produce its hypotensive effects by direct relaxation of vascular smooth muscle, particularly the arterioles, with little effect on veins, which results in a reduction in peripheral resistance. Consequently, renal blood flow is increased, providing an advantage to clients with renal failure. Hydralazine also maintains cerebral blood flow and produces sodium and water retention. However, the resultant hypotension is thought to stimulate the baroreceptor reflex, causing an increase in heart rate and cardiac output. Unfortunately, this response offsets the antihypertensive effects of the drug.

Tolerance to the antihypertensive action may be offset by the addition of a diuretic to the drug regimen. The diuretic enhances the antihypertensive effect and reduces the potential for increased cardiac output and fluid retention. Hydralazine decreases diastolic pressure more than systolic. It also increases plasma renin activity.

An oral dose of hydralazine has an onset of action in 45 minutes or by IV within 10 to 20 minutes. Its peak effect is within 1 hour (orally) or 15 to 30 minutes (IV); half-life is between 3 and 7 hours; duration of action is 3 to 8 hours. It is metabolized in the liver and excreted by the kidneys.

The side/adverse effects of hydralazine include diarrhea, nausea, vomiting, tachycardia, anorexia, headache, facial flushing, stuffy nose, and edema.

The adult oral dose is 40 mg daily PO for 2 to 4 days, then 100 mg in divided doses for the remainder of the first week. The maintenance dose is 50 mg four times a day or the lowest effective dosage. Children receive 0.75 mg/kg divided into two to four doses, increased slowly over 1 to 4 weeks as necessary to a maximum of 7.5 mg/kg. For parenteral administration for hypertension, the adult dose is 10 to 40 mg given intramuscularly or intravenously. Repeat if necessary. Pediatric dosage is 1.7 to 3.5 mg/kg divided into four to six daily doses.

▪ Nursing Management

Hydralazine Therapy

Assessment. Hydralazine hydrochloride is administered with caution to clients with coronary artery disease, in which anginal attacks may be intensified; aortic aneurysm; rheumatic mitral valvular disease, which may increase pulmonary artery pressure and precipitate congestive heart failure; and hypersensitivity to hydralazine. Clients with cerebrovascular disease may be at risk for increased cerebral ischemia, and those with advanced renal disease may need lower dosages of hydralazine.

Before initiation of hydralazine therapy, a baseline blood pressure is obtained.

If hydralazine and diazoxide or other hypotension-producing agents are used concurrently, a severe hypotension may result; monitor the client for at least several hours for this effect.

Nursing diagnosis. With the administration of hydralazine, the client may experience the following nursing diagnoses: risk for injury related to hypotension (dizziness, lightheadedness); fluid volume excess related to sodium and water retention (swelling of feet or lower legs); altered comfort (headache, nasal congestion, flushing of face, skin rash, anorexia, nausea, and vomiting); altered bowel elimination (diarrhea or constipation); and the collaborative problems of lupus erythematosus–like syndrome (malaise, sore throat, fever, arthralgia); peripheral neuritis (tingling, numbness, and weakness in hands or feet); lymphadenopathy; and an allergic response.

Implementation

Monitoring. Check the blood pressure and pulse of clients receiving parenteral hydralazine every 5 minutes until stabilized; continue to check frequently (about every 10 to 15 minutes) during parenteral therapy. Monitor intake and output during parenteral therapy; output may be increased with improved renal blood flow. With simultaneous use of parenteral diazoxide, observe the client for several hours to assess for profound hypotension.

Weigh the client daily to check for fluid retention. Report to the prescriber any gain in weight. Also, advise the client to reduce salt intake.

Observe the mental status of the client. Report to the prescriber any signs of anxiety or mental depression; this condition may indicate cerebral ischemia.

Complete blood count, lupus erythematosus (LE) cell preparation, and antinuclear antibody (ANA) titer tests are indicated if the client develops fever, sore throat, arthralgia, chest pain, and chronic malaise. Repeat these tests periodically if the client is receiving prolonged therapy. Systemic lupus erythematosus (SLE)-like syndrome may occur in clients receiving higher doses (more than 200 mg/day), in slow acetylators, and in clients with renal impairment. Discontinue the drug if tests are positive.

Intervention. Administer the parenteral form as quickly as possible after drawing it through a needle. The drug changes color after contact with a metal filter. Most clients can be changed to oral dosage forms after 24 to 48 hours of parenteral therapy. Administer drugs with meals or food; this minimizes first-pass metabolism of drug in the intestinal wall, thereby enhancing bioavailability.

Education. Teach the client the importance of taking medication at the same time each day and to take it exactly as prescribed, even when feeling well. Inform the client that the drug should not be discontinued even if side effects occur; instead, the prescriber should be contacted. This agent should be discontinued gradually; otherwise abrupt withdrawal will precipitate a sudden rise in blood pressure and heart failure.

Emphasize to the client the importance of keeping clinical appointments, including those involving laboratory studies. After long-term administration of hydralazine, drug tolerance may develop, necessitating adjustment of the drug regimen.

Inform the client that palpitations and headache may occur during the early stages of oral administration, but these symptoms usually subside with continued therapy. Usually, a beta blocker such as propranolol may be prescribed to prevent reflex tachycardia.

Instruct the client to report any signs of peripheral neuritis (numbness, tingling, and paresthesias) so that pyridoxine (vitamin B_6) may be prescribed to combat the antipyridoxine response of hydralazine.

Since orthostatic hypotension may occur, advise the client to make position changes slowly. Also, instruct the client to avoid standing still for long periods of time, taking hot baths or showers, or doing strenuous exercise. Warn the client against operating potentially hazardous machinery, since dizziness or faintness may occur. Instruct the client to carry a medical identification card or Medic Alert bracelet or pendant. As with other antihypertensive medications, instruct the client in nonpharmacologic therapies to reduce blood pressure (see Figure 27-4).

Evaluation. The client will maintain a blood pressure within normal limits and not experience any adverse effects of hydralazine.

minoxidil [mi nox' i dill] (Loniten)

Minoxidil (Loniten) is an orally effective direct-acting peripheral vasodilator. It reduces blood pressure by decreasing peripheral vascular resistance in the arteriolar vessels with little effect on veins. It does not cause orthostatic hypotension. It is a potent vasodilator and also causes a reflex increase in cardiac output, induces sodium retention, promotes development of edema, and increases plasma renin activity.

Minoxidil is reserved for *severe* hypertension unresponsive to traditional agents, i.e., severe hypertension associated with chronic renal failure. Concomitant administration of a beta-adrenergic blocking agent such as propranolol (Inderal) is necessary to prevent severe reflex tachycardia. Administration of a diuretic agent is also essential to counteract sodium and water retention.

Minoxidil has an onset of action in 30 minutes; peak effect in 2 to 3 hours (after a single dose); half-life of the drug and metabolites is 4.2 hours. Its duration of effect is between 1 and 2 days. It is metabolized by the liver and excreted mostly by the kidneys.

The side/adverse effects of minoxidil include nausea, vomiting, tachycardia, anorexia, headaches, excessive hair growth, red flushing of skin, angina, and pericarditis.

For children 12 years and older and adults, the dose is 5 mg PO daily, increased in 100% increments as necessary (10 mg, 20 mg, 40 mg, etc.). It is usually recommended that dosage increases be on a minimum 3 day schedule, but in selected cases increases can be made every 6 hours with close monitoring of the client. For children up to 12 years old the dose is 0.2 mg/kg/day.

■ Nursing Management
Minoxidil Therapy

Assessment. Inquire if the client is pregnant or has plans for pregnancy, since studies are inconclusive about the risk to the fetus. Hypertrichosis has been reported in newborns following maternal therapy with minoxidil. Do not use in clients with pheochromocytoma, because minoxidil may stimulate catecholamine secretion from the tumor. Use minoxidil cautiously in clients with recent myocardial infarction (of 1 month or less), pericardial effusion, coronary insufficiency, or congestive heart failure not due to hypertension, since the drug may further limit blood flow to myocardium. Clients with renal function impairment may require lower dosages.

A baseline assessment of the client should include blood pressure and weight determinations.

Review the client's current medication regimen for significant drug interactions. Interactions may occur when minoxidil is given with the following drugs:

Drug	Possible effect and management
guanethidine (Ismelin)	**This combination is not recommended, since antihypertensive effects may be potentiated. Avoid or a potentially serious drug interaction may occur.**
diazoxide (Hyperstat IV), nitrates, or nitroprusside (Nitropress)	**This combination may result in severe hypotensive reaction. Avoid or a potentially serious drug interaction may occur. If administered, monitor client closely for several hours.**

Nursing diagnosis. With the administration of minoxidil, the client may experience the following nursing diagnoses: excess fluid volume related to sodium and water retention (dependent edema, rapid weight gain); body image disturbance related to hypertrichosis; altered comfort (headache, rash, itching, paresthesia, and chest pain); and the collaborative problems of allergic reaction, angina, cardiac effusion, Stevens-Johnson syndrome, and reflex sympathetic activation (tachycardia, flushing of skin).

Implementation

Monitoring. When minoxidil is first administered, clients, particularly those who have been receiving guanethidine, should be monitored in a hospital setting to prevent too rapid a decrease in blood pressure. Take blood pressure and pulse rate before administering minoxidil, and use these parameters as a guideline to determine progress. During therapy, monitor blood pressure and pulse rate regularly. Report to the prescriber any sharp drop in blood pressure, which can precipitate cerebrovascular accident and myocardial infarction.

Monitor weight gain, intake and output, and presence of edema. Inform prescriber of an increase in weight (kilogram/day) so that fluid retention can be corrected. The client also should monitor weight at home.

Monitor electrolyte balance, especially potassium level if the client is receiving a diuretic, which may produce hypokalemia. Potassium replacement therapy should be prescribed. Watch for pericardial effusion with or without tamponade, since this may occur in about 3% of clients not receiving dialysis. This requires more vigorous diuretic therapy, or if pericardiocentesis does not alleviate the condition, discontinuation of minoxidil is necessary.

Observe for anginal symptoms or tachycardia, which can then be relieved by concomitant administration of a beta-adrenergic blocker.

Intervention. Closely monitor clients with renal failure or those receiving dialysis, to prevent exacerbation of renal failure or precipitation of cardiac failure. Lower doses of minoxidil are indicated for these clients. It is recommended that a 3-day interval occur between dosage adjustments. In an acute care setting, more rapid dosage changes may occur with careful monitoring of the blood pressure.

Education. Instruct the client to count the radial pulse rate for 1 minute before taking minoxidil and to report to the prescriber an increase of 20 or more beats/min above baseline. Advise the client receiving combination therapy to take each medication at the proper time and not to mix them. A diuretic is given to reduce salt and fluid retention, and a beta blocker is given to control reflex tachycardia. Combined therapy is indicated to increase the drug's effectiveness and to minimize side effects by lowering the dose of minoxidil. Advise the client to weigh daily and to report any sharp increase in weight to the prescriber.

Inform the client that if a dose is missed, it may be taken a few hours later. However, a missed dose should not be made up the next day; instead, the regular dosing schedule should be resumed. Consult the prescriber if there is any question.

Emphasize the importance of drug compliance despite uncomfortable side effects. Inform the client that minoxidil is a powerful drug for reducing blood pressure and that by relaxing small blood vessels, more blood flow protects vital organs (heart, kidney, and brain). Alert the client not to discontinue the drug without notifying the prescriber, since abrupt withdrawal will cause rebound hypertension.

Inform the client that hypertrichosis will likely occur (incidence is 80%) 3 to 6 weeks after starting therapy. This involves elongation, thickening, and increased pigmentation of fine body hair over the temples, eyebrows, sideburns, malar area, shoulders, back, legs, and forearms. This side effect is particularly troublesome to women. Advise the client that this condition is reversible within 2 to 6 months following discontinuation of therapy. No endocrine abnormalities have been found to account for this distressing effect. Hair remover (depilatory creams) or shaving may be effective in removing unwanted hair.

Instruct the client that minoxidil may be taken with or without food. Advise the client against increasing salt intake, and request that a dietitian provide information regarding appropriate dietary choices. Inform the client that if difficulty in breathing occurs, especially when lying down, to notify the prescriber since this may indicate impending congestive heart failure.

Advise the client not to take other drugs, including OTC agents, without first consulting the prescriber. Instruct the client to carry a medical identification card or Medic Alert bracelet or pendant.

Evaluation. The client will maintain a blood pressure within normal limits and not experience any adverse reactions of minoxidil.

Arterial and Venous Dilator Drugs

▲ **nitroprusside** [nye troe pruss' ide] (Nipride, Nitropress) Nitroprusside is a potent and fast direct-acting vasodilator agent that greatly reduces arterial blood pressure. It relaxes both arterial and venous smooth muscles but is more active on veins. Therefore, nitroprusside reduces cardiac load; that is, the decrease in systemic resistance results in a reduction in preload and afterload improving cardiac output in the client with congestive heart failure. It is indicated for rapid reduction of blood pressure in hypertensive emergencies, adjunct therapy in myocardial infarction and valvular regurgitation, and also as an antidote for ergot alkaloid toxicity.

Sodium nitroprusside has an onset of action and peak effect almost immediately (within minutes) after administration by IV infusion. The half-life of nitroprusside is 2 minutes; the half-life of thiocyanate, a possible toxic metabolite, is 3 days. The duration of effect is between 1 and 10 minutes after the discontinuance of the infusion. Metabolism is by erythrocytes (to cyanide) and the liver (cyanide to thiocyanate). The drug is excreted by the kidneys.

The side/adverse effects of nitroprusside include dizziness, excessive sweating, headaches, anxiety, abdominal cramps, tachycardia, and muscle twitching. See the Management of Drug Overdose box at right for treatment of nitroprusside overdose.

For adult dosage, mix contents of vial in dextrose 5% injection only and administer by intravenous infusion. Initial dose is 0.0003 mg/kg/min, which is slowly increased in increments of 0.3 μg according to client response. The usual dose is 0.003 mg (or 3 μg)/kg/minute. For the pediatric antihypertensive dose, see the recommended adult dose.

■ Nursing Management
Sodium Nitroprusside Therapy

Assessment. Do not use the drug in clients with inadequate cerebral circulation because there is a reduced tolerance for hypotension. Sodium nitroprusside should be used cautiously with clients with renal or hepatic function impairment, Leber's hereditary optic atrophy, vitamin B_{12} deficiency, or tobacco amblyopia, because these conditions influence the metabolism and excretion of the drug. Clients with encephalopathy and other conditions in which they are at risk for increased intracranial pressure may experience increases in that pressure. A baseline blood pressure should be obtained.

If the client is also on dobutamine, it may result in higher cardiac output and lower pulmonary wedge pressure. Concurrent use of other antihypertensive agents is an indication for closer monitoring of the blood pressure, because there may be an additive effect.

Nursing diagnosis. With the administration of sodium nitroprusside, the client may experience the following nursing diagnoses: risk for injury related to rebound hypertension upon abrupt withdrawal of the drug, or hypotension (dizziness, restlessness, tachycardia); impaired tissue integrity (pain at infusion site); altered comfort (headache, abdominal cramping); and the collaborative problems of thiocyanate toxicity (ataxia, blurred vision, delirium, dizziness, nausea and vomiting, ringing of the ears) and cyanide toxicity (decreased consciousness progressing to coma).

⚠ MANAGEMENT OF DRUG OVERDOSE

Nitroprusside

- For severe hypotension, slow or discontinue the infusion. Placing the client supine with the legs elevated on pillows will maximize venous return.

Cyanide toxicity

- Discontinue nitroprusside and administer sodium nitrite (3% solution) in dose of 4 to 6 mg/kg IV over 2 to 4 minutes. If IV sodium nitrite is not immediately available, amyl nitrite inhalation should be utilized.
- Nitrites buffer the cyanide by converting about 10% of the client's hemoglobin to methemoglobin.
- After administration of sodium nitrite, administer sodium thiosulfate (150 to 200 mg/kg) IV in order to convert the cyanide to thiocyanate.
- Thiocyanate is less toxic and rarely a problem, but if thiocyanate toxicity occurs, use hemodialysis. Be aware, however, that hemodialysis does not remove cyanide.
- If necessary, this regimen (nitrite and thiocyanate) may be repeated after 2 hours, in one-half the original dose.

Alternate method for prophylaxis of nitroprusside-induced cyanide

- Investigators report that if thiosulfate is mixed in the nitroprusside infusion at a 10:1 ratio (such as 500 mg thiosulfate to 50 mg nitroprusside) during administration of the nitroprusside, the less toxic thiocyanate will be formed and excreted. This method reduces the potential for cyanide accumulation and toxicity.

From Hall and Guest (1992).

Implementation

Monitoring. Monitor blood pressure every 30 seconds when the infusion is first started, to avoid rapid hypotension. Later, check it every 5 minutes. Facilities and personnel must be adequate for this purpose; intensive care facilities are recommended. Observe the client for any precipitous drop in blood pressure, which may occur if large doses are given. Do not allow the infusion rate to exceed 10 μg/kg/min. If adequate reduction in blood pressure does not occur in 10 minutes, the drug will be discontinued.

Monitor intake and output. Monitor the client for thiocyanate toxicity (tinnitus, blurred vision, and delirium). Because sodium nitroprusside is converted to thiocyanate, monitor the blood thiocyanate level when infusion is continued for more than 72 hours, especially in clients with renal dysfunction.

Intervention. After preparing an intravenous solution, promptly wrap the container in the supplied opaque sleeve or aluminum foil or other opaque material to protect the drug from light. Use fresh solution and do not keep longer than 24 hours. Freshly prepared solution has a faint brown tinge; discard if it is highly colored (e.g., blue, green, or dark red).

Administer the infusion using a microdrip regulator or an automatic infusion pump. These devices must be available to allow precise measurement of the prescribed flow rate. Do not add other drugs to the nitroprusside infusion. Avoid extravasation, since it results in tissue damage.

If the blood thiocyanate level exceeds 10 mg/dl, the infusion should be discontinued or decreased to prevent toxicity. With prolonged treatment and overdosage, a potential for cyanide intoxication exists. (Note that nitroprusside is metabolized first to cyanide, then to thiocyanate.) In the event of cyanide toxicity (coma, dilated pupils, pink color, shallow respirations, imperceptible pulse rate, distant heart sounds, hypotension, and absent reflexes), discontinue nitroprusside. The Management of Drug Overdose box at left describes the treatment for overdosage. Continue to observe the client for several hours to prevent the recurrence of signs of overdosage.

Be aware that the client's therapy will be changed to oral antihypertensive agents as soon as a response occurs. As oral therapy is instituted, the client will require lower doses of nitroprusside.

Education. Keep the client advised as to the care that is taking place.

Evaluation. The client will maintain a blood pressure within normal limits without experiencing any adverse effects of the sodium nitroprusside.

SUMMARY

Hypertension is the most common cardiovascular health problem, affecting over 30 million Americans. Ninety percent of such cases are considered to be essential, idiopathic, or primary hypertension—that is, the specific cause of the hypertension is not known. Because hypertensive individuals are at higher risk of cardiovascular injury, they are treated nonpharmacologically and/or pharmacologically to reduce their blood pressure and therefore reduce their risk of premature death or disability.

Nonpharmacologically, clients are encouraged to modify their lifestyles to include weight reduction, sodium restriction, elimination or limited consumption of alcohol and tobacco, reduction of dietary saturated fats, regular exercise, and behavior modification to promote relaxation.

Pharmacologically, a stepped-care approach is recommended by the Joint Committee on the Detection, Evaluation, and Treatment of High Blood Pressure. This plan is a progressive approach that begins therapy with the administration of a single drug, increases the dosage of that drug, and then, in sequential order, gradually adds more potent agents as the need for more intensive therapy is indicated.

Diuretic drugs play an important role in the management of hypertension. Their administration results in the loss of excess salt and water from the body by renal excretion. This volume depletion, plus a direct effect on the arterioles that produces vasodilation, results in a decrease in blood pressure. These drugs are discussed primarily in Chapter 34.

Although adrenergic inhibiting agents were discussed in Chapter 22, in terms of their modification of the effects of the sympathetic nervous system, they are the most effective antihypertensive drugs. The centrally acting drugs clonidine, methyldopa, guanabenz, and guanfacine are effective as stage 3 antihypertensives of the stepped-care regimen, especially when combined with a diuretic. The peripheral adrenergic inhibitors, guanethidine, guanadrel, and *Rauwolfia* derivatives, are also used an antihypertensives. Alpha-adrenergic blocking agents such as doxazosin, prazosin, and terazosin lower blood pressure by preventing norepinephrine from activating $alpha_1$ receptors on vascular smooth muscle to produce vasoconstriction. Beta-adrenergic blocking agents are also used successfully in the treatment of hypertension (see Chapter 22).

Vasodilators act on the smooth muscle walls of the arterioles and veins, lowering peripheral resistance and blood pressure. Arteriolar dilator agents commonly administered for hypertension are diazoxide, hydralazine, and minoxidil. Sodium nitroprusside is a direct-acting vasodilator that relaxes both arteriolar and venous smooth muscle, which greatly reduces arterial blood pressure. Captopril, enalapril, and doxazosin are angiotensin II antagonists that inhibit the action of the renin-angiotensin-aldosterone system, a disturbance of which may cause hypertension.

Nurses have a major role in the administration of antihypertensive agents when involved in the direct care of the client. But the greatest contribution of nursing by far is client education to sustain adherence to the accurate and safe self-administration of antihypertensive agents. This guidance will assist the client in changing his or her lifestyle to incorporate the modifications to promote a decrease in hypertension and thus a healthier life.

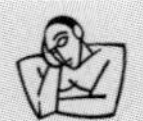

Critical Thinking

1. Tim Rogers, age 46, has mild primary hypertension for which his health care provider prescribed reserpine 0.1 mg PO daily. As part of a drug history to be taken before Mr. Rogers begins his reserpine therapy, what past medical conditions would the nurse specifically ask about?
2. Stella Parr, age 52, expresses her relief now that her prescriber has placed her on a diuretic as part of her antihypertensive medications: "Now I won't have to struggle with all that tasteless food without salt. If I get water retention, the diuretic will take care of it." How should the nurse respond? What other lifestyle issues will you need to explore with Ms. Parr?

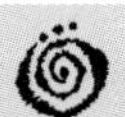

Collaborative Learning Activities

1. The students will imagine that they were receiving antihypertensive therapy for primary hypertension. What issues would foster noncompliance within their own medication regimen and health maintenance? Other students will relate an approach to foster compliance with the antihypertensive regimen.

BIBLIOGRAPHY

American Hospital Formulary Service (1996). *AHFS drug information '96*. Betheseda, MD: American Society of Hospital Pharmacists.

Anderson, et al. (Eds.) (1994). *Mosby's medical, nursing, & allied health dictionary* (4th ed.). St. Louis: Mosby.

Carter BL, Furmaga EM, & Murphy CM (1995). Essential Hypertension. In Young LY & Koda-Kimble MA (Eds.). *Applied therapeutics* (6th ed.). Vancouver: Applied Therapeutics.

Desmond S, et al. (1992). Perceptions of hypertension in black and white adolescents, *Health Values 16*(2):3-10.

Hall VA & Guest JM (1992). Sodium nitroprusside-induced cyanide intoxication and prevention with sodium thiosulfate prophylaxis, *Amer J Crit Care I*(2):19-27.

Hawkins DW et al. (1993). Hypertension. In DiPiro JT, et al. *Pharmacotherapy* (2nd ed.). Norwalk, CT: Appleton & Lange.

Hoffman BB & Lefkowitz RF (1996). Catecholamines, sympathomimetic drugs, and adrenergic receptor antagonists. In Hardman JG & Limbird LE (Eds.). *Goodman & Gilman's the pharmacological basis for therapeutics* (9th ed.). New York: McGraw-Hill.

Joint National Committee on Detection, Evaluation, and Treatment of High Blood Pressure (JNC V) (1992). *The fifth report of the JNC*. Washington, DC: National Heart, Lung, and Blood Institute, National Institutes of Health.

Levy RA (1993). *Ethnic and racial differences in response to medicines: Preserving individualized therapy in managed pharmaceutical programs*. Reston, VA: National Pharmaceutical Council.

Mann KV (1989). Promoting adherence in hypertension: A framework for patient education, *Can J Cardiovasc Nurs 1*(1):8.

Miller CA (1992). $Alpha_1$ adrenergic blockers, *Geriatr Nurs 13*(1):55.

Oates JA (1996). Antihypertensive agents and the drug therapy of hypertension. In Hardman JG & Limbird LE (Eds.). *Goodman and Gilman's the pharmacological basis of therapeutics* (9th ed.) New York: McGraw-Hill.

Olin BR (Ed.) (1996). *Facts and comparisons*. St. Louis: Facts and Comparisons.

Porsche R (1995). Hypertension: Diagnosis, acute antihypertension therapy, and long-term management, *AACN Clin Issues: Adv Pract Acute Crit Care* 6(4):515-25.

Pulaski Cuddy R (1993). Treating the hypertensive patient: A guide, *Advance Nurs Practit* (June): 17-21.

Sagraves R, Letassy NA, & Barton TL (1995). Obstetrics. In Young LY & Koda-Kimble MA (Eds.). *Applied therapeutics* (6th ed.). Vancouver: Applied Therapeutics.

Strong AG (1988). Pharmacologic management of black hypertensive patients, *J Cardiovasc Nurs* 2(4):20.

United States Pharmacopeial Convention (1996). *USP DI: Drug information for the health care professional* (16th ed.). Rockville, MD: The Convention.

Wolfe SM (1995). Widely used calcium channel blocking drugs, *Worst Pills, Best Pills News* 1(9):1,4.

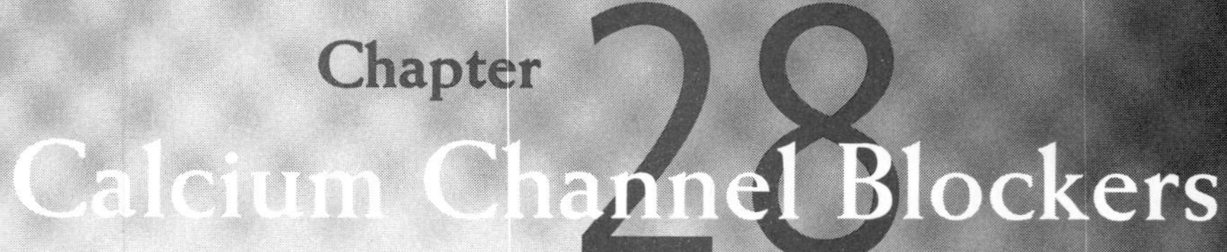

Chapter 28 Calcium Channel Blockers

Chapter Focus

Calcium channel blockers are indicated for a variety of cardiovascular conditions. They are used primarily for their antianginal, antiarrhythmic, and antihypertensive properties. Because they are increasingly prescribed the nurse must be knowledgeable about calcium channel blockers so as to administer them safely and provide guidance for clients to self-administer these drugs. The following objectives and key terms are important for a good understanding of this chapter.

Key Terms

automaticity (p. 551)
calcium channel blocker (p. 551)
peripheral vascular resistance (p. 551)

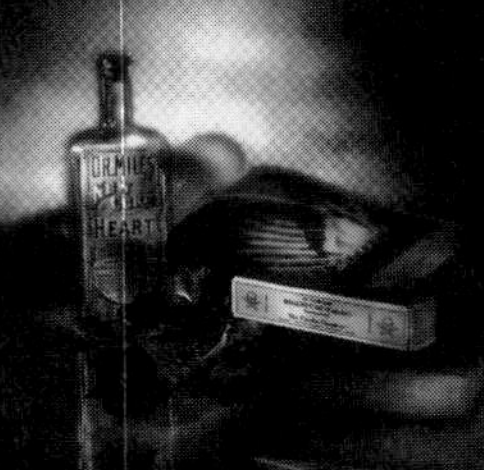

Key Drugs [▲]

verapamil

Objectives

1. State the mechanism of action of calcium channel blockers on cardiac muscle, the cardiac conduction system, and the smooth muscle cells in the walls of blood vessels.
2. Compare and contrast the therapeutic effects of the calcium channel blockers: amlodipine, bepridil, diltiazem, felodipine, isradipine, nicardipine, nifedipine, nimodipine, nisoldipine, and verapamil.
3. Describe specific nursing interventions that may inhibit side effects associated with calcium channel blockers.
4. Identify specific client education measures necessary when calcium channel blockers are prescribed.
5. Implement the nursing management of the care of a client receiving calcium channel blocker therapy.

The **calcium channel blockers,** with diverse chemical structures, all share a basic electrophysiologic property—they block the inward movement of calcium through the slow channels of the cell membranes of cardiac and smooth muscle cells. (See Chapter 24 for a discussion of the physiology of fast and slow channels of cardiovascular fibers.) This activity, however, varies according to the specific type of cardiovascular cells involved. The three types of tissues or cells are:

1. Cardiac muscle or myocardium
2. Cardiac conduction system—SA node and AV junction
3. Vascular smooth muscle

ACTION

Cardiac muscle or myocardium. Calcium channel blockers decrease the force of myocardial contraction by blocking the inward flow of calcium ions through the slow channels of the cell membrane during phase 2 (or plateau phase) of the action potential. (See Figure 24-2 on p. 482.) The diminished entry of calcium ions into the cells thereby fails to trigger the release of large amounts of calcium from the sarcoplasmic reticulum within the cell. This free calcium is needed for excitation-contraction coupling, an event that activates contraction by allowing cross-bridges to form between the actin and myosin filaments of muscle. The force of the heart's contraction is determined by the number of actin and myosin cross-bridges formed within the sarcomere. Decreasing the amount of calcium ion released from the sarcoplasmic reticulum causes fewer actin and myosin cross-bridges to be formed, thus decreasing the force of contraction and resulting in a negative inotropic effect.

Cardiac conduction system (SA node and AV junction). In these tissues calcium channel blockers decrease automaticity in the SA node and decrease conduction in the AV junction. **Automaticity** means that a cell depolarizes spontaneously and initiates an action potential without an external stimulus. Automaticity is a normal characteristic of the SA nodal cells. Depolarization (phase 0) of the action potential is normally generated by the inward calcium ion current through the slow channels. Thus the agents that can block the inward calcium ion current across the cell membrane of SA junction tissue decrease the rate of depolarization and depress automaticity. The result is a decrease in heart rate (negative chronotropic effect). Similarly, an agent that decreases calcium ion influx across the cell membrane of the AV junction slows AV conduction (negative dromotropic effect) and prolongs AV refractory time. When AV conduction is prolonged, fewer atrial impulses reach the ventricles, thus slowing the rate of ventricular contractions. Diltiazem (Cardizem) depresses SA nodal automaticity, while verapamil (Calan, Isoptin) slows AV conduction; therefore verapamil is preferred to treat supraventricular tachycardia.

Vascular smooth muscle. The smooth muscle of the coronary and peripheral vessels has a significant influence on the hemodynamics of circulation. Calcium channel blockers effectively inhibit calcium ion influx through the slow channels of the membrane of smooth muscle cells. The depressed interaction between actin and myosin results in a decreased force of smooth muscle contraction. As a consequence, coronary artery dilation occurs, which lowers coronary resistance and improves blood flow through collateral vessels, as well as oxygen delivery to ischemic areas of the heart. Hence drugs with these actions are useful in the treatment of angina pectoris.

Calcium channel blockers also inhibit the contraction of smooth muscle of the peripheral arterioles. This results in widespread reduction in **peripheral vascular resistance** (resistance to blood flow through the body determined by the tone of the vascular musculature and the diameter of the blood vessels) and blood pressure. The hemodynamic change reduces afterload, which also decreases oxygen demands of the heart. This indirectly provides a beneficial effect in the management of angina.

■ ■ ■

The calcium channel blockers include amlodipine (Norvasc), bepridil (Bepadin, Vascor), diltiazem (Cardizem), felodipine (Plendil), isradipine (DynaCirc), nicardipine (Cardene), nifedipine (Procardia), nisoldipine (Sular), nimodipine (Nimotop), and verapamil (Calan, Isoptin). Flunarizine (Sibelium), indicated for migraine prophylaxis, is only marketed in Canada. These agents dilate coronary arteries and arterioles, inhibit coronary artery spasm, and/or dilate peripheral arterioles and reduce total peripheral resistance (afterload), thus lowering arterial blood pressure at rest and during exercise. Table 28-1 shows a comparison of the effects of calcium channel blockers.

TABLE 28-1 Calcium channel blocking agents: comparison of effects

Effects	amlodipine	bepridil	diltiazem	felodipine	nifedipine nicardipine isradipine	verapamil
Contractility	↑	↓	↓	↑	0/↓	↓↓
Vasodilation						
Coronary	↑	↑↑↑	↑↑↑	↑	↑↑↑	↑↑
Peripheral	↓↓↓	↓	↓	↓↓↓	↓↓↓	↓↓
Heart rate	+/−	↓	0/↓	↑	↑	↑↓
Cardiac output	↑	0	0/↑	↑	↑↑	↑↓

↑—slight increase; ↓—slight decrease; ↑↑—intermediate increase; ↓↓—intermediate decrease; ↑↑↑—significant increase; ↓↓↓—significant decrease; +/−—minimal effect; ↑↓—slight effect; 0—no effect.

Therapeutically, the calcium antagonists have been used to treat angina pectoris, supraventricular tachycardia, hypertension, Raynaud's phenomenon, posthemorrhagic cerebral vasospasm, and vascular headache. Investigationally, verapamil is used to treat hypertrophic cardiomyopathy and vascular headaches. Because these agents differ in specificity and their individual effects on cardiac and peripheral tissues, see Table 28-2 for FDA-approved indications (*USP DI*, 1996).

TABLE 28-2 FDA-approved indications for calcium antagonists

Antianginal	amlodipine, bepridil, diltiazem, nicardipine, nifedipine, verapamil
Antiarrhythmic	diltiazem (parenteral), verapamil
Antihypertensive	amlodipine, diltiazem, felodipine, isradipine, nicardipine, nifedipine, nisoldipine, verapamil
Therapy for subarachnoid hemorrhage	nimodipine

Bepridil is only indicated for chronic stable angina. Its use is limited by its potentially serious adverse effects, serious ventricular arrhythmia and agranulocytosis. The action of diltiazem is largely restricted to dilating the coronary and peripheral blood vessels. Felodipine and isradipine are indicated for the treatment of essential hypertension. Nicardipine is a very potent peripheral vasodilator that does not affect the sinoatrial (SA) node or atrioventricular (AV) junction. Because of its pronounced effect on the peripheral vascular bed, nifedipine causes the greatest hypotensive effect. However, it exerts minimal cardiac depressant action. Nimodipine, which is highly lipophilic, crosses the blood-brain barrier and has a greater effect on the cerebral arteries than other arteries in the body. It is indicated for the treatment of cerebral arterial spasm after subarachnoid hemorrhage. It also inhibits platelet aggregation. The adult dose is 60 mg every 4 hours, starting within 96 hours after the subarachnoid hemorrhage and continuing for 3 weeks. See Table 28-3 for pharmacokinetics of the calcium channel blocking agents.

The side/adverse effects associated with the calcium antagonists include headaches, nausea, hypotension, dizziness, skin flushing or rash, edema, and tachycardia. See the boxes on p. 553 for the geriatric implications of the use of the calcium channel blockers and for overdose treatment.

TABLE 28-3 Calcium channel blocking agents: pharmacokinetics

Drug	Onset of action (min)	Time to peak concentration (hr)	Duration of action (hr)	Metabolism	Excretion
amlodipine (Norvasc)	2-5 (IV)	6-12	N/A	Liver	Kidneys
bepridil (Vascor)	60	2-3	24	Liver	Kidneys (70%); feces
diltiazem (Cardizem)	30	2-3	4-8	Liver—has active metabolite desacetyldiltiazem	Kidneys and bile
Extended release	30-60	6-11	12	Same	Same
felodipine (Plendil)	120-300	2.5-5	24	Liver	Kidneys
isradipine (DynaCirc)	120	1.5	12	Liver	Kidneys
nicardipine (Cardene)	—	½-2	8	Liver	Kidneys
nifedipine (Procardia)	Oral: 20 (more rapid when given sublingually)	½-1	4-8	Liver	Kidneys (80%), feces (20%)
nimodipine (Nimotop)	—	1	Variable	Liver	Bile, feces, kidneys
nisoldipine (Sular)		N/A	24	Liver	Kidneys
verapamil (Calan, Isoptin)	Oral: 60-120 IV: 1-5	1-2	IV: 2 Oral regular: 8-10 Oral extended release: 24	Liver—has active metabolite norverapamil	Kidneys and feces

*Nanograms per milimeter.
N/A, not available.

Geriatric Implications

Calcium channel blockers

The elderly are more susceptible to these agents and the side effects of increased weakness, dizziness, fainting episodes, and falls.

While nitroglycerin (or other nitrates) may be taken concurrently with these agents, the client should be advised to report any increase in frequency or intensity of angina attacks to his or her physician.

Nicotine may reduce the effectiveness of these agents; thus reduction or avoidance of tobacco smoking is advisable (Long, 1990).

Alcohol consumption may result in hypotensive episodes in some clients. Whenever possible, the use of alcohol should be avoided.

Diltiazem, nimodipine, and verapamil half-lives may increase because of accumulation from decreased elimination in the elderly.

The risk of hypotension is increased with use of nimodipine.

These agents should not be discontinued abruptly, since severe rebound angina attacks may result (gradual drug withdrawal is recommended).

MANAGEMENT OF DRUG OVERDOSE

Calcium Blockers

- For symptomatic hypotension administer IV fluids plus IV dopamine or dobutamine, metaraminol, isoproterenol, calcium chloride, or norepinephrine. Use Trendelenburg position for parenteral verapamil-induced hypotension.
- Direct-current cardioversion, IV lidocaine, or IV procainamide is used for tachycardia, rapid ventricular rate in clients with antegrade conduction, in atrial flutter or fibrillation, and accessory pathway with Wolff-Parkinson-White syndrome.
- For bradycardia use IV atropine, isoproterenol, norepinephrine, or calcium chloride. In some instances an electronic cardiac pacemaker may be necessary.

DOSING OF SPECIFIC AGENTS

amlodipine (Norvasc). Adult antihypertensive dose is 5 mg PO daily while angina dose is 5 to 10 mg daily. Maximum dose is 10 mg daily. Geriatric or compromised clients should be started on 2.5 mg daily, with the prescriber titrating the dose as necessary.

bepridil (Vascor). Adult oral dose for chronic stable angina is 200 mg/day adjusted as necessary after 10 days of therapy. Most clients are maintained at 300 mg daily (maximum daily dose is 400 mg/day). Geriatric clients may start at usual adult dosages but require closer monitoring.

diltiazem (Cardizem). Adult oral dose is 30 mg four times daily before meals and at bedtime, increased to 180 to 360 mg daily (in divided doses) at 1 to 2 day intervals until a therapeutic response is achieved. Sustained-release initial dosage is 60 to 120 mg twice a day, adjusted as necessary. Parenteral dose is 0.25 mg/kg bolus over 2 minutes (usual dose 20 mg). If necessary a second prescribed dose of usually 0.35 mg/kg may be repeated after 15 minutes (usual dose 25 mg). In clients with atrial fibrillation or atrial flutter a continuous IV infusion of 5 to 10 mg/hr (maximum 15 mg/hr) may be administered for up to 24 hours with close monitoring of blood pressure and a continuous ECG. The pediatric dose (oral and IV) has not been established.

felodipine (Plendil) extended-release tablet. Adult antihypertensive oral dose is 5 mg daily with dosage adjustments if necessary at 2 week intervals. The usual dosage range is 5 to 10 mg daily; the maximum daily dose is 20 mg. Geriatric clients should be closely monitored; their maximum dose is usually 10 mg per day.

isradipine (DynaCirc). Adult antihypertensive oral dose is 2.5 mg twice a day. Dosage adjustments are implemented at 2 to 4 week intervals; maximum daily dose is 20 mg.

nicardipine (Cardene). Adult dose for angina and hypertension is 20 mg orally three times a day. Dose adjustments may be necessary after 3 days of therapy.

nifedipine (Procardia, Adalat). Adult dose initially is 10 mg PO three times a day for angina, gradually increased over 7 to 14 days as needed and tolerated. Elderly clients may be more sensitive to this drug and should be monitored closely. Maximum daily dosage is 180 mg daily, although daily dosages greater than 120 mg are rarely necessary. Pediatric dosage has not been established. In clients unable to swallow, the contents of a nifedipine capsule may be administered buccally or sublingually by piercing the capsule and squirting the medication under the tongue. This method of administration may result in slightly earlier peak blood levels of the drug (*USP DI,* 1996). Dosage is equivalent to the oral dosage.

nisoldipine (Sular). Nisoldipine (Sular) is an extended release tablet that is used for the management of hypertension in adults. The adult dose is 20 mg PO daily, increased if necessary in increments of 10 mg daily at usually weekly intervals. The usual maintenance dose is 20 to 40 mg daily. Maximum dose is 60 mg daily.

nimodipine (Nimotop). The adult oral dose to treat subarachnoid hemorrhage (SAH) (should be started within 96 hours) is 60 mg every 4 hours for 21 consecutive days. Medication can be extracted from the capsule via a syringe and administered via nasogastric tubing to unconscious persons.

▲ **verapamil (Calan, Isoptin).** Adult parenteral dose for angina pectoris, supraventricular tachyarrhythmias, and hypertension is initially 5 to 10 mg IV bolus administered over a 2 minute period. If ineffective, 10 mg (or 0.15 mg/kg) may be administered 30 minutes after the first dose. In older (geriatric) clients, administer slowly (over a minimum of 3 minutes). In children up to 1 year the dose is 0.1 to 0.2 mg/kg over 2 minutes; for children 1 to 15 years the dose is 0.1 to 0.3 mg/kg (usual single dose is 2 to 5 mg) over 2 minutes. Repeat dose if necessary 30 minutes afterward.

The adult oral dose initially is 80 to 120 mg PO three times daily, increased daily or weekly as necessary. The total daily dosage needed to maintain a therapeutic effect is usually between 240 and 480 mg. Elderly clients may be more sensitive to this drug and need to be monitored closely. Geriatric recommended oral dose is 40 mg tid initially. For infants less than 12 months and children to 15 years old, the dose is 4 to 8 mg/kg/day PO in divided doses.

Verapamil extended-release tablet (Covera-HS) was released to correlate with an individual's circadian rhythm. It is dosed at bedtime so serum levels peak in the morning and provide 24 hours protection. The most common side effect is constipation, which is usually mild and transient. It is available in 180 and 240 mg tablets (Searle, 1996).

Several combination products for the treatment of hypertension have been approved. They include Tarka, a combination of verapamil (calcium channel blocker) and trandolapril (angiotensin-converting enzyme [ACE] inhibitor) and Teczem, which combines diltiazem (calcium channel blocker) and enalapril (ACE inhibitor). These products are reserved for hypertensive clients that do not respond to the maximum dose of either drug alone or if further increasing the dose of one of these agents cannot be done because of unacceptable side effects (FDA News and Product Notes, 1997).

Nursing Management

Calcium Channel Blocker Therapy

Assessment. The client's health status should be reviewed for conditions that contraindicate the use of calcium channel blockers or indicate that special caution is required with their administration. Do not administer these drugs to individuals who have severe hypotension (less than 90 mm Hg systolic). Bepridil, diltiazem and verapamil are contraindicated for clients with heart block, sick sinus syndrome, and Wolff-Parkinson-White syndrome unless the client has a functioning artificial ventricular pacemaker because these drugs may cause severe bradycardia or arrhythmias. Calcium channel blockers should be administered with caution to clients with severe aortic stenosis, bradycardia, heart failure, cardiogenic shock, acute myocardial infarction, and mild-to-moderate hypotension because these conditions will be worsened.

Clients with renal or hepatic function impairment may have reduced clearance of the drugs, which results in prolonged half-life. Intolerance to the prescribed calcium channel blockers is also a contraindication for the drug. Ask a female client if she is pregnant or plans to be. Tests on laboratory animals have resulted in teratogenic effects to the fetus (FDA pregnancy category C).

Elderly clients may require more caution in the dosage of calcium channel blockers because of age-related renal impairment. (See the box on Geriatric Implications of Calcium Channel Blockers.) The half-life of diltiazem, nimodipine, verapamil, and other calcium channel blockers may be increased because of decreased clearance; the half-life of nicardipine has shown no difference in clients over 65 and young adults.

The client's current medication regimen should be reviewed for potential significant drug interactions. The following interactions may occur when calcium channel blocking agents are given with the drugs listed below.

Drug	Possible effect and management
beta-adrenergic blocking agents, systemic and ophthalmic	Although advantageous in some clients, this combination should be closely monitored because adverse cardiac effects may occur (bradycardia, hypotension, and heart failure caused by prolonged AV conduction). In clients with impaired cardiac function, avoid concurrent use if possible.
carbamazepine, cyclosporine, or quinidine	Diltiazem and verapamil may inhibit liver metabolism (cytochrome P450) resulting in increased serum levels and toxicity of these drugs. Nifedipine with quinidine may result in reduced serum levels of quinidine. Monitor such combinations closely because dosage adjustments may be necessary.
digitalis glycosides	Increased serum levels of digoxin reported, especially when administered with verapamil (occur to a lesser degree with other calcium antagonists); monitor digoxin serum levels closely whenever a calcium-blocking agent is started or discontinued or when dosage is changed. Monitor for prolonged AV conduction, bradycardia, or AV blocks, especially during the initial week of therapy because digoxin dose may need to be changed.
disopyramide (Norpace)	**Do not administer disopyramide within 48 hours before or 24 hours after verapamil because additive negative inotropic effects may result in serious reactions including death. Use extreme caution when administering calcium antagonists with disopyramide. If possible, avoid this combination. Caution is also necessary when flecainide is given concurrently with calcium antagonists.**
hypokalemia-producing drugs, such as corticosteroids and potassium-depleting diuretics	**Increases the risk of bepridil-induced arrhythmias occurring.**
procainamide, quinidine and any drugs that prolong QT interval	**Both drug classifications have negative inotropic effects and when given concurrently, may result in serious adverse effects (such as hypotension, bradycardia, tachycardia, AV block, and pulmonary edema). Avoid such combinations if possible.**

A baseline assessment should include pulse, blood pressure, lung sounds, and ECG readings. If long term therapy is anticipated, liver and renal function studies are recommended.

Nursing diagnoses. With the administration of calcium channel blockers, the client may be at risk for the following nursing diagnoses: altered mucous membranes (gingival hyperplasia); altered comfort (skin rash, flushing, dizziness, headache, chest pain, and nausea); fluid volume excess related to sodium and water retention evidenced by swelling of feet, ankles, and lower legs; activity intolerance related to lethargy and weakness; altered sleep pattern (drowsiness); altered bowel elimination (constipation, diarrhea); and the collaborative problems of allergic reaction, angina, congestive heart failure, and altered cardiac output related to hypotension, arrhythmias, or tachycardia.

Implementation

Monitoring. Monitor blood pressure and pulse rate, particularly if the drug is coadministered with a beta-adrenergic blocking agent. Observe ECG for prolonged P-R interval, which is caused by slowing of AV conduction. Congestive heart failure may occasionally occur after initiation of calcium channel blocker therapy, particularly in those also receiving beta blocking agents. Assess intake, output, and weight and assess for edema. If beta blockers are withdrawn before calcium channel blocker therapy, taper dosage gradually. Abrupt withdrawal may provoke angina, especially when nifedipine is started. During long-term therapy with calcium channel blockers, hepatic and renal function studies may be required. Periodic potassium levels are recommended during bepridil therapy.

Intervention. Administer oral dosage on an empty stomach to promote rapid absorption. However, if nausea occurs with bepridil, administer with meals or at bedtime. Take the client's pulse before each dose (diltiazem or verapamil); withhold dose and report to the prescriber if the pulse rate is 50 or below.

For verapamil injection, inspect the parenteral drug preparation; discard if cloudy. Administer initial intravenous dosage in a treatment center with appropriate facilities for monitoring and resuscitation. Give slowly as a direct injection over at least 2 minutes (in the elderly, over at least 3 minutes). Monitor with ECG. Avoid repeated doses in clients with hepatic or renal failure, since intravenous dose may prolong duration of effects. If repeated injections are required, closely monitor blood pressure and P-R interval and use smaller doses as prescribed. If bolus therapy is successful, the client may be placed on continuous IV administration. Use a controlled infusion device for precise dosage. Maximum effects of verapamil occur in 15 to 30 minutes, so adjustments in infusion rates are made at 30 minute intervals (Swavely et al, 1993). Monitor the client carefully for a return of abnormal ECG readings for several hours after the discontinuance of the IV verapamil because the drug is excreted over 2 to 5 hours.

Clients receiving IV diltiazem should be monitored continuously on telemetry with frequent blood pressure determination (Paul, 1993). Emergency equipment should be readily available. If the client becomes hypotensive, the diltiazem rate should be slowed or discontinued.

Education. Instruct the client to perform meticulous daily dental hygiene with regular dental examinations and cleaning, because this may reduce the incidence or severity of gingivitis and gingival hyperplasia (a rare side effect).

Because calcium channel blockers may be coadministered with sublingual nitroglycerin and other nitrates, instruct the client to keep a record of nitroglycerin administration and anginal episodes and report promptly if changes occur in previous pattern (increased frequency, duration, and severity of anginal attacks). The symptoms may develop when starting calcium channel blockers or increasing dosages. (Nitroglycerin is used to abort acute angina attacks.)

Caution the client against smoking because the effectiveness of calcium channel blockers is reduced in smokers (Jackson, 1993).

Instruct the client to move from a sitting or lying position to a standing position cautiously to avoid orthostatic hypotension. Advise the client to avoid alcohol to prevent dizziness and hypotension.

Emphasize the importance of regular visits to a health care provider to monitor progress during therapy.

Teach the client to take a pulse and report a heart rate of less than 50. Instruct the client to report headaches, rashes, nausea, and vomiting, as well as edema and weight gain (more than 1 kg/day) because these symptoms may indicate congestive heart failure.

If a dose is missed, advise the client to take it as soon as remembered, unless it is almost time for the next dose, in which case it should be omitted.

If calcium channel blockers are being taken as antihypertensives, instruct the client to take the medication even if feeling well, since lifelong therapy may be required. Compliance may be ascertained by monitoring refill frequency. Advise the client regarding the hazards of untreated hypertension and the need for decreased sodium intake, smoking cessation, and weight control. Instruct the client in procedure of periodic blood pressure determination; have the client report results to the prescriber at follow up visits. Caution the client to check with the prescriber before taking other medications, particularly OTC sympathomimetics such as commonly found in cold remedies.

For verapamil injection, instruct the client to remain recumbent following IV bolus for at least 1 hour to reduce hypotensive effects.

Evaluation. The client will demonstrate a regular sinus rhythm on ECG and have a blood pressure within the normal limits. If the drug is taken for angina, the client will report a decrease in the frequency and severity of angina, and the client's tolerance for activity will increase. The client will have a sufficient understanding of his or her condition and medications and will be able to self-administer medications safely and accurately.

SUMMARY

Calcium channel blockers are one of the newest groupings of cardiac drugs. Their action is to block the inward movement of calcium through the slow channels of the cell membranes of cardiac and smooth muscle cells. In cardiac muscle this action decreases the force of myocardial contraction; in vascular smooth muscle, it decreases the force of the smooth muscle contraction and in particular inhibits the contraction of smooth muscle of the peripheral arterioles. Within the cardiac conduction system, calcium channel blockers decrease the automaticity in the SA node and decrease conduction in the AV node.

At present a number of calcium channel blockers have been approved by the FDA for the treatment of angina pectoris and hypertension. However, each has distinctive properties. Diltiazem is generally restricted to coronary blood vessel dilatation. Nicardipine and nifedipine are potent peripheral vasodilators but do not affect the cardiac conduction system; this makes them effective as antihypertensive agents and in the treatment of Raynaud's phenomenon. Nimodipine has a greater effect than other calcium channel blockers on the cerebral arteries. Verapamil is also effective as an antiarrhythmic because it prolongs AV conduction time and depresses the contractibility of cardiac muscle.

The goals for the administration of calcium channel blockers and client teaching include: a decrease in the frequency and intensity of the client's angina attacks; blood pressure within the normal range; increased activity tolerance; and sufficient client understanding of his or her condition and medications to enable the safe and accurate self-administration of medications.

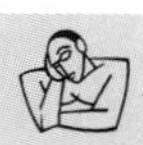

Critical Thinking

1. John Samuels, age 56, developed a supraventricular tachycardia during a stress test and was transferred to the coronary care unit. He is prescribed verapamil (Calan, Isoptin) 5 mg IV push stat. Besides Mr. Samuels' ECG, what other assessments should the nurse be concerned with during the administration of the drug?
2. Alice Hooker, age 62, has angina. She has been prescribed nifedipine (Procardia) 10 mg PO tid. What laboratory values should the nurse monitor during the nifedipine therapy?

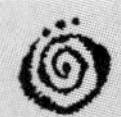

Collaborative Learning Activities

1. A student team will represent each of the various calcium channel blockers. Each team will present to the class the unique action of its drug as well as those in common. Each team will discuss to compare the side/adverse effects of its drug, reactions in common, and those unique to the team's particular agent. The teams will follow up by presenting the nursing management, comparing for unique implications for specific agents.

BIBLIOGRAPHY

American Hospital Formulary Service (1996). *AHFS drug information '96*. Bethesda, MD: American Society of Hospital Pharmacists.

Anderson KN, et al. (Eds.) (1994). *Mosby's medical, nursing, & allied health dictionary* (4th ed.). St Louis: Mosby.

Clem JR (1995). Pharmacotherapy of ischemic heart disease, *AACN Clin Issues Adv Crit Care* 6(3):404-17, 493-4.

FDA News and Product Notes (1997). New formulations/combinations-Tarka. *Formulary* 32 (1):24.

Fleury J (1992). Long-term management of the patient with stable angina, *Nurs Clin North Am* 27(1):205-30.

Foley JJ (1994). Treatment of calcium-channel blocker overdose, *J Emerg Nurse* 20:314-5.

Jackson G (1993). The management of stable angina, *Hosp Pract* 28(1):59.

Kayser SR (1995). Pharmacology news. Calcium channel blocker's —is vasoselectivity relevant? *Prog Cardiovasc Nurs* 10(1):35-9.

Kelly T (1993). Medical management of calcium channel blocker overdoses, *Drug newsletter* 12(3)18.

Long JW (1990). *The essential guide to prescription drugs*. New York: Harper Collins.

Olin BR (Ed.) (1996). *Facts and comparisons: Drug information*. St Louis: Facts and Comparisons.

Paul SC (1993). New pharmacologic agents for emergency management of supraventricular tachydysrhythmias, *Crit Care Nurs Q* 16(2):35-45.

Salerno SM, et al. (1994). Calcium channel antagonists: What do the second-generation agents have to offer? *Postgrad Med* 95(1):181-8, 190, 201-2.

Searle (1996). Brief summary of Covera-HS. Searle advertisement P96CV12022V.

Sikes PJ & Nolan S (1993). Pharmacologic management of cerebral vasospasm, *Crit Care Nurs Q* 154:78-87.

Swavely DA, Molchany CA, & Jozefiak E (1993). Continuous verapamil infusion: The nurse's role in monitoring patient outcomes, *Dimensions Crit Care Nurs* 12(4):186-93.

Talbert RL (1993). Ischemic heart disease. In DiPiro JT et al. *Pharmacotherapy* (2nd ed.). Norwalk, CT: Appleton & Lange.

United States Pharmacopeial Convention (1996). *USP DI: Drug information for the health care professional* (16th ed.). Rockville, MD: The Convention.

Chapter 29
Vasodilators and Antihemorrheologic Agents

Chapter Focus

Nitrates have been prescribed for over 100 years to treat ischemic heart disease, but because these drugs have a short duration of action and poor bioavailability, manufacturers are continuously working on new forms to improve the therapeutic effect (Yakabowich, 1992). The antihemorrheologics are relatively new therapeutic agents to improve microcirculatory flow. The following objectives and key terms are important for a good understanding of this chapter.

Key Terms

angina pectoris (p. 558)
hemorrheology (p. 564)
nitrates (p. 558)

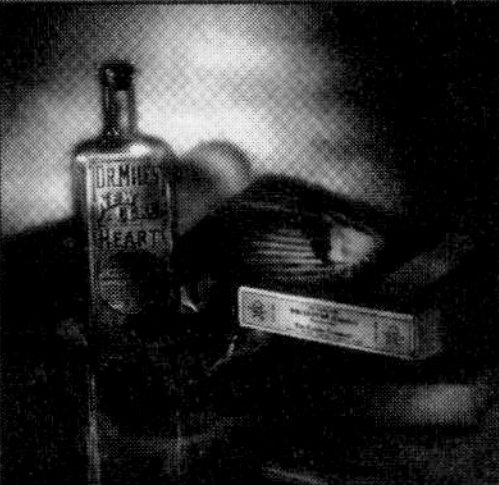

Key Drugs [▲]

nitroglycerin
pentoxifylline

Objectives

1. Identify the three therapeutic objectives for the use of antianginal agents.
2. Compare the effects of nitrates, beta blockers, and calcium blocking agents on the heart.
3. Discuss the mechanism of action, side effects/adverse reactions, significant drug interactions, and dosages for nitrates.
4. Instruct a client in the self-management of a transdermal system for the administration of nitroglycerin.
5. Discuss isoxsuprine as an agent used in the treatment of peripheral vascular disease.
6. Implement nursing management of the care of a client receiving vasodilators.
7. Define the science of hemorrheology.
8. Implement nursing management of the care of a client receiving pentoxifylline.

Vasodilators are used for the treatment of vascular disorders, including peripheral vascular conditions. These agents produce peripheral vasodilation by relaxing smooth muscle in the blood vessel walls. Some drugs act primarily on veins or arterioles while others dilate both type blood vessels.

Vasodilators utilized to treat hypertension are reviewed in Chapter 27. This chapter addresses the use of vasodilators for angina and peripheral occlusive arterial disease and the use of antihemorrheologic agents for the treatment of peripheral vascular disease. The action for the antihemorrheologic drugs is to improve microcirculatory blood flow to ischemic tissues.

ANGINA

The term **angina pectoris** refers to temporary interference with the flow of blood, oxygen, and nutrients to heart muscle, or intermittent myocardial ischemia. Angina is characterized by pain behind the sternum. The pain usually occurs with exercise or stress and is relieved by rest. Angina pectoris occurs when the work load on the heart is too great and oxygen delivery is inadequate. Coronary flow is very responsive to oxygen requirements of the heart. Inadequate oxygenation of the heart implies that coronary blood flow is less than the amount actually needed.

Therefore angina pectoris is usually associated with myocardial ischemia. When coronary blood flow is inadequate, hypoxia causes an accumulation of pain-producing substances such as lactic acid (anaerobic metabolite) and other chemical irritants such as potassium ions, kinins, and prostaglandins. These products then stimulate the cardiac sensory nerve endings, which transmit impulses to the central nervous system to produce the typical anginal pain response.

Inadequate oxygenation may be caused by coronary atherosclerosis or vasomotor spasm of the coronary vessels. Other causes of anginal pain may be pulmonary hypertension and valvular heart disease. Individuals with severe anemia, even with minimal coronary artery disease, may suffer from anginal attacks because of inadequate oxygen supply. The presence of carbon monoxide hemoglobin (carboxyhemoglobin) in smokers, who have reduced amounts of available blood oxygen, is another factor in causing angina pectoris.

Drug therapy of angina pectoris is based on the belief that relaxation of coronary smooth muscle will bring about coronary vasodilation, which in turn will improve blood flow to the heart. However, coronary arteries narrowed by disorders such as sclerosis and calcification cannot respond to any coronary vasodilator. Nitrates are the primary drugs prescribed for the treatment of angina.

VASODILATORS

The **nitrates** are very effective drugs for the treatment of angina pectoris because of their dilating effect on the veins and arteries. The pooling of blood in the veins (capacitance blood vessels) decreases the amount of blood returned to the heart (preload), which reduces left ventricular end-diastolic volume. This decrease in blood return may help reduce the myocardial oxygen demand. Chest pain induced by angina pectoris largely results from an inadequate supply of oxygen to the heart (Box 29-1).

BOX 29-1

Types of Angina Pectoris

Classic angina (stable or effort)
Pain usually associated with coronary arteriosclerosis. The attack can be precipitated by exertion or stress (e.g. , cold, fear, emotion) and by eating. The pain lasts about 15 minutes and disappears with rest or nitrates.

Unstable angina (crescendo or preinfarction)
A progressive form of angina whereby pain occurs more frequently and becomes more severe in time. The attack may appear during rest and may last longer, with less relief with antianginal drugs. These individuals eventually show signs and symptoms of impending myocardial infarction or coronary failure.

Variant angina (Prinzmetal's or vasospastic)
Pain that may be associated with spasms of the coronary arteries and that usually occurs in the presence of coronary stenosis. The pain often happens during rest without any cause. Its occurrence follows a regular pattern (e.g., it appears at the same time during the night). Dysrhythmias often accompany the attack, and the ECG shows an elevation in the S-T segment during the anginal episode.

The ideal antianginal drug would (1) establish a balance between coronary blood flow and the metabolic demands of the heart; (2) have a local rather than a systemic effect (it would act directly on coronary vessels to promote coronary vasodilation with no effects on other organ systems; (3) promote oxygen extraction by the heart from arterial flow; (4) be effective when taken orally and have sustained action; and (5) have absence of tolerance.

Currently, no drug meets these criteria. Drugs presently available provide only temporary relief. Evidence is increasing that the nitrates exert their effect not so much by coronary vasodilation but by lowering blood pressure and decreasing venous return and cardiac work. Box 29-2 gives a comparison of the effects of nitrates, beta blockers, and calcium blocking agents.

Nitrates

The nitrate drug category contains a variety of drug entities and dosage forms, such as amyl nitrite inhalant; erythrityl tetranitrate (Cardilate); isosorbide dinitrate (Isordil, Sorbitrate); nitroglycerin (NTG) sublingual tablet (Nitrostat); NTG extended-release buccal tablet (Nitrogard SR); NTG lingual aerosol (Nitrolingual); NTG extended-release capsules (Nitrocap); NTG parenteral injection (Nitro-Bid, Nitrol);

BOX 29-2

Comparison of Effects of Nitrates, Beta Blockers, and Calcium Blocking Agents

	Nitrates	Beta blockers	Calcium blocking agents
Systolic blood pressure	(−)	(−)	(−)
Ventricular volume	(−)	(+)	(−) or (0)
Heart rate	(+)	(−)	(−),(+), or (0)
Myocardial contractility	(0)	(−)	(−)
Coronary blood flow	(+)	(+) or (0)	(+)
Coronary vessel resistance	(−)	(+) or (0)	(−)
Coronary spasms	(−)	(+) or (0)	(−)
Collateral flow of blood	(+)	(0)	(−)

(−), decreased; (+), increased; (0), no change.

TABLE 29-1 Nitrates: pharmacokinetics

Drug	Onset of action (min)	Duration of action (hr)	Metabolism	Excretion
erythrityl tetranitrate				
Oral tablet	15-30	Up to 6	Liver	Kidneys
Sublingual tablet	5	2-3		
isosorbide dinitrate				
Oral tablet/capsule	15-40	4-6	Liver	Kidneys
Chewable tablet	2-5	1-2		
Extended-release	30	12		
Sublingual	2-5	1-2		
▲ nitroglycerin				
Sublingual	1-3	½-1	Liver	Kidneys
Extended-release (buccal)	3	5		
Lingual aerosol	2-4	—		
IV infusion	Immediate	Several minutes		
Ointment	30	4-8		
Transdermal	30	8-24		
Extended-release tablet/capsule	—	8-12		
pentaerythritol tetranitrate				
Tablet	30	4-5	Liver	Kidneys
Extended-release tablet and capsule	Slow	12		

NTG ointment (Nitro-Bid, Nitrostat); NTG transdermal topical systems (Nitrodisc, Transderm-Nitro, Nitro-Dur); pentaerythritol tetranitrate tablet (Peritrate); pentaerythritol tetranitrate extended-release capsules (Duotrate); and others.

Mechanism of action. Nitrates dilate venous capacitance and arterial resistance vessels, which results in reduced myocardial oxygen demand and a more efficient distribution of blood in the myocardium. The antihypertensive effect of nitrates also is a result of peripheral vasodilation.

Indications. Amyl nitrite has been used to treat acute angina attacks, but it has been replaced by the other, safer nitrate dosage forms. Although not approved by FDA labeling in the United States, amyl nitrite has been used as an antidote for cyanide poisoning and in cardiac function tests to assess reserve cardiac function. It has also been abused and used as a sexual stimulant or euphoric agent, but such applications are dangerous and should be avoided.

Nitrates are used to reduce or prevent the pain of angina, to treat congestive heart failure associated or not associated with myocardial infarction, and as an antihypertensive (nitroglycerin injection).

Pharmacokinetics are listed in Table 29-1. Side effects include dizziness, headaches, nausea or vomiting, agitation, facial flushing, and an increased pulse rate. Adverse reactions are rare or infrequent; they include dry mouth, rash, prolonged headaches, and blurred vision.

For dosage and administration, see Table 29-2. Pregnancy safety is FDA category C.

■ Nursing Management

Nitrate Therapy

Assessment. Although it is rare, clients intolerant of one nitrate may show intolerance to other nitrates. Nitroglycerin injection is not considered appropriate for use for clients with cerebral hemorrhage or other head injury because of its tendency to increase cerebrospinal fluid pressure or for clients with pericardial tamponade or constrictive pericarditis. In addition, caution should be used in administering nitrates to clients with recent myocardial infarction (resultant hypotension may aggravate ischemia); glaucoma (may increase intraocular pressure); severe anemia; or hyperthyroidism. Any hypovolemia should be corrected before the administration of nitroglycerin by injection because it may precipitate severe hypotension and shock.

The client's current medication regimen should be reviewed for significant drug interactions, such as with other va-

TABLE 29-2 Nitrates: dosage and administration

Drug	Adults	Children
erythrityl tetranitrate	*Tablets:* 5-10 mg PO, SL, or buccally, three or four times daily. Adjust dosage as necessary, to a maximum of 100 mg/day.	Not established
isosorbide dinitrate	*Capsules and tablets:* 5-20 mg PO every 6 hr. Adjust dosage as necessary. (Range is usually 5-40 mg four times daily.) *Chewable tablets:* 5 mg, chewed well and swallowed, every 2 or 3 hr. Adjust dosage as necessary. Hold chewed tablet in mouth 1-2 min before swallowing. *Sublingual tablets:* 2.5-5 mg sublingually or buccally, every 2 or 3 hr as needed. *Extended-release tablets or capsules:* 40-80 mg PO every 8-12 hr.	Not established
nitroglycerin	*Sublingual tablet:* 150-600 μg (0.15-0.6 mg) sublingually or buccally, repeated at 5 min intervals if necessary. If relief is not obtained after administering three tablets, immediately contact physician or transport individual to a hospital. Maximum dose is 10 mg/day. *Extended-release buccal tablet:* 1 mg dissolved bucally every 5 hr during waking hours. Adjust dosage as necessary. *Lingual aerosol:* Apply one or two metered doses on or under tongue. Dose may be repeated at 5 min intervals up to a total of three doses. If relief is not obtained, contact a physician or transport individual to a hospital. Maximum daily dose is 1.2 mg. Each metered dose is equivalent to 400 μg (0.4 mg). *Oral, extended-release capsules:* 2.5, 6.5, 9 mg PO every 12 hr. Dosage may be increased to every 8 hr, if necessary. *Oral, extended-release tablets:* 1.3, 2.6, or 6.5 mg every 12 hr. Dosage may be increased to every 8 hr if necessary. *Parenteral injection:* Intravenous infusion—initial 5 μg/min increased in increments of 5 μg/min at 3 or 5 min intervals until desired effect is obtained. If no response is seen at 20 μg/min, increase by 10 μg/min and then 20 μg/min. When partial blood pressure response is observed, reduce size of dosage increments and lengthen interval between increases. (This preparation is not for direct injection. Follow manufacturer's instructions carefully.) *Ointment:* Apply 1-2 inches (15-30 mg) to skin every 8 hr and at bedtime. If angina occurs between doses, drug may be applied every 6 hr. Maximum is 5 inches (75 mg) per application. *Transdermal topical system:* Apply a transdermal unit to intact skin every 24 hr. To reduce development of tolerance, it is recommended the patch be applied for 12 to 14 hr and removed for 10 to 12 hr each day. See the package insert for additional information.	
pentaerythritol tetranitrate	*Tablet:* 10-20 mg PO four times daily. Increase dosage as necessary to a maximum of 160 mg/day. *Extended-release capsules/tablets:* 30-80 mg PO twice daily. Increase dosage as necessary to a mamixum of 160 mg/day.	Not established

sodilators, because concurrent use may exaggerate the orthostatic hypotensive effects of the drugs, necessitating dosage adjustments. Concurrent use of any drug with hypotensive effects such as alcohol, opioid analgesics, or antihypertensive agents should be avoided if at all possible for the same reasons. If it is not possible to avoid concurrent administration, monitor closely because dosage reductions may be necessary.

Nursing diagnosis. With the administration of nitrates, the client may experience the following nursing diagnoses: altered comfort related to dry mouth, flushing, headache, rash, dizziness, and nausea and vomiting; risk for injury related to orthostatic hypotension or blurred vision; and impaired skin integrity (erythema) related to the application of topical dosage forms.

Implementation

Monitoring. Assess the client's chest pain on a scale of 1 to 10 before administration and 5 minutes after the sublingual dose to determine effectiveness. Monitor pulse and blood pressure before and after administration. Over the course of therapy, monitor for orthostatic hypotension, and take blood pressure in both arms and in sitting and standing positions.

For ointment administration, take baseline blood pressure and heart rate with the client in a sitting position, after the client has been at rest for 10 minutes. Repeat the vital signs 1 hour after drug administration and report them to the prescriber. An appropriate dosage produces a 10 mm Hg fall in blood pressure or a 10 beat rise in heart rate with the client in a resting position.

To titrate intravenous dosage for desired hemodynamic function, monitor blood pressure, heart rate, and pulmonary capillary wedge pressure continuously until the correct dose is obtained. Clients with normal or low capillary wedge pressure are likely to be sensitive to the hypotensive effects of intravenous nitroglycerin. Dosage after long-term or high-dose therapy should be reduced gradually to minimize withdrawal rebound angina.

Tolerance has been reported and is manifested by a lack of pain relief following the usual dose. Nitrates may be discontinued for several days until tolerance is lost and then the drug is reinstated. To help prevent tolerance clients need to have an 8 to 12 hour "no nitrate" time. The paste and patches should be removed after 12 hours. If the client experiences pain during the day, the nitrate should be used during the day and removed at night, whereas if the pain occurs at night, the nitrate should be removed during the day (Kuhn, 1992).

Intervention. Dosage must be adjusted by the prescriber to the needs and tolerance of the individual client.

Store stock supply of drug in the original container, tightly closed with a metal screw cap. Federal regulation requires that the sublingual form of nitroglycerin be dispensed in the original unopened manufacturer's container. A supplementary stainless steel container has been approved for carrying small amounts of nitroglycerin. The pendant-like container may be worn on a chain around the neck for a convenient supply of the drug when it is needed.

Intravenous infusion. Use special nitroglycerin disposable infusion sets provided by the manufacturer. They are made of non–polyvinyl chloride plastic to minimize the loss of nitroglycerin. Polyvinyl chloride (PVC) plastic may adsorb up to 40% to 80% of the nitroglycerin from a diluted solution of infusion; therefore use glass intravenous bottles or the administration set provided by the manufacturer.

The drug is not to be used with a direct intravenous infusion. Dilute with 5% dextrose injection USP or 0.9% sodium chloride injection USP before infusion. Because the concentration and/or volume of the drug varies, carefully follow the dosage instructions of the manufacturer. Be aware that switching from a standard (PVC) set to a special (non-PVC) set is likely to affect the dosage—the PVC set requires a higher dosage, which would be excessive if changed to a non-PVC set. In addition, *do not mix nitroglycerin with other medications*.

Ointment. Squeeze the prescribed dose onto a specially designed dose-measuring applicator supplied with the package. Wash off the last application. *Avoid the use of fingers* to spread ointment. Apply in a thin, uniform layer to premarked 6-square-inch surface on clean, dry, nonhairy skin area of chest, abdomen, anterior aspect of thigh, or forearm. Rotate sites to prevent inflammation. Do not massage or rub in ointment because rapid absorption will interfere with the drug's sustained action. Cover the area with a transparent wrap and secure it with tape.

Transdermal systems. Rotate sites. Wash skin when the patch is removed. Remove the patch for 8 to 12 hours daily. Patches with aluminum backings should be removed before defibrillation because the electric current may cause it to burn (Figure 29-1).

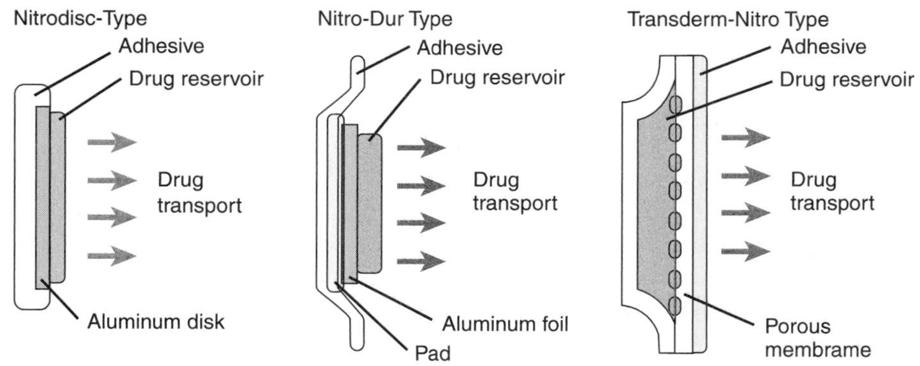

Figure 29-1 Transdermal system.

Education. Instruct the client to avoid alcoholic beverages while taking nitrates because of a shocklike syndrome (flushing, weakness, pallor, hypotension, and syncope) that may occur. Inform the client about the importance of learning to identify stressful situations that precipitate anginal attacks. These include emotional stress, overeating, smoking, temperature extremes, and sudden increase in physical activity. Explain the need to pace activities and to plan for rest periods. The client should receive support to modify behaviors that precipitate anginal attacks.

When nitrates are used to prevent angina in the buccal, lingual, sublingual, and chewable oral forms, instruct the client to take the drug 5 to 10 minutes before the occurrence of the anticipated stressor.

Dizziness, lightheadedness, and slight headache may occur. Have client sit and rest until symptoms pass. Advise changing positions slowly to avoid dizziness. Headache may be treated with a mild analgesic. However, instruct client to report to prescriber if blurring of vision, dry mouth, or severe headaches occur. These are signs of overdosage that require immediate attention.

Inform client about the inactivation of nitroglycerin by exposure to air, heat, and moisture. It is generally recommended that unused tablets be discarded 6 months after the bottle is opened. The length of time of potency appears to vary with the manufacturer. Read the drug insert and check the expiration date. After the bottle is opened, do not leave the cotton or package insert in the container; these articles may absorb some of the drug, which results in less potent tablets.

If handling the drug, be sure hands are dry, since moisture hastens deterioration of the drug. Nitroglycerin is affected by cold and heat. Do not store in the refrigerator or in the bathroom medicine cabinet.

Instruct the client not to change dosage or medication without consulting the prescriber and to report regularly for cardiac function monitoring.

Sublingual tablets. Instruct the client to sit or lie down and take the medication on the first indication of an oncoming anginal attack. This prevents postural hypotension that results from the drug. The signs and symptoms include dizziness, syncope, and weakness.

Explain to the client that the tablet should be placed under the tongue or in the buccal pouch and allowed to dissolve; tablet is not to be swallowed. Avoid eating, drinking, or smoking while the drug dissolves. Usually the potency of drug is indicated by a burning or stinging sensation under the tongue. However, the newer, more stable preparations may not produce this effect.

Dosage may be repeated at 5 minute intervals for three doses if necessary. If pain is not relieved in 15 minutes, the prescriber should be notified. For a hospitalized individual, a specific number of tablets (about 25) may be prescribed to be placed at the bedside in an appropriate container and properly labeled for the client's use. Instruct the client to keep a record of frequency of anginal attacks, precipitating factors, number of tablets used, and occurrence of side effects. Warn the client of transient headaches, which usually last 5 to 20 minutes after sublingual administration of nitroglycerin. The prescriber should be notified if the headache persists. Headaches may disappear within several days to weeks if the drug is continued and may be relieved by aspirin, acetaminophen, or a temporary reduction of the nitrate dosage.

Buccal extended-release tablets. Instruct the client to place the tablet between the upper lip and gum to dissolve or above the incisors if food or drink is to be taken within the 3 to 5 hours it takes to dissolve. Caution against using at bedtime, since aspiration is a risk. The tablet may be replaced if it is accidentally swallowed.

Chewable tablets. Instruct the client to chew the tablet well and to hold it in the mouth for 2 minutes before swallowing.

Oral sustained-release tablets or capsules. Administer on an empty stomach (1 hour before or 2 hours after meals) with a full glass of water and swallow medication whole. Alert the client to notify the prescriber if undigested tablets are found in stools.

Lingual aerosol. When administering, do not shake the can. Hold the can vertically and spray it onto or under the client's tongue. Instruct the client not to inhale the spray and not to swallow immediately.

Ointment. Instruct the client in the application of ointment as described previously. Instruct the caregiver not to get ointment on hands because the medication may precipitate a headache. Tell the client to store nitroglycerin ointment in a cool place and in the original container with the tube tightly capped.

Transdermal system. Remove the old system and apply the new one at the same time each day. The system should be applied to clean, dry, and hairless skin areas of the chest, shoulder, or inside of the upper arm. Avoid skin folds, areas distal to the knee or elbow, and irritated or excessively scarred areas. Rotate application sites to prevent irritation. Apply a new system if the current one becomes loosened. Do not trim the units, since this will alter the dosage (Box 29-3). Alert the client to use caution near microwave ovens when wearing a transdermal system that has a metallic backing, because leaking radiation may heat the backing and cause a burn.

Evaluation. The client will report a decrease in the frequency and severity of angina attacks along with increased activity tolerance. If nitrates are administered for congestive heart failure, the client will demonstrate a clearing of peripheral edema and the lung fields, urinary output of more than 30 ml/hr, and blood pressure, pulmonary artery pressure, and pulmonary wedge pressure within normal limits.

PERIPHERAL VASCULAR DISEASE

Peripheral vascular disease that results in coolness or numbness of the extremities, intermittent claudication, and leg ulcers is a common problem in the elderly. The primary pathophysiologic factor is atherosclerosis or hyperlipidemia. The use of various direct-acting vasodilators for peripheral occlusive arterial disease have generally been very disappointing.

BOX 29-3

Transdermal Nitroglycerin Systems

Since the transdermal nitroglycerin delivery systems are quite popular, the nurse should be familiar with several issues and concerns associated with these products. Three systems are currently available, and the actual amount of nitroglycerin delivered by each system can vary depending on the system and the individual client's skin absorption of the nitroglycerin.

Each system has a different mechanism of drug delivery. For example, Nitrodisc contains nitroglycerin mixed in a solid polymer similar to silicone. The drug is absorbed through the skin from this polymer, which also contains a cosolvent to enhance skin penetration.

Nitro-Dur contains a gel-like matrix surrounded by fluid. Nitroglycerin moves from the matrix to the fluid to the skin.

Transderm-Nitro contains a semipermeable membrane between the drug supply and the skin. The membrane is actually the controlling factor for the drug delivery (see Figure 29-1).

Drug absorption in all systems is by passive diffusion and is based on processes relating to heat transfer (or Fick's law of diffusion).

The three systems are not interchangeable, since the patch size, nitroglycerin content, and average amount of nitroglycerin delivered in 24 hours can differ. Although many individuals are reportedly controlled or have responded to this dosage form, other clients do not achieve adequate therapeutic blood levels or a clinically significant therapeutic response. Some researchers believe maintaining stable nitroglycerin serum levels over 24 hours is not always desirable, since tolerance to the drug and the need to increase dosages would occur. The intermittent use of transdermal products, such as application for 12 to 16 hours and then removal for the night, results in prolonged clinical results without the development of significant drug tolerance.

Research and studies are ongoing in this area, and manufacturers are continuing their search for better methods of delivering their drug products.

Because cyclandelate (Cyclospasmal) has been classified as ineffective by the FDA, it is not reviewed in this section. Papaverine (Cerebid, Pavabid) is an old drug that was exempted from the FDA's review on drug effectiveness. However, the advisory committee of the FDA, the Peripheral and Central Nervous System Drug Review Committee, concluded after reviewing studies and open hearings that papaverine has vasodilator effects but was not proved to be effective for its claimed indication, smooth muscle relaxation (Olin, 1996; *USP DI*, 1996).

The FDA requires substantial evidence of effectiveness in order to grade a drug "effective." The following drug lacks this information and is rated only "possibly effective" by the U.S. Food and Drug Administration.

isoxsuprine hydrochloride [eye sox' syoo preen] (Vasodilan)

Isoxsuprine produces a direct relaxation effect on the smooth muscles of peripheral arterial walls located within skeletal muscle; it has little effect on cutaneous blood flow. It also causes an increase in heart rate, contractility and cardiac output and uterine relaxation (Olin, 1995).

Isoxsuprine is considered "possibly effective" for the treatment of symptoms of cerebrovascular insufficiency and peripheral vascular disease and may relieve symptoms of Raynaud's disease, arteriosclerosis obliterans, and thromboangiitis obliterans (Buerger's disease).

Isoxsuprine has an onset of action of 10 minutes when given intravenously or 1 hour when administered orally. In adults, half-life is 1.25 hours. It is partially metabolized in the blood and excreted via the kidneys. Side effects include nausea or vomiting, or, rarely, chest pain, rash, and respiratory difficulties. No significant drug interactions are reported with isoxsuprine.

It is administered in 10 to 20 mg tablets orally three or four times a day. The dose to inhibit premature labor is 5 to 10 mg IM 2 to 3 times daily. Pregnancy safety has not been established although in near-term neonates the drug has a half-life of 1.5 to 3 hours.

■ Nursing Management

Isoxsuprine Therapy

Assessment. Before administration of isoxsuprine, it should be ascertained that the client does not have severe cerebrovascular disease and has not recently had a myocardial infarction or severe coronary artery disease. Because it has a greater vasodilating effect on peripheral vessels than on those of coronary or cerebral areas, isoxsuprine may reduce blood flow and so increase ischemia in those areas. Intravenous administration is not recommended for clients with hypotension or tachycardia; use caution if the drug is administered intramuscularly. If isoxsuprine is used for the management of premature labor, it should not be used immediately postpartum or if any of the following conditions exist: maternal cardiac disorders or hyperthyroidism (arrhythmias may occur); intrauterine infection or fetal death or hemorrhage (immediate delivery is indicated); eclampsia, severe preeclampsia; or pulmonary hypertension.

Nursing diagnosis. With the administration of isoxsuprine the client should be assessed for the potential occurrence of the following nursing diagnoses: altered comfort related to gastrointestinal effects such as nausea and vomiting (more frequent with parenteral dosing), chest pain; altered peripheral tissue perfusion related to the client's underlying condition and ineffectiveness of the drug; and risk for injury related to hypotension (dizziness, syncope). The potential complications of pulmonary edema and allergic reaction may also occur.

Implementation

Monitoring. Monitor blood pressure in lying, sitting, and standing positions to detect hypotension. Monitor peripheral pulses during drug administration to evaluate its effectiveness. For isoxsuprine use with clients with premature labor, monitor fetal and maternal heart rate, maternal blood pressure, and uterine activity. With prolonged intravenous administration for premature labor, assess blood glucose and fluid and electrolyte status.

Intervention. Administer with milk, food, or antacids to prevent gastrointestinal distress.

Education. Instruct the client to move slowly upright from a sitting or lying position because of the drug's hypotensive effects. Advise clients to avoid smoking, since nicotine's vasoconstrictive properties are counterproductive to the use of isoxsuprine. Caution the client with premature labor to contact her health care provider if her water breaks or her contractions begin again.

Evaluation. The client with vascular insufficiency will experience an improvement in pulse volume, skin color, and temperature; report decreased extremity pain; report improved mental status; and demonstrate increased activity tolerance. For other clients, premature labor will cease.

HEMORRHEOLOGY

Hemorrheology is a science that deals with the deformation and flow properties of blood under physiologic and pathophysiologic conditions. Because arteriosclerosis reduces blood flow to tissues distal to the obstruction, blood viscosity is elevated, thereby diminishing the flow of blood still further. In addition, the impaired blood flow at the microcirculatory level affects the normal capacity of the red blood cells to flex as they enter the narrowed capillary lumen, which has a mean diameter smaller than the erythrocytes. A major function of red blood cells is to transport hemoglobin that carries oxygen, which during the metabolic process is converted to energy for muscle movement such as walking.

Accordingly, the decreased flexibility of the red blood cells and the elevated blood viscosity are responsible for diminishing tissue oxygenation. Hence, during exercise the demand for an increase in blood flow and tissue oxygenation may result in claudication, thereby limiting the distance a person can walk.

Intermittent claudication is a syndrome that results from an insufficient blood supply to skeletal muscles in the legs. Reduced microcirculatory blood flow causes ischemia and pain. This syndrome is a common complication of atherosclerosis and is characteristic of Buerger's disease. While walking, affected individuals experience first pain and then cramps and weakness in muscles.

Antihemorrheologic Agent

▲ **pentoxifylline** [pen tox i' fi leen] (Trental)

Pentoxifylline represents an important concept in the therapy for peripheral vascular disorders, because the ability of vasodilators to improve blood flow by dilation of rigid, arteriosclerotic blood vessels is somewhat limited. Furthermore, because capillary walls lack smooth muscle, dilation by this group of drugs is often unlikely to occur.

Pentoxifylline improves hemorrheologic disorders in the microcirculation, which involves the flow of blood through the fine vessels (arterioles, capillaries, and venules). Although the mechanism of action of pentoxifylline is not completely understood, current evidence shows that the drug possesses several properties to improve microcirculatory blood flow to ischemic tissues:

1. It restores red blood cell flexibility, probably by its inhibition of phosphodiesterase, which results in an increase in cyclic AMP in red blood cells.
2. It lowers blood viscosity by decreasing fibrinogen concentrations and inhibiting aggregation of red blood cells and platelets.

The result is increased microcirculatory blood flow and oxygenation of tissues.

Pentoxifylline is indicated as an adjunct to surgery for the treatment of intermittent claudication caused by occlusive arterial disease of the limbs. It is administered orally and on absorption binds to erythrocyte membranes. It has a half-life of 0.4 to 0.8 hours for the primary drug, 1 to 1.6 hours for the metabolites. Peak concentration in the blood occurs in 2 to 4 hours, and the onset of action with chronic dosing is between 2 and 4 weeks. It is metabolized by red blood cells and in the liver and is excreted primarily by the kidneys.

The less frequent side effects reported are dizziness, headaches, abdominal distress, nausea, and vomiting. Rare adverse reactions are chest pain and an irregular heart rate. With an overdose the client experiences increased sedation, flushing of skin, feeling of faintness, increased excitability, or convulsions. No significant drug interactions have yet been reported with this drug.

For adult dosage give 400 mg orally three times daily with meals. If undesirable side effects occur, such as gastrointestinal upset or CNS disturbances, the dosage should be decreased to 400 mg twice daily. Pregnancy safety for pentoxifylline has been established as FDA category C.

■ Nursing Management

Pentoxifylline Therapy

Assessment. Because pentoxifylline is a xanthine derivative, do not administer it to clients who have an intolerance to other xanthine derivatives such as caffeine, theophylline, or theobromine; excessive CNS stimulation may result. Pentoxifylline should also be used with caution in clients with hepatic and renal function impairment because the drug may accumulate and dosages may need to be lowered. Because pentoxifylline enhances microcirculation, careful monitoring would be required for any client who was at risk for bleeding, particularly a cerebral or retinal hemorrhage.

Nursing diagnosis. With the administration of pentoxifylline, the client may be at risk for altered comfort related to gastrointestinal effects such as nausea and vomiting and abdominal cramping, and the CNS effects of dizziness, drowsiness, and headache. The potential complications may be angina and dysrhythmias.

Implementation

Monitoring. Monitor blood pressure periodically in clients receiving concurrent antihypertensive therapy. Small decreases in blood pressure have been noted in clients receiving pentoxifylline alone, so a reduction of the hypotensive agent might be indicated. Monitor the client with peripheral vascular disease for an improvement in walking distance and duration. Monitor pulses, color, and temperature of affected extremities.

Intervention. Administer with food, milk, or antacids to decrease gastrointestinal distress. If gastrointestinal side effects persist, notify the prescriber to consider a reduction in the dosage.

Education. Instruct client to swallow extended-release tablets whole without crushing or chewing. Instruct the client that improvement in the clinical status may not occur before 8 weeks of therapy and that it is essential for the medication to be taken as prescribed until it is discontinued by the prescriber. Advise smoking cessation because nicotine constricts the blood vessels and defeats the purpose of the medication. The client should receive support in smoking avoidance through group or individual counseling.

Evaluation. The client will experience an improvement in pulse volume, and skin color and temperature; report decreased pain; and demonstrate increased activity tolerance.

SUMMARY

Vasodilators and antihemorrheologics are both used in the treatment of vascular disorders. Vasodilators produce vasodilation by relaxing smooth muscle in the blood vessel walls, whereas antihemorrheologic agents improve microcirculatory blood flow to ischemic tissues by lowering blood viscosity and increasing cyclic AMP in red blood cells. Vasodilators have been more effective in the treatment of angina and intermittent myocardial ischemia than they have been for peripheral vascular disease.

The goals of therapy with nitrates, the classic antianginal agents, are to decrease the duration and intensity of pain during an attack, decrease the frequency of attacks, and improve work capacity even though angina may occur. Nursing management of the client taking nitrates is to assist, through medication administration and evaluation, in the determination of the appropriate dosages for the client, based on symptom control. The nurse also prepares the client for safe and accurate self-administration of nitrates.

Chronic occlusive arterial disease has been less successfully treated with vasodilating agents. The FDA has indicated that vasodilators are only possibly effective in the treatment of peripheral vascular disease because dilation of rigid, arteriosclerotic blood vessels is limited and capillaries lack smooth muscle. The antihemorrheologic agent pentoxifylline increases microcirculatory blood flow and thereby oxygenation of the tissues. It is a valuable new adjunct in the treatment of occlusive arterial disease of the limbs, such as Buerger's disease.

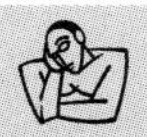

Critical Thinking

1. Mr. Scott has been taking sublingual nitroglycerin for years. He has now been prescribed a transdermal patch. How will Mr. Scott have to modify his therapeutic regimen?
2. In taking a drug history from Mr. Slattery, who is about to begin pentoxifylline therapy, you determine that he has an intolerance for milk and coffee and smokes a pack of cigarettes a day. What action would you take?

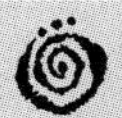

Collaborative Learning Activities

1. Student teams will be designated for each of the dosage forms of nitrates. The teams will identify important nursing considerations and the variation in client teaching required for each dosage form.

BIBLIOGRAPHY

American Hospital Formulary Service (1996). *AHFS drug information '96*. Bethesda, MD: American Society of Hospital Pharmacists.

Anderson HK, et al. (Eds.) (1994). *Mosby's medical, nursing, & allied health dictionary* (4th ed.). St. Louis: Mosby.

Jackson G (1993). The management of stable angina, *Hosp Pract* 28(1):59.

Kuhn JK & McGovern M (1992). Peripheral vascular assessment of the elderly client, *J Gerontol Nurs* 18(12):35-8.

Kuhn M (1992). Nitrates, *AACN* 3(2):09.

Olin BR (Ed.) (1996). *Facts and comparisons: Drug information*. St Louis: Facts and Comparisons.

United States Pharmacopeial Convention (1996). *USP DI: Drug information for the health professional* (16th ed.). Rockville, MD: The Convention.

Yakabowich M (1992). Administering nitrates, *Nursing* 22(9):52-5.

Chapter 30

Overview of the Blood

Chapter Focus

Because cells in the body are metabolically active, the blood plays an important role in maintaining hemostasis by providing constant nutrition and waste removal. Because the blood affects every other body system, it is a consideration in the assessment and care of most clients. Many drugs have adverse effects that cause disorders of the blood such as thrombocytopenia or agranulocytosis. The nurse therefore needs to be knowledgeable about hematology. The following objectives and key terms are important for a good understanding of this chapter.

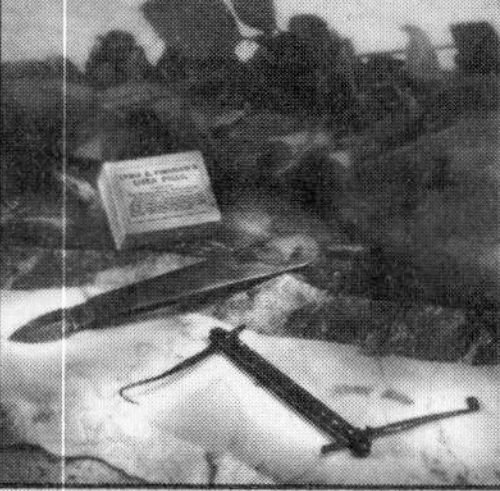

Key Terms

albumin (p. 568)
anemia (p. 567)
erythrocytes (p. 567)
erythropoietin (p. 567)
fibrinogen (p. 569)
globulin (p. 568)
hematocrit (p. 567)
hemoglobin (p. 567)
hemostasis (p. 569)
leukocytes (p. 567)
leukocytosis (p. 567)
leukopenia (p. 567)
phagocytosis (p. 568)
plasma (p. 567)
platelets (p. 568)
thrombocytes (p. 568)
thrombocytopenia (p. 568)

Objectives

1. Describe the functions of blood.
2. List the three types of blood cells and their functions.
3. Compare and contrast the five types of white blood cells.
4. Describe the role of platelets in blood clotting.
5. Name the three major blood proteins and their functions.

Blood is the major transport system in the body. It is also vitally important for the proper functioning and regulation of the human body. Pumped by the heart, blood carries nutrients and oxygen from the digestive and respiratory systems to cells throughout the entire body. In addition, it picks up waste products from body cells and delivers them to the proper system for excretion, usually the liver, kidneys, and lungs. Hormones, enzymes, buffers, and many other biochemical substances are also transported by the blood from one site in the body to the receptors or target cells. Blood also helps to regulate body heat by absorbing and transporting heat from the body core where it can be more easily dispersed.

BLOOD VOLUME

Blood is composed of billions of cells and **plasma,** a fluid portion in which the cells are suspended. Although blood volume can vary from person to person, the average blood volume in a normal adult is approximately 5000 ml (5 L). Of this volume, 3000 ml is usually plasma and the remainder is primarily red blood cells. **Hematocrit** is the packed cell volume of the red blood cells expressed as a percentage of the total blood volume, or the blood viscosity. Hematocrit is measured by a laboratory test performed on a blood sample. The higher the hematocrit, the greater the blood viscosity. For example, persons with polycythemia may have a hematocrit of 60 or 70 because of an excessive number of red blood corpuscles. Increased blood viscosity can retard blood flow through blood vessels, resulting in headaches, fatigue, weakness, dyspnea, and perhaps an enlarged spleen and increased basal metabolism.

BLOOD COMPOSITION

Blood is composed of three types of blood cells: (1) red blood cells, or **erythrocytes,** which transport oxygen and carbon dioxide; (2) **leukocytes,** or white blood cells, which defend the body against bacteria and infections; and (3) platelets, or thrombocytes, which are necessary for blood coagulation. Proteins such as serum albumin, globulins, and fibrinogen are also present in the blood.

Plasma may contain thousands of other substances, such as glucose, electrolytes, vitamins, hormones, and waste products. This discussion on blood, however, is limited to blood cells, blood proteins, and blood groups, or types.

Blood Cells

Red Blood Cells

Red blood cells (RBCs, erythrocytes) are small and disk shaped. They are the cells present in the largest quantities in the bloodstream. Their life span is approximately 120 days. The major function of red blood cells is to carry **hemoglobin** within the cell. Each hemoglobin molecule contains four iron atoms, which combine with four oxygen molecules to transport oxygen from the lungs to the tissues. Hemoglobin can also combine with carbon dioxide and carry it from the cells to the lungs for excretion. It also serves as an acid-base buffering system in whole blood.

After birth, red blood cells are produced by the bone marrow. They are manufactured by most bones in early life, but after 20 years of age most red blood cells are produced in the bone marrow of the vertebrae, sternum, ribs, and ilia.

Males have more hemoglobin in their blood than females do. Generally, most normal men have between 14 and 16 g/dl, while women have a range of 12 to 14 g/dl. A person with a hemoglobin below 10 is usually diagnosed as having **anemia.** Anemias are classified according to both the size and the number of functional red blood cells in the blood.

Red blood cells are rapidly formed and destroyed in the body. It has been estimated that over 100 million red blood cells are produced every minute during adulthood. The normal healthy adult has between 4.5 and 5.5 million cells/mm^3 of blood. The body balances production versus destruction of these cells to maintain a relatively constant body level of red blood cells. The exact body mechanism for this is unknown.

It is known that the rate of red blood cell production can be increased if a considerable decrease in red blood cells occurs or tissue hypoxia develops. Then the kidneys will be stimulated to increase secretion of **erythropoietin,** a hormone that acts to stimulate the production of red blood cells by the bone marrow. With maximum bone marrow stimulation, red blood cell production can be increased to nearly seven times over normal.

The bone marrow needs adequate supplies of vitamin B_{12}, iron, and other substances to make new red blood cells. A deficiency in absorption of vitamin B_{12} from the gastric tract, caused by a lack of intrinsic factor (see Chapter 68), can lead to pernicious anemia.

Anemias can also be induced by increased red cell destruction, such as occurs in infections, cancer, or from bone marrow suppression caused by radiation therapy and many cancer chemotherapeutic agents (Box 30-1).

Leukocytes. There are five types of leukocytes found in the blood. They are classified according to the presence or absence of granules in the cell cytoplasm. The granular leukocytes are neutrophils, eosinophils, and basophils; the nongranular leukocytes are lymphocytes and monocytes. The granular leukocytes have two or more nuclear lobes, so they are referred to as polymorphonuclear leukocytes or "polyps."

Blood in the normal person usually contains between 5000 and 9000 leukocytes per cubic milliliter (Box 30-2). A differential count may be ordered by the physician or health care provider to aid in diagnosis. For example, in acute appendicitis, the percentage of neutrophils increases, as does the total leukocyte count.

Leukocytes are produced primarily in the bone marrow. Lymphocytes are produced mainly in lymph tissues and organs, such as the spleen, thymus, tonsils, and various other lymphoid tissue in the bone marrow, gastrointestinal tract, and elsewhere. Several terms are important to understand. **Leukopenia** refers to an abnormal decrease in the number of leukocytes to fewer than 5000/mm^3; **leukocytosis** refers to an abnormal increase in the number of leukocytes.

BOX 30-1

Drugs That Cause Bone Marrow Depression

amphotericin B, systemic (Fungizone)
antithyroid medications
azathioprine (Imuran)
busulfan (Myleran)
carmustine (BCNU; BiCNU)
chlorambucil (Leukeran)
chloramphenicol (Chloromycetin)
cisplatin (Platinol, Platinol-AQ ♣)
colchicine
cyclophosphamide (Cytoxan, Procytox ♣)
cytarabine (Ara-C, Cytosar ♣)
dacarbazine (DTIC ♣, DTIC-Dome)
dactinomycin (Actinomycin-D, Cosmegen)
daunorubicin (Cerubidine)
doxorubicin (Adriamycin RDF)
etoposide (VePesid, VP-16)
floxuridine (FUDR)
flucytosine (Ancobon, 5-FC, Ancotil ♣)
fluorouracil, systemic (5-FU, Adrucil)
hydroxyurea (Hydrea)
interferon (Roferon-A, Intron A)
lomustine (CCNU, CeeNU)
mechlorethamine, systemic (Mustargen, nitrogen mustard)
melphalan (Alkeran, L-PAM)
mercaptopurine (Purinethol)
methotrexate (Mexate)
mitomycin (Mutamycin)
pentamidine (Pentam)
plicamycin (Mithracin, mithramycin)
procarbazine (Matulane, Natulan ♣)
sodium iodide I 131 (Iodotope)
sodium phosphate P 32
streptozocin (Zanosar)
thioguanine (Lanvis ♣)
thiotepa
uracil mustard
vinblastine (Velban, Velbe ♣)
vincristine (Oncovin)
zidovudine (Retrovir)

Neutrophils, monocytes, lymphocytes, and basophils are very mobile. They can leave the capillaries and migrate to organisms or foreign particles that have entered the body. The neutrophils and monocytes ingest and destroy the invaders, a process known as **phagocytosis.** Lymphocytes defend the body against bacteria, fungus, and viruses by forming B-lymphocytes or T-lymphocytes. (See Chapter 62 for an overview of the immune system.)

Eosinophils are considered weak phagocytes and have limited mobility. An increased level is usually seen with allergic reactions or a cell injury caused by parasites (e.g., hookworm).

BOX 30-2

Differential Normal Leukocyte Count

Neutrophils (polymorphonuclear)	62%
Eosinophils (polymorphonuclear)	2.3%
Basophils (polymorphonuclear)	0.4%
Monocytes	5.3%
Lymphocytes	30%

From Guyton, 1990.

The life span of granulocytes is estimated to be 4 to 8 hours in the bloodstream and 3 to 5 days in body tissues. If involved in ingestion of invading organisms, this life span can be reduced to only a few hours, because during this process they are also destroyed. Monocytes also have a short life span in blood, but in the body tissues they can live for months or even years if not destroyed by phagocytosis. Monocytes in the tissues often increase in size to become tissue macrophages, so they often provide a first line of defense against tissue infections.

Platelets. **Platelets** or **thrombocytes** are small, round, or oval colorless cells produced by the bone marrow. They have a life span of 5 to 8 days. A normal platelet level in the blood is between 150,000 and 350,000/mm^3.

Platelets are key substances for blood clotting in the body. If a blood vessel is injured and blood is escaping, platelets will quickly congregate at the site and clump together to form a plug to stop the bleeding. If the wound is large, platelets will set off a series of chemical reactions within the body to form a clot and seal the injury (Figure 30-1).

Persons with a low quantity of platelets have **thrombocytopenia.** Such persons tend to bleed and their skin usually displays small purple spots, hence the name *thrombocytopenia purpura.* Bleeding problems usually do not occur until the platelets are below 50,000/mm^3. Thrombocytopenia is often induced by irradiation injury to the bone marrow or from aplasia of the bone marrow induced by specific drugs.

Blood Proteins

The blood contains three major proteins: albumin, globulins, and fibrinogen. **Albumin** is responsible for the osmotic pressure gradient produced at the capillary membrane. This prevents plasma fluid from leaving the capillaries to enter the interstitial spaces.

Globulins are divided into alpha, beta, and gamma globulins. Gamma globulin and perhaps beta globulin (to a lesser extent) help to protect the body against infections. Gamma globulin is involved with humoral immunity. Alpha and beta globulins are also believed to perform other functions, such as transportation of certain substances in the blood by reversibly combining with them. They may also be a substrate to form other substances.

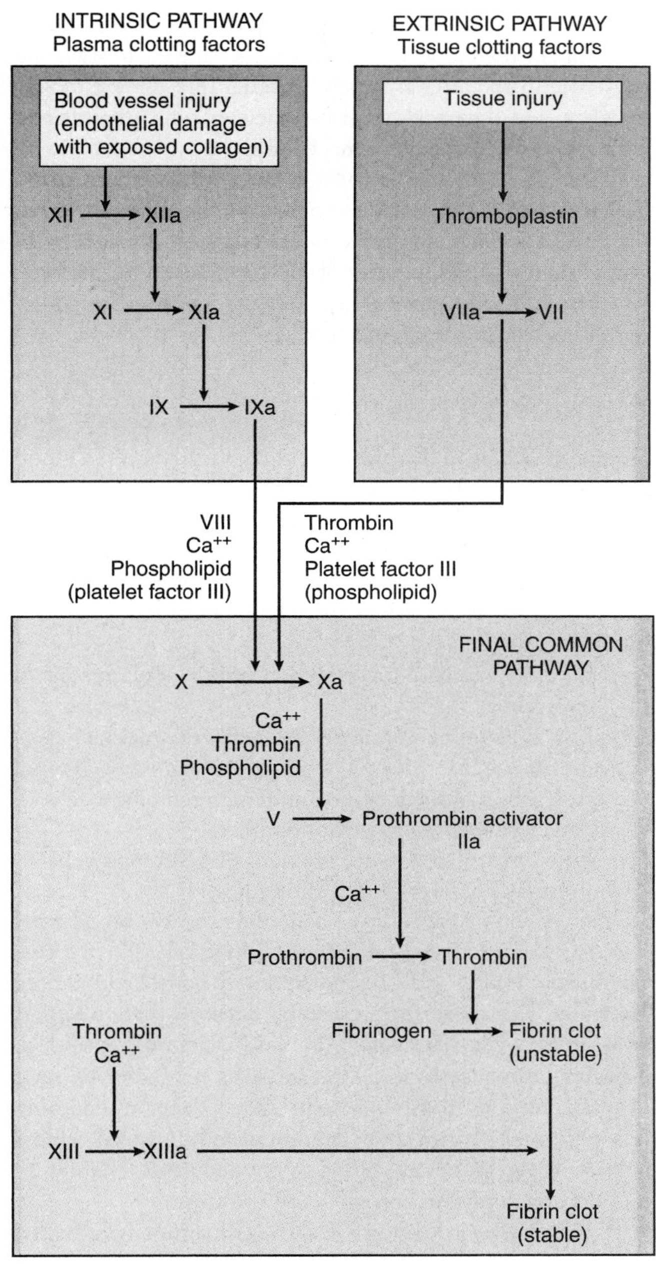

Figure 30-1 Coagulation mechanisms for intrinsic and extrinsic pathways for blood clotting. Final pathway (activation of factor X) is common to both the intrinsic and extrinsic coagulation systems.

Fibrinogen, a plasma protein that is converted to fibrin by thrombin in the presence of calcium ions, is necessary for coagulation.

COAGULATION

Hemostatic Mechanism

Hemostasis is a process that spontaneously stops bleeding from damaged blood vessels. Blood is normally fluid while circulating in the vessels, but with vessel injury, it rapidly clots at the site of injury.

After any injury to a blood vessel, hemostasis is achieved by three sequential steps: (1) blood vessels constrict to retard blood flow from the injured area; (2) platelet plugs form to temporarily seal the leaking small arteries and veins; and (3) blood coagulates to plug openings within the damaged vessels and wounds to prevent further bleeding.

Blood vessel constriction. Immediately after a blood vessel is injured, vascular constriction occurs as a reflex response. This response instantly slows the flow of blood from the ruptured vessel.

Platelet plug formation. After injury to a blood vessel, interruption of the continuity of its endothelial lining exposes the collagen (a fibrous protein) in the underlying connective tissue. Platelets immediately adhere to the exposed collagen to form a dense aggregate, a process known as *platelet adhesion*. This attachment triggers the release of adenosine diphosphate (ADP), which causes the outer surface of the platelets to become extremely sticky so that other adjacent platelets adhere to one another at the damaged site. This process eventually forms the platelet plug. Because this plug is relatively unstable, it can stop bleeding quickly as long as the damage to the vessel is minute. However, for long-term effectiveness the platelet plug must be reinforced with fibrin. This involves a chemical mechanism called *blood coagulation*.

Blood coagulation. Blood coagulation is the final stage of a complex series of events in hemostasis. The process ultimately results in the formation of a stable fibrin clot, which is composed of a meshwork of fibrin threads that entraps platelets, blood cells, and plasma. Thus the physical formation of a blood clot or thrombus plays a key role in hemostasis by permanently closing the hole in the injured vessel to prevent further bleeding.

The chemical events in the blood coagulation mechanism involve two distinct pathways: the intrinsic pathway and the extrinsic pathway.

Intrinsic pathway. Because all the chemical substances involved in coagulation are normally found in the circulating blood, this pathway is referred to as the *intrinsic system of coagulation*. In this pathway, activation of specific blood coagulation factors is initiated by injury to the endothelial lining of the blood vessel wall. When blood contacts the exposed underlying collagen, the Hageman factor (factor XII) is activated by enzymatically converting it to the active form (factor XIIa). The simultaneous damage of platelets also causes the release of platelet phospholipid (platelet factor 3), which is required later in the coagulation process. Factor XIIa then activates factor XI to XIa. The reaction of factor XIa with factor IX requires calcium ions to form activated factor IX. In the presence of calcium ions and platelet phospholipid, factor IXa interacts with factor VIII and thrombin to form a complex. This combination then speeds up the activation of factor X. Factor Xa combines with factor V, calcium ions, and platelet phospholipid to form a complex known as the *prothrombin activator (factor IIa)*. Factor IIa initiates the cleavage of prothrombin to form thrombin, which then enzymatically converts fibrinogen into fibrin,

TABLE 30-1 Blood coagulation factors and synonyms

Factor	Name or synonym
I	Fibrinogen
II	Prothrombin
III	Tissue thromboplastin
IV	Calcium
V	Proaccelerin (labile factor, accelerator globulin)
VII	Proconvertin (stable factor, serum prothrombin conversion accelerator [SPCA])
VIII	Antihemophilic factor (AHF)
IX	Plasma thromboplastin component, Christmas factor
X	Stuart-Power factor
XI	Plasma thromboplastin antecedent (PTA)
XII	Hageman factor
XIII	Fibrin stabilizing factor

forming an unstable clot. The final step involves the action of factor XIII (a fibrin-stabilizing factor), thrombin, and calcium ions, which catalyze the formation of a stronger, stable fibrin clot. See Figure 30-1 for a summary of the main events of the intrinsic pathway.

Extrinsic pathway. The extrinsic pathway is activated by trauma to the vascular wall or to the tissues outside the blood vessels. In this pathway, clotting occurs when products of tissue damage gain access to the blood. The tissue factor thromboplastin is released and becomes part of a complex with factor VII and calcium ions. This combination of components activates factor X, which is the step at which the extrinsic pathway converges with the intrinsic pathway; coagulation then continues through a common route with the resultant formation of a final stable clot. (See Figure 30-1 for the extrinsic pathway; Table 30-1 lists blood coagulation factors.)

The final pathway common to both the intrinsic and the extrinsic coagulation systems begins with the activation of factor X and ends in the formation of fibrin. Both systems function simultaneously in the body. The lack of a normal factor in either system will usually result in a blood disorder.

Blood Coagulation Abnormalities

Diseases associated with abnormal clotting vessels cause many deaths. It is estimated that over a million persons suffer from thrombosis or embolism in the United States each year. Diseases caused by intravascular clotting include some of the major causes of death from cardiovascular sources—coronary occlusion and cerebrovascular accidents. Drugs that inhibit clotting are therefore important.

Local trauma, vascular stasis, and systemic alterations in the coagulability of blood are considered the main factors in the initiation of thrombosis. Basically, coagulation mechanisms are responsible for forming two kinds of thrombi: arterial thrombi and venous thrombi. Arterial thrombi are most frequently associated with atherosclerotic plaques, high blood pressure, and turbulent blood flow that damages the endothelial lining of the blood vessel and causes platelets to stick and aggregate in the arterial system. Arterial thrombi are mostly platelets, and their formation is associated with the intrinsic pathway of the coagulation mechanism.

Venous thrombi occur most often in areas where blood flow is reduced or static. This appears to initiate clotting and produces a thrombus in the venous system. Its formation involves the extrinsic pathway of the coagulation mechanism. Current anticoagulants are more effective in preventing venous rather than arterial thrombi.

BLOOD TYPES

Blood type refers to the type of antigen located on red blood cell membranes. Although many antigens have been identified, antigens A, B, and Rh are the most important blood antigens involved with blood transfusions and newborn survival. Every person belongs to one of the four blood groups and in addition is also Rh positive or Rh negative. The ABO blood groups are:

- Type A: A antigen on red blood cells (the plasma has antibody B)
- Type B: B antigen on red blood cells (the plasma has antibody A)
- Type AB: A antigen and B antigen on red blood cells (the plasma contains no antibodies)
- Type O: neither A nor B antigens on red blood cells (plasma contains A and B antibodies)

Persons with type A blood can safely receive blood from A and O donors. Persons with type B blood can safely receive blood from type B and O donors. People with AB blood are known as the universal recipients, because their blood is compatible with types AB, A, B, and O. Before transfusion, however, crossmatching of the blood is necessary because other agglutinins may be present. Type O persons can only receive type O blood, but they are called universal donors because they can donate blood to anyone. (See Chapter 31 for additional information on blood transfusion.)

A person who is Rh-positive carries Rh antigen on the red blood cells. One who is Rh-negative does not have any Rh antigens on the red blood cells. Approximately 85% of the population is Rh-positive. Rh factor is particularly important when an Rh-negative woman is impregnated by an Rh-positive man. The mother may have antibodies against the Rh-antigen that can cross the placenta and attack the fetus should its blood be Rh-positive. If this occurs, the infant may develop jaundice or be dead on delivery.

An Rh-negative woman could acquire Rh antibodies via blood transfusions. It is also possible for her to develop them if fetal blood enters her bloodstream during childbirth or miscarriage. Regardless, the first pregnancy usually has less risk associated with it than subsequent pregnancies.

Physicians can reduce this danger by administering an anti-Rh antibody (Gamulin Rh, RhoGAM, or HypRho-D) to Rh-negative women after each pregnancy. This will prevent their systems from making antibodies to Rh-positive blood.

Rh-negative women who have a spontaneous or induced abortion or a termination of an ectopic pregnancy of up to and including 12 weeks' gestation are given a microdose of immune globulin (MICRhoGAM or Mini-Gamulin Rh) if the father is Rh-positive.

SUMMARY

The role of blood is to transport cellular requirements and products from one part of the body to another. The continuous exchange between the interstitial fluid and the blood serves to maintain a cellular environment that fluctuates only within narrow limits. An appreciation of the role of blood in the body's homeostasis is essential.

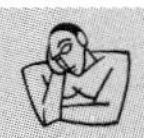

Critical Thinking

1. Many medications have the adverse effect of depressing bone marrow production of various blood cells. What symptoms would you expect to see if a client had diminished production of platelets? red blood cells? white blood cells?
2. Mrs. Chandler has type AB blood. At one time individuals with this blood type were considered to be universal recipients. Why was that so? Why might that term be misleading?

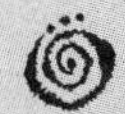

Collaborative Learning Activities

1. Pairs of students will represent to the class: (1) a description of the functions of blood in the body; (2) the three types of blood cells and their functions; (3) a comparison and contrasting of the five types of white blood cells; (4) a description of the role of platelets in blood coagulation; and (5) the three major blood proteins and their functions.

BIBLIOGRAPHY

Anderson KN, et al. (Eds.) (1994). *Mosby's medical, nursing, & allied health dictionary* (4th ed.). St Louis: Mosby.

Guyton AC (1990). *Textbook of medical physiology* (8th ed.). Philadelphia: WB Saunders.

Guyton AC (1987). *Human physiology and the mechanism of disease* (4th ed.). Philadelphia: WB Saunders.

Olin BR (Ed.) (1996). *Facts and comparisons.* St Louis: Facts and Comparisons.

Thibodeau G & Patton K (1996). *Anatomy and physiology* (3rd ed.). St Louis: Mosby.

United States Pharmacopeial Convention (1996). *USP DI: Drug information for the health care professional* (16th ed.). Rockville, MD: The Convention.

Van Wynsberghe D, Noback CR, & Carola R (1995). *Human anatomy and physiology* (3rd ed.). New York: McGraw-Hill.

Chapter 31

Anticoagulants, Thrombolytics, and Blood Components

Chapter Focus

Blood affects every body system because it transports gases, nutrients, metabolic wastes, blood cells, immune cells, and hormones throughout the body. The nurse must manage the client's therapeutic regimen for anticoagulants, thrombolytics, and blood components effectively to ensure the most positive outcome possible for clients with a wide variety of illnesses and injuries. The following objectives and key terms are necessary for a good understanding of this chapter.

Key Terms

embolus (p. 573)
fibrinolytic activity (p. 574)
hemophilia (p. 586)
thrombus (p. 573)
thrombolytic drugs (p. 583)

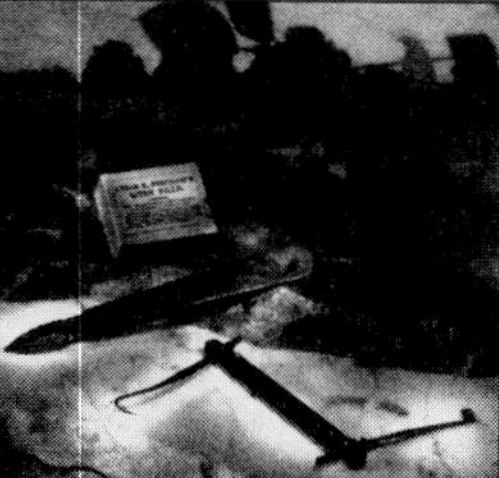

Key Drugs [▲]

heparin
streptokinase
warfarin

Objectives

1. Identify the disease processes that require the administration of drugs to inhibit clotting.
2. Differentiate between the mechanisms of action of parenteral and oral anticoagulant agents.
3. Implement the nursing management of the care of a client with anticoagulant therapy.
4. Discuss the use of protamine sulfate and vitamin K as anticoagulant antagonists.
5. Differentiate between the actions of thrombolytic and anticoagulant drugs on blood clots.
6. Discuss drugs that may be successfully used in treating hemophilia.
7. Implement the nursing management of the care of a client receiving blood components.

This chapter reviews drugs and substances that affect hemostasis or blood clotting, preformed thrombi, and blood administration. While normal blood clotting is a defense mechanism constantly available for protection against excessive hemorrhage, the development of a **thrombus** (an aggregation of platelets, fibrin, clotting factors, and the cellular elements of the blood that becomes attached to the inner wall of a blood vessel or blood clot) in a blood vessel can obstruct blood flow and cause an infarction with resultant tissue necrosis. An **embolus,** a mass of undissolved matter that breaks off from the thrombus, can travel in the blood vessel and lodge in areas of the body; this can cause death. By contrast, a defect in the blood clotting mechanism may lead to excessive bleeding or hemorrhage, even after a minor injury. Both thrombotic and hemorrhagic disorders can be treated with drugs. The following discussion describes the rationale for use of various groups of therapeutic agents.

ANTICOAGULANT DRUGS

Anticoagulant drug therapy is primarily prophylactic because these agents act by preventing (1) fibrin deposits, (2) extension of a thrombus, and (3) thromboembolic complications. While long-term anticoagulant therapy remains controversial, there is evidence that anticoagulant therapy reduces the incidence of thrombosis and therefore prolongs life.

Anticoagulation therapy is directed toward preventing intravascular thrombosis by decreasing blood coagulability. This therapy has no direct effect on a blood clot that has already formed or on ischemic tissue injured by an inadequate blood supply because of the clot. The two main groups of anticoagulant drugs are (1) parenteral anticoagulant drugs and (2) oral anticoagulant drugs. For effective anticoagulant therapy the manner of use for both groups is important. They have been utilized to complement each other, and in some instances the administration of both a rapidly acting parenteral anticoagulant (heparin) and one of the synthetic oral anticoagulants is started simultaneously. Heparin is usually discontinued as soon as the prothrombin time has been sufficiently reduced and the oral compound is producing a full therapeutic effect.

■ Nursing Management

Anticoagulant Therapy

The role of the nurse with the client receiving anticoagulant therapy is primarily one of assessing the client for altered protection related to the increased tendency for bleeding and educating the client for the safe and accurate self-administration of the particular anticoagulant agent.

Assessment. Before anticoagulation therapy is initiated the client should be assessed for any preexisting health conditions that would contraindicate anticoagulation or would indicate the need for caution in the use of anticoagulant therapy. Instances in which bleeding would be imminently life-threatening, such as threatened abortion, cerebral or aortic aneurysm, cerebrovascular hemorrhage, active hemorrhage, severe hypertension, hemophilia, thrombocytopenia, pericarditis, and recent or contemplated ophthalmic surgery or neurosurgery would contraindicate anticoagulation.

Caution would be required if the client had any of the following conditions in which increased risk of hemorrhage is present: recent childbirth; severe diabetes; severe renal function impairment; severe trauma, especially CNS; severe vasculitis; and active ulcers or lesions of the GI, GU, or respiratory tract. The nurse should also be concerned if the client has any condition that might increase the client's response to anticoagulant therapy, such as visceral carcinoma, severe hepatic impairment, and vitamin C or K deficiency; or if the client were to undergo a procedure that presented the risk of bleeding and a risk for injury, such as regional or lumbar block anesthesia or spinal puncture. See the Pregnancy Safety box on p. 590 for FDA classifications of the various anticoagulant agents.

The client's current medication regimen should be reviewed for significant drug interactions. In addition to the specific drug interactions listed within the discussion of heparin and the oral anticoagulants, the nurse should consider that the risk of hemorrhage may be increased by the concurrent use of any medication that inhibits platelet aggregation or causes hypoprothrombinemia, thrombocytopenia, or gastrointestinal ulcers.

The appropriate laboratory tests to determine coagulation times, as well as a hematocrit and complete blood count, including platelets, should be done before the initiation of anticoagulant therapy.

Nursing diagnosis. The client receiving anticoagulant therapy is at risk for altered tissue perfusion (cardiopulmonary, cerebral, gastrointestinal, peripheral, renal) related to the client's underlying condition and the complication of bleeding and excessive bruising related to the anticoagulant effect of the drugs.

Implementation

Monitoring. The nurse needs to remain vigilant to the early signs of bleeding in the client receiving anticoagulant therapy. The skin should be assessed for signs of overdose such as ecchymosis, petechiae, hematomas, nosebleeds, and unusual bleeding from gums, cuts, wounds, and tube insertion sites. Internal bleeding would reveal itself as abdominal pain or swelling, backache, bloody or black tarry stools, dizziness, headache, hematemesis, hematuria, hemoptysis, or joint pain. The client's urine and stool should be checked periodically for occult blood.

Laboratory values should be monitored before the drug is administered to ensure that the client's values are in the therapeutic, not dangerous, range.

For heparin, the activated partial thromboplastin time (APTT) and/or the activated clotting time (ACT) is used to measure the drug's effect on clotting; for the oral anticoagulants, prothrombin time (PT) determinations are used. These tests report the value in seconds along with the control value in seconds. The control value may vary somewhat from day to day because the reagents used may vary. Some laboratories report values as ratios or percentages of normal activity, since the client's results are compared with the control. Normally the client's value is 85% to 100%. However, in anticoagulant therapy where the goal is to prevent thrombus formation, the therapeutic range desired is higher than the control, a prolonged coagulation time. The therapeutic range for the APTT is 1.5 to 2.5 times the control value in seconds, for the ACT it is 2 to 3 times, and for the PT it is 1.3 to 1.5 times for prevention and 2 to 2.5 times (or 20% to 30%) for clients who are at especially high risk (Pagana & Pagana, 1992).

Intervention. The dosage of anticoagulants is individualized and adjusted according to the appropriate laboratory test.

Education. Clients need to recognize and report signs of bleeding: excessive bruising, bleeding gums, nosebleeds, cuts that do not stop bleeding, red or brown urine, and red or black bowel movements. Instruct the client to use a soft toothbrush for oral hygiene and an electric razor to shave and to avoid activities that have a potential for injury. Female clients who have heavy menstrual flow should be cautioned; however, treatment is not contraindicated unless bleeding is excessive. Advise the client to alert any other health care providers, such as dentists, that the drug is being taken. A medical alert bracelet or card should be carried. Medications containing ibuprofen, aspirin, and other salicylates should not be taken while the client is receiving anticoagulant therapy. Instruct client in how to read labels for OTC drugs that may contain these products. In addition, nonpharmacologic measures such as the following should be reinforced with the client: avoiding constrictive clothing, crossing legs at knees, sitting or standing for long periods of time, and pressure on ischemic areas; smoking cessation; regular exercise; and prevention of injury. The client should limit alcohol consumption to not more than an occasional drink or two. Encourage the client to have a normal, balanced diet and not to change dietary patterns radically or to take vitamins or dietary supplements without consulting the prescriber because of the possibility of altering the effect of anticoagulant therapy by changes in the intake of vitamin K. Stress the importance of follow-up visits to the health care provider for laboratory testing and clinical monitoring.

Evaluation. Appropriate coagulation testing will show values in the therapeutic range and the client will not show any signs or symptoms of bleeding or thrombus formation.

Parenteral Anticoagulant Drugs

▲ **heparin sodium** [hep' a rin] (Liquaemin, Hepalean♣)
Heparin is formed in especially large amounts in the mast cells of the liver, lungs, and intestinal mucosa. The source for heparin for injection is bovine lung and the mucosal lining of pig intestines. It is a rapidly acting injectable anticoagulant.

Heparin produces its anticoagulant effect by combining with antithrombin III (heparin cofactor), a naturally occurring anticlotting factor in the plasma. This compound is unrelated to factor III (tissue thromboplastin), a factor in the process of blood coagulation. The binding of heparin with antithrombin III forms a complex that acts at multiple sites in the normal coagulation system, inactivating factors IXa, Xa, XIa, and XIIa. Inactivation of factor Xa of the intrinsic and extrinsic pathways prevents the conversion of prothrombin to thrombin, thereby inhibiting the formation of fibrin from fibrinogen. Furthermore, by preventing the activation of factor XIII (fibrin stabilizing factor), heparin also prevents the formation of a stable fibrin clot. As fibrin is associated with venous thrombi, heparin is useful in preventing venous thrombosis. The drug does not have **fibrinolytic activity.** This means that it will not dissolve existing clots but can prevent the extension of existing clots.

The normal function of antithrombin III is to maintain intravascular fluidity of the blood. Thromboembolism frequently occurs in individuals with acquired or congenital deficiency of this plasma protein. Therefore, in the absence of antithrombin III, heparin is unable to perform its anticoagulating effect.

Heparin is used to prevent and treat all types of thromboses and emboli. It is used prophylactically to prevent blood clotting in surgery of the heart or blood vessels, during blood transfusion, in clients with disseminated intravascular coagulation (DIC), and in the hemodialysis process. It is considered the drug of choice for sudden arterial occlusion, since its action is immediate and can be readily reversed if surgery is necessary.

Heparin is superior to the coumarin drugs in preventing pulmonary complications in cases of thrombophlebitis. It is also preferred for the treatment of thrombophlebitis during pregnancy, since it does not cross the placental barrier and is not excreted in breast milk. When rapid anticoagulation is necessary, it is used before the oral anticoagulants (Table 31-1).

It is administered via the parenteral route of administration because its large molecular size and polarity prevent any gastrointestinal absorption. By intravenous injection its onset of action is immediate. Subcutaneous injection usually

TABLE 31-1 Anticoagulant drugs: comparison of characteristics

	Heparin	Coumarins/indanediones
Onset of action	Immediate	Slow (24 to 48 hours)
Route of administration	Parenteral	Oral
Duration of action	Short (less than 4 hours)	Long (approximately 2 to 5 days)
Laboratory test for dosage control	APTT, ACT	Prothrombin time
Antidote	Protamine sulfate	Vitamin K, whole blood, or plasma

APTT, activated partial thromboplastin time; *ACT,* activated clotting time.

results in an onset of action within 20 to 60 minutes. The half-life is dose dependent but averages 1.5 hours (range is 1 to 6 hours). It is highly protein bound, metabolized in the liver, and excreted via the kidneys. For side effects/adverse reactions, see Table 31-2.

Dosage and administration. Dosage is expressed in USP heparin units/ml in the United States. In Canada, dosage may be expressed in USP units or in International Units (IU). USP heparin units are not equivalent to International Units. Because the potency may vary between USP and IU, the student should review the current package insert for dosage instructions whenever packages are labeled in International Units. The following recommended dosages will be given in USP units.

Heparin sodium adult dose is 10,000 to 20,000 USP units subcutaneously or 10,000 USP units intravenously initially or 5,000 to 10,000 units intravenously every 4 to 6 hours. Pediatric dose is usually 50 USP units/kg initially, followed by 50 to 100 units/kg every 4 hours.

Heparin dosage is closely monitored with coagulation tests such as the activated partial thromboplastin time (APTT), the activated clotting time (ACT), or other tests as ordered. For consistency it is recommended that a single laboratory be used to monitor a client on heparin therapy.

■ Nursing Management

Heparin Therapy

In addition to the nursing management of anticoagulant therapy already discussed, consider the following in relation to heparin therapy.

Assessment. The client should be assessed to determine that heparin is not contraindicated by preexisting conditions such as those discussed in the previous discussion of the nursing management of anticoagulant therapy. Caution must be used in administering heparin to clients who have any condition in which hemorrhage is possible. Clients over the age of 60, especially women, are more susceptible to the hemorrhagic effects of heparin. Heparin is the anticoagulant of choice for use during pregnancy because it does not cross the placenta and affect clotting mechanisms in the fetus. However, because of the risk of maternal bleeding, it is only cautiously used in the last trimester of pregnancy and the postpartum period.

TABLE 31-2 Anticoagulant drugs: side effects/adverse reactions

Drug	Side effects*	Adverse reactions†
heparin		Less frequent or rare: chest pain, chills, elevated temperature, respiratory difficulties, wheezing, rash, pruritus, hives, increase in nasal secretions (allergic reaction), anaphylaxis, paresthesia of hands or feet, blue tinge on arms or legs, increased or persistent erections, thrombocytopenia Early signs of overdosage: increased bruising, nosebleeds, excessive bleeding from minor cuts, wounds, brushing of teeth, or menstrual period Internal bleeding signs: stomach pain or swelling; backaches; bloody urine, bloody or black stools; dizziness; severe persistent headaches; swollen, stiff, or painful joints; vomiting or coughing up of blood Following 6 months or more of therapy: rib or back pain, height decrease (osteoporosis), alopecia At site of injection: hematoma or blood accumulation under the skin, pain, local skin reaction such as irritation, peeling, or sloughing
anisindione		The following effects, though not yet reported with this drug, were reported with phenindione, another indanedione derivative, and may also be seen with this product: edema of face or lower extremities, unexpected weight gain, leukopenia, agranulocytosis, liver toxicity, diarrhea, nausea, vomiting, severe abdominal distress
dicumarol	More frequent: stomach gas Less frequent: anorexia, alopecia	More frequent: diarrhea Less frequent or rare: leukopenia, liver toxicity, nausea, vomiting, mouth sores, agranulocytosis
warfarin	Less frequent: alopecia	Less frequent or rare: leukopenia, nausea, vomiting, abdominal cramps or distress

*If side effects continue, increase, or disturb the patient, inform the prescriber.
†If adverse reactions occur, contact the prescriber, because medical intervention may be necessary.

A baseline assessment should consist of an activated partial thromboplastin time (APTT), a platelet count, and a hematocrit evaluation. Anticipate that each dose of heparin will be individualized after the prescriber has evaluated the APTT or provided a sliding scale or protocol by which specific doses will be administered based on the laboratory values. Check to be sure that these tests are performed as ordered (before each IV or SC injection or daily) and the results are reported promptly. If no dosage adjustments have been required for 2 weeks, further monitoring need not be as frequent. The exception is pregnant women, who need to be monitored throughout therapy because heparin requirements increase as the client's blood volume increases as the pregnancy progresses.

The client's medication regimen needs to be reviewed for significant drug interactions, such as those that can occur when heparin is given with the drugs listed below.

Drug	Possible effect and management
aspirin, sulfinpyrazone (Anturane), NSAIDs, or other platelet aggregation inhibitors	**Increased risk of bleeding because of platelet inhibition by these drugs. Also, large doses of aspirin may produce hypoprothrombinemia. All drugs increase the risk of toxicity because of their potential to produce gastrointestinal ulceration and bleeding. Avoid or a potentially serious drug interaction may occur.**
cefamandole (Mandol), cefoperazone (Cefobid), cefotetan (Cefotan), plicamycin (Mithramycin), or valproic acid (Depakene)	**Increased risk of bleeding and hemorrhage possible with these drugs. These agents can cause hypothrombinemia and platelet inhibition. Avoid or a potentially serious drug interaction may occur.**
methimazole (Tapazole) or propylthiouracil (PTU)	**May produce a hypoprothrombinemic effect that can increase the anticoagulant effect of heparin. Avoid or a potentially serious drug interaction may occur. If necessary to give concurrently, monitor closely for bleeding.**
probenecid (Benemid)	**May prolong and enhance heparin's anticoagulant effects. Avoid or a potentially serious drug interaction may occur. If necessary to give concurrently, monitor coagulation tests closely.**
thrombolytics, such as alteplase, anistreplase, streptokinase, or urokinase	**Increased risk of bleeding and hemorrhage possible with this combination. Avoid or a potentially serious drug interaction may occur. Some studies indicate that heparin may be given with low doses of thrombolytic agents via the intracoronary route of administration. Also, heparin may be administered before or after thrombolytic therapy.**

Nursing diagnosis. With the administration of heparin, clients are at risk for the following nursing diagnoses: impaired tissue perfusion related to the underlying condition and ineffectiveness of the drug; risk for injury related to increased bleeding tendencies; altered comfort such as irritation, pain, or redness at the injection site related to parenteral administration; altered self-concept related to unusual hair loss (long-term therapy); and the potential complications of allergic reaction, thrombocytopenia, and osteoporosis with long-term therapy. The Nursing Care Plan at right lists other selected nursing diagnoses for clients receiving anticoagulant therapy.

Implementation

Monitoring. Adjust heparin dosage to maintain the APTT between 1½ and 2½ times normal control level and the ACT between two and three times the control value, while observing that the client remains free of signs of hemorrhage as discussed in the section on the nursing management of anticoagulant therapy. Any value under or over this range should be reported to the prescriber immediately.

Test stools and urine for occult blood daily to determine hidden bleeding. Monitor platelet count for any possible thrombocytopenia, which may be associated with arterial thrombosis or "white clot" syndrome. Perform hematocrit tests frequently.

There is the possibility of "heparin resistance" in conditions associated with infection, thrombophlebitis, fever, pleurisy, cancer, myocardial infarction, and extensive surgery. Also be aware that abrupt withdrawal of heparin may precipitate an increase in coagulability; usually a full dose of heparin is followed by oral anticoagulants for prophylaxis. Thus there generally is an overlap of both drugs for 3 to 5 days while heparin is being tapered off.

Intervention. Heparin comes in many concentrations: carefully check the vial and the prescriber's order. Errors have been known to occur between the 1000 USP units/ml and the 10,000 USP units/ml vials and the 2500 USP units/ml and the 25,000 USP units/ml vials; watch those decimal points. Be alert, too, that the heparin-lock flush solution maintains patency of the indwelling venipuncture unit and that the solution is not used for systemic anticoagulation. The nurse working with premature neonates should be aware that some heparin sodium injections contain benzyl alcohol as this preservative and so should not be administered to these babies.

For subcutaneous administration, use the smallest gauge (25 to 27) ⅜- to ⅝-inch needle to prevent hematoma at the injection site. Use a "bunching" technique (pulling the fatty layer away from the underlying tissue). Inject the heparin deep into the fatty tissue above the iliac crest or into the abdominal fat layer. Avoid the umbilical veins by avoiding a 2-inch radius around the umbilicus. This distance should also be maintained from scars and lesions. Do not aspirate and *do not massage the injection site.* Hold the needle in place for 10 seconds after administration and withdraw it gently to minimize bruising. Apply direct pressure for 1 to 2 minutes if needed. Rotate sites to prevent the formation of hematomas.

Document the location of injection sites graphically. Intramuscular injection is not recommended because it causes hematomas, irritation, and pain at the injection site and because it causes erratic absorption.

Nursing Care Plan

Selected Nursing Diagnoses for Clients Receiving Anticoagulant Therapy

Nursing diagnosis	Outcome criteria	Nursing interventions
Tissue perfusion, alteration in: reduced blood flow (prevention and treatment of thromboembolic disorders)	Clotting studies are maintained within therapeutic range; APPT is prolonged to 1.5-2 times the control (heparin). PT is prolonged to 1.5-2 times the control (warfarin). Extension of the thrombus or embolization of thrombi does not occur.	Monitor clotting studies as ordered. Administer anticoagulant therapy and assess effectiveness. Monitor vital signs and blood pressure every 4 hours. Report immediately any change in vital signs or decrease in blood pressure. Ausculate breath sounds every 4 hours. Report the development of rales. Assess for other developments of pulmonary emboli, in addition to above, such as dyspnea, cough, or hemoptysis. Apply antiembolism stockings as ordered. Measure calf dimension, bilaterally; compare and record every 8 hours.
Injury, risk for hemorrhage	No signs of hemorrhage occur.	Administer heparin SC rather than IM to prevent hematoma formation. Inject into lower abdomen using a small-gauge needle (25-27); do not massage injection sites. Rotate sites. All personnel should be alerted that the client is on anticoagulant therapy. Venipunctures and injections should be kept to a minimum and pressure applied to prevent bleeding when they are done. Observe client for excessive bruising, bleeding gums, nosebleed, blood in urine, feces, and/or secretions, and report.
Knowledge deficit related to medication regimen	Client will describe underlying condition and how the drug relates to the condition, how and when to take the medication, common drug interactions, safety precautions, common side effects, and which of these warrant reporting. Self-administer warfarin safely and accurately.	Assess learning needs and learning readiness. Plan with client for the achievement of realistic goals. Provide information to meet outcome criteria. Caution the client to use a soft toothbrush and an electric razor. Recommended to client that all health care personnel be informed of anticoagulant therapy before treatment. Advise on the importance of having blood studies done as ordered. Instruct client on the need to report any signs of bleeding.

For IV dosage a loading dose usually precedes a continuous infusion or heparin may be administered intermittently via a heparin lock. This IV dose may be given undiluted over at least a minute. Many clinicians prefer continuous intravenous infusions for the administration of heparin because it provides a more constant blood level of the drug and the risk for bleeding complications is decreased. For continuous IV infusion of heparin, use an infusion pump or a volume control unit so that the flow rate and fluid volume of the drug can be controlled precisely. Check the system frequently to prevent overdosage or underdosage. Never add other drugs to the heparin infusion or piggyback other drugs into an intravenous line containing heparin—many other drugs inactivate heparin.

For clients receiving intermittent heparin dosage, subcutaneously or by heparin lock, the blood samples for the APTT should be drawn 30 minutes before the next dose to avoid a falsely high APTT. This false reading can also be avoided for the client with a continuous heparin infusion by drawing the sample from the arm opposite the infusion site.

Although controversy exists on whether normal saline or diluted heparin solutions (10 to 100 units of heparin sodium/ml) should be used to irrigate and maintain patency of an indwelling venipuncture device, the nurse should be aware that the purpose of the device is to maintain an open intravenous line so that ordered intermittent drugs, intravenous solutions, or both may be administered through this line.

Nursing Research

Heparinized versus nonheparinized intravascular lines

Controversy over the use of heparinized saline as opposed to normal saline as a flush solution in intermittent intravenous (IV) sets in acute-care settings has developed in recent years throughout the country. The question centers around whether heparin mixed in variable dilutions in saline is necessary to maintain the patency of an IV site that is used for intermittent infusions (McMullen, 1993). Peterson and Kirshhoff (1991) performed an analysis of the research about heparinized versus nonheparinized intravascular lines and concluded that there is no significant difference in duration of patency between intravascular catheters flushed with saline solution and those flushed with a heparinized solution. Given the cost savings of discontinuing the use of heparin and client well-being in the prevention of heparin-related complications, many hospitals decided to change their practice (McAllister et al, 1993), although the *Intravenous Nursing Standards of Practice* established by the Intravenous Nurses' Society supports the use of heparinized saline as the accepted solution for the maintenance of intermittent IV locks (Fry, 1992).

A large-scale multicenter trial has found that heparin does make a difference in keeping arterial pressure monitoring lines open, although other factors are also important (American Association of Critical Care Nurses, 1990). In the 3-year "Thunder Project" conducted by the American Association of Critical Care Nurses, clinicians at 198 institutions randomly assigned 5139 individuals on arterial pressure monitoring lines to flush solutions with or without heparin. Lines stayed clear more often when heparin was used—94% versus 88% of nonheparinized lines—and were more likely to remain clear over time. Several other variables figured into whether lines stayed patent. Lines were more likely to stay clear among clients receiving other anticoagulants or thrombolytics than among clients receiving no anticoagulants. Catheters greater than 2 inches in length also enhanced the probability of patency. The researchers also found greater patency in femoral catheters than in other sites, and lines, whether heparinized or not, were slightly more likely to remain open in men.

Critical thinking questions

- If you were assigned a client with an intermittent IV lock, what would be your preferred flush solution? Why?
- If you were assigned a client with an arterial pressure monitoring line who was intolerant of heparin, what recommendations would you make to maximize its patency?

The Nursing Research box above discusses research comparing heparinized versus nonheparinized intravascular lines.

Therefore, within each clinical practice setting, obtain information about the accepted (usually medically approved) practices or policies concerning the solution to be used and how often the device should be flushed if not in frequent use; then closely monitor the unit for patency.

If heparin solution is being used to maintain the patency of an indwelling peripheral venipuncture device, usually 1 ml of heparin lock flush solution will be effective for 4 to 8 hours. If the device is being used to administer a drug that is incompatible with heparin, the device should be flushed with sterile water or 0.9% sodium chloride for injection before and after the drug is given. Inject the heparin-lock flush solution after the second flush. If the device is being used to obtain blood samples for laboratory analysis and heparin might alter the results of the test, the heparin solution should be cleared from the device by aspirating and discarding 1 ml of solution from the device before the blood sample is taken. After the blood sample is drawn, the device is again filled with 1 ml of heparin-lock flush solution.

Heparin is to be stopped immediately if the client complains of a chill, low back pain (a sign of abdominal bleeding), or spontaneous bleeding. Notify the prescriber and have protamine sulfate on hand. In some cases it may be necessary to give whole blood or plasma.

Alert other staff members that the client is receiving heparin (i.e., place a sign over the client's bed). Pressure should be applied to venipuncture and injection sites to minimize bruising. These invasive procedures should be avoided if at all possible. Consult the prescriber regarding a change from intramuscular administration of other drugs to other routes of administration while the client is receiving heparin (see the case study at right).

Education. In addition to the client education information discussed in Nursing Management: Anticoagulant Therapy, inform the client of the potential for diuresis beginning 36 to 48 hours after the initial dose of heparin and lasting 36 to 48 hours after termination of therapy.

Advise the client that alopecia may occur several months after heparin therapy and that the condition is reversible on discontinuation of drug.

Evaluation. The client's APTT will show values 1½ to 2½ times the control value in seconds, or ACT values 2 to 3 times the control value in seconds, and the client will not evidence any signs or symptoms of bleeding or thrombus formation.

Low Molecular Weight (LMW) Heparins

The low molecular weight heparins are new antithrombins with the potential of being more effective than heparin. They have longer half-lifes, require less laboratory monitoring, and are safe and effective for the management of thromboembolic disease (Turpie, 1995).

Case Study

The Client with Deep Vein Thrombosis

John Tucker is a 53-year-old construction worker who has been admitted to the hospital with a diagnosis of deep vein thrombosis of the right leg. Mr. Tucker experienced increasing pain and swelling of the right lower leg over several days. He has received an intravenous bolus of 5000 units of heparin followed by a continuous infusion of heparin (25,000 units in 1000 ml of 0.9% sodium chloride).

1. What measures should the nurse implement to ensure accurate administration of the continuous heparin infusion?
2. What data are used by the nurse to evaluate the client's response to the heparin therapy?
3. In preparation for discharge in 4 days Mr. Tucker is started on warfarin sodium (Coumadin) at the same time as he is started on the intravenous heparin. What is the reason for administering two anticoagulants?
4. The nurse carefully questions Mr. Tucker about his use of over-the-counter medications. The client admits to using aspirin for headaches and assorted muscle aches from his job. He also takes a multiple vitamin daily. How should the nurse respond to this information?
5. What additional information does the client need for safe self-administration during anticoagulant therapy?

enoxaparin [en ox' uh pear in] (Lovenox)
Enoxaparin is the first low molecular weight heparin (LMWH) released in the United States for the prevention of postsurgical deep vein thrombosis (DVT) after hip and knee-replacement surgery. The low molecular weight heparins appear to have the advantage of having slightly fewer hemorrhagic complications than standard heparin.

Mechanism of action is similar to the standard heparin although it appears to have a higher ratio of anti-Factor Xa to anti-Factor IIa and less lipase release activity than heparin (Olin, 1996). It binds to antithrombin III, which inhibits the synthesis of factor Xa, thus reducing thrombin formation.

Significant side/adverse effects are few with enoxaparin and include local irritation effects such as erythema, hematomas, urticaria, and pain. Thrombocytopenia and bleeding episodes have also been reported (Olin, 1996).

Usual adult dose is 30 mg subcutaneously twice a day for 7 to 14 days postsurgically, with the first dose administered as soon as possible (not more than 24 hours) after the surgery. Treatment is continued throughout the postoperative period until the risk for deep vein thrombosis declines.

Nursing management for enoxaparin therapy is as for heparin therapy.

dalteparin [dalt' ta pear in] (Fragmin)
Dalteparin is an LMW heparin used for the prevention of pulmonary thromboembolism and deep vein thrombosis. It is administered once a day, which makes it more convenient for the client. This product produces its antithrombotic effects by potentiating inhibition of Factor Xa and thrombin by antithrombin.

It does not affect platelet aggregation, lipase, fibrinolysis, or the standard blood clotting tests, such as prothrombin time (PT), thrombin time (TT) or activated partial thromboplastin time (APTT).

A significant side/adverse effect of dalteparin is hematoma at the injection site. Less commonly reported are bleeding episodes, allergic type reactions, and thrombocytopenia. Usual adult dose is 2500 units SC 1 to 2 hours before abdominal surgery. This dose is repeated daily for 5 to 10 days afterward (*USP DI,* 1996).

Nursing management is as for heparin therapy.

Parenteral Anticoagulant Antagonist

protamine sulfate [proe' ta meen] (Heparin Antidote)
Protamine sulfate, a protein-like substance derived from the sperm and mature testes of salmon and other fish, is an antidote for a heparin overdose. Protamine is a very weak anticoagulant alone, but when given in conjunction with heparin a combination is formed that dissociates the heparin–antithrombin III complex, thus reducing the anticoagulant action of heparin. Because protamine is a basic protein (many free amino groups), it is able to combine with the sulfuric acids of heparin and inactivate them.

Protamine is indicated for the treatment of a severe heparin overdose that has resulted in hemorrhaging. Blood transfusions may also be necessary. It is also used to neutralize the effects of heparin administered during dialysis or cardiac or arterial surgery.

Administered intravenously it has an onset of action within 30 to 60 seconds and a duration of effect of usually 2 hours. When protamine is administered too rapidly, respiratory difficulties, bradycardia, and a sudden hypotensive effect may result. Less often reported are bleeding problems and, rarely, coughing spells, facial edema, or a rash, which should be reported to the prescriber immediately. Less frequent and usually less troublesome side effects include sensations of heat, flushing, nausea, vomiting, or feelings of increased weakness. No significant drug interactions have been reported with protamine.

Protamine is administered by slow intravenous injection at a rate of 1 mg/min. One milligram of protamine is necessary to neutralize approximately 100 USP units of heparin. It is recommended that not more than 50 mg of protamine be given in any 10 minute period and no more than 100 mg be administered over a 2 hour period. Close monitoring with blood coagulation tests is required.

■ Nursing Management

Protamine Sulfate Therapy

Assessment. Protamine is used as an antidote to severe heparin overdose evidenced by frank hemorrhaging or abnormally high values on APTT or ACT. It is not used in instances of minor heparin overdose, which could be treated by withholding the doses of heparin.

Nursing diagnosis. The client receiving protamine sulfate is at risk for impaired tissue perfusion and fluid volume deficit related to the underlying hemorrhage; and altered comfort (back pain, feelings of warmth and flushing, and nausea or vomiting). The potential complications exist of cardiovascular collapse related to too rapid administration; anaphylaxis; bleeding related to protamine overdose or rebound heparin activity; and pulmonary edema.

Implementation

Monitoring. Frequent assessment of vital signs is essential as is some estimation of blood loss. Observe the client for spontaneous bleeding or heparin "rebound" (the effects of heparin last longer than the effects of protamine) after procedures involving extracorporeal circulation such as cardiac or arterial surgery or dialysis. This may occur as long as 18 hours after the initial neutralization of the heparin. Monitor APTT to determine protamine efficacy and dosage.

Intervention. Protamine sulfate should be administered by a physician. The drug should be administered slowly intravenously—over 1 to 3 minutes—not more than 50 mg in any 10 minute period. Too rapid administration may cause injury, dyspnea, and shock. Emergency equipment should be available.

Evaluation. The client will not evidence bleeding, the hemoglobin and hematocrit will have stabilized, and the APTT or ACT will be within normal, or therapeutic, limits.

Oral Anticoagulant Drugs

There are two major types of oral anticoagulant drugs: coumarins and indanediones.

Coumarins

dicumarol [dye koo' ma role]
▲ **warfarin sodium** [war' far in] (Coumadin)

Indanediones

anisindione [an iss in dye' one] (Miradon)

Both the coumarin and the indanedione derivatives interfere with liver synthesis of the vitamin K–dependent clotting factors. Thus they depress the synthesis of factors X, IX, VII, and II (prothrombin). Factor VII is depleted quickly; the sequential depletion of factors IX, X, and II follows. These agents do not affect established clots but do prevent further extension of formed clots, thereby diminishing the potential for secondary thromboembolic complications.

The oral anticoagulant drugs are used for the prophylaxis and treatment of deep venous thrombosis and pulmonary thromboembolism. They are also used for the prophylaxis of thromboembolism associated with chronic atrial fibrillation or myocardial infarction. The major advantages of these drugs are that they are effective orally and that they need to be given only once daily, after the maintenance dose has been established (Table 31-3).

With the exception of dicumarol all the oral anticoagulants are well absorbed from the gastrointestinal tract. The

TABLE 31-3 Oral anticoagulants: pharmacokinetics and dosage and administration

Generic/trade name	Onset of action (days)	Duration of action (days)	Half-life (days)	Dosage and administration
Coumarins				
dicumarol*	1-5	2-10	1-4 (dose dependent)	Adult: 25-200 mg daily orally as indicated by prothrombin time Children: not established
warfarin sodium (Coumadin)	.5-3	2-5	1.5-2.5	Adult: 10-15 mg orally for 2-4 days; then 2-10 mg daily as indicated by prothrombin time Children: not established Injectable dosage form: same dosage as oral
Indanediones				
anisindione (Miradon)	2-3	1-3	3-5	Adult: 25-250 mg orally daily as indicated by prothrombin time Children: not established

*Dicumarol activity is variable.

absorption of dicumarol is slow, incomplete, and erratic from the gastrointestinal tract. Oral anticoagulants are highly protein bound (99%), metabolized in the liver, and excreted via the kidneys.

For side effects/adverse reactions, pharmacokinetics, and dosage and administration, see Tables 31-2 and 31-3. Fetal abnormalities and facial anomalies have been reported. If an anticoagulant is necessary during pregnancy, heparin is usually the drug of choice because it does not cross the placenta.

■ Nursing Management

Oral Anticoagulant Therapy

In addition to the nursing management of anticoagulant therapy described at the beginning of the chapter, consider the following for oral anticoagulant therapy.

Assessment. The client should be assessed for health conditions for which oral anticoagulant therapy is contraindicated or for which the client might be at risk of adverse effects. Review the assessment content within the discussion of nursing management of anticoagulant therapy in general. Before initiating therapy, inquire if client is pregnant and inform her of the potential risk of congenital malformations. See also the discussion in the Geriatric Implications box at right.

The client's current medication regimen should be reviewed for significant drug interactions. Although all interactions between coumarin and indandione and other medications have not been identified, a listing of the medications that are known to cause interactions can be found in the Box 31-1.

A baseline assessment should consist of a prothrombin time (PT) determination, a platelet count, and a hematocrit evaluation. Anticipate that the dosage of these drugs will be individualized after the prescriber has evaluated the client's PT.

Nursing diagnosis. With the administration of oral anticoagulant therapy, clients are at risk for the following nursing diagnoses: impaired tissue perfusion related to the underlying condition; risk for injury related to increased bleeding tendencies; altered protection related to agranulocytosis or leukopenia (chills, fever, sore throat, excessive fatigue); impaired skin integrity related to allergic dermatitis; altered comfort (bloated stomach or gas); altered bowel elimination related to gastrointestinal effects (diarrhea); altered self-concept related to unusual hair loss (long-term therapy); and the potential complications of acute adrenal insufficiency (diarrhea, nausea with or without vomiting, abdominal cramps) and hepatotoxicity (dark urine, yellow sclera and skin).

Implementation

Monitoring. Anticipate that dosage is based on prothrombin time. Check to be sure that this test is performed as ordered, and report results to the prescriber immediately. The therapeutic aim for clients undergoing anticoagulant therapy is to produce a prolongation of the prothrombin time within 1.3 to 1.5 times the control. If the client is at higher risk for thrombus, then a prolongation of the prothrombin time within 1.5 to 2 times the control is the therapeutic level sought. Once maintenance dosage has been determined, further monitoring need not be as frequent. Review the section on client monitoring within the discussion on the general nursing management of anticoagulant therapy. In addition to those observations related to hemorrhage, clients receiving anisindione will need to be observed for nephrotoxicity, hepatotoxicity, and blood dyscrasias.

Intervention. Be aware that the onset of action of oral anticoagulants is slow; therefore heparin sodium is usually given during the first few days of treatment. Blood for prothrombin time should be drawn just before or 5 hours after the intravenous heparin administration.

Geriatric Implications

Anticoagulants

The elderly may be more susceptible to the effects of anticoagulants, such as warfarin (Coumadin) and dicumarol; thus a lower maintenance dose is usually recommended for the geriatric client along with very close supervision and monitoring.

The primary adverse effects of excessive drug usage are prolonged bleeding from gums when brushing teeth or from small shaving cuts, excessive or easy skin bruising, blood in urine or stools, and unexplained nosebleeds. These may be early signs of overdose that indicate the need for medical intervention.

Caution clients to carry an identification card indicating the use of an anticoagulant. Also, remind client to always consult his or her prescriber before starting any new drug, including OTC medications and vitamins, or if changing a medication dose or when any drug product is discontinued. Many medications can change the effects of an anticoagulant in the body.

Be aware that administration of concurrent drug therapy that may induce gastric irritation increases the risk for gastrointestinal bleeding. Drugs such as the nonsteroidal antiinflammatory agents (NSAIDs such as ibuprofen, indomethacin) that are commonly prescribed for the elderly client often cause gastrointestinal effects.

Alcohol consumption can alter the effect of this medication in the body. Clients should be instructed to avoid alcohol or at the least limit their daily alcohol intake to one alcoholic drink a day. Alcohol may cause liver damage, which increases the individual's sensitivity to anticoagulants (*USP DI*, 1996.)

The nurse should be aware that diet can interfere with the anticoagulant effect. In a previously stabilized person, vitamin C deficiency, chronic malnutrition, diarrhea, or other illnesses may result in an increased anticoagulant effect, while increased intake of green leafy vegetables (such as broccoli, cabbage, collard greens, lettuce, spinach, and others) or the consumption of a nutritional supplement or multiple vitamin containing vitamin K can result in decreased anticoagulant effectiveness.

BOX 31-1

Significant Drug Interactions of Oral Anticoagulants

The oral anticoagulants have a great potential for causing drug interactions; therefore clients must be cautioned against taking any drug and/or making significant dietary changes without prior consultation with their prescriber. Check a current *USP-DI* for major drug interactions.

Agents that may increase the anticoagulant effect, often necessitating a dosage reduction

allopurinol	clofibrate	indomethacin	propylthiouracil
amiodarone	danazol	mefenamic acid	quinidine
anabolic steroids	dextran	meperidine	salicylates
androgens	dextrothyroxine	mezlocillin	streptokinase
aspirin	diflunisal	methimazole	sulfinpyrazone
azlocillin	dipyridamole†	metronidazole	sulfonamides
cefamandole	disulfiram	nalidixic acid	sulindac
cefoperazone	erythromycins	phenytoin‡	thyroid hormone
chloral hydrate*	fenoprofen	piperacillin	ticarcillin
chloramphenicol	gemfibrozil	plicamycin	urokinase
cimetidine			

Agents that may decrease the anticoagulant effect, often necessitating an increase in anticoagulant dosage

oral antidiabetic agents§	colestipol	ethchlorvynol	primidone
barbiturates	contraceptives, oral	glutethimide	rifampin
carbamazepine	estramustine	griseofulvin	vitamin K
cholestyramine	estrogens		

*Usually occurs during first 2 weeks of therapy. With chronic concurrent therapy, the anticoagulant effect may return to normal or be decreased.
†With doses of dipyridamole over 400 mg/day.
‡Increased anticoagulant effect occurs initially. With chronic concurrent therapy decreased activity may occur. May also see a decrease in metabolism of phenytoin, possibly leading to increased serum levels and toxicity.
§May initially increase anticoagulant effects, but with long-term concurrent therapy, such effects may decrease. Also, the decrease in metabolism of the antidiabetic agent may increase serum levels and cause prolonged half-life, hypoglycemia, and toxicity.

Oral anticoagulant therapy is usually terminated gradually over a 3 or 4 week period to prevent rebound thromboembolic complications.

Education. In addition to the points discussed in Nursing Management: Anticoagulant Therapy, instruct the client to carry an identification card that lists the client's and prescriber's names and phone numbers and the name and dosage of the oral anticoagulant drug. Emphasize the importance of not taking any other medication, especially ibuprofen, aspirin, or other salicylates, without checking with the prescriber, since so many drugs interact with anticoagulant agents. Also, alcoholic individuals should be closely monitored because of the risk for ineffective management of the therapeutic drug regimen.

Once maintenance therapy is established and the client is discharged, stress the importance of adherence to the schedule of laboratory procedures and prescriber's appointments. Prothrombin time should be performed from intervals of 1 to 4 weeks, depending on dosage. Periodic urinalysis, blood counts, stool guaiac, and liver function tests should also be performed. Ensure that the client is aware of different dosage tablets as the prescriber may vary the dosage by phone on the basis of the prothrombin time.

Vitamin K_1 (phytonadione) should be readily accessible if bleeding occurs. Outpatients should carry vitamin K_1 with them and, after first consulting with the prescriber, take 1 to 10 mg at once if bleeding occurs. Statistics show that bleeding occurs in approximately 10% of all patients on long-term anticoagulant therapy; however, fatalities are rare.

Evaluation. The client's PT will show values 1.3 to 1.5 or 2 times the control value in seconds and the client will not evidence any signs or symptoms of bleeding or thrombus formation.

Oral Anticoagulant Antagonists

Vitamin K

menadiol sodium diphosphate [men a dye' ole] (Synkayvite)
phytonadione [fye toe na dye' one] (Mephyton, AquaMephyton)

Vitamin K is essential to the hepatic synthesis of prothrombin (factor II) and factors VII, IX, and X. It contributes to the activation of an enzyme necessary to the formation of prothrombin. Deficiency of vitamin K leads to hypoprothrombinemia and hemorrhage.

Vitamin K is used to prevent and treat hypoprothrombinemia. Prothrombin deficiency may occur because of inadequate absorption of vitamin K from the intestine (usually caused by biliary disease in which bile fails to enter the intestine) or because of destruction of intestinal organisms, which may occur with antibiotic therapy. It is also seen in the newborn, in which case it is probably caused by the fact that the intestinal organisms have not yet become established. It may result from therapy with certain medications, such as salicylates, sulfonamides, quinine, quinidine, or broad spectrum antibiotics.

Vitamin K is useful only in conditions in which the prolonged bleeding time is caused by a low concentration of prothrombin in the blood and not by damaged liver cells. Vitamin K is routinely administered to newborns to help prevent hemorrhage. Although prothrombin levels may be normal at birth, they decline until about the sixth to the eighth day, when the liver is able to form prothrombin. Phytonadione is usually the preferred agent.

Vitamin K is also indicated in the preoperative preparation of individuals with deficient prothrombin, particularly those with obstructive jaundice. In addition, it is given as an antidote for overdosage of oral anticoagulants.

It is important to measure prothrombin activity of the blood frequently when the client is receiving a preparation of vitamin K. Parenteral preparations should be administered if intestinal absorption is impaired. Natural vitamin K is normally synthesized by the intestinal flora. When synthetic forms of vitamin K are administered, the absorption is good, but phytonadione requires the presence of bile salts.

The onset of action for menadiol sodium diphosphate injection is 8 to 24 hours; for oral phytonadione it is 6 to 12 hours; for the injectable form it is 1 to 2 hours. Vitamin K is metabolized in the liver and excreted via the kidneys and in the bile.

Infrequent side effects reported are facial flushing, taste alterations, and redness or pain at the injection site.

The dose of menadiol (vitamin K) as a nutritional supplement for hypoprothrombinemia is 5 mg/day orally, or 5 to 15 mg IM or SC once or twice daily. As an antidote for drug-induced hypoprothrombinemia, the oral dose is 5 to 10 mg daily; the intramuscular or subcutaneous dose is 5 to 15 mg PO or IM daily.

■ Nursing Management

Vitamin K Therapy

Assessment. The client should be assessed for preexisting conditions for which vitamin K therapy would entail some risk, such as hepatic function impairment in which large doses of vitamin K might increase the impairment, or glucose-6-phosphate dehydrogenase (G6PD) deficiency in which menadiol might induce erythrocyte hemolysis.

Drug interactions with vitamin K in the client's current medication regimen need to be identified. When vitamin K is given concurrently with the oral anticoagulants, a decrease in anticoagulation effect is reported. If other hemolytics are used concurrently with vitamin K, especially menadiol, the potential for toxic side effects may increase.

Nursing diagnosis. Administration of vitamin K may place the client at risk for altered comfort (facial flushing, unusual taste, and discomfort and redness at the injection site) and the potential complications of hemolytic anemia or a rare hypersensitivity-like reaction.

Implementation

Monitoring. Monitor prothrombin time as a baseline measurement and throughout vitamin K therapy to evaluate response. During intravenous infusion, observe for signs of side effects such as flushing, weakness, and hypotension, and report them to the prescriber.

Intervention. Because vitamin K has a delayed onset, the administration of plasma or fresh whole blood may be necessary with severe bleeding. Although intravenous administration is not recommended because of the risk of hypersensitivity reactions, if necessary, administer the drug by slow intravenous infusion over 2 to 3 hours and protect the infusion container from light by wrapping it in aluminum foil.

Education. Generally, dietary supplements for vitamin K are not necessary because a normal diet and intestinal bacterial synthesis supply sufficient amounts. However, green leafy vegetables, meats, and dairy products are the best sources of vitamin K with little nutritional loss of the vitamin during ordinary cooking. The client's intake of dietary vitamin K should be considered in determining therapeutic dosages for long-term use.

Evaluation. The client's prothrombin time will be within 2 seconds of the control time and the client will not evidence bleeding.

THROMBOLYTIC AGENTS

Thrombolytic (fibrinolytic) **drugs** are used to treat acute thromboembolic disorders. Unlike anticoagulants, they dissolve clots and are used in a hospital setting only by health care providers who are experienced in the management of diseases caused by thrombosis. These agents alter the hemostatic capability of the client more profoundly than does anticoagulant therapy. Consequently, when bleeding occurs, it is more severe and very difficult to control.

alteplase [al ti plase'] (Activase)
anistreplase [an eye' strep lase] (Eminase)
▲ **streptokinase** [strep toe kye' nase] (Streptase)
urokinase [yoor oh kin' ase] (Abbokinase)

These agents dissolve clots via the endogenous fibrinolytic system. All four drugs have similar biochemical mechanisms of action on the fibrinolytic system—converting plasminogen in the blood to plasmin. Plasmin, a fibrinolytic enzyme, digests or dissolves fibrin clots wherever they exist and can be reached by plasmin. Streptokinase is a key drug because it was the first thrombolytic agent released. Alteplase, streptokinase and urokinase are indicated for the treatment of acute pulmonary thromboembolism; currently only streptokinase is indicated for the treatment of an acute, deep venous thrombosis (*USP DI*, 1996). All four drugs can be used to treat an acute coronary arterial thrombosis associated with an acute myocardial infarction.

These agents are administered intravenously and/or intraarterially. Alteplase has an elimination half-life of 35 minutes; streptokinase and urokinase half-lives are 23 minutes and up to 20 minutes, respectively. Anistreplase, which is an acylated complex of streptokinase and human plasminogen, has a long half-life of approximately 90 minutes. Peak effect after IV injection is from 20 minutes to 2 hours. Duration of thrombolysis effect is approximately 4 hours for alteplase, streptokinase and urokinase; anistreplase thrombolysis effect is in 6 hours. Table 31-4 lists side effects/adverse reactions.

In an acute coronary artery thrombosis evolving into a transmural myocardial infarction, thrombolytic therapy is most effective when started within 3 to 4 hours after the onset of symptoms. Usually alteplase is given at 1.25 mg/kg IV in divided doses over 3 hours for clients weighing less than 65 kg, or 100 mg intravenously for clients 65 kg or over (in divided doses over 3 hours). See current literature for recommended dosages over each of the 3 hours.

The dose of anistreplase is 30 units in solution administered by IV injection over 2 to 5 minutes. For streptokinase, the dose is 1,500,000 IU IV administered within an hour. Smaller doses of 20,000 IU initially followed by an additional 2000 IU/min are used for intraarterial administration. Urokinase 6000 IU/min is administered intraarterially until the artery is opened. For other indications, refer to a current package insert or *USP DI* for dosing information. Pediatric dosages are not established.

antithrombin III (Human) [an' tee throm bin] (ATnativ)

Antithrombin III is prepared from pooled human plasma of healthy donors. It is indicated for the treatment or prevention of thromboembolism associated with a hereditary antithrombin III deficiency. Heparin and antithrombin III will enhance each others effects, thus they have been administered concurrently, depending on the situation.

Side/adverse effects includes diuresis, hypotension, chest pain, fever, hives, and shortness of breath in some persons. The usual adult dose is 50 to 100 IV/min intravenous, titrated to desired effect.

Nursing Management

Thrombolytic Therapy

Assessment. Note that thrombolytic therapy is contraindicated for clients in whom there is the risk of uncontrollable bleeding because of preexisting conditions such as aneurysm or arteriovenous malformation, active bleeding, brain tumor, cerebrovascular accident, intracranial or intraspinal surgery within the last 2 months, recent thoracic surgery, or recent CNS trauma. Such therapy is also contraindicated in severe uncontrolled hypertension because of the risk of cerebral hemorrhage. Use with caution in high-risk clients who have experienced major surgery, childbirth, serious gastrointestinal bleeding, organ biopsy, previous puncture of noncompressible blood vessels, or severe trauma other than CNS within the past 10 days. Use with caution with any condition in which the risk of bleeding is present or would be difficult to control because of its location. In addition to those already listed are coagulation defects secondary to severe hepatic and renal disease, neurosurgical procedures within the last 2 months, suspected left heart thrombus involving mitral stenosis with atrial fibrillation, subacute bacterial endocarditis, and diabetic hemorrhagic retinopathy. If the client has been treated previously with anistreplase or streptokinase, the formation of antibodies to the drug may either cause a resistance to the therapeutic effects of the drug or a severe allergic reaction.

TABLE 31-4 Thrombolytic agents: side effects/adverse reactions

Drug	Side effects/adverse reactions*
alteplase	More frequent: bleeding episodes (cuts, wounds, gums); elevated temperature Less frequent: allergic reactions of facial flushing, headache, arthralgia, nausea, rash, pruritus, and respiratory difficulties; easy bruising
anistreplase	More frequent: bleeding episodes; hypotension; arrhythmias; allergic reactions of rash, pruritus, and facial flushing Less frequent: chills, fever, headaches, nausea, vomiting, tremors, paresthesia, irritability, and respiratory difficulties
streptokinase and urokinase	Most frequent: stomach pain or swelling; backache; bloody urine; bloody or black stools; constipation; coughing up of blood; severe headaches; dizziness; swollen stiff, or painful joints; painful or stiff muscles; nosebleeds; excessive bleeding from vagina; vomiting of blood or substances that look like coffee grounds; tachycardia; bradycardia; oozing of blood from cuts or scratches. Elevated temperature is more frequent with streptokinase than urokinase. Less frequent with streptokinase but rare with urokinase are flushed red skin, mild headaches or muscle pain, nausea, rash, pruritus, hives, respiratory difficulties. Rare (for streptokinase only) severe and/or sudden hypotension; shortness of breath; chest tightness; severe wheezing; or edema of eyes, face, lips, or tongue (anaphylaxis or a severe allergic reaction)

*If adverse reactions occur, contact physician because medical intervention may be necessary.

Before thrombolytic therapy, coagulation tests, such as thrombin time (TT), activated partial thromboplastin time (APTT), prothrombin time (PT), fibrin/fibrinogen degradation product (FDP/fdp) titer, and fibrinogen concentration must be performed, as well as an ECG, and hematocrit and platelet counts.

The client's current medication regimen should be reviewed for significant drug interactions (Table 31-5).

Nursing diagnosis. With the administration of thrombolytic agents the client is at risk for the following nursing diagnoses: risk for injury related to increased bleeding tendencies, altered comfort (chest pain), impaired tissue perfusion related to cardiac arrhythmias, hyperthermia, and the potential complication of embolism. In addition, with streptokinase the client is at risk for the complication of an allergic reaction.

Implementation

Monitoring. Observe client carefully during the early phase of therapy for allergic reactions. With urokinase, relatively mild reactions (e.g., bronchospasm, skin rash) are reported. Streptokinase may produce more serious reactions and possibly anaphylaxis. See allergic effects under side effects/adverse reactions. If allergic manifestations occur, discontinue infusion and treat with epinephrine, antihistamines, and corticosteroids. If fever occurs, it should be treated symptomatically with acetaminophen.

Monitor vital signs frequently (i.e., pulse rate, temperature, respiratory rate, and blood pressure), at least every 4 hours. To avoid possible dislodgement of deep vein thrombi, do not take blood pressure in the lower extremities. Monitor client carefully for bleeding: every 15 minutes for the first hour, every 30 minutes for the next 8 hours, and every 4 hours until therapy is discontinued. The prescriber should be notified immediately if bleeding occurs. Therapy should be discontinued if bleeding occurs that is not controlled by local pressure. In addition to observing for overt bleeding, observe client for internal bleeding—bloody sputum, hematuria, hematemesis, dark stools (i.e., guaiac positive), flank and abdominal pain, and neurologic changes and mental status (intracranial bleeding). For uncontrollable bleeding, stop treatment and be ready to administer whole blood (fresh blood if available), packed red cells, cryoprecipitate or fresh-frozen plasma, and aminocaproic acid.

Observe extremities and palpate pulses of affected extremities every hour. The prescriber should be notified immediately if there are signs of circulatory impairment. Observe the client carefully for dysrhythmias during and after intracoronary infusion of streptokinase. Rapid lysis of coronary thrombi has caused atrial and ventricular dysrhythmias. ECG monitoring is recommended.

Continue to observe the client for bleeding during and after treatment. Coagulation tests, such as APTT, PT, and TT are used to assess fibrinolytic activity. Because the thrombolytic effects of the drug last for several hours, the sites of invasive devices are common areas for hematoma formation.

After therapy, monitor fibrinogen levels—which are decreased by thrombolytic agents—until they return to normal.

Intervention. Thrombolytic therapy is administered only by personnel who are experienced in the management of thrombotic diseases and where skilled personnel and laboratory resources are available. Also, typed and crossmatched whole blood and packed red cells should be available in case of hemorrhage. Follow manufacturer's instructions when reconstituting and diluting drug to minimize fibrin formation:

- *alteplase.* Reconstitute using the diluent supplied with the drug (sterile water for injection); do not use bacteriostatic water for injection. It may be used as is or diluted further. If it is diluted further, use only 0.9% sodium chloride solutions or 5% dextrose injection without preservatives. Mix gently to prevent foaming. Leave the solution undisturbed for a few minutes; any bubbles created will dissipate.

TABLE 31-5 Thrombolytic agents: drug interactions

Drug	Possible effect and management
aminocaproic acid or other antifibrinolytic drugs	May inhibit effectiveness of thrombolytic agents. Reserve such drugs to treat severe bleeding induced by the thrombolytic agents.
anticoagulants, oral or heparin	Increased risk of bleeding and hemorrhage. Heparin has been administered with thrombolytic agents to treat an acute coronary arterial occlusion. Monitor closely when concurrent therapy is prescribed.
antiinflammatory agents, nonsteroidal, aspirin,* sulfinpyrazone	**Inhibition of platelet aggregation may increase potential for gastrointestinal ulceration and bleeding. Avoid or a potentially serious drug interaction may occur.**
carbenicillin, dextran, dipyridamole, divalproex, ticarcillin	**These drugs inhibit platelet aggregation; if used concurrently with the thrombolytic agents, they may increase the risk of severe bleeding and hemorrhage. Avoid or a potentially serious drug interaction may occur.**
cefamandole, cefoperazone, cefotetan, plicamycin, or valproic acid	**May cause hypoprothrombinemia and inhibit platelet aggregation. Use of these drugs is not recommended because of increased risk of hemorrhage. Avoid or a potentially serious drug interaction may occur.**

*Low doses of aspirin have been given concurrently with thrombolytic therapy, especially with streptokinase. This combination is reported to decrease the risk of reocclusion, stroke, and death more significantly than streptokinase alone (*USP DI,* 1996).

- *anistreplase*. Slowly add 5 ml of sterile water for injection to the vial, aiming the stream of diluent at the side of the vial. The vial should be rolled, not shaken, to dissolve the drug. The reconstituted solution should be used within 30 minutes. Any unused solution needs to be discarded because it contains no preservative.
- *streptokinase*. Slowly add 5 ml of sodium chloride injection or 5% dextrose injection, directing the stream toward the side of the vial rather than into the powder. Do not shake the vial but gently roll and tilt it for reconstitution. Note that shaking may cause foaming and increase flocculation (small thin fibers). Then slowly dilute the entire contents of the vial to a total of 45 ml or, if necessary, up to 500 ml in 45-ml increments. The solution may be used if there is slight flocculation, but it should be discarded if it is extensive. If reconstituting for arteriovenous cannula obstruction clearance, use 2 ml of sodium chloride injection or 5% dextrose injection for each 250,000 IU of streptokinase. If solution is not used soon after reconstitution, store at 2° to 4° C, and use within 24 hours. Note that a client with a recent streptococcal infection may require a higher loading dose because of higher resistance levels.
- *urokinase*. For intracoronary arterial administration, add 5 ml of sterile water without preservatives (not bacteriostatic water) for injection to each of three 250,000 IU vials immediately before use. Roll and tilt, but do not shake for reconstitution. Further dilute by adding the 500 ml of 5% dextrose solution to the three vials to make a solution of 5000 IU/ml. For intravenous infusion, see the manufacturer's instructions. For IV catheter clearance (for the 250,000 IU size only), add 5 ml of sterile water (without preservatives) to the vial. Add 1 ml of the reconstituted solution to 9 ml of sterile water for injection to make a solution of 5000 IU/ml. Discard the unused portion of the reconstituted material.

Do not add any other medication to the container of alteplase, anistreplase, streptokinase, or urokinase solution or administer other medications through the same intravenous line. Do not administer by intramuscular injection because of the danger of hematoma. In addition, use venipuncture sites as seldom as possible, and perform this procedure with care. Maintain pressure dressings at the site for at least 30 minutes, and check frequently for bleeding.

Start thrombolytic therapy as soon as possible after the thrombotic event: coronary thrombosis, 3 to 4 hours; arterial thrombus, 3 days; deep vein thrombosis, 3 to 4 days; and pulmonary embolus, 5 to 7 days. If after 4 hours of therapy thrombin time is less than one and one-half times the normal control value, discontinue therapy. Administer using a constant infusion pump.

For arteriovenous cannula occlusion, administer heparinized saline solution to clear the cannula. If adequate flow is not reestablished, use streptokinase.

To prevent bruising during therapy, avoid unnecessary handling of client. The side rails of the client's bed should be padded.

After completion of thrombolytic therapy, begin continuous intravenous infusion of heparin (without a loading dose) when thrombin time has decreased to less than twice the normal control value (usually within 4 hours after completion of the infusion). Use an infusion pump for heparin. Later give the client oral anticoagulant therapy, a procedure that prevents the recurrence of thrombosis.

Evaluation. When used for the emergency treatment of coronary artery thrombosis, the client will experience cessation of chest pain, improved ECG values, and absence of coronary occlusion upon cardiac catheterization. When administered for treatment of venous thrombosis, pulmonary embolism, and arterial thrombosis and embolism, the client will demonstrate increased tissue perfusion evidenced by absence of ischemic pain, return of normal peripheral pulses, good capillary refill; and for pulmonary embolus, normal blood gases and lung scan.

ANTIHEMOPHILIC AGENTS

Hemophilia is a hereditary disorder caused by a deficiency of one or more plasma protein clotting factors. This condition usually leads to persistent and uncontrollable hemorrhage after even minor injury. The symptoms include excessive bleeding from wounds and hemorrhage into joints, the urinary tract, and on occasion the central nervous system. There are two types of hemophilia: hemophilia A, the classic type, in which factor VIII activity is deficient, and hemophilia B, or Christmas disease, in which factor IX complex activity is deficient. In recent years a correct diagnosis of the coagulation disorder has led to specific factor replacement therapy, and this medical advance has resulted in effective management of the client at home.

factor VIII (Koate-HP, Recombinate)

Factor VIII or the antihemophilic factor (AHF) is a glycoprotein necessary for hemostasis and blood clotting. In the intrinsic pathway of the coagulation mechanism, the antihemophilic factor is required for the transformation of prothrombin to thrombin. In the treatment or prevention of hemophilia A, factor VIII administration is based on replacing the missing plasma clotting factor to control and prevent bleeding.

When administered intravenously, factor VIII has a distribution half-life of 2.4 to 8 hours and an elimination half-life of 8.4 to 19.3 hours. Time to peak effect is between 1 to 2 hours after IV administration. Mild to severe allergic reactions have been reported, such as bronchospasm, elevated temperature, chills, or rash. Other side/adverse effects, which may be related to the rate of infusion, include headache, increased heart rate, tingling of fingers, fainting, lethargy, sedation, hypotension, back pain, nausea or vomiting, visual disturbances, and chest constriction. No significant drug interactions are reported with factor VIII.

Dosage of factor VIII must be individualized according to the client's weight, severity of the deficiency, and the amount of blood loss. During hemorrhage the dosage is adjusted so that a level of 25% of normal levels of factor VIII can produce hemostasis. Clients who develop inhibitors to factor VIII may not respond to factor VIII therapy. After careful evaluation of the client, the administration of antiinhibitor coagulant complex, which reduces factor VIII inhibitors, may be indicated to correct this condition.

Two recombinant DNA–derived factor VIII preparations (Recombinate and Kogenate) were marketed in 1993. Before these products, concentrates were prepared from donor plasma pools; thus some concentrates have been the source of transmission of various viruses, such as hepatitis, HIV, and others. The recombinant products are essentially free of viruses because they are prepared by genetic engineering in a controlled laboratory setting. They appear to be as effective as the plasma source concentrates, although presently they are much more expensive than the other products (Abramowicz, 1993).

■ Nursing Management

Factor VIII Therapy

Assessment. Obtain baseline values of coagulation studies and vital signs before administering antihemophilic factor. If the pulse increases significantly, reduce the rate of the administration or stop the drug.

Nursing diagnosis. The client may experience altered comfort (headache, dermatitis, chills, fever, back pain, nausea and vomiting) related to mild allergic reaction, and ineffective airway clearance (bronchospasm) also related to allergic response.

Implementation

Monitoring. Monitor vital signs over the course of the drug's administration. Adverse effects are related to the rate of administration. Slow the rate of flow or stop the infusion until the symptoms of flushing, headache, and alterations of blood pressure and pulse disappear. Periodic coagulation studies will determine the efficacy of the drug with each client.

Intervention. Refrigerate the concentrate until ready for use, but do not freeze it. Do not refrigerate after reconstitution, since the active ingredient may precipitate. Warm the concentrate and diluent to room temperature before reconstitution. Gently rotate (do not shake) the vial containing the concentrate and diluent until it is completely dissolved. This may take as long as 5 to 10 minutes. Because the antihemophilic factor is filtered before administration, the active components would be filtered out if it is not fully dissolved. Although antihemophilic factor remains stable for 24 hours at room temperature after reconstitution, it should be used within 3 hours. Do not mix it with other medications.

Antihemophilic factor is for intravenous infusion only. Use only plastic syringes to prepare for administration, since the solution adheres to the ground surfaces of glass syringes.

Education. Instruct the client to wear a Medic Alert ID to alert medical personnel in an emergency situation that factor VIII may be required.

Evaluation. The client's clotting tests will be within the normal range and the client will not experience any abnormal bleeding.

antiinhibitor coagulant complex (Autoplex, Feiba VH Immuno)

Antiinhibitor coagulant complex is made from pooled human plasma. It contains variable quantities of clotting factors and kinin system factors and has been standardized to help correct clotting time in factor VIII-deficient individuals or to treat factor VIII-deficient individuals who have plasma-containing inhibitors to factor VIII.

Antiinhibitor coagulant complex is indicated for clients with factor VIII inhibitors who are bleeding or if they are being prepared for surgery. Approximately 10% of factor VIII-deficient individuals have inhibitors to factor VIII present. Clients with factor VIII inhibitor levels greater than 10 Bethesda units are usually treated with this product.

Allergic reactions and hypersensitivity (fever, chills, rash, hypotension) reactions have been reported. If antiinhibitor coagulant complex is administered too rapidly, the recipient may experience flushing, headache, and changes in blood pressure and heart rate. These are indications to slow the rate of flow or stop the infusion until the symptoms disappear.

Concurrent administration with epsilon-aminocaproic acid or tranexamic acid is not recommended. Antiinhibitor coagulant complex is administered only by intravenous infusion. The recommended dose varies from 25 to 100 units/kg depending on the site and severity of the hemorrhage. Check current package insert or *USP DI* for specific recommendations.

In addition to the nursing management for factor VIII, weigh the benefits of the antiinhibitor complex against the risk of hepatitis associated with its administration.

Vaccinate the client against hepatitis B, as ordered, using hepatitis B vaccine inactivated. Because this complex is prepared from human plasma, the risk of transmitting hepatitis exists.

factor IX complex (Konȳne 80, Proplex T)

Factor IX complex is a purified plasma fraction prepared from pooled units of plasma. It contains factors II, VII, IX, and X, which are known as the vitamin K coagulation factors. This agent is used for therapy in individuals with a deficiency of these factors during hemorrhage or before surgery. It is also indicated for hemophilia B in which factor IX (Christmas disease) is deficient. Factor IX complex is used to prevent or control bleeding in individuals with factor IX deficiency. It is also used to treat clients with bleeding problems who have inhibitors to factor VIII and will reverse hemorrhage induced by coumarin anticoagulants.

Factor IX has an elimination half-life of 18 to 32 hours; time to peak effect after IV administration is 10 to 30 minutes. Side/adverse effects include chills and fever, especially when large doses are given. Also, if the intravenous infusion is given too rapidly, headache, flushing, rash, nausea, vomiting, sedation, lethargy, elevated temperature, and tingling have been reported. The infusion should be stopped; in most clients it can be resumed at a much slower rate.

Thrombosis and disseminated intravascular coagulation (DIC) have occurred as a result of the administration of factor IX. Myocardial infarction, pulmonary embolism, and anaphylaxis have also been reported. It should not be used in individuals undergoing elective surgery, since they are at a greater risk for thrombosis. No significant drug interactions have been reported to date.

Factor IX should be administered slowly by intravenous injection or by intravenous infusion. The dosage is individualized according to the client's coagulation assay, which is performed before treatment. Check current references for specific dosing recommendations.

■ Nursing Management
Factor IX Therapy

The considerations for factor IX therapy are the same as for factor VIII; only the instructions for preparation differ. Factor IX is administered intravenously or by intravenous infusion only, at a rate not to exceed 3 ml/min. Warm the diluent to room temperature before reconstitution. Gently rotate the mixture in the vial until it is completely dissolved, or the active components will be filtered out when it is administered through the filter needle. Although stable for 12 hours at room temperature, it should be used within 3 hours of reconstitution. Do not refrigerate the reconstituted preparation, since the active ingredients may precipitate.

The risk of hepatitis exists as for antiinhibitor coagulant complex because it is also derived from pooled plasma.

ANTIPLATELET AGENTS

The antiplatelet drugs or drugs that inhibit platelet aggregation include aspirin, dipyridamole (Persantine), ticlopidine (Ticlid), and abciximab (ReoPro). Aspirin inhibits cyclooxygenase, an enzyme necessary for thromboxane A_2 synthesis. As mentioned previously, thromboxane A_2 promotes platelet aggregation and vasoconstriction, and thus aspirin suppresses these actions (see Chapter 14). The other three drugs are discussed in this chapter.

The composition of arterial thrombi is primarily platelet aggregates; venous thrombi are usually composed of fibrin and red blood cells. Therefore the anticoagulant drugs are used to reduce the risks or complications of venous thrombi whereas the antiplatelet agents are used for arterial thrombi.

dipyridamole [dye peer id' a mole] (Persantine)

The mechanism of action for dipyridamole has been postulated to be inhibition of:

1. thromboxane A_2 formation, a potent platelet activator;
2. phosphodiesterase, which results in an increase in cyclic-3', 5' monophosphate in the platelets; and
3. red blood cell uptake of adenosine, a platelet aggregation inhibitor.

Dipyridamole is used in combination with coumarin anticoagulants for the prevention of postsurgical thromboembolic complications after cardiac valve replacement.

After an oral dose, dipyridamole reaches peak serum levels in about 75 minutes, is highly protein bound, metabolized in the liver, and excreted in bile. Significant side/adverse effects include headache, dizziness, abdominal upset, and rash. The usual adult (adjunctive) dose is 75 to 100 mg orally four times daily.

ticlopidine [tye kloe' pih deen] (Ticlid)

Ticlopidine is believed to produce an irreversible, adenosine diphosphate–induced inhibition of platelet-fibrinogen binding. It is indicated to decrease the risk of stroke in clients who have had warnings of a thrombotic stroke or those who have had a thrombotic stroke.

Administered orally, it reaches peak serum levels in about 2 hours and peak effect with repeated dosing in 8 to 11 days. It is metabolized by the liver and excreted by the kidneys. Significant side/adverse effects include nausea, stomach cramps, bloating or gas, dizziness, skin rash, and diarrhea. Less frequently reported effects include bleeding, pruritus, neutropenia, agranulocytosis, thrombocytopenia, and purpura. Serum cholesterol levels have also reportedly increased by approximately 8% to 10% in persons receiving ticlopidine. The recommended adult dose is 250 mg PO twice daily with food.

abciximab [ab six' i mab] (ReoPro)

Abciximab, a monoclonal antibody fragment, inhibits platelet aggregation by binding or blocking the glycoprotein (GPIIb/IIIa) receptor involved in the pathway for platelet aggregation. It is indicated as adjunct therapy (to aspirin and heparin) for prevention of acute cardiac vessel ischemic complications in persons undergoing percutaneous transluminal coronary angioplasty or atherectomy (PTCA).

Significant side/adverse effects include major bleeding episodes and hypotension. The recommended adult dose is 0.25 mg/kg administered 10 to 60 minutes before the procedure. Maintenance dose by IV infusion is 0.01 mg/minute for up to 12 hours.

■ Nursing Management
Antiplatelet Agent Therapy

Assessment. Antiplatelet therapy is contraindicated for clients with hematopoietic disorders such as neutropenia and thrombocytopenia. Because these drugs prolong bleeding times, they are also contraindicated for clients with a hemostatic disorder, a history of bleeding within the last 6 weeks, or active bleeding, such as peptic ulcer or intracranial bleeding; or for clients with hepatic dysfunction, who may be prone to bleeding. Use with caution with clients who are at risk for trauma, surgery, or lesions that might bleed, such as intracranial aneurysm, arteriovenous malformation, or neoplasm; severe uncontrolled hypertension; and a CVA in the last 2 years. With dipyridamole, clients with unstable angina will experience an increased risk of myocardial ischemia, which may lead to hypotension, ventricular arrhythmias, and cardiac arrest. Hypotensive and asthmatic clients may have their conditions aggravated. With abciximab, clients over 65 years old, weight greater than 75 kg, and those with a failed percutaneous transluminal coronary angioplasty (PTCA), PTCA lasting more than 70 minutes, or a

PTCA within 12 hours of the onset of symptoms for acute myocardial infarction are at an increased risk for bleeding.

The client's current medication regimen should be reviewed for significant drug interactions. With dipyridamole and abciximab, all of the drugs listed on Table 31-5 plus the thrombolytic agents would result in additive bleeding effects, as well as the other antiplatelet agents. For ticlopidine, an increased risk of bleeding exists if the client is also administered cimetidine, anticoagulants, thrombolytic agents, or aspirin; antacids decrease its absorption.

A baseline assessment of the client receiving antiplatelet therapy should include ECG, a complete blood count including white cell differential and platelet count, and coagulation studies (ACT, APTT, and PT).

Nursing diagnosis. The client receiving antiplatelet therapy may be at risk for: altered comfort (headache [12.2% with IV dipyridamole], flushing, nausea, dyspepsia, and GI cramping); ineffective airway clearance related to bronchospasm (shortness of breath, dyspnea, wheezing); risk for injury related to dizziness (13.6% with dipyridamole); impaired skin integrity (rash [5.1% with ticlopidine], pruritus, or purpura); altered bowel elimination (diarrhea [12.5% with ticlopidine]); and altered protection related to neutropenia and thrombocytopenia. The potential complications of angina pectoris or its exacerbation (>19% with dipyridamole), bleeding, ECG changes, and arrhythmias.

Implementation

Monitoring. With ticlopidine, monitor the CBC every 2 weeks until the third month of therapy; monitor more frequently if the neutrophil count is declining or is 30% less than the baseline count. After the third month obtain a CBC only if the client has signs and symptoms of an infection.

With dipyridamole, monitor ECG tracings and vital signs, particularly the blood pressure.

With abciximab, platelet counts are recommended 2 to 4 hours after the initial IV injection and at 24 hours or at discharge, whichever comes first. Monitor also for hypersensitivity reactions.

All platelet aggregate inhibitor therapy should be discontinued if the platelet count is less than 80,000 cells/mm^3. Monitor the client for bleeding—epistaxis, hematuria, conjunctival hemorrhage, GI bleeding, excessive bruising, catheter insertion sites, arterial and venous puncture sites, cutdown sites, and needle puncture sites; coagulation studies should also be performed.

Intervention. Administer with food to minimize gastrointestinal distress. With abciximab, administration is with a continuous infusion pump with an in-line filter. Be aware that hypersensitivity or anaphylaxis may occur at any time during abciximab administration.

Education. With ticlopidine, advise the client on the importance of the routine blood testing and of any symptoms of infection that may indicate neutropenia, such as fever, chills, and sore throat, which should be reported to the prescriber. Symptoms of hepatic dysfunction, such as yellowing skin and sclera, and darker urine and lighter stools, should also be reported.

Advise the client on dipyridamole and abciximab to report any symptoms of chest pain, palpitations, or edema to the prescriber.

Instruct the client to apply direct pressure to the site if bleeding does occur and to seek medical attention for any unusual bleeding. Encourage the client to wear a medical identification indicating this medication and alert other health care providers that antiplatelet therapy is being taken. Other medications should not be taken without consultation with the prescriber.

Evaluation. The client will not experience any thrombotic episodes, such as stroke, and will not experience adverse effects of the drug.

HEMOSTATIC AGENTS

Hemostatic agents are compounds used to hasten clot formation to reduce bleeding. The purpose of these agents is to control rapid loss of blood.

Systemic Hemostatics

aminocaproic acid [a mee noe ka proe' ik] (Amicar)
Aminocaproic acid is a synthetic compound that inhibits fibrinolysis when excessive bleeding occurs. This drug acts as a competitive antagonist of plasminogen, therefore reducing the conversion of plasminogen to plasmin or fibrinolysin. To a lesser degree, it directly inhibits plasmin (fibrinolysin) by noncompetitive mechanisms.

It is used in the treatment of hyperfibrinolysis-induced hemorrhage such as fibrinolytic bleeding after heart surgery, prostatectomy, nephrectomy, and for hematologic disorders such as aplastic anemia, hepatic cirrhosis, and neoplastic disease states. Although not an approved indication, it has also been used as a specific antidote for an overdose of thrombolytic drugs.

Aminocaproic acid is absorbed orally and reaches a peak concentration within 2 hours. The therapeutic serum concentration is 130 μg/ml to inhibit systemic hyperfibrinolysis, or 150 to 300 μg/ml to prevent recurrent subarachnoid hemorrhage. It is excreted mainly by the kidneys. Side effects reported with this drug include nausea, diarrhea, menstrual difficulties, and increased weakness. Adverse reactions include weakness or severe muscle pain; a decrease in urination; edema of face, feet, or lower legs; unusual weight gain; slow or irregular heart rate; abdominal pain; rash; stuffy nose; tinnitus; bloodshot eyes; and thrombosis.

The adult recommended dose is 5 g orally or parenterally (IV infusion) initially, followed by 1 g/hour for up to 8 hours or until the desired response is achieved. Maximum dose is 30 g/24 hours. The pediatric dose (oral or parenteral) is 100 mg/kg body weight the first hour, followed by 33.3 mg/kg/hour up to 18 g/m^2/24 hours.

■ Nursing Management

Aminocaproic Acid Therapy

Assessment. Aminocaproic acid is contraindicated for use in clients with active intravascular clotting because of the risk of serious thrombus formation. It is used cautiously in individuals with cardiac (may cause hypotension and bradycardia), hepatic (may make diagnosis of cause of bleeding more difficult), or renal disease (may accumulate) or those with a predisposition to thrombosis. Assess the female client's current drug regimen for estrogen or estrogen-containing contraceptives because they will increase the risk for thrombus formation if administered concurrently with aminocaproic acid.

Assess baseline vital signs and coagulation studies initially and periodically during administration.

Nursing diagnosis. With the administration of aminocaproic acid, the client is at risk for the development of the following nursing diagnoses: altered comfort (headache, myopathy, tinnitus, stuffy nose, rash, nausea, abdominal cramping, or unusual menstrual cramping); altered bowel elimination (diarrhea); altered urinary pattern related to bladder obstruction caused by blood clot formation; fatigue; sexual dysfunction (dry ejaculation); risk for injury related to hypotension; and the potential complications of renal failure (sudden decrease in urinary output, edema) or thromboembolism (sudden headache, pains in chest, groin, or legs, sudden shortness of breath, slurred speech, vision changes, or weakness of arm or leg).

Implementation

Monitoring. Monitor client for signs of thromboembolic complications such as thrombophlebitis, pulmonary embolus, myocardial infarction, and cerebrovascular accident. Monitor for the signs and symptoms of the above nursing diagnoses. Aminocaproic acid therapy is usually discontinued when the bleeding stops or when lab values of fibrinolysis indicate the drug is no longer necessary.

Intervention. Dilute before administering intravenously. However, dilution with sterile water for injection is not recommended for clients with subarachnoid hemorrhage. Administer slowly, since too rapid infusion may result in hypotension or bradycardia. Take care with insertion and positioning of the infusion needle to minimize thrombophlebitis.

Education. Inform the client of the purpose of the medication and subjective symptoms to report, such as headache, dizziness, tinnitus, and abdominal cramping.

Evaluation. The client's laboratory values for fibrinolysis will be within normal limits and the client will have no signs of bleeding.

tranexamic acid [tran ex am' ik] (Cyklokapron)

Tranexamic acid is a competitive inhibitor of plasminogen activation; at high doses, it is a noncompetitive inhibitor of plasmin. Its effects are similar to aminocaproic acid but it is approximately 5 to 10 times more potent in vitro. It is used after dental surgery in clients with hemophilia to reduce or prevent bleeding episodes.

Peak plasma level is reached 3 hours after oral administration; peak plasma level is 8 μg/ml after a 1 g dose. Duration of action in serum is 7 to 8 hours, and excretion is by the kidneys.

Significant side/adverse effects include nausea, vomiting, and diarrhea. Visual disturbance, thrombosis, and menstrual discomfort have been infrequently reported. No significant drug interactions have been reported.

The oral adolescent and adult dose before dental surgery in hemophiliacs is 25 mg/kg three or four times daily, starting a day before the planned dental procedure. Clotting factors VIII or IX should also be given before surgery. Postsurgically the dose is 25 mg/kg orally three or four times daily for 2 to 8 days. By injection the dose is 10 mg/kg IV before surgery and 10 mg/kg postsurgically three or four times daily for 2 to 8 days. The parenteral postsurgical dose is usually reserved for persons unable to take the oral product.

■ Nursing Management

Tranexamic Acid Therapy

See nursing management of aminocaproic acid. In addition to those nursing measures, tranexamic acid places the client at risk for visual disturbances. For this reason ophthalmologic examinations (visual acuity, color vision, eye grounds, and visual fields) are suggested before and periodically during therapy. It is recommended that administration of the drug be discontinued if visual changes occur or if thromboembolic complications occur.

Tranexamic acid, as an intravenous medication, should not be administered at a rate greater than 100 mg/min, or the client may experience hypotension.

aprotinin [aye pro' tin in] (Trasylol)

Aprotinin is a proteinase inhibitor obtained from bovine lung that directly prevents fibrinolysis by inhibiting plasmin and kallikrein, an enzyme of the renal cortex. It is used in cardiopulmonary bypass surgery to reduce blood loss and the need for blood transfusions.

Significant side/adverse effects are rare but include allergic type reactions and anaphylaxis. The recommended adult dose is 10,000 KIU (1 ml) as a test IV dose first, administered at least 10 minutes before the loading dose. If no allergic type reaction occurs, all other dosages should be administered via a central venous line and no medications

Pregnancy Safety

Category	Drug
B	aprotinin, dalteparin, dipyridamole, enoxaparin, ticlopidine, tranexamic acid, urokinase
C	abciximab, alteplase, aminocaproic, anistreplase, antiinhibitor coagulant complex, antithrombin III, factor IX, heparin, protamine, streptokinase

Pregnancy safety is not established for warfarin and anisindione but they both cross the placenta and should not be used during pregnancy.

should be given in this line. See current *USP DI* or package insert for dosing recommendations.

■ Nursing Management

Aprotinin Therapy

Assessment. Determine if the client is allergic to aprotinin by history and/or test dose. The drug is contraindicated in first time CABG surgery. Assess the client's pulse, blood pressure, respirations, breath sounds, and skin for color, temperature, and other indicators of peripheral perfusion. A baseline ECG, renal and hepatic function studies should be done.

Review the client's medication profile to determine drug-drug interactions, such as heparin which with concurrent administration will increase the risk for hemorrhage.

Nursing diagnosis. The client receiving aprotinin has the potential for the following nursing diagnoses/collaborative problems: risk for injury related to hypotension; ineffective airway clearance related to asthma; and the potential complications of atrial fibrillation, myocardial infarction, congestive heart failure, arrhythmias, and allergic reactions.

Implementation

Monitoring. Continue to monitor the client by the indicators in the baseline assessment.

Intervention. After a loading dose over 20 to 30 minutes, a continuous infusion of 50 ml/hr is used. Administer other drugs through a separate line. Do not administer aprotinin in solution with heparin, corticosteriods, tetracyclines, amino acids, and fat emulsions.

Education. Inform the client of the purpose of aprotinin and any subjective symptoms that should be reported, such as palpitations and beginning dyspnea.

Evaluation. Clients receiving aprotinin will not evidence blood loss, and the pulse, blood pressure, and ECG will remain within normal limits for the client.

Topical Hemostatics

absorbable gelatin sponge (Gelfoam)

Absorbable gelatin sponge is specially prepared nonantigenic gelatin capable of holding many times its weight in whole blood. It is used in thin strips to control capillary bleeding and may be left in place in a surgical wound because it is completely absorbed in 4 to 6 weeks. It should be well moistened with isotonic saline solution or thrombin solution before it is applied to a bleeding surface. Its presence does not induce excessive scar formation. Sterile technique must be used to avoid infection.

When inserted into cavities or tissue spaces, the gelatin sponge reduces bleeding by acting as a tampon. The contact with the sponge damages platelets, liberating the thromboplastin needed for clot formation. This product completely dissolves within 2 to 5 days when applied to bleeding areas on skin or in the nose, rectum, or vagina.

It is indicated in surgical procedures as an adjunct to hemostasis when bleeding is not controlled by ligature or when such methods are impractical. It is also used by dentists to aid in hemostasis.

Insertion of the gelatin sponge in the prostatic cavity promotes hemostasis in open prostatic surgery. The gelatin sponge may provide a site for infection. Monitor the surgical incision and implantation site closely for redness, swelling, or discomfort, as well as for signs of recurrent bleeding.

No significant drug interactions have been reported. This product is available in different sizes and diameters. Application instructions and size depend on the area to be treated.

absorbable gelatin film (Gelfilm)

A sterile absorbable gelatin film (Gelfilm) is also available for specific indications, as in neurosurgery or thoracic or ocular surgery. When it is implanted in tissues, the rate of absorption could range from 2 to 5 months, depending on the site of implantation and the size of the film implanted. This product is useful as a dural substitute (neurosurgery) or to repair pleural defects during thoracic surgery.

absorbable gelatin powder (Gelfoam)

A sterile absorbable gelatin powder (Gelfoam) is also available to promote hemostasis. This powder can be made into a paste to control bleeding from bone areas when standard procedures such as ligatures are ineffective or not practical. It is also used to treat chronic leg ulcers and decubitus ulcers.

oxidized cellulose (Oxycel, Surgicel)

Oxidized cellulose is a specially treated form of surgical gauze or cotton that exerts a hemostatic effect but is absorbable when buried in the tissues. The hemostatic action is caused by the formation of an artificial clot by cellulosic acid. Absorption of oxidized cellulose occurs between the second and the seventh days following implantation, although absorption of large amounts of blood-soaked material may take 6 weeks or longer. Oxidized cellulose is valuable in controlling bleeding in surgery of organs such as the liver, pancreas, spleen, kidney, thyroid, and prostate. Its hemostatic action is not increased by the addition of other hemostatic agents. It should not be used as a surface dressing except for the control of bleeding, because cellulosic acid inhibits the growth of epithelial tissue. It also interferes with bone regeneration, so it should not be implanted in fractures.

No significant drug interactions are reported. Do not moisten it, and use sterile techniques in applying or inserting the cellulose. Serious adverse reactions are related to site of application, amount used, and pressure applied to blood vessel or specific area. Careful application and monitoring are necessary to reduce complications such as obstruction, necrosis, and stenosis. When used after nasal polyp removal or hemorrhoidectomy, a burning sensation has been reported. Headache, stinging, and sneezing may also occur.

microfibrillar collagen hemostat (Avitene)

This is an absorbable topical hemostatic substance that, when placed on a bleeding surface, will attract platelets and platelet aggregation in the area, forming thrombi. It is used as an adjunct to hemostasis during surgery when ligature or standard procedures are ineffective or impractical.

Adhesions, allergic or foreign body reactions, hematomas, or infections such as abscesses may occur. Monitor the client closely because these conditions may cause serious problems. No significant drug interactions have been reported.

Generally Avitene is applied directly on the source of bleeding in a dry form. Do not moisten or wet this substance, and do not resterilize it. Apply pressure over the area with a dry sponge for a minute or more. Use dry forceps to handle it because it will adhere to wet gloves or instruments. Do not use gloved fingers to apply the necessary pressure.

thrombin (Thrombinar, Thrombostat)

Thrombin is a hemostatic agent prepared as a sterile powder obtained from bovine prothrombin that has been treated with thromboplastin in the presence of calcium. Thrombin catalyzes the conversion of fibrinogen to fibrin. It has several additional mechanisms, which may include stimulating the release, reaction, and aggregation of platelets. It is used topically to treat capillary bleeding. It has also been used during various surgeries with absorbable gelatin sponge for hemostasis.

Febrile and an allergic type of reaction has been reported when thrombin was used for epistaxis. No significant drug interactions are reported.

Thrombin may be applied topically as a powder or solution. Concentration of the preparation varies with its use—see the package insert.

■ **Nursing Management**

Thrombin Therapy

Assessment. Ascertain whether the client is sensitive to bovine products.

Nursing diagnosis. The client may be at risk for infection and the potential complications of an allergic reaction and bleeding related to the ineffectiveness of the thrombin therapy.

Implementation

Monitoring. Monitor client for recurrent bleeding, infection, and allergic reaction.

Intervention. Do not inject thrombin into large blood vessels, since extensive intravascular clotting and even death may result. Sponge—do not wipe—all blood from recipient surface before applying the thrombin as a powder or a solution. If applied as a powder, thrombin may need to be pulverized with a sterile instrument before use. To avoid disturbing the clotting, do not sponge once the thrombin is applied. Thrombin may be used in association with absorbable gelatin foam. In this case the saturated sponge is applied to the bleeding area for 10 to 15 seconds to promote hemostasis.

Use the solution within a few hours of reconstitution or freeze and use within 48 hours.

Evaluation. The client will not evidence bleeding.

BLOOD AND BLOOD COMPONENTS

The bloodstream is the main mode of transport and distribution in the body. As such, it functions to deliver vital nutrients, water, and oxygen from the digestive and respiratory systems to all body parts. Wastes are retrieved for excretion by the bloodstream. In the kidneys, the bloodstream provides the hydrostatic pressure necessary to create urine as an excretory vehicle for those waste products. It conveys hormones from endocrine glands and enzymes, vitamins, buffers, and other biochemical substances to target areas. The bloodstream buffers and regulates the body's heat exchange processes by absorbing and transferring core body heat to the surface for dissipation, and it buffers the body's acid-base balance. The bloodstream also carries components such as platelets, blood cells, and antibodies to sites where a sudden need for these exists, as in hemorrhage, inflammation, or infection.

It creates oncotic or colloid osmotic pressure to regulate the volume of interstitial fluids. It also transports therapeutic additives such as medications, fluids, electrolytes, and nutrients to their respective sites of action.

Abnormal States of Blood Components

Normally, a thrifty bodily balance is maintained between the production and loss, attrition, or excretion of all components that comprise the bloodstream. Pathologic conditions result from a disturbance in production or an excessive loss or excretion of one or more components. Hemorrhage results in a generally impoverished bloodstream and may significantly alter many body functions. Impaired production or increased destruction of any one component may impinge on one or more functions. All this is a matter of degree. If the impairment is minor or is detected early, correction of the cause and replenishment by natural or therapeutic means may restore functioning.

Naturally harmful or foreign substances also may build up in the bloodstream when excretory systems fail (e.g., renal failure) or when metabolizing capabilities fail (e.g., liver failure). Some examples of abnormal states of blood components follow.

Depending on the individual's size and preexisting blood integrity, acute whole blood loss of more than 500 ml is manifested by signs of anemia. Chronic, gradual, unnoticed blood loss from gastrointestinal tract malignancy, ulcers, or hemorrhoids may be compensated for naturally, or iron deficiency anemia may develop. Signs of anemia usually reflect the true importance of red blood cell loss. Deficiencies in intake or functioning of certain essential nutritional elements may result in iron deficiency anemia or one of the megaloblastic anemias, which usually are caused by deficiencies in vitamin B_{12} or folic acid. A pathologic overabundance of erythrocytes can be compensation for long-standing hypoxia from pulmonary or cardiac disease, certain tumors, or polycythemia vera. Delayed or disordered production of erythrocytes (aplastic anemia) may result from disorders of the reticuloendothelial system, primarily the bone marrow, which is responsible for their systematic production. The bone marrow is particularly vulnerable to certain drugs, poisons, and antineoplastic agents. On the other hand, too-rapid destruction of erythrocytes can lead to hemolytic anemia.

Leukocytes also are lost in hemorrhage, but reductions in their numbers most often are associated with certain specific conditions. Each of the five types of white blood cells—neutrophils, eosinophils, basophils, lymphocytes, and monocytes—is associated with different disorders. For example, abnormally low neutrophil counts are associated with certain aplastic diseases, as well as with acute reactions to such drugs as sulfonamides, propylthiouracil, and chloramphenicol. Excessively high neutrophil counts primarily are found with bacterial infections, as well as with some inflammatory disorders, leukemia, and hyperplastic disorders.

Thrombocytes also may be present in inadequate numbers because of their rapid destruction, typically caused by idiopathic thrombocytopenia purpura. Conversely, excessive platelet counts are associated most often with hyperplastic disorders, iron deficiency anemia, splenectomy, and chronic inflammatory conditions such as tuberculosis. Other factors crucial to the clotting process may be absent in hemophilia and similar disorders.

Losses of the liquid portion of the blood can create dehydration problems, impede metabolic processes that function only through use of hydrogen or oxygen molecules, or subvert hydrodynamic and hydraulic processes.

In addition to hemorrhage, plasma proteins may be lost through burn wounds or wound drainage or may be insufficient because adequate available substrates such as amino acids are lacking. The results vary, depending on the type of plasma protein, and may include deficiencies in immune status, blood viscosity, or colloid osmotic pressure (oncotic pressure).

Replacement Therapies

Therapy to replace all or certain components of the bloodstream is a common practice in most health facilities. Since blood is considered a tissue, transfusions are technically tissue transplants. The usual treatment of choice is replacement of the sole blood component that is deficient rather than whole blood, since the body is better able to replace intravascular fluids than formed elements of the blood. Transfusing only the depleted blood fraction serves two other purposes: (1) it prevents the fluid overload in high-risk individuals such as the elderly and those with cardiovascular or renal disease, and (2) it more efficiently uses the remaining blood fractions for other clients' needs. Table 31-6 outlines indications for

TABLE 31-6 Indications for common blood component therapies

Component	Indications
Whole blood	Hemorrhage, hypovolemic shock
Fresh whole blood	Multiple transfusions, exchange transfusions; priming agent for hemodialysis machines (normal saline also may be used)
Packed red blood cells	Transfused when whole blood could result in circulatory overload
Deglycerolized or washed red cells	Transfused when hypersensitivity reactions are likely; as in immunosuppressed clients and those with history of reactions or extreme hypersensitivity
Fresh-frozen plasma (FFP)	Clotting deficiencies, especially factors V and VII; blood volume expansion in burns, shock, or protein deficiencies (believed to be overused for these deficiencies)
Plasma exchange (plasmapheresis): blood drawn off, cleansed, and components returned	Immune-related disorders: multiple myeloma, glomerulonephritis, systemic lupus erythematosus, rheumatoid arthritis, myasthenia gravis
Plasma expanders (Dextran—large polysaccharide polymer)	Temporary volume expansion in hemorrhagic shock states (sole use for Dextran 70 or 75); not a substitute for blood or plasma
Granulocytes	Granulocyte counts below 500
Platelets	Platelet counts at or below 20,000/mm^3
Cryoprecipitate (fresh-frozen plasma precipitate; contains factors I and VIII)	Hemophilia, fibrinogen deficiency, von Willebrand's disease
Antihemophilic factor (AHF) concentrate	Treatment of hemophilia; preferred over FFP
Factor VII	
Factor IX complex	Hemophilia B; deficiencies of clotting factors II, VII, X; coumarin overdose
Plasma protein fraction (PPF)	Hypovolemic shock; protein replacement; burns; adult respiratory distress syndrome, dehydration, and hypoalbuminemia; as additive to complement packed cells when necessary
Fibrinogen	When fibrinogen levels insufficient for adequate control of bleeding
Albumin	Blood volume expansion by oncotic pressure; prevention and treatment of cerebral edema
Gamma globulins	Exposure to hepatitis; to prevent complications of mumps

this therapy. When a client is to receive blood, the nurse is largely responsible for its safe administration.

■ Nursing Management

Blood and Blood Component Replacement Therapies

Assessment. Take client history regarding previous transfusions and the client's response to them. Report any history of an adverse reaction to the prescriber and the blood bank. Assess the client for adequacy of venous access. Gather baseline data about the client's blood studies and vital signs before administration and observe the general appearance and demeanor of the client.

Nursing diagnosis. The client is at risk for injury related to a hemolytic or allergic reaction (anaphylactic shock), volume overload (pulmonary congestion, circulatory overload), or response to aged blood (hyperkalemia).

Implementation

Monitoring. As administration begins, observe the client closely for reactions for 15 minutes or more while the flow rate is kept at 20 to 30 drops/min. Assess and record vital signs several times during the first 15 minutes. If reactions occur, stop the transfusion and administer prescribed corrective measures. Observe the client for the development of the following:

- Apprehension; restlessness; flushed skin; increased pulse and respiratory rates; burning sensations; fever; chills; dyspnea; chest, head, or back pain; shock—hemolysis (possible blood type incompatibility)
- Rash; swellings of the skin, face, or throat; pruritus; shock—allergic reaction
- Fever and chills starting 1 hour after administration and lasting up to 10 hours—febrile reaction
- Nausea, weakness, jaundice considerably later—possible viral hepatitis
- Fever and chills, hypotension, vomiting, abdominal pain, bloody diarrhea—bacterial contamination
- Dyspnea, tight chest, cough with basilar rales, pulmonary edema—circulatory overload
- Cyanosis, dyspnea, abrupt onset of localized pain, shock—air embolism

Frequent assessment of the needle insertion site is essential because absorption of infiltrated blood is very slow. If no symptoms of reactions appear after the first 15 minutes, the flow rate may be calculated and set so that therapy is concluded in ½ to 2 hours (volumes usually are between 250 and 500 ml). Continue monitoring vital signs and observing for symptoms throughout administration.

Intervention. Administer blood components promptly to ensure that the transfused product is fresh, uncoagulated, and without toxic breakdown products. Before administration, the product should remain out of the blood bank's refrigerator and untransfused for no longer than 30 minutes. Refrigeration in the standard hospital units or home refrigerator will not prevent deterioration. Blood and blood components must not lie unused at the nursing station but must be returned to the blood bank refrigerator if administration has not started within half an hour. A unit of whole blood or packed RBCs cannot be returned to a blood bank if it has been out of a monitored environment (1° to 6° C) for more than 30 minutes. Whole blood or packed red blood cells should be transfused within 2 hours, 4 hours at the most.

Because incompatibility is a possibility, especially after multiple doses of these products, take precautions such as scrupulously comparing the product ordered with the label on the product before administration. Often the worst adverse reactions to blood transfusions result from misidentification of the blood or client. Although procedures of various institutions vary, at least two persons, often two registered nurses, must verify the identification of blood product and client. This will vary with the administration of blood products in the home (see the Home Health Care box below). Client identification must match, as well as

Home Health

Blood Component Administration

It is becoming increasingly common for whole blood, blood components, or expanders to be administered in the home setting. The administration of these substances allows for the restoration of blood volume or the replacement of serum, plasma, RBCs, platelets, or albumin in a more cost effective and comfortable environment for the client.

The client and caregiver(s) need to understand the purpose of the blood administration. Ask them if they understand the procedure and why it is being done. Assess the client's allergy history and ascertain any previous reactions to blood products.

Make the client comfortable in bed or in a reclining chair. Have the client void before the procedure begins. Check the blood bag information with the client identification with at least one other person. Check the bag for leaks. Select an appropriate site and perform the venipuncture using aseptic technique. See the discussion of nursing management for infusion techniques. Determine the drip rate per minute and time for blood completion. Administer the blood slowly for the first 15 minutes and monitor the client and vital signs carefully during this time. Monitor vital signs every hour while the blood is infusing; check the drip rate every 15 minutes. Assess the infusion site for infiltration. Assess the client for symptoms of transfusion reaction as discussed in the text. Change the blood tubing and filter if more than one unit is to be administered. Remove the intravenous needle or cannula after transfusion and ensure that it is intact. Document the procedure as described in the text.

If the client experiences any untoward symptoms, stop the transfusion and transfuse normal saline. Follow the health care agency protocols for emergency action. Stay with the client until the situation is resolved.

the prescriber's name, blood type, Rh factor, and unit number. Note the Venereal Disease Research Laboratories' (VDRL) information and expiration date. Compare the client's identifying armband or tag with the label on the container.

Nurses should be aware of transfusion hazards in certain blood-type combinations. Careful typing and crossmatching help to prevent serious complications. ABO antigen-antibody reactions result from the following and must be avoided:

Recipient's blood type	Should not receive
A	Type B or AB
B	Type A or AB
O	Any except type O

Recipient's blood type	Reactions with multiple transfusions
A	Type O
B	Type O
AB	Type A, B, or O

Immediately report to the blood bank any discrepancies between the information on the compatibility tag, the unit of blood, and the prescriber's order on the clinical record; blood that is past its expiration date; or any signs of contamination.

Hypersensitivity is also common, since most of these products are essentially foreign proteins. Exceptions include autologous transfusions collected previously from the client's own blood or transfusions of inert, synthetic products. Diphenhydramine (Benadryl) 25 mg, taken orally or injected into blood transfusion tubing before the transfusion is recommended to prevent mild allergic reactions.

Return the product to the blood bank or laboratory if the contents appear unusual because of discoloration, gas bubbles, or an overfull (gaseous) appearance. Mix the contents by gently upending the container once or twice; take care not to bruise or damage blood cells or other fragile components by squeezing or agitating the bag carelessly.

Note that many of these agents require the concomitant use of a 170-µg filter incorporated into the transfusion tubing to remove the debris and tiny clots found in the blood. Check the filter often to ensure that it is not clogged and slowing the transfusion. If the rate of transfusion is too slow, it may be necessary to use a filter with a larger surface area. This may also be necessary when administering packed RBCs because of the viscosity of the product. Access to the vein should be provided by a needle no smaller than 19 gauge and fresh tubing. For adults with small veins and for children, a 22- or 23-gauge needle is recommended. A normal saline solution should be hung in tandem with the blood product using a Y-set multiple lead tubing. Use the saline solution to flush the tubing before connecting it to the insertion site. Using straight tubing limits the possibility of stopping the transfusion while keeping the vein open if the client has an untoward response to the blood. Piggybacking on an established intravenous line increases the risk of contamination, especially with the administration of multiple units of blood. Change filter and administration set at least every 4 hours; do not transfuse more than 2 units per administration set.

Infuse approximately 60 ml of saline through the tubing before and after the transfusion. Do not use dextrose and other solutions with red blood cell products, since they may react with the product in the tubing to clump cells and cause hemolysis. When inserting the spike of the administration set into the port of the blood bag, guide it straight into the container to avoid puncturing the side of the bag. Note that infusion pumps intended specifically for maintaining transfusion rates are safe and reliable when used with appropriate tubing and filters. Raising the height of the container or applying a pressure sleeve to the bag (at pressures up to 300 mm Hg) is also useful to maintain transfusion flows at prescribed rates. Higher pressures may burst the bag.

To maintain the prescribed infusion rate, agitate the blood by inverting the bag frequently during administration. If a rapid transfusion is to be made through a CVP line, a blood-warming device (up to 37° C or 98.6° F) will be necessary. Do not administer any medications through the same tubing while any blood products are being infused.

Documentation should include the client's baseline vital signs before the transfusion was started; the signatures of the two persons who identified the client and the blood product; the blood product administered; the time the transfusion was started and completed; the total volume of fluid transfused, listing the starter solution separately; the client's response to the transfusion; and any nursing intervention taken in response to an adverse response to the blood.

Be aware that the risks of nursing personnel contracting diseases such as hepatitis when accidentally injected with pooled blood, especially repeatedly, are not entirely known. Therefore take care when manipulating these products and their equipment. Use universal precautions.

If the client experiences any of the untoward symptoms discussed above, stop the transfusion; infuse normal saline. Notify the prescriber. Continue to monitor vital signs, monitor intake and output, observe the client, and follow the health agency's emergency measures. Obtain a blood sample and first voided urine specimen after the reaction.

Education. Explain the transfusion procedure to the client, especially the reason why it has been ordered. Many elderly clients associate blood transfusion with being critically ill and may be upset about the need for a blood transfusion. Ensure that a consent form for the procedure has been signed (Box 31-2).

Instruct the client to report any symptoms of an adverse reaction, such as nausea, chills, burning sensations, or headache.

Evaluation. The client will experience increased hemoglobin and hematocrit levels. One unit of whole blood typically raises the average adult's hemoglobin level by 1 to 1.5 g/dl and the hematocrit by 2% to 3%.

BOX 31-2

Legal Implications: Consent for Transfusion

The law is clear that ordinarily a physician has the sole and exclusive right to obtain his or her client's informed consent to surgery. However, who bears the responsibility to obtain the client's informed consent to a blood transfusion? Whose duty is it to apprise the client of all of the risks attendant to the transfusion of donated blood? Must the client be informed that there are several options, including donations from "anonymous" sources, direct donations (usually from family or friends), or an autologous donation (in which the client donates blood before surgery) for use during surgery?

In *Jones v. Philadelphia Coll. of Osteo. Med.* (813 F. Supp. 1125-PA [1993]) informed consent was at issue. On October 6, 1986, J. Jones was admitted to the hospital by his primary treating physician to undergo a lumbar myelogram to diagnose the cause of his severe low back pain. Following this examination his physician recommended surgery in order to alleviate his condition. During surgery Mr. Jones lost blood and received 9 units of packed cells and 2 units of fresh frozen plasma. One of the units of fresh frozen plasma came from an "anonymous" donor who was infected with the HIV virus. Before his transfusion Mr. Jones was never advised by the physicians or the hospital of the potential risk of contracting AIDS as a result of the use of contaminated blood products. He brought suit against the hospital and physicians involved in the surgery, alleging that he received HIV-contaminated blood during the surgery.

The United States District Court for the Eastern District of Pennsylvania held that informed consent was necessary for blood transfusions. The law of Pennsylvania is that consent is valid only if the individual grants it after being fully apprised of such important matters as the nature of the therapy, the seriousness of the situation, the disease and organs involved, and the potential results of the treatment. In determining whether a client's consent was "informed," the standard is whether the physician disclosed all the facts, risks, and alternatives that a reasonable person in the situation would deem significant. In this state the doctrine of informed consent is limited to cases involving surgery or operative procedures. However, the Court held that a physician cannot inform a client of all of the risks of a surgical procedure without also informing him or her of the risks associated with blood transfusion when transfusion is a potential part of the procedure.

Although the Court held that only the primary treating physician could be held liable for failure to obtain informed consent, there was also a basis for liability on the part of the hospital. Because the hospital was bound by FDA regulations requiring it to obtain informed consent and because the hospital could also be held liable for battery (lack of informed consent) since it intended that the client come in contact with a foreign substance as a part of a planned procedure, the hospital had Mr. Jones sign two documents for informed consent for transfusion. In doing so the hospital "gratuitously undertook an obligation to obtain informed consent." Because of this the Court concluded that Mr. Jones may indeed have a valid claim against the hospital as well as the physician.

How would this knowledge of informed consent influence your nursing practice in relation to clients receiving blood transfusion?

From Tammelleo AD (Ed.) (1993). Must hospitals obtain "consent" for transfusions? *Reagan Report* 33(12):1.

SUMMARY

This chapter reviewed substances that concern anticoagulant therapy, thrombolytic therapy, and blood and blood component administration.

Anticoagulant therapy is primarily prophylactic; it acts to prevent fibrin deposits, thrombus extension, and thromboembolic complications by decreasing blood coagulability. Anticoagulants may be administered parenterally or orally. Heparin (the parenteral drug) acts immediately but has a short duration of action (less than 4 hours). Coumarin and the indanedione derivatives are administered orally; the onset of action is slow (24 to 48 hours) and the duration is long (2 to 5 days). This allows heparin and coumarin to be used in a complementary fashion. They may be started simultaneously, heparin being used when an immediate anticoagulant effect is needed, with its dosage being tapered off as the oral agent is producing its full therapeutic effect. In the administration of both types of anticoagulants, the client has potential for injury related to increased bleeding tendencies, so nursing care focuses on observation, protection, and education of the client to prevent injury. There are specific antidotes for both parenteral and oral anticoagulants: protamine sulfate is the antidote for heparin, vitamin K for the oral anticoagulants.

Whereas anticoagulants are used prophylactically, thrombolytic agents are used to dissolve clots in the treatment of acute thromboembolic disorders. Thrombolytic enzyme therapy with streptokinase, urokinase, alteplase, or anistreplase alters the hemostatic capability of the client to a greater extent than anticoagulant therapy; therefore when bleeding does occur, it is more severe and more difficult to control.

Hemostatic agents are compounds used to hasten clot formation to reduce bleeding and therefore control rapid blood loss. Aminocaproic acid, a hemostatic agent, has been used as an antidote for the thrombolytic agents, but this use is not approved.

The antihemophilic agents are specific factors within the clotting process that can be used in replacement therapy for clients who have a hemophilia, a deficiency of one or more plasma protein clotting factors. With accurate diagnosis of the specific missing factor, this replacement therapy has allowed for successful management of these clients at home.

Blood and blood components may need to be replaced as the result of impaired production, excessive loss, or increased destruction of any of the components. Since blood is considered a tissue, transfusions are essentially tissue transplants. The preferred therapy is replacement of the sole blood component that is deficient rather than whole blood. However, the nurse needs to be alert to the many responses that clients may have to such transfusions. Careful typing and crossmatching helps to prevent many serious complications, but careful observation of the client is essential during transfusion of blood and blood components.

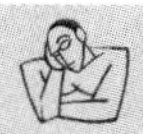

Critical Thinking

1. Mary Brickland, age 58, is admitted to a general medical unit for the treatment of acute thrombophlebitis in her right calf. Strict bed rest and heparin 5000 U by IV bolus followed by 1000 U/hr are prescribed. Why would heparin be the anticoagulant of choice? How would you best monitor the effectiveness of the heparin therapy?

   In preparation for discharge, the prescriber adds coumadin to Ms. Brickland's medication regimen. How will this affect her response to the heparin therapy?
2. George Thomas, age 45, has been admitted to the emergency department with an acute myocardial infarction. In the brief medical history that was obtained, it was determined that Mr. Thomas was seeing his primary care physician for an active peptic ulcer for which he was taking antacids and cimetidine. The ED physician decides to administer streptokinase IV. What will be of major concern for the client's safety? What assessments will he require to monitor his condition?
3. What is the informed consent policy for the transfusion of blood products within your practice setting? What part do you play in this policy as a nursing student? What will your role be as a graduate nurse?

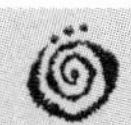

Collaborative Learning Activities

1. The students will have 10 minutes to review the first part of the case study on p. 579 and write answers to questions 1 and 2. Share solutions. The students will respond to question 3 and incorporate appropriate nursing interventions. The students will write answers to questions 4 and 5. Share these answers.
2. Write the 7 groups of symptoms on p. 594 on separate slips of paper. The class will be divided into seven teams and each team will be given a slip of paper with a group of symptoms. Each team will determine the adverse reaction described and what nursing interventions they would take in response to their assigned adverse reaction.

BIBLIOGRAPHY

Abramowicz M (Ed.) (1993a). Recombinant antihemophilic factor, *Med Lett* 35(898):51.

Abramowicz M (Ed.) (1993b). Enoxaparin: A low-molecular-weight heparin, *Med Lett* 35(903):75.

Abramowicz M (Ed.) (1993). Ticlopidine for prevention of stroke, *Med Lett* 34(874):65.

Agnelli G (1995). Anticoagulation in the prevention and treatment of pulmonary embolism, *Chest* 107(1 Suppl):39S-44S.

American Association for Critical Care Nurses (1990). Nationwide practice survey results announced, *AACN News* Aug:3.

American Hospital Formulary Service (1996). *AFHS drug information '96*. Bethesda, MD: American Society of Hospital Pharmacists.

Anderson KN, et al. (Eds.) (1994). *Mosby's medical, nursing, & allied health dictionary* (4th ed.). St Louis: Mosby.

Aragon D & Martin M (1993). What you should know about thrombolytic therapy for acute MI, *Amer J Nurs* 93(9):24.

Bick RL & Strauss J (1995). Thrombolytic therapy and its uses, *Lab Med* 26(5):330-7.

Burns D (1993). Review of thrombolytic use in acute myocardial infarction, pulmonary embolism, and cerebral thrombosis, *Crit Care Nurs Q* 15(4):1.

Clem JR. (1995). Pharmacotherapy of ischemic heart disease, *AACN* 6(3):404-17, 493-4.

Danek GD & Noris EM (1992). Pediatric IV catheters: Efficacy of saline flush, *Pediatr Nurs* 18(2):111.

Do benefits of antiplatelet and fibrinolytic drugs really outweigh risks? (1992). *Amer J Nurs* 92(7):45.

Dunn SM & Senerchia CB (1993). Bleeding complications in the patient with cardiac disease following thrombolytic and anticoagulant therapies, *Crit Care Nurs Clin North Amer* 5(3):511-23.

Fry B (1992). Intermittent heparin flushing protocols: A standardization issue, *J Intrav Nurs* 15(3):160.

Gilman AG, et al. (Eds.) (1990). *Goodman and Gilman's the pharmacological basis of therapeutics* (8th ed.). New York: Macmillan.

Gonterman R, Kiracofe S, & Owens P (1994). Administering, documenting, and tracking blood products and volume expanders, *MEDSURG Nurs* 3(4):269-76.

Jaffee MS & Skidmore-Roth L (1988). *Home health nursing care plans*. St Louis: Mosby.

Kleiber C et al. (1993). Heparin vs. saline for peripheral IV locks in children, *Pediatr Nurs* 19(4):405.

Majoros KA (1993). Comparisons and controversies in clot buster drugs, *Crit Care Nurs Q* 16(2):46-69.

McAllister CC et al. (1993). Changing from heparin to saline flush solutions: A research utilization model for implementation, *Emerg Nurs* 19(4):306.

McCloskey JC & Bulechek GM (Eds.) (1996). *Nursing interventions classification (NIC)*. St Louis: Mosby.

McMullen A, et al. (1993). Heparinized saline or normal saline as a flush solution in intermittent intravenous lines in infants and children, *MCN* 18(2):78.

National Blood Resource Education Program's Nursing Education Working Group (1991). Transfusion nursing: Trends and practices for the '90s, *Amer J Nurs* 91(6):42.

Olin BR (Ed.) (1996). *Facts and comparisons*. St Louis: Facts and Comparisons.

Pagana KD & Pagana TJ (1997). *Mosby's diagnostic and laboratory test reference* (3rd ed.). St Louis: Mosby.

Peterson FY & Kirshoff KT (1991). Analysis of the research about heparinized versus nonheparinized intravascular lines, *Heart & Lung* 20(6):631.

Tootill DM (1995). Thrombolytic therapy: Nursing strategies for successful outcomes, *Prog Cardiovasc Nurs* 10(1):3-12.

Turpie AGG (1995). Management of deep vein thrombosis: Prevention and treatment, *P & T Journal* 20(6S):7S-15S.

United States Pharmacopeial Convention (1996). *USP DI: Drug information for the health care professional* (16th ed.). Rockville, MD: The Convention.

Workman ML (1994). Anticoagulants and thrombolytics: What's the difference? *AACN* 5(1):26-35.

Chapter 32

Antihyperlipidemic Drugs

Chapter Focus

A strong link exists between coronary artery disease and elevated plasma lipoprotein concentrations. These elevated lipids, or hyperlipidemia, may develop as the result of high dietary fat intake, systemic disease, or genetic factors. The nurse needs to be knowledgeable about drugs that lower serum lipids, as well as factors that increase lipid levels, in order to provide appropriate information to clients to prevent the coronary artery disease that might result from hyperlipidemia. The following objectives and key terms are important for a good understanding of this chapter.

Key Terms

atherosclerosis (p. 599)
chylomicrons (p. 599)
high-density lipoproteins (HDLs) (p. 599)
hyperlipidemia (p. 599)
lipoprotein (p. 599)
low-density lipoproteins (LDLs) (p. 599)
very low-density lipoproteins (VLDLs) (p. 599)

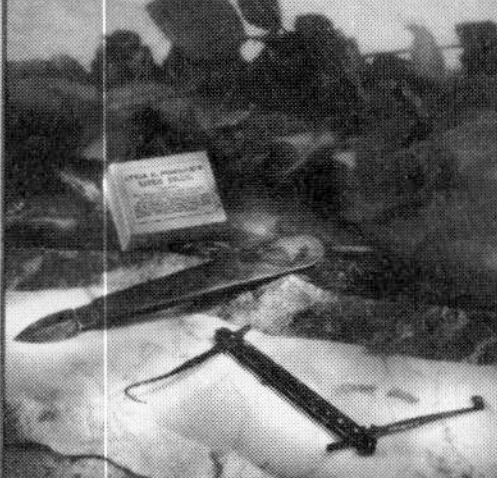

Key Drugs [▲]

cholestyramine
lovastatin

Objectives

1. Define hyperlipidemia and describe the pathophysiology of this condition.
2. Identify the four types of lipoprotein and differentiate them according to their lipid content.
3. Discuss the importance of combining dietary modifications with drug therapy to treat hyperlipidemia.
4. Implement nursing management of the care of clients receiving antihyperlipidemic agents.

Hyperlipidemia is a metabolic disorder characterized by increased concentrations of cholesterol and triglycerides, two of the major serum lipids in the body. Antihyperlipidemic or antilipidemic drugs are used along with dietary modifications to treat hyperlipidemia. Clinical and experimental studies offer evidence that an important relationship exists between high levels of circulating triglycerides and cholesterol and atherosclerosis. **Atherosclerosis,** a disorder that involves large- and medium-sized arteries, is characterized by lipid deposits in the lining of the blood vessels, eventually producing degenerative changes and obstructing blood flow.

Atherosclerosis is a causative factor in coronary artery disease (CAD), which may result in angina, heart failure, and myocardial infarction; cerebral arterial disease that results in senility or cerebrovascular accidents; peripheral arterial occlusive disease (which may cause gangrene and loss of limb), and in renal arterial insufficiency. It is also a factor in hypertension. Therefore there is intensive research to develop more effective and safer antihyperlipidemic drugs. If serum lipid or blood lipid levels could be controlled within normal limits, the development and progression of atherosclerosis might be inhibited or prevented.

HYPERLIPIDEMIC DISORDERS

Lipid compounds do not circulate freely in the bloodstream but rather are bound to plasma proteins (albumin, globulin), which act as carriers. These complexes are called **lipoproteins.** The lipoprotein has a protein shell and interior composed of a core lipid (cholesterol, triglycerides) (Table 32-1). Hyperlipoproteinemia is always associated with an increased concentration of one or more lipoprotein, particularly cholesterol.

Classification of lipoprotein. Lipoprotein complexes are classified according to their densities and electrophoretic mobilities. The three primary lipoproteins found in the blood of fasting individuals are very-low density lipoproteins (VLDLs), low-density lipoproteins (LDLs), and high-density lipoproteins (HDLs).

TABLE 32-1 Lipoproteins: core lipids and transport/function

Lipoproteins	Core lipid	Transports/function
chylomicrons	dietary triglycerides	dietary triglyceride
chylomicron remnants	dietary cholesterol	dietary cholesterol
VLDL	endogenous cholesterol	endogenous triglyceride
IDL	endogenous cholesterol & triglycerides	endogenous cholesterol
LDL	endogenous cholesterol	endogenous cholesterol
HDL	endogenous cholesterol	removes cholesterol

The **very low-density lipoproteins (VLDLs)** contain a large amount of triglycerides (50% to 65%) and 20% to 30% cholesterol, which are formed in the liver from endogenous fat sources. These lipoproteins contain 15% to 20% of the total blood cholesterol and most of the triglyceride found in the body (McKenney, 1995). Because these particles are quite large, they are not believed to be involved in atherosclerosis.

After secretion from the liver, the VLDL particles will in time become smaller particles as the triglyceride content is removed. Two enzymes, lipoprotein lipase and hepatic lipase are involved with triglyceride removal. The VLDL is eventually broken down into intermediate-density lipoprotein (IDL), which contains 50% each of cholesterol and triglycerides. About 50% of this substance is converted to the cholesterol-rich lipoprotein, or LDL. Therefore medications that increase the action of lipoprotein lipase will lower triglyceride levels.

The triglyceride depleted lipoprotein now is smaller and contains a higher quantity of cholesterol. These smaller remnant VLDL particles now include VLDL, IDL, and LDL. These lipoproteins can now be involved in the development of atherosclerosis.

The **low-density lipoproteins (LDLs)** contain the major portion of cholesterol in the blood and are considered to be the most harmful. They carry 60% to 70% of total blood cholesterol and elevated LDL levels suggest that an individual has a greater potential for developing atherosclerosis.

The **high-density lipoproteins (HDLs)** are the smallest and most dense lipoproteins. Their function is to transport cholesterol from peripheral cells to the liver where they are metabolized and excreted. Thus high levels of HDL are considered beneficial. The higher the HDL levels, the lower the potential risk for developing cardiovascular disease. This transport mechanism prevents the accumulation of lipids in the arterial walls, thereby providing protection against the development of coronary artery disease.

Chylomicrons are large particles that transport cholesterol and fatty acids from diet and/or the GI tract to the liver. This is known as the *exogenous* system of transport. The lipoproteins transporting cholesterol to and from the liver to peripheral cells are known as the *endogenous* system. Chylomicrons consist mainly of triglycerides (85% to 95%). In a normal person they are produced in the small intestine during absorption of a fatty meal and are cleared from the bloodstream by the enzyme lipoprotein lipase after 12 to 14 hours. A deficiency of the enzyme is rare, but when present it results in increased levels of chylomicrons, causing a disease called *exogenous hyperlipoproteinemia.* This condition is usually found in children, but it may also be induced by alcoholism. Therapy is aimed at keeping the diet low in fat.

Apoliproteins

Lipoproteins contain proteins on their surface called apoliproteins. These proteins have a number of functions that include helping the lipoprotein bind with cell receptors, activating the enzyme system, and providing structure for the lipoprotein. If apoliproteins metabolism is impaired, an

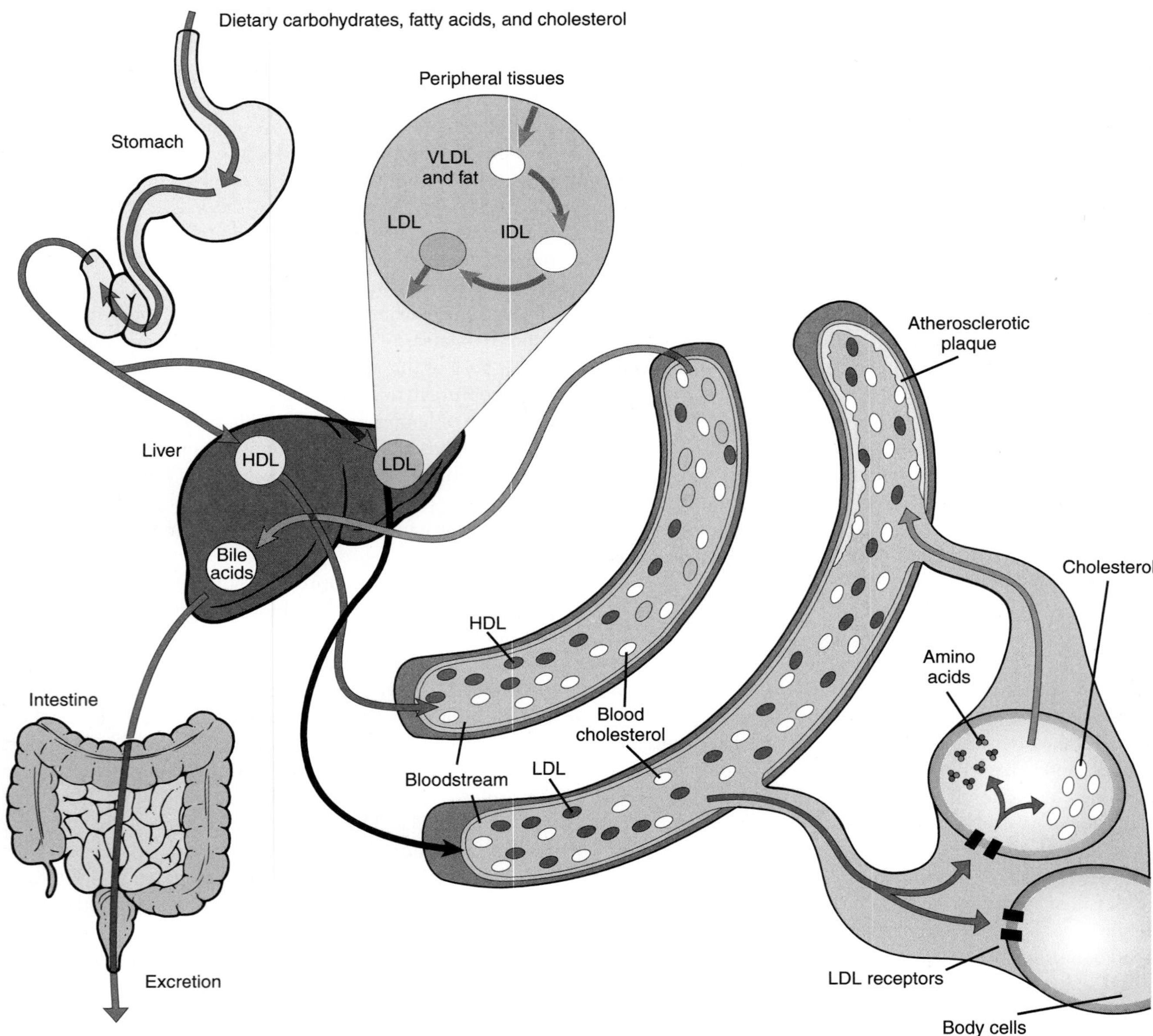

Figure 32-1 Dietary carbohydrates, fatty acids, and cholesterol: conversion sites and processes.

increased risk of atherosclerosis exists. Thus blood levels of apoliproteins are important in evaluating lipid disorders. The clinically important apoliproteins are A-I, A-II, B-100, C-II, and E. For example, a deficiency of the C-II apoliprotein in VLDL particles results in impaired triglyceride metabolism and hypertriglyceridemia. The quantity of apoliprotein B present is used to determine the number of VLDL and LDL substances in circulation. High levels of apoliprotein A-I in HDL correlates with a lower coronary heart disease association than HDL particles that have both A-I and A-II (McKenney, 1995).

Figure 32-1 reviews the normal lipid transport system. Dietary fats and cholesterol are orally consumed and transported into the system by bile acids; in the endogenous transport, the liver converts excess calories from carbohydrates and fatty acids into triglycerides. The liver ultimately produces both HDL or the "good" cholesterol and LDL or the "bad" cholesterol. The function of HDL is to carry about 25% of blood cholesterol to the liver, where it is processed into bile acids. Thus the cholesterol it carries is for ultimate excretion. LDL carries more than 50% by weight of cholesterol and this LDL-cholesterol combination can penetrate arterial walls, resulting in atherosclerotic plaques. Therefore, in excess it is referred to as the "bad" cholesterol.

Usually plasma lipoproteins are in a state of dynamic equilibrium because LDL needed to transport fats such as fatty acids and cholesterol is throughout the body. When cells outside the liver need cholesterol, they produce LDL receptors on their surfaces (see Figure 32-1). These receptors are necessary for LDL to enter the cell, where it is broken down into amino acids and free cholesterol. When the cellular need for

TABLE 32-2 Drug treatment for lipid disorders

Lipid disorder	Tests	Drug therapy recommendations
hypercholesterolemia	LDL TG <200 mg/dl	bile acid sequestering agent, niacin, or reductase inhibitor
hypertriglyceridemia		niacin, gemfibrozil, or reductase inhibitor
combined hyperlipidemia	LDL TG 200-400 mg/dl	niacin, reductase inhibitor, or gemfibrozil
low HDL (<35 mg/dl)	LDL } increased	niacin, reductase inhibitor, or gemfibrozil
	TG } increased	niacin, gemfibrozil, or reductase inhibitor
	alone, with CAD	niacin, reductase inhibitor

(Expert Panel, 1993)
TG, Triglycerides.

cholesterol is met, the production of LDL receptors stops and the excess cholesterol is discarded into the plasma. LDL receptors are also located in the liver where they function to monitor the plasma levels and LDL; and when the appropriate level of LDL is present in the plasma, the liver will suppress its production. This is essentially a feedback system that functions like a thermostat in the home; it maintains adequate plasma levels of LDL in order to provide cholesterol to body cells on demand.

Table 32-2 describes the approach for drug treatment of lipid disorders, as recommended by the Adult Treatment Panel II (Expert Panel, 1993). Dietary modifications are important in the treatment of high LDL-cholesterol levels.

Dietary management consists of a two-step plan. The Step I diet limits (a) saturated fat to 8% to 10% of total calories; (b) up to 30% of total calories obtained from fat; and (c) less than 300 mg of cholesterol intake per day. If adherence to the Step I diet does not meet the goal of lowering cholesterol, the Step II diet plan is instituted. The Step II diet limits saturated fat to 7% or less of total calories and cholesterol to 200 mg/day. Persons with CHD are usually started on the Step II diet. Dietary evaluation and consultation are highly recommended for the client. If dietary changes fail to decrease hyperlipidemia, there may be a genetic cause, which usually requires drug treatment; dietary noncompliance indicates the need for pharmacologic intervention.

Many drugs may affect serum levels of LDL cholesterol, HDL cholesterol, and triglycerides; Table 32-3 contains a listing of drugs affect on lipids.

Treatment guidelines. Treatment recommendations are based on the client's cholesterol level and the presence of CAD or two other risk factors, such as current cigarette smoking; hypertension; family history of premature CAD (i.e., myocardial infarction or sudden death before 55 years of age in father or other male first-degree relatives, or before the age of 65 in mother or other female first-degree relatives); male 45 or older, female 55 or older, or postmenopausal woman without estrogen replacement; low HDL cholesterol level (<35 mg/kl); and diabetes mellitus. A negative risk factor was added to the list: clients with an HDL cholesterol greater than 60 mg/dl would reduce their total risk factors by one.

Total serum cholesterol and HDL cholesterol should be evaluated in a nonfasting state at least every 5 years in adults 20 years and older (Table 32-4). As noted in Table 32-4, an

TABLE 32-3 Drugs' effects on serum lipids

Drug	Effect on lipids* LDL cholesterol	Triglycerides	HDL cholesterol
Beta-blockers			
nonselective	N/C	I	D
selective	N/C	I	D
Corticosteroids	I	I	—
Diuretics			
thiazides	I	I	I
loop	N/C	N/C	D
Ethyl alcohol	N/C	I	—
Oral contraceptives			
monophasics	I	I	I/D
triphasics	I	I	I

(McKenney, 1995; *USP DI*, 1996)
I, Increased; *D*, decreased; *N/C*, no change; —, unknown.

LDL cholesterol level of 130 to 159 mg/dl is classified as borderline/high-risk, whereas 160 mg/dl and over is considered a high-risk level. Assessment by a prescriber includes a clinical evaluation to determine if high LDL cholesterol levels are secondary to other risk factors or causes and also to evaluate for familial disorders.

The primary goals are as follows:

- Individuals without CAD and less than two risk factors, with LDL cholesterol levels >160 mg/dl, should receive dietary instructions and be reevaluated in 1 year. If such a person has an LDL cholesterol level >190 mg/dl, drug therapy should be initiated.
- Individuals with no CHD but with two or more risk factors and an LDL cholesterol level >130 mg/dl should receive a complete clinical evaluation plus dietary instructions. Further treatment will be based on evaluation findings. If the LDL cholesterol is >160 mg/dl, then drug therapy is indicated.
- Individuals with CHD and LDL cholesterol of >100 mg/dl receive dietary instructions; if LDL cholesterol is 130 mg/dl or over, drug therapy should be instituted.
- If a negative response to dietary alterations is noted, then drug therapy may be indicated.

TABLE 32-4 Cholesterol levels recommended by NIH

Risk	Total cholesterol (mg/dl)	LDL cholesterol (mg/dl)
Desirable	<200	<130
Borderline/high risk	200-239	130-159
High risk	≥240	≥160

Hormone replacement therapy with estrogen in postmenopausal women to reduce menopause symptoms and osteoporosis may have the benefit of also reducing the risk of CHD by up to 50%. Doses of estrogen (e.g., 0.625 mg conjugated estrogen or 2 mg micronized estradiol per day) may reduce LDL cholesterol by 25% and increase HDL cholesterol by approximately 15%. Clinical studies have not been performed to evaluate the risk-to-benefit ratio of estrogen; thus if it is used for its primary indications of treatment for menopausal symptoms or prevention of osteoporosis in women with hypercholesterolemia, the lipoprotein cholesterol levels should also be monitored to evaluate the potential additional effect of estrogen (McKenney, 1993).

The student is referred to the reference by McKenney (1993) and the Expert Panel on Detection, Evaluation and Treatment of High Blood Cholesterol in Adults (1993) for a detailed review of drug application, current drug application, and management.

Antihyperlipidemic agents offer the client a pharmacologic method for reducing serum lipid levels and ideally reducing the risk of atherosclerosis with its many complications. Use of antihyperlipidemic agents is reserved for clients who have specifically been identified to be at significantly increased risk and are unable to lower their serum lipid levels satisfactorily through exercise, diet, and other nondrug methods. Drug therapy for these clients augments the therapy aimed at lowering serum lipids and cardiovascular risk. See the box at right for Geriatric Implications.

Geriatric Implications

Antihyperlipidemic drugs

Dietary modifications and recommendations are vital to a successful lipid reduction program. When goals are not obtainable by diet alone, drug therapy should be considered.

The elderly often take multiple medications for their illnesses in addition to antihyperlidemia medications. Therefore the nurse should take a thorough drug history to determine if the client is taking medications that can increase lipid levels. For example, thiazides can increase triglycerides by 30% to 50%; nonselective beta blockers by 20% to 50%; ethanol by up to 50%; and so on (McKenney, 1995).

A common side effect, constipation (sometimes severe), has been reported in geriatric clients taking cholestyramine and colestipol. Encourage the client to increase daily fluid intake to help reduce the constipating effects of this drug.

Be aware that long-term use of cholestyramine or colestipol may lead to vitamins A, D, E, K, folic acid, and calcium deficiencies. Additional nutritional supplementation may be necessary (Long, 1990).

Administer the antihyperlipidemic drugs before or with meals (follow manufacturer's instructions) because the drugs are generally not effective if not administered with food. Lovastatin is often given with supper to obtain its maximum beneficial effects, because the highest rate of cholesterol production occurs from midnight to 5 AM (Long, 1990).

BILE ACID SEQUESTERING AGENTS

▲ **cholestyramine** [koe less' tir a meen] (Questran)
colestipol [koe les' ti pole] (Colestid)

Cholestyramine and colestipol are nonabsorbable anion-exchange resins that are also called bile acid sequestrants. These drugs are used for their cholesterol-lowering effects. Cholesterol is the major precursor of bile acids that normally are secreted from the gallbladder and liver into the small intestine. Here the bile acids perform two functions: they (1) emulsify fat present in food to facilitate chemical digestion, and (2) are required for absorption of lipids (including fat-soluble vitamins, A, D, E, and K). After their physiologic performance, the major portion of the bile acids is returned to the liver.

The anion-exchange resins bind bile acids in the intestine, thus preventing their absorption and producing an insoluble complex that is excreted in the feces. To compensate for the loss of bile acids removed by the drugs, the liver increases the rate of oxidation of cholesterol by converting more sterol to bile acids. Subsequently, the long-term fecal loss of bile acids causes a reduction of serum cholesterol levels and low-density lipoprotein (LDL) cholesterol.

Both cholestyramine and colestipol are used in the treatment of hyperlipidemia of the primary hypercholesterolemia. Cholestyramine is also used to treat pruritus induced by bile acid deposits in dermal tissues (from partial biliary obstruction). While not approved indications, cholestyramine is also used as an antidiarrheal agent for diarrhea caused by bile acids (not for common diarrhea), and as an antidote for negatively charged drugs and other medications (e.g., digoxin, oral penicillin, tetracyclines, and thyroid medication).

Plasma cholesterol levels usually decrease within 1 to 2 weeks after initiation of therapy. With cholestyramine, plasma cholesterol levels may continue to fall for up to a year. After the initial decrease, plasma cholesterol levels in some individuals may increase to previous levels or even exceed these levels with continued therapy. Close monitoring for effectiveness is necessary. Diarrhea induced by increased bile acids will respond to cholestyramine within 24 hours, whereas it usually takes 1 to 3 weeks of therapy before a response is noted in cases of pruritus caused by cholestasis.

Colestipol's peak effect is noted within 1 month. After the initial decrease in cholesterol, some clients may exhibit an increased cholesterol level that equals or surpasses the previous level.

After withdrawal of colestipol and cholestyramine, plasma cholesterol levels will increase in about 2 to 4 weeks. Pruritus will return in about 1 to 2 weeks after discontinuance of the medication. Side/adverse effects include constipation, indigestion, abdominal pain, nausea, and vomiting.

Dosage and administration. Cholestyramine is available as Questran and Questran Light (sugar free), powders for oral suspension. Adult dose is 4 g once or twice daily before meals; maintenance dose is 8 to 24 g in 2 to 6 divided doses daily as necessary. Pediatric dose is 4 g/day in two divided doses initially, then 8 to 24 g in two or more divided doses as necessary.

Colestipol adult dose is 15 to 30 g orally before meals in two to four divided dosages. Pediatric dosage has not been established.

■ Nursing Management

Cholestyramine and Colestipol Therapy

Assessment. Ascertain whether the client has a preexisting condition for which the drug would be used with great caution or contraindicated. The risk of cholestyramine and colestipol therapy should be considered in clients with constipation because it may induce fecal impaction. Because of its tendency to enhance constipation, it should be used with caution in individuals with medical conditions that could be aggravated by severe constipation, such as hemorrhoids or coronary artery disease. Use with caution in clients with peptic ulcer, gallstones, steatorrhea, bleeding disorders, and impaired renal function and with the elderly. Clients with complete biliary obstruction or complete atresia will have no bile acids in the GI tract to bind with cholestyramine and colestipol. These drugs are contraindicated for use in clients who have an allergy to bile acid sequestrants. Clients with phenylketonuria will be sensitive to phenylalanine in aspartame in the sugar-free preparation of cholestyramine. Colestipol is contraindicated in clients with primary biliary cirrhosis because it may further increase serum cholesterol concentrations. Safety of these drugs is not established for use by pregnant women and lactating mothers (see the Pregnancy Safety box on p. 605 for FDA classifications). However, the drugs are almost totally unabsorbed after ingestion and so there is the risk of impaired maternal absorption of vitamins and other nutrients.

The client's current medication regimen should be reviewed for significant drug interactions.

Drug	Possible effect and management
oral anticoagulants, coumarin, or indanediones	Concurrent use significantly decreases absorption of oral anticoagulants and vitamin K; thus anticoagulant effect may be increased or decreased. It is suggested that oral anticoagulants be given 6 hours before these drugs. Also monitor prothrombin times closely because dosage adjustments may be necessary.
digitalis glycosides, especially digitoxin	Half-life of digitalis glycosides, as well as gastrointestinal absorption, may be reduced. It is recommended that cholestyramine or colestipol be administered at least 8 hours after digoxin to reduce the potential for interactions. Also, if cholestyramine or colestipol is discontinued in a client also taking a digitalis product, monitor the individual closely for digitalis toxicity.
thiazide diuretics (oral), phenylbutazone, oral propranolol, oral penicillin G, oral tetracyclines, or oral vancomycin	Decreased absorption of these medications has has been reported. Give such medications several hours before or after cholestyramine or colestipol. Whenever possible, give these medications before cholestyramine or colestipol.
thyroid hormones	Decreased absorption of thyroid products is reported. Give thyroid first on the medication administration schedule, then give cholestyramine or colestipol several hours later.

Before cholestyramine and colestipol therapy the client should have serum cholesterol and triglyceride concentration determinations done as a baseline by which to evaluate therapy.

Nursing diagnosis. Be aware that clients receiving cholestyramine and colestipol are at risk for the following nursing diagnoses: altered bowel elimination (constipation in about 10% of clients, mild to severe, and possible fecal impaction); altered comfort (headache, belching, bloating, heartburn, nausea or vomiting, and abdominal discomfort); and the potential complications of gallstones or pancreatitis (severe stomach pain with nausea and vomiting), GI bleeding or peptic ulcer (black, tarry stools), or steatorrhea or malabsorption syndrome (sudden loss of weight).

Implementation

Monitoring. Continue to monitor serum cholesterol and triglyceride levels in relation to baseline periodically at regular intervals. (Table 32-5 gives a comparison of the antilipidemic effects of these drugs.) In addition, prothrombin-time values are recommended because vitamin K deficiency may occur with the chronic use of both drugs, which would put the client at risk for increased bleeding tendencies. With the chronic use of cholestyramine, serum calcium concentration should be monitored because of decreased absorption of calcium.

Monitor cardiac glycoside levels in clients receiving both drugs simultaneously. To avoid toxicity, adjust dosage of cardiotonic glycoside before discontinuing anion-exchange resin.

The client should be placed on a fluid balance record to monitor hydration and bowel status in relation to the drug effect of constipation.

Intervention. Administer the drug before meals. Mix powder by sprinkling it on the surface of 2 oz of a preferred liquid or semiliquid, such as cold beverages, hot cereals, thin soups (tomato, chicken noodle), or pulpy fruit (fruit cocktail,

TABLE 32-5 Summary of comparison of antihyperlipidemic effects

Drug	Effect on lipids*		Effect on lipoproteins			Typical response	Indications with diet control
	Cholesterol	Triglycerides	VLDL	LDL	HDL		
cholestyramine	−	0 or slight +	0 or +	−	0 or +	Decreases cholesterol 20%-40%	Type IIa
colestipol	−	0 or slight +	+	−	0 or +	Decreases cholesterol 20%-40%	Type IIa
clofibrate	−	− (greatest effect)	−	0 or −	0 or +	Lowers triglycerides; only slight decrease in cholesterol	Type III
dextrothyroxine	−	0	0 or −	−	0		Type IIa
gemfibrozil	−	−	−	0 or −	+	Decreases triglycerides; only slight decrease in cholesterol; increases HDL	Type IV
niacin	−	−	−	−	+	Decreases triglycerides and cholesterol 10%-20%	Types II, III, IV, and V
probucol	−	0 or +	+ or −	−	−	Decreases cholesterol 12%-25%; also decreases HDL	Type IIa
lovastatin	−	−	−	−	+	LDL cholesterol levels reduced 19%-39%, total cholesterol levels reduced 18%-34%	Types IIa and IIb

* +, Increased; −, decreased; 0, no change. Typical response was approximated with individual taking drug while concurrently on specified diet.

pears, peaches, or pineapple), to increase palatability of the drug. Allow the drug to sit on the surface of the liquid for 1 to 2 minutes before stirring vigorously to prevent lumpiness. Then add an additional 2 to 4 oz of diluent and shake vigorously again. Be sure the drug is thoroughly mixed, since it does not dissolve. Incomplete mixing of the dry form may result in mucosal irritation and esophageal impaction, or it may be accidentally inhaled. Rinse the glass or cup with a small amount of liquid and have the client drink it to ensure that the complete dose is taken.

Concurrent administration of a laxative or stool softener may help to prevent constipation. The client should also increase fluid intake to 2500 ml if not contraindicated.

Because resins interfere with absorption of other drugs when taken concurrently, administer the other drugs 1 hour before or 4 to 6 hours after cholestyramine or colestipol.

Education. Instruct the client in preparation of medication for administration as discussed above. Warn the client that sudden withdrawal of resins could lead to uninhibited absorption of other drugs taken concomitantly, resulting in overdosage or toxicity.

Usually, supplemental parenteral or water-miscible vitamins A, D, E, and K and also folic acid are prescribed to prevent vitamin deficiencies in clients receiving long-term therapy. Instruct individual to report early symptoms of bleeding immediately: petechiae, ecchymoses, bleeding from mucous membranes of gums or nose, or tarry stools (which indicate hypoprothrombinemia). Administration of vitamin K_1 (parenteral) and vitamin K_2 (oral) may be necessary.

Encourage the client to observe bowel elimination patterns and to adhere to a high-fiber diet (e.g., grains, fruits, raw vegetables) and an increased fluid intake as adjunctive therapy to the drug. If constipation occurs, dosage may be lowered to prevent fecal impaction, or a stool softener or laxative may be prescribed. Instruct the individual to report gastrointestinal symptoms to the prescriber: gastric distress, nausea and vomiting (pancreatitis), and unusual weight loss (steatorrhea).

Evaluation. The client will have a reduction of serum cholesterol and low-density lipoprotein (LDL) levels to within normal range. Drug is usually withdrawn if response is unsatisfactory after 3 months of therapy.

ADDITIONAL ANTIHYPERLIPIDEMIC AGENTS

clofibrate [kloe fye' brate] (Atromid-S, Claripex ♣)

The results of several large studies raise specific warnings concerning the use of clofibrate. First, there is possibly an increased risk of inducing malignancy and cholelithiasis in humans with the use of this product. Individuals taking clofibrate

Pregnancy Safety

Category	Drug
B	dextrothyroxine, probucol
C	clofibrate, gemfibrozil
X	fluvastatin, lovastatin, pravastatin, simvastatin
Unclassified	cholestyramine, colestipol, niacin

had twice the risk for cholelithiasis and cholecystitis that required surgery than nonusers. Second, there is no evidence of reduced cardiovascular mortality with its use. In fact, studies reported an increase in cardiac arrhythmias, angina, and thromboembolic episodes (Olin, 1996). As a result, the clinical use of clofibrate has declined tremendously.

Clofibrate is more effective in reducing very low-density lipoproteins (VLDLs) rich in triglycerides than in lowering low-density lipoproteins (LDLs) high in cholesterol. The exact mode of action of the drug is unknown although VLDL breakdown may contribute to its effect.

Clofibrate is indicated for the treatment of hyperlipidemia. It is slowly but completely absorbed from the intestines, is highly protein bound (96%), and reaches peak plasma levels in 2 to 6 hours after a dose. Peak effect with continued therapy is seen in approximately 3 weeks. A reduction in plasma VLDL concentrations is seen within 2 to 5 days. The half-life of this drug ranges from 6 to 25 hours for a single dose or 54 hours at steady state in normal healthy individuals. It is metabolized in the liver and gastrointestinal tract and excreted by the kidneys.

The side/adverse effects of clofibrate include diarrhea, nausea, muscle pain or cramps, fatigue, headache, weight gain, abdominal pain, gas, nausea, and vomiting. Adult dose is 1.5 to 2 g orally daily in two to four divided doses. A pediatric dose has not been established.

■ Nursing Management

Clofibrate Therapy

Assessment. A complete health assessment should be obtained to ensure that the client does not have a preexisting condition for which the administration of clofibrate would be contraindicated or entail risk. The presence of primary biliary cirrhosis precludes the use of clofibrate because the drug may further raise the serum cholesterol levels. Hepatic dysfunction may require a reduced dosage of clofibrate because protein binding of the drug is reduced but the half-life is not changed, which leads to increased side/adverse effects. With renal dysfunction the reduced protein-binding and clearance of the drug also leads to increased incidence of side effects, especially myopathy. Hypothyroidism may also predispose the client to drug-induced myopathy. Reactivation of peptic ulcer has been reported as well as an increased risk of biliary complications in the presence of gallstones with clofibrate.

Obtain a family health history as well; because of the genetic tendency of the disease, children and other family members should be screened for abnormal lipid levels.

As a baseline assessment, a complete blood count, liver function tests, and serum cholesterol and triglyceride levels should be determined.

Inquire if the client is pregnant. Strict birth control measures must be observed to prevent pregnancy and thus fetal damage. The drug must be withdrawn at least 2 months before conception.

Review the client's medication regimen to detect significant drug interactions. When clofibrate is given with oral anticoagulants, coumarin or indanedione-type, an increased anticoagulant effect is reported. Monitor prothrombin times closely because the anticoagulant dosage may need to be decreased significantly.

Nursing diagnosis. While taking clofibrate the client is at risk for the development of the following nursing diagnoses: altered comfort (nausea, vomiting, flu-like syndrome, headache, heartburn, and abdominal discomfort); diarrhea; altered mucous membranes (stomatitis); sexual dysfunction (decreased sexual ability); and the potential complications of myopathy (muscle aches or cramps); angina (chest pain, shortness of breath), cardiac arrhythmias, anemia or leukopenia (abnormal blood counts and signs of infection—fever or chills, cough, painful urination), pancreatitis or gallstones (severe stomach pain with nausea and vomiting), and renal toxicity (blood in urine, decreased urinary output, pedal edema).

Implementation

Monitoring. In addition to clinically monitoring the client for signs and symptoms of side/adverse effects, monitor complete blood counts for signs of anemia or leukopenia, and serum cholesterol and triglyceride levels for the drug's effectiveness. Because clofibrate may increase the risk of biliary diseases such as cholelithiasis and cholecystitis, appropriate diagnostic tests should be performed if signs and symptoms of biliary disease occur. In diabetic individuals the drug may produce hyperglycemia and glycosuria, so serum glucose levels should be monitored. Consult with the prescriber to withdraw the drug if any of the test results are abnormal.

Intervention. Administer drug with meals to prevent gastric distress.

Education. Before initiating clofibrate therapy, advise client to adhere to diet recommended by prescriber. The diet is usually low in fats, cholesterol, and/or sugars. Encourage weight reduction and physical exercise.

A decrease in serum lipid levels during the first and second months of therapy indicates a therapeutic response. Warn the client that a paradoxic rise in levels may occur in 2 or 3 months, but afterward a further decrease is customary.

Instruct the client to keep clinical appointments for laboratory studies and reevaluation by the prescriber. If serum cholesterol and triglyceride levels are not lowered within 3 months, drug therapy is usually discontinued.

Advise the client to report any flu-like symptoms (muscular aching, soreness, cramping). This condition may be remedied by dosage reduction. Instruct the individual to check with the prescriber about alcohol intake because alcohol may be restricted to prevent hypertriglyceridemia.

The client should be aware that there is no substantial evidence that the drug reduces the incidence of coronary artery disease or fatal myocardial infarction. Furthermore, increased incidences of cardiac dysrhythmias, thromboembolism, intermittent claudication, and angina have been reported in clients treated with clofibrate.

Evaluation. The client will evidence a reduction in serum lipid levels to within normal limits.

gemfibrozil [jem fi' broe zil] (Lopid)

Gemfibrozil is an agent that primarily decreases serum triglycerides found in very low-density lipoprotein (VLDL) and increases high-density lipoprotein (HDL). The mechanism of this action has not been established but it may involve an inhibition of peripheral lipolysis and a decrease in hepatic extraction of free fatty acids, which result in reduction of triglyceride production. In addition, the drug may accelerate turnover and removal of cholesterol from the liver, which is ultimately excreted in the feces.

Gemfibrozil is indicated for the treatment of hyperlipidemia. Orally, well absorbed from the gastrointestinal tract; reaches peak levels in 1 to 2 hours; onset of action in reducing serum VLDL levels is within 2 to 5 days; peak effect is seen in 4 weeks. It is metabolized in the liver and excreted by the kidneys and with the feces.

The side/adverse effects of gemfibrozil include muscle aches and cramps, nausea, vomiting, rash diarrhea, gas, and abdominal distress. When gemfibrozil is given with oral anticoagulants, coumarin or indanedione-type, an increased anticoagulant effect is reported. Monitor prothrombin times closely because the anticoagulant dose may need to be decreased significantly. If administered with lovastatin, an increase risk of rhabdomyolysis and myoglobinuria may result in acute renal failure. This has been reported in 3 weeks to several months of combined drug therapy. If possible avoid concurrent drug administration.

The adult dose is 1.2 g daily in two divided doses, preferably before breakfast and supper. Pediatric dosages have not been established.

Gemfibrozil has chemical, pharmacologic, and clinical effects that are similar to those of clofibrate. See the discussion of clofibrate for nursing management.

dextrothyroxine [dex tro thy rox' seen] (Choloxin)

Dextrothyroxine's mechanism of action as an antihyperlipidemic agent is not fully understood. Dextrothyroxine appears to act in the liver to increase formation of LDL and, to a greater extent, to increase the breakdown of LDL. The result is an increased excretion of cholesterol and bile acids via bile into the feces, which results in a decrease in serum cholesterol and LDL.

A definite relationship exists between thyroid function and serum cholesterol levels. Hypothyroidism is associated with high serum cholesterol levels, and administration of thyroid hormones lowers serum cholesterol. Dextrothyroxine apparently stimulates the liver to increase the rate of oxidation of cholesterol, and it promotes biliary excretion of cholesterol and its byproducts.

Dextrothyroxine is used as an adjunct to diet and other measures to reduce elevated serum cholesterol (LDL) levels in persons with no evidence of heart disease. Other antihyperlipidemic agents have replaced this drug because significant cardiac side effects are associated with its use. Dextrothyroxine is approximately 25% absorbed from the gastrointestinal tract; is highly protein bound with a half-life of 18 hours, and reaches its peak effect as an antihyperlipidemic agent in 1 to 2 months. Duration of action after the drug is withdrawn is 6 weeks to 3 months. It is metabolized in the liver and excreted by the kidneys and in feces.

The side/adverse effects of dextrothyroxine are rare and include nausea, vomiting, chest pain, abdominal pain, and irregular heart rate. Adult dose for antihyperlipidemic effect is 1 to 2 mg daily orally, increased monthly if necessary, to achieve desired effect. Maximum recommended dose is 8 mg/day. For children 2 yrs and older, the dose is 0.05 mg/kg daily, titrated monthly as necessary to achieve desired effect. Maximum recommended dose is 4 mg/day.

■ Nursing Management
Dextrothyroxine Therapy

Assessment. Do not administer drug to clients with cardiovascular disease, such as angina pectoris, coronary artery disease, history of myocardial infarction, cardiac dysrhythmias, congestive heart failure, or rheumatic heart disease, because of the risks associated with the increased metabolic demands caused by thyroid hormone administration. Dextrothyroxine should be used with caution for clients with liver or kidney disease, diabetes mellitus (may increase need for antidiabetic agent), or history of iodism. Use with caution with elderly clients, who may be more sensitive to thyroid hormones. Monitor therapy closely.

When dextrothyroxine is given with oral anticoagulants (coumarin or indanediones), depending on the thyroid status of the client, the anticoagulant effects may be increased or decreased. Monitor prothrombin times closely because oral anticoagulant dosage may need to be adjusted. If given concurrently with cholestyramine or colestipol, dextrothyroxine absorption is reduced, unless the dextrothyroxine is taken approximately 4 to 5 hours before or after these drugs.

Nursing diagnosis. Clients receiving dextrothyroxine should be monitored for altered comfort (headache, rash, itching, sweating, flushing); and the potential complications of myocardial infarction and angina (chest pain, shortness of breath), gallstones (severe stomach pain with nausea and vomiting), and hyperthyroidism (irritability, nervousness, insomnia, sweating, increased sensitivity to heat, weight loss, tremors).

Implementation

Monitoring. Serum cholesterol and triglyceride levels are determined for a baseline and then monitored every 2 months to determine effectiveness of therapy. Laboratory values will show that a decrease in cholesterol levels may not occur until 2 to 4 weeks after initiation of drug therapy; maximum decrease occurs about 2 or 3 months later. If response is inadequate after 3 months of therapy, discontinue drug. Vital signs and weight loss should be monitored at clinical visits to determine if hyperthyroidism is a problem.

With pediatric clients receiving long-term therapy, measurements of bone age, growth, and psychomotor development should be monitored periodically.

Intervention. Dextrothyroxine should be discontinued at least 2 weeks before surgery to reduce the potential for precipitating cardiac dysrhythmias during the operative procedure. In clients receiving digitalis, do not give more than 4 mg/day of dextrothyroxine to prevent danger of increasing myocardial oxygen requirement. Also, closely monitor the effects of both drugs.

Diabetes mellitus should be controlled if present. The drug may increase blood sugar levels, and therefore an increase in antidiabetic drugs or a decrease in dextrothyroxine may be required. Loss of diabetic control is noted by the following symptoms: glycosuria, polydipsia, and polyuria.

Education. Before initiating dextrothyroxine therapy, advise the client to adhere to the diet recommended by the prescriber. The diet is usually low in fats, cholesterol, and/or sugars. Encourage weight reduction and physical exercise.

Instruct the client to keep clinical appointments so that prescriber can check progress.

Advise client to immediately report the following side effects: chest pain, palpitation, headache, sweating, diarrhea, nocturnal coughing, and dyspnea. Also, report promptly signs of iodism: stomatitis, bronchitis, laryngitis, coryza, brassy taste, conjunctivitis, acneiform rash, and pruritus. Side effects may not occur for 6 weeks.

Evaluation. The client will evidence serum lipid levels within normal limits.

niacin [nye' a sin] (nicotinic acid, Nicobid)

Niacin is a water-soluble vitamin that can lower total cholesterol and triglyceride levels by inhibiting VLDL synthesis and also, increases HDL cholesterol serum level. It is used as an adjunct to other therapies because its vasodilating and other side effects limit its usefulness. Because nicotinic acid inhibits lipolysis in adipose tissue, it lowers the plasma concentration of free fatty acids, which usually is the main sources of synthesis of triglycerides in the liver.

Niacin is used as adjunctive therapy in the treatment of both hypertriglyceridemias and hypercholesterolemia (types IIa, IIb, III, IV, or V). It is also used to prevent and treat niacin (vitamin B_3) deficiency. It is well absorbed orally and has a half-life of approximately 45 minutes.

It reduces cholesterol levels several days after therapy is started; reduction in triglyceride levels occurs within several hours after oral doses are begun. Metabolism occurs in the liver and the drug is excreted via the kidneys.

The side/adverse effects of niacin include increased feelings of warmth, flushing or red skin on face and neck, headache, pruritus, and skin rash. No significant drug interactions have been reported to date. The adult dose for antihyperlipidemic effect is 1 g orally three times daily. Dosage may be increased to 500 mg/day every 2 to 4 weeks as necessary. Maximum dose is 6 g/day.

■ Nursing Management

Niacin Therapy

Assessment. The drug should be used cautiously in individuals with allergies and with peptic ulcers, since nicotinic acid causes a release of histamine and stimulates hydrochloric acid secretion. Niacin should be used with caution in individuals with arterial bleeding and hypotension (vasodilating effects of drug may worsen these conditions), hepatic dysfunction (may cause hepatic damage), glaucoma (may worsen the condition), diabetes mellitus (may impair glucose tolerance), and gout (may cause hyperuricemia).

Nursing diagnosis. With the administration of niacin, the client may experience altered comfort (flushing of the skin of the head and neck and headaches, dizziness, nausea, and vomiting); altered bowel elimination (diarrhea); impaired skin integrity (pruritus); and the potential complications of peptic ulcer (stomach pain), hyperglycemia (frequent urination, unusual thirst), hyperuricemia (joint pain, flank pain), or myalgia (fever, muscle aching, or cramping).

Implementation

Monitoring. Serum cholesterol levels should be monitored periodically to evaluate effectiveness of drug therapy as well as blood glucose, uric acid, and hepatic function studies to determine adverse effects. Monitor for orthostatic hypotension, especially if the client is also on antihypertensive agents. Prolonged treatment with niacin has resulted in hepatic disease.

Intervention. Giving the drug with meals or with antacids may reduce the incidence and severity of gastric distress.

Education. Instruct client to swallow the extended-release form whole, without chewing or crushing. The powder within the capsule may be mixed with jam or applesauce for ease of administration. Advise the client to adhere to the dietary regimen—low cholesterol and low saturated fats. Instruct the client to maintain clinical appointments so that serum cholesterol and triglycerides may be monitored on a periodic basis.

Alert the client that numerous and often disagreeable side effects may occur from nicotinic acid. Common side effects include severe gastrointestinal upset, flushing, pruritus, nervousness, and urticaria. Although tolerance to the flushing, pruritus, and gastrointestinal effects usually occurs within 2 weeks, these effects may be minimized by starting the client's therapy with a low dose and increasing the dosage slowly. If flushing continues to be a discomfort for the client 300 mg of aspirin may be taken 30 minutes before each dose of niacin.

Evaluation. The client's serum lipid levels will be within the normal limits.

probucol [proe byoo' kole] (Lorelco)

Probucol is an antihyperlipidemic agent for persons with primary hypercholesterolemia that have not responded to other measures. It lowers both LDL-cholesterol and the desired HDL-cholesterol levels which limits the usefulness of this product. In addition to lowering cholesterol levels, though, probucol also induces regression of xanthomas in persons with homozygous familial hypercholesterolemia and inhibits atherosclerosis as result of its antioxidant properties (Witztum, 1996).

Probucol is administered orally and it has a variable absorption pattern. It tends to accumulate in fatty tissues with chronic therapy. Peak serum levels increase slowly and reach steady state after 3 or 4 months of treatment, whereas the peak effect usually occurs in 20 to 50 days after initiation of the drug. Half-life ranges from 12 to 500 hours. Probucol is excreted as bile in the feces.

The side/adverse effects of probucol include gas, diarrhea, nausea, vomiting, abdominal distress, and, rarely, angioneurotic edema. It has no reported significant drug interactions. The adult dose is 500 mg orally twice daily with breakfast and supper. A pediatric dose has not been established.

■ Nursing Management

Probucol Therapy

Assessment. The drug is usually administered to individuals who do not respond adequately to dietary management and weight reduction. Do not give probucol to clients with primary biliary cirrhosis because it may further raise cholesterol levels, or to clients with QT interval prolongation because the risk of additive QT interval may increase the risk of ventricular tachycardia. The drug should be used with caution with evidence of myocardial damage and unresponsive congestive heart failure and only with ECG monitoring because these conditions may be exacerbated.

A baseline assessment should include serum cholesterol and serum triglycerides.

Nursing diagnosis. With the administration of probucol, the client may experience altered comfort related to gastrointestinal irritation (bloating, nausea, vomiting, abdominal discomfort), dizziness, headache, and tingling of the fingers and toes. Potential complications include eosinophilia, anemia, thrombocytopenia, and QT interval prolongation and ventricular arrhythmias.

Implementation

Monitoring. Serum cholesterol and triglyceride levels should be obtained periodically during therapy to determine the efficacy of treatment. A baseline and periodic ECG readings should be monitored, especially for QT prolongation. Observe for syncope and pulse irregularities.

Intervention. If syncope occurs, probucol should be discontinued and the client monitored with ECG. If the client's response is not adequate after 4 months of therapy, probucol is usually discontinued. When the drug is discontinued, continue to monitor serum lipids because serum cholesterol levels may rise up to or above the original base.

Education. If medication is given, adherence to a low-cholesterol and low-fat diet and physical exercise should continue. Instruct the individual to take drug with food to minimize gastric irritation.

Evaluation. The client will evidence serum lipid concentrations within normal limits.

REDUCTASE INHIBITORS

fluvastatin [floo' va sta tin] (Lescol)
▲ **lovastatin** [loe' va sta tin] (Mevacor)
pravastatin [pra' va sta tin] (Pravachol)
simvastatin [sim va stat' in] (Zocor)

Reductase inhibitors are competitive inhibitors of HMG-CoA reductase, an enzyme necessary for cholesterol biosynthesis. These drugs convert HMG-CoA reductase to mevalonate, which results in an increase in HDL cholesterol and a decrease in LDL cholesterol, VLDL cholesterol, and plasma triglycerides.

These agents are indicated as adjuncts for the treatment of primary hypercholesterolemia (types IIa and IIb) caused by an elevated LDL-cholesterol level not controlled by diet or other treatment measures.

On absorption they have extensive first-pass hepatic extraction; all but pravastatin are highly protein bound; peak serum levels are reached in 0.5 to 0.7 hour for fluvastatin, 2 to 4 hours for lovastatin, 1 hour for pravastatin, and 1.3 to 2.4 hours for simvastatin. Lovastatin and simvastatin are converted by the liver to several active metabolites. Initial response is seen within 1 to 2 weeks, with the maximum therapeutic response occurring within 4 to 6 weeks of chronic drug administration. Excretion is primarily fecal.

The side/adverse effects of reductase inhibitors include gas, stomach cramps or pain, rash, constipation or diarrhea, nausea, and headaches. A significant drug interaction may occur if the drugs are administered with cyclosporine (Neoral, Sandimmune), gemfibrozil (Lopid), or niacin (B_3). An increased risk of rhabdomyolysis (necrosis of skeletal muscle with the release of myoglobulin, which may result in myopathy and acute renal failure) may occur. At the present time such effects have only been reported with lovastatin but the potential of inducing these effects exists with all four agents. Monitor closely if concurrent administration is necessary.

The recommended adult dose for fluvastatin is 20 mg PO daily at bedtime, titrated monthly as necessary and tolerated. Lovastatin adult dose is 20 mg daily with the evening meal, increased monthly as necessary according to the client's response to therapy, up to a maximum of 80 mg/day. Pravastatin adult dose is 10 to 20 mg at bedtime, with dosage adjustments at monthly intervals as needed. Simvastatin adult dose is 5 to 10 mg in the evening, titrated monthly as necessary and tolerated. The maximum dose is 40 mg/day.

■ Nursing Management

Reductase Inhibitor Therapy

Assessment. Do not administer to clients with active liver disease or unexplained persistent elevations of serum transaminase. Use with caution in clients with organ transplant with immunosuppressant therapy because of the increased risk of rhabdomyolysis and renal failure. Administer with caution in those conditions in which there is increased risk of secondary renal failure if rhabdomyolysis occurs, such as hypotension, severe infection, uncontrolled seizures, major surgery, trauma, and severe metabolic, endocrine, or electrolyte disorders. A baseline assessment should include serum cholesterol, serum creatine kinase (CK), and liver function studies.

Nursing diagnosis. Clients receiving reductase inhibitor therapy are at risk for the following nursing diagnoses: altered comfort related to myalgia or myositis (fever, muscle aches), headache, and nausea; risk for injury related to blurred vision and dizziness; disturbed sleep pattern (insomnia-lovastatin only); sexual dysfunction (impotence-lovastatin only) and impaired skin integrity (rash).

Implementation

Monitoring. Liver function studies should be done periodically because reductase inhibitors may elevate transaminase levels as well as serum creatine concentrations. If the client develops muscular tenderness, serum creatine kinase levels should be determined. Serum cholesterol levels will determine the efficacy of treatment.

Intervention. Discontinue reductase inhibitor therapy if serum transaminase concentrations increase to 3 times the upper limit of normal or if creatine kinase (CK) concentrations markedly increase or myositis occurs.

Education. As with other antihyperlipidemic medications, an appropriate diet, exercise, and weight reduction in obese clients should be instituted along with drug therapy.

Evaluation. The client's serum lipid concentrations will be within the normal limits.

SUMMARY

Along with dietary modifications, antihyperlipidemic agents are used to treat hyperlipidemia, a metabolic disorder characterized by increased serum concentrations of cholesterol and triglycerides. High levels of these serum lipids have been associated with atherosclerosis, in which lipids are deposited in the linings of medium- and large-sized arteries. Box 32-1 gives a summary of the drug treatment goals and selected drug therapies.

Atherosclerosis is a causative factor in hypertension, coronary artery disease, cerebral artery disease, peripheral artery occlusive disease, and renal arterial insufficiency. Although atherosclerosis has many causes, such as dietary saturated fats, faulty fat metabolism, genetic influences, and others, some clinicians believe that if serum lipid levels can be controlled, the progression of atherosclerosis can also be controlled. At the present time, however, the available antihyperlipidemic agents remain controversial.

The bile acid sequestering agents, cholestyramine and colestipol hydrochloride, combine with bile acids in the intestine, preventing their absorption and promoting their loss from the body in feces. To compensate for their loss, the liver increases its rate of oxidation of cholesterol to replace the bile acids, which causes a reduction of serum cholesterol levels. Clofibrate is more effective in lowering serum triglyceride levels; it appears to block the synthesis of triglycerides in the liver. Dextrothyroxine and probucol enhance the excretion of cholesterol. Gemfibrozil and niacin lower both triglyceride and cholesterol levels. As enzyme inhibitors, fluvastatin, lovastatin, pravastatin, and simvastatin inhibit liver synthesis of cholesterol and so are effective for clients with primary hypercholesterolemia. Each agent is indicated for specific instances of hyperlipidemia (see Table 32-2).

Nursing management focuses on client education for compliance with lifestyle changes, particularly adherence to a low-fat dietary regimen as a long-term commitment, and in the short term for most clients, adherence to the prescribed medication regimen until the hyperlipidemia is resolved.

BOX 32-1

Summary of Drug Treatment Goals and Selected Drug Therapies

Drug treatment goals

Primary: reduce risk of coronary heart disease

Approaches: lower LDL cholesterol and triglyceride serum levels; increase HDL cholesterol serum level

Selected drug therapies

Bile acid sequestering agents to lower high LDL cholesterol levels

Niacin to lower total and LDL cholesterol levels, increase HDL cholesterol level

Reductase inhibitors are very potent drugs that lower LDL cholesterol and triglyceride levels; increase HDL serum levels

Gemfibrozil lowers triglycerides

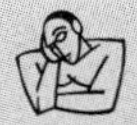

Critical Thinking

1. Mr. Clark has been on cholestyramine for 6 months. In this office visit he indicates that he increasingly has been experiencing nosebleeds. What might be happening?
2. How would the nurse counter the common belief of clients that drug therapy replaces dietary restrictions in the management of hyperlipidemia?

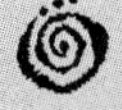

Collaborative Learning Activities

1. Four student teams will present thumbnail sketches of each type of hyperlipidemic disorder (see Table 32-2) and the appropriate treatment for each. Ensure that the mechanisms of action are presented so that the rationale for the use of each drug is presented.
2. Discuss Critical Thinking question 2 in the text. The students will plan ways to incorporate diet and exercise into client education. They could consider their own lifestyles to consider what changes they would need to make if they were prescribed an antilipidemic agent. How difficult would they find this and why?

BIBLIOGRAPHY

American Hospital Formulary Service (1996). *AHFS drug information '96.* Bethesda, MD: American Society of Hospital Pharmacists.

American Medical Association (1995). *Drug evaluations: Annual 1995.* Chicago: The Association.

Anderson KN, et al. (Eds.) (1994). *Mosby's medical, nursing, & allied health dictionary* (4th ed.). St Louis: Mosby.

Clark J (1995). Lipid-lowering drugs in heart disease prevention, *Community Nurse 1*(2 Nurse Prescriber):3-4.

Hardman JC & Limbird LE (Eds.) (1996). *Goodman & Gilman's the pharmacological basis of therapeutics* (9th ed.). New York: Macmillan.

Long JW (1990). The essential guide to prescription drugs. New York: HarperCollins.

McKenney JM (1995). Dyslipidemias. In Young LY & Koda-Kimble MA. *Applied therapeutics* (6th ed.). Vancouver: Applied Therapeutics.

Mishkel M (1992). Dyslipidemia: Practical goals and guidelines, *Medicine North America 4*(36):4476-9.

National Cholesterol Program (1993). *Second report of the expert panel on detection, evaluation, and treatment of high blood cholesterol in adults (adult treatment panel II): Executive summary.* Washington, DC: National Institutes of Health, NIH Publication No. 93-3096.

Olin BR (Ed.) (1996). *Facts and comparisons.* St Louis: Facts and Comparisons.

Smith DA (1994). Hypercholesterolemia: A guide to primary and secondary prevention, *Consultant 34*(6):844-50, 852.

United States Pharmacopeial Convention (1996). *USP DI: Drug information for the health care professional* (16th ed.). Rockville, MD: The Convention.

Wilson BA (1994). Understanding management of hyperlipidemia, *MEDSURG Nursing 3*(4):319-21.

Witztum JL (1996). Drugs used in the treatment of hyperlipoproteinemias. In: Hardmon JG & Limbird LE (Eds.). *Goodman & Gilman's the pharmacological basis of therapeutics* (9th ed.). New York: McGraw-Hill.

Chapter 33

Overview of the Urinary System

Chapter Focus

The urinary system functions with other organs to regulate the volume and composition of fluid within the body, retaining essential materials and excreting waste. Because of this function, the urinary system affects other body systems and the client's general health. As many pharmacologic effects are diminished or enhanced by the activity of the urinary system, the nurse is required to be knowledgeable of its anatomy and physiology. The following objectives and key terms are important for a good understanding of this chapter.

Key Terms

electromagnetic gradient (p. 613)
glomerular filtration (p. 612)
glomerulus (p. 612)
hypertonic (p. 613)
hypotonic (p. 613)
isotonic (p. 613)
osmotic gradient (p. 613)
threshold concentration (p. 613)
tubular transport maximum (p. 613)

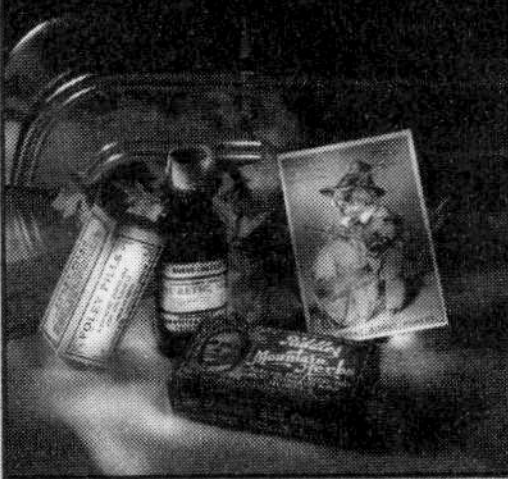

Objectives

1. Describe the anatomy and physiology of the urinary system.
2. Identify the functions of the various segments of the nephron.
3. Describe the major functions of the kidneys.
4. Describe the sites of action and primary effects of the antidiuretic hormone, vasopressin, and aldosterone on the nephrons.

The urinary system is composed of organs that manufacture and excrete urine from the body: two kidneys, two ureters, the bladder, and the urethra (Figure 33-1). Urine formed in the kidneys flows through the ureters to the bladder, where it is stored. When approximately 250 ml of urine is collected, the bladder expansion will result in a feeling of distention and a desire to void. The urine flows from the bladder into the urethra to be expelled from the body.

In the male the urethra is surrounded by the prostate gland; it then passes through fibrous tissue connected to the pubic bones and terminates at the urinary meatus, or tip of the penis (Figure 33-2). The male urethra serves a dual purpose, the elimination of urine from the body and semen transport. In the female the urethra is the final vehicle for urination (Figure 33-3).

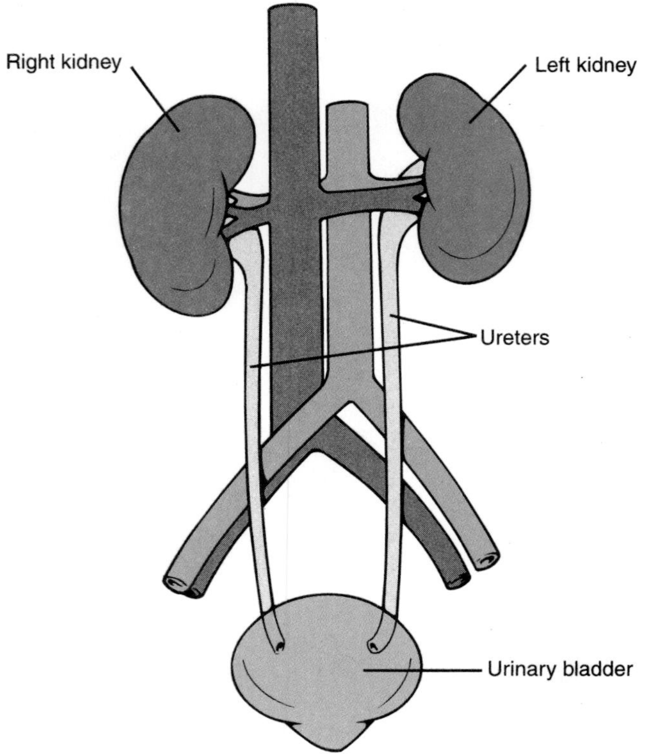

Figure 33-1 Urinary system.

The kidneys regulate homeostasis in the body; they are responsible for the maintenance of body fluids, electrolytes, and acid-base balance in addition to elimination of body waste, urea, and urine. The primary focus of this chapter is the kidneys.

ANATOMY AND PHYSIOLOGY OF THE KIDNEY

The kidney is composed of millions of individual units called nephrons. Each nephron consists of a glomerulus and a tubular system. The volume and composition of urine as a result of concentration and dilution depend on three major processes in the kidney: glomerular filtration, tubular reabsorption, and tubular secretion.

Glomerular filtration. **Glomerular filtration** occurs as a result of plasma flowing across a cluster of capillary blood vessels and into the urinary space of the Bowman's capsule. This capillary cluster is enveloped within a thin wall, giving off uriniferous tubules, and is called the **glomerulus.** The heart works to create pressure in the blood vessels, which in turn provides the force necessary to accomplish glomerular filtration. Blood flow to the kidney is 1200 ml/min, which is 20% to 25% of cardiac output. The blood pressure within the glomerular capillaries is about 60% of arterial pressure. Systemic blood pressure has to be significantly reduced before glomerular filtration is greatly altered. Usually some degree of filtration will exist if the mean blood pressure remains above 50 mm Hg. Maintenance of glomerular hydrostatic pressure is aided by the ability of the afferent and efferent arterioles to alter vessel resistance effectively. In the absence of disease the glomerular membrane does not filter plasma proteins greater than 100 angstroms, such as hemoglobin and albumin and the small amount of protein-bound substances.

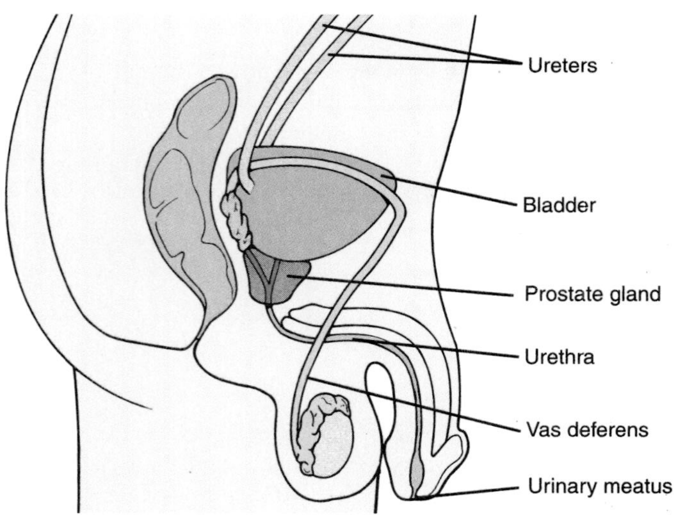

Figure 33-2 Sagittal section of male pelvis.

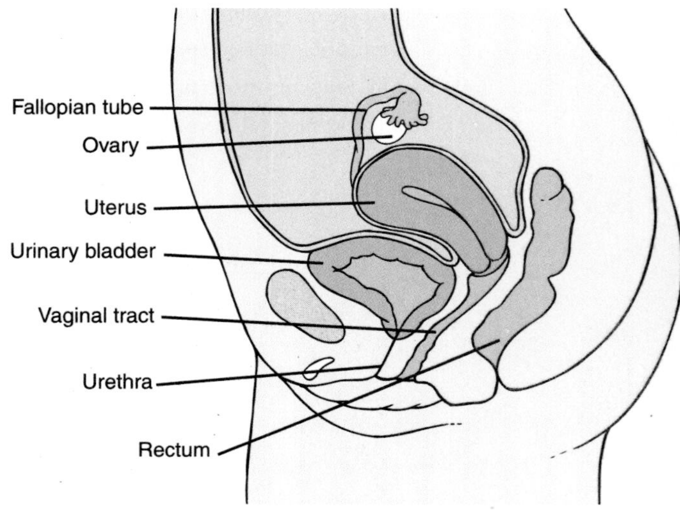

Figure 33-3 Sagittal section of female pelvis.

The glomerular filtrate is otherwise almost identical to plasma. The rate of filtration in an average adult is approximately 125 ml/min; 99% of this tubular filtrate is ultimately reabsorbed throughout the tubule.

Tubular reabsorption. Tubular reabsorption involves both active and passive transport of substances into the tubular epithelial cell and into the extracellular fluid compartment. Passive transport, or diffusion, through the tubular membrane occurs because of a difference in concentration of particles (**osmotic gradient**) or electrical charge (**electromagnetic gradient**).

In the proximal tubule, sodium is *actively* transported across the tubular cell membrane from tubule filtrate. Chloride follows passively because of an electromagnetic gradient. Water, in turn, follows passively in response to an osmotic gradient established by sodium chloride solute. Then diffusion of 60% of urea content occurs to maintain a chemical gradient. Depending on the amount of a drug in ionized or nonionized form and the pH of the tubular fluid, weak acids and weak bases may be reabsorbed by diffusion.

For almost every substance that is actively transported across the membrane, there is a maximum rate at which the transport mechanism can function, after which the excess substance will not be reabsorbed and the substance will appear in the urine. This is called the **tubular transport maximum.** For example, the tubular transport maximum for glucose averages 320 mg/min for most adults. If the tubular load becomes greater than 320 mg/min, then the excess will not be reabsorbed but will appear in the urine. Every substance that has a tubular transport maximum also has a **threshold concentration,** the plasma concentration below which none of the substance appears in the urine and above which progressively larger quantities appear.

Tubular secretion. Tubular secretion affects the composition of urine by allowing compounds such as penicillin, histamine, probenecid, methotrexate, and thiazides to enter into tubular fluid from peritubular or interstitial capillaries. This is accomplished via specific transport mechanisms for secretion of organic compounds. Other very important examples of tubular secretion include that of the hydrogen ions, ammonia, and potassium ions.

Proximal tubule. Most of the glomerular filtrate is reabsorbed in the proximal tubule and returned to the bloodstream. Approximately 70% of salt and water is reabsorbed rapidly, maintaining nearly the same osmolality between tubular fluid and interstitial fluid at the end of the proximal tubule (**isotonic**). The general mechanism for sodium, chloride, water, and urea reabsorption is under tubular reabsorption with respect to gradient transport. There are *no* dilutional or concentration changes of these ions in the proximal tubule.

Other substances reabsorbed in the proximal tubule include glucose, amino acids, phosphate, uric acid, and a major portion of potassium. Nearly 90% of bicarbonate in tubular filtrate is reabsorbed as carbon dioxide if hydrogen ion is secreted in the tubular lumen. Plasma carbon dioxide is hydrolyzed in the tubular cell to form carbonic acid, which dissociates to give bicarbonate and hydrogen ion. This reversible reaction is catalyzed by carbonic anhydrase. The hydrogen ion secreted into the lumen combines with bicarbonate of the glomerular filtrate to form carbonic acid in the lumen. This again dissociates to give water and carbon dioxide, which are reabsorbed. This reaction is catalyzed at both steps by carbonic anhydrase. Proximal tubule reabsorption is usually constant in spite of moderate changes in the glomerular filtration rate.

Descending loop of Henle. This portion of the nephron is permeable to water; water is passively taken up to equilibrate medullary interstitial osmolality. This produces a **hypertonic** (more concentrated) filtrate at the tip of the loop of Henle, the papilla. There is very low sodium and urea permeability in this segment.

Ascending loop of Henle. Water permeability is almost nil in the ascending limb of the loop of Henle, whereas sodium and chloride permeability is high. Approximately 20% to 25% of sodium load in glomerular filtrate is reabsorbed and chloride follows *passively*. Consequently, two very important situations occur. The concentration of tubular filtrates becomes very dilute, or **hypotonic**; this is often termed "free water production." Meanwhile, the medullary interstitium becomes hypertonic, which is necessary to the concentration capacity of the countercurrent multiplier. The concentration gradient established across the tubular epithelium becomes multiplied in a longitudinal direction, resulting in a large osmotic gradient between the isosmotic renal cortex and the hyperosmotic medulla and papilla. The ascending limb of the loop of Henle is not responsive to any hormones as are other segments.

Distal convoluted tubule. Between 5% and 10% of sodium reabsorption *actively* takes place in the distal tubule. This uptake is largely determined by the presence of a hormone called aldosterone. When the extracellular fluid volume is decreased, the renin-angiotensin system is involved, stimulating the release of aldosterone. Increased levels of aldosterone act to increase the active reabsorption of sodium. Although an increase in potassium secretion is seen, a simple sodium-potassium exchange pump is no longer recognized.

Collecting duct. The hypotonic fluid entering the collecting duct may be altered in the medullary portion by the presence of antidiuretic hormone (ADH), vasopressin. The released ADH will act at the distal tubule and collecting duct to reabsorb water to increase plasma volume, thus lowering plasma osmolality. Urinary output is more concentrated, or fluid is lost because of the osmotic gradient set up by hypertonic medullary interstitium. Thus the collecting duct is responsible for urine concentration.

PHYSIOLOGIC REGULATION BY THE KIDNEY

The kidneys excrete metabolic byproducts of the body, especially nitrogenous-type substances such as urea. They maintain electrolyte homeostasis (sodium, potassium, chloride, etc.) and body fluids. Sodium is actively reabsorbed in the proximal tubules (approximately 65%) and ascending

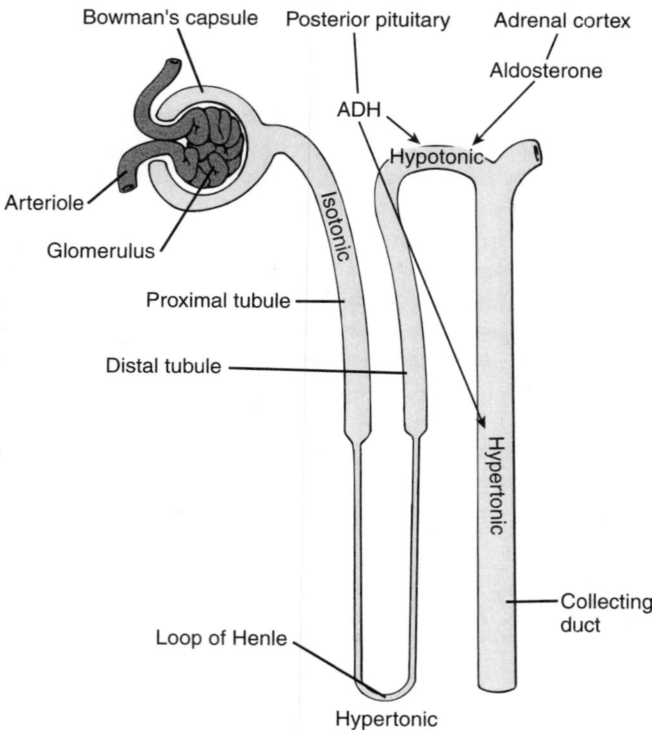

Figure 33-4 Components of a nephron.

BOX 33-1

Nephron Functions

Site	Major functions
Glomerulus	Filtration
Proximal tubule	Reabsorption of glucose, potassium, sodium, amino acids, water, and nutrients; remaining fluid isotonic
Loop of Henle	Sodium and chloride reabsorbed in ascending loop. Countercurrent mechanism produces decrease in osmolality of filtrate in ascending loop of Henle; i.e., sodium chloride is transported into the body but not water. Filtrate leaves loop of Henle as hypotonic urine.
Distal tubule	Sodium and bicarbonate reabsorbed. Potassium, hydrogen, and ammonia may be secreted. ADH necessary to reabsorb water at this site. Filtrate leaves distal tubule as hypotonic urine.
Collecting duct	ADH, if present, will reabsorb water at this site. Urine may be hypertonic. If ADH is unavailable or not functioning, dilute urine (hypotonic) may be excreted.

loop of Henle (27%). Approximately 8% of sodium reaches the distal tubules, and the rate of reabsorption here depends on the presence of aldosterone. If large quantities of aldosterone are present, sodium is reabsorbed. A lack of aldosterone will result in elimination of sodium in the urine. Generally, healthy kidneys excrete the daily sodium intake. Figure 33-4 and Box 33-1 explain nephron functions. Potassium is also reabsorbed from the proximal tubules and loop of Henle in percentages equivalent to sodium. Thus approximately 8% of the filtered potassium reaches the distal tubules. Aldosterone controls potassium secretion; in its presence, sodium is reabsorbed and potassium is secreted in the distal tubules. The daily potassium intake is generally excreted daily in the kidneys.

Antidiuretic hormone (ADH), or vasopressin, is a water-conserving hormone synthesized in the hypothalamus and stored in the posterior pituitary gland. When plasma osmolarity increases as a result of dehydration or water deprivation, osmoreceptors in the supraoptic area of the hypothalamus will stimulate the release of ADH. The released ADH will act at the distal tubule and collecting duct to reabsorb water to increase plasma volume, thus lowering plasma osmolality. Urine output is decreased and more concentrated.

Acid-base balance is partially controlled in the kidneys. The kidneys are one of three pH control mechanisms in the body; the others are blood buffering and the respiratory adjustment mechanism. As the blood pH becomes more acidic, the kidneys will respond by increasing the renal tubule excretion of hydrogen and ammonia, which results in an increase in blood bicarbonate and an increase in pH (toward normal). This is an effective method of adjusting hydrogen ions within the system.

The hormone erythropoietin is synthesized in the kidneys. A decrease in red blood cells below normal, or tissue hypoxia, will stimulate an increased release of erythropoietin from the kidneys. The increased serum concentration of erythropoietin will stimulate the bone marrow to increase its production of red blood cells so that the red blood cell average is restored to normal.

SUMMARY

The kidneys as part of the urinary system participate with other body organs to regulate the volume and composition of interstitial fluid within a narrow range of values. They remove waste products from the blood and are important in controlling blood volume, the concentration of ions in the blood, and the pH of the blood. The kidneys also function in the control of red blood cell production. As the major excretory organs in the body the kidneys are essential in maintaining a normal environment for the body cells.

Critical Thinking

1. Sally Bownes ate a large box of salty pretzels. What effect would this have on her urine concentration and volume? Why?
2. For the past week your client in the extended-care facility, Mrs. Jones, has indicated that she has a worsening burning sensation in "the spot where my catheter goes in." You check her temperature and find that it is 100.2° F. What do you suspect is occurring? What laboratory values would you expect to find on Mrs. Jones' urinalysis to confirm your suspicions? Why would Mrs. Jones be more likely to have this condition than Mr. Smith, another client with an indwelling catheter?
3. Mr. Smith has had a course of acyclovir for a week at the high level of the dosage range and needs continued encouragement to drink fluids. Knowing that a potential complication of this drug is renal toxicity, what laboratory values would you be monitoring? How would you expect them to change if Mr. Smith began to develop toxicity and why?

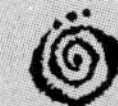

Collaborative Learning Activities

1. Four teams of students will present the function of each part of the nephron (glomerulus, proximal tubule, Loop of Henle, and distal tubule) using the transparency titled "Nephron Function"

BIBLIOGRAPHY

Anderson KN, et al. (Eds.) (1994). *Mosby's medical, nursing, & allied health dictionary* (4th ed.). St Louis: Mosby.

Martini F, et al. (1992). *Fundamentals of anatomy and physiology* (2nd ed.). Englewood Cliffs, NJ: Prentice Hall.

Seeley RR, Stephens TD, & Tate P (1995). *Anatomy & physiology* (3rd ed.). St Louis: Mosby.

Thibodeau GA & Patton K (1996). *Anatomy and physiology* (3rd ed.). St Louis: Mosby.

Van Wynsberghe D, Noback CR, & Carola R (1995). *Human anatomy and physiology* (3rd ed.). New York: McGraw-Hill.

Wingard LB, et al. (1991). *Human pharmacology*. St Louis: Mosby.

Chapter 34

Diuretics

Chapter Focus

Diuretics play a leading role in many therapies, including congestive heart failure and hypertension. Although diuretics can be beneficial, they may also result in many side effects and drug interactions. With appropriate nursing assessment and intervention, diuretic therapy can have positive effects in the treatment of hypertension and edemas and cause a minimum of adverse effects. The following objectives and key terms are important for the understanding of this chapter.

Key Terms

diuretic (p. 617)
loop diuretics (p. 623)
osmotic diuretics (p. 626)
potassium-sparing diuretics (p. 625)
proximal tubule diuretics (p. 617)
thiazide-type diuretics (p. 619)

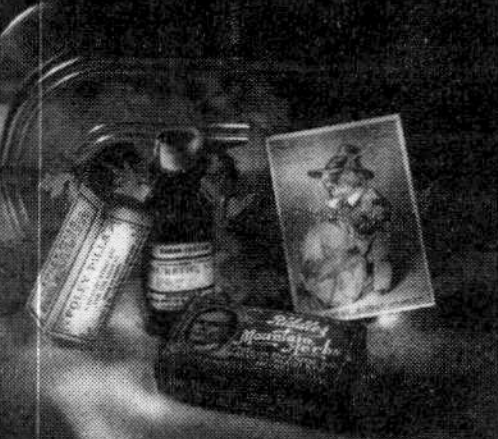

Key Drugs [▲]

furosemide
hydrochlorothiazide
spironolactone

Objectives

1. Compare and contrast the five classifications of diuretics.
2. Identify the most common agents within the five classifications of diuretics and the site within the nephron where the action of each classification occurs.
3. Identify signs and symptoms of fluid and electrolyte imbalances associated with diuretic therapy.
4. Explain nursing care and client education required for clients receiving potassium-depleting diuretics and those receiving potassium-sparing diuretics.
5. Implement the nursing management of the care of a client receiving diuretic therapy.

Diuretics modify renal function to induce diuresis, or the loss of body water by urination. In addition to water, diuretics increase the excretion of electrolytes, primarily sodium chloride. Understanding their action requires knowledge of the events that take place along each of the tubular segments (see Chapter 33). Diuretics are among the most commonly used medications. They represent the mainstay in the treatment of hypertension (see also Chapter 27) and are an integral part of drug therapies in edematous conditions such as cirrhosis, nephrotic syndrome, chronic renal failure, and acute and chronic congestive heart failure.

Therapeutically, drug selection is best understood if each diuretic is presented according to their major site of action. This approach does not preclude drug effect at other sites in the nephron. Figure 34-1 shows the various sites of action of diuretic drug groups by means of water and electrolyte transport system in a kidney nephron.

PROXIMAL TUBULE DIURETICS

Carbonic Anhydrase Inhibitors

acetazolamide [a set a zole' a mide] (Diamox, Acetazolam ♣)

Acetazolamide, a sulfonamide, is the prototype of the **proximal tubule diuretics,** which act primarily to reduce the volume of sequestered fluids, especially of the aqueous humor. It inhibits the action of the enzyme carbonic anhydrase, which in turn prevents the reabsorption of bicarbonate ions from the proximal tubules. These bicarbonate ions then act to increase tubular osmotic pressure, causing osmotic diuresis. With long-term use, however, the diuretic effect of these drugs is lost.

Acetazolamide is widely used as an antiglaucoma agent because it lowers intraocular pressure by decreasing the production of aqueous humor by more than 50%; this is discussed in Chapter 43. Acetazolamide is indicated for

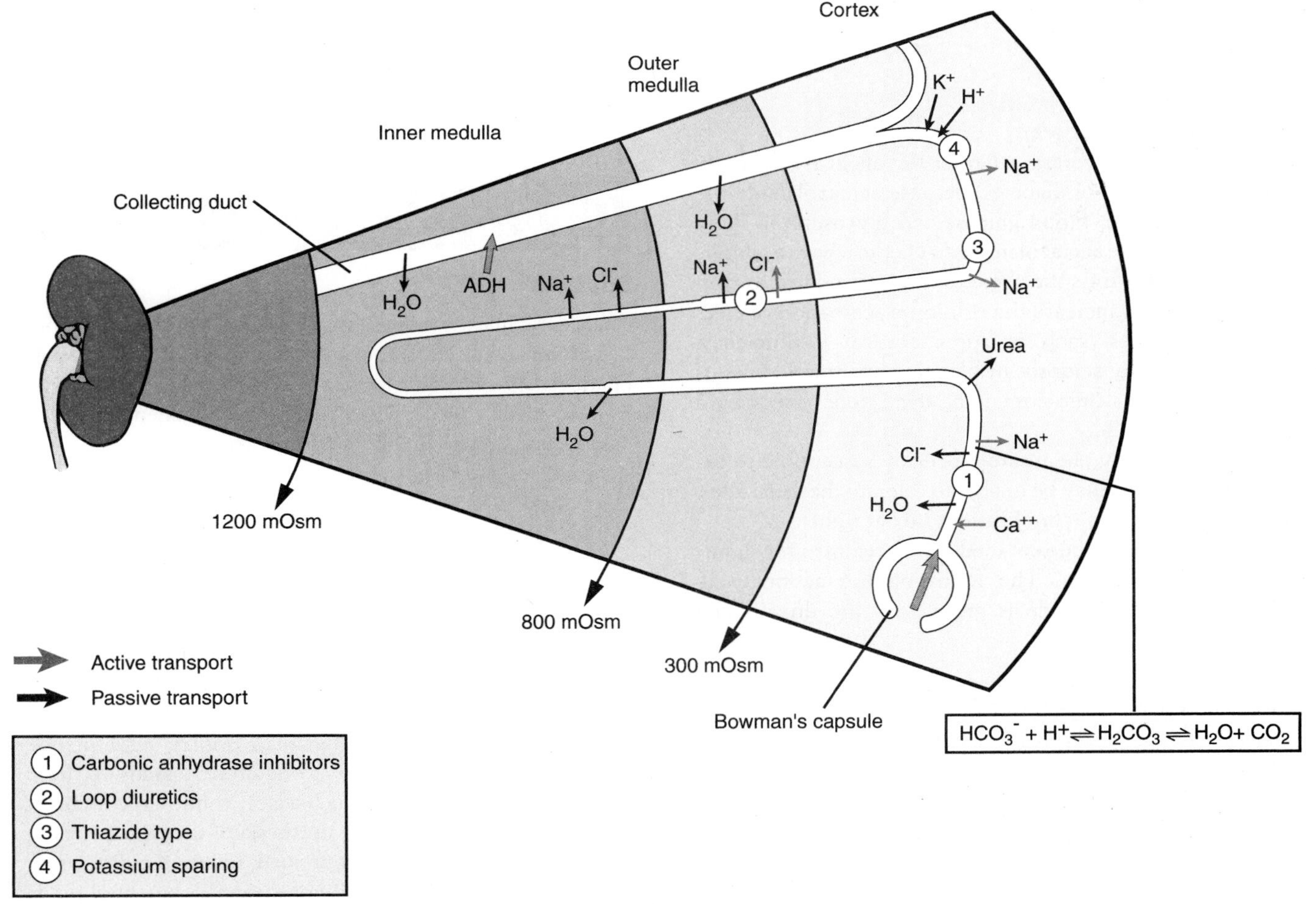

Figure 34-1 Site of action of diuretics by means of water and electrolyte transport.

the treatment of open-angle glaucoma and is also used as adjunct treatment with anticonvulsants to manage absence seizures (petit mal), generalized tonic-clonic seizures (grand mal), mixed seizure patterns, and myoclonic seizures. It has been found especially useful for women who experience an increase in seizures during their menstrual periods. When acetazolamide is taken orally, it has been found to decrease the incidence and severity of symptoms of altitude sickness in mountain climbers. In addition, acetazolamide produces an alkaline urine, which may help increase excretion of weakly acidic drugs in cases of drug overdose.

Acetazolamide is well absorbed orally, reaches a peak level in 2 to 4 hours after a 500 mg dose or 8 to 12 hours after a 500 mg extended-release capsule. Its half-life is 10 to 15 hours, and excretion is mainly by the kidneys. Side/adverse effects include headaches, increased nervousness, anorexia, nausea, vomiting, depression, tremors, rash, alopecia, ataxia, and chest, groin, or leg pain.

Adult oral dose for glaucoma is 250 mg orally one to four times daily. Anticonvulsant dose is 4 to 30 mg/kg orally divided into four doses per day. For altitude sickness the dose is 250 mg orally two to four times daily. Pediatric dose for glaucoma is 8 to 30 mg/kg orally per day in divided doses. Acetazolamide is also available as a parenteral injection for intravenous or intramuscular use. See current package insert for dosing instructions.

▪ Nursing Management

Acetazolamide Therapy

Assessment. Ascertain whether the client has diabetes or a familial history of diabetes, because acetazolamide has caused elevations of blood glucose and glycosuria in these clients. Do not give acetazolamide to clients who are allergic to sulfonamides. Assess the client for preexisting health conditions that might increase the risk for exacerbation of electrolyte imbalances, such as adrenocortical insufficiency, renal or respiratory acidosis, or hepatic impairment. Clients with a history of calcium-containing renal stones may have a recurrence of calculi.

Note that elderly clients are especially susceptible to excessive diuresis and may be unable to tolerate the usual adult doses (see the Geriatric Implications box at right).

Review the client's current medication regimen for significant drug interactions. The following interactions may occur when acetazolamide is given with the drugs listed below.

Drug	Possible effect and management
amphetamines, mecamylamine (Inversine), or quinidine	Because of alkalinization of urine, the excretion of these drugs is decreased. Therefore increased serum levels and toxicity may be seen. Avoid concurrent drug administration with mecamylamine. Dosage adjustments may be necessary with the other two drugs whenever a carbonic anhydrase inhibitor is started, dosage is changed, or medication is discontinued.
methenamine mandelate (Mandelamine)	Alkaline urine will reduce the effectiveness of methenamine. Avoid concurrent use. A baseline assessment of the client's underlying condition should be obtained; the neurologic status of the client with seizures, the presence of edema in clients with congestive heart failure, and the eye comfort and intraocular pressure of clients with glaucoma should be determined.

Nursing diagnosis. With the administration of acetazolamide, clients are at risk for the following nursing diagnoses: altered comfort (headache, bitter taste, nausea, vomiting, and numbness or tingling of fingers, toes, lips, or tongue); altered urinary elimination pattern with an increase and frequency of urination; disturbed sleep pattern related to polyuria; altered bowel elimination (diarrhea or constipation); fatigue; altered thought processes (confusion, depression); and the potential complications of decreased cardiac output (ventricular dysrhythmias secondary to hypokalemia); electrolyte imbalance, such as hypokalemia (dry mouth, increased thirst, irregular heartbeats, muscle cramps, fatigue); renal calculi or nephrotoxicity (hematuria, lower back pain, burning on urination); and blood dyscrasias (fever, sore throat, unusual bleeding or bruising).

Implementation

Monitoring. Observe the client for signs of allergic reaction and photosensitivity. Weigh the client daily. A rapid

Geriatric Implications

Diuretics

The elderly may be more sensitive to diuretic-induced hypotension and electrolyte disturbances than the average adult.

Pharmacologically, the elderly client is started with the lowest dose possible, generally one-half the recommended adult dose and titrated slowly to effect (Menscer, 1992).

Advise clients to drink sufficient fluids. Diuretics are often referred to as "water pills" with many persons believing fluid intake is restricted with this drug category. This erroneous belief should be discussed with the client.

Avoid or use *extreme* caution and close monitoring if concurrent potassium supplementation or a potassium chloride salt substitute is ordered for persons receiving a potassium-sparing diuretic. Hyperkalemia and fatality have been reported with this combination.

Be aware that all diuretics will increase urinary incontinence.

Report any signs and symptoms of diuretic toxicity to the prescriber, such as anorexia, nausea, vomiting, confusion, increased weakness, and paresthesia of the extremities.

When a diuretic is to be discontinued, reduce the drug gradually to avoid the possibility of the development of fluid retention and edema.

loss of body water (which may cause hypotension) will be reflected in a rapid weight loss. Monitor blood pressure for indications of hypotension. Monitor intake and output and electrolytes, especially serum potassium levels. Do complete blood cell counts periodically to monitor for blood dyscrasias. Monitor blood and urine sugar levels for clients with diabetes or those at risk for diabetes.

Intervention. Reconstituting acetazolamide with at least 5 ml sterile water is necessary before parenteral use. Discard it after 24 hours of reconstitution, since it contains no preservatives.

Administer the oral forms of acetazolamide with meals or with antacids to decrease gastrointestinal distress. For clients who are unable to tolerate tablets for oral administration, crush acetazolamide tablets and mix with a flavored syrup such as chocolate or cherry. Although up to 500 mg may be prepared in 5 ml syrup, it is more palatable if only 250 mg/5 ml is used. Refrigeration also increases the palatability but not the stability of the preparation; use within a week of preparation. Mixing the drug with fruit juices and elixirs is not as satisfactory.

Planning a high fluid intake for the client with gout or hypercalciuria (excessive calcium in the urine) is necessary because of the risk of renal calculi. Establish dosing schedules that minimize the inconvenience of diuresis that results from altered urinary elimination patterns. When this drug is used in diuretic therapy, consult the prescriber and the dietitian to provide a high-potassium diet.

Acetazolamide is used to prevent or minimize high-altitude sickness, but it is not a substitute for rapid descent if the climber manifests signs of pulmonary or cerebral edema.

Education. Oral and intravenous routes of administration are preferred, but if the drug is to be given intramuscularly, alert the client that the injection will be painful because of the drug's alkalinity.

Alert the client that constipation is common with diuretic therapy and may be prevented or minimized by adequate fluid intake, high-fiber diet, and moderate exercise if these are not contraindicated by the client's health status. High fluid intake, 2500 to 3000 ml/day, is necessary to reduce the risk of renal calculi.

Instruct the client to move gradually from a sitting or lying position to a more upright one to prevent lightheadedness caused by orthostatic hypotension. Caution the client that the ability to accomplish tasks requiring mental alertness or physical coordination may be impaired.

Advise the client that dryness of the mouth may occur, but its discomfort may be minimized by the use of sugarless hard candies and frequent mouth rinses. Advise the client to get regular dental checkups to monitor caries and gum disease development that may occur as the result of xerostomia.

Although the sensation of "not feeling well" is common with the drug, malaise should be reported to the prescriber so that monitoring for acidosis, blood dyscrasias, or hypokalemia may be done. Advise the client to notify the prescriber if paresthesias (numbness, tingling, or burning) of the mouth, fingers, or toes occur.

Instruct the client and the family member who shops for and prepares the food about a high-potassium diet in keeping with the client's usual dietary patterns.

Advise the client to consult the prescriber before switching brands or using a generic formulation of acetazolamide because bioequivalence problems have been noted.

Evaluation. The client receiving acetazolamide to reduce intraocular pressure in glaucoma will have intraocular pressure readings within the normal limits when measured with a tonometer. If the drug is administered for the prevention of seizures, the client will be free of seizures. If taken for altitude illness, the client will not evidence signs of an attack, such as shortness of breath, headache, or syncope.

DILUTING SEGMENT DIURETICS

Thiazide and Thiazide-Type Drugs

bendroflumethiazide [ben droe floo me thy' a zide] (Naturetin)
benzthiazide [benz thy' a zide] (Exna, Hydrex)
chlorothiazide [klor oh thy' a zide] (Diuril)
chlorthalidone [klor' tha li done] (Hygroton)
cyclothiazide [sye kloe thy' a zide] (Anhydron)
▲ **hydrochlorothiazide** [hydro klor oh thy' a zide] (HydroDiuril, Esidrix)
hydroflumethiazide [hye droe flu me thy' a zide] (Diucardin, Saluron)
metolazone [me toe' la zone] (Zaroxolyn)
polythiazide [pol ee thy' a zide] (Renese)
trichlormethiazide [try klor me thy' a zide] (Metahydrin, Naqua)

Thiazide diuretics are the major diuretics active in the diluting segments of the kidney. They are synthetic drugs that are chemically related to the sulfonamides. Hydrochlorothiazide is one of the most commonly used thiazides. Because these agents are similar, all the diluting segment diuretics will be described collectively as the **thiazide-type diuretics** with important differences mentioned later. Table 34-1 lists selected diuretic pharmacokinetics and dosages.

The primary action and site of action appear to be inhibition of sodium reabsorption in the early distal tubules in the nephron, the cortical diluting segment. These drugs are less potent than the loop diuretics, since the maximum portion of the sodium load they can affect at the distal tubule is less than 10% of the glomerular filtrate. The thiazide-type diuretics therefore primarily promote the renal excretion of water, sodium, chloride, potassium, and magnesium; they also may increase serum levels of calcium, glucose, and uric acid.

An especially important feature of the thiazides is their ability to impair free water clearance with no effect on concentration ability. The initial natriuretic effect lasts for about 1 week and then resets at a lower level. This diuretic tolerance occurs because of increased aldosterone levels and a decreased sodium load at the distal tubule. The mechanisms of antihypertensive action are believed to be initially due to the

TABLE 34-1 Selected diuretic pharmacokinetics and dosages*

Category/generic (trade name)	Onset of action (hr)	Peak effect (hr)	Duration of action (hr)	Initial dose	
				Adults	Children
Thiazide diuretics					
chlorothiazide (Diuril)	PO 2	4	6-12	250 mg q6-12h	6 months & older, 10-20 mg/kg/day
chlorthalidone (Hygroton)	PO 2	2	48-72	25-100 mg/day	2 mg/kg/day
hydrochlorothiazide (Esidrix)	PO 2	4	6-12	25-100 mg/day	1-2 mg/kg/day
metolazone (Zaroxolyn)	PO 1	2	12-24	5-20 mg/day	Not established
Loop diuretics					
bumetanide (Bumex)	PO 0.5-1	1-2	4-6	0.5-2 mg/day	Not established
	IV min	0.25-0.5	0.5-1		
ethacrynic acid (Edecrin)	PO 0.5	2	6-8	50-100 mg/day	25 mg/day
	IV within 5 min	0.25-0.5	2		
furosemide (Lasix)	PO ⅓-1	1-2	6-8	20-80 mg/day	2 mg/kg/day
	IV within 5 min	0.5	2		
torsemide (Demadex)	PO 0.5-1	1-2	6-8	10-20 mg/day	Not established
	IV within10 min	0.5-1	6-8		
Potassium-sparing diuretics					
amiloride (Midamor)	PO 1-2	6-10	24	5-10 mg/day	Not established
spironolactone (Aldactone)	PO 24-48	48-72	48-72	25-200 mg/day	1-3 mg/kg/day
triamterene (Dyrenium)	PO 2-4	24-72	7-9	25-100 mg/day	2-4 mg/kg/day
Osmotic diuretics					
glycerin (Osmoglyn)	PO 20 min	1-1.5	5	1-1.5 g/kg initially, then 0.5 g q6h	Same initial dose; may repeat in 4-8 hr.
isosorbide (Ismotic)	PO 10-30 min	1-1.5	5-6	1.5 g/kg 2-4 times/ day	Not established
mannitol (Osmitrol)	IV 0.5-1	1	6-8	50-100 g as 5%-25% IV infusion	0.25-2 g/kg as 15%-20% IV infusion
urea (Ureaphil)	IV 20 min	1-2	3-10	0.5-1.5 g/kg as 30% IV infusion	2 years and older, see adult dose

*Doses are titrated as needed and tolerated (Olin, 1996; *USP DI*, 1996).

reduction in plasma and extracellular fluid volume, which results in a decrease in cardiac output. In time, the cardiac output returns to normal. The thiazides also decrease peripheral resistance by a direct action on the peripheral blood vessels.

When an increased sodium load is presented to the distal tubule, there is a corresponding increase in potassium secretion. In addition, as the extracellular fluid volume decreases, plasma renin activity and aldosterone levels increase, with resulting potassium loss (Figure 34-2). Potassium is one of the most common electrolytes lost, with loss occurring in 14% to 60% of ambulatory hypertensive clients. This loss is dose related, occurring early in treatment (first month) and more frequently with the larger diuretic doses or with the long-acting type of diuretics (e.g., chlorthalidone) and in individuals with a high sodium intake (Tang & Lau, 1995). However, in many cases the loss is intermittent and neither harmful nor clinically observable. Potassium loss may be a serious threat in those who are taking digitalis preparations, since it can precipitate serious dysrhythmias as a result of digitalis toxicity. Hypokalemia may predispose the client with cirrhosis to hepatic encephalopathy and coma.

Health care providers should caution clients with prescribed thiazide therapy to increase their dietary intake of potassium (Box 34-1). If hypokalemia occurs, the prescriber may order oral potassium preparations; if urgent replacement is necessary, intravenous potassium chloride administration may be performed. Potassium loss may also be reversed by the addition of a potassium-sparing diuretic that acts to inhibit potassium loss at the distal tubule. However, potassium replacement is usually not necessary in 80% to 90% of individuals taking the thiazide diuretics, particularly for the treatment of nonedematous states. Potassium replacement may be dangerous in the elderly, in renal dysfunction, or when used in combination with potassium-sparing diuretics, since dangerously high serum potassium levels may occur.

Clients receiving the thiazide-type diuretics may have an increase in serum uric acid. The 1 to 2 mg/dl increase in serum uric acid level is persistent and probably results from inhibition of tubular secretion of uric acid. However, this

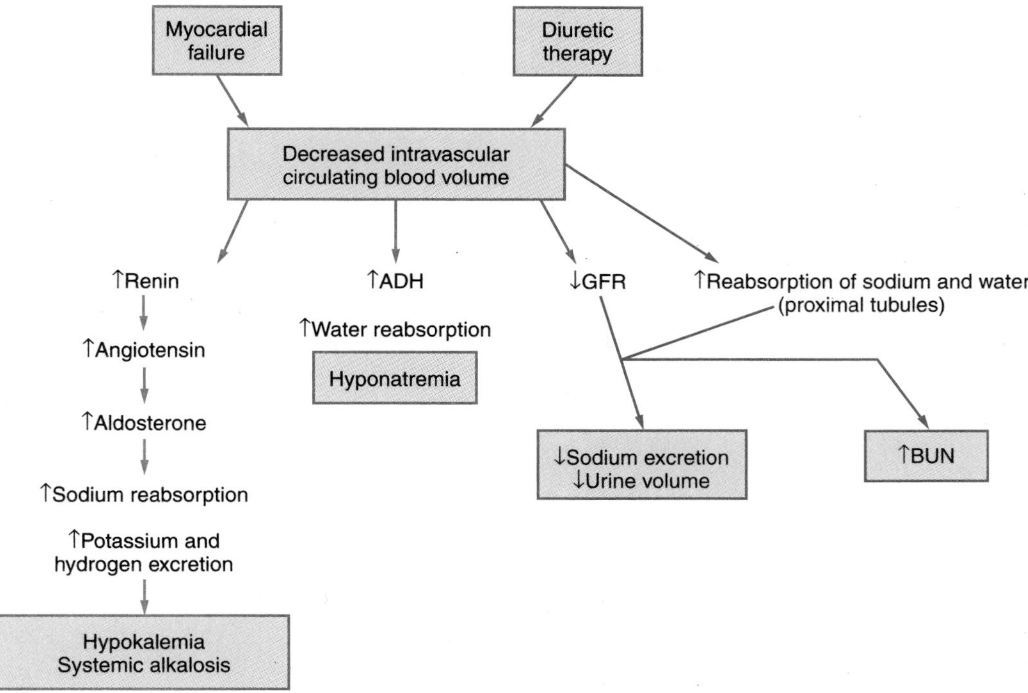

Figure 34-2 Body adaptation to extracellular volume depletion.

effect is reversible when the drugs are discontinued. In the absence of gout or genetic predisposition, the hyperuricemia is usually asymptomatic and requires no treatment. However, in a client with a history of gout the use of allopurinol or probenecid is suggested to counteract any elevation of serum uric acid.

Hyperglycemia or impaired glucose tolerance has also been reported with the thiazide-type and loop diuretics. This effect is reported most often in the elderly. The thiazides can precipitate diabetes in individuals with overt or subclinical disease patterns. Thiazide diuretics are not contraindicated for use in diabetic clients because if hyperglycemia is noted it can usually be controlled by diet alterations or by increasing the insulin dose. When hyperglycemia does occur in the nondiabetic client, many prescribers may try another type of diuretic such as furosemide to see if the problem can be reduced or alleviated.

The thiazide diuretics and perhaps furosemide have been associated with increasing serum levels of cholesterol and triglycerides. Because elevated serum lipid levels are associated with an increase in coronary heart disease, it is important that serum lipids be monitored and perhaps a specific dietary approach or weight loss program be implemented if necessary.

The indications for the thiazide diuretics include treating hypertension, edema associated with congestive heart failure, cirrhosis with ascites, and some types of renal impairment, such as nephrotic syndrome, acute glomerulonephritis, and chronic renal failure. These agents are well absorbed orally and are usually excreted unchanged by the kidneys. For pharmacokinetics and dosages, see Table 34-1.

■ Nursing Management

Thiazide and Thiazide-Type Diuretic Therapy

Assessment. Thiazide diuretics are given with caution to clients with severe renal impairment (may be ineffective or precipitate azotemia), hepatic impairment (may precipitate hepatic coma), diabetes mellitus (the dosages of hypoglycemic agents may need to be altered), or electrolyte imbalances (may be exacerbated). They are contraindicated or given carefully to pregnant women, since they cross the placental barrier (see the Pregnancy Safety box on p. 622). Check creatinine clearance for elderly clients to ensure adequate renal function before administering thiazide-type diuretics. About 60% of all adverse drug reactions in geriatric clients are due to diuretics (Kellick, 1992).

Review the client's current medication regimen for significant drug interactions. The following interactions may occur when thiazide or thiazide-type diuretics are given with the drugs listed below.

Drug	Possible effect and management
cholestyramine (Questran) or colestipol (Colestid)	Concurrent administration may reduce GI absorption of thiazide diuretics. Schedule administration of diuretics 1 hour before or 4 hours after administration of these drugs.
digitalis glycosides	Increased risk of digitalis toxicity in presence of hypokalemia. Monitor pulse and ECG closely.
lithium	**Not recommended. Increased risk of lithium toxicity possible because of decreased lithium excretion. Also, lithium has potential for nephrotoxic side effects. Avoid this combination.**

A baseline assessment of the client's underlying condition should be obtained: the blood pressure in hypertension and

BOX 34-1

Foods Rich in Potassium

Food	Amount	Potassium (mg)	Food	Amount	Potassium (mg)
Apricots			Prunes		
Fresh	1	105	Juice, canned or bottled	1 cup	706
Canned in water	1 cup	409	Dried	1 cup	1200
Dried, uncooked	1 cup	1791	Raisins	1 cup	1089
Avocado	1	1097	Lima beans, frozen, cooked	1 cup	694
Banana	1	451	Beets, sliced, cooked	1 cup	532
Figs			Brussels sprouts, cooked	1 cup	494
Fresh	1	116	Peanuts roasted in oil	1 ounce	200
Canned in heavy syrup	1 cup	258	Potato		
Dried, uncooked	1 cup	1418	Baked	1	610
Grapefruit			Boiled	1	515
Canned in water	1 cup	322	Spinach		
Fresh	½	312	Cooked, fresh	1 cup	838
Juice, canned, unsweetened	1 cup	378	Canned	1 cup	709
Melon, fresh cantaloupe	1 cup	494	From frozen	1 cup	566
Orange			Squash		
Fresh	1	237	Acorn, baked	1 cup	896
Juice, frozen, diluted	1 cup	474	Hubbard, mashed	1 cup	504
Peaches			Winter, mashed	1 cup	895
Fresh	1	171	Zucchini, canned	1 cup	622
Canned in water	1 cup	241	Sweet potato, baked	1	397
Dried	1 cup	1594	Tomato	1	297
Pears			Tomato juice, canned	1 cup	535
Fresh	1	208			
Canned in juice	1 cup	238			
Dried	1 cup	959			

Wardlaw et al (1994).

Pregnancy Safety

Category	Drug
B	amiloride, chlorothiazide, chlorthalidone, ethacrynic acid, hydrochlorothiazide, isosorbide, mannitol, methyclorthiazide, metolazone, torsemide, triamterene
C	acetazolamide, bendroflumethiazide, benzthiazide, bumetanide, cyclothiazide, furosemide, glycerin, hydroflumethiazide, trichlormethiazide, urea
Not established	spironolactone

the extent and severity of edema in clients with congestive heart failure.

Nursing diagnosis. Clients receiving thiazide or thiazide-like diuretics are at risk for the following nursing diagnoses: altered comfort (nausea); altered urinary elimination pattern (frequency and amount); altered bowel elimination (diarrhea or constipation); risk for injury related to orthostatic hypotension; and the potential complications of electrolyte imbalances (hypokalemia, hyponatremia, and hypochloremic alkalosis); allergic reaction; agranulocytosis (fever, lower back pain, dysuria); gout; hepatotoxicity; and thrombocytopenia (unusual bleeding and bruising, petechiae, and blood in urine or stools).

Implementation

Monitoring. Take the client's blood pressure before administering the diuretic to ensure that the client is not hypotensive. Daily weight and fluid balance monitoring will assist in determining the progress of the diuretic therapy. Because electrolyte imbalances are possible, monitor laboratory reports, particularly serum potassium levels. Monitoring is particularly important when digitalis compounds are part of the regimen, since hypokalemia primes clients taking digitalis preparations for toxic cardiac effects of the digitalis, such as bradycardia or ventricular irritability. Latent diabetes or gout may occasionally occur; laboratory reports should be monitored for hyperglycemia or hyperuricemia. Observe the client for signs and symptoms of fluid and electrolyte imbalances: hypovolemia, hyponatremia, hypokalemia, hypocalcemia, hypochloremia, or hypomagnesemia (Box 34-2).

Intervention. To reverse hypokalemia, add foods rich in potassium to the diet. Liquid potassium for oral use, although unpleasant tasting, may be disguised in cold juices and taken with food. Regular tomato juice is not recommended for this purpose because its sodium content is high, but low-sodium juices will do well to disguise the taste of potassium. Enteric-coated potassium tablets should be avoided because they have been implicated in ulcerations of the lining of the gastrointestinal tract.

Discontinue thiazides before parathyroid function tests are performed, since they may alter serum calcium concentrations.

As with other diuretics, plan dosing schedules to minimize the inconvenience of diuresis for the client.

Education. Teach clients that thiazides may make them feel unusually tired. Because of the potential for digitalis toxicity when these drugs are taken in combination with digitalis, clients also need to know how to take their pulse rate before taking digitalis medications. If the pulse rate is less than 60 beats/min or is irregular, digitalis medications should be discontinued and the prescriber notified. Nausea, vomiting, and anorexia are even earlier signs of digitalis toxicity that nurses and clients should recognize.

Clients should understand that diuretic drugs, if prescribed for a chronic condition, need to be taken as an integral part of their lifestyles.

As with acetazolamide, the client should receive instruction related to the prevention and minimization of the effects of xerostomia, constipation, and orthostatic hypotension. Signs and symptoms of electrolyte imbalances and blood dyscrasias should be taught, with proper referral to the prescriber.

Instruct clients to eat foods rich in potassium if a supplement is not prescribed.

Evaluation. Because these diuretics are indicated for hypertension and fluid volume excess, an expected outcome is that the client's blood pressure would decrease or be within normal limits and that, if fluid volume excess is evident, the client would experience an increased urinary output, weight loss, and an absence of rales and edema.

BOX 34-2

Signs and Symptoms of Fluid and Electrolyte Imbalances Associated with Diuretic Therapy

Hypovolemia: hypotension, weak pulse, tachycardia, clammy skin, rapid respirations, and reduced urinary output

Hyponatremia: low serum sodium levels (normal range 135 to 145 mEq/L), lethargy, disorientation, muscle tenseness, seizures, and coma

Hypokalemia: low serum potassium levels (normal range 3.5 to 5.0 mEq/L), weakness, abnormal ECG, postural hypotension, and flaccid paralysis

Hypocalcemia: low serum calcium levels (normal range 8.4 to 10.2 mg/dl), irritability, vomiting, diarrhea, twitching, hyperactive reflexes, cardiac dysrhythmias, tetany, and seizures

Hypochloremia: low blood chloride levels (normal range 100 to 110 mEq/L)

Hypomagnesemia: low serum magnesium levels (normal range 1.3 to 2.1 mEq/L), nausea and vomiting, lethargy, muscle weakness, tremors, and tetany

With potassium-sparing diuretics, be alert for:

Hyperkalemia: above-normal values for potassium serum levels, nausea, diarrhea, muscle weakness, postural hypotension, and ECG changes

LOOP DIURETICS

bumetanide [byoo met' a nide] (Bumex)
ethacrynic acid [eth a krin' ik] (Edecrin)
▲ **furosemide** [fur os' e myd] (Lasix, Furoside♣)
torsemide [tore' seh mide] (Demadex)

These agents are **loop diuretics,** so called because they inhibit reabsorption of sodium and water in the ascending loop of Henle. Agents that work here at the Na^+-K^+-$2Cl^-$ cotransport (or carrier transfer site) in the ascending limb are most effective because the diuretic effect is greater than that reported with the other diuretic sites (Jackson, 1996). These drugs for the most part are very similar to the thiazide-type diuretics in pharmacology and in the side effects they produce. Hyperglycemia, hyperuricemia, and increases in LDL cholesterol and triglycerides with a decrease in HDL cholesterol plasma levels are reported. The loop diuretics also increase excretion of magnesium and calcium, which may result in hypomagnesemia and hypocalcemia; thus they are administered with a normal saline infusion to treat hypercalcemia (Jackson, 1996).

Bumetanide inhibits sodium reabsorption in the ascending limb of the loop of Henle, as shown by marked reduction of free-water clearance during hydration and tubular free-water reabsorption during dehydration. Reabsorption of chloride in the ascending loop is also blocked by bumetanide, which may have an additional action in the proximal tubule. Because phosphate reabsorption takes place largely in the proximal tubule, phosphaturia during bumetanide-induced diuresis indicates this additional reaction. Bumetanide does not appear to have a noticeable action on the distal tubule.

The indications for loop diuretics include treatment of edema associated with congestive heart failure, cirrhosis, or renal disease. Furosemide is also used to treat hypertension.

These agents are also used as adjunct therapy in clients with acute pulmonary edema and in clients who are refractory to the other diuretics. The loop diuretics have fair-to-good absorption orally, are highly protein bound, are metabolized in the liver, and are excreted by the kidneys and in bile. For pharmacokinetics and dosage information see Table 34-1.

The side/adverse effects of loop diuretics include postural hypotension, blurred vision, headaches, abdominal distress, diarrhea, anorexia, anxiety, confusion, and ototoxicity. Photosensitivity has been reported with furosemide.

■ Nursing Management

Loop Diuretic Therapy

Assessment. The use of loop diuretics is not recommended in the presence of anuria or severe renal impairment because of decreased effectiveness. However, if they are used, the reduced clearance with renal function impairment may require higher doses but at more prolonged dosing intervals to reduce accumulation and the resultant risk of ototoxicity. With liver dysfunction, the use of loop diuretics increases the risk of dehydration and electrolyte imbalance.

The client's current medication regimen should be assessed for significant drug interactions. The following interactions may occur when loop diuretics are given with the drugs listed below.

Drug	Possible effect and management
amphotericin B injectable	**Increases risk for ototoxicity, nephrotoxicity, and electrolyte imbalance (especially hypokalemia). Avoid or a potentially serious drug interaction may occur.**
anticoagulants; coumarin (Coumadin), indanedione-type, or heparin	**Anticoagulant effects may be decreased with concurrent therapy. With ethacrynic acid the anticoagulant effects may be enhanced because of displacement of the anticoagulant from its protein binding sites. Gastrointestinal ulcers or bleeding is a possible adverse reaction to ethacrynic acid, which may increase the risk for hemorrhage. When possible, avoid giving ethacrynic acid to clients receiving anticoagulants. Avoid or a potentially serious drug interaction may occur. If loop diuretics are given concurrently, monitor clients closely for increased or decreased anticoagulant effectiveness.**
hypokalemia-causing drugs	Increased risk of hypokalemia when loop diuretics are administered concurrently. Monitor serum potassium levels and ECGs carefully; potassium supplements may be required.
lithium	Increased risk of lithium toxicity because of reduced renal clearance. Monitor closely.
nephrotoxic medications or other ototoxic medications	**Increases risks for ototoxicity and nephrotoxicity, especially in clients with renal impairment. Avoid or a potentially serious interaction may occur.**

A baseline assessment of the client's underlying condition should be obtained: the blood pressure in clients with hypertension and the extent and severity of edema in clients with congestive heart failure, cirrhosis, and renal disease.

Nursing diagnosis. Clients receiving loop diuretics should be assessed for the development of the following nursing diagnoses: altered comfort related to headache, local irritation at site of injection, and abdominal cramping; altered urinary elimination pattern (frequency and amount); altered bowel elimination (diarrhea or constipation); sensory-perceptual alterations (visual—blurred vision); risk for injury related to orthostatic hypotension (most frequent adverse effect); and the potential complications of allergic reaction (rash), ototoxicity evidenced by tinnitus (deafness), gout (joint pain, back pain), hepatotoxicity (yellow eyes or skin), pancreatitis (severe abdominal pain with nausea and vomiting), thrombocytopenia (unusual bleeding or bruising, black stools, hematuria, petechiae), and agranulocytosis or leukopenia (fever, chills, cough, dysuria).

Implementation

Monitoring. Weigh the client at the initiation of therapy and periodically thereafter to monitor fluid loss. When these diuretics are administered for acute excess fluid volume, it may be necessary to weigh the client on a daily basis. Weigh the client at the same time each day, preferably before breakfast, in similar clothing, and on the same scale for the most accurate readings. Weight loss and reduction in the extent of the edema would indicate effectiveness of the drug. Monitor blood pressure on a periodic basis; a reduction in blood pressure to values within normal limits is also sought. Closely monitor clients, especially the elderly, for extreme blood pressure changes; postural hypotension; dehydration (e.g., body weight loss of more than 2 pounds/day); allergic reactions (rashes); nausea, vomiting, and diarrhea; ototoxicity (tinnitus, hearing loss); and serum potassium deficiency.

Monitor carefully clients who may be experiencing potassium loss through other causes, such as vomiting, diarrhea, diaphoresis, gastrointestinal drainage, or paracentesis, for signs and symptoms of hypokalemia.

Be aware that hyperuricemia may occur; reversible elevation of BUN and creatinine levels may occur, especially in association with dehydration and particularly in clients with renal insufficiency.

Check reports of serum electrolytes, uric acid, blood and urine glucose tests, and BUN levels for abnormalities. Excessive doses or too-frequent administration can lead to prolonged water loss, electrolyte depletion, dehydration, reduction in blood volume, and circulatory collapse, with the possibility of vascular thrombosis and embolism, especially in elderly clients.

Be aware that hypokalemia can occur. Prevention of hypokalemia requires particular attention to the following conditions: individuals receiving digitalis and diuretics for congestive heart failure, hepatic cirrhosis, or ascites; states of aldosterone excess with normal renal function; potassium-losing nephropathy; and certain diarrheal states. Monitor serum potassium levels periodically; potassium supplements or potassium-sparing diuretics may be necessary. Periodic determination of other electrolytes is advised in clients who are on high doses for prolonged periods, particularly in clients on low-salt diets.

Periodically determine blood sugar, particularly in clients with diabetes or suspected latent diabetes.

Intervention. Use of the intramuscular route can produce temporary pain at the site, so oral or intravenous routes are preferable. Administer these drugs so that onset and peak of action will coincide with access to toilet facilities. Administer with food if gastrointestinal upset occurs with oral forms. When administering oral solutions, use the calibrated dropper provided by the manufacturer for accurate dosages.

For bumetanide and furosemide, administer intravenous injection slowly over 2 minutes. Administer ethacrynic acid intravenously at a controlled rate over 30 minutes; if a second dose is required use a different injection site to prevent thrombophlebitis.

Because many glass ampules have to be broken to prepare large dosages of furosemide intravenous infusions, there is the possibility of glass fragments occurring in the solution. Use a filter to remove these particles while drawing the drug into the syringe and also during intravenous administration.

Education. Caution the client to move carefully from sitting or lying positions to upright ones because of positional hypotension. Alcohol ingestion, hot weather, and standing or lying for long periods also increase the risk of orthostatic hypotension. Instruct the client in the symptoms of electrolyte imbalances (Box 34-2), particularly hypokalemia. Provide dietary counseling so the client will know which foods are rich in potassium.

Checking refills of the medication prescription provides a basis for client counseling for compliance with the regimen and also provides the opportunity for appropriate feedback.

Photosensitivity is a problem for some clients taking furosemide; caution them to avoid prolonged exposure to the sun or sunlamps. Encourage clients to use sunblocking lotion and to cover themselves with clothing.

Evaluation. The client will experience diuresis, absence of rales and edema, and blood pressure, central venous pressure (CVP), and pulmonary artery pressure (PAP) within normal limits.

DISTAL TUBULE DIURETICS/ POTASSIUM-SPARING DIURETICS

amiloride [a mill' oh ride] (Midamor)
▲ **spironolactone** [speer on oh lak' tone] (Aldactone)
triamterene [trye am' ter een] (Dyrenium)

The **potassium-sparing diuretics** are similar in action to other diuretics and are generally considered to be weak diuretics that act at the distal renal tubules. They block sodium reabsorption in the distal tubule thus increasing sodium and water excretion while conserving potassium. Generally they are primarily considered useful when combined with other potassium-losing diuretics.

Amiloride and triamterene directly inhibit reabsorption of sodium and water while spironolactone is an aldosterone antagonist. Any of the three agents may be used when it is necessary to restore or preserve the normal serum potassium level if other concurrent diuretic therapy challenges it and when potassium supplementation by medication or diet is inappropriate. These agents are highly effective for this purpose. If prescribed singly, however, their efficacy may actually result in an undesirable and rapidly developing hyperkalemia.

Spironolactone, a synthetic steroidal compound, antagonizes aldosterone effect by binding competitively to the protein that permits potassium secretion at the distal tubule. This response is directly related to the amount of circulating aldosterone in the serum. Spironolactone produces a very mild diuresis of sodium and water at the distal tubule by means of this mechanism. It does not interfere with renal tubule transport of sodium and chloride and does not inhibit carbonic anhydrase. Triamterene directly depresses the renal tubular transport of sodium in the distal tubule independent of the presence of aldosterone.

The potassium-sparing diuretics are indicated for the prevention and treatment of hypokalemia. They are also used as adjunct therapy in the treatment of edema and hypertension, and spironolactone is indicated in the diagnosis and treatment of primary hyperaldosteronism. These agents have low (amiloride), moderate (triamterene), or good (spironolactone) absorption from the gastrointestinal tract. Spironolactone and triamterene are metabolized in the liver, and amiloride and spironolactone are excreted mainly by the kidneys. Triamterene is excreted primarily in bile. For pharmacokinetics and dosages, see Table 34-1.

The side/adverse effects of potassium-sparing diuretics include abdominal cramps, diarrhea, nausea, vomiting, dry mouth, sedation, and hyperkalemia. Photosensitivity is reported with triamterene.

■ Nursing Management

Distal Tubule and Potassium-Sparing Diuretic Therapy

Assessment. Before giving these compounds, ascertain that the client has no related drug history of allergy or hyperkalemia because the potassium-sparing diuretics may further increase serum potassium levels. For clients who are at risk for developing hyperkalemia because of preexisting conditions such as impaired renal or hepatic function or diabetes mellitus, for severely ill patients, and for those with decreased urine volumes, which might aggravate electrolyte imbalances, greater caution is required in the administration of these diuretics.

The client's current medication regimen should be reviewed for significant drug interactions. The following interactions may occur when potassium-sparing diuretics are given with the drugs listed below.

Drug	Possible effect and management
anticoagulants	Anticoagulant effects may be decreased when used concurrently with potassium-sparing diuretics as a result of plasma volume reduction concentrating procoagulant factors in the blood. Dosage adjustment of anticoagulants may be necessary.
lithium	Concurrent use increases the risk of lithium toxicity by reducing renal clearance.
blood from bank, angiotensin-converting enzyme (ACE) inhibitors, cyclosporine, other potassium-sparing diuretics, low-salt milk, potassium-containing medications, or potassium supplements	May increase potassium levels and result in hyperkalemia. Monitor serum electrolytes closely.

A baseline health assessment, in addition to an assessment of the client's underlying condition for which the diuretic was prescribed, should include blood pressure, BUN and/or serum creatinine levels, and for triamterene a platelet and WBC count.

Nursing diagnosis. With the administration of distal tubule and potassium-sparing diuretics, the client should be assessed for the following nursing diagnoses: altered comfort related to muscle cramps, headache, dizziness, and gastrointestinal effects (nausea, vomiting, and abdominal cramping); altered bowel elimination (constipation or diarrhea); altered self-concept related to decreased libido, gynecomastia in males, and hirsutism in females; and the potential complications of hyperkalemia (confusion, dysrhythmias, paresthesia, fatigue), allergic reaction (shortness of breath, rash), nephrolithiasis (flank pain), agranulocytosis (fever, chills, dysuria), and thrombocytopenia (unusual bleeding or bruising, black stools, hematuria, petechiae).

Implementation

Monitoring. Monitor blood pressure, weight loss, and fluid balance to evaluate effectiveness of diuretic. Evaluate compliance with the client frequently. Especially at first, be alert to an irregular heartbeat (often the first clinical sign of hyperkalemia) or peaked T waves on ECG. Other warning signs of hyperkalemia are confusion, tingling in the extremities, difficulty in breathing, unexplained anxiety, fatigue, and physical weakness. Serum electrolyte determinations and an ECG are probably indicated if these occur.

Check laboratory reports closely, especially if the client is taking other similar drugs or potassium-rich foods. Rapidly increased serum potassium levels may occur. Act immediately to reverse hyperkalemia if serum potassium level exceeds 6 to 6.5 mEq/L and anticipate treatment with sodium bicarbonate, with glucose and regular insulin preparations, or with other therapy.

If the client is receiving spironolactone, remain sensitive to cues that he or she may be concerned about body image changes that may threaten sexual identity.

Note that when triamterene is being given, a complete blood count is probably indicated if the client has an unexplained sore throat, mouth ulcerations, or fever, which are all indications of a possible blood dyscrasia.

Intervention. Administering these drugs with food or milk may allay some gastrointestinal symptoms and possibly enhance bioavailability. Deal with unpleasant side effects such as dry mouth, thirst, or drowsiness if they arise.

Plan nursing measures common to diuretic agents, for example, measurements of fluid intake and output, daily weight changes, vital signs and heart rhythm, assessment of postural hypotension, weakness, or confusion. Monitor closely for hyperkalemia when transfusing blood. Whole blood may contain up to 30 mEq of potassium per liter; this may be doubled if blood has been stored for more than 10 days.

Education. The client should be counseled to avoid excessively stringent low-salt diets and relatively concentrated potassium intake in the form of citrus juices, cola beverages, low-sodium milk, some salt substitutes, and other potassium supplements.

Evaluation. The client will experience diuresis, absence of rales and edema, and blood pressure and serum potassium values within normal limits.

OSMOTIC DIURETICS

glycerin [gli' ser in] (Osmoglyn)
isosorbide [eye sew sore' bide] (Ismotic)
mannitol [man' i tole] (Osmitrol)
urea [yoor ee' a] (Ureaphil)

Osmotic diuretics include the parenteral agents, mannitol and urea, and the oral agents, glycerin and isosorbide. The two parenteral agents cause diuresis by adding to the solutes already present in the tubular fluid; they are particularly effective in increasing osmotic pressure because they are not reabsorbed by the tubules. Thus more water is pulled into tubular fluid, and less sodium, chloride, and water are reabsorbed by the kidneys in an effort to equalize the higher solute content. These excesses are then excreted in the urine. The oral agents are primarily used to reduce intraocular pressure before and after intraocular surgery and to interrupt an acute attack of glaucoma.

Parenteral agents (mannitol and urea) are used to treat cerebral edema and secondary glaucoma when other methods have been unsuccessful. Mannitol has also been used to increase urinary excretion of toxic substances (salicylates, barbiturates, lithium, bromides), as an irrigating preparation to prevent hemolysis and hemoglobin accumulation during transurethral prostatic resection, and as an adjunct to other therapies in the treatment of edema in acute renal failure.

Very little if any mannitol is metabolized in the liver. Urea is partially metabolized in the gastrointestinal tract to ammonia and carbon dioxide, which may be resynthesized into urea. Both mannitol and urea are excreted by the kidneys. Glycerin is metabolized in the liver and excreted by the kidneys. See Table 34-1 for pharmacokinetics and dosing.

The side/adverse effects of parenteral agents (mannitol, urea) include nausea, vomiting, dry mouth, headache, increased urination, and weakness. Mannitol may also cause visual disturbances, dizziness, and rash. Glycerin and isosorbide may induce nausea, vomiting, headache, increased thirst, dry mouth, diarrhea, and confusion.

Nursing Management

Osmotic Diuretic Therapy

Assessment. Ascertain that the client does not have preexisting severe dehydration, anuria, or severe pulmonary congestion for which osmotic diuretics are contraindicated. Intracranial bleeding, except during craniotomy, would negate the use of mannitol and urea. Caution should be used in their administration in clients with significant renal dysfunction or severe cardiopulmonary impairment because the sudden increase in extracellular fluid might lead to circulatory overload and congestive heart failure. The concurrent use of osmotic diuretics with digitalis glycosides may increase the risk of digitalis toxicity associated with hypokalemia.

Recommend that baseline serum electrolyte and renal function determinations be performed if they have not been done, and monitor the results.

Note that mannitol is different from the drug mannitol hexanitrate; do not confuse them.

Nursing diagnosis. Clients receiving osmotic diuretics should be assessed for the following nursing diagnoses: altered comfort (dry mouth, nausea, vomiting, headache, dizziness, rash, chest pain, and blurred vision); hyperthermia; altered urinary elimination pattern (frequency and amount); and the potential complications of electrolyte imbalance, pulmonary congestion, and thrombophlebitis.

Implementation

Monitoring. Because these are potent osmotic drugs, it is essential to be alert to rapidly changing client conditions; frequently assess urinary output and vital signs for changing intravascular volume, pulmonary edema, or hemoconcentration. Monitor fluid and electrolyte balance, particularly serum and urine potassium and sodium levels. When urea is administered, BUN determinations should be done before and frequently during intravenous administration. If the BUN exceeds 75 mg/dl or if there is no diuresis within 1 to 2 hours, slow or stop the infusion and have the client reevaluated. If the osmotic diuretics are administered for reduction of intraocular pressure, monitor the pressure closely.

Intervention. If the adequacy of renal function is suspect before the administration of mannitol, a test dose is usually ordered prescribed. It is given as an intravenous infusion over 3 to 5 minutes. Urine flow should increase to at least 30 to 50 ml/hr for 2 to 3 hours after this or a second test dose. If it does not, mannitol should be withheld and the client should be reevaluated. Infuse mannitol and urea separately from other drugs and blood. Crystallization in solution is common; it may be countered by warming the solution until crystals are invisible and by inserting a filter in the line whenever this drug is infused. Avoid extravasation of urea and mannitol; observe the intravenous site periodically for tissue inflammation, irritation, and necrosis.

Infuse urea into large veins. For both urea and mannitol, avoid using lower extremity intravenous sites because phlebitis and thrombosis may occur, particularly in the elderly. Do not infuse urea more rapidly than 4 ml/min because hemolysis and cerebral vasomotor symptoms may occur.

To assist in the prevention and relief of headache caused by cerebral dehydration, have the client lie down during and after the administration of these drugs.

Use an indwelling catheter with comatose clients to ensure urinary drainage. The use of a urometer that allows for precise measurement of output is important because the therapy is based on evaluation of accurate intake and output.

When these drugs are administered preoperatively, the dosing schedule should be: glycerin, isosorbide, and mannitol, ½ to 1 hour before surgery; urea, 1 hour before surgery if administered for the reduction of intraocular pressure or at the time of scalp incision during intracranial surgery.

Glycerin and isosorbide may be mixed with iced unsweetened fruit juice and sipped through a straw to increase palatability. With repeated doses of these drugs, maintain adequate fluid and electrolyte balance.

Education. Prepare the client for the diuresis that will occur with these drugs. Provide for the convenience, comfort, and privacy of the client.

Advise client taking glycerin and isosorbide for the reduction of intraocular pressure to visit the physician regularly for intraocular pressure monitoring.

Evaluation. If osmotic diuretics are administered for increased intracranial pressure, the client should have an ICP monitor value within an acceptable range. If the indication for the drugs is increased intraocular pressure, the client should demonstrate a reduced intraocular pressure value upon tonometer measurement. If these drugs are being given for acute renal failure, the client should have diuresis and an improvement in BUN and serum creatinine values.

DIURETIC COMBINATIONS

As mentioned previously, a thiazide diuretic may be combined with a potassium-sparing diuretic. Fixed-dose combinations, which are commercially available, may provide additional diuretic activity and decrease the potassium depletion characteristic of the thiazide diuretics. Additionally, diuretics are combined with antihypertensive agents to simplify medication regimens for clients whose hypertensive status has somewhat stabilized (Box 34-3).

BOX 34-3

Examples of Fixed-Dose Diuretic Combinations

Trade name	Contents
Aldactazide 25/25	spironolactone, 25 mg; hydrochlorothiazide, 25 mg
Aldactazide 50/50	spironolactone, 50 mg; hydrochlorothiazide, 50 mg
Capozide 50/15, 25/25, & 50/25	captopril 25 or 50 mg with hctz* 15 or 25 mg
Dyazide	triamterene, 50 mg; hydrochlorothiazide, 25 mg
Hydropres-50	reserpine 0.125 mg with hctz* 50 mg
Hyzaar	losartan 50 mg with hctz* 12.5 mg
Inderide LA 80/50, 120/50, or 160/50	propranolol 80, 120, or 160 mg with hctz* 50 mg
Lopressor HCT 50/25, 100/25, or 100/50	metroprolol 50 or 100 mg with hctz* 25 or 50 mg
Maxzide	triamterene, 75 mg; hydrochlorothiazide, 50 mg
Timolide 10-25	timolol 10 mg with hctz* 25 mg
Ziac	bisoprolol fumarate 2.5, 5, or 10 mg with hctz* 6.25 mg

*hctz, hydrochlorothiazide.

SUMMARY

Diuretics are valuable assets in the therapeutic regimen for the treatment of hypertension and other conditions in which fluid volume excess is an issue, such as congestive heart failure, cirrhosis, and nephrotic syndrome. These drugs act on the tubular function of the kidneys and inhibit solute reabsorption; water reabsorption is affected because water diffuses passively across the tubular membrane when sodium transport occurs. Diuretics are therefore generally grouped by the major site of their action along the tubule: proximal tubule diuretics, diluting segment diuretics, loop diuretics, and distal tubule diuretics. Osmotic diuretics act by adding to the solutes already present in tubular fluid; since they are not reabsorbed, more water is pulled into tubular fluid and less sodium, chloride, and water are reabsorbed by the kidneys in an effort to equalize the higher solute volume that is excreted in the urine.

Nursing management focuses on the education of the client for safe and accurate self-administration of diuretics, particularly in the early recognition of adverse reactions. Hypokalemia is common, except in clients taking potassium-sparing diuretics, and clients should understand the importance of including potassium-rich foods in their diet if a potassium supplement has not been prescribed. Evaluation of the effectiveness of the therapeutic regimen through the accurate measurement of the client's blood pressure, fluid balance, and weight is essential.

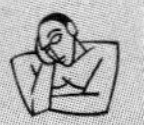

Critical Thinking

1. What conditions will place clients receiving loop diuretics at higher risk for hypokalemia? What observations by the nurse would be particularly important for these clients?
2. What conditions will place clients receiving distal tubule and potassium-sparing diuretics at higher risk for hyperkalemia? What observations by the nurse would be particularly important for these clients?
3. Mrs. Williams, an 82-year-old woman, lives alone in substandard urban housing. Although she has hypertension and chronic congestive heart failure, she maintains her independence with the assistance of members of her church shopping for her, bringing her meals occasionally, and taking her for visits to her doctor. Her current medication regimen is: digoxin 0.25 mg PO daily; furosemide 20 mg PO bid; K-Dur 20 mEq PO daily; verapamil SR 240 mg PO daily; and isosorbide dinitrate 10 mg PO qid. For what nursing diagnoses/collaborative problems is Mrs. Williams at risk? Why? As her home health care nurse, what will be your plan of care?

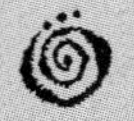

Collaborative Learning Activities

1. Student teams will present each of the various classifications of diuretics, including the mechanism of action, differing indications, and side/adverse effects. Discuss the effect of each with regard to nursing care and client instruction.

BIBLIOGRAPHY

American Hospital Formulary Service (1996). *AHFS drug information '96*. Bethesda, MD: American Society of Hospital Pharmacists.

American Medical Association (1995). *Drug evaluations: Annual 1995*. Chicago: The Association.

Anderson KN, et al. (Eds.) (1994). *Mosby's medical, nursing, & allied health dictionary* (4th ed.). St Louis: Mosby.

FDA (1994). Regulatory actions, Demadex, *Hosp Formul* 29(4):226.

Jackson EK (1996). Diuretics. In Hardman JG & Limbird LE (Eds.). *Goodman & Gilman's the pharmacological basis of therapeutics* (9th ed.). New York: McGraw-Hill.

Kollick KA (1992). Diuretics, *AACN* 3(2):472.

Mendyka BE (1992). Fluid and electrolyte disorders caused by diuretic therapy, *AACN* 3(3):672.

Menscer D (1992). Hypertension. In Ham RJ & Sloane PD. *Primary care geriatrics: A case-based approach* (2nd ed.). St Louis: Mosby.

Olin BR (Ed.) (1996). *Facts and comparisons*. St Louis: Facts and Comparisons.

Tang I & Lau AH (1995). Fluid and Electrolyte Disorders. In Young LY & Koda-Kimble MA (Eds). *Applied therapeutics: The clinical use of drugs* (6th ed.). Vancouver, WA: Applied Therapeutics.

United States Pharmacopeial Convention (1996). *USP DI: Drug information for the health care professional* (16th ed.). Rockville, MD: The Convention.

Wardlaw GM, et al. (1994). *Contemporary nutrition: Issues and insights* (2nd ed.). St Louis: Mosby.

Williams SR (1993). *Nutrition and diet therapy* (7th ed.). St Louis: Mosby.

Chapter 35

Uricosuric Drugs

Chapter Focus

Gout, a disorder of uric acid metabolism in the body, affects nearly a half million Americans. While it can affect both males and females, nearly all those with gout are men, with less than 5% of diagnosed cases being postmenopausal women, probably because estrogen promotes excretion of uric acid (McCance & Huether, 1994). The nurse manages care during the acute episodes but primarily provides teaching and counseling for clients to self-manage the therapeutic regimen to prevent the painful attacks of gout. The following objectives and key terms are important for a good understanding of this chapter.

Key Terms

gout (p. 630)
hyperuricemia (p. 630)
urate nephropathy (p. 632)

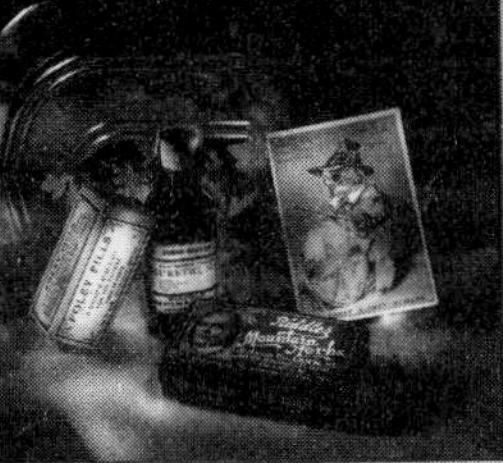

Key Drugs [▲]

allopurinol
colchicine

Objectives

1. Recall the process of production of uric acid in the body.
2. Describe the classic symptoms of gout and the objectives for the treatment of gout.
3. Identify other diseases in which a secondary hyperuricemia may occur and common drugs that may increase or decrease a client's uric acid level.
4. List the common side effects/adverse reactions and the significant drug interactions for uricosuric drugs.
5. Implement the nursing management for the care of a client receiving a uricosuric drug.

Hyperuricemia and gout occur in persons with an abnormality in uric acid production and/or excretion.

GOUT

Gout is a disease associated with an inborn error of uric acid metabolism that increases production or inhibits the excretion of uric acid. The hallmark of gout is **hyperuricemia**, or high levels of uric acid in the blood.

Gout is characterized by a defective purine metabolism and manifests itself by attacks of acute pain, swelling, and tenderness of joints, such as those of the big toe, ankle, instep, knee, and elbow. The amount of uric acid in the blood becomes elevated, and tophi, which are deposits of uric acid or urates, form in the cartilage of various parts of the body. These deposits tend to increase in size. They are seen most often along the edge of the ear. Chronic arthritis, nephritis, and premature sclerosis of blood vessels may develop if gout is uncontrolled.

Treatment goals for gout are to (1) end the acute gouty attack as soon as possible, (2) prevent a recurrence of acute gouty arthritis, (3) prevent the formation of uric acid stones in the kidneys, and (4) reduce or prevent disease complications that result from sodium urate deposits in joints and kidneys.

The drugs used to treat an acute gout attack include colchicine, nonsteroidal antiinflammatory drugs (NSAIDs), and corticosteroids. The NSAIDs are primarily used to treat the acute inflammation and have no effect on the underlying metabolic problem. They are often prescribed to relieve an acute gout attack while colchicine is reserved for persons that are not responsive to these agents or individuals that cannot tolerate them (*USP DI*, 1996). The NSAIDs are reviewed in Chapter 14. Colchicine, specifically used to treat gout, is reviewed in this chapter. To treat chronic gouty arthritis or to prevent gout attacks, allopurinol, probenecid, sulfinpyrazone, and salicylates have all been used. Salicylates require very high daily dosages, such as 4 to 6 g/day. Because few individuals can tolerate such high dosages on a long-term basis, they are not commonly prescribed for gout.

The nurse should be aware that low doses of aspirin can interfere with uric acid excretion, resulting in exacerbation of gout, and that a secondary hyperuricemia may occur from neoplastic diseases or cancer, psoriasis, Paget's disease, and other common and rare disease states. Many drugs have also been reported to cause an increase or a decrease in uric acid levels (Table 35-1). It is preferable for the prescriber to identify the cause of the hyperuricemia and then to decide whether or not to treat it. Asymptomatic hyperuricemia in an elderly person may or may not be drug induced and often is not treated by the prescriber because of the potential adverse drug reactions and the cost of the medications (Figure 35-1). However, if symptoms are present or a treatable disease state is identified, then specific treatments would be indicated.

▲ colchicine (kol' chi seen)

Colchicine's mechanism of action for gout is unknown although it is reported to have antiinflammatory effects in gout. It also decreases phagocytosis, leukocyte motility, lactic acid production, and the release of a glycoprotein produced during urate crystal phagocytosis. This results in a decrease in urate deposits and inflammation even though the drug does not affect levels of uric acid in the circulatory system.

Colchicine is used in the treatment and prophylaxis of acute gouty arthritis and in the treatment of chronic gouty arthritis. In acute gouty arthritis it has an onset of action within 12 hours after oral administration and intravenous injection. The peak effect for relief of pain and inflammation is reached in 1 to 2 days, but reduction of swelling may require 3 days or more. Colchicine is metabolized in the liver and excreted mainly in bile.

The side/adverse effects with oral administration of colchicine include diarrhea, nausea, vomiting, abdominal pain, anorexia, and, with chronic therapy, alopecia.

The adult antigout dosage for prophylaxis is 0.5 to 0.6 mg orally daily, increased if necessary to twice daily. The dose for acute gouty attacks is 0.5 to 1.2 mg (1 to 2 tablets) initially, followed by one tablet every 1 to 2 hours until pain is relieved or the side effects of nausea, vomiting, or diarrhea have occurred or until the maximum dose of 6 mg has been reached. Pediatric dosage has not been established. The adult IV dose for prophylaxis is 0.5 mg to 1 mg once or twice daily. For use in acute gouty attacks, the dosage is 2 mg IV initially followed by 0.5 mg every 6 to 12 hours until the desired effect is achieved.

■ Nursing Management

Colchicine Therapy

Assessment. Caution should be used when this drug is given to elderly persons because they have diminished renal function and are more likely to have cumulative toxicity, as are those with cardiac, renal, or gastrointestinal disease. Because colchicine is excreted primarily through the biliary route, caution should be used if the client has hepatic function impairment. Obtain a baseline assessment of the client's uric acid levels, complete blood count, and joint pain and stiffness before therapy.

TABLE 35-1 Medications affecting serum uric acid levels

Increase levels	Decrease levels
alcohol	acetohexamide
aminoglycosides	ACTH hormone
cancer chemotherapeutic agents	allopurinol
diuretics (thiazides, furosemide)	chloramphenicol
ethambutol	probenecid
levodopa	radiopaque dyes
methyldopa	salicylates (more than 3 g/day)
pancrelipase	streptomycin
salicylates (less than 2 g/day)	tetracycline (outdated)

(Pagana & Pagana, 1992; *USP DI*, 1996; Young & Comagna, 1995.)

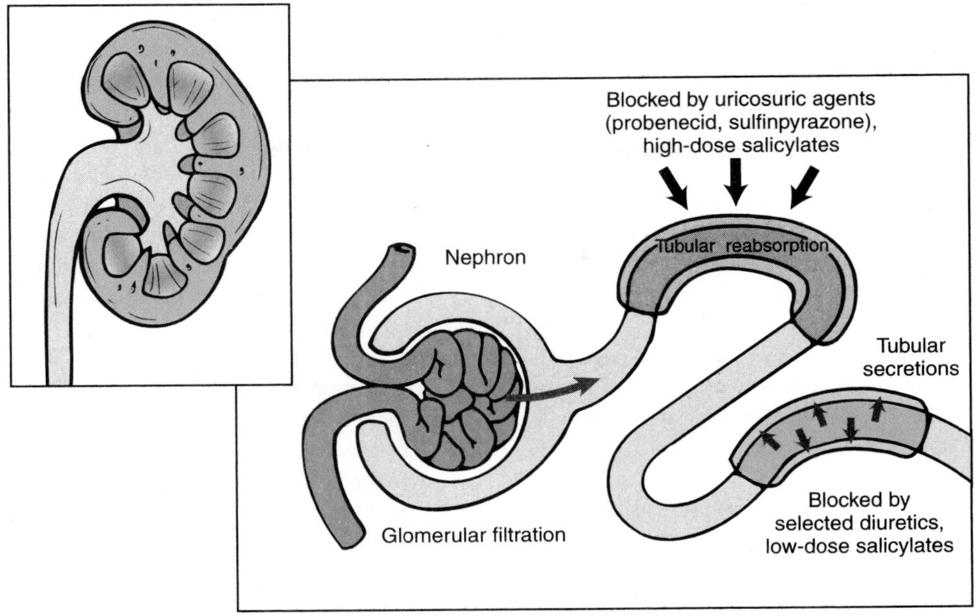

Figure 35-1 Drug effects on uric acid excretion in the kidney.

When colchicine is given concurrently with radiation therapy or drugs that induce blood dyscrasia or bone marrow depression (such as phenylbutazone [Alka Butazolidine], chloramphenicol [Chloromycetin], antineoplastics, and others) the risk of inducing bone marrow depression or other serious, toxic, hematologic effects may be increased.

A baseline assessment should include the client's general health status, the frequency and severity of gout symptoms, and complete blood counts.

Nursing diagnosis. Assessment of the client receiving colchicine should include consideration of the following selected nursing diagnoses: altered comfort related to pain at injection site (thrombophlebitis), rash, stomach pain, anorexia, nausea, and vomiting; hyperthermia; altered protection related to leukopenia; altered thought processes related to mood and mental changes; disturbance of self-concept related to hair loss; altered urinary elimination pattern related to renal effects evidenced by decreased urinary output; and the potential complications of thrombocytopenia (increased tendency to bleed), seizures, aplastic anemia, respiratory depression, pulmonary edema, and peripheral neuritis (numbness and tingling of the hands and feet).

Implementation

Monitoring. The nurse should monitor the client's affected joints for range of motion, pain, and swelling. Because of the risk of bone marrow depression, the client's complete blood count as well as serum uric acid levels should be monitored. Monitor fluid intake and output to assess adequacy of urinary output. The drug should be discontinued as soon as the pain of the acute gout episode is relieved, if gastrointestinal symptoms occur, or if the maximum dosage is reached.

Intervention. To be effective, colchicine must be given properly at the first indication of an oncoming attack, and the dosage must be adequate. Once the dose that will cause diarrhea has been determined, it is often possible to reduce subsequent doses to prevent diarrhea and still achieve satisfactory relief of pain. To avoid the toxic effects of accumulation the drug should not be administered for 3 days after being administered for the acute episode.

Oral colchicine may be administered with food to prevent gastrointestinal distress. Oral administration is preferred for prophylaxis; however, administration via the IV route is preferable for alcoholic clients because they are more susceptible to gastrointestinal toxicity, which is more likely to occur with oral administration.

Colchicine cannot be given subcutaneously or intramuscularly because it is highly irritating and will cause tissue necrosis. When given intravenously, extravasation must be avoided. Colchicine is incompatible with and will precipitate if mixed with or injected into intravenous tubing containing 5% dextrose solution, solutions containing a bacteriostatic agent, or any solution that would change the pH of the colchicine solution. To dilute colchicine, use 0.9% sodium chloride injection or sterile water for injection. Change the needle before administration. Administer the intravenous injection over a period of 2 to 5 minutes.

Fluid intake needs to be encouraged to ensure a urinary output of at least 2000 ml daily.

Education. Alert the client to start the medication at the earliest sign of an attack, but to discontinue it when the pain is relieved, at the first sign of diarrhea, nausea or vomiting, or stomach pain, or when the maximum dosage is reached; the course of therapy should not be repeated for at least 3 days unless otherwise instructed by the prescriber. Because colchicine has such a narrow margin of safety, alert the client to report to the prescriber as soon as possible any signs of nausea, vomiting, diarrhea, sore throat, unusual bleeding or bruising, or unusual tiredness. Advise the client to visit the health care provider regularly so that progress can be monitored.

Caution the client not to drink alcoholic beverages while taking colchicine since alcohol increases the risk of gastrointestinal toxicity and decreases the effectiveness of the medication by increasing uric acid levels.

Instruct the client to inform other health care providers that colchicine is being taken before any surgical or dental procedures are performed.

Evaluation. The client on colchicine therapy will experience relief of pain associated with the gout attack or will not experience an acute episode of gout.

▲ **allopurinol** [al oh pure' i nole] (Zyloprim, Purinol ♣)
Allopurinol decreases the production of uric acid by inhibiting xanthine oxidase, the enzyme necessary to convert hypoxanthine to xanthine and xanthine to uric acid (Figure 35-2). It also increases the reutilization of both hypoxanthine and xanthine for nucleic acid synthesis, thus resulting in a feedback inhibition of purine synthesis. The result is a decrease of uric acid in both the serum and urine.

This decrease of uric acid will prevent or decrease urate deposits, thus preventing or reducing both gouty arthritis and **urate nephropathy**. The reduction in urinary urate levels prevents the formation of uric acid or calcium oxalate calculi in the kidneys.

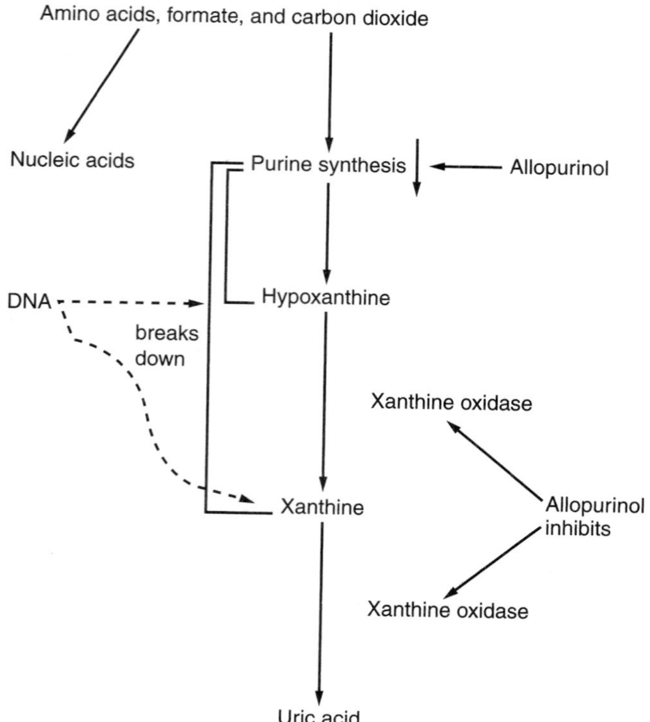

Figure 35-2 Uric acid production and allopurinol effects in the body.

Allopurinol is indicated for the treatment of chronic gouty arthritis and for the prophylaxis and treatment of hyperuricemia, uric acid nephropathy, and renal calculi. It is well absorbed orally; the onset of action in reducing serum uric acid is 2 to 3 days. Approximately 70% of a dose is metabolized in the liver to an active metabolite, oxipurinol. Reduction of uric acid to a normal range occurs in 1 to 3 weeks, whereas a decrease in frequency of acute gout attacks may require several months of drug therapy. Excretion is via the kidneys.

The side/adverse effects of allopurinol include pruritus, allergic reaction, rash, hives, diarrhea, abdominal distress, nausea, and vomiting.

The adult antihyperuricemic dosage is 100 mg daily initially, increased by 100 mg/day at 7 day intervals if necessary. The maximum daily dosage should not exceed 800 mg. The maintenance dosage is 100 to 200 mg two to three times daily or 300 mg once daily. For treatment of hyperuricemia (from antineoplastic therapy), initially administer 600 to 800 mg orally daily, beginning 2 to 3 days before chemotherapy or radiation therapy. For maintenance therapy, adjust dosage according to serum uric acid levels, which are analyzed about 2 days after the initiation of allopurinol and periodically thereafter. Discontinue allopurinol during the period of tumor regression.

To treat uric acid calculi, give 100 to 200 mg orally one to four times daily or 300 mg daily as a single dose. For the pediatric dosage as an antihyperuricemic agent in antineoplastic therapy, see a current package insert or *USP DI*.

■ Nursing Management

Allopurinol Therapy

Assessment. If the client has impaired renal function or any illness that may predispose to a change in renal function, such as diabetes mellitus or hypertension, a reduction in dosage and monitoring of renal function may be necessary because allopurinol may accumulate and increase the risk of allergic reactions and other adverse effects.

The client's medication regimen should be reviewed for significant drug interactions, which may occur when allopurinol is given concurrently with the drugs listed below:

Drug	Possible effect and management
anticoagulants, oral (coumarin or indanedione)	Allopurinol may inhibit metabolism of the oral anticoagulant resulting in an increase in serum levels, activity, and perhaps toxicity. Monitor prothrombin levels closely because dosage adjustment may be necessary.

Pregnancy Safety

Category	Drug
C	allopurinol
D	colchicine
Unclassified	probenecid, sulfinpyrazone

Drug	Possible effect and management
azathioprine (Imuran) or mercaptopurine (Purinethol)	Allopurinol's effect of inhibiting xanthine oxidase may result in decreased metabolism of these medications, leading to an increased potential for therapeutic and/or toxic effects (especially bone marrow depression). Monitor closely because interventions or dosage adjustments may be necessary.

A baseline assessment of the client should include serum uric acid levels, complete blood counts, hepatic and renal function determinations, and joint stiffness and pain.

Nursing diagnosis. Assessment of the client receiving allopurinol should include consideration of the following nursing diagnoses: altered comfort (headache, stomach pain, anorexia, nausea, and vomiting); impaired skin integrity (exfoliative dermatitis); altered bowel elimination (diarrhea); disturbance of self-concept related to hair loss; altered urinary elimination related to renal effects evidenced by decreased urinary output; and the potential complications of peripheral neuritis (numbness and tingling of the hands and feet), allergic dermatitis (rash, hives, itching), hepatitis, thrombocytopenia (increased tendency to bleed), erythema multiforme (chills, fever, sores in mouth, skin rash), and Stevens-Johnson syndrome, or toxic epidermal necrolysis (chills, fever, muscle ache, peeling of skin).

Implementation

Monitoring. For proper dosing, serum uric acid levels should be monitored. CBCs and renal and hepatic function studies are recommended at periodic intervals during therapy, particularly in the first few months. Monitor the client's intake to ensure an adequate fluid intake. Observe the client's pain level and the mobility status of affected joints.

Intervention. Administer with food to minimize gastrointestinal distress. For ease of administration for clients who have difficulty swallowing, the tablets may be crushed and mixed with a small amount of applesauce or jelly.

A high fluid intake (80 to 96 oz daily to produce 2 L of urine) and alkalinization of the urine are necessary to lessen the risk of stone formation and sluding of the tubules with urates.

Any single dose of allopurinol should not exceed 300 mg; it may be given in divided doses.

Education. Encourage the client to comply with the medication regimen. The client should be advised that allopurinol helps prevent, but does not relieve, acute gout episodes.

Caution the client not to drink alcoholic beverages because alcohol increases uric acid concentrations. Alert the client that drowsiness may occur and that hazardous activities requiring mental alertness, such as driving, need to be avoided until the response to the medication has been determined. Stress the importance of the large amount of fluid intake necessary to ensure adequacy of fluid output.

To minimize the formation of calcium oxalate stones, the client should maintain a diet that enhances the alkalinity of the urine, such as milk, fruits (except plums, prunes, and cranberries), carbonated beverages, vegetables (except corn and lentils), molasses, and baking soda and baking powder. Aspirin and large doses of vitamin C should be avoided.

The client should be advised to report to the prescriber immediately any signs of a skin rash or other adverse reactions. Skin rash usually precedes severe hypersensitivity reactions. Regular visits to the prescriber are necessary to monitor progress through periodic blood testing and assessment for side effects/adverse reactions.

Evaluation. The client on allopurinol therapy will experience fewer or no acute gout attacks.

probenecid [proe ben' e sid] (Benemid, Benuryl)

Probenecid is indicated for the treatment of hyperuricemia, chronic gouty arthritis, and as an adjunct to antibiotic therapy. It lowers serum levels of uric acid by competitively inhibiting the reabsorption of urate at the proximal renal tubule, thus increasing the urinary excretion of uric acid. It has no antiinflammatory action or analgesic effects.

As an adjunct to antibiotic therapy, probenecid competitively inhibits the secretion of weak organic acids, such as penicillin and some of the cephalosporins, at both the proximal and distal renal tubules in the kidneys. The result is an increase in blood concentrations and duration of action of these antibiotics. This combination is used to treat sexually transmitted diseases (e.g., gonorrhea, acute pelvic inflammatory disease [PID], and neurosyphilis).

Probenecid is well absorbed orally and is highly bound to plasma proteins, especially to albumin. The therapeutic serum level for uricosuric effect is 100 to 200 μg/ml; for suppression of penicillin excretion, 40 to 60 μg/ml. Peak uricosuric effect is reached within 30 minutes, whereas peak suppression of penicillin excretion is noted in 2 hours and lasts nearly 8 hours. Probenecid is metabolized in the liver and excreted by the kidneys.

The side/adverse effects of probenecid include headaches, anorexia, mild nausea or vomiting, sore gums, pain and/or blood on urination, and lower back pain. The adult dose is 250 mg twice daily for 7 days, then increased to 500 mg twice a day. As an adjunct to penicillin/cephalosporin drug therapy the dose is 500 mg four times daily. Pediatric dosage as an antihyperuricemic agent is not established. As an antibiotic adjunct, check a current drug reference for recommended dosing schedules.

■ Nursing Management

Probenecid Therapy

Assessment. Probenecid is well tolerated by most clients, except those with peptic ulcer disease, glucose-6-phosphate dehydrogenase deficiency, acute intermittent porphyria, blood dyscrasias, and a history of uric acid kidney stones, because their conditions may be exacerbated.

The client's drug history should be taken to detect significant drug interactions such as those that may occur when probenecid is given concurrently with the drugs listed below:

Drug	Possible effect and management
indomethacin (Indocin), ketoprofen (Orudis), and other NSAIDs	**Probenecid decreases the renal excretion of ketoprofen by 66%, protein binding by 28%, and the formation of ketoprofen conjugates. This leads to an increase in ketoprofen serum levels and, possibly, toxicity. Avoid or a potentially serious drug interaction may occur.** Probenecid may also decrease excretion of indomethacin and possibly other NSAIDs from the body, thus leading to increased serum levels, extended half-life, and an increased potential for NSAID toxicity. Monitor closely because the prescriber may need to lower the daily dose of NSAID if adverse effects are reported.
antineoplastic cytolytic drugs	**Increases potential toxicity of uric acid nephropathy. Also, the rapidly acting antineoplastic drugs may increase plasma uric acid levels and interfere with any control of the previous hyperuricemia and gout. Avoid or a potentially serious drug interaction may occur.**
aspirin or salicylates	**Not recommended because salicylates in moderate to high doses given chronically will inhibit the effectiveness of probenecid. Also, if high doses of salicylates are being given for their uricosuric effects, probenecid may lower the excretion of salicylates, which may result in elevated serum salicylate levels and toxicity. Avoid or a potentially serious drug interaction may occur.**
cephalosporins, penicillins	Probenecid decreases the renal tubular secretion of penicillin and selected cephalosporins, which may result in an increased serum level and prolonged duration of action of the antibiotic. An increased risk of toxicity may also be present. Monitor serum levels closely if given concurrently. Cephalosporins not affected by probenecid include cefoperazone (Cefobid), ceforanide, ceftazidime (Fortaz), ceftriaxone (Rocephin).
heparin	**The anticoagulant effects of heparin may be enhanced and prolonged. Avoid or a potentially serious drug interaction may occur.**
methotrexate (Folex, Mexate)	Probenecid may decrease the renal excretion of methotrexate, which may increase the risk of serious toxicity with methotrexate. If used concurrently, administer a lower dose of methotrexate and monitor closely for toxicity or monitor methotrexate serum levels.
nitrofurantoin (Furadantin)	Probenecid may decrease the renal tubular secretion of nitrofurantoin, resulting in an increase in serum levels and possibly toxicity. This may reduce the urinary levels and effectiveness of nitrofurantoin. A reduction in probenecid dosage may be necessary to use nitrofurantoin in urinary tract infections. Monitor effectiveness closely.
zidovudine (AZT)	Concurrent drug administration may lead to inhibition of zidovudine metabolism and secretion, resulting in elevated serum levels and an increased risk of zidovudine toxicity. The administration of probenecid may permit a reduced daily dose schedule for zidovudine. In one trial, a high incidence of skin rash was reported.

A baseline assessment of the client should include serum uric acid determinations, acid-base balance determinations, and joint pain and stiffness.

Nursing diagnosis. Assessment of the client receiving probenecid should include consideration of the following selected nursing diagnoses: altered comfort (headache, stomach pain, anorexia, nausea, and vomiting); hyperthermia; disturbance of self-concept related to hair loss; altered urinary elimination related to renal effects evidenced by decreased urinary output; and the potential complications of allergic dermatitis, uric acid renal calculi (low back pain), thrombocytopenia (increased tendency to bleed), or anemia.

Implementation

Monitoring. The nurse should monitor the client's involved joints for range of motion, pain, and swelling during the course of medication, as well as serum uric acid levels and CBCs, and if urinary alkalizers are used, then acid-base balance values. Fluid intake and output are monitored to ensure adequacy of urinary output (2000 to 3000 ml daily) to minimize urate stone formation.

Intervention. Probenecid may be administered with an antacid or food to minimize gastrointestinal distress. A high fluid intake (2500 ml of water daily) to produce copious volumes of urine is recommended to minimize formation of uric acid stones and occurrence of renal colic and hematuria.

Alkalinization of the urine may be required to minimize the formation of kidney stones. Sodium bicarbonate, potassium citrate, and acetazolamide are agents recommended for the alkalinization of urine. Diet therapy is also recommended as with allopurinol therapy.

Education. Encourage the client to comply with the medication regimen. Variations in the dosage may precipitate an acute episode of gout. It is important for the client to understand that this drug helps to prevent attacks, but it does not relieve acute episodes of gout. Regular visits to the prescriber are necessary to monitor progress.

Stress the importance of maintaining adequate fluid intake. Alert clients with diabetes who test urine for glucose with copper sulfate tests (Clinitest) that a false-positive result may result while taking this medication. Enzymatic tests (Ketodiastix, Tes-Tape) should be used to assess urine glucose levels.

Caution the client not to drink alcohol because it increases uric acid levels. Aspirin and other salicylates should be avoided because they decrease the effectiveness of probenecid and may precipitate a gout attack. Advise the client to read the labels of OTC medications carefully because aspirin and other salicylates are common ingredients of OTCs.

The client should be cautioned to report to the prescriber any symptoms of hypersensitivity (skin rash), renal stones (hematuria, dysuria, low back pain), or blood dyscrasias (sore throat, fever, unusual bleeding or bruising, unusual fatigue).

Evaluation. The client will not experience attacks of gout, or they will be diminished in frequency and severity.

sulfinpyrazone [sul fin peer' a zone] (Anturane)
The mechanism of action is similar to probenecid, i.e., it inhibits reabsorption of urate at the proximal renal tubule thus increasing urinary uric acid excretion. It is indicated for the treatment of chronic gouty arthritis and hyperuricemia. Sulfinpyrazone is well absorbed orally and is highly bound to plasma proteins. It is metabolized in the liver into four active metabolites; the p-hydroxy-sulfinpyrazone metabolite produced contributes between 33% to 50% of the uricosuric effect of sulfinpyrazone. The duration of effect for the uricosuric effect is usually 4 to 6 hours. Sulfinpyrazone is excreted by the kidneys.

The side/adverse effects of sulfinpyrazone include nausea, vomiting, abdominal pain, and rash or allergic reaction. The adult antigout dosage is 100 to 200 mg orally twice daily initially, increased gradually at 2 day intervals if necessary until it is sufficient to control the elevated serum uric acid levels (usually 400 to 800 mg/day). Maintenance dosage is 200 to 400 mg daily. Pediatric dosage has not been established.

■ Nursing Management

Sulfinpyrazone Therapy

Assessment. Sulfinpyrazone is used with caution in clients with a history of blood dyscrasias, peptic ulcer, renal stones, or renal function impairment.

The client's current medication regimen should be reviewed to detect significant drug interactions such as those that may occur when sulfinpyrazone is given concurrently with the drugs listed below:

Drug	Possible effect and management
anticoagulants (coumarin or indanedione, heparin) or thrombolytics (streptokinase or urokinase)	Sulfinpyrazone may increase the anticoagulant effect by displacing coumarin or indanedione from their protein-binding sites and by inhibiting their metabolism. Monitor prothrombin time closely because dosage adjustments may be necessary. **An increase in bleeding episodes or hemorrhage may result from concurrent administration of sulfinpyrazone and anticoagulant or thrombolytic therapy. The potential for this reaction is caused by the inhibitory effect of sulfinpyrazone on platelet aggregation and its possibility of causing gastrointestinal ulceration or hemorrhage. Avoid or a potentially serious drug interaction may occur.**
alprostadil (Prostin VR), anagrelide, aspirin, dextran, carbenicillin (parenteral), dipyridamole (Persantin), divalproex (Depakote), moxalactam, NSAIDs, plicamycin (Mithramycin), ticarcillin (Ticar), ticlopidine (Ticlid), or valproic acid (Depakene)	These drugs inhibit platelet aggregation; therefore concurrent drug administration may increase the potential of bleeding episodes. Monitor closely for early signs of bleeding.
antineoplastic agents, rapidly cytolytic	**Increased risk of inducing uric acid nephropathy or losing control of uric acid serum levels (preexisting levels) and gout is possible. Avoid or a potentially serious drug interaction may occur.**
aspirin or salicylates	**When salicylates are given long term in moderate to high doses, the uricosuric effect of sulfinpyrazone may be inhibited. See comments about probenecid. Avoid or a potentially serious drug interaction may occur.**
cefotetan (Cefotan), cefamandole (Mandole), cefoperazone (Cefobid), or plicamycin (Mithramycin)	**These drugs can cause platelet function inhibition and hypoprothrombinemia. Monitor closely for bleeding tendencies. Avoid or a potentially serious drug interaction may occur.**
nitrofurantoin (Furadantin)	**Sulfinpyrazone may decrease kidney excretion of nitrofurantoin, which may increase the risk of nitrofurantoin toxicity and reduce the effectiveness of nitrofurantoin as a urinary tract anti-infective agent. Avoid or a potentially serious drug interaction may occur.**

A baseline assessment of the client should include serum uric acid determinations, blood counts, renal function determinations, and joint pain and stiffness.

Nursing diagnosis. Assessment of the client receiving sulfinpyrazone should include consideration of the following selected nursing diagnoses: altered comfort (stomach pain, anorexia, nausea, and vomiting); hyperthermia (allergic reaction); activity intolerance related to anemia; altered bowel elimination (diarrhea); altered urinary elimination related to renal effects evidenced by decreased urinary output; and the potential complications of thrombocytopenia (increased tendency to bleed), allergic dermatitis, and uric acid renal calculi (low back pain).

Implementation

Monitoring. CBCs, uric acid determinations, and renal function studies should be performed at intervals during therapy. Monitor fluid intake and output to ensure that intake is adequate for sufficient urinary output (2 to 3 L/day) to help prevent urinary stones. Monitor the client's mobility and discomfort in affected joints.

Intervention. Sulfinpyrazone may be administered with an antacid or food to minimize gastrointestinal distress. Clients should maintain adequate fluid intake (8 oz 10 to 12 times daily) and urinary alkalinization by the administration of sodium bicarbonate, potassium citrate, or acetazolamide if necessary, because sulfinpyrazone is a potent uricosuric agent that may cause urolithiasis and renal colic, especially in the initial stages of therapy.

Education. Encourage the client to comply with therapy. This is essential because optimal effectiveness of the drug may not be reached for several months. Advise the client that sulfinpyrazone helps prevent gout attacks but does not relieve an acute episode. Regular visits to the health care provider should be maintained to monitor progress. Stress the importance of adequate fluid intake in the prevention of the formation of stones.

Caution the client not to use alcohol because it increases uric acid levels. Aspirin and other salicylates should be avoided because they decrease the effectiveness of sulfinpyrazone and may precipitate a gout attack.

Evaluation. The client on sulfinpyrazone therapy will experience diminished attacks of gout.

■ ■ ■

The nonsteroidal antiinflammatory agents naproxen (Naprosyn), phenylbutazone (Butazolidin), and sulindac (Clinoril) are also used in the treatment of acute gouty arthritis. For information on these drugs, see Chapter 14.

SUMMARY

Gout is a metabolic disorder characterized by hyperuricemia. The aims of therapy for gout are to end the acute attack quickly, to prevent a recurrence, to prevent uric acid renal calculi, and to prevent or minimize complications of sodium urate deposits in the joints. Agents used for these purposes are colchicine, allopurinol, probenecid, and sulfinpyrazone.

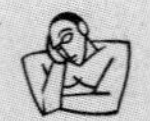

Critical Thinking

1. Mr. Stevens, 56 years old, comes to the clinic with a red, swollen big toe on his left foot. He is accompanied by his wife. He indicates that the pain, redness, and swelling that he has had for about a week have been unrelieved by aspirin. For what risk factors of gout will you assess Mr. Stevens? How will his medical diagnosis be confirmed? Given what Mr. Stevens has already said, what health teaching does he require?
2. Why is a diet that enhances alkalinity of the urine recommended for clients with gout? What should be included in such a diet? What dietary limitations are prescribed for these clients?

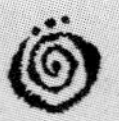

Collaborative Learning Activities

1. Four teams of students will be administered an identical, simplified case study of a client with gout. Each team will design a nursing plan for the administration of one of the following drugs: colchicine, allopurinol, probenecid, or sulfinpyrazone. Each nursing care plan must incorporate side/adverse effects and significant drug interactions into the assessment, nursing diagnoses, implementation, and evaluation components.

BIBLIOGRAPHY

Anderson KN, et al. (Eds.) (1994). *Mosby's medical, nursing, & allied health dictionary* (4th ed.). St Louis: Mosby.

Abrams WB & Berkow R. (1990). *The Merck manual of geriatrics.* Rahway, NJ: Merck Sharp & Dohme Research Laboratories.

American Hospital Formulary Service (1996). *AHFS drug information '96.* Bethesda, MD: American Society of Hospital Pharmacists.

American Medical Association (1995). *Drug evaluations: Annual 1995.* Chicago: American Medical Association.

McCance KL & Huether SE (1994). *Pathophysiology: The biologic basis for disease in adults and children* (2nd ed.). St Louis: Mosby.

Olin BR (Ed.) (1996). *Facts and comparisons.* St Louis: Facts and Comparisons.

Pagana KD & Pagana TJ (1997). *Mosby's diagnostic and laboratory test reference* (3rd ed.). St Louis: Mosby.

PDR (1996). *Physicians' desk reference* (50th ed.). Montvale, NJ: Medical Economics.

Seeley RS & Tate P (1995). *Anatomy and physiology* (3rd ed.). St Louis: Mosby.

Thibodeau GA & Patton KT (1996). *Anatomy and physiology* (3rd ed.). St Louis: Mosby.

United States Pharmacopeial Convention (1996). *USP DI: Drug information for the health care professional* (16th ed.). Rockville, MD: The Convention.

Young LY & Campagna KD (1995). Gout and hyperuricemia. In Young LY & Koda-Kimble MA. *Applied therapeutics: The clinical use of drugs* (6th ed.). Vancouver: Applied Therapeutics.

Chapter 36

Drug Therapy for Renal System Dysfunction

Chapter Focus

Renal dysfunction can alter the bioavailability, distribution, and protein binding of drugs by modifying systemic pH, altering the configuration and amount of albumin, and altering body hydration and renal excretion. Even for drugs that are not excreted renally, renal dysfunction may cause toxic metabolites to accumulate. In addition, drug-induced nephrotoxicity may occur. The nurse needs to be acutely aware of the effects of renal system dysfunction on drug therapy and vice versa. The following objectives and key terms are important for a good understanding of this chapter.

Key Terms

acute renal failure (p. 638)
azotemia (p. 638)
chronic renal failure (p. 638)
end-stage renal disease (p. 640)
hemodialysis (p. 638)
peritoneal dialysis (p. 638)

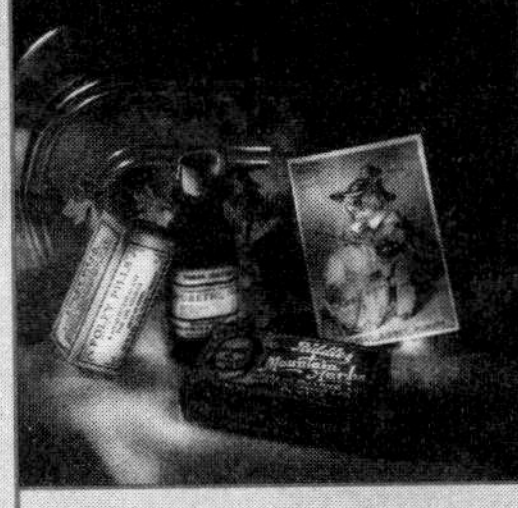

Objectives

1. Differentiate between acute renal failure and chronic renal failure.
2. Describe two laboratory tests used to evaluate renal impairment.
3. Explain why dietary protein, fluid intake, potassium, magnesium, and phosphorus are restricted in chronic renal failure.
4. Describe the differences between and advantages of the drug dosage reduction method and the interval extension method of treatment.
5. Implement nursing management of drug therapy for the client with renal system dysfunction.

As many potentially toxic drugs are excreted by the kidneys, individuals with impaired renal function receiving standard drug dosages on a regular schedule may experience drug accumulation and toxicity. Therefore it is important for the health care provider to monitor and evaluate clients with impaired renal function because drug dosages or time intervals frequently need to be adjusted.

ACUTE VERSUS CHRONIC RENAL FAILURE

Acute renal failure, a condition characterized by oliguria and by the rapid accumulation of nitrogenous wastes in the blood, a rapid decline in renal function, occurs in 2% to 5% of all hospitalized individuals and up to 1% of hospital admissions from the community (Bailie, 1995). Primary causes include trauma, pregnancy, renal ischemia as a result of surgery, severe hemorrhage, severe volume depletion, and shock. In some instances, nephrotoxic agents such as heavy metals and aminoglycosides may also induce acute renal failure. If recognized early and treated promptly, acute renal failure may be reversed before acute tubular necrosis or permanent damage occurs.

Chronic renal failure (CRF) is a progressive disease usually caused by an irreversible kidney injury that results in permanent nephron or renal mass loss. It is a major health concern in North America. In 1991, nearly 215,000 persons in the U.S. Medicare program had end-stage renal disease (Ateshkadi & Johnson, 1995). The most common causes of CRF are glomerulonephritis, diabetes mellitus, hypertension, polycystic kidney disease, and other diseases that may lead to destruction or impaired functioning of the kidneys. Individuals with CRF may be treated conservatively initially, but in end-stage renal disease (ESRD), hemodialysis, peritoneal dialysis, or organ transplantation may be necessary. **Hemodialysis** is a procedure in which impurities or wastes are removed from the blood, shunting the blood from the body through a machine for diffusion and ultrafiltration, then returning it to the client's circulation. **Peritoneal dialysis** is another form of dialysis, but one in which the peritoneum is used as the diffusible membrane. A solution, known as dialysate, is placed via a catheter into the peritoneal cavity and retained for a specified time while osmosis, diffusion, and filtration pass needed electrolytes into the bloodstream and remove wastes into the dialysate, which is then drained by gravity from the abdominal cavity.

Since the focus of this book is pharmacology, this chapter concentrates on the therapeutic regimen and recommendations for drug dosage adjustments in clients with impaired renal function.

SIGNS AND SYMPTOMS OF RENAL FAILURE OR INSUFFICIENCY

One of the more common signs of acute renal failure is a marked alteration in the expected urine output, usually a significant reduction (<400 ml/day). Thus the first phase is the oliguric phase. Phase two is the diuretic phase; in this phase the individual has an increase in their urine volume for a few days but they are still **azotemic**, retaining excessive amounts of nitrogenous compounds (blood urea nitrogen and creatinine) in the blood. Phase three is considered the recovery phase as azotemia decreases and renal function is recovering. The recovery phase may occur over weeks to months, depending on the damage caused by the original insult to the kidneys (Bailie, 1995). Signs of acute renal failure, in the presence of reduced urine production, are usually the result of fluid overload: edema, weight gain, weakness, hypertension, and tachycardia.

The most common complaints with chronic renal failure are increasing weakness, fatigue, and lethargy. Gastrointestinal signs include anorexia, gastrointestinal distress, nausea, vomiting, thirst, and weight loss. Paresthesias, peripheral neuropathy, convulsions, and neuromuscular irritability may also occur. On examination, the client may appear pale and dehydrated and have an increased respiratory rate and uremic breath. Hypertension with retinopathy, cardiac hypertrophy, pulmonary edema, or pericarditis may often be present.

A detailed client history, thorough physical examination, urinalysis, and blood chemistry levels are important for assessment, diagnosis, and determination of an appropriate treatment plan. The degree of renal impairment is usually estimated by reviewing the serum creatinine and blood urea nitrogen (BUN) levels. Elevated levels indicate a decrease in renal clearance, which, of course, predisposes the individual to drug toxicity.

MEASUREMENT OF RENAL FUNCTION

Many formulas and nomograms are available to determine the client's approximate creatinine clearance and the appropriate drug dosage adjustment necessary to minimize the possibility of toxicity. Normal values may vary from laboratory to laboratory, but in general a normal BUN ranges between 5 and 20 mg/dl, while the range of serum creatinine, which varies with age, is usually between 0.5 and 1.2 mg/dl. The most reliable test is the creatinine clearance test; but since accurate collection of all urine excreted for a 24 hour period is difficult, many clinicians use a formula to estimate creatinine clearance and others may prefer to use a nomogram. The formulas most commonly used are noted in Box 36-1. The mean endogenous creatinine clearance in an adult is usually between 90 and 130 ml/min/1.73 m^2 body surface per 24 hours. Therefore reductions in this quantity signify impairment of renal function (Box 36-2).

Another important factor in evaluating drug blood levels in clients with renal failure or renal impairment is an assessment of serum albumin and total protein for the client. Serum protein is decreased in individuals with renal insufficiency, which can alter the interpretation of serum levels of drugs that are protein bound (90% or more) in the normal person. Individuals with a lower albumin or protein value may have a

BOX 36-1

Formulas for Estimating Creatinine Clearance

Adult male =

$$\frac{(140 - \text{age}) \times (\text{ideal body weight in kg})}{72 \times \text{serum creatinine (mg per dl)}}$$

Adult female =

$$\frac{(140 - \text{age}) \times (\text{ideal body weight in kg})}{72 \times \text{serum creatinine (mg per dl)}} \times 0.85$$

Ideal body weight calculations

IBW (males) = 50 kg + (2.3 kg × inches over 5 feet)

IBW (females) = 45 kg + (2.3 kg × inches over 5 feet)

From *USP DI*, 1996.

BOX 36-2

Typical Grading for Renal Impairment Using Creatinine Clearance

Degree of renal failure	Creatinine clearance
Normal	Men: 90-139 ml/min Women: 80-125 ml/min
Mild impairment	50-80 ml/min
Moderate impairment	10-50 ml/min
Severe impairment	<10 ml/min

Data from Bennett WM, et al. (1983). *Am J Kidney Dis* 3(3):155.

drug concentration in the low range that appears to be therapeutic. This is possible if the laboratory does not differentiate between the bound and unbound drug in the testing. Lower protein levels may lead to a higher unbound concentration of the drug (the active form), thus producing an adequate therapeutic response.

SPECIAL NEEDS OF THE CRF CLIENT

The individual in CRF has special dietary, electrolyte, and fluid requirements. In general, dietary protein is usually restricted to 0.5 to 1 g/kg of lean body weight daily. This limitation will reduce the incidence of azotemia, hyperkalemia, and acidosis. Fluid intake is based on daily losses and metabolic needs. Dietary sodium is restricted to approximately 2 g or 90 mEq/day. Potassium, magnesium, and phosphorus are also restricted. Often, an aluminum hydroxide gel is prescribed to decrease phosphate absorption from the gastrointestinal tract. The reduced excretion of phosphates, magnesium, and potassium from the kidneys in chronic renal failure can lead to elevated serum levels or hypermagnesemia, hyperkalemia, and hyperphosphatemia, which in turn lead to hypocalcemia and osteodystrophy.

Thus dietary restrictions are absolutely necessary. Calcium supplements and vitamin D are often prescribed for these clients to reduce or prevent hyperparathyroidism and bone disease. Magnesium levels are kept somewhat in check by client avoidance of magnesium-containing antacids and laxatives.

Production of red blood cells (erythropoiesis), which is usually decreased in CRF, leads to anemia, weakness, and fatigue. Iron therapy may be prescribed for those clients with iron deficiency anemia resulting from chronic blood loss; folic acid, vitamin C, and soluble B-complex vitamins are often given to replace substances usually lost during dialysis. Therefore it is not unusual to care for CRF clients with many dietary and fluid restrictions, as well as prescriptions for vitamins, calcium, specific antacids, and additional drugs as necessary. A drug specifically used to stimulate erythropoiesis in CRF is epoetin alfa.

epoetin alfa, recombinant [eh poh' ee tin] (Epogen)

Epoetin alfa is a glycoprotein chemically identical to human erythropoietin. It is indicated for the treatment of anemia associated with renal failure and severe anemia associated with acquired immunodeficiency (AIDS) syndrome but should not be considered a substitute for blood or blood transfusions.

Epoetin alfa has the same biologic action as the endogenous hormone; it stimulates erythropoiesis in the bone marrow and also induces the release of reticulocytes from bone marrow. Since endogenous erythropoietin is manufactured mainly in the kidneys, anemia resulting from chronic renal failure is caused by an inadequate production of the hormone. With the use of epoetin, the initial increase in reticulocytes is seen within 7 to 10 days while an increase in red cell count, hematocrit, and hemoglobin occurs within 2 to 6 weeks. This product reaches peak serum level within 15 minutes after intravenous administration and within 5 to 24 hours after a subcutaneous dose. Half-life is between 4 and 13 hours after intravenous or subcutaneous administration. When therapy is discontinued, the hematocrit decreases in approximately 2 weeks (duration of action).

The most common adverse reactions to epoetin alfa include clotting of the arteriovenous (AV) shunt and/or dialyzer, hypertension, and polycythemia. More frequent side effects include arthralgias or bone pain, asthenia (severe muscle weakness), nausea and vomiting, increased weakness, and diarrhea. The most frequent side effects include chest pain, edema of extremities or face, weight gain, tachycardia, headache, and hypertension. No significant drug interactions have been reported.

The initial adult dose (IV, SC) is 50 to 100 units/kg three times a week. If hematocrit has not increased after 2 months of therapy by at least 5 to 6 points and the client is still below the desired range of 30% to 33%, then dosage increments of 25 units/kg may be instituted. For maintenance, decrease the dose gradually by 25 units/kg monthly to the lowest dose that maintains hematocrit at the desired level. Dosage has not been determined for children below 12 years of age. Pregnancy safety has been established at FDA category C.

■ Nursing Management

Epoetin Alfa Therapy

Assessment. The client with hypertension is at risk with the administration of epoetin alfa because its resultant increase in hematocrit increases blood viscosity and peripheral vascular resistance, leading to a rise in blood pressure.

Clients with poorly controlled hypertension should have epoetin alfa therapy delayed until it is controlled. Even then, the client's (and the previously normotensive client's) blood pressure should be monitored closely because of the increased risk of hypertension, which may lead to hypertensive encephalopathy. The drug should not be used if the client is hypersensitive to human albumin or to mammalian cell–derived products, such as beef and pork insulin.

Nursing diagnosis. Clients receiving epoetin alfa may be at risk for the following selected nursing diagnoses/collaborative problems: altered comfort related to arthralgias (11%), headache (16%), chest pain (7%), nausea (10.5%), and flu-like syndrome; fatigue (9%); fluid volume excess (weight gain, swelling of face, fingers, feet, and ankles (9%); impaired skin integrity (skin reaction at administration site, 7%); altered bowel elimination, diarrhea (8.5%); and the potential complications of polycythemia (increased clotting tendency), seizures (1.1%), and hypertension (24%).

Implementation

Monitoring. As mentioned, the blood pressure should be monitored. CBCs, as ordered by the prescriber, should be assessed for change. Hematocrit values are particularly important with baseline and twice weekly frequencies being recommended as a guide for dosage and efficacy. A rise in the hematocrit of more than four points in a 2 week period or a value over 36%, which is considered the safety limit for the prevention of adverse reactions, should be brought to the prescriber's attention.

It is recommended that the client's iron stores status be monitored to determine the need and the amount of iron supplementation for the client. Since iron is incorporated into hemoglobin as a result of the drug's effectiveness, the client's iron stores may be depleted causing a decrease in the epoetin alfa's efficacy.

Neurologic assessments for premonitory signs for the risk of seizures should be done periodically, particularly during the first 90 days of therapy and at times when the hematocrit rises rapidly. Renal function studies should be monitored since the need to begin or increase dialysis may occur with the administration of epoetin alfa. Weight should be taken daily and the client's fluid balance monitored by intake and output measurements.

Intervention. Each vial of epoetin alfa should be used to administer one dose only because the injection contains no preservative. Discard any unused portion of the drug. Do not shake the vial; shaking may denature the substance and render it biologically inactive. Do not mix with other medications.

Education. Alert the client to avoid activities that may be hazardous if seizures would occur, especially during the first 90 days of therapy. The client should be instructed in dietary sources of iron, folic acid, and B_{12} as an adjunct to iron and other vitamin supplementation. Dietary restrictions as part of the antihypertensive regimen and those pertinent to clients with chronic renal failure should be reviewed with the client. The correction of the anemia may result in an increased appetite, making it more difficult for the client to maintain compliance with the dietary restrictions required. Keeping prescriber and dialysis appointments should be encouraged.

Evaluation. A clinically significant increase in the red cell count, hematocrit, and hemoglobin should be seen in 2 to 6 weeks of initiation of epoetin alfa therapy. The hematocrit should stabilize in the 30% to 33% range. With the correction of the client's anemia, the client will demonstrate an improved activity tolerance; decreased fatigue; improved appetite, sleep pattern, and cognitive function; and an improved sense of well-being.

SELECTED DRUG MODIFICATIONS IN RENAL FAILURE

As previously mentioned, BUN and serum creatinine are waste products to be excreted by the kidneys. Serum levels of these substances are used to measure renal function. Unfortunately, neither test is useful in discovering early renal impairment because abnormal levels do not appear until 50% or more of renal function is impaired. Fortunately, human kidneys are functional even if 90% of the glomerular filtration rate is lost. However, the continuing progressive loss may result in **end-stage renal disease,** renal loss necessitating hemodialysis, peritoneal dialysis, kidney transplantation, and other interventions discussed in this chapter.

In individuals with renal insufficiency or impairment, the drug dosage may be decreased (dosage reduction method) while maintaining the usual interval, or if the dose is the usually prescribed one, the interval between doses is lengthened (interval extension method). Usually the dosage reduction method is preferred for drugs that require a constant blood therapeutic level. For most clients receiving a loading dose, the dose is similar to the dose given to a client without renal impairment. This permits a therapeutically desirable blood level that is then maintained by one of the above dosing methods. Table 36-1 gives typical dosing recommendations for selected medications along with a list of drugs that may or may not be removed by hemodialysis or peritoneal dialysis. The reader is referred to the current package inserts or renal failure dosing guides for specific data.

TABLE 36-1 Selected medication dosing for adults in renal insufficiency

	Creatinine clearance (ml/min)*			
	Normal dose	Renal failure		
Medication	>50	10-50	<10	t½ (hr)
acyclovir (Zovirax)	5 mg/kg q8h	5 mg/kg q12-24h	2.5 mg/kg q24h	N: 2.5 A: 20
ampicillin (Omnipen-N)	1-2 g q4-6h	1-1.5 g q6h	1 g q8-12h	N: 0.8-1.5 A: 20
cefazolin (Ancef)	1-2 g q8h	0.5-1.5 g q12h	0.5-1 g q24h	N:1.8-2.6 A: 12-40
ciprofloxacin (Cipro)	250-750 mg PO q12h	250-500 mg q12h	250-750 mg q24h	N: 4 A: 8.5
fluconazole (Diflucan)	100-200 mg q24h	50-200 mg q24h	50-100 mg q24h	N: 20-50 A: 98
gentamicin (Garamycin)	1 mg/kg q8h	0.25-0.5 mg/kg q8h	0.1 mg/kg q8h	N: 1.5-3 A: 20-54
meperidine (Demerol)	50-100 mg IV/IM q3-4h	75%-100% of dose q6h	50% of dose q6-8h	N: 3-7 A: ?
vancomycin (Vancocin)	500 mg q6h	1 g q3-7days	1 g q1-2wk	N: 4-9 A: 129-190

(Aweeka, 1995; *USP DI*, 1996; *PDR*, 1996)
T½, Half-life; *N*, normal; *A*, anuric.
*Creatinine clearance or glomerular filtration rate.

Nursing Management

Pharmacologic Therapies for Clients with Renal System Dysfunction

Assessment. The initial assessment should include a history of recent weight changes, edema, malaise, increasing irritability or mental changes, metallic taste in the mouth, polyuria and nocturia (caused by reduced ability to concentrate urine), headache, dizziness, gastrointestinal disturbances, and hypertension.

Because other body systems may be affected by renal dysfunction, a thorough multisystem assessment should be conducted. A baseline assessment of the client's lab values should include BUN, serum creatinine, serum electrolytes, CBC, and urinalysis. The client's current drug regimen requires review to determine the risk for drug toxicities related to drug accumulation. If the client is receiving medications with significant toxicities, the appropriate serum drug levels should be carefully monitored to help prevent overdosing the client. Table 36-2 lists the medications that are most commonly associated with inducing renal dysfunction.

Nursing diagnosis. The client is at risk for the following selected nursing diagnoses/collaborative problems: fluid volume excess related to inability to adequately excrete fluids and electrolytes and/or excessive fluid intake during periods of decreased renal function; ineffective breathing pattern related to circulatory volume overload and/or metabolic acidosis leading to hyperventilation; altered nutrition: less than body requirements related to anorexia, nausea, and vomiting; fatigue secondary to anemia and uremia; and risk for infection related to debilitated state and the use of indwelling catheters and other invasive procedures. The potential complications exist of decreased cardiac output related to dysrhythmias from renal failure; anemia related to bone marrow suppression, increased hemolysis and bleeding tendencies; and altered levels of consciousness related to electrolyte imbalances, accumulation of waste products in the blood and hypoxia.

Implementation

Monitoring. Daily weights should be taken at the same time of day, with the same amount of clothing, and with the same scale. The client at home may be better able to establish a routine by weighing first thing in the morning after the first voiding and before dressing or eating. The daily weight can be evaluated in light of the 24-hour intake and output balance for determination of fluid volume excess or fluid volume deficit.

The fluid intake and output of the client should be accurately recorded on a 24-hour basis. The 24-hour balance should be calculated by subtracting the output from the intake. The balance, whether positive or negative, should relate to weight loss or gain at approximately 500 ml to the pound. BUN and serum creatinine levels should be monitored to ascertain the client's end-stage renal disease and to anticipate clinical signs and symptoms of physiologic injury that would require nursing intervention and client education.

Serum potassium levels should be monitored daily. When the level exceeds 6 mEq/L, cardiovascular monitoring should

TABLE 36-2 Medications associated with renal toxicity or dysfunction

Medications	Possible toxicity or dysfunction
kanamycin, colistin, amikacin (rare), tobramycin (rare), gentamicin, cephalothin, cephaloridine, lithium, amphotericin B, cisplatin, rifampin, bacitracin, tetracycline, nitrofurantoin, kanamycin, neomycin, polymixin B, colistin, streptozocin, cyclosporin	Renal tubule damage and/or necrosis
penicillins, methoxyflurane, cephalothin, sulfonamides, nonsteroidal antiinflammatory drugs, allopurinol	Acute interstitial nephritis
trimethadione, paramethadione, gold, probenecid, lithium, heroin	Glomerular damage
Injectable antihypertensive drugs given to elderly, excessive dosages of low molecular weight dextran, diuretics, opioid medications	May induce acute ischemic renal failure

From Douglas S (1992). Acute tubular necrosis: Diagnosis, treatment, and nursing implications, *AACN* 3(3):688.

become more intense. In addition to blood pressure and apical heart rate determinations, assessment by cardiac monitor is required. Serum levels of calcium and phosphate should be monitored every 3 to 4 days, and the client should be clinically assessed for hypocalcemia and hyperphosphatemia as evidenced by irritability, muscular twitching, and tetany.

The client's arterial blood gases should be monitored. Clinically, the client should be observed for increased respiratory rate and depth and changes in mental status that would indicate impending metabolic acidosis. CBCs should be taken periodically, and the client should be assessed for signs and symptoms of anemia that might necessitate interventions such as iron supplements and anabolic steroids or, in the extreme, transfusion of packed or frozen RBCs.

Intervention. Fluid intake may be restricted. If so, fluid allotments should be planned with the client regarding the type of fluids and time of intake to enhance the regimen's acceptability by the client and to maintain the client's feeling of control. Dietary sodium is usually restricted, and intake will need to be planned with the client based on the degree of restriction. Drug therapy is based on each client's particular form of dysfunction and its cause. Because of the many body systems that are affected by renal dysfunction, several medications may be used. The more common agents are diuretics for control of fluid balance, edema, and hypertension and antibiotics to treat infection. Because altered renal function also alters pharmacokinetics of many drugs, dosages and dose intervals are adjusted based on the drug and degree of renal system dysfunction.

Education. As with any condition, particularly those with multisystem consequences, knowledge deficit is likely. The client should be instructed in the purpose of the medications, such as antihypertensives, diuretics, calcium supplements, vitamin D, and phosphate binders. In addition, the client should be told of the side effects and adverse reactions of any medications being taken because with increasing renal insufficiency the margin of safety with any medication is diminished. Multiple drug therapy increases the chance of a drug interaction. The stressors placed on the client with increasing renal insufficiency are multiple. Changes in lifestyle, body image, and the impact of the disease on the client require the nurse to exercise skill in the roles of support and education for the client and family to minimize the potential for ineffective coping.

Evaluation. The client will adhere to the prescribed fluid restrictions and will be normovolemic as evidenced by stable weight, normal breath sounds, absence of edema, and blood pressure and pulse within the client's normal range. In addition, the client will verbalize orientation to person, place, and time and a decrease in fatigue and will increase participation in activities. The client will be free of infection, as evidenced by normothermia, WBC within normal limits, clear urine, normal breath sounds, and absence of drainage at catheter sites.

SUMMARY

Renal system dysfunction may be a source of tremendous stress for the client and family, and it also presents a challenge for the nurse. Therapy is complicated by multiple drug therapy and altered pharmacokinetics. Drug interactions or adverse reactions may appear at any time and make close monitoring of drug effects and renal function by the nurse essential. In addition, nondrug therapy, such as diet modification and fluid restriction, and involvement of other body systems, present additional areas for nursing intervention.

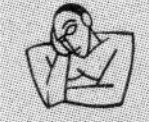

Critical Thinking

1. Mrs. Defrees, a 54-year-old female client, height 5'3", weight 175 pounds, has been admitted to your unit for congestive heart failure. She has been prescribed digoxin 0.25 mg daily for her condition. However, she has indicated that she has a history of renal failure, and you are concerned about the level of her renal function with the administration of digoxin. You are aware that a creatinine clearance is the best indicator of renal function, but it is a 24-hour test. The lab has just called to the unit with her serum creatinine value of 3.2 mg/dl. Estimate her creatinine clearance to determine the severity of her renal impairment. What action would you take based on your findings?

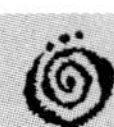

Collaborative Learning Activities

1. Teams of students will identify medications that can cause one of the following dysfunctions: (1) damage and/or necrosis to renal tubules; (2) acute interstitial nephritis; (3) glomerular damage; and (4) acute ischemic renal failure. Each group should elaborate on simple definition by describing each dysfunction. Work up a client assessment, monitoring, and education plan that incorporates implementation and evaluation strategies.

BIBLIOGRAPHY

Anderson KN, et al. (Eds.) (1994). *Mosby's medical, nursing, & allied health dictionary* (4th ed.) St Louis: Mosby.

Ateshkadi A & Johnson CA (1995). Chronic renal failure. In Young LY & Koda-Kimble MA. *Applied therapeutics: The clinical use of drugs* (6th ed.). Vancouver: Applied Therapeutics.

Aweeka FT (1995). Dosing of drugs in renal failure. In Young LY & Koda-Kimble MA. *Applied therapeutics: The clinical use of drugs* (6th ed.). Vancouver: Applied Therapeutics.

Baer C & Lancaster LE (1992). Acute renal failure, *CCNQ* 14(4):1.

Bailie GR (1995). Acute renal failure. In Young LY & Koda-Kimble MA. *Applied therapeutics: The clinical use of drugs* (6th ed.). Vancouver: Applied Therapeutics.

Brundage DJ (1992). *Renal disorders*. St Louis: Mosby.

Chambers JK (1993). Renal insufficiency: Implications for care of the medical-surgical patient, *MEDSURG Nurs* 2(1):33.

Douglas S (1992). Acute tubular necrosis: Diagnosis, treatment, and nursing implications, *AACN* 3(3):688.

Pagana KD & Pagana TJ (1997). *Mosby's diagnostic and laboratory test reference* (3rd ed.). St Louis: Mosby.

Thibodeau GA & Patton KT (1996). *Anatomy & physiology* (3rd ed.). St Louis: Mosby.

United States Pharmacopeial Convention (1996). *USP DI: Drug information for the health care professional* (16th ed.). Rockville, MD: The Convention.

Chapter 37

Overview of the Respiratory System

Chapter Focus

Because the respiratory system functions to maintain the exchange of oxygen and carbon dioxide in the lungs and cells and to regulate the pH of body fluids, a change within this system affects other body systems. The reverse is also true; disorders of other body systems may increase the body's need for oxygen, such as with fever, and so increase the work of respiration. Many clients that you will encounter in your practice will have respiratory problems that will require the provision of direct nursing care and education of the client and caregivers for effective management of the therapeutic regimen at home. This chapter provides a review of anatomy and physiology as background for understanding the drugs affecting the respiratory system. The following objectives and key terms will assist you to gain a good understanding of this chapter.

Key Terms

bronchial glands (p. 645)
bronchoconstriction (p. 646)
bronchodilation (p. 646)
cellular respiration (p. 645)
gas transport (p. 645)
goblet cells (p. 645)
mucokinesis (p. 645)
pulmonary ventilation (p. 645)

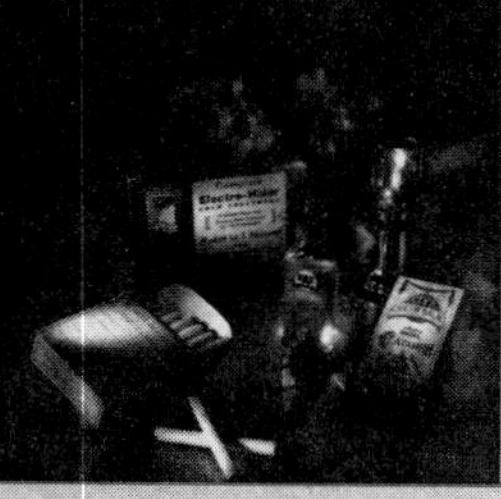

Objectives

1. Explain the three interrelated processes of respiration.
2. Name the two sources of respiratory secretions.
3. Describe the $beta_2$ receptor theory of bronchodilation.
4. Describe the parasympathetic effect on the respiratory system.
5. Discuss the central and peripheral control of respiration.

The respiratory system includes all structures involved in the exchange of oxygen and carbon dioxide, such as the airway passages, the lungs, nasal cavities, pharynx, larynx, trachea, bronchi, bronchioles, pulmonary lobules with their alveoli, the diaphragm, and all muscles concerned with respiration itself.

The most urgent and critical need for maintaining life is a continued, uninterrupted supply of oxygen. Oxygen is supplied to the body through the process of respiration. *Respiration* is a term loosely used to describe three distinct but interrelated processes:

- **Pulmonary ventilation,** which involves the movement of air into and out of the lungs
- **Gas transport,** which involves the exchange of gases between the air in the lungs, the blood, and the cell
- **Cellular respiration,** which involves the utilization of oxygen in the catabolism of energy-yielding substances for the production of energy

Respiration, one of the body's regulating systems, helps maintain physiologic dynamic equilibrium. It also compensates for rapid adjustment to changes in metabolic states.

The air passages permit air to flow from the external environment to pulmonary blood and modify the air taken in by warming and moistening it and removing noxious substances. Airway efficiency is determined by the following factors:

- Shape and size of each portion of the respiratory tract (nasal cavity, pharynx, larynx, trachea, bronchi, bronchioles, alveolar sacs)
- Presence of a ciliated, mucus-secreting, epithelial lining throughout most of the respiratory tract
- Character and thickness of respiratory tract secretions
- Compliance of the cartilaginous and bony supports
- Pressure gradients
- Traction on airway walls
- Absence of foreign substances in the lumen of the respiratory tract

Any alteration of any of these factors will affect the ease with which air flows through the air passages, or effective airway clearance. Congenital anomalies, injuries, allergies, or disease will cause air flow resistance if these factors are abnormally affected. For example, resistance occurs if there is stenosis or narrowing of any portion of the respiratory tract, loss of cilia that ordinarily sweep out foreign substances, any thick or tenacious secretions, loss of elasticity, or presence of foreign objects.

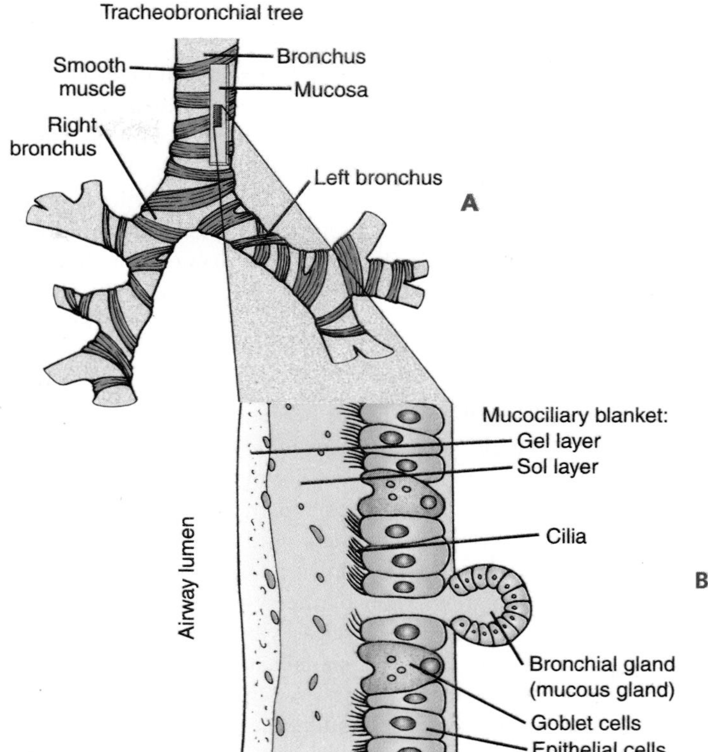

Figure 37-1 Tracheobronchial tree and bronchial smooth muscle. **A,** Diagram of tracheobronchial tree. **B,** Cut-out section of inner lining of bronchus.

RESPIRATORY TRACT SECRETIONS

The tracheobronchial tree, made up of repeated branching tubes, is a tubular airway that serves as a conduit for passage of air from the external environment to the alveolar-capillary exchange unit. The inner surface of the tracheobronchial tree is lined with ciliated columnar epithelium interspersed with **goblet cells.** The gelatinous mucus (gel layer) produced by goblet cells is normally discharged into the tubular lumen. In some obstructive pulmonary diseases, mucus secretion is greatly increased, thus making it difficult for the cilia to transport secretions along the airway (Figure 37-1).

The **bronchial glands,** which are located in the submucosa of the tracheobronchial tree, secrete a relatively watery fluid (sol layer) through ducts leading to the surface of the ciliated epithelium. Under vagal (parasympathetic) control, the glands can be stimulated by irritant agents or aerosol drugs to release their contents into the lumen of the airway (see Figure 37-1, *B*).

The products of these two sources—goblet cells and bronchial glands—form the sol-gel film that makes up the mucociliary blanket. This protective blanket of fluid bathes the ciliated epithelium of the tracheobronchial tree. In addition, the cilia continuously propel the sol-gel film up toward the larynx along the respiratory tree. The normal adult produces approximately 100 ml of respiratory secretions per day and swallows this material without being aware of it. The process of moving mucus along the tracheobronchial tree is called **mucokinesis.** The mucociliary blanket is a basic concern in most chronic obstructive pulmonary disease. The cilia must sustain appropriate function; a dry atmosphere causes the respiratory secretions to become thick and tenacious, which tends to interfere with ciliary movements. Thus adequate humidity should be maintained to prevent the change in the normal consistency of the respiratory secretions.

BRONCHIAL SMOOTH MUSCLE

Smooth muscle arrangement. An important structure of the tracheobronchial tree is the smooth muscle. The mass of muscle fibers along the bronchi progressively increases as it extends down toward the distal bronchioles. Isolated muscle fibers may be found as far down as the alveolar ducts. The smooth muscle fibers are arranged along the length of the tubular tree in a double helical or spiral pattern, and this formation profoundly influences the diameter or the lumen of the airways. Because of this structural feature, the effect of muscle contraction reduces both the diameter and the length of the bronchus (see Figure 38-1, *C*).

Nerve supply. The airway or tracheobronchial tree is innervated by the autonomic nervous system. The bronchial smooth muscle tone is influenced by the balance maintained between parasympathetic and sympathetic stimuli during rest. Activation of the parasympathetic fiber (vagus nerve) releases acetylcholine, which results in **bronchoconstriction,** a narrowing of the lumen of the bronchial airway. By contrast, the stimulation of the sympathetic fiber and the sympathoadrenal system releases epinephrine and norepinephrine from the adrenal medulla into circulation. Their action on the beta$_2$ receptor sites in the bronchial smooth muscle produces **bronchodilation** by means of smooth muscle relaxation, which improves ventilation to the lungs.

Receptors. Several kinds of receptors are found along the bronchial airway. The release of acetylcholine activates muscarinic receptors during stimulation of the parasympathetic system, whereas the sympathetic system affects adrenergic receptors. Most of the adrenergic receptors present in the bronchial smooth muscle are beta$_2$ receptors that are stimulated mainly by epinephrine released from the adrenal medulla. Beta$_1$ receptors are also found, although the ratio of beta$_2$ to beta$_1$ receptors is approximately 3:1. Thus bronchial smooth muscle is supplied primarily by beta$_2$ receptors. The sympathomimetic drugs used principally as bronchodilators stimulate the beta$_2$ receptors. Because many of these agents are not purely selective in their pharmacologic effect, they also stimulate the beta$_1$ receptors in the heart, as well as alpha receptors in the lungs and peripheral arterioles. The side effects on the heart are increased cardiac output, tachycardia, and dysrhythmia. The presence of alpha receptors on the bronchial smooth muscle is relatively scarce, and their stimulation results in only mild bronchoconstriction.

Bronchodilation. The beta$_2$-adrenergic receptors mediate bronchodilation. This mechanism presumably is initiated by epinephrine released from the adrenal medulla and norepinephrine released from the peripheral sympathetic nerves. Also located in the cell membrane is an enzyme system known as adenyl cyclase. In the presence of magnesium ions, adenyl cyclase catalyzes the action of adenosine triphosphate (ATP) in the cytoplasm of the cell to produce cyclic 3'5' adenosine-monophosphate (cyclic 3'5' AMP or c 3'5' AMP). Cyclic 3'5' AMP then performs its important function, inducing relaxation of bronchial smooth muscle or bronchodilation. The hormone epinephrine is designated as the "first messenger" and cyclic 3'5' AMP as the "second messenger." As a final action, cyclic 3'5' AMP is inactivated by an enzyme, phosphodiesterase, which catalyzes it to the inactive 5' AMP. This results in a fall in the cyclic 3'5' AMP level. The action of phosphodiesterase may be inhibited by a xanthine drug such as theophylline. As a consequence, the cyclic 3'5' AMP level remains elevated, thereby affecting smooth muscle dilation (see Figure 38-4).

Circulating catecholamines can exert their effects on beta$_1$, beta$_2$, and alpha receptors. Clients with asthma may have a normal reaction to both alpha and beta stimulation through a reduced cyclic AMP response, by an abnormally sensitive response to alpha stimulation, and by an exaggerated response to the muscarinic agonists via the vagal pathways. This exaggerated bronchoconstrictive airway response may result from the effects of a decrease in cyclic AMP, histamine effects on smooth muscle, the vagal reflex pathway, an increase in cyclic guanylic acid secondary to calcium influx, and histamine-induced release of the contents of mast cells. Bronchodilation is induced by circulating catecholamines or administration of a sympathomimetic agent.

Circulating catecholamines reach the lung via circulation and interact with the beta$_2$-adrenergic receptors in the cell membrane of the bronchial smooth muscle cell.

Bronchoconstriction. The bronchial smooth muscle is innervated by the parasympathetic fibers from the vagus nerve. Acetylcholine released from the terminal interacts with the muscarinic receptors on the membrane of the cell. Stimulation of the muscarinic receptor increases the activity of the enzyme guanylate cyclase in the membrane, thereby promoting the rate of formation of cyclic 3'5' guanosine monophosphase (cyclic 3'5' GMP) from guanosine triphosphate (GTP) (see Figure 38-4). The cyclic 3'5' GMP level affects the bronchial muscle by producing bronchoconstriction. In addition, alpha receptors found on the bronchial smooth muscle have a similar involvement with this mechanism. On activation, the alpha receptors also increase the cyclic GMP level. Further, cyclic 3'5' GMP stimulates the release of chemical mediators from the mast cell during an asthmatic attack, and these mediators are responsible for causing bronchoconstriction.

CONTROL OF RESPIRATION

Central control. The basic rhythm for respiration is initiated and maintained in the medullary rhythmicity area located beneath the lower part of the floor of the fourth ventricle in the medial half of the medulla. Neurons that control inspiration and expiration intermingle and discharge, or fire impulses alternately. However, signals from the spinal cord, the cerebral cortex and midbrain, the apneustic area of the pons, and the pneumotaxic area of the upper pons can enter the medullary rhythmicity area, modify the rhythm of respiration, and contribute to the normal pattern of respiration.

Normally, the human organism is unaware of the respiratory process. However, voluntary influence and control of breathing are possible. This is important when a client must learn to voluntarily control breathing patterns.

Peripheral control. The medullary rhythmicity area is also influenced by various sensory and peripheral stimuli, the vasomotor center, reflex mechanisms (e.g., the Hering-Breuer reflex), the chemoreceptors in the carotid and aortic bodies, and the baroreceptors in the carotid sinus and aortic arch. Fear, pain, stress, blood pressure, body temperature, and blood levels of oxygen and carbon dioxide can all modify the activity of the respiratory centers.

Humoral regulation of respiration is achieved primarily through changes in the concentrations of oxygen, carbon dioxide, or hydrogen ions in body fluids. In a healthy individual, carbon dioxide is the chief respiratory stimulant. An increase in the carbon dioxide tension of the blood directly stimulates the inspiratory and expiratory centers, which increases both the rate and depth of breathing. This results in a blowing off of carbon dioxide to keep the carbon dioxide tension of the blood constant. The pH of the blood is determined by the ratio of bicarbonate ion (HCO_3) to carbon dioxide. When the carbon dioxide content of the blood is increased, there is a subsequent increase in the formation of carbonic acid in the blood. This alters the bicarbonate/carbonic acid ratio from the normal value of 20:1 and results in acidosis. Conversely, a decrease in the carbon dioxide content of the blood results in alkalosis. Therefore respiration is important for regulating the pH of the blood by controlling the carbon dioxide tension of the blood.

Basically, changes in arterial oxygen concentration have little, if any, direct effect on the respiratory center. However, if the arterial oxygen concentration falls below normal, the chemoreceptors in the carotid and aortic bodies are stimulated and in turn stimulate the respiratory center to increase alveolar ventilation. This mechanism operates primarily under abnormal conditions such as chronic obstructive pulmonary disease.

SUMMARY

The highest priority for the survival of the human organism is an adequate, uninterrupted supply of oxygen. Oxygen is supplied to the various body tissues by the processes of pulmonary ventilation, gas transport, and cellular respiration. Although it is possible to influence and control the respiratory pattern voluntarily, the rhythm and depth of pulmonary ventilation are generally initiated and maintained centrally in the medulla and influenced peripherally by reflex mechanisms, chemoreceptors, and baroreceptors.

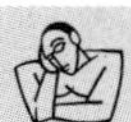

Critical Thinking

1. You are caring for Tommy, a three-year-old, who threatens to hold his breath. What effect will holding his breath have on his blood pH? What would happen to his blood pH if he hyperventilated?
2. It is known that smoking decreases the number of cilia in the respiratory airway. What will occur as the result of this change?

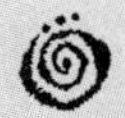

Collaborative Learning Activities

1. Student teams will present demonstrations on: (1) the three interrelated processes of respiration; (2) bronchial smooth muscle components and functions; and (3) central and peripheral control of respiration.

BIBLIOGRAPHY

Anderson KN, et al. (Eds.) (1994). *Mosby's medical, nursing, & allied health dictionary* (4th ed.). St Louis: Mosby.

Guyton AC (1990). *Textbook of medical physiology* (8th ed.). Philadelphia: WB Saunders.

Martini F, et al. (1992). *Fundamentals of anatomy and physiology* (2nd ed.). Englewood Cliffs, NJ: Prentice Hall.

McCance KL & Huether SE (1994). *Pathophysiology: The biological basis for disease in adults and children* (2nd ed.). St Louis: Mosby.

Seeley RR, Stephens TD, & Tate P (1995). *Anatomy & physiology* (3rd ed.). St Louis: Mosby.

Thibodeau GA & Patton K (1996). *Anatomy and physiology* (3rd ed.). St Louis: Mosby.

Van Wynsberghe D, Noback CR, & Carola R (1995). *Human anatomy and physiology* (3rd ed.). New York: McGraw-Hill.

Wingard LB, et al. (1991). *Human pharmacology*. St Louis: Mosby.

Chapter 38

Mucokinetic and Bronchodilator Drugs

Chapter Focus

Clients using mucokinetic and bronchodilator drugs may have ineffective breathing patterns, ineffective airway clearance, or impaired gas exchange. Nurses involved in caring for clients with these nursing diagnoses use a variety of technologies with which the nurse must be knowledgeable. These agents are used with clients who have respiratory disorders and with clients who have respiratory problems caused by nonrespiratory disorders. The following objectives and key terms are important for a good understanding of this chapter.

Key Terms

aerosol therapy (p. 650)
expectorants (p. 651)
mucokinetic agents (p. 649)
mucolytics (p. 651)
mucus (p. 649)
nebulizer (p. 650)
sputum (p. 649)
xanthine derivative (p. 662)

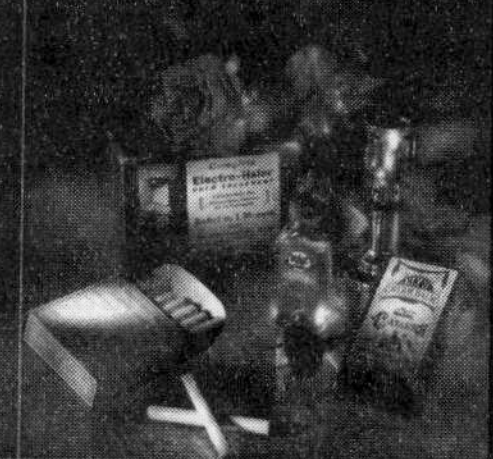

Key Drugs [▲]

albuterol
cromolyn
ipratropium
theophylline

Objectives

1. Describe effective aerosol therapy, including number and size of droplets, side effects, and resultant quality of client breathing.
2. Compare the advantages and disadvantages of water and saline as diluents.
3. Identify the therapeutic goals of mucolytic and bronchodilator drugs.
4. Compare and contrast the sympathomimetic bronchodilator drugs.
5. Identify drugs and beverages in the xanthine group.
6. Discuss the use of the xanthine derivatives, cromolyn, sympathetic agonists, and corticosteroid drugs in the treatment of asthma.
7. Implement the nursing management of the care of clients receiving mucokinetic and bronchodilator drug therapy.

Mucokinetic and bronchodilator drugs help to maintain patency of the respiratory tract. They are the two main groups of drugs discussed in this chapter.

Mucokinetic Drugs

Mucokinetic agents promote the removal of abnormal or excessive respiratory tract secretions by thinning hyperviscous mucus, which allows for a more effective ciliary action. These agents prevent sputum retention, which may result from abnormal ciliary activity, defects in airflow, or modification in cough effectiveness. **Sputum** (or phlegm) may be defined as an abnormal, viscous secretion that is an excretory production of the lower respiratory tree. It consists mainly of **mucus,** a proteinaceous material having a mucopolysaccharide as its major component. In addition, sputum contains deoxyribonucleic acid (DNA) molecules, which are derived from the breakdown of mucosal cells, leukocytes, and bacteria. These products are responsible for the characteristic heavy quality and yellow color of the sputum. The terms *sputum* and *mucus* should not be used interchangeably. Sputum is an abnormal secretion originating in the lower respiratory tract, whereas mucus is a normal secretion produced by the surface cells in the mucous membrane.

Individuals with respiratory disorders such as chronic bronchitis develop disturbances of the mucociliary blanket, resulting in a significant impairment of the mucus clearance process (Figure 38-1). Consequently, mucus plugging and pathogenic colonization of microorganisms occur in the lower respiratory tract. These changes lead to overproduction of thick, tenacious sputum. Thus the advantage provided by the mucokinetic drugs is that they alter the consistency of the sputum, thereby promoting the eventual expectoration, or expulsion, of these secretions.

DILUENTS

Water

The most commonly used agent to dilute respiratory secretions is water. Persons with chronic obstructive pulmonary disease (COPD) frequently suffer from dehydration; thus respiratory secretions are retained. These secretions then become highly viscous in consistency and lead to widespread plug formation in the respiratory tree. Water may be administered by ultrasonic nebulizer. Small amounts

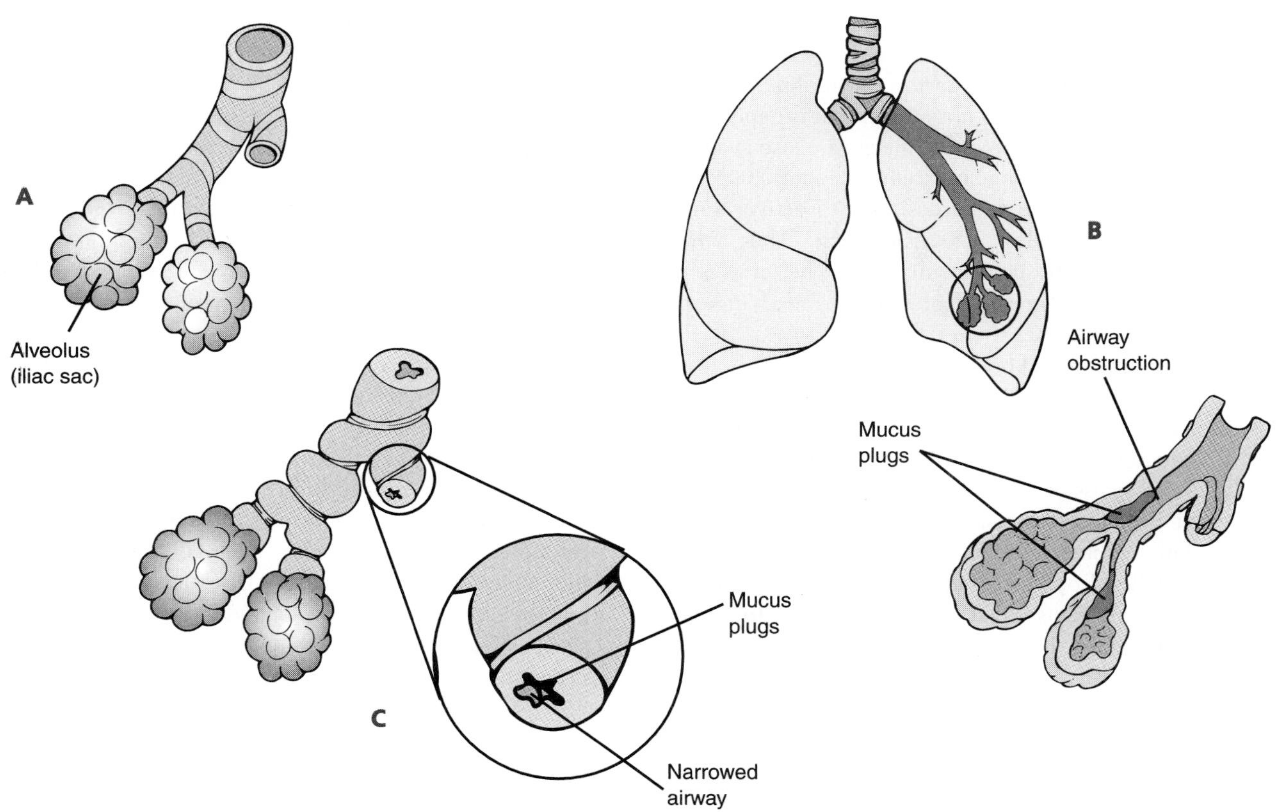

Figure 38-1 Bronchiole in, **A**, normal state and, **B**, during an asthma attack. An asthmatic attack is illustrated by bronchial muscle spasms, inflammation, and excessive mucus, resulting in mucus plugs, edema, and trapped air in the air sacs (alveoli), which causes airway obstruction, **C**. Total amount of air inhaled and exhaled is decreased because of air trapped in the lungs after expiration.

of water deposited on the gel layer of the respiratory tree appear to reduce the adhesive characteristics and general viscosity of the gelatinous substances found in this layer. Care is needed with clients receiving restricted fluid intake, since water can be absorbed through the inhalation route. If fluid intake is being measured, water added to the nebulizer and absorbed through the inhalation route must be added to the client's intake record. If a client's fluid intake is not restricted, large amounts of water are usually encouraged to liquefy the respiratory secretions.

Saline Solutions

Normal saline (0.9% sodium chloride) is physiologic (isotonic) salt solution that exerts the same osmotic pressure as plasma fluids. Therapy by nebulization is well tolerated, resulting in hydration of respiratory secretions. Hypotonic solution (0.45% sodium chloride) is thought to provide deeper penetration into the more distal airways or in the alveoli via the inhalation route, whereas inhalation of hypertonic solution (1.8% sodium chloride) stimulates a productive cough since the particles deposited on the respiratory mucosa are irritating. Hypertonic solution osmotically attracts fluid out of the mucosa and into the respiratory secretions, thereby promoting their excretion.

AEROSOL THERAPY

Aerosol therapy is a form of inhaled, topical pulmonary treatment. An aerosol is a suspension of fine liquid or solid particles dispersed in a gas or in solution that is deposited in the respiratory tract. Dry powder inhalers are also available. Liquid or solid particles range in size from about 0.005 to 50 μm in diameter. **Nebulizers** are designed to deliver a maximum number of particles of a desired size. Thus aerosol therapy is delivered through nebulization. The terms *aerosol therapy* and *nebulization therapy* are often used interchangeably. Aerosol therapy promotes the following:

- Bronchodilation and pulmonary decongestion
- Loosening of secretions
- Topical application of corticosteroids and other drugs
- Moistening, cooling, or heating of inspired air

The effectiveness of nebulization therapy depends on the number of droplets that can be suspended in an inhaled aerosol. This number is directly related to the size of the droplets. Smaller droplets can be suspended in greater numbers than large droplets. Small droplets (about 2 to 4 μm in diameter) are more likely to reach the periphery of the lungs—the alveolar ducts and sacs. Larger droplets (8 to 15 μm in diameter) will be deposited primarily in the bronchioles and bronchi. Droplets of more than 40 μm will be deposited primarily in the upper airway (mouth, pharynx, trachea, and main bronchi).

Rate and depth of breathing are other factors that determine effectiveness of nebulization therapy. Rapid or shallow breathing decreases the number, as well as the retention, of droplets reaching the periphery of the lungs. Rapid breathing permits escape of significant amounts of fine droplets during expirations, although few droplets will escape if the breath is held long enough after deep inspiration to permit droplet deposit in the lung periphery. Small droplets are more effective for absorption of bronchodilators.

Almost all large droplets will be retained somewhere in the larger air passages. Large droplets are used for keeping large airways (nose, trachea) moist and for loosening secretions. Slow and deep breathing is required for proper lung aeration and penetration of the mist into peripheral lung areas. The breath should be held for a few seconds after a full inspiration.

Droplet size can be controlled by the amount of pressure used to force oxygen or room air through the solution to produce a mist. The nebulizer tubing diameter, its length, and its number of bends affect turbulent flow and mist temperature. With most nebulizers maximum density of the inhaled mist is achieved by making the flow of mist as smooth and direct as possible. Nebulizers commonly used in hospitals produce similar mists. *A note of precaution:* drug reconcentration can occur with both jet and ultrasonic nebulizers if a humidity deficit occurs. Evaporation of water molecules causes a gradual increase in drug concentration in the droplets, thus increasing the risk of drug toxicity. Control of temperature and humidity can prevent this toxicity.

The main groups of drugs conventionally administered by aerosol include bronchodilators, cromolyn (Intal), nedocromil (Tilade), and steroid preparations. It is important to remember that the lung is an absorptive organ and thus is a route of access for drugs to enter the systemic circulation. For example, after inhalation anesthetic agents enter the blood, they exert their main effect on the central nervous system. Aerosol therapy, when used as a method of administering drugs, is supposed to minimize systemic absorption and side effects. Yet certain bronchodilator aerosols do produce cardiovascular effects simply because the drug may possess a property that adversely influences cardiac action after absorption into the bloodstream.

When combination inhalation aerosols are prescribed for a client without specific prescriber instructions about a sequence of administration, the nurse should be aware of the proper recommendations for drug administration. For example, if corticosteroids (Beclovent, Vanceril) or cromolyn (Intal) or nedocromil (Tilade) are prescribed to be administered with ipratropium (Atrovent), the ipratropium should be administered 5 minutes before either of the other drugs to promote bronchodilation. Whenever a beta agonist (Alupent, Proventil) is prescribed with ipratropium (Atrovent), the beta agonist is always administered first with a 5 minute wait before administration of the second drug. Do not administer both aerosols in rapid sequence, because of the possibility of inducing fluorocarbon toxicity; also, this rapid administration decreases drug effectiveness. Box 38-1 lists additional therapeutic tips.

> **BOX 38-1**
>
> **Therapeutic Tips**
>
> Selective, $beta_2$ drugs such as albuterol, terbutaline, and others provide the most rapid relief of acute asthmatic symptoms. Subcutaneous injection is not more effective than inhalation therapy and it often causes more side effects/adverse reactions; therefore its use is usually reserved for persons with a very severe dyspnea that prevents them from responding to inhalation therapy.
>
> Oral, selective $beta_2$ drugs are considered less effective than the same agents administered by inhalation. They also have a longer onset of action time and frequently cause more tremor than inhaled preparations.
>
> Corticosteroid inhalation products are less toxic than oral preparations. Oral candidiasis can occur with use if proper preventive measures such as rinsing and/or gargling with water after each use are not employed. Other adverse effects may occur with continuous, long-term use; check current drug reference for information.
>
> Theophylline is considered a less potent bronchodilator than inhaled adrenergic drugs; thus it has limited usefulness in acute, intermittent asthma. Theophylline is more useful in chronic asthma.
>
> Cromolyn decreases airway hyperreactivity. It has no bronchodilator effects and thus should not be used for the treatment of acute asthma.
>
> Ipratropium is usually reserved for persons with acute asthmatic symptoms that have not responded to a course of $beta_2$ agonists. When added to the $beta_2$ agonist therapy, it contributes an additive bronchodilating effect. Some prescribers also use it to suppress symptoms in chronic asthma (Abramowicz, 1991).

MUCOLYTIC DRUGS

Mucolytics are drugs that exert a disintegrating effect on mucus. These agents, also called **expectorants,** promote coughing or spitting and thereby the removal of mucus or other exudates from the lung, bronchi, or trachea. One of the more commonly used mucolytics is acetylcysteine.

acetylcysteine [a se teel sis' tay een] (Mucomyst, Airbron♣)

Acetylcysteine reduces the thickness and stickiness of purulent and nonpurulent pulmonary secretions by decreasing the viscosity of the respiratory mucoprotein molecules into smaller, more soluble, and less viscous strands. In addition, this drug also effects similar changes in the DNA molecule and cellular debris. The decrease in viscosity of bronchial secretions aids their removal by coughing, postural drainage, or suctioning.

Acetylcysteine is indicated as an adjunct treatment for thick or abnormal mucus in bronchopulmonary disease, cystic fibrosis, or atelectasis caused by a mucus obstruction. It is also used as a diagnostic aid in a variety of bronchial studies, such as bronchospirometry and bronchograms.

When administered systemically, it is a specific antidote for an acetaminophen overdose. Acetylcysteine reduces the extent of liver injury after acetaminophen overdose by altering hepatic metabolism; it maintains or restores glutathione concentrations. Glutathione is necessary for the inactivation of an intermediate metabolite of acetaminophen that on accumulation is believed to be hepatotoxic.

In inhalation therapy, some acetylcysteine is absorbed from the pulmonary epithelium, although its primary effects are local on the mucus in the lungs. When inhaled it produces an effect within 1 minute, although direct instillation via an intratracheal catheter produces an immediate effect. The peak response from inhalation occurs within 5 to 10 minutes. Acetylcysteine is metabolized in the liver.

Less frequently reported side effects of acetylcysteine include fever, nausea, vomiting, runny nose, throat or lung irritation, clammy skin, and sore mouth. Its less frequent adverse reactions include hemoptysis and respiratory difficulties. No significant drug interactions have been reported with acetylcysteine when administered by inhalation.

The usual adult and pediatric dose by nebulization using a face mask, mouthpiece, or tracheostomy is 3 to 5 ml of a 20% solution or 6 to 10 ml of a 10% solution inhaled three or four times daily. To treat an acetaminophen overdose, acetylcysteine is administered orally in a dose of 140 mg/kg initially, then 70 mg/kg every 4 hours for 17 additional doses.

■ Nursing Management

Acetylcysteine Therapy

Assessment. Use acetylcysteine with caution in the elderly and debilitated and those with asthma or severe respiratory insufficiency, because the drug may increase airway obstruction; bronchospasm may occur in susceptible clients.

Nursing diagnosis. With the administration of acetylcysteine, the client is at risk for the following nursing diagnoses: altered comfort related to the drug's unpleasant odor during administration or facial stickiness after nebulization by face mask, nausea or vomiting, rash, rhinorrhea, and throat irritation; hyperthermia; altered mucous membranes (stomatitis); ineffective airway clearance; and the collaborative problems of allergic dermatitis, bronchospastic allergic reaction, and hemoptysis.

Implementation

Monitoring. The frequency of the client's cough and its character should be monitored and documented. The character and quantity of expectorated material should be observed. Percussion and auscultation of the chest should be accomplished on a periodic basis.

Intervention. Ultrasonic nebulizers are recommended for administration of the drug. Hand nebulizers are discouraged because the output is too small and the fluid particles too large. The nebulized drug may be inhaled either directly or by the use of a plastic face mask, face tent, mouthpiece, or oxygen tent. The nebulizer may be used with an intermittent positive pressure breathing (IPPB) apparatus. IPPB apparatus is a ventilator that assists or controls respiration by delivering compressed gas under positive pressure into a person's airways until a preset pressure is reached. Passive exhalation is allowed through a valve, and the cycle begins again as the flow of gas is triggered by inhalation. When the drug is nebulized using a dry gas, it may become concentrated because of evaporation of the solution. The last remaining quarter of the drug can be diluted with an equal part of sterile water for injection to continue nebulization so the client is ensured the appropriate dosage. After nebulization, the face should be washed with water to remove the sticky coating left by the drug. The equipment should be cleaned immediately after use to prevent blockage of the fine parts and corrosion of the metal ones. In many health care agencies, respiratory therapists administer these treatments, but nurses may be responsible for them at night and with the client in the home.

Some clients may develop nausea and vomiting, but this may be from the disagreeable odor of the nebulized drug and quantity of respiratory secretions eliminated. With the aid of these agents and postural drainage, most individuals can expectorate pulmonary secretions without further assistance; however, in the elderly or debilitated, suctioning may be indicated.

Because of release of hydrogen sulfide, solutions of acetylcysteine will harden rubber and become discolored on contact with certain metals. Acetylcysteine solutions should be used with equipment made of glass, plastic, or stainless steel. If the vacuum seal has been broken on the bottle, the solution should be refrigerated to retard oxidation and then used within 48 hours.

When acetylcysteine is administered orally, it may be diluted in soft drinks or citrus juices. The diluted solution should be used within the hour.

Education. The client should clear the airway by coughing before the drug is administered by aerosol. Instruction should be given on the correct use of the nebulizer.

Evaluation. The client will experience increased sputum production and expectoration and a clearing of the lung fields.

Antidotal use. When acetylcysteine is administered as an antidote for acetaminophen overdose, it is most beneficial when started within 10 to 12 hours after the ingestion of the overdose, but it is still beneficial if started within the first 24 hours. The client should be supported through gastric lavage or induced emesis and other appropriate therapies. The greatest risk of acetaminophen overdose is hepatotoxicity, the potential for which can be assessed from plasma acetaminophen concentrations, so monitoring these and liver function studies are essential. Liver function studies should be performed every 24 hours for at least 96 hours after the ingestion of the overdose. Monitor fluid and electrolyte balances, renal function, and cardiac function. Nursing care is provided for the client with knowledge deficit or a high risk for self-harm.

Other Expectorants

Over the years, many other products have been used as expectorants in both prescription and over-the-counter medications. Guaifenesin, the only expectorant listed by the FDA in Category I (safe and effective) is reviewed in Chapter 11. A prescribed respiratory inhalant product is recombinant human DNase or dornase alfa (Pulmozyme). This product is used to increase expectoration in cystic fibrosis.

dornase alfa (Pulmozyme)

Cystic fibrosis is a respiratory disease associated with thick secretions from an accumulation of DNA from degenerating neutrophils and inflammation. Dornase alfa is an enzyme that digests extracellular DNA, thus improving pulmonary function and reducing the risk of respiratory tract infections common with cystic fibrosis. The use of this product has resulted in a decrease in respiratory infections, hospitalizations, and medical costs (Franz et al, 1994).

Significant improvement in pulmonary function is seen within 3 to 7 days, the decrease in respiratory infections between weeks to several months. The side/adverse effects of dornase alfa include chest pain, sore throat, laryngitis, skin rash, conjunctivitis, and hoarseness.

The usual dose for children 5 years and older and adults is 2.5 mg daily inhaled via nebulization.

▪ Nursing Management

Dornase Alfa Therapy

Assessment. It should be determined that the client does not have a sensitivity to dornase alfa, Chinese hamster ovary cell products, or any other component of the product. Although drug interactions have not been studied with dornase alfa, it has been administered safely to clients with cystic fibrosis with other medications that they commonly take such as bronchdilators, antibiotics, corticosteroids, enzymes, vitamins, and analgesics. Establish a baseline assessment of the client's respiratory status.

Nursing diagnosis. The client receiving dornase alfa has the potential for the following nursing diagnoses: altered comfort (chest pain, sore throat, conjunctivitis); impaired skin integrity (rash); and disturbed body image (hoarseness, voice changes).

Implementation

Monitoring. The client's respiratory status should be carefully monitored for cough, breath sounds, sputum, forced expiratory volume, vital capacity, and tidal volume.

Intervention. Dornase alfa is administered via nebulizer. See package literature for recommended devices. Wash hands thoroughly before assembling nebulizer and mouthpiece. Do not mix or dilute dornase alfa with other agents. It should be administered every day; a decrease in pulmonary function occurs within 48 hours after therapy is stopped.

Education. Instruct the client on the appropriate nebulizer and ensure its correct use with dornase alfa. Advise the client not to use a face mask but only a mouthpiece. Do not use the medication if it is cloudy or discolored.

Evaluation. The client's airway is patent; the breathing pattern is effective without fatigue or dyspnea. Breath sounds are clear.

DRUGS THAT ANTAGONIZE BRONCHIAL SECRETIONS

Anticholinergic agents decrease secretions and also make them hard to expectorate. While not generally used for this purpose, atropine may be given cautiously to decrease secretions and excessive expectoration in certain forms of bronchitis. Many remedies used to treat colds contain atropine, an anticholinergic.

▲ **ipratropium** [i pra troe' pee um] (Atrovent)
Ipratropium is an anticholinergic drug that produces a local bronchodilation after inhalation. It is indicated for maintenance (not for acute episodes) therapy in clients with COPD (chronic bronchitis or emphysema). After administration, onset of action is between 5 and 15 minutes, and peak effect is in 1 to 2 hours with duration of action between 3 and 6 hours.

More frequently reported side effects of ipratropium include dry mouth or throat, coughing, headache, anxiety, and gastrointestinal distress. Although rarely occurring, the following side effects should be reported immediately to the prescriber: hives, skin rash, or stomatitis. The usual adolescent or adult dose is 1 or 2 inhalations 3 or 4 times daily, administered every 4 hours. Shake unit well before using.

■ Nursing Management
Ipratropium Therapy

Assessment. Because ipratropium has primarily a local, site-specific effect, the risk benefit is minimal. However, this anticholinergic drug may precipitate or exacerbate urinary retention and angle-closure glaucoma. Concurrent use with other anticholinergic drugs might have an additive effect. An accurate baseline status of the client's respiratory status should be documented.

Nursing diagnosis. The client receiving ipratropium therapy may be at risk for the following nursing diagnoses: altered mucous membranes (stomatitis); altered comfort (rash, cough/dryness of mouth or throat, headache, metallic taste, nausea); disturbed sleep pattern (insomnia); altered urinary elimination (urinary retention); activity intolerance; ineffective breathing pattern; and risk for injury related to blurred vision or hypotension (weakness, syncope). Potential complications might be paralytic ileus or increased bronchospasm, which may be due to other agents in the preparation such as benzalkonium chloride.

Implementation

Monitoring. Continuing assessment of the client should include lung sounds, respirations, pulse, and blood pressure before and after each inhalation therapy until the client's response has stabilized.

Intervention. A gas flow of 6 to 10 L/min of oxygen or compressed air is necessary for nebulization of ipratropium. A face mask or mouthpiece may be used, but the mouthpiece is preferable to reduce the risk of the drug getting into the eyes. If more than one inhalation is necessary, allow 1 minute between inhalations for the most effective results. Consult with the prescriber immediately if the client's symptoms do not improve within 30 minutes. If the client also uses a beta agonist inhalation aerosol, it should be used 5 minutes before the ipratropium. For clients also using a corticosteroid or cromolyn inhalation aerosol, the ipratropium should be used 5 minutes before its use. Do not mix ipratropium and cromolyn in a nebulizer—they will form a precipitate.

Education. Caution the client to avoid contact with the eyes because temporary irritation will occur. As an anticholinergic, the drug may cause dryness of the mouth and throat; tell the client about the use of sugarless candies and gum or ice chips for relief. Instruct the client to inspect the oral cavity for candidiasis and seek regular dental attention for the detection of caries.

Evaluation. The client receiving ipratropium therapy will experience a decrease or absence in respiratory distress; respiratory rate and effort will be within the normal limits for the client.

Bronchodilator Drugs

Bronchodilator drugs are primarily used to treat chronic pulmonary diseases such as asthma, chronic bronchitis, and emphysema. Major causes of ineffective airway clearance include (1) bronchial smooth muscle contraction (asthma), (2) mucus hypersecretion (chronic bronchitis), and (3) mucosal edema or inflammation (chronic bronchitis). Bronchial asthma may appear with some or all of these symptoms (see Figure 38-1).

In the past asthma was classified on the basis of the stimuli that may induce an attack, such as intrinsic asthma caused by emotional factors or exercise and extrinsic asthma caused by pollens, molds, dust, or animal hair. Because many asthmatics have a combination type asthma, this type of classification is not considered useful. The National Institute of Health (NIH) defines asthma as a lung disease that has reversible airway obstruction, airway inflammation, and increased airway sensitivity to stimuli (Self & Kelly, 1995). Therefore clients are classified according to the frequency and severity of their asthma attacks (mild, moderate, or severe) because this information is the most useful when considering pharmacologic interventions.

- mild: intermittent attacks of less than 1 to 2 a week or nocturnal asthma <1 to 2 times monthly. PEF* >80%; normal after bronchodilator use; PEF variability <20%.
- moderate: attacks more than 1 to 2 times weekly, nocturnal asthma symptoms more than twice a month and the use of a beta agonist inhaler nearly daily. PEF 60% to 80%; normal after bronchodilator use; PEF variability 20% to 30%.
- severe: frequent and continuous asthmatic symptoms including nocturnal asthma plus having been hospitalized for asthma in the previous year.

*PEF, Peak Flow Meter: objectively measures peak expiratory flow rate and daily variability determinations before and after use of medications, especially bronchodilators.

The major drugs used in treatment of asthma include sympathomimetic drugs, theophylline, cromolyn, nedocromil, and the corticosteroids while on a cellular level. Figure 38-2 gives an overview of the effects of antiasthmatic medications. Figure 38-3 illustrates the primary action sites for these drugs. The principal agents used in the treatment of airway obstruction include sympathomimetic drugs and xanthine derivatives. Prophylactic antiasthmatic agents also prevent airway obstruction in individuals with certain types of asthma. Most of these drugs enhance the production of cyclic 3'5' AMP in bronchial smooth muscle cells to effect bronchodilation (Figure 38-4).

Nursing Management

Bronchodilator Drug Therapy

Assessment. Bronchodilators are primarily indicated for the treatment of chronic pulmonary conditions, such as asthma, chronic bronchitis, and emphysema. A baseline assessment of the client should include a description of the respiratory status—respiratory rate and effort; use of accessory muscles; nasal flaring or lip pursing; breath sounds per auscultation; circumoral pallor or cyanosis; presence of cough and/or sputum; activity intolerance; and signs of impaired gas exchange such as anxiety, confusion, and irritability. In addition, the following diagnostic tests are usually done: arterial blood gas (ABG) values, chest x-ray, sputum culture, CBC, pulmonary function studies, and ECG.

Nursing diagnosis. Because these diseases interfere with the basic human need for air, expect the client to exhibit anxiety, not only during acute episodes but also in anticipation of such events. Ineffective airway clearance, ineffective breathing pattern, impaired gas exchange, and activity intolerance are nursing diagnoses that are common to clients receiving bronchodilator therapy. See the Nursing Care Plan on p. 656 for other selected nursing diagnoses.

Implementation

Monitoring. The client's respiratory status should be monitored on an ongoing basis to evaluate the drug's effectiveness. Monitor for side effects of bronchodilators, including tachycardia and dysrhythmias. Depending on the specific drug, serum levels may be monitored.

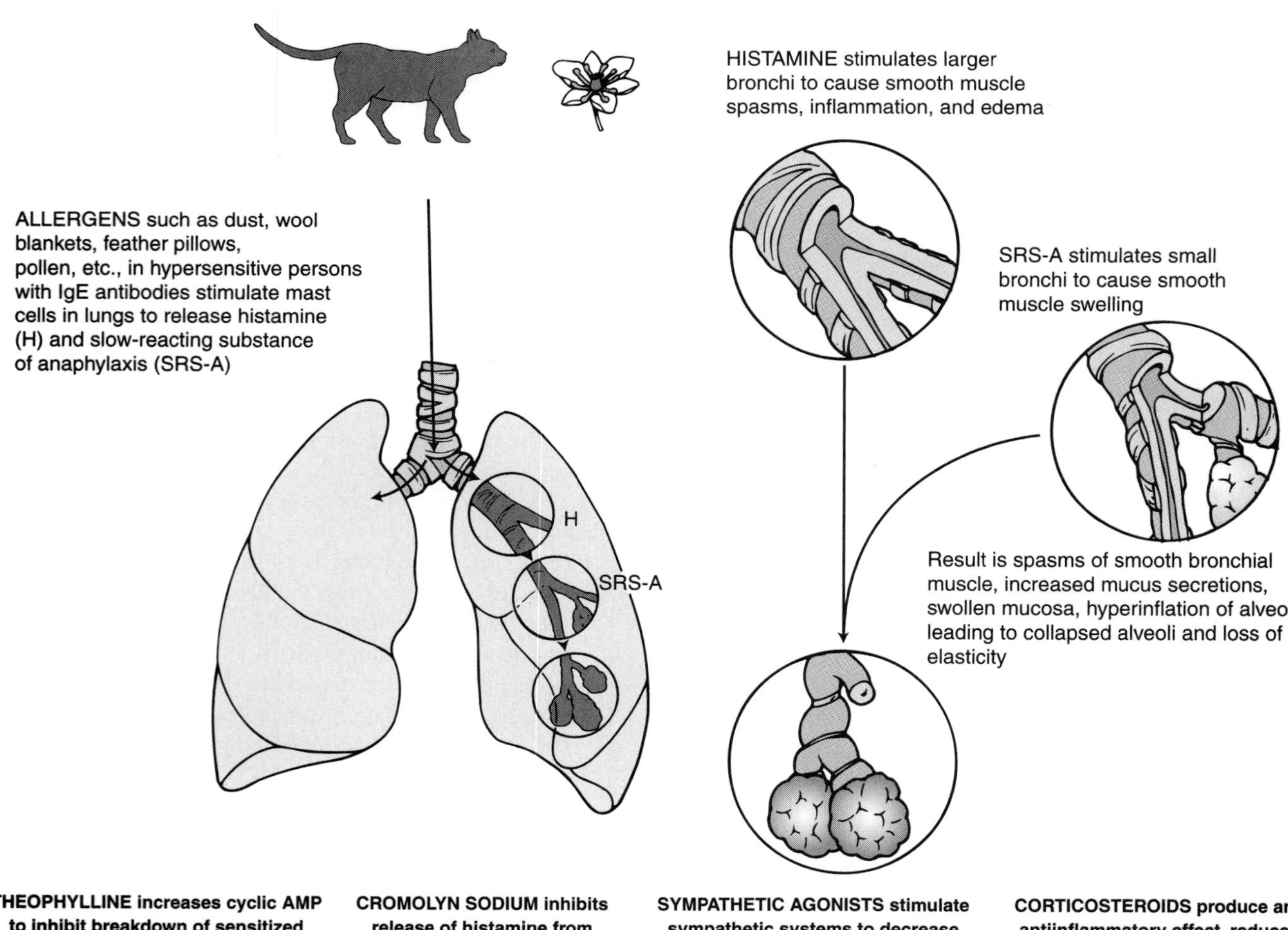

Figure 38-2 Overview of the effects of various antiasthmatic medications.

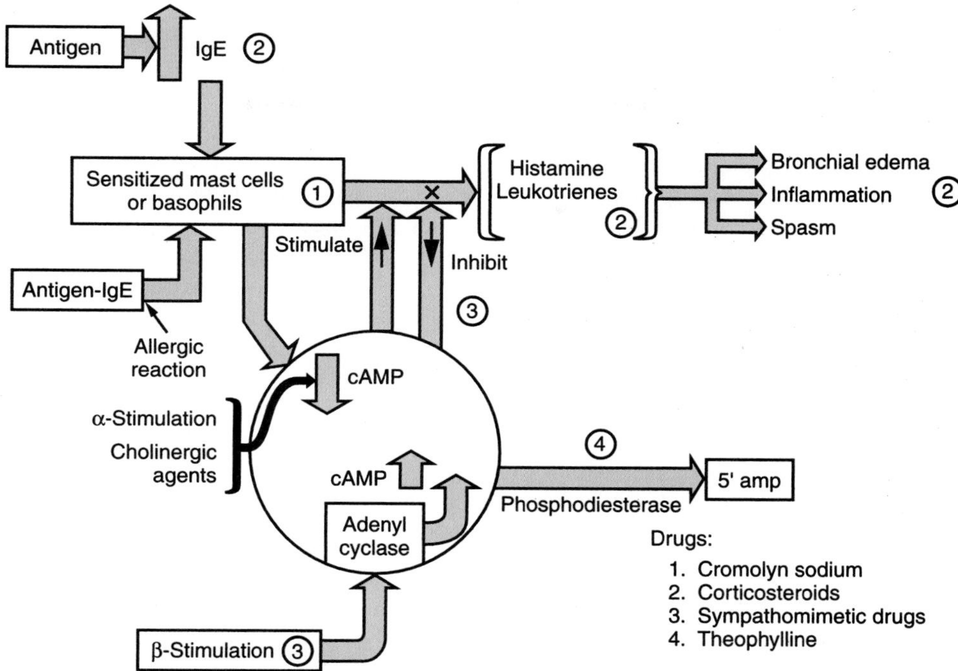

Figure 38-3 Major sites of action of drugs used to treat asthma.

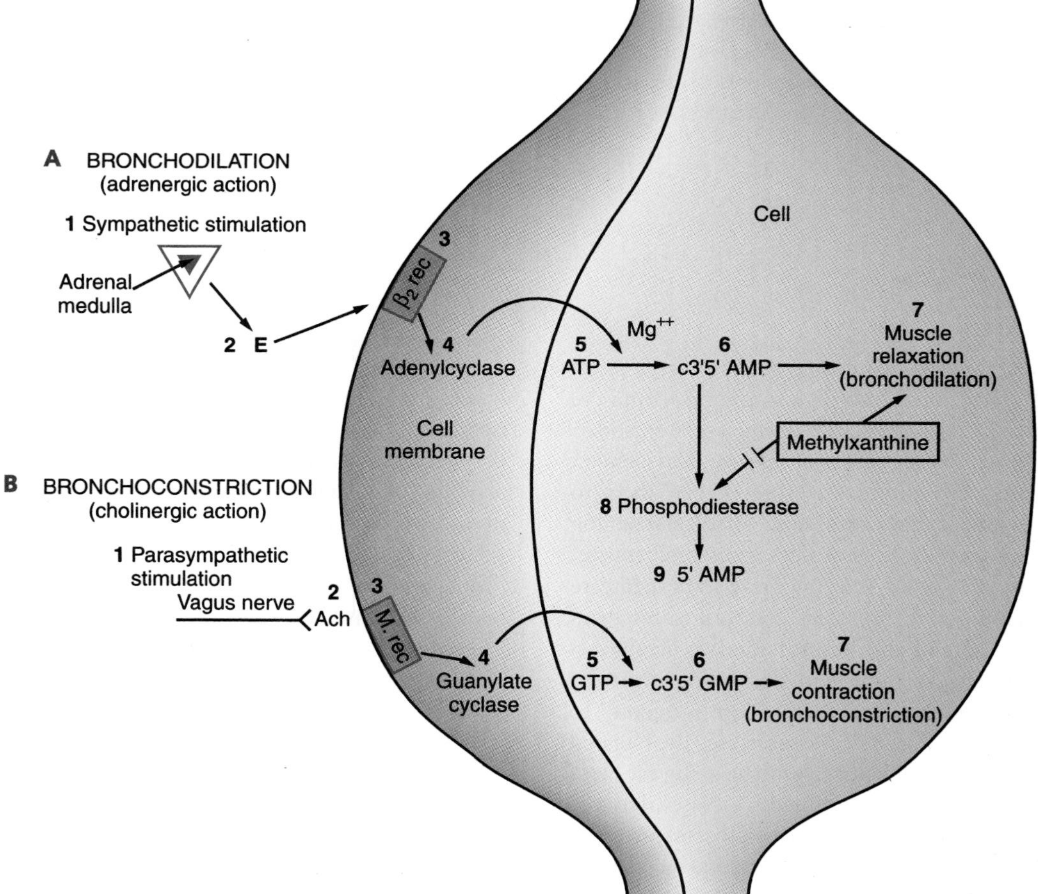

Figure 38-4 Mechanism of bronchial smooth muscle action. **A,** Bronchodilation pathway. **B,** Bronchoconstriction pathway. (*E,* epinephrine; *Ach,* acetylcholine; β_2 *rec,* β_2 receptor; *M. rec,* muscarinic receptor)

Nursing Care Plan

Selected Nursing Diagnoses Related to Bronchodilators

Nursing diagnosis	Outcome criteria	Nursing interventions
Airway clearance, ineffective, related to reversible airway obstruction	Coughs effectively and expectorates sputum Absence of abnormal breath sounds Absence of sputum production	Assess respiratory status every 4 hours Assist client to turn, cough, and deep breathe as necessary Provide adequate humidification as ordered Monitor characteristics of sputum every 8 hours and record
	Fluid intake of at least 3000 ml/24 hours unless contraindicated	Encourage fluids to at least 3000 ml daily
Activity intolerance related to reversible airway obstruction	Increasing level of activity Pulse, respiration, and blood pressure remain within acceptable limits during activity	Plan with client for increasing levels of activity including activities that have priority for client Identify and limit the factors that decrease the client's tolerance for activity Monitor pulse rate, respiration, and blood pressure while increasing the level of activity
Knowledge deficit related to medication regimen	Client will describe underlying condition and how the drug relates to the condition, how and when to take the medication, common drug interactions, safety precautions, common side/adverse effects and which of those warrant reporting Self-administer medication safely and accurately	Administer oral forms with food to minimize gastrointestinal distress Emphasize the need for drug to be taken as prescribed around the clock Caution the client not to self-administer any over-the-counter drugs without prescriber consultation Advise the client to notify the prescriber if the usual dose fails to be therapeutic or if condition worsens after treatment Instruct the client to minimize ingestion of foods and beverages containing xanthine (coffee, chocolate, colas) Emphasize the need for ongoing contact with the prescriber for serum levels and evaluation

Intervention. Provide supportive nursing care with oxygen and fluid replacement to bring respiration within the normal range for rate, depth, and effort during acute episodes.

Education. An important aspect of nursing management is to provide clients with information that enables them to maintain some measure of the control over what is happening to them and so decrease their anxiety. Education for clients receiving bronchodilators should be an integral part of their care and include instruction on factors that tend to precipitate an acute episode. They should also be instructed to maintain a diary of symptoms and the time and dose of medications during attacks; to explain their medication program; to demonstrate how to take inhaled medications (see the Nursing Research box on p. 657) and inhaler care; to describe the measures to take during an attack; and to identify those signs and symptoms that need to be reported to the health care provider.

Evaluation. The client will have an adequate respiratory status as evidenced by the absence of adventitious breath sounds, ABGs within normal limits (PaO_2 > 60 mm Hg, $PaCO_2$ 35 to 45 mm Hg), pH 7.35 to 7.45, and a respiratory rate of 12 to 20 breaths/min.

SYMPATHOMIMETIC DRUGS

Based on their receptor action, three types of sympathomimetic drugs are recognized: (1) nonselective adrenergic drugs that have alpha, $beta_1$ (cardiac), and $beta_2$ (respiratory) activities (e.g., epinephrine); (2) nonselective beta adrenergic drugs with $beta_1$ and $beta_2$ effects (e.g., isoproterenol); and (3) selective $beta_2$ agents (e.g., albuterol [Proventil], bitolterol [Tornalate], isoetharine [Bronkosol], metaproterenol [Alupent], pirbuterol [Maxair], salmeterol [Serevent], terbutaline [Brethine]) that act primarily on $beta_2$ receptors with minor activity at $beta_1$ receptors in the lungs (bronchial smooth muscle).

Nonselective Adrenergic Drugs

Nonselective adrenergic drugs such as epinephrine, ephedrine, and others possess both alpha- and beta-receptor stimulating properties. Alpha activity appears to mediate vasoconstriction to reduce mucosal edema, while $beta_2$ stimulation produces bronchodilation and vasodilation. In contrast, $beta_1$ receptor action causes unwanted cardiac side effects such as increases in heart rate and force of myocardial contraction.

Nursing Research

Teaching the use of inhalers

Many clients don't know how to use a metered dose inhaler and depend on their health care providers to instruct them. It may be that nurses and physicians need more skill themselves.

Two investigators from Baylor College of Medicine reached that conclusion after surveying 100 asthmatic clients and 170 health professionals, evaluating their ability to complete the 6 steps that should be followed when using the device. Their findings were that 65% of the clients, 82% of the nurses, and 39% of the house medical staff received a "poor" rating. This rating means that they were unable to perform more than 2 steps correctly. Respiratory therapists, however, performed the best—85% of them knew at least 5 of the 6 steps.

The investigators concluded that better training is essential for both clients and health care providers, so that everyone is familiar with the following procedure:

- Remove the inhaler cap and shake.
- Exhale normally.
- Administer the medication at the beginning of the next inhalation.
- Slowly inhale.
- Hold your breath for up to 10 seconds.
- Wait at least 30 seconds before inhaling a second puff.

Critical thinking questions

- Why is it essential for clients to use an inhaler correctly?
- How could you effectively evaluate the client's/nurse's ability to correctly use an inhaler?

From Interiano B and KK Guntupalli (1993). Metered-dose inhalers: Do health care providers know what to teach? *Arch Intern Med* 153(1):81.

Undesirable effects on $beta_2$ receptors include skeletal muscle tremors, tachycardia, palpitations, increased CNS stimulation, hypokalemia (after large doses are administered), glycogenolysis, and gluconeogenesis.

epinephrine [ep i nef' rin] (Adrenalin)

Epinephrine induces relaxation of bronchial smooth muscle (by stimulating $beta_2$ receptors in the lungs), thus relieving bronchospasm, increasing vital capacity, and reducing airway resistance. It also inhibits the bronchoconstriction induced by the release of histamine and substances released during anaphylaxis.

Epinephrine is indicated for the treatment of bronchial asthma, bronchitis, and other pulmonary disease states and the prevention of bronchospasm and bronchial asthma. By inhalation, only slight absorption occurs, but if large doses of epinephrine are administered, systemic absorption increases. Systemic absorption is rapid by intramuscular or subcutaneous administration.

The onset of action is within 3 to 5 minutes by inhalation, between 6 and 15 minutes by subcutaneous injection, and variable by IM injection. The duration of action is between 1 and 3 hours by inhalation or 1 to 4 hours by the parenteral routes. It is metabolized at sympathetic nerve endings and other tissues with a small amount of excretion in the kidneys.

The side effects of epinephrine most frequently reported are nervousness, insomnia, tachycardia, dizziness, headaches, hypotension, anorexia, nausea, a pounding tachycardia, sweating, vomiting, dry mouth and throat (especially with inhalation), and difficulty in urination.

Many drug interactions have been reported with epinephrine. For example, when it is given concurrently with a corticosteroid (or other) inhaler that also contains a fluorocarbon propellant, fluorocarbon toxicity may result. Teach the client to allow at least a 5 minute interval between the use of such inhalants. Also alpha-adrenergic blocking agents (e.g., prazosin, tolazoline) or other medications with alpha-blocking properties (e.g., phenothiazines, haloperidol) or the fast-acting vasodilators (nitrates), may block the alpha-stimulating effects of epinephrine, which may result in severe hypotension and tachycardia. Monitor closely because medical interventions may be necessary. The vasodilator effects of nitrites may also be decreased with concurrent drug administration.

Concurrent use of epinephrine with anesthetics, such as chloroform, cyclopropane, and halothane, may increase the risk for severe arrhythmias. Tricyclic antidepressants or cocaine and epinephrine may increase the risk of cardiac arrhythmias, tachycardia, hypertension, and hyperpyrexia. Such combinations should be avoided.

Beta-adrenergic blocking agents (oral, parenteral, and ophthalmic) may reduce the therapeutic effects of both agents. In addition, adverse cardiovascular side effects (e.g., hypertension, bradycardia, and heart block) may be enhanced. Whenever possible, avoid concurrent administration. With the digitalis glycosides (digoxin, digitoxin), an increase in the risk for cardiac arrhythmias may occur. If concurrent therapy is necessary, monitor with an electrocardiogram.

Ergotamine and the ergoloid mesylates may result in peripheral vascular ischemia, gangrene, or with ergotamine, severe hypertension. This drug combination should be avoided.

Various forms of epinephrine are available for example, epinephrine (Bronkaid Mist, Primatene Mist), epinephrine bitartrate (AsthmaHaler, Medihaler-Epi), and racepinephrine (AsthmaNefrin, Vaponefrin). By inhalation, the adult dose is usually 10 drops of a 1% solution or a diluted racepinephrine solution (2.25%) in a nebulizer. Generally one inhalation of the former or 2 or 3 inhalations of the latter preparation is administered. Doses may be repeated at sufficient intervals as stated in the current package inserts or *USP DI*. With the aerosol preparations, one inhalation is administered, which if necessary may be repeated in 1 minute if needed. Subsequent doses are usually administered in 3 to 4 hours. Pediatric doses are individualized by the prescriber according to response.

Many other adrenergic bronchodilators are available. In choosing a beta-receptor agonist, the $beta_2$ selectivity, potency, and duration of action of the drug are considered.

The high incidence of undesirable cardiotoxic effects caused by the $beta_1$ property of sympathomimetic agents (nonselective agents) led to the search for a more specific $beta_2$ receptor agonist such as isoetharine and the noncatecholamine $beta_2$ receptor agonists, albuterol, metaproterenol, and terbutaline.

■ Nursing Management

Epinephrine Therapy

The nursing management of clients receiving epinephrine is discussed in detail in Chapter 22, p. 426. This selection should be consulted because the drug has far-reaching systemic effects. In addition, the general nursing management of clients receiving bronchodilators should also be consulted. However, some nursing management relates specifically to epinephrine administration by inhalation.

Epinephrine and other beta-adrenergic agents may be used interchangeably during inhalation therapy. Do not administer concurrently; allow 4 hours between doses when changing from one to another. Instruct the client in the use of the metered dose nebulizer. Teach the client to take pulse rate before inhalation therapy. Allow 2 minutes between doses, and do not administer more frequently than required to relieve symptoms, because excessive use may cause paradoxical bronchospasm. The client should not receive more than 12 bronchodilator inhalations in 24 hours. Symptoms should be relieved within 20 minutes. The prescriber should be notified if symptoms are not relieved with the usual dosage, since this may indicate a worsening of bronchospasm, which requires reassessment of therapy. Advise the client to rinse the mouth with water to prevent mucosal absorption of the drug. In case of emergency, the client should be taught to self-inject epinephrine subcutaneously.

Nonselective Beta-Adrenergic Drugs

Nonselective beta-adrenergic drugs exhibit both $beta_1$ and $beta_2$ agonist activity. Their main action is on the bronchial smooth muscle as well as the heart. Isoproterenol is the prototype example for this drug category.

isoproterenol solution [eye soe proe ter' e nole] (Vapo-Iso, Isuprel)

Isoproterenol is indicated for the treatment of bronchial asthma, bronchitis, and other pulmonary disease states. Onset of action by inhalation is within 2 to 5 minutes; sublingually (SL) within 15 to 30 minutes; and by intravenous injection, immediately. Its duration of action is 0.5 to 2 hours by inhalation, 1 to 2 hours SL, and less than 1 hour by IV injection. It is metabolized in the liver, lungs, and other body tissues and excreted by the kidneys.

The side/adverse effects of isoproterenol include restlessness, anxiety, insomnia, pink or red colored saliva, and a dry mouth or throat after inhalation usage. Dizziness, flushing of the skin, headache, tremors, palpitations, sweating, tachycardia, weakness, vomiting, and hypertension or hypotension have also been reported.

Significant drug interactions are similar to those of epinephrine, except for the interactions noted with parenteral local anesthetics, alpha blocking agents, and the ergoloid mesylates or ergotamine. These exceptions are due to the fact that isoproterenol does not have alpha effects.

The adult bronchodilator inhalation dose is 6 to 12 inhalations of a 0.25% nebulized solution, which may be repeated at 15 minute intervals, if needed, for three doses. The maximum number of treatments recommended in a 24 hour period is 8. In an acute asthmatic attack, 5 to 15 deep inhalations of a 0.5% nebulized solution or 3 to 7 inhalations of 1% nebulized solution are administered. The sequence is repeated once after waiting 5 to 10 minutes if needed. Up to 5 subsequent doses per day may be administered, if necessary. For bronchospasm in chronic obstructive lung disease (COPD), a nebulizer of IPPB drug administration may be used. Pediatric dosage recommendations are similar to an adult with the exception of using the 1% solution.

Isoproterenol injection is used IV as a bronchodilator for bronchospasm during anesthesia at a dose of 10 to 20 μg. If necessary, the dose may be repeated.

■ Nursing Management

Isoproterenol Therapy

Assessment. The nursing management of clients receiving isoproterenol, as well as the nursing management of bronchodilator therapy, is discussed in detail in Chapter 22, p. 429. These selections should be consulted because the drug has both bronchodilating and cardiotonic effects. However, some interventions relate specifically to its administration by inhalation. Instruct the client to use the nebulizer correctly. The client should allow 1 to 5 minutes between first and second inhalations. Advise the client of the number of doses permitted in a 24 hour period, based on the literature for the particular form or delivery device of the drug. If this limit is reached within a 24 hour period, the prescriber should be notified. This frequency of treatment may indicate that other medications may need to be added to the therapeutic regimen. Advise the client that sputum and saliva may turn pink with use of the drug. Isoproterenol needs to be stored in a tight, light-resistant container and is not to be used if a precipitate or discoloration occurs.

Selective $Beta_2$ Receptor Drugs

Catecholamine $Beta_2$ Agents

isoetharine inhalation [eye soe eth' a reen] (Bronkosol)

Isoetharine is a direct-acting sympathomimetic catecholamine that selectively stimulates $beta_2$ receptors to relax bronchial smooth muscle. Since it possesses a weak $beta_1$ response, less risk of cardiotonic side effects exists than with epinephrine and isoproterenol. Its $beta_2$ adrenergic-receptor activity relieves bronchospasm, increasing vital capacity, and decreasing resistance of bronchial airways. It may also inhibit antigen-induced release of histamine by stimulating the production of cyclic 3'5' AMP, which stabilizes the mast cell.

Isoetharine has the same indications as epinephrine. This drug has an onset of action of 1 to 6 minutes and a peak effect between 15 and 60 minutes. Its duration of action is 1 to 4 hours. It is metabolized in the liver, lungs, gastrointestinal tract, and other body tissues and is excreted by the kidneys. Side/adverse effects include dizziness, headaches, dry mouth, and a foul taste in the mouth or throat after use of the inhalation product; nausea, anxiety, palpitations, tremors, insomnia, tachycardia, weakness, and vomiting have also been reported. For significant drug interactions, see those for isoproterenol.

Adult bronchodilator dose with a hand nebulizer is 4 inhalations of an undiluted 0.5% or 1% solution, usually administered every 4 hours. For intermittent positive pressure breathing (IPPB) or oxygen aerosolization dosage, see current package insert or *USP DI*. Dosage in children has not been established.

■ Nursing Management
Isoetharine Therapy

Assessment. Determine initially if the client has a preexisting condition that would indicate cautious use of the drug: cardiovascular disease, such as hypertension, coronary artery disease, or limited cardiac reserve; hyperthyroidism; pheochromocytoma; or sensitivity to sympathomimetics. Baseline assessments are the same as those discussed in the nursing management of bronchodilator drugs.

Nursing diagnosis. With the administration of isoetharine, the following nursing diagnoses should be considered for the client: altered comfort (dryness of the mouth and throat, headache, nausea, nervousness, trembling, and palpitations); altered sleep pattern (insomnia); anxiety; activity intolerance (weakness) related to overdosage; ineffective airway clearance related to paradoxical bronchospasm (increase in wheezing and difficulty breathing); and the collaborative problem of altered cardiac output related to tachycardia.

Implementation

Monitoring. The client's respiratory status should be monitored on an ongoing basis to evaluate the drug's effectiveness. Monitor for side effects of isoetharine, including tachycardia and arrhythmias.

Intervention. Isoetharine may be administered by hand nebulizer, IPPB, and oxygen aerosolization. The use of IPPB is currently limited as a method of aerosol deposition in that the amount of drug lost in the room air and the apparatus is approximately 40% to 65%, and the amount of drug deposited in the lower airways is about 5% to 15%. However, it is a convenient procedure for helping clients with airway obstruction to breathe deeply. IPPB is generally administered by the respiratory therapist.

Education. Instruct client in the use of the inhaler (Box 38-2). Warn the client to avoid contact of spray with eyes and to rinse mouth after therapy to prevent dryness and throat irritation. Advise the client to use inhalation therapy as prescribed since rapid relief encourages overuse. Thus tolerance to a bronchodilator agent may occur, with a potential for causing cumulative drug toxicity (e.g., palpitations, tachycardia, headache, dizziness, and nausea).

Repeated use of the inhaler may cause paradoxical airway resistance, which produces sudden dyspnea. To relieve possible bronchospasm, the prescriber may discontinue therapy and use another drug. Instruct client to take no more than 2 inhalations at a time and to allow 1 to 2 minutes between inhalations. Encourage an increase in fluid intake to adequately hydrate the client, which will also aid in liquefying bronchial secretions. Inform client that sputum may be rust-colored because of oxidation of medication.

Evaluation. The client will have an adequate respiratory status as evidenced by the absence of adventitious breath sounds, ABGs within normal limits (PaO_2 >60 mm Hg, $PaCO_2$ 35 to 45 mm Hg), pH 7.35 to 7.45, and a respiratory rate of 12 to 20 breaths/min or within the client's baseline.

Noncatecholamine Beta$_2$ Receptor Drugs

Noncatecholamine drugs have two advantages over the catecholamine type agents: they are longer acting and have fewer cardiovascular side effects.

Albuterol and metaproterenol will represent this category, although salmeterol (Serevent) is the first long-acting bronchodilator inhaler approved for twice daily dosing.

▲ **albuterol** [al byoo' ter ole] (Proventil, Ventolin)

Albuterol, a sympathomimetic bronchodilator, possesses a relatively selective specificity for beta$_2$-adrenergic receptors in the lungs and therefore is less likely to cause unwanted cardiovascular effects. Its interaction with the beta$_2$ receptor in the cell membrane of the bronchial smooth muscle stimulates the enzyme adenyl cyclase to produce cyclic 3'5' AMP, which results in relaxation of the smooth muscle of the bronchi (see Figure 38-4), thus relieving bronchospasm and decreasing airway resistance. In addition, this mechanism causes relaxation of the smooth muscle of the uterus and blood vessels of skeletal muscle. However, it has been reported that high doses of the drug administered intravenously would be required to inhibit uterine contractions to delay premature labor (see the Pregnancy Safety box on p. 661). This drug has the same indications as epinephrine.

By inhalation, albuterol has an onset of action between 5 and 15 minutes, peak effect in 1 to 1½ hours after two inhalations, and a duration of action of 3 to 6 hours. Orally, its onset of action is between 15 and 30 minutes, peak effect is in 2 to 3 hours, and it has a duration of action of 8 hours or more (12 hours for the sustained-release dosage form). The drug is metabolized in the liver and excreted by the kidneys and in feces.

The side/adverse effects of albuterol include nausea, increased anxiety, palpitations, tremors, tachycardia, sedation, hypokalemia, difficulty in urination, dizziness, headaches, heartburn, muscle cramping, insomnia, increased sweating, vomiting, increased weakness, hypotension or hypertension, and an unusual taste in the mouth.

The adult bronchodilator dosage for inhalation is 200 to 400 μg every 4 to 6 hours. Oral dosage is 2 to 6 mg orally, three or four times daily. This dose may be increased to a maximum of 8 mg four times daily if necessary. Extended-release tablets are administered 4 or 8 mg orally every 12 hours. See package insert for pediatric dosage schedule.

BOX 38-2

Client Education: Using an Inhaler

It is important that the client be instructed in the correct use of a metered dose nebulizer before it is needed to relieve an asthma attack. The prescriber will indicate whether the Closed-Mouth or the Open-Mouth Technique is to be used. If it is optional, encourage the client to use the Open-Mouth Technique for better inhalation of the drug. If used incorrectly, the dose may be dispersed into the air or even swallowed. Since only 10% of an inhaled dose reaches the lungs under the best of conditions, the ability to use the metered dose nebulizer appropriately is essential for the client.

A placebo nebulizer should be used for demonstration. This will enable the client to repeat the demonstration a number of times until the nebulizer can be easily and correctly used.

The closed-mouth technique

1. Shake the container for 2 to 5 seconds.
2. Hold the nebulizer with the drug container upside down.
3. Place the mouthpiece in the mouth, closing lips tightly around it.
4. Exhale steadily and completely through nose.
5. Inhale slowly and deeply, and at the same time press the container down on the mouthpiece.
6. Hold breath for as long as possible before exhaling and remove mouthpiece from your mouth.
7. Wait 15 seconds.
8. Repeat steps 1 through 6 above.
9. If no relief is achieved after 5 minutes and condition worsens, contact prescriber.

The open-mouth-technique

1. Shake the container for 2 to 5 seconds.
2. Hold the nebulizer with the drug container upside down.
3. Hold the mouthpiece two fingerwidths (about 1½ inches) in front of widely opened mouth. Hold container upright.
4. Exhale deeply, then inhale slowly through mouth and at the same time press down firmly on the container. Continue to breathe deeply.
5. Hold breath for a few seconds, then exhale slowly. Wait approximately 15 seconds, and then repeat steps 3 to 5 for second inhalation. (Keep eyes closed—temporary blurring of vision may occur if the aerosol is sprayed into the eyes.)

Many practitioners are now advising the use of a spacer, a small tube which fits into the inhaler mouthpiece and goes into the client's mouth, to enhance the delivery of nebulized agent to the bronchioles.

■ ■ ■

Advise client that rinsing the mouth after using the nebulizer prevents systemic absorption and minimizes dryness of the mouth. The mouthpiece should be rinsed at least once daily to avoid clogging. Stress the importance of keeping the equipment clean to prevent infection. If using a refillable nebulizer, do not place more than a day's supply of drug in nebulizer. Change solution daily.

Clients with asthma benefit greatly from the use of sympathomimetic inhalers; however, they should be discouraged from using over-the-counter inhalers because of the non-selective beta-agonist drug effect of the epinephrine base. The nurse needs to recognize the possibility of misuse and the consequences of abuse in order to successfully help the client with inhalant drug therapy.

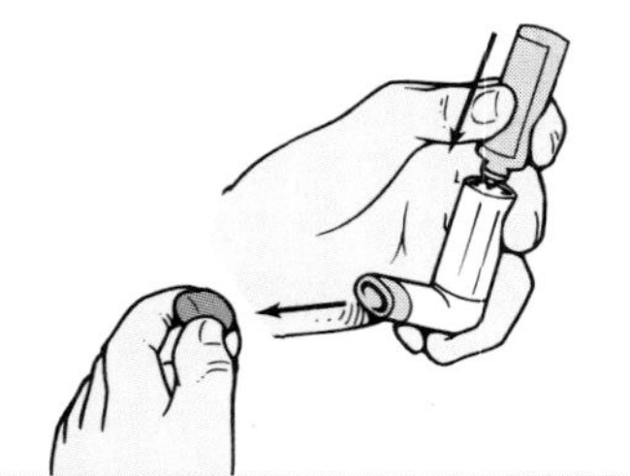

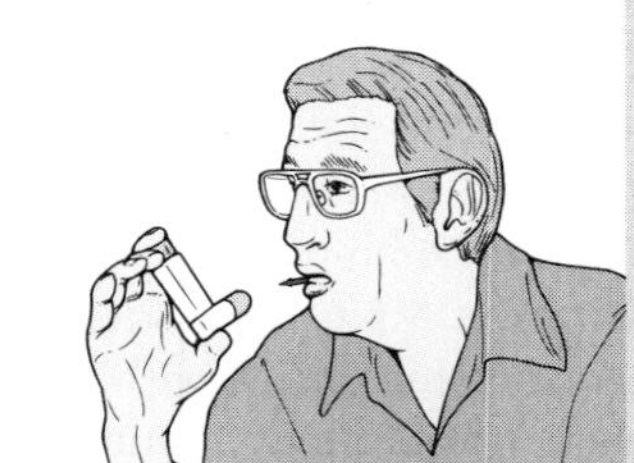

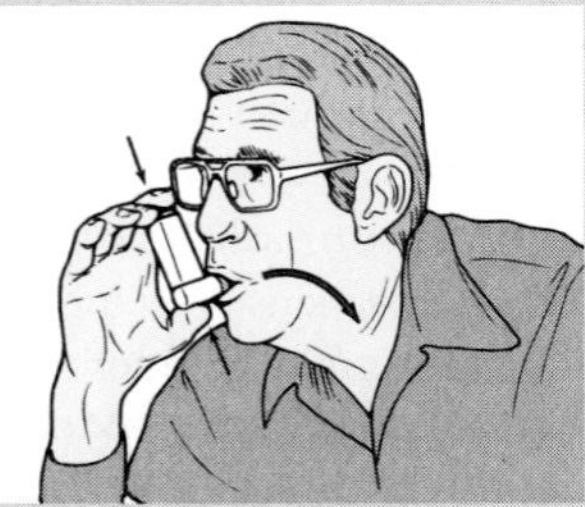

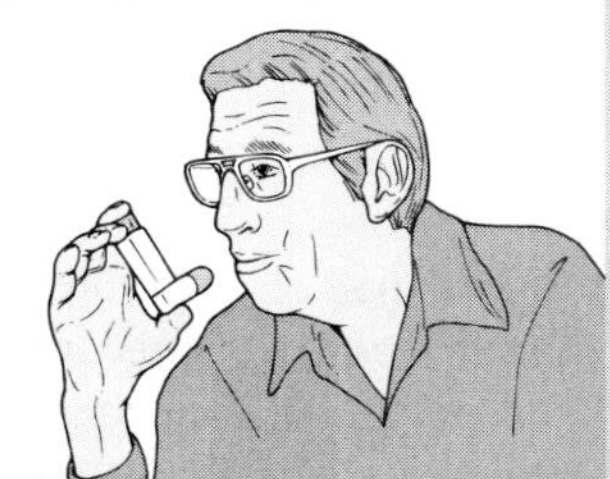

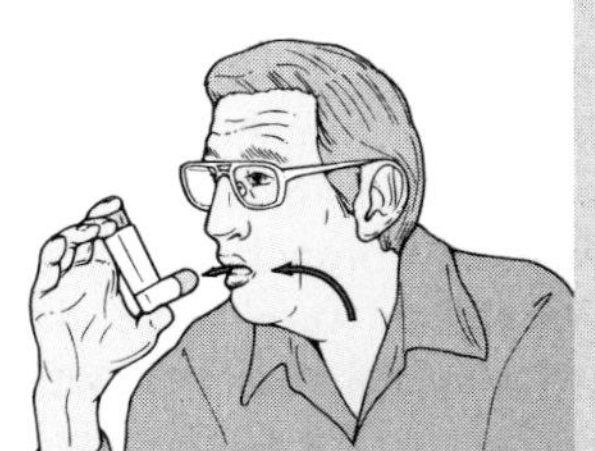

BOX 38-2

Client Education: Using an Inhaler—cont'd

Cleaning

1. Once a day clean the inhaler and cap by rinsing it in warm running water. Let it dry before you use it again. Have another inhaler to use while it is drying.
2. Twice a week wash the plastic mouthpiece with mild dishwashing soap and warm water. Rinse and dry well before putting it back.

Checking how much medicine is left in the canister

1. If the canister is new, it is full.
2. An easy way to check the amount of medicine left in your metered dose inhaler is to place the canister in a container of water and observe the position it takes in the water. *Note:* This method does not work for all inhalers. Please ask your doctor if you can check *your* inhaler this way.

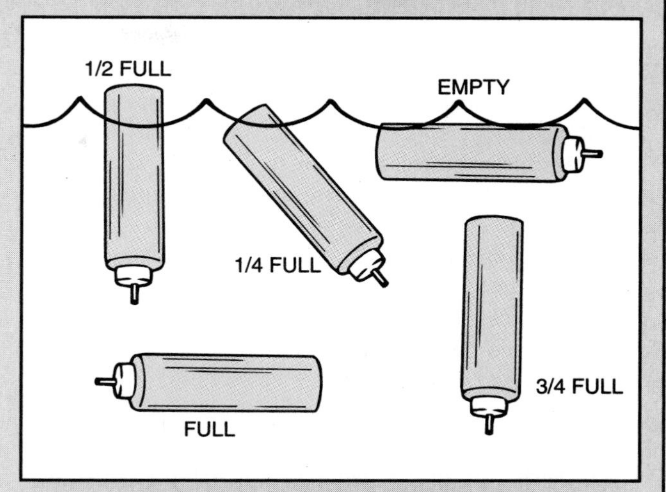

Pregnancy Safety

Category	Drug
B	cromolyn, ipratropium, terbutaline
C	albuterol, beclomethasone, flunisolide, isoetharine, isoproterenol, metaproterenol, theophylline
D	triamcinolone

■ Nursing Management

Albuterol Therapy

Assessment. Initially clients should be assessed for a previous intolerance to other sympathomimetic agents, since this may indicate an intolerance to albuterol. Albuterol should be used with caution in clients having cardiac arrhythmias, coronary insufficiency, hypertension, or pheochromocytoma. Clients with diabetes mellitus may need an increased dosage of insulin when receiving albuterol because of drug-induced hyperglycemia. Clients with hyperthyroidism may have an exaggerated response to albuterol. Elderly clients are more susceptible to the drug's effects and usually require lower dosages.

Determine interactions with the client's medication regimen. Significant drug interactions are similar to those of isoproterenol, with the exception of the interactions noted with alpha-adrenergic blocking agents, ergoloid mesylate, and ergotamine. Albuterol also has a significant drug interaction with MAO inhibitors; the effects of albuterol on the vascular system may be enhanced.

A baseline assessment is as previously discussed in the nursing management of the client receiving/taking bronchodilator drugs.

Nursing diagnosis. With the administration of albuterol, the client should be assessed for the following nursing diagnoses: altered comfort (dryness of the mouth and throat, unusual taste, coughing, flushing of the face and increased sweating, nausea and vomiting, heartburn, headache, weakness, muscle cramps, nervousness, trembling, palpitations, and chest pain); anxiety; altered sleep patterns (drowsiness or insomnia); and the collaborative problems of paradoxical bronchospasm (increase in dyspnea and wheezing) and altered cardiac output related to hypertension and tachycardia.

Implementation

Monitoring. Monitor as discussed for other bronchodilating drugs.

Intervention. A mouthpiece or a face mask may be used to administer the inhalation solution through a nebulizer. The nebulizer may be used with compressed air or oxygen, 6 to 10 L/min. A typical treatment lasts about 10 minutes.

Education. The client should be taught the correct use of the inhaler. Inform client that after long-term use, the drug may have a shorter duration of action (1 to 2 hours). The client should report to the prescriber a failure to respond to usual dose, which may mean the development of drug tolerance or worsening of the disease state. The development of tolerance may stimulate adverse reactions such as cardiac arrest if the dose continues to be increased. Advise the client to rinse mouth after inhalation therapy to prevent dryness, throat irritation, and systemic absorption. Any foul taste that occurs as a result of treatment will gradually disappear with repeated usage.

Warn client that excessive use of aerosol may be harmful, causing paradoxical (rebound) bronchospasm, which means that the effects of the drug are no longer therapeutic. Stress the importance of not changing dosage or frequency of albuterol without consulting prescriber. Chest pain, extreme dizziness and lightheadedness, severe headache, palpitations, continuing tachycardia, dysrhythmias, and hypertensive episodes should be reported to the prescriber.

Evaluation. Signs of the client's anxiety should decrease as breathing becomes more effective. Wheezing, if present, should also decrease. Signs of respiratory distress such as increased effort to breathe, increased use of accessory muscles, contraction of the abdominal muscles on expiration, and diaphoresis will decrease as the medication becomes effective. The client will respond subjectively if relief from the respiratory distress is felt.

metaproterenol [met a pro ter' e nole] (Alupent, Metaprel)

The metaproterenol mechanism of action is the same as for albuterol, while its indications are the same as epinephrine. Metaproterenol inhalation has an onset of action within 1 minute, a peak effect in 1 hour, and a duration of action of 1 to 5 hours after a single dose. Orally its onset of action is within 15 to 30 minutes, its peak effect occurs in an hour, and duration of action is up to 4 hours. It is metabolized in the liver and excreted in the kidneys.

The side/adverse effects of metaproterenol include anxiety, restlessness, dizziness, headaches, hypertension, muscle cramps, nausea, vomiting, palpitations, tremors, sweating, tachycardia, and weakness. Respiratory difficulties are a rare adverse reaction seen with this drug. Significant drug interactions are similar to those for albuterol.

Adult bronchodilator inhalation dose is 1.3 to 2.25 mg (2 or 3 inhalations) every 3 to 4 hours, not to exceed 9 mg (12 inhalations) in 24 hours. The oral dose is 20 mg three or four times daily. Dosage is not established for children under 6 years. For children 6 to 9 years old who weigh up to 27 kg, the oral dosage is 10 mg three or four times daily. For children over 9 years old weighing at least 27 kg, apply the adult dosage scale. For nursing management, see the discussion for albuterol.

terbutaline aerosol [ter byoo' ta leen] (Brethaire)
terbutaline tablets and injection (Brethine, Bricanyl)

The mechanism of action of terbutaline is similar to albuterol and indications are the same as epinephrine. Terbutaline's onset of action by inhalation is within 5 to 30 minutes, peak effect within 1 to 2 hours, and duration of action within 3 to 6 hours. Orally its onset of action is within 1 to 2 hours, peak effect in 2 to 3 hours, and duration of action in 4 to 8 hours. Parenterally, its onset of action is within 15 minutes, peak effect in 0.5 to 1 hour, and duration of action in 1.5 to 4 hours. Terbutaline is metabolized in the liver and excreted in the kidneys.

The side/adverse effects of terbutaline include tremors, increased anxiety, restlessness, dizziness, sedation, headaches, hypertension, muscle cramps, nausea, vomiting, palpitations, insomnia, sweating, tachycardia, weakness, dry mouth or throat, and an unusual taste in the mouth. Rare adverse reactions include chest pain and an increase in respiratory difficulties.

Adult bronchodilator dose is 1 to 2 inhalations (200 to 500 μg), the second inhalation at least 1 minute after the first, then dosed every 4 to 6 hours. Orally a 2.5 to 5 mg tablet three times daily every 6 hours is recommended. For children 12 to 15 years, give 2.5 mg orally 3 times a day. Parenterally, a 250 μg subcutaneous dose is administered, which may be repeated in 15 to 30 minutes. A total dose of 500 μg is the maximum in a 4 hour period.

BOX 38-3

Leukotriene Receptor Antagonist

Zafirlukast (Accolate) is a selective, competitive leukotriene receptor antagonist (D_4 and E_4), which are components of slow-reacting substance of anaphylaxis. It is used for the prophylaxis and chronic treatment of asthma. It is not indicated for acute asthma attacks although its use can be continued during an acute asthma exacerbation.

Pharmacokinetics

Zafirlukast is administered orally, peak serum levels are reached in 3 hours, and half-life is approximately 10 hours. It is metabolized in the liver and excreted in urine. Side/adverse effects include headache, nausea, diarrhea, and infection. Infections primarily affect the respiratory tract, are dose-related, and have also been associated with concurrent use of corticosteroid inhalers.

Dose for adults and children 12 years and older is 20 mg twice a day, before meals or 2 hours after a meal (Olin, 1997).

For nursing management information, see the discussion under albuterol, p. 661.

zileuton (Zyflo) [zye loo' ton]

Zileuton is the first lipoxygenase inhibitor approved in the United States. By blocking lipoxygenase, it interferes with the formation of substances that cause mucus plugs and constriction of bronchial airways. Liver enzyme testing is recommended before therapy, monthly for the first 3 months and then every 2 to 3 months for the first year of zileuton therapy. The recommended dose is 600 mg four times daily (McCann, 1997).

See Box 38-3 for the first drug in a new drug classification, leukotriene receptor antagonist.

XANTHINE DERIVATIVES

The xanthine group of drugs includes caffeine, theophylline, and theobromine. Beverages from the extracts of plants containing these alkaloids have been used by humans since ancient times. **Xanthine derivatives** relax smooth muscle (particularly bronchial muscle), stimulate cardiac muscle and the central nervous system, and also produce diuresis, probably through a combined action of increased renal perfusion and increased sodium and chloride ion excretion.

The drugs in this category are methylated forms of xanthines or methylxanthines. The effectiveness of these preparations as bronchodilators depends on their conversion to theophylline, which is the active constituent. Therefore, with the exception of dyphylline, the action of xanthine depends on the content of theophylline. Xanthines inhibit mast cell degranulation and the release of histamine and other mediators that are responsible for bronchoconstriction. Because the methyxanthines impede enzymatic action, they are also called phosphodiesterase inhibitors (see Figures 38-3 and 38-4).

Theophylline products, especially slow-release products, can vary in their rate of absorption and therapeutic effects even if they have the same strength and active ingredient (*USP DI*, 1996). Some states, such as Florida, do not permit generic substitution for theophylline slow-release products.

While theophylline toxicity may occur in some persons at 15 μg/ml, the upper therapeutic level is 20 μg/ml. Dosage adjustment with theophylline is also necessary under certain conditions especially when concurrent factors affecting therapeutic effects are present. See Box 38-4 for factors affecting theophylline's therapeutic effects.

BOX 38-4

Factors Affecting Theophylline's Therapeutic Effects

May be increased by:
Age: elderly and newborn
Drugs: erythromycin, cimetidine, ciprofloxacin
Disease states: cirrhosis, pulmonary edema, congestive heart failure, and severe COPD
Diet: high carbohydrate

May be decreased by:
Substances: tobacco, marijuana
Drugs: phenobarbital, phenytoin
Diet: high protein
Age: adolescence

aminophylline [am in off' i lin] (Aminophylline, Palaron ♣)
oxtriphylline [ox trye' fi lin] (Choledyl, Apo-Oxtriphylline ♣)
▲ **theophylline** [thee off' i lin] (Bronkodyl, Elixophyllin, and others)

Theophylline is the prototype of the xanthine derivatives. It competitively inhibits the action of phosphodiesterase, the enzyme that degrades cyclic 3'5' AMP, which results in bronchodilation, as discussed previously (see Figure 38-4). These drugs are used for the prevention and treatment of bronchial asthma, and treatment of bronchitis, pulmonary emphysema, and chronic obstructive pulmonary diseases.

Oral liquids and uncoated tablets of aminophylline, oxtriphylline, and theophylline are rapidly absorbed, whereas enteric-coated tablets have a delayed and at times an unreliable absorption pattern. Extended-release dosage forms are slowly absorbed and sometimes unreliable. The retention enema is rapidly absorbed, whereas rectal suppositories are slow and unreliable. Dyphylline has good oral absorption. Theophylline peak level is reached in 1 to 2 hours with the oral solution, immediate release capsules, or tablets; in approximately 4 hours with delayed release tablets; and 4 to 13 hours for extended release products. Theophylline half-life varies by age and concurrent illness. For example, with premature newborns, the half-life is approximately 30 hours during the first 15 days of life; for children 1 to 4 years of age, it is 3.4 hours; for the adult nonsmoker with uncomplicated asthma, it is 8.2 hours; and for the elderly, the half-life is nearly 10 hours. In clients with acute hepatitis half-life is 19 hours; cirrhosis 32 hours; hyperthyroidism 4.5 hours (*USP DI*, 1996). The theophylline half-life in an adult smoker is only 3 to 4 hours (Self & Kelly, 1995).

Aminophylline, oxtriphylline, and theophylline salts all release free theophylline in vivo. Theophylline is metabolized by the liver to caffeine. Caffeine concentrations may average about 30% of the theophylline concentration in adults, but in neonates it may be much more. Caffeine does not accumulate in adults.

The therapeutic serum levels for bronchodilator effects with theophylline are usually stated to be between 10 and 20 μg/ml. Some studies, however, have indicated that therapeutic response may be seen at the 5 to 15 μg serum level while some clients have minimal gain, and some experience toxicity in the 15 to 20 μg/ml range (Kelly & Hill, 1993).

Therefore close supervision with dosage adjustments according to client's therapeutic response or the presence of toxic effects is necessary. As a respiratory stimulant, theophylline serum level is between 5 and 10 μg/ml. Theophylline is metabolized in the liver and excreted by the kidneys.

Side/adverse effects include nausea, increased anxiety, restlessness, gastric upset, and vomiting.

Dosage and administration. The dosage of theophylline preparations must be tailored to the medical circumstances in each case. The usual efficacy of a theophylline preparation depends on the attainment of a serum concentration of 10 to 20 μg/ml (see previous comments on serum levels). The rapid intravenous administration of theophylline and its derivatives has caused severe and even fatal acute circulatory failure; therefore the drug should be administered slowly, over 20 to 30 minutes. (Table 38-1 lists the xanthine parenteral preparations and dosages.) Since theophylline has a low therapeutic index, using caution when determining the dosage is essential. See the box on p. 664 for management of xanthine overdose. The various xanthine preparations contain the following:

Drug	Percent of anhydrous theophylline present
aminophylline anhydrous	86
aminophylline dihydrate	79
oxtriphylline	64
theophylline monohydrate	91

■ Nursing Management

Xanthine Derivative Therapy

Assessment. Use with caution in individuals with active gastritis, or active or a history of peptic ulcers, since theophylline products may cause local gastric irritation or act centrally to stimulate gastric acid secretion. This condition can be aggravated when the serum theophylline level

TABLE 38-1 Xanthine: dosage and administration

Drug	Dosage
aminophylline injection	Adult dose in an acute attack for persons not receiving theophylline: IV infusion of the equivalent of 5 mg of anhydrous theophylline/kg administered over 20 to 30 min. If person was receiving theophylline, then obtain a serum level and dose according to theophylline instructions below. For specific instructions on maintenance, children's doses, etc., see a current package insert
theophylline in dextrose injection	For children and adults, the dose in acute attack for persons not receiving theophylline: 5 mg/kg administered over 20 to 30 min. If client is receiving a theophylline product, obtain a theophylline serum level and dose appropriately. Each 0.5 mg of theophylline/kg of lean body weight provides a 1 μg/ml increase in serum theophylline

! MANAGEMENT OF DRUG OVERDOSE

Theophylline (Xanthine)

- Treatment is supportive and symptomatic because there is no known specific antidote.
- To decrease drug absorption, administer an activated charcoal preparation orally or via a nasogastric tube. Charcoal should be premixed with sorbitol or a single dose of sorbitol should follow the charcoal dose. Sorbitol is considered to be more effective than magnesium-containing laxatives.
- Gastric lavage if instituted early (within an hour of ingestion) or whole bowel irrigation with a polyethylene glycol and electrolyte solution are useful for very large overdoses of theophylline.
- If the client has seizures, establish an airway and administer oxygen. Diazepam or phenobarbital IV may be administered to control the seizures.
- Charcoal hemoperfusion may be necessary when theophylline serum concentration is very high (greater than 40 μg/ml in chronic overdose or if other risk factors are present, such as an elderly client, concurrent illnesses, etc.). Hemodialysis and peritoneal dialysis are less or ineffective, respectively, for theophylline toxicity (*USP DI*, 1996).
- Monitor vital signs and provide supportive care as required.

exceeds 20 μg/ml. Use cautiously with clients who have severe cardiac disease, acute myocardial injury, cardiac dysrhythmias, congestive heart failure (CHF), or cor pulmonale, since circulatory impairment may cause very slow serum xanthine clearance and xanthines are potentially cardiotoxic. Also, individuals with severe hypoxemia, hypertension, hyperthyroidism, prostatic hypertrophy, and renal and hepatic disease require cautious use of aminophylline, oxtriphylline, and theophylline. Aminophylline and sodium chloride solutions potentially may lead to sodium retention. Xanthines are contraindicated in individuals with hypersensitivity to any of its components. In addition, use xanthine derivatives cautiously with young children and the elderly.

Theophylline crosses the placenta; since teratogenic effects have been demonstrated in mice, the risk-benefit to the fetus and mother must be considered. Also, dangerous levels of caffeine concentration in the neonate may occur, since the newborn is unable to metabolize this compound. The xanthines are excreted in breast milk and can produce toxicity in the neonate. Symptoms include tachycardia, jitteriness, irritability, gagging, and vomiting.

Smoking one to two packs of cigarettes a day decreases the serum half-life of theophylline. Consequently, smokers require larger doses of xanthines than nonsmokers. This effect may persist for months to years, even after the person has stopped smoking (see the case study on p. 665).

Review the client's current drug regimen for significant drug interactions. Such drug interactions occur when xanthine products are given with the following:

Drug	Possible effect and management
phenytoin (Dilantin)	Increased metabolism of xanthines occurs. Decreased absorption of phenytoin, leading to low serum levels, may be seen with concurrent administration. Serum levels of both drugs should be closely monitored, since dosage adjustments may be necessary.
beta-adrenergic blocking agents, systemic or ophthalmic	Therapeutic effects of both drugs may be inhibited. Concurrent use may also decrease theophylline excretion. Monitor closely because dosage adjustments may be necessary.
cimetidine (Tagamet), erythromycin (Erythrocin), ranitidine (Zantac), or troleandomycin (Tao)	May decrease theophylline metabolism, resulting in elevated serum levels of theophylline and possible toxicity. Monitor closely because dosage adjustments may be necessary.
ciprofloxacin (Cipro), norfloxacin (Noroxin)	Concurrent drug administration may reduce theophylline excretion, resulting in an increase in theophylline half-life, serum level, and potential toxicity. Monitor serum levels closely because a dosage adjustment may be indicated.

Case Study

The Client with Asthma

Christine Newman is a 32-year-old woman with a long history of bronchial asthma. She is currently being maintained on theophylline (Theo-Dur) 200 mg twice a day. When respiratory wheezing increases, she uses an albuterol (Proventil) inhaler, two puffs every 4 hours until her breathing improves. In spite of her history of asthma, Christine continues to smoke at least half a pack of cigarettes a day. She is making an effort to quit smoking but finds it is hard to stop.

1. What is the pharmacologic effect of the Theo-Dur in the management of the client with asthma?
2. Explain the effect the Proventil inhaler has on the client's wheezing.
3. Why is it especially important to support Christine's effort to stop smoking, in light of her drug therapy and her asthmatic condition?

One evening Christine is brought to the emergency room by her family. She is having an acute asthma attack. She has difficulty talking because of respiratory distress. Her breathing is extremely labored, with accessory muscle use. She has audible wheezing. Her family tells the nurse that Christine's breathing became more difficult the day before. She began using the Proventil inhaler but found that it did not provide any relief.

After a brief examination she is given metaproterenol (Alupent) by nebulization. She has some decrease in respiratory distress, but the wheezing continues. A continuous intravenous infusion of aminophylline is started. She is admitted to the hospital. The Alupent nebulizer treatments continue at 4 hour intervals.

4. What will you include in your assessment (subjective, objective, and laboratory data) of Christine while she is receiving aminophylline intravenously?
5. Compare the actions of Alupent and Proventil in the treatment of asthma.

Christine is to be discharged with the following medications: Theo-Dur, 200 mg twice a day; Proventil inhaler, two puffs every 6 hours; and beclomethasone (Vanceril) inhaler, two puffs every 6 hours.

6. Christine asks why she needs a second inhaler. How will you respond to her need for this information about the use of the Vanceril inhaler?
7. What does Christine need to be taught about the combined use of the Vanceril and Proventil inhalers?

Drug	Possible effect and management
smokers of tobacco or marijuana	May result in increased metabolism of xanthines (except dyphylline), which may result in low serum theophylline levels. Dosage adjustments of 50% to 100% greater dosage has been required in smokers.
nicotine chewing gum, or other smoking deterrents	Smoking cessation may increase the therapeutic effects of the xanthines (except dyphylline) by decreasing metabolism; however, nonsmoking normalization of xanthines levels may not occur for 3 months to 2 years after smoking cessation.

A baseline assessment of the client's respiratory status should be accomplished as discussed in the nursing management of the client receiving bronchodilator therapy.

Nursing diagnosis. With the administration of the xanthine derivatives, the client should be assessed for the following nursing diagnoses: risk for aspiration related to the drug's ability to induce gastroesophageal reflux in those clients who may have impaired gag reflex, infants under 2 years of age, and elderly, debilitated, or stuporous clients; altered comfort (flushing of the face, headache, nausea, nervousness, and palpitations); altered mucous membranes (rectal irritation with rectal dosage forms of the drug); and the collaborative problems of allergic reaction and drug toxicity.

Implementation

Monitoring. Anticipate adverse effects if the serum theophylline level exceeds the normal serum therapeutic range of 10 to 20 μg/ml. Because of the variation in the metabolism of xanthines, monitoring of serum theophylline concentration and client response is necessary to prevent toxicity.

Be sure that intravenous administration is given slowly with an infusion pump. Monitor vital signs and observe the client for signs of toxicity such as hypotension, tachycardia, ventricular dysrhythmias, or convulsions. Earlier, less severe signs of toxicity may not occur. Have oxygen, respirator, and IV diazepam (for convulsions) available during initiation of therapy. Maintain airway, hydration, and normal temperature by tepid water sponges or hypothermic blanket for hyperpyrexia (Potter & Perry, 1993). An unconscious client may require gastric lavage if the drug was ingested. Serum levels obtained immediately before the next dose (trough concentrations) tend to be more consistent than peak serum levels.

Pulmonary studies are done to assess the client's progress while taking the drug. Intake and output should also be monitored.

Observe children closely because they are more susceptible than adults to CNS effects (nervousness, restlessness, insomnia, hyperactive reflexes, twitching, and convulsions).

Monitor the client during a change from one route of administration to another until dosage is regulated. Wait 4 to 6 hours after changing from intravenous to oral therapy and 12 hours when changing from rectal administration, since its absorption tends to be less consistent.

If a client with status asthmaticus does not respond quickly to bronchodilating agents, additional medication such as corticosteroids will be required. Note positive responses to the medication, such as increased ease of respiration, decreased wheezing, and a decrease in the client's anxiety regarding the dyspnea.

Intervention. Be aware of the following intravenous admixture incompatibilities:

- Do not mix theophylline in a syringe with other drugs; add it separately to the intravenous solution.
- When administering "piggyback," turn off the other intravenous solution already in place while giving theophylline or start another IV line.
- Do not mix with alkali-labile drugs such as epinephrine, norepinephrine, dopamine, dobutamine, isoproterenol, or penicillin G.

Administer oral dosage on an empty stomach to promote faster absorption; however, to lessen local gastrointestinal irritation, the drug may be given with food. Whether it is given with food or not, it is important that the drug be administered consistently with or without food and at approximately the same time each day. For chewable tablet form, the client should chew tablets before swallowing; for enteric-coated tablet or extended release form, the client should swallow the tablet whole without crushing, breaking, or chewing. Also, the contents of the capsule form may be mixed with 1 teaspoon of jelly, jam, or applesauce if too large to swallow. The elixir dosage forms have a high alcohol content (20%), so the alcohol-free liquid forms are generally preferred. These liquid forms, however, contain sorbitol, which may cause diarrhea and hyperglycemia.

To enhance absorption, schedule administration of rectal preparations of theophylline when rectum is free of feces. Have the client remain in recumbent position for 15 to 20 minutes after rectal administration of the drug. Administer before meals to enhance retention. Rectal suppositories are irritating to tissues, and absorption is unreliable. Although rectal retention enema provides rapid and more reliable absorption, it should be used only if the client is unable to take oral preparations. Rectal preparations are also contraindicated if irritation or infection of the rectum or lower colon is present. If enemas are used, they should not be administered for more than 24 to 36 hours because of the irritating effect of the alkaline solution on the bowel wall.

Store medication in a tightly closed container at room temperature. Also follow manufacturer's directions regarding storage of suppositories, since some are stored at room temperature and others refrigerated.

Education. Caution the client not to take over-the-counter remedies that contain ephedrine or other sympathomimetics for treatment of asthma or cough. Instruct the client to limit intake of xanthine-containing beverages, such as coffee, tea, chocolate, cocoa, and cola beverages because these may increase the CNS stimulant effects of the xanthine derivatives. Also inform the client to limit charcoal-broiled foods because charcoal increases theophylline metabolism, resulting in decreased serum concentrations of the drug.

Warn elderly clients of possible dizziness during therapy and have them take necessary precautions for safety.

If the client is taking the extended-release form of the drug, advise against changing brands unless prescribed to do so, since the various brands may not be bioequivalent.

The client should notify the prescriber of any fever, flu-like symptoms, or diarrhea as the prescribed dosage may need to be changed. Advise the client to keep medical and laboratory appointments to check the progress of therapy.

The client should maintain some consistency in dietary patterns because a high protein, low carbohydrate diet increases the metabolism of theophylline and so decreases serum concentrations, whereas a low protein, high carbohydrate diet inhibits the metabolism of the drug and increases serum concentrations.

Evaluation. The client will have an adequate respiratory status as evidenced by: the absence of adventitious breath sounds, ABGs within normal limits (PaO_2 > 60 mm Hg, $PaCO_2$ 35 to 45 mm Hg), pH 7.35 to 7.45, and a respiratory rate of 12 to 20 breaths/min or return to baseline rate.

PROPHYLACTIC ASTHMATIC DRUGS

▲ **cromolyn** [kroe' moe lin] (Intal, Novo-Cromolyn 🍁)
nedocromil [ned o kroe' mill] (Tilade)

Cromolyn and nedocromil are antiinflammatory agents that inhibit the release of histamine, leukotrienes, and other mediators of inflammation from mast cells, macrophages, and other cells associated with asthma. Neither drug has any bronchodilator effect nor do they have any effect on any inflammatory mediators already released in the body. Nedocromil appears to be more effective than cromolyn (Serafin, 1996) and in some persons is therapeutically effective in twice daily dosing (*USP DI*, 1996).

Both drugs are indicated for prevention of bronchospasms and bronchial asthmatic attacks. Administered by oral inhalation, cromolyn has approximately 8% to 10% absorption in the lungs, an onset of action within 4 weeks, and is excreted in the kidneys and bile. Nedocromil has systemic absorption of 7% to 9%, a half-life of 1.5 to 3.3 hours, onset of action as maintenance therapy is between 2 to 4 weeks. It is excreted by the kidneys. It can also prevent bronchospasm if given up to ½ hour before exposure to allergens or exercise.

Side/adverse effects include cough, hoarseness, dry mouth or throat, nasal congestion, sneezing, and bad taste in mouth from inhalation device.

The adult oral inhalation dose to prevent bronchial asthma for cromolyn is 2 inhalations (1.6 or 2 mg) four times daily at 4 or 6 hour intervals. To prevent exercise-induced or allergen-induced bronchospasms, the dose is 2 oral inhalations approximately 10 to 15 minutes before exercise or exposure. A dose is not established for children under 5 years old. For 5 years and older, see adult dosage.

The usual adult and adolescent dose for nedocromil is initially 2 oral inhalations four times daily. Reduction of doses to three and then twice daily may be attempted in persons whose symptoms are under good control.

■ Nursing Management

Prophylactic Asthmatic Drug Therapy

Assessment. During the initial assessment, determine that the client does not have a sensitivity to cromolyn or nedocromil.

Nursing diagnosis. With the administration of cromolyn and nedocromil, the client has the potential for the following nursing diagnoses: ineffective airway clearance related to increased bronchospasm; altered comfort (unpleasant taste, dryness of mouth and throat, sneezing and watering of eyes, dizziness, nausea, headache, rash); and the collaborative problems of eosinophilic pneumonia and allergic response (angioedema, arthalgia, bronchospasm, anaphylactic reaction, laryngeal edema).

Implementation

Monitoring. The client should be monitored for the frequency and intensity of asthma attacks or other symptoms of allergy.

Intervention. Cromolyn and nedocromil help prevent but do not relieve asthma or bronchospasm attacks. If used during an acute attack, they may actually worsen the client's symptoms. If the client is also using a bronchodilator inhaler, it should be used 15 minutes before the cromolyn or nedocromil inhalation.

Education. The client should be taught to rinse the mouth and gargle after an inhalation treatment to relieve the dryness of the mouth and throat and the unpleasant aftertaste.

A client using the aerosol, capsule, or solution dosage form for inhalation should be aware that instructions come with each preparation. The nurse should make sure the client can administer the drug correctly. Demonstration kits are available for the inhalation capsule dosage form of cromolyn. Caution clients using the aerosol form to avoid medication contact with the eyes. Inhalation capsules are to be used with a special inhaler; they are not effective if swallowed. The inhalation solution is to be used with a power-operated nebulizer, since the hand-held nebulizers do not provide sufficient force to administer the medication. Instruct the client not to float the canister to test fullness but to keep a record of sprays.

The client should be advised that it may be as long as 4 weeks before the drug is fully beneficial. Compliance with the regimen is necessary to achieve these results. It is also important to maintain any concurrent therapies, such as adrenocorticoids, until discontinued by the prescriber. If the client's condition does not improve or worsens, the prescriber should be notified.

Evaluation. A satisfactory response to prophylactic therapy is indicated by a reduction in the number of attacks, reduced cough, decreased sputum production, and/or a decreased need for other antiasthma drugs. Some clients show improvement in pulmonary function. These responses occur in 4 weeks of treatment. Only those clients showing improvement should continue to receive cromolyn and nedocromil.

Corticosteroid Drugs

Corticosteroid drugs are used in chronic asthma to decrease airway obstruction. As antiinflammatory agents, they stabilize the membranes of lysosomes, thus preventing the release of hydrolytic enzymes that produce the inflammatory process in the tissues. The exact mechanism in asthma is still poorly understood, but it does involve suppression of antibody formation that is responsible for provoking the asthmatic attack. In addition, corticosteroids inhibit the leukotriene synthesis, thus reducing bronchoconstriction and secretion of mucus (Wingard et al, 1991).

Daily administration of systemic corticosteroid therapy provides great therapeutic benefits, but the high incidence of side effects has led to the use of the alternate-day schedule of treatment. This regimen provides the best benefit/risk ratio for prolonged therapy because it minimizes the likelihood of unwanted side effects. The corticosteroids generally used have an intermediate-acting duration of action. These corticosteroids include prednisone, prednisolone, and methylprednisolone; see Chapter 49 for details of these drugs.

Chronic use of the steroid aerosols has resulted in a decrease in bronchial hyperreactivity and symptom prevention. Inhaled corticosteroids have been reported to be more effective than alternate-day therapy with oral steroids (Abramowicz, 1991). Topical corticosteroid therapy offers the possibility of limiting action at the site of application and thereby avoiding systemic effects. By chemically modifying the structural arrangement of the steroid molecule, compounds were developed to diminish systemic absorption from the respiratory tract. The products available are beclomethasone (Vanceril, Beclovent), budesonide (Pulmicort), flunisolide (AeroBid), and triamcinolone (Azmacort).

They offer the advantage of producing few systemic adverse effects, including that of limited or no adrenal suppression. This category also includes dexamethasone (Decadron), but it is less often used today because of a higher incidence of side effects than the other agents. (Box 38-5 explains the step approach to therapeutic management of asthma for the current recommendations for corticosteroids.) The aerosols are rapidly absorbed from pulmonary tissues with limited gastrointestinal absorption. The maximum improvement in pulmonary function may take 1 to 4 weeks.

The side/adverse effects of corticosteroid drugs include abdominal distress, anorexia, cough without infection, dizziness, headache, unpleasant taste in mouth, and oral fungal infection or candidiasis.

Beclomethasone (Vanceril, Beclovent) adult dosage is 2 oral inhalations three or four times daily. For severe asthma, use 12 to 16 sprays initially a day, then decrease dosage according to client response. For children under 6 years of age,

BOX 38-5

Step Approach for Therapeutic Management of Asthma

Step 4, severe	For long-term prophylaxis control, a high dose corticosterioid inhaler *plus* a long-acting beta$_2$ agonist tablet, or inhaler or a long-acting theophylline *plus* corticosteriod oral (2mg/kg/day, not exceeding 60 mg/day) daily should be utilized. A short-acting beta$_2$ agonist inhaler is available for symptom control.
Step 3, moderate	Intermediate dose corticosteroid inhaler *plus* a long-acting beta$_2$ agonist inhaler, tablets or long-acting theophylline daily. A short-acting beta$_2$ agonist inhaler is available for symptom control.
Step 2, mild (persistent)	Low dose corticosteroid inhaler or nedocromil daily. Children may start with cromolyn or nedocromil. Zafirlukast, zileuton or a long-acting theophylline product are alternatives for clients 12 years old or older. A short-acting beta$_2$ agonist inhaler is available for symptom control.
Step 1, mild (intermittent)	Short-acting beta$_2$ agonist inhaler is available for symptom control. If inhaler is used more than twice weekly, consider Step 2 therapy.

(Expert Panel Report II: Guidelines for the Diagnosis and Management of Asthma, National Asthma Education and Prevention Program, February, 1997)

dosage is not established; for 6 to 12 years old, administer 1 or 2 metered sprays three or four times daily.

The initial adult dosage of budesonide inhalation powder (Pulmicort) for severe asthma is 0.2 to 2.4 mg daily, divided in 2 to 4 doses. Maintenance dose is 0.2 to 0.4 mg twice daily, adjusting dosage based on individual's response. This product is not recommended for children under 6 years old; for children 6 to 12 years old with severe asthma, 0.1 to 0.2 mg twice daily.

For flunisolide (Aerobid), the dose is two oral inhalations twice daily, morning and night, for children 4 years and older and adults.

Triamcinolone (Azmacort) adult dosage is 2 inhalations three or four times daily. In very severe asthma, 12 to 16 inhalations per day may be used. For children 6 to 12 years old, 1 or 2 inhalations three or four times a day is recommended. Do not exceed 12 inhalations per day in children.

■ Nursing Management

Inhalation Corticosteroid Therapy

Assessment. These drugs are contraindicated when the client has bronchiectasis or when clients are intolerant of fluorocarbon propellants because these preparations also contain fluorocarbons. Inhalation corticosteroid therapy is not indicated in clients with status asthmaticus or nonasthmatic bronchial conditions. Its use is not appropriate for asthma controlled by other medications, such as bronchodilators or other noncorticosteroids. Do not use for acute attacks. It should also be determined if the client has diabetes mellitus because a significant drug interaction may occur when these agents are given with oral antidiabetic agents or insulin; serum glucose levels may increase, requiring dosage adjustments in either or both drugs. Whenever these corticosteroids are discontinued in a diabetic client, a dosage adjustment of the antidiabetic agent may be required. In addition, clients with cardiac disease, hypertension, osteoporosis, peptic ulcer, inflammatory processes of the GI tract, or myasthenia gravis may have their condition exacerbated with chronic use of inhalation doses of dexamethasone and triamcinolone or higher doses of the other inhalation aerosols. Tuberculosis may be reactivated with long-term corticosteroid inhalation therapy; asthmatic clients with a positive Mantoux test should be monitored carefully.

A baseline assessment of the client's respiratory status should be completed; see assessment within the general nursing management of the bronchodilator drugs. Drug interactions are unlikely to occur with the usual doses of inhalation corticosteroids.

Nursing diagnosis. With the administration of corticosteroids by inhalation the client is at risk for the following nursing diagnoses: altered comfort (unpleasant taste, dry/ irritated mouth and throat, and cough and hoarseness without signs of infection); and the collaborative problems of oral candidiasis (creamy, white patches within the mouth), monilial esophagitis (difficulty in swallowing), upper respiratory tract infection, bronchospasm, and allergic reaction.

Implementation

Monitoring. The client's respiratory status should be monitored on an ongoing basis to evaluate the drug's effectiveness. Monitor for side effects of corticosteroid therapy.

Intervention. If the client also uses a bronchodilator, it should be used 15 minutes before the corticosteroid inhalation. If the client's response to the corticosteroid begins to diminish, the prescriber should be notified so that the dosage can be adjusted. Box 38-6 gives a nursing review of inhalants used for the treatment of asthma.

Education. Stress the importance of self-management. Assess the client's ability to hold and manipulate a metered dose nebulizer. Provide instruction on inhaler use. The nurse should ensure that the client is able to use the inhaler. After inhaling, the client should hold the inhaled drug for a few seconds before exhaling and allow a minute to elapse between each inhalation to increase its effectiveness. In addition to verbal discussion, written instructions should also be provided.

BOX 38-6

Nursing Review: Inhalants for Asthma Treatment

With the wide variety of medications that may be used concurrently for the treatment of asthma, the nurse should be aware of the following.

- For prophylactic use, the antiinflammatory inhalation drugs cromolyn (Intal) or nedocromil (Tilade) are recommended. These drugs have no role in the treatment of acute asthmatic attacks.
- Corticosteroid inhalers such as beclomethasone (Beclovent, Vanceril), flunisolide (Aerobid), etc., are for preventive use only, and they may cause localized fungal infections in the mouth and pharynx. Advise client to rinse mouth with water or mouthwash after each use and also to thoroughly rinse and dry the inhaler tip after each use. This will help reduce the incidence of dry, sore throat and oropharyngeal candidiasis.
- $Beta_2$ agonist inhalers have no antiinflammatory effects but are considered the most effective drugs for treatment of acute bronchospasm and asthma. Subcutaneous injection of beta agonists has not been found to be more effective than inhalation, and it has been reported to cause more systemic adverse effects (Abramowicz, 1993). Examples include albuterol (Proventil, Ventolin), bitolterol (Tornalate), pirbuterol (Maxair), terbutaline (Brethaire), and salmeterol (Serevent), a drug that acts twice as long as albuterol (Dyer, 1993).

Clients with asthma often have multiple inhalers prescribed, such as ipratropium (Atrovent), an anticholinergic; beclomethasone (Vanceril), a corticosteroid; and albuterol (Ventolin), a $beta_2$ agonist.

What instructions would you offer the client with asthma?

If the prescriber has not given specific dosing instructions, generally the order of administration to obtain optimal drug effects is as follows:

1. The beta agonist is used first to open the airways.
2. The anticholinergic agent is administered.
3. The corticosteroid is administered.

Instruct client to wait approximately 5 minutes between each medication and to rinse mouth thoroughly without swallowing the rinse, after the corticosteroid dose.

Encourage use of a diary to record administration of as needed (prn) medications and the client's response. The diary should be reviewed routinely by a health care provider to monitor for continued beneficial effects or the presence of side effects/adverse reactions and early treatment failures. This information may be the first warning that indicates incorrect use of the medication or failure to take early preventive measures, or it may indicate the need for a change in dosage, for a change in medication, or for additional medication.

BOX 38-7

Environmental Allergens

While some allergens may be impossible to avoid, many occupational or environmental allergens may be reduced or eliminated. For example, smoking is an irritant to many asthmatics, especially children; asthmatic attacks may be precipitated or aggravated by dust, dust mites, cat or dog hair, hairspray, perfumes, temperature changes, and physical exertion. Whenever possible, changes that can reduce or eliminate the irritants should be attempted, such as keeping the house as dust free as possible and avoiding shag carpeting, heavy draperies, dust on silk flower arrangements, use of perfumed soap and products, and smokers or smoke-contaminated areas.

The client should be told that fungal infections of the mouth may occur with inhalation of corticosteroids. The mouth should be thoroughly examined daily for the presence of infection. In addition, tell the client that rinsing the mouth after each treatment and washing and drying the inhaler thoroughly after use will help prevent infection.

Instruct the client in ways to control known risk factors whenever possible to support the treatment plan and help prevent recurrences (Box 38-7).

Evaluation. The client with asthma will experience fewer asthmatic episodes of lesser severity without adverse drug effects. If the inhalation therapy has been for rhinitis, the client will have decreased nasal secretions and sneezing.

SUMMARY

In clients with ineffective airway clearance, nursing interventions and mucokinetic and bronchodilator drugs are used together to prevent or minimize the client's condition. Mucokinetic agents promote the removal of abnormal or excessive respiratory tract secretions by thinning hyperviscous secretions, thereby enhancing the ciliary action of the respiratory tract. Bronchodilators diminish airway obstruction by bronchial smooth muscle relaxation. Mucokinetic agents are either diluents of respiratory secretion or mucolytic by dissolving linkages of mucoprotein molecules of the respiratory secretions. Bronchodilators may be sympathomimetic drugs, either nonselective adrenergic, nonselective beta-adrenergic, or selective $beta_2$ agents. Use of the nonselective adrenergic drugs (e.g., epinephrine) not only results in bronchodilation and vasodilation but also in unwanted side effects such as increased heart rate, muscle tremors, CNS stimulation, glycogenolysis, and gluconeogenesis. The nonselective beta-adrenergic agents (e.g., isoproterenol) act upon bronchial smooth muscle, as well as the heart, whereas the selective $beta_2$ receptor agents (e.g., isoetharine and albuterol) have less cardiotonic effect and act primarily to relieve bronchospasm. Xanthine derivatives are also used as bronchodilators. Cromolyn and nedocromil are used as a prophylactic asthmatic agent. Corticosteroids are also used in chronic asthma to prevent or minimize inflammation.

Nursing management of the care of the client receiving mucokinetic and bronchodilator drugs is focused on the client experiencing increased ease of respiration, decreased wheezing, and a decrease in medication usage. The nurse should stress the need for responsible self-management of the therapeutic medication regimen. Nurses can play a crucial role in reducing the morbidity and mortality of asthma by, first, keeping current on the guidelines and treatment of asthma and, second, taking an active role in applying their clinical skills of assessment, intervention, client education, and evaluation to their clients.

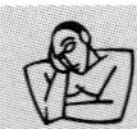

Critical Thinking

1. John Holt, age 62, was admitted to the hospital with the symptoms of fatigue, weakness, dyspnea, malaise, and a persistent nonproductive cough. He was diagnosed as having a viral upper respiratory tract infection. Would a mucolytic drug be appropriate for this client? Why or why not?
2. What nursing interventions would be considered appropriate to the nursing management of a client receiving either a mucolytic or bronchodilating drug?
3. Stanley Myers, age 22, a college student with a history of asthma, has come to the clinic for a regularly scheduled visit. In reviewing his inhalant therapy with him, he indicates that he takes the medications in any order "just to get it over with." What should be the response of the nurse?

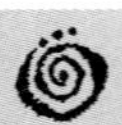

Collaborative Learning Activities

1. Students will pair off to teach each other how to use an inhaler. If demonstration inhalers are not available, the students will roll up paper to simulate the inhaler mouthpiece. Demonstrate both the closed and open mouth technique.
2. Form three teams. Each team will briefly present the differences in indication and nursing management for clients receiving mucolytic, bronchodilator, and corticosteroid agents.

BIBLIOGRAPHY

Abramowicz M (1991). Drugs for ambulatory asthma, *Med Lett Drugs Ther* 33(837):9.

Abramowicz M (1993). Drugs for ambulatory asthma, *Med Lett Drugs Ther* 35(889):11.

American Hospital Formulary Service (1996). *AHFS drug information '96*. Bethesda, MD: American Society of Hospital Pharmacists.

Anderson KN, et al. (Eds.) (1994). *Mosby's medical, nursing, & allied health dictionary* (4th ed.). St Louis: Mosby.

Centers for Disease Control and Prevention (CDC), US Department of Health and Human Services (1992). Asthma—United States, 1980-1990, *JAMA* 268(15):1995.

Dyer J (1993). Drug watch: New long-lived bronchodilator knocks out albuterol, *Amer J Nurs* 93(5):53.

Franz MN & Cohn RC (1994). Management of children and adults with cystic fibrosis: one center's approach, *Hosp Formul* 29(9):364-78.

Ip M, Lam K, Kung A, & Ng M (1994). Decreased bone mineral density in premenopausal asthma patients receiving long-term inhaled steroids, *Chest* 105(6):1722-7.

Kelly HW & Hill MR (1993). Asthma. In DiPiro JT, et al. *Pharmacotherapy* (2nd ed.). Norwalk, CT: Appleton & Lange.

Mathewson HS & Kovac AL (1994). Update on inhaled steroids, *Resp Care* 39(8):837-40.

McCann J (1997). First in new class of drugs cleared for asthma, *Drug Topics* 141(1):27.

McFadden ER & Gilbert IA (1992). Asthma, *New Engl J Med* 327(27):1928.

New Drugs & Devices (1994). Serevent for asthma, *Amer Pharm* NS34(4):9.

Olin BR (Ed.) (1996, 1997). *Facts and comparisons: Drug information*. St Louis: Facts and Comparisons.

Potter PA & Perry AG (1997). *Fundamentals of nursing: Concepts, process, and practice* (4th ed.). St Louis: Mosby.

Public Health Service, US Department of Health and Human Services (1991). *Executive summary: Guidelines for the diagnosis and management of asthma*. National Institutes of Health Publication No. 91-3042A.

Self TH & Kelly HW (1995). Asthma. In Young LY & Koda-Kimble MA. *Applied therapeutics: The clinical use of drugs* (6th ed.). Vancouver: Applied Therapeutics.

Serafin WE (1996). Drugs used in the treatment of asthma (p 659-682). In Hardman JG & Limbird LE (Eds.). *Goodman & Gilman's the pharmacological basis of therapeutics* (9th ed.). New York: McGraw-Hill.

Wingard LB, et al. (1991). *Human pharmacology*. St Louis: Mosby.

Wordell CJ (1993). Recombinant human DNase for treatment of cystic fibrosis, *Hosp Pharmacy* 28(12):1226.

United States Pharmacopeial Convention (1996). *USP DI: Drug information for the health care professional* (16th ed.). Rockville, MD: The Convention.

Chapter 39

Oxygen and Miscellaneous Respiratory Agents

Chapter Focus

An understanding of oxygen therapy and other associated therapies is essential to the delivery of effective respiratory care. The following objectives and key terms are important for a good understanding of this chapter.

Key Terms

analeptics (p. 677)
hypercapnia (p. 674)
hypoxemia (p. 672)
hypoxia (p. 672)
pulse oximetry (p. 675)

Key Drugs [▲]

cyproheptadine
diphenhydramine

Objectives

1. Describe how the body uses oxygen and the result of oxygen deprivation.
2. Implement nursing interventions applicable to each of the various methods of oxygen administration.
3. Discuss the effects of carbon dioxide.
4. Implement the nursing management of the care of clients receiving respiratory stimulants and depressants.
5. Discuss antitussive agents and the proper method of administration.
6. Explain the three actions of histamine in the body.
7. Implement nursing management of the care of clients receiving antihistamine therapy.
8. Discuss serotonin's pharmacokinetics, pharmacologic effects, and its relationship to drugs and several disease states.

DRUGS THAT AFFECT THE RESPIRATORY CENTER

Therapeutic Gases

Oxygen

Oxygen—a gas that is essential for life—is colorless, odorless, and tasteless. It is not flammable, but it supports combustion much more vigorously than does air.

Inspired air normally contains 20.9% oxygen, which, at an atmospheric pressure of 760 mm Hg, exerts a partial pressure (PO_2) or tension of 159 mm Hg. However, as oxygen passes through the bronchial airway, the inspired air becomes saturated with water vapor, which then reduces the PO_2 in the alveoli to approximately 100 mm Hg. Finally, the oxygen appears in dissolved form in the arterial blood. The PO_2 of arterial blood is normally above 80 mm Hg.

Oxygen must be continuously supplied to tissue cells, since no fiber or cell can remain without oxygen, or hypoxic, for very long and survive. The adult human brain consumes from 40 to 50 ml of oxygen per minute. The cortex consumes more than the centers in the medulla or spinal cord. Cerebral oxygen consumption proceeds without pausing, and the replenishment of oxygen by the blood must be maintained continuously. Whenever any circulatory stress exists, cerebral blood flow tends to be preserved at the expense of other less vital organs. Of all the tissues affected by **hypoxia** (inadequate cellular oxygen), the brain is most susceptible to disruption of normal function and irreversible damage. An acute reduction of the PO_2 to 50 mm Hg decreases mental functioning, emotional stability, and finer muscular coordination. Further reduction of the PO_2 to 40 mm Hg produces impaired judgment, decreased pain perception, and impairment of muscular coordination. When the PO_2 is reduced to 32 mm Hg or less, unconsciousness and a progressive descending depression of the central nervous system ensue.

The kidneys are vital organs in which there must be considerable constancy of blood flow and oxygen supply. Oxygen consumption is greater in the renal cortex; renal medullary tissue has an oxygen consumption that is 15% less than that of the renal cortex. This difference is related to the variation in pressure gradient and to the fact that cortical flow is rapid while the medullary flow is slower. The renal cortex is highly dependent on oxygen, whereas the renal medulla can function relatively independently of the oxygen supply.

The rate of oxygen consumption by the kidneys is approximately 0.06 ml/g/min, more than most other tissues. For each 100 ml of blood entering the kidney, 1.4 ml of oxygen is consumed. The oxygen consumed by the kidneys is primarily used for sodium reabsorption.

When the renal arterial content falls to less than 55% of normal, renal vasoconstriction occurs. This response is believed to be mediated by chemoreceptors, which stimulate the vasomotor center to produce renal vasoconstriction. Renal vasoconstriction also occurs as a result of the action of ether, barbiturates, and other anesthetics. Renal blood flow is also decreased during periods of exercise. It is important to note that autoregulation of renal perfusion does occur.

In skeletal muscles oxygen consumption is related to blood flow. Oxygen consumption and blood flow are decreased when muscle is at rest and significantly increased during exercise.

Reduction of oxygen supply to the intestinal tract is regarded by some investigators as a key factor for inadequate splanchnic vasoconstriction during hypotension. Inadequate oxygen supply impairs myocardial metabolism and function.

Arterial blood pressure determinations, when used alone, are unreliable indicators of the adequacy of tissue perfusion. Therefore arterial blood gas determinations should be obtained, since these results provide a more accurate and reliable indication of shifts in the partial pressures of oxygen and carbon dioxide. Severe hypoxia may produce changes in the ST segment and T wave of the ECG, dysrhythmias, ectopic beats, and myocardial infarction.

Indications. Oxygen is used chiefly to treat hypoxia and **hypoxemia** (diminished oxygen tension in the blood). Basically, the four types of hypoxia are the following:

1. Hypoxic hypoxia—produced by any condition causing a decrease in PO_2
2. Ischemic hypoxia—inadequate blood flow to an organ or tissue in the presence of a normal PO_2 and hemoglobin content
3. Anemic hypoxia—inadequate hemoglobin to carry O_2 in the presence of a normal PO_2
4. Histotoxic hypoxia—adequate PO_2 and hemoglobin but inability of tissues to use oxygen delivered because of a toxic agent

Clinically, hypoxic hypoxia is the most common form of hypoxia. A variety of pathologic conditions result in hypoxic hypoxia, which makes the use of oxygen treatment necessary. Some of these conditions are hypoventilation, increased airway resistance, pneumothorax, respiratory center depression, abnormal ventilation perfusion ratio, congenital cyanotic heart disease, decreased pulmonary compliance, and breathing oxygen-poor air. The use of oxygen is also indicated in cardiac failure or decompensation and coronary occlusion, and anesthesia administration (to increase the safety of general anesthesia).

Administration. Oxygen is administered by inhalation. Various methods are used, each having advantages and disadvantages (Figure 39-1).

A *nasal catheter* is made of soft plastic. When used, it should be lubricated with water-soluble K-Y Jelly and passed through the nose until the tip is just above the epiglottis. This distance is usually the same as the distance from an individual's external nares to the tragus of the ear, minus 1 cm. The catheter should not be inserted so far that the client swallows oxygen, since this will cause stomach distention and abdominal discomfort. The catheter is fastened with tape to the forehead and/or nose. Flow rate varies according to individual need, but 4 to 8 L/min of a 25% to 40% concentration of oxygen is commonly used. Since this form of therapy is very drying to the mucous membrane, the oxygen should be humidified. In addition, nasal and oral hygiene are important to maintain cleanliness and intact mucous membrane

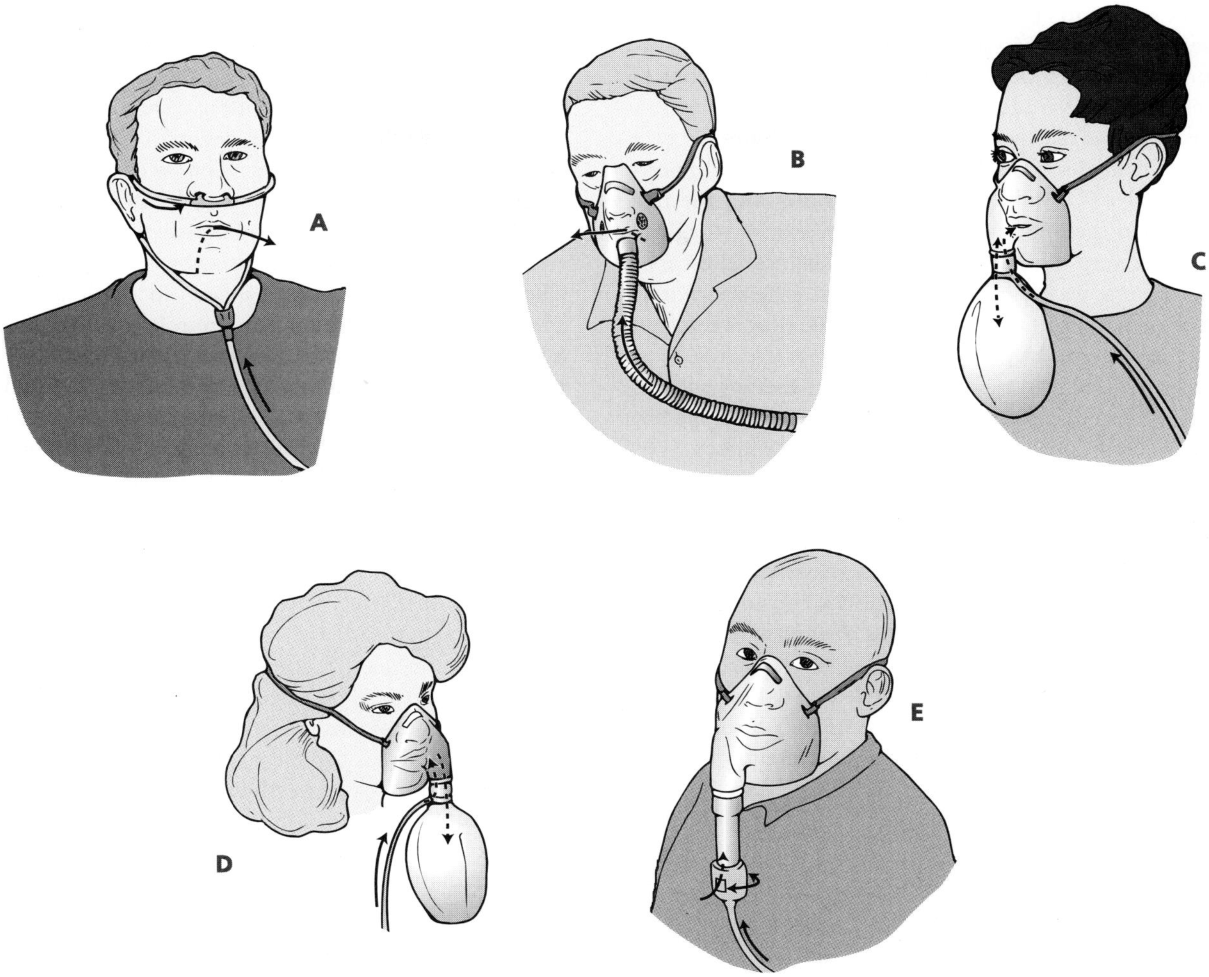

Figure 39-1 Various oxygen delivery systems. **A,** Nasal cannula. **B,** Simple face mask. **C,** Partial rebreathing mask. **D,** Nonbreathing mask. **E,** Venturi mask.

and to prevent infection and discomfort. Most clients receiving oxygen therapy are mouth breathers, and frequent mouth care is required to prevent sores. Nasal catheters become obstructed with encrusted secretions and must be removed and cleaned or replaced several times a day.

A *nasal cannula* is much more comfortable for the client than is a catheter. Cannulas have either single or double short prongs that are inserted into the lower part of the nostrils. They are less likely to become obstructed with secretions. Nasal and oral mucosa still require frequent attention. A flow of 1 to 6 L/min of a 23% to 40% concentration of oxygen is adequate for many clients.

An *oxygen mask* is the most effective means of delivering needed oxygen. Oxygen concentrations up to 90% can be administered by mask. To be effective, the mask must fit well over the nose and mouth; high flow rates can compensate to some extent for a poor fit. Masks are better tolerated when used intermittently or when disposable plastic masks are used. Only absolutely clean and uncontaminated rubber masks should be used, since they can be a source of nosocomial infection. There are two main types of oxygen masks: those that deliver low concentrations of oxygen and those that deliver high concentrations of oxygen.

A *simple face mask,* which is lightweight and disposable, is useful for short-term therapy of oxygen administration, such as in the early postoperative period or when intermittent oxygen therapy is required. The flow rate is only 6 to 10 L/min at a low oxygen concentration of 35% to 60%. Since the mask is loose-fitting and can leak, simple face masks are suitable for individuals with carbon dioxide retention. It is also indicated for clients who cannot use a nasal cannula—for example, those who have a nasal obstruction.

A *partial rebreathing mask* is a disposable, light-weight plastic face mask consisting of a reservoir bag and a partial rebreathing valve. It is commonly used by individuals who require oxygen. On expiration, only a portion of the exhaled air enters the reservoir, so it roughly conserves one third of the client's exhaled air. Because it comes from the trachea and bronchi and doesn't participate in gas exchange in the lungs, it is rich in oxygen.

Accordingly, to prevent the rebreathing of carbon dioxide, the reservoir bag should deflate only slightly on inhalation. By this method a concentration of 60% to 90% of oxygen can be delivered at a flow rate of 10 L/min.

A *nonrebreathing mask* is designed to fit tightly over the face and is usually made of rubber with a reservoir bag and a nonbreathing valve. On inhalation, oxygen flows into the bag and mask, and the one-way valve prevents exhaled air from flowing back into the bag. The expired air instead escapes through the one-way flap valve in the mask. The concentration of oxygen is 95%, which is high, and the flow is adjusted to keep the reservoir bag fully inflated.

This type of mask is used for short-term therapy such as counteracting smoke inhalation. The rubber can become hot and sticky so that prolonged use can cause discomfort.

An *oxygen tent* is of limited value, particularly when it is necessary to open the canopy for monitoring vital signs and administering care to the client. The rate of flow is 20 L/min at an oxygen concentration of 60%. Obviously, the oxygen concentration falls, making the flow difficult to control each time the tent is opened. Consequently, oxygen tents are now used less frequently.

The *Ventimask (Mix-O-Mask)* is a development originating from the Venturi mask. It is used for clients with chronic alveolar hypoventilation and carbon dioxide retention. Exact low-flow concentrations of oxygen are delivered to the individual. The Ventimask provides an air-oxygen mixture with the desired oxygen concentration. The size of the orifice to the mask determines the concentration of oxygen—24%, 28%, 35%, and 40% with flow rates of 4, 6, 8, and 10 L/min, respectively. A thin elastic band holds the Ventimask in position and tends to press into the skin behind the ears. A gauze padding under each side of the elastic band will alleviate this discomfort. The device must be removed when the client eats and may give the client a feeling of being smothered.

Most of the oxygen administered in hospitals for therapy is provided from a central source where it is stored as a gas or liquid oxygen. The gas is piped into a client's room at a standard pressure of 50 pounds per square inch (psi) at the gauge. Compressed oxygen is marketed in steel cylinders that are fitted with reducing valves for the delivery of the gas. The cylinders are usually color coded; green is used in the United States. Since the gas is under considerable pressure, the tanks must be handled carefully to prevent falling or jarring.

The effectiveness of oxygen administration depends on the carbon dioxide content of the blood. Individuals with chronic obstructive pulmonary disease (COPD) have difficulty with carbon dioxide and oxygen exchange and are subject to **hypercapnia** (high carbon dioxide content in the blood). Because of chronic hypercapnia, the medullary center of these individuals is relatively insensitive to stimulation of carbon dioxide; rather, a low PaO_2 serves as a stimulant to respiration. Therefore, oxygen flow rates are kept low (1 to 2 L/min) for clients with COPD. Nursing care should also be used to prevent a greater accumulation of carbon dioxide by encouraging the improvement of gas exchange. This involves having the client turn, deep breathe, and use pursed lip breathing periodically. Toxic carbon dioxide levels may result in further depression of respiration and respiratory acidosis. The nurse should be alert to neurologic symptoms that indicate an accumulation of carbon dioxide. Symptoms may include drowsiness, mental confusion, paresthesias, and visual disturbances. The occurrence of carbon dioxide narcosis may be prevented by gradually increasing the concentration of oxygen administered.

Oxygen administration in the premature infant. Nurses caring for premature infants in incubators must be constantly aware of the danger of retrolental fibroplasia. This is a vascular proliferative disease of the retina that occurs in some premature infants who have had high concentrations of oxygen at birth.* The oxygen concentration should be kept between 30% and 40%. Higher concentrations can be administered to cyanotic infants without increasing the danger of retrolental fibroplasia because it is PaO_2, not inspired PO_2, that is implicated in this disease. Therefore careful monitoring of arterial blood gases is essential. Some incubators are equipped with a safety valve that automatically releases any excess oxygen outside the chamber. When orders for an infant include oxygen prn, the nurse must make certain that it is administered only as needed and at low concentrations rather than continuously. Frequently, the removal of a very small plug of mucus can clear the airway, thus enabling the infant to breathe oxygen without assistance.

Hyperbaric oxygen. In recent years hyperbaric oxygen has been used in the treatment of various conditions. In the treatment of infections caused by *Clostridium welchii*, the anaerobic bacillus producing gas gangrene, the intermittent use of hyperbaric oxygen has been valuable. It is believed that an increased oxygen pressure in the tissue may exert an inhibitory effect on enzyme systems of these bacteria. This same inhibitory effect may be implicated in the use of hyperbaric oxygen on other anaerobic microorganisms.

Hyperbaric oxygen has also been used in certain circulatory disturbances, such as air or gas embolism, decompression sickness, carbon monoxide and cyanide poisoning, and exceptional blood loss. It has also been used in certain local circulatory disturbances such as necrotizing soft-tissue infections; acute traumatic ischemia, crush injury and compartment syndrome; compromised (ischemic) grafts and flaps; radiation necrosis; refractory osteomyelitis; and enhancement of healing in selected problem wounds (Weaver, 1992).

Helium-oxygen mixtures. Helium-oxygen mixtures have been used to treat obstructive types of dyspnea. Helium is an inert gas and so light that a mixture of 80% helium and 20% oxygen is only one third as heavy as air. Helium is only slightly soluble in body fluids and has a high rate of diffusion. Because of its low specific gravity, mixtures of this gas with oxygen can be breathed with less effort than either oxygen or air alone when air passages are obstructed.

---

*Excessive oxygen constricts the developing retinal vessels of the eye. Consequently, normal vascularization is suppressed; since the endothelial cells become disorganized, they cause destruction of the immature retina. The result is blindness.

These mixtures are recommended for individuals with status asthmaticus, bronchiectasis, and emphysema, as well as during anesthesia for a client with respiratory tract obstruction.

Oxygen toxicity. Exposure to 100% oxygen for a period of 6 hours causes an inflammatory response with subsequent destruction of the alveolocapillary membrane of the respiratory tract. Toxicity is often difficult to recognize, but the most common symptoms are substernal distress (ache or burning sensation behind the sternum), increase in respiratory distress, nausea, vomiting, restlessness, tremors, twitching, paresthesias, convulsions, and a dry, hacking cough.

■ Nursing Management

Oxygen Therapy

Assessment. Dyspnea or increased respiratory rate, may indicate the need for oxygen therapy. The best means of gauging the need for oxygen or the effectiveness of oxygen therapy is via arterial blood gas evaluations or pulse oximetry before and during therapy (Box 39-1). In addition, the nurse should document the client's blood pressure and pulse, level of consciousness, and respiratory status, including respiratory rate, effort, adventitious breath sounds, cyanosis, and activity intolerance.

The nurse should know normal blood gas values and recognize deviations (Box 39-2). The goal of oxygen therapy is to achieve a PaO_2 range between 60 and 80 mm Hg or oxygen saturation greater than 90%.

In chronic carbon dioxide retention, the PaO_2 may range from 55 to 60 mm Hg. Arterial blood gas analysis is required 30 minutes after the oxygen dosage is changed unless the oxygen saturation is being monitored.

Oxygen should be given with extreme caution to some clients. The client with chronic hypoxemia has central chemoreceptors that no longer act as the primary stimulus for breathing. The peripheral chemoreceptors which are sensitive to changes in PaO_2 maintain respiratory drive. Therefore, if oxygen therapy causes PaO_2 to exceed 60 mm Hg, the stimulus to breathe is lost and apnea results. Low-flow oxygen is administered to these clients and arterial blood gas evaluations should be checked frequently.

Nursing diagnosis. The client receiving oxygen therapy may be experiencing the following: ineffective airway clearance, ineffective breathing pattern, and impaired gas exchange. In addition, oxygen therapy places the client at risk for these nursing diagnoses: impaired skin integrity of the face related to the mask, infection related to contamination of the oxygen equipment, injury related to the combustibility of oxygen, altered mucous membranes related to the drying effects of oxygen, and the potential complications of oxygen toxicity and, for infants, retrolental fibroplasia.

Implementation

Monitoring. Monitor the client's vital signs—pulse rate, blood pressure, and respiratory rate and pattern. Also, observe level of consciousness, skin temperature, and color. Report any abnormal findings to the prescriber. Examine the client and the equipment frequently to see if skin and mucous membrane in contact with the equipment are intact and without irritation; the equipment is patent, without leaks, and properly positioned; the flow rate is at the prescribed level; the humidifier contains solution; and, if an oxygen cylinder is being used, that it is stabilized and contains enough oxygen. Pulse oximetry, as well as blood gases, may be required on a periodic basis.

Intervention. To prevent dryness of nose and throat and respiratory complications, add sterile, distilled water to the humidifying device, and administer oxygen concentration and liter flow as prescribed. Because oxygen is a dry gas, adequate humidification is essential to the client and must be monitored frequently.

BOX 39-1

Pulse Oximetry

An advance in monitoring for tissue hypoxia is the development of **pulse oximetry.** It has been called one of the most significant technologic advances ever made in monitoring the respiratory function of clients. Simply explained, pulse oximetry works by passing light of differing wavelengths through living tissue and analyzing the differences in absorption. Oxygenated hemoglobin absorbs light differently, and these variations in absorption serve as the basis of calculations that determine the presence and amount of oxygenated hemoglobin compared to nonoxygenated hemoglobin. This provides a continuous reading of arterial blood oxygen saturation. A saturation of 90% or greater is desired for clients. (This correlates with a PaO_2 of 60.)

Current pulse oximeters work with a small probe (light source and detector), which may be placed on a client's ear, finger, toe, bridge of the nose, nasal septum, or temple. Pulse oximetry monitors are relatively inexpensive, noninvasive, safe, extremely accurate, require no calibration, and provide almost instantaneous results. While initially used with clients during anesthesia, recovery, and critical care, the use of pulse oximetry is rapidly expanding as an immediate and safe method of determining tissue oxygenation in any client having respiratory difficulties.

BOX 39-2

Normal Values for Arterial Blood Gases

pH	7.36-7.44
$PaCO_2$	36-44 mm Hg
PaO_2	80-100 mm Hg
O_2 saturation	95% or above
HCO_3	22-26 mEq/L

Since oxygen supports combustion and combustible materials (linens, wooden furniture, plastic articles) burn with greater ease and intensity, smoking and using matches, woolen blankets, clothing, or electric equipment (radios, electric razors, hair dryers) that may cause sparks are strictly forbidden in rooms where oxygen is being administered. Also, post "no smoking" signs on the individual's door and above the bed, even though smoking is not permitted in most health care agencies.

Because oxygen therapy is frequently administered to debilitated clients, take special care to prevent contamination of the equipment used in the administration of oxygen to prevent nosocomial infection. Nasal cannulas, Ventimasks, other masks, tubing, nebulizers, and other equipment exposed to moisture need to be changed daily. Nasal catheters should be changed every 8 to 12 hours. Remove an oxygen mask periodically, if the client's condition permits, to dry, powder, and massage the skin around the mask.

Education. The equipment for oxygen administration should be shown to the client and family. Explain the procedure and the benefits of oxygen therapy. Point out the importance of not smoking in the client's room to the client and visitors. (Since oxygen supports combustion, the possibility of fire always exists.) Prepare the client and caregivers for oxygen use in the home (see the Home Health box below).

Evaluation. The client will have adequate gas exchange as evidenced by a respiratory rate of 12 to 20 breaths/min or a rate in keeping with the client's baseline and blood gas values of PaO_2 >60 mm Hg, $PaCO_2$ 35 to 45 mm Hg, and pH 7.35 to 7.45.

Carbon Dioxide

Carbon dioxide is a colorless, odorless gas that is heavier than air. Carbon dioxide used as a pharmacologic agent affects respiration, circulation, and the central nervous system. Inhalation of carbon dioxide for a short period of time increases both rate and depth of respiration unless the respiratory center is depressed by narcotics or disease.

Carbon dioxide stimulates cells of the sympathetic nervous system, the respiratory center, and the peripheral chemoreceptors. Carbon dioxide also depresses the cerebral cortex, myocardium, and smooth muscle of the peripheral blood vessels. Carbon dioxide may also interfere with nerve conduction and transmission. When carbon dioxide increases the rate and force of respiration, venous return to the heart is usually enhanced as a result of decreased peripheral resistance; there is improved rate and force of myocardial contraction and less likelihood of myocardial irritability and dysrhythmias.

Too much carbon dioxide has a depressant effect and results in acidosis and unresponsiveness of the respiratory center to the gas. Therefore it is important that carbon dioxide be administered with caution.

Indications. The following are indications for use of carbon dioxide.

Carbon monoxide poisoning. A 5% to 7% concentration of carbon dioxide in oxygen is sometimes used in the treatment of carbon monoxide poisoning. Physiologically, carbon dioxide increases the rate of separation of carbon monoxide from carboxyhemoglobin.

General anesthesia. Most general anesthetics cause a reduction in response to carbon dioxide, which is reflected in

Home Health

Home Management of Oxygen Therapy

For home use of oxygen, the client and family must understand how the system works, how to determine that the system is not functioning, and how to "troubleshoot" the system, how to contact the supplier, and what to do in an emergency. Essentially there are three methods of delivery for home oxygen systems. (1) The liquid oxygen system in which liquid oxygen is provided in large reservoir canisters with smaller portable units that can be transfilled by the client. It has the advantage of delivering 100% oxygen on all flow rates so higher liter flow is achievable. The disadvantages are that the stationary unit must be refilled periodically (a small amount evaporates), and it may be the most costly method. (2) The oxygen concentrator system, which extracts oxygen from ambient air, is inexpensive and convenient, but the main unit is not portable so the client also needs a portable unit. It is heavy and the client must have a backup system in case of power failure. (3) Compressed oxygen tanks deliver 100% oxygen on all flow rates so a higher liter flow is achievable. But it is heavy and unsightly, a safety hazard if not stored properly, and it must be replaced by periodic delivery (Pedersen, 1992).

Whatever the system, it should be checked by the client or caregiver daily. The assessment should include proper function of the equipment, prescribed flow rates, remaining liquid or compressed gas content, and backup supply to meet the client's needs. The supplier's name and phone number need to be in a handy place for reordering or in case of emergency. Fire hazards should be prevented by instructing the client and family not to smoke or use an open flame in the room where and when the oxygen is on. Electrical appliances, such as razors and electric blankets, should not be used in the vicinity of the administration of the oxygen. No oil (vaseline, hair oils, body oils), wool blankets, or flammable liquids (alcohol) should be used in the area. "No smoking" signs should be posted as reminders. The local fire department should be alerted to the presence of oxygen tanks in the house.

A respiratory care practitioner or nurse should visit at least monthly to clinically assess the client and to reinforce appropriate practices and performance by the client and caregivers and assure that the equipment is being maintained in accordance with the manufacturer's recommendations (AARC, 1992).

central nervous system depression. The degree of depression is directly related to the depth of anesthesia. The more deeply the individual is anesthetized, the greater the depression of the central nervous system. Carbon dioxide initially speeds up anesthesia by increasing pulmonary ventilation. By lessening the sense of asphyxiation, it reduces struggling. In the post-anesthesia period, it hastens the elimination of many anesthetics. Inhalation of 5% to 7% carbon dioxide increases cerebral blood flow by approximately 75%, primarily by dilation of cerebral vessels.

Respiratory depression. The use of carbon dioxide as a respiratory stimulant in the presence of depressed respiration is limited. When used, close monitoring of pulse oximetry and PaO_2 is important; if desired results are not obtained, it should be discontinued. Mechanical assistance to respiration and oxygen administration is the usual treatment in cases of respiratory depression.

Postoperative use. Occasionally, carbon dioxide is used postoperatively to increase ventilation and prevent atelectasis. Most investigators think the use of deep breathing exercises, coughing, frequent turning, tracheal suction, and intermittent positive pressure breathing produce better results.

Carbon dioxide administration has also been used in the treatment of postoperative hiccups. Relief of hiccups is apparently accomplished by stimulating the respiratory center, causing large excursions of the diaphragm that suppress spasmodic contractions of that muscle, thereby promoting regular contractions.

Administration. Carbon dioxide is kept in metal cylinders and vaporizes as it is delivered from the cylinder. When carbon dioxide is used for medical purposes, it is administered in combination with oxygen. A 5% to 10% concentration of carbon dioxide delivered through a tight-fitting face mask is inhaled by the client until the depth of respiration is definitely increased, which usually occurs within 3 minutes. For the postoperative individual, the procedure would be repeated every hour or two for the first 48 hours and then several times a day for several days.

Another way of administering carbon dioxide is to allow the client to hyperventilate with a paper bag held over the face. Reinhaling expired air causes the carbon dioxide content to be continually increased.

Signs of carbon dioxide overdosage are dyspnea, breath-holding, markedly increased chest and abdominal movements, nausea, and increased systolic blood pressure. Administration of the gas should be discontinued when these symptoms appear. The administration of 5% carbon dioxide may produce severe mental depression if given over an hour, and a 10% concentration can lead to loss of consciousness within 10 minutes. The administration should be stopped as soon as the desired effects on the client's respiration have been obtained.

Direct Respiratory Stimulants

Direct respiratory stimulants come under a broader classification of central nervous system stimulants and are often referred to as **analeptics** (see Chapter 18). These drugs act directly on the medullary center to increase respiratory rate and tidal exchange. Although these drugs are available for stimulating depth of respiration and rate of respiration, airway management and support of ventilation are more effective in the treatment of respiratory depression. The mechanical support of ventilation is often superior to the use of drugs, since respiratory stimulants in large doses can cause convulsions.

Respiratory stimulants (analeptics) have in the past been advocated in the treatment of drug-induced respiratory depression, but since these drugs are not specific antagonists to sedatives or narcotics, their use in drug-induced respiratory depression is now considered obsolete. Indeed, repeated doses of an analeptic may potentiate the depressant effects of central nervous system depressants. For information on the direct respiratory stimulant doxapram, see Chapter 18.

Reflex Respiratory Stimulants

Aromatic ammonia spirit is given by inhalation for its action as a reflex respiratory stimulant. In cases of fainting, it is administered by inhaling the vapor. Reflex stimulation of the medullary center occurs through peripheral irritation of sensory nerve receptors in the pharynx, esophagus, and stomach. The rate and depth of respiration are then increased through afferent messages to the respiratory control centers. Reflex stimulation of the vasomotor center results in a rise in blood pressure.

Respiratory Depressants

The most important respiratory depressants are opium and its derivatives and barbiturates. These agents depress the respiratory center, thereby making breathing slower and more shallow and lessening the irritability of the respiratory center. Respiratory depression, however, is seldom desirable or necessary, although it is sometimes unavoidable. It is a side/adverse effect of otherwise very useful drugs.

Occasionally an opiate such as codeine is administered to inhibit the rate and depth of respiration for a painful or harmful cough. Concentrations of carbon dioxide that are too high in inhalation mixtures may paradoxically act to depress respiration.

COUGH SUPPRESSANTS

The OTC cough suppressants are reviewed in Chapter 11, and prescription-requiring cough suppressants are discussed in this chapter. The prescribing of these agents is usually reserved for the nonproductive cough that is inadequately controlled or nonresponsive to the OTC medications.

Treatment of the cough is secondary to treatment of the underlying disorder; that is, the therapeutic objective is to decrease the intensity and frequency of the cough yet permit adequate elimination of tracheobronchial secretions and exudates.

Opioid Antitussive Drugs

Opioids such as morphine and hydromorphone are potent suppressants of the cough reflex, but their clinical usefulness is limited by side effects. They inhibit the ciliary activity of the respiratory mucous membrane, depress respiration, and may cause bronchial constriction in allergic or asthmatic clients. In addition, they can cause drug dependence. Codeine and hydrocodone exhibit less pronounced antitussive effects, but they also have fewer side effects. They are widely used. (See Chapter 14 for opioid agents.)

Nonopioid Antitussive Drugs

The nonnarcotic drugs in this group have fewer gastrointestinal side effects than do codeine and related compounds.

benzonatate [ben zoe' na tate] (Tessalon)
Benzonatate, chemically related to the local anesthetic tetracaine, relieves coughing by peripherally anesthetizing the stretch or cough receptors in the lungs and respiratory passages, and it may also have a central effect on the cough reflex.

Benzonatate is indicated for the symptomatic treatment of nonproductive cough. After oral administration, the onset of action is within 15 to 20 minutes with duration of action up to 8 hours. Side effects reported include drowsiness, headaches, dizziness, tightness or numbness in chest, nausea, constipation, abdominal upset, skin eruptions, nasal congestion, and a vague sensation of chill.

Dosage for adults and children over 10 years old is 100 mg three times a day; maximum daily dose is 600 mg.

■ Nursing Management

Benzonatate Therapy

Assessment. Assess from the client's history that there is no known hypersensitivity to benzonatate or related compounds (local anesthetics). Also determine the cause of the cough, since the cough could indicate congestive heart failure or other disease. Benzonatate is contraindicated in a productive cough because secretions would be retained if the cough were suppressed. No significant drug interactions have been reported with this drug. A baseline assessment of the client's respiratory status and cough should be obtained.

Nursing diagnosis. With the administration of benzonatate, the client should be assessed for the following nursing diagnoses: ineffective airway clearance; altered comfort related to the gastrointestinal effects (nausea, heartburn) and nasal congestion; constipation; altered skin integrity related to the occurrence of rash; risk for injury related to CNS effects (sedation, dizziness); and the potential complication of an allergic reaction.

Implementation

Monitoring. Clients should be observed for drowsiness and dizziness, nausea, gastrointestinal distress, constipation, and rash. Assess the client's cough regarding whether it is productive or nonproductive. Chest pain associated with the cough should be noted.

Intervention. Nursing actions supportive of antitussives are deep breathing exercises, frequent change of position, limitation or cessation of smoking, maintenance of adequate humidity in the environment, and adequate hydration. The nurse should attempt to pinpoint the cause of the cough and then direct nursing measures toward the cause. Infections should be treated with pulmonary hygiene (e.g., cough, deep breathing, as discussed above). If a specific stimulus for the cough can be identified, such as dust, smoking, or pollen, then attempts should be made to minimize exposure to these substances.

Education. The capsule should be swallowed whole. If it is chewed or dissolved in the mouth, temporary local anesthesia of the oral mucosa would result. Caution the client about operating a car or other machinery, since the drug may cause drowsiness or dizziness. Advise the client to report a cough that persists longer than a week.

Evaluation. The intensity and frequency of the client's cough should diminish with the administration of the antitussive.

▲ **diphenhydramine** [dye fen hye' dra meen] (Benylin, Benadryl, and others)
Diphenhydramine, available OTC and by prescription, depresses the cough center in the medulla of the brain (antitussive effect). It is reviewed in the antihistamine section of Chapter 11.

The adult dose for antitussive effect (syrup) is 25 mg orally every 4 to 6 hours; antihistamine dose is 25 to 50 mg orally every 4 to 6 hours when necessary; and as a sedative-hypnotic, the dose is 50 mg given 20 to 30 minutes before bedtime. Antidyskinetic or antiparkinson effect dosage is 50 to 150 mg orally daily in divided doses. For antiemetic or antivertigo effects, the dose is 25 to 50 mg orally 30 minutes before traveling and before each meal as necessary. The elderly may be more sensitive to the effects of this drug; therefore, lower adult doses should be prescribed with close monitoring for any adverse effects. The maximum daily dosage recommended is 300 mg in divided doses.

For children, the antihistamine dose is 1.25 mg/kg orally every 4 to 6 hours. Maximum daily dosage is 300 mg. Do not use diphenhydramine in premature or full-term neonates.

The adult dose of diphenhydramine injection used as an antihistamine or antidyskinetic is 10 to 50 mg IM or IV every 2 to 3 hours. As an antiemetic or antivertigo agent, the dose is 10 mg initially IM or IV, which may be increased to 20 to 50 mg every 2 or 3 hours. In children the antihistamine or antidyskinetic dose is 1.25 mg/kg IM four times daily. Do not use in premature or full-term neonates.

For a discussion of nursing management, see benzonatate therapy above and the nursing management discussion of antihistamine therapy later in this chapter.

For information on dextromethorphan, another nonopioid antitussive drug, see Chapter 11.

HISTAMINE

Distribution

Histamine is a chemical mediator that occurs naturally in almost all body tissues. It is present in highest concentration in the skin, lung, and gastrointestinal tract. These structures are frequently exposed to environmental assaults and require protection against damage. When liberated from its cells, the free form of histamine plays an early transient role in the inflammatory process that defends the exposed tissues against injury.

In many tissues the chief site of production and storage of histamine occurs in the cytoplasmic granules of the mast cell or, in the case of blood, the basophil that closely resembles the mast cell in function. The mast cells are small, ovoid structures widely distributed in the loose connective tissue. They are especially abundant along small blood vessels and along the bronchial smooth muscle cell, which appears to have the highest concentration of mast cells of any organ in the body. Both the mast cells and basophils make up the mast-cell histamine pool. A second major site of histamine production is known as the nonmast pool, where the amine is stored in the cells of the epidermis, gastrointestinal mucosa, and the central nervous system. Although histamine is present in various foods and is synthesized by intestinal flora, the amount absorbed does not contribute to the body's stores of this amine.

Pharmacologic Actions

The reactions mediated by histamine are attributed to receptor activity, which involves two distinct populations of receptors called H_1 and H_2 receptors. The principal actions of histamine are listed in Table 39-1.

Vascular effects. In the microcirculatory component of the cardiovascular system (arterioles, capillaries, venules) the liberation of histamine has been shown to involve both the H_1 and H_2 receptors. Stimulation of these receptors dilates the capillaries and venules, producing an increased localized blood flow, increased capillary permeability, erythema, and edema. By activating the H_1 and H_2 receptors on the smooth muscles of the arterioles, histamine is also capable of eliciting a systemic response, that is, vasodilation of the arterioles, which can result in a profound fall in blood pressure.

Smooth muscle effects. Although histamine exerts a powerful relaxing effect on the smooth muscle of the arterioles, it produces a contractile action on smooth muscles of many nonvascular organs, such as the bronchi and gastrointestinal tract. In sensitized individuals, activation of the H_1 receptors of the lungs can cause marked bronchial muscle contraction that often progresses to dyspnea and airway obstruction.

Exocrine glandular effects. While histamine stimulates the gastric, salivary, pancreatic, and lacrimal glands, the main effect is seen in the gastric glands. Stimulation of H_2 receptors in the exocrine glands of the stomach increases production of gastric acid secretions. Its high hydrochloric acid concentration is attributed to the activity of the parietal cells of the stomach and is implicated in the development of peptic ulcers.

Central nervous system effect. Histamine is also known to be present throughout the tissues of the brain. Its effects seem to involve both H_1 and H_2 receptor mediation. The activation of H_1 receptors of the semicircular canals is associated with motion sickness.

TABLE 39-1 Histamine: receptor-mediating effects

Structure	Histamine receptors	Pharmacologic effects
Vascular system		
Capillary (Microcirculation)	H_1 and H_2	Dilation; Increased permeability
Arteriole (Smooth muscle)	H_1 and H_2	Dilation
Smooth muscle		
Bronchial, bronchiolar	H_1	Contraction
Gastrointestinal	H_1	Contraction
Exocrine glands		
Gastric	H_2	Gastric acid secretion (HCl)
Epidermis	H_1	Triple response (flush, flare, wheal)
Adrenal medulla	—	Epinephrine and norepinephrine release
Central nervous system	H_1	Motion sickness

Pathologic Effects

Histamine as a chemical mediator is implicated in many pathologic disorders. Conditions for which drugs are used to counteract this compound are concerned with the hypersensitivity response known as the allergic reaction. Although four different types of hypersensitivity responses to immunologic injury exist, the type I anaphylactic reaction is the one associated with the disorders caused by histamine release.

Individuals with type I-mediated hypersensitivity develop allergies as a result of sensitization to a foreign agent that may be ingested, inhaled, or injected. An incalculable number of these agents acting as antigens exist. They vary widely in that seasonal exposure to pollens, grasses, and weeds or nonseasonal agents such as house dust, feathers, molds, and other similar substances can develop different forms of allergic reactivity.

Hypersensitivity to a variety of foods such as shellfish or strawberries requires ingestion of the antigen. Insects such as bees or wasps and even drugs, particularly penicillin, also possess allergic properties that may induce a severe response in hypersensitive individuals.

Thus type I anaphylactic hypersensitivity accounts for a substantial number of allergic disorders, and it involves a complex series of anomalies that range from mild urticaria to anaphylactic shock. The mechanism of type I anaphylactic reaction involves the attachment of an antigen (Ag) to an antibody (Ab), specifically immunoglobulin E (IgE), and this complex in turn becomes fixed to the mast cell. The pathologic manifestations of Ag-IgE interaction are caused by mast cell degranulation, resulting in the release of histamine and other mediators responsible for producing the allergic symptoms. The type I anaphylactic reaction is responsible for various disorders, such as urticaria, atopy (allergic rhinitis, hay fever), food allergies, bronchial asthma, and systemic anaphylaxis.

Urticaria. Urticaria is a vascular reaction of the skin characterized by immediate formation of a wheal and flare accompanied by severe itching. Contact with an external irritant such as drugs or foods produces the Ag-IgE mediated response with resultant release of histamine from the mast cell into the skin. The local vasodilation produces the red flare, and the increased permeability of the capillaries leads to tissue swelling. These swellings are called "hives," and when giant hives occur, they are known as angioneurotic edema. Antihistaminic drugs administered before exposure to the antigen will prevent this response.

Atopy. Atopy occurs in genetically susceptible individuals and is usually caused by seasonal pollen. This condition is manifested as an upper respiratory tract disorder known as allergic rhinitis (hay fever)(Box 39-3). See Chapter 11 for additional information. After the interaction of Ag-IgE antibody on the surface of the bronchial mast cells, histamine is released, producing local vascular dilation and increased capillary permeability. This change produces a rapid fluid leakage into the tissues of the nose, resulting in swelling of the nasal linings. In certain individuals antihistaminic therapy can prevent the edematous reaction if the drug is administered before antigenic exposure.

Food allergies. Food allergies involve intestinal immunoglobulin E (IgE)—mast cell responses to ingested antigens. If the upper gastrointestinal tract is affected, vomiting results; if the lower gastrointestinal tract is invaded, cramps and diarrhea occur. This condition also has been known to produce systemic anaphylaxis following ingestion of a large amount of antigen.

Bronchial asthma. When the inhaled antigen combines with the IgE antibody, stimulation of the mast cells triggers the release of mediators in the lower respiratory tract, usually in the bronchi and bronchioles. Histamine plays a minor role in this response because the slow-reacting substance of anaphylaxis (SRS-A) is a more potent mediator, causing long-term contraction of the bronchiolar smooth muscle. The difficulty in breathing may be relieved by a bronchodilator such as epinephrine. The administration of antihistaminic drugs actually has no value in relieving this condition, since more potent chemical mediators than histamine are responsible for causing the reaction.

Systemic anaphylaxis. Systemic anaphylaxis is a generalized reaction manifested as a life-threatening systemic condition. The Ag-IgE mediator response involves the basophils of the blood and the mast cells in the connective tissue. The most common precipitating causes of this response are drugs, particularly penicillin; insect stings (wasps and bees); and occasionally certain foods. The release of massive amounts of histamine into the circulation causes widespread vasodilation, resulting in a profound fall in blood pressure. The excessive dilation also allows plasma to leave the capillaries, and a loss of circulatory volume ensues. When the reaction is fatal, death is usually caused not only by shock but also by laryngeal edema. The symptoms of the latter condition include smooth muscle contraction of the bronchi and pharyngeal edema, which usually leads to asphyxiation. Since the mediator, SRS-A, also is released from the cells, spasm of the smooth muscle of the bronchioles elicits the asthma-like attack.

Antihistaminic drugs are less effective against systemic anaphylaxis because these agents do not antagonize the SRS-A mediator that causes the severe bronchoconstriction. Accordingly, a drug such as epinephrine, a bronchodilator, is indicated for this life-threatening situation. The relief produced by this drug results from the $beta_2$-receptor action that relaxes bronchial smooth muscles.

Drug allergies frequently develop in susceptible individuals who show no adverse effects after the first dose of drug administration. However, a second or subsequent reexposure to even a minute amount of this same antigen may elicit an exaggerated IgE response either locally or systemically. Individuals who exhibit such reactions are said to be allergic to the drug. The IgE-mediated response, particularly with penicillin, may occur either in the skin,

BOX 39-3

Colds, Allergic Rhinitis, and Influenza: Signs or Symptoms

Signs or symptoms	Common cold	Allergic rhinitis	Influenza
Fever	Rare	Absent	Common—sudden onset, may range 102-104°F
Aches and pains	Slight	Absent	May be severe
Sneezing	Usual	Common	Infrequent
Pruritus	Absent or rare	Common	Absent
Cough	Mild-moderate	Uncommon	Common
Headaches	Rare	Can occur	Prominent
Causative	Usually viruses	Usually allergens	Usually viruses
Occurrence	Anytime	Usually seasonal	Anytime
Complications	Sinus congestion, earache	Uncommon	Bronchitis, pneumonia

producing severe urticaria, or in the respiratory tract, causing bronchial asthma.

On the other hand, even limited contact in certain sensitized individuals can produce a fatal systemic anaphylaxis. Some of the drugs that elicit an allergic response include penicillin, chloramphenicol, streptomycin, sulfonamides, aspirin, and phenacetin. Allergic reactions to penicillin account for nearly 100 deaths per year in the United States. Therefore, if an individual exhibits even the mildest sign of an allergic response, such as a slight skin rash, this symptom should be reported immediately to the prescriber. In all probability the drug will be discontinued to avoid the possibility of an exaggerated type I hypersensitivity reaction.

Histamine Testing: Gastric Function

Histamine is used to test for gastric acid secretory functions. If achlorhydria is the response to histamine, then the person may have pernicious anemia, gastric polyps, gastric carcinoma, or atrophic gastritis. If gastric acid hypersecretion occurs after the histamine, then a duodenal ulcer of Zollinger-Ellison syndrome may be the problem.

This test is contraindicated in clients with a history of hypersensitivity to the drug, bronchial asthma, vasomotor instability, urticaria, or severe cardiac, pulmonary, or renal disease. Histamine should be used cautiously in individuals with pheochromocytoma. Histamine H_2 receptor antagonists, such as cimetidine and ranitidine, are not to be administered for the 24 hours before the test because they will antagonize the effects of the histamine. Antacids and anticholinergics are also withheld before the examination. The procedure and any anticipated effects of the histamine test should be explained to the client.

The client should fast for a minimum of 12 hours and be at rest under basal conditions. Use a nasogastric tube to empty the stomach contents before the examination and to obtain specimens during the examination. The client may swallow 300 ml of water; then the histamine dose of 0.01 mg/kg (equal to histamine phosphate 0.0275 mg/kg) is given subcutaneously. If the side effects of flushing, headache, nasal stuffiness, dizziness, faintness, and nausea become too severe, epinephrine or ephedrine may be administered. These drugs antagonize the effects of histamine except for those on gastric secretion.

Monitor pulse rate and blood pressure closely. Prevent the client from swallowing saliva; its alkalinity may interfere with test results. Obtain four samples for volume and acidity of gastric contents, 15 minutes apart for analysis. The maximum effect from the histamine is usually seen in about 30 minutes. *This test should be performed by or under the direction of a physician.*

Other drugs are also used to induce gastric secretion. Besides histamine, Histalog, an analogue of histamine, is used as well as pentagastrin, a synthetic compound. Pentagastrin is currently the drug of choice because it has fewer side effects (Watson & Jaffe, 1995).

ANTIHISTAMINES

Antihistamines are drugs that compete with histamine for its receptor sites. With the discovery of two histamine receptors, H_1 and H_2, the antihistamines should be divided into the H_1 receptor antagonists and the H_2 receptor antagonists. The H_2 receptor blocking agents, which include cimetidine (Tagamet), ranitidine (Zantac), and others, are discussed in Chapter 41, while the OTC antihistamines are reviewed in Chapter 11. This section reviews the prescription antihistamines.

H_1 Receptor Antagonists

Antihistamines prevent the physiologic action of histamine by preventing histamine from reaching its site of action; thus the H_1 antihistamines have the greatest therapeutic effect on nasal allergies. They do not inhibit histamine already attached to receptors; therefore, these drugs are more effective if given before histamine is released. They relieve symptoms better at the beginning of the hay fever season than during its height but fail to relieve the asthma that frequently accompanies hay fever. These preparations are palliative and do not immunize the individual or protect him over time against allergic reactions. They do not replace other remedies such as epinephrine, ephedrine, and others.

In acute asthmatic reactions the antihistamine drugs serve only as supplements to these remedies, and relief of various symptoms of allergy is obtained only while the drug is being taken. Dozens of antihistamine drugs are available and generally differ from each other by potency, duration of action, and incidence of side effects, particularly sedation. It is often necessary to try different types of antihistamines to determine the appropriate one for a client.

Antihistamines are indicated for the treatment of allergies, vertigo, motion sickness, antitussive effect (diphenhydramine), and sedative and local anesthetic effects in dentistry. Generally, their oral absorption pattern is good, and onset of action is within 15 to 60 minutes for most of them. With astemizole (Hismanal), the onset of action is 2 to 3 days. Dimenhydrinate (Dramamine) rectally has an onset of action within 30 to 45 minutes. The time to peak effect can vary with each individual preparation. For example, astemizole's peak effect occurs within 9 to 12 days while triprolidine (Myidil) is within 2 to 3 hours. Duration of action is also variable with dimenhydrinate between 3 and 6 hours, azatadine at 12 hours, and loratadine (Claritin) at least 24 hours. These agents are primarily metabolized in the liver and excreted in the kidneys with the exception of astemizole, which is mainly excreted fecally.

For side effects/adverse reactions, see the previous section on diphenhydramine.

The antihistamine dosage varies with each drug's chemical classification and pharmacokinetic profile. The newer agents released generally are longer-acting drugs with fewer sedative side effects, such as loratadine (Claritin), which is taken once a day and has few, if any, sedative and anticholinergic side effects.

The older agents that usually exhibit these side effects carry warnings about the drug use in the elderly; the geriatric client is usually more sensitive to the effects of these drugs and may require a reduction in dosage. The adult and pediatric dosages are noted in Table 39-2.

Fexofenadine (Allegra), an antihistamine approved in 1996, is a metabolite of terfenadine (Seldane) that was chemically altered to eliminate the serious and potentially fatal cardiovascular drug interactions associated with terfenadine (Seldane). It is indicated for the treatment of seasonal allergic rhinitis (Rxtra Facts, 1996).

Many prescription antihistamine-decongestant formulations are also available, for example acrivastine-pseudoephedrine (Semprex-D), brompheniramine and pseudoephedrine (Bromfed), and others. The trend, however, is for more antihistamines and antihistamine combinations

TABLE 39-2 Antihistamines: recommended dosages

Antihistamine	Adult dosage	Children's dosage
astemizole (Hismanal)	10 mg daily	6-12 yr, 5 mg/day
azatadine (Optimine)	1-2 mg every 8-12 hr	12 yr and older, 0.5-1 mg twice daily
brompheniramine (Dimetane)	4 mg every 4-6 hr up to maximum of 24 mg/day	0.5 mg/kg in 3 or 4 divided doses
	Extended release: 8 mg every 8-12 hr or 12 mg every 12 hr as necessary	6 yrs and older, 8 or 12 mg every 12 hr as necessary
	Parenteral IM, IV, or SC: 10 mg every 8-12 hr as necessary	12 yr and under, 0.125 mg/kg 3 or 4 times daily as needed
cetirizine (Reactine ✤)	5-10 mg daily	2-6 yr, 5 mg daily 6-11 yr, 10 mg daily
chlorpheniramine (Chlortrimeton)	4 mg every 4-6 hr as needed	6-12 yr, 2 mg 3 or 4 times a day as needed
	Parenteral IM, IV, SC: 5-40 mg as single dose as necessary	SC: 87.5 μg/kg every 6 hr as needed
clemastine (Tavist)	1.34 mg twice daily or 2.68 mg 1 to 3 times a day as needed	6-12 yr, 670 μg to 1.34 mg twice a day as necessary
cyproheptadine (Periactin)	4 mg every 8 hr, increase as necessary (range 4 to 20 mg/day)	0.125 mg/kg every 8-12 hr as needed
dexchlorpheniramine (Polaramine)	2 mg every 4-6 hr as needed	150 μg/kg in 4 divided doses
	Extended release: 4 or 6 mg every 8-12 hr as needed	Not recommended
dimenhydrinate (Dramamine)	50-100 mg every 4 hr as necessary	5 mg/kg in 4 divided doses
	Parenteral, IM, IV: 50 mg IM or 50 mg in 10 ml normal saline for IV every 4 hr (administer IV slowly)	1.25 mg/kg IM or IV, every 6 hr as necessary (maximum 300 mg/day)
diphenhydramine (Benadryl)	25-50 mg every 4-6 hr	6-12 yr, 12.5-25 mg every 4 to 6 hr
doxylamine (Unisom)	12.5-25 mg every 4-6 hr as necessary	6-12 yr, 6.25-12.5 mg every 4 to 6 hr as necessary
fexofenadine (Allegra)	60 mg PO twice daily	Not available
loratadine (Claritin)	10 yr old and adults: 10 mg daily, before eating	2-9 yr: 5 mg daily before eating
phenindamine (Nolahist)	25 mg every 4-6 hr as necessary	6-12 yr, 12.5 mg every 4-6 hr as necessary
tripelennamine (Pyribenzamine)	25-50 mg every 4-6 hr as necessary	1.25 mg/kg every 6 hr as needed (maximum 300 mg/day)
	Extended-release: 100 mg every 8-12 hr as necessary	Not recommended
triprolidine (Myidil)	2.5 mg every 4-6 hr as necessary	4 to 24 mo, 312 μg every 6-8 hr; 2-4 yr, 625 μg every 6-8 hr; 4 to 6 yr, 937 μg every 6-8 hr; 6 to 12 yr, 1.25 mg every 6-8 hr as needed

to be allowed OTC marketing status in the future. For a discussion on antihistamine combinations, see Chapter 11.

■ Nursing Management

Antihistamine Therapy

Assessment. Use antihistamines with caution in clients with the following: asthma, since the drying effect may thicken secretions and diminish expectoration; prostatic hypertrophy or predisposition to urinary retention, because the urinary retention may be aggravated; or a predisposition to narrow-angle glaucoma, since the drug may precipitate an acute episode. Astemizole may induce arrhythmias in clients with a history of QT interval prolongation or in clients with hepatic impairment because increased plasma concentrations will occur. Hypokalemia should be corrected before astemizole and terfenadine therapy because of the risk of ventricular arrhythmias.

Review the client's health history to determine if there is a previous intolerance to antihistamines and the current medication regimen to determine significant drug interactions such as when antihistamines are given with:

Drug	Possible effect and management
alcohol, CNS depressants	Concurrent use may enhance CNS depressant effects. If CNS depressant also has anticholinergic side effects, enhanced anticholinergic side effects may be seen. Monitor closely since interventions may be necessary.
anticholinergic medications, psychotropics, and others	Enhanced CNS depressant and anticholinergic side effects may be noted. Monitor closely because intervention may be necessary.
erythromycin (Erythrocin)	**If administered concurrently with astemizole, an increased risk of cardiotoxic effects has been reported. Avoid or a potentially serious drug interaction may occur.**
ketoconazole (Nizoral)	**If administered concurrently with astemizole and loratadine, increased levels of antihistamines may result, which increases the potential for cardiotoxicity. Avoid or a potentially serious drug interaction may occur.**
monoamine oxidase (MAO) inhibitors	**Prolonged anticholinergic and CNS depression effects may result. Avoid or a potentially serious drug interaction may occur.**

A baseline assessment of the condition for which the antihistamine is being administered should be obtained.

Nursing diagnosis. With the administration of antihistamines, the client should be assessed for the following nursing diagnoses: altered sleep pattern (drowsiness); altered comfort related to dryness of mouth and throat, rash, and/or tinnitus; risk for injury related to blurred vision and hypotension (fainting); altered thought processes (confusion); altered urinary elimination pattern (difficult or painful urination); and the potential complications of blood dyscrasias (unusual bleeding or bruising, sore throat, fever) and paradoxical reaction (excitement, restlessness, nightmares).

Implementation

Monitoring. With IV administration, monitor the client's blood pressure before and after dosing. Observe the client for drowsiness that might be hazardous. Clients on long-term antihistamine therapy should have periodic blood counts to monitor for the development of blood dyscrasias. Tolerance to some antihistamines may occur. If a tolerance develops, another antihistamine may be prescribed.

In the older child a paradoxical response to the drug may occur and the child may exhibit hyperexcitability rather than the drowsiness that is usually seen. With the elderly client, sedation and hypotension are more likely to occur, as well as the antimuscarinic effects of the drug, resulting in dryness of the mouth or urinary retention, particularly in the male.

Closely monitor individuals with hypertension or cardiac or renal disease who are taking antihistamines. See the Pregnancy Safety box below for FDA ratings.

Intervention. Administer oral dosage form with food, water, or milk to minimize gastric irritation. Do not break, crush, or chew sustained-release capsules or long-acting tablets.

Education. Advise the client who will be using antihistamines on a long-term basis to maintain dental hygiene by brushing and flossing because the diminished salivary flow resulting from antihistamines will contribute to caries and gum disease. Regular dental checkups should also be advised. The discomfort of the dryness of the mouth may be minimized by using ice, sugarless gum, or hard candy.

Drowsiness is a common effect of antihistamines. Caution the client about driving or using other hazardous equipment until the response to the drug has been ascertained. When the effect is known, then the client may modify lifestyle accordingly. Also, if the drowsiness is severe, another antihistamine may be prescribed.

Alert the client to the symptoms of blood dyscrasias, such as sore throat, fever, unusual bruising and bleeding, and tiredness, since these should be reported to the prescriber. Caution the client about ingesting alcohol or CNS depressants because the effects of the drugs will be potentiated.

If the client is taking antihistamines as prophylaxis for motion sickness, the dose should be taken 30 minutes to 1 to 2 hours before its effect is needed. The client taking antihistamines should alert the allergist if scheduled for allergy skin tests because these drugs interfere with the results.

Pregnancy Safety

Category	Drug
B	azatadine, brompheniramine, chlorpheniramine, clemastine, cyproheptadine, dexchlorpheniramine, dimenhydrinate, diphenhydramine, loratadine, triprolidine
C	astemizole, benzonatate, terfenadine
Unclassified	doxylamine, hydroxyzine, tripelennamine

Evaluation. If antihistamines are taken for an antitussive effect, the client will report a decrease in coughing. If taken for symptoms of allergy, the client will demonstrate relief from itching, sneezing, and nasal secretions. If taken for the prevention of motion sickness, the client will report an absence or a decreased frequency or intensity of nausea episodes. If taken for sleep, the client will report having slept well.

Inhibitor of Histamine Release

Cromolyn sodium provides a local protective effect in the mucosal airways by inhibiting the granulation of pulmonary mast cells and thereby preventing the release of histamine and SRS-A. See the section on cromolyn sodium in Chapter 38.

SEROTONIN

As with histamine, serotonin (5-hydroxytryptamine or 5-HT) has no therapeutic application; however, its importance is related to the action of other drugs and several disease states. Serotonin is widely distributed in nature, occurring in both plants (pineapples, bananas, strawberries, tomatoes, nuts) and animals. In human beings, serotonin occurs in various body tissues, but primarily in three tissue types: (1) The largest fraction (90%) is synthesized and stored in the enterochromaffin cells of the gastrointestinal tract mucosa, particularly in the pylorus of the stomach and in the upper region of the small intestine. (2) A much smaller fraction is stored but not synthesized in platelets; on disintegration this fraction is released in serum and in the spleen. (3) In the CNS the greatest concentration occurs in the hypothalamus, midbrain, reticular formation, raphe (midline) regions of medulla and pons, and pineal gland. A neuron that releases serotonin is termed a serotoninergic or tryptaminergic fiber. Only a very low concentration of serotonin appears in cells.

Pharmacologic Actions

Serotonin appears to possess multiple pharmacologic actions, but because of discrepant experimental findings, this variability has caused much controversy. Despite the need for additional experimental analysis, it is now known that the primary function of serotonin is exerted on various smooth muscles and nerves. As previously stated, serotonin is not a therapeutic agent, but its more prominent effects are associated with its influence on other drugs and some disease states.

Gastrointestinal tract. Serotonin is secreted from specialized cells of the stomach and intestine that are responsible for contraction of the gastrointestinal smooth muscle, thereby producing the peristaltic response.

Carcinoid syndrome is a condition elicited from carcinoid tumors causes and overproduction of serotonin; bradykinin and histamine may also be released. Serotonin is responsible for causing this syndrome, which is characterized by paroxysmal flushing, hyperperistalsis, diarrhea, bronchoconstriction, and cardiac valvular lesions. The diagnosis of carcinoid syndrome is confirmed by the presence of excess 5-HT, which eventually is excreted in the urine.

Blood platelets. Serotonin is released from platelets during their breakdown within the circulation. This compound then activates receptors on the surface of other blood platelets, thereby promoting platelet aggregation. It has been suggested that through this mechanism the discharge of serotonin from platelets may contribute to the formation of pulmonary embolism.

Central nervous system. Serotonin is manufactured and stored in the neurons in the brain. The central action of the neuronal system appears to elicit primarily an inhibitory response from the specific nuclei of the brain. Researchers now postulate that altered function of serotoninergic pathways is a factor in various CNS dysfunctions.

Sleep. Serotonin-synthesizing cells are required for the induction of non–rapid eye movement (NREM) sleep (quiet brain, potentially excitable muscles) and the onset of REM sleep (active brain, rapid eye movements, dreams, atonic muscles). Normal sleep depends on serotonin along with the combined functions of norepinephrine and cholinergic systems. The basic sleep pattern consists of four to six cycles that alternate between NREM and REM sleep. Destruction of the raphe nuclei results in insomnia. Other disorders of sleep are quite common; for example, narcolepsy is characterized by a sudden change from wakefulness directly to REM sleep.

Sleep hypnotics such as barbiturates tend to decrease REM sleep, which is an essential component of restful sleep. Also, the drug *p*-chlorophenylalanine inhibits formation of serotonin, and this depletion can cause prolonged wakefulness when administered to animals.

Pain perception. The serotoninergic neurons located in the raphe nuclei of the brainstem have axons that project to the spinal cord and forebrain. One important system related to the brain involves a substance called beta-endorphin, which is associated with neurons that interconnect various nuclei in the hypothalamus, limbic system, and thalamus. The beta-endorphin neurons mediate euphoric and emotional behavior. The thalamic nuclei mediates poorly localized deep pain, which is best influenced by opiates. The density of opiate receptors in the brain appears to be much greater in the medial and lateral thalamus. The extent of opiate addiction and withdrawal are influenced by the quantity of opiate receptors involved.

Serotonin also is implicated in the action of morphine. Studies suggest that as tolerance develops toward this narcotic, the synthesis but not the accumulation of serotonin doubles. In addition, a decrease in brain serotonin level increases a person's sensitivity to painful stimuli, thus decreasing the analgesic effect of morphine.

Mental illness. CNS depression correlates with low levels of total brain serotonin. The enzyme monoamine oxidase metabolizes serotonin, resulting in a lower level of the transmitter (Figure 39-2). Accordingly, a monoamine oxidase inhibitor (MAOI) blocks the degradation of serotonin and thereby increases the concentration level of the neurotransmitter in the

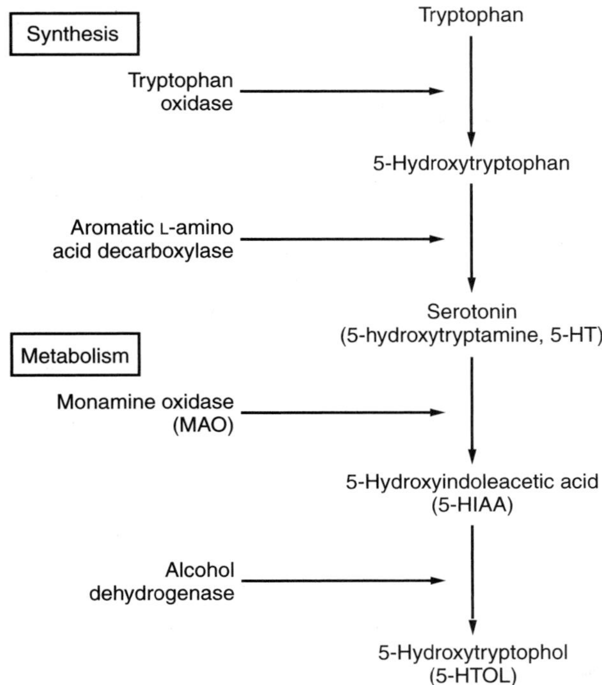

Figure 39-2 Synthesis and metabolism of serotonin.

brain. (The antidepressant effects of MAOI drugs are discussed in Chapter 19.) The tricyclic compounds also act as antidepressants, blocking the reuptake of serotonin and norepinephrine at the membrane of the neuron and thereby potentiating the action of the synapse.

ANTISEROTONINS

Antiserotonins, or serotonin antagonists, are considered complex compounds because they possess varying degrees of specificity, and thus the exact mechanism of action is unknown. In addition to performing serotonin-blocking activity, many other pharmacologic actions are involved in inhibiting responses to serotonin.

▲ **cyproheptadine** [si proe hep' ta deen] (Periactin)
Cyproheptadine blocks serotonin activity in the smooth muscle of blood vessels and the intestine and also has antihistaminic and possibly anticholinergic properties. It may produce weight gain by blocking serotonin activity in the appetite center in the hypothalamus; in other words, cyproheptadine then stimulates appetite. Although not approved by the FDA, it has also been used to treat vascular headaches. It is administered primarily for allergic disorders. (See Antihistamines, p. 681.)

lysergic acid diethylamide (LSD)
The basic mechanism underlying LSD's hallucinogenic properties is not known. Experts agree, however, that its profound effects on behavior are mediated through the central neurotransmitter, serotonin. Studies in the 1970s suggested that the more powerful hallucinogenic drugs exert a dual function in the brain: they inhibit the action of serotonin and stimulate the norepinephrine system. See Chapter 9 for a discussion of LSD as a drug of abuse.

methysergide maleate [meth i ser' jide] (Sansert)
Although its mechanism of action in preventing vascular headaches is unknown, methysergide is both a potent antiserotonin and a vasoconstrictor agent. These properties apparently help to relieve migraine and other vascular headaches (see Chapter 22, p. 446).

SUMMARY

The drugs in this chapter cover a wide range of therapeutic effects on the respiratory system. Oxygen, a therapeutic gas, is essential to sustain life, and its administration is required for many clients. Although most acute care facilities have a respiratory therapy department, the nurse is responsible for evaluating the client's response to oxygen and, in some circumstances, initiating oxygen therapy.

Cough suppressants are generally used for nonproductive coughs in which prolonged coughing is annoying, exhausting, and painful. (Opioid antitussive drugs are discussed in Chapter 14.) However, nonnarcotic antitussive drugs may be effective and have fewer gastrointestinal side effects.

Histamine is a chemical mediator naturally occurring in most body tissues and has been implicated in a number of pathologic conditions, such as urticaria, atopy, food allergies, bronchial asthma, and systemic anaphylaxis. This makes antihistamines, which compete at receptor sites with histamines to prevent their physiologic actions, invaluable as medications. Antihistamines are contained in numerous antitussive preparations, cold-cough products, OTC sleeping compounds, and oral analgesic products. Serotonin is also a naturally occurring substance with no therapeutic application. However, it is related to the action of other drugs, such as the opiates. CNS depression also correlates with low levels of total brain serotonin. The antiserotonin methysergide maleate may be used to relieve vascular headaches.

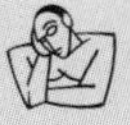

Critical Thinking

1. Mr. Hodges, a 72-year-old with COPD, has been receiving low-flow oxygen therapy at 2 L/min per nasal cannula. When you check the flowmeter, you discover it is set at 6 L/min. What assessment do you need to make of Mr. Hodges immediately? Why?
2. You are preparing Mr. Hodges and his wife for his return home, where he will be continuing his oxygen therapy. Although Mr. Hodges has given up smoking since he has become so ill, you have noticed that both his wife and his son, with whom he lives, smoke. What action will you take?

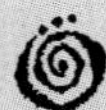

Collaborative Learning Activities

1. The instructor will demonstrate each method of oxygen administration, asking students to suggest advantages and disadvantages of each. The students will suggest nursing assessments and intervention strategies.

BIBLIOGRAPHY

AARC Clinical Practice Guideline (1992). Oxygen therapy in the home or extended care facility, *Resp Care* 37(3):918-20.

Abramowicz M (1994). Acrivastine/pseudoephedrine (Semprex-D) for seasonal allergic rhinitis, *Med Lett* 36(930):78.

American Hospital Formulary Service (1996). *AHFS drug information '96*. American Society of Hospital Pharmacists.

Anderson KN, et al. (Eds.) (1994). *Mosby's medical, nursing, & allied health dictionary* (4th ed.). St Louis: Mosby.

Branson RD (1993). The nuts and bolts of increasing arterial oxygenation: Devices and techniques, *Resp Care* 38(6):672-83.

Crocco JA & Francis PB (1991). Acute oxygen therapy—when and how? *Patient Care* 25(14):69-74.

Feldman EG & Davidson DE (1990). *Handbook of nonprescription drugs* (9th ed.). Washington, DC: American Pharmaceutical Association and The National Professional Society of Pharmacists.

Olin BR (Ed.) (1996). *Facts and comparisons: Drug information*. St Louis: Facts and Comparisons.

Rxtra Facts (1996). *Supplement to Facts and Comparisons* 1(3):1.

Somerson SJ & Sicilia MR (1992). Emergency oxygen administration and airway management, *Crit Care Nurse* 12(4):23-9.

United States Pharmacopeial Convention (1996). *Drug information for the health care professional* (16th ed.). Rockville, MD: The Convention.

Weaver LK (1992). Hyperbaric treatment of respiratory emergencies, *Resp Care* 37(7):720-30.

Wilson SF & Thompson JM (1990). *Respiratory disorders*. St Louis: Mosby.

Overview of the Gastrointestinal Tract

Chapter Focus

The gastrointestinal (GI) system, responsible for the digestive processes of the body, supplies nutrients to fuel the body. This function contributes to the client's wellness by influencing overall health. The nurse should assess every client's nutritional-metabolic need. This assessment requires a thorough knowledge of the anatomy and physiology of the GI system and provides the background for the nurse to plan and deliver appropriate care for clients with GI disorders. This chapter provides a review of that anatomy and physiology. The following objectives and key terms are important for a good understanding of this chapter.

Key Terms

acute gastritis (p. 689)
cholecystitis (p. 690)
cholelithiasis (p. 690)
chronic gastritis (p. 689)
digestion (p. 688)
peptic ulcer disease (p. 689)
peristaltic process (p. 689)

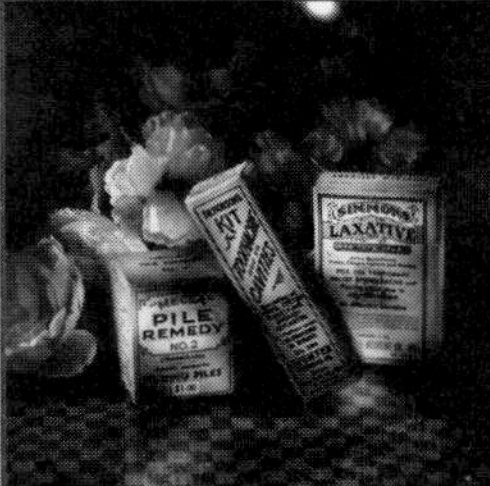

Objectives

1. Identify the major parts of the GI tract.
2. Describe the functions of individual components of the GI tract.
3. List the effects of parasympathetic and sympathetic innervation on the GI tract.
4. Describe common disorders affecting the GI tract.

Disorders of the gastrointestinal (GI) tract such as indigestion, gastritis, constipation, and peptic ulcers are very common problems reported by large numbers of the population. Since the cause of many GI diseases remains unclear, pharmacologic management is often directed at relieving symptoms rather than at control or cure. In this chapter the anatomy and functions of the GI tract are reviewed.

The GI system itself is made up of the alimentary canal or digestive tract, the biliary system, and the pancreas (Figure 40-1). The alimentary canal extends from the mouth to the anus. Food substances entering the canal undergo mechanical and chemical changes called **digestion.** These changes permit nutrients to be absorbed and undigestible materials to be excreted by the body. Absorbed nutrients may be used as an energy source or stored (glycogen for glucose or fat for carbohydrate). Movements by the smooth muscle fibers surrounding the canal (1) mix the contents by segmental contractions and (2) move the mass through the tract by peristalsis.

The secretory and muscular activities of the GI system are regulated by neural mechanisms. An interconnecting network of neurons is located in smooth muscle and secretory cells. This system is self-regulating; it is capable of controlling exocrine gland secretions and muscular contractions without any external influence.

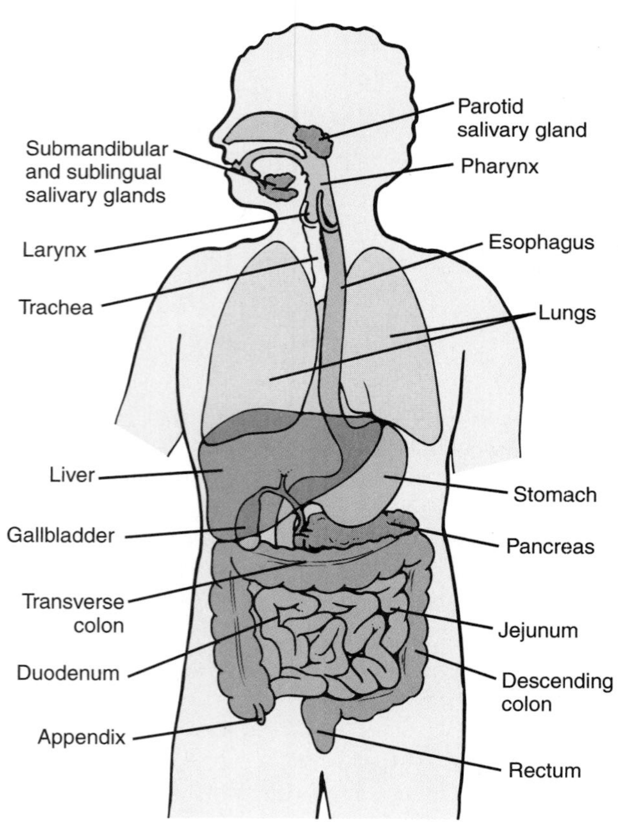

Figure 40-1 Gastrointestinal and respiratory systems.

By contrast, the external innervation of the GI system is supplied by the divisions of the autonomic nervous system. Their major function is to correlate activities between different regions of the GI system and also between this system and other parts of the body. The influence of the parasympathetic division mediated by two branches of the vagus nerve exerts an excitatory action, which increases digestive secretions and muscular activity. By contrast, the splanchnic nerves of the sympathetic division are primarily inhibitory, depressing digestive secretions and muscular activity. Under normal conditions, the two divisions of the autonomic nervous system maintain a delicate balance of control of functions.

Drugs affecting the GI tract exert their action mainly on muscular and glandular tissues. The action may be directly on the smooth muscle and gland cells or indirectly on the autonomic nervous system. Drugs also may cause increased or decreased function, tone, emptying time, or peristaltic action of the stomach or bowel. In addition, they may be used to relieve enzyme deficiency, to counteract excess acidity or gas formation, to produce or prevent vomiting, or as diagnostic aids.

MOUTH (ORAL CAVITY)

The mouth, or oral cavity, functions as the starting point of the digestive process. Food is taken in, chewed, and mixed with saliva that contains the enzyme amylase (ptyalin), which begins the process of chemical digestion.

Three pairs of salivary glands secrete saliva into ducts emptying into the mouth. The sublingual and submandibular salivary glands are located beneath the tongue; the largest pair, the parotid glands, are found in front of and slightly below the ears. When the food bolus has been chewed and reduced in the mouth, it is swallowed. Swallowing (deglutition) is a complex process that begins as a voluntary movement but is continued as an involuntary muscular reflex as the food is propelled through the GI tract.

Disorders affecting the mouth. Systemic diseases, nutritional deficiencies, and mechanical trauma can cause irritation or inflammation of buccal structures. Dental disorders (e.g., caries, gingivitis, and pyorrhea) and bacterial, viral, or fungal infections (e.g., candidiasis or herpes simplex) can affect the structures of the oral cavity, causing such symptoms as mouth blistering or other lesions, swelling, pain, and inflammation.

Agents acting on the oral cavity are discussed in Chapter 41.

PHARYNX

The pharynx (throat), a tubelike passageway connecting the mouth and the esophagus, is important in swallowing. Food and fluid pass through the pharynx into the esophagus. During this passage the trachea is closed to prevent aspiration into the lungs.

Disorders affecting the pharynx. Like the mouth, the pharynx can be affected by various systemic diseases. It can become irritated and inflamed (e.g., from sinusitis or the "common cold") and treated symptomatically with an antiinflammatory agent. It can also become a locus of infection (e.g., with strep throat), requiring systemic antibiotic therapy.

ESOPHAGUS

The esophagus is a pliable muscular structure approximately 25 cm long that extends from the pharynx to the cardiac end of the stomach. It extends through the diaphragm as it drops from the thoracic cavity into the abdominal cavity.

The esophagus is considered the beginning of the digestive system proper, since the rest of the GI tract organs function only in digestion and/or excretion. The esophagus continues the process of swallowing and begins the **peristaltic process,** or the squeezing of the food bolus down the GI tract by band contraction. The peristaltic band wave stimulates the lower esophageal sphincter, which closes to prevent gastroesophageal reflux and then returns the esophagus to its normal resting state.

Disorders affecting the esophagus. Esophageal disorders are characterized by retrosternal pain (heartburn) and difficulty in swallowing (dysphagia). The sources of the pain are numerous; some potential causes include diffuse esophageal spasm, achalasia, pyloric or duodenal ulcers, scleroderma, postural changes (bending forward), excessive alcohol ingestion, and nonspecific dysmotility.

However, heartburn commonly results from reflux esophagitis, in which the incompetent lower esophageal sphincter permits gastric contents to flow back into the esophagus; or from hiatal hernia, in which a part of the stomach protrudes into the diaphragm. One type of hiatal hernia, paraesophageal hernia, may be associated with esophageal obstruction and strangulation. Difficulty in swallowing can be a symptom of esophageal obstruction, mechanical interference with or paralysis of the muscles of deglutition, neuromuscular incoordination, achalasia, carcinoma of the esophagus, anxiety states, hysteria, or schizophrenic hallucinations.

Inflammation of the esophagus can have many causes: reflux esophagitis associated with hiatal hernia, irritant ingestion, infection, peptic ulceration, prolonged gastric intubation, and uremia.

STOMACH

The stomach, a pouchlike structure lying below the diaphragm, has three divisions: the fundus, the body, and the pylorus. Two sphincter muscles—the cardiac sphincter and the pyloric sphincter—regulate the stomach opening. Gastric glands secrete mucus and gastric juice composed of enzymes and hydrochloric acid. They also produce intrinsic factor, a protein essential for absorption of vitamin B_{12}. Vitamin B_{12} in turn is needed for erythropoiesis (red blood cell formation).

The stomach functions as a temporary storage site for food as it is being digested. It also manufactures gastrin, a hormone that regulates enzyme production to facilitate digestion. The stomachs of men and women differ, both in food storage capacity and size. Females have smaller and more slender stomachs. The stomach is capable of holding 1500 to 2000 ml. It distends after eating and gradually collapses as the food bolus moves out into the small intestine. Its churning action further breaks down the food bolus and mixes it with gastric juice to continue chemical digestion. A limited amount of nutrient and drug absorption takes place in the stomach.

The time required for digestion in the stomach depends on the amount of food eaten. Normal emptying time is 2 to 6 hours. However, the gastric emptying time may be affected by drug administration, physical activity of the individual, and body position during digestion. Gastric emptying time is a factor to consider in the timing of drug administration, since the presence of food may block the absorption of some drugs.

Disorders affecting the stomach. **Acute gastritis** is an inflammatory response of the stomach lining to ingestion of irritants, such as ethanol or nonsteroidal antiinflammatory agents, including aspirin. Symptoms include epigastric discomfort, nausea, abdominal tenderness, and gastrointestinal hemorrhage. Treatment consists of lifestyle modifications and drugs such as antacids, antiemetic agents, anticholinergics, and antihistamines (see Chapter 41).

Chronic gastritis is a long term inflammation of the stomach lining, generally with degeneration of the gastric mucosa, but its causes are not well established. It is more common in women, and the incidence increases with age, excessive smoking, and ethanol use. Symptoms are nonspecific but may include flatulence, epigastric fullness after meals, diarrhea, and bleeding. Treatment is the same as for acute gastritis. Iron deficiency anemia and pernicious anemia may result from chronic gastritis. Treatment of symptoms with antacids, anticholinergics, and sedatives, as well as vitamin B_{12} if pernicious anemia is present, and elimination of possible causative or aggravating factors (e.g., aspirin use) comprise the usual therapeutic regimen.

Peptic ulcer disease is a broad term encompassing both gastric and duodenal ulcers. Although both types of ulcers produce a "break" in the gastric mucosa, the causes differ. With gastric ulcers, the ability of the gastric mucosa to protect and repair itself seems to be defective; in duodenal ulcers hypersecretion of gastric acid is responsible for the erosion of the gastric mucosa. Gastric colonization with *Helicobacter pylori,* a gram-negative bacilli, has been identified as a causative agent in clients with peptic ulcer disease that was not caused by the nonsteroidal antiinflammatory drugs. Treatment with various antibacterial combinations has resulted in healing and a low peptic ulcer recurrence rate (Abramowicz, 1994). *H. pylori* has been identified in nearly all persons with duodenal ulcer and also, in nearly 75% of persons with gastric ulcers (Berardi & Dunn-Kucharski, 1993).

Duodenal ulcers are more common than gastric ulcers, accounting for nearly 80% of all peptic ulcers. Duodenal ulcers usually occur more frequently in younger persons.

Overall, the reported incidence of peptic ulcers is much lower in females. In addition to antibacterial combination therapies, pharmacologic treatment of peptic ulcer disease may also include the use of antacids, H_2 receptor antagonists, and sucralfate. However, nondrug treatment (diet and lifestyle modifications) is equally important (see Chapter 41). Hereditary factors, use of some drugs (e.g., aspirin and corticosteroids), psychic factors, stress, and diet have been implicated in the development of peptic ulcer disease.

LIVER

Immediately under the diaphragm and above the stomach is the largest gland in the body, the liver. It weighs approximately 1.5 kg and is an extremely active and important organ that performs over 100 different functions.

The liver consists of two lobes composed of multitudes of lobules that function to remove toxins from the bloodstream, store nutrients such as iron and some vitamins, and secrete bile. Bile is transported via the hepatic ducts to the gallbladder for storage. In the intestine, bile aids in digestion, emulsification, and absorption of fat. Because it is normally alkaline, bile also functions to neutralize gastric acid in the duodenum.

Venous blood goes directly to the liver from the intestinal tract, so nutrients and absorbed drugs pass through the liver before reaching the systemic circulation. Thus the liver plays an active role in absorbing and metabolizing fats, carbohydrates, and proteins. It also stores vitamins A, B_{12}, and D and iron. Some drugs are taken up by the liver, released into the bile, and then excreted in the feces. Other drugs move from the bile into the small intestine, where they are reabsorbed and recirculated. Still other drugs are transformed by the liver and excreted in the urine. In all of these cases the liver metabolizes the drug to make it more water soluble. This biotransformation changes the parent compound to a metabolite that may have greater, lesser, or equal activity. Cytochrome P-450 in the liver is responsible for biotransformation. There are also drugs that pass through the body and are secreted unchanged in the urine.

Disorders affecting the liver. Viral hepatitis, Läennec's and postnecrotic cirrhosis, carcinoma, or chronic alcoholism causes damage to the liver and liver cell dysfunction.

GALLBLADDER

Lying on the undersurface of the liver is the gallbladder, a pear-shaped organ 7 to 10 cm long and 2.5 to 3.5 cm wide. The gallbladder can hold 30 to 50 ml of bile. It concentrates the bile and stores it until it is needed for digestion in the stomach and small intestine.

Disorders affecting the gallbladder. **Cholecystitis,** inflammation of the gallbladder, is often associated with the presence of gallstones (**cholelithiasis**). The stones lodge in the gallbladder neck or ducts, causing congestion and edema as bile builds up. This may be an acute or a chronic condition. Treatment of cholecystitis and cholelithiasis includes administration of analgesics, antispasmodics, and chenodeoxycholic acid. Malignant tumors of the gallbladder are infrequent.

PANCREAS

The pancreas is a gland about 15 to 20 cm long and 5 cm wide that weighs approximately 75 g. The gland has three major segments: the head (found in the curve of the duodenum), the body, and the tail (which touches or nearly touches the spleen). The role of the pancreas is twofold: the exocrine cells secrete the digestive enzymes found in pancreatic juice, and the endocrine cells help control carbohydrate metabolism with their production of glucagon and insulin.

Disorders affecting the pancreas. With the exception of diabetes mellitus, many pancreatic diseases have symptoms that are not readily diagnosed. Inflammation of the pancreas may be acute or chronic. Among the many causes are blockage of the pancreatic ducts, trauma to the pancreas, alcohol consumption, drug use, and tumors, cysts, or abscesses. Symptoms are nonspecific but ultimately include severe pain. Carcinoma of the pancreas is as difficult to diagnose as other pancreatic disorders.

SMALL INTESTINE

The small intestine is a coiled tube approximately 21 feet long. It consists of the duodenum, jejunum, and ileum. Within the small intestine the food bolus is thoroughly mixed with the digestive juices to complete the "breakdown" process. The intestinal mucosa then absorbs nutrients and drugs, which are filtered through the liver before entering the circulatory and lymphatic systems.

Disorders affecting the small intestine. Two disorders affecting the entire lower gastrointestinal tract are diarrhea and constipation. These are discussed in Chapters 11 and 41 along with the drugs used in their treatment.

Other disorders affecting the small intestine include obstruction, malabsorption syndrome, and blind loop syndrome. Symptomatic treatment is customary while the underlying causative factors are investigated.

LARGE INTESTINE

The cecum, colon, and rectum make up the large intestine. The distal 2.5 cm of the rectum is known as the anal canal. The large intestine is approximately 5 feet long. It completes the digestive and absorptive processes. The large intestine is involved mainly with water absorption (from 1800 to 3000 ml/day) and synthesis of vitamin K. The lining of the large intestine secretes mucus to coat the undigested residue and protect the bowel lining. The undigestible residue is expelled through the reflex action known as defecation.

Disorders affecting the large intestine. Diarrhea and constipation, discussed in Chapters 11 and 41, also affect the large intestine. Other disorders include diverticular disease, which has no specific therapy; ulcerative colitis, treated with lifestyle modifications, antidiarrheals, and steroids; carcinoma;

and irritable bowel syndrome. Hemorrhoids (varicosities of the external or internal hemorrhoidal veins) are common.

SUMMARY

Food sustains life and determines nutritional status, which contributes to an individual's state of health, levels of achievement, and resistance to and ability to handle disease. The primary function of the gastrointestinal tract is to provide the body cells with nutrients, electrolytes, and water through the processes of ingestion, digestion, and absorption of food and fluid and elimination of waste products and residue. Drugs affect the gastrointestinal tract by acting primarily on muscular and glandular tissue. Although some drugs are prescribed primarily for their effect on the gastrointestinal tract, the nurse needs to be aware that most drugs prescribed for other reasons also have gastrointestinal side effects and/or adverse reactions.

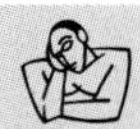

Critical Thinking

1. Imagine being a bolus of food progressing through the gastrointestinal tract; describe what the journey would be like.
2. Patty Smith has been diagnosed as having achlorhydria, a condition in which the stomach stops producing hydrochloric acid. What effect will this have on her digestion? On her red blood cell count?

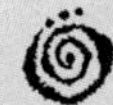

Collaborative Learning Activities

1. Discuss Critical Thinking questions in class. Each of the digestive organs will be represented by a student indicating its particular effect on the bolus of food.

BIBLIOGRAPHY

Abramowicz M (Ed.) (1994). Drugs for the treatment of peptic ulcers, *The Medical Letter* 36(927):65-67.

Anderson KN, et al. (Eds.) (1994). *Mosby's medical, nursing, & allied health dictionary* (4th ed.). St Louis: Mosby.

Berardi RR & Dunn-Kucharski VA (1993). Peptic ulcer disease: An update, *Amer Pharmacy NS*33(6):26-34.

Feldman M, et al. (1992). Treating ulcers and reflux: What's new? *Patient Care* 26(13):53.

McCance KL & Huether SE (1994). *Pathophysiology: The biological basis for disease in adults and children* (2nd ed). St Louis: Mosby.

Melmon KL, et al. (1992). *Clinical pharmacology: Basic principles in therapeutics* (3rd ed.). New York: McGraw-Hill.

Richter JE (1992). Gastroesophageal reflux: Diagnosis and management, *Hosp Practice* 27(1):39.

Thibodeau GA & Patton KT (1996). *Anatomy and physiology* (3rd ed.). St Louis: Mosby.

Van Wynsberghe D, Noback CR, & Carola R (1995). *Human anatomy and physiology* (3rd ed.). New York: McGraw-Hill.

Wingard Jr LB, et al. (1991). *Human physiology: Molecular-to-clinical.* St Louis: Mosby.

Chapter 41

Drugs Affecting the Gastrointestinal Tract

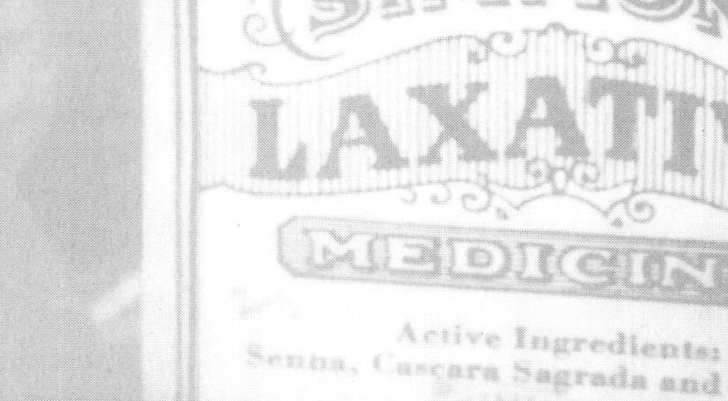

Chapter Focus

The gastrointestinal (GI) tract affects the overall health of the individual because it has the essential task of supplying necessary nutrients to fuel the physiologic processes of other vital organs, the brain, lungs, and heart, and the elimination of the body's wastes. Many GI disorders, too, are evidenced by pain, nausea, constipation, and diarrhea, which negatively affect the client's quality of life. The nurse then needs to be knowledgeable and skillful in the management of the pharmacologic therapeutic regimen related to the GI tract in order to assist clients toward self-management and optimal health. The following objectives and key terms are necessary for a good understanding of this chapter.

Key Terms

adsorbents (p. 722)
antiemetic (p. 699)
cathartic (p. 716)
chemoreceptor trigger zone (p. 699)
constipation (p. 715)
diarrhea (p. 715)
emetic center (p. 699)
laxatives (p. 716)

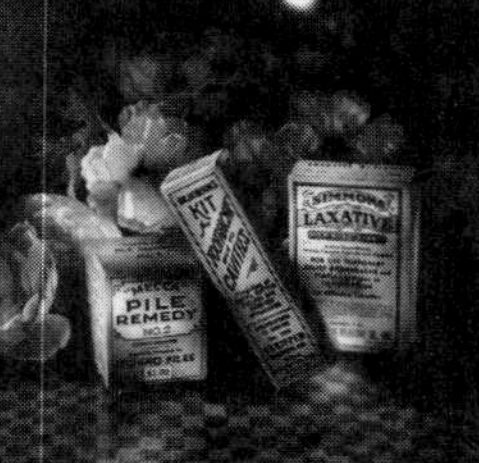

Key Drugs [▲]

cimetidine
metoclopramide
misoprostol
omeprazole
ondansetron

Objectives

1. Discuss the use and side effects of antacids.
2. List four drugs administered to promote digestion.
3. Differentiate the five classes of antiemetic medications and their sites of action.
4. Describe the emetic agents and their use.
5. Discuss the effect of H_2 receptor antagonists on gastric acid secretion.
6. Implement nursing management for the care of clients receiving agents affecting the gastrointestinal tract.

Drugs Affecting the Upper Gastrointestinal Tract

AGENTS THAT AFFECT THE MOUTH

Medications generally have little effect on the mouth. Good oral hygiene, which includes brushing properly after meals and at bedtime, flossing, and gum stimulation, has more influence on the tissues of the mouth than most medicines. Many mouth and throat preparations are available containing steroids, anesthetics, and antiseptics for various disorders of the oral cavity, including chapped lips, sun and fever blisters, inflammatory lesions, ulcerative lesions secondary to trauma, gingival lesions, teething pain, toothache, irritation caused by orthodontic appliances or dentures, and oral cavity abrasions.

Most agents that affect the mouth may be purchased over-the-counter.

Mouthwashes and Gargles

Mouthwashes and gargles are dilute aromatic solutions that contain a sweetener and an artificial coloring agent. They may also contain an antiseptic (e.g., alcohol, cetylpyridinium chloride, phenol), anesthetic (eugenol, clove oil), astringent (zinc chloride), and anticaries agent (sodium fluoride). Mouthwashes with a high alcohol content may be problematic in special populations (Box 41-1).

Although several products claim to contain ingredients that reduce plaque formation, clinical trials have demonstrated some success with volatile oils and cetylpyridinium chloride alone or in combination with domiphene bromide. Commercial products that contain at least one of these active ingredients include Cepacol (cetylpyridinium chloride), Listerine (volatile oils), and Scope (cetylpyridinium chloride and domiphene bromide). A detergent-type product to lessen plaque (Plax) is also available on the market. The client should be informed that these products do not replace good oral hygiene but instead are recommended as an adjunct to proper brushing and flossing of the teeth (Flynn, 1996).

Mouthwashes are often used for halitosis, or "bad breath," or as gargles to treat colds or sore throats. They are generally not considered effective for such problems. Mouthwashes may improve mouth odor briefly, but if such a problem persists, the underlying cause needs to be identified and treated, such as poor dental hygiene, various gum diseases, and many other potential causes.

Sore throats are usually caused by infection, most often viral rather than bacterial. Gargling cannot reach the site of infection, which is usually deep in the throat tissues. Sodium chloride solution (½ tsp of salt to an 8 oz glass of warm water) has been recommended for use as a gargle and mouthwash and is probably as effective as some of the remedies sold today.

> **BOX 41-1**
>
> **Alcoholic Mouthwash Warnings**
>
> *Pediatric alert*
>
> The leading mouthwashes usually contain from 14% to 27% alcohol. Because safety closures are not generally used with mouthwashes, parents of young children should be cautioned to store these products in a safe area, preferably a locked cabinet. The use of mouthwash in young children is not recommended since children often swallow the mouthwash rather than expectorate it.
>
> *Alcohol abuse*
>
> Alcohol-containing products such as mouthwashes and cough-cold preparations may be substituted by alcoholics when beverage alcohol is not readily available. The health care professional should be alert for ingestion abuse of alcohol-containing products in persons with a history of alcohol abuse (Katzung, 1992).

Oxygen-Releasing Agents

Hydrogen peroxide is a weak antibacterial agent used to clean wounds topically and orally. The antibacterial effect depends on the liberation of oxygen, which occurs when the peroxide comes in contact with the tissue enzyme catalase. The resulting effervescence (bubbling action) loosens pus and tissue debris, which helps reduce bacterial content. Hydrogen peroxide is usually used in a 1.5% to 3% solution for cleaning wounds or as a mouthwash. As a gargle, the 3% solution should be diluted with an equal amount of water before use.

A number of other oxygen-releasing products are commercially available. Perimax Perio Rinse (hydrogen peroxide) is used for treatment of canker sores, denture irritation, and irritation following orthodontic intervention. The solution is expectorated. Hydrogen peroxide gel (Peroxyl) is also available for minor mouth irritation and is applied and expectorated after use.

Fluoridated Mouthwash

A number of fluoride-containing preparations, including mouthwash (Fluorigard), toothpaste, tablets, and solutions, are available for use as anticaries agents. The exact mechanism of action of fluoride in preventing caries is not fully understood; however, fluoride ions appear to exchange for hydroxyl or citrate (anion) ions and then settle in the anionic space in the surface of the enamel (Marcus, 1996). This results in a harder outer layer of tooth enamel (a fluoridated hydroxyapatite) that is more resistant to demineralization. Fluoridated mouthwashes have been used in communities with both limited fluoridated and unfluoridated water supplies, and their use has been associated with a significant decrease (between 17% and 47%) in tooth decay (Flynn, 1996).

BOX 41-2

Fluoride Toxicity

Fluoride is capable of producing an acute toxic reaction that may be fatal if not treated promptly. A chronic toxic state resulting in mottling or discoloration of the tooth enamel and possible osteosclerosis has been reported. This effect may occur when excessive fluoride is consumed during childhood. In severe cases, the teeth appear as brown- to black-stained corroded areas. Fluoridated water supplies usually contain 1 ppm (part per million) of fluoride, which is accepted as a safe level that is effective in reducing the incidence of caries in permanent teeth. Health care professionals, particularly in primary health care settings, need to be aware of the amount of fluoride in their water supplies and to recommend and/or closely supervise the use of additional fluoride products by their clients. Fluoride supplements are recommended when community drinking water contains less than 0.7 ppm of fluoride (*USP DI*, 1996).

Mouthwashes are generally used once a day (rinsed for a minute and expectorated), preferably after brushing and flossing. The client should be taught to avoid taking anything by mouth for approximately 30 minutes after usage (Box 41-2).

Antiseptic Mouthwash

Phenol penetrates plaque and is a local anesthetic and antimicrobial agent. Chloraseptic mouthwash contains phenol and sodium phenolate. Teething preparations that provide temporary relief of sore gums caused by teething often contain phenol or benzocaine. Phenol or phenol-type compounds are also present in several OTC lozenges, liquids, and sprays for the treatment of sore throat. The liquid is diluted with equal parts of water or may be sprayed full strength.

Dentifrices

A dentifrice is a substance used to aid in cleaning teeth. Ordinary dentifrice contains one or more mild abrasives, a foaming agent, and flavoring materials made into a powder or paste (toothpaste) to be used as an aid in the mechanical cleansing of accessible parts of the teeth. Fluoride dentifrices are effective anticaries agents. These products carry the American Dental Association Council on Dental Therapeutics seal to indicate its endorsement.

Dentifrices are also available for the treatment of hypersensitive teeth, which usually occur from exposed root areas at the cement-enamel junction. This exposed area allows pain stimuli access to the nerve fibers in the pulp area. Dentists often suggest desensitizing dentifrices that contain potassium nitrate, such as Promise, Mint Sensodyne, or Denquel.

Oral Antifungal Agents

clotrimazole [kloe trim' a zole] (Mycelex)
ketoconazole [kee toe koe' na zole] (Nizoral)
nystatin [nye stat' in] (Mycostatin, Nilstat)

Clotrimazole, ketoconazole, and nystatin inhibit synthesis of sterols in the fungal wall, increasing permeability of the cell membrane, which results in the loss of important cellular contents. Ketoconazole and clotrimazole also inhibit oxidative enzyme activity, which may increase intracellular hydrogen peroxide to toxic levels and thus contribute to the destruction of the fungal cells and their contents. In addition, they inhibit fungal synthesis of triglycerides and phospholipids. These agents are indicated for the treatment of candidiasis or fungal infections caused by *Candida* species. Fluconazole (Diflucan) and itraconazole (Sporanox) are more potent drugs used to treat candida infections. Table 41-1 lists dosage and administration information.

■ Nursing Management
Oral Antifungal Agent Therapy

See also Chapter 60, Antifungal and Antiviral Drugs, for information related to systemic use of antifungal agents.

Assessment. Inspect the oropharynx using a tongue depressor and a flashlight. Ask the client to remove any partial or complete dentures. Poorly fitting dentures can be a source of inflammation. Clients who have AIDS or are taking antineoplastic or immunosuppressive drugs, such as steroids, are particularly at risk for oral candidiasis. Normal mucosa is pink, although dark-skinned clients may have bluish or patch-type pigmented mucosa. Candidiasis will present as cream-colored or bluish white patches of exudate on the tongue, mouth, or pharynx that reveal bloody engorgement when scraped. A culture of the fungus may be obtained before antifungal therapy begins.

Nursing diagnosis. Clients receiving oral antifungal agents for candidiasis may experience altered mucous membranes related to the underlying condition and the ineffectiveness of the oral antifungal drug or altered comfort related to the gastrointestinal effects of the drug evidenced by nausea or vomiting, diarrhea, and, perhaps, abdominal cramping.

Implementation

Monitoring. Inspect and document daily the size and condition of the affected areas of the mouth, using a tongue blade and flashlight.

Intervention. Brush teeth or have the client brush teeth and cleanse the area carefully before each dose is administered. For infants and dependent clients, gently swab the medication on the oral mucosa. Clients with partial or full dentures will need to soak them nightly in the oral suspension to eliminate the fungus.

When administering the oral suspension, shake well to ensure consistency in dosing. Protect the suspension

TABLE 41-1 Selected oral antifungal agents: dosage and administration

Drug	Adults	Children
clotrimazole troches	Dissolve one 10 mg lozenge slowly orally five times daily for approximately 2 weeks, longer in immunosuppressed individuals	Same as adult
ketoconazole	200 mg to 400 mg daily	Same as adult
nystatin		
tablets	500,000 to 1 million units orally three times daily	Children 5 yr and older: 500,000 units four times daily
suspension	400,000-600,000 units four times daily	Premature/low birth weight infants: 100,000 units four times daily Older infants: 200,000 units four times daily Older children: see adult dose
lozenges	Adult & children 5 yr & older; 1 to 2 lozenges dissolved in mouth 4 or 5 times a day up to 2 weeks	

from freezing. When preparing the oral suspension from powder, shake well and use immediately, since it contains no preservatives.

To improve retention within the mouth, nystatin can be administered in the form of flavored frozen water on a stick. The nystatin vaginal tablet may also be used as a lozenge since its slow rate of dissolution prolongs contact with the oral mucosa.

Education. Instruct the client in good oral hygiene techniques. Inform the client that a yearly dental examination is recommended.

When using the oral suspension forms of the antifungals, instruct the client to swish the medication around in the mouth and maintain contact with the mucosa as long as possible before swallowing. The client may also gargle the solution. Provide a careful explanation to the client using the troche form (clotrimazole) or lozenge form (nystatin) that it is to be dissolved slowly (15 to 30 minutes) in the mouth. It is not to be chewed or swallowed whole. The client is to swallow the saliva. The troche may be cut in half to facilitate administration. Avoid the use of troches or lozenges with children under 5 years of age because they may be unable to safely manage that form of the medication.

Instruct the client to continue the medicine for the full time of prescription and report to the prescriber if symptoms persist. Inform the client that therapy is continued for 48 hours after symptoms have disappeared to prevent relapse.

Before an initial course of antineoplastic chemotherapy, instruct the client to consult a dentist to complete any care needed to help prevent oral complications.

Evaluation. The client will experience normal colored, intact oropharyngeal mucous membranes.

Saliva Substitutes

Saliva substitutes (Orex, Xero-Lube, Moi-stir, Salivart) are used for the relief of dry mouth and throat in xerostomia. They are available as solutions in squirt bottles and as pump or aerosol sprays. They contain electrolytes (potassium phosphate, magnesium chloride, potassium chloride, calcium, and sodium), sodium fluoride, sorbitol, and carboxyymethylcellulose as the base.

Drugs Used to Treat Mouth Blistering

Acute and chronic diseases contribute to mouth blistering and erosions. Acute viral diseases such as herpes simplex, herpes zoster, and varicella have previously been treated only symptomatically. Acyclovir (Zovirax), an antiviral agent, is effective against herpes simplex virus and varicella zoster virus, the viruses associated with skin manifestations. It acts to reduce viral shedding, time to crusting, duration of local pain, and severity of symptoms (*AHFS,* 1996). Acyclovir is available in topical, oral, and parenteral dosage forms. It and other antivirals are covered in Chapter 60.

Mouth lesions or blistering (acute or chronic) may be caused by local irritation, medications, radiation, dental manipulations, or systemic disease. To properly treat, one must first identify the causative factor and then institute appropriate treatment.

DRUGS THAT AFFECT THE STOMACH

Conditions of the stomach requiring drug therapy include hyperacidity, hypoacidity, ulcer disease, nausea, vomiting, and hypermotility. Some of the drugs used for these conditions are not unique in their treatment of gastric dysfunction but are members of other major groups of drugs, such as anticholinergic preparations, antihistamines, and antidepressants.

Drugs Used to Treat Gastric Hyperacidity

Antacids

Antacids are chemical compounds that buffer or neutralize hydrochloric acid in the stomach and thereby increase the gastric pH. The major ingredients in antacids include aluminum salts, calcium carbonate, magnesium salts, and sodium bicarbonate, alone or in combination. Most antacids may be purchased as over-the-counter preparations.

Traditionally, the antacids have been termed nonsystemic or systemic. Nonsystemic indicates the almost negligible amount of drug absorbed into the circulation; activity occurs only locally within the gastrointestinal tract. The nonsystemic metal ion, however, is absorbed to some degree. The aluminum ion is absorbed the most and magnesium the least; calcium is absorbed slightly more than magnesium. Long-term chronic use of antacids or their use in the presence of impaired renal function may result in increased adverse effects from metal ion absorption, especially of calcium carbonate or magnesium hydroxide.

Antacids are indicated for the relief of symptoms associated with hyperacidity related to the diagnosis of peptic ulcer, gastritis, gastric esophageal reflux disease (GERD), gastric hyperacidity, heartburn, or hiatal hernia. Antacids generally have a rapid onset of action. When administered in a fasting state, the antacid effect lasts from 20 to 40 minutes. If administered 1 hour after meals, though, the effects may be extended for up to 3 hours. A small amount of absorbable antacid is absorbed (15% to 30%), but the remainder is broken down via the digestive process and excreted via the feces. For side effects/adverse reactions of antacids, see Table 11-2.

Altered drug solubility, stability, and absorption. Many drugs are either weak acids or weak bases, and the pH of the stomach is an important factor in their absorption. Drugs that are weak acids are nonionized in the acidic environment of the stomach, are lipid soluble, and are absorbed by simple diffusion across the gastric mucosal cells. The administration of an antacid either with a weak acidic drug or shortly before or after its administration will raise the pH of the stomach contents, causing the formation of a more ionized drug that will not be absorbed to the degree the nonionized, lipid-soluble form was absorbed. A weakly basic drug is absorbed in a more alkaline medium. Changes in pH modify drug solubility and stability, which also affect absorption. Consider then that antacids will affect the absorption of most drugs to some degree.

Drugs that are weak bases include morphine sulfate, quinine, pseudoephedrine, antihistamines, amphetamines, theophylline, tricyclic antidepressants, and quinidine. Examples of weak acids are isoniazid, barbiturates, nalidixic acid, nonsteroidal antiinflammatory agents, sulfonamides, salicylates, nitrofurantoin, and coumarins.

Additional drug interactions. Antacids have been reported to reduce the absorption of many drugs, such as quinolone antibiotics, tetracyclines, ketoconazole, sucralfate, digoxin; therefore the nurse should carefully schedule the majority of medications hours apart from the administration time for an antacid. Close monitoring for both therapeutic response and possible side effects is also recommended. For dosage and administration, see Chapter 11.

■ Nursing Management

Antacid Therapy

Although antacids are considered to be over-the-counter preparations, and so are discussed in Chapter 11, these medications are commonly administered by nurses in a variety of health care settings. In addition, the nurse is ideally placed within the health care delivery system to offer clients instruction on the safe use of antacids as OTC medications.

Assessment. A baseline assessment of the client receiving antacids should include the client's discomfort or pain and nutritional status. Sensitivity to antacids should be determined.

All antacids should be carefully considered with the client with renal function impairment. However, clients with renal failure receiving magnesium-containing antacids are particularly at risk of hypermagnesemia. If such antacids are given to clients with renal dysfunction, low doses (50 mEq magnesium/day) should be administered under close monitoring by a health care provider. Antacids that contain magnesium may also cause diarrhea, so caution should be used with any condition that might be worsened by diarrhea, such as ulcerative colitis, diverticulitis, or with the client with an ostomy. On the other hand, aluminum- and calcium-containing antacids tend to be constipating and so should be administered with caution to clients with constipation or hemorrhoids, which might be aggravated. Clients with hypercalcemia should not receive calcium-containing antacids. Cautious use of antacids is recommended if the client has symptoms of appendicitis, undiagnosed gastrointestinal bleeding, and intestinal obstruction because the laxative or constipating effects may worsen the condition. Aluminum-containing antacids may exacerbate Alzheimer's disease and calcium ones may effect hypothyroidism and sarcoidosis. Consult with the prescriber about low sodium antacids for clients having sodium restrictions.

Review the client's current medication regimen keeping in mind that antacids have an effect on most oral forms of drugs. In particular, consider the following significant drug interactions that may occur when antacids are given with the drugs listed below.

Drug	Possible effect and management
fluoroquinolones	Aluminum- and magnesium-containing antacids may reduce absorption of these drugs; advise taking fluoroquinolones at least 2 hours before or 2 hours after antacid for norfloxacin (Chibroxin, Noroxin) and ofloxacin (Floxin); 6 hours after antacid for ciprofloxacin (Cipro) and lomefloxacin (Maxaquin) and 8 hours after antacid for enoxacin (Penetrex).

ion-exchange resin (e.g., sodium polystyrene sulfonate)	When calcium- or magnesium-containing antacids are given concurrently with this agent, neutralization of gastric acid may be impaired. The binding of the calcium and magnesium may result in anion absorption and systemic alkalosis. Avoid oral administration of this combination.
isoniazid (INH)	Aluminum antacids interfere with the absorption of isoniazid. Separate the administration of these drugs by at least an hour or administer a non–aluminum-containing antacid to prevent this interaction.
ketoconazole (Nizoral)	Increased gastric pH may decrease absorption of ketoconazole. Advise clients to take antacids at least 3 hours after ketoconazole.
mecamylamine (Inversine)	Effects of mecamylamine may be prolonged because an alkaline urine decreases its excretion. Concurrent administration should be avoided.
methenamine (Mandelamine, Hiprex)	An alkaline urine may decrease methenamine's effectiveness by prohibiting its conversion to formaldehyde. Concurrent administration is not recommended. Because urine alkalinization may occur with antacids, monitor client for increased risk of crystalluria and nephrotoxicity.
tetracyclines, oral	Antacids may combine with tetracyclines, decreasing their absorption in the gastrointestinal tract. Advise clients to take antacids at least 3 to 4 hours before or after tetracycline.

Nursing diagnosis. With the administration of antacids, the client may experience pain related to the underlying condition and the ineffectiveness of the antacid or noncompliance related to their chalky taste. Other concerns for the client are related to the type of antacid administered. With aluminum- or calcium-containing antacids, constipation may be the alteration of bowel function, whereas diarrhea may result from magnesium-containing antacids. Excessive use of calcium- and sodium bicarbonate-containing antacids may place the client at risk for the complication of metabolic alkalosis (mood/mental changes; muscle twitching, decreased respiratory rate, unpleasant taste, fatigue). With long-term use of aluminum- and sodium bicarbonate–containing antacids, hypercalcemia associated with milk-alkali syndrome (headache, urinary frequency, anorexia, nausea/vomiting, fatigue) and osteomalacia/osteoporosis caused by phosphate depletion (bone pain; wrist or ankle joint swelling) may occur.

Implementation

Monitoring. Assess epigastric discomfort at the time of each dose and record the client's progress. Evaluation of antacid therapy is important. The client's subjective response to antacid therapy and the nurse's objective observations (e.g., frequency with which the client takes the antacid) can help determine the effectiveness of therapy.

Note the frequency and consistency of stools. If diarrhea occurs, it may be advantageous to change to another antacid, such as magnesium hydroxide with magnesium trisilicate or aluminum hydroxide. If constipation occurs, a magnesium hydroxide antacid or an increase in the intake of bran and roughage in the diet may be instituted.

Monitor clients undergoing long-term aluminum antacid therapy regularly for serum phosphate levels because phosphate depletion may result in osteoporosis and serum calcium levels for milk-alkali syndrome.

Intervention. The scheduling of dosing of antacid therapy is important. Antacids given immediately after meals will delay gastric emptying and the buffering effect. When given at 1 and 3 hours after meals and at bedtime, the gastric pH remains at about 3 throughout the day. Because of their ability to interact with numerous medications, scheduling in relation to other medications should be considered. Administer antacids 1 hour before or 2 hours after digoxin, tetracyclines, phenothiazines, and all enteric-coated medications. However, antacids combined with ibuprofen, indomethacin, phenylbutazone, potassium chloride supplements, reserpine, sulindac, and tolmetin can help to reduce the gastric distress that these drugs can cause.

Shake liquid preparations vigorously before administration to achieve a uniform suspension. When administering antacids via a nasogastric tube, assess the placement and patency of the tube before giving the medication and follow the dose with sufficient water to clear the tube. Refrigerate antacids to make them more palatable. (Do not freeze.)

Do not administer calcium carbonate antacids with milk, milk products, or other foods or vitamin supplements high in vitamin D, since milk-alkali syndrome may occur.

Education. Discuss the sodium content and side effects of various antacids with the client (see Table 11-2 for side/adverse effects). Inform clients that antacids differ in their sodium content, which can be significant for clients who are on low-sodium diets or who take antihypertensive drugs or diuretics. Instruct clients with hypertensive, cardiac, or renal disease to avoid antacids containing sodium, particularly if antacids are used frequently.

Inform clients that liquid antacids have superior neutralizing properties compared with tablets. However, clients who must frequently take liquid antacids may lose their desire for food or drink. For this reason chewable tablets may be advised. Instruct clients taking chewable antacid tablets to chew or pulverize the tablets thoroughly. The tablets may not mix well with water. A full glass of water will facilitate the action of the antacid tablets.

Stress adherence to antacid therapy schedules. Allow clients to take their own antacids while they are hospitalized to encourage effective management of the therapeutic regimen. Caution clients about side effects, and instruct them to consult their prescriber if these occur. Alert clients to check the expiration dates of the antacids, since the effectiveness of antacids decreases with age. Alert clients to carefully check the name when purchasing OTC antacids. Names may be similar (Mylanta versus Mylanta II), but dosage requirements will differ. Advise clients who self-medicate with antacids for recurring gastrointestinal symptoms to seek medical care, since they are treating the symptoms rather than the cause of the problem. Since antacids are OTC drugs and there is no medically supervised restriction, clients may abuse or misuse antacids through self-medication.

Help clients to identify sources of gastric discomfort, such as overeating, smoking, tension, anxiety, or other emotional stress, since this may teach them to avoid the causes of discomfort and eliminate the need for antacid therapy.

Evaluation. The client receiving antacid therapy will experience decreased discomfort or absence of pain without adverse effects (i.e., constipation or diarrhea) of antacid therapy.

Digestants

Digestants are drugs that promote the process of digestion in the gastrointestinal tract. Problems with digestion may be caused by a deficiency of hydrochloric acid, digestive substances, enzymes, or bile salts; organic disease states (stomach cancer, pernicious anemia, cholecystectomy); or, possibly, a reaction to emotional situations or stress.

Digestive enzymes secreted by the mouth, stomach, small intestine, pancreas, and liver are necessary for the digestion of food. Pepsin is the stomach enzyme that reduces protein to smaller particles. It can be given alone or in combination with a hydrochloric acid source in hypochlorhydric or achlorhydric clients.

Hydrochloric acid keeps the gastric pH level below 4 and protects the proteolytic activity of pepsin. A pH level of 1.5 to 2.5 is usually the optimal range. Pepsin is not considered a critical enzyme because proteolytic enzymes released from the pancreas and intestine cause the same effects.

pancreatin [pan' kree a tin] (Entozyme, Donnazyme)
pancrelipase [pan kre li' pase] (Pancrease, Viokase)

The pancreas releases digestive enzymes and bicarbonate into the duodenum to help in the digestion of fats, carbohydrates and proteins. Bicarbonate neutralizes acid and thus helps to protect the enzymes from both acid and pepsin. When acid chyme enters the duodenum, vagal stimulation regulates pancreatic secretion, so that enzyme replacement therapy may be necessary for clients who have had vagal fibers surgically severed or had surgical procedures that cause food to bypass the duodenum.

Both pancreatin and pancrelipase contain the enzymes amylase, trypsin, and lipase, but pancrelipase has greater enzyme activity in the neutral or alkaline media of the gastrointestinal tract. It has about 12 times the lipolytic and 4 times the proteolytic and amylolytic activities of pancreatin. These agents are not interchangeable because they are not bioequivalent.

Both pancreatin and pancrelipase aid in the digestion and absorption of fats, carbohydrates, and triglycerides. In addition, replacement therapy is usually necessary in exocrine pancreatic enzyme deficiency states, chronic pancreatitis, cystic fibrosis, pancreatic tumors, pancreatic obstruction, and pancreatectomy.

Both products are available in enteric-coated capsules to avoid destruction in the stomach. The enteric-coated microsphere formulation resists gastric inactivation, so enzymes reach the duodenum to hydrolyze fats into glycerol and fatty acids, proteins into proteases, and starch into dextrins and sugars. The usual adult pancreatin dose is 1 to 2 tablets with meals or snacks, while the dose for pancrelipase is one to three capsules or tablets or one or two packets before or with meals or snacks. Dosage should be adjusted as necessary. In extreme deficiency the dosage interval may be changed to hourly if no nausea or diarrhea develops.

The side/adverse effects of pancreatin and pancrelipase include nausea, abdominal cramps, and loose stool.

■ Nursing Management

Digestant Therapy

Assessment. A baseline assessment should include the client's discomfort levels associated with eating, bowel status, and serum and urine uric acid levels. Treatment with pancrelipase is contraindicated if the client has acute pancreatitis or a sensitivity to pork protein, pancrelipase, or pancreatin. Consideration should be given to clients whose religious beliefs prohibit the use of pork products.

Review the client's medications for drug interactions. The most significant drug interaction occurs when calcium and magnesium antacids negate pancrelipase enzyme action. Serum iron response to oral iron therapy is decreased by pancreatic extracts.

Nursing diagnosis. The client receiving digestant therapy may experience altered comfort (nausea and abdominal cramps); altered mucous membranes (oral) related to enzymatic digestion of mucous membranes when tablet dosage form is held in the mouth; altered bowel elimination (diarrhea); and potential complications related to an allergic reaction (rash), sensitization induced by inadvertent inhalation of powder dosage form (dyspnea, nasal congestion, wheezing), hyperuricemia, or hyperuricouria.

Implementation

Monitoring. Monitor for discomfort associated with eating, diarrhea, irritated mouth, respiratory status, and elevated serum and urine uric acid levels.

Intervention. Because pancreatin is inactivated by gastric pepsin and acid pH, cimetidine or antacids (except for those containing calcium and magnesium) may be prescribed to be taken with it. For children or adults who cannot swallow the capsules or tablets, sprinkle the powder from the opened capsule or the powdered form on food. Avoid inhalation of capsule contents.

Education. Instruct the client to swallow enteric-coated tablets whole; do not crush or allow them to be chewed or irritation of the mouth may occur. Instruct the client on the rationale for taking the pancreatic enzyme preparations. Also instruct client not to stop taking the medication without prescriber approval. Urge the client to adhere to the prescribed diet, since the dosage for pancrelipase is individualized and determined by the client's indigestion and malabsorption and the fat content of the diet.

If capsules need to be opened to be administered, advise the client to be careful not to spill the contents on hands or to inhale them, since this substance is very irritating to nasal membranes, respiratory tract, and skin. If the capsules contain enteric-coated spheres, they should be taken with liquids or small amounts of foods which do not need chewing. Tablet forms should be followed with 1 or 2 mouthfuls of food to decrease the risk of esophageal irritation, particularly in recumbent clients. If side effects such as nausea, abdominal cramping, and diarrhea occur, have the client contact the prescriber.

Evaluation. The client receiving digestant therapy will experience normal digestion and effectively manage the digestant therapy without experiencing any side/adverse effects.

Emetic (Vomiting) Reflex

The vomiting or **emetic center** located in the medulla oblongata may be stimulated by smells, strong emotion, severe pain, increased intracranial pressure, labyrinthine disturbances (motion sickness), endocrine disturbances, toxic reactions to drugs, gastrointestinal disease, radiation treatments, and chemotherapy (Figure 41-1). The stimuli may involve neurotransmitters and vagal and/or sympathetic afferent nerve transmission.

The **chemoreceptor trigger zone** (CTZ) is an area of sensory nerve cells activated by chemical stimuli that relays messages to the emetic center. It has various receptors (serotonin, dopamine, opiate) that detect irritating drugs or toxins in the blood to stimulate or mediate emesis. The chemoreceptor trigger zone itself is not able to induce vomiting.

Since the CTZ is located close to the respiratory center in the brain, it is difficult to completely control vomiting initiated from this site without affecting respiration. The cerebral cortex area is involved in anticipatory nausea and vomiting, a conditioned response caused by a stimulus connected with a previous unpleasant experience. For example, unpleasant memories, such as a client receiving cancer chemotherapy that has resulted in vomiting, might vomit at the sight of the hospital, doctor, or nurse, even before treatment is given (Koda-Kimble & Young, 1995). See the discussion in Chapter 56, Antineoplastic Chemotherapy.

If the emetic center is activated by stimuli, it sends impulses (via efferent nerves) to the diaphragm, stomach muscles, esophagus, and salivary glands, resulting in vomiting.

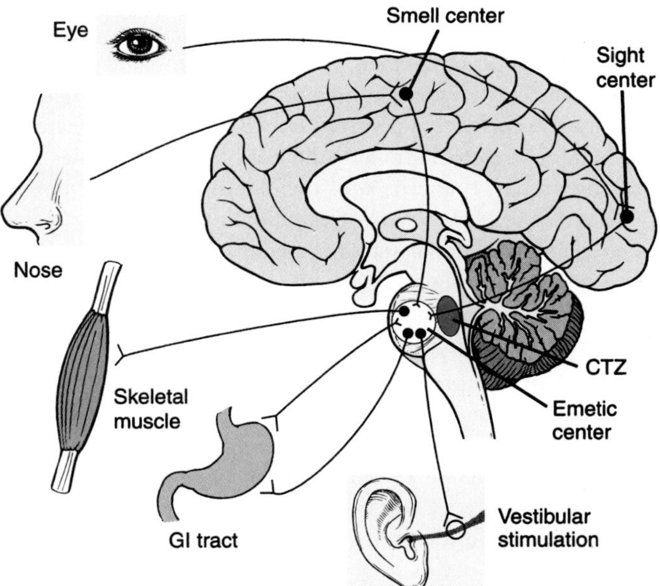

Figure 41-1 CTZ (chemoreceptor trigger zone) and other sites activating the emetic center.

Antiemetics

Antiemetics are drugs given to prevent or relieve nausea and vomiting. Control of vomiting is important and at times may be difficult. Numerous preparations have been used, but effective treatment usually depends on treating the cause. The primary pathways for the vomiting reflex are:

1. Higher CNS or cerebral cortex stimulation
   a. Emotional or anticipatory vomiting
2. Peripheral or central nerve transmission secondary to body tissue or organ alterations
   a. Irritation of GI tract
   b. Increased intracranial pressure
   c. Vestibular stimulation
3. Stimulation from the chemoreceptor trigger zone
   a. Toxins circulating in blood

Antiemetics may exert their effects on the vomiting center, the cerebral cortex, the CTZ, or the vestibular apparatus (Box 41-3).

The neurotransmitters and pharmacologic agents used to control and/or prevent nausea and vomiting include:

1. *Neurotransmitter:* dopamine (D_2) receptors located in the GI tract and CTZ.

   Pharmacologic agents: Phenothiazines, such as chlorpromazine (Thorazine) and promethazine (Phenergan), and metoclopramide (Reglan) are dopamine antagonists. They act on the chemoreceptor trigger zone, GI tract, and other dopamine neurotransmitter areas. These are the most effective antiemetics and often the drugs of choice.
2. *Neurotransmitter:* acetylcholine (ACh) receptors in vestibular and vomiting center. Overstimulation of the labyrinth (inner ear) results in the nausea and vomiting of motion sickness.

   Pharmacologic agents: Anticholinergics, such as scopolamine, reduce the excitability of labyrinth receptors, depress conduction in the vestibular cerebellar pathways, or prevent impulses from stimulating the CTZ.
3. *Neurotransmitter:* histamine (H_1) receptors in vestibular and vomiting centers.

   Pharmacologic agents: H_1 antihistamines affect neural labyrinth pathways; examples include cyclizine (Marezine), dimenhydrinate (Dramamine), and diphenhydramine (Benadryl). Many antihistamines have anticholinergic side effects (see #2 above).

BOX 41-3

Proposed Sites of Action for Antiemetic Drugs

Proposed sites	Drugs
Emetic center	anticholinergic antihistamines thiethylperazine maleate*
Chemoreceptor trigger zone	benzquinamide hydrochloride butyrophenones dephenidol hydrochloride* metoclopramide* phenothiazine thiethylperazine maleate* trimethobenzamide HCl
Cerebral cortex	cannabinoids (THC, nabilone, dronabinol) diazepam lorazepam scopolamine* antihistamines
Peripheral	diphenidol hydrochloride* metoclopramide* scopolamine*
Unknown	corticosteroids

*Dual action.

4. *Neurotransmitter:* serotonin ($5HT_3$) receptors in GI tract, CTZ, and vomiting centers (Lichter, 1993).

   Pharmacologic agents: Ondansetron (Zofran) and granisetron (Kytril) are selective serotonin receptor antagonists approved for prevention of nausea and vomiting induced by cancer chemotherapy.
5. *Miscellaneous agents:* Antacids relieve gastric irritation; diphenidol (Vontrol) acts on the vestibular apparatus, and benzquinamide (Emete-Con) acts on the CTZ to reduce nausea and vomiting. Steroids (dexamethasone, methylprednisolone) and cannabinoids (nabilone, THC) are also used.

Cancer-chemotherapy–induced vomiting. Vomiting from cancer chemotherapy can be serious enough to limit the dosages of chemotherapeutic agents given to a client. Since antiemetics are usually more effective in preventing vomiting than they are in treating it, they should be administered prophylactically before chemotherapy administration. Also, chemotherapy-induced vomiting may require several antiemetic agents with different sites of action for effectiveness—for example, metoclopramide (Reglan) and lorazepam (Ativan), metoclopramide and dexamethasone, or prochlorperazine (Compazine) and dexamethasone. A number of persons respond well to the serotonin receptor antagonists alone if properly scheduled according to the manufacturer's recommendations (see the Nursing Research box below).

Nursing Research

Antiemetic drug therapy

Despite recent advances, antineoplastic drug–induced nausea and vomiting remain a serious problem for clients with cancer. Not only can these effects be physically harmful, but they may also directly contribute to client noncompliance. It has been suggested that up to 50% of clients with potentially curable cancers refuse treatment and/or are noncompliant in some treatment programs.

New antiemetic agents are being evaluated with the hope of decreasing the incidence of nausea and vomiting associated with cancer chemotherapy on a continuing basis. However, none of the single antiemetic agents currently being used block a combination of receptor sites. In a randomized open crossover study, Plezia et al (1990) examined the antiemetic efficacy of a five-drug antiemetic regimen consisting of metoclopramide, dexamethasone, diazepam, diphenhydramine, and thiethylperazine compared with one of high dose metoclopramide. Thirteen clients treated with cisplatin combination chemotherapy regimens were evaluated. However, the study was terminated before accrual of the planned number of individuals because of the statistically significant difference in efficacy between treatments found at interim analysis. The duration of nausea and number of vomiting episodes on the day of chemotherapy were significantly less ($p<0.01$) after receiving the five-drug combination. After receiving the five-drug regimen, 77% of the clients did not experience any episodes of vomiting on day 1, and 8% of clients had only one episode. In contrast, only 31% of clients treated with high dose metoclopramide did not have any episodes of vomiting on day 1, and 61% of the clients had five or more episodes. None of the clients treated with the five-drug regimen required additional antiemetic administration. Although both regimens were, in general, well tolerated, when given the choice of continuing antiemetic therapies, 92% of the clients preferred the five-drug antiemetic combination.

Critical thinking questions

- How could a combination of drugs be expected to function more effectively than a single agent? Although the client is receiving a greater number of drugs, why might combination therapy be safer for the client?
- What ethical considerations might have contributed to the termination of this study before the accrual of the planned number of participants?

From Plezia et al (1990).

■ Nursing Management
Antiemetic Therapy

Assessment. A baseline assessment should include allergy history in relation to the antiemetic, fluid balance data, the degree of nausea reported by the client, and the frequency of vomiting. Do not give antiemetics until the underlying cause of nausea has been established. For example, overdosage of drugs or increased intracranial pressure may cause nausea.

Nursing diagnosis. With the administration of antiemetic therapy, the client may experience: altered comfort (nausea) related to the underlying health condition, chemotherapy, and/or ineffectiveness of the antiemetic agent; fluid volume deficit or altered nutrition, less than required, related to vomiting secondary to chemotherapy and ineffectiveness of the antiemetic drug; or altered sleep pattern (drowsiness).

Implementation

Monitoring. Monitor for nausea and vomiting, general sense of well-being, and fluid balance.

Intervention. Give antiemetics, such as prochlorperazine maleate (Compazine), thiethylperazine maleate (Torecan), and metoclopramide (Reglan), before the administration of chemotherapeutic agents. The time of administration of the antiemetic agent will depend on the chemotherapeutic regimen prescribed. If antiemetic therapy is unavailable or cannot be given, or to support the administration of antiemetics, provide a quiet environment, make the client comfortable, and give ice chips, a carbonated beverage, or, if allowed, hot tea to drink.

Education. Instruct the client that any hypersensitivity to these drugs necessitates discontinuance of the drug and reporting the effects to the prescriber.

Most antiemetics cause drowsiness as a side effect. Caution clients against performing hazardous tasks until the effects of the drug have subsided. Also caution clients against combining antiemetics with alcohol or any CNS depressants. The CNS depressant effects of the drug can be potentiated when these drugs are combined.

Vomiting during pregnancy or as the result of cancer chemotherapeutic agents can cause serious electrolyte imbalance and a nutritional deficit. Instruct the pregnant client to take small frequent meals or small nutritional snacks between meals.

Evaluation. The client receiving antiemetic therapy will experience diminished or no nausea and vomiting.

▲ **metoclopramide** [met oh kloe' pra mide] (Reglan, Maxeran♣)
cisapride [sis' a pride] (Propulsid)

Metoclopramide has both a central and peripheral action in preventing or relieving nausea and emesis. Centrally it blocks dopamine receptors in the CTZ while peripherally it increases motility of the upper GI tract, increases peristalsis, and overcomes the immobility, dilation, and reverse motility that occurs with the vomiting reflex. Cisapride is chemically similar to metoclopramide although it lacks any dopamine receptor activity. Cisapride has been postulated to increase acetylcholine release from postganglionic nerves located in the myenteric plexus, which decreases esophageal reflux; it also enhances gastric and duodenal emptying by increased contractility. Therefore it increases transit in both the small and large intestine.

Metoclopramide is used for diabetic gastroparesis, gastroesophageal reflux, and parenterally for the prevention of nausea and vomiting secondary to emetogenic cancer chemotherapeutic agents, radiation, and opioid medications. It is also used as an adjunct for GI radiologic examination because it hastens barium's transit through the upper GI tract by its stimulation of gastric emptying and acceleration of intestinal transit. Parenteral metoclopramide may be used to facilitate intestinal intubation. Cisapride is used to prevent or treat, gastroesophageal reflux (*USP DI*, 1996).

Metoclopramide onset of action is ½ to 1 hour after oral administration, 10 to 15 minutes after an intramuscular dose, and within 3 minutes after an intravenous dose. Duration of action is 1 to 2 hours; half-life is 4 to 6 hours. It is metabolized by the liver and excreted in the kidneys. Most common side effects include diarrhea, sleepiness, restlessness, and increased weakness. Extrapyramidal (parkinsonian) effects, hypotension, hypertension, tachycardia, and agranulocytosis are rare adverse effects reported.

Cisapride onset of action is ½ to 1 hour; peak serum concentration is reached in 1 to 2 hours; and half-life is 7 to 10 hours. It is metabolized by the liver and excreted by the kidneys and in feces. The side/adverse effects of cisapride include stomach cramps, constipation or diarrhea, headache, nausea, and drowsiness. Convulsions, a rare adverse effect, have also been reported.

Metoclopramide. To treat diabetic gastroparesis or gastroesophageal reflux in an adult, the oral dose is 10 mg 30 minutes before each meal and at bedtime (up to four times daily). Check package insert for further instructions. The IV dose is 10 mg as a single dose. Antiemetic adult dose (for chemotherapy-induced emesis) is 2 mg/kg by IV infusion 30 minutes before chemotherapy; the dose may be repeated every 2 to 3 hours as necessary.

The oral pediatric dose is 0.1 to 0.2 mg/kg per dose 30 minutes before meals and at bedtime to increase peristalsis. See current references for additional dosing recommendations.

Cisapride. Adult dose to prevent gastroesophageal reflux is 10 mg PO twice a day, before breakfast and at bedtime. To treat reflux, the dose is 5 to 10 mg 3 to 4 times daily, 15 minutes before meals and at bedtime. Pediatric dose is 0.15 to 0.3 mg/kg body weight PO 3 or 4 times daily before meals.

■ Nursing Management
Metoclopramide and Cisapride Therapy

In addition to the previous discussion of nursing management of antiemetics, consider the following for metoclopramide and cisapride therapy.

Assessment. Do not give metoclopramide or cisapride to clients with epilepsy (isolated seizures have been reported) or to those in whom stimulation of gastrointestinal motility is hazardous (e.g., those with gastrointestinal hemorrhage, perforation, or mechanical obstruction) because these conditions may be aggravated by increased bowel motility. Clients with liver or renal dysfunction may have a decreased clearance of these agents. Extrapyramidal effects may be increased if metoclopramide is administered to clients with chronic renal failure. With metoclopramide, clients with pheochromocytoma are at risk for hypertensive crisis. With both agents, assess for sensitivity. Clients with an intolerance to procaine and procainamide may experience cross-sensitivity to metoclopramide.

Review the client's medication regimen for significant drug interactions that may occur when metoclopramide and cisapride are given with the drugs listed below.

Drug	Possible effect and management
alcohol and CNS depressant medications	Concurrent administration may increase the CNS depressant effects of either or both drugs. It may also result in an increased rate of absorption of alcohol from the small intestine. Avoid or a potentially serious drug interaction may occur.
anticholinergic agents and opioid analgesics	Concurrent administration of these agents may antagonize motility effects of metoclopramide and cisapride and increase the sedative effects of all the agents.
itraconazole (Sporanox), IV miconazole (Monistat IV), and troleandomycin (TAO)	**Concurrent administration of these agents markedly increases cisapride plasma concentrations because of inhibition of the hepatic enzymes responsible for cisapride metabolism. Avoid or a potentially serious drug interaction may occur.**
oral ketoconazole (Nizoral)	**Concurrent use may result in markedly elevated cisapride plasma concentrations and prolonged QT interval associated with ventricular arrhythmia. Avoid or a potentially serious drug interaction may occur.**

Obtain a baseline assessment of blood pressure, mental status, and underlying nausea and vomiting.

Nursing diagnosis. With the administration of metoclopramide, the client may experience altered sleep patterns (drowsiness—about 10%); altered comfort (headache, dryness of the mouth, breast tenderness and swelling, and dizziness); altered thought processes (confusion, agitation, restlessness—about 10%, depression); fatigue (about 10%); altered protection related to agranulocytosis (chills, fever, sore throat, fatigue); altered cardiac output related to tachycardia and hypertension; risk for injury related to postural hypotension; altered bowel function (constipation or diarrhea); and the potential complications of parkinsonian extrapyramidal effects and tardive dyskinesia.

With the administration of cisapride, the client may experience: altered bowel pattern (constipation or diarrhea [14.2%]); altered comfort (nausea, headache, abdominal cramping); fatigue; and sleep pattern disturbance (drowsiness). The complication of seizures has only been reported in clients with a history of seizures.

Implementation

Monitoring. For metoclopramide, monitor CBCs, blood pressure, mental status, bowel status, for the presence of extrapyramidal effects and tardive dyskinesia, and the incidence of nausea and vomiting. For cisapride, monitor bowel status and the incidence of nausea and vomiting.

Intervention. For metoclopramide, administer oral preparations 30 minutes before meals and at bedtime; for cisapride, 15 minutes.

Administer metoclopramide intravenous injections slowly over 1 to 2 minutes; if administered more rapidly, a brief episode of anxiety and restlessness will occur followed by drowsiness. For infusion, dilute in 50 ml of appropriate IV solution and infuse for a period of time, not less than 15 minutes.

Solutions of parenteral metoclopramide may be kept for 48 hours after dilution. Protect from light and discard unused portions after 48 hours.

Be aware that extrapyramidal side effects may be seen at therapeutic doses and are more likely to occur in children and young adults.

Education. Because these drugs can cause drowsiness, caution the client against operating any potentially hazardous equipment. Caution the client against using alcohol or other CNS depressants with this drug. Instruct client on symptoms to report to prescriber.

Evaluation. Approximately 20% to 30% of clients experience mild and reversible side effects after these drugs are withdrawn. If the drug therapy has been successful, the client should report that nausea is relieved without any side/adverse effects and there are no vomiting episodes.

diphenidol hydrochloride [di phen' i dol] (Vontrol)
Diphenidol may decrease vestibular stimulation and have a potential effect on the medullary chemoreceptive trigger zone. It is used to prevent and control vertigo (Meniere's disease, labyrinthitis following middle or inner ear surgery, and motion sickness), nausea, and vomiting.

Diphenidol is well absorbed orally, reaches peak serum levels in 1.5 to 3 hours, has a half-life of 4 hours, and is excreted by the kidneys. The reported side effects of diphenidol include drowsiness, dry mouth, headache, insomnia, weakness, rash, dizziness and indigestion. Rare adverse effects include disorientation, delusion, and hallucinations.

When diphenidol is given with alcohol or other CNS depressants, the effects of either drug may be potentiated. One must monitor closely for enhanced CNS depressant effects.

Adult dosage for antiemesis and antivertigo is 25 to 50 mg orally every 4 hours as needed.

■ Nursing Management

Diphenidol Therapy

In addition to the previous discussion of nursing management of antiemetics, consider the following for diphenidol therapy:

Assessment. Use diphenidol cautiously in clients with glaucoma (may increase intraocular pressure), or gastrointestinal or urinary obstruction (may decrease tone and motility). Clients with hypotension may have an additional decrease in blood pressure. Do not use diphenidol in the presence of renal failure (systemic accumulation of diphenidol).

Because diphenidol may cause hallucinations, disorientation, and confusion within the first 3 days of administration, its administration should be limited to clients in the hospital setting.

Nursing diagnosis. Clients receiving diphenidol may experience: disturbed sleep patterns (drowsiness, more frequent); altered thought processes (confusion, less than 5%); sensory/perceptual alterations (hallucinations less than 5%, blurred vision); and risk of injury related to postural hypotension.

Implementation

Monitoring. Assess the client's mental status before and during therapy. Monitor blood pressure.

Intervention. Administer diphenidol with food, water, or milk to decrease gastric irritation. Do not administer concurrently with alcohol or other CNS depressants.

Education. Caution the client to consult the prescriber if drowsiness or blurred vision occurs.

Evaluation. If diphenidol therapy is successful, the client will state that nausea is relieved without any side/adverse effects and there will be no vomiting episodes.

thiethylperazine maleate [thye eth il per' a zeen] (Torecan)

Thiethylperazine is a phenothiazine derivative with antiemetic effects, probably by an inhibition action on the chemoreceptor trigger zone and vomiting center. It is used to prevent nausea and vomiting caused by toxins, surgery, chemotherapy, and radiation therapy. For pharmacokinetics see the discussion of phenothiazines in Chapter 19. The reported side effects of thiethylperazine include sleepiness, dizziness, dry mouth, skin rash, fever, ringing of the ears, and headache. Adverse effects are less common or rare and are mainly related to the phenothiazine structure, extrapyramidal effects (parkinsonism in the elderly and dystonia in younger persons), and also agranulocytosis and cholestatic jaundice. Confusion, seizures, and peripheral edema have also been noted.

The adult dose is 10 mg one to three times daily orally, intramuscularly, or rectally. Thiethylperazine is not recommended for children.

■ Nursing Management
Thiethylperazine Therapy

In addition to the previous discussion of nursing management of antiemetics, consider the following for thiethylperazine therapy.

Assessment. Clients with preexisting severe cardiovascular disease or CNS depression or comatose states may have their condition worsen with the administration of thiethylperazine. Hepatic dysfunction may decrease the metabolism of the drug and enhance its CNS effects. Clients with active alcoholism increase their risk of hypotension and CNS depression with the drug. Because of the anticholinergic effects of thiethylperazine, clients with a predisposition to angle-closure glaucoma may experience an acute episode.

The client's medications should be reviewed to detect significant drug interactions such as the ones that may occur when thiethylperazine is given with the drugs listed below.

Drug	Possible effect and management
alcohol and CNS depressants	Concurrent use may result in increased CNS and respiratory depression. Dosages reductions of either drug may be necessary.
epinephrine (Adrenalin)	**Avoid use of epinephrine to treat severe hypotension induced by thiethylperazine. Avoid or a potentially serious drug interaction may occur. Norepinephrine and phenylephrine are drugs of choice for this purpose.**
levodopa (L-dopa)	Concurrent administration may cancel the therapeutic antiparkinson's effect of levodopa. Avoid concurrent drug administration.
metrizamide, intrathecal (Amopaque)	Concurrent drug administration may result in an increased risk of seizures because thiethylperazine lowers the seizure threshold. Avoid or a potentially serious drug interaction may occur. Thiethylperazine should be discontinued at least 48 hours before metrizamide is administered.
phenothiazines, other extrapyramidal causing medications	Monitor for increased potential and severity of extrapyramidal reactions.
quinidine	An increase in adverse cardiac effects may result with this combination. Avoid or a potentially serious drug interaction may occur.

Nursing diagnosis. With the administration of thiethylperazine, the client may experience: altered sleep patterns (drowsiness—more frequent); altered bowel patterns (constipation) related to anticholinergic effects of drug; altered comfort (headache, decreased sweating, nasopharyngeal dryness); risk of injury related to postural hypotension and dizziness; sensory/perceptual alterations (ringing in ears); altered protection (agranulocytosis); and the complications of paradoxical reaction, cholestatic jaundice (fever and chills, fatigue, abdominal discomfort, nausea, yellow skin or eyes), convulsions, and extrapyramidal effects.

Implementation

Monitoring. Blood pressure and CBCs should be monitored. Depending on the client's preexisting health condition, cardiovascular status, hepatic function, neurologic tests, or ophthalmologic exams may be required.

Intervention. It may be taken with food or milk to decrease gastric irritation. After long-term therapy, gradual dosage reduction is recommended to prevent withdrawal symptoms. (See additional nursing management for phenothiazine drugs in Chapter 19.)

Education. Dryness of the mouth may be relieved by ice chips and sugarless gum or candy. Instruct the client to avoid alcohol and other CNS depressants and to use caution when driving until the effects of the drug are known. Caution the client about sitting or standing abruptly because of thiethylperazine's hypotensive effects.

Evaluation. The client receiving thiethylperazine should experience a reduction in nausea and vomiting without any side/adverse effects of the drug.

trimethobenzamide [trye meth oh ben' za mide] (Tigan)

Trimethobenzamide may depress the chemoreceptor trigger zone in the medulla rather than the vomiting center directly. As an antiemetic, it is not as effective as metoclopramide (Brunton, 1996). Trimethobenzamide is metabolized in the liver and excreted in the urine. The reported side effects include sleepiness, blurred vision, diarrhea, dizziness, headache, and muscle cramps. Rare adverse reactions include allergic reactions, seizures, blood dyscrasias, impaired liver function, tremors, Reye's syndrome, and depression (*USP DI*, 1996).

The oral adult dose of trimethobenzamide is 250 mg three or four times per day. Rectally or intramuscularly, 200 mg is given three or four times per day. For children 15 mg/kg is given orally per day, divided into three or four doses. See a current drug reference for additional recommendations.

■ Nursing Management

Trimethobenzamide Therapy

In addition to the previous discussion of nursing management of antiemetics, consider the following for trimethobenzamide therapy.

Assessment. Trimethobenzamide is not recommended for use in children with viral illness, since it may contribute to development of Reye's syndrome, an acute encephalopathy. Administer with caution to clients with dehydration, electrolyte imbalance, high fever, gastroenteritis, or encephalitis because of the increased risk for adverse CNS reactions such as convulsions, coma, and extrapyramidal symptoms. Suppositories contain 2% benzocaine; use with caution in allergic clients.

A baseline assessment should include determining the etiology of the underlying nausea and vomiting, blood pressure, and neurologic status.

Nursing diagnosis. The client receiving trimethobenzamide may experience the following: altered sleep pattern (drowsiness); altered comfort (headache, muscle cramps); altered bowel elimination (diarrhea); sensory-perceptual alterations (blurred vision, dizziness); altered thought processes (depression); altered protection related to blood dyscrasias; and the potential complications of allergic reactions (rash), convulsions, hepatic function impairment, Parkinson-like syndrome, or Reye's syndrome.

Implementation

Monitoring. Monitor closely if trimethobenzamide is given concurrently with CNS-depressing drugs, because these effects may be potentiated. Hypotension can occur in the surgical client when trimethobezamide is administered parenterally. Assess blood pressure before administering the medication and frequently after it has been given. Administration of trimethobenzamide may mask symptoms of appendicitis or signs of ototoxicity (tinnitus, dizziness) secondary to large doses of salicylates.

Intervention. Inject the drug deeply into the upper outer quadrant of the gluteal area to minimize injection site irritation.

Education. Caution the client against using alcohol or other CNS depressants with this drug. Use caution when driving or doing other activities requiring alertness because the drug may cause dizziness and drowsiness.

Evaluation. The client will experience relief from nausea and vomiting without experiencing side/adverse effects.

scopolamine transdermal (Transderm-Scop)

Scopolamine is an anticholinergic agent used to prevent motion-induced nausea and vomiting by depressing conduction in the labyrinth of the inner ear. Overstimulation in this area is responsible for the nausea and vomiting of motion sickness. Scopolamine is metabolized in the liver and excreted by the kidneys. The side/adverse effects with scopolamine are related to its anticholinergic effects: decreased sweating, sleepiness, dry mouth, nose, throat, or skin. In the elderly, impaired memory and insomnia (paradoxical reaction) have been reported.

Scopolamine transdermal is recommended for use in adults only. In the United States, the product is a four-layered film that releases 0.5 mg of scopolamine over a 3 day period. It is applied on the skin behind the ear usually 4 hours before the antiemetic effect is desired. In Canada, it is formulated to release 1 mg of scopolamine over the 3 day period, and it should be applied 12 hours before the antiemetic effect is desired.

■ Nursing Management

Scopolamine Transdermal Therapy

In addition to the previous discussion of nursing management of antiemetics, consider the following for scopolamine transdermal therapy.

Assessment. Take precautions when clients have asthma, narrow-angle glaucoma, pyloric or intestinal obstruction, urinary tract obstruction, or diminished renal or hepatic function. Elderly clients are more susceptible to scopolamine's effects. Do not use in children because of adverse effects. Use cautiously, if at all, during pregnancy or for women who are breastfeeding.

Drug interactions may result from the decreased gastrointestinal tract motility and the delay of gastric emptying time, which may decrease the absorption of other medications. Also, anticholinergic/antimuscarinic drugs or CNS depressants may be potentiated.

Nursing diagnosis. The client using a transdermal patch may experience the following: altered sleep patterns (drowsiness); altered comfort (headache, nasal congestion, dry mouth); altered bowel status (constipation); altered urinary pattern (urinary hesitancy and retention); and risk for injury related to blurred vision.

Implementation

Monitoring. The client may have a dilated pupil on the side that the patch is worn. Be aware that clients can develop tolerance to the drug after prolonged use.

Intervention. Apply the system at least 4 hours or 12 hours before the antiemetic effect is desired depending on the type of patch. Wash and dry the hands thoroughly before and after application of the system. Apply to intact skin in the hairless area behind the ear.

Education. Warn the client that operating machinery or driving a motorized vehicle is hazardous because of drowsiness, disorientation, confusion, and blurred vision.

Evaluation. The client will not experience motion sickness, nausea, and vomiting or any side/adverse effects of the drug.

▲ **ondansetron hydrochloride** [on dan' si tron] (Zofran)
granisetron [gran iz' e tron] (Kytril)

Ondansetron was the first of a new class of serotonin receptor (5-HT_3) antagonists approved by the FDA for the prevention of nausea and vomiting associated with the use of antineoplastic agents. Granisetron, released in 1995, is also a selective serotonin antagonist. Serotonin (5-HT_3) receptors are located peripherally on the vagus nerve terminal, and centrally, in the CTZ. It is believed that antineoplastics cause the release of stored serotonin from the enterochromaffin cells of the GI tract (*USP DI,* 1996). The serotonin stimulates serotonin receptors located in the vagus nerve in the GI tract, which then stimulates serotonin receptors in the CTZ, inducing vomiting. When ondansetron or granisetron are administered before antineoplastic therapy, they block serotonin receptors in the brain stem and GI tract. As a result, serotonin released in response to the administration of antineoplastic agents cannot bind with the serotonin receptors and so prevents vomiting.

Ondansetron administered orally peaks in 1 to 2 hours; elimination half-life is 3 to 4 hours, and it is metabolized in the liver and excreted primarily by the kidneys. Pharmacokinetic information on granisetron is limited; elimination IV half-life in clients may range from 9 to 12 hours, it is metabolized in the liver and excreted in the urine and feces.

The most common side effects of granisetron include stomach pain, diarrhea or constipation, headache, and increased weakness. Rarely reported adverse effects include cardiac arrhythmias, fainting, and hypersensitivity or allergic type reactions. The most common side effects of ondansetron include fever, headache, constipation, and diarrhea. Rare adverse effects reported are anaphylaxis, chest pain, and bronchospasm.

Dosage for IV ondansetron to prevent cancer-chemotherapy–induced nausea and vomiting in adults and children 4 to 18 years is 0.15 mg/kg infused over 15 minutes beginning 30 minutes before the start of chemotherapy, followed by 0.15 mg/kg at 4 and 8 hours after the first dose of ondansetron. Oral adult dose is 8 mg 30 minutes before cancer chemotherapy, then 8 mg at 8 hours after the first dose, followed by 8 mg every 12 hours for several days.

Dosage for IV granisetron to prevent cancer-chemotherapy–induced nausea and vomiting in children 2 years and older and adults is 10 µg/kg given over 5 minutes, 30 minutes before the chemotherapy or radiotherapy. Oral dosage is 1 mg twice a day with the first dose administered an hour before chemotherapy and the second dose 12 hours after the first dose (*USP DI,* 1996; Olin, 1996).

■ Nursing Management

Ondansetron and Granisetron Therapy

In addition to the previous discussion of nursing management of antiemetics, consider the following for ondansetron and granisetron therapy.

Assessment. Sensitivity to ondansetron or granisetron contraindicates its use. Ondansetron is contraindicated at its standard dosage and schedule for clients with hepatic impairment because it may increase hepatic enzymes. Except in rare instances, it is contraindicated for pregnant women (FDA pregnancy safety category B) and nursing mothers. Use with caution in children under 3 years of age. Use granisetron with caution in children under 2 years of age.

A baseline assessment should include a description of the client's previous experience with antiemetic therapy, nutritional status, bowel status, serum electrolytes, and respiratory status.

Nursing diagnosis. The client receiving ondansetron and granisetron therapy may experience the following: altered comfort (headache, abdominal cramping, dry mouth, rash); fatigue; altered sleep pattern (drowsiness); and altered bowel elimination (diarrhea or constipation). With ondansetron, there is the potential complication of bronchospasm; with granisetron, weakness.

Implementation

Monitoring. Monitor the client's fluid and electrolytes, and bowel status for diarrhea or constipation. Monitor the client's respiratory and comfort status.

Intervention. With ondansetron, dilute the IV injection in 50 ml of 5% dextrose or 0.9% NaCl solution before administering; infuse each of the three separate doses over 15 minutes. With granisetron, infuse over 5 minutes, 30 minutes before the administration of cancer chemotherapy.

Education. Alert the client that headache may occur, which can be relieved by an analgesic.

Evaluation. The client will not experience antineoplastic drug–induced nausea and vomiting or any adverse effects of ondansetron or granisetron.

Cannabinoids

dronabinol [droe nab' i nol] (Marinol)

Dronabinol is the synthetic derivative of THC (delta-9-tetrahydrocannabinol) indicated for the treatment of nausea and vomiting related to cancer chemotherapy. Dronabinol is indicated as a second line agent to prevent nausea and vomiting associated with chemotherapy when other antiemetics are ineffective. It is also used as an appetite stimulant to treat anorexia and weight loss in persons with acquired immunodeficiency syndrome (AIDS).

It reaches peak serum levels in 2 to 4 hours; duration of action is 4 to 6 hours for psychic effects and 1 day or longer for appetite stimulating effects. It is metabolized in the liver and excreted mainly in the feces.

Less frequent side effects of dronabinol include ataxia, lightheadedness, nausea, vomiting, blurred vision, dry mouth, restlessness, weakness, and drowsiness. Adverse reactions reported include tachycardia or bradycardia and CNS side effects, such as confusion, delusions, hallucinations, depression, mood alterations, restlessness, and anxiety. The elderly are particularly prone to the CNS adverse reactions.

The adult oral dose is 5 mg/m^2 of body surface 1 to 3 hours before chemotherapy, then every 2 to 4 hours afterward for 4 to 6 doses daily. If the initial dose is ineffective, it may be increased in increments of 2.5 mg/m^2 (maximum dose is 15 mg/m^2). The appetite stimulant dose is 2.5 mg twice daily before lunch and supper, which may be increased if necessary up to a maximum of 20 mg/day. Pediatric dosage is similar to adult dose.

nabilone [na' bi lone] (Cesamet ✤)

Nabilone is a synthetic derivative of cannabinoid (not THC) approved for selected persons receiving emetogenic chemotherapy nonresponsive to other first line antiemetic agents. It has an onset of action within ½ to 1 hour and peak effect is in 2 hours; it is metabolized in the liver and excreted primarily in feces. Side effects include ataxia, sedation, dry mouth, euphoria, headache, and difficulty in concentration.

The adult dose is 1 or 2 mg twice daily. Pediatric dose is not established.

▪ Nursing Management

Cannabinoid Therapy

In addition to the previous discussion of nursing management of antiemetics, consider the following for cannabinoid therapy.

Assessment. Sensitivity to other marijuana products or sesame oil may preclude the use of these agents. These agents should be used with caution with clients with cardiac disorders and hypertension because with an increase in sympathomimetic activity, arrhythmias and hypertension may occur. Clients with mental disorders such as manic, depressive, and schizophrenic states may have increased symptoms. Clients with a history of substance abuse may tend to abuse these agents. Assess the client's mental status before therapy.

Nursing diagnosis. The client receiving cannabinoid therapy may experience the following nursing diagnoses: altered sleep patterns (drowsiness); altered thought patterns as a result of the drug's psychotomimetic effects (mood swings, confusion, inability to think, depression, anxiety, hallucinations); altered mucous membranes (dry mouth); risk for injury related to blurred vision and lightheadedness; and the potential complication of altered cardiac output (tachycardia, hypertension).

Implementation

Monitoring. Monitor the client's vital signs and mental status. Some clients report feelings of well-being and euphoria; others have transient psychoses characterized by hallucinations and depersonalization.

Intervention. These agents should be administered in an in-house setting where the client may be observed. Administer 1 to 3 hours before chemotherapy. The amount dispensed should be limited to that necessary to accompany a single cycle of chemotherapy. Clients may experience withdrawal (irritability, insomnia, restlessness, diarrhea, sweating, anorexia) when the drugs are abruptly discontinued after 12 to 16 days of therapy; clients should be weaned gradually from the drug.

Education. Alert the client to make position changes slowly, particularly from the recumbent to upright position, to prevent dizziness and fainting, symptoms of orthostatic hypotension. Caution the client to avoid alcoholic beverages and other CNS depressants while taking cannabinoids. Use caution when driving or doing other activities that require alertness.

Evaluation. The client will not experience nausea and vomiting or any adverse effects of the cannabinoid therapy.

Corticosteroids

Corticosteroids have been reported to be effective for chemotherapy-induced nausea and vomiting alone or when used in combination with other antiemetics (Koda-Kimble & Young, 1995). The mechanism of action is unknown, but it has been proposed that these drugs may inhibit prostaglandin synthesis, which may be involved in cancer-chemotherapy–induced vomiting. Research has indicated that certain prostaglandins (especially the PGE series) can induce nausea and vomiting.

Many studies with corticosteroids have involved the use of dexamethasone and methylprednisolone although corticotropin and hydrocortisone may also be used. Their effectiveness as antiemetics was a serendipitous discovery—clients receiving various chemotherapeutic regimens had less nausea and vomiting when prednisone was one of the agents administered. Thus the corticosteroids are used as antiemetics in cancer chemotherapy, especially for persons not responsive to other drug therapies. Discussion related to cortico-steroids may be found in Chapter 49, Drugs Affecting the Adrenal Cortex.

Emetic Agents

Emetic drugs exert their effects on the same centers as antiemetic drugs but with the opposite effect. They are used to induce vomiting as part of the treatment for certain drug overdoses and poisonings.

ipecac syrup [ip' e kak]

Ipecac syrup is an OTC drug for home emergency treatment; it is the emetic of choice. Its major alkaloids are emetine and cephaeline, which stimulate the chemoreceptor trigger zone and irritate the gastric mucosa to induce vomiting (Box 41-4).

Approximately 80% to 90% of clients vomit within a half hour after oral drug administration; the average time for vomiting is 20 minutes. Although this product is generally

BOX 41-4

Ipecac Syrup Precaution

Ipecac syrup is the only product to be used as an emetic. *Do not use ipecac fluidextract*; it is 14 times more concentrated than the syrup, and its use has resulted in serious injury and sometimes death. Although the fluidextract is no longer commercially produced in the United States, this product may still be on the shelves of some older pharmacies.

given in the home, a poison control center or health care provider should be called for advice before administration. However, if medical help is not available, one could still use this product. Vomiting-induced gastrointestinal contents recovered may range up to 78% (mean 28%). Therefore clients need further monitoring and/or treatment, since not all the toxic substances are recovered from the gastrointestinal tract.

Ipecac syrup has the advantage of oral administration. The active alkaloid emetine is a cardiotoxic substance. Although administration of a single dose does not usually lead to major problems, serious complications including fatalities have resulted from chronic use of this product by persons with an eating disorder, such as anorexia or bulimia. Emetine is excreted very slowly, so with repeated doses, it will accumulate in the body. It may produce systemic effects for months, even after the drug is discontinued.

Myopathy or muscle aching and weakness, especially in the muscles of the neck and extremities, hyporeflexia, slurred speech, and dysphagia have been reported. Cardiotoxicity has caused some fatalities. Cardiac and muscle effects are due to emetine toxicity and are usually symptoms associated with misuse or overdose of this drug.

For adults and children over 12 years old, dose is 15 to 30 ml (1 oz) orally. Children 1 to 12 years are given 15 ml orally. For adults, follow each dose of ipecac syrup with 8 oz (240 ml) of water; for children 4 to 8 oz of water is given. If vomiting does not occur in 20 to 30 minutes, a second dose may be given. If vomiting does not occur then, gastric lavage should be implemented.

■ Nursing Management

Ipecac Therapy

See Chapter 73, Poisons and Antidotes, for a detailed discussion of nursing management of the client with poisoning.

Assessment. Assess the client's vital signs, level of consciousness, and determine the substance ingested. Call the poison control center or emergency department before administering ipecac.

CAUTION: Vomiting should never be induced in the client who is unconscious, has swallowed corrosive substances or petroleum distillates, or who has depressed gag or cough reflexes. Vomiting may result in aspiration of gastric contents into the lungs, which may be fatal.

Ipecac use in strychnine poisoning may precipitate seizures.

Nursing diagnosis. The client receiving ipecac therapy is at risk for the complication of cardiotoxicity if vomiting does not occur within 30 minutes of the second dose.

Implementation

Monitoring. Monitor for vomiting and document the amount and character of the vomitus. Monitor vital signs and ECG before and after the drug is given. Monitor for drug toxicity if the client does not vomit (abdominal pain, hypotension, dyspnea, cardiac disturbances, shock, seizures, coma). Daily bowel activity and consistency should be noted. Monitor fluid balance and for signs of dehydration (dry mucous membranes, poor skin turgor).

Intervention. Follow the administration of ipecac syrup with water as described above. Sometimes giving the water before the medication is more helpful in young or frightened children. If a child will not drink water, dilute, clear juice (apple) may be substituted. Do not give milk, since it will delay the emetic effect of the drug.

If the client is conscious, drug-induced vomiting is usually preferable to gastric lavage, particularly in children, since aspiration of vomitus is less likely to occur. Nurses should employ the necessary measures to reduce the likelihood of aspiration of vomitus (e.g., proper positioning of client).

Education. Parents should be encouraged to keep ipecac syrup in their home first aid kit and be aware of its proper use.

Evaluation. The client will vomit the noxious agent without aspiration or cardiotoxicity.

Drugs Used to Treat Peptic Ulcers

Treatment of peptic ulcer disease may include a variety of drugs—antimicrobials, antacids, anticholinergics, antidepressants, anxiolytics, H_2 receptor antagonists, and cytoprotective agents (substances that protect cells from damage) such as sucralfate. This section is limited to the more specific agents: the cytoprotective agents and the H_2 receptor antagonists. See the box on p. 708 for Geriatric Implications of the anti-ulcer therapies.

Heliobacter pylori has been found in persons with gastritis and gastric and duodenal peptic ulcers. It has been reported that persons who have a colony of this bacteria in the stomach are more prone to gastritis and gastric and duodenal ulcers (Fedotin, 1993). It has been recommended that all persons with non–drug-induced peptic ulcer be treated with a combination of antibacterials to eradicate *H. pylori*. Controlling or eradicating this bacteria vastly improves the chances of nonrecurrence of the ulcer. The drug regimen usually includes a bismuth preparation (Pepto-Bismol), tetracycline, and metronidazole (Flagyl) plus an H_2 blocking agent. Some resistance has been reported to metronidazole in addition to side effects with all three drugs, which has lead to the use of other combinations, such as bismuth and amoxicillin or amoxicillin and omeprazole (Abramowicz, 1994; Graham, 1993; Smith, 1995).

Several combination medications were also released in 1996. Ranitidine bismuth citrate (Tritec) is used in combination with clarithromycin while bismuth subsalicylate, metro-

Geriatric Implications

Antiulcer therapies

Gastrointestinal symptoms are very common in elderly clients. Every symptom should be properly evaluated before instituting drug therapy.

Acid secretion reaches its peak during sleep, between the hours of 10 PM and the early morning hours (Covington, 1995). Therefore, H_2 receptor antagonists prescribed as a daily dose should be administered at bedtime.

Cigarette smoking, which increases the amount of acid produced in the stomach, may decrease the effect of H_2 blockers. Clients should be advised to stop smoking if possible, or at least not to smoke after the last daily dose of medication is taken (*USP DI*, 1996).

With the routine administration of H_2 blockers, confusion and dizziness are more commonly reported by the elderly than in younger adults (*USP DI*, 1996). With cimetidine, famotidine, and ranitidine, mental status changes have been reported, especially in elderly persons that have impaired liver or renal function or are severely ill. Acute mental changes in the elderly may indicate the need for lowering the drug dose or discontinuing the medication.

Antacids effectively neutralize gastric acid while food also serves as a buffer for gastric acid. Thus antacids are most beneficial if administered between meals and at bedtime.

When H_2 receptor antagonists are prescribed with antacids, schedule medications at least 1 hour apart, administering antacid first.

---

nidazole, and a tetracycline combination (Helidac) may also be used to treat active duodenal ulcers associated with *H. pylori* infection (Olin, 1997). Combining individual agents in a single product helps to simplify a complicated drug schedule.

Cytoprotective Agents

sucralfate [soo kral' fate] (Carafate, Sulcrate♣)

Sucralfate is a local topical agent composed of sulfated sucrose and aluminum hydroxide that in the presence of albumin and fibrinogen forms a protective, acid-resistant shield in the ulcer crater. This barrier hastens the healing of the peptic ulcer by protecting the mucosa for up to 6 hours. It is administered orally with minimal systemic absorption (up to 5%). Excretion is primarily by the fecal route. This product is indicated for short-term (up to 8 weeks) duodenal ulcer treatment (see the case study on p. 709).

The side effects of sucralfate are minimal; the most common one reported is constipation. Other possible effects include diarrhea, nausea, gastric discomfort, dry mouth, dizziness, drowsiness, back pain, rash, and itching.

The adult dose for treatment of a duodenal ulcer is 1 g four times daily an hour before each meal and at bedtime. The dose for prophylaxis of duodenal ulcer is 1 g twice daily on an empty stomach.

■ Nursing Management

Sucralfate Therapy

Assessment. A baseline assessment should include the client's underlying condition, sensitivity to sucralfate, and renal status. Obtain a serum aluminum level in clients with renal failure. Sucralfate should be used with caution in clients with renal failure because the absorption of the aluminum in the drug may cause aluminum toxicity, especially with long-term use.

Review the client's current medications for significant drug interactions, which may occur when sucralfate is administered with the following drugs.

Drug	Possible effect and management
antacids	Concurrent use may interfere with sucralfate binding, thus reducing its effect. Administer antacids either 30 minutes before or 1 hour after sucralfate administration.
ciprofloxacin (Cipro) norfloxacin (Noroxin) or ofloxacin (Floxin)	Sucralfate is reported to decrease absorption and serum levels of these antibiotics. Advise clients to take antibiotics 2 to 3 hours before sucralfate.
digoxin (Lanoxin) or theophylline (Elixophyllin)	Sucralfate interferes with absorption of digoxin and theophylline. Advise clients to take digoxin or theophylline 2 hours before or after sucralfate.
phenytoin (Dilantin)	Concurrent administration with sucralfate may decrease phenytoin serum levels, resulting in a loss of seizure control. Advise clients not to take sucralfate within 2 hours of phenytoin administration.

Nursing diagnosis. The client receiving sucralfate may experience the following: altered bowel elimination (constipation or diarrhea); altered sleep pattern (drowsiness); altered mucous membranes (dry mouth); and altered comfort (nausea, itching, indigestion, dizziness).

Implementation

Monitoring. Monitor the client's bowel elimination for constipation or diarrhea. The ulcer will be monitored by x-ray or endoscopic examination.

Intervention. Administer to the client with water on an empty stomach 1 hour before meals and at bedtime. If the client's regimen also includes antacids, they may be administered ½ hour before or 1 hour after the sucralfate.

Education. Instruct the client not to chew the tablet. If the client is unable to swallow tablets, an oral suspension may be made by placing the tablets in distilled water and allowing them to stand for 15 to 20 minutes. A flavoring agent and 70% sorbitol may be added for palatability. Encourage compliance with the regimen for at least 4 to 8 weeks, until healing has been documented by x-ray or endoscopic examination. Sucralfate therapy is not recommended for longer than 8 weeks.

Evaluation. The client's duodenal ulcer will heal within 8 weeks as evidenced by x-ray or endoscopic examination.

▲ **misoprostol** [mye soe prost' ole] (Cytotec)

Misoprostol, a gastric mucosa-protecting agent, is indicated for the prevention of gastric ulcers associated with the use

Case Study
The Client with Duodenal Ulcer

Annette Jones, a 24-year-old white female, has been diagnosed as having duodenal ulcer disease. After an initial attack, the prescriber prescribed antacids. However, recurrent symptoms have caused her family physician to hospitalize her. You are told that Annette is an exceptionally bright young woman but "very sensitive and childish." She entered law school last year at the insistence of her father, Arthur Jones, a prominent trial attorney. An only child, Annette lives with her parents, who are very demanding of her and do not appear to tolerate mistakes. She is treated medically and her symptoms again resolve.

When she is discharged this time, the prescriber puts her on sucralfate (Carafate) 1 g qid PO.

1. How does sucralfate work differently from other agents used in the treatment of duodenal ulcer?
2. You are teaching Annette the most common side effects of sucralfate, of which constipation is the most common. What are other side effects she should be told about?
3. What other important information will Annette need to know about sucralfate?
4. Considering Annette's health history, what other drug issues should be included in her health instruction?
5. If Annette experiences a recurrence of her ulcer, what other drug regimens are available for her treatment?

of nonsteroidal antiinflammatory drugs (NSAIDs), especially in persons at increased risk of developing complications from gastric ulcers. Normally, prostaglandins protect the stomach by decreasing gastric acid secretion and increasing gastric cytoprotective mucus and bicarbonate. The NSAIDs inhibit prostaglandin synthesis, which reduces the protective mechanisms and may result in gastric ulcers. Misoprostol, a synthetic prostaglandin E_1 analog, suppresses gastric acid secretion and thus helps to heal gastric ulcers (Brunton, 1996).

Misoprostol is rapidly absorbed orally, reaching a peak serum level in approximately 15 minutes with a duration of action of 3 to 6 hours. It is metabolized to an active metabolite that is later metabolized to inactive metabolites in various body tissues. It is primarily excreted by the kidneys. The most frequent side effects associated with its use are stomach distress and diarrhea, which are dose related. Less frequent side effects include constipation, gas, headache, nausea, or vomiting. At the present time, no significant drug interactions have been noted with misoprostol.

The adult dose is 0.2 mg four times daily after meals and at bedtime or 0.4 mg twice daily, taking the last dose at bedtime. Pediatric dosage has not been established.

■ Nursing Management
Misoprostol Therapy

Assessment. Determine if the client is sensitive to other prostaglandins or prostaglandin analogs because there may be cross-sensitivity. Use misoprostol with caution with clients with cerebrovascular or coronary artery disease because, although it has not been reported with this drug, prostaglandins have caused hypotension, which would worsen these conditions. Use the drug cautiously with clients with epilepsy because prostaglandins administered by other than oral route have been reported to have caused seizures, although this effect has not been reported with misoprostol itself. It should be determined whether the client is pregnant, because the drug increases the frequency and intensity of uterine contractions and may cause miscarriages.

Nursing diagnosis. The client receiving misoprostol may experience the following: altered bowel elimination (diarrhea, 13% to 40%; constipation, 1.1%); altered comfort (mild abdominal pain, flatulence, 2.9%; headache, 2.4%); and fluid volume deficit related to nausea and vomiting; and the potential complication of uterine stimulation and vaginal bleeding.

Implementation

Monitoring. Monitor the client for gastrointestinal distress and discomfort and the stools for type, amount, color, and guaiac.

Intervention. Administer to the client with or after meals. The course of therapy should be started at the same time as the nonsteroidal antiinflammatory drugs (NSAIDs). Misoprostol may be administered with antacids, but magnesium-containing antacids are not recommended because they may aggravate any misoprostol-induced diarrhea.

Therapy should continue for 4 weeks unless healing has been documented by endoscopic examination.

Education. Alert the client to report any diarrhea episode lasting more than 1 week to the prescriber. Misoprostol is not to be taken longer than 4 weeks unless otherwise prescribed, and then only for another 4 weeks if necessary. Instruct the client not to give the drug to any other person. Misoprostol has an expiration date of 18 months after manufacture.

Evaluation. The client will maintain ulcer free as evidenced by endoscopic examination without any side/adverse effects of misoprostol.

Proton Pump Inhibitors

Proton pump inhibitors suppress gastric acid secretion by inhibiting the hydrogen/potassium ATPase enzyme system at the secretory surface of the gastric parietal cells. Therefore they block the final step of acid production, inhibiting both basal and stimulated gastric acid secretion. Omeprazole binds irreversibly at this site while lansoprazole's effects are dose related.

lansoprazole [lan soe' pra zole] (Prevacid)
▲ **omeprazole** [oh me' pray zol] (Prilosec)
Omeprazole, the prototype drug, and lansoprazole are indicated for the treatment of severe erosive esophagitis that occurs with gastroesophageal reflux; treatment of duodenal ulcer; and for the long-term treatment of hypersecretory gastric conditions.

Administered orally, omeprazole's onset of action is within 1 hour, peak effect is in 2 hours, and duration of action is 3 to 4 days (time needed for production of new enzyme). It is metabolized in the liver and excreted by the kidneys. Lansoprazole's onset of action is within 1 to 3 hours (depending on dose) and has a duration of action greater than 24 hours. It is metabolized in the liver and excreted in bile and feces primarily.

The most frequent side effects reported are stomach colic or pain for omeprazole, diarrhea for lansoprazole. Other potential side effects include abdominal distress, increased weakness, muscle aches, dizziness, headache, sedation, chest pain, heartburn, constipation or diarrhea, gas, nausea, vomiting, or skin rash. Rare adverse reactions reported with omeprazole include anemia, neutropenia, pancytopenia, thrombocytopenia, and urinary tract infections.

The adult oral dose for omeprazole for gastroesophageal reflux is 20 mg (delayed release capsule) daily for 1 to 2 months. For the gastric hypersecretory conditions, the oral dose is 60 mg daily, adjusting dose as necessary. For elderly clients the dosage should not exceed 20 mg/day. Pediatric dosage has not been established.

Lansoprazole adult dose for duodenal ulcer is 15 mg orally before breakfast for up to 1 month; for erosive esophagitis 30 mg daily before breakfast for up to 2 months; for hypersecretory conditions 60 mg before breakfast daily. The pediatric dose has not been established.

■ Nursing Management

Proton Pump Inhibitor Therapy

Assessment. It should be determined whether the client has a sensitivity to the drug or a history of or current chronic hepatic disease that would require a reduced dosage because of the increased half-life in hepatic dysfunction. Review the concurrent medications of the client because these drugs increase gastric pH and so have the potential to affect the bioavailability of medications that have pH-dependent absorption. Omeprazole may interact and cause an inhibition of the liver-metabolizing enzyme system (P-450), thus decreasing the metabolism of the coumarin and indandione anticoagulants, diazepam, or phenytoin. Serum levels of these agents can rise, resulting in toxicity.

Nursing diagnosis. The client receiving proton pump inhibitor therapy may experience the following nursing diagnoses: altered comfort (heartburn, flatulence, abdominal pain, itching, headache, chest pain); altered protection related to blood dyscrasias; fatigue; altered bowel elimination (diarrhea or constipation); risk for injury related to CNS disturbance (dizziness); and the potential complications of urinary tract infection (frequency, urgency, and burning on urination, hematuria, proteinuria).

Implementation

Monitoring. Monitor the client for decreased GI reflux or heartburn. Record stools as to frequency, character, and color. Monitor CBCs, urinalysis, and hepatic function studies. Monitor concurrent therapy closely.

Intervention. Therapy should continue for at least 4 to 6 weeks but rarely beyond 8 weeks. Administer immediately before meals, preferably in the morning. Omeprazole may be taken with antacids to minimize gastric discomfort.

Education. Instruct the client in administration times and about swallowing the capsule whole; it is not to be crushed or chewed.

Evaluation. The client's hyperacidity is alleviated without side/adverse effects of omeprazole.

H_2 Receptor Antagonists

Histamine, found in the mucosal cells of the GI tract, activates H_2 receptors to increase gastric acid secretion. The major components of the gastric secretion include hydrochloric acid (HCl) and intrinsic factor (IF), produced by the parietal (acid-forming) cells; pepsinogen, synthesized by the chief cells; and mucus. The principal function of mucus is to protect the epithelial cells of the gastrointestinal tract from attack by pepsin and irritation by the HCl secreted by the stomach. Pepsinogen, an enzyme, is the precursor of pepsin; HCl catalyzes the cleavage of pepsinogen to active pepsin by providing a low pH environment in which pepsin can initiate the digestion of proteins.

Gastric secretion is regulated by a neural mechanism, parasympathetic (vagus) fibers, and a hormonal mechanism, gastrin. Activation of the vagus nerve causes secretion of vast quantities of pepsinogen and HCl. In contrast, the hormonal mechanism involves the actual presence of food, which distends the stomach and stimulates the antral mucosa to release gastrin. This hormone is then absorbed into the blood and carried to the parietal cells and chief cells secreting HCl and pepsinogen, respectively. Histamine is believed to activate the gastric mucosa much the same as gastrin does. In addition, caffeine and alcohol are potent stimuli for gastrin release. When the acidity of the gastric juice is increased to a pH of 2, a negative feedback mechanism helps to block production of gastric secretion from the parietal and chief cells. Thus inhibition of gastric gland secretion plays an essential role in protecting the stomach against excessively acidic secretions, which are responsible for causing peptic ulcerations.

Normally the mucosal surface of the stomach and upper duodenum is protected from the irritation of gastric acid by a layer of mucus. If a circumscribed area of the mucosal surface is damaged and fails to repair rapidly, it may become eroded, forming an ulcer at one of these sites. When gastric acid comes in contact with this inflamed region, pain may result. Moreover, clinical studies have suggested that esophageal, gastric, and duodenal ulcers (peptic ulcers) are associated with the excessive production of gastric acid.

Clinical evidence has shown that histamine released by severe injuries, particularly burns, may lead to the formation of peptic ulcers.

The H_2 receptor blocking agents include cimetidine (Tagamet), ranitidine (Zantac), famotidine (Pepcid), and nizatidine (Axid). They act to prevent histamine from stimulating the H_2 receptors located on the gastric parietal cells, thus resulting in a reduction in the volume of gastric acid secretion (from stimuli such as food, pentagastrin, histamine, caffeine, and insulin) and the concentration (acid content) of the secretions. All four drugs are presently considered to be equally potent and effective, although pharmacokinetics, side effects/adverse reactions, and drug interactions may differ.

▲ **cimetidine** [sye met' i deen] (Tagamet)
ranitidine [ra nye' te deen] (Zantac)
famotidine [fa moe' ti deen] (Pepcid)
nizatidine [ni za' ti deen] (Axid)

These agents are used to treat and prevent duodenal ulcer, and to treat gastric ulcer, gastroesophageal reflux, and hypersecretory gastric states. For pharmacokinetics, see Table 41-2. The side effects of H_2 receptor blockers include diarrhea, constipation, headache, stomach cramps or pain, dizziness, and rash. Breast swelling or pain in males and females has also been reported. Famotidine may also cause dry mouth or skin, anorexia, and tinnitus. Less common and rare adverse effects include confusion, neutropenia, bradycardia, tachycardia, and agranulocytosis.

For treatment of duodenal and benign active gastric ulcer, the adult dosage is:

- cimetidine: 300 mg orally 4 times daily with meals and at bedtime, or 600 mg twice a day, or 800 mg at bedtime. Adult dose by IM, IV, or IV infusion is 300 mg every 6 to 8 hours.
- famotidine: 40 mg at bedtime. Parenteral adult dose is 20 mg IV or IV infusion every 12 hours.
- nizatidine: 300 mg at bedtime.
- ranitidine: 150 mg twice a day or 300 mg at bedtime. Parenteral dose is 50 mg IM, IV, or IV infusion every 6 to 8 hours.

See a current reference for additional dosing recommendations. In addition, see also the case study below.

■ Nursing Management

H_2 Receptor Antagonist Therapy

Assessment. Determine sensitivity to H_2 receptor blockers. Note that clients with impaired renal function may require a reduction in dosage for cimetidine, famotidine, ranitidine, or nizatidine because of delayed excretion,

TABLE 41-2 H_2 receptor antagonists: pharmacokinetics

Drug	Absorption	Time to peak plasma level	Plasma half-life (hr)	Duration of action (hr)	Metabolism/excretion
cimetidine (Tagamet)	Very good orally, 60%-70%	45-90 min after oral dose	2	4-5 basal 6-8 nocturnal	Liver/kidneys
famotidine (Pepcid)	Fair orally, 40%-45%	1-3 hr after oral dose	2.5-3.5	10-12 basal & nocturnal	Liver/kidneys
nizatidine (Axid)	Very good orally, 90%	0.5-3 hr after oral dose	1-2	Up to 8 basal Up to 12 nocturnal	Liver (has active metabolite)/ kidneys
ranitidine (Zantac)	Good orally, 50%	2-3 hr after oral dose	2-2.5	Up to 4 hr basal; up to 13 hr (nocturnal)	Liver/kidneys

Case Study

The Client with Peptic Ulcer Disease

Henry Blake is a 47-year-old electronic engineer who has had a gastric ulcer for 3 years. The prescriber is seeing him because his symptoms have worsened. The nursing history reveals that Mr. Blake has had increased gastric pain after he eats, and the pain was relieved by antacids. He smokes a pack of cigarettes a day and has a drink of wine before dinner occasionally. He has been using two aspirin three to four times a day to treat pain in his elbow that he has when he plays racquetball. His prescriber is placing him on cimetadine (Tagamet) 300 mg PO qid.

1. What is the mechanism of action for histamine H_2-blocking agents?
2. What are the side effects of cimetadine Henry should be aware of?
3. What is important to teach Henry about his smoking habit? Considering Mr. Blake's health history, what other issues should be included in his health instruction?

risking increased side effects, particularly CNS effects. In clients with impaired liver function, a further reduction in dosage may be necessary. For clients undergoing hemodialysis, adjust the time of dosage so that the medication is administered at the end of the procedure, thus preventing a decrease in blood level of the drug. These agents are dialyzable.

Assess the underlying condition. These drugs are not to be used for minor digestive complaints. Before administering, the potential existence of malignant gastrointestinal neoplasm should be ruled out. Assess smoking history. Do not administer to nursing mothers, pregnant women, women of childbearing potential, and children under 16 years of age.

A baseline assessment of the client's GI pain should be obtained, along with a CBC.

Review the client's medications for significant drug interactions. Since cimetidine, unlike the other H_2 receptor antagonists, inhibits the liver drug metabolism systems, the major drug interactions noted are with cimetidine. All of the H_2 receptor antagonists, though, may exhibit a similar effect with ketoconazole and antacids.

Drug	Possible effect and management
anticoagulants (coumarin, indanedione); antidepressants, tricyclic; metoprolol (Lopressor); phenytoin (Dilantin); propranolol (Inderal), or xanthines (exception: dyphylline)	When administered with cimetidine, a decrease in metabolism and excretion of these medications may occur. Since dosage adjustments may be necessary, blood concentration (for phenytoin and xanthines), prothrombin time (for anticoagulants), and blood pressure monitoring (for metoprolol and propranolol) are indicated.
antacids	Concurrent use is often prescribed, but if the H_2 receptor antagonist (all four agents) is given concurrently with an antacid, absorption of the antagonist may be decreased. Antacids should not be administered within 1 hour of administration of the H_2 receptor antagonist.
ketoconazole (Nizoral)	An increase in gastrointestinal pH induced by the H_2 receptor antagonist (all four agents) may result in a reduced absorption of ketoconazole. Advise clients to take the H_2 receptor antagonist at least 2 hours after ketoconazole.

Nursing diagnosis. With the administration of H_2 receptor antagonists, the client may experience the following nursing diagnoses: altered comfort (headache, nausea or vomiting, rash, and dizziness); altered bowel function (constipation or diarrhea); altered sleep pattern (drowsiness); altered thought processes (confusion); hyperthermia; altered protection related to blood dyscrasias; and the potential complications of allergic reaction, bradycardia or tachycardia, and bronchospasm.

Pregnancy Safety

Category	Drug
B	cimetidine, famotidine, granisetron, lansoprazole, metoclopramide, ondansetron, ranitidine, sucralfate, ursodiol
C	cisapride, difenoxin and atropine, diphenoxylate and atropine, dronabinol, ipecac, monoctanoin, nizatidine, omeprazole, pancreatin, pancrelipase, scopolamine
X	chenodiol, misoprostol
Not established	diphenidol, trimethobenzamide; thiethylperazine is not recommended for use during pregnancy

Implementation

Monitoring. Assess client regularly for GI pain. Periodic evaluation of blood counts, gastric acid secretion tests, and renal and hepatic function tests are required during therapy. The use of ranitidine, which is metabolized in the liver, may cause elevated hepatic enzyme levels, especially serum glutamic-pyruvic transaminase (SGPT) levels. Since ranitidine is potentially hepatotoxic, perform periodic hepatic studies.

Be aware that after long-term treatment (1 month or more), mild bilateral gynecomastia in males and galactorrhea in females have been observed in some clients taking cimetidine. This drug also may cause a reversible decline in sperm count or impotence. No such problems have been reported with ranitidine.

Intervention. Administer drug with meals, since food slows gastric emptying and prolongs the drug's effect. If prescribed, a bedtime dose protects the stomach from nocturnal hypersecretion of gastric acid. Give concomitant antacids to relieve acute ulcer pain 1 hour before or after administration of H_2 antagonist to prevent drug interaction. Although the symptoms of duodenal ulcers may diminish in a week or two, therapy should be continued for 4 to 6 weeks but rarely beyond 8 weeks.

Note that the parenteral form of the drug is stable for 48 hours at room temperature. The intravenous solutions in which cimetidine, ranitidine, and famotidine are compatible for dilution are 0.9% sodium chloride and dextrose 5%. Rapid intravenous bolus administration (less than 2 minutes) may result in cardiac dysrhythmias and hypotension.

Education. Warn the client that intramuscular administration may be painful. Instruct the client to keep clinical and laboratory appointments as scheduled.

Encourage the client with peptic ulcer disease to discontinue smoking or at least to discontinue smoking after the last dose of the day, since the effectiveness of H_2 antagonists to inhibit nocturnal gastric acid secretions is diminished by smoking.

Evaluation. The client receiving H_2 antagonist therapy will report diminished or absence of pain and demonstrate healing or absence of ulceration by endoscopic examination or x-ray.

DRUGS AFFECTING THE GALLBLADDER

chenodiol [kee noe dye' ole] (Chenix, Chendol♣)

Chenodiol (chenodeoxycholic acid) is a normal bile acid synthesized in the liver. Cholesterol is broken down by bile acids and lecithin, so when the amount of cholesterol exceeds the capacity of bile acids and lecithin to perform this effect, crystallization and gallstones may result. Chenodiol blocks liver synthesis of cholesterol, thus reducing biliary cholesterol levels, leading to gradual dissolving of floating, radiolucent cholesterol gallstones.

Chenodiol is indicated for the client with radiolucent stones who has a well-opacified, functioning gallbladder, but who is at increased risk with elective surgery because of systemic disease, age or cardiovascular, renal, or respiratory disease.

Chenodiol is absorbed in the small intestine, metabolized by the liver, and excreted in feces. Dose-related diarrhea has been reported in clients taking chenodiol. It may occur with initial therapy or any time during the treatment period. Most cases of diarrhea are mild and tolerated, so they do not interfere with therapy. In some clients, a dosage decrease and/or an antidiarrheal agent may be required.

Other side effects of chenodiol include fecal urgency, cramps, heartburn, constipation, nausea, vomiting, anorexia, flatulence, and nonspecific abdominal pain. No significant drug interactions have been reported.

The adult oral dose is 13 to 16 mg/kg/day in two divided doses taken with milk or food in the morning and at night. The initial dose is 250 mg twice daily for 2 weeks and increased by 250 mg/day each week thereafter until either maximum tolerated dose or recommended dose is attained.

■ Nursing Management

Chenodiol Therapy

Assessment. Ultrasonography is a screening procedure for gallstone detection, but initiation and continuation of therapy are based on the result of oral cholecystogram. Contraindications to chenodiol therapy should be determined, such as allergy to chenodiol and other bile products, pregnancy, and lactation. Use of the drug should be evaluated for clients with bile duct abnormalities and cholelithiasis complications because surgery may be more appropriate given the length of treatment time. Bile acid metabolism may be further impaired in clients with hepatic dysfunction. A baseline assessment of the client's gastrointestinal distress, food intolerances, and bowel status should be obtained.

Nursing diagnosis. The client receiving chenodiol may experience the following: altered bowel elimination (frequently diarrhea, rarely constipation), and altered comfort (gas, indigestion, abdominal cramping, nausea).

Implementation

Monitoring. Serum aminotransferase levels are taken each month for 3 months and every 3 months thereafter. Chenodiol is discontinued if elevations over three times normal upper limits occur. Oral cholecystogram or ultrasonogram is needed at 6 and 9 month intervals to monitor response. The response to therapy may be noted on a cholecystogram or ultrasonogram taken 1 month after therapy is begun. Success usually occurs within 12 to 18 months. If no therapeutic response is achieved by 18 months, the drug is discontinued; use beyond 24 months is not recommended. Stones recur within 5 years in about 50% of clients. Clients are monitored annually for possible recurrence. Radiolucency and gallbladder function must be established before initiating another course of treatment. Serum cholesterols are monitored at 6 month intervals and therapy discontinued if cholesterol values exceed the client's age-acceptable limit.

Bowel status is monitored for diarrhea, which is usually dose-related. GI symptoms such as gas, anorexia, and indigestion usually cease after 2 to 4 weeks of therapy.

Intervention. Administer with food or milk, since the presence of bile and pancreatic juice in the intestine enhances dissolution.

Education. Instruct the client about a high-fiber, low-fat diet and a weight reduction program if necessary. Because therapy is long term, compliance may be a problem. Encourage the client through a relationship of trust and confidence.

Evaluation. The client receiving chenodiol therapy will experience dissolution of the gallstones and relief from gastrointestinal distress.

monoctanoin [mon oh ock' ta noyn] (Moctanin)

Monoctanoin is a solubilizing agent (dissolves cholesterol stones) indicated for the treatment of cholesterol gallstones in the bile duct or after a unsuccessful cholecystectomy. It is more effective for a single radiolucent stone than for multiple gallstones. Monoctanoin is administered directly into the common bile duct.

This product is absorbed by the portal vein and metabolized by pancreatic lipases to fatty acids and glycerol. The most common side effect reported is abdominal irritation and pain. Less frequently reported side effects include diarrhea, anorexia, nausea, or vomiting.

The adult dose via catheter (continuous perfusion) is 3 to 5 ml/hour administered at a pressure of 10 cm of water for 1 to 3 weeks. Do not administer this drug by IM or IV administration.

■ Nursing Management

Monoctanoin Therapy

Assessment. It should be determined that the client does not have a condition for which the administration of monoctanoin is contraindicated, such as severe biliary tract infection, obstructive jaundice, recent duodenal ulcer, or pancreatitis, which might be aggravated. Hepatic dysfunction might interfere with the metabolism of the fatty acids generated from monoctanoin and result in adverse reactions. It might also increase the risk of ulceration and hemorrhage in jejunitis or duodenal ulcer. The drug should be used with caution with clients sensitive to monoctanoin or vegetable oils and those with biliary duct obstruction.

A baseline assessment of pulse, blood pressure, and temperature, hepatic function studies, and a cholangiogram is obtained.

Nursing diagnosis. The client receiving monoctanoin may experience the following nursing diagnoses: altered comfort (abdominal pain, backache, flushing of the face, metallic taste); altered bowel elimination (diarrhea); fluid volume deficit related to nausea and vomiting; altered protection related to leukopenia; and the potential complication of acidosis.

Implementation

Monitoring. Monitor the client's blood pressure, pulse, temperature, and comfort status every 4 to 6 hours during the perfusion. An elevated temperature with increasing upper abdominal pain might be indicative of ascending cholangitis. Monitor WBC for leukopenia. Hepatic function studies are suggested.

After placement of a percutaneous T-tube or nasobiliary tube directly into the common bile duct by endoscopy, an infusion pump with an overflow manometer is used to regulate the continuous perfusion of monooctanoin into the duct. Monitor perfusion flow pressure to prevent exceeding 15 cm of water. Adjust if necessary; gastrointestinal side effects, such as nausea and diarrhea, are more apt to occur if the rate is too fast.

A cholangiogram is recommended every 3 days to monitor stone dissolution. If endoscopy or x-ray does not show a significant decrease in stone size after 10 days, therapy will be discontinued. Complete stone dissolution is variable from 7 to 21 days.

Intervention. The perfusion may be interrupted for 1 to 2 hours at mealtime to reduce GI effects. Hourly aspiration of bile will reduce pressure and distention in the biliary and may decrease abdominal and back discomfort.

Education. Instruct the client to alert the nurse to any nausea, diarrhea, or discomfort that may occur. Provide counseling related to low-fat, high-fiber dietary changes if required.

Evaluation. The client's gallstone will be dissolved with monoctanoin therapy.

ursodiol [yoos oh dye' ole] (Actigall)

Ursodiol, an analog of chenodiol, is an oral product used to dissolve cholesterol gallstones in clients with uncomplicated gallstone disease. It is more effective against small, floatable stones and is not indicated for the treatment of calcified cholesterol stones, radiopaque (calcium-containing) stones, or radiolucent bile pigment type stones or when surgery is clearly necessary.

While its exact mechanism of action is unknown, ursodiol inhibits intestinal absorption of cholesterol and also decreases cholesterol synthesis and secretion in the liver. It concentrates in bile. A decrease in cholesterol saturation allows for the gradual dissolution of cholesterol from the gallstones. Ursodiol also increases bile flow in the body. Be aware, however, that gallstone dissolution may necessitate 6 to 24 months of oral therapy, depending on the composition and size of the stone. This therapy is monitored by performing ultrasonograms at 6 month intervals during the first year. If partial effectiveness is not recorded after 1 year of treatment, then ursodiol is usually determined to be ineffective and drug therapy is discontinued. If successful, ursodiol is recommended for at least 3 months after complete dissolution of the stones to ensure the removal of small particles that are not visible via the ultrasonogram.

Administered orally, ursodiol is absorbed from the small intestine; reaches peak concentration in 1 to 3 hours and is metabolized by the liver to taurine and glycine conjugates that are secreted in bile. Excretion is mainly in the feces. An infrequent side effect reported with ursodiol is diarrhea. Ursodiol may cause hepatotoxicity, but to date, liver injuries have not been reported.

No significant drug interactions have been reported with ursodiol, but the nurse should keep in mind that antacids (containing aluminum), cholestyramine, or colestipol may decrease absorption and effectiveness of ursodiol when administered concurrently. Space such medications at least 2 hours apart from ursodiol.

The oral dose is 8 to 10 mg/kg daily, divided into two or three doses taken with meals. A pediatric dose has not been established.

■ Nursing Management

Ursodiol Therapy

Assessment. Although ursodiol is indicated for the dissolution of cholesterol gallstones, it is administered with caution if the client's health status is further compromised with bile duct abnormalities, complications of gallstones such as cholecystitis or pancreatitis, or chronically impaired hepatic function. The client will usually have ultrasonogram and/or hepatic function studies to determine if these conditions exist before beginning a regimen of ursodiol. Hepatic function studies are done to rule out preexisting liver disease. A nursing baseline assessment would include ursodiol sensitivity, comfort, and bowel status.

Nursing diagnosis. During the course of ursodiol therapy the client may experience altered bowel elimination (diarrhea) as an adverse response to the drug.

Implementation

Monitoring. Ultrasonogram and/or hepatic function studies are usually done periodically over the course of drug therapy to determine the dissolution of gallstones and the development of hepatotoxicity. Monitor the client's bowel elimination for frequency and character of stools.

Intervention. Administer with meals. If partial dissolution has not occurred after 12 months of therapy, then the drug is considered ineffective and is discontinued.

Education. The client should be instructed to take ursodiol with meals because it dissolves more rapidly when bile and pancreatic enzymes are present. Compliance is encouraged and the client is cautioned to be patient because gallstone dissolution may take 6 months to 2 years, depending on the size and number of stones.

Evaluation. If ursodiol therapy is successful, the client's gallstones should diminish in size and number as evidenced by ultrasonogram, without any adverse effects of the drug occurring.

Agents Affecting the Lower Gastrointestinal Tract

Bowel elimination is often a major concern of clients, particularly constipation in the older client and diarrhea in children and immunosuppressed clients. The nursing diagnosis "altered bowel elimination" provides a framework for supportive nursing care to accompany the pharmacologic intervention that may be required for clients with conditions affecting the lower gastrointestinal tract. Most of the agents that affect the lower gastrointestinal tract may be purchased over-the-counter and so are discussed in Chapter 11. However, clients admitted to various health care agencies for short stays in acute care institutions, or for extended stays in long-term care facilities, frequently experience altered bowel elimination, constipation, or diarrhea.

Constipation is defined as difficult fecal evacuation as a result of degree of hardness and perhaps infrequent movements. Each person has regular bowel movements that may range from three per day to three per week. The Eighth National Conference on the Classification of Nursing Diagnoses further classified the condition into colonic and rectal constipation (Box 41-5). A subjective aspect of constipation is the individual's feeling or attitude of dissatisfaction regarding bowel function or pattern of elimination or perceived constipation. Chronic constipation is sometimes caused by organic disease, such as from tumors; bowel obstruction; megacolon; metabolic abnormalities such as diabetes mellitus or hypercalcemia; rectal disorders; diseases of the liver, gallbladder, or muscles; neurologic abnormalities, such as multiple sclerosis and Parkinson's disease; and pregnancy. Persons that suffer from disorders of the gastrointestinal tract frequently complain of constipation. On the other hand, many persons complain of constipation when no organic disease or lesion can be found.

When not a result of organic factors, constipation is generally attributable to faulty eating habits, failure to respond to defecation impulses, insufficient fluid intake or exercise, or being hospitalized, off the usual routine, and in a strange place. For example, diet that provides inadequate bulk and residue will contribute to the development of constipation. The gastrointestinal tract should function normally if fluids and residue are supplied in sufficient quantities to keep the stool formed but soft.

Another common cause of constipation is a failure to respond to the normal defecation impulses and insufficient time to permit the bowel to produce an evacuation. In addition, sedentary habits and insufficient exercise may be factors.

BOX 41-5

Nursing Diagnoses (NANDA) Related to Altered Bowel Elimination

Colonic constipation is a state in which an individual's pattern of elimination is characterized by hard, dry stool that results from a delay in passage of food residue. Its major defining characteristics are decreased frequency, hard, dry stool, painful defecation, abdominal distention, and a palpable mass. Minor characteristics are rectal pressure, headache, appetite impairment, and abdominal pain. Related factors are less than adequate fiber, less than adequate dietary intake, immobility, lack of privacy, emotional disturbance, chronic use of medications and enemas, stress, change in daily routine, and metabolic problems, such as hypothyroidism, hypocalcemia, and hypokalemia (NANDA, 1988).

Perceived constipation is a state in which an individual makes a self-diagnosis of constipation and ensures a daily bowel movement through the use of laxatives, enemas, and suppositories. The defining characteristic is an expectation of a daily bowel movement, which may be expected at the same time every day, with the resulting overuse of laxatives, enemas, and suppositories. Related factors are cultural and family health beliefs, faulty appraisal, and impaired thought processes (NANDA, 1988).

Rectal constipation is a state in which an individual's pattern of elimination is characterized by stool retention, normal stool consistency, and delayed elimination that results from biopsychosocial disruptions. There is also abdominal discomfort, rectal fullness, and a change in flatus. Related factors are weak pelvic floor muscles, painful anorectal lesions, self-care deficits, environmental constraints, altered mobility, low or no social support, impaired communication, altered awareness, and emotional disturbances (NANDA, 1992).

Diarrhea is the frequent passage of loose, watery stools, generally the result of increased motility in the colon. The cause of the condition includes stress and anxiety; dietary intake; the side effects of medications; inflammation, toxins, contaminants, or radiation. The defining characteristics include abdominal pain, cramping, increased frequency of elimination, increased frequency of bowel sounds, loose or liquid stools, urgency of defecation, and a change in the color of the feces (NANDA, 1975).

From Carpenito (1995)

Clients with impaired physical mobility may be constipated because of inactivity or unnatural position for defecation, such as using a bedpan.

Another causative factor is the effect of drugs. The use of antacids, diuretics, morphine, tricyclic antidepressants, codeine, aluminum hydroxide, and anticholinergics often leads to constipation as a side effect. Constipation can also be a symptom of both functional and organic disorders, such as febrile states, psychosomatic disorders, anemias, and tension headaches. Finally, a third less frequent cause of constipation may be atonic and hypotonic conditions of the musculature of the colon. These may result from habitual use of **cathartics,** substances that produce a liquid or fluid evacuation of the bowel.

LAXATIVES

Laxatives are drugs given to induce defecation. Laxatives may be classified according to their source, site of action, degree of action, or mechanism of action (see Chapter 11). Box 41-6 summarizes the types of laxatives discussed in Chapter 11. Although the nursing management of laxative therapy is discussed in this chapter, only the monographs for the prescription laxatives, Lactulose and GoLYTELY, are in this section (Table 41-3).

BOX 41-6

Selected Types of Laxatives

Saline laxatives retain and increase water content of feces by virtue of osmotic qualities

Stimulant laxatives increase peristalsis in the colon by irritating intramural sensory nerve plexi endings in the mucosa

Bulk laxatives absorb water and increase the volume, bulk, and moisture of nonabsorbable intestinal contents, thereby distending the bowel and initiating reflex bowel activity

Intestinal lubricants mechanically lubricate feces to facilitate defecation

Emollients, or fecal softening agents act as dispersing wetting agents, facilitating mixture of water and fatty substances within the fecal mass; when a homogeneous mixture is produced, the feces become soft

Hyperosmotic agents increase the intraluminal osmotic pressure in the bowel; because they are not absorbed, they draw water into the intestine, resulting in an increased volume that stimulates peristalsis

lactulose [lak' tyoo lose] (Chronulac, Duphalac♣)
Lactulose is composed of galactose, fructose, and other sugars, and in the GI tract, the normal colonic bacteria (*Lactobacillus* and *Bacteroides, Escherichia coli; Streptococcus faecalis*) metabolize lactulose syrup to organic acids, primarily lactic, acetic, and formic acids. These acids produce an osmotic effect, an increase in fluid accumulation, distention, peristalsis, and bowel movement within 24 to 72 hours. Lactulose is also used to decrease blood ammonia levels in persons with hepatic encephalopathy secondary to chronic liver disease.

After oral administration absorption is minimal and it is excreted via the kidneys. Lactulose syrup is used in clients

TABLE 41-3 Prescription laxative overview

	Lactulose syrup/PEG 3350*
Disadvantages with repeated frequent (long-term) administration	Early, transient flatulence and cramps; nausea reported
Increases rate of transit in small bowel	Possibly
Causes net secretion of water and electrolytes in small bowel	No
Inhibits absorption in small bowel	Not reported
Increases mucosal permeability in small bowel	No
Causes mucosal damage in small bowel	No
Acts only in colon (not small bowel)	Yes
Indicated for long-term treatment	Yes—lactulose No—PEG
Examples of type	Chronulac (lactulose) CoLyte GoLYTELY (PEG 3350)
Physical or chemical property responsible for action	Colon-specific increase in stool water content and stool softening by increase in osmotic pressure (hyperosmotic) and colon acidification

**PEG 3350,* Polyethylene glycol electrolyte solution.

with a history of chronic constipation that generally do not respond sufficiently to the bulk laxatives. It increases the number of bowel movements daily and the number of days on which bowel movements occur. Dose-related flatulence and intestinal cramps, gas, and belching are reported. Excessive doses may produce some diarrhea (hypokalemic) and nausea (caused by the sweet taste).

The effectiveness of lactulose may be reduced if it is used concomitantly with an antibiotic that destroys the normal colonic bacteria. A nonabsorbed antibiotic such as neomycin destroys enough luminal colonic bacteria to interfere with lactulose. Most systemic, highly absorbable antibiotics do not affect the colonic bacteria in the lumen.

Adult dose is 1 to 2 tablespoons (15 to 30 ml) daily, increased in 5 and 10 ml increments to 60 ml daily after breakfast.

polyethylene glycol (PEG) and electrolytes (GoLYTELY)

This powder consists of a mixture of polyethlylene glycol (nonabsorbable osmotic substance) with sodium salts (sulfate, bicarbonate, and chloride) and potassium chloride that is isotonic with body fluids. Because it is isotonic, fluids and electrolytes will be neither absorbed nor secreted in the GI tract, thus it can be used in dehydrated persons and in individuals with renal impairment or cardiac disease. The drug acts as an osmotic agent.

GoLYTELY is used for bowel cleansing before colonoscopy and before administration of a barium enema for radiologic examination. There is a low incidence of nausea, vomiting, bloating, cramps, and abdominal fullness with GoLYTELY.

Nursing Management

Laxative Therapy

Assessment. Determine the client's bowel status by careful assessment. Occurrence of last bowel movement, quality of bowel sounds, defecation habits, dietary patterns, fluid intake, level of daily activity, and use of laxatives are important components of the nurse's assessment. Review the client's medical history for causative factors. Assess the client's current medication regimen for drugs that might contribute to the constipation as well as any significant drug interactions. These include the following:

- High-fiber and bulk-forming laxatives may decrease the effects of tetracycline, anticoagulants, digitalis glycosides, or salicylates by binding with the drug or delaying its absorption. Separate administration by at least 2 hours.
- Saline or osmotic laxatives that contain calcium may interact with the same drugs as the magnesium-containing antacids. Calcium or magnesium salts may interact with tetracycline, forming a nonabsorbable complex when administered within 1 to 2 hours of tetracycline. The diarrhea produced by these drugs may interfere with absorption.
- Stimulant/contact/irritant laxatives such as bisacodyl oral tablets, which contain an enteric coating, will be prematurely released in the stomach when administered with antacids or dairy products, producing severe cramping in the stomach and duodenum.
- Lubricant/emollient laxatives such as mineral oil may interfere with absorption of antibiotics, anticoagulants, oral contraceptives, digitalis glycosides, and fat-soluble vitamins when concurrently administered, thereby reducing their therapeutic effectiveness.
- Mineral oil is not recommended for children under the age of 6 years or for bedridden elderly, because they are more at risk for aspiration of droplets coating the pharynx, which may result in lipid pneumonia. Do not give mineral oil routinely to pregnant women, since it decreases vitamin K availability to the fetus, resulting in hypoprothrombinemia and hemorrhagic disease. Chronic use of mineral oil in any client may decrease vitamin K absorption leading to an increased potential for bleeding.
- Stool softener/surfactant or wetting agent laxatives may increase the absorption of mineral oil if administered together. Granuloma formation or tumor-like deposits in tissues are also reported.
- Phenolphthalein may have increased absorption with the concurrent use of docusate, a stool softener.
- Use of lactulose during pregnancy has not been evaluated. Lactulose use in diabetic clients may cause elevations in blood glucose levels; another type of laxative without galactose or lactose may be better. Elderly and debilitated clients receiving lactulose for 6 months or more should have serum electrolytes (potassium, chloride, and carbon dioxide) periodically evaluated. Because lactulose contains galactose (less than 2.2 g/15 ml), it is contraindicated in low-galactose diets.
- Do not use laxatives when an emergency surgical condition in the abdomen might be suspected, such as appendicitis, bowel obstruction, hemorrhage, or intussusception.

Nursing diagnosis. Clients receiving laxatives have the potential for the following nursing diagnoses: colonic constipation related to the ineffectiveness of the laxative or intestinal obstruction (bulk laxatives); diarrhea related to misuse of laxatives; altered comfort (abdominal cramping, flatulence, nausea); and the potential complications of allergic reaction or electrolyte imbalance (weakness, muscle cramping, confusion).

Implementation

Monitoring. Observe the client's stools for frequency, consistency, and color. Determine the client's comfort during defecation.

Intervention. Encourage nonpharmacologic interventions to relieve constipation. Depending on the client's health assessment, measures to relieve constipation include adding fresh fruits, vegetables, and whole grains to increase bulk to the diet; allowing for a calm, adequate, and routine time for defecation; ensuring a daily fluid intake of eight to ten glasses of water for adequate hydration; and increasing the amount of daily exercise. When laxatives are indicated, use the mildest laxative necessary.

Lactulose. To make lactulose more palatable, mix it in water, juice, or milk. Results may occur 24 to 36 hours after administration of lactulose. The solution may darken on exposure to high temperature, but this will not change its therapeutic effect. Freezing does not alter the therapeutic effect.

GoLYTELY. GoLYTELY is given orally, 4 L at a rate of 240 ml every 10 minutes (rapidly swallowed). Fasting 3 to 4 hours before use is necessary. Generally a midmorning examination permits 3 hours for consumption, followed by a 1 hour period for bowel movement. Less stool is retained after its use, but the water or electrolyte balance does not change. Only clear liquids are permitted after its administration and before examination.

After reconstitution of the powder, refrigerating the solution improves palatability. The reconstituted solution must be used within 48 hours.

Castor oil. Castor oil may be unpleasant and nauseating. This may be overcome by emulsifying it in a blender or mixing it with cold orange or other fruit juices and having the client drink the mixture immediately after mixing to disguise the taste of the oil. Neoloid is a preemulsified preparation. Castor oil is contraindicated in pregnancy. Its administration often results in engorgement of the pelvic area, which may reflexively stimulate the gravid uterus.

Bulk-forming laxative (Metamucil and others). Because there is a possibility of impaction or obstruction if fluid intake is not substantial, avoid use of bulk-forming laxatives in clients with stenosis, adhesions, or dysphagia. Administer with a full glass of liquid (240 ml) plus additional liquid every day to avoid intestinal impaction. Some preparations contain sugar and sodium and so may not be used with clients for whom these substances are restricted.

Education. Instruct clients on the measures to prevent constipation appropriate to the lifestyle information obtained in your assessment.

Encourage clients to avoid the laxative habit. Inform them that misuse or overuse may result in dependence on laxatives for routine bowel function. Instruct clients not to take laxatives unnecessarily. For example, some individuals believe that laxatives are to be taken to "clean out" the system, as a tonic, in the case of colds, or at the change of seasons. (See the case study below.)

Bisacodyl (Ducolax). Because bisacodyl tablets are enteric coated, instruct clients not to chew them or administer them when they are chipped. Instruct clients to swallow bisacodyl tablets whole no sooner than 1 hour before or after ingestion of dairy products or antacids. Milk or antacids can break down the enteric coating, which can lead to gastric irritation, cramping, and vomiting. See Chapter 11 for additional information on bisacodyl.

Phenolphthalein (Ex-Lax, Feen-a-Mint Gum, and others). Clients taking phenolphthalein laxatives may experience belching, cramping, loose stools, nausea, mucus secretion, fluid and electrolyte loss, and rectal mucosal irritation. Phenolphthalein discolors alkaline (red, violet, brown) and acid (yellow, brown) urine; this information should be shared with the client. Alert parents to secure the candylike and gum forms of this laxative away from children.

Case Study

Drug Therapy for Bowel Elimination

Margaret Gordon, a 73-year-old widow, is recovering at home from an internal fixation of a fractured left hip. Mrs. Gordon is recovering well from the surgery. She continues with physical therapy, but she does not go out much and spends most of the day sitting in a chair watching television. Her primary meal of the day is delivered to her home by a voluntary agency. The remainder of her food intake includes snack foods and occasionally soup and crackers.

The medications for Mrs. Gordon include the following:

Colace, 100 mg orally at bedtime as needed
Milk of Magnesia, 1 tbsp at bedtime as needed
Metamucil, 2 tsp daily
Kaopectate, 2 tbsp after each loose stool

A review of the client's history by the community health nurse reveals that Mrs. Gordon takes the Colace daily. When questioned, she reports that this is the same way it was given to her in the hospital. Her physician routinely orders Colace for all clients who have orthopedic surgery. If she goes more than one day without a bowel movement, she takes the Milk of Magnesia as she has done for years. She has been taking Metamucil daily for several years. When she returned home from the hospital she began using the Metamucil again. Several weeks later she developed diarrhea. She began taking the Kaopectate without consulting her physician.

Mrs. Gordon readily admits that she believes "normal" bowel habits are essential to her health. She believes that one well-formed stool daily is her normal pattern. Any deviation from this pattern she calls diarrhea or constipation and promptly treats the problem with any or all of the above medications, which she purchases over the counter. The physician's office renews the prescription for Colace at her request.

1. What factors during Mrs. Gordon's postoperative recovery may have contributed to the present situation?
2. What effect does each medication have on Mrs. Gordon's bowel elimination?

Polycarbophil calcium (Mitrolan). Instruct the client to follow each dose of polycarbophil calcium for constipation with at least 8 oz of water or other liquid. If the drug is being used to treat diarrhea, administer less fluid with each dose. Also instruct the client to thoroughly chew polycarbophil tablets before swallowing.

Caution clients to forbid children free access to laxative preparations that are in a candylike form, chewing gum, or mint, because they are likely to regard them as ordinary candy or gum and take an overdose of the drug. Deaths have been reported from such accidents.

Evaluation. The client reports bowel movements of soft stools without straining or pain.

ANTIDIARRHEALS

This section focuses on the prescription drugs with a direct pharmacologic effect on the gastrointestinal tract. Although many antidiarrheal preparations may be purchased over-the-counter, as were discussed in Chapter 11, the nurse may be administering these same preparations within a health agency setting.

■ Nursing Management

Antidiarrheal Therapy

Assessment. The objectives of treatment are to (1) replenish fluid and electrolyte loss, (2) ascertain, if possible, the cause or causes of diarrhea, (3) reduce the frequency of evacuation, (4) absorb toxins, (5) restore the intestinal flora, and (6) treat the underlying cause or causes.

It is important to determine the cause of the diarrhea through careful individual client evaluation. Such evaluative questions for discovering the cause or causes may be used in assessing the following criteria:

- Age of the client
- Occupation
- Duration of diarrhea (precipitating factors tantamount to onset)
- Stool description (frequency of evacuation, rectal bleeding or black stool appearance, foul odor, light color, or greasy consistency)
- Medication profile (prescribed and self-administered as OTC drugs)
- Presence or absence of anorexia, weight reduction (involuntary), fever, abdominal tenderness, dehydration
- Ingestion of foods, toxic substances, milk intake, alcohol use
- Travel outside the United States or Canada
- Symptom description (location)
- Relief obtained, if any, and treatment modality
- Chronic diseases, presence of acute or concurrent illness, emotional or behavioral problems

Nursing diagnosis. The client may experience: altered bowel pattern (diarrhea) related to underlying cause and ineffectiveness of the antidiarrheal agent; altered comfort related to abdominal cramping; and the potential complications of hypovolemia and electrolyte imbalances.

Implementation

Monitoring. Fluid and electrolyte loss may cause tachycardia, postural hypotension, elevated hematocrit or blood urea nitrogen, and poor skin turgor. The stool specimen may reveal occult blood (gastrointestinal bleeding), fecal leukocytes, parasites, or fat.

Intervention. Nonspecific treatment is directed at the increased stool frequency, which burdens daily lifestyle; the alleviation of abdominal cramps; the prevention of dehydration and metabolic acidosis from fluid and electrolyte loss; and the minimization of weight loss and nutritional deficits resulting from malabsorption. Specific treatment is directed at the cause or condition creating the diarrhea, as demonstrated by the Nursing Care Plan on p. 720.

Hospitalization is needed for dehydration that would compromise a client with congestive heart failure or chronic renal disease, since this complicates fluid replacement efforts. If a child or infant is unable to consume oral replacement fluid, hospitalization is needed to replace fluids and maintain urine flow. Bed rest alone may reduce stool frequency. In addition to the child or infant, the elderly client with a poor medical history, a client with chronic illness (heart disease, asthma), and pregnant women are at risk from acute or chronic diarrhea.

Maintenance of fluid and electrolyte balance is the most important goal of supportive therapy in acute diarrhea. If left untreated, a loss of anions (bicarbonate, organic anions as short-chain fatty acids) will create a gain of hydrogen ions, resulting in metabolic acidosis. This gain will be exacerbated by the (often) concomitant ketoacidosis of starvation and the acidosis of prerenal azotemia. As volume increases in diarrhea, a rise in sodium and chloride develops with a decrease in potassium concentration. The decreased contact time of the luminal contents with the mucosal surface decreases the passive secretion of potassium. The electrolyte composition of stool water will then be close to that of plasma. The electrolyte loss of sodium, potassium, chloride, and bicarbonate is the basis of therapy.

It is recommended that clear liquids (noncarbonated soft drinks, fruit juice, diluted and flavored gelatin, and apple juice) and a bland diet be continued for 1 to 2 days. According to the cause of the diarrhea, several different medications can be given along with bed rest. These include activated charcoal, absorbents, anticholinergic drugs, and many other drug products.

Over-the-counter antidiarrheals may contain the following ingredients: limited amounts of opiates; adsorbents, such as bismuth salts, aluminum salts, attapulgite, kaolin, pectin, activated charcoal, and belladonna alkaloids (hyoscyamine, hyoscine, scopolamine, atropine); and calcium salts. Inactive ingredients vary, but the nurse should be aware of the variation in alcohol content (1.5% to 18%).

Antidiarrheal products have a warning stating that they are not to be used for longer than 2 days, not to be used if a fever is present, and not to be used in infants or children

Nursing Care Plan

Selected Nursing Diagnoses: Antidiarrheal Medication Administration

Nursing diagnosis	Outcome criteria	Nursing interventions
Altered bowel elimination (diarrhea)	Decrease in number of stools to less than three per day Formed stools	Record frequency, number, consistency of stools Encourage bland diet and liquids Administer antidiarrheal agents as prescribed
Potential complications: hypovolemia and electrolyte imbalance	The client will: Maintain electrolytes within normal limits Maintain normal fluid balance Experience less diarrhea Maintain normal body weight	Monitor client's intake and output Monitor bowel movements, recording diarrhea as output Weigh client daily Administer antidiarrheal agents as prescribed Assess client for signs of dehydration and hypokalemia Encourage high fluid intake Monitor serum electrolyte determinations
Risk for alteration in comfort related to abdominal cramping and diarrhea	The client will: Verbalize comfort or pain relief Maintain ADL without disruption because of discomfort	Assess comfort status of client Instruct client in appropriate diet to minimize intestinal cramping Provide suggestions for nondrug pain management (positioning, activities, distraction) Administer antidiarrheal medications as prescribed Consult prescriber if additional pain relief is needed

under 3 years of age. The prescriber may modify these instructions.

The intractable diarrhea of infancy is traditionally treated with clear liquids and gradual reintroduction of milk or formula, with the addition of oral elemental diets or total parenteral nutrition. The infant syndrome is described as loose stools, resulting in dehydration and a failure to thrive. Because a newborn's total body weight is usually 75% water, a 10% or greater weight loss may occur if the infant has severe diarrhea. If an infant has eight to ten bowel movements in a 24-hour period, the fluid loss may cause circulatory collapse and renal impairment. Diarrhea in infants should be considered serious enough to warrant referring the client to a prescriber for evaluation.

Persistent diarrhea in the elderly can result in fluid and electrolyte loss, dehydration, and perhaps more serious medical complications. Such clients should be referred to a prescriber.

Education. Explain the effects of diarrhea on hydration and electrolytes. Instruct the client on interventions to prevent future episodes.

Evaluation. The client will experience a decrease in the number, frequency, and fluidity of stools.

Prescription Antidiarrheal Agents

Opioids

The opioids (codeine and paregoric—Rx C-III) act by virtue of their constipative and sedative action. They lower the propulsive motility of the bowel, reduce pain, and relieve tenesmus (rectal spasms). The delay in transit time of food permits contact time of intestinal contents with the absorptive surface of the bowel, which increases the reabsorption of water and electrolytes and reduces stool frequency and net volume.

The anticholinergics and opium derivatives decrease the motility of the bowel. They should not be used when the cause of diarrhea is an invading organism (as toxigenic bacteria or pseudomembranous enterocolitis) because these drugs decrease intestinal motility and subsequently lower excretion of the organisms and their toxins, resulting in epithelial penetration and multiplication of the organisms.

Codeine and paregoric cause depression and sedation. This factor must be considered if the client is taking other CNS depressant drugs because of the additive effects. The opiates are short acting; frequent administration (4 to 6 hour intervals) is needed to control the gastrointestinal smooth muscle function. The opiates are discussed in greater detail in Chapter 14, Analgesics.

opium tincture, deodorized

Tincture of opium, a hydroalcoholic (19% alcohol) solution, contains 10% opium, with an average dosage of 0.6 ml four times daily. This is a class II prescription under the Controlled Substances Act.

paregoric

Paregoric (camphorated opium tincture although camphor is no longer required in the United States in this formulation) requires a prescription. It is a class III drug that is equivalent to 2 mg of morphine/5 ml. It is important that the nurse not confuse opium tincture, deodorized (10 mg morphine equivalent/1 ml), and camphorated opium tincture (0.4 mg morphine equivalent/1 ml), because opium tincture, deodorized, has 25 times more morphine equivalent than camphorated opium tincture. Addiction liability has been reported with these preparations. When paregoric is combined with another drug, it becomes a class V product if the combination contains no more than 100 mg of opium or 25 ml of paregoric/100 ml of the mixture. The adult antidiarrheal dose is 5 to 10 ml one to four times daily. The pediatric dosage is 0.25 to 0.5 ml/kg one to four times daily.

Synthetic Opioids

The synthetic opioids used to treat diarrhea include diphenoxylate and difenoxin.

diphenoxylate and atropine [dye fen ox' i late] (Lomotil)

Diphenoxylate, a class V product, inhibits intestinal propulsive motility by acting directly on intestinal smooth muscles and thus decreases transit time. It is indicated as an adjunct to fluid and electrolyte replacement for the treatment of acute and chronic diarrhea in adults. It is not recommended for use in children.

The onset of diphenoxylate effect is between 45 to 60 minutes; half-life is 2.5 hours; duration of action is 3 to 4 hours. It is metabolized in the liver and excreted primarily by the kidneys. Side effects include drowsiness, dizziness, tachycardia, dry mouth, hyperthermia, abdominal distress, rash, and agitation.

For adults and children 12 years and older, dosage is 1 to 2 tablets orally three or four times daily.

▪ Nursing Management

Diphenoxylate Therapy

Assessment. The client's health status should be assessed for conditions that would contraindicate diphenoxylate therapy or determine that its use would indicate risk. For example, the drug should not be used with clients with pseudomembranous colitis (*Clostridium difficile* toxin) secondary to broad-spectrum antibiotic therapy because slowing of the peristalsis would inhibit the evacuation of toxins from the bowel, thereby worsening the client's diarrhea. The risk associated with diphenoxylate use in dehydration, particularly in children, requires caution because it may predispose the client to delayed diphenoxylate intoxication. Antidiarrheal agents (e.g., diphenoxylate, loperamide, or narcotics) should be carefully considered in instances of acute diarrhea or traveler's diarrhea caused by bacteria (enterotoxin-producing strains of *Escherichia coli, Campylobacter jejuni, Salmonella*, or *Shigella*), parasites (*Giardia lamblia*), and viruses (parvovirus or rotavirus), because these penetrate the intestinal wall if retained in the intestine and must be eliminated in the feces. Cautious use of antidiarrheals is also true of diarrhea that is caused by poisoning until the toxic materials have been eliminated from the gastrointestinal tract.

Diphenoxylate may precipitate hepatic coma in clients with impaired hepatic function. Pediatric and geriatric clients are more susceptible to the respiratory depressant effects of diphenoxylate. Toxic megacolon may develop as the result of inhibition of intestinal motility in clients with acute ulcerative colitis. The client's current drug regimen should be reviewed for significant drug interactions; these include the following:

- The CNS depressant effects are potentiated by alcohol and other CNS depressant drugs.
- Concurrent use with monoamine oxidase inhibitors (MAOIs) may precipitate hypertensive crisis because of the chemical similarity to meperidine.
- Additive effects are seen with drugs that have anticholinergic/antimuscarinic effects because of the atropine present.

A baseline assessment of the client's bowel disorder should be obtained, including gastrointestinal status and the frequency of diarrhea.

Nursing diagnosis. The client is at risk for the following nursing diagnoses: altered bowel elimination, diarrhea related to the ineffectiveness of the drug regimen or constipation related to the drug's side effects; altered breathing pattern related to the drug's effect of respiratory depression; altered thought processes related to CNS effects of drug; and altered comfort (blurred vision, dry mouth, flushing of skin) related to the drug's anticholinergic effects.

Implementation

Monitoring. Monitor hepatic function in the client receiving long-term therapy. Dehydration in clients may cause a variability in the response to diphenoxylate. Clients can have a delayed toxic response; observe for bloating, constipation, abdominal pain, and diminished bowel sounds indicative of paralytic ileus or toxic megacolon. If abdominal distention occurs, discontinue the drug. In hospitalized clients electrolytes must be monitored and dehydration corrected. If the client is not hospitalized, fluid intake should be increased to prevent dehydration. Weigh client daily until diarrhea is controlled to monitor fluid loss. Maintain client on intake and output.

Frequency and character of stools should be carefully monitored to observe if constipation, a potential side effect, occurs or if diarrhea is diminishing, indicating the efficacy of therapy.

Intervention. Modify the client's diet to support hydration and help control diarrhea. Provide good skin care to the perianal area.

Education. Caution clients about taking alcohol and CNS depressants with the drug. Instruct about its habit-forming potential. Dizziness and drowsiness are common side effects. Caution the client regarding tasks that involve alertness. Refer the client to the prescriber if diarrhea increases or fever develops.

Evaluation. The client will experience a decrease in or absence of diarrhea without side/adverse effects of the drug.

difenoxin [dye fen ox' in] (Motofen)

A third product in this category is difenoxin with atropine (Motofen). Difenoxin is the active metabolite derived from diphenoxylate, therefore it is effective at ⅕ the dose of diphenoxylate. It is indicated for the treatment of acute nonspecific diarrhea and acute exacerbations of chronic diarrhea. Peak serum levels are reached between 40 to 60 minutes. It is metabolized in the liver and primarily excreted by the kidneys and in feces.

The adult oral dose is 2 tablets initially, then 1 tablet after each loose stool or 1 tablet every 3 to 4 hours as needed. Maximum daily dose is 8 tablets.

Nursing management is as for diphenoxylate.

Adsorbents

Adsorbents are substances that take up or attach to (adsorb) another substance. They act by coating the wall of the gastrointestinal tract, absorbing the bacteria or toxins causing the diarrhea, and passing them out with the stools. Examples of drugs in this class requiring a prescription are the anion exchange resins, colestipol, and cholestyramine.

cholestyramine [koe less' tir a meen] (Questran)
Cholestyramine has a direct adsorbent affinity for acidic materials (e.g., bile acids). It is indicated as adjunctive therapy to diet in the treatment of hypercholesterolemia. Although not an FDA approved indication, cholestyramine has been used to treat diarrhea. For nursing management of cholestyramine, see Chapter 32, Antihyperlipidemic Drugs.

SUMMARY

Drugs and agents that affect the mouth are usually used for the provision of good oral hygiene. Dentifrices are helpful as mechanical aids for brushing teeth. Clotrimazole, ketoconazole, and nystatin are specific agents for the treatment of oral candidiasis.

Drugs that affect the stomach are classified as antacids, antiflatulents, digestants, antiemetics, emetics, and those used in the treatment of peptic ulcer. Antacids are used to neutralize hydrochloric acid in the stomach and may be composed of aluminum salts, calcium carbonate, magnesium salts, or sodium bicarbonate, alone or in combination. Digestants are administered to promote the process of digestion in instances of the deficiency of some substance essential to that process. Antiemetics are given for the relief of nausea and vomiting, but it is essential to determine the cause of the gastric distress, since these drugs may mask symptoms of more serious illnesses when they are administered. Emetics are administered to induce vomiting, usually as a part of drug overdoses or poisonings. Drugs used in the treatment of peptic ulcer are cytoprotective agents, which act locally to promote healing, and H_2receptor antagonists, which prevent histamine from stimulating the H_2 receptor and so reduce gastric acid secretion.

Chenodiol and ursodiol, which affect the gall bladder, are administered to dissolve radiolucent cholesterol gallstones of clients who may be surgical risks because of preexisting conditions.

Drugs affecting the lower gastrointestinal tract are either laxatives or antidiarrheal agents. Laxatives are given to relieve or prevent constipation, to expel parasites or poisonous substances, to obtain a specimen, or to cleanse the bowel for diagnostic examination. They are usually classified by their mechanism of action: saline, stimulant, bulk-forming, emollient, or lubricant laxatives, or bowel evacuants. The goal is to return the client to a normal, adequate bowel pattern.

The antidiarrheals are administered to reduce the frequency of evacuations. This is only part of a treatment plan that should also include replenishment of fluid and electrolyte loss, diagnosis and treatment of the underlying cause, and restoration of the intestinal flora. Again the goal of treatment is to return the client to a normal, adequate bowel pattern.

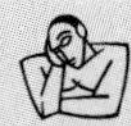

Critical Thinking

1. Given the efficacy of the products, why are advertising monies spent for mouthwashes and gargles?
2. Why is it important to establish the underlying cause of vomiting before administering any antiemetic?
3. How would you use ipecac syrup for a 2-year-old who has ingested half a bottle of baby aspirin?
4. What lifestyle teaching would be important to be supportive of H_2 receptor antagonist therapy?
5. What would be the laxative of choice for Mr. Preston, a 56-year-old client, 3 days after his myocardial infarction? For Jimmy Tyrone, 7 years old, whose last bowel movement was 4 days ago? For Mrs. White, a 42-year-old client being prepared for a colonoscopy? Why would it be the drug of choice and what disadvantages are involved in its use?
6. Alice Reagan, a 27-year-old teacher, has just returned from a week's vacation in Mexico with severe diarrhea of 3 days' duration. What criteria should be considered in the selection of an antidiarrheal agent?

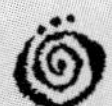

Collaborative Learning Activities

1. Form teams to discuss the case study of the client with peptic ulcer disease, p. 711. Each team will develop and present a plan related to health instruction for Mr. Blake.
2. Discuss the case study on drug therapy for bowel elimination, p. 718. If admitting Margaret Gordon to the home health agency, what plan of care should be established? What would be appropriate care outcomes for Ms. Gordon and how would the class intervene to achieve these goals?

BIBLIOGRAPHY

Abramowicz M (1994). Drugs for treatment of peptic ulcers, *Med Lett* 36(927):65-7.

Ahronheim JC (1992). *Handbook of prescribing medications for geriatric patients.* Boston: Little, Brown.

Allison OC, et al. (1994). Chronic constipation: Assessment and management in elderly, *J Amer Acad Nurs Pract* 6(7):311-7.

American Hospital Formulary Service (1996). *AHFS drug information '96*. Bethesda, MD: American Society of Pharmacists.

Anastasi JK (1993). Caring for clients with diarrhea, *Nursing* 23(8):68.

Anderson KN, et al. (Eds.).(1994). *Mosby's Medical, nursing, & allied health dictionary* (4th ed.). St Louis: Mosby.

Brunton LL (1996). Agents affecting gastrointestinal water flux and motility; emesis and antiemetics; bile acids and pancreatic enzymes. In Hardman JG & Limbird LE (Eds.). *Goodman & Gilman's the pharmacological basis of therapeutics* (9th ed.). New York: McGraw-Hill.

Canty SL (1994). Constipation as a side effect of opioids, *Oncol Nurs Forum* 21(4):739-45.

Carpenito LJ (1995). *Nursing diagnosis: Application to clinical practice* (6th ed.).Philadelphia: JB Lippincott.

Carpenito LJ. (1989-90). *Nursing diagnosis: Application to clinical practice.* (3rd ed.). Philadelphia: JB Lippincott.

Cerda JJ, et al. (1994). A revolution in peptic ulcer disease, *Patient Care* 28(9):18-22, 24, 25-8.

Covington TR (Ed.) (1996). *Handbook of nonprescription drugs: Product updates* (11th ed.). Washington DC: The American Pharmaceutical Association.

Egan AP, et al. (1992). Management of chemotherapy-related nausea and vomiting using a serotonin antagonist, *Oncol Nurs Forum* 19(5):791.

Fedotin MS (1993). Helicobacter pylori-associated ulcer disease: Current treatment options, *Hosp Formul* 28(7):632-4, 636, 639-40.

Flynn AA.(1996). Oral Health Products. In Covington TR (Ed.). *Handbook of nonprescription drugs* (11th ed.). Washington, DC: American Pharmaceutical Association.

Graham DY (1993). Treatment of peptic ulcers caused by *Helicobacter pylori, New Engl J Med* 328(5):349-350.

Hall GR, et al. (1995). Managing constipation using a researched-based protocol, *MedSurg Nurs* 44(1):11-20.

Hamacher DR (1993). Mouthwash, *NARD Journal* 115(6):57.

Katzung BG (1992). *Basic and clinical pharmacology* (5th ed.). Norwalk, CT: Appleton & Lange.

Koda-Kimble MA & Young LY (1995). Nausea and vomiting. In Young LY & Koda-Kimble MA. *Applied therapeutics* (6th ed.). Vancouver: Applied Therapeutics.

Lichter I (1993). Forum: Which antiemetic? *J Palliat Care* 9(1):42.

Long K, et al. (1994). Treating gastroesophageal reflux disease, *Nurs Pract Forum* 5(2):63-4.

Marcus R (1996). Agents affecting calcification and bone turnover. In Young LY & Koda-Kimble MA. *Applied therapeutics* (6th ed.). Vancouver, WA: Applied Therapeutics.

Ofman J, et al. (1994). Peptic ulcer disease dealing with *H. pylori*-induced ulceration, *Consultant* 34(7):987-90, 992-4.

Olin BR (Ed.) (1996-1997). *Facts and comparisons.* St Louis: Facts and Comparisons.

Plezia PM, et al. (1990). Randomized crossover comparison of high-dose intravenous metoclopramide versus a five-drug antiemetic regimen, *J Pain Sympt Management* 5(2):101.

Smith C (1995). Upper gastrointestinal disorders. In Young LY & Koda-Kimble MA. *Applied therapeutics* (6th ed.). Vancouver, WA: Applied Therapeutics.

United States Pharmacopeia Convention (1996). *USP DI: Drug information for the health care professional* (16 ed.). Rockville, MD: The Convention.

Williams SG & DiPalma JA (1992). Medication-induced digestive system injury in the elderly, *Geriatr Nurs* 13(1):39.

Chapter 42

Overview of the Eye

Chapter Focus

Approximately 70% of all sensory information is perceived through the eyes. Visual impairment, which often accompanies ophthalmic disorders, affects the client's ability to function independently and diminishes his or her perception of the environment. Disorders of the eye are becoming increasingly common as our population ages. To appropriately assess and care for clients with ophthalmic problems, the nurse needs an understanding of the anatomy and physiology of the eye. The following objectives and key terms are important for a good understanding of this chapter.

Key Terms

accommodation (p. 725)
cataract (p. 725)
cornea (p. 725)
cycloplegia (p. 726)
miosis (p. 725)
mydriasis (p. 725)

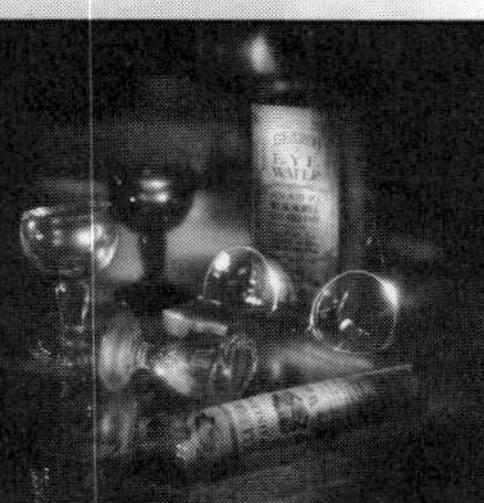

Objectives

1. Describe the anatomy and physiology of the eye.
2. Identify the muscles involved with miosis and mydriasis and explain their functions.
3. Define accommodation and cycloplegia.
4. Name four protective mechanisms associated with the eye.

The eye is the receptor organ for one of the most delicate and valuable senses—vision. Figure 42-1 shows the parts of the eye.

The eyeball has three layers or coats: the protective external layer (cornea and sclera), the middle layer (which contains the choroid, iris, and ciliary body), and the light-sensitive retina.

The eyeball is protected in a deep depression of the skull called the orbit. It is moved in the orbit by six small extraocular muscles.

The anterior covering of the eye is the **cornea**. The cornea is normally transparent, so it allows light to enter the eye. The cornea has no blood vessels and receives its nutrition from the aqueous humor and its oxygen supply by diffusion from the air and surrounding structures. The corneal surface consists of a thin layer of epithelial cells, which are quite resistant to infection. However, an abraded cornea is very susceptible to infection. The cornea is also supplied with 60 to 80 sensory fibers that elicit pain whenever the corneal epithelium is damaged. Seriously injured corneal tissue is replaced by scar tissue, which is usually not transparent. Increased intraocular pressure results in loss of transparency.

The sclera, which is continuous with the cornea, is nontransparent; it is the white fibrous envelope of the eye.

The conjunctiva is the mucous membrane lining the anterior part of the sclera and the inner surfaces of each eyelid.

The iris gives the eye its brown, blue, gray, green, or hazel color. It surrounds the pupil; the sphincter and dilator muscles in the iris alter pupil size. The sphincter muscle, which encircles the pupil, is parasympathetically innervated; the dilator muscle, which runs radially from the pupil to the periphery of the iris, is sympathetically innervated. Contraction of the sphincter muscle, either alone or with relaxation of the dilator muscle, causes constriction of the pupil, or **miosis.** Contraction of the dilator muscle and relaxation of the sphincter muscle causes dilation of the pupil, or **mydriasis** (Figure 42-2). Drugs producing miosis (miotics) act by (1) interfering with cholinesterase activity or (2) acting like acetylcholine at receptor sites in the sphincter muscle. Drugs producing mydriasis (mydriatics) act by (1) interfering with the action of acetylcholine or (2) stimulating sympathetic or adrenergic receptors. Pupil constriction normally occurs in bright light or when the eye is focusing on nearby objects. Pupil dilation normally occurs in dim light or when the eye is focusing on distant objects.

The lens is situated behind the iris. It is a transparent mass of uniformly arranged fibers encased in a thin elastic capsule. Its protein concentration is higher than that of any other tissue of the body.

The function of the lens is to ensure that the image on the retina is in sharp focus. The lens does this by changing shape (**accommodation**) to adjust to variations in distance. This occurs readily in young persons, but with age the lens becomes more rigid. The ability to focus on close objects is then lost, and the *near point* (the closest point that can be seen clearly) recedes. With age the lens may also lose its transparency and become opaque; this is known as a **cataract.** Unless it can be treated or removed surgically, blindness can occur. However, if the opaque (cataract) portion is located peripherally in the lens, vision is not compromised.

The lens has suspensory ligaments called zonular fibers around its edge, which connect with the ciliary body. Their tension helps to change the shape of the lens. In the unaccommodated eye the ciliary muscle is relaxed and the zonular fibers are taut. When zonular fibers contract, the pupil dilates, resulting in sharp distant vision and blurred

Posterior chamber
Anterior chamber (aqueous humor)
Conjunctiva
Cornea
Pupil
Iris
Canal of Schlemm
Zonular fibers
Ciliary body
Sclera
Choroid
Fovea
Optic nerve
Retina
Vitreous body

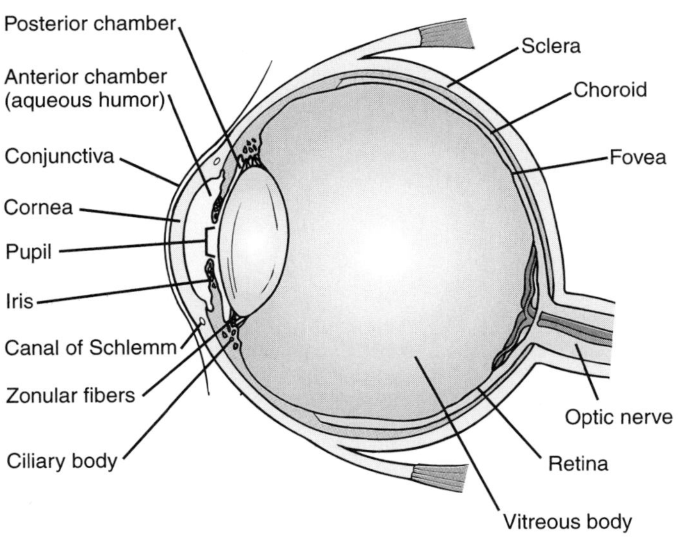

Figure 42-1 Parts of the eye.

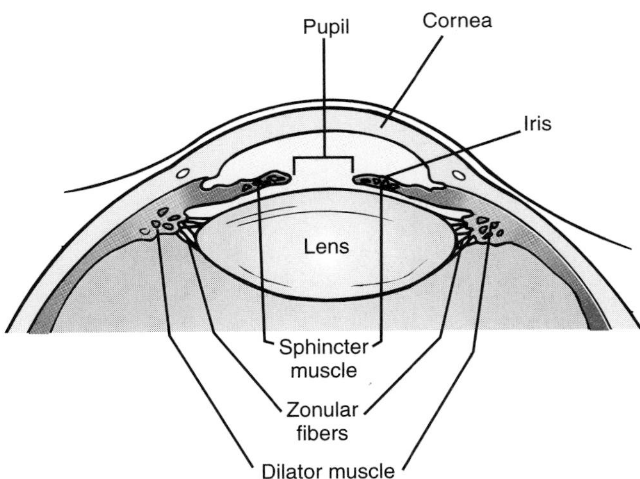

Figure 42-2 Accommodation and pupillary alterations. When zonular fibers contract, the pupil dilates, resulting in sharp distant vision and blurred near vision (unaccommodated eye). Parasympathetic stimulation accommodates the eye for near vision; the pupil constricts in response to contraction of the sphincter muscle. The zonular fibers are relaxed. *Pupillary diameter:* Constriction (miosis): contraction of sphincter muscle (parasympathetic stimulation) alone or with relaxation of dilator muscle. Dilation (mydriasis): contraction of dilator muscle (sympathetic stimulation) alone or with relaxation of dilator muscle.

near vision (unaccommodated eye). Parasympathetic stimulation accommodates the eye for near vision; the pupil constricts in response to contraction of the sphincter muscle. The zonular fibers are relaxed.

Accommodation depends on two factors: (1) ciliary muscle contraction and (2) the ability of the lens to assume a more biconvex shape when tension on the ligaments is relaxed. The ciliary muscle is innervated by parasympathetic fibers. Paralysis of the ciliary muscle is termed **cycloplegia.**

Aqueous humor is formed by the ciliary body. It bathes and feeds the lens, iris, and posterior surface of the cornea. After it is formed, it flows forward between the lens and the iris into the anterior chamber. It drains out of the eye through drainage channels located near the junction of the cornea and sclera. A trabecular meshwork called the canals of Schlemm drains the aqueous humor into the venous system of the eye (Figure 43-2).

The retina contains nerve endings plus the rods and cones that function as visual sensory receptors. It is connected to the brain by the optic nerve, which leaves the orbit through a bony canal in the posterior wall.

Eyelashes, eyelids, blinking, and tears all serve to protect the eye. Each eye has about 200 eyelashes. A blink reflex occurs whenever a foreign body touches the eyelashes. The lids close quickly to prevent the foreign substance from entering the eye. Blinking, which is bilateral, occurs every few seconds during waking hours. It keeps the corneal surface free of mucus and spreads the lacrimal fluid evenly over the cornea. Tears are secreted by lacrimal glands and contain lysozyme, a mucolytic enzyme with bactericidal action. Tears provide lubrication for lid movements. They wash away noxious agents. By forming a thin film over the cornea, tears provide it with a good optical surface. Tear fluid is lost by evaporation and by draining into two small ducts (the lacrimal canaliculi) at the inner corners of the upper and lower eyelids.

SUMMARY

The eyes provide much of the information of the world around us. These delicate structures are protected from direct sunlight, damaging particles, and dryness of the environment by accessory structures such as eyelids, eye muscles, and tear glands.

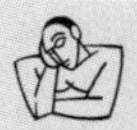

Critical Thinking

1. Mrs. B. has come to have her eyes examined. During the examination her pupils will be dilated. As part of your post-examination instructions to her, you tell her she will be unable to drive home. Why?
2. One of your classmates can't see the whiteboard during class and moves to the front row, but still gets headaches. What do you think is happening and what causes this?

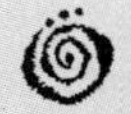

Collaborative Learning Activities

1. Pairs of students will present the main components of the eyeball. They will incorporate functions of both major and related minor components and to include applicable disorders.

BIBLIOGRAPHY

Anderson KN, et al. (Eds.) (1994). *Mosby's medical, nursing, & allied health dictionary* (4th ed.). St Louis: Mosby.

Seeley RR, et al. (1995). *Anatomy and physiology* (3rd ed.). St Louis: Mosby.

Thibodeau GA & Patton K (1996). *Anatomy and physiology* (3rd ed.). St Louis: Mosby.

Van Wynsberghe D, Noback CR, & Carola R (1995). *Human anatomy and physiology* (3rd ed.). New York: McGraw-Hill.

Wingard LB, et al. (191). *Human pharmacology.* St Louis: Mosby.

Chapter 43

Ophthalmic Drugs

Chapter Focus

Eye disorders and the sensory/perceptual alterations that occur can cause varying degrees of disability. Early detection and treatment of eye disorders can minimize limitations of vision. Ophthalmic drugs make a significant contribution to the treatment of disorders of the eye and the preservation of vision. The following objectives and key terms are important for a good understanding of this chapter.

Key Terms

glaucoma (p. 731)
miotics (p. 733)
mydriasis (p. 736)

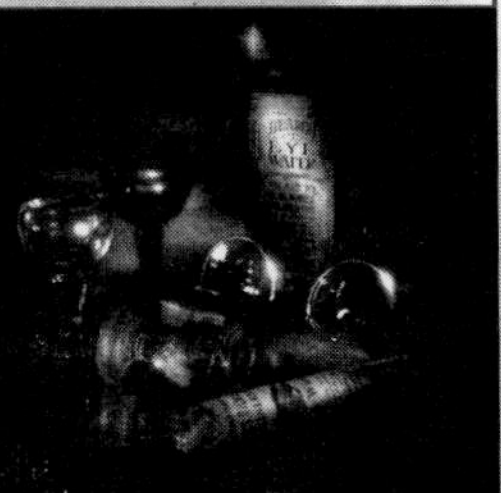

Objectives

1. Discuss nursing management of ophthalmic drug administration.
2. Compare and contrast the antiglaucoma agents.
3. Discuss systemic effects of ophthalmic drugs.
4. List antiinfective and antiinflammatory ophthalmic agents.
5. Implement the nursing management of the care of clients receiving ophthalmic agents.

Drugs used to treat eye disorders can be divided into three major groups: the antiglaucoma agents, the mydriatics and cycloplegics, and the antiinfective/antiinflammatory agents. There are many eye preparations available, including ophthalmic diagnostic products, enzymes, irrigating solutions, eye washes, and hyperosmolar preparations. This chapter discusses the major groups and selected other eye preparations, along with their major dosage and administration considerations and nursing management.

Nursing Management

Drugs Affecting the Eye

Assessment. Assess the eyes for redness, swelling, tearing, discharge, decrease in visual acuity, and pain. In the case of glaucoma, the client will demonstrate increased intraocular pressure on tonometry.

Nursing diagnosis. Once clients have begun a course of therapy with ophthalmic preparations, they should be evaluated for the following possible nursing diagnoses: knowledge deficit related to the self-administration of the medication and the condition for which it is administered; risk for the development of hypersensitivity, superinfections, and systemic effects of the drug; and risk for injury related to blurred vision as the result of the instillation of drops or ointment into the eye. For other selected nursing diagnoses to consider for clients receiving ophthalmic conditions, see the Nursing Care Plan below.

Implementation

Monitoring. Monitor the affected eye(s) on a daily basis for improvement of the condition for which the medication was prescribed. Assess for redness, itching, swelling, and burning sensation that was not present before therapy started and so might be indicative of a hypersensitivity. Systemic absorption may occur with eyedrops and cause adverse systemic reactions (Table 43-1). Assess the client for ocular side/adverse effects related to administration of systemic medications as outlined in Table 43-2.

Intervention. In addition to developing a working knowledge of the ophthalmic agents available, the nurse must be especially aware of the special considerations in administering these drugs. Ocular drugs are administered by topical application of a solution or ointment (Box 43-1).

Nursing Care Plan

Selected Nursing Diagnoses Related to Ophthalmic Drugs

Nursing diagnosis	Outcome criteria	Interventions
Knowledge deficit related to new ophthalmic drug regimen	Client will: Express understanding of purpose, function, side effects/adverse reactions Demonstrate proper handling and administration Discuss possible drug interactions	Assess client's level of understanding. Determine educational needs of client. Instruct client in: Purpose and function of medicine Side effects/adverse reactions that may occur and appropriate response Proper storage and handling Correct method of administration Systemic reactions that may occur with topically applied eye preparations Provide client with a list of possible drug interactions.
Anxiety related to possible decrease in or loss of vision	Client will: Verbalize fears and concerns	Assess client for perceptions and fears related to eye disorder. Encourage open communication about fears. Provide emotional support. Provide information related to effectiveness of drug therapy. Allay unwarranted fears.
Alteration in comfort related to ophthalmic disorder	Client will: Express a decrease in discomfort	Closely assess the client's symptoms and level of comfort. Provide rest and limiting of eye activity (reading, etc.). Provide emotional support and encouragement.
Risk for injury related to impaired vision	Client will: Maintain activity appropriate for level of vision without injury Discuss necessary lifestyle adjustments	Assess level of vision impairment. Provide safety measures as needed. Encourage client to adjust activities in accordance with client's level of vision.

TABLE 43-1 Ophthalmic drugs: adverse systemic effects

Ophthalmic drug	Reported adverse effect
Antimicrobial agents	
chloramphenicol eyedrops	Aplastic anemia
sulfacetamide eyedrops	Stevens-Johnson syndrome, systemic lupus erythematosus
Anticholinergic drugs	
atropine eyedrops	Tachycardia, elevated temperature, fever, delirium
cyclopentolate	Convulsions, hallucinations
scopolamine eyedrops	Acute psychosis
Antiglaucoma medications	
beta blocking agents (timolol)	Bradycardia, syncope, low blood pressure, asthmatic attack, congestive heart failure, hallucinations, loss of appetite, headaches, nausea, weakness, depression
anticholinesterase (echothiophate)	Asthmatic attack, systemic cholinergic effects
parasympathomimetic (pilocarpine)	Nausea, stomach pain, increased sweating, salivation, tremors, bradycardia, lightheadedness
Adrenergic medications	
phenylephrine (10%)	Severe hypertension, cerebral hemorrhage, dysrhythmias, myocardial infarction
epinephrine eyedrops	Tremors increased sweating, headaches, hypertension

TABLE 43-2 Ocular side effects induced by systemic medications

Drug	Possible ocular side effect induced	Drug	Possible ocular side effect induced
allopurinol	Retinal hemorrhage, exudative lesions	indomethacin	Mydriasis, retinopathy
aspirin	Allergic dermatitis including keratitis and conjunctivitis	isoniazid	Optic neuritis
barbiturates	Nystagmus	lithium carbonate	Exophthalmos
busulfan	Cataracts	nitroglycerin	Transient elevation in intraocular pressure
cannabis, marijuana	Nystagmus, conjunctivitis, double vision	opiates	Miosis, nystagmus
chloral hydrate	Eyelid edema, conjunctivitis, miosis	phenothiazines	Corneal and conjunctival deposits, cataracts, retinopathy, oculogyric crisis
chloroquine	Lenticular and corneal opacity, retinopathy	phenytoin	Nystagmus
clomiphene citrate	Blurred vision, light flashes	quinine	Blurring of vision, optic neuritis, blindness (reversible)
clinidine	Miosis	thiazide diuretics	Acute transient myopia, yellow coloring of vision
corticosteroids	Cataracts, increased intraocular pressure, papilledema	vincristine	Ptosis, paresis of extraocular muscles
diazoxide	Oculogyric crisis	vitamin A overdose or toxicity	Papilledema, increased intraocular pressure
digitalis glycosides	Scotomas, optic neuritis	vitamin D toxicity	Calcium deposits in cornea
ethyl alcohol	Nystagmus		
guanethidine	Miosis, ptosis, blurred vision		
hydralazine	Lacrimation, blurred vision		
ibuprofen	Altered color vision, blurred vision		

BOX 43-1

Guidelines for Instillation of Eyedrops and Ointments

To instill eyedrops

Wash your hands and put on gloves if necessary.

Gently cleanse exudate from the eye, if necessary.

Ask the client to tilt the head toward the side of the affected eye.

Gently pull the lower eyelid down and ask the client to look up.

Instill the correct number of drops in the sac formed by the lower eyelid (Figure 43-1).

Take care not to touch the dropper to the eye or eyelashes.

Gently apply pressure for 30 seconds to 1 minute over the inner canthus next to the nose to prevent absorption through the tear duct and premature drainage of the medication away from the eye.

Ask the client to gently close the eye, which distributes the solution. Warn against squeezing the eye tightly, which will force out the medication.

Wipe away any excess medication.

If both eyes are to be medicated, do the second instillation quickly before the patient begins to blink and tear as a reaction to the burning sensation occurring in the first eye medicated.

To instill eye ointment

The procedure is the same except the ointment is expressed directly onto the exposed conjunctival sac from inner to outer canthus with a small individual tube and close eye; gently massage to distribute the medication.

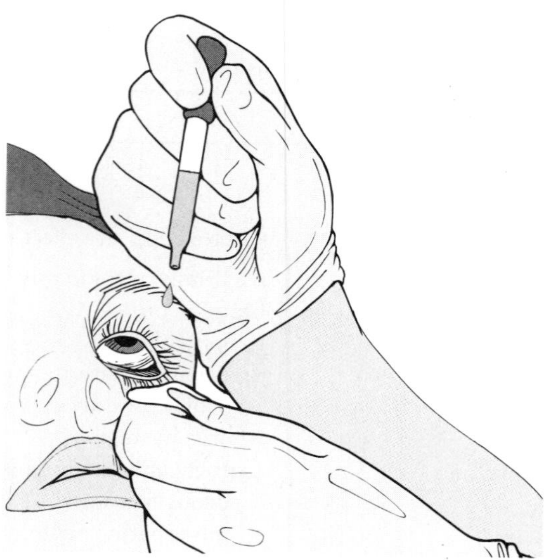

Figure 43-1 Instillation of drops into the conjunctiva of the lower lid of the eye.

Ocular solutions are sterile and easily administered, and usually do not interfere with vision. Their main disadvantage is the short time that the drug is in contact with the eye. Ocular ointments have the advantages of being quite comfortable on instillation and keeping the drug in longer contact with the eye for more prolonged effects. However, ointments form a film or haze over the eye that interferes with vision and causes a higher incidence of contact dermatitis than do solutions. In addition, most ointments are not sterile.

Packs may also be used to apply drugs to the eye. These are cotton pledgets saturated with an ophthalmic solution and inserted into the inferior or superior cul-de-sac. Ocular drugs may also be physician-administered by iontophoresis, subconjunctival (sub-Tenon's) injection, retrobulbar injection, or injection directly into the vitreous or anterior chamber of the eye.

Ocular gel formulations and Ocuserts provide new delivery systems for pilocarpine and perhaps other medications as well. The newer systems were developed to overcome some of the problems with conventional eyedrops or ointments. Their longer duration of action improves client management of the therapeutic regimen and avoids the peak and valley response associated with the previous solutions and ointments. A steady pilocarpine release or range should reduce drug-induced adverse reactions and improve treatment outcome.

Education. Instruct the client and/or home caregiver in proper administration of eye medications (see Figure 43-1 and Box 43-1). Caution the client to always check the bottle label for correct medication and concentration, such as 0.1% or 1%. Checking labels is increasingly important because many beauty aids and home products (glues) are now packaged in similar containers (Box 43-2). Discard solutions that have become cloudy or darkened.

Store medications as directed on the label; some may need refrigeration. Once opened, most medications have a limited life (3 months or the end of the current illness). If stored longer, the medication is more likely to become contaminated and lead to an infection of the eye (see the Nursing Research Box on p. 731). To avoid such contamination from the outset, the sterility of the preparation and/or dropper must be maintained. Do not allow the tube tip or dropper to touch anything, including the skin. Hold the dropper with the tip down. Never allow medication to flow into the bulb of the dropper. Keep the container closed when not in use. If two or more family members are using eye medications, each should have a separate vial to prevent cross-contamination.

BOX 43-2

Eyedrops and Look Alikes

Containers that are facsimiles are the culprits behind many ophthalmic emergencies. Thinking they are instilling eyedrops, adults and children have instead dropped in superglue, contact lens cleaners, ear drops, and perfumes. These products are often sold in bottles that are similar in shape, size, and color. The elderly who may have poor eyesight are particularly at risk for mistaking one product for another.

In most cases, the injured eye responds to copious flushing to dilute and wash out the offending agent, followed by topical antibiotics, lubricants or cycloplegics, and patching, if needed. If the client has instilled glue in the eye and has no significant pain, irrigation and a sterile eyepatch soaked in tap water and left overnight are sufficient. The solvents to dissolve the glue are too toxic for the eye, so if the conservative approach does not work, the client may need to be referred to an ophthalmologist, who may cut the eyelids apart to prevent corneal abrasion.

Advise all clients to keep their eyedrops in one particular place away from other chemicals. Recommend that they check the labels on the container while still wearing their glasses or contact lenses to ensure they have the right medicine before administering their eyedrops.

Critical thinking questions

- What other ways could eye instillations of inappropriate solutions be prevented for visually impaired clients?
- Should there be regulation of the packaging to prevent such accidents? If so, what would be the social and economic effects of such regulation?

From O'Boyle & Enzenauer (1992).

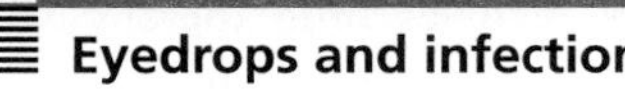

Nursing Research

Eyedrops and infection

A study was done at the Massachusetts Eye and Ear Infirmary to examine the incidence of contamination of eyedrops and ointments in use by clients. Schein et al (1992) cultured 220 eye medications in use by 101 patients who had nonmicrobial ocular surface disease at the Infirmary. Conjuctival cultures were taken from the study patients and from 50 age-matched controls without eye surface disease or infection. Potentially pathogenic organisms were cultured from 64 medications (29%) and from 34 study patients (34%), compared with only 5 of 50 control patients. The commonest contaminants were gram-negative organisms. Coagulase-negative staphylococci and diphtheroides—the usual conjuctival flora—were also found frequently in the eyedrops and ointments, as were small numbers of gram-positive organisms and fungi.

Medication caps had the highest rate of bacterial colonization. The contents then become colonized by contamination from the dropper or ointment drip. Contamination of the dropper or medication itself is clinically important because it guarantees delivery of the organism to the ocular surface.

Clients should be advised to discard old bottles of eye medications. They should be carefully instructed in the administration of eye medications so that the tip of the dropper or ointment tube does not come in contact with the skin, eye, or eyelashes. They should promptly cap the medication after use.

Critical thinking questions

- How would this research influence your assessment of a client using eye medications? How would it influence your health teaching?
- Try administering eyedrops or eye ointment with garden gloves on to simulate impaired mobility of the hands which might occur with aging. How might this limitation affect contamination of the medication?

From Schein et al (1992).

Inform the client of signs of side effects/adverse reactions, as well as signs of progress. Advise the client when to contact or return to the prescriber for assessment.

Evaluation. The client will experience a decrease in or absence of the symptoms for which the agent was prescribed.

ANTIGLAUCOMA AGENTS

Glaucoma is an eye disease characterized chiefly by abnormally elevated intraocular pressure (IOP) that may result from excessive production of aqueous humor or diminished ocular fluid outflow. Increased pressure, if sufficiently high and persistent, may lead to irreversible blindness. Although it is primarily a disease of middle age, occurring in approximately 2% of all persons 40 years and older, it has also been diagnosed in younger adults and children. There are three major types of glaucoma—primary, secondary, and congenital.

Primary glaucoma includes angle-closure (acute congestive) glaucoma and open-angle (chronic simple) glaucoma (Figure 43-2). Persons with angle-closure glaucoma have closure of the angle of the anterior chamber, possibly because of a physiologic or anatomic predisposition. Drugs are needed to control the acute attack associated with angle-closure glaucoma, followed usually by surgery, such as iridectomy or laser surgery. Open or wide-angle glaucoma is more common, occurring in approximately 90% of the individuals with primary glaucoma. The increased IOP is secondary to an increased production of aqueous humor or a decreased outflow caused by degenerative changes in the outflow system. It has a gradual insidious onset, and its control depends on drug therapy or perhaps a peripheral iridectomy.

Secondary glaucoma may result from previous eye disease or may follow cataract extraction (Abel, 1995). Therapy for secondary glaucoma usually involves drug therapy while congenital glaucoma requires surgical treatment.

Primary medications used to treat glaucoma include beta-adrenergic blocking agents, cholinergics, and sympathomimetics; selection of a drug is determined largely by the requirements and individual response of the person.

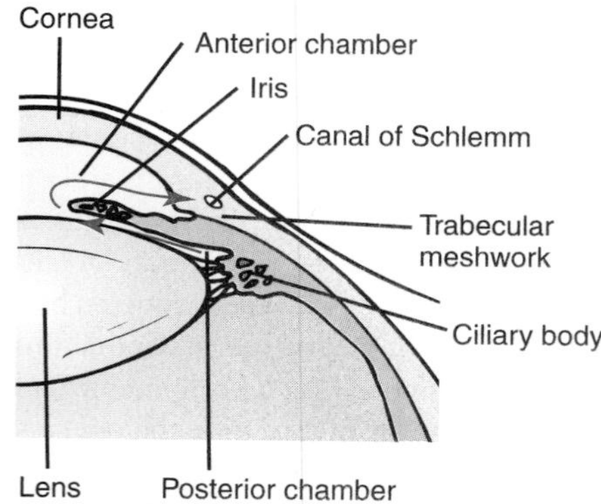

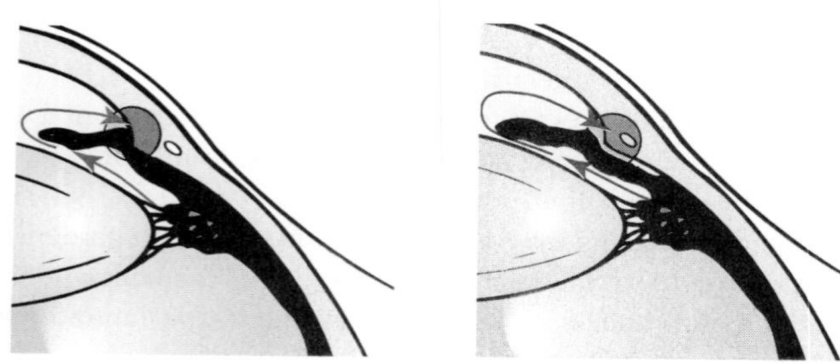

Figure 43-2 Main structures of the eye and enlargement of the canal of Schlemm showing aqueous flow in normal, angle-closure, and open-angle glaucoma.

Beta-Adrenergic Blocking Agents

The beta-adrenergic blocking agents include betaxolol (Betoptic), carteolol (Ocupress), levobunolol (Betagen C Cap), metipranolol (OptiPranol), and timolol (Timoptic). Betaxolol is a cardioselective ($beta_1$) blocking agent, whereas all the other beta blockers are noncardioselective—they block both $beta_1$ and $beta_2$ adrenergic receptors. These agents work alone or in combination with other drugs to decrease the production of aqueous humor, thus reducing intraocular pressure in open-angle glaucoma. The exact mechanism of action for these agents though is unknown.

Timolol is also used to treat glaucoma in selected cases of secondary glaucoma. Betaxolol is indicated for the treatment of open-angle glaucoma and ocular hypertension and may be a drug of choice for clients with pulmonary disease because of its selective $beta_1$ blocking effects, although the nurse should still monitor for respiratory difficulties.

The side/adverse effects of the beta-adrenergic blocking ophthalmic agents are primarily local reactions, such as burning, stinging, or eye irritation. Rare effects include eye inflammation, visual disturbance, pruritus, or allergic reaction. These agents can be systemically absorbed to cause bradycardia or tachycardia, confusion, insomnia, weakness, wheezing, respiratory difficulties, depression, ataxia, edema of lower extremities, nausea, and vomiting. Hallucinations have been reported with timolol only. Table 43-3 lists beta-adrenergic blocking agents, pharmacokinetics, and dosing information.

▪ Nursing Management

Beta-Adrenergic Blocking Agent Ophthalmic Therapy

Assessment. Use caution in administering beta-adrenergic blocking agents to clients who have bronchial asthma, heart disease, sinus bradycardia or greater than first-degree heart block, cardiogenic shock, right ventricular failure caused by pulmonary hypertension, or congestive heart failure. There is sufficient absorption from the conjunctiva and nasopharynx to produce systemic nonselective beta-adrenergic ($beta_1$ and $beta_2$) effects such as cardiopulmonary

TABLE 43-3 Beta-adrenergic blocking agents: pharmacokinetics and dosing

Drug	Onset of action (hr)	Peak effect (hr)	Duration of action (hr)	Usual adult dosage
betaxolol (Betoptic)	0.5	2	12	0.25%, 0.5%—instill one drop twice daily
carteolol (Ocupress)	N/A	2	6-8	1%—instill one drop twice daily
levobunolol (Betagan C Cap B.I.D.)	1	2-6	up to 24	0.25%—instill one drop 1-2 times daily; 0.5%, instill one drop daily
metipranolol (OptiPranolol)	0.5	2	24	0.3%—instill one drop twice daily
timolol (Timoptic)	0.5	1-2	up to 24	0.25%,0.5% instill one drop 1-2 times daily

N/A, not available.

complications and exacerbation of asthma. If these agents are used with clients with diabetes mellitus, symptoms of hypoglycemia may be masked.

Because the drug may be absorbed systemically, review the client's current medication regimen for drug interactions such as those listed in Chapter 22 for systemic beta-adrenergic blocking agents.

Obtain baseline determinations for the client's vision, intraocular pressure, and vital signs.

Nursing diagnosis. The client has the potential for the following selected nursing diagnoses: sensory/perceptual alterations (visual) related to the client's underlying condition or the development of ocular irritation, altered comfort related to eye pain, and the collaborative problem of decreased cardiac output related to systemic absorption of the drug.

Implementation

Monitoring. Assess the client's vision and intraocular pressure periodically. Monitor the eye for inflammation because although these agents are usually well tolerated, occasional signs of mild ocular irritation may occur. Local hypersensitivity (rash) occurs rarely. Monitor the client's vital signs because a slight reduction of resting heart rate may occur, and acute bronchospasm in clients with bronchospastic disease has been reported.

Intervention. Use nasolacrimal occlusion to minimize systemic absorption.

Education. Instruct the client in the proper administration technique. Alert clients with diabetes that symptoms of hypoglycemia may be masked, such as tachycardia and trembling. Instruct the client to alert health practitioners to the drug if surgery is considered, since some prescribers recommend that these agents be gradually withdrawn 48 hours before surgery. Encourage regular consultation with the prescriber to check intraocular pressure.

Evaluation. The client will experience therapeutic reduction in intraocular pressure without systemic beta-adrenergic blocking effects.

Also see nursing management of beta-adrenergic blocking agents in Chapter 22.

Cholinergic Agents

Cholinergic medications or **miotics,** so called because they cause pupillary constriction, are topically applied agents useful in treating open-angle and angle-closure glaucoma. Cholinergic miotics (direct acting) are chemically related to acetylcholine, the neurotransmitter that mediates nerve impulse transmission at all cholinergic or parasympathetic nerve sites. Applied topically to the eye, cholinergic drugs cause contraction of the sphincter muscle of the iris, resulting in pupil constriction (miosis), and contraction of the ciliary muscle attached to the trabecular meshwork, thus opening the spaces in the meshwork increasing the outflow of aqueous humor. The ciliary muscle effect leaves the eye in accommodation of near vision.

Anticholinesterase drugs (indirect acting), such as carbachol (Carboptic) and pilocarpine (IsoptoCarpine), inhibit the enzymatic destruction of acetylcholine by inactivating cholinesterase. This permits acetylcholine to act on the iris sphincter and ciliary muscles, producing pupil constriction (miosis) and ciliary muscle contraction (accommodation).

The irreversible anticholinesterase drugs, (echothiophate [Phospholine Iodide] and isoflurophate [Floropryl]), form stable complexes with cholinesterase and thus irreversibly impair the destructive function of the enzyme. Destruction of acetylcholine then depends on synthesis of new enzymes. Demecarium (Humorsol) is more toxic than the other agents in this category, so it is not as commonly used. Although it is a reversible inhibitor, its prolonged action has results similar to the irreversible inhibitors.

The cholinesterase inhibitors, though, are usually reserved for persons that inadequately respond to the first line agents, such as beta blockers, cholinergics (pilocarpine), and sympathomimetics (epinephrine).

Cholinergic side/adverse effects include visual blurring, irritation, myopia, ciliary spasm, brow pain, and headache resulting from stimulation of accommodative ancillary muscles. Miosis also makes it difficult to adjust quickly to changes in illumination. This may be serious in elderly persons, since their light adaptation and visual acuity are often reduced. Nighttime is particularly hazardous for these individuals.

Cysts of the iris, synechiae, retinal detachments, obstruction of tear drainage, and even cataracts may develop with prolonged use, especially with the long-acting anticholinesterases. Generally direct-acting cholinergic side effects are less severe and occur less frequently than those caused by anticholinesterase agents. Systemic side effects include salivation, nausea, vomiting, diarrhea, precipitation of asthmatic attack, fall in blood pressure, and other symptoms of parasympathetic stimulation. Table 43-4 lists Cholinergic Agents: Pharmacokinetics and Dosing.

Sympathomimetic Agents

The primary sympathomimetic agents are dipivefrin (Propine), which is converted to epinephrine by enzyme hydrolysis in the eye, and epinephrine, a direct acting sympathomimetic agent. Dipivefrin's chemical modification results in a more lipophilic compound that facilitates absorption and penetration through the cornea into the anterior chamber of the eye. The penetration and absorption of dipivefrin is greater than epinephrine. The mechanism of action is unknown although it appears they lower intraocular pressure by decreasing aqueous humor production and increasing its outflow. They are indicated for the treatment of open-angle glaucoma.

Side/adverse effects are rarely troublesome; they include burning, stinging or eye irritation, headache, brow pain, and watering of the eyes. The signs and symptoms of systemic absorption include tachycardia, palpitations, hypertension, increased sweating, tremors, and lightheadedness.

TABLE 43-4 Cholinergic agents: pharmacokinetics and dosing

Drug	Onset of action (hr)	Peak effect (hr)	Duration of action (hr)	Usual adult dosage
Miotics—direct acting				
carbachol (Carboptic)	0.25	Miosis: 2-5 min IOP: within 4	24	0.75%-3%—one drop topically 3 times daily
pilocarpine (Isopto Carpine)	up to 0.5	1-1.25	4-8	0.25%-4%—1 drop topically up to 4 times daily
Miotics—cholinesterase inhibitors				
demecarium (Humorsol)	Miosis: <1 IOP: 4	2 within 24	24-48	0.125%-0.25%—1 drop topically once or twice daily
echothiophate (Phospholine Iodide)	Same as demecarium			0.03%-0.25%—1 drop topically once or twice daily
isoflurophate (Floropryl)	Same as demecarium			0.025% ointment—thin strip topically once every 3 days to 3 times daily

Epinephrine has an onset of action within an hour, peak effect is reached in 4 to 8 hours, and duration of action is up to 24 hours. Available in 0.1% to 2% strengths, the usual adult dose is 1 drop topically, once or twice daily. Dipivefrin has an onset of action within 30 minutes and reaches peak effect in 1 hour. The pediatric and adult dose is 1 drop (0.1%) topically every 12 hours.

■ Nursing Management

Sympathomimetic Ophthalmic Therapy

Assessment. Sympathomimetic agents are contraindicated in clients with narrow-angle glaucoma because pupil dilation may aggravate the condition. In aphakic clients (those devoid of a crystalline lens), dipivefrin or epinephrine may cause macular edema. Ophthalmic epinephrine should be administered with caution to clients with hypertension or other cardiovascular disease, hyperthyroidism, parkinsonism, asthma, or diabetes mellitus.

The client's drug history should be reviewed to determine the risk for drug interactions. Epinephrine may be absorbed systemically to interact with beta blockers, digitalis glycosides, or MAO inhibitors.

A baseline assessment of the client should include the client's ocular pressure, pupil size, vision status, and vital signs.

Nursing diagnosis. Clients receiving these ophthalmic solutions may be at risk for altered comfort related to possible photophobia and burning, stinging, or other eye irritations. If the agent is absorbed systemically, the client may experience the collaborative problem of altered cardiac output (tachycardia, hypertension).

Implementation

Monitoring. The client's condition should be evaluated periodically by the prescriber throughout therapy by fundus and intraocular pressure examinations to ensure the effectiveness of therapy. Assess for decreased visual acuity and ocular discomfort. Obtain periodic pulse and blood pressure determinations to assess for systemic effects such as tachycardia and elevated blood pressure.

Intervention. If dipivefrin is administered with other antiglaucoma ophthalmic solutions, review the regimen carefully. When dipivefrin is to replace epinephrine, the epinephrine should be discontinued when the dipivefrin is started. If the antiglaucoma agent to be replaced is something other than epinephrine, that agent should be discontinued on the second day of dipivefrin administration. If administered in addition to other antiglaucoma agents, dipivefrin is given at the usual adult dose.

To minimize systemic absorption, pressure should be maintained on the lacrimal sac during and for 1 to 2 minutes after instillation of the drug. Discoloration or precipitation of epinephrine indicates oxidation to inactive products, and the solution should be discarded.

Education. Review with the client the safe and accurate techniques for the self-administration of ophthalmic

TABLE 43-5 Antiglaucoma agents: pharmacokinetics and dosing

Drug	Onset of action (hr)	Peak effect (hr)	Duration of action (hr)	Usual adult dosage
Carbonic anhydrase inhibitors				
Oral				
acetazolamide (Diamox)				
capsules	2	8-12	18-24	500 mg PO twice daily, morning and evening
tablets	1-1.5	2-4	8-12	250 mg PO 1 to 4 times daily
IV	2 min	15 min	4-5	500 mg IV
dichlorphenamide (Daranide)	0.5-1	2-4	6-12	100-200 mg initially, then 100 mg every 12 hours; maintenance dose 25-50 mg 1 to 3 times daily
methazolamide (Neptazane)	2-4	6-8	10-18	50-100 mg 2 or 3 times daily
Eyedrops				
dorzolamide (Trusopt)	N/A	N/A	N/A	2% solution—one drop 3 times daily
Prostaglandin agonist				
latanoprost (Xalatan)	N/A	2	N/A	One drop in affected eye(s) in the evening

N/A, not available.

agents. See Nursing Management: Drugs Affecting the Eye, p. 728.

Alert the client that pigment deposits in the conjunctiva may occur after prolonged use of epinephrine. The client should seek medical advice regarding the use of contact lens during therapy. Instruct the client on which symptoms to report to the prescriber.

Evaluation. The client will experience therapeutic mydriasis and a reduction in intraocular pressure without adverse systemic effects.

Carbonic Anhydrase Inhibitor Agents

The oral carbonic anhydrase inhibitors include acetazolamide (Diamox), dichlorphenamide (Daranide), and methazolamide (Neptazane). Acetazolamide, the most widely used drug of this class, is the focus of this discussion. The carbonic anhydrase inhibitors are sulfonamides (nonbacteriostatic) with an undetermined mechanism of action, but they appear to lower intraocular pressure by decreasing the aqueous production to about half of its baseline measurement. The topical sulfonamide dorsolamide, a carbonic anhydrase inhibitor, is systemically absorbed to produce its antiglaucoma effects. The 2% eyedrop solution tid is approximately equivalent to an oral 2 mg dose bid in effect.

The oral drugs are used for the treatment of open-angle, secondary, and angle-closure glaucoma while the eyedrop is indicated for open-angle glaucoma and ocular hypertension. Side effects with the oral agents include diarrhea, discomfort; diuresis; anorexia; metallic taste in mouth; nausea; vomiting; tingling or numbness (paresthesia) of fingers, hands, and toes; and weight loss. Prescriber intervention is necessary if the client has the signs and symptoms of acidosis, blood dyscrasias, or hypokalemia. Eyedrop side effects include topical allergic reaction of the eye, bitter taste in mouth, photosensitivity, and superficial punctate keratitis. Table 43-5 lists Antiglaucoma agents: Pharmacokinetics and Dosing.

■ Nursing Management

Carbonic Anhydrase Inhibitor Ophthalmic Therapy

Assessment. The client's health status should be assessed for conditions that might indicate that carbonic anhydrase inhibitors should be administered cautiously, such as clients with adrenocortical insufficiency who would be more inclined to electrolyte imbalances. Reactions to sulfonamide agents (thiazide diuretic, oral sulfonylureas) will raise suspicion for cross-allergenicity and hypersensitivity. Contraindications include clients with decreased sodium/potassium serum levels or hepatic or renal dysfunction (potential for renal calculi formation).

Review the client's current medication regimen for significant drug interactions. The following interactions may occur when carbonic anhydrase inhibitors are given with the drugs listed below.

Drug	Possible effect and management
amphetamines, quinidine, mecamylamine (Inversine)	Carbonic anhydrase inhibitors decrease excretion of these drugs because of alkalinization of the urine, which may result in a prolonged duration of drug action and possibly increased side effects. Avoid concurrent use of mecamylamine. Monitor other agents closely because dosage adjustments are usually necessary.
methenamine (Mandelamine)	Alkalinization of the urine prevents conversion of methenamine to formaldehyde, thus reducing the effectiveness of methenamine. Concurrent drug administration is not recommended.

Obtain a baseline assessment of the client's vision, intraocular pressure, ocular pain, vital signs, urinalysis, complete blood cell count, platelet count, and serum electrolytes.

Nursing diagnosis. The client is at risk for altered comfort in a variety of ways, including metallic taste; anorexia; nausea and vomiting; numbness or tingling of the fingers, toes, mouth, and tongue; and feelings of malaise. In addition, the client may experience altered patterns of bowel elimination, such as diarrhea, and an altered urinary elimination pattern, or polyuria. Fluid volume deficit may occur. The client's feelings of malaise should be carefully assessed because he or she may also be at risk for collaborative problems related to the development of crystalluria, hypokalemia, blood dyscrasias, and acidosis.

Implementation

Monitoring. These drugs cause some decrease in renal blood flow and glomerular filtration rate, which produces an increased excretion of sodium, potassium, bicarbonate, and water alkaline diuresis. Monitor appropriate serum concentrations for electrolyte imbalances. To monitor for fluid volume depletion, maintain an accurate record of intake and output and daily weights and assess skin turgor and mucous membranes. Monitor the affected eye(s) on a daily basis for improvement.

Intervention. Administer with meals to minimize gastrointestinal distress. Schedule doses early in the day to minimize nocturia. If potassium supplements are required, assess serum chloride levels, which may be elevated, requiring a potassium preparation that does not contain chloride.

Education. Instruct the client in a high-potassium, low-sodium diet. Advise a fluid intake of 2 L daily to reduce the risk of renal calculi. Encourage the client to monitor weight daily and instruct him or her about the signs and symptoms of fluid and electrolyte imbalances.

Evaluation. The client will experience a decrease in intraocular pressure without any adverse effects from the carbonic anhydrase inhibitors (see the case study below).

Prostaglandin Agonist

Latanoprost (Xalatan) is the first prostaglandin agonist approved to treat open-angle glaucoma and ocular hypertension. It reduces intraocular pressure by increasing aqueous humor outflow.

Osmotic Agents

Osmotic agents are given intravenously or orally to reduce the intraocular pressure. These agents generally do not cross the blood aqueous barrier into the anterior chamber of the eye and are rarely found in ocular humor. The osmotic agents are discussed in Chapter 34, Diuretics.

MYDRIATIC AND CYCLOPLEGIC AGENTS

Adrenergic agonists cause pupil dilation (**mydriasis**) while cycloplegic agents paralyze ciliary muscle (accommodation). These agents are primarily used for diagnosis of ophthalmic disorders. The effects of these agents depend on the client's age, race, and color of iris. For example, mydriatic agents evoke less of a response in persons with heavily pigmented (dark) irides than in those with lighter-pigmented (blue) irides. Thus blacks tend to respond less to the agents than whites. Anticholinergic agents produce both mydriasis and cycloplegia via blockade of muscarinic receptors.

Case Study

The Client with Glaucoma

James Gibson, a 70-year-old male, has been having difficulty with his peripheral vision and has been diagnosed with closed-angle glaucoma. The doctor prescribes pilocarpine (Isopto Carpine) 1 gtt tid and Diamox 250 mg PO qid for him. The nurse's major responsibility becomes client teaching.

1. What are important issues related to teaching Mr. Gibson how to instill his eyedrops?
2. How does pilocarpine affect glaucoma?
3. Why sould the physician place him on a carbonic anhydrase inhibitor (Diamox) in addition to the eyedrops?
4. Mr. Gibson has been on furosemide (Lasix) 40 mg PO daily. What side effects does he need to watch for while he is taking the Diamox?

Contraction of the iris sphincter leads to relaxation and possibly, an increase in intraocular pressure. This discussion focuses on anticholinergic agents and adrenergic agonists.

Anticholinergic Agents

Anticholinergic agents are indicated for the treatment of inflammations such as uveitis and keratitis to relieve ocular pain by relaxing inflamed intraocular muscles. They are also used for relaxation of ciliary muscle for accurate measurement of refractive errors, which permits proper lens determination for eyeglasses, and for preoperative and postoperative use in intraocular surgery.

Local side/adverse effects reported with the use of anticholinergic ophthalmic agents include stinging or an increase in intraocular pressure. With chronic use, allergic lid reactions, red eye, and various eye irritation injuries may be induced. If absorbed systemically, mild to serious adverse reactions may result, such as dryness of the mouth, inhibition of sweating, flushing, tachycardia, ataxia, hallucinations, psychiatric and behavioral problems, fever, delirium, convulsions, respiratory depression, and coma. Deaths have been recorded in children after systemic absorption.

Pupillary dilation from either local or systemic administration can precipitate acute glaucoma in predisposed persons. If unrecognized or untreated, this can result in blindness. Table 43-6 lists Anticholinergic Agents: Pharmacokinetics and Dosing.

Combination eyedrops include Cyclomydril, Murocoll-2, and Paremyd. These agents in combination produce a greater mydriasis than either drug alone. Table 43-6 gives indications and dosage.

■ Nursing Management

Anticholinergic Ophthalmic Therapy

Assessment. Anticholinergic therapy with atropine is contraindicated with clients with a history of severe systemic reaction to atropine. It is used with caution in clients with primary glaucoma. Dilation of the pupil causes a narrowing of the iridocorneal angle where the canal of Schlemm is located. This restricts drainage of intraocular fluids, although secretion continues and intraocular pressure rises. This may precipitate an attack of acute glaucoma.

Obtain a baseline assessment of the client's vision status and intraocular pressure.

Nursing diagnosis. The client receiving anticholinergic ophthalmic therapy is at risk for the following nursing diagnoses: sensory-perceptual alterations related to blurred vision and increased sensitivity of the eyes to light; impaired tissue integrity related to eye irritation not present before therapy and swelling of the eyelids; and risk for injury related to systemic absorption (confusion, dizziness, dryness of skin, fever, slurred speech, tachycardia, drowsiness, dryness of the mouth).

Implementation

Monitoring. The client's intraocular pressure and vision should be monitored periodically over the course of therapy. The potential for systemic side effects is more pronounced in infants, young children, children with blond hair or blue eyes, clients with Down syndrome, children with brain damage, and the elderly. Monitor these clients for fast, irregular pulse, skin dryness, confusion, slurred speech, dry mouth, fever, and unusual drowsiness or weakness.

Intervention. If the ointment form is to be used for refraction, it should be applied several hours before the vision

TABLE 43-6 Anticholinergic agents: pharmacokinetics and dosing

Drug	Time to maximal mydriasis (min)	Recovery (days)	Time to maximal cycloplegia (min)	Recovery (days)	Usual adult dose
atropine	30-40	7-10	60-180	6-12	1%—1 drop
cyclopentolate	30-60	1	25-75	6-24 hr	0.5%-2%—1 drop
homatropine	40-60	1-3	30-60	1-3	2%-5%—1 drop
scopolamine	20-130	3-7	30-60	3-7	0.25%—1 drop
tropicamide	20-40	6 hr	30	6 hr	1%—1 drop

	Indication	Usual adult dosage
Combination eyedrops		
cyclopentolate & phenylephrine (Cyclomydril)	mydriasis	1 drop in each eye every 5-10 min as necessary; do not exceed 3 doses
scopolamine & phenylephrine (Murocoll-2)	mydriasis, cycloplegia, and for posterior synechiae in iritis	mydriasis—1-2 drops in eye, repeated in 5 minutes if necessary
tropicamide & hydroxyamphetamine (Paremyd)	mydriasis with partial cycloplegia	1-2 drops in conjunctival sac

(Moroi & Lichter, 1996; Olin, 1996; *USP DI*, 1996)

exam to minimize any impairment of the transparency of the cornea.

Although 2 drops are the recommended dose by some manufacturers, the conjunctival sac will usually only hold 1 drop. To minimize systemic absorption, the lacrimal duct should be compressed during and for 2 to 3 minutes after the administration of the drops.

Education. Instruct clients that the next instillation should be omitted if side effects (dryness of mouth, tachycardia) are present. Alert the client that during therapy he or she may be unable to focus (blurred vision) on nearby objects and will be unusually sensitive to light. Dark glasses should be worn to decrease this photophobia. The eye will be accommodated for distant vision. Because atropine is highly toxic, it should be stored in a safe place out of the reach of children.

Evaluation. The client on anticholinergic ophthalmic therapy will experience cycloplegia and, if administered for uveitis, the condition will be alleviated as evidenced by a lack of discomfort, redness, and drainage from the eye.

Adrenergic Agonist Agents

Topical adrenergic agents mimic (direct acting) or potentiate (indirect acting) the action of epinephrine on the dilator muscle of the iris resulting in mydriasis and decreased congestion of conjunctival blood vessels. The primary adrenergic drugs used in ophthalmology include epinephrine (Epifrin, Glaucon), phenylephrine (Ak-Nefrin, Prefin, Neo-Synephrine), oxymetazoline (Ocuclear), hydroxyamphetamine (Paredrine), naphazoline (Allerest, VasoClear), and tetrahydrozoline (Murine Plus, Visine).

Adrenergic drugs applied topically to the eye elicit the following sympathetic responses: vasoconstriction, pupil dilation, an increase in outflow of aqueous humor plus a decrease in aqueous humor formation, and relaxation of the ciliary muscle. Exactly how these effects are produced remains uncertain, but there is some evidence that alpha-adrenergic receptors are present in the outflow mechanism of the eye. When stimulated, they increase outflow of aqueous humor. It has also been shown experimentally that vasoconstriction decreases the rate of aqueous humor formation (Abel, 1992).

Adrenergic drugs are used to treat wide-angle glaucoma and glaucoma secondary to uveitis, to produce mydriasis for ocular examination, and to relieve congestion and hyperemia. Adrenergic drugs are contraindicated in the treatment of narrow-angle glaucoma or abraded cornea because dilation of the pupil will further restrict ocular fluid outflow, which may cause an acute attack of glaucoma. See the discussion of pharmacokinetics of adrenergic agents in Chapter 22.

Serious systemic side effects from these drugs are unusual and include local pain and brow ache. Systemic absorption, though, is a concern, especially in clients with cardiovascular disease because tachycardia and elevated blood pressure can occur with these agents. Sweating, tremors, and confusion may also occur. As with other ophthalmic drugs, the potential for systemic drug interactions exists if significant absorption occurs.

Apraclonidine (Iopidine) reduces intraocular pressure (IOP) in glaucoma and also in clients after laser trabeculoplasty or iridotomy. This drug is a selective alpha agonist that does not have any local anesthetic action.

The onset of action is usually within 60 minutes; maximum IOP reduction occurs within 3 to 5 hours. After topical application, apraclonidine is absorbed and may induce systemic side/adverse effects such as stomach pain, diarrhea, vomiting, and dry mouth; ophthalmic side effects include burning, pruritus, dryness, blurred vision, conjunctival

TABLE 43-7 Adrenergic ophthalmic agents

Drug	Duration of action (hr)	Market availability	Usual adult dosage
epinephrine (Epifrin, Glaucon)	V+—<1 IOP—12-24	Rx	0.5%-2%—1 drop once or twice daily
hydroxyamphetamine (Paredrine)	1-3	Rx	1%—1 or 2 drops for dilation of pupil
naphazoline			
(Allerest, VasoClear)	3-4	OTC	0.012%-0.03%—1 drop up to 4 times daily
(Albalon, Vasocon)	3-4	Rx	0.1%—1 drop every 3-4 hr as necessary
oxymetazoline (OcuClear)	4-6	OTC	0.025%—1 drop every 6 hr as necessary
phenylephrine			
(Ak-Nefrin, Prefin)	0.5-1.5	OTC	0.12%—1 or 2 drops up to 4 times daily as necessary
(Neo-synephrine)	1-7	Rx	2.5%, 10%—1 drop as necessary
tetrahydrozoline (Murine Plus, Visine)	1-4	OTC	0.05%—1 or 2 drops up to 4 times daily

(Olin, 1996; *USP DI*, 1996)
V+, Vasoconstriction; *IOP*, reduction in intraocular pressure; *Rx*, prescription.

blanching, and mydriasis. Table 43-7 lists adrenergic ophthalmic drugs, duration of action, market availability, and usual adult dosage.

ANTIINFECTIVE/ ANTIINFLAMMATORY AGENTS

To treat ocular infections, the drug of choice and the dose required should be determined by laboratory isolation of the offending organism. The initial culture from the infected area is obtained before any ophthalmic agent is applied. However, treatment is not withheld if the time required to make these determinations may cause increased severity of infection and if the type of infection (e.g., most cases of conjunctivitis, which tend to be self-limiting) does not warrant the expense of laboratory analysis.

Prophylactic use of antiinfective/antiinflammatory agents in general is useless, wasteful, and potentially dangerous because a large proportion of the inflammatory diseases seen in ophthalmology are caused by viruses or other agents that are not susceptible to any currently available antiinfective agents. Systemic medications that can induce ocular side effects need to be considered before an antiinfective or antiinflammatory agent is introduced. See Table 43-2 for drugs that induce ocular side effects.

Most antiinfective agents do not readily penetrate the eye when applied. However, some drugs will penetrate the inflamed eye when the blood-aqueous barrier is decreased by injury or inflammation. Topically applied antiinfective agents can cause sensitivity reactions (stinging, itching, angioneurotic edema, urticaria, dermatitis). Individuals sensitized to one drug may show cross reactions to chemically related drugs. Topical application of antiinfective agents may also interfere with the normal flora of the eye, which may encourage growth of other organisms.

Eye infections require prompt treatment to help prevent spread of infection because severe infections may damage the eye and impair vision. Solutions are preferred for treatment of eye infections, since ointment bases often tend to interfere with healing.

Antibacterials

Antibiotics

To avoid possible sensitization to systemic antiinfective drugs and to discourage development of resistant strains of offending organisms, the antibiotic of choice is not given systemically. Rather, these agents are administered topically, subconjunctivally, or intrauveally. Selection of an antibiotic for ocular infection is based on (1) clinical experience, (2) the nature and sensitivity of the organisms most commonly causing the condition, (3) the disease itself, (4) the sensitivity and response of the client, and (5) laboratory results.

Some of the common ocular infections treated with antibiotics include the following:

- *Conjunctivitis*—Acute inflammation of the conjunctiva resulting from bacterial invasion or viral infection. It is a common sign in severe colds. "Pink eye" is the acute contagious epidemic form of conjunctivitis usually caused by *Hemophilus* organisms. Symptoms include redness and burning of the eye, lacrimation, itching, and at times photophobia. Conjunctivitis is usually self-limiting. The eye should be protected from light.
- *Hordeolum* (sty)—An acute localized infection of the eyelash follicles and the glands of the anterior lid margin, resulting in the formation of a small abscess or cyst.
- *Chalazion*—Infection of the meibomian (sebaceous) glands of the eyelids. A hard cyst may form from blockage of the ducts.
- *Blepharitis*—Inflammation of the margins of the eyelid resulting from bacterial infection or allergy. Symptoms are crusting, irritation of the eye, and red and edematous lid margins.
- *Keratitis*—Corneal inflammation caused by bacterial infection; herpes simplex keratitis is caused by viral infection.
- *Uveitis*—Infection of the uveal tract, or the vascular layer of the eye, which includes the iris, ciliary body, and choroid.
- *Endophthalmitis*—Inner eye structure inflammation caused by bacteria.

Antibiotic ophthalmic preparations include bacitracin, chloramphenicol, ciprofloxacin, erythromycin, gentamicin, norfloxacin, ofloxacin, polymyxin B, and tobramycin. Combination preparations usually contain various combinations of these ingredients and/or neomycin, gramicidin, oxytetracycline, or trimethoprim. The following are examples of selected antibiotic ophthalmic products.

triple antibiotic ophthalmic ointment

(neomycin, polymyxin B sulfate, and bacitracin ophthalmic ointment) [nee oh mye' sin, pol i mix'in, bass i tray'sin] (Mycitracin, Neosporin)

Bacitracin is rarely used systemically because of its nephrotoxic effects. It is particularly useful in treating surface superficial infections caused by gram-positive bacteria (it inhibits protein synthesis). Bacitracin does penetrate the conjunctiva or the cornea slightly, but in therapeutic amounts it is nonirritating to the eye, is excreted in the nasolacrimal system, and produces no systemic effects.

A broader spectrum of antimicrobial activity is produced when bacitracin is used in combination with other antibiotics, than when it is used alone. Although all three of these agents have been or are available as single ophthalmic drugs, reports of sensitization to the individual drug have somewhat limited their usefulness. The combination dosage form provides a bactericidal effect against many gram-positive and gram-negative organisms. It is indicated for the treatment of superficial ocular infections caused by susceptible organisms. A small amount (1 cm) of ointment is usually applied to the conjunctiva every 3 to 4 hours.

■ Nursing Management

Triple Antibiotic Ophthalmic Therapy

Assessment. The use of this agent is contraindicated if the client has had a previous allergic reaction to the drug. A baseline assessment of the ocular infection is required. A specimen for culture and sensitivity should be obtained before therapy is initiated.

Nursing diagnosis. The client should be assessed for the following nursing diagnosis: risk for injury related to the ineffectiveness of the drug and the collaborative problem of a hypersensitivity response (burning, itching, redness, and swelling not present before therapy).

Implementation

Monitoring. The status of the infected eye(s) should be monitored as to pain, redness, swelling, and drainage.

Intervention. The presence of exudate interferes with the effectiveness of the medication; it should be removed before the medication is applied. A thin strip (about 1 cm) of ointment is placed in the conjunctival sac. Be careful not to touch the tip of the tube to the surface of the eye. Keep ophthalmic ointments exclusive for each client.

Education. Instruct the client and caregiver in the application of the ointment. Alert them to symptoms of hypersensitivity that need to be reported to the prescriber.

Evaluation. The client's ocular infection will be resolved as evidenced by the absence of pain, redness, swelling, and drainage.

chloramphenicol [klor am fen' i kole] (Chloroptic)
A bacteriostatic, chloramphenicol prevents peptide bond formation and protein synthesis in a wide variety of gram-positive and gram-negative organisms. Thus it is an extremely useful drug for superficial intraocular infections.

Side effects are usually rare. Burning and stinging on instillation have been reported. Irreversible aplastic anemia has not been reported with this form of chloramphenicol, although it would be prudent to monitor for blood dyscrasias.

When treating adults, apply a thin strip of ointment (1% solution) to the conjunctiva every 3 hours or more often if necessary. The solution dosage for adults is 1 drop into the conjunctiva every 3 hours.

In addition to the nursing management discussed earlier for triple antibiotic, avoid prolonged (more than 3 days) or frequent use. Chloramphenicol has been implicated in the development of aplastic anemia after prolonged use; monitor CBCs. Monitor the client for pallor, sore throat and fever, unusual bleeding or bruising, and unusual tiredness, which may indicate irreversible bone marrow depression associated with aplastic anemia. See Table 43-1 for systemic effects from a variety of ophthalmic agents.

erythromycin [er ith roe mye' sin] (Ilotycin)
Erythromycin ophthalmic ointment is a bacteriostatic agent, but in high concentrations against very susceptible organisms it may be bactericidal. It is indicated for the treatment of neonatal conjunctivitis caused by *Chlamydia trachomatis* and for the prevention of ophthalmia neonatorum (against *Neisseria gonorrhoeae* or *C. trachomatis*) and other ocular infections caused by susceptible organisms.

Eye irritation not present before therapy is rarely reported with this drug. For adults and children with ocular infections apply a thin ointment strip to conjunctiva daily or more often (up to 6 times daily) if necessary.

Aminoglycosides

gentamicin [jen ta mye' sin] (Garamycin, Genoptic)
Gentamicin is effective against a wide variety of gram-negative and gram-positive organisms. It is particularly useful against *Pseudomonas, Proteus,* and *Klebsiella* organisms and *Escherichia coli,* as well as staphylococci and streptococci that have developed resistance to other antibiotics. It is applied as an ointment two or three times daily, or 1 drop of solution every 4 hours. For nursing management, see triple antibiotic ophthalmic therapy.

tobramycin [toe bra mye' sin] (Tobrex)
This water-soluble aminoglycoside is used topically on a wide variety of gram-positive and gram-negative external ophthalmic pathogens and is particularly valuable for treating gentamicin-resistant infections. Adverse reactions include ocular toxicity and hypersensitivity, including lid itching, swelling, and conjunctival erythema. When topical aminoglycosides are used concurrently with systemic aminoglycosides, the total serum concentration will be affected and should be monitored. Systemic toxicity from absorption may occur from excessive use.

The dose for mild to moderate infection is 1 drop in the affected eye every 4 hours. For nursing management, see triple antibiotic ophthalmic therapy.

Sulfonamides

sulfacetamide [sul fa see' ta mide] (Bleph-10, Sulamyd)
sulfisoxazole [sul fi sox' a zole] (Gantrisin)
Ophthalmic bacteriostatic antiinfective agents block the synthesis of folic acid in susceptible bacterial organisms. The action of sulfonamides, though, is reduced by the presence of paraaminobenzoic acid (PABA) or its derivatives, procaine and tetracaine, and also by the presence of purulent drainage or exudate (purulent matter contains PABA). Therefore, lid exudate should be removed before the drugs are instilled.

Because the activity of sulfacetamide may be inhibited by concurrent administration of ophthalmic anesthetics, such-drugs are applied 30 to 60 minutes apart. Sulfonamides are physically incompatible with thimerosal and silver preparations.

Before administration the client should check to see that the solution has not darkened in color; if so, discard it. Solutions are instilled at a rate of 1 drop every 1 to 3 hours during the day, with increased time intervals during the night. Instillation of the drops may cause some mild pain and discomfort. For nursing management, see triple antibiotic ophthalmic therapy.

Antifungal Agents

natamycin [na ta mye' sin] (Natacyn)
Natamycin ophthalmic suspension is used to treat fungal blepharitis, conjunctivitis, and keratitis. By binding to steroids in the cell membrane of the fungus, natamycin produces an altered membrane permeability causing a loss of the cellular constituents. Because it is mainly retained in the conjunctival

area, significant drug levels in the ocular fluids are not achieved. It is not systemically absorbed. Natamycin may cause irritation of the eye. For fungal keratitis, 1 drop of the 5% solution is instilled into the conjunctiva at 1 to 2 hour intervals initially for 3 or 4 days followed by 6 to 8 times daily dosing afterward. For fungal blepharitis and conjunctivitis, 1 drop 4 to 6 times daily is usually adequate. See triple antibiotic ophthalmic therapy for nursing management.

Antiviral Agents

Antiviral ophthalmic preparations include idoxuridine, trifluridine, and vidarabine.

idoxuridine [eye dox yoor' i deen] (Stoxil, Herplex)
Idoxuridine resembles thymidine, a substance necessary for viral DNA; thus it replaces it and inhibits the replication of the viral DNA. It is indicated for the treatment of herpes simplex virus keratitis. Less frequent side/adverse effects include hypersensitivity (eye redness, pruritus, irritation), visual disturbance, and photosensitivity that were not present before therapy.

Adult dosage of idoxuridine solution for treatment of herpes simplex virus keratitis is 1 drop hourly during waking hours and every 2 hours during the night. For ointment, apply a thin strip every 4 hours (five times daily) during waking hours.

trifluridine [trye flure' i deen] (Viroptic)
For mechanism of action and indications, see idoxuridine. In addition, trifluridine is used to treat herpes simplex virus keratoconjunctivitis. A frequent side effect reported is burning or stinging on application. Rare side/adverse effects include increased intraocular pressure, blurred vision, and hypersensitivity reaction, evidenced by redness, swelling, or eye irritation not present before therapy.

The usual adult dose is 1 drop (1% solution) into conjunctiva every 2 hours during waking hours. Maximum daily dose is 9 drops. Continue therapy until cornea has recovered then reduce dosage to 1 drop every 4 hours during waking hours (minimum of 5 drops per day) for 1 week.

vidarabine [vye dare' a been] (Vira-A)
The antiviral mechanism of action is due to vidarabine conversion to substances intracellularly that inhibit viral DNA polymerase or other virus DNA specific enzymes. It is indicated for the treatment of herpes simplex virus keratitis and keratoconjunctivitis. Systemic absorption is not expected after ocular administration.

The side/adverse effects of vidarabine include increased tear flow and a sensation of something being in the eye. The prescriber should be contacted if photosensitivity, redness, eye swelling, or increased eye irritation not present before treatment occurs.

The usual adult dose is application of a thin strip of ointment to the conjunctiva every 3 hours five times daily. Therapy is continued until cornea is completely reepithelialized, then the dose is decreased to twice daily for 7 to 10 days.

Antiseptics

Many antiseptics that were used to treat surface infections of the eye before the advent of antibiotics are now obsolete. Inorganic mercuric salts such as yellow mercuric oxide ophthalmic ointment (1% to 2%), thimerosal (Merthiolate), and ammoniated mercury formerly served as bacteriostatic agents. They are seldom used today because they do not completely sterilize, spores are resistant to them, and they are irritating to the eye.

silver nitrate
Two drops of a solution of 1% silver nitrate is routinely instilled in each eye immediately after birth as a prophylaxis against gonorrheal ophthalmia neonatorum. In many states this is required by law. The gonococci are particularly susceptible to silver salts. Liberated silver ions precipitate bacterial proteins. Silver nitrate is preferred over effective antibiotic agents, since these may sensitize the client and silver nitrate has stood the test of time.

Silver nitrate ophthalmic solution is available in collapsible capsules containing about 5 drops of a 1% solution. The solution should be in contact with the conjunctival sac for not less than 30 seconds to produce a mild chemical conjunctivitis. Irrigation after use is not recommended.

Corticosteroids

Many corticosteroids are available for ophthalmic use as topical solutions, suspensions, or ointments. They include betamethasone (Betnesol), dexamethasone (Maxidex, Decadron), fluorometholone (FML S.O.P., FML), hydrocortisone (Cortamed), medrysone (HMS Liquifilm]) and prednisolone (Pred-Forte, Predair-A). These are available in varying strengths and in combination with various antibiotics or mydriatics. They are indicated for the treatment of allergic and inflammatory ophthalmic disorders of the conjunctiva, cornea, and anterior segment of the eye.

Rare side/adverse effects of corticosteroids include burning or lacrimation; blurred vision or visual disturbances, eye pain, headaches, ptosis, or enlarged pupils should be reported to the prescriber. For dosage and administration, see *USP DI* or current package inserts.

■ Nursing Management

Ophthalmic Corticosteroid Therapy

Assessment. Ophthalmic corticosteroid therapy is not used for pyogenic (pus-producing) inflammations of the eye because corticosteroids decrease defense mechanisms and reduce resistance to pathogenic organisms. Corticosteroid therapy is not recommended for minor corneal abrasions. Steroids may actually increase ocular susceptibility to fungal infection. When steroids are used for various eye conditions, they should be used for a limited time only and the eye should be checked for increased intraocular pressure. Corticosteroids may diminish the resistance to infection and may also mask the allergic reactions or hypersensitivity reactions to other drugs. A baseline assessment of the client's ocular inflammation and vision should be noted.

Nursing diagnosis. The client should be assessed for the following nursing diagnoses: risk for injury related to the ineffectiveness of the drug, the potential complications of hypersensitivity and the long-term effects of the drug (open-end glaucoma, optic nerve damage, cataracts, defects in vision).

Implementation

Monitoring. Periodic examination by a physician by tonometry and slit-lamp examination should be performed to monitor client progress. The eye should be assessed periodically for infection and reported to the prescriber if it occurs.

Intervention. The glucocorticoids used in ophthalmology may be applied topically, injected into the conjunctiva, or given systemically to diminish leukocyte infiltration where inflammation exists.

Education. Alert the client that temporary stinging may occur after application. Instruct the client to shake the ophthalmic suspensions well before use for adequate dispersion of the active ingredients. Contact lenses should not be used during and for some time after corticosteroid therapy because of the risk of infection. Caution the client not to stop the medication without consulting the prescriber. Inflammation recrudescence secondary to abrupt cessation of ophthalmic steroid administration may be overcome by dose frequency reduction (from every 3 hours, to every 6 hours, to 3 times daily, to twice daily, to once daily, and to every other day) or by decreasing the percentage strengths and using the above schedule.

Evaluation. The client's inflammation will be resolved without the occurrence of infection.

TOPICAL ANESTHETIC AGENTS

Local anesthetics stabilize neuronal membranes so that they become less permeable to ions; this prevents initiation and transmission of nerve impulses. It is theorized that sodium ion permeability is limited by these agents.

Local anesthetics are used to prevent pain (deep anesthesia) during surgical procedures (removal of sutures and foreign bodies) and tonometry examinations. The local anesthetics have rapid onset (within 20 seconds) and last for 15 to 20 minutes.

proparacaine [proe par' a kane] (Ophthaine, Ophthetic)

Proparacaine is similar to tetracaine. A 0.5% solution is administered by topical instillation. Anesthesia is produced within 20 seconds and lasts for 15 minutes. It is relatively free from the burning and discomfort of other anesthetics, but it is highly toxic if it enters the systemic circulation. Side/adverse effects include allergic contact dermatitis, softening and erosion of corneal epithelium, pupillary dilation, cycloplegia, conjunctival congestion and hemorrhage, and stromal edema.

tetracaine [tet' ra kane] (Pontocaine)

Tetracaine is a widely used anesthetic used topically for rapid, brief, superficial anesthesia. One to two drops of a 0.5% solution of tetracaine will produce anesthesia within 30 seconds; the client may feel a burning or stinging sensation. The anesthetic effect lasts for 10 to 15 minutes. Tetracaine can cause epithelial damage and systemic toxicity; therefore it is not recommended for prolonged home use by clients. It is physically incompatible with the mercury or silver salts often found in ophthalmic products.

■ Nursing Management
Topical Anesthetic Agents

Assessment. Question the client about past experiences with anesthetics to determine if a hypersensitivity reaction occurred. Note the condition of the eye and vision status as a baseline assessment.

Nursing diagnosis. The client receiving topical anesthetic agents should be assessed for the following nursing diagnoses: altered comfort related to ineffectiveness of the drug; and the potential complications of hypersensitivity, loss of sensation in the eye (delayed wound healing, perforation of the cornea, accidental trauma), and long-term effects of the drugs (permanent corneal opacification).

Implementation

Monitoring. Clients receiving local anesthetics that produce systemic toxicity should be monitored for central nervous system excitation (blurred vision, dizziness, trembling, nervousness, restlessness) followed by CNS depression (drowsiness, dyspnea) and cardiovascular depression (arrhythmias). The appearance of the eye and vision status should also be monitored.

Intervention. The practice of repeatedly applying such an anesthetic to an eye after removal of a foreign body is to be condemned. Besides delaying wound healing, this can produce sensitivity, permanent corneal opacification, visual loss, or perforation of the cornea.

Patching the anesthetized eye is prudent, since the blink reflex is lost and protection of the cornea from debris and irritants is then needed.

Education. The client should be instructed not to touch or rub the eye until the anesthesia has worn off to prevent damage to the eye.

Evaluation. The client will remain without discomfort and without any adverse reactions or injuries.

OTHER OPHTHALMIC PREPARATIONS

Artificial Tear Solutions and Lubricants

Lubricants or artificial tears are used to provide moisture and lubrication in diseases in which tear production is deficient, to lubricate artificial eyes and moisten contact lenses, to remove debris, and to protect the cornea during procedures on the eye. These agents are also incorporated in ophthalmic preparations to prolong the contact time of topically applied drugs.

Such products have a balanced salt solution (equivalent to 0.9% sodium chloride), buffers to adjust pH, highly viscous agents (methylcellulose, propylene glycol, and others) to extend eye contact time, and preservatives to maintain sterility. These products are usually administered three or four times a day.

An artificial tear insert (Lacrisert) was devised to extend the effect of the preparation. It is usually inserted daily or at most twice a day for selected clients.

Ointment preparations are also used as ocular lubricants. They will help to protect the eye (such as during and after eye surgery) and to lubricate the eye. They are particularly valuable for clients who have an impaired blink reflex and for nighttime use. Examples include Lacri-Lube, Duratears, and Hypo Tears.

Antiallergic Agents

Three antiallergic ophthalmic agents are available—cromolyn, levocabastine, and lodoxamide tromethamine.

cromolyn sodium (Opticrom)

Cromolyn sodium inhibits degranulation of sensitized mast cells occurring after exposure to a specific antigen. This mast cell release inhibition prevents the mediators of inflammation (histamine and slow-releasing substance of anaphylaxis) from producing their characteristic effects. The drug is used for allergic eye disorders (vernal and allergic keratoconjunctivitis, papillary conjunctivitis, keratitis) that have symptoms of itching, tearing, redness, and discharge.

The side/adverse effects of cromolyn sodium include stinging and burning sensation in the eyes. Concomitant corticosteroids may be necessary. In adults and children (over 4 years old), instill 1 drop in each affected eye four to six times a day at regular intervals.

■ Nursing Management

Cromolyn Sodium Therapy

Assessment. Assess the client for itching, tearing, redness, and discharge from eyes.

Nursing diagnosis. The client receiving this agent should be assessed for the following nursing diagnoses: risk for injury related to the ineffectiveness of the drug and the potential complications of hypersensitivity or chemosis (severe swelling of the conjunctiva).

Implementation

Monitoring. Note that signs and symptoms of relief will appear within days but that treatment at regular intervals for as long as 6 weeks may be required.

Intervention. Refrigerate the drug, keep it out of direct sunlight, and discard any unused portion after 4 weeks.

Education. Remind client to remove soft contact lenses before the first instillation of drops and to resume wearing them only after the drug has been discontinued.

Evaluation. The client's eye will not evidence an allergic reaction; itching, tearing, redness, and discharge will not be present.

levocabastine (Livostin)

Levocabastine is a topical antihistamine indicated for allergic conjunctivitis. The side effects are mild, such as burning, stinging, visual alterations, eye pain, red eyes, and headaches. The usual adult dose is 1 drop in eyes four times a day.

Pregnancy Safety

Category	Drug
B	cromolyn, dipivefrin, erythromycin, lodoxamide, tobramycin
C	acetazolamide, atropine, betaxolol, carbachol, carteolol, cyclopentolate, dichlorphenamide, dorzolamide, echothiophate, epinephrine, homatropine, idoxuridine, lantanoprost, levocabastine, levobunolol, methazolamide, metipranolol, naphazoline, natamycin, norfloxacin, phenylephrine, pilocarpine, polymyxin B, proparacaine, sulfonamides, tetracaine, timolol, trifluridine, vidarabine
X	demecarium, isoflurophate
Unclassified	chymotrypsin, gentamycin, hydroxyamphetamine, oxymetazoline, scopolamine, tetrahydrozoline, tropicamide

lodoxamide [loe dox' a mid] (Alomide)

Lodoxamide ophthalmic, an antiallergic and mast cell stabilizer, is used for the treatment of vernal conjunctivitis, vernal keratitis, and several other eye disorders. Lodoxamide inhibits Type I immediate hypersensitivity reactions by interfering with histamine release, and inhibits the release of SRS-A (slow reacting substance of anaphylaxis) and eosinophil chemotaxis.

The side/adverse effects of lodoxamide include a transient burning of the eye. Less frequently reported are blurred vision, pruritus of the eye, tearing, or eye irritation. The usual dose for children 2 years and older and adults is 1 drop to the conjunctiva four times daily for up to 3 months (*USP DI,* 1996). Nursing management is as for cromolyn sodium therapy.

Diagnostic Aids

fluorescein [flure' e sceen] (Fluorescite, Fluor-I-Strip)

Fluorescein is a nontoxic water-soluble dye that is used as a diagnostic aid. When applied to the cornea, it stains corneal lesions or ulcers a bright green; foreign bodies appear to be surrounded by a green ring. These effects permit detection of corneal epithelial defects caused by injury or infection and location of foreign bodies in the eye. The dye is also used in fitting hard contact lenses. Areas that lack fluorescein-stained tears will appear black under ultraviolet light, indicating that the contact lens is touching the cornea at those areas. Fluorescein is used in retinal photography to determine retinal vascular status and to identify defects in the retinal pigment epithelium. In addition, it may be used to test lacrimal apparatus patency; if after the dye is instilled into the eye it appears in the nasal secretions, the nasolacrimal drainage system is open.

Injection is used in ophthalmic angiography to examine the fundus, vasculature of the iris, and aqueous flow, to make differential diagnosis of cancerous and noncancerous tumors, and to determine time for circulation in the eye. Side/adverse effects after injection include nausea, headache, abdominal distress, vomiting, hypotension, hypersensitivity reactions, and anaphylaxis.

Topical solution to detect foreign bodies and corneal abrasions; instill 1 or 2 drops of the 2% solution. For strip application and injection, check a current drug reference for instructions.

Enzyme Preparation

chymotrypsin [kye moe trip' sin] [Catarase]

Chymotrypsin, a proteolytic enzyme, is used in selected cases to facilitate cataract extraction. Injected behind the iris into the posterior chamber, it dissolves the filaments or zonules that hold the lens, thereby facilitating intracapsular lens extraction. This effect is usually obtained in 5 to 15 minutes with total lysis of the entire zonular membrane reported within 30 minutes. Side/adverse effects include a transient postoperative glaucoma lasting about 1 week, which can be relieved by the use of pilocarpine.

Hyperosmolar Preparation

sodium chloride ointment (Muro-128) and solution (Adsorbonac)

This 5% ointment and 2% or 5% solution are used to reduce the corneal edema that occurs in certain corneal dystrophies and after cataract extraction. The dose is 1 to 2 drops or a small amount of ointment in affected eye(s) every 3 to 4 hours as directed.

Nonsteroidal Antiinflammatory Agents

Flurbiprofen, suprofen, diclofenac, and ketorolac tromethamine are available topically for ophthalmic use. These agents are nonsteroidal antiinflammatory drugs (NSAIDs). They have the following indications:

- flurbiprofen [flure bee proe' fen] (Ocufen) and suprofen [sue' proe fen] (Profenal) are used to inhibit intraoperative miosis.
- diclofenac [dye kloe' fen ak] (Voltaren) is used to treat postoperative inflammation after a cataract extraction.
- ketorolac [kee' toe role ak] (Acular) is used to treat conjunctivitis and seasonal allergic ophthalmic pruritus.

These agents, if absorbed, may produce a systemic effect. Because they have the potential to cause increased bleeding, monitor their use closely in clients who are known to have bleeding tendencies. The most common side effect reported is transient burning or stinging on application. Other minor symptoms of ocular irritation have also been reported, such as itching, redness, discomfort, allergic reaction. For dosing recommendations, see a current package insert or drug reference.

Irrigating Solutions

The sterile isotonic external irrigating solutions are used in tonometry, fluorescein procedures, and removal of foreign material, and to cleanse and soothe the eyes of clients wearing hard contact lenses. These external products do not require a prescription and are available as drops, irrigations, and eyewashes. Examples of irrigating solutions include BSS Plus, Surgisol, and Lavoptik Eye Wash.

SUMMARY

Although there are myriad ophthalmic preparations, the drugs to treat eye disorders can be divided into three major groups: the antiglaucoma agents, the mydriatics and cycloplegics, and the antiinfective/antiinflammatory agents. Antiglaucoma agents may be miotics. These cause pupillary constriction by direct action (cholinergic) to minimize the effects of acetylcholine at autonomic synapses or the neuroeffector junction of the parasympathetic nervous system, or by indirect action (anticholinesterase), inactivating the enzyme cholinesterase by preventing hydrolysis of acetylcholine. Antiglaucoma drugs may also be sympathomimetic agents that decrease aqueous humor production (beta-adrenergic effect) and increase its outflow (alpha-adrenergic effect). Beta-adrenergic blocking agents, carbonic anhydrase inhibitor agents, and osmotic agents are also used in the treatment of glaucoma.

Mydriatic and cycloplegic agents used for ophthalmic disorders are topically applied autonomic drugs that cause dilation of the pupils (mydriasis) and paralysis of accommodation (cycloplegia). In addition to being used for specific treatment of ophthalmic disorders, they are also used during eye examinations and in preparation of the client for intraocular surgery.

Antiinfective/antiinflammatory agents used in the treatment of ocular infections may be antibacterial, antifungal, or antiviral agents, as well as corticosteroids.

The role of the nurse in the clinical management of the client receiving ophthalmic drugs focuses on safe administration and the preparation of the client for self-administration of such drugs.

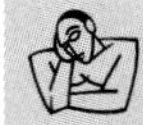

Critical Thinking

1. How would the teaching plan for the self-administration of ophthalmic agents vary between antiglaucoma agents, antiinfective agents, and corticosteroids?
2. Steve Cameron has had his ophthalmic medication changed from an optic solution to an optic ointment. What instruction will you provide Mr. Cameron to prepare him for safe self-administration of the new form of medication?

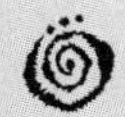 Collaborative Learning Activities

1. Student teams will demonstrate the instillation of eyedrops, one for each of the following age groups; infant, toddler, school age child, and adult.
2. One team will role play the teaching of an elderly client to self-administer epinephrine eyedrops. The student playing the part of the elder could wear glasses, the lenses of which have been coated with Vaseline, and gardening gloves to inhibit fine movement to simulate some of the impairments that may be found with elderly clients. That student will discuss his or her experience and suggest what actions by the nurse might have been more assistive.

BIBLIOGRAPHY

Abel SR (1995). Eye disorders. In *Applied therapeutics* (6th ed.). Vancouver: Applied Therapeutics.

American Hospital Formulary Service (1996). *AHFS drug information '96*. Bethesda, MD: American Society of Hospital Pharmacists.

Anderson KN, et al. (Eds.) (1994). *Mosby's medical, nursing, & allied health dictionary* (4th ed.). St. Louis: Mosby.

DiPiro JT, et al. (1993). *Pharmacotherapy: A pathophysiologic approach* (2nd ed.). Norwalk, CT: Appleton & Lange.

Eye drops and infection: The solution may be the problem (1992). *Emerg Med* 24(4):142.

Hahn K (1989). Administering eye medications, *Nursing* 19(9):80.

Moroi SE & Lichter PR (1996). Ocular pharmacology. In Hardman JG & Limbird LE (Eds.). *Goodman & Gilman's the pharmacological basis of therapeutics* (9th ed.). New York: McGraw-Hill.

Newhouse J (1994). Opening your eyes to intraocular drug administration, *Nursing* 24(6):44-5.

O'Boyle JE & Enzenaur RW (1992). "Super glue" in the eye, *Emerg Med* 24(6):59-60, 62.

Olin BR (Ed.) (1996). *Facts and comparisons.* St Louis: Facts and Comparisons.

Schein OD, et al. (1992). Eye drops and infection, *Arch Ophthamol* 110:82.

United States Pharmacopeial Convention (1996). *USP DI: Drug information for the health care professional* (16th ed.). Rockville, MD: The Convention.

Chapter 44

Overview of the Ear

Chapter Focus

Disorders of the ear can be painful and impair the client's ability to hear and maintain balance. Pharmacologic interventions for the ear are somewhat limited, however, many systemic drugs have ototoxic effects. The nurse requires a thorough understanding of the anatomy and physiology of the ear to appropriately assess and care for clients with disorders of the ear. The following objectives and key terms are important for a good understanding of this chapter.

Key Terms

auditory ossicles (p. 747)
cochlea (p. 747)
eustachian tube (p. 747)
external ear (p. 747)
inner ear (p. 747)
middle ear (p. 747)
otitis media (p. 747)
tympanic membrane (p. 747)

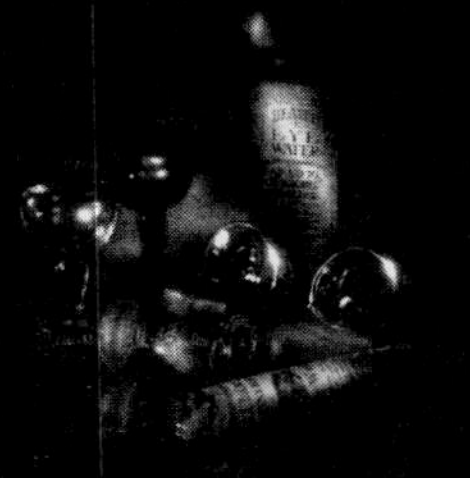

Objectives

1. Differentiate between the external, middle, and inner ear.
2. Name the three bones of the inner ear.
3. Describe the function of the eustachian tube.
4. List common ear disorders.

ANATOMY AND PHYSIOLOGY

The ear consists of three sections or parts: external ear, middle ear, and inner ear (Figure 44-1).

The **external ear** has two divisions, the outer ear, or pinna, and the external auditory canal. The external auditory canal leads to the eardrum, or **tympanic membrane,** a thin, transparent partition of tissue between the canal and the middle ear. The function of the external ear is to receive and transmit auditory sounds to the eardrum. The tympanic membrane protects the middle ear from foreign substances and transmits sound to the bones of the middle ear.

The **middle ear** is an air-filled cavity in the temporal bone that contains three small bones called the **auditory ossicles.** The ossicles are the malleus (hammer), incus (anvil), and stapes (stirrup). The tip of the malleus is attached to the surface of the tympanic membrane. Its head is attached to the incus, which in turn is attached to the stapes. The ossicles amplify and transmit sound waves to the inner ear. The middle ear is also directly connected to the nasopharynx by the **eustachian** (auditory) **tube.** The eustachian tube is usually collapsed except when the individual swallows, chews, yawns, or moves the jaw. This tube joins the nasopharynx and the tympanic cavity, which allows for the equalization of the air pressure in the inner ear with atmospheric pressure to prevent the tympanic membrane from rupturing. On airline flights pressure changes are relieved by action of the eustachian tube when the individual chews gum, yawns, or deliberately swallows.

The **inner ear** is the complex structure of the ear that communicates directly with the acoustic nerve, which transmits sound vibrations from the middle ear. The inner ear, also referred to as the labyrinth because of its series of canals, has two main divisions. The bony labyrinth consists of the vestibule, cochlea, and semicircular canals, and the membranous labyrinth consists of a series of sacs and tubes within the bony labyrinth. The **cochlea,** through which passes fibers of the cochlear division of the acoustic nerve, is the primary organ of hearing, and the vestibular apparatus is necessary to maintain equilibrium and balance (see Figure 44-1).

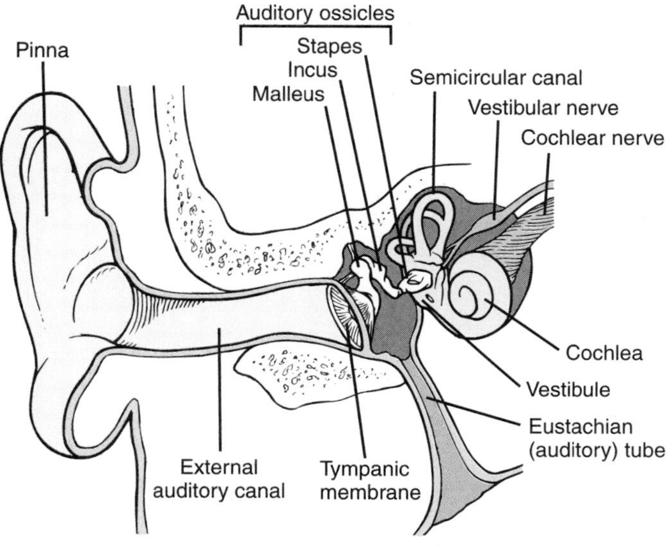

Figure 44-1 Anatomy of the ear.

COMMON EAR DISORDERS

The most common ear disorders include infections of the ear (bacterial or fungal), earwax accumulation, and various other painful or distressing conditions. Many ear disorders are minor and easily treated or are self-limiting. Persistent pain or ear problems should be professionally evaluated because some untreated disorders can lead to hearing loss.

External ear disorders usually include trauma, such as lacerations or scrapes to the skin. These are often minor and heal with time. If the injury results in bleeding and perhaps a hematoma, referral to a primary health care provider is necessary. Localized infections of the hair follicles resulting in boils may occur. Clients with recurring boils and small boils that do not respond to good hygiene and topical compresses should be referred to a provider for evaluation and possibly systemic antibiotics.

Dermatitis of the ear, itching, local redness, weeping, or drainage are also reported. Such conditions must be individually evaluated, since the causes can vary from inflammation induced by seborrhea, psoriasis, or contact dermatitis to head trauma producing ear discharge. Self-medication should be discouraged when infection is suspected or in the presence of known injuries of the ear or whenever drainage, pain, and dizziness are present.

Middle ear disorders are not to be treated with OTC medications. The most commonly reported problem is middle ear inflammation, **otitis media.** This most often occurs in children, although chronic otitis media may be caused in adults by a nasopharyngeal tumor. Pain, fever, malaise, pressure, a sensation of fullness in the ear, and hearing loss are common symptoms. Clients with such conditions should be treated promptly by a prescriber. Acute tympanic membrane perforation from foreign objects or from water sports (such as diving or water skiing) will result in a multitude of symptoms, if untreated. Pain at the time of injury that subsides, diminished hearing acuity, tinnitus, nausea, vertigo, and otitis media or mastoiditis may be noted. A physician's examination is vital when a perforated tympanic membrane is suspected.

Loss of hearing, especially unilateral hearing loss, may result from viral infection of the inner ear. Hearing deficits may be caused by genetic diseases or slowly progressive diseases such as otosclerosis or Meniere's disease. Untreated external and middle ear infections may also affect hearing and the functioning of the inner ear.

In addition the nurse needs to be aware of drugs that have as an adverse effect ototoxicity, which results in impaired hearing for the client (see Chapter 45).

SUMMARY

Pharmacologic interventions for the ear are limited, but the nurse requires a thorough understanding of the anatomy and physiology to appropriately assess and care for clients receiving otic agents.

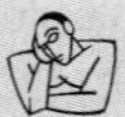

Critical Thinking

1. When airplanes begin their descent and the cabin pressure changes, it is not uncommon to hear infants on board begin to cry. Why does this occur and what action would you recommend to the caregivers to minimize this response?
2. Mr. Jones has worked with heavy equipment at construction sites for a number of years before OSHA regulations made ear protection required. He admits to having difficulty hearing. Why do you think this has happened?
3. Mrs. Harris, 84 years old, has come to the emergency room with a broken arm from a fall in her home. She indicates that she has had increasing problems maintaining her balance. Why might this be so?

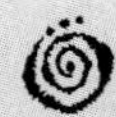

Collaborative Learning Activities

1. Student teams will discuss the Critical Thinking questions above and present their conclusions to the class.

BIBLIOGRAPHY

Anderson KN, et al. (Eds.) (1994). *Mosby's medical, nursing, & allied health dictionary* (4th ed.). St Louis: Mosby.

Guyton AC (1987). *Human physiology and mechanisms of disease* (4th ed.). Philadelphia: WB Saunders.

Thibodeau GA & Patton KT (1996). *Anatomy and physiology* (3rd ed.). St Louis: Mosby.

Chapter 45

Drugs Affecting the Ear

Chapter Focus

Persons with ear disorders may experience impaired communication related to hearing loss, or difficulty with balance and vertigo. Otic drugs may be prescribed for the former; however, systemic drugs may result in ototoxicity, causing both a loss of hearing and balance. The nurse needs not only to be concerned about the client's comfort, auditory perception, and risk of injury related to vestibular dysfunction, but also to be knowledgeable regarding drugs affecting the ear in order to provide client instruction for effective self-management of the therapeutic drug regimen. The following objectives and key terms are important for a good understanding of this chapter.

Key Terms

cerumen (p. 750)
ototoxicity (p. 751)
tinnitus (p. 751)
vertigo (p. 751)

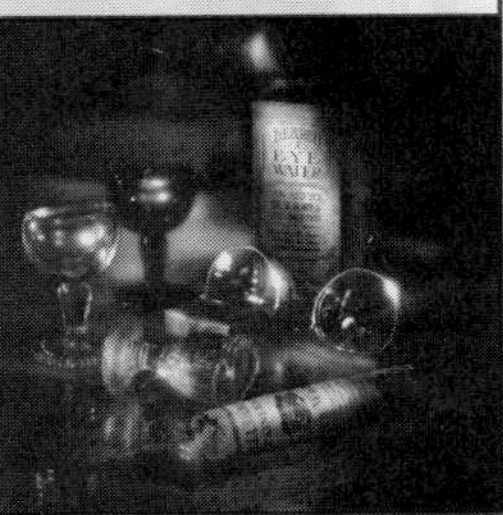

Objectives

1. List drugs commonly used to treat ear infections.
2. Discuss the various preparations used to treat ear ailments.
3. List five drugs reported to cause ototoxicity.
4. Implement the nursing management of the client receiving drugs affecting the ear.

Disorders and infections of the external ear canal are treated with antibiotic solutions, corticosteroids, and miscellaneous preparations such as wax emulsifiers, antibacterials, antifungals, local anesthetics, antiinflammatory agents, and local analgesic-type preparations. The potent systemic medications that may adversely affect the client's hearing and/or balance are also reviewed in this chapter.

ANTIBIOTIC EAR PREPARATIONS

Antibiotic ear preparations are used to treat infections of the external auditory canal surface as a topical agent. For serious inner ear infections, systemic antibiotics are indicated.

Chloramphenicol [klor am fen' a kole] (Chloromycetin Otic), a broad-spectrum antibiotic (bacteriostatic) solution is used to treat external ear infections caused by *Staphylococcus aureus, Escherichia coli, Pseudomonas aeruginosa, Enterobacter aerogenes, Haemophilus influenzae,* and other susceptible organisms.

The possible side effects produced by chloramphenicol are burning, redness, rash, swelling, or other signs of topical irritation that were not present before the start of therapy. The medication should be discontinued if this hypersensitivity reaction occurs. Usual dosage for adults and children is 2 or 3 drops inserted in the ear canal every 6 to 8 hours.

Gentamicin sulfate otic solution [jen ta mye' sin] (Garamycin), a bactericidal antibiotic, is another antibiotic that is not presently available in the otic preparation in the United States but is available in Canada. Although it is not FDA approved, prescribers sometimes use the ophthalmic preparation marketed in the United States for otic infections.

Side effects are similar to chloramphenicol. The dose is 3 or 4 drops inserted in the ear canal three times daily.

CORTICOSTEROID EAR PREPARATIONS

Corticosteroid otic solutions include betamethasone and hydrocortisone, only available in Canada (Betnesol ♣ and Cortamed ♣) and dexamethasone (Decadron), available in both countries. Hydrocortisone combinations with acetic acid (VoSol HC, Acetasol HC), with alcohol (EarSol-HC), or with acetic acid and benzethonium (AA-HC Otic) are also available. Acetic acid, boric acid, benzalkonium chloride, benzethonium, and aluminum acetate (Burow's solution) are used for their antibacterial or antifungal effects. Hydrocortisone is included for its antiinflammatory, antipruritic, and antiallergic effects (Olin, 1996; *USP DI,* 1996).

Corticosteroid may be combined with the antibiotics neomycin and polymyxin B to treat external ear canal infections and mastoidectomy cavity infections. Many such products are available that may also include other ingredients, such as those included in the OTC otic preparations. These are prescription otic solutions such as AK-spore HC, Cort-Biotic, Cortisporin, Cortomycin, and others (*USP DI,* 1996).

OTHER OTIC PREPARATIONS

Over-the-counter otic preparations often contain acidified (acetic acid) solutions of alcohol, glycerin, or propylene glycol to help restore the normal acid pH to the ear canal, especially after the person swims or bathes. Glycerin, mineral oil, and olive oil (sweet oil) are used as emollients to help relieve itching and burning in the ear while propylene glycol enhances the antibacterial effect and acidity of acetic acid. Carbamide peroxide (urea hydrogen peroxide) is an antibacterial agent that releases oxygen to help remove **cerumen** (ear wax) accumulations. Thus combinations of these ingredients are often included in OTC otic solutions (Covington, 1993).

A wide variety of both single and combination products is used to treat impacted cerumen, inflammation, bacterial or fungal infections, ear pain, and other minor or superficial problems associated primarily with the external ear canal. More serious problems such as an earache secondary to an upper respiratory tract infection, ear discharge or drainage, persistent or recurrent otitis, or ear pain caused by recent injury or head trauma require a health care provider's thorough evaluation and intervention to prevent complications. In such cases systemic medications with or without ear preparations are usually necessary.

Although most OTC otic preparations are considered safe and effective, clients should be advised to see a provider if symptoms do not improve within several days of using these preparations or if an adverse reaction occurs. Table 45-1 for selected examples of OTC otic solutions.

■ Nursing Management

Drugs Affecting the Ear

Assessment. Before initiation of therapy, assess hearing and extent of symptoms (earache, pain, erythema, vertigo, drainage, and others) that may be present. Before instilling the ear drops, assess that the ear canal is clear and not impacted with cerumen and that the tympanic membrane is intact.

To identify areas for education, assess the client for improper hygiene or health practices that may contribute to the development of infections, such as cleaning the ear canal with a cotton swab.

Nursing diagnosis. The client is at risk for the following nursing diagnoses: impaired communication related to hearing loss; altered comfort; risk for injury related to vertigo secondary to vestibular dysfunction; risk for infection related to the underlying condition; and the potential complication of deafness.

Implementation

Monitoring. Monitor the client's affected ear(s) for improvement of the condition for which the ear drops are being administered. Monitor for possible hypersensitivity to the ear drops, evidenced by burning, redness, and swelling that were not present when the medication was started. If hypersensitivity occurs, discontinue drops and notify the prescriber. Monitor the client's level of comfort, hearing, and temperature periodically.

TABLE 45-1 Selected examples of OTC otic solutions

Ingredients (trade names)	Use/indications
carbamide peroxide (Auro Ear Drops)	ear wax
isopropyl alcohol (Auro-Dri Ear Drops)	swimmer's ear
boric acid & isopropyl alcohol (Aurocaine 2)	swimmer's ear
isopropyl alcohol in glycerin (Swim-Ear Drops)	swimmer's ear
carbamide peroxide & glycerin (Dent's Ear Wax Drops, E.R.O. Ear Drops, Ear Wax Removal System)	ear wax
hydrocortisone, propylene glycol, alcohol, benzyl benzoate (Earsol-HC Drops)	antiinflammatory, antipruritic

Modified from *Nonprescription products: formulations & features '97–'98* (1997). Washington, DC: American Pharmaceutical Association.

Intervention. Ear drops are more comfortably tolerated if they are warmed (if not contraindicated) before instillation. This can be achieved by running warm water over the side of the bottle without the label or immersing the bottle in warm water in a medicine cup. Even carrying the bottle in a pocket for half an hour or so will take the chill off the drops.

Let an irritable child get comfortable before attempting to administer ear drops. To prepare for the instillation of ear drops cleanse any drainage present from the ear and position the client so that the ear to be medicated is facing upward.

The instillation of ear drops requires a knowledge of anatomic structure across the life span because the shape of the auditory canal of a young child is different from that of an adult. In children 3 years of age or younger, gently pull the pinna of the ear slightly down and back to instill ear drops. In older children and adults, hold the pinna up and back. Gentle massage of the area immediately anterior to the ear will facilitate the entry of the drops into the ear canal (see Figure 7-3).

Education. Instruct the client to remain on his or her side for 5 minutes. A small cotton pledget may be gently inserted into the ear canal if desired. Alert the client to the hazard of impaired hearing related to the drops, the cotton pledget, or the ear ailment itself. Instruct the client and/or family member in the appropriate method of ear drop instillation based on the client's age.

Evaluation. The client will evidence no clinical signs of infection (fever, pain, redness, heat, odor, drainage) or hearing loss and will have a normal WBC count. Cultures of the ear canal will be negative for pathogenic growth.

DRUG-INDUCED OTOTOXICITY

Many medications have reportedly caused **ototoxicity** in humans. The ototoxicity may affect the person's hearing (auditory or cochlear function), balance (vestibular function), or both. The most common symptom reported is **tinnitus**, a ringing or buzzing sound in the ears.

Cochlear ototoxicity causes a progressive or continuing hearing loss. High pitched tinnitus or the loss of the highest tones occurs first, then progresses to affect the lowest tones. Because of this slow progression, most clients are not aware that it is occurring. Vestibular toxicity may start with a severe headache of 1 to 2 days duration, followed by nausea, vomiting, dizziness, ataxia, and difficulty with equilibrium. The person may feel as though the room is in motion (**vertigo**). Ototoxicity is usually bilateral and may be reversible, but it can become irreversible if not recognized early enough to stop the offending medications. Most drug-induced ototoxicity is associated with the use of aminoglycosides, such as streptomycin, gentamicin, tobramycin and others. Table 45-2 lists selected drugs reported to induce ototoxicity.

■ Nursing Management

Drugs That Induce Ototoxicity

Assessment. Assess hearing function before starting therapy with an ototoxic drug. Concurrent administration of more than one ototoxic drug may increase the potential for hearing loss. Use caution when administering ototoxic drugs in clients who have any condition that may increase their risk of adverse reaction from otic drugs. An example is the client with renal failure, a condition that alters the elimination of aminoglycosides and may result in ototoxic serum levels.

Take a thorough drug history, particularly of a client with sudden hearing loss or tinnitus. Aspirin is the most widely used drug that causes tinnitus, but keep in mind nonsteroidal antiinflammatory drugs, aminoglycosides, quinine and its synthetic substitutes, diuretics, and antineoplastics (see Table 45-2).

Nursing diagnosis. The client who is taking drugs that cause ototoxicity is at risk for: sensory/perceptual alterations related to ototoxicity (auditory deficit, tinnitus); injury related to vestibular dysfunction (ataxia, dizziness); and the potential complication of deafness.

Implementation

Monitoring. Serum levels of some drugs may be monitored to help detect the development of dangerously high blood levels. Monitor the client's ability to hear by observing for cues indicative of increasing hearing loss (inappropriate responses to others' conversation, speaking loudly, moving closer to others when they speak) and noting any comments by the client of not being able to hear or understand what others are saying. Report indications of increased hearing loss to the prescriber.

Intervention. When given intravenously, aminoglycosides should be administered over 30 to 60 minutes to avoid high peak levels.

TABLE 45-2 Selected drugs reported to cause ototoxicity

Drug	Comments
Analgesics	
aspirin and NSAIDs	Salicylates, especially in high doses, can cause tinnitus, vertigo and hearing loss. It is generally reversible if drug is reduced or discontinued, although some cases of irreversible hearing loss are documented. With NSAIDs, hearing disturbances and loss are reported.
Antibiotics	
aminoglycosides	Incidence of ototoxicity is 1%-5% and may be irreversible.
clarithromycin	Hearing loss reported (usually reversible). Occurs more often in elderly women.
erythromycin	Reversible hearing loss has been reported in persons with liver and/or kidney impairment; in persons 50 years and older and in individuals that received high doses (>4 g/day) IV erythromycin has resulted in irreversible ototoxicity.
vancomycin	Hearing loss reported especially in persons with kidney impairment or those receiving another ototoxic medication concurrently.
Antineoplastic agents	
cisplatin	Ototoxicity with tinnitus, hearing loss, and possible deafness has been reported. This effect is especially severe in children (younger than 12 years old). This effect is accumulative; therefore audiometric testing is recommended.
mechlorethamine	Tinnitus and, less frequently, hearing loss reported.
Loop diuretics	
bumetanide, ethacrynic acid, furosemide	Reversible and irreversible hearing loss reported, usually with too rapid IV injection, high diuretic dosages, concurrent use with other ototoxic medications, and in renal impairment.

(Olin, 1996)

Education. Instruct clients to report tinnitus or any other hearing impairment immediately. Auditory damage is usually reversible if the causative drug is discontinued early.

Evaluation. The client states being able to understand others and expresses satisfaction with sensory input.

SUMMARY

Drugs that affect the ear may relate to the treatment of inflammation, excess cerumen, bacterial or fungal infection, or ear discomfort, or they may cause ototoxicity as an adverse effect of being administered for some other condition. In both instances the nurse needs to be concerned about the client's comfort and auditory perception and the risk for injury from the adverse effects of the drugs or as an extension of the client's symptoms.

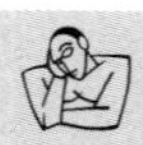

Critical Thinking

1. Joan Stevens is a 10-month-old white infant who is brought to the clinic by her mother because of irritability, tugging at her ear, and a fever of 101° F. What would the nurse consider to be essential to her assessment of Joan?
2. What clients would be particularly at risk for drug-related ototoxicity and why?

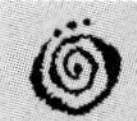

Collaborative Learning Activities

1. The class will be divided into teams to plan their responses to Critical Thinking questions 1 and 2. Compare answers.

BIBLIOGRAPHY

Anderson KN, et al. (Eds.) (1994). *Mosby's medical, nursing, & allied health dictionary* (4th ed.). St Louis: Mosby.

Covington TR (1993). *Handbook of nonprescription drugs* (10th ed.). Washington, DC: American Pharmaceutical Association.

Covington TR (1995). *Product update, handbook of nonprescription drugs* (10th ed.). Washington, DC: American Pharmaceutical Association.

Olin BR (Ed.) (1996). *Facts and comparisons: Drug information.* St Louis: Facts and Comparisons.

Semia TP, et al. (1993). *Geriatric dosage handbook: American Pharmaceutical Association.* Hudson, OH: Lexi-Comp.

United States Pharmacopeial Convention (1996). *USP DI: Drug information for the health care professional* (16th ed.). Rockville, MD: The Convention.

Zivic RC & King S (1993). Cerumen-impaction management for clients of all ages, *Nurse Pract* 18(3):29.

Chapter 46

Overview of the Endocrine System

Chapter Focus

The endocrine and nervous systems serve as the body's communication system. The endocrine glands respond to signals from the internal and external environment by synthesizing and releasing hormones into the circulation. To provide care to clients with disorders of this complex system, it is essential that the nurse be knowledgeable about the anatomy and physiology of the endocrine system. The following objectives and key terms are important to a good understanding of this chapter.

Key Terms

aldosterone (p. 760)
androgens (p. 760)
cretinism (p. 758)
diabetes mellitus (p. 761)
glucagon (p. 761)
glucocorticoid (p. 760)
goiter (p. 758)
hormone (p. 754)
insulin (p. 760)
mineralocorticoid (p. 760)
myxedema (p. 759)
negative feedback (p. 754)
oxytocin (p. 756)
thyrotoxicosis (p. 759)
vasopressin (antidiuretic hormone) (p. 756)

Objectives

1. Define hormones and explain their functions.
2. List the primary hormones released from the anterior and posterior pituitary.
3. Describe the effects of the thyroid hormones on the body.
4. Discuss the functioning of the parathyroid glands in relationship to calcium and vitamin D.
5. Describe the functions of the three hormones released from the adrenal glands.
6. Compare the effects of insulin and glucagon on blood sugar levels.

HORMONES

Hormones are active, natural chemical substances secreted into the bloodstream from the endocrine glands that initiate or regulate the activity of an organ or group of cells in another part of the body. They have specific, well-defined physiologic effects on metabolism. The list of major hormones includes the products of the secretions from the anterior and posterior pituitary glands, the thyroid hormones, parathyroid hormone, pancreatic insulin and glucagon, epinephrine and norepinephrine from the adrenal medulla, several potent steroids from the adrenal cortex, and the gonadal hormones of both sexes (Figure 46-1).

The major types of hormones are the steroid hormones and the amino-acid–derived hormones. Steroid hormones are those substances secreted by the adrenal gland and the sex glands. They transport proteins in the plasma, their physiologic effect beginning when the steroid enters the cell, with subsequent binding to the specific cytosol or nuclear protein receptor.

Hormones from the various endocrine glands work together to regulate vital processes, including the following:

1. Secretory and motor activities of the digestive tract
2. Energy production
3. Composition and volume of extracellular fluid
4. Adaptation, such as acclimatization and immunity
5. Growth and development
6. Reproduction and lactation

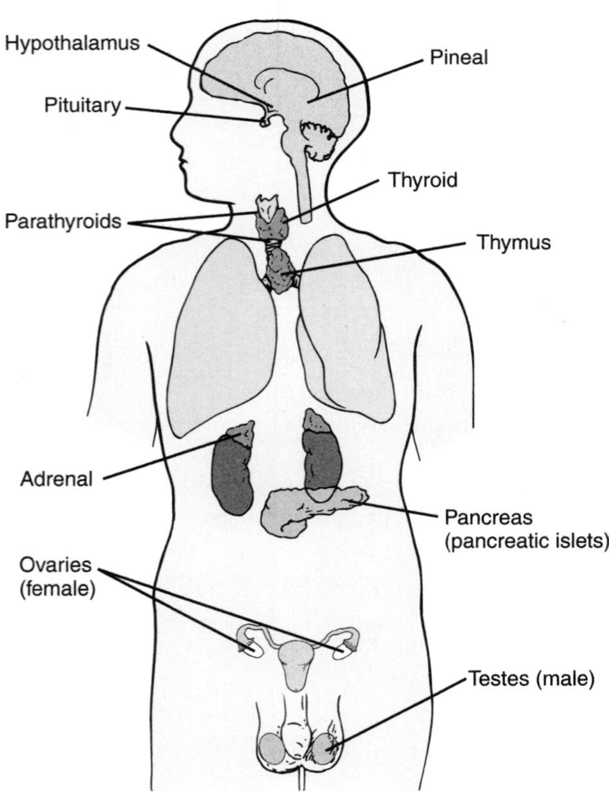

Figure 46-1 Locations of the major endocrine glands.

Hormones may exert their effects by controlling the formation or destruction of an intracellular regulator cyclic 3'5' adenosine monophosphate (cyclic AMP), controlling protein synthesis, or controlling membrane permeability and the movement of ions and other substances. The effect of a hormone depends on its interaction with a receptor and is determined by the level of the circulating active hormone.

To maintain the internal environment, hormone secretion must be controlled. This is achieved by a self-regulating series of events known as **negative feedback**; that is, a hormone produces a physiologic effect that, when strong enough, inhibits further secretion of that hormone, thereby inhibiting the physiologic effect. Increased hormonal secretions may be evoked in response to stimuli from the external environment; cessation of external stimuli ends the internal secretion response (Figure 46-2).

Hormones are not "used up" in exerting their physiologic effects but must be inactivated or excreted if the internal environment is to remain stable. Inactivation occurs enzymatically in the blood or intercellular spaces, in the liver or kidney, or in the target tissues. Excretion of hormones is primarily via the urine and, to a lesser extent, the bile. Most hormones are destroyed rapidly, having a half-life in blood of 10 to 30 minutes. However, some, such as the catecholamines, have a half-life of seconds, and thyroid hormones have a half-life measured in days. Some hormones exert their physiologic effects immediately; others require minutes or hours before their effects occur. In addition, some effects end immediately when the hormone disappears from the circulation. Other responses may persist for hours after hormone concentrations have returned to basal levels. The exposure of a tissue to an

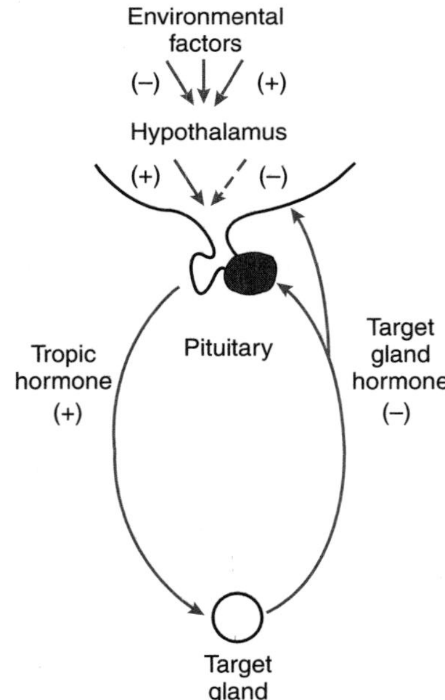

Figure 46-2 Various internal and external factors may inhibit or stimulate the hypothalamus to secrete inhibitory (–) or releasing (+) factors to control output of hormones from anterior pituitary and ultimate hormone release from target glands.

active hormone also is controlled by that hormone's pathway for metabolism, including molecular alterations, consumption at the site of action, and hepatorenal excretion. This wide range of onset and duration of hormonal activity contributes to the flexibility of the endocrine system.

One of the major developments of this century in the fields of biology and medicine has been the recognition, isolation, purification, and chemical and cellular understanding of most known hormones. In addition, once their chemical structure is known, duplicating hormones by chemical synthesis becomes theoretically possible. This has been accomplished for some but not all hormones.

In medicine, hormones generally are used in three ways: (1) for replacement therapy, exemplified by the use of insulin in diabetes or of adrenal steroids in Addison's disease; (2) for pharmacologic effects beyond replacement, as in the use of larger-than-endogenous doses of adrenal steroids for their antiinflammatory effects; and (3) for endocrine diagnostic testing.

Research in endocrinology has advanced the concept of specific receptors within or on the surface of cells. This has led to knowledge of hormone specificity and the essential cellular mechanisms involved in the hormone-receptor complex. The recognition and activation properties found in the hormone-receptor complex come from different receptor molecular sites. Only specific receptor material binds a hormone and begins its activity; the hormone has no effect on other tissues that do not carry specific receptors.

Alterations in either hormone secretion or hormone receptor responses may culminate in endocrine disease states. Certain cell surface receptors may become antigenic and develop antibodies that accelerate receptor destruction, block receptor function, or mimic the action of the target tissue. Among the receptor-like disorders, referred to as *antireceptor autoimmune diseases,* are myasthenia gravis, Graves' disease, insulin-resistant diabetes mellitus, and bronchial asthma.

PITUITARY GLAND

The hormones of the pituitary gland exert an important effect in regulating the secretion of other hormones. The pituitary body is about the size of a pea and occupies a niche in the sella turcica of the sphenoid bone. It consists of an anterior lobe (adenohypophysis), a posterior lobe (neurohypophysis), and a smaller pars intermedia composed of secreting cells. The anterior lobe is particularly important in sustaining life. The function of the pars intermedia is not well understood. Figure 46-3 shows the major pituitary hormones and their principal target organs.

Regulation of Anterior Pituitary Function

The pituitary and target glands have a negative feedback relationship. A trophic hormone from the pituitary stimulates the target gland to secrete a hormone that inhibits further secretion of the trophic hormone by the pituitary. When the serum concentration of the target gland hormone falls below a certain level, the pituitary again secretes the trophic hormone until the target gland produces enough hormone to inhibit the pituitary secretion. However, the negative feedback concept alone is not enough to account for changes in serum levels of target gland hormones, especially those caused by changes in the external environment. Thus the central nervous system is believed to play a decisive role in regulating pituitary function to meet environmental demands.

The discovery of various hypothalamic-releasing factors is of great research interest. These factors cause the release of inhibition of the various hormones from the anterior pituitary. Among these releasing factors are thyroid-stimulating hormone releasing factor, corticotropin-releasing factor, growth hormone releasing hormone, growth hormone pituitary hormone (somatostatin), luteinizing hormone releasing hormone, and prolactin inhibitory factor.

Anterior Pituitary Hormones

The number of hormones secreted by the anterior pituitary gland is unknown, but at least seven extracts have been prepared in a relatively pure state, and they have definite specific action.

1. A growth factor influences the development of the body. It promotes skeletal, visceral, and general growth. Acromegaly, gigantism, and dwarfism are associated with pathologic conditions of the anterior lobe of the pituitary gland.

   Growth hormone (GH) (somatotropin, somatropin, somatotropic hormone, STH) has been obtained as a small crystalline protein, but thus far the growth hormone has found no established place in medicine except in documented clinical and laboratory evidence of growth hormone deficiency associated with chronic renal insufficiency (Olin, 1996). Its use in various clinical conditions is largely experimental. See Chapter 47 for further discussion on growth hormone.
2. Follicle-stimulating hormone (FSH) stimulates the growth and maturation of the ovarian follicle, which in turn brings on the characteristic changes of estrus (menstruation in women). This hormone also stimulates spermatogenesis in the male. FSH appears to be a protein or is associated with a protein, but this human pituitary gonadotropin has not yet been obtained in a highly purified form.
3. Luteinizing hormone (LH), also known as the *interstitial cell-stimulating hormone (ICSH),* together with FSH (Pergonal), causes maturation of the graafian follicles, ovulation, and the secretion of estrogen in the female. It causes spermatogenesis, androgen formation, and growth of interstitial tissue in the male. Luteinizing hormone also promotes the formation of the corpus luteum in the female.
4. Thyrotropic hormone (TSH) is necessary for normal development and function of the thyroid gland. If too much is present, it is known to produce hyperthyroidism and increase the size of the gland in laboratory animals.

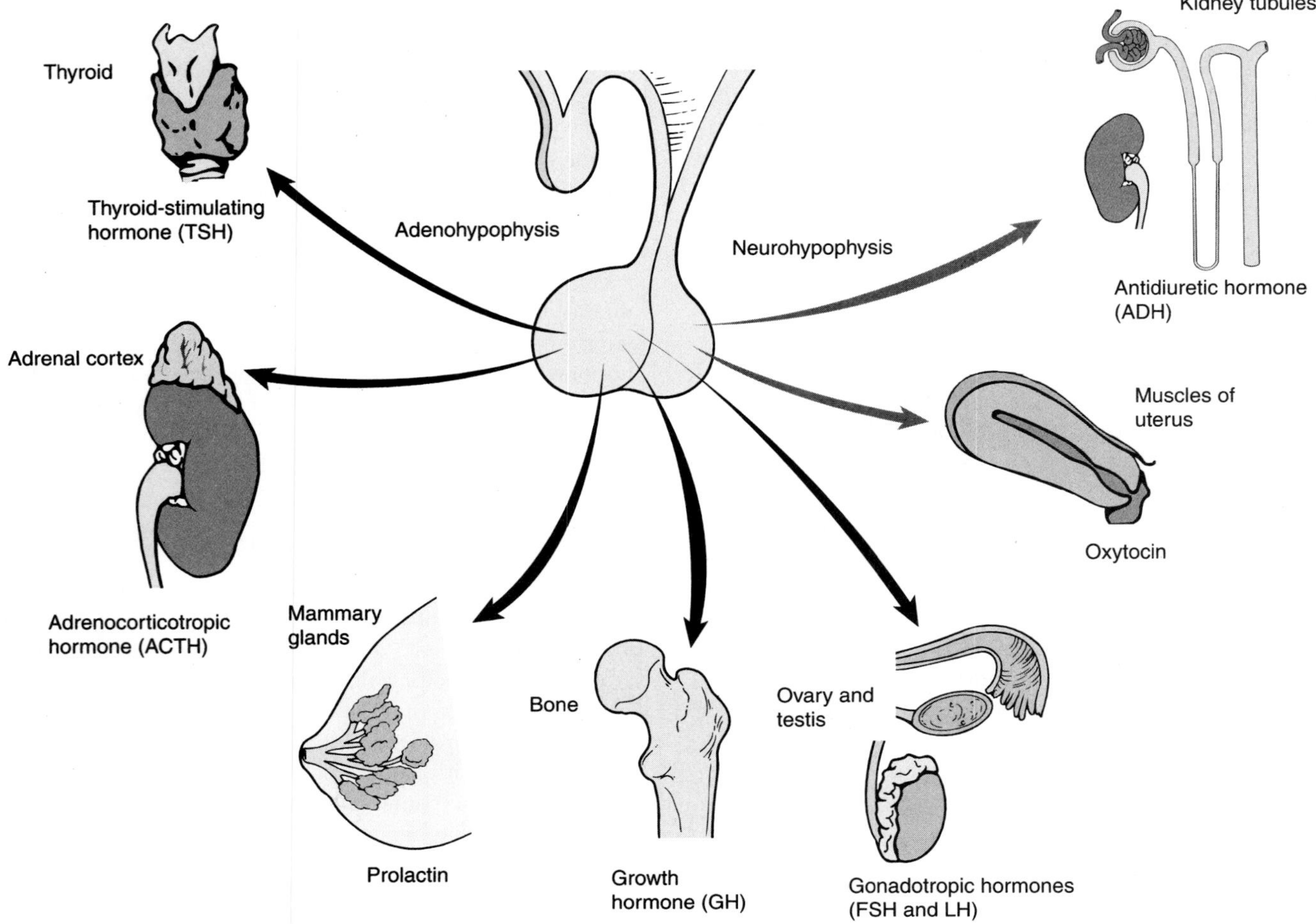

Figure 46-3 Pituitary hormones. Some of the major hormones of the adenohypophysis and neurohypophysis and their principal target organs.

5. A lactogenic factor (prolactin or mammotropin) plays a part in the proliferation and secretion of the mammary glands of mammals. This may be identical to the hormone responsible for the development of the corpus luteum. In its absence the corpus luteum fails to produce progesterone.
6. Adrenocorticotropic hormone (corticotropin or ACTH) stimulates the cortex of the adrenal gland.
7. Melanocyte-stimulating hormone (intermedin or MSH) is probably produced in the intermediate lobe. Its physiologic role is unknown, but when injected in human beings it darkens the skin.

The hormones produced by the anterior lobe of the pituitary gland are important physiologically, but recently purified preparations became available, at least for clinical study; such preparations are both expensive and limited in supply. They may become useful in combating certain disorders in the future, however, as chemically defined preparations become available.

Posterior Pituitary Hormones

Two hormones obtained from the posterior lobe of the pituitary gland have been identified and chemically analyzed. These compounds, **oxytocin** (a hormone that stimulates the smooth muscle of the uterus to contract) and **vasopressin** (the **antidiuretic hormone**), are both peptides, and each contains eight amino acids. It has proved possible to synthesize them chemically. Availability of these hormones in pure form has clarified their mechanism of action and has allowed better control of their therapeutic use. For example, a certain overlap of pharmacologic action exists even in the pure preparation; pure oxytocin has some vasopressor activity, and vice versa. The antidiuretic potency of vasopressin is much greater than its pressor potency.

Although vasopressin is available in a natural state, synthetic formulations, such as lypressin and desmopressin, have been developed, and they act primarily as ADH. They have very little, if any, pressor or oxytocic activity.

Oxytocin is discussed in Chapter 53.

THYROID GLAND

The thyroid gland, one of the most richly vascularized tissues of the body, secretes three hormones essential for proper regulation of metabolism: thyroxine (T_4), triiodothyronine (T_3), and calcitonin. Because of its role in calcium metabolism, calcitonin is discussed in greater detail in the section on parathyroid gland hormones (see Chapter 48).

The thyroid gland is composed of at least two types of cells: follicular, which produce T_3 and T_4; and parafollicular, the source of calcitonin.

Thyroid Hormones

The large amount of iodine in thyroid hormones and the availability of radioactive iodine have led to detailed knowledge about thyroid physiology and its role in metabolism. Iodine is essential for thyroid hormone synthesis. About 1 mg of iodine is required per week, most of which is ingested in food, water, and iodized table salt. About two thirds of this iodine is reduced in the gastrointestinal tract, enters the circulation as iodide, and is excreted into the urine. The remaining third is taken up by the thyroid gland for hormone synthesis. This process is aided by the "iodide pump," which takes up the iodide from the extracellular fluid, traps it, and concentrates it to many times that found in plasma. The ratio of iodide in the thyroid gland to that in the serum is expressed as the T/S ratio; normally this ratio is 20:1. In hypoactivity the ratio may be 10:1; in hyperactivity it may be as great as 250:1.

Thyroglobulin is synthesized first. It contains tyrosine, an amino acid that reacts with iodine to form thyroid hormones. The thyroglobulin-thyroid hormone complex is stored in the follicles of the thyroid gland and is called "colloid." About 30% of the thyroid mass is stored thyroglobulin, which contains enough thyroid hormone to meet normal requirements for 2 to 3 months without any further synthesis.

Normally, thyroglobulin is not released into the circulation but undergoes proteolytic digestion (a coupling reaction), which releases the active thyroid hormones T_3 and T_4. Hormone synthesis—iodine trapping, iodination and proteolysis of thyroglobulin, and hormone release—is controlled by the thyroid-stimulating hormone (thyrotropin, TSH) from the beta cells of the anterior pituitary gland. Thyroid secretion is maintained by this TSH secretion. Decreased serum levels of T_3 and T_4 stimulate thyrotropin-releasing hormone (TRH) from the hypothalamus, which stimulates the pituitary gland to secrete TSH; this in turn stimulates release of thyroxin from thyroglobulin.

TSH secretion is negatively regulated by T_3 and T_4, which directly inhibit the pituitary gland's thyrotropic cells. An increase in free, unbound thyroid hormone causes a decrease in TSH secretion and inhibits TRH production, and a decrease in the free unbound hormone causes an increase in TSH secretion and stimulates TRH production—a negative feedback mechanism.

Physiologic Effects of Thyroid Hormones

The precise physiologic role of the thyroid hormones is not yet known, although several hormonal actions have been identified and studied. Three generalizations can be made about thyroid hormones:

1. They have a diffuse effect and do not seem to have any specific target organ effect; no special cells or tissues appear to be particularly affected by the thyroid hormones.
2. Their long delay in onset of action and their prolonged action rule them out as minute-to-minute regulators of physiologic function. Instead, their role is more likely to be that of establishing and maintaining long-term functions such as growth, maturation, and adaptation.
3. They are not necessary for survival, although reduced levels can affect quality of life.

Thyroxine and triiodothyronine appear to have the same physiologic actions, although T_3 is far more potent than T_4.

Growth and maturation. A normal, functioning thyroid is essential for normal growth. Thyroid hormones stimulate production of messenger ribonucleic acid (RNA) molecules, which are involved in the synthesis of various proteins, thus facilitating growth and development. The hormones must be present in the right amounts for growth to occur at the normal rate. In children who are hypothyroid the rate of growth is retarded, which may lead to shortness of stature. Conversely, children who are hyperthyroid may have excessive skeletal growth and become taller than they otherwise would. If there is premature closing of the epiphyses because of accelerated bone maturation, however, stunting of growth results. In the adult, excess thyroid hormone causes increased demineralization of bone and increased loss of calcium and phosphate.

Cells in the interstitial tissue between follicles of the thyroid gland produce calcitonin; the effect of this hormone is to reduce the blood calcium ion concentration, an effect that is the exact opposite of that of parathyroid hormone. Calcitonin is essential for bone formation in children because it promotes deposition of calcium. In the adult, calcitonin has a very weak effect on plasma concentration because absorption and deposition of calcium are slow in the adult and calcitonin effects are rapidly overridden by parathyroid hormone.

Central nervous system function. From the time of birth through the first year of life, thyroid hormone must be present for normal development of the cerebrum; if the hormone is not present, irreversible mental retardation occurs. In the adult, hypothyroidism causes listlessness, a general dulling of mental capacity, decreased sensory capacity, slow speech, impaired memory, and somnolence. Hyperthyroidism in the adult results in hyperexcitability, irritability, restlessness, exaggerated responses to environmental stimuli, and emotional instability. Psychosis can occur in either hypothyroidism or hyperthyroidism.

Basal metabolic rate. Thyroid hormones increase oxygen consumption in most cells of the body with the exception of the lungs, spleen, gastric smooth muscle, the gonads, and accessory sex organs. In hypothyroidism the basal metabolic rate is subnormal; in hyperthyroidism it may be 40% to 60% above normal.

Carbohydrate and lipid metabolism. Thyroid hormones accelerate glucose catabolism, increase cholesterol synthesis, and enhance the liver's ability to excrete cholesterol in the bile. Because the effect on cholesterol excretion is greater than that on cholesterol synthesis, the result is a decrease in plasma cholesterol level. The hormones also stimulate the mobilization of fatty acids from adipose tissue. The hypothyroid individual will have an elevated serum cholesterol level and increased blood levels of phospholipids and triglycerides.

Protein metabolism. Thyroid hormones are essential for the development of protein mass. In hypothyroidism both the synthesis and the breakdown of protein are diminished, but the effect on protein synthesis is more profound. In addition, deposition of mucoproteins occurs in subcutaneous spaces, which osmotically attract water, causing "puffiness." In hyperthyroidism increased catabolism of protein, or breakdown of muscle mass, and increased nitrogen excretion occur.

Gastrointestinal function. Thyroid hormones increase gastrointestinal motility, absorption of food, and secretion of digestive juices. Hypothyroidism decreases both intestinal absorption and secretion of pancreatic enzymes. Constipation also may occur.

Water and electrolyte balance. In thyroid hormone deficiency, water and electrolytes accumulate in subcutaneous spaces; administering thyroid hormone results in diuresis and a loss of fluid and electrolytes from the subcutaneous spaces.

Cardiovascular function. Because the thyroid hormones increase metabolism, the tissues have an increased need for oxygen and nutrients, which in turn demands increased blood flow. In hyperthyroidism these effects cause increased cardiac output, increased pulse pressure, and tachycardia. If these effects are prolonged, cardiac hypertrophy and even high-output myocardial failure may occur. The opposite effects occur in hypothyroidism.

Muscle function. Moderate increases in thyroid hormone makes muscle react with vigor; large increases result in muscle weakness because of excess protein catabolism. A characteristic sign of hyperthyroidism is a fine muscle tremor. Hypothyroidism causes the muscles to be sluggish.

Temperature regulation. Thyroid hormones must be present for an increase in heat production or a decrease in heat loss to occur. Although the hormones do not initiate the physiologic response to cold, they appear to magnify the body's response to catecholamine effects, which innervate the sympathetic system during cold exposure. Hypothyroidism causes decreased tolerance to cold.

Lactation. Thyroid hormone is necessary for normal milk production; without thyroid hormone, the fat content of milk and total milk production are greatly reduced.

Reproduction. Thyroid hormone is required for normal rhythmicity in the reproductive cycle.

Thyroid Gland Disorders

Goiter

The synthesis of the thyroid hormones and their maintenance in the blood in adequate amounts depend largely on an adequate intake of iodine. Iodine ingested by way of food or water is changed into iodide and is stored in the thyroid gland before reaching the circulation. Prolonged iodine deficiency in the diet results in enlargement of the thyroid gland, known as a simple **goiter.** When thyroid hormones fail to be synthesized because of a lack of iodine, the anterior lobe of the pituitary is stimulated to increase the secretion of thyrotropic hormone, which in turn causes hypertrophy and hyperplasia of the gland. The enlarged thyroid then removes residual traces of iodine from the blood. This type of goiter (simple or nontoxic) can be prevented by providing an adequate supply of iodine for young persons. Iodine is not abundant in most foods except fish and seafood, and iodized salt is frequently the primary source of iodine in areas where seafood is expensive or not readily available.

Hypothyroidism

Clients with primary hypothyroidism have decreased T_3 and T_4 levels and an elevated TSH level. Those with pituitary (secondary) hypothyroidism and hypothalamic (tertiary) hypothyroidism have decreased levels of T_3, T_4, and TSH.

The TSH test, the most sensitive index of hypothyroidism, is elevated in primary hypothyroidism and depressed in secondary hypothyroidism. The free thyroxine index ($FTI = TT_4 \times RT_3U$) is depressed in clients with both primary and secondary hypothyroidism but elevated in clients with hyperthyroidism. The T_3 resin uptake (RT_3U) is depressed in pregnancy and in clients with primary and secondary hypothyroidism but elevated in clients with hyperthyroidism. The serum T_3 level is depressed in both secondary and primary hypothyroidism but elevated in hyperthyroid states and T_3 thyrotoxicosis. The total T_4 (TT_4 Murphy-Pattee) is elevated in pregnancy and hyperthyroidism but depressed in both primary and secondary hypothyroidism. The free T_4 (unbound) is depressed in both primary and secondary hypothyroid states but is elevated in hyperthyroid states.

In children, normal skeletal growth is evidence of adequate therapy; an increase in serum alkaline phosphatase indicates that growth will occur. In cretinism, thyroid hormone levels equal to or above those required for the adult must be established immediately after birth to prevent permanent mental and physical retardation. Treatment of the older cretin will not reverse the mental retardation that has already occurred. Clients with hypothyroidism need to be informed of their lifelong need for replacement therapy.

Hypothyroidism in the young child is known as **cretinism** and is characterized by cessation of physical and mental development, which leads to dwarfism and mental retardation. Clients with cretinism usually have thick, coarse skin; a thick tongue; gaping mouth; protruding abdomen; thick, short legs; poorly developed hands and feet; and weak musculature. This condition may result from faulty development or atrophy of the thyroid gland during fetal life. Failure of development of the gland may be caused by lack of iodine in the mother.

Severe hypothyroidism in the adult is called **myxedema** (acid mucopolysaccharide accumulation). When it is the last stage of a long-standing, inadequately treated, or untreated hypothyroidism, coma sets in, accompanied by hypotension, hypoventilation, hypothermia, bradycardia, hyponatremia, and hypoglycemia. The development of myxedema is usually insidious and causes gradual retardation of physical and mental functions. There is gradual infiltration of the skin and loss of facial lines and facial expression (resulting in a puffy, expressionless face). The formation of subcutaneous connective tissue causes the hands and face to appear puffy and swollen. The basal metabolic rate becomes subnormal, the skin is cold and dry, the hair becomes scant and coarse, movements become sluggish, cardiac output is reduced, and the client becomes hypersensitive to cold.

Hyperthyroidism (Thyrotoxicosis)

Excessive formation of the thyroid hormones and their escape into the circulation result in a toxic state called **thyrotoxicosis.** This occurs in the condition known as *diffuse toxic goiter,* or *exophthalmic goiter (Graves' disease),* or in some forms of adenomatous goiters.

Primary hyperthyroidism is characterized by elevated levels of T_3 and T_4 and decreased level of TSH. In pituitary (secondary) hyperthyroidism levels of T_3, T_4, and TSH increase. Hyperthyroidism leads to symptoms quite different from those seen in myxedema. The metabolic rate is increased, sometimes as much as 60% or more. The body temperature frequently is above normal, the pulse rate is fast, and the client complains of feeling too warm. Other symptoms include restlessness, anxiety, emotional instability, muscle tremor and weakness, sweating, and exophthalmos. The increased thyroxine levels may cause cardiomegaly, tachycardia, congestive heart failure, hepatic alterations (necrosis, dysfunction, fatty changes), lymphoid hyperplasia, osteoporosis, pretibial myxedema, and neurologic irritability. In thyroid storm, sudden onset of hyperthyroid symptoms occurs, especially those affecting the nervous and cardiovascular systems, because of elevated thyroxine levels. Before the advent of antithyroid drugs, treatment was limited to a subtotal resection of the hyperactive gland. Propylthiouracil is the most commonly used antithyroid medication. However, antithyroid drugs provide less rapid control of hyperthyroidism than do surgical measures. Radioactive therapy is used primarily in treatment of middle-aged and elderly clients.

PARATHYROID GLANDS

Lying just above and behind the thyroid gland are bean-shaped glands known as the parathyroids. Humans have two pairs. The adult glands consist of encapsulated masses of cells, between which are abundant adipocytes and vascular channels. The primary function of the parathyroids is to maintain adequate levels of calcium in the extracellular fluid. Parathyroid hormone has multiple effects, ultimately culminating in mobilization of calcium from bone. It also reduces phosphate concentration, permitting more calcium to be mobilized.

Parathyroid Hormones

Parathyroid hormone (PTH) is a polypeptide. The active component has a half-life of 30 minutes, the inactive component of 7 to 10 days. PTH circulates in elevated concentrations in clients with hyperplastic parathyroid glands as a result of diminished calcium levels, as found in persons with impaired renal function or intestinal malabsorption. These elevated PTH levels may cause metabolic bone disease, including osteoporosis and osteomalacia.

The mechanism of PTH action in the bone or kidney is incompletely understood. Some researchers suggest that PTH receptor-binding and adenylate cyclase activity are coupled events subject to down regulation of the receptors. Clients with hyperparathyroidism may be resistant to PTH action on kidney and bone. The decreased number of these receptors, not their altered affinity, produces a reduction in PTH-stimulated adenylate cyclase activity.

Cholesterol-derived provitamin D is converted to vitamin D_3 by the action of sunlight on the skin. The vitamin is also present as a milk additive. Along with PTH, vitamin D_3 is converted to its active form in the kidney. It is involved in calcium, phosphate, and magnesium metabolism in bone and the gastrointestinal tract. Primary hyperparathyroidism is the most common parathyroid disorder. Generally it is caused by adenomas, chief cell hyperplasia, or hypertrophy. PTH elevations produce altered function of renal tubular cells, bone cells, and gastrointestinal tract mucosa. Elevated levels of calcium and increased bone resorption with the development of renal calculi occurs generally in hyperparathyroidism. In secondary hyperparathyroidism, an overactive parathyroid gland causes increased calcium excretion and possibly kidney stones, but serum calcium levels generally remain stable because of an effective feedback mechanism.

Hypoparathyroidism leads to manifestations of hypocalcemia and tetany, the symptoms of which include muscle spasms, convulsions, gradual paralysis with dyspnea, and death from exhaustion. Before death, gastrointestinal hemorrhages and hematemesis frequently occur. At death the intestinal mucosa is congested, and the calcium content of the heart, kidney, and other tissues is increased.

The symptoms of tetany are relieved by administration of calcium salts. Large doses of vitamin D also help to relieve tetany and to restore the normal calcium level in the blood. The client is hospitalized because frequent assessment of blood calcium and phosphate levels is essential.

ADRENAL GLANDS

The adrenal glands are located just above the kidneys. They consist of two parts, the inner medulla and the outer cortex. The adrenal cortex synthesizes three important classes of hormones: the glucocorticoids (cortisol), mineralocorticoids (primarily aldosterone), and androgens (primarily dehydroepiandrosterone). The **glucocorticoids,** adrenocortical steroid hormones that increase glyconeogenesis, exert an antiinflammatory effect, and influence many body functions, are synthesized primarily in the zona fasciculata and are under the control of ACTH from the pituitary gland.

Although the basal production rate averages 30 mg every 24 hours, under stressful conditions (trauma, major surgery, infection) there is a reserve capacity production of up to 300 mg daily. Increases in glucocorticoid production may be related to proportional increases in the release of ACTH by the pituitary. See the discussion of steroid abuse in Chapter 9.

The **mineralocorticoids** are synthesized specifically in the zona glomerulosa of the adrenal cortex. Production is primarily under the control of both the renin-angiotensin axis system (discussed later) and the blood potassium level. The production of aldosterone is stimulated by salt depletion and causes sodium retention in the kidney at the distal convoluted tubule to preserve the extracellular fluid volume. Mineralocorticoids also increase the urinary excretion of potassium and hydrogen ions and maintain normal blood volume.

The **androgens** are synthesized in the zona fasciculata and the zona reticularis and essentially enhance male characteristics and control growth of the hair follicles in the skin.

Normally a reaction to serious stress causes a prompt and noticeable increase in cortisol and aldosterone production; these hormones operate together to maintain the cardiovascular tone essential for survival. A client under stress who has impaired ability to produce these hormones incurs the risk of developing acute adrenal crisis. The production of cortisol is under the control of a continuous feedback mechanism involving the pituitary and ACTH production, which is in turn inhibited by the circulating cortisol levels. Stress is a stimulus to override this inhibition and initiates secretion of corticotropin-releasing factor, which culminates in ACTH release and activation of the adrenal cortex, leading to an increased production of cortisol.

Mineralocorticoids: Aldosterone

Aldosterone is the primary mineralocorticoid to regulate sodium and potassium balance in the blood. It is synthesized in the adrenal zona glomerulosa, which is the outer edge of the adrenocortical tissue below the adrenal capsule. Aldosterone production is maintained primarily by the renin-angiotensin system and the concentration of circulating serum potassium. A drop in the circulating arterial volume stimulates volume receptors in the juxtaglomerular apparatus. As a result, renin (a proteolytic enzyme) is produced and acts on angiotensinogen, which is synthesized by the liver to form angiotensin I. When the angiotensin I passes through the pulmonary circulation, two amino acids are cleared from it to form angiotensin II. Angiotensin II stimulates the adrenal zona glomerulosa to produce aldosterone. Aldosterone promotes sodium reabsorption in the kidney at the distal convoluted tubule to preserve extracellular fluid volume. In the normal client, aldosterone secretion is stimulated by a decrease in circulating volume (loss of blood, excessive diuresis, low salt intake, etc.) and increased potassium levels. Aldosterone secretion is suppressed by an elevation of sodium levels in the blood (e.g., by excessive dietary salt intake). It restricts the loss of sodium and its accompanying anions, chloride and bicarbonate, and thereby helps to maintain extracellular fluid volume. It also maintains acid-base and potassium balance.

In adrenal insufficiency, aldosterone deficit occurs, sodium reabsorption is inhibited, and potassium excretion decreases. Hyperkalemia and mild acidosis occur. In adrenalectomy the loss of aldosterone leads to an overall reduction of sodium reabsorption and a powerful and uncontrolled loss of extracellular fluid. Plasma volume drops, and a state of hypovolemic shock may ensue. This may cause death unless a mineralocorticoid, salt, and water are administered. In excessive doses aldosterone increases potassium excretion, and unless dietary intake compensates for the loss, hypokalemia results. Acidification of the urine then occurs, leading to metabolic alkalosis.

Aldosterone is much more potent in its electrolyte effects than desoxycorticosterone, although it has not yet established a therapeutic status comparable to that of desoxycorticosterone. Its use has been limited because of its cost and relative unavailability and because it must be administered intramuscularly.

The amount of aldosterone secreted by the adrenal cortex apparently is affected by the concentration of sodium in body fluids rather than by the stimulation of the adrenal cortex by ACTH.

PANCREAS

The pancreas is a gland that lies transversely across the posterior wall of the abdomen. It secretes a limpid, colorless fluid that digests proteins, fats, and carbohydrates. It also produces internal secretions—insulin and glucagon—that affect blood sugar levels.

Insulin is a hormone secreted by the beta cells of the islets of Langerhans in the pancreas in response to increased levels of glucose in the blood. On hydrolysis, this hormone yields several amino acids. In its crystalline state it appears to be chemically linked with certain metals (zinc, nickel, cadmium, or cobalt). Normal pancreatic tissue is rich in zinc, which may be significant to the natural storage of the hormone. Insulin consists of two polypeptide chains and contains 48 amino acids, the exact sequence of which is known. Insulin is stored in the beta cells as a larger protein known as *proinsulin.* Because relatively small amounts of insulin are necessary in the body tissues, it is thought that insulin acts as a catalyst in cellular metabolism.

Carbohydrate metabolism is controlled by a finely balanced interaction of several endocrine factors (adrenal, anterior pituitary, thyroid, insulin), but the particular phase of carbohydrate metabolism that is affected by insulin is not entirely known. When insulin is injected subcutaneously, however, it produces a rapid lowering of the blood sugar. This effect is produced in both diabetic and nondiabetic persons. Moderate amounts of insulin in the diabetic animal promote the storage of carbohydrate in the liver and also in the muscle cells, particularly after the feeding of carbohydrate. In the normal animal the deposit of muscle glycogen also increases, but apparently the level of liver glycogen does not. In both diabetic and nondiabetic persons the oxygen consumption increases and the respiratory quotient rises.

Glucagon, like insulin, is a pancreatic extract and is thought to oppose the action of insulin. Glucagon is a product of the alpha cells of the islets of Langerhans. Glucagon acts primarily by mobilizing hepatic glycogen and converting it to glucose, which produces an elevation in the concentration of glucose in the blood.

Diabetes Mellitus

Diabetes mellitus is a heterogenous complex disorder of carbohydrate, fat, and protein metabolism that is primarily a result of a relative or complete lack of insulin or defects of the insulin receptors. Insulin action is ineffective at the tissue site, or not enough insulin is available. Obesity, certain drugs, viruses, autoimmune phenomena, genetic predisposition, and age may have roles in its development. The blood sugar becomes elevated, and when it exceeds a certain amount, the excess is secreted by the kidney (glycosuria). Symptoms include increased appetite (polyphagia), thirst (polydipsia), weight loss, increased urine output (polyuria), weakness (fatigue), and itching such as pruritus vulvae.

In diabetes mellitus, glycogen fails to store in the liver, although the conversion of glycogen back to glucose or the formation of glucose from other substances (gluconeogenesis) is not necessarily impaired. As a result, the level of blood sugar rapidly rises. This derangement of carbohydrate metabolism results in an abnormally high metabolism of proteins and fats. The ketone bodies, which result from oxidation of fatty acids, accumulate faster than the muscle cells can oxidize them, resulting in ketosis and acidosis.

The course of untreated diabetes mellitus is progressive. The symptoms of diabetic coma and acidosis are directly or indirectly the result of the accumulation of acetone, beta-hydroxybutyric acid, and diacetic acid. Respirations become rapid and deep, the breath has an odor of acetone, the blood sugar is elevated, the client becomes dehydrated, and stupor and coma develop unless treatment is started promptly.

The long-term complications of diabetes mellitus can lead to an increase in morbidity and mortality. Some of the most commonly associated problems are peripheral atherosclerosis, which may result in coronary artery disease, infections, gangrene, or strokes; and diabetic retinopathy, which can include vitreal hemorrhage, retinal detachment, and blindness. Renal disease, peripheral sensory neuropathy, and cardiomyopathy leading to heart failure are also reported.

Diabetes mellitus usually is treated with exogenous insulin, diet, and exercise. Glucose and insulin promote the formation and retention of glycogen in the liver, and the oxidation of fat in the liver is arrested. Therefore the rate of formation of acetone bodies is slowed and the acidosis is checked. Other supportive measures, such as restoring the fluid and electrolyte balance of the body, are very important in its treatment.

Recent advances in diabetic therapy include (1) the synthesis of human insulin by bacteria genetically altered by recombinant DNA technology, (2) islet-cell and/or pancreas transplantation, and (3) external and implanted continuous insulin infusion pumps.

SUMMARY

The endocrine system carries out integrative and regulatory functions within the body through the actions of hormones. Hormones regulate mechanisms that allow the body as a whole to meet needs. The endocrine system consists of specialized glands and their hormones, which act on specific target cells and stimulate various responses. The overproduction or underproduction of hormones results in pathologic conditions. Hormonal replacement therapy is the major concern in the underproduction of hormones by the endocrine system.

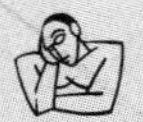

Critical Thinking

1. Given that the hospital laboratory has the ability to determine blood levels of TSH, T_3, and T_4, create a methodology for determining whether hyperthyroidism in an individual is the result of a pituitary abnormality or the production of a nonpituitary thyroid-stimulating substance.
2. A client is admitted into the emergency department with polydipsia (thirst), polyuria (excess urine production), and urine with low specific gravity. The prescriber wants to reverse these symptoms. Which of the following substances will he or she ask you to administer: insulin, glucagon, ADH, or aldosterone? Explain why.
3. A client arrives at the emergency department unconscious. His Medic-Alert bracelet indicates that he has diabetes. The client may be in diabetic coma or insulin shock. How could you tell which, and what treatment would you recommend for each condition? (Seeley, 1992).

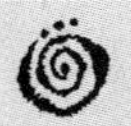

Collaborative Learning Activities

1. A pair of students will present a role play of clients with thyroid dysfunction, one with hypothyroidism, the other with hyperthyroidism. "Freeze" the action to allow students to "diagnose" these disorders and discuss the pathophysiologic etiology of their symptoms.

BIBLIOGRAPHY

Anderson KN, et al. (Eds.) (1994). *Mosby's medical, nursing, & allied health dictionary* (4th ed.). St Louis: Mosby.

Hershman JM, et al. (1992). A savvy approach to thyroid testing, *Patient Care* 26(3):134.

Kessler CA (1992). An overview of endocrine function and dysfunction, *AACN* 3(2):289.

Melmon KL, et al. (1992). *Clinical pharmacology: Basic principles in therapeutics* (3rd ed.). New York: McGraw-Hill.

Olin BR (Ed.) (1996). *Facts and comparisons.* St Louis: Facts and Comparisons.

Seeley RR, et al. (1995). *Anatomy and physiology* (3rd ed.). St Louis: Mosby.

Thibodeau GA & Patton KT (1996). *Anatomy and physiology* (3rd ed.). St Louis: Mosby.

Toto KH (1994). Endocrine physiology: A comprehensive review, *Crit Care Nurs Clin North Amer* 6(4):637-53, 655-9.

Wingard LB, et al. (1991). *Human pharmacology: Molecular to clinical.* St Louis: Mosby.

Chapter 47

Drugs Affecting the Pituitary

Chapter Focus

Although the pituitary secretes numerous hormones, this chapter discusses only the growth hormones and the antidiuretic hormone, vasopressin. Other hormones are discussed in chapters more directly related to the endocrine glands that they affect. Although disorders involving these two hormones are not common, the nurse is expected to appropriately assess and care for clients with pituitary dysfunction. The following objectives and key terms are important for a good understanding of this chapter.

Key Terms

diabetes insipidus (p. 766)
dwarfism (p. 764)
gigantism (p. 765)
growth hormone-inhibiting hormone (somatostatin) (p. 764)
growth hormone-releasing hormone (GHRH) (p. 764)

Key Drugs [▲]

somatrem
vasopressin

Objectives

1. Describe the primary functions of the anterior and posterior pituitary hormones.
2. Describe the effects of somatrem, somatropin, and octreotide.
3. List the effects of vasopressin.
4. Implement the nursing management of the care the client receiving drugs affecting the pituitary.

The variety of preparations available that affect the pituitary gland are generally used as replacement therapy for hormone deficiency, drug therapy for specific disorders using such preparations to produce a therapeutic hormonal response, and diagnostic aids to determine hypofunctional or hyperfunctional hormone states.

A number of hormones have been identified, and many have been synthesized, including the following: growth hormone-releasing hormone (GRH), growth hormone-inhibiting hormone (somatostatin), thyrotropin-releasing hormone (TRH), corticotropin-releasing hormone (CRH), gonadotropin-releasing hormone (GnRH), and prolactin inhibiting hormone (PIH or dopamine). Six anterior pituitary hormones and two posterior pituitary hormones have also been identified. The anterior pituitary hormones include growth hormone (GH), thyrotropin (TSH), adrenocorticotropin (ACTH), follicle-stimulating hormone (FSH), luteinizing hormone (LH), and prolactin. The posterior pituitary hormones are vasopressin and oxytocin. This chapter covers specific agents affecting the pituitary.

Of the above-mentioned hormones, gonadotropin-releasing hormone (gonadorelin) is discussed in Chapter 52 and thyrotropin-releasing hormone (TRH) and corticotropic-releasing hormone (CRH) are discussed in Chapters 48 and 49, respectively. While a true hormone with prolactin-inhibiting effects has not been identified, the substance is believed to be dopamine. Bromocriptine, a drug with dopamine-agonist properties, is reviewed in Chapters 23 and 53.

Of the remaining two substances, the **growth hormone-releasing hormone (GHRH)** has been identified in vivo but is still under investigation. This substance has been found to stimulate the release of growth hormone after intranasal application. It is currently listed as an orphan drug, manufactured by Fujisawa. Information on orphan drug availability may be obtained from the Office of Orphan Products Development (HF-35), 5600 Fishers Lane, Rockville, MD 20857 (Olin, 1996).

The **growth hormone-inhibiting hormone (somatostatin)** was obtained from human cadaver pituitaries, but its distribution in the United States was stopped in 1985. Creutzfeldt-Jakob disease (a neurotropic virus), which is very rare in young people, was diagnosed in some clients and resulted in the death of several persons 5 to 7 years after receiving this product. Several biosynthetic hormones grown through recombinant DNA technology are available in the United States. Growth hormone preparations include somatrem and somatropin while octreotide is used to inhibit the release of growth hormone.

ANTERIOR PITUITARY HORMONES

▲ **somatrem** [soe' ma trem] (Protropin)
Somatrem contains the identical sequence of the pituitary-derived human growth hormone plus one additional amino acid, methionine. In tests it has been demonstrated to be therapeutically equivalent to somatropin, the pituitary human growth hormone.

As a mechanism of action, somatrem's anabolic effects are due to indirect effect of other hormones, known as somatomedin-C or insulin-like growth factors (IGFs) (Ascoli & Segaloff, 1996). IGF-1 is directly responsible for skeletal and soft tissue growth and it also increases cell numbers in the body rather than cell size. Therefore a major pharmacologic consequence of somatrem use is an increase in longitudinal growth, whereas a deficiency in growth hormone usually results in **dwarfism**.

Somatrem also has metabolic effects—it decreases insulin sensitivity and may also affect glucose transport; it increases lipolysis; it promotes cellular growth by retaining phosphorus, sodium, and potassium and enhances protein synthesis by increased nitrogen retention.

Somatrem is indicated for the treatment of growth failure in children caused by a pituitary growth hormone deficiency. It is sometimes abused by athletes seeking increased size and strength (Box 47-1).

BOX 47-1

Growth Hormone Abuse

Some athletes are using growth hormone to either increase their size and strength or their ultimate height, depending on the age of the user. Although the effects of short-term usage are difficult to predict, they are at risk for the adverse effects of the drug—acromegalic syndrome, with symptoms such as increased size of facial bones, thickened hands and fingers, osteoporosis, long-term cardiac failure, diabetes, impotence, and amenorrhea. In addition, because the drug is injectable there is the added risks of hepatitis and AIDS as the result of shared needles and syringes.

Under an amendment to the Food, Drug, and Cosmetic Act, "whoever knowingly distributes, or possesses, human growth hormone for any use in humans other than the treatment of disease or other recognized medical condition, or such use as has been authorized by the Secretary of Health and Human Services under Section 505 and pursuant to the order of a physician, is guilty of an offense punishable by not more than 5 years in prison, such fines as are authorized by Title 18, United States Code, or both." This legislation clearly defines growth hormone distribution as a serious federal offense, and federal authorities are authorized to investigate these practices.

Fortunately, the abuse of growth hormone is limited by its cost and the fact that anabolic steroids are simply more enticing to the athlete. However, there are adverse effects with which many athletes are unfamiliar and education of the potential consequences of growth hormone excess is important in counseling athletes considering its use.

From Haupt, 1993.

While the half-life of parenteral (IV) somatrem is 20 to 30 minutes (IM and SC is 3 to 5 hours), duration of action is 12 to 48 hours, and it is metabolized in the liver and excreted by the kidneys.

Antibodies to somatrem have been reported in 30% to 40% of treated clients during the first 3 to 6 months of therapy, but only 5% of the clients develop neutralizing antibodies. It is rare that a client does not respond to therapy. However, pain and edema have been reported at the site of injection and, rarely, an allergic type reaction (rash, itching). Excessive doses may produce **gigantism,** an abnormal condition characterized by excessive size and stature, in children. So before the drug is used, growth failure must be carefully documented and dosages and individual responses closely monitored. Hypothyroidism has been rarely reported.

When somatrem is given concurrently with adrenocorticoids, glucocorticoids, or corticotropin (ACTH), the growth response effects of somatrem may be impaired. ACTH should not be given concurrently, and if it is necessary to treat with an adrenocorticoid agent, the daily dosages should be limited. For example, the total daily dose per square meter of body area should not be greater than the following: cortisone (12.5 to 18.8 mg); hydrocortisone (10 to 15 mg); methylprednisolone (2 to 3 mg); prednisone or prednisolone (2.5 to 3.75 mg); betamethasone (300 to 450 μg) and dexamethasone (250 to 500 μg).

The dosage and administration of somatrem for injection (Protropin) for children, is up to 0.1 mg/kg IM or SC (preferred) three times weekly. Monitor growth rate response in 3 to 6 months to determine if dosage adjustment is necessary. Therapy is usually continued until epiphyseal closure occurs or there is no further response. If therapy is unsuccessful (<2 cm per year), the treatment should be discontinued and the child reevaluated (Olin, 1996; *USP DI,* 1996).

■ Nursing Management

Somatrem Therapy

Assessment. It should be ascertained that the client does not have a malignancy, especially an intracranial tumor. Somatrem is also contraindicated in clients with closed epiphyses or those with a known sensitivity to benzyl alcohol such as neonates. Use with caution in clients with untreated hypothyroidism because the growth response will be adversely affected.

Review the client's current medication regimen to ensure the client is not receiving adrenocorticoids, glucocorticoid, or corticotropin, which inhibit the growth response to somatrem.

Nursing diagnosis. The client receiving somatrem therapy has the potential for the following nursing diagnoses/collaborative problems: altered growth and development related to underlying lack of endogenous growth hormone secretion and ineffective response to drug, impaired tissue integrity (pain and swelling at injection site), and the potential complications of allergic reaction (rash), slipped capital femoral epiphysis (limp, pain in hip or knee), and hypothyroidism.

Implementation

Monitoring. Obtain baseline data from bone age determinations, thyroid function studies, and anti-growth hormone antibody. Monitor these data periodically during therapy. If growth rate does not exceed its pretreatment rate by 2 cm per year, the client should be monitored for noncompliance or other factors such as antibody formation, hypothyroidism, or malnutrition. After several months of therapy, antibodies to somatrem may be formed in some clients. These rarely reduce the response to therapy.

Observe the injection site; pain and swelling has occurred at the site of injection.

Monitor for signs of hypothyroidism such as lethargy, intolerance to cold, weight gain, dry skin, and brittle, lackluster hair, which have been reported in less than 5% of clients with hypopituitarism receiving somatrem therapy.

Intervention. Prepare the drug for parenteral use by diluting with 1 to 5 ml of bacteriostatic water for injection. Do not shake the vial; rotate it gently between the palms of the hands until the solution is clear. Cloudy solution should not be used. Store in the refrigerator.

Education. Advise the client of the importance of regular visits to the pediatric endocrinologist for the monitoring of blood and urine studies, thyroid function studies, and growth rate and bone age determinations.

Evaluation. Increases in the growth pattern should occur by which to evaluate the efficacy of the therapy, minimally 2.5 cm in 6 months. Therapy is usually continued as long as the client is responsive, until a mature adult stature is reached or the client's epiphyses close.

somatropin, recombinant [soe ma troe' pin] (Humatrope)

Somatropin is a DNA recombinant product that is identical to the amino acid sequence of human growth hormone. It is used to stimulate linear growth in clients who lack sufficient endogenous growth hormone, thus resulting in increased skeletal growth (an increased length of the epiphyseal plates of long bones reported). The number and size of muscle cells, organs, and red cell mass are also increased. An increase in cellular protein synthesis and lipid mobilization resulting in a decrease in body fat stores is also reported.

The mechanism of action, indications, and other properties of somatropin are similar to somatrem. The recommended dosage is individualized up to 0.06 mg/kg SC or IM three times weekly (Olin, 1996).

For nursing management, see the discussion of somatrem.

octreotide [ok tree' oh tide] (Sandostatin)

Octreotide is a long acting agent with an effect similar to somatostatin, the growth hormone-inhibiting hormone, although it is a more potent inhibitor of growth hormone, glucagon, and insulin (Olin, 1996). It is indicated to lower blood levels of growth hormone and IGF-1 to normal in persons with acromegaly that are unable or have not responded to other therapies, such as surgery, radiation, and bromocriptine. It is also used to treat the symptoms associated with carcinoid tumors, such as flushing and severe diarrhea. It also has many unapproved uses, including the treatment of AIDS-associated diarrhea. See a current reference for additional indications, approved and unapproved.

It is rapidly absorbed after SC injection, reaching a peak serum concentration in about 25 minutes with a half-life of 1.7 hours. Its duration of action is variable but depending on the tumor can be up to 12 hours. The IV and SC doses of octreotide are considered equivalent in effect.

The side/adverse effects of octreotide include pain, swelling, and pruritus at the injection site; sinus bradycardia in acromegalics; diarrhea, stomach distress in acromegalics (30% to 58%) and other disorders (5% to 10%); headache, arrhythmias, and cold-like symptoms. Hyperglycemia, hypoglycemia, and hypothyroidism are also reported primarily in acromegalics. Check a current reference for list of other potential side/adverse effects.

Dose in acromegaly is 50 µg three times a day, SC or IV, adjusted according to client's response and the presence of side/adverse effects.

■ Nursing Management

Octreotide Therapy

Assessment. It should be determined that the client does not have a history of or active gallbladder disease or gallstones because there is an increased risk of cholelithiasis because of the decrease gallbladder motility and alteration of fat absorption with the administration of octreotide. A baseline and periodic ultrasonograms may be necessary to assess the presence of gallstones.

Review the client's current medication regimen for oral antidiabetic agents, insulin, glucagon, or growth hormone because the use of these medications in combination with octreotide may result in hypoglycemia or hyperglycemia. Baseline determination of blood glucose concentrations is recommended.

A detailed assessment of the condition for which the octreotide is administered should be recorded before therapy is begun.

Nursing diagnosis. The client receiving octreotide has the potential for the following nursing diagnoses/collaborative problems: altered comfort (abdominal cramping, headache, flushing of face, nausea and vomiting); impaired tissue integrity (pain and redness at injection site); diarrhea; fatigue; and the potential complications of hypoglycemia or hyperglycemia.

Implementation

Monitoring. Monitor blood glucose determinations, particularly during dosage changes in the medication regimen. Observe the client for hypoglycemia (anxiety; cool, pale skin; headache; hunger; nausea; difficulty in concentration; nervousness; shakiness; weakness; unconsciousness) and hyperglycemia (drowsiness; red, dry skin; anorexia; acetone-like breath; thirst; nausea and vomiting; rapid weight loss; lethargy; unconsciousness).

Intervention. Octreotide is administered subcutaneously with the hip, thigh, and abdomen being the preferred sites. Administer octreotide slowly at room temperature and rotate injection sites to prevent tissue irritation. To minimize gastrointestinal symptoms of ocetreotide, administer between meals and at bedtime.

Education. Counsel the client on the importance of close monitoring by the prescriber. Instruct the client to rotate and select injection sites and to report any signs of irritation at injection sites or symptoms of hyperglycemia or hypoglycemia.

Evaluation. If the client is receiving octreotide as an antidiarrheal for gastrointestinal tumors or AIDS, the client will experience fewer, firmer stools or a normal bowel elimination pattern for that client. If octreotide is administered for a pituitary tumor, there will be a reduction in secretion of the growth hormone evidenced by suppressed tumor growth and a decrease in the client's symptoms of acromegaly.

POSTERIOR PITUITARY HORMONES

The posterior pituitary gland hormones are oxytocin and vasopressin (ADH, or antidiuretic hormone). Oxytocin is discussed in Chapter 53 with the drugs related to labor and delivery. Vasopressin is obtained from natural sources while lypressin and desmopressin are synthetic derivatives of vasopressin. Desmopressin has a longer duration of activity than the other agents.

▲ **vasopressin** [vay soe press' in]) (Pitressin)
desmopressin [des moe press' in] (DDAVP, Stimate)
lypressin [lye press' in] (Diapid)

The antidiuretic hormone effect is the result of increasing water reabsorption in the collecting ducts of the nephron, resulting in a decreased urine volume with a higher osmolarity. At higher than physiologic dosages, vasopressin stimulates peristalsis through a direct effect on gastrointestinal motility, increases secretion of corticotropin, growth hormone, and follicle-stimulating hormone (FSH), and may increase blood pressure secondary to a vasoconstriction effect.

Vasopressin (Pitressin) is used to treat **diabetes insipidus,** a metabolic disorder characterized by extreme polyuria and polydipsia caused by the deficient production or secretion of the antidiuretic hormone centrally. It is not effective for polyuria induced by renal impairment, nephrogenic diabetes insipidus, psychogenic diabetes insipidus, or drug-induced (lithium or demeclocycline) diabetes insipidus.

The synthetic formulations (desmopressin [DDAVP], lypressin [Diapid]) act as ADH with little vasopressor activity. Lypressin is used to treat persons that are either nonresponsive or unable to tolerate other interventions. Desmopressin intranasal is used for primary nocturnal enuresis. The oral, intranasal, and parenteral dosage forms are used to treat central diabetes insipidus, while only the parenteral dosage form of desmopressin is used for hemostasis in hemophilia A and von Willebrand's disease clients.

Vasopressin administered intramuscularly or subcutaneously has a half-life of 10 to 20 minutes; the duration of effect is 2 to 8 hours. It is metabolized in the liver and kidneys and excreted by the kidneys.

Lypressin nasal spray has an immediate onset of antidiuretic activity; peaks in 1/2 to 1 1/2 hours and has a duration of action between 3 to 8 hours. Desmopressin nasal has a half-life of approximately 3.5 hours and peak serum concentration is reached in 40 to 45 minutes; oral and intranasal dosage forms reach peak serum level in 1 to 1 1/2 hours. The onset of antidiuretic effects with the tablets is within 1 hour while the maximum effect is reached between 4 to 7 hours.

Table 47-1 lists the side effects/adverse reactions for these agents. No significant drug interactions have been reported.

The adult dosage of aqueous vasopressin injection (Pitressin) is 5 to 10 units intramuscularly or subcutaneously two or three times a day when needed to treat central diabetes insipidus. In children the dosage for treatment of central diabetes insipidus is 2.5 to 10 units three or four times daily.

The adult lypressin nasal spray dose is 1 or 2 sprays to one or both nostrils when urination frequency increases or a significant thirst sensation occurs. The usual pediatric and adult dose is 1 or 2 sprays in each nostril 4 times a day.

For children 6 years and older and adults, the desmopressin intranasal dose for primary nocturnal enuresis is 10 μg (0.2 ml) intranasal at bedtime, adjusted as necessary. The central diabetes insipidus adult dose is 0.1 to 0.4 mg daily as a single dose or in divided doses. Parenteral dose is 0.5 to 1 ml SC or IV daily in two divided doses. Oral adult dose starts with 0.05 mg twice daily and is adjusted according to response.

■ Nursing Management

Antidiuretic Hormone Therapy

Assessment. Use vasopressin with caution in clients with inadequate coronary circulation because it may precipitate anginal pain and myocardial infarction, and in clients with hypertension because the drug may increase blood pressure. Use with caution in elderly clients because of the risk of water intoxication and hyponatremia. Its use should be avoided if at all possible in clients with chronic nephritis with nitrogen retention. Obtain a baseline ECG and fluid and electrolyte status determinations.

Lypressin and desmopressin have fewer pressor effects than vasopressin so cardiovascular precautions are not as great. However, clients with allergic rhinitis, nasal congestion, or upper respiratory infection may experience less efficacy because of a decrease in the absorption in the nasal dosage of these drugs.

Nursing diagnosis. The client receiving antidiuretic agents has the potential for the following nursing diagnoses: fluid volume excess related to water intoxication (confusion, drowsiness, increasing headache, weight gain, seizures); altered tissue integrity at injection site (pain); ineffective airway clearance with nasal dosage forms (runny or stuffy nose); altered comfort (abdominal cramping); and the potential complications of altered cardiac output related to increased fluid volume and the drug's vasopressor effect; and the potential complications of angina and myocardial infarction (chest pain, shortness of breath).

Implementation

Monitoring. Obtain fluid and electrolyte determinations periodically during therapy. Monitor the specific gravity of the client's urine, as well as the intake and output and daily weights, to evaluate the drug's effectiveness. Monitor blood pressure; hypertension may occur, or in the case of nonresponse to the drug, hypotension. If desmopressin is used with clients with hemophilia A or Willebrand's disease, then Factor VIII coagulant concentrations and other bleeding factors should be monitored.

TABLE 47-1 Posterior pituitary hormones: side/adverse effects

Drug	Side effects*	Adverse reactions†
desmopressin (DDAVP, Stimate)	Less frequent: headache, nausea, mild stomach cramps, vulval pain. Injection: local redness, burning or swelling, facial flush, slight increase or decrease blood pressure.	Rare: severe allergic reaction including anaphylaxis with parenteral.
lypressin (Diapid)	Less frequent: abdominal distress, headache, heartburn, eye pain, nasal irritation or itching, runny nose, increase in bowel movements.	Rare: continuous coughing, chest pain, shortness of breath, difficult breathing.
vasopressin (Pitressin)	Less frequent: abdominal distress, gas, sweating, nausea, vomiting, tremors, increased pressure for bowel evacuation, headache.	Rare: chest pain due to angina or myocardial infarction; allergic reaction; increased or continuing headaches, confusion, coma, convulsions, weight gain, drowsiness, urinary difficulties (usually the result of water retention or intoxication).

*If side effects continue, increase, or disturb the client, inform the prescriber.
†If adverse reactions occur, contact the prescriber because medical intervention may be necessary.

Be alert for early signs of water toxicity such as confusion, headache, drowsiness, weight gain, and seizures. Withdraw the drug and restrict fluid intake until specific gravity of urine is at least 1.015 and polyuria occurs. Notify the prescriber immediately.

Intervention. Vasopressin may be administered intramuscularly, subcutaneously, intravenously, or intraarterially. To allow for a precise intravenous or intraarterial flow rate, administer the vasopressin aqueous injection by an infusion pump. Avoid extravasation because tissue necrosis and gangrene may result.

Lypressin is administered intranasally; it is not to be inhaled. If lypressin is not effective with 3 sprays, it is recommended that the frequency of administration be increased, rather than the number of sprays per dose.

Desmopressin is administered in a parenteral form for IV or SC use and an intranasal dosage to be administered as a spray or through a flexible catheter known as a rhinyle.

Education. Alert the client to the importance of taking the medication as prescribed and to maintain supervision by the prescriber. Instruct the client to hold the medication and report symptoms of water intoxication, such as weight gain, headache, confusion, and drowsiness. Fluid intake may need to be adjusted to decrease the risk for water intoxication, particularly in pediatric and geriatric clients.

With lypressin, whenever the frequency of urination increases, the client may administer 1 to 2 sprays. If the daily dosage does not control the client's nocturia, an additional dose may be taken at bedtime.

Desmopressin dosage is adjusted to the diurnal pattern of response with morning and evening doses being adjusted separately. The initial goal is to control nocturia.

Evaluation. If antidiuretic agents are administered for diabetes insipidus, the client will experience a decreased urinary output and the client's urinalysis will evidence an increased osmolality and specific gravity. If desmopressin is administered for bleeding disorders, hemostasis will be maintained.

SUMMARY

Drugs affecting the pituitary are generally used as replacement therapy for hormone deficiency, drug therapy for a specific disorder, or diagnostic aids to diagnose hypofunctional or hyperfunctional hormone states. Somatrem is therapeutically equivalent to somatropin, or the human growth hormone from the anterior pituitary, and is used for the treatment of growth failure in children caused by a deficiency of that hormone. Octreotide is used as a growth-hormone–inhibiting agent. The two posterior pituitary hormones are oxytocin and vasopressin. Oxytocin is discussed in the chapter on labor and delivery. Vasopressin and the other antidiuretic agents, lypressin and desmopressin, are used for the treatment of diabetes insipidus, which results from a deficiency of ADH. The pituitary gland serves a major role in the regulation of the endocrine system.

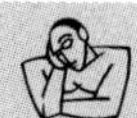

Critical Thinking

1. Timmy Johnson is receiving somatrem to enhance his growth process. In the last 6 months he has grown 3 cm; would you consider the drug to be effective? His current x-ray indicates epiphyseal closure. What impact will this have on his therapy?
2. Your client, Polly Jones, has been receiving vasopressin for her diabetes insipidus. Now she is disoriented, irritable, and short of breath. On assessment, her vital signs are stable: BP 124/70, pulse 82, respirations 24, and temperature 96.8° F (36° C). Her laboratory results are as follows:

Client	Normal values
sodium, 116 mEq/L	135-145 mEq/L
chloride, 86 mEq/L	100-108 mEq/L
potassium, 3.6 mEq/L	3.5-5.0 mEq/L
blood urea nitrogen, 10 mg/d	8-20 mg/dl
serum creatinine, 1 mg/dl	0.5-1.1 mg/dl for women
serum osmolality, 243 mOsm/kg H_2O	275-295 mOsm/kg H_2O
urine osmolality 1.541 mOsm/kg H_2O	300-1000 mOsm/kg H_2O
urine sodium, 320 mEq/24 hr	130-280 mEq/24 hr
urine specific gravity, 1.04	1.025-1.032

What is happening to Ms. Jones? How should the nurse intervene?

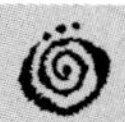

Collaborative Learning Activities

1. Role play a conference between a nurse, a parent whose child is about to start a course of somatrem therapy, and the child, who is small in stature for his age. What client education is essential in this first interview? What questions might the parent have? What questions might the boy have?

BIBLIOGRAPHY

Ascoli M & Segaloff DL (1996). Adenohypophyseal hormones and their hypothalamic releasing factors. In Hardman JG & Limbird LE (Eds.). *Goodman & Gilman's the pharmacological basis of therapeutics* (9th ed.). New York: McGraw-Hill.

American Hospital Formulary Service (1996). *AHFS drug information '96.* Bethesda, MD: American Society of Hospital Pharmacists.

Anderson KN, et al. (Eds.) (1994). *Mosby's medical, nursing, & allied health dictionary* (4th ed.). St. Louis: Mosby.

Batcheller J (1992). Disorders of antidiuretic hormone secretion, *AACN* 3(2):370.

Blevins LS Jr & Wand GS (1992). Diabetes insipidus, *Crit Care Med* 20(1):669-79.

Haupt HA (1993). Anabolic steroids and growth hormone, *AM J Sports Med* 21(3):468.

Jaffe CA & Barkan AL (1994). Acromegaly: recognition and treatment, *Drugs* 47(3):425-45.

Olin BR (Ed.) (1996). *Facts and comparisons.* St Louis: Facts and Comparisons.

United States Pharmacopeial Convention. (1996). *USP DI: Drug information for the health care professional* (16th ed.). Rockville, MD: The Convention.

Chapter 48

Drugs Affecting the Parathyroid and Thyroid

Chapter Focus

Disorders of the thyroid and parathyroid have far-reaching effects because as part of the endocrine system they influence growth and development, metabolic rate, energy level, and reproductive systems. The nurse needs to be knowledgeable about the various preparations of drugs that affect the parathyroid and thyroid system in order to provide direct care to clients, as well as client education for the safe and accurate self-management of the therapeutic regimen. The following objectives and key terms are important for a good understanding of this chapter.

Key Terms

iodine (p. 776)
myxedema (p. 772)
primary hyperparathyroidism (p. 770)

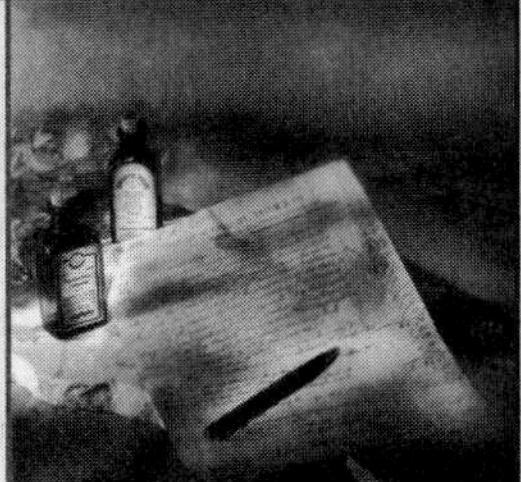

Key Drugs [▲]

propylthiouracil
thyroid

Objectives

1. Describe the clinical complications associated with hypothyroidism, hyperthyroidism, hypoparathyroidism, and hyperparathyroidism.
2. Describe the dose and action of calcium and vitamin D products in the treatment of hypoparathyroidism.
3. Describe the primary therapy and the agents available to treat hypothyroidism.
4. Name two diagnostic agents used to assess thyroid function.
5. Describe the actions of iodine (iodide ion), radioactive iodine, and thioamide drugs in treating hyperthyroidism.
6. Implement nursing management of clients receiving drugs affecting the parathyroid or thyroid gland.

A variety of medications are available to treat the various conditions of the thyroid and parathyroid glands.

PARATHYROID

In idiopathic hypoparathyroidism, serum calcium levels are decreased while serum phosphate levels are increased. Usually vitamin D levels are low. The administration of vitamin D and calcium supplements usually will restore the calcium and phosphorus levels to normal (Box 48-1). Calcitriol (Rocaltrol) is an active metabolite form of vitamin D that is also used to elevate serum calcium levels. Table 48-1 lists drugs used to treat hypocalcemia.

Primary hyperparathyroidism is a hyperactivity of the parathyroid glands with excessive secretion of parathyroid hormone that results in increased resorption of calcium from the skeletal system and increased absorption of calcium by the kidneys and the gastrointestinal system. The urine phosphate is high (serum level is low to normal), which can lead to renal stones, bone pain with skeletal lesions, and possibly pathologic fractures. Since adenomas or tumors may cause this syndrome, surgery is usually the primary treatment. In clients with mild hypercalcemia or mild hyperparathyroidism, a thorough examination by a physician determines whether or not surgery is indicated. High serum levels of calcium may require immediate treatment. Table 48-2 describes typical recommendations for treatment of hypercalcemia.

Calcitonin and other synthetic drugs are used to treat hypercalcemia, osteoporosis, and Paget's disease. Two calcitonin products are available, salmon calcitonin (Calcimar) and human calcitonin (Cibacalcin), and both products produce the same effect although the salmon calcitonin has a slightly longer half-life (70 to 90 minutes versus 60 minutes).

Calcitonin is indicated for the treatment of hypercalcemia (parenteral), Paget's disease (parenteral), and postmenopausal osteoporosis (nasal and parenteral) (Olin, 1996).

The side/adverse effects (nasal spray; Miacalcin) include rhinitis, nasal irritation and redness, muscle and back pain, epistaxis, and headache; the parenteral dosage form may cause flushing or a tingling sensation of the face, ears, hands and feet; gastric distress, anorexia, nausea, vomiting, and pain or swelling at the injection site.

The usual salmon calcitonin adult dose for Paget's disease is 100 IU daily, decreasing to 50 IU daily, every other day and then three times weekly. For hypercalcemia, see Table 48-2.

TABLE 48-1 Hypocalcemia treatment

Drug	Usual adult dose
calcium gluconate	IV: 970 mg given slowly at rate not exceeding 5 ml (47.5 mg) per minute
Vitamin D analogs	
calcifediol (Calderol)	Oral: 50 μg daily per week; adjust dose monthly if necessary
calcitriol (Rocaltrol)	Oral: 0.25 μg daily, increased every 2 to 4 weeks if necessary IV: 0.5 μg three times a week, increased every 2 to 4 weeks if necessary
dihydrotachysterol (Hytakerol)	Oral: 0.125 to 2 mg daily
ergocalciferol (Calciferol)	Oral: individualized dosing; prophylaxis dose is 5 to 10 μg daily

BOX 48-1

Calcium Supplements

The activity of calcium depends on calcium ion (elemental) content. The following calcium salts are listed by milligrams per gram, milliequivalents per gram, and percent of calcium in the preparations.

Preparation	Calcium mg/g	Calcium mEq/g	Percent of calcium
calcium carbonate	400	20.0	40
calcium chloride	272	13.6	27.2
calcium citrate	211	10.5	21.1
calcium gluceptate	82	4.1	8.2
calcium gluconate	90	4.5	9
calcium lactate	130	6.5	13
calcium phosphate			
dibasic	230	11.5	23
tribasic	400	20	38

When low-percentage preparations are used, larger quantities of the drug are necessary to provide adequate calcium supplementation. For example, if the prescriber desired 1 g of elemental calcium from either calcium carbonate or calcium lactate preparations, it would require 2.5 g of calcium carbonate or nearly 7 g of calcium lactate to provide the calcium ordered. Other considerations would indicate client acceptance—taste, tolerance, side effects, and other factors.

Bisphosphonates

Alendronate (Fosamax), etidronate (Didronel), and pamidronate (Aredia) are bisphosphonates that act by inhibiting normal and abnormal resorption of bone. In addition, etidronate reduces bone formation while alendronate and pamidronate inhibit bone resorption without inhibiting bone formation.

Their action is postulated to be due to binding to hydroxyapatite in bone, decreasing dissolution of mineral bone content or their effect on bone resorbing cells. They are indicated for treatment of Paget's disease and hypercalcemia, and alendronate also is used for osteoporosis in postmenopausal women.

The side/adverse effects with alendronate include gas, acid regurgitation, esophageal ulcer, gastritis, dysphagia, muscleskeletal pain, headaches, and seizures; with etidronate nausea, diarrhea, metallic taste, and rarely, hypersensitivity; with pamidronate, fever, nausea, vomiting, anorexia, leukopenia, psychosis, hypokalemia, hypomagnesemia, and uremia (Olin, 1996).

TABLE 48-2 Hypercalcemia: treatment recommendations

Increase calcium excretion	
saline diuresis	Infuse normal saline (100 to 200 ml/hr) to increase calcium excretion. Monitor fluid intake, output, and electrolytes. Watch closely for evidence of fluid overload.
furosemide (Lasix)	Often used with the administration of normal saline as above. Usual dose is 20 to 40 mg IV bid to qid.
Inhibit bone resorption	
calcitonin-salmon (Calcimar)	IM or SC: 4 to 8 IU/kg every 6 to 12 hours. Tolerance can develop in 24 to 72 hours; therefore corticosteroids may be prescribed concurrently.
etidronate (Didronel)	IV infusion: 7.5 mg/kg in 250 ml normal saline, administered over 2 hours daily until calcium level is normal or for a maximum of 1 week.
pamidronate (Aredia)	IV infusion: 60-90 mg in liter of normal saline infused over 24 hours. The advantage of this product is that it is effective in a single dose.
plicamycin (Mithramycin)	More toxic than other agents. Reserve for individuals that do not respond to other therapies. Usual dose is 25 µg/kg in 500 ml dextrose in water administered IV over 4 to 60 hours.

(Tang & Lau, 1995; Woodley & Whelan, 1992)

The usual adult dose for Paget's disease for alendronate is 40 mg daily for 6 months; for etidronate, 5 mg/kg PO daily for 6 months or 7.5 mg/kg by IV infusion daily for 3 consecutive days; and pamidronate, 30 mg/day on 3 consecutive days by IV infusion up to 30 mg weekly for 6 weeks (90 to 180 mg total dose per treatment) given at a rate of 15 mg/hour. For other dosages, see a current reference. For treatment of hypercalcemia, see Table 48-2.

■ Nursing Management

Bisphosphonate Therapy

Assessment. Bisphosphonate therapy is contraindicated in clients with renal insufficiency and women who are pregnant or lactating. Clients with preexisting hypocalcemia or vitamin D deficiency should have these conditions corrected before bisphosphonate therapy begins.

Review the client's current drug regimen for potential drug interactions, such as would occur with calcium supplements and antacids, which decrease the absorption of the bisphosphonates.

A baseline assessment of the client with osteoporosis should include bone studies to determine bone mass and serum calcium levels. Clients with Paget's disease require documentation of their symptoms (bone pain, headache, skull size) and serum alkaline phosphatase before beginning therapy. With etidronate, assess for bone pain, weakness, and loss of function.

Nursing diagnosis. Clients receiving bisphosphonate therapy may experience the following nursing diagnoses/collaborative problems: risk for injury related to the preexisting condition and the ineffectiveness of therapy; altered comfort (headache, abdominal discomfort, nausea, heartburn, musculoskeletal pain); altered bowel elimination (diarrhea or constipation); impaired skin integrity (rash, erythema); and the potential complications of hypercalcemia (nausea, vomiting, anorexia, weakness, constipation, thirst, cardiac arrhythmias); hypocalcemia (paresthesia, muscle twitching, colic, cardiac arrhythmias); and gastritis or esophageal ulceration.

Implementation

Monitoring. Bone scans for bone density and serum calcium determinations should be done periodically for those clients being treated for osteoporosis. Clients with Paget's disease require alkaline phosphatase determinations periodically.

Intervention. Administer the drug first thing in the morning with 8 oz of water 30 minutes before meals or other medications. Have the client sit upright for 30 minutes after ingesting the drug to minimize esophageal irritation.

Education. Instruct the client to take the drug as above. Beverages other than water will decrease the absorption of the drug. Encourage the client to engage in supportive lifestyle changes, such as smoking cessation, reduction of alcohol intake, participation in regular exercise with weight-bearing on the long bones such as walking. Consult with the prescriber about calcium and vitamin D supplementation.

Evaluation. The client will experience a decrease in the progression of the osteoporosis or Paget's disease. Serum calcium determinations will be within the normal limits for age.

THYROID

Thyroid Preparations

Individuals with hypothyroidism require thyroid replacement therapy. For many years, natural or desiccated thyroid was used for replacement therapy but the synthetic thyroids available today are more standardized and stable formulations and so are generally prescribed. Thyroid USP is derived mainly from hog thyroid glands, although cattle and sheep thyroid glands have also been used.

The thyroid produces two iodine-containing active hormones, thyroxine (T_4) and triiodothyronine (T_3), which are essential for human growth and development and also maintain metabolic homeostasis. These hormones have been synthesized and are available as liothyronine (for T_3), levothyroxine (for T_4), and liotrix (both T_3 and T_4). See Chapter 46 for further information on the functioning of the thyroid gland. Table 48-3 illustrates equivalent and usual adult dose of thyroid products.

The goal of treatment of clients with hypothyroidism or **myxedema** (adult hypothyroidism) is to eliminate their

TABLE 48-3 Thyroid preparations: equivalent and usual adult dose

Drug	Equivalent dose	Usual adult dose
levothyroxine (Synthroid)	100 μg (0.1 mg)	Orally: 12.5 to 50 μg daily (geriatric or those with cardiovascular disease, dose range is 12.5 to 25 μg daily), adjusting dose every 2 to 3 weeks as necessary. Injection: 50 to 100 μg IM or IV daily. For myxedema, stupor, or coma, the dose is 200 to 500 μg IV initially, even in geriatric clients. If improvement is not noted by the second day, additional 100 to 200 μg (0.1 to 0.3 mg) may be given. Switch to oral dose form as soon as possible.
liothyronine (Cytomel)	25 μg (0.025 mg)	Orally: 25 to 50 μg daily, adjusting dose every 1 to 2 weeks as needed. For myxedema and simple, nontoxic goiter, dose is 2.5 to 5 μg daily (increasing at 5 to 10 μg increments every 7 to 14 days) as necessary. Maintenance myxedema dose is 25 to 50 μg/day; for simple goiter, it is 50 to100 μg/daily.
liotrix (Thyrolar)	50 to 60 μg of levothyroxine and 12.5 to 15 μg liothyronine	Orally: myxedema, 50 to 60 μg of levothyroxine and 12.5 to 15 μg of liothyronine daily; increase monthly if necessary. Geriatric dose is 25% to 50% of the usual adult dose, adjusted as necessary at 6 to 8 week intervals.
▲ thyroid	60 mg	Orally: 60 to 120 mg daily. For myxedema or hypothyroidism with cardiovascular disease, initial dose is 15 mg daily, increased as necessary every 2 weeks. Geriatric: 7.5 to 15 mg daily, doubled every 6 to 8 weeks if necessary

Pregnancy safety for all thyroid products has been established at FDA category A.

BOX 48-2

Hyperthyroidism vs. Hypothyroidism: Clinical Features

	Hyperthyroidism	Hypothyroidism
Eyes	Prominent	Eyelids edematous, ptosis
Hair	Thin, fine texture	Dry, brittle, thin
Temperature	Intolerance to heat	Intolerance to cold
Weight	Appetite increases, weight loss	Appetite decreases, weight gain
Emotional	Increased nervousness, irritability, insomnia	Lethargic, depressed, increase in sleeping needs
Gastrointestinal	Diarrhea	Constipation
Neuromuscular	Fast deep-tendon reflexes	Slow or delayed deep-tendon reflexes
Extremities	Hot, moist skin	Cold, dry skin

symptoms and to restore them to a normal emotional and physical state (Box 48-2 lists clinical features of hyperthyroidism versus hypothyroidism). Clinical response is more important than blood hormone level; however, laboratory assessments of T_3, T_4, serum cholesterol, and TSH levels are used as criteria for adequacy of therapy.

Thyroid hormone concentrations are regulated by the hypothalamic-anterior pituitary and thyroid body feedback mechanism (Box 48-3). Thyroid supplements are indicated for the treatment of hypothyroidism, treatment and prevention of goiter, treatment and prevention of thyroid carcinoma, and thyroid function diagnostic tests.

Thyroid and levothyroxine are incompletely absorbed from the gastrointestinal tract (50% to 75%), whereas liothyronine is nearly completely absorbed (95%). They are highly protein bound with peak effect in 3 to 4 weeks and duration of action of 1 to 3 weeks for thyroid, thyroglobulin, and levothyroxine after withdrawal of chronic therapy. Liothyronine peaks in 2 to 3 days and has a duration of action of up to 3 days after withdrawal. These agents are metabolized the same as endogenous thyroid hormone, some in peripheral tissues, smaller amounts in the liver and excreted in bile.

Side effects are dose related and may occur more rapidly with liothyronine than with the other products mainly because it has a faster onset of action. The general signs of underdosage or hypothyroidism are dysmenorrhea, ataxia, coldness, dry skin, constipation, lethargy, headaches, drowsiness, tiredness, weight gain, and muscle aching. During the early period of treatment, hair loss may occur in children but with chronic therapy, normal hair growth will resume.

A rare adverse reaction is an allergic skin rash. Overdose with thyroid products results in hyperthyroidism—alterations in appetite and menstrual periods, elevated temperature, diarrhea, hand tremors, increased irritability, leg cramps, increased nervousness, tachycardia, irregular heart rate, increased sensitivity to heat, chest pain, respiratory difficulties, increased sweating, vomiting, weight loss, and insomnia.

BOX 48-3

Thyroid Feedback Mechanism

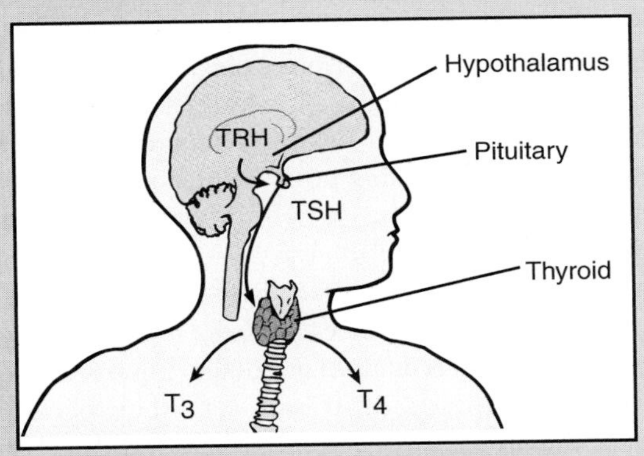

Physiology of influences on the thyroid

When serum levels of T_3 and T_4 are increased, the release of TRH from the hypothalamus and TSH from the anterior pituitary gland is reduced, thus inhibiting their effects on the thyroid gland.

When serum levels of T_3 and T_4 are decreased, TRH release triggers the release of TSH from the pituitary. TSH effects on the thyroid are an increase in the size and number of follicular cells in the thyroid, thus increasing their ability to absorb iodide, and an increase in thyroglobulin breakdown, which releases T_3 and T_4 hormones from the thyroid gland into the bloodstream, thus increasing blood levels of the thyroid hormones.

▪ Nursing Management

Thyroid Preparation Therapy

Assessment. Use with care in elderly clients, because they are more sensitive to the effects of thyroid hormones. A 25% reduction in the dose of the thyroid hormone replacement may be required for clients over 60 years of age (see the Geriatric Implications box on p. 774). The use of thyroid hormonal therapy is carefully considered if the client has preexisting adrenocortical or pituitary insufficiency (thyroid hormonal replacement increases the physiologic need for adrenocortical hormone), cardiovascular disease (too rapid thyroid hormonal replacement increases metabolic demand), history of hyperthyroidism, or thyrotoxicosis. In cases of chronic hypothyroidism or myxedema, an increased sensitivity may exist.

Before thyroid hormone preparations are given, the client's drug regimen should be reviewed for significant drug interactions such as those that may occur when they are given with the drugs listed below.

Drug	Possible effect and management
anticoagulants, oral (coumarin or indanedione)	May alter the therapeutic effects of oral anticoagulant. An increase in thyroid hormone may require a decrease in anticoagulant oral dosage. Monitor coagulation time closely using the prothrombin time (PT) test.
cholestyramine (Questran) or colestipol (Colestid)	May bind thyroid hormones, delaying or decreasing their absorption from the gastrointestinal tract. A 4 to 5 hour interval is recommended between administration of these drugs.
sympathomimetics	The effects of one or both medications may be increased. May result in an increased risk of coronary insufficiency if individual has coronary artery disease, or, if a thyroid preparation is given with tricyclic antidepressants, an increase in cardiac arrhythmias may result. Monitor closely, since dosage adjustments may be necessary.

Geriatric Implications

Thyroid hormones

Since the elderly are usually more sensitive to and experience more adverse reactions to thyroid hormones than other age groups, it is recommended that thyroid replacement doses be individualized. In some clients, the dose should be 25% lower than the usual adult dose.

Hypothyroidism, the second most common endocrine disease in the elderly, is often misdiagnosed. Only one third of the geriatric clients exhibit the typical signs and symptoms of cold intolerance and weight gain. Most often the symptoms are nonspecific, such as failing to thrive, stumbling and falling episodes, incontinence, and, if neurologic involvement has occurred, the client may be misdiagnosed as having dementia, depression, or a psychotic episode (*USP DI*, 1996; Rizzolo, 1992).

Laboratory tests for serum T_4 and TSH are used to confirm hypothyroidism.

Levothyroxine (Synthroid, others) is usually the drug of choice for thyroid replacement.

Nursing diagnosis. The client receiving thyroid hormones is at risk for the following complications related to underdosage (hypothyroidism) or overdosage (hyperthyroidism). Selected nursing diagnoses associated with hypothyroidism are fluid volume excess, edema related to retention of fluids secondary to slowed metabolism; activity intolerance related to weakness and fatigue secondary to decreased metabolic rate; altered nutrition, more than body requirements related to decreased need; constipation related to decreased peristalsis; risk for ineffective breathing pattern, hypoventilation related to decreased respiratory drive; and the potential complication of myxedema coma. Selected nursing diagnoses related to hyperthyroidism are these: altered nutrition, less than body requirements related to hypermetabolism; disturbed sleep pattern; anxiety related to sympathetic nervous system stimulation; and the potential complication of thyrotoxic crisis. See the Nursing Care Plan on p. 775 for greater detail.

Implementation

Monitoring. Assess the client for a decrease in the symptoms of hypothyroidism: weight loss, loss of constipation, and increased activity levels, appetite, sense of well-being, and pulse rate should be seen. Laboratory reports should indicate normal T_3, T_4, and TSH levels.

Monitor thyroid function studies before and throughout therapy. Such studies may include free T_4 index determinations, TSH determinations, T_3 or T_4 resin uptake determinations, and total serum T_3 and T_4 determinations. Assess pediatric clients periodically for growth, bone age, and psychomotor development. Monitor baseline apical pulse and blood pressure before and periodically during therapy.

Clients are at risk for altered cardiac output related to the thyroid's cardiovascular effects. If the resting pulse is over 100, hold the dose and notify the prescriber. For clients with preexisting cardiovascular disease, observe closely for cardiac ischemia and tachyarrhythmias.

Intervention. Since clients with hypothyroidism respond rapidly to replacement doses, the client is started on the lowest possible dosage, with increases in the dosage titrated over several weeks in accordance with the client's clinical response and laboratory data until the optimal clinical response is obtained. Once the maintenance dosage has been established, it is taken or given daily, preferably before breakfast.

Levothyroxine is preferred for thyroid replacement therapy. It is recommended that levothyroxine be taken on an empty stomach. In its parenteral form, levothyroxine sodium is reconstituted with sodium chloride injection (without preservative) to a solution of 100 µg (0.1 mg)/ml. It should be reconstituted immediately before use.

Education. Lifelong therapy is a possibility with thyroid hormonal replacement. Counsel the client accordingly. This means regular consultations with the prescriber to monitor effectiveness of the therapy, as well as compliance with the prescribed regimen. To simulate the natural process of the body, the client should take the medication at the same time every day. Morning administration will help to prevent insomnia.

Inform the client that if a dose is missed, it is to be taken as soon as possible. If it is close to the next day's dose, caution the client not to take the dose, since this will have the effect of doubling doses. Contact the prescriber if two or more consecutive doses are missed.

Tell the client to alert other health care providers about the thyroid hormonal replacement, particularly if any kind of surgery is required, including dental surgery. A medical identification should be worn. Advise the client to consult with the prescriber before taking other medications concurrently with thyroid replacement.

Advise the client to inform the prescriber if the pulse rate increases or if palpitations or chest pain occur. Irritability, nervousness, heat intolerance, and excessive sweating may indicate a need for a reduction in dosage; however, insomnia is usually the earliest sign. If such symptoms occur, withdrawal of the drug may be indicated for a few days before it is resumed at a lower dose.

Alert parents of a pediatric client that partial hair loss sometimes occurs during the first few months of therapy with children, but it is temporary and the hair will usually return, even if hormonal replacement is continued.

Advise the client not to change brands of thyroid replacement therapy, since different brands of the same drug are not bioequivalent.

Evaluation. The client is able to be independent in activities of daily living without becoming overtired. The client maintains a euthyroid state.

Diagnostic Testing for Hypothyroidism

Protirelin (Thypinone, Relefact TRH) and thyrotropin (thyroid-stimulating hormone, TSH) are diagnostic agents used to assess thyroid function. The thyroid-stimulating hormone

Nursing Care Plan

Selected Nursing Diagnoses Related to Thyroid Therapy

Nursing diagnosis	Outcome criteria	Nursing interventions
Knowledge deficit related to thyroid dysfunction	Client will: Express understanding of normal thyroid function and the effects of altered thyroid function	Assess client's level of understanding. Determine educational needs of client and family. Instruct client in function of the thyroid gland and thyroid hormones. Instruct client in specific effects related to client's alteration in thyroid function. Provide opportunity for client to ask questions and verbalize concerns.
Knowledge deficit related to drug regimen (thyroid drug)	Client will: Relate the purpose of drug therapy and identify side effects/adverse reactions of the medication	Teach the client: Purpose and action of the drug Proper administration The need for continued therapy throughout lifetime, even after euthyroid state is obtained Signs and symptoms of hypothyroidism and hyperthyroidism Side effects/adverse reactions Provide the client with a list of drugs or conditions that interact with or alter the drug requirements. Explain the benefit of wearing or carrying a medical identification tag, bracelet, or card.
Body image disturbance related to thyroid dysfunction	Client and family will: Express concerns regarding body image changes State the basis for body changes related to thyroid function and identify the benefit of drug therapy	Assess the client and family for perceptions and concerns related to body image. Encourage open communication and talking about perceived body image. Encourage adequate rest periods. Adjust calorie intake and diet to changing client needs. Encourage a high-bulk diet, fluids, and exercise to prevent or limit constipation. Encourage good grooming and attractive dress to promote self-confidence and positive self-image.
Altered nutrition related to altered metabolic needs	Client will: Maintain a stable body weight Show evidence of maintaining a well-balanced diet	Assess normal dietary patterns. Instruct client to monitor his or her weight weekly. Instruct client to adjust diet to match caloric needs. Assist client in planning meals and dietary modifications. Administer thyroid drugs as prescribed.
Risk for impaired skin integrity related to altered thyroid function	Client will: Maintain intact skin Demonstrate proper skin care	Assess skin for dryness, itching, or altered integrity. Monitor client for development of skin disruption. Keep skin clean and well lubricated. Apply moisturizer as needed. Use skin massage and position changes. Instruct client in proper skin care.

(TSH) stimulation test is a very sensitive test used to diagnose hypothyroidism. The thyroid-releasing hormone (TRH) is administered to measure the pituitary's response to TRH. For example, in hypothalamic hypothyroidism, the pituitary responds slowly to exogenous TRH and produces a slow but rising TSH. In clients with primary hypothyroidism, TSH basal levels are increased, and the pituitary is hyperreactive to TRH stimulation. If the client has hypothyroidism resulting from hypopituitarism, no response to TRH is expected. Therefore the TSH stimulation test can differentiate a primary from a secondary hypothyroidism and also differentiate hypopituitary from hypothalamic hypothyroidism. See Box 48-3 for an illustration of this thyroid feedback mechanism.

Antithyroid Agents

An antithyroid drug is a chemical agent that lowers the basal metabolic rate by interfering with the formation, release, or

Case Study

The Client Receiving Thyroid Replacement Therapy

Helen Hanson, a 47-year-old teacher, has been admitted to the hospital for a thyroidectomy. A year before admission she noticed a lump in her neck. When she finally sought treatment, she was given a trial of sodium levothyroxine (Synthroid) 0.1 mg for 2 weeks, then 0.2 mg for 5 weeks. This treatment did not result in any decrease in the size of the nodule. Helen, a thin, active woman, did not note any changes in her weight, skin, or eyes. The only "hyperthyroid" symptoms noted were a heightened sense of "nervousness" and a fine tremor of her hands.

Helen and her health care provider decided on the surgical procedure because of the lack of definitive success with medical treatment and the need to identify the nature of the nodule. Before the surgery, the provider tried a short course of antithyroid medication, propylthiouracil.

1. Initially, why would the provider prescribe a thyroid replacement for Helen if her thyroid is already enlarged?
2. What are some of the key points that Helen needs to know about taking propylthiouracil?
3. What are the normal effects of propylthiouracil, and what side effects should she look for?
4. After surgery Helen will receive thyroid replacement therapy. What will be important to teach her about lifelong replacement therapy?

action of thyroid hormones. Those that interfere with the synthesis of the thyroid hormones are known as goitrogens. A variety of compounds are included in this category of antithyroid drugs, but only iodine (iodide ion), radioactive iodine, and thioamide derivatives are discussed here.

Iodine, Iodides

Iodine, an essential micronutrient, almost 80% of which in the body is in the thyroid gland, is the oldest of the antithyroid drugs. Although a small amount of iodine is necessary for normal thyroid function and to synthesize thyroid hormones, the response of the client with thyrotoxicosis to iodine administration is inhibition of thyroid hormone synthesis and thyroid release from the hyperfunctioning thyroid gland.

Thyroid-Iodide Pump

Iodide from diet is rapidly absorbed into the bloodstream. Approximately one third of it is removed from the blood by the iodide pump in the thyroid. The initial iodide removed from the blood is usually sodium or potassium iodide. The enzyme peroxidase converts the iodides to iodine, which is then used to form monoiodotyrosine (MIT) and diiodotyrosine (DIT), which are the components of T_3 and T_4. The synthesized hormones (T_3, T_4) are stored within thyroglobulin until they are released into the blood circulation. These activities involve a complex negative feedback mechanism between the thyroid gland and the hypothalamus-pituitary gland. Low levels of circulating thyroid hormone increase the release of thyroid-stimulating hormone (TSH) from the pituitary and appear to influence the secretion of thyrotropin-releasing factor (TRF) from the hypothalamus. Increased levels of TSH increase iodide trapping by the gland, which results in an increase in synthesis and circulating thyroid hormones. As thyroid hormone levels increase, the hypothalamic and pituitary centers stop the release of TRF and TSH. This process is repeated if thyroid hormone levels decrease again, in response to the declining levels of circulating thyroid hormones. See Box 48-3.

The inhibition of thyroid hormone release for several weeks leads to an increase in TSH secretion that can overcome this blockade. Thus, large doses of iodides are generally used for 7 to 14 days before thyroid surgery in order to decrease the thyroid's size and vascularity, resulting in diminished blood loss and a less complicated surgical procedure.

Radioactive iodine (RAI) is preferred for clients who are poor surgical risks, such as debilitated clients, those with advanced cardiac disease, and the elderly. It is also used for clients who have not responded adequately to drug therapy or who have had recurrent hyperthyroidism after surgery. The primary disadvantage of using surgery or RAI therapy, in addition to the risk involved with surgery and postsurgical complications, is the induction of hypothyroidism.

Iodine Products

strong iodine solution (Lugol's solution; Thyro-Block)
potassium iodide

Iodine is indicated to protect the thyroid gland from radiation before and after the administration of radioactive isotopes of iodine or in radiation emergencies and may be used with an antithyroid drug in clients with hyperthyroidism in preparation for thyroidectomy. Therapeutic effects may be noted within 24 hours with maximum effects achieved within 10 to 14 days of continuous therapy. Table 48-4 lists side effects/adverse reactions.

Strong iodine solution is a combination of 5% iodine and 10% potassium iodide. The iodine is converted to iodide in the GI tract before systemic absorption. Adult oral dose is 2 to 6 drops three times daily.

Potassium iodide liquid or tablets are also commonly known as KI or SSKI. The adult oral dose is 100 to 150 mg 24 hours before radiation, then daily for 3 to 10 days after-

TABLE 48-4 Antithyroid agents: significant side effects/adverse reactions

Drug(s)	Side effects*	Adverse reactions†
iodine or iodide products	Diarrhea, nausea, vomiting, abdominal pain	Most frequent: skin rash, swelling or tenderness of the salivary gland Rare: bloody or black colored stools (due to GI bleeding), irregular heart rate, paresthesias of hands or feet, increased tiredness, leg weakness, confusion (due to potassium toxicity), increased temperature (hypersensitivity), edema of neck or throat With prolonged usage: severe headaches, sore gums or teeth, increased salivation, burning in mouth or throat, metallic taste in mouth
sodium iodide ^{131}I (Iodotope)	Less frequent: sore throat, neck swelling or pain, loss of taste (temporary), nausea, vomiting, painful salivary glands	After treatment for hyperthyroidism: increased or unusual irritability or tiredness After treatment of thyroid carcinoma: fever, sore throat, and chills (due to leukopenia), increased bleeding episodes (due to thrombocytopenia) Signs of hypothyroidism may follow treatment, including changes in menstrual cycle, increased clumsiness, cold feelings, sedation, dry, puffy skin, headaches, muscle aching, temporary dryness or thinning of hair, increased weakness, and unusual weight gain
thioamide derivatives: methimazole tablets, propylthiouracil tablets	Most frequent (3% to 5%): rash or pruritus Less frequent: dizziness, loss of taste, nausea, vomiting, paresthesias, abdominal pain	Less frequent: elevated temperature, chills or sore throat, overall feelings of discomfort or weakness (may be agranulocytosis, leukopenia, or lupus-like syndrome), jaundice of skin and eyes (due to cholestatic hepatitis) Rare: edema of feet or lower legs, backache, unusual increases or decreases in urination (nephritis), joint pain, swollen lymph nodes, increased bleeding tendencies or bruising Signs of overdosage or hypothyroidism: see above Signs of thyrotoxicosis or subtherapeutic therapy: fever, diarrhea, increased irritability, weakness, tachycardia, vomiting

*If side effects continue, increase, or disturb the patient, inform the prescriber.
†If adverse reactions occur, contact prescriber since medical intervention may be necessary.

ward. Children 1 year and older are given a 130 mg oral dose daily for 10 days after exposure to radioactive iodine.

While unclassified regarding pregnancy safety, potassium iodide does cross the placenta and may produce abnormal thyroid function in infants.

■ Nursing Management

Iodine Product Therapy

Assessment. Iodine products are contraindicated in clients sensitive to them. Initial assessment should determine if the client is allergic to seafood, since this may be indicative of a cross-sensitivity to iodine. Skin testing is recommended before administering parenteral doses. The earliest symptoms of the hypersensitivity are irritation and swelling of the eyelids.

Be aware that iodine products are contraindicated in hyperkalemia as it might be exacerbated; checking serum potassium levels is advisable before administering iodine products. Pulmonary edema, acute bronchitis, and pulmonary tuberculosis are also contraindications to the use of iodines because these drugs cause irritation and increase secretions. Ensure that the client has adequate renal function for potassium excretion. Iodine therapy during pregnancy can cause abnormal thyroid function or goiter in the newborn.

Review the client's current medication regimen because iodide products may have significant drug interactions when administered with the following drugs:

Drug	Possible effect and management
antithyroid drugs	May increase the hypothyroid and goitrogenic effects of the drugs. Monitor closely for decreased metabolic activity.
diuretics, potassium-conserving type	If these diuretics are used concurrently with potassium iodide, increased levels of potassium may result in hyperkalemia, cardiac arrhythmias, or cardiac arrest. Monitor serum potassium levels closely.
lithium	The hypothyroid and goitrogenic effects of both drugs may be potentiated. Obtain and monitor baseline thyroid status periodically to plan appropriate interventions.

As part of a baseline assessment, serum potassium concentrations and thyroid function studies should be ascertained.

Nursing diagnosis. The client receiving iodide therapy is at risk for the following nursing diagnoses: altered bowel elimination pattern (diarrhea); altered comfort (nausea and stomach cramps); and the potential complications of allergic reactions (angioedema, arthalgia, urticaria), hyperkalemia (confusion, arrhythmias, tiredness, and weakness), and iodism (burning of the mouth and throat, gastric upset, increased salivation, metallic taste, headache, rhinitis).

Implementation

Monitoring. As well as monitoring the determinations of periodic serum potassium and thyroid function studies, assess the client's vital signs for return to normal and the client's comfort status related to the gastrointestinal and dermatologic effects of iodine.

Intervention. Dilute Lugol's solution and saturated solutions of sodium or potassium in 240 ml of fruit juice, carbonated beverage, broth, or another substance to improve taste. Tablet dosage forms should be dissolved in 120 ml of liquid before administering. Since the medication evaporates rapidly, do not leave open to air for long periods before administration. Do not use if the solution has turned brownish yellow. Administer iodides through a straw to prevent discoloration of the teeth. Administer after meals to minimize gastric irritation.

Education. Instruct the client to discontinue use and notify the prescriber if any of the following occur: fever, skin rash, metallic brassy taste, swelling of the neck and throat, burning soreness of gums and teeth, head cold symptoms, or severe gastrointestinal distress. These symptoms are characteristic of iodism, chronic iodide poisoning. Stress the need to maintain regular visits to prescriber to monitor progress.

Advise the client to consult with the prescriber regarding the use of iodized salt and seafood in the diet. Iodine-rich foods, such as soybeans, cabbage, kale, and other green leafy vegetables may need to be restricted.

Caution the client to maintain the prescribed dosage. Missing doses may precipitate a thyroid storm. Instruct the client to consult with the prescriber before taking OTC cold remedies, because some contain iodides.

Evaluation. The client will experience a decrease in the symptoms of hyperthyroidism. For clients receiving the drug as part of a preoperative course of therapy, there should be a decrease in the size and vascularity of the thyroid.

sodium iodide (^{131}I, Iodotope)

Sodium iodide, a radioactive isotope of iodine, accumulates in thyroid tissue and selectively damages or destroys it. It is indicated for the treatment of hyperthyroidism and thyroid carcinoma.

Administered orally, it has an onset of effect within 2 to 4 weeks; peak therapeutic effect occurs between 2 and 4 months; and it is mainly excreted by the kidneys. Up to 20% of the dose may appear in breast milk within 24 hours. It has a radionuclide half-life of approximately 8 days; principal types of radiation are beta and gamma rays. For side effects/adverse reactions, see Table 48-4.

While no significant drug interactions are noted with this product, many drugs are capable of interfering with test results. See a current reference for possible drug interferences and current dosage recommendations. Pregnancy safety is classified as FDA category X.

■ Nursing Management
Sodium Iodide ^{131}I Therapy

Assessment. Thyroid function studies should be performed before and after therapy. Do not give radioactive iodine to pregnant women or nursing mothers. With a woman with childbearing potential, therapy begins the first few days after the onset of menses.

Nursing diagnosis. Most clients will experience anxiety and knowledge deficit related to the administration of radioactive materials. The client may also experience temporary altered comfort following a course of ^{131}I therapy, evidenced by loss of taste, nausea and vomiting, and tenderness of the salivary glands. In addition, with therapeutic dosages there is the potential complication of hypothyroidism, the incidence of which should be 100% if the regimen has been successful. Potential complications may include leukopenia, evidenced by fever, chills, and sore throat, and thrombocytopenia, evidenced by unusual bleeding or bruising.

Implementation

Monitoring. Assess post-therapy thyroid function with serum thyroxine examinations.

Intervention. The client should take nothing by mouth after midnight before a morning dose, because food slows the absorption of the drug. Increase the fluid intake of the client to 2500 ml/daily to enhance excretion of the isotope.

If the dose is administered for hyperthyroidism, institute full radiation precautions for 24 hours. If the dose is for cancer of the thyroid, isolate the client for 3 days. Check the institution's protocol for radiation precautions. Pregnant women, be they personnel or visitors, should not have contact with the client. Use disposable utensils with the client. Consult with nuclear medicine personnel about limitations for individual staff contact with the client. To avoid exposure to the radioactive products of the iodine, wear rubber gloves when giving ^{131}I to clients and when disposing of their excreta. Limit exposure of individuals by limiting time of contact to and increasing distance from the source of radiation.

Education. To prevent radiation contamination of others and the environment, instruct the client in appropriate methods for disposal of urine and feces, such as double-flushing toilet and washing hands after using toilet, until radiation precautions are no longer needed. If the client is discharged but radiation precautions are still necessary, ensure that the client receives specific instructions for visitor contact and disposal of utensils and excreta from the personnel in the nuclear medicine department.

If the client received a dose of ^{131}I for the treatment of hyperthyroidism or thyroid carcinoma, these 48- to 72-hour precautions may include the following: avoiding close contact with others, especially children; not kissing anyone or sharing other persons' eating or drinking utensils; not engaging in sexual activities; sleeping alone; washing sink and tub after use; and using and washing clothes, towels, and linens separately.

Evaluation. The client will experience a euthyroid state.

Thioamide Derivatives

methimazole [meth im' a zole] (Tapazole)
▲ **propylthiouracil** [proe pill thye oh yoor' a sill] (Propyl-Thyracil ♣)

Thioamide derivatives, or antithyroid agents, inhibit thyroid hormone synthesis by inhibiting incorporation of iodide into tyrosine and the coupling of iodotyrosines. They do not affect exogenous thyroid hormones.

Propylthiouracil (not methimazole) also inhibits the conversion of thyroxine (T_4) to triiodothyronine (T_3), which may make it more effective for treatment of thyroid crisis or storm. They are indicated for the treatment of hyperthyroidism, before surgery or radiotherapy, or as adjunct therapy for treatment of thyrotoxicosis or thyroid storm (propylthiouracil preferred for latter indication).

Half-life of methimazole is 5 to 6 hours, propylthiouracil 1 to 2 hours. Peak effect is 7 weeks with methimazole; 17 weeks with propylthiouracil. They are metabolized in the liver and excreted by the kidneys. For side effects/adverse reactions, see Table 48-4.

Methimazole oral adult dosage is 15 to 60 mg daily for hyperthyroidism. The maintenance dosage is 5 to 30 mg daily in 1 or 2 divided doses. To treat thyrotoxic crisis, the dosage is 15 to 20 mg every 4 hours for 24 hours used as an adjunct to other therapies. Pediatric dose for hyperthyroidism is 0.4 mg/kg daily; maintenance dose is 0.2 mg/kg daily.

Propylthiouracil oral adult dosage is 300 to 900 mg daily in divided doses. Children between 6 and 10 years old receive 50 to 150 mg daily, while children over 10 years old receive 50 to 300 mg daily. For neonatal thyrotoxicosis, the dosage is 10 mg/kg daily in divided doses. Pregnancy safety has been established at FDA category D; both drugs cross the placenta and can cause fetal hypothyroidism and goiter.

■ Nursing Management

Thioamide Derivative Therapy

Assessment. The client's health status should be reviewed to ascertain that the client does not have a condition for which the administration of these drugs would entail greater risk such as infection, bone marrow depression, or hepatic function impairment. Monitor thyroid function studies before and periodically during therapy, as well as monitoring leukocyte counts. Concomitant thyroid administration during thioamide therapy in the hyperthyroid pregnant woman may avert hypothyroidism in the mother and fetus.

The following drug interactions may occur when methimazole or propylthiouracil is administered with the drugs listed below.

Drug	Possible effect and management
amiodarone, iodinated glycerol, lithium, or potassium iodide	Amiodarone contains 37% iodine by weight. Increased or excess amounts of amiodarone, iodide, or iodine may result in a decreased response to the antithyroid drugs. Iodine deficiency, however, may result in an increased response to the antithyroid medications. Monitor closely.
anticoagulants (coumarin or indanedione)	As thyroid status approaches normal, the response to anticoagulants may decrease, or, if thiomide produces a drug-induced hypoprothrombinemia, the anticoagulant response may increase. Monitor closely because anticoagulant doses are adjusted based on prothrombin time test results.
digitalis glycosides	As thyroid status decreases, serum levels of digoxin and digitoxin may increase. Monitor closely; dosage adjustments may be necessary.
sodium iodide ^{131}I	Thyroid uptake of ^{131}I may be decreased by the antithyroid agents. Monitor closely.

Nursing diagnosis. The client receiving these antithyroid medications is at risk for the following nursing diagnoses: altered comfort (nausea, loss of taste, itching, stomach cramping, dizziness), and altered protection related to the bone marrow depressant effects of the drug (delayed healing, gingival bleeding, leukopenia); and the potential complications of arthalgias, lupus-like syndrome, and peripheral neuropathy, as well as hyperthyroidism as a result of the ineffectiveness of the therapeutic regimen or hypothyroidism due to overdosage with the drug.

Implementation

Monitoring. Observe the complete blood count periodically during therapy to detect blood dyscrasias such as agranulocytosis, leukopenia, or thrombocytopenia. Propylthiouracil may reduce thrombin and result in bleeding; monitor prothrombin time during therapy.

The client should be assessed for the effectiveness of the therapeutic regimen. Signs of thyrotoxicosis, such as fever, tachycardia, irritability, weakness, diarrhea, and vomiting, indicate inadequate therapy; signs of hypothyroidism, such as intolerance to cold, constipation, lethargy, and weight gain, indicate overdosage. TSH and T_4 assays are important in monitoring the client's status.

Intervention. Administer with meals to minimize gastric irritation. Use the smallest effective dose (less than 300 mg daily) for pregnant clients. Propylthiouracil crosses the placental barrier; therefore large doses can cause goiter in the newborn or cretinism in the fetus.

Because therapy to obtain a prolonged remission may last from 6 months to several years, client adherence may become an issue. To be most effective the doses should be divided into evenly spaced intervals throughout the day. However, to improve compliance and decrease the incidence of side effects, a once- or twice-a-day dosage schedule may be used, although it is less effective. Propylthiouracil needs to be taken at the same time every day in relation to meals, because food may alter the response to the drug by affecting its absorption.

Because of the risk of thyroid storm, the client should consult with the prescriber if his or her health status changes from infection, injury, or other illness, or if surgery, dental surgery, or emergency treatment is required.

Education. Instruct clients that if they develop sore throat, head cold, skin eruptions, or malaise, they should report these symptoms immediately to their prescriber, since these symptoms signal the onset of agranulocytosis. It may occur too quickly to be determined by periodic blood testing. Instruct the client to consult with the prescriber about the restriction of iodized salt and seafood. Caution against taking OTC medications because many contain iodine preparations. Alert breastfeeding mothers to take these drugs with caution and ensure thyroid function monitoring for their infants, since the drugs are excreted in the milk.

Evaluation. The client will experience a euthyroid state.

SUMMARY

As with other endocrine glands, parathyroid and thyroid functioning may be increased or decreased, resulting in pathologic conditions for the client. With hypoparathyroidism, the administration of vitamin D and calcium supplements will usually restore the calcium and phosphorus levels to normal. However, with hyperparathyroidism, surgery is usually the primary treatment.

In hypothyroidism, the clinical goal is to eliminate the client's symptoms by thyroid replacement therapy, for which a number of preparations are available. Hyperthyroidism is managed by large doses of iodides, which inhibit thyroid hormone release and decrease the thyroid's size; by thioamide derivatives, which inhibit the synthesis of thyroid hormone; by radioactive iodine; or by surgery.

Through all the therapies associated with hormonal replacement or inhibition, the client requires support and explanation to understand the many changes of body and mood that may occur with these therapies. Because clinical manifestations of the therapies are as important as the laboratory studies in determining the efficacy of treatment, ongoing skilled assessment of the client's health status is essential.

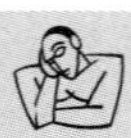

Critical Thinking

1. Grace Smith examines the label on the OTC calcium supplement she takes each day. It indicates that two tablets taken daily provide 3000 mg of calcium carbonate. How much elemental calcium is Grace taking?
2. Why is clinical response more important than blood hormone level in thyroid preparation therapy? What signs and symptoms should the nurse be monitoring to determine the effectiveness of the therapy?

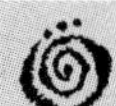

Collaborative Learning Activities

1. Groups of students will take about 15 minutes to identify goals of therapy for clients with hypercalcemia, hypoparathyroidism, hyperthyroidism, and myxedema and draw up appropriate nursing plans including specifics for possible drugs of choice. Ensure coverage of geriatric implications.

BIBLIOGRAPHY

Angelucci PA (1995). Caring for patients with hypothyroidism, *Nursing* 25(5):60-1.

American Hospital Formulary Service (1996). *AHFS drug information '96*. Bethesda, MD: American Society of Hospital Pharmacists.

American Medical Association (1995). *Drug evaluations; annual 1995*. Chicago: The Association.

Anderson KN, et al. (Eds.) (1994). *Mosby's medical, nursing, & allied health dictionary* (4th ed.). St Louis: Mosby.

Baker KH & Feldman JE (1993). Thyroid cancer: A review, *Oncol Nurs Forum* 20(1):95.

Katzung BG (1992). *Basic and clinical pharmacology* (5th ed.). Norwalk, CT: Appleton & Lange.

Kim TS (1994). Primary hyperparathyroidism, *Orthopaedic Nurs* 13(3):17-28.

Kovacs CS, MacDonald SM, Chik CL, & Bruera E. (1995). Hypercalcemia of malignancy in the palliative care patient: A treatment strategy, *J Pain & Sympt Manag* 10(3):224-32.

McCance KL & Huether SE (1994). *Pathophysiology: The biological basis for disease in adults and children* (2nd ed.). St Louis: Mosby.

Melmon KL, et al. (1992). *Clinical pharmacology: Basic principles in therapeutics* (3rd ed.). New York: McGraw-Hill.

Olin BR (Ed.) (1996). *Facts and comparisons*. St Louis: Facts and Comparisons.

Rizzolo P (1992). Thyroid. In Ham RJ & Sloane PD. *Primary care geriatrics: A case-based approach* (2nd ed.). St. Louis: Mosby.

Tang I & Lau AH (1995). Fluid and electrolyte disorders. In Young LY & Koda-Kimble MA. *Applied therapeutics* (6th ed.). Vancouver, WA: Applied Therapeutics.

Toft AD (1994). Thyroxine therapy, *New Engl J Med* 331(3):174-80.

United States Pharmacopeial Convention (1996). *USP DI: Drug information for the health care professional* (16th ed.). Rockville, MD: The Convention.

Woodley M & Whelan A (1992). *Manual of medical therapeutics* (27th ed.). Boston: Little, Brown.

Chapter 49

Drugs Affecting the Adrenal Cortex

Chapter Focus

A number of pathologic conditions associated with hyposecretion or hypersecretion of the adrenal cortex are pharmacologically managed. In addition, the glucocorticoids, in pharmacologic doses, are widely used for their antiinflammatory and immunomodulating effects. However, clients receiving systemic corticosteroid preparations for nonendocrine disorders are at risk of developing adverse effects. Nurses need to be skillful at assessment of not only the steroid-responsive disorder but also the client's individual responses to corticosteroid therapy.

Key Terms

circadian rhythm (p. 782)
corticosteroids (p. 782)
glucocorticoid (p. 782)
mineralocorticoid (p. 782)
septic shock (p. 783)
ultradian rhythm (p. 782)

Key Drugs [▲]

cortisone
fludrocortisone

Objectives

1. Compare and contrast glucocorticoids and mineralocorticoids.
2. Describe the major pharmacologic effects of the corticosteroids.
3. Discuss five significant drug interactions of the glucocorticoids.
4. Describe the advantages for an alternate-day regimen schedule.
5. Discuss a recommended method for corticosteroid drug withdrawal.
6. Name four major adverse reactions associated with the use of adrenocorticoids.
7. Implement the nursing management of drug therapy for the care of clients receiving agents affecting the adrenal cortex.

The term **corticosteroids** refers to the adrenocortical hormones and the higher-potency, synthetic formulations. Some corticosteroids, such as cortisol, have a profound effect on carbohydrate metabolism, whereas aldosterone primarily affects mineral (or electrolyte) and water metabolism. Therefore corticosteroids are divided into two classes, **glucocorticoids** and **mineralocorticoids** (halogenated glucocorticoids).

Cholesterol, which is used for the biosynthesis of corticosteroids, is synthesized and stored in the adrenal cortex. Corticosteroid synthesis depends on pituitary ACTH, which is governed by the corticotropin-releasing hormone (CRH) from the hypothalamus. Evidence suggests that increased levels of corticosteroids can inhibit the adrenal glucocorticoid system by inhibiting the release of CRH from the hypothalamus and by inhibiting the release of ACTH from the pituitary.

GLUCOCORTICOIDS

Two rhythms appear to influence glucocorticoid function: circadian (daily) rhythm and ultradian rhythm. **Circadian rhythm,** a pattern based on a 24-hour cycle, with the repetition of certain physiologic phenomena, is controlled by the dark/light and sleep/wakefulness cycles. Normal persons sleeping in the dark at night will have increased plasma cortisol levels in the early morning hours that reach a peak after they are awake. These levels then slowly fall to very low levels in the evening and during the early phase of sleep. The importance of this rhythm is emphasized by the finding that corticosteroid therapy is more potent when given at midnight than when given at noon.

Ultradian rhythms are periodic or intermittent functions with frequencies greater than once every 24 hours. In human beings, four to eight adrenal glucocorticoid bursts occur each 24 hours, which may follow bursts in CRH and ACTH releases. These bursts are clustered close together and are very pronounced during the circadian rise in plasma glucocorticoid levels in the early hours of the morning. At other times they may be so widely spaced that adrenal secretion is zero. Consequently the adrenal cortex secretes glucocorticoids only about 25% of the time in unstressed individuals.

Glucocorticoids have the following pharmacologic actions:

- *Antiinflammatory action.* Glucocorticoids, especially cortisol in larger than normal dosages, can stabilize lysosomal membranes and prevent release of proteolytic enzymes during inflammation. They can also potentiate vasoconstrictor effects.
- *Maintenance of normal blood pressure.* Glucocorticoids potentiate the vasoconstrictor action of norepinephrine. When glucocorticoids are absent, the vasoconstricting action of the catecholamines is diminished and blood pressure falls.
- *Carbohydrate and protein metabolism.* Glucocorticoids help to maintain the blood sugar level and liver and muscle glycogen content. They facilitate breakdown of protein in muscle and extrahepatic tissues, which leads to increased plasma amino acid levels. Glucocorticoids increase the trapping of amino acids by the liver and stimulate the deamination of amino acids. They also increase the activity of enzymes important to gluconeogenesis and inhibit glycolytic enzymes. This can produce hyperglycemia and glycosuria. They are diabetogenic. These effects can aggravate diabetes, bring on latent diabetes, and cause insulin resistance. Inhibition of protein synthesis can delay wound healing and cause muscle wasting and osteoporosis. In young persons these effects can inhibit growth.
- *Fat metabolism.* Glucocorticoids promote mobilization of fatty acids from adipose tissue, increasing their concentration in the plasma and their use for energy. Despite this effect, clients taking glucocorticoids may accumulate fat stores (rounded face, buffalo hump). The effect of glucocorticoids on fat metabolism is complex and little known.
- *Thymolytic, lympholytic, and eosinopenic actions.* Glucocorticoids can cause atrophy of the thymus and decrease the number of lymphocytes, plasma cells, and eosinophils in blood. By blocking the production and release of cytokines, corticosteroids interfere with the T and B lymphocytes, macrophages, and monocytes integrated role in immune response (Schimmer & Parker, 1996). These effects ultimately interfere with the immune and allergic responses. This, along with their antiinflammatory action, makes them useful immunosuppressants for delaying rejection in clients with organ or tissue transplants, as well as useful antiallergenics for the treatment of acute allergic reactions such as urticaria, bronchial asthma, and anaphylactic shock. However, steroids can also be a source of danger in infections by limiting useful protective inflammation. These hormones also inhibit activity of the lymphatic system, causing lymphopenia and reduction in size of enlarged lymph nodes.
- *Stress effects.* During stressful situations (injury, major surgery, etc.), corticosteroids are suddenly released or are necessary to help maintain homeostasis. This sudden release is believed to be a protective mechanism for the individual. Without steroid administration, hypotension and shock may occur (Figure 49-1). During stress, epinephrine and norepinephrine also are released from the adrenal medulla, and these catecholamines have a synergistic action with the corticosteroids.
- *Central nervous system.* Corticosteroids effect mood, behavior and possibly cause neuronal or brain excitability. Some persons report euphoria, insomnia, anxiety, depression, increased motor activity, or may become psychotic.

Glucocorticoids are used in replacement therapy for adrenocortical insufficiency and also to treat severe allergic reactions; anaphylactic reactions not responsive to other therapies; collagen disorders such as systemic lupus erythematosus; treatment of dermatologic conditions, hematologic disorders, adjunct treatment for neoplastic disease, ophthalmic disorders, respiratory disorders, rheumatic disorders, and treatment of shock and other conditions (Box 49-1).

The glucocorticoids are well absorbed orally; parenterally (IM) the soluble esters (sodium phosphate, sodium succinate) are rapidly absorbed while the poorly soluble agents (acetate, acetonide, diacetate, hexacetonide, tebutate) are slowly but completely absorbed. Topically, the soluble esters

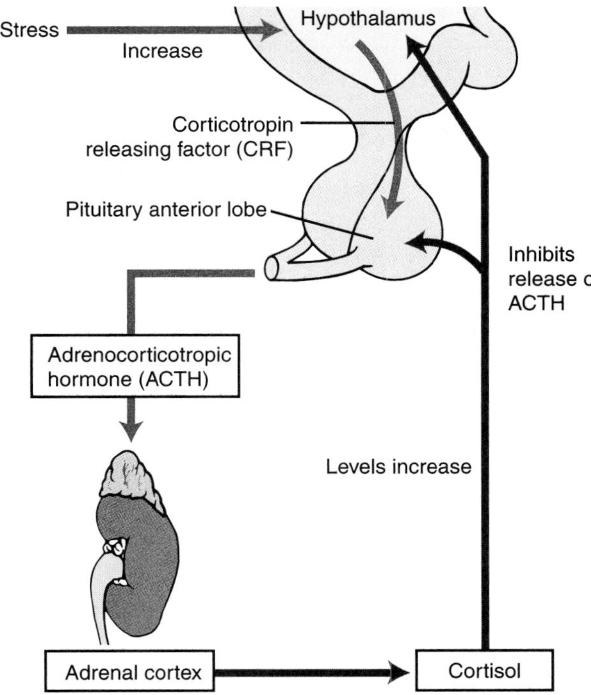

Figure 49-1 Glucocorticoid secretion.

> **BOX 49-1**
>
> **Septic Shock**
>
> **Septic shock** usually results from a gram-negative bacteremia that leads to circulatory insufficiency. The inadequate tissue perfusion generally results in hypotension, oliguria, tachycardia, elevated temperature, and tachypnea.
>
> Mechanism
>
> Septic shock may be caused by bacterial substances that interact with body cell membranes and systems, especially coagulation and the complement system, resulting in injury to cells and alterations in blood flow in the body.
>
> Treatment
>
> Treatment may consist of volume replacement, antibiotics, surgery (if the client has an abscessed or necrotic bowel or organs/tissues), vasoconstricting agents (dopamine, norepinephrine, or levarterenol), diuretics, and glucocorticoids (steroids). Use of steroids is somewhat controversial, but several published studies have reported a benefit with their use if used early in the treatment of shock.
>
> Steroid beneficial effects
>
> Beneficial effects of steroids include protecting cellular membranes from injury, decreasing platelet aggregation, reducing extracellular release of leukocyte enzymes, and preventing the formation of vasoactive substances in the body.

are less rapidly absorbed while the poorly soluble agents are slowly but completely absorbed. Rectally about 20% of the drug is absorbed normally, but if the rectum is inflamed, absorption may increase up to 50%.

These agents are mainly metabolized in the liver and excreted by the kidneys. Cortisone and prednisone are inactive until metabolized to hydrocortisone and prednisolone, respectively. The fluorinated adrenocorticoids are more slowly metabolized than the other drugs.

For onset of action, peak effect, duration of action, see Table 49-1. For the relative potency of the major short-acting, intermediate-acting, and long-acting adrenocorticoids, see Table 49-2. For side effects/adverse reactions, see Table 49-3. See Table 49-4 for corticosteroid preparations and dosing.

Nursing Management

Glucocorticoid Therapy

Assessment. Do not give glucocorticoids to clients with systemic fungal infections or tuberculosis because these infections may be exacerbated. The prescriber should carefully consider risk-benefit before administering systemic corticosteroids to clients with or a predisposition to acquired immunodeficiency syndrome (AIDS) or human immunodeficiency virus (HIV) because of the risk of uncontrollable infection. Clients with diabetes mellitus may find their condition exacerbated. Clients with active or latent esophagitis, gastritis, or peptic ulcer may have symptoms of progression or reactivation masked and may bleed without warning. Clients for whom edema may be hazardous, such as those with cardiac disease, congestive heart failure, hypertension, or renal function impairment should be monitored very carefully. Note that myasthenic crisis may be induced if these drugs are administered to clients with myasthenia gravis. Clients with ocular herpes simplex are at risk for corneal perforation with this therapy. Use of glucocorticoids with clients with measles or chickenpox, existing or recent, including recent exposure, run the risk of a generalized (potentially fatal) course of the disease.

Use cautiously in pregnant women also, since adrenal insufficiency in both mother and child is possible at delivery. Fetal abnormalities also can occur. If the drug is administered maternally to help prevent neonatal respiratory distress syndrome, there is an increased risk of maternal infection (tuberculosis, herpes type II), uterine bleeding, placental insufficiency, and premature membrane rupture. Geriatric clients are more likely to develop hypertension during glucocorticoid therapy, and postmenopausal women are also more likely to develop osteoporosis.

If the corticosteroid is for intraarticular injection, the joint should not be infected, bleeding, fractured, or have had recent surgery because the condition will be aggravated and/or healing in these instances will be inhibited.

Rectal administration of the drug should be avoided in instances of bowel obstruction, recent gastrointestinal surgery, or infection because healing will be delayed.

Because there is a risk for fluid volume excess related to sodium and fluid retention, obtain baseline weight before therapy. Also obtain baseline data for hematologic values,

TABLE 49-1 Adrenocorticoids/corticotropin: pharmacology

Drug (route)	Onset of action	Peak effect	Duration of action
betamethasone (PO)	—	1-2 hr	3.25 days
(IM, IV)	Rapid	—	—
acetate/sodium phosphate (IM)	1-3 hr	—	7 days
corticotropin repository (IM)	—	—	12-24 hr
cortisone acetate (PO)	Rapid	2 hr	30-36 hr
(IM)	Slower	20-48 hr	—
dexamethasone (PO)	—	1-2 hr	66 hr
(IM)	—	8 hr	6 days
(IV)	Rapid	—	—
hydrocortisone (PO)	—	1 hr	30-36 hr
(IM)	—	4-8 hr	—
rectal enema (retention)	3-5 days	—	—
rectal foam	5-7 days	—	—
cypionate (PO)	Slow	1-2 hr	
(IM)	Rapid	1 hr	Varies
methylprednisolone (PO)	—	1-2 hr	30-36 hr
(IM)	6-48 hr	4-8 days	1-4 wk
(IA) (IL) (ST)	Very slow	7 days	1-5 wk
sodium succinate (IV, IM)	Rapid	—	—
prednisolone (PO)	—	1-2 hr	30-36 hr
acetate/sodium phosphate (IM)	—	—	Up to 4 wk
(IB, IS, IA, ST)	—	—	3-28 days
sodium phosphate (IV, IM)	Rapid	1 hr	—
prednisone (PO)	—	1-2 hr	30-36 hr
triamcinolone (PO)	—	1-2 hr	52 hr
(IM)	1-2 days	—	1-6 wk

—, Not available; *PO*, orally; *IA*, intraarticularly; *IB*, intrabursal; *IL*, intralesion; *IM*, intramuscularly; *IS*, intrasynovial; *ST*, in soft tissue.
(*USP DI*, 1996)

TABLE 49-2 Major adrenocorticoids: relative potency and half-life

Adrenocorticoids	Equivalent glucocorticoid dose (mg)*	Relative glucocorticoid potency†	Relative mineralocorticoid potency‡	Half-life (hr)	
				Serum	Tissue
Short-acting					
cortisone	25	0.8	2	0.5	8-12
hydrocortisone	20	1	2	1.5-2	8-12
Intermediate					
methylprednisolone	4	5	0§	>3.5	18-36
prednisolone	5	4	1	2.1-3.5	18-36
prednisone	5	4	1	3.4-3.8	18-36
triamcinolone	4	5	0§	2->5	18-36
Long-acting					
betamethasone	0.6	20-30	0§	3-5	36-54
dexamethasone	0.5-0.75	20-30	0§	3-4.5	36-54

*Approximate dosages, applies to oral and IV only.
†Refers to antiinflammatory, immunosuppressant, and metabolic-type effects.
‡Potassium excretion, sodium and water retention.
§Some hypokalemia and/or sodium and water retention may occur, depending on dose and individual response.

TABLE 49-3 Adrenocorticoids/corticotropin: side effects/adverse reactions

Side effects*	Adverse reactions†
Most frequent: Euphoria, increase in appetite, insomnia, restlessness, increased anxiety, gas. With triamcinolone: anorexia Less frequent/rare: Hyperpigmentation or hypopigmentation (the latter most likely at injection sites), hypotension, headache, increased hair growth on body or face. After intranasal administration—red flushing of face, nosebleeds. After intraarticular injection—increase in joint pains that may persist for 48 hours.	Lowers resistance to infections (bacterial, viral, fungal, and parasitic). May also mask symptoms of infections making it difficult to diagnose (at pharmacologic dosages). At replacement dosages for adrenocorticoid insufficiency, major adverse effects rarely occur if client is closely monitored and dosage is adjusted according to individual's need (at physiologic dosages). Less frequent: Visual disturbances (cataracts, diabetes), increased urination or thirst (diabetes), decreased growth in children. Rectal dosage form—bleeding, blistering, pain, or itching caused by local irritation or allergic reaction. Rare: Mental changes including depression, mania, psychoses, paranoia, disorientation, and other psychic disturbances possible. At injection site—redness, swelling, rash caused by allergic reaction, or pain, tingling, or numbness at site injection. If "pulse" therapy, i.e., rapid IV administration of high dosages, is used: seizures, severe hypotension, rash or hives, respiratory difficulties, wheezing, shortness of breath. Hypertension, tachycardia, and redness of face are also reported. Chronic or long-term therapy: abdominal pains (may be caused by peptic ulcer formation or pancreatitis), acne, black tarry stools (GI bleeding), round face (Cushing's syndrome), hip or shoulder pain. Hypertension, edema of feet or lower legs and weight gain reported because of sodium and water retention. Muscle cramping or pain, increased weakness, irregular heart rate caused by potassium loss. Nausea, vomiting, muscle weakness, menstrual alterations, bone pain, increased bruising, wounds difficult to heal.

*If side effects continue, increase, or disturb the client, the prescriber should be informed.
†If adverse reactions occur, contact the prescriber, since medical intervention may be necessary.

TABLE 49-4 Corticosteroid preparations and dosing

Drug	Usual dosage: Adult	Usual dosage: Child
betamethasone (Celestone, Betnelan🍁)	Oral: 0.6 to 7.2 mg/day as single dose or in divided doses	Adrenocortical insufficiency; 17.5 μg/kg in 3 divided doses Other conditions: 65.5 to 250 μg/kg in 3 to 4 divided doses
	IM/IV/intraarticular/intralesional/soft tissue injections: up to 9 mg daily	Adrenocortical insufficiency (IM):17.5 μg/kg in divided doses every third day Other conditions (IM): 20.8 to 125 μg/kg every 12 to 24 hr
corticotropin (Acthar)	Diagnostic aid: 10 to 25 units in 500 ml D_5W. Therapeutic IM or SC: 40 to 80 units/day.	IV/IM/SC: 1.6 units/kg per 24 hr in divided doses
repository corticotropin (Acthar Gel)	Therapeutic IM or SC: 40 to 80 units every 24 to 72 hr	IM or SC: 0.8 units/kg per 24 hr
▲ cortisone (Cortone)	Oral: 25 to 300 mg daily	Adrenocortical insufficiency: 0.7 mg/kg daily in divided doses Other conditions: 2.5 to 10 mg/kg daily

Continued

TABLE 49-4 Corticosteroid preparations and dosing—cont'd

Drug	Usual dosage: Adult	Usual dosage: Child
dexamethasone (Decadron and others)	Oral: 0.5 to 9 mg daily	Adrenocortical insufficiency is 23.3 μg/kg daily in three divided doses
	Dexamethasone suppression test for Cushing's syndrome: 1 mg at 11 PM or 0.5 mg every 6 hr for 2 days	Other indications: 83.3 to 333.3 μg/kg/day in divided doses
	Cerebral edema in recurrent or inoperable brain tumors: 2 mg two or three times daily after use of injectable dexamethasone	
hydrocortisone (Cortef and others)	Oral/IM: 15 or 20 mg up to 240 mg daily	Oral: 0.56 mg/kg/day IM: 0.56 to 4 mg/kg/day
enema (Cortenema)	Rectal: 100 mg retention enema nightly for 3 weeks	Not established
aerosol (Cortifoam)	Rectal: 90 mg once or twice daily for 14 to 21 days	Not established
methylprednisolone (Medrol)	Oral: 4 to 48 mg daily	Adrenocortical insufficiency: 117 μg/kg daily in three divided doses Other conditions: 417 μg to 1.67 mg/kg in three or four divided doses
prednisolone (Delta-Cortef and others)	Oral: 5 to 60 mg daily (maximum 250 mg/day)	Adrenocortical insufficiency: 140 μg/kg daily in three divided doses
prednisone (Deltasone and others)	Oral: 5 to 60 mg daily	Dose varies according to indication and age; check current reference
triamcinolone (Aristocort, Kenacort)	Oral: 4 to 48 mg/day	Adrenocortical insufficiency: 117 μg/kg daily Other conditions: 416 μg to 1.7 mg/kg daily

Dexamethasone, methylprednisolone, prednisolone, and triamcinolone are also available in short-acting and long-acting preparations; see current reference for dosing information.

Pregnancy Safety

Category	Drug
C	corticotropin, fludrocortisone, metyrapone
D	aminoglutethimide
X	trilostane
Not established	other glucocorticoids

serum electrolytes, and serum and urine glucose. Check stool for occult blood. If therapy is anticipated to last more than 6 weeks, the client should obtain a baseline ophthalmologic examination for the presence of cataracts, glaucoma, and ocular infections. These determinations should be monitored during therapy. Obtain a baseline assessment of the underlying condition for which the glucocorticoid is being prescribed.

Assess children for growth before and periodically during therapy, since there is a risk for altered growth and development with glucocorticoid therapy.

Review the client's current medication regimen for significant interactions that may occur when corticosteroids are given with the drugs listed below.

Drug	Possible effect and management
aminoglutethimide (Cytadren)	Suppresses adrenal function; therefore do not administer corticotropin concurrently. When aminoglutethimide is given, glucocorticoid supplements are often prescribed. Be aware that aminoglutethimide can increase the metabolism of dexamethasone, reducing its half-life significantly. Hydrocortisone is recommended, though, because its metabolism does not appear to be affected by aminoglutethimide.
amphotericin B parenteral (Fungizone)	May result in severe hypokalemia. If given concurrently, monitor serum potassium levels closely. May also decrease the adrenal gland response to corticotropin.
antacids	When given concurrently with prednisone or dexamethasone, a decrease in steroid absorption may result. Monitor closely; steroid dosage adjustments may be necessary.
antidiabetic drugs (oral) or insulin	Glucocorticoids may elevate serum glucose levels (both during therapy and after, if the glucocorticoid is stopped); therefore a dosage adjustment of one or both drugs may be necessary.
digitalis glycosides	May result in increased potential for toxicity (dysrhythmias) associated with hypokalemia.

Drug	Possible effect and management
diuretics	The sodium and fluid-retaining effects of the adrenocorticoids may reduce the effectiveness of the diuretic agents. Monitor closely for edema and fluid retention. Potassium-depleting diuretics given with adrenocorticoids may result in severe hypokalemia. Monitor potassium serum levels. The effects of potassium-sparing diuretics may be decreased. Monitor serum potassium levels and client response closely.
hepatic enzyme-inducing agents	Barbiturates, carbamazepine, phenytoin, and others may decrease the adrenocorticoid effect because of increased metabolism. Dosage adjustment may be necessary. Monitor serum cortisol levels closely.
mitotane (Lysodren)	Mitotane will decrease the adrenal gland's response to corticotropin. Avoid concurrent use. Adrenocorticoids are usually necessary during mitotane administration because mitotane suppresses adrenocortical function. Usually higher than normal doses of glucocorticoids are needed.
potassium supplements	These reduce the effect of either one or both medications on serum potassium levels. Monitor serum levels if given concurrently.
ritodrine (Yutopar)	When ritodrine is given to inhibit premature labor in the pregnant woman and the long-acting glucocorticoids are given to enhance fetal lung maturity, the result may be pulmonary edema in the mother. Monitor pregnant women closely for first signs of pulmonary edema (shallow, rapid, difficult breathing; anxiety; restlessness; increased heart rate and blood pressure; enlarged peripheral and neck veins; edema of extremities; lung rales; and diaphoresis); early detection and treatment are necessary to prevent a potentially serious adverse effect or fatality.
sodium-containing foods or medications	Concurrent usage may result in edema and hypertension. Monitor weight, intake and output, and blood pressure closely.
somatrem or somatropin	The growth response to somatrem or somatropin may be inhibited with concurrent chronic therapy with corticotropin or with daily doses of glucocorticoids above certain levels, such as daily doses of prednisone or prednisolone above 2.5 to 3.75 mg/m^2 of body surface. For dosages for other glucocorticoids, refer to a current *USP DI.*
vaccines, live virus, and other immunizations	**Generally, immunizations are not recommended for clients receiving pharmacologic or immunosuppressant doses of glucocorticoids. Since corticosteroids inhibit antibody response, the immunization effect will be reduced or ineffective and the client may develop neurologic complications. Avoid or a potentially serious drug interaction may occur.** **If live virus vaccines are given to individuals receiving immunosuppressant glucocorticoid therapy, the client may develop the viral disease or at least have a reduced response to the vaccine. Avoid or a potentially serious drug interaction may occur. Also, do not administer the oral polio vaccine to persons in close contact with a person receiving immunosuppressant glucocorticoid therapy.**

Nursing diagnosis. Clients are at risk for the following nursing diagnoses: sleep pattern disturbance due to drug-induced insomnia; body image disturbance related to physical changes with long term therapy (moon face, central obesity, striae, acne, hirsutism); activity intolerance related to muscle wasting; sexual dysfunction related to physiologic limitations secondary to abnormal hormone levels; risk for infection related to immunosuppression; risk for trauma related to osteoporosis; altered thought processes related to the CNS effects (euphoria, psychotic behavior, restlessness); altered nutrition: more than body requirements related to increased appetite; fluid volume excess related to sodium and water retention; and the potential complications of congestive heart failure and hypertension related to cardiovascular effects, peptic ulcer related to GI effects, and hypokalemia, hyperglycemia, and hyperlipidemia related to metabolic effects.

Implementation

Monitoring. Weigh daily; report any sudden increases, which would indicate fluid retention, to the prescriber. Monitor intake and output daily. Correlate with physical findings of edema. Check stool for occult blood. Assess for the following when long-term or excessive doses are given: CNS symptoms (anxiety, depression/stimulation), elevated blood pressure, hematologic values, serum electrolytes, and Cushing's syndrome. If therapy is more than 6 weeks, the client should obtain an ophthalmologic examination at periodic intervals.

Closely monitor the blood sugar of clients taking glucocorticoids, since these drugs can cause hyperglycemia. Diabetic clients may need changes in diet or insulin dosage to maintain blood sugar control.

Remember that not only the total daily dose, but also frequent individual doses during the day must be adjusted to meet the client's needs. Notify the prescriber of the client's varying responses to the drugs.

Intervention. Note that an alternate-day regimen may be valuable when considering the long-term use of glucocorticoids in less severe disease processes, especially when an intermediate range-acting agent (methylprednisolone, prednisolone, prednisone) is used, since it diminishes hypothalamic-pituitary-adrenal (HPA) axis suppression. The alternate-day dose given every other morning before 9 AM is at least twice the daily dose equivalent. This therapy requires that a client possess a responsive pituitary axis and be stabilized initially on the alternate-day schedule.

Give glucocorticoids as a single daily dose in the morning before 9 AM if possible, with food or milk. They suppress adrenal activity the least when it is at its peak, which is early morning.

Administer IM injections of suspensions deep in the gluteal muscle to avert local tissue atrophy at the injection sites. Note that injections into the deltoid muscle can cause atrophy.

Note that clients taking cortisone who require surgery should receive a preoperative dose of a rapid-acting corticosteroid. The drug is continued postoperatively in decreasing doses for several days. Clients with atrophy of the adrenal gland may be unable to cope with the stress of surgery if cortisone treatment is interrupted.

Be prepared to do an HPA axis suppression test after high doses or long-term therapy to determine level of suppression. Know that withdrawal should be carried out slowly and under close supervision to avoid adrenal insufficiency. Note that the usual rate of withdrawal of systemic corticosteroids is the steroid equivalent of 2.5 mg prednisone every 4 days, when the client is under close and continuous medical supervision. When this is not possible, withdrawal of systemic corticosteroids is slower, approximately 2.5 mg prednisone (or equivalent corticosteroid dosage) every 10 days. When withdrawal symptoms such as weakness, lethargy, hypoglycemia, depression, anorexia, and nausea appear, the previous dose may be resumed for 7 days before continuing the decrease. If a medical-surgical emergency or stressful event occurs, the drug may be increased again to prevent the possibility of acute adrenal insufficiency.

Clients may require sodium restriction or potassium supplementation based on their serum electrolyte levels. An increased protein intake may also be necessary during long term drug therapy because the drug promotes protein catabolism. Weight-bearing exercises, such as walking, and the administration of calcium and vitamin D may help reduce the risk of drug-induced osteoporosis.

Education. After intraarticular injection, instruct the client not to overuse the injected joint. Weight-bearing joints should be rested 24 to 48 hours after injection.

With systemic administration, instruct clients to report any signs of infections, such as sore throat, fever, and poor wound healing. Corticosteroids can mask infection and increase its spread. The client should avoid individuals with known contagious illnesses. Also advise clients to avoid any immunizations while taking glucocorticoids, since these agents impair the antibody response.

Instruct clients to report any visual disturbances. Long-term glucocorticoid therapy can cause cataracts, glaucoma, or optic nerve damage.

Since these drugs can cause gastric distress, instruct clients to report any persistent symptoms and instruct them to take the drug with meals or milk in the morning.

Warn the client and family that disturbances in self-concept may occur as the result of changes in appearance (Box 49-2). The nurse should assist the client and family in dealing with the changes that occur, as well as reassure them that they will disappear when the drug is stopped.

Most clients receiving glucocorticoids should be on a high-potassium, low-sodium diet to counter the potassium-depleting and sodium-retaining effects of the drug. Clients should limit alcohol, caffeine, aspirin, and other gastric irritants to minimize peptic ulceration.

Inform female clients that they may experience menstrual irregularities while taking glucocorticoids and that the following drugs are unsafe to take during pregnancy because of their effects on the fetus: cortisone, dexamethasone, hydrocortisone, methylprednisolone, and prednisolone. Have clients carry a card describing their medical condition and drug therapy.

BOX 49-2

Body Image Alterations with Glucocorticoid Therapy

Alterations in body image may be a major concern in clients receiving glucocorticoid therapy. Among the body changes that may occur are the following:

- Abdominal distention
- Acneiform eruptions
- Fat deposits on upper back ("buffalo hump")
- Fluid retention
- Hirsutism
- Hyperpigmentation
- Loss of muscle mass
- Lupus erythematosus–like lesions
- Petechiae and ecchymosis
- Purpura
- Round face ("moon face")
- Striae
- Thin fragile skin
- Thinning of extremities, thickening of torso
- Weight gain

Remember that any client who has received a significant amount of cortisone or related glucocorticoids is likely to have some atrophy of the adrenal cortex. The amount of hormone that will produce atrophy is unknown, as is how long the atrophy will persist, but acute adrenal insufficiency may result from too rapid withdrawal of therapy. Instruct the client to report withdrawal symptoms including weakness, lethargy, malaise, restlessness, hypoglycemia, psychologic despondency, anorexia, and nausea.

Because altered thought processes may occur, have the client report changes in mental status (euphoria, mood swings, depression, insomnia) to the prescriber. Also caution the client to report to the physician any symptoms of abdominal pain, infection, bone pain, tiredness, bruising, or tarry stools.

Evaluation. The client will experience an improvement in the signs and symptoms of the underlying condition for which the glucocorticoid was administered without any adverse effects of the drug.

MINERALOCORTICOIDS

Mineralocorticoids such as aldosterone, are secreted by the adrenal cortex to increase the rate of sodium reabsorption by the kidneys, thereby increasing blood levels of sodium. This results in increased water reabsorption by the kidneys and increases blood volume. They also increase potassium and hydrogen ion excretion into the urine, thereby decreasing blood levels of potassium and hydrogen ions. In adrenal cortex insufficiency, replacement of a glucocorticoid and in some individuals, a mineralocorticoid such as fludrocortisone is necessary.

▲ fludrocortisone [floo droe kor' ti sone] (Florinef)
Fludrocortisone has potent mineralocorticoid activity with some moderate glucocorticoid effects although it is used primarily for its mineralocorticoid effects. It primarily acts on the renal distal tubule to reabsorb sodium and enhance excretion of potassium and hydrogen and is indicated for the treatment of Addison's disease (chronic primary adrenocortical insufficiency) and congenital adrenogenital syndrome.

Fludrocortisone has good oral absorption, a half-life of about 3.5 hours in the plasma with a biologic half-life of activity in the body of 18 to 36 hours. Duration of action is 24 to 48 hours with metabolism in the liver and kidneys and excretion by the kidneys.

The less frequent/rare adverse effects of fludrocortisone include severe or persistent headaches, hypertension, dizziness, edema of lower extremities, joint pain, hypokalemia, increased weakness, tingling or numbness in legs that may progress to arms, trunk, and face, congestive heart failure, and anaphylaxis. Such adverse reactions should be reported immediately to the prescriber.

The adolescent and adult oral dose is 0.1 mg daily. The usual pediatric dose is 50 to 100 μg daily.

■ Nursing Management
Fludrocortisone Therapy

Assessment. Determine that the client does not have hypertension, congestive heart failure, cardiac disease, or renal function impairment except for Type IV renal tubular acidosis, conditions for which mineralocorticoid therapy is administered with caution.

Because clients receiving mineralocorticoid therapy are at risk for fluid volume excess related to sodium and fluid retention, establish the client's baseline serum electrolytes, weight, and blood pressure.

The following significant drug interactions may occur when fludrocortisone is given concurrently with the drugs listed below:

Drug	Possible effect and management
digitalis glycosides	Hypokalemic effect may potentiate the risk for cardiac dysrhythmias or digitalis toxicity. Monitor closely with ECG and pulse readings.
diuretics	Effectiveness of diuretics may be decreased with these medications. Concurrent use of potassium-depleting diuretics or hypokalemic-inducing medications may produce severe hypokalemia. Monitor serum potassium levels closely.
hepatic enzyme inducers	Increased metabolism of mineralocorticoids may result in a decrease in the effectiveness of these drugs.
sodium in food or medications	In type IV renal tubular acidosis, concurrent use of sodium with fludrocortisone may result in hypertension, hypernatremia, and edema. Monitor sodium intake closely and advise clients on safe consumption of foods and medications to avoid hypernatremia. Instruct clients to read labels on both foods and medication.

Nursing diagnosis. Clients receiving fludrocortisone are at risk for the following nursing diagnoses: altered comfort (headache); fluid volume excess (peripheral edema); and the potential complication of altered cardiac output related to congestive heart failure; anaphylaxis; and hypokalemic syndrome (weakness, anorexia, nausea, arrhythmia, muscle cramps).

Implementation

Monitoring. Weigh daily and report weight increases to the prescriber. Monitor intake and output. Periodically assess the client's blood pressure and check for evidence of edema. If hypertension develops, adjust the salt intake and consult with the prescriber to modify the dosage of the steroid.

Periodic serum electrolyte determinations are recommended. Because there is a potential for hypokalemia, be aware that excessive loss of potassium can cause dysrhythmias and sudden weakness, palpitations, paresthesia, or nausea.

Intervention. Provide the client a diet that is low in sodium and high in potassium and protein.

Education. Advise the client to arrange periodic checking of the serum electrolyte levels, especially during prolonged therapy, and to implement dietary salt restrictions. Use of a potassium supplement may be necessary.

Instruct the client to take daily weight measurements and to report a sudden weight gain to the prescriber. Consult with the prescriber for specific weight-gain limitations for each individual client.

Advise the client to carry a medical identification and to notify health care providers of the medication regimen.

Evaluation. The client will not evidence any signs of fluid volume deficit and other signs and symptoms of mineralocorticoid insufficiency or any adverse effects of fludrocortisone therapy.

ANTIADRENALS (ADRENAL STEROID INHIBITORS)

Aminoglutethimide, metyrapone, and trilostane are antiadrenals or adrenal steroid inhibitors. They inhibit or suppress adrenal cortex function.

aminoglutethimide [a mee noe gloo teth' i mide] (Cytadren)
Aminoglutethimide inhibits the enzyme conversion of cholesterol or pregnenolone, thereby blocking the synthesis of adrenal steroids. It also may have other suppression effects in the synthesis and metabolism of the steroids. It also inhibits estrogen production from androgens by blocking an enzyme in the peripheral tissues and may also enhance estrone metabolism; thus it is investigationally used to treat breast cancer. It is indicated for the treatment of Cushing's syndrome associated with adrenal carcinoma, ectopic adrenocorticotropic hormone tumors, or adrenal gland hyperplasia.

Aminoglutethimide is absorbed orally and has a half-life of 13 hours, which is reduced to 7 hours after chronic therapy. Time to peak concentration is 1.5 hours with adrenal function suppression occurring within 3 to 5 days of therapy. Aminoglutethimide is metabolized in the liver and excreted by the kidneys. Table 49-5 lists side effects/adverse reactions.

The adult oral dosage is 250 mg two or three times daily for approximately 14 days; maintenance dose is 250 mg every 6 hours four times daily. A pediatric dose has not been established.

■ Nursing Management

Aminoglutethimide Therapy

Assessment. Because of the cortical hypofunction, use antiadrenals cautiously in clients undergoing stress such as surgery, infection, trauma, and acute illness. Aminoglutethimide should not be administered to clients with or recent exposure to chickenpox and herpes zoster or other infections because the disease may become more generalized.

Do not give to pregnant women, since aminoglutethimide causes increased fetal deaths and teratogenic effects. Geriatric clients may be more sensitive to the CNS effects of the drug and become lethargic.

Obtain baseline lying and standing blood pressures, serum electrolyte levels, thyroid function studies, and AST (SGOT) concentrations.

The only significant drug interaction reported in the *USP DI* (1996) is with dexamethasone. Aminoglutethimide increases the metabolism of dexamethasone, thus reducing its effectiveness. If a glucocorticoid is necessary for a client receiving aminoglutethimide, hydrocortisone is usually the drug of choice.

Nursing diagnosis. The client receiving aminoglutethimide is at risk for the following nursing diagnoses: injury related to the CNS effects of hypotension, drowsiness, dizziness, and clumsiness; altered nutrition related to gastrointestinal effects, evidenced by anorexia and nausea (12%); body image disturbance related to masculinization and hirsutism in females; altered comfort related to dermatologic effects (measles-like rash), headache, and muscle pain; and the potential complications of allergic response, hypothyroidism and goiter, thrombocytopenia, leukopenia, and agranulocytosis.

Implementation

Monitoring. Monitor thyroid function studies periodically during therapy. Since this drug can cause blood dyscrasias and liver and electrolyte abnormalities, routinely monitor serum electrolytes and hematologic and liver function studies. Since hypotension (weakness, dizziness) is caused by aldosterone suppression, monitor blood pressure. If the aminoglutethimide is administered for adrenal disorders, plasma cortisol or 24-hour urinary 17-hydroxycorticosteroid concentrations should be monitored to determine if steroid supplementation is required. In prostatic carcinoma, serum acid phosphatase concentrations will indicate the client's response to therapy; concentrations should decrease.

Intervention. Clients receiving this drug should be under the care of an oncologist or endocrinologist. Consult with the physician about lowering the dosage if CNS side effects occur.

Education. Because the client may experience orthostatic hypotension, advise the client to change position or to stand slowly to minimize this effect. Alert the client to avoid activities that require alertness until response to the drug has been determined.

Instruct the client to alert other health care providers that the drug is being taken and to carry a medical identification card indicating such. The prescriber should be notified if injury, infection, or illness occurs because a steroid supplement may be needed.

TABLE 49-5 Antiadrenal drugs: side effects/adverse reactions

Drug	Side effects*	Adverse reactions†
aminoglutethimide (Cytadren)	Most frequent: Ataxia, dizziness, sedation, loss of energy, uncontrolled eye movements (CNS effects are usually dose related; effects may decline in 2-6 weeks of continuous therapy but if severe, drug may need to be stopped); anorexia, nausea, vomiting, measle-like rash on face and/or palms of hands Rare: Dark skin, depression, dizziness, headaches, pain in muscles	Rare: Increased temperature, chills, sore throat (caused by leukopenia or agranulocytosis), fever or jaundice of eyes and skin (hypersensitivity), increased bleeding episodes or unusual bruising (thrombocytopenia)
trilostane (Modrastane)	Most frequent: Diarrhea, abdominal distress Less frequent: Muscle aches, headache, increased temperature, flushing, increased salivation, nausea, dizziness, gas, burning sensation in mouth or nose, watery eyes	Rare: Dark skin, sedation, anorexia, vomiting, rash, depression

*If side effects continue, increase, or disturb the client, the prescriber should be informed.

†If adverse reactions occur, contact the prescriber, since medical intervention may be necessary.

Evaluation. The client will experience an improvement in the signs and symptoms of the underlying condition without any adverse effects of the drug.

metyrapone [me tyr' a pone} (Metopirone)
Metyrapone inhibits synthesis of cortisol and corticosterone in the adrenal cortex. It is indicated to test the hypothalamic-pituitary ACTH function.

Metyrapone is administered orally and has a half-life of 20 to 26 minutes; peak diagnostic effect is within 24 hours with liver metabolism and renal excretion. Its major side effects include nausea, stomach distress, dizziness, headache, drowsiness, and rash.

While no significant drug interaction has been reported with metyrapone, a number of drugs may interfere with its laboratory test results. Estrogens, corticosteroids, and hepatic enzyme inducers have been reported to produce significant interference with laboratory measurements (*USP DI*, 1996). All corticosteroid drugs should be discontinued 24 to 48 hours before and during testing with this drug. Because there are several recommended dosing methods for testing of pituitary function, the student is referred to a current package insert or reference for specific instructions. The adult dosage of metyrapone is 750 mg orally every 4 hours for six doses.

■ Nursing Management
MetyraponeTherapy

Assessment. The ability of the adrenal gland to respond to exogenous ACTH should be determined before the test, since acute adrenal insufficiency is precipitated in clients with reduced adrenal secretory capacity. Note that metyrapone testing requires that all corticosteroid therapy be stopped before and during testing. It should not be used with hypopituitarism because of the possibility of precipitating acute adrenal insufficiency or hypoglycemia.

Nursing diagnosis. The client is at risk for the following nursing diagnoses: altered protection related to bone marrow depression (sore throat or fever, unusual bleeding, weakness, lethargy); fluid volume excess (edema); altered comfort (headache, anorexia, and nausea); altered thought processes (confusion); disturbed body image related to hirsutism or alopecia; and the potential complications of hypokalemic alkalosis (weakness, arrhythmias, muscle cramps) and acute adrenal insufficiency (confusion, thirst, arrhythmias, decreased consciousness).

Implementation

Monitoring. Monitor the client's blood pressure, pulse, and serum electrolyte levels. Plasma determinations of ACTH and cortisol may be monitored, as well as urinary free cortisol, to titrate the dose and to indicate continued effectiveness.

Intervention. Administer with milk or food to decrease gastrointestinal distress.

There is a 2-day test for pituitary functioning in which oral metyrapone is administered at 2300 hours, and then at 0800 the following morning a blood sample is collected for plasma 11-deoxycortisol and/or corticotropin (ACTH) concentrations. There is also a 6-day test for which the reader should consult the institutional protocol.

Education. Explain to the client the purpose and procedures for this test. Alert the client to symptoms of drowsiness, dizziness, and lightheadedness and the need to modify activities until the client's response to the drug has stabilized.

Evaluation. The client will experience decreased signs and symptoms of secondary adrenocortical insufficiency or Cushing's syndrome.

trilostane [trye' loe stane] (Modrastane)
Trilostane suppresses synthesis of adrenal steroids by inhibiting specific enzymes in the adrenal cortex. It is indicated for the treatment of Cushing's syndrome.

Trilostane has a half-life of 8 hours and is metabolized by the liver. For side effects/adverse reactions, see Table 49-5.

The oral adult dosage is 30 mg four times daily increased as necessary according to patient response. Maximum dose is 480 mg/day. Pediatric dosage has not been established.

■ Nursing Management
Trilostane Therapy

Assessment. Trilostane is contraindicated in clients with adrenal insufficiency, severe renal disease, or hepatic disease. Because trilostane may prevent physiologic responses to stress, it may be discontinued briefly before surgery or in times of physiologic stress, such as trauma, infection, or shock. It has no significant drug interactions.

Nursing diagnosis. Clients are at risk for the nursing diagnoses of altered comfort (abdominal cramping, headache, nausea, and flushing); altered bowel elimination pattern (diarrhea); and the potential complication of adrenal insufficiency evidenced by anorexia, tiredness, nausea, vomiting, rash, depression, and darkening of the skin.

Implementation

Monitoring. Monitor the blood pressure periodically and alert the prescriber if hypotension becomes a concern for the client. Monitor serum electrolytes for imbalances. Clinical response is usually assessed by 8 AM plasma cortisol or 24-hour urinary 17-hydroxycorticosteroid determinations.

Intervention. Clients receiving this drug should be under the care of a clinical endocrinologist. The client is usually hospitalized, or monitored frequently on an outpatient basis, until the dosage is adjusted to produce the desired level of adrenal suppression.

Education. Because orthostatic hypotension may occur with the drug, alert the client to change positions or come to a standing position slowly. Stress the importance of carrying medical identification stating that the medication is being used. Alert the client to check with the prescriber immediately if injury, infection, or other illness occurs, because of the risk of adrenal insufficiency.

Evaluation. The client will evidence the desired level of adrenal suppression.

SUMMARY

Drugs affecting the adrenal cortex—corticosteroids—are divided into glucocorticoids and mineralocorticoids. Glucocorticoids have many pharmacologic actions: antiinflammatory action; maintenance of blood pressure; fat, carbohydrate, and protein metabolism; thymolytic, lympholytic, and eosinopenic actions; and stress effects. Mineralocorticoids act on the renal distal tubules to reabsorb sodium and enhance the excretion of potassium and hydrogen. Because the actions of both of these groups of agents affect all aspects of the body's physiology, evaluation of the client for therapeutic effects and adverse reactions of their administration is particularly important. Of the antiadrenals or adrenal steroid inhibitors, aminoglutethimide and trilostane are used for the treatment of Cushing's syndrome, whereas metyrapone is used as an agent to test hypothalamic-pituitary ACTH function.

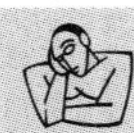

Critical Thinking

1. A 28-year-old man is brought to the emergency department 2 hours after a motorcycle accident. The client is conscious upon admission, with stable vital signs and with minimal abrasions to the left side of his body. A neurologic examination reveals an absence of light touch and pinprick sensation in both lower extremities, lower-extremity paralysis, and no reflexes below the groin. He is started on high-dose intravenous methylprednisolone. Why is a corticosteroid indicated? What observations and interventions by the nurse will be necessary?
2. Bella (1992) reports that misunderstanding about steroid use generated by recent publicity about steroid abuse by athletes has contributed to a widespread "steroid phobia." Why would that be so? How would you counter this impression in a newly diagnosed asthmatic client who has been prescribed corticosteroid inhalers?

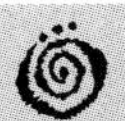

Collaborative Learning Activities

1. Groups of students will collaborate in the development of nursing care plans related to the glucocorticoid therapy for different clinical situations: (1) a 28-year-old woman undergoing treatment for cerebral edema; (2) a 72-year-old man being administered a dexamethasone suppression test for Cushing's syndrome; (3) a 37-year-old woman with acute exacerbation of multiple sclerosis; and (4) a 9-year-old boy with adrenocortical insufficiency.

BIBLIOGRAPHY

American Hospital Formulary Service (1996). *AHFS drug information '96*. Bethesda, MD: American Society of Hospital Pharmacists.

Anderson KN, et al. (Eds.) (1994). *Mosby's medical, nursing, & allied health dictionary* (4th ed.). St. Louis: Mosby.

Buckley S & Kudsk KA (1994). Metabolic response to critical illness and injury, *AACN Clin Issues Crit Care Nurs* 5(4):443-9.

Epstein CD (1992). Adrenocortical insufficiency in the critically ill patient, *AACN* 3(3):705-13.

Greenberger PA (1992). Corticosteroids in asthma: Rationale, use, and problems, *Chest* 101(6):418S.

Hilton G & Frei J (1991). High-dose methylprednisolone in the treatment of spinal cord injuries, *Heart Lung* 20(6):675.

Katzung BG (1992). Basic and clinical pharmacology (5th ed.). Norwalk, CT: Appleton & Lange.

Melmon KL, et al. (1992). *Clinical pharmacology* (3rd ed.). New York: McGraw-Hill.

Olin BR (Ed.) (1996). *Facts and comparisons*. St Louis: Facts and Comparison.

Schimmer BP & Parker KL (1996). Adrenocorticotropic hormone: Adrenocortical steroids and their synthetic analogs; inhibitors of the synthesis and actions of adrenocortical hormones. In Hardman JG & Limbird LE (Eds.). *Goodman & Gilman's the pharmacological basis of therapeutics* (9th ed.). New York: McGraw-Hill.

United States Pharmacopeial Convention (1996). *USP DI: Drug information for the health care professional* (16th ed.). Rockville, MD: The Convention.

Chapter 50

Drugs Affecting the Pancreas

Chapter Focus

Diabetes mellitus is the most important disease involving the pancreas. It affects approximately 5% of the United States population, half of whom are undiagnosed. The incidence is equal in males and females and increases with age. Clients with diabetes have to effectively manage their lives to maintain a balance between lifestyle and treatment. To assist them in this process, nurses need to be knowledgeable about diabetes mellitus and the drugs affecting the disease process. The following objectives and key terms are necessary for a good understanding of this chapter.

Key Terms

glucagon (p. 794)
gluconeogenesis (p. 807)
glycogenesis (p. 794)
glycogenolysis (p. 794)
insulin (p. 795)
insulin-dependent diabetes mellitus (IDDM) (p. 794)
non–insulin-dependent diabetes mellitus (NIDDM) (p. 794)

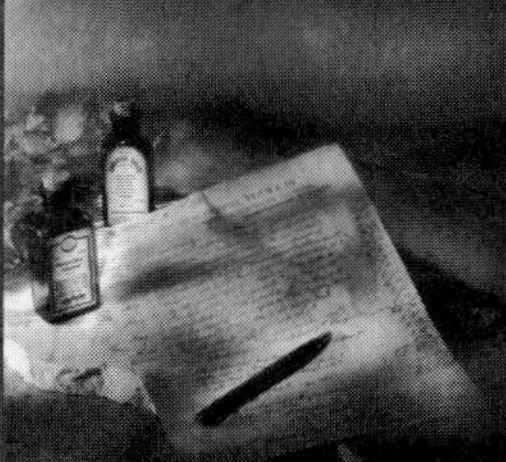

Key Drugs [▲]

acarbose
glucagon
insulin
tolbutamide

Objectives

1. Describe insulin-dependent diabetes mellitus (type I) and non–insulin-dependent diabetes mellitus (type II).
2. Compare and contrast the different insulin preparations.
3. Discuss oral hypoglycemic agents and related nursing management of the client's therapeutic regimen.
4. List hyperglycemic agents and their mechanisms of action.
5. Implement nursing management of clients receiving agents affecting the pancreas.

The primary hormones released by the pancreas are insulin and glucagon. When serum blood glucose declines, **glucagon,** which is synthesized in the alpha cells of the pancreatic islets, facilitates the catabolism of stored glycogen in the liver. The result is **glycogenolysis** or the conversion of glycogen to glucose, resulting in an increase in blood glucose (Figure 50-1). The release of glucagon stimulates insulin secretion, which then inhibits the release of glucagon. Thus the feedback mechanism serves to keep glucose within a desired serum level. When blood glucose increases, glycogenesis, or the conversion of excess glucose to glycogen for storage on skeletal muscle and the liver, occurs.

The most important disease involving the endocrine pancreas is diabetes mellitus, a disorder of carbohydrate metabolism that involves either an insulin deficiency, insulin resistance, or both. All causes of diabetes lead to hyperglycemia (see Chapter 46, Overview of the Endocrine System).

HYPERGLYCEMIA

The two general classifications for diabetes mellitus are **type I** or **insulin-dependent diabetes mellitus** (**IDDM**) and **type II, non–insulin-dependent diabetes mellitus** (**NIDDM**). Clients with type I diabetes have very little or usually no endogenous insulin capacity. This type of diabetes usually occurs before the age of 30 and was previously called juvenile-onset diabetes. The client with type I diabetes is prone to ketosis and requires exogenous insulin therapy for survival.

Type II diabetes was previously known as maturity-onset diabetes because the age of onset is usually over 40 years old. About 90% of the diabetic population is type II (Koda-Kimble & Carlisle, 1995). Generally, clients with this type of diabetes have some insulin function, so they are not fully dependent on insulin for survival. Often weight reduction through dietary adjustments will help reduce hyperglycemia in clients with type II diabetes. The vast majority of individuals with type II diabetes are obese, and ketosis is rare.

Diet, exercise and, if necessary, an oral hypoglycemic agent or insulin is necessary to control blood glucose levels.

Although insulin resistance may occasionally occur with type I diabetes, it is believed to be more common in type II diabetes because of receptor and postreceptor defects. Box 50-1 gives a comparison of the primary features of both types of diabetes.

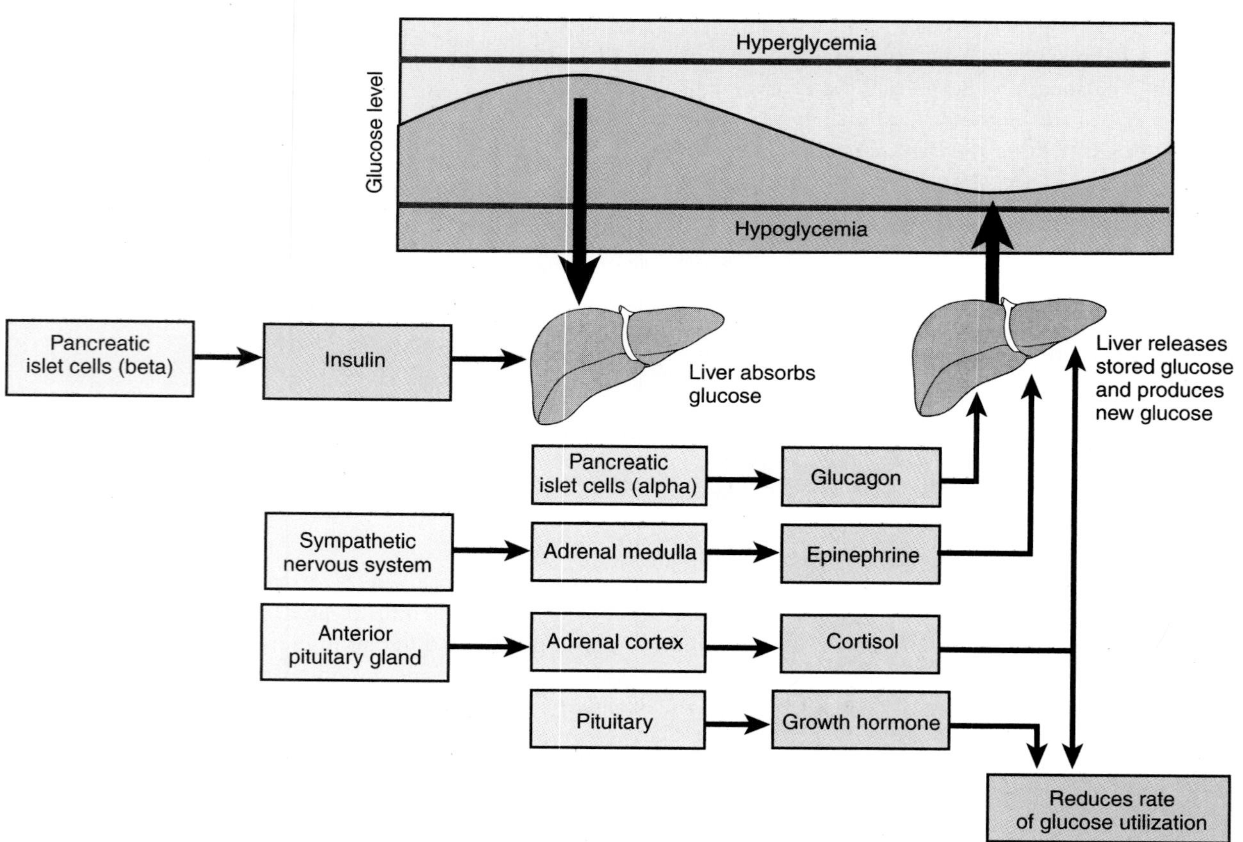

Figure 50-1 Insulin causes the liver to absorb excess blood glucose; when blood glucose levels are low, the alpha cells in the islets of Langerhans secrete glucagon, which stimulates liver glycogenolysis and gluconeogenesis. The sympathetic nervous sytem signals the adrenal medulla to secrete epinephrine while the anterior pituitary gland affects the adrenal cortex to release cortisol. Both substances enhance gluconeogenesis while epinephrine also increases glycogenolysis and cortisol slows down the rate of glucose utilization and also increases the plasma level of amino acids available for glucose production. The pituitary secretes growth hormone that decreases cellular glucose utilization and promotes glycogenolysis.

INSULIN PREPARATIONS

▲ **Insulin,** which is normally synthesized and secreted by the beta cells of the pancreas, is composed of two amino acid chains, A (acidic) and B (basic), joined together by disulfide linkages.

Insulin preparations are derived from animals (extracted from beef or pork pancreas) or synthesized in the laboratory from either an alteration of pork insulin or recombinant DNA technology using strains of *E. coli* to form human insulin (a biosynthetic human insulin). Beef insulin differs from human insulin by three amino acids, whereas the pork insulin differs from human insulin by only a single amino acid. The human (or recombinant) insulin is identical to the insulin produced by the pancreas.

Many diabetics do well on the beef-pork combination insulins if they have not developed insulin resistance, insulin allergies, or lipoatrophy (a breakdown of subcutaneous fat occurring after repeated injections) at the same insulin injection sites. The beef-only insulins were indicated mainly for clients who are allergic to pork or for use in clients who must avoid the use of pork for religious reasons. There is a higher degree of immunogenicity reported with beef and beef-pork insulin than with pork insulin (Koda-Kimble & Carlisle, 1995).

Pork insulin has been found to be useful for clients who have local or systemic allergies, insulin resistance, or lipoatrophy or for clients who have a short-term need for insulin. The pure pork insulin is closer to human insulin, and in many instances its use has resulted in reduction of the insulin dose (in insulin resistance) and in the improvement of local allergy (erythema, induration, and pruritus at injection site) in approximately 80% of the clients with insulin allergies.

Human insulin can be substituted for the same reasons as pork insulin, especially in persons allergic to pork, because it is much less antigenic than the animal-based insulin. Subcutaneous human insulin may also be absorbed faster and have a shorter duration of action than the animal insulins. It is standard practice now to prescribe human insulin whenever possible. Clients switched from an animal to human insulin should be closely monitored initially because a dosage adjustment may be necessary. As a result of the decreased allergenic effects, skin allergies, and resistance reported with human insulin, it is a commonly prescribed insulin for newly diagnosed diabetics and pregnant women (Davis & Granner, 1996; Melmon et al, 1992).

A new, fast-acting insulin analog, insulin lispro (Humalog) was approved for release in 1996. This insulin utilizes regular human insulin and reverses the sequence of two amino acids in it. The primary advantage of the new insulin is it has a more rapid onset of action than regular insulin, therefore it can be administered 15 minutes before a meal. It also has an earlier peak effect and a shorter duration of action, therefore insulin dependent diabetics will usually require concurrent use of a long acting insulin product (Rodgers, 1996).

Insulin controls the storage and metabolism of carbohydrate, protein, and fat binding to receptor sites on cellular plasma membranes, especially in the liver, muscle, and adipose tissues. While insulin's exact molecular mechanism of action is still being investigated, it is known that insulin influences cell membrane transport, cell growth, enzyme activation and inhibition, and the metabolism of protein and fats.

Insulin is indicated for the treatment of diabetes mellitus, insulin-dependent (Type I, IDDM) and for treatment in non–insulin-dependent diabetes mellitus during emergencies or in specific situations, such as supplementation in the client with low physiologic endogenous insulin during high fevers, severe infection, ketoacidosis, severe burns, after major surgery and severe trauma, or during pregnancy.

The wide variety of insulins (including combination mixtures) available allow for sufficient blood glucose control to meet a diabetic's individual need and lifestyle. Maintaining glucose levels as close to normal as possible will

BOX 50-1

Features of Insulin-Dependent (IDDM) and Non–Insulin-Dependent (NIDDM) Diabetes

	IDDM	NIDDM
Synonym	Type I	Type II
Age of onset	Usually <30 years	Usually >35 years
Onset of symptoms	Sudden (symptomatic)	Gradual (usually asymptomatic)
Body weight	Usually nonobese	Obese (80%)
Family history	Usually negative	Often positive
Incidence	10%	90%
Insulin levels	Low then absent	May be low, normal, or high (insulin resistance)
Insulin dependent	Yes	Usually not required
Insulin resistance	No	Yes
Receptors	Normal	Usually decreased or defective
Plasma insulin	Decreased	Normal or increased
Complications	Frequent	Frequent
Ketoacidosis	Prone to	Usually resistant
Dietary modifications	Mandatory	Mandatory

TABLE 50-1 Characteristics of insulin preparations after subcutaneous administration

Insulins*	Onset (hr)	Peak effect (hr)	Duration of action (hr)
Rapid acting			
insulin injection (Regular Insulin, Humalin R)†	½-1	2-4	5-7
Intermediate acting			
isophane insulin suspension (NPH Insulin)	3-4	6-12	18-28
insulin zinc suspension (Lente Insulin)	1-3	8-12	18-28
Long acting			
extended insulin zinc suspension (Ultralente)	4-6	18-24	36
Combinations			
isophane human insulin (50%) & human insulin (50%) (Humalin 50/50)	½	3	22-24
isophane human insulin (70%) & human insulin (30%) (Humalin 70/30, Novalin 70/30)	½	4-8	24

*Semilente insulin is available in Canada but is no longer available in the United States. Onset of action of Semilente insulin is 1-3 hr, peak effect is in 2-8 hr, and duration of action is 12-16 hr.
†These insulins may be administered intravenously. Intravenously, the onset of action is within ⅙ to ½ hr, peak effect within ¼ to ½ hr, and duration of action within ½ to 1 hr.

BOX 50-2

Symptoms of Hypoglycemia and Hyperglycemia

Persons administering insulin should be aware of the symptoms of hypoglycemia and hyperglycemia and know what action to take if they occur.

Hypoglycemia: Increased anxiety, blurred vision, chilly sensation, cold sweating, pallor, confusion, difficulty in concentrating, drowsiness, headache, nausea, increased pulse rate, shakiness, increased weakness, increased appetite

Hyperglycemia: Drowsiness; red, dry skin; fruity breath odor; anorexia; abdominal pain; nausea, vomiting; dry mouth; increased urination; rapid, deep breathing; unusual thirst; rapid weight loss

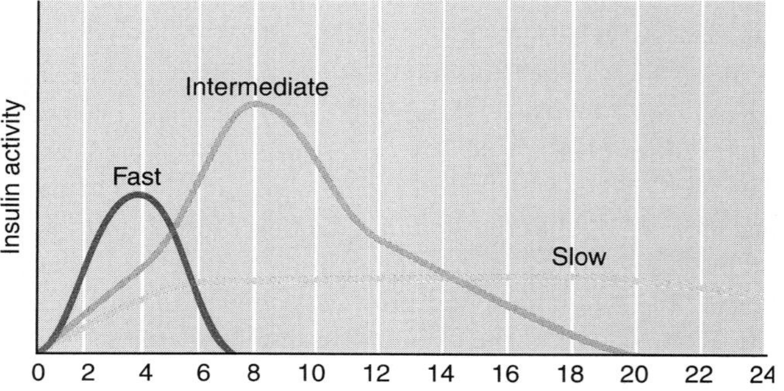

Figure 50-2 Insulin pharmacokinetics (see Table 50-1).

help to improve the person's quality of life and also reduce the progression of complications associated with diabetes (Campbell, 1992).

Table 50-1 describes insulin pharmacokinetics.

There is no average dose of insulin for the diabetic person; each client's needs must be determined individually to attain euglycemia and to avoid hypoglycemia and hyperglycemia. Box 50-2 lists the symptoms of these adverse effects of ineffective management of the therapeutic regimen. To maintain euglycemia, blood glucose levels are frequently determined by blood glucose monitoring, which has been simplified by the availability of both visual test strips and strips used in blood glucose meters or instruments. Such devices allow clients to monitor their diabetes and make the necessary adjustments with medication, diet, and exercise, as instructed by their physician or health care provider. The visual glucose testing strips are less expensive than the testing instruments, but the meter readings are much more precise (assuming they are properly calibrated). Thus clients with visual problems or a need for a more accurate blood glucose reading will benefit from using a blood glucose meter instrument.

Insulin dosage is expressed in units rather than in milliliters. Insulin injection is standardized so that each milliliter contains 100 USP units. Insulin is classified according to its duration of action (short- or rapid-acting, intermediate-acting, and long-acting (Figure 50-2). Generally meals should occur at the same time that administered insulin reaches its peak effect. Insulin requirements can vary widely among individuals, so dosages must be adjusted to an individual's needs.

Clients with diabetes who become hyperglycemic, perhaps because of hospitalization or an infection, may need insulin coverage in addition to their regular insulin. The amount of insulin given will vary with the blood glucose values or (in some instances) with the glucose in the urine; this titration is known as "sliding-scale" administration of in-

Nursing Research

The effect of long-term intensified insulin treatment on the development of microvascular complications of diabetes mellitus

Microvascular complications develop in many clients with insulin-dependent diabetes mellitus (IDDM), and the effect of intensified insulin treatment on these complications has not been established.

This study randomly assigned 102 individuals with IDDM, nonproliferative retinopathy (a noninflammatory eye disorder resulting from changes in the retinal blood vessel), normal serum creatinine concentrations, and unsatisfactory blood glucose control to intensified insulin treatment (48 participants) or standard insulin treatment (54 participants). The participants were then evaluated for microvascular complications after 18 months and 3, 5, and 7.5 years.

The results of the study were as follows: Mean (± SD) glycosylated hemoglobin values were reduced from 9.5 ± 1.3% to 7.1 ± 0.7% in the group receiving intensified treatment and from 9.4 ± 1.4% to 8.5 ± 0.7% in the group receiving standard treatment (P = 0.001). In 12 of the participants receiving intensified treatment (27% of those included in the analysis) and 27 of those receiving standard treatment (52%), serious retinopathy requiring photocoagulation developed (P = 0.01). Visual acuity decreased in 6 participants receiving intensified treatment (14%) and in 18 receiving standard treatment (35%) (P = 0.02). Nephropathy (urinary albumin excretion, >200 μg/minute) developed in one participant in the group receiving intensified treatment compared with 9 participants in the group receiving standard treatment (P = 0.01). No one in the intensified treatment group had neuropathy with subnormal glomerular filtration rates, as compared with 6 participants in the standard treatment group (P = 0.02). The conduction velocities of the ulnar, tibial, peroneal, and sural nerves decreased significantly more in the standard treatment group than in the intensified treatment group. The odds ratio for serious retinopathy was 0.4 (95% confidence interval, 0.2 to 1.0; P = 0.04) in the intensified treatment group as compared with the standard treatment group. The corresponding odds ratio for nephropathy was 0.1 (95% confidence interval, 0 to 0.8; P = 0.04).

The investigators concluded that long-term intensified insulin treatment, as compared with standard treatment, retards the development of microvascular complications in clients with IDDM.

Critical thinking questions

- How does this study support a "tight control" approach to the management of IDDM? What is its contribution to the importance of self-management of care by the client?
- What was the difference in the treatment of the intensified versus the standard treatment groups all other things being equal?
- What else may have been occurring during this study that might contribute to the findings?

From Reichard P, Nilsson BY, & Rosenquist U (1993). The effect of long-term intensified insulin treatment on the development of microvascular complications of diabetes mellitus, *N Engl J Med* 329:304.

sulin. The latter method of testing urine may be used in some health care settings, but it is rarely used now to monitor blood glucose. If at all possible, urine glucose tests should not be used to determine insulin dosages. There may be variations between urine glucose tests; therefore they should not be used interchangeably for urine glucose monitoring. The specific instructions for testing urine for glucose using a particular reagent is included with the testing kit.

Dietary intake, physical activity, ability to manage the therapeutic regimen, and the client's glucose tolerance are all taken into consideration when insulin dosages are established. Insulin dosages should not be considered to be a fixed regimen; the dosage may need to be adjusted as a result of physical growth (child growing into adulthood), illness, stress, the development of antiinsulin antibodies, concomitant administration of certain medications, or changes in exercise and diet. Specific instructions should be obtained regarding insulin administration for the preoperative client because of the alteration in the client's dietary patterns and metabolic requirements as the result of the surgical procedure. Treatment programs need to be reviewed and adjusted as necessary, with the prescriber, nurse, and client working closely to manage hypoglycemia and hyperglycemia and, if possible, avoid their complications. Recent research is supporting closer management for euglycemia (see the Nursing Research box above).

Insulin is given subcutaneously (or intravenously, regular insulin only). It cannot be given by mouth because it is destroyed by digestive enzymes. Regular insulin is usually given about 15 to 30 minutes before meals.

Portable insulin pumps have improved the metabolic state of some type I clients who did not have adequate diabetic control after intensive dietary restrictions and multiple daily injections of insulin. The insulin pump is battery-operated and connected to a small computer that is programmed to release small amounts of insulin per hour. It does not analyze the blood glucose level, however; it is programmed based on the individual's daily insulin needs, diet, and physical exercise. The client can also push a button that releases a bolus dose to cover each meal consumed.

Although the pumps are effective and useful in clients who are properly trained, health care professionals need to be aware of several problems associated with them. Malfunction of the insulin infusion may occur because of battery failure, and defects in the tubing may cause leakage of insulin solution or may block the infusion tubing. Therefore it is vitally important to teach the client to change the infusion set and battery. Clients must be highly motivated and educated in the handling of insulin pumps. The client should be capable of keeping records and following specific procedures and should be willing to perform blood tests daily or more often. Also, these pumps are very expensive. Therefore insulin pumps currently are not recommended for every type I diabetic.

Needleless injectors, such as the Vitajet, Medi-jector, and Precijet 50, are also available. These devices are expensive and appear to have limited usefulness in practice. Many devices are also available for the visually impaired client with diabetes. Information on injection aids for the blind may be obtained from state and national associations, such as the American Foundation for the Blind and the American Diabetic Association.

During pregnancy, insulin is the drug of choice to control diabetes. Insulin requirements may drop for 24 to 72 hours after delivery and slowly return to prepregnancy levels in about 6 weeks.

Nursing Management

Insulin Therapy

Assessment. A comprehensive nursing history is necessary for the nurse to help the client manage the diabetic state. This assessment is as essential for the newly diagnosed client with diabetes as it is for clients who are seeking reassurance that they are managing their diabetes appropriately or readjustment of insulin dosage because of stress, illness, change of lifestyle, or ineffective management of the therapeutic regimen. A baseline assessment of the client's blood glucose level is obtained before beginning or changing dosages with insulin therapy.

Determine the client's ideal body weight, present weight, daily exercise, dietary management and preferences, and understanding of diabetes and its control. Also note any physical impairments, such as decreased manual dexterity and limitations of vision, that would impede the self-administration of insulin. Because the cost of insulin, injection equipment, and blood testing equipment can be considerable, assess the client's financial status and health insurance coverage and locate alternative resources if necessary. Clients with certain religious affiliations (such as Jewish or Islamic clients) prefer not to use pork insulin because their dietary codes involve the avoidance of pork.

The client's current medication regimen should also be reviewed for significant drug interactions (Box 50-3). In addition, many commonly abused substances can be very problematic in the client with diabetes (Box 50-4). Box 50-5 lists sugar-free OTC medications. The following interactions may occur when insulin is given concurrently with the drugs listed below.

BOX 50-3

Drugs Reported to Cause Hyperglycemia or Hypoglycemia

Hyperglycemia	Hypoglycemia
baclofen	anabolic steroids
corticosteroids	beta-adrenergic blocking agents
diuretics	disopyramide
estrogens (oral contraceptives)	ethanol
glucagon	monoamine oxidase inhibitors (MAOIs)
NSAIDs	NSAIDs
pentamidine (toxic to pancreatic islet cells)	pentamidine (increases insulin release)
phenytoin	salicylates
sympathomimetics	sulfonamides
thyroid hormones	

(*USP DI*, 1996)

Drug	Possible effect and management
adrenocorticoids, glucocorticoids	Adrenocorticoids and glucocorticoids may increase blood glucose levels. A dosage adjustment of insulin may be necessary. Monitor closely.
alcohol	May increase the hypoglycemic effect of insulin. Monitor closely, since dosage adjustments may be necessary. If possible, avoid the concurrent use of alcohol.
beta-adrenergic blocking agents (including eye preparations)	These agents may mask symptoms of hypoglycemia, such as increased pulse rate and decreased blood pressure. May also prolong hypoglycemia by blocking gluconeogenesis. Dosage adjustments of insulin may be necessary. Selective beta blockers in low dosages, such as metoprolol and atenolol, cause fewer problems than the other beta-adrenergic blocking agents. Propranolol may cause hyperglycemia or hypoglycemia when given concurrently with insulin. Periodic blood glucose tests are recommended to monitor the combined effects and allow for adjustment of insulin dose, if necessary.

A baseline assessment would include: skin (lesions and color); ophthalmologic testing; orientation, peripheral sensation, reflexes; blood pressure, pulse, respirations, lung sounds; urinalysis; and blood glucose levels.

Nursing diagnosis. See the Nursing Care Plan on p. 800.

Implementation

Monitoring. Monitor effectiveness by obtaining blood glucose levels frequently in the client with diabetes, more frequently if the client is under stress, is pregnant, or is recently diagnosed. Glucose-monitoring devices, such as Chemstrip and Dextrostix, which allow for blood glucose monitoring at home, are much more reliable than urine glucose tests and facilitate tighter control of blood sugar levels.

BOX 50-4

Effects of Commonly Abused Drugs on Diabetic Management

Many drugs can increase or decrease blood glucose levels, but rarely are the commonly abused drugs reviewed in relation to diabetes. Because substance abuse by the client with diabetes can be very problematic, the most commonly abused drugs are reviewed here.

Alcohol

Alcohol promotes hypoglycemia; blocks the formation, storage, and release of glycogen. It also may interact with many other drugs, including oral hypoglycemic agents such as chlorpropamide. In alcoholics who have decreased their food intake, alcohol can cause a serious drop in blood glucose levels, leading to a need for acute intervention.

CNS stimulants

Amphetamines, sympathomimetics, anorexics, cocaine, psychedelic drugs, and others may result in hyperglycemia and an increase in liver glycogen breakdown. Large amounts of caffeine in products such as coffee, tea, and cola drinks can also increase blood glucose levels.

Marijuana

Marijuana may increase appetite and food consumption. Heavy use may produce a glucose intolerance leading to hyperglycemia.

Cigarettes

Nicotine in cigarettes is a potent vasoconstrictor. It can decrease the absorption of subcutaneous insulin or increase the person's insulin requirements by 15% to 20%. Cigarette smoking can cause a drop of 1 to 2 degrees in skin temperature. It also is a risk factor for the development of diabetic nephropathy.

Abuse of CNS-acting drugs

CNS-acting drugs (such as stimulants, depressants, sedative-hypnotics, opiates, marijuana, alcohol) can impair judgment and alter perceptions (time, place) and thus interfere with the individual's control of the diabetic state.

Urine glucose testing is less commonly performed because it is an indirect measurement of the client's glycemic status secondary to individual differences in the renal threshold for glucose. Usually glucose spillage into the urine occurs at blood levels of 160 to 180 mg/100 ml, but it may be higher in elderly clients or lower in children and pregnant women. Therefore it may not correlate well with serum glucose levels. The maintenance of euglycemia (70 to 140 mg/100 ml) indicates the appropriate dosage of insulin for the client.

BOX 50-5

Sugar-Free Over-the-Counter Medications

Advise clients to always read bottle labels or check with their pharmacists before purchasing medications. The sugar contents of OTC medications are changed often by the manufacturers, so the best advice is to check the list of contents every time medication is purchased. The following is a select listing of medications currently listed as sugar-free.

Antacids, antiflatulents

Maalox Anti-Gas
Maalox Extra Strength
Mylanta
Riopan
Titralac Extra Strength Antacid
Titralac Plus Tablets/Liquids

Antipyretics

Acetaminophen Solution
Bayer Aspirin
Cama-In-Lay Tablets
Motrin IB
Panadol Children's Liquid
Tempra 3 chewable tablets
Tylenol Children's Fruit Flavor

Cough-cold preparations

Benadryl cold
Benylin Expectorant
Diabetic Tussin DM
Diabetic Tussin EX
Naldecon Senior DX and EX
Tussar-SF

From Covington, 1996.

Glycosylated hemoglobin determinations are done to more comprehensively evaluate the adequacy of diabetic control and give information not available in individual blood and urine glucose tests. Clients with diabetes may have undetected periods of hyperglycemia alternating with post-insulin periods of euglycemia or hypoglycemia. High Hb A_{1c} determinations indicate inadequate diabetic control for the previous 3 to 5 weeks (Watson & Jaffe, 1995).

Monitor the client for signs and symptoms of hyperglycemia and hypoglycemia. Observe injection sites for impaired tissue integrity, such as lipoatrophy or lipohypertrophy (a buildup of subcutaneous fat tissue).

In the primary care setting clients are evaluated periodically for the complications of diabetes mellitus related to the ineffectiveness of insulin therapy including: visual impairment (ophthalmic exam); nephropathy (complete urinalysis [including protein], blood urea nitrogen, serum creatinine); neuropathy (neurologic exam); increased atherosclerotic disease (serum cholesterol, high-density lipoprotein cholesterol,

Nursing Care Plan

Selected Nursing Diagnoses for Clients Receiving Insulin

Nursing diagnosis	Outcome criteria	Nursing interventions
Knowledge deficit related to newly diagnosed diabetes	Client and family will: Demonstrate an understanding of diabetes, its therapy and complications, and measures to minimize or prevent complications	Assess the understanding and learning ability of client and family. Determine educational needs and desires. Provide information regarding the pathophysiology of diabetes and the function of insulin. Explain methods and goals of diet and drug therapy. Explain function and purpose of tests. Answer questions and clarify misconceptions. Provide resources for further learning and support (American Diabetes Association [ADA], Juvenile Diabetes Foundation [JDF], and others).
Knowledge deficit related to newly prescribed diabetic medication (insulin)	Client and family will: Demonstrate correctly appropriate storage, handling, and administration of insulin Be familiar with the signs and symptoms of insulin reaction/hypoglycemia reaction and appropriate response State the different insulin preparations and appropriate adjustment of drug therapy Be aware of possible side effects or adverse reactions to insulin	Teach the client and family: The function and importance of therapy; name and dosage of insulin Technique of blood (or urine) glucose monitoring and adjusting insulin appropriately Proper technique of administration Need for lifelong dietary and drug management The differences between the three forms of insulin How to correctly calculate dosages Proper storage and handling of insulin Importance of rotating sites to minimize adverse local reactions Signs and symptoms of insulin/hypoglycemic reaction and appropriate management Help client establish and maintain a monitoring record of blood (or urine) glucose and insulin administration. Advise client to wear or carry a medical identification tag, bracelet, or card. Provide client with a list of drugs and conditions that may alter insulin requirements.
Risk for injury related to hyperglycemia or hypoglycemia due to insulin administration	Client will: Achieve control of blood glucose and maintain desired nutritional intake Client and family will: Demonstrate knowledge of appropriate diabetic diet and modifications of dietary practices	Administer insulin as prescribed Teach client and family: Correct method of blood (or urine) glucose monitoring Signs, symptoms, and treatment for hyperglycemia and hypoglycemia Importance of balanced diabetic diet to control diabetes Provide dietary instruction and counseling in appropriate diet/refer to dietitian. Assist client and family in planning a sample diet.
Body image disturbance related to insulin dependence	Client and family will: Verbalize feelings and concerns Understand disease and measures of control Client will: Maintain, as much as possible, prediagnosis activities	Encourage client and family to express feelings and concerns. Determine assets and strengths. Determine, with client and family, strategies for managing areas of difficulty or concern. Provide resources for further learning and support (ADA, JDF, others). Be alert for signs of nonacceptance or difficulties such as ineffective management of therapeutic regimen or denial.

Nursing Care Plan

Selected Nursing Diagnoses for Clients Receiving Insulin–cont'd

Nursing diagnosis	Outcome criteria	Nursing interventions
Feelings of powerlessness related to perceived lack of personal control	Client and family will: Identify those areas of diabetes that are possible to control and participate in decision making related to diabetic management	Assess client and family coping patterns and support mechanisms. Assess client and family perceptions related to diagnosis. Allow and encourage expression of concerns and fears. Encourage client and family participation in therapy planning and implementation.

serum triglycerides, ECG, peripheral pulses, bruits); and foot and skin exam for problem areas (ADA, 1990).

Intervention. Note that all insulin preparations are stable as long as the vials are protected from heat or cold; store in a cool place, but do not freeze. Regular (concentrated) Iletin I is available as U-500 for clients who have developed insulin resistance and require large doses. Take care not to store U-500 insulin in the same area as other insulin preparations because of the possibility of massive overdose if it is accidentally administered to a client.

Vials of insoluble preparations (all except regular insulin) should be rotated between the hands and inverted end-to-end several times before a dose is withdrawn. A vial should not be shaken vigorously or the suspension made to foam. Do not interchange human, beef, or pork insulins, since species differences may require a dosage change, or use insulin that has become clumped or granular in appearance.

Use a properly calibrated syringe for insulin. For doses of less than 50 units of U-100, use a low-dose syringe (50 units of U-100/0.5 ml). The decreased diameter of the barrel of the syringe results in the calibrations being further apart, which enhances accuracy of measurement. Avoid bubbles in the solution because the displacement of a few units of insulin, particularly with U-100 insulin, can alter the actual dose that the client receives.

Administer the insulin subcutaneously, using a 25- or 26-gauge needle, with the length of the needle determined by the client's size. A ⅜- to ⅝-inch needle is usually used, and the injection is administered at a 90-degree angle in a large fold of skin that has been gently pinched up. Alternately, the injection may be inserted at a 30- to 45-degree angle at the base of the fold of skin. Apply pressure but do not rub the site after injection because it alters the absorption rate. Rotate injection sites. Because of the differences in absorption from different anatomic sites, rotate injections with a pattern, e.g., morning injections rotated within the abdominal region, evening injections in the thighs.

Understand that only the regular form of insulin may be injected by the intravenous route. Insulin adsorption onto plastic intravenous infusion administration sets removes up to 80% of an insulin dose; most often not less than 20% to 50% of a dose is removed by adsorption. The adsorption on the tubing surface occurs within 1 hour and requires individual client monitoring of insulin needs. Saturation of the adsorption sites on the tubing requires special care when changing the tubing for reexposure to the insulin and further monitoring of client needs. Adsorption can be minimized by injecting directly into the vein, using an intermittent infusion device, or using a port close to the IV access site. When insulin is administered as an infusion, use an intravenous pump for accurate administration.

Education. Instruct clients on the relationship of diabetes to the administration of insulin, blood glucose monitoring, and the necessity to maintain euglycemia. Teach clients about blood glucose monitoring so they can adjust insulin doses when their blood levels are above normal limits. To help prevent soreness from daily finger sticks, instruct the client to use the left thumb on Monday, the left index finger on Tuesday, and so on through Friday. The right thumb can be used on Saturday and the right index finger on Sunday. The other three fingers can be used as alternates in case of an unsuccessful finger stick on another day. If finger sticks are done twice a day, instruct the client to use the left thumb on Monday morning, the left index finger on Monday afternoon, the left middle finger on Tuesday morning and so on. The client will use all of the fingers this way, and by Saturday can start the sticks with the left thumb again (Vibulbhan, 1993).

Instruct the client in the administration of insulin, including the type of insulin, the proper storage of insulin, the disposal of syringes, and rotation of injection sites.

Have the client agitate the vial, unless using regular insulin, and properly cleanse the top with 70% isopropyl alcohol. To draw any insulin out of a vial, inject the vial with an amount of air equal to the insulin dose. This prevents a negative pressure from occurring in the vial, which would make the withdrawal of the insulin difficult. Teach the client to eliminate air bubbles from the syringe because they decrease the insulin dosage.

When mixing insulins, inject air equal to the dose to be withdrawn into the vial of NPH insulin first. Then inject air into the vial of the regular insulin. Keep the needle in the vial, draw the regular insulin into the syringe first to avoid contamination of the regular insulin vial with the other insulin admixture. Then return to the NPH vial and withdraw the dose of NPH insulin. The onset of the action of regular insulin is delayed when mixed with other insulins. This interaction of regular and NPH insulin occurs within 15 minutes after mixing and then will remain at this stability for 30 days at room temperature and 90 days if refrigerated. Regular and lente mixtures require up to 24 hours for the interaction to reach a stable level of consistent response; if premixed in the same syringe, their activity is also 30 days at room temperature and 90 days under refrigeration. Clients stabilized on this premixed insulin will have a different response if they inject the insulin separately from each component. See the Home Health box at top left on Prefilling of Insulin by Home Health Nurses. Different brands of syringes have sufficient differences in "dead space" (the unmeasured volume between the needle point and the bottom calibration) to cause improper dosages. Dosage errors are avoided by not changing the injection order of mixing insulins or changing the model of needles, brands of syringes, or sources of insulins.

Instruct the client in the planned rotation of injection sites and to observe for lipodystrophies, the occurrence of which may be minimized by rotation. Note that insulin is most rapidly absorbed from the abdomen, followed by the upper arm, then the thigh. Physical activity in the client accelerates absorption, especially in the injected limb; alert joggers and walkers. Teach client that alternating the insulin injection sites from the leg to the abdomen or arm has the effect of accelerating the absorption of insulin and diminishing the postprandial rise in plasma glucose. Varying the insulin injection sites within the same anatomic region rather than between different regions may diminish daily fluctuations or variations in insulin absorption and in metabolic control in insulin-dependent diabetic patients. For example, if the abdomen is used for a morning injection, subsequent morning injections should also be given in the abdomen. Injections at another time of day should always be given in the same part of the body, for example, use thigh sites for before dinner injections. Each injection should be administered an inch away from any previously used site and any site should not be used more frequently than once a month (Box 50-6).

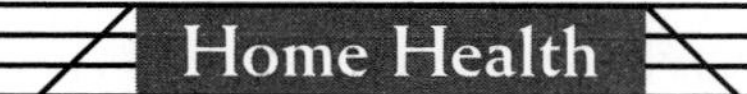

Prefilling of Insulin Syringes by Home Health Nurses

The timing of the chemical interaction following the combination of different types of insulins modifies the clinical effectiveness of the insulins by delaying the onset of action of regular insulin. Home health nurses who prefill insulin syringes with different insulins in the same syringe for their clients for future use in the home should ensure that the client is not administered insulin mixed the same day. The insulin should be administered so there will be consistency of dosage in the insulin therapy. Administering a "fresh" syringe, one mixed within the previous 15 minutes, will be as though the insulins were administered separately and may significantly alter the client's blood glucose levels.

BOX 50-6

Intrasite Rotation of Insulin Injection Sites

A good approach is to instruct the client to mark the first injection site with a spot bandage and give future injections around the bandage. Imagine each circle as a clock, administering injections at 12 o'clock, 3 o'clock, 6 o'clock, and 9 o'clock points before starting a new circle more than an inch away from the previous sites, as shown below.

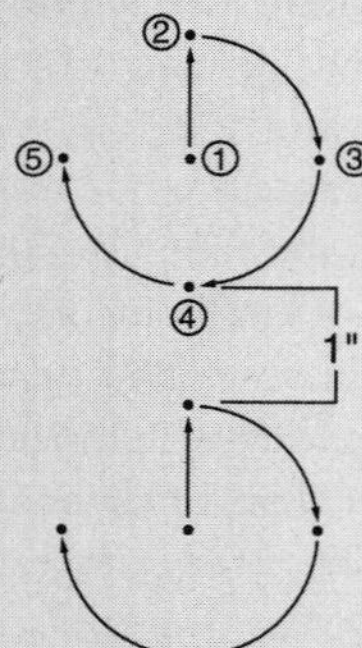

Following this plan, your client can administer five injections per circle. The spot bandage works too as a convenient memory jogger. After having been through 2 or 3 showers, the bandage is usually ready to be removed and a new one applied about the time the circle is complete.

From Drass, 1992.

BOX 50-7

Quick Fixes for Clients with Mild Hypoglycemia

Clients who have the potential to develop hypoglycemia should have ready access to a source of rapid-acting carbohydrate. The following substances contain 10 to 15 g of such a carbohydrate, which will stabilize a client who is having a mild hypoglycemic reaction—usually within 15 minutes. Some forms are easier to carry on a daily basis, such as the glucose tablets and cake frosting below.

- 3 glucose tablets
- 4 oz orange juice
- 6 oz regular soda
- 6-8 oz 2% fat or skim milk
- 6-8 Lifesavers
- 3 graham cracker squares
- 6 jelly beans
- 2 tablespoons raisins
- 1 small (2 oz) tube of cake frosting

From Macheca (1993).

Be sure the client understands that frequent serum glucose monitoring is necessary to achieve insulin control. Stress compliance with the understanding that insulin helps to control hyperglycemia but is not a cure for diabetes.

Instruct clients about signs and symptoms of hypoglycemia that can occur secondary to insulin dosage. A dosage adjustment downward may be necessary to prevent repeated episodes of hypoglycemia. The hypoglycemic individual should have a carbohydrate with a high sugar content promptly, and the prescriber should be notified. If the individual is conscious, orange juice, candy, or a lump of sugar, or a complex carbohydrate such as milk or cheese and crackers can be given (Box 50-7). Early symptoms of hypoglycemia are fatigue, headache, drowsiness, lassitude, tremulousness, or nausea. Late symptoms are weakness, sweating, tremors, or nervousness. Observe the client at night for excessive restlessness and profuse sweating.

Teach clients to assess for signs of hyperglycemia: thirst, polyuria, drowsiness, flushed skin, fruity odor to breath, and unconsciousness. Instruct the family to have regular insulin available for administration and to observe the client closely after insulin has been given.

Discuss the following with the client and family to prevent recurrences of ketoacidosis:

- Use a regimented pattern of diabetic control.
- Never omit antidiabetic drugs, particularly when a secondary illness is manifested.
- Consume clear liquids and eat smaller meals when illness occurs.
- When ill, frequently test blood for glucose levels.
- Notify the prescriber of secondary illness, nausea and vomiting, fever, inability to eat, or inability to control blood glucose levels.

Inform the family and client that the following factors may lead to diabetic ketoacidosis: insulin-dependent diabetes mellitus, omission of insulin, infections, cerebrovascular accidents (stroke), myocardial infarction, pregnancy, trauma, surgery, and stress (especially emotional).

Inform the client that an important part of glucose control is diet therapy. The dietitian and the meal preparer must be included in the total care of the client with diabetes. Before clients are discharged, they must be able to verbalize an understanding of their diet therapy and be willing to participate in meal planning.

Caution clients against the ingestion of alcohol, since hypoglycemia could result. If alcohol is consumed, their insulin dosage may need to be reduced since alcohol potentiates the hypoglycemic effect of insulin.

If the client is using urine testing to assess blood glucose, emphasize that it is important in determining correct insulin dosage. Whichever method of urine testing is used, the client should test the second voided specimen. Urine should be tested before each meal.

At all times the client should carry a medical identification that identifies him or her as a diabetic and describes the therapeutic regimen.

For other aspects of education for the client with diabetes not directly related to insulin therapy, such as skin care, foot care, stress reduction, and dietary regimen, the reader is referred to a general nursing text.

Evaluation. The client's blood glucose level will remain within normal limits and the client will effectively manage the therapeutic insulin regimen. See the case study on p. 807.

ORAL HYPOGLYCEMIC AGENTS

Non–insulin-dependent (type II) diabetics are treated with the oral hypoglycemics, diet, exercise and when necessary, insulin. Currently there are three classifications of oral agents, first and second generation sulfonylureas and a miscellaneous group that includes acarbose and metformin (biguanide classification). Although these drugs are sometimes called "oral insulins," this description is incorrect since chemically they are completely different from insulin. They also differ from insulin in mode of action. See Table 50-2 for pharmacokinetics and usual adult dose.

The first generation sulfonylureas include acetohexamide (Dymelor), chlorpropamide (Diabinese), tolazamide (Tolinase) and tolbutamide (Orinase), which are considered to be, equally effective although they may differ in pharmacokinetics and perhaps, side/adverse reactions. The second generation includes glipizide (Glucotrol) and glyburide (DiaBeta, Micronase), which are much more potent than the previous generation but have not proven to be more therapeutically or clinically effective (Koda-Kimble & Carlisle, 1995).

The advantages in using the second generation are that they have a long duration of action and have less side/adverse effects. In the first generation, tolazamide also has similar advantages.

The sulfonylureas enhance the release of insulin from the beta cells in the pancreas, decrease liver **glycogenolysis** (the breakdown of glycogen stored in the liver to glycogen) and **gluconeogenesis** (the conversion of excess glucose to glycogen for storage in the skeletal muscle and liver), and increase the cellular sensitivity to insulin in body tissues. Therefore they reduce blood glucose concentration in persons with a functioning pancreas (Figure 50-3). In addition, chlorpropamide has an antidiuretic effect; it increases the effect of low levels of antidiuretic hormone present in persons with central diabetes insipidus.

Oral hypoglycemic agents are indicated for the treatment of uncomplicated non–insulin-dependent diabetes mellitus (type II) in persons whose diabetes cannot be controlled by diet only. See Table 50-3 for side effects/adverse reactions.

Miscellaneous Hypoglycemics

▲ **acarbose** [ah car' bohse] (Precose)

Acarbose is the first alpha-glucosidase inhibitor released for the treatment of non–insulin-dependent diabetes mellitus (type II). Inhibition of this enzyme delays carbohydrate digestion and absorption in the small intestine. This product does not increase insulin secretion or cause hypoglycemia, lactic acidosis, or weight gain. It may be given

TABLE 50-2 Hypoglycemic agents: pharmacokinetics and usual adult dose

Generic (brand name)	Onset of action (hr)	Peak effect (hr)	Duration of action (hr)	Usual adult dose	
Sulfonylureas					
First generation					
acetohexamide (Dymelor, Dimelor ♣)	1	1.5-6*	8-24	250-1000 mg/day	Use with caution in elderly and clients with renal insufficiency.
chlorpropamide (Diabinese)	1	2-4	24-72	250-500 mg/day	Longest acting hypoglycemic. More reported side effects than other agents.
tolazamide (Tolinase)	4-6	3-4	10-20	100-500 mg with breakfast	Active metabolites may be increased in renal impairment.
▲ tolbutamide (Orinase, Mobenol ♣)	1	3-4	6-12	250-2000 mg daily in divided doses	Shortest acting agent. Rapidly metabolized to inactive metabolites.
Second generation					
glipizide (Glucotrol)	1-1.5	1-3	12-24	5-40 mg before meals in divided doses	Dose 30 min before meals.
glipizide extended release (Glucotrol XL)	—	6-12	24	5-20 mg with breakfast	
glyburide nonmicronized (Diabeta, Micronase)	2-4	4	24	1.25-20 mg with breakfast, divide dosages >10 mg	Use with caution in elderly clients in renal failure.
glyburide micronized (Glynase PresTab)	1	3	24	0.75-12 mg/day. Doses over 6 mg divided and given with meals	Micronized formula has increased bioavailability, thus lower dose required.
Miscellaneous					
acarbose (Precose)	Not absorbed			50-100 mg with meals	Most effective if given with high-fiber diet.
metformin (Glucophage, Novo-Metformin ♣)	—	2-3	6-12	500 mg or 850 mg bid or tid.	Take with food to reduce nausea & vomiting.

(Davis & Granner, 1996; Koda-Kimble & Carlisle, 1995; Olin, 1996; *USP DI*, 1996.)
*Includes active metabolite, hydroxyhexamide.

alone or in combination with a sulfonylurea to lower blood glucose. This drug is poorly absorbed and may cause dose related side effects of malabsorption, abdominal gas, and bloating (Davis & Granner, 1996). See Table 50-2 for additional information.

metformin [met fore' man] (Glucophage)
Another non-sulfonylurea antihyperglycemic agent for the treatment of type II diabetes is metformin, a biguanide chemical classification. The first drug released in this chemical category was phenformin but due to its association with lactic acidosis, it was withdrawn from the market. Metformin has been associated only rarely with this complication (Davis & Granner, 1996).

Metformin decreases glucose absorption from the intestines, glucose production in the liver, and also improves insulin sensitivity in peripheral tissues. It does not affect the pancreatic beta cells; therefore, it does not increase insulin release nor cause hypoglycemia. For pharmacokinetics and dosing, see Table 50-2. Most commonly reported side/adverse reactions include anorexia, abdominal gas or pain, headache, nausea, and vomiting.

Nursing Management

Oral Hypoglycemic Agent Therapy

Assessment. The client's level of knowledge for health maintenance related to diabetes mellitus and the prescribed oral hypoglycemic agent should be assessed. Information is to be provided or reinforced related to compliance with the appropriate ADA diet for ideal weight attainment, weight monitoring, activity program, stress man-

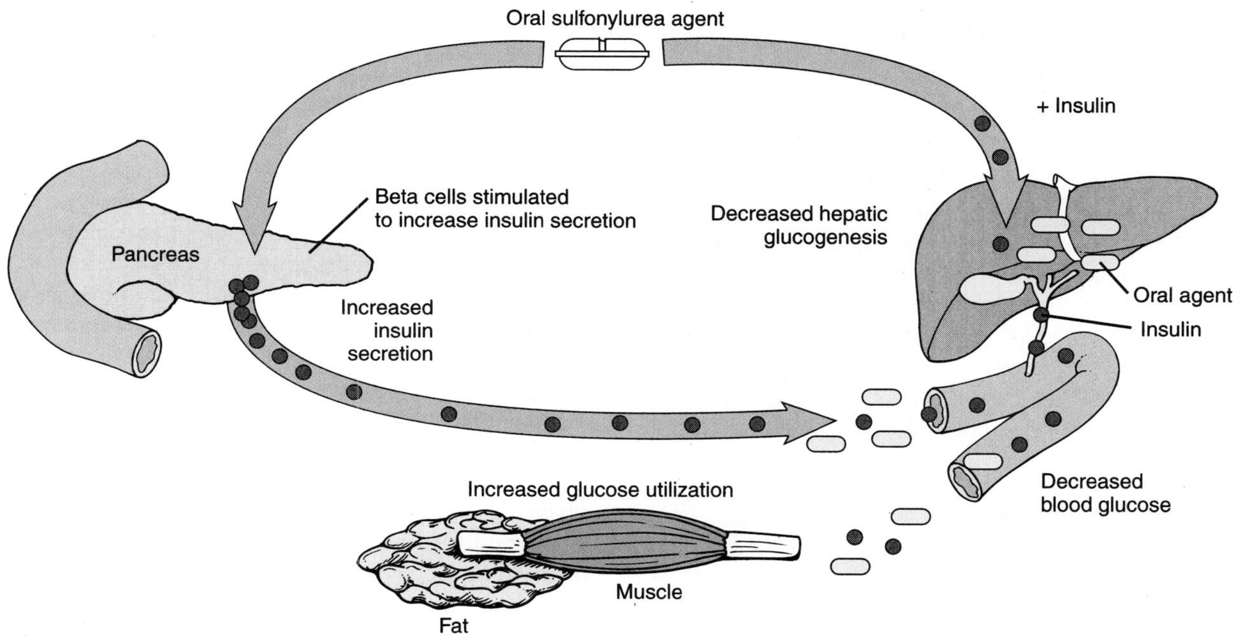

Figure 50-3 Mechanism of action of oral sulfonylurea agents.(From Beare PG & Myers JL [1994]. *Principles and practice of adult health nursing* [2nd ed.]. St. Louis: Mosby.)

TABLE 50-3 Hypoglycemic oral agents: side effects/adverse reactions

Side effects*	Adverse reactions†
Most frequent: Diarrhea or constipation, dizziness, gas, anorexia, headache, nausea, vomiting, abdominal distress	Less frequent: Chlorpropamide only—respiratory difficulties (CHF in persons with cardiac problems). Sedation; cramping of muscles; convulsions; edema of face, hands, or ankles; comatose, increased weakness (antidiuretic effect).
Less frequent/rare: Photosensitivity, rash	Rare: Pruritus, jaundice, light colored stools, dark urine (impairment of liver function). Increased fatigue, sore throat, increased temperature, increased bleeding or bruising (blood dyscrasias).
	Overdosage: Symptoms of hypoglycemia (see insulin side effects/adverse reactions).

*If side effects continue, increase, or disturb the client, the prescriber should be informed.
†If adverse reactions occur, contact the prescriber because medical intervention may be necessary.

agement, and adverse signs and symptoms to report to the health care provider.

These agents are not administered to clients who require close control by titration of insulin such as those with diabetic coma, ketoacidosis, significant ketosis or acidosis, severe burns, infection, or trauma or those undergoing major surgery. They are to be used with caution with clients with adrenal or pituitary insufficiency; high fever; prolonged nausea and vomiting; thyroid, renal, or hepatic function impairment; or debilitated or malnourished clients because these clients are predisposed to hypoglycemia. Consideration should be given to use of oral hypoglycemic agents other than chlorpropamide with clients with cardiac impairment or fluid retention because of chlorpropamide's antidiuretic effects. The client's sensitivity to oral antidiabetic agents, sulfonamides, or thiazide-type diuretics needs to be determined because of their cross-sensitivity.

A baseline assessment of the client is the same as it would be for insulin administration.

The client's current medication regimen should be reviewed for significant drug interactions (see Box 50-3). The following may occur when the oral hypoglycemic agents are given with the drugs listed below:

BOX 50-8

Troglitazone (Rezulin)

Troglitazone is the first agent in a new class of drugs that lowers insulin resistance in poorly controlled, type II or non–insulin-dependent diabetes mellitus. This product appears to resensitize the body to its own insulin, thus it may reduce and in some instances eliminate the need for insulin injections. Troglitazone enters fat and muscle cells to stimulate the release of proteins that work with insulin to transfer sugar molecules from the bloodstream into body cells. This mechanism of action is totally different from all the other hypoglycemic agents. *Be aware, though, that this medication is not indicated for diabetics that cannot produce insulin (type I diabetics).*

In studies that compared troglitazone to placebo, reported side/adverse effects were minimal. It is currently available in 200 mg (and soon to be released 400 mg) tablets (Pfeiffer, 1997). This is a significant breakthrough drug because it treats the cause and not just the symptom associated with insulin resistance in type II diabetics.

Pfeiffer N (1997). Newsbreaks: So long, insulin shots? *Drug Topics* *144*(4):16

Drug	Possible effect and management
alcohol	**May result in disulfiram (Antabuse)-type reaction, primarily with chlorpropamide (Diabinese). The reaction may include stomach pain, nausea, vomiting, facial flushing, lowered blood glucose levels, and headaches. Avoid or a potentially serious drug interaction may occur. This problem is reported less often with glipizide (Glucotrol) and glyburide (Diabeta, Micronase).**
anticoagulants, oral, (coumarin or indanedione)	Initially, increased serum levels of both drugs may be seen but with chronic therapy a reduction in plasma levels and effectiveness of the anticoagulant is reported. An increased serum level of the oral hypoglycemic agent may result in increased effects and toxicity because of a decrease in liver metabolism. Monitor closely because one or both drugs may require a dosage adjustment.
chloramphenicol (Chloromycetin), guanethidine (Ismelin), insulin, monoamine oxidase (MAO) inhibitors, salicylates or sulfonamides	May result in an increase in hypoglycemic effect. Monitor closely, since dosage adjustments may be necessary.
beta-adrenergic blocking agents (including ophthalmics)	Increase risk of hyperglycemia or hypoglycemia. See drug interaction for insulin for further information.

Nursing diagnosis. Clients receiving oral hypoglycemic agents may experience the following nursing diagnoses: altered bowel patterns of either diarrhea or constipation; altered comfort such as headache, heartburn, nausea, vomiting, abdominal discomfort, rash, and photosensitivity; and the potential complications of hypoglycemia, agranulocytosis, aplastic or hemolytic anemia, eosinophilia, thrombocytopenia, and hepatic function impairment. With chlorpropamide only, the client is at risk for fluid volume excess and altered cardiac output related to the drug's antidiuretic effect, evidenced by weight gain, difficulty in breathing, oliguria, and edema of the face, hands, and feet.

Implementation

Monitoring. Remember that the client with diabetes requires close supervision, especially when an oral hypoglycemic agent is tried for the first time. When converting from insulin to an oral hypoglycemic agent for control of the diabetic status, monitor the client's blood for glucose three times a day before meals. No transition period is usually required when changing from one hypoglycemic agent to another one, except with chlorpropamide. In the case of chlorpropamide caution should be exercised in the first week because of its prolonged half-life, 25 to 60 hours.

Elderly persons tend to be more sensitive to the effects of the oral hypoglycemic agents. Because hypoglycemia may be more difficult to recognize in these clients, they require lower dosages and closer monitoring.

Observe for hypoglycemia in the client who has irregular meal patterns, exercises more than usual, or ingests significant amounts of alcohol; hypoglycemia is more likely in these clients. A moderate lifestyle is essential to diabetes management. Periods of physiologic or psychologic stress may necessitate a temporary use of insulin.

See monitoring for insulin administration.

Intervention. For recommended administration times, see Table 50-2.

Education. Recognize that the need for instruction stressing dietary restriction is even greater for clients receiving oral hypoglycemic agents than for those taking insulin. Clients weighing more than 20% over their ideal weight may not respond to oral hypoglycemic agents. The client should weigh in once a week at the same time using the same scale and keep a weight record. Remember that these clients should be taught how to test for blood glucose levels, proper skin care, and the signs and symptoms of hypoglycemia and hyperglycemia.

Caution clients about excessive alcohol intake (and medications containing alcohol) when oral antidiabetic therapy is begun. Alcohol can increase the rate of metabolism of these drugs when there is long-term consumption of excessive quantities of these drugs. In addition, a disulfiram-like reaction may occur with the sulfonylureas.

Blood glucose testing should be performed frequently during the transition period when clients are switched from insulin to oral antidiabetic agents. Teach clients to carry or have access to forms of glucose at all times.

Have the client administer the initial dosage in the morning to decrease nocturnal hypoglycemia. Drugs given with food will decrease any gastric upset. If the client is taking divided doses of oral antidiabetic agents and omits a dose, advise that it should be taken as soon as it is remembered, but they should not be taken together. Administration before meals will maximize postprandial insulin release.

Make the client aware that the administration of these agents has been associated with increased incidence of death from cardiovascular disease compared with treatment with diet alone or diet plus insulin.

Evaluation. The client's blood glucose level will remain within normal limits and the client will effectively manage the therapeutic oral hypoglycemic regimen.

HYPERGLYCEMIC AGENTS

▲ **glucagon** [gloo' ka gon]

Glucagon (for injection) is a natural polypeptide hormone secreted by pancreatic alpha cells in response to hypoglycemia. It is released to maintain plasma levels of glucose by stimulating hepatic glycogenolysis and **gluconeogenesis** (the conversion of glycerol and amino acids to glucose) and by inhibition of glycogen synthesis. Glucagon's effect is accelerated by stimulation of the synthesis of cyclic AMP (cAMP). Hepatic and adipose tissue lipolysis is enhanced by activation of adenyl cyclase, producing free fatty acids and glycerol, which stimulate ketogenesis and gluconeogenesis.

Glucagon is indicated for the treatment of severe hypoglycemia in clients with diabetes and as an adjunct for gastrointestinal radiography. It is useful in hypoglycemia only if liver glycogen is available; thus it is ineffective in chronic hypoglycemia, starvation, and adrenal insufficiency.

Glucagon is also used as an adjunct to barium in gastrointestinal radiography. It produces relaxation of the esophagus, stomach, duodenum, small bowel, and colon (hypotonicity) and decreases peristalsis, thus improving outcome of the exam.

Parenterally administered (IM, IV or SC), it has a half-life of 10 minutes and an onset of action (hyperglycemic) according to route of administration: IV, 5 to 20 minutes; IM, 15 minutes; SC, 30 to 45 minutes. Duration of action is 1.5 hours. It is metabolized in the liver and excreted by the kidneys.

The side effects/adverse reactions of glucagon are not usually severe and may include nausea or vomiting and an allergic reaction. No significant drug interactions have been reported.

The adolescent and adult dose in hypoglycemia is 0.5 to 1 mg intramuscular, intravenous, or subcutaneous, repeated in 20 minutes when necessary. Pediatric dose is 0.025 mg/kg up to a maximum dose of 1 mg (IM, IV, or SC).

Case Study

The Client with IDDM

Edward Milton is 25 years old. He was recently diagnosed with insulin-dependent diabetes mellitus. In addition to a 2300 calorie ADA diet, Mr. Milton was started on an insulin administration program that includes 5 U of regular insulin and 10 units of NPH insulin each morning with 5 U of regular insulin and 5 U of NPH before the evening meal. He is also instructed in the procedure for self-monitoring blood glucose. Mr. Milton is advised to check his blood sugar in the morning before his insulin dose and in the late afternoon before supper.

One month after beginning treatment, he came to the emergency room at 6:00 in the evening with profuse sweating, tremors, headache, and an elevated blood pressure. His blood sugar by fingerstick was 45 mg/dl. A serum blood sample confirmed the diagnosis of hypoglycemia. Mr. Milton was given an intravenous bolus of 50 cc of 50% dextrose. In interviewing Mr. Milton before he was released from the ER, you discover that he had not eaten his usual meals that day because of vague feeling of nausea, anorexia, and mild diarrhea. He also admits that he has not been testing his blood sugar at home because he is too rushed in the morning. He frequently eats out in the evening with friends and is too embarrassed to test his blood sugar "in front of my friends." Mr. Milton says he does follow his diet and finds no problems in balancing his food intake.

1. What is the significance of the time of day that Mr. Milton experienced his hypoglycemia?
2. Outline the instructions you will give Mr. Milton about managing his diabetes on days when he is sick.
3. Explain the importance of self-monitoring of blood glucose for diabetes management.

After his first hypoglycemic episode, Mr. Milton began monitoring his blood glucose twice a day as he had been instructed. One year later he reports that his sugars have been increasing both in the morning and the afternoon. He denies any change in food intake or activity. He says he follows his diet faithfully. His insulin regimen is changed to add 5 units of regular insulin to the morning dose of NPH. He is also to take 10 units of NPH and 5 units of regular insulin in the evening, before supper. Although Mr. Milton agrees to the twice-a-day insulin injections, he asks why he can't take pills for diabetes the way his grandfather did for his diabetes.

4. How will you respond to Mr. Milton's questions about taking pills for his diabetes?
5. What are the differences between NPH and regular insulin that Mr. Milton needs to learn?
6. List the steps you will teach Mr. Milton about preparing the two insulins for injection.

Pregnancy Safety

Category	Drug
B	acarbose, glucagon, metformin
C	acetohexamide, chlorpropamide, diazoxide, glipizide, glyburide, tolazamide, tolbutamide

■ Nursing Management

Glucagon Therapy

Assessment. It is important for the nurse to recognize the symptoms of hypoglycemia: anxiousness, irritability, altered mood, nervousness, weakness, shakiness, inability to concentrate; perspiring, cool, pale skin; hunger, nausea, headache; and unconsciousness. A rapid blood glucose level may be obtained to confirm the hypoglycemia.

If glucagon is being used for testing purposes, there is a risk of hyperglycemia in the client with diabetes mellitus. Risk versus benefit will need to be considered if the client has a history of insulinoma (paradoxical decrease in blood glucose may occur) or pheochromocytoma (may cause hypertension as the result of the release of catecholamines).

Nursing diagnosis. The client may develop altered comfort (nausea and vomiting) as a result of the underlying hypoglycemia or overdose of the glucagon, and the potential complication of allergic reaction or severe hypoglycemia due to the ineffectiveness of the drug.

Implementation

Monitoring. Check the client's blood glucose level throughout the hypoglycemic episode, after administration, and for 3 to 4 hours after the client regains consciousness. Note the client's clinical response. Monitor the client's vital signs and level of consciousness.

Intervention. Glucagon is administered for hypoglycemia in the unconscious client as directed by the prescriber. After administering, turn the individual on one side to prevent choking and/or aspiration. Emergency medical assistance should be obtained as quickly as possible. Inform the prescriber of the client's status. If the client has not regained consciousness in 5 to 20 minutes, give a second dose and transport the client to the hospital. Intravenous glucose will need to be started if the individual does not respond to the second dose of glucagon. Glucagon and glucose may be given at the same time.

If the client does regain consciousness and can swallow, offer some oral form of sugar followed by a more complex carbohydrate, such as crackers and cheese or a glass of milk. This will help prevent a recurrence of the hypoglycemia before the next meal. If the client is experiencing nausea and vomiting that prevent food intake for more than an hour after the administration of the glucagon, seek medical assistance.

Replace the client's supply of glucagon as soon as possible. Medical follow up is necessary for all clients having a hypoglycemic episode as a result of oral antidiabetic agents.

Education. Teach the family and the client how to mix the drug and how to inject properly before the need arises to use glucagon. A standard insulin syringe may be used for injection unless the dose is greater than the capacity of the syringe. However, the injection should be made at a 90-degree angle instead of the usual subcutaneous approach. Advise the client and family to keep supplies on hand and check the expiration dates frequently.

Instruct the client and family about the symptoms of hypoglycemia and the importance of ingesting some form of sugar, such as orange juice, honey, syrup, hard candy, sugar cubes, or milk, when symptoms first occur.

Evaluation. The client's blood glucose level will be within normal limits. The client and family will state an understanding of effective management of glucagon therapy and successfully demonstrate administration techniques.

diazoxide [dye az ox' ide] (Proglycem)

Oral diazoxide produces a prompt, dose-related increase in blood glucose levels by inhibition of pancreatic insulin release. It may also have an extrapancreatic effect. It is indicated for the treatment of hypoglycemia caused by hyperinsulinism, secondary to an inoperable islet cell adenoma or carcinoma, an extrapancreatic malignancy, or an islet cell hyperplasia. It is not indicated for treatment in functional hypoglycemia. It is also available in parenteral dosage form to treat hypertensive emergencies.

Diazoxide is rapidly absorbed orally, has an onset of action within 1 hour, duration of effect less than 8 hours, and a half-life of between 20 and 36 hours in normal individuals. It is highly protein bound, metabolized in the liver, and excreted by the kidneys. Side effects reported include taste alterations, constipation, anorexia, nausea, vomiting, and abdominal pain. With chronic use it may cause increased hair growth on arms, legs, back, and forehead (hypertrichosis). The most frequently reported adverse reactions include a decrease in urine output resulting in edema of hands, feet, or lower extremities, weight gain, and possibly congestive heart failure in susceptible individuals. Hyperglycemia or ketoacidosis are typical symptoms reported with a diazoxide overdose.

The adult diazoxide dose is 1 mg/kg every 8 hours; adjusting dosage as necessary. Maintenance dosage is 3 to 8 mg/kg orally daily; divide into two or three equal doses and administer every 12 or 8 hours. Maximum dose is usually 15 mg/kg/day.

■ Nursing Management

Diazoxide Therapy

Assessment. Determine whether the client has a sensitivity to thiazide diuretics or other sulfonamide medication because he or she may also be sensitive to diazoxide.

Carefully consider the use of diazoxide in clients with cardiovascular problems, such as acute aortic dissection, compensatory hypertension, coronary or cerebral insufficiency, or inadequate cardiac reserve, because of the potential for fluid volume excess resulting from the drug's tendency to increase water and sodium retention.

A baseline assessment of the client's urine and serum glucose and blood pressure should be obtained before the initiation of diazoxide therapy.

The client's current medication regimen should be reviewed for significant drug interactions. The following may occur when diazoxide is given with the drugs listed below:

Drug	Possible Effect and Management
anticonvulsants, hydantoin (phenytoin)	May decrease or nullify the action of both drugs. Monitor effects of both drugs and adjust doses accordingly.
medications that induce hypotension (alcohol, diuretics, calcium channel blocking agents, beta-adrenergic blocking drugs) and peripheral vasodilators	Concurrent use may cause enhanced severe, hypotensive effect. Monitor closely, since dosage adjustments may be necessary.

Nursing diagnosis. Clients receiving diazoxide may experience the following nursing diagnoses: fluid volume excess (rapid weight gain, swelling of feet and ankles); altered comfort (change in taste, nausea, vomiting, and abdominal pain); altered bowel pattern (constipation); altered self-concept related to hypertrichosis; impaired physical mobility related to the drug's extrapyramidal effects, evidenced by stiffness of limbs, and trembling and shaking of fingers and hands; and the potential complications of allergic reaction, angina pectoris, myocardial ischemia or infarction, thrombocytopenia, and transient cerebral ischemic attacks.

Implementation

Monitoring. Monitor blood glucose at least daily. Monitor the client's blood pressure, intake and output, and weight daily. Observe clients for swelling of the feet and lower legs, increased weight gain, and decrease in urinary output as signs of fluid retention. Diuretics are sometimes given concurrently to avert these side effects. Observe for signs and symptoms of hyperglycemia.

Intervention. Dosage forms vary in their ability to produce blood concentrations of diazoxide. The oral suspension dosage form produces higher concentrations than those of the capsule form. Caution needs to be taken when changing the client from one to the other.

There is usually a transient hyperglycemia (24 to 48 hrs) after the IV administration of diazoxide, but it rarely progresses to ketoacidosis.

Education. Instruct clients in the importance of diet, testing of blood for glucose, regular visits to the prescriber, symptoms of hypoglycemia and hyperglycemia, and of not taking other medications unless discussed with the prescriber.

Advise the client to change position from lying to sitting or standing position slowly to minimize lightheadedness and fainting.

Evaluation. The client's blood glucose level will return to normal limits, and the client will not have fluid or sodium retention. The client and family will state an understanding of effective management of diazoxide therapy. If the drug is not effective within 2 to 3 weeks in managing hypoglycemia, then its use needs to be reevaluated.

glucose [gloo' koes] (Glutose, Insta-Glucose)
Glucose is a monosaccharide that is absorbed from the intestine and then either utilized or stored by the body. It is indicated to treat or manage hypoglycemia. Glucose provides 4 calories/g. The only side effects have been some reports of nausea. No significant drug interactions have been reported.

In adults approximately 10 to 20 g are administered orally and repeated in 10 minutes if necessary.

SUMMARY

The two primary hormones released by the pancreas are insulin and glucagon. When the blood glucose falls, glucagon is released, facilitating the catabolism of glycogen stored in the liver, which increases blood glucose. The release of glucagon stimulates the secretion of insulin, inhibiting the release of glucagon, and maintaining homeostasis of carbohydrate metabolism. Diabetes mellitus is a disorder of carbohydrate metabolism that is the result of an insulin deficiency or resistance or both. Diabetes mellitus is classified as insulin-dependent diabetes mellitus (type I), previously called juvenile-onset diabetes, and non–insulin-dependent diabetes mellitus (type II), maturity-onset diabetes. Although type II may require insulin at some time, it is usually managed by dietary treatment, weight reduction, client, and, if necessary, oral hypoglycemic agents.

Insulin may be rapid, intermediate, or long-acting. Therapeutic dosages are not fixed but are set in response to blood glucose levels, considering the client's dietary intake, and physical activity. Client education is essential in order for the client to participate in ascertaining the insulin dosage needed through blood testing and to self-administer insulin safety and accurately. See the selected nursing diagnoses for clients receiving insulin on p. 800.

Oral hypoglycemic agents encourage the release of insulin from the pancreas, decrease glycogenolysis and gluconeogenesis, increase the sensitivity of body tissues to insulin, and are used for type II diabetes mellitus.

Hyperglycemic agents are used in the treatment of hypoglycemia in which the client is unable to ingest sufficient amounts of glucose to meet body requirements.

Critical Thinking

1. Sally Milton, age 59, has been diagnosed with diabetes mellitus for 6 years. In the past, her blood glucose control has been managed by weight loss and diet. She has just started treatment with glyburide (Glucotrol XL) 2.5 mg PO daily. She confides in you, "I'm pleased to be starting on the pills. I was tired of watching my diet." How should you respond?
2. Loretta Baxter, age 45, has been recently diagnosed with insulin-dependent diabetes mellitus. When admitted to the hospital for additional testing, she weighed 240 pounds. She is placed on a 1500 calorie ADA diet and prescribed 30 U of NPH insulin to be taken at 7 AM each morning. At 4 PM, she becomes diaphoretic, weak, and pale. What action should you take? What explanation will you provide Ms. Baxter about what has occurred?

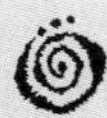

Collaborative Learning Activities

1. The students, without looking at their books, will write the differences between the two types of diabetes, including: (1) usual age of onset; (2) timing of onset of symptoms; (3) typical client body weight; (4) incidence; (5) family history; (6) insulin levels; (7) insulin dependence; (8) insulin resistance; (9) condition of receptors: (10) occurrence and types of complications; and (11) dietary modifications required. Draw a chart on the board and have the students fill it in, discussing related issues as they go along.
2. Incorporate case study questions 1, 2, and 3 with the general discussion of insulin types. The students will provide the answers in the discussion.
3. Incorporate case study questions 4, 5, 6, and 7 with general discussion of insulin therapy. The students will provide the answers in the discussion.
4. The students will discuss what they would do if during a home visit they discovered an unconscious client who had a history of diabetes.

BIBLIOGRAPHY

American Diabetic Association (ADA) (1990). *Physician's guide to non–insulin-dependent (type II) diabetes: Diagnosis and treatment.* Alexandria, VA: American Diabetic Association.

American Hospital Formulary Service (1996). *AHFS drug information '96.* Bethesda, MD: American Society of Hospital Pharmacists.

Anderson KN, et al. (Eds.) (1994). *Mosby's medical, nursing, & allied health dictionary* (4th ed.). St Louis: Mosby.

Beaulieu JA (1989). Nursing diagnoses co-occurring in adults with insulin-dependent diabetes mellitus, *Classif Nurs Diagn Proc Eighth Conf* (p. 199). St Louis: Mosby.

Betz JL (1995). Pharmacy update: Fast-acting human insulin analogues: A promising innovation in diabetes care, *Diabetes Educator* 21(3):195, 197-8, 200.

Campbell RK (1992). The clinical use of insulin, *US Pharmacist*, Diabetes Supplement, November.

Covington TR (Ed.) (1996). *Handbook of nonprescription drugs* (11th ed.). Washington, DC: American Pharmaceutical Association.

Davis SN & Granner DK (1996). Insulin, oral hypoglycemic agents, and the pharmacology of the endocrine pancreas. In Hardman JG & Limbird LE (Eds.). *Goodman & Gilman's the pharmacological basis of therapeutics* (9th ed.). New York: McGraw-Hill.

Diabetes update '93. (1993). *Nursing* 23(8):59-60.

Drass J (1992). What you need to know about insulin injections, *Nursing* 22(11):40-3.

Katzung BG (1992). *Basic and clinical pharmacology* (5th ed.). Norwalk, CT: Appleton & Lange.

Koda-Kimble MA & Carlisle BA (1995). Diabetes mellitus. In Young LY & Koda-Kimble MA (Eds.). *Applied therapeutics: The clinical use of drugs* (6th ed.). Vancouver: Applied Therapeutics.

Kupecz D (1995). Metformin: An antihyperglycemic drug for non–insulin-dependent diabetes mellitus, *Nurse Practit* 20(7):70-2.

Macheca MJK (1993). Diabetic hypoglycemia: How to keep the threat at bay, *Amer J Nurs* 93(4):26-30.

Melmon KL, et al. (1992). *Melmon and Morrelli's clinical pharmacology* (3rd ed.). New York: McGraw-Hill.

Olin BR (Ed.) (1996). *Facts and comparisons.* St Louis: Facts and Comparisons.

Rodgers K (1996). New Ammon: Faster-acting insulin set to debut in August, *Drug Topics* 140(13):59.

United States Pharmacopeial Convention (1996). *USP DI: Drug information for the health professional* (16th ed.). Rockville, MD: The Convention.

Vibulbhan S (1993). Blood glucose sticks: A finger a day, *Nursing* 23(5):22.

Watson J & Jaffe MS (1995). *Nurse's manual of laboratory and diagnostic tests.* Philadelphia: FA Davis.

Wilson BA (1994). What nurses don't know about managing NIDDM, *MEDSURG Nursing* 3(2):152-4.

Chapter 51

Overview of the Female and Male Reproductive Systems

Chapter Focus

Because secrecy and cultural sensitivity often influence perceptions of reproductive disorders, care for clients with dysfunctions of the reproductive system is particularly challenging for the nurse. The client may experience disturbance of self-esteem, altered sexual patterns, and sexual dysfunction, requiring the nurse to apply knowledge of reproductive anatomy and physiology and associated drugs for sensitive and appropriate teaching and counseling. This chapter will serve to review your knowledge of the anatomy and physiology of the female and male reproductive systems as groundwork for the next four chapters, which discuss the drugs affecting the reproductive system. The following objectives and key terms are important for a good understanding of this chapter.

Key Terms

androgen (p. 812)
estrogen (p. 812)
follicle-stimulating hormone (FSH) (p. 812)
luteinizing hormone (LH) (p. 812)
ovulation (p. 812)
progestogen (p. 812)
testosterone (p. 816)

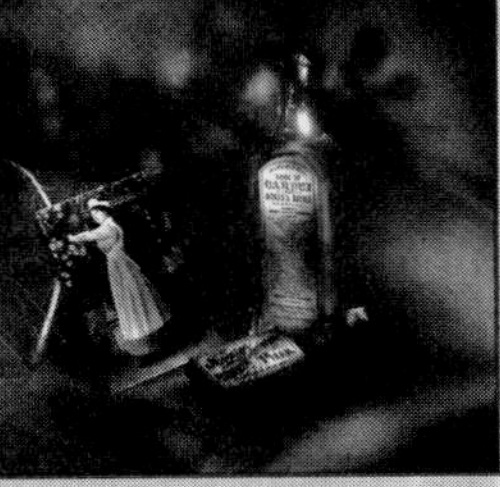

Objectives

1. Identify the anterior pituitary gland hormones that influence the female and male reproductive systems.
2. Describe hormonal influences on uterine function during the menstrual cycle.
3. Identify the primary male and female hormones.
4. Describe the effects of estrogen and progesterone during the proliferative stage.
5. Trace the transport of sperm in the male body from production to ejaculation.

Reproduction is the sum of genetic and hormonal influences originating from the sexes of a species to perpetuate the species. In human beings, the reproductive process in both sexes is highly complex, involving **follicle-stimulating hormone (FSH)**, which stimulates the growth and maturation of graafian follicles in the ovary and spermatogenesis in the testes, and **luteinizing hormone (LH)**, which stimulates the secretion of sex hormones by the ovary and the testes and is involved in the maturation of the spermatozoa and ova; both hormones are secreted from the anterior pituitary gland. The hormones from the reproductive systems of the male (**androgens**) and the female (**estrogens** and **progestogens**) are also involved in the reproductive process.

ENDOCRINE GLANDS

The reproductive system of the human female consists of the ovaries, fallopian tubes, uterus, and vagina. The male reproductive system consists of the testes, seminal vesicles, prostate gland, bulbourethral glands, and penis. The reproductive organs of both male and female are mainly under the control of the endocrine glands. The ovaries and testes, known as gonads, not only produce ova and sperm cells but also form endocrine secretions that initiate and maintain the secondary sexual characteristics in men and women. The structure and physiologic functions of the pituitary gland are reviewed in Chapter 47; the discussion of the pituitary gland in this chapter is limited to its effect on the female and male reproductive systems.

PITUITARY GONADOTROPIC HORMONES

The gonadotropins or pituitary hormones responsible for the development and maintenance of sexual gland functions are the following:

1. Follicle-stimulating hormone (FSH), which stimulates the development of the ovarian (graafian) follicles up to the point of ovulation in the female; in the male, FSH stimulates the development of the seminiferous tubules and promotes spermatogenesis.
2. Luteinizing hormone (LH), or interstitial cell-stimulating hormone (ICSH), which acts in the female to promote the growth of the interstitial cells in the follicle and the formation of the corpus luteum; in the male, ICSH stimulates the growth of interstitial cells in the testes and promotes the formation of the hormone androgen, testosterone.
3. Luteotropic hormone, or luteotropin, which is identical to the lactogenic hormone, or prolactin.

In the female, FSH initiates the cycle of events in the ovary. Under the influence of both FSH and LH the graafian follicle grows, matures, secretes estrogen, ovulates, and forms the corpus luteum. LH promotes the secretory activity of the corpus luteum and the formation of progesterone. In the absence of LH the corpus luteum undergoes regressive changes and fails to make progesterone.

FEMALE REPRODUCTIVE SYSTEM

Figure 51-1 illustrates the effects of the pituitary hormones, ovarian hormones, and uterine functions during the menstrual cycle.

Day 1 of the menstrual cycle is the onset of menses, and Day 5 usually signifies the end of menstruation. During this time, FSH is stimulating follicular growth in the ovary and also stimulating the ovary to produce estrogen, which is low at the beginning of the cycle. As estrogen levels increase, FSH levels decrease. The rising estrogen levels are preparing the uterus for a fertilized ovum, which is known as the proliferative stage of the uterus and results in the following:

1. The growth of glandular surface of the endometrium, or inner lining of the uterus.
2. The production, by the endocervical glands, of a more plentiful, viscous mucus that contains nutrients that can be used by the sperm.

The increasing levels of estrogen also stimulate the pituitary gland to release LH. As FSH is decreasing, LH is increasing. At this time (day 14), **ovulation** occurs when the mature follicle ruptures and releases its ovum. The ovum travels through the fallopian tube to the uterus. Female pelvic organs are shown in Figure 51-2.

The increasing levels of LH will affect the ruptured follicle by changing the follicle capsule into the corpus luteum. Under the influence of LH, the corpus luteum releases estrogen and progesterone. In the second phase, or secretory phase, both uterine hormones increase secretion of the glands of the endometrium. If the ovum is fertilized and reaches this area on approximately the eighteenth day of the cycle, it will be able to thrive on the nutrient secretions of the endometrium.

But if fertilization does not occur, the pituitary will respond to the increased levels of estrogen and progesterone by shutting off the release of FSH and LH. Without the central stimulation, the corpus luteum cannot produce estrogen or progesterone, so the surface layer of the endometrium will slough off, resulting in menstruation. Figure 51-3 depicts the feedback mechanism of FSH and LH and their main effects on the ovaries.

Most women demonstrate month-to-month variations in their menstrual cycles; therefore ovulation is not always predictable. The previous description of the menstrual cycle is based on a 28-day cycle, but ovulation varies and occurs on different days in different length cycles. Physiologically, this is the primary reason for the unreliability of the rhythm method of contraception, which depends on predicting the day of ovulation based on previous menstrual cycles.

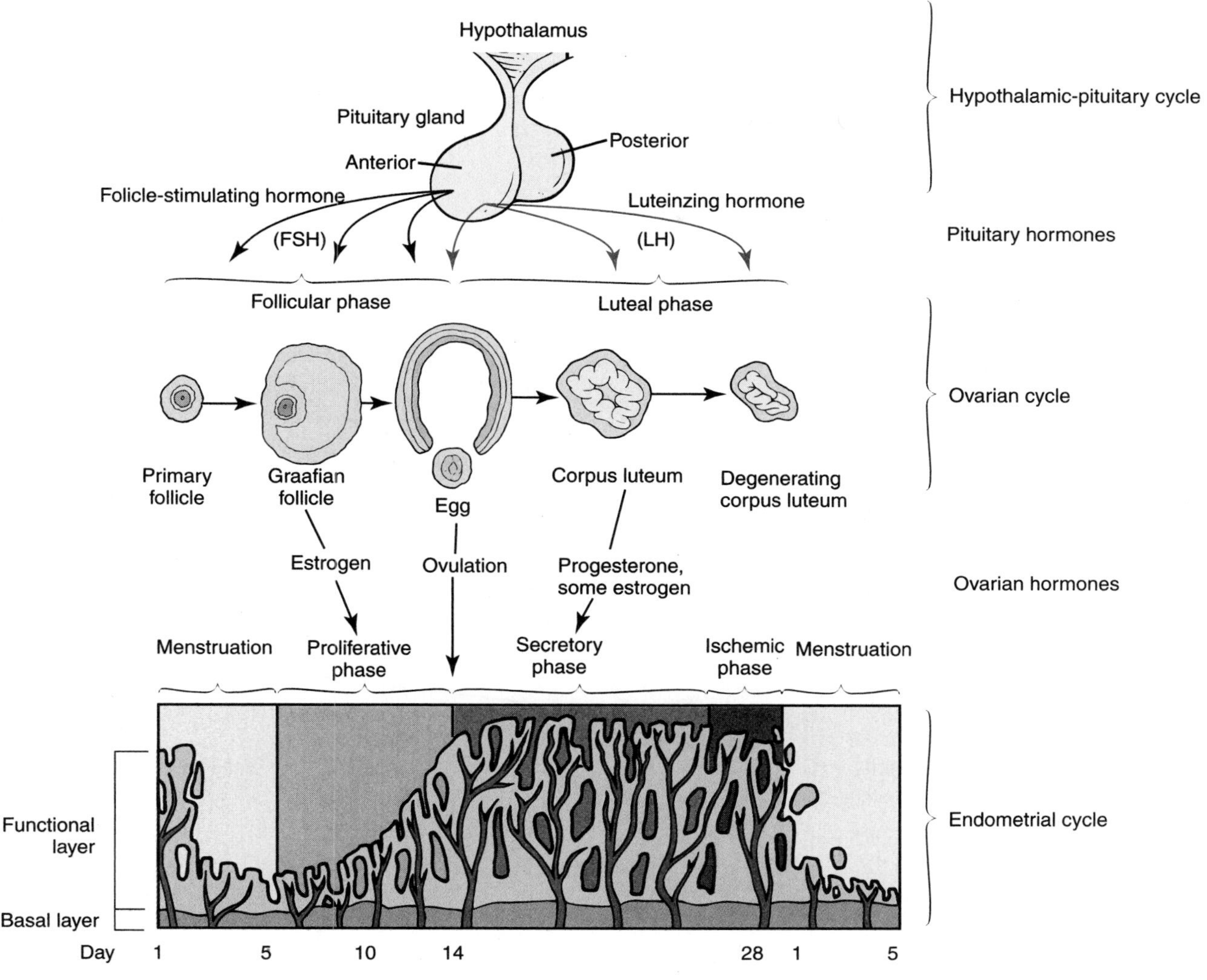

Figure 51-1 Menstrual cycle.(Modified from Lowdermilk DL, Perry SE, & Bobak IM [1997]. *Maternity and women's health care* [6th ed.]. St. Louis: Mosby.)

Female Sexual Response

For both males and females, psychic stimulation and local sexual stimulation are necessary for a satisfactory sexual experience. Psychic stimulation may be aided by an individual's erotic thoughts, although sexual desire is also affected by increasing levels of estrogen secretion, especially during the preovulatory period.

Local sexual stimulation causes similar responses in both sexes; that is, massage, increasing stimulation or irritation of the perineal region or sexual organs, can result in an enhancement of sexual sensations. In the female, the clitoris is very sensitive, and its stimulation can initiate a sexual sensation. Erectile tissue is located in the introitus (vaginal opening) and clitoris areas. This tissue is under parasympathetic nerve control; therefore in early stimulation, the parasympathetic nerves dilate the arteries located in the erectile tissues. Blood collects in the erectile tissue in the area so that the introitus will tighten around the penis, which aids male satisfaction for sexual stimulation, thus leading to ejaculation.

The parasympathetic nerves also signal the Bartholin's glands situated near the labia minora, which results in increased mucus secretion inside the introitus. This secretion, in addition to mucus from the vaginal epithelium, serves as a lubricant during sexual intercourse.

The female climax, or orgasm, is reached when the local sexual stimulation reaches the maximum sensation or intensity. It is considered similar to emission and ejaculation in the male and may also help to promote fertilization of the ovum. It has been theorized that orgasm produces a rhythm in the female tract from spinal cord reflexes that increase both uterine and fallopian tube motility and may result in cervical

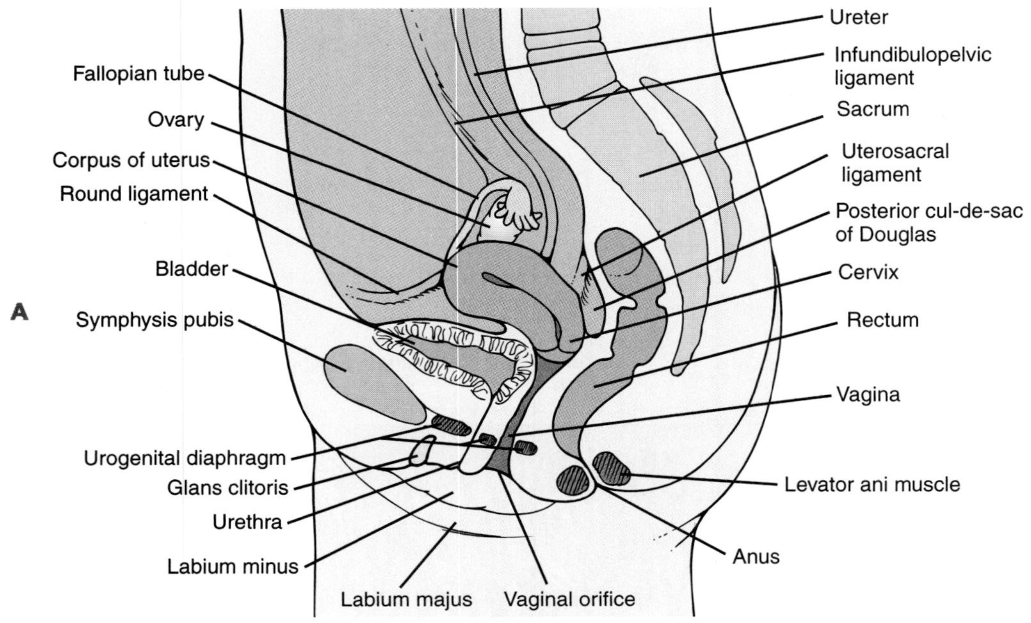

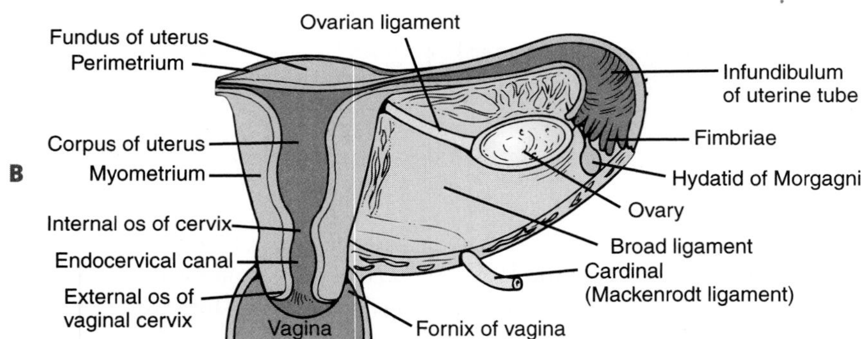

Figure 51-2 A, Female reproductive system. B, Cross section of uterus, adnexa, and upper vagina. (**B** Modified from Beare PG & Myers JL [1994]. *Principles and practice of adult health nursing* [2nd ed.]. St. Louis: Mosby.)

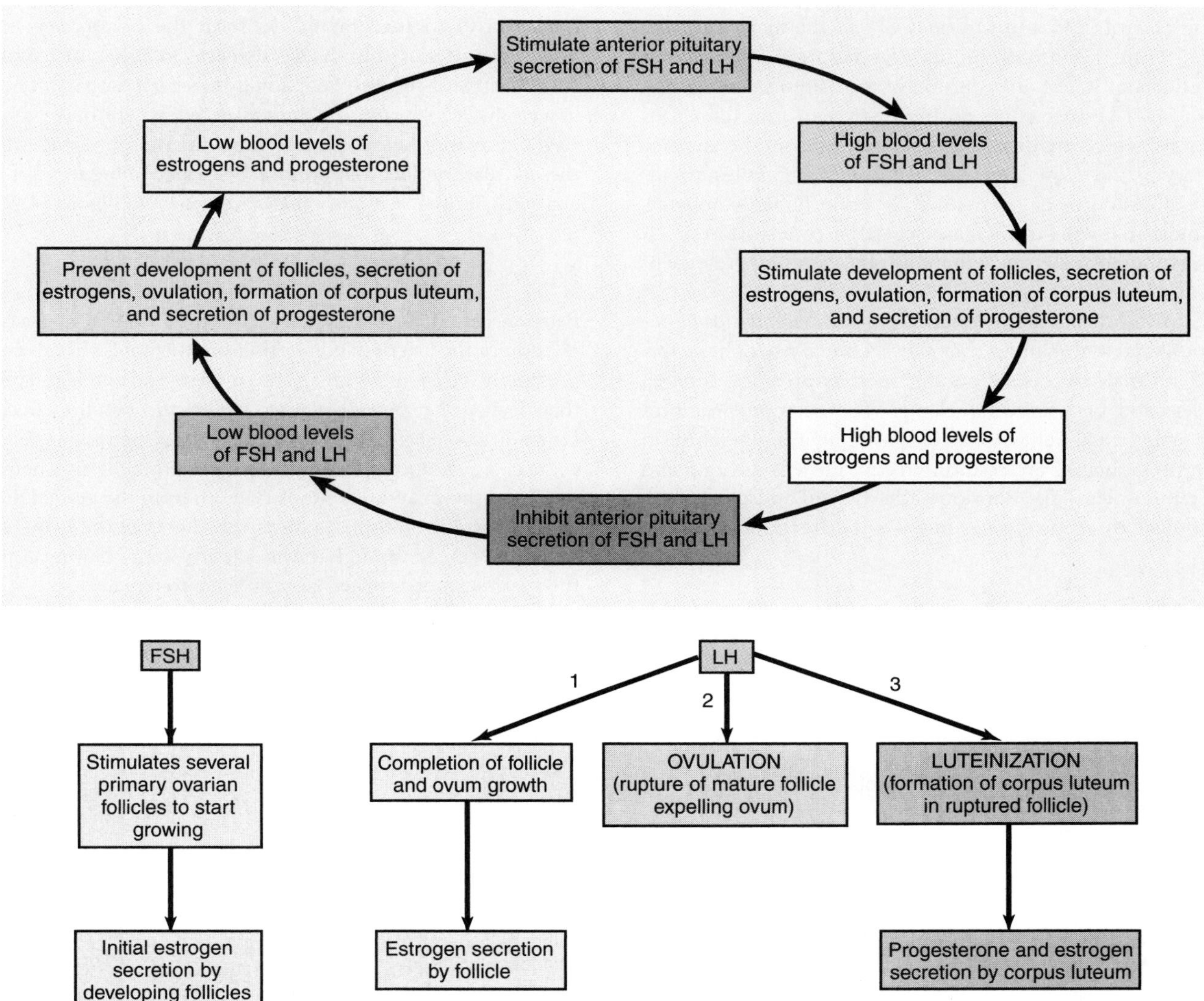

Figure 51-3 Feedback mechanism of follicle-stimulating hormone (FSH) and luteinizing hormone (LH) and their main effects on the ovaries. (Modified from Anthony C & Thibodeau G [1987]. *Textbook of anatomy and physiology* [12th ed.]. St. Louis: Mosby.)

canal dilation for up to 30 minutes. This will allow for easy sperm transport in the female.

The intense sexual sensations that develop during orgasms also result in an increase in muscle tension throughout the body. After the sexual act, this tension subsides into relaxation or feelings of satisfaction, sometimes referred to as resolution.

MALE REPRODUCTIVE SYSTEM

The effects of FSH and LH or ICSH in the male were described in the section on pituitary gonadotropic hormones. The effects of ICSH on secretion of testosterone are seen in Figure 51-4. **Testosterone,** an androgen, performs numerous functions, which are described below. FSH from the anterior pituitary gland stimulates the seminiferous tubules to increase production of spermatozoa, while ICSH stimulates the interstitial cells to increase secretion of testosterone. A high level of testosterone will inhibit the pituitary's release of FSH and ICSH.

Testosterone has many functions in the male. It aids in developing and maintaining the male secondary sex characteristics and male accessory organs, such as prostate, seminal vesicles, and bulbourethral glands. Testosterone promotes adult male sexual behavior, as well as regulating metabolism and protein anabolism, resulting in the growth of bone and skeletal muscles. This hormone affects fluid and electrolyte metabolism by reabsorbing sodium and water and increasing excretion of potassium. FSH and ICSH secretion are also inhibited from the anterior pituitary by testosterone.

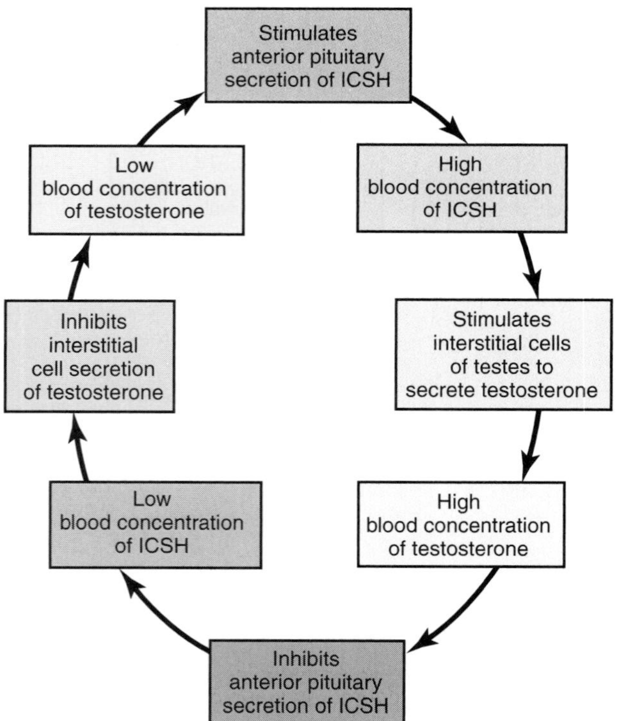

Figure 51-4 Effect of interstitial cell-stimulating hormone (ICSH) on testosterone. (Modified from Anthony C & Thibodeau G [1987]. *Textbook of anatomy and physiology* [12th ed.]. St. Louis: Mosby.)

Transport of Sperm in the Male

Sperm produced in the testes mature by spending 1 to 3 weeks in the epididymis of the male. The sperm, in seminal fluid, then travels through the epididymis (ducts that lie around the top of the testes) to the vas deferens. The vas deferens, a duct extension of the epididymis, extends over the bladder surface (posteriorly) to the ampulla to form the ejaculatory duct. Sperm can be stored in the vas deferens in excess of 1 month without loss of fertility depending on sexual activity. Thus a vasectomy, or severing of the vas deferens will make a man sterile primarily because it interrupts the journey of sperm to the ejaculatory duct and urethra. Male pelvic organs and the anatomy of the ejaculatory ducts are shown in Figure 51-5.

Male Sexual Response

Penile erection is a parasympathetic response that consists of dilation of the arteries and arterioles in the penis, which compresses the veins in this area. Thus more blood enters the penis than leaves, the penis becomes larger, and erection occurs. Emission and ejaculation of the sperm or semen is a reflex response. The stimulus that initiated erection will also help to move the sperm and secretions (semen) from the genital ducts to the prostatic urethra. Orgasm, the climax of the sexual act, moves the semen through the ejaculatory ducts. During coitus, the sperm can be transferred from male to female.

Later in life gonadal function ceases. Women undergo menopause or cessation of menses, and men have a decrease in sex hormone production, which is sometimes called the male climacteric.

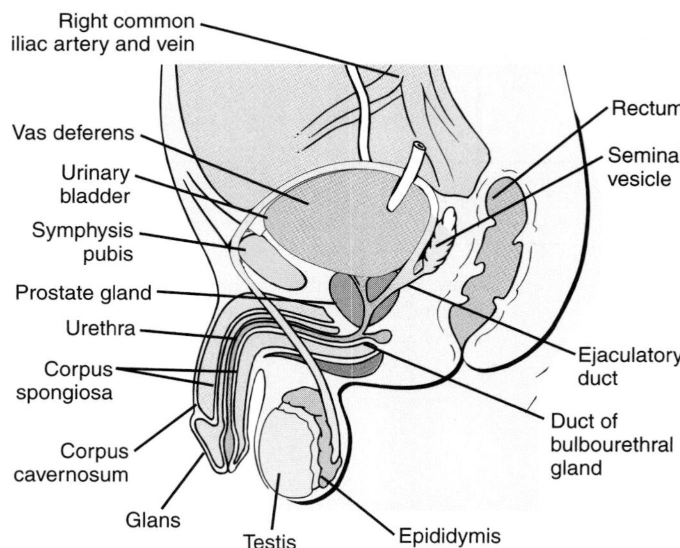

Figure 51-5 Male reproductive system.(Modified from Anthony C & Thibodeau G [1987]. *Textbook of anatomy and physiology* [12th ed.]. St. Louis: Mosby.)

SUMMARY

Disorders of the reproductive system of men and women result in acute and chronic physical and emotional stress. The nurse requires a sound knowledge of the anatomy and physiology of the reproductive system to assess clients for health adaptations and alterations and to assist clients with complex health issues in this domain.

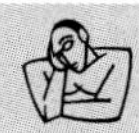

Critical Thinking

1. If you wanted to develop a birth control pill for men, how would you want that pill to influence the male hormonal system?
2. Because of the positive-feedback mechanism of hormonal influences in the menstrual cycle, what hormonal changes will occur if fertilization does not occur?

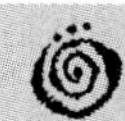

Collaborative Learning Activities

1. The class will be divided into teams to plan their responses to the critical thinking questions. Compare answers.

BIBLIOGRAPHY

Anderson KN, et al. (Eds.) (1994). *Mosby's medical, nursing, & allied health dictionary* (4th ed.). St Louis: Mosby.

Gray M (1992). *Genitourinary disorders.* St Louis: Mosby.

Guyton AC (1990). *Textbook of medical physiology* (8th ed.). Philadelphia: WB Saunders.

Seeley RR, et al. (1995). *Anatomy and physiology.* (3rd ed.). St Louis: Mosby.

Thibodeau GA & Patton KT (1996). *Anatomy and physiology* (3rd ed.). St Louis: Mosby.

Van Wynsberghe D, Noback CR, & Carola R (1995). *Human anatomy and physiology* (3rd ed.). New York: McGraw-Hill.

Chapter 52

Drugs Affecting the Female Reproductive System

Chapter Focus

Drugs that affect the female reproductive system therapeutically are synthetic or natural analogues of homogenous hormones. They are administered to mimic the biologic effects of endogenous hormones: supplement inadequate production (e.g., menopause), correct hormonal balance (e.g., dysfunctional bleeding), reverse an abnormal process (e.g., hirsutism), and for contraception. Whatever the indication, the nurse needs to be knowledgeable about these drugs to support the client's need for intervention and instruction. The following objectives and key terms are important for a good understanding of this chapter.

Key Terms

anovulation (p. 831)
biphasic (p. 827)
estrogen (p. 822)
monophasic (p. 827)
oral contraception (p. 826)
progestogen (p. 822)
triphasic (p. 827)

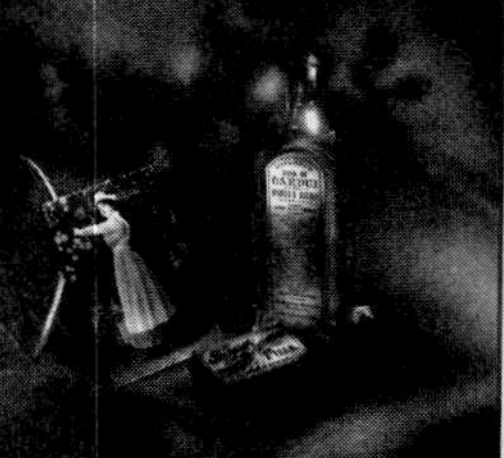

Key Drugs [▲]

estrogen
progestin

Objectives

1. List drugs affecting the female reproductive system.
2. Describe the source and action of chorionic gonadotropin.
3. Discuss the function of the primary female sex hormones.
4. Discuss side/adverse effects of estrogens and progestins.
5. Compare and contrast monophasic, biphasic, and triphasic oral contraceptives.
6. Implement nursing management of the care of clients receiving drug therapy affecting the female reproductive system.

Synthetic and natural substances that affect the female reproductive system include gonadotropin-releasing hormones, nonpituitary chorionic gonadotropin, menotropins, female sex hormones, oral contraceptives, ovulatory stimulants, and drugs used for infertility.

GONADOTROPIN-RELEASING HORMONE (GnRH)

Five preparations of GnRH are available, leuprolide (Lupron) and goserelin (Zoladex), which are reviewed in Chapter 57, Antineoplastic Agents; and gonadorelin, nafarelin, and histrelin, which are discussed in this chapter.

gonadorelin [goe nad oh rell' in] (Factrel)

Gonadorelin is a synthetic gonadotropin-releasing hormone used as an adjunct to other tests to diagnose hypogonadism in males and females. It is chemically identical to the natural luteinizing gonadotropin-releasing hormone; it stimulates the synthesis and release of luteinizing hormone (LH) and to a lesser extent follicle-stimulating hormone (FSH) from the anterior pituitary. In the diagnosing of hypogonadism, multiple dosing may be more valuable than a single dose test in differentiating between hypothalamic function impairment and pituitary function impairment.

Intravenously it has an initial half-life of 2 to 10 minutes followed by a terminal half-life of 10 to 40 minutes. It is metabolized rapidly in the body and excreted by the kidneys. No significant drug interactions are reported with its use. Adverse effects of gonadorelin include anaphylaxis, pain or inflammation at injection site, and multiple pregnancies.

In children 12 years and older and adults, the dose to diagnose hypogonadism is 100 μg SC or IV. In females, the drug should be administered in the early follicular phase of the menstrual cycle, preferably within the first week.

■ Nursing Management

Gonadorelin Therapy

Assessment. Before the initiation of gonadorelin testing, it should be determined that the client is in good general health and is not allergic to gonadorelin.

Nursing diagnosis. Once gonadorelin has been administered, the client should be assessed for the following nursing diagnoses: altered comfort (abdominal discomfort, transient flushing, headaches, nausea); impaired skin integrity related to generalized skin rash or itching and swelling at injection site; and the potential complication of sensitization following multiple doses (anaphylaxis).

Implementation

Monitoring. To determine a baseline serum concentration of luteinizing hormone, samples of venous blood are drawn 15 minutes before and immediately before the administration of gonadorelin and the results averaged. After administration of the drug, multiple blood samples are drawn at regular intervals, such as 15, 30, 45, 60, and 120 minutes for diagnostic purposes.

Intervention. Add the diluent supplied by the manufacturer immediately before use. Any unused reconstituted solution should be discarded.

Education. Explain the test procedure to the client. Alert the client to signs and symptoms of hypersensitivity reaction, such as hives, wheezing, and dyspnea and indicate these are to be reported immediately.

Evaluation. In postpubertal males and females and in premenopausal females, normal baseline serum LH concentrations are usually 5 to 25 mIU/mL depending on the laboratory. The test will determine the client's functional capacity and response to gonadotropic hormones without the client experiencing any untoward effects of the procedure.

GONADOTROPIN-RELEASING HORMONE AGONIST

nafarelin [naf' a re lin] (Synarel)

Nafarelin is a potent agonist of gonadotropin-releasing hormone that initially stimulates the release of LH and FSH but with continued dosing results in a decreased secretion of the gonadotropins. The continuous stimulation of the GnRH receptors results in desensitization and ultimately decreased production of LH and FSH. It is indicated for the treatment or management of endometriosis.

This product is administered nasally with maximum serum levels reported in 10 to 40 minutes. It has a half-life of 3 hours with maximum effect within 1 month. There are no recorded significant drug interactions with nafarelin usage. Side/adverse effects include hot flashes, decreased libido, vaginal dryness, headaches, insomnia, oily skin, acne, edema, hirsutism, hypersensitivity, and paresthesia.

The dosage is one nasal spray of 200 μg in one nostril in the morning and one spray in the other nostril at night. It is usually administered for a period of 6 months.

■ Nursing Management

Nafarelin Therapy

Assessment. It should be determined before therapy that the client is not pregnant, breastfeeding, or experiencing any undiagnosed abnormal vaginal bleeding.

Because some bone density loss has been demonstrated with use of the drug, caution should be used if more than one 6 month course is considered for women who are at high risk for osteoporosis (women with a strong family history of osteoporosis, chronic alcohol or tobacco use, or chronic use of drugs that can reduce bone mass [anticonvulsants or corticosteroids]). A baseline assessment of the client's endometriosis should be obtained before therapy.

Nursing diagnosis. The client should be assessed for the development of the following nursing diagnoses/collaborative problems related to the adverse reactions of nafarelin: altered comfort (hot flashes, headaches, and nasal irritation); altered sexuality related to libido increase or decrease, and vaginal dryness; altered sleep patterns (insomnia); ineffective individual coping related to emotional lability or depression; altered self-image related to acne, weight gain or loss, and hirsutism; and the potential complications of osteoporosis, arthralgia, and breakthrough bleeding, menorrhagia, or amenorrhea.

Implementation

Monitoring. The client should be regularly assessed for improvement of the endometriosis. Assess for discomfort of nasal passages, dryness, and irritation related to administration of the drug.

Intervention. Treatment is initiated between days 2 and 4 of the menstrual cycle. One spray of nafarelin is administered into one nostril in the morning and one spray into the other nostril in the evening.

Dietary calcium and calcium supplements have not been shown to help prevent bone calcium loss associated with the administration of GnRH.

Education. The client should be alerted that menstruation will cease with effective nafarelin therapy, so if regular menstruation continues, the prescriber needs to be notified. Although nafarelin will usually inhibit ovulation and inhibit menstruation, advise the client that it is not a reliable contraceptive, and a nonhormonal or barrier form of contraception should be used. The client should discontinue the drug and notify her prescriber immediately if she suspects she is pregnant.

If the client develops rhinitis during therapy, the prescriber may also recommend a nasal decongestant. In that case, the client should be instructed to use the decongestant at least 30 minutes after the nafarelin spray to minimize the possibility of decreasing drug absorption.

Evaluation. If therapy is successful, the client will have pain relief and reduction of her endometrial lesions.

histrelin [his' tre lin] (Supprelin)

Histrelin is a synthetic gonadotropin-releasing hormone agonist that is more potent than the natural hormone. It controls pituitary gonadotropins secretion which results in a decrease in sex steroid levels and regression of secondary sexual characteristics in children with precocious puberty. It is used only with clients with centrally mediated precocious puberty before the age of 8 in girls and 9.5 years in boys. In females, it decreases estradiol levels; in males it inhibits testosterone. Decreases in LH, FSH, and sex steroid serum levels are noted within 3 months of therapy.

Side/adverse effects of histrelin include vasodilation, vaginal dryness, breast edema and pain, gastric distress, headaches, fever, arthralgia, anxiety, and reactions at the site of injection. Vaginal bleeding usually occurs once in 1 to 3 weeks of therapy.

The usual dose for central precocious puberty is 10 μg/kg by daily SC injection.

▪ Nursing Management
Histrelin Therapy

Assessment. Before histrelin therapy is initiated a thorough physical and endocrinologic evaluation should be performed. This would include height and weight, hand and wrist x-ray for bone age determination, and total sex steroid level (estradiol or testosterone) as baseline for monitoring therapy. The nurse should assess whether the child/parents will be able to maintain a daily regimen of injections.

Nursing diagnosis. The child receiving histrelin therapy may experience the following nursing diagnoses/collaborative problems: impaired tissue integrity at the injection site (redness, swelling, itching [45%]); disturbance of body image related to vaginal bleeding (usually only one episode after starting histrelin [22%]); pyrexia (14%); altered comfort (headache [22%], arthalgia [4%], abdominal discomfort [3% to 10%]); and the potential complications of hypersensitivity (2%), vasodilation (35%), and vaginal dryness (12%).

Implementation

Monitoring. The child is monitored after 3 months and every 6 to 12 months during therapy with height measurements, bone age determinations (yearly), and GnRH testing to ensure that the responsiveness of the pituitary remains prepubertal while on therapy. Clinical evaluation of the secondary sex characteristics should be documented.

Intervention. Histrelin for injection contains no preservative; it is to be kept refrigerated. Inspect the vial for discoloration or particulate matter. Vials are used once and any unused drug is discarded.

Education. Stress the importance of the daily injection being given at the same time each day and compliance with daily administration. The pubertal process may be reactivated if injections are not daily. Instruct the client and family on proper storage of the drug. The solution should come to room temperature before administration. Injection sites should be rotated between the upper arms, abdomen, and thighs.

Alert the client that she may experience a light menstrual flow within the first month of therapy because of withdrawal of estrogen support from the endometrium. Advise the client that redness, swelling, and itching may occur at the injection site and to report it to the prescriber if the injection site reactions become severe. The client should be instructed to stop the drug and seek medical attention immediately if any signs of sensitivity occur.

Evaluation. With histrelin therapy for girls, menses ceases, serum estradiol levels are decreased to prepubertal levels, linear growth velocities decrease, skeletal growth is slowed, and adult height predictions increase. In boys, growth is also slowed, serum testosterone levels are decreased to prepubertal levels, and testicular volume is decreased.

NONPITUITARY CHORIONIC GONADOTROPIN

Certain gonadotropic substances formed by the placenta during pregnancy are extracted from the urine of pregnant women. The action of human chorionic gonadotropin is nearly equivalent to the pituitary's luteinizing hormone (LH) with little or no follicle-stimulating effects. A discussion of nonpituitary chorionic gonadotropin and menotropins is in this chapter.

gonadotropin, chorionic [goe nad' oh troe pin] (A.P.L., Pregnyl)

This drug is administered to make up for a deficiency in luteinizing hormone. Chorionic gonadotropin is indicated for:

- Prepubertal cryptorchidism and hypogonadotropic hypogonadism: stimulation of androgen production in the testes may enhance testes descent and increase development of the secondary male sex characteristics.

- Treatment of male and female infertility. In females it is combined with other drugs, such as menotropins. Men may receive it alone or in combination.
- Used in conjunction with other procedures to help in the stimulation of multiple oocytes in ovulatory women.

Administered IM, the drug has a half-life of between 11 and 23 hours, and ovulation usually occurs within 32 to 36 hours of administration. It is excreted by the kidneys within 24 hours. It has no significant drug interactions. The side/adverse effects of chorionic gonadotropin therapy include headaches, anxiety, depression, breast enlargement, weakness, abdominal bloating/pain, increase in multiple births, and possibly arterial thrombolism.

The adult dosage for male hypogonadotropic hypogonadism is 1000 to 4000 U IM two to three times a week for several weeks to months or in some cases indefinitely. For induction of ovulation, a dose of 5000 to 10,000 U IM is administered after the last dose of menotropins or from 5 to 9 days after the last dose of clomiphene.

For children with prepubertal cryptorchidism, 1000 to 5000 U IM two or three times a week for a maximum of 10 doses or the therapy is stopped when the desired response is achieved.

■ Nursing Management

Chorionic Gonadotropin Therapy

Assessment. It should be determined whether the client has a preexisting pituitary hypertrophy or tumor, because the medication will stimulate growth of the tumor. The drug should not be used with individuals with precocious puberty, prostatic cancer, abnormal vaginal bleeding, fibroids, ovarian cysts, or active thrombophlebitis. An ultrasound examination is recommended before therapy to determine a baseline assessment of the ovaries. For male clients, baseline serum testosterone levels are determined.

The drug should be used with careful monitoring in clients with asthma, cardiac disease, epilepsy, migraine headaches, or renal dysfunction, because of the potential for fluid volume excess due to fluid retention.

Nursing diagnosis. The following nursing diagnoses may occur with the client receiving chorionic gonadotropin: altered comfort (nausea, abdominal discomfort and distention, headache, or pain at the injection site); disturbance in self-concept related to physical changes in the secondary sexual characteristics of young male clients, such as precocious puberty (rapid increase in height, acne, growth of pubic hair, enlargement of penis or testes); altered thought processes related to depression or irritability; excess fluid volume evidenced by oliguria, rapid weight gain, shortness of breath, swelling of feet and lower legs; and altered bowel patterns, diarrhea. The potential complication of ovarian cysts or ovarian hyperstimulation syndrome (OHS) may also occur.

Implementation

Monitoring. The client's progress should be assessed periodically. Because the regimen is lengthy and time-consuming, the client should continue to be supported and encouraged to cooperate over the course of therapy.

To monitor the female client receiving the drug for induction of ovulation, measurement of estradiol serum determinations should be done. Hyperstimulation of the ovaries may be indicated by abdominal or pelvic pain and should be reported to the prescriber immediately. A pelvic examination and/or ultrasound examination may be done to evaluate ovarian size and minimize the risk of ovarian hyperstimulation syndrome.

To monitor the male client receiving the chorionic gonadotropin therapy for hypogonadism, inspect the genitalia for signs of puberty. Serum testosterone may be measured periodically to assess progress. If the drug is administered for male infertility, testosterone levels, sperm counts, and determinations of sperm mobility should also be done.

Intervention. Reconstitute with the diluent provided by the manufacturer.

Education. When used to treat infertility, provide support for the client and spouse throughout their attempt to achieve fertility. Societal and familial pressures create stress for them as a couple and individually. They should be advised that gonadotropin-induced ovulation is expensive and may result in multiple births. Since success is difficult to achieve, the couple should be counseled on alternatives such as adoption.

If the prescriber has requested daily recording of the woman's temperature, inform the client about the relationship of temperature to ovulation and its importance for the appropriate timing of intercourse to enhance the chance of pregnancy. Daily or every other day intercourse should be attempted beginning the day after chorionic gonadotropin is given until ovulation is thought to have occurred. Therapy should be reconsidered after three cycles of nonovulatory menses.

In treating prepubertal cryptorchidism, prepubertal males receiving chorionic gonadotropin should be prepared for an acceleration in sexual development and supported through self-image changes.

Evaluation. The client's underlying condition for which the drug is administered will be improved or corrected.

MENOTROPINS

Menotropin is a human pituitary gonadotropin, a purified preparation of follicle-stimulating hormone (FSH) and luteinizing hormone (LH) obtained from the urine of postmenopausal women. It is sometimes called human menopausal gonadotropins (HMG).

menotropins [men oh troe' pins] (Pergonal)

The mechanism of action is equivalent to effects produced by FSH and LH; menotropin stimulates the development of the ovarian follicle, causes ovulation, and may stimulate corpus luteum development. In males, it stimulates sperm production.

Menotropin is indicated in the treatment of the following conditions:

- Female infertility caused by ovulatory dysfunction, administered in combination with chorionic gonadotropin.

Menotropins are considered the treatment of choice for clients with hypothalamic hypogonadism or in those who did not respond to clomiphene.
- Male infertility, used in combination with chorionic gonadotropin to stimulate spermatogenesis in primary or secondary hypogonadotropic hypogonadism (male infertility).
- Used in combination with chorionic gonadotropin to stimulate multiple oocyte development in ovulatory clients who are using other technologies in order to conceive, such as gamete intrafallopian transfer or in vitro fertilization.

Menotropins are administered IM with excretion via the kidneys. There are no reported significant drug interactions. Side/adverse effects include gastric distress, severe pelvic pain, weight gain, edema, shortness of breath, decreased urine output, abdominal bloating or pain (usually in females); breast enlargement and erythrocytosis in males.

The adult menotropin dosage for induction of ovulation is 1 ampule (75 units of FSH and LH activity) IM daily for a week or more, followed by 5000 to 10,000 U of chorionic gonadotropin, a day after the last menotropin dose. If necessary, ampule dose may be increased every 4 to 5 days, up to a maximum of 6 ampules. For treatment of male infertility, administer 1 ampule IM three times weekly (in addition to chorionic gonadotropin twice a week) for a minimum of 4 months after pretreatment with chorionic gonadotropin for 4 to 6 months.

Nursing management is similar to that for chorionic gonadotropin except that this preparation is reconstituted with 1 to 2 ml of sodium chloride injection USP.

FEMALE SEX HORMONES

The ovaries, in addition to providing ova, manufacture and secrete female hormones that control secondary sex characteristics, the reproductive cycle, and the growth and development of the accessory reproductive organs in the female. Two main types of hormones are secreted by the ovary: (1) the follicular of estrogenic hormones **(estrogens)** produced by the cells of the developing graafian follicle and (2) the luteal or progestational hormones **(progestogens)** derived from the corpus luteum that is formed in the ovary from the ruptured follicle. The periodic cycling of the female sex hormones depends on an interaction between FSH and LH with the ovarian hormones estrogen and progesterone. This results in a menstrual cycle that normally continues throughout life, except for pregnancy, until menopause. While estrogens are primarily secreted by the ovarian follicles, some may also be secreted by the adrenals, corpus luteum, placenta, and testes.

Estrogens

Estrogens are available from natural sources (the urine of pregnant mares) in conjugated dosage forms and have been synthetically formulated. Examples of natural steroidal estrogens include estradiol, estrone, esterified estrogens, and estrone; nonsteroidal estrogens include diethylstilbestrol (DES), dienestrol, and chlorotrianisene.

▲ **estrogen** [ess' troe jen] (various manufacturers)
Estrogen increases the synthesis of DNA, RNA, and protein in estrogen-responsive tissues. Elevated estrogen serum levels inhibit secretion of FSH and LH from the pituitary, which results in inhibition of lactation, ovulation, and the development of a proliferative endometrium. Estrogen is indicated for the following conditions:
- Treatment of estrogen deficiency; atrophic vaginitis; female hypogonadism; insufficient primary ovarian function; abnormal uterine bleeding; severe vasomotor symptoms in menopause and postmenopausal osteoporosis.
- Treatment of cancer: breast carcinoma in selected metastatic breast carcinomas in postmenopausal women with tumor estrogen-negative receptors; also in selected male breast carcinomas and treatment of advanced prostatic carcinomas.

The use of estrogen therapy in postmenopausal women has resulted in reports of a significant decrease in the risk of heart disease (Pharmacy Practice News, 1995), including a reduction in the death rate in women with coronary artery disease (Belchetz, 1994). The American College of Physicians (1992) issued new guidelines for the counseling of postmenopausal women about hormone therapy. These include recommending that the individual with coronary heart disease (CHD) or at a greater risk of having CHD be advised about the benefits of hormone therapy. Counseling should include a review of the risks and benefits of long-term hormonal therapy.

Estrogen is protein bound, metabolized in the liver, and excreted by the kidneys. The side/adverse effects include stomach cramps or gas, anorexia, chloasma, headaches, nausea, vomiting, change in female libido and decrease in male sex drive, edema of lower extremities, breast pain and enlargement, and changes in menstrual bleeding.

Precautions

1. The risk of endometrial cancer increases with prolonged use of estrogens in postmenopausal women. However, low-dose estrogen given cyclically or the use of a progestin (concurrently or sequentially) may reduce the risk of inducing endometrial cancer.
2. Estrogens, especially DES, should not be administered during pregnancy because of an increased risk of congenital malformations, (FDA category X).
3. Estrogens are excreted in breast milk and will also inhibit lactation; therefore administration of estrogens to nursing women is not recommended.

Dosage and administration

1. The lowest effective dose of estrogens should be administered for the shortest time period to reduce the possibility of serious adverse effects. When continuous therapy is required, the prescriber should reevaluate the client at least annually.

2. To avoid overstimulation of estrogen-sensitive tissues, a cyclic dosing schedule of 3 weeks of estrogen administration and 1 week off or the addition of a progestin for the last 10 to 13 days of the cycle will most closely approximate the natural hormonal cycle. This is not the schedule for oophorectomized individuals or clients with cancer who are receiving hormonal therapy.
3. Estradiol and estrone are naturally occurring steroidal estrogens that are principal endogenous estrogens. Estradiol is available alone or synthetically as estradiol cypionate, estradiol valerate, ethinyl estradiol, and polyestradiol phosphate. The primary pharmacologic effects of all estrogens are similar.
4. Conjugated estrogens (Premarin) a mixture of estrogenic substances (especially estrone and equilin), are available in oral, parenteral, and vaginal cream dosage formulations. Dosage must be individualized according to diagnosis and therapeutic response, for example, vasomotor symptoms associated with menopause. The usual oral adult dose for esterified estrogens is 0.3 to 1.25 mg daily cyclically or continuously. Some women may require higher dosages.
5. Diethylstilbestrol (DES) is a synthetic nonsteroidal estrogen primarily used as an antineoplastic agent.
6. Transdermal estradiol (Estraderm) is used for women with estrogen deficiency. Applied topically to intact skin, 50 μg (0.05 mg) or 100 μg (0.1 mg) daily is released from the transdermal patch. It should be replaced twice weekly and is usually worn continuously.

■ Nursing Management

Estrogen Therapy

Assessment. The drug is contraindicated if breast cancer is known or suspected because there is the possible promotion of tumor growth, or if the client has abnormal or undiagnosed vaginal bleeding, which may indicate endometrial hyperplasia or carcinoma, which would be promoted by estrogen use.

Estrogens are to be used with caution with the client who has hypercalcemia associated with metastatic breast disease, endometriosis, uterine fibroids, active thrombophlebitis, or a history of thrombophlebitis secondary to estrogen use because these conditions may be aggravated by estrogen use. In males for whom estrogens may be administered for the treatment of prostatic or breast cancer, there is an increased risk of myocardial infarction, pulmonary embolism, and thrombophlebitis, so care should be exercised in clients with a past or active history of these conditions.

Given the individual health status of the client, some of the following assessment will be accomplished as a baseline before therapy: a physical examination to include blood pressure, Pap smear and breast examination, mammogram, and serum lipid profile, and hepatic function determinations.

The client's current medication regimen should be reviewed for significant drug interactions that may occur when estrogens are given, such as with the drugs listed below.

Drug	Possible effect and management
bromocriptine (Parlodel)	**Concurrent use may result in amenorrhea and may also interfere with bromocriptine's therapeutic effect. Avoid or a potentially serious drug interaction may occur.**
cyclosporine (Sandimmune)	Metabolism is inhibited, which may result in increased cyclosporine plasma levels and increased risk of hepatotoxicity and nephrotoxicity. Use concurrently only with very close monitoring of cyclosporine serum levels and liver and kidney function.
hepatotoxic drugs, especially dantrolene	**Estrogens increase risk of inducing hepatotoxicity: females over 35 years old are at increased risk. Avoid or a potentially serious drug interaction may occur.**
smoking tobacco	**Tobacco smoking increases the risk of serious cardiac adverse reactions, such as cerebrovascular accident (CVA), transient ischemic attacks (TIAs), thrombophlebitis, and pulmonary embolism. The risk is higher in women over 35 years old who smoke. Avoid or a potentially serious drug interaction may occur.**

Nursing diagnosis. Clients receiving estrogen therapy may experience the following nursing diagnoses: altered comfort related to anorexia, nausea, vomiting, abdominal cramping, breast tenderness, headaches, or skin irritation (transdermal patches); impaired skin integrity related to the development of acne; impaired vision related to a steepening of the corneal curvature contributing to an intolerance of contact lenses; fluid volume excess (peripheral edema, sudden weight gain); disturbance in self-concept related to melasma (brown, blotchy skin changes), gynecomastia (men), change in libido (women), or decreased libido (men); as well as the potential complications of thrombophlebitis, thromboembolism, hepatitis, hypercalcemia, chorea, irregular menses, and breast tumors.

Implementation

Monitoring. Blood pressure should be monitored periodically. Hepatic function studies should be done every 6 to 12 months for clients with hepatic dysfunction. Males treated with estrogens should be checked regularly for the development of breast carcinomas. Females should have, at least annually, a physical examination including Pap test, mammogram, and serum lipid profile.

Bone age determinations are recommended every 6 months for children and adolescents.

Intervention. Estrogens are usually administered on a cycle of 3 weeks on and 1 week off the medication, except for males. Administer the intramuscular forms slowly to minimize client discomfort. Large muscles, such as gluteus maximus, should be used to maximize absorption. For oil-based preparations use at least a 21-gauge needle and a dry syringe.

Administer intravenous estrogens slowly; vaginal burning occurs if administered too rapidly.

Vaginal forms should be administered at bedtime to enhance absorption. Sanitary napkins or panty shields may be used to protect clothing from stains.

Clients who have been taking oral estrogens should wait a week before starting transdermal dosage forms.

Education. Assist the client in exploring her concerns about the risks of taking estrogens. Provide her with information regarding the occurrence of cardiovascular disease and cancer in relationship to her age, smoking habits, and other health characteristics. Encourage the client to read the package insert carefully and then discuss any concerns she might have. Advise the client to have regular physical examinations, which should include a pelvic and breast examination, mammogram, and a Pap smear, every 6 to 12 months during treatment. Instructions should be provided for monthly self-examination of the breasts and any lumps found should be reported to the prescriber. The client should be advised to stop the medication immediately and contact her prescriber if she suspects she is pregnant.

Caution the client that smoking increases the incidence of serious side effects of the drug, particularly in women over 35. Instruct the client to notify her health provider in the instance of severe headache, blurred or lost vision (which may signal possible stroke), or symptoms of chest pain, shortness of breath, or leg pain, which may indicate thromboemoblism elsewhere in the body. The prescriber should also be informed of severe abdominal pain or mass, jaundice, severe mental depression, or unusual bleeding.

Nausea, frequently occurring at the beginning of therapy, usually ceases after 1 or 2 weeks. Seldom severe, it can be controlled by taking the medication with meals.

Advise the client to weigh one or two times weekly and report a sharp increase in weight or other signs of fluid retention, such as swollen ankles, puffy eyelids, and "tight" rings. A low-sodium diet and diuretic may be prescribed to control these symptoms.

Encourage the client to maintain a program of good oral hygiene, including teeth cleaning by a professional and thorough brushing and plaque control by the client to minimize any gingival hyperplasia that may occur during estrogen therapy. Warn the client that exposure to the sun or tanning devices may result in brown, blotchy discoloration of skin. Bleeding after estrogen withdrawal is expected. Explain to postmenopausal women that such bleeding does not indicate that a state of fertility has returned.

Instruct users with diabetes to report positive urine or blood sugar tests so the dosage of their antidiabetic medications can be adjusted.

Forewarn male clients of estrogen-induced feminization and impotence, which will disappear when therapy terminates. Advise clients of the increased risk of myocardial infarction, pulmonary embolism, and thrombophlebitis while undergoing estrogen therapy.

Instruct clients taking prescribed conjugated estrogens and esterified estrogens for osteoporosis prophylaxis to increase their intake of calcium and vitamin D and to engage in regular weight-bearing exercise such as walking.

When applying the transdermal form of the drug, the client should wash her hands before and after application of the patch. The system should be applied immediately after removal from the pouch and its protective liner. It should be applied to the abdomen on clean, dry, intact skin without hair. The sites on the abdomen should be rotated to prevent application to any site more frequently than every 7 days. The patch should not be applied to the breasts or to the waistline where clothing might cause the patch to become loose. The patch should be pressed into place for 10 seconds and then examined to ensure all the edges are tight. If the patch becomes loose, it may be reapplied or a new one may be applied.

Evaluation. The client will demonstrate an improvement in the underlying condition for which the drug was prescribed without experiencing any adverse effects related to drug therapy.

Progesterone and Progestins

Progesterone produced by the ovaries is a naturally occurring progestin. The anterior pituitary luteinizing hormone stimulates the synthesizing and secretion of progesterone from the corpus luteum, mainly during the latter half of the menstrual cycle. Progesterone may also be formed from steroid precursors available in the ovaries, testes, adrenal cortex, and placenta.

Progesterone and synthetic progestins have similar pharmacologic effects in the body. Progestins were developed because progesterone was not always therapeutically satisfactory. The advantages with progestins were: (a) greater potency that lowered the dose necessary to produce an equivalent response to progesterone; (b) a longer duration of action; and (c) some products have an effective oral/sublingual dosage form.

progesterone [proe jess' ter one]
▲ **progestin** [proe jess' tin] (various manufacturers)

Progesterone and progestins (hydroxyprogesterone, norethindrone and others) produce biochemical changes in the endometrium to prepare for the implantation and nourishment of the embryo. They also: (a) supplement the action of estrogen in its effects on the uterus and mammary glands; (b) cause suppression of ovulation during pregnancy; (c) cause relaxation of the uterine smooth muscles; (d) increase the synthesis of DNA and RNA; and (e) inhibit, in large doses, the secretion of luteinizing hormone (LH) from the anterior pituitary.

Progesterone/progestins are indicated for the treatment of female hormonal imbalance of amenorrhea and dysmenorrhea, endometriosis and specific carcinomas. They are also used to diagnose endogenous estrogen deficiency and to prevent pregnancy. They are metabolized primarily in the liver and excreted by the kidneys. Side/adverse effects include weight gain, stomach pain/cramps, swelling of face, and lower extremities, headache, mood alterations, anxiety, increased weakness, amenorrhea, breakthrough bleeding, hyperglycemia, menorrhagia, galactorrhea, rash, acne, insomnia, and breast pain.

Dosage and administration. Because dosage and method of administration for progestins can vary according to indications and current standards of practice, the student is referred to a current package insert or *USP DI* for the most recent recommendations. The following are examples of selected progestins and dosing regimens.

Hydroxyprogesterone [hye drox ee proe jess' ter one] Hylutin and others). Indicated for amenorrhea, dysfunctional bleeding of the uterus; administer 375 mg IM.

Megestrol [me jess' trole] (Megace). For breast cancer, the dose is 40 mg PO four times daily or 160 mg as a single dose; to treat endometrial cancer, dose is 40 to 320 mg daily in divided doses. Allow 2 months of therapy with megestrol before evaluating its effectiveness.

Norethindrone [nor eth in' drone'] (Micronor, Norlutate). Contraceptive dose is 0.35 mg/day; for amenorrhea or dysfunctional uterine bleeding the dose is 2.5 to 10 mg PO from day 5 through day 25 of the menstrual cycle. For endometriosis, the dose is 5 mg initially, increased by 2.5 mg daily at 2-week intervals until 15 mg/day is reached. This dose is continued for 6 to 9 months.

Progesterone [proe jess' ter one] (Gesterol and others). When used to treat amenorrhea caused by female hormone imbalance, progesterone is 5 to 10 mg IM daily for 6 to 10 days. Bleeding will usually occur within 2 to 3 days after the last injection; normal menstrual cycles may then follow. Discontinue injections if menstrual bleeding occurs during the series of injections.

■ Nursing Management

Progesterone/Progestin Therapy

Assessment. It should be determined that the client does not have preexisting cancer of the breast or reproductive tract, suspected pregnancy, incomplete abortion, abnormal and undiagnosed vaginal bleeding, a history of or active thrombophlebitis or thromboembolic disorder, hepatic dysfunction, or conditions for which progestins are contraindicated. Because of the tendency of progestins to cause fluid retention that might aggravate these conditions, these drugs should be used cautiously in clients with asthma, migraine headaches, epilepsy, cardiac insufficiency, or renal dysfunction. Clients with a history of ectopic pregnancy or diabetes should also be monitored carefully for any unusual symptoms. Because some progestins elevate LDL levels, hyperlipemia may be aggravated. Mental depression may worsen.

Congenital anomalies have been reported with the use of progestins during the first 4 months of pregnancy. They should not be used as diagnostic tests for pregnancy (see the Pregnancy Safety box above). Progestins are also excreted in breast milk; therefore they are not recommended for use by nursing women either.

When progestins are given concurrently with bromocriptine, the result may be amenorrhea and/or excessive lactation, which will interfere with bromocriptine's therapeutic effect. Concurrent use is not recommended.

Pregnancy Safety

Category	Drug
B	gonadorelin
C	chorionic gonadotropin, clomiphene
D	hydroxyprogesterone, progesterone
X	estrogens, histrelin, levonorgestrel, megestrol suspension, menotropins, nafarelin, norethindrone, norgestrel, oral contraceptives, urofollitropin

Nursing diagnosis. Clients on progestin therapy are at risk for the following nursing diagnoses: altered comfort (headache, nausea, breast tenderness, or irritation at injection site); fluid volume excess (peripheral edema, weight gain); sleep pattern disturbance (insomnia); fatigue; disturbance in self-concept related to increased facial and body hair, loss of scalp hair, weight gain, or melasma; impaired skin integrity (acne); altered thought pattern (mental depression); and visual disturbances related to neuro-ocular lesions (double vision or loss of vision); and for the complications of changed vaginal bleeding pattern, hepatitis, thrombophlebitis, retinal thrombosis, or thromboembolism.

Implementation

Monitoring. Undesirable effects are usually mild or absent during short-term use. However, as the duration of progestin therapy increases, the number and severity of adverse reactions also increase. Evaluation for these effects must continue as long as therapy continues. A physical examination at least every 6 to 12 months should include a breast and pelvic examination, Pap test, and hepatic function studies.

Intervention. Give oil preparations by deep IM injection. A low-sodium diet and diuretic may be prescribed to control symptoms of fluid retention, such as swollen ankles and puffy eyelids.

Education. Regulations require that a patient package insert be given to every client who is dispensed a progestin unless the drug is being used as an antineoplastic adjunct. Encourage the client to read the package insert carefully and then discuss with the health care provider any concerns she might have. Advise the client to have regular physical examinations as described previously.

Instruct the client to notify her prescriber in the instance of severe headache, blurred or lost vision (which may possibly signal stroke), and symptoms of chest pain, shortness of breath, or leg pain, which may indicate thromboembolism elsewhere in the body. The prescriber should also be informed of severe abdominal pain or mass, jaundice, severe mental depression, or unusual bleeding. Changes in vaginal bleeding may include irregular cycle time, spotting, breakthrough bleeding, or a complete lack of bleeding.

Instruction should be provided for monthly self-examination of the breasts, and any new lumps found should be reported.

Since progestins may cause glucose intolerance, instruct users with diabetes to report positive urine tests so that an adjustment in their insulin or oral hypoglycemic dosage may be prescribed.

If progestins are used for contraceptive purposes, instruct the client to take the drug at same time of the day, every day of the year. The tablets need to be kept in their original containers. It is best to keep an extra month's supply, replacing it with the new container of tablets purchased each month. This will always ensure a fresh supply.

The client should be advised to discontinue the medication immediately and notify the prescriber if she suspects she is pregnant. Pregnancy should be avoided during the first month of administration of progestins and for at least 3 months after they have been discontinued. Barrier contraceptives should be used during this time.

Evaluation. The client will demonstrate improvement in the underlying condition for which the drug was prescribed without experiencing untoward effects. If the drug is taken for the prevention of pregnancy, that will occur.

ORAL CONTRACEPTIVES

The most effective form of birth control presently available is **oral contraception**. Millions of women have used oral contraceptives, and through experience an enormous amount of information about effectiveness, estrogen-progestin combination, the relationship of risk factors to major side effects and mortality has been collected. For example, the newer, low-dose oral contraceptives have: (a) a lower risk for adverse cardiovascular effects; (b) increased risk for a myocardial infarction, especially in smokers and women over 35 years old; (c) lower risk for stroke or thromboembolic disease than with the older oral contraceptives although there is still a higher risk than with nonusers; (d) decreased rate for ectopic pregnancies; (e) decreased risk for ovarian cysts, epithelial ovarian cancer, and endometrial cancer; (f) increased risk for cervical cancer, liver cancer, and possibly earlier onset of breast cancer after long term use (Kenyon, 1995). See the Nursing Research box on p. 827.

Performing a thorough history and physical examination, selecting an appropriate contraceptive method with the individual/couple, plus instituting a client teaching and monitoring program are basic for the development of a good family planning program.

estrogens and progestins (oral contraceptives)
(various manufacturers)

The combination oral contraceptives inhibit ovulation by increasing serum levels of estrogens and progestins which in turn, inhibits secretion of FSH and LH from the pituitary. In addition, changes in the endometrium impairs ova implantation and an increase in cervical mucus impedes the passage of sperm.

Estrogens and progestins are indicated for the prevention of pregnancy and for treatment of hypermenorrhea. The oral contraceptives are protein bound, metabolized mainly in the liver, and excreted primarily by the kidneys.

Side effects/adverse reactions. Hormone-related side effects are caused by an excess or a deficiency in estrogen or progestin or by an androgen excess. Androgen effects are more common with norgestrel and levonorgestrel than with the other progestins. Reporting side effects to the prescriber is useful because it then allows the choice of a more appropriate oral contraceptive for the individual.

Excesses and deficiencies of estrogen and progestins elicit a variety of symptoms. Estrogen excess side effects include nausea, dizziness, abdominal bloating, leg pain, chloasma, hypertension, cyclic weight gain, hypertension, breast tenderness, and an increase in breast size. A deficiency in estrogen may produce an increase in anxiety, hot flashes, midcycle spotting, decrease in menstrual flow and a possible decrease in libido. An excess in progestins may result in alopecia, oily skin (acne) and scalp, increased fatigue, increased appetite and weight gain that is noncyclic, decrease in length of menstrual flow, breast tenderness, and increased breast size. A progestin deficiency may manifest itself as dysmenorrhea, heavy menstrual flow, weight loss, and/or a delayed onset of menses. An androgen excess may result in hirsutism, oily skin or skin rash, acne, pruritus, increased appetite and weight gain (noncyclic), and cholestatic jaundice.

Dosage and administration

1. Although the use of exogenous estrogenic substances alone will inhibit ovulation, undesirable bleeding frequently occurs during the latter phase of the cycle. If estrogen levels are increased to prevent this, severe nausea and breast tenderness may occur. This is why estrogens are combined with progestins in oral contraceptives.
2. Since naturally occurring progesterone is inactivated or extremely weak in its effect when taken orally and must be given by injection to be effective, progestins (steroidal compounds related to progesterone) were developed. The majority of the oral contraceptives contain a synthetic progestin, usually norethynodrel, norethindrone, or norgestrel.
3. Norethynodrel is a basic progestin, norethindrone is a more androgenic progestin, and norgestrel is a synthetic progestogen similar to norethindrone. Norethindrone is sometimes recommended for clients having excess side effects from estrogen, such as greater weight gain and amenorrhea. Norethynodrel is good for clients with oily skin, acne, hirsutism, and breakthrough bleeding.
4. Several methods of oral contraception are available: combination estrogen and progestin, low-dosage progestogens (minipill), and phasic (bi- and tri-) oral contraceptives with varying amounts of progestin (and

Nursing Research

The controversy surrounding oral contraceptive use

The oral contraceptive pill has been a source of controversy, intense study, and media attention since its introduction. It has probably been studied more extensively than any other medication. Despite this scrutiny, or perhaps because of it, "the pill" is widely misunderstood and feared.

Over the years numerous studies have indicated that problems with the pill are dose related and that some underlying health problems can be potentiated with their use. As these studies were released, the media began reporting negative aspects of oral contraceptives directly to the public without balanced coverage indicating the improvements in oral contraceptive safety. As bad news captures far more attention than good, many women now fear estrogen use and mistrust information given by the health care provider. The issue that many adverse reactions have been greatly diminished by low-dose estrogen formulas has not been appreciated (Dirubbo, 1992). For example, for women under the age of 35 who smoke a pack and a half or less a day, the use of the pill is safer than having a baby. For nonsmokers, the risk of death from oral contraceptive use is one in 63,000, whereas one in 14,300 women will die from continuing a pregnancy (Hatcher, 1993).

Many clients believe that the use of estrogen increases the risk for cancer, particularly breast cancer. Henrich (1992) examined the postmenopausal estrogen/breast cancer controversy by reviewing 24 original articles and three meta-analyses, as well as five studies that minimized the influence of detection bias on risk estimates. Henrich concluded that there is no compelling evidence that women who have ever used postmenopausal estrogens are at increased risk of breast cancer. Reports of women with a surgical menopause, benign breast disease, or a family history of breast cancer, or women who use estrogens over prolonged periods are at increased risk are inconclusive and not consistent across studies. The reported risk in current users only, with the observation that estrogen effects predominate in lower-stage tumors and are associated with decreased mortality, may reflect unique biologic characteristics of estrogen-associated tumors, or be due to detection bias in studies that reported these effects. Detection bias relates to the issue that women diagnosed with breast cancer who had used estrogens were under closer medical surveillance and were more likely to have their disease detected at an earlier stage than women with breast cancer who had not used estrogens. Women who do not use estrogens are less likely than estrogen-treated women to be engaged in health promotion and disease prevention activities, such as breast cancer surveillance (Barrett-Connor, 1991). Henrich recognized that further research is required because the validity of the summary risk estimates obtained are limited by the quality of the published data, some of which is based on the observation of antiquated medical knowledge and practice that involved unopposed, oral, conjugated estrogen use.

The pill offers protection against pelvic inflammatory disease, a major cause of infertility. Women who use the pill have a reduction in functional ovarian cysts, benign breast cysts, fibroadenomas of the breast, and iron-deficiency anemia. The incidence of ectopic pregnancy and rheumatoid arthritis is reduced (Dirubbo, 1992). Kritz-Silverstein & Barrett-Connor (1993) have examined the long-term consequences of prior contraceptive use for bone density in postmenopausal women. They found that women who had used oral contraceptives for 6 or more years had significantly higher bone density of the lumbar spine and femoral neck that was not explained by age, body mass index, parity, cigarette smoking, years postmenopausal, or use of estrogen and thiazide medications, than women who had never used oral contraceptives.

As nurses, we play an important role in the prevention of unintended pregnancies and the use of hormonal replacement therapy by older women, therapies that might be influenced by misconceptions about estrogen use. Counseling and education are necessary to teach women of all ages about the effective management of estrogen therapy.

Critical thinking questions

- How might you use this information on estrogen use to assist your client in assessing adverse risks associated with estrogen use?
- If the use of oral contraceptives for 6 or more years reduces the risk of postmenopausal bone loss, what might be the impact on public health?

sometimes estrogen) administered in 2 or 3 phases. The purpose of the phasic dosing was a belief it might be less apt to interfere with women's normal metabolism. Clinically though, this has not been substantiated. Table 52-1 lists the composition, doses, and brand names, or oral contraceptives used in these three methods.

5. Combination estrogen and progestin contraceptives are divided into three types:
   - **Monophasic** oral contraception is a fixed ratio of estrogen and progestin that is taken for 21 days of the normal menstrual cycle.
   - **Biphasic** oral contraception supplies two different amounts of progestin during the first and second phases of the menstrual cycle; that is, low levels of progestin in the follicular phase (first 7 to 10 days), which is increased during the next 11 to 14 days of the luteal phase of the menstrual cycle. The 28-day biphasic cycle has placebo tablets of a third color so that the proper sequence is clearly marked to reduce any possibility of confusion.
   - **Triphasic** oral contraception most closely simulates the normal estrogen and progesterone levels during

TABLE 52-1 Selected oral contraceptives

Brand name	Content of estrogen (μg)	Progestin (mg)
Monophasic*		
Brevicon (21 & 28†)	ethinyl estradiol 35	norethindrone 0.5
Ovcon-35 (21 & 28†)	ethinyl estradiol 35	norethindrone 0.4
Demulen (21 & 28†)	ethinyl estradiol 35	ethynodiol diacetate 1
Lo/Ovral (21 & 28†)	ethinyl estradiol 30	norgestrel 0.3
Biphasic		
Ortho-Novum 10/11	Phase 1, ethinyl estradiol 35 (10 tabs)	norethindrone 0.5
	Phase 2, ethinyl estradiol 35	norethindrone 1
Triphasic		
Ortho-Novum 7/7/7	Phase 1, ethinyl estradiol 35	norethindrone 0.5
	Phase 2, ethinyl estradiol 35	norethindrone 0.75
	Phase 3, ethinyl estradiol 35	norethindrone 1
Triphasil	Phase 1, ethinyl estradiol 30	levonorgestrel 0.05
	Phase 2, ethinyl estradiol 40	levonorgestrel 0.075
	Phase 3, ethinyl estradiol 30	levonorgestrel 0.125

*Low-dose combination oral contraceptives.
†28s have 7 placebo tablets.

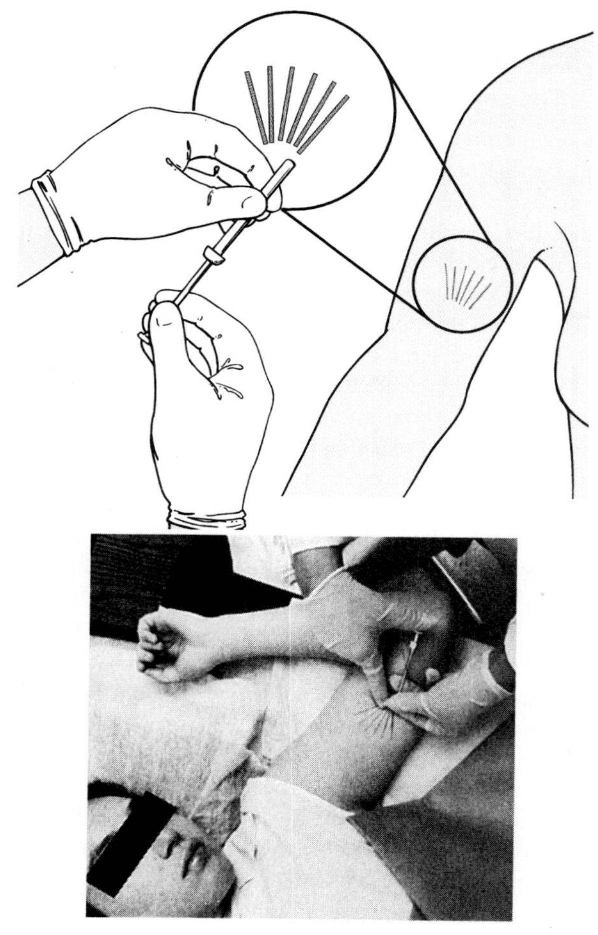

Figure 52-1 Norplant is another form of contraceptive therapy. Porous capsules containing progestin are placed just under the skin on the inside of the upper arm. (From Haas K & Haas A [1993]. Understanding sexuality [3rd ed.]. New York: McGraw-Hill.)

the menstrual cycle. The dose of estrogen is kept at a low and constant level during the 21-day dosing period while the progestin is progressively increased (three times) to mimic the natural release of hormones in the female. Because the lowest dosages of hormones possible are used in this type formulation, the incidence and severity of adverse reactions reported are considerably lower than with the monophasic or biphasic formulations.

6. Low-dosage progestogens (minipill) oral contraceptives do not contain estrogen. They are generally prescribed for 28 days of the menstrual cycle and are usually less effective than the combination products, and have a higher incidence of spotting and breakthrough bleeding. An advantage is that they generally do not cause the more serious adverse reactions associated with estrogen therapy.
7. Long-acting progestin-only contraceptives include levonorgestrel implants (Norplant), intrauterine progesterone (Progestasert), and medroxyprogesterone injection (Depo-Provera). Side/adverse effects include vaginal bleeding, muscle pain, stomach distress, vaginitis, melasma, breast discharge, and weight gain. Rarely reported is thrombus formation or thromboembolism.

The levonorgestrel system is a set of six silastic capsules that contains 36 mg each of levonorgestrel; it is implanted under the skin of the medial aspect of the upper arm (Figure 52-1). The progestin is released at a constant rate for approximately 5 years. It is then removed and a new set is inserted if continuing contraceptive action is desired. Fertility will return after removal of the implants.

Intrauterine progesterone system is a unit containing 38 mg progesterone that is inserted in the uterine cavity. It is indicated for women in a stable, monogamous relationship that have had at least one child and do not have any history of pelvic inflammatory disease (PID). This system releases an average of 65 mcg/day of progesterone for 1 year.

Medroxyprogesterone IM is administered to women every 3 months to inhibit gonadotropin secretion resulting in contraception.

TABLE 52-2 Recommendations for selection of an oral contraceptive (OC)

Conditions	Contraceptive management
Age	
Sexually active teenagers to 35 years old	low estrogen (30-35 µg)/low progestin discourage smoking
Heavy smokers* and women >35 years old and nonsmokers >40 years old	increased risk of serious cardiovascular side effects use alternate methods of contraception
Concurrent disease states	
Cancer (breast, uterus, cervix, liver)	oral contraceptives contraindicated
Cerebrovascular disease, coronary artery disease, and thromboembolic disorders	
Liver impairment; smokers >35 yrs old; history of CVA, uncontrolled hypertension, and migraine	progestin only mini-pill
Management of side effects	
Acne, oily skin, hirsutism, sebaceous cysts, weight gain	trial with OCs with lower progestin dose
Breakthrough bleeding	early to mid-cycle bleeding or bleeding that never completely stops after menses is usually due to estrogen deficiency, while late breakthrough bleeding is due to progestin deficiency; prescribers often continue with same OC for 3 to 4 months because intermenstrual bleeding usually decreases with continued use; if bleeding continues, estrogen and/or progestin dosage may be adjusted to minimize effects
Withdrawal bleeding absent	first rule out pregnancy; if not pregnant, then an OC with a lower progestin dose may be prescribed; some prescribers use ethinyl estradiol 20 µg for 3 months in addition to the OC (Ruggiero, 1995)

(Data from Olin, 1996; Ruggiero, 1995; *USP DI*, 1996.)
*>15 cigarettes/day.

Table 52-2 lists recommendations for selection of an oral contraceptive.

New Combination Oral Contraceptive

Estrostep is a graduated estrophasic dosage form of an oral contraceptive. It contains norethindrone acetate and ethinyl estradiol that contains 20 µg of estrogen/1 mg progestin for the first 5 days and then 30 µg/1 mg for days 6 through 12 and 35 µg/1 mg for days 13 through 21 of the cycle. A second formulation is a 28-day regimen that contains an additional 7 days of ferrous fumarate, taken on days 22 through 28. The manufacturer reports clinical studies found that this product was more effective (greater than 99%) than other combination oral contraceptives (FDA News and Product Notes, 1997).

■ Nursing Management

Oral Contraceptive Therapy

Assessment. See assessment in previous sections on estrogens and progestins.

Nursing diagnosis. In addition to the nursing diagnoses and collaborative problems previously cited in the material for estrogens and progestins, see the Nursing Care Plan on p. 830.

Implementation

Monitoring. Clients should be monitored for the development of side effects or adverse reactions. Among the more commonly seen reactions are fluid retention, breakthrough bleeding, thromboembolic disorders, hypertension, and nausea. If significant adverse reactions occur, a different birth control pill formula or alternate birth control method should be used. See other monitoring needed from previous discussion within the nursing management of progesterone/progestin therapy.

Education. Instruct the client to take the medications as prescribed. The tablets should be taken at the same time each day, preferably in association with another daily routine, i.e., brushing of teeth, cleansing of face in the morning or at night. Nighttime administration may be preferable to decrease nausea. Nausea occurs in some clients during the first cycle but tends to subside after the third or fourth month. It may be prevented or reduced by taking the medication with food.

Caution clients never to let their tablet supply run out and to keep an extra month's supply on hand. The packages should be rotated by using the extra package after the pills currently being used and replacing the extra supply each month on a regular basis.

Nursing Care Plan

Selected Nursing Diagnoses Related to Hormone Therapy and Oral Contraceptive Use

Nursing diagnosis	Outcome criteria	Nursing interventions
Knowledge deficit related to female hormone therapy	Client will be able to verbalize action, use, dose, and side effects/adverse reactions of hormonal therapy. Client will demonstrate a reduction in symptoms without side effects/adverse reactions.	Instruct client to take medication as prescribed. Advise client taking dosage in vaginal cream form to administer at bedtime to increase absorption. Use a sanitary napkin, not tampons, to protect clothing. Advise client that the medication may be taken with food to minimize or prevent nausea. Alert client to stop taking her medication and consult with the prescriber if she suspects she is pregnant. Advise client to report to the prescriber any symptoms of thromboembolism (sudden, severe headache, sudden change in vision, sudden pain, weakness, or numbness); liver impairment (yellow eyes or skin, dark urine, pale stools); or mental depression. Alert client that cigarette smoking while on this medication increases the risk of thromboembolism (deep-vein thrombosis, pulmonary embolism, heart attack, stroke), particularly after age 35. Stress the importance of regular visits to the prescriber for follow-up care every 6-12 months.
Knowledge deficit related to oral contraceptive regimen	Client will demonstrate compliance with medication regimen (oral contraception) without side effects/adverse reactions	Instruct client to take medication as prescribed. Advise client to use an additional method of birth control during the 3 weeks of the initial cycle. Encourage client to take the medication at the same time each day, not more than 24 hours apart. Alert client that although nausea may occur in the first few weeks of therapy, it is usually temporary and may be minimized by taking the dose with food. Advise client to always keep a month's supply on hand. Replace the extra supply each month. Provide specific information regarding appropriate action to be taken by the client when "missed" doses occur. Stress the importance of regular visits to the prescriber for follow-up care every 6 to 12 months. Advise client to alert other health care providers that she is taking oral contraceptives, since they may cause serious symptoms and interact with other drugs to less contraceptive effectiveness. Alert client to stop taking her medication and consult with the prescriber if she suspects she is pregnant. Advise client to report to the prescriber any symptoms of thromboembolism (sudden severe headache, sudden change in vision, sudden pain, weakness, or numbness); liver impairment (yellow eyes or skin, dark urine, pale stools); or mental depression. Alert client that cigarette smoking while on this medication increases the risk of thromboembolism (deep-vein thrombosis, pulmonary embolism, heart attack, stroke), particularly after age 35.

Case Study

The Client Taking Oral Contraceptives

Linda Cosgrove is a 35-year-old woman who has been taking oral contraceptives for 5 years. She is currently using Ortho-Novum 7/7/7-28. On a recent routine physical examination the nurse noted that Linda's blood pressure has increased to 154/90 from a previous range of 122/70-134/80. She has also experienced a recent 10-pound weight gain without a change in eating habits or activity.

1. Why might these symptoms be significant for this client?
2. What additional assessment data does the nurse need to gather from this client related to her drug therapy and her current status?
3. What elements of the physical examination are important for this client?
4. What information should the nurse provide this client about adverse reactions to oral contraceptives and her options for contraception?

Instruct the client to use the pills in the same sequence that they appear in the container.

Instruct the client beginning to use oral contraceptives to use a barrier method of birth control for the first cycle until the body adjusts to the medication. If she misses a dose of the medicine for 1 day of the 21-day schedule, she should take it as soon as she remembers. If she does not remember until the next day, tell her to take the missed tablet and the regularly scheduled one together. If she does not remember a dose for 2 days in a row, she should take 2 tablets a day for each of the next 2 days. In addition, she should use a second method of birth control for full protection. If she misses 3 doses or more in a row, then she should stop taking the medicine and use another method of birth control until she menstruates or until it is determined she is not pregnant. Then she may restart the medication with the appropriate cycle.

If the client is using a 28-day schedule and misses any of the first 21 tablets, instruct her to follow the preceding instructions. If she misses any of the last 7 tablets, which are inactive, there is no hazard of pregnancy; however, the first tablet of the next month's series must be taken on the regularly scheduled day. Be sure to review the literature provided with the medication with the client to ensure understanding.

Assist the client in exploring her concerns about the risks of taking oral contraceptives. Provide her with information regarding the occurrence of cardiovascular disease and cancer in relationship to her age, smoking habits, and other health characteristics. Encourage the client to read the patient package insert carefully and then to discuss with her health care provider any concerns she might have.

Advise the client to have physical examinations, which should include a pelvic and breast examination and a Pap smear, every 6 to 12 months during the treatment.

Instruct the client to notify her prescriber immediately in the instance of severe headache, blurred or lost vision (which may signal possible stroke), and symptoms of chest pain, shortness of breath, or leg pain, which may indicate thromboembolism elsewhere in the body. The health care provider should also be informed of severe abdominal pain or mass, jaundice, severe mental depression, or unusual bleeding. Instructions should be provided for monthly self-examination of the breasts, and any lumps found should be reported to the prescriber.

Medical intervention is necessary for various changes in menstrual bleeding pattern, increased and painful urination, jaundice, abdominal cramping, ocular changes (double vision, partial or complete loss of vision, bulging eyes), increased blood pressure, breast alterations (lumps, secretions), depression, or pain or numbness in fingers or toes.

Compliance with therapy is especially important if oral contraceptives are to be effective. Periodically review with the client the appropriate use and importance of taking the drug on a daily schedule. Ensure that the client knows the proper procedure to follow should one or more doses be missed.

Evaluation. The client will not get pregnant and will not evidence any untoward effects of the oral contraceptive. For further analysis of the client taking oral contraceptives, see the case study above.

OVULATORY STIMULANTS AND DRUGS USED FOR INFERTILITY

Anovulation, the absence of ovulation, is physiologic in women who are pregnant, breastfeeding, or postmenopausal. It becomes a suspected pathologic condition in individuals with abnormal bleeding or infertility. The incidence of anovulation is unknown and cannot be ascertained, but diagnostic tests may determine its presence. Clomiphene and urofollitropin are ovulation stimulants used to treat infertility in the female.

clomiphene citrate [kloe' mi feen] (Clomid, Serophene) Clomiphene has antiestrogenic effects with some estrogen effects. Although its exact mechanism of action is unknown, it has been postulated that its competition with estrogen for receptor sites in the hypothalamus causes an increased secretion of FSH and LH. The result is ovarian stimulation, maturation of the ovarian follicle, and development of the corpus luteum.

Clomiphene is indicated to treat female infertility. It is well absorbed orally and recirculated in the enterohepatic system, which may account for its prolonged duration of action in the body. It has a plasma half-life of 5 to 7 days with ovulation usually occurring between 4 to 10 days after the first day of treatment. Clomiphene is metabolized in the liver and excreted in the feces and bile. It has no known significant drug interactions. Side/adverse effects include hot flashes, abdominal pain or gas, visual disturbances, headache, nausea, vomiting, depression, anxiety, and weakness.

The adult dose for female infertility is 50 mg PO daily for 5 days, starting on the fifth day of the menstrual period if bleeding occurs or at any time in women who have no recent uterine bleeding. This cycle is repeated until conception occurs, up to three or four cycles. If ovulation does not occur, the dose is increased to 75 to 100 mg a day for 5 days, which may be repeated if necessary.

■ Nursing Management

Clomiphene Therapy

Assessment. It should be determined whether the client has preexisting conditions for which clomiphene would be contraindicated, such as abnormal and undiagnosed vaginal bleeding, endometriosis, fibroid tumors, mental depression, active or a history of hepatic dysfunction, or thrombophlebitis. If the client has ovarian cysts, clomiphene may cause enlargement of them. Clients with polycystic ovary syndrome may experience an exaggerated response to the drug.

Nursing diagnosis. Clients receiving clomiphene therapy are at risk for the following nursing diagnoses: altered comfort related to premenstrual syndrome (over 5%), hot flashes (10%), headache, breast tenderness, nausea and vomiting; sleep pattern disturbance (insomnia); visual disturbances (blurred vision, after-images, diplopia, floaters, phosphenes, scotoma, or photophobia); altered thought processes (depression); and for the following potential complications of development or enlargement of ovarian cysts, enlargement of uterine fibroids, hepatotoxicity, or thromboembolism.

Implementation

Monitoring. A pelvic examination to assess ovarian size should be completed before each course of the drug. Immunologic assay for human chorionic gonadotropin (HCG) is recommended for detection of pregnancy if menses does not occur before the next course of clomiphene is to begin. Urinary luteinizing hormone surge testing may be used to predict pregnancy. If treatment with clomiphene is continued for more than a year, or if visual disturbances occur, an ophthalmologic examination is recommended.

Intervention. Women who have been hypoestrogenic for a long time may require pretreatment with estrogen therapy to ensure a better environment for ovum implantation. A single injection of 5000 to 10,000 USP units of human chorionic gonadotropin may be given 5 to 9 days after the last dose of clomiphene to simulate the midcycle LH surge that results in ovulation to increase the efficacy of clomiphene. If three or four cycles of clomiphene therapy do not result in pregnancy, or pregnancy does not occur after a treatment interval of 3 to 6 months with documented ovulation, review the course of therapy with the client and her spouse to ensure understanding. If the regimen is being effectively managed by the client, then the client's diagnosis should be reconsidered.

Education. Coitus should occur at or around the time ovulation is anticipated, usually about 7 days (range 5 to 10 days) after the last dose of clomiphene to enhance fertilization.

If the medication is to start on day 5, count the first day of the menstrual period as day 1. Advise the client that taking the medication at the same time every day maintains drug levels and helps her remember the daily dose. If a dose is missed, advise the client to take it as soon as possible. If the dose is not remembered until time for the next dose, both should be taken together. If more than one dose is missed, the prescriber should be consulted.

Inform the client and her spouse of the possibility of multiple births with this drug. Advise her that abdominal pain is an indication for immediate medical attention, since this may be symptomatic of ovarian cyst or enlargement. Counsel her to report visual disturbances to the prescriber at once. Alert her to be cautious with tasks that require alertness, since clomiphene may cause visual disturbances, vertigo, and lightheadedness.

Evaluation. The client will become pregnant without any adverse effects of the drug.

urofollitropin [yur oh foe li troe pin] (Metrodin)
Urofollitropin, obtained from the urine of postmenopausal women, contains follicle stimulating hormone (FSH). Human chorionic gonadotropin (action is very similar to LH) is administered after urofollitropin to simulate natural ovulation. Urofollitropin is used to treat female infertility.

The most commonly reported side/adverse effects of urofollitropin are ovarian cysts or ovarian enlargement. Pain and redness may occur at injection site. Less common or rare adverse effects include severe stomach pain, bloating, decrease in urination, severe nausea, vomiting or diarrhea, weight gain, swelling of the lower extremities, breathing difficulties, severe pelvic pain as a result of the syndrome of severe ovarian hyperstimulation. Skin rash, elevated temperature, and chills have also been reported.

Usual adult dose is 75 units daily for a week or more, followed by 5000 to 10,000 units of human chorionic gonadotropin a day after the last dose of urofollitropin.

■ Nursing Management

Urofollitropin Therapy

Assessment. It should be ascertained that the client does not have a medical condition for which urofollitropin would be contraindicated, such as undiagnosed vaginal bleeding, ovarian cyst or enlargement not associated with polycystic ovary syndrome, or sensitivity to urofollitropin or other gonadotropins. No significant drug interactions have been reported with its use. A baseline ultrasound examination is recommended to determine the number and size of mature follicles.

Nursing diagnosis. The woman receiving urofollitropin is at risk for the following nursing diagnoses/collaborative problems: altered comfort (breast tenderness, nausea, vomiting, chills, rash, mild diarrhea); pyrexia; impaired tissue integrity (pain, swelling, and tenderness at injection site); and the complications of ovarian enlargement or ovarian cysts (20%) and severe ovarian hyperstimulation syndrome.

Implementation

Monitoring. Serum estradiol concentrations are monitored to determine the best dosing levels and to decrease the risk of ovarian hyperstimulation syndrome. Periodic ultrasound examination to follow follicular development is recommended. Daily basal body temperatures may be taken to determine if ovulation has occurred.

Intervention. Dosage varies considerably and is based on the client's clinical response.

Education. Intercourse or insemination should be performed daily beginning the day after the drug is administered, until ovulation is thought to have occurred.

Instruct the client to take basal body temperature daily and record it on a flow chart. This determines when ovulation occurs and assists in properly timing coitus so as to enhance fertilization. Easy-to-read oral thermometers are available that register 96° to 100° F; however, some prescribers prefer rectal temperatures for accuracy. The temperature is taken from day 1 of the menstrual period and every morning upon awakening and before the client engages in any activity, such as drinking coffee, brushing teeth, smoking, or intercourse. The body temperature is low (approximately 97.5° F) and stable for 2 weeks after menstruation. At ovulation there is a slight decrease, followed the next day by an increase (approximately 98.5° F), which continues if progesterone levels are normal. The temperature decreases again just before menstruation. If this decrease does not occur, the client may be pregnant.

Evaluation. The client will become pregnant without any ill effects of the drug.

SUMMARY

Drugs used for diagnostic purposes, to treat disorders, or to alter the normal functioning of the female reproductive system include many substances, such as gonadotropin-releasing hormone, nonpituitary chorionic gonadotropin, menotropins, female sex hormones, oral contraceptives, ovulatory stimulants, and drugs used for infertility. Gonadotropin-releasing hormone, or gonadorelin, is used for the diagnosis of hypogonadism in both males and females and, investigationally, for the treatment of primary hypothalamic amenorrhea. The gonadotropin-releasing hormone agonist, nafarelin, is used in the management of endometriosis. A deficiency in luteinizing hormone is the indication for chorionic gonadotropin. Menotropins are used in the treatment of both male and female infertility.

Estrogens, progesterone, and progestins are the more commonly used drugs in this group. Estrogen is used for hormonal replacement therapy, the treatment of breast and prostatic carcinomas, and prevention of osteoporosis in postmenopausal women. Progesterone/progestins are indicated for hormonal replacement, the treatment of endometriosis and specific carcinomas, and the prevention of pregnancy.

Oral contraception with combinations of estrogen and progestin is the most effective form of birth control currently available. Because these drugs are primarily for self-administration, the emphasis for the nurse is on client education for accurate and safe administration and for early recognition of adverse reactions, particularly thromboembolism. Clomiphene and urofollitropin, on the other hand, are indicated for the treatment of infertility.

Since all of these drugs affect sexual identity, the nurse must be sensitive to the client's needs as a sexual being and alert to cues that reflect problems such as a disturbance of self-concept.

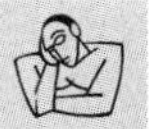

Critical Thinking Questions

1. Lillian Taylor, a college freshman, was seen in the University Health Center in September by the nurse practitioner, who prescribed Ortho-Novum birth control pills for her. In February, Ms. Taylor calls the Center and states that she thinks she is pregnant even though she has consistently taken her birth control pills. What instructions should the nurse give her?
2. Mary Ann Gilbert, age 51, has been experiencing distressing menopausal symptoms for which her health care provider has prescribed estrogen replacement. As she is leaving the office, she seems concerned about filling her prescription because her neighbor said "those pills cause cancer." What action should the nurse take?

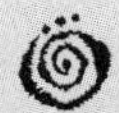

Collaborative Learning Activities

1. The students will write on slips of paper the various myths they have heard about different methods of contraception. Collect them and then read each in turn. Count a show of hands as to how many also have heard each statement. Discuss the reality of each myth.
2. Two teams of students will debate the pros and cons of oral contraception. The audience will pose different client profiles for their consideration during the debate.

BIBLIOGRAPHY

American Hospital Formulary Service (1996). *AHFS drug information '96*. Bethesda, MD: American Society of Hospital Pharmacists.

American College of Physicians (1992). Guidelines for counseling postmenopausal women about preventive hormone therapy, *Amer Coll Physicians 117*(12):1038-1041.

Anderson KN, et al. (Eds.) (1994). *Mosby's medical, nursing, & allied health dictionary* (4th ed.). St Louis: Mosby.

Belchetz PE (1994). Hormonal treatment of postmenopausal women, *New Engl J Med 330*(15):1062-1071.

Dirubbo N (1992). Oral contraceptives still misunderstood, *Nurs Pract 17*(8):7.

FDA News and Product Notes (1997). New Formulations/Combinations, *Formulary, 32*(1):23.

Gordon L (1995). Cardiac benefits of ERT confirmed, *Med Trib for Family Physician 36*(1):17.

Henderson BE, et al. (1991). Postmenopausal estrogen and prevention bias, *Arch Intern Med 155*:455-456.

Henrich JB (1992). The postmenopausal estrogen/breast cancer controversy, *JAMA 268*(14):1900-1902.

Kenyon J (Ed.) (1995). Assessment of long-term risks and benefits of combined oral contraceptives, *Drugs & Ther Perspect* 6(10):9-11.

Kritz-Silverstein D & Barrett-Connor E (1993). Bone mineral density in postmenopausal women as determined by prior oral contraceptive use, *Amer J Public Health* 83(1):100-2.

Maddox MA (1992). Women at midlife: Hormone replacement therapy, *Nurs Clin North Amer* 27(4):959.

Marten SK (1993). Complications of menopause and the risks and benefits of estrogen replacement therapy, *J Amer Acad Nurse Pract* 5(2):55-61.

McKeon VA (1994). Hormone replacement therapy: Evaluating the risks and benefits, *J Obs Gyn & Neonatal Nurs* 23(8):647-57.

Melmon KL, et al. (1992). *Clinical pharmacology* (3rd ed.). New York: McGraw-Hill.

Moore AA & Noonan MD (1996). A nurse's guide to hormone replacement therapy, *J Obs Gyn & Neonatal Nurs* 25(1):24-31.

Olin BR (Ed.) (1996). *Facts and comparisons.* St Louis: Facts and Comparisons.

Pharmacy Practice News (1995). Hormone replacement scores in landmark trial, *Pharm Pract News* 22(4):43.

Ruggiero R (1995). Contraception. In Young LY & Koda-Kimble MA. *Applied therapeutics* (6th ed.). Vancouver, WA: Applied Therapeutics.

Sobel NR (1994). Progestins in preventive hormone therapy, including pharmacology of the new progestins, desogestrel, norgestimate, and gestodene: Are there advantages?, *Obstet & Gyn Clin North Amer* 21(2):299-319.

United States Pharmacopeial Convention (1996). *USP DI: Drug information for the health care professional* (16th ed.). Rockville, MD: The Convention.

Wehrle KE (1994). The Norplant system: Easy to insert, easy to remove, *Nurse Pract* 19(4):47-54.

Youngkin EQ (1993). Progestogens: A look at the "other" hormone, *Nurse Pract* 18(11):28-40.

Chapter 53

Drugs for Labor and Delivery

Chapter Focus

Labor and delivery are the culmination of the childbearing cycle and constitute an intense experience for all involved. To implement nursing care, the nurse must understand the essential processes of labor, maternal and fetal adaptations, and the effects of the drugs used for labor and delivery. The following objectives and key terms are necessary for a good understanding of this chapter.

Key Terms

oxytocics (p. 836)
tocolytics (p. 836)

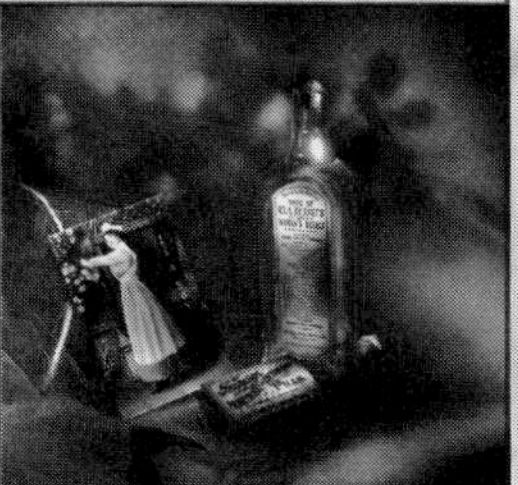

Key Drugs [▲]

oxytocin
ritodrine

Objectives

1. Describe the altered pharmacokinetic pattern of drugs during labor and delivery.
2. Discuss the pharmacologic action of oxytocics on the uterus.
3. Identify the three primary indications for the use of oxytocin.
4. Explain the two primary actions of ergonovine.
5. Discuss the mechanism of action and use of ritodrine.
6. Explain the action of lactation inhibitors.
7. Implement nursing management of the drug therapy of a client experiencing labor and delivery.

Since many drugs are available for use during labor and delivery, it is important to consider the benefit versus risk to the fetus. The pharmacokinetics of drugs may be altered during labor and delivery, e.g., during labor, gastric emptying is delayed and vomiting may result, which would alter drug absorption. Vomiting may also be exacerbated by the use of opioid analgesics. Because oral drug absorption is unpredictable at this time, parenteral routes should be used. Drug metabolism and excretion may be altered and prolonged during labor; and although clinical data are currently sparse, the potential for inducing adverse or undesirable effects is always a concern. If a drug such as an opioid analgesic or sedative may be potentially harmful to the fetus, then the smallest possible dose should be used if alternate methods are not available.

Complications in pregnancy may also dictate the use of additional medications, such as those to treat diabetes, hypertension, preeclampsia, eclampsia, and systemic infections. These medications and their proper use are discussed in the appropriate pharmacologic sections of this book. For example, magnesium sulfate for toxemia of pregnancy is reviewed in Chapter 17, Anticonvulsants. Discussion in this chapter is limited to the drugs used to induce labor (**oxytocics**), inhibit premature labor (**tocolytics**), and suppress lactation.

DRUGS AFFECTING THE UTERUS

The uterus is a highly muscular organ that exhibits a number of characteristic properties and activities. The smooth muscle fibers extend longitudinally, circularly, and obliquely in the organ. The uterus has a rich blood supply; however, when the uterine muscle contracts, blood flow is diminished. Profound changes occur in the uterus during pregnancy: it increases in weight from about 50 g to approximately 1000 g, its capacity increases tenfold in length, and new muscle fibers may be formed. These changes are accompanied by changes in response to drugs.

Drugs that act on the uterus include oxytocics, those that increase uterine contractility, and tocolytics, those that decrease it.

Oxytocics

Agents that stimulate contraction of the smooth muscle of the uterus, resulting in contractions and spontaneous labor are oxytocics. The most commonly used oxytocics are alkaloids of synthetic oxytocin and ergot, although many other drugs may have some effect on uterine contractility.

▲ **oxytocin** [ox i toe' sin] (Pitocin, Syntocinon)
Oxytocin is one of two hormones secreted by the posterior pituitary; the other hormone is vasopressin, or antidiuretic hormone (ADH). Oxytocin means "rapid birth," a term derived from its ability to contract the pregnant uterus. It also facilitates milk ejection during lactation.

The nonpregnant uterus is relatively insensitive to oxytocin, but during pregnancy uterine sensitivity to oxytocin gradually increases, with the uterus being most sensitive at term. Oxytocin secretion may precede and possibly trigger delivery of the fetus. Large amounts of oxytocin have been detected in the blood during the expulsive phase of delivery. A positive feedback mechanism may be operant; more forceful contractions of uterine muscle and greater stretching of the cervix and vagina result in more oxytocin release. Oxytocin acts directly on the myometrium, having a stronger effect on the fundus than on the cervix.

Oxytocin also transiently impedes uterine blood flow and stimulates the mammary gland to increase milk excretion from the breast, although it does not increase the production of milk. This product is indicated for induction of labor, for control of postpartum and postabortion hemorrhage, and for stimulation of lactation. For side/adverse effects of oxytocin, see Table 53-1.

This product is available parenterally and in a rapidly absorbed nasal dosage form (Syntocinon). Because the intranasal product may be erratic, it is primarily used before nursing or pumping of the breasts.

Oxytocin has a half-life of 1 to 6 minutes and an onset of action as follows: nasal, within a couple of minutes; intramuscular, within 3 to 5 minutes; intravenous, immediate, although uterine contractions increase gradually over 15 to 60 minutes before they stabilize. Duration of action is as follows: nasal, 20 minutes; IM, 30 to 60 minutes; IV, within an hour after the infusion is stopped. Oxytocin is metabolized and excreted via the kidneys.

The dose to induce labor is 0.5 to 2 mU/min by IV infusion, increased every 15 to 60 minutes by 1 to 2 mU/min every 15 to 30 minutes until a contraction pattern is established that simulates normal labor (up to a maximum of 20 mU/min).

For control of postpartum uterine bleeding, the dose is 10 units at a rate of 20 to 40 mU infused intravenously after birth of the infant. The dose for the nasal solution is 1 spray in one or both nostrils 2 or 3 minutes before nursing or pumping of breasts.

■ Nursing Management

Oxytocin Therapy

Assessment. Before administering oxytocin ascertain that the client in labor is not experiencing any contraindications to a vaginal delivery, such as cord presentation or prolapse, placenta previa or vasa previa, or fetal distress. Oxytocin is also contraindicated for those with a history of allergy to the drug and those with hypertonic uterine patterns. Prolonged use of oxytocin is not recommended for clients with uterine inertia, only a 6 to 8 hour course.

Oxytocin should be used cautiously if the client in labor exhibits grand multiparity (several prior births), over distention of the uterus, past history of trauma or major surgery on the cervix or uterus because of the predisposition for uterine rupture; invasive cervical carcinoma (vaginal delivery is contraindicated), partial placenta previa, prematurity of the fetus, or an unfavorable fetal position. Caution is also recommended in women over 35 years of age or those having an abortion using hypertonic saline because of the higher risk for water intoxication. When oxytocin is used as an adjunct to drugs that cause abortion, such as intraamniotic sodium chloride or urea, or other oxytoxics, it should not be administered until the oxytocic effect of the abortifacient has diminished to decrease the risk of uterine hyperactivity and cervical laceration.

Before administering the drug, it should be determined that there is pelvic adequacy of the client in labor and that there is fetal maturity. Record baseline data, including blood pressure and other vital signs, characteristics, frequency and duration of contractions, and fetal heart rate. If the nasal spray is indicated for pain related to postpartum breast engorgement, obtain a baseline assessment of the client's breastfeeding status before therapy begins.

Nursing diagnosis. Clients receiving oxytocin have a potential for the following nursing diagnoses: fluid volume excess related to the drug's antidiuretic effect (hypertension, water intoxication); altered comfort with nasal use related to nasal irritation and tearing of the eyes; altered cardiac output (hypertension or hypotension); and the collaborative problems of anaphylaxis and other allergic reactions, cardiac dysrhythmias, or postpartum hemorrhage. The fetus may also be at risk because of the potential for injury related to fetal trauma (cardiac arrhythmias, intracranial hemorrhage, asphyxia), fetal bradycardia, and neonatal jaundice.

Implementation

Monitoring. During the infusion, check the client's blood pressure and pulse at least every 15 minutes, and also assess the frequency, duration, and force of uterine contractions. Assess the myometrium for tonus during and between contractions and report hypertonic uterine contractions or a period of uterine relaxation. Continuous fetal monitoring should be done while the client is receiving oxytocin, and the infusion should be discontinued at any sign of uterine hyperactivity or fetal distress. Dosage is individualized for each client depending on maternal and fetal response.

Fluid intake and output determinations and assessment of breath sounds are needed since oxytocin has a slight antidiuretic effect, which, with prolonged intravenous infusion, could result in severe water intoxication. Hypochloremia and hyponatremia may occur in the client because of water intoxication.

When the nasal spray is used for postpartum breast engorgement, monitor milk ejection and the client's comfort level.

Intervention. Administration should be only in a hospital setting and under medical supervision. Intravenous infusion is preferred for induction or stimulation of labor because absorption from intramuscular administration is difficult to regulate and could result in uterine hyperactivity and fetal distress. Accurate administration by infusion pump or microdrip regulator is mandatory, as is using a Y connection so that the oxytocin solution may be discontinued while access to the vein is maintained. When preparing an oxytocin infusion, distribute the drug throughout the solution by gently rotating the bottle. Administer oxytocin for no longer than 6 to 8 hours in instances of uterine inertia.

When oxytocin is administered by nasal spray, instruct the client to clear nasal passages. Then, with the client's head in a vertical position and the bottle upright, spray the solution into the nostril. Use the spray before breastfeeding or pumping breasts. Do not administer oxytocin by more than one route simultaneously.

Education. If oxytocin is being administered as a lactation stimulant, the client should be taught the proper technique for self-administration. She should also be aware that there is the possibility that oxytocin may not be effective.

Evaluation. When oxytocin is administered for postpartum breast engorgement, the client will express relief from pain and diminished swelling. When it is given to induce or stimulate labor, then the client's labor will progress normally without indications of fluid volume excess. When oxytocin is administered after the expulsion of the placenta, postpartum bleeding will be reduced. For further analysis, see the case study below.

Pregnancy Safety

Category	Drug
B	ritodrine
X	oxytocin

Case Study

The Client in Labor

Karen Evans has spent 12 hours in labor with her first pregnancy and has made little progress. She is becoming exhausted and the uterine contractions have decreased in strength. Oxytocin is being considered as an alternative to improve the progress of labor.

1. How might the oxytocin be administered?
2. What are the associated risks of the drug for both the mother and the fetus?
3. What physiologic signs and symptoms should be monitored in this client?
4. How should the nurse describe the drug therapy to this client?

ergonovine [er goe noe' veen] (Ergotrate)

Ergonovine increases the force and frequency of uterine contractions by direct stimulation of the smooth muscle of the uterine wall. It is indicated to prevent and treat postpartum hemorrhage.

Administered orally or parenterally, ergonovine has an onset of action orally within 6 to 15 minutes, intramuscularly within 2 to 3 minutes, and intravenously within 1 minute. Duration of uterine contraction: orally and intramuscularly, approximately 3 hours; intravenously, about 45 minutes, but rhythmic contractions can persist for up to 3 hours. The drug is metabolized in the liver excreted via the kidneys. Ergonovine has no significant drug interactions. Side effects/adverse reactions are listed in Table 53-1.

Orally the dosage for ergonovine maleate tablets is 0.2 to 0.4 mg two to four times a day (on a schedule of every 6 to 12 hours). The usual treatment course is 48 hours. Parenterally, 0.2 mg is administered intramuscularly or intravenously and repeated in 2 to 4 hours if necessary, for up to five doses. The intravenous route is usually only recommended in emergencies or in cases of excessive uterine bleeding.

■ Nursing Management

Ergonovine Therapy

Assessment. If the client does not tolerate other ergot derivatives, the client may not tolerate ergonovine. Its use is contraindicated in clients with unstable angina or recent myocardial infarction as ergonovine-induced vasospasm may precipitate another attack. Because it causes coronary vasospasm, the drug should be used cautiously with clients who have coronary artery disease; ergonovine increases susceptibility to angina and myocardial infarction. Clients with occlusive peripheral vascular disease or Raynaud's phenomenon may have their ischemia exacerbated. Ergonovine may also increase blood pressure; thus its use should be limited in clients with hypertension, preeclampsia, eclampsia, and a history of transient ischemic attacks and cerebrovascular accidents. As with most drugs, ergonovine is to be administered with care to clients with hepatic or renal function impairment. Septic clients may have an increased sensitivity to the drug.

The administration of ergonovine is contraindicated before delivery of the placenta, since it may result in the entrapment of the placenta. It is not to be used for the induction of labor or in cases of threatened spontaneous abortion.

A baseline standard should be determined for the pulse, blood pressure, and uterine response. If indicated for the diagnosis of variant angina pectoris, a baseline blood pressure and electrocardiogram should be obtained.

Nursing diagnosis. Clients receiving ergonovine have the potential for the development of the following nursing diagnoses: altered comfort (severe uterine cramping, dizziness, nausea and vomiting); altered bowel pattern (diarrhea); perceptual disturbances (ringing in the ears); and the collaborative problems of severe hypertension, coronary vasospasm (chest pain), bradycardia, myocardial infarction, peripheral vasospasm, allergic reaction, and overdose (ergotism), with such symptoms as severe headache, diarrhea, nausea and vomiting, peripheral vasospasm, respiratory depression, seizures.

Implementation

Monitoring. Blood pressure and pulse should be monitored, as well as fundal tone and placement; the character and amount of vaginal bleeding should also be assessed. If the client has chest pain, the physician or nurse midwife should be notified immediately and an ECG obtained. ECG monitoring is essential if the drug is used for the diagnosis of variant angina pectoris.

If the client does not respond to the drug, tests to determine serum calcium levels should be done. Correction of hypocalcemia with intravenous calcium salts will restore the oxytocic action of the drug.

The client should be observed for signs of ergotism, such as headache, nausea and vomiting, peripheral ischemia, and paresthesia.

Intervention. When given intravenously, the drug should be administered slowly over a minimum of 1 minute.

Education. Clients should be instructed to avoid smoking because nicotine enhances the effects of ergonovine. Caution the client about exposure to cold because the body's ability to respond may be diminished. The client should be alerted that discomfort may result from ergonovine-related uterine contractions and instructed in appropriate analgesics and nonpharmacologic methods to alleviate the discomfort.

Evaluation. The client will experience a reduction in or absence of uterine bleeding and will have stable vital signs.

methylergonovine [meth ill er goe noe' veen] (Methergine)

The mechanism of action is direct stimulation of the smooth muscle of the uterine wall, which results in hemostasis. Methylergonovine is indicated to prevent and treat postpartum hemorrhage. It may be administered orally or parenterally, with a postpartum uterine contraction effect noted within 5 to 10 minutes (PO), 2 to 5 minutes (IM), or immediately (IV). Duration of action orally and intramuscularly is approximately 3 hours, while with intravenous administration the effect lasts about 45 minutes. The drug is metabolized in the liver and excreted by the kidneys. It has no reported significant drug interactions; for side/adverse effects, see Table 53-1.

The oral dose is 200 to 400 μg orally two to four times daily (spaced every 6 to 12 hours) until uterine bleeding and atony are under control. Usually oral dosing follows the administration of an initial parenteral dose. See the discussion of nursing management for ergonovine therapy.

Premature Labor Inhibitors

Preterm labor, or labor that occurs before the thirty-seventh week of pregnancy, is a major problem in obstetrics. It occurs in approximately 10% to 15% of all pregnancies. Premature birth increases the possibility of neonatal morbidity and mortality. Ritodrine is the prototype for premature

TABLE 53-1 Labor and delivery drugs: side effects/adverse reactions

Drug	Side effects	Adverse reactions
Oxytocics (stimulate uterine contractions)		
oxytocin (Pitocin)	Rare or infrequent: With parenteral use only—nausea, vomiting, tachycardia, irregular heart rate	May occasionally cause nausea, vomiting, premature ventricular contractions, fetal bradycardia, dysrhythmias, neonatal jaundice, postpartum excessive bleeding Rarely: Hematoma in the pelvic area, increased loss of blood, and afibrinogenemia Allergic and anaphylactic reactions have also occurred Prolonged therapy may result in water intoxication and possible maternal death because of its slight antidiuretic effects. Monitor clients closely during prolonged use, since hypertensive episodes and subarachnoid hemorrhage may result When given in excessive dosages to hypersensitive clients, uterine spasms and tetanic contractions can occur, which may lead to uterine rupture, abruptio placentae, reduction in blood flow to the uterus, amniotic fluid embolism, and trauma to the fetus (resulting in dysrhythmias, intracranial hemorrhage, and asphyxia)
ergonovine (Ergotrate)	Most frequent: Nausea or vomiting, seen mostly after IV administration Less frequent: Diarrhea, dizziness, tinnitus, increased sweating, confusion, hypertension Dose-related effect: Abdominal cramping	Less frequent: Coronary vessel spasms resulting in chest pain Rare: Respiratory difficulties (allergic effect); hypertensive episode (client complains of sudden, very severe headache); pruritus; pain in arms, legs, or lower back; cold hands or feet; leg weakness
methylergonovine maleate (Methergine)	Same as ergonovine	Same as ergonovine
Tocolytic (premature labor inhibitor)		
ritodrine (Yutopar)	With IV dosage form, nearly 80% to 100% of the clients have increased maternal heart rate and increased systolic and decreased diastolic maternal blood pressure. Oral dosage forms may cause small increases in maternal heart rate but do not affect maternal blood pressure or fetal heart rate.	
	Most frequent: Orally—trembling or tremors; IV—trembling or tremors, erythema, nausea, vomiting, headaches Less frequent: IV—increased anxiety or nervousness and restlessness; Orally—rash, jitteriness	Most frequent (10% to 15% with oral dosage forms, 35% with IV administration): Tachycardia, irregular heart rate Rare (1% to 2% after IV use): Chest pain, respiratory difficulties Signs of excessive dosing: Severe nausea, vomiting, nervousness, trembling, shortness of breath, tachycardia or irregular heart rate With IV, monitor closely as some cases of maternal pulmonary edema resulting in death have occurred. Cause is unknown but contributing factors include concurrent corticosteroids, hypokalemia, twin gestations, a sustained rapid heartbeat of over 140 beats/min and perhaps undiagnosed cardiac disease

labor inhibitors, but see Box 53-1 and the Home Health box at right for discussions of the use of terbutaline in premature labor and for the home care of the pregnant woman with premature labor using terbutaline.

▲ **ritodrine** [ri' toe dreen] (Yutopar)

Ritodrine, a beta$_2$-adrenergic stimulant that relaxes the uterine muscle by inhibiting uterine contractions, is indicated to prevent and treat premature labor (uncomplicated) in pregnancies of 20 or more weeks gestation.

It is available orally and parenterally. After oral administration the drug has an onset of action within ½ to 1 hour; intravenously, within 5 minutes. The time to peak serum concentration by both routes is within 1 hour. Half-life orally is biphasic, 1.3 and 12 hours (in male testing); IV half-life has three phases: 6 to 9 minutes, 1.7 to 2.6 hours, and 15 to 17 hours in nonpregnant females. The drug is metabolized in the liver and excreted by the kidneys. For side effects/adverse reactions, see Table 53-1.

Adult oral dose is 10 mg initially ½ hour before the intravenous infusion is stopped, then 10 mg every 2 hours for 24 hours. Maintenance dose is 10 to 20 mg orally every 4 to 6 hours until birth or as directed by the prescriber. Maximum recommended daily dosage is 120 mg.

Adult dose is 50 to 100 µg/min intravenously increased every 10 minutes if necessary by increments of 50 µg to an effective dosage. Maintenance dose is 150 to 350 µg/min intravenously, which is continued for 12 to 24 hours after labor contractions have stopped. Oral therapy is then instituted.

■ Nursing Management

Ritodrine Therapy

Assessment. The length of gestation should be determined, since ritodrine is not recommended for use before the twentieth week of pregnancy. Preterm labor should not have progressed more than 4 cm of cervical dilation or 80% effacement or the drug may be ineffective. Use in clients with ruptured membranes may lead to intrauterine infection. Risk to the fetus must be considered because ritodrine crosses the placenta. Neonatal hypoglycemia, ketoacidosis, and tachycardia have been reported.

BOX 53-1

Update: Terbutaline in Premature Labor

Terbutaline, a beta$_2$-adrenergic stimulant (betamimetic) is used investigationally for the inhibition of premature labor. Studies indicate that parenterally terbutaline is as effective as ritodrine although the incidence of side/adverse effects is significantly higher with terbutaline. The adverse effects with terbutaline, though, may be dose-related. To prevent recurrent labor, oral terbutaline (30 mg/d) was more effective than oral ritodrine (120 mg/d) (Sagraves, Letassy, & Barton, 1995).

Home Health

Home Care of the Pregnant Woman Using Terbutaline

The technologic advance of the terbutaline pump, along with home uterine monitoring, has allowed some women with recurrent preterm labor, who might otherwise have faced prolonged hospitalization, to be managed at home.

Terbutaline pump therapy is begun in the hospital after the acute episode of preterm labor has been stabilized. Transition to the pump requires 1 to 3 days additional hospitalization to develop the most effective basal rate and bolus schedule combination. Preparation of the client for home use of the pump includes operation of the pump, changing the pump syringe, rotation of the subcutaneous infusion site every 3 to 4 days, and reading the various displays on the pump and how to make changes based on those displays. Safety factors that are taught include checking the pulse before the boluses are delivered, keeping prefilled syringes cool and protected from light when stored, and protecting the pump from moisture and from being dropped. Proper disposal of used syringes and infusion sets are also covered.

Once home, the client is usually visited once or twice a week by a home health care nurse for assessment and intervention related to the client's physiologic, psychosocial, and educational needs. Because the use of terbutaline may result in tachycardia, the client is usually taught to hold boluses for maternal pulses over 110 or 120. Bolus schedules are based on the client's 24-hour circadian pattern, with dose frequency occurring every 4 hours or more during quiescence, and every 2 to 3 hours during peak activity periods. The standard bolus of terbutaline is 0.25 mg, and daily totals of the drug should be less than 3 to 5 mg. A review of the client's log of drug administration and uterine activity is done. Assessment of the client includes an examination of the infusion site and may include cervical examination. Bowel status should be assessed because terbutaline may decrease maternal intestinal tone, which (compounded by bed rest) may result in constipation. Instruct the client regarding adequate fluid and fiber intake for the prevention of constipation.

In addition, the nurse needs to evaluate the client's stress related to the high-risk pregnancy, coping with home treatment, and the restrictions of bed rest. Educational needs of the client include reinforcement of preterm birth prevention principles and warning signs of early labor. Other informational needs may include prepared childbirth, parenting information, and newborn care. Such information is usually available in the community to all childbearing clients.

Technologic advances such as the terbutaline pump require the adaption of acute care skills of nurses for the provision of quality client care in the home setting.

From Cowan, 1993.

Ritodrine is contraindicated when the client has cardiac disorders or hyperthyroidism because arrhythmias or heart failure may occur. It is also contraindicated in clients with eclampsia, severe preeclampsia, or pulmonary hypertension. Immediate delivery is required for clients with intrauterine infection, hemorrhage, or intrauterine fetal death. Caution is indicated if the client has diabetes or preeclampsia.

The client's current medication regimen should be reviewed for potential significant drug interactions such as those that may occur when ritodrine is given with the selected drugs listed below.

Drug	Possible effect and management
beta-adrenergic blocking agents (labetalol, nadolol, propranolol, and others)	Usage is not recommended because the two drugs are antagonistic toward each other. Drugs with greater $beta_1$ selectivity may be less antagonistic.
corticosteroids, long-acting (betamethasone, dexamethasone, paramethasone)	**Concurrent drug use has resulted in pulmonary edema and death in pregnant women. Avoid or a potentially serious drug interaction may occur. If concurrent drug administration is absolutely necessary, monitor closely and discontinue both drugs at first sign of pulmonary edema.**

A baseline assessment of the client's labor patterns should be obtained before ritodrine therapy is initiated. A determination should be made of the client's beliefs, attitudes, and values regarding the possible premature birth to enhance the educational and emotional support to be provided by the nurse. See the Cultural Aspects box above for a cultural perspective of premature birth.

Nursing diagnosis. Clients receiving ritodrine have the potential for the development of the following selected nursing diagnoses: fluid volume excess (pulmonary edema); altered comfort related to headache (10% to 15% with IV use), trembling (10% to 15%), or nausea and vomiting (10% to 15% with IV use, 5% to 8% with oral use); impaired skin integrity related to rash (3% to 4% with oral use); anxiety (5% to 8%); and the collaborative problems of altered cardiac output (tachycardia), which could result in angina (1% to 2% with IV use); pulmonary edema (1% to 2% with IV use); or hepatic function impairment.

Implementation

Monitoring. The client's blood pressure, heart rate, and uterine activity should be monitored periodically, as well as the fetal heart rate. Increases in maternal heart rate and systolic blood pressure are common with intravenous ritodrine. Oral dosages do not affect maternal blood pressure. If the maternal heart rate is greater than 120 or the fetal heart rate greater than 170 or 180, the IV rate may be slowed or the dose decreased without reducing ritodrine's effectiveness. However, if labor persists after the administration of the maximum dosage, it is recommended that ritodrine therapy be discontinued.

For those clients receiving prolonged intravenous therapy, blood glucose level, lung sounds, and fluid and electrolyte balance should be monitored. Closely monitor fluids to prevent circulatory overload. Tachycardia and dyspnea may indicate impending pulmonary edema. Other side effects for which to observe are headache, nausea and vomiting, erythema, and trembling.

Intervention. A controlled infusion device should be used when administering ritodrine intravenously to better enable dosage titration. Avoid the use of sodium chloride for infusion because of the risk of pulmonary edema. The client is placed on her left side to reduce blood pressure changes. Intravenous administration is usually continued for 12 to 24 hours after contractions stop and then followed by oral dosage.

Education. The client should be cautioned to notify the prescriber if her water breaks or if her contractions begin again. If the client's contractions do not recur, she may gradually resume ambulation and other activities of daily living after 36 to 48 hours.

Evaluation. The client evidences the absence of premature labor.

Cultural Aspects — A Cultural View of Premature Birth

In a recent article, Corrine and others describe a situation involving Lily, a 30-year-old Haitian woman who had had a series of more than 11 miscarriages. A nurse visited her after her most recent miscarriage and found her very sad. Lily said, "I was almost seven months pregnant. I've never gotten that close before. I really thought I was going to have this baby." She continued: "You know, my husband's mother hated me from day one. She promised that I would never have a child while she was alive. She sold my womb to the devil. But I kept praying to God that this condition be reversed."

Many Haitian people are Catholic but also practice Voodoo, a religion of African origin in which the faithful congregate to worship the gods or spirits, known as *loa*. These spirits are believed to be angels who had rebelled against God; they are thought to have great powers and provide favors related to protection, wealth, and health. Those who practice Voodoo believe their sicknesses or problems are the result of an evil spirit. Western health services may be bypassed initially or are a second choice. The childbearing experience may be particularly culture bound.

Critical thinking question

- How would such a belief system as Lily's influence the instruction the nurse would provide related to ritodrine and the premature birth experience?

From Corrine L et al (1992).

LACTATION INHIBITORS

Estrogens such as chlorotrianisene (Tace) and bromocriptine (Parlodel) have been used to treat postpartum breast engorgement and to inhibit lactation, respectively. The use of estrogens for breast engorgement has declined over the years, mainly because the incidence of painful engorgement is considered low and studies have indicated that analgesics or other supportive therapies are quite effective. The prescriber must also weigh the benefit of using estrogens for this purpose against the risk, particularly that of inducing a thromboembolism.

Bromocriptine directly inhibits the release of prolactin from the anterior pituitary gland, resulting in suppression of lactation. For further information on bromocriptine, see the drug monograph for dopamine agonist in Chapter 23.

SUMMARY

Although many drugs are available for use during the labor and delivery process, it is essential to consider possible alteration of drug pharmacokinetics during labor and to weigh the risks and benefits to the fetus. The drugs discussed in this chapter focus on uterine contractility. This contractility controls the labor process. Therefore drugs that increase or decrease the contractility of the uterus also enhance or inhibit labor.

Oxytocics are drugs that increase uterine motility to induce labor, augment labor, control postpartum hemorrhage, and facilitate milk ejection during lactation. The most commonly used oxytocics are oxytocin, ergonovine, and methylergonovine. When oxytocics are used to induce or augment labor, the nurse should perform a baseline assessment of fetal heart tones, uterine status, and maternal vital signs. These indicators should be monitored every 15 to 30 minutes during the administration of these drugs.

Premature labor, occurring before the thirty-seventh week of pregnancy, increases the possibility of neonatal morbidity and mortality. Once a determination is made that it is in the best interest of the mother and the fetus to halt the labor process, ritodrine may be prescribed. Ritodrine, a beta$_2$-adrenergic stimulant that relaxes uterine muscle and inhibits uterine contractions, is used to prevent and treat premature labor in pregnancies of 20 weeks or more gestation.

The role of the nurse in the administration of these drugs is to facilitate healthy outcomes for both the fetus and the mother.

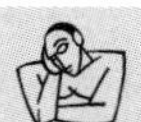

Critical Thinking

1. Shirley Demas is admitted to labor and delivery in possible preterm labor at 30 weeks gestation. She is to be treated with ritodrine. What observations will be most relevant to determine maternal side effects of this drug? Mrs. Demas' contractions do not abate, and betamethasone is ordered for her. The client asks you why she is receiving this drug. What is your response?

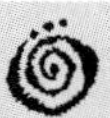

Collaborative Learning Activities

1. Teams of students will reach a consensus on nursing care plans for either labor induction, labor inhibition, or the client education dilemma outlined in the Cultural Aspects box without using their texts.

BIBLIOGRAPHY

American Hospital Formulary Service (1996). *AHFS drug information '96*. Bethesda, MD: American Society of Hospital Pharmacists.

Anderson KN, et al. (Eds.) (1994). *Mosby's medical, nursing, & allied health dictionary* (4th ed.). St Louis: Mosby.

Bobak IM, Lowdermilk DL, & Jensen MD (1995). *Maternity nursing* (4th ed.). St Louis: Mosby.

Corrine L, et al. (1992). The unheard voices of women: Spiritual interventions in maternal-child health, *MCN 17*(3):141-5.

Cowam M (1993). Home care of the pregnant woman using terbutaline, *MCN 18*(2):99-105.

Faller HS (1992). Among women: Characteristics and birth outcomes, 1990, *Birth 19*(3):144-50.

Papke KR (1993). Management of preterm labor and prevention of premature delivery, *Nurs Clin North Amer 28*(2):279-88.

Sagraves R, Letassy NA, & Barton TL (1995). Obstetrics. In Young LY & Koda-Kimble MA. *Applied therapeutics* (6th ed.). Vancouver, WA: Applied Therapeutics.

United States Pharmacopeial Convention (1996). *USP DI: Drug information for the health care professional* (16th ed.). Rockville, MD: The Convention.

Chapter 54

Drugs Affecting the Male Reproductive System

Chapter Focus

Although androgens are usually prescribed for androgen deficiency, when they are prescribed for other indications their most common undesirable effect is virilism, the development of masculine characteristics. Body image disturbance, because of androgen deficiency or effect, then may be of concern for clients receiving androgen therapy. The nurse must be prepared to encourage the client to express perceptions of self and provide reliable information about the client's health concerns. The following objectives and key terms are important for a good understanding of this chapter.

Key Terms

anabolic agents (p. 844)
androgens (p. 844)
hypogonadism (p. 844)
testosterone (p. 844)

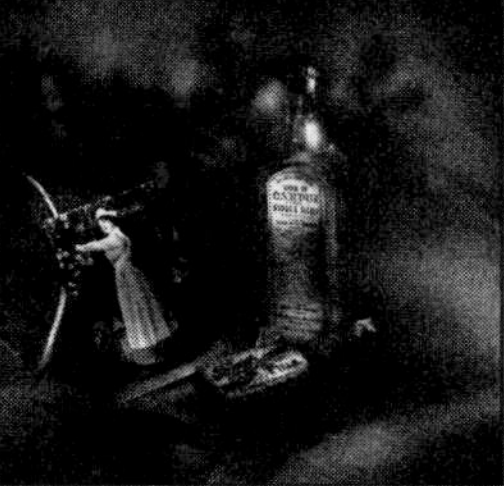

Key Drugs [▲]

testosterone

Objectives

1. Compare the pharmacokinetics of three preparations of testosterone.
2. Discuss the approved indications for androgen (testosterone) therapy.
3. List the side effects/adverse reactions of androgen therapy.
4. Discuss appropriate nursing management in the care of clients undergoing androgen therapy.
5. Discuss the use of finasteride for benign prostatic hypertrophy.
6. Implement nursing management for the care of clients receiving finasteride therapy and other drugs affecting the male reproductive system.

Androgens, primarily testosterone, are male sex hormones necessary for the normal development and maintenance of male sex characteristics. Testosterone, its derivatives and synthetic agents are commonly used as replacement therapy for males who lack the hormone. In individuals with **hypogonadism** or eunuchoidism (a deficiency of male hormone), the androgens produce marked changes in growth of the male sex organs, body contour, voice, and other secondary sex characteristics.

Hypertrophy of the glandular and connective tissue in the portions of the prostate that surround the urethra or benign prostatic hypertrophy (BPH), is considered a normal age-related change in men. Finasteride (Proscar) is a welcome addition to the treatment of BPH, which has been almost exclusively surgical.

TESTOSTERONE

Testosterone, a naturally occurring androgenic hormone produced primarily by the testes, regulates male development. It is available in combination with esters to prolong the medication's duration of action. For example, testosterone propionate is formulated in an oily solution that produces hormonal effects for 2 or 3 days, whereas testosterone cypionate and testosterone enanthate in oil are much longer acting. They are usually administered once every 2 to 4 weeks. Testosterone pellets are available for subcutaneous implantation. This form will also provide an extended duration of action; depending on the number of pellets used, it may extend from 2 to 6 months before replacement pellets are necessary.

In 1996, a transdermal testosterone system (Testoderm) was marketed. This is applied to scrotal skin where testosterone is highly absorbed at a rate at least five times greater than other skin sites. A second transdermal testosterone (Androderm) is also available and it is applied to nonscrotal skin. This system requires the application of two patches nightly, every 24 hours. Either system requires approximately 10 PM nightly application so that maximum serum concentrations are achieved in the morning, which simulates the normal circadian rhythm in healthy young males (Olin, 1996).

Oral testosterone is absorbed but is highly metabolized by the liver before it reaches systemic circulation. Administering methyltestosterone by the buccal route of administration increases its serum level and effectiveness. Fluoxymesterone is a synthetic androgen that is effective orally in tablet form.

Mechanism of action. As a natural hormone in normal males, androgens are responsible for the stimulation of spermatogenesis, the development of male sex characteristics (secondary) and, at puberty, sexual maturity. Testosterone also stimulates the synthesis and activity of RNA, which results in an increased protein production. Androgens are also potent **anabolic agents**; they stimulate the formation and maintenance of muscular and skeletal protein. They bring about retention of nitrogen (essential to the formation of protein in the body) and enhance storage of inorganic phosphorus, sulfate, sodium, and potassium. Athletes have used androgens to increase weight, musculature, and muscle strength. Weight gains may be caused by fluid retention, a side effect of androgen therapy. The potential risk of developing the major serious adverse reactions from androgens far outweighs the advantages to be gained in athletic events. Many major sporting events disqualify athletes whose use of such products is documented. Additional information on the abuse of androgens can be found in Chapter 9.

Indications. Testosterones are indicated for the following:

1. Treatment of androgen deficiency, such as testicular failure caused by cryptorchidism (failure of one or both testes to descend into the scrotum), orchitis (inflammation of the testes), orchidectomy (surgical removal of one or both testes), or pituitary-hypothalamic insufficiency
2. Treatment of delayed male puberty when not induced by a pathologic condition
3. Treatment of breast carcinoma: palliative or secondary treatment for inoperable metastatic breast cancer in postmenopausal women who have demonstrated a previous response to hormone therapy
4. Anemia: androgens stimulate erythropoiesis, the production of erythrocytes, in certain types of anemia (refractory to other therapies primarily), although this is not an approved indication for these products in the United States

Pharmacokinetics. The half-life of testosterone (IM) in plasma is 10 to 20 minutes; fluoxymesterone, 9.2 hours; methyltestosterone, between 2.5 and 3.5 hours. The time to peak concentration for methyltestosterone, buccal tablet, is 1 hour; oral tablet, 2 hours. The duration of action depends on the dose and the ester formulation administered. The longest duration of testosterone preparations is with enanthate, then cypionate, propionate, and base form is the shortest. Testosterone is metabolized in the liver and excreted by the kidneys.

Side effects/adverse reactions. In females the most frequent adverse reactions are an increase in oily skin or acne, deepening of the voice, increased hair growth or alopecia, enlarged clitoris, and irregular menses. The deep voice or hoarseness may not be reversed, even when medication is stopped. The most frequent adverse reactions reported in males are urinary urgency, breast swelling or tenderness (gynecomastia), and frequent or continuous erections. Less frequent side effects occurring in both sexes include abdominal pain, insomnia, diarrhea or constipation, dizziness, increased weakness, red skin or changes in skin color, redness at the site of injection, mouth soreness, frequent headaches, confusion, respiratory difficulties, depression, nausea, vomiting, pruritus, edema of lower extremities, jaundice, an increase in bleeding episodes, and an unusual increase or decrease in libido.

Dosage and administration

1. Choice of dosage and length of therapy depend on the diagnosis, the client's age and sex, and the intensity of the side effects/adverse reactions.
2. Usually in delayed puberty and hypogonadal (a decrease in androgen secretion from gonads) males,

dosage regimens are started in the lower ranges and gradually increased according to the individual's needs and response. In delayed puberty, after 4 to 6 months of therapy, the androgens are discontinued for 1 to 3 months while x-ray examinations are evaluated to determine the drug's effect on bone growth. The hypogonadal male will receive the androgens through puberty with dosage adjustments as required. Usually lower maintenance dosages are used after puberty.
3. Androgen antineoplastic therapy usually requires a 3-month period to evaluate effectiveness.
4. Temporary withdrawal of the drug is required if the male experiences priapism (persistent, abnormal penis erection). This is an indication of excessive dosing of the androgen.
5. Women with metastatic breast cancer should receive a shorter-acting androgen, especially during the initial therapies. It has been reported that androgens occasionally increase the extension of breast cancer.

Sterile testosterone suspension. The adult usual dose is 25 to 50 mg IM two or three times a week. Antineoplastic therapy for metastatic breast carcinoma in females is 50 to 100 mg three times a week. Pediatric dosage IM for delayed puberty in males is 100 mg monthly for 4 to 6 months.

Testosterone enanthate injection. The usual adult dose is 50 to 400 mg IM every 2 to 4 weeks. For antineoplastic therapy for inoperable breast cancer in females, the dose is 200 to 400 mg every 2 to 4 weeks. Pediatric dosage for delayed puberty in males is 100 mg monthly for approximately 4 to 6 months.

Methyltestosterone capsules (Metandren). The adult oral dosage for replacement therapy (hypogonadism, climacteric, or impotence) is 10 to 50 mg daily; for cryptorchidism, 10 mg PO three times a day; and for metastatic breast carcinoma in females, 50 mg one to four times a day. The pediatric dose for delayed puberty in males is 5 to 25 mg/day for approximately 4 to 6 months.

Methyltestosterone buccal tablets (Metandren). Dose is one half the capsule dosage previously noted.

Fluoxymesterone tablets (Halotestin). The usual adult dose is 5 mg one to four times a day. For metastatic breast carcinoma in females, it is 20 to 50 mg daily for 2 to 6 months. Pediatric dosage for treatment of delayed puberty in males is 2.5 to 10 mg daily for approximately 4 to 6 months.

■ Nursing Management

Testosterone Therapy

Assessment. Assess whether the male client has breast cancer or known or suspected prostatic cancer, since androgens are contraindicated in both conditions. These drugs should be used with caution in clients with severe cardiorenal disease because they may cause fluid retention. Those clients with prostatic hypertrophy may experience further enlargement. Impaired hepatic dysfunction may result in an increased half-life and so increase the incidence of gynecomastia. Because of the drugs' hypercholesterolemic effects, those with a history of myocardial infarction or coronary artery disease may experience a worsening of their condition.

Significant drug interactions have been reported when testosterone was given concurrently with oral anticoagulants (coumarin or indanedione) or with other hepatotoxic medications. In the former, the anticoagulant effects are enhanced or increased; in the latter, the risk of inducing hepatotoxicity is increased.

For pediatric clients, a baseline assessment should include height, weight, and a description of their sexual development. For adult clients, a baseline description of the underlying condition for which the testosterone is being prescribed should be obtained.

Nursing diagnosis. The client receiving androgen therapy is at risk for the following nursing diagnoses: disturbance in self-concept related to virilism in female clients and prepubertal males, gynecomastia and priapism in male clients, increased or decreased libido in both sexes; fluid volume excess (rapid weight gain, edema of feet and lower legs, shortness of breath); altered comfort (nausea, vomiting, and abdominal pain); altered sleep pattern; altered skin integrity (acne); altered tissue integrity (pain, redness, and swelling at the injection site); and the potential complications of erythrocytosis, hepatic impairment, hypercalcemia, and polycythemia.

Implementation

Monitoring. Monitor the client's serum calcium carefully. Promptly report indications of hypercalcemia: nausea and vomiting, lethargy, loss of muscle tone, polyuria, and increased urine and serum calcium levels. Hypercalcemia in clients with metastatic breast cancer usually indicates bone metastasis.

Serum cholesterol levels should be monitored to ascertain the client's risk of cardiovascular disease as the result of androgen administration. Hepatic function should also be monitored; hemoglobin and hematocrit should be evaluated for polycythemia. Bone age determinations should be done every 6 months to assess the rate of bone maturation in children and adolescents. Tumor growth should be monitored by radiography. Elderly men should be observed for increasing difficulty or frequency of urination, which may indicate enlargement of the prostate secondary to the drug.

If androgens are administered for gender change androgen therapy, the determination of luteinizing hormone serum levels is suggested every 6 months to monitor success of therapy, and ALTs to monitor for adverse hepatic effects.

Intervention. Administer the oral preparations with food to minimize gastric distress. Administer intramuscular testosterone deep within the gluteal muscle. The nurse should be aware that testosterone cypionate and testosterone enanthate are not interchangeable with testosterone propionate and suspension forms of the drug because of the difference in duration and action. With testosterone cypionate, the preparation may be warmed and shaken to dissolve the crystals. It may also turn cloudy if a wet needle or syringe is used, but this does not affect its potency.

The client should be encouraged to drink 3 to 4 L or more of fluids to ensure adequate urinary output to prevent urinary calculi. Active clients should be encouraged to include weight-bearing exercise, such as walking daily. Clients confined to bed should have range-of-motion exercises at least daily. This exercise inhibits mobilization of calcium from bone.

The nurse should be sensitive to the emotional responses of clients taking androgens. Female clients may have changes in secondary sex characteristics such as unnatural hair growth or heightened libido, which will subside with the cessation of the drug. Other changes that may occur, such as enlarged clitoris or hoarseness or deepening of the voice, may not be reversible. Male clients may need support to deal with deepening of the voice and rapid changes in height, size of sex organs, and hair growth patterns. Frequent or continuing erection may be a concern.

Education. Work with the client and/or responsible family member to develop a diet high in protein, calories, vitamins, and minerals that is individualized to the client's food preferences. Monitor the client with diabetes closely. Antidiabetic agents may require dosage adjustment with concurrent administration of androgens. Instruct the client to weigh daily to monitor for fluid retention. Sodium restriction and/or diuretics may be required if edema occurs. Advise the client to maintain regular visits to the prescriber for monitoring progress.

Instruct the male client using the transdermal patch dosage form that the patch should be applied to a clean, dry, and dry-shaved skin area of the scrotum. Advise him also that there is the potential for transfer of testosterone to his female sexual partner that might result in mild virilization.

Evaluation. The client's underlying condition for which the testosterone is prescribed will show improvement.

BENIGN PROSTATIC HYPERPLASIA

Benign prostatic hypertrophy (BPH), the hypertrophy of the glandular and connective tissue in the portions of the prostate that surround the urethra, is considered a normal age-related change that begins around the age of 40 years in men. By the age of 75, about half of all men will notice a decrease in the force of their urinary stream as the result of BPH (Miller, 1993). BPH obstructs the bladder neck and compresses the urethra, which results in urinary retention, increasing the risk of bacteriuria. If untreated, it may affect the ureters and kidneys and result in hydroureter, hydronephrosis, and renal impairment. The symptoms of BPH include hesitancy (difficulty starting urinary stream), a decrease in the diameter and force of the stream, inability to terminate urination abruptly resulting in postvoid dribbling, and a sensation of incomplete bladder emptying resulting in frequency and nocturia.

Because the pathophysiology of BPH may also include impaired detrusor contractility, sensory abnormalities of the bladder wall, and contractility of the smooth muscle of the prostatic urethra with functionally important alpha$_1$ adrenergic receptors, pharmacologic treatment of BPH with nonselective adrenergic blockers was tried. While prazocin (Minipress) is used investigationally for this purpose, terazocin (Hytrin) is approved for the treatment of BPH (*USP DI*, 1996). (See Chapter 22 for a discussion of adrenergic blockers.) Finasteride, a 5-alpha reductase inhibitor, is also available for the treatment of BPH.

finasteride [fin ass' te ride] (Proscar)

Finasteride inhibits 5-alpha reductase, the enzyme that converts testosterone into the potent androgen 5-alpha dihydrotesterone (DHT), a substance responsible for prostate gland growth. Finasteride decreases serum DHT by nearly 70%, thus causing shrinkage of the enlarged prostate gland. It is the first of a new class of drugs approved by the FDA indicated for the treatment of symptomatic BPH. Gormley (1992) reports men treated with a daily dose of 5 mg of finasteride had a significant decrease in their urinary symptoms, an increase in their urinary flow rate, and a 19% decrease in prostate volume.

Finasteride is 90% protein bound to plasma proteins, with maximum plasma concentrations being reached in 1 to 2 hours after oral administration. No dosage adjustments are required for elderly clients. Side/adverse effects of finasteride include decreased libido, impotency, and decreased amount of ejaculate. The drug is administered orally, 5 mg daily.

■ Nursing Management

Finasteride Therapy

Assessment. Finasteride is contraindicated in individuals with a hypersensitivity to any component of the drug. There is no indication for use in women and children. It should be used with caution in clients with liver function impairment. Determine if the client has been evaluated for prostate cancer because finasteride may interfere with the serum PSA test, a screening test for that type of cancer. Drugs such as anticholinergics or those with anticholinergic activity, adrenergic bronchodilators, and xanthine-derivative bronchodilators, may precipitate or worsen urinary retention and so reduce the effectiveness of finasteride.

A baseline assessment of the client should include liver function studies, prostatic status, and an evaluation of the client's urinary elimination pattern.

Nursing diagnosis. The client receiving finasteride is at risk for sexual dysfunction related to impotence and decreased libido.

Implementation

Monitoring. Continue to monitor the client's urinary hesitancy, force of his urinary stream, postvoid dribbling, nocturia, and frequency, urgency, and burning upon urination. Periodic liver function studies should be accomplished. A periodic digital rectal examination will assist to detect possible prostate cancer.

Intervention. Finasteride may be given with or without meals because the bioavailability is not affected by food. Women who are or may become pregnant should avoid handling the crushed tablets to avoid the possibility of transdermal absorption.

Education. Inform the client that 6 months of treatment may be necessary before the drug becomes effective in

Pregnancy Safety

Category	Drug
C	terazosin
X	androgens, finasteride

relieving symptoms. Alert the client that if his sexual partner is pregnant or to become pregnant, he should avoid exposing her to his semen because a small amount of the drug is present in his semen (see the Pregnancy Safety box above). Finasteride helps to control but not cure BPH. Lifelong therapy may be necessary. All clients with BPH should avoid drinking fluids, especially coffee and alcohol, in the evening to minimize nocturia.

Evaluation. The client's prostate will decrease in size, and the client will not experience urinary hesitancy, urinary dribbling, nocturia, or frequency and urgency of urination.

SUMMARY

Androgens, the male sex hormones, are responsible for the normal development and maintenance of male sex characteristics. Testosterone is most commonly used for hormonal replacement therapy in males, as well as being indicated for the treatment of breast carcinoma and anemia. Clients receiving androgen therapy require additional support for their risk of experiencing a disturbance in self-concept because of the drug's effects upon secondary sex characteristics. Although testosterone may be essential for an improvement in health status, the development of virilism in female clients, gynecomastia and priapism in male clients, and a change in libido may be distressing for clients of both sexes.

A relatively new drug, finasteride, is being used in the treatment of benign prostatic hypertrophy, with some positive results.

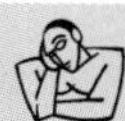

Critical Thinking

1. Althea Johnson, 54 years old and 3 years postmenopause, has an estrogen-dependent tumor. The physician has prescribed testosterone for her condition. What do you need to teach Ms. Johnson about the effects of testosterone in women?
2. Ed Taylor, 56 years old and a widower of 2 years, has just been placed on finasteride. What assessments of his sexuality and sexual functioning pattern will be necessary?

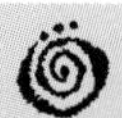

Collaborative Learning Activities

1. The students will develop a plan of care for a male client receiving testosterone therapy, and a female receiving the same. How would the client teaching vary in each plan?

BIBLIOGRAPHY

American Hospital Formulary Service (1996). *AHFS drug information '96*. Bethesda, MD: American Society of Hospital Pharmacists.

Anderson KN, et al. (Eds.) (1994). *Mosby's medical, nursing, & allied health dictionary* (4th ed.) St Louis: Mosby.

Gilman AG, Rall TW, Nies AS, & Taylor P (Eds.) (1990). *Goodman and Gilman's the pharmacological basis of therapeutics* (8th ed.). New York: Macmillan.

Gromley GJ, et al. (1992). The effect of finasteride in men with benign prostatic hypertrophy, *New Engl J Med* 327(17):1185-91.

Miller CA (1993). New medication for the treatment of benign prostatic hyperplasia, *Geriatr Nurs* 14(2):111-2.

Monda JM & Oesterling JE (1994). Medical management of prostatic obstruction, *J Urolog Nurs* 13(2):717-38.

Olin BR (1996). *Facts and comparisons*. St Louis: Facts and Comparisons.

United States Pharmacopeial Convention (1996). *USP DI: Drug information for the health care professional* (16th ed). Rockville, MD: The Convention.

Chapter 55

Drugs Affecting Sexual Behavior

Chapter Focus

Sexuality is an integral part of one's identity; it is a reflection of how one feels about oneself and how one interacts with others. *Sexual function* refers to the ability to perform in a sexually satisfying manner, with or without a partner (Carpenito, 1995). Drugs can influence both sexuality and sexual function. The nurse should be able to discuss sexual health with the client and provide information about medications and their side effects that affect sexual behavior. The following objectives and key terms are important for a good understanding of this chapter.

Key Terms

impotence (p. 849)
libido (p. 849)
premenstrual syndrome (PMS) (p. 851)

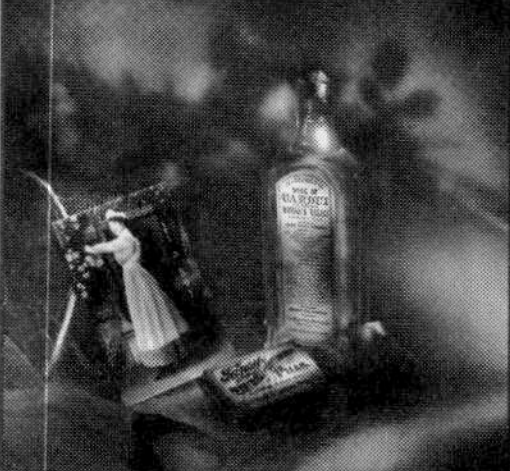

Objectives

1. Describe the effect of drugs on sexual behavior.
2. Identify the effect of commonly prescribed drugs, such as antihypertensives, antihistamines, antispasmodics, sedatives and tranquilizers, antidepressants, ethyl alcohol, barbiturates, steroid hormones, and methadone, on the libido.
3. Discuss drugs that may affect sexual behavior to enhance libido or sexual gratification.
4. Identify client cues about problems related to drug use and sexuality.
5. Provide appropriate client education about drugs with the potential for causing sexual dysfunction.

Sexuality and sexual behavior have psychologic, social, and physiologic dimensions that reflect a complexity beyond drug-related effects. Contributing factors include self-esteem, general health, availability of a partner, appropriate environment, and perhaps age. Since drugs can affect sexual activities or sexual identity, nurses must be sensitive to their clients' needs as sexual beings and alert to cues that reflect problems. Clients may present these cues if given the chance—for example, confusion, or embarrassment about lack of interest in sexual activities, about lack of arousal despite desire, or about other phenomena they consider unusual.

Certain drug therapies can produce one or more side or adverse reactions; among these are decreased levels of testosterone, which is normally present in both sexes and enhances **libido** or sexual drive; increased levels of estrogen; emotional depression that effectively limits interest or response to sexual stimuli; or autonomic nervous system blockade, which may interfere with tumescence, lubrication, erection, or ejaculation. The references at the end of this chapter and information in Chapter 51 provide a better understanding of the structure and function of the reproductive systems.

Many physiologic functions significant to sexual pleasure are controlled by the psyche and the autonomic nervous system (see also Chapter 20). This system comprises two parts—the sympathetic (adrenergic) and parasympathetic (cholinergic) systems—and its functional units are nerves, nerve plexuses, and ganglia. Although viewed as physiologic antagonists, the two systems often have synergistic effects on sexual functioning. The male and female sexual organs are composed of homologous tissues; although the shapes of the organs differ, they correspond, part for part, in structure, position, and embryologic origin. In the embryo the genital protuberance appears identical in both sexes. The embryo is characteristically female initially and does not differentiate until fetal androgens begin to masculinize tissues (seventh to twelfth weeks of pregnancy). Thus it is not surprising that the mature analogous organs function similarly.

In the male, sympathetic (adrenergic) impulses produce ejaculation by causing contraction of the prostate and seminal vesicles along with effects on the bulbocavernosus and ischiocavernosus muscles. **Impotence** or impotency is the inability of the adult male to achieve or maintain a penile erection and decreased sexual function.

Drugs that block adrenergic impulses may affect ejaculatory function through sympathetic blockade. Parasympathetic (cholinergic) stimulation controls penile erection. This response results from congestion of the vascular sinuses in the penile corpora caused by parasympathetic nerve action in the venous channels. Drugs that interfere with parasympathetic nerve transmitters (cholinergic nerves) can cause defects in erection. In addition, ganglionic blocking agents, which may block both sympathetic and parasympathetic nerve transmission, can cause complete impotence and impaired sexual functioning.

In the female, parasympathetic (cholinergic) impulses cause arterial dilation and venoconstriction, which produce clitoral erection and vasocongestion of the vulva, transudation (oozing of a fluid through pores) of lubricating secretions from the vaginal walls, and swelling of the introitus (vaginal opening). Continued stimulation of the clitoris and/or the Graefenberg spot, which is located on the anterior wall of the vagina, may then produce orgasm and, for some, a miniature facsimile of ejaculation from glands that surround the female urethra.

DRUGS THAT IMPAIR LIBIDO AND SEXUAL GRATIFICATION

Antihypertensives

Central acting alpha$_2$ agonists such as methyldopa (Aldomet), clonidine (Catapres), guanabenz (Wytensin), and guanfacine (Tenex) have been associated with more frequent reports of impotency and sexual dysfunction. Difficulty in ejaculation has been reported with guanethidine (Ismelin) while reserpine (Serpasil) may induce impotency or a decreased interest in sex.

Anticholinergic drugs, especially those with ganglionic blocking activity, may also produce impotence and other untoward effects on sexual function. Guanethidine falls into this category. Other agents include mecamylamine (Inversine) and trimethaphan (Arfonad), which are used as antihypertensive agents. Since these drugs may block both sympathetic and parasympathetic innervation of the sex organs, both erectile capability and ejaculatory function may be affected during their use.

Diuretics

The thiazide diuretics may induce sexual dysfunction and spironolactone (Aldactone) has been associated with a decrease in libido, impotency, and gynecomastia. Spironolactone has considerably more sexual dysfunction reports than the thiazides; this effect appears to be dose related.

Antihistamines

Antihistaminic drugs act as competitive inhibitors of histamine at physiologic receptor sites to prevent histamine effects. Well-known examples of such drugs include diphenhydramine (Benadryl), promethazine (Phenergan), and chlorpheniramine (Chlor-Trimeton). These drugs are consumed by millions as antiemetics, as mild sedatives, and for the control of allergy symptoms. Most antihistamines display anticholinergic effects such as dry mouth, urinary retention, and constipation. Continuous use of these drugs may interfere with sexual activity. This effect is presumably mediated by the blockade of parasympathetic nerve impulses to the sex glands and organs.

Antianxiety and Psychotropic Drugs

A wide variety of central acting agents affect sexual interest and capability both directly and indirectly. The benzodiazepines, phenothiazines, and short-acting barbiturates are often associated with sexual dysfunction.

Phenothiazines such as chlorpromazine (Thorazine), prochlorperazine (Compazine), thioridazine (Mellaril), and mesoridazine (Serentil) are commonly prescribed agents that often induce a sedative effect that may partly account for decreased sexual interest of persons undergoing phenothiazine therapy.

In addition to their central nervous system effects, the peripheral effects of phenothiazines may contribute to inhibition of sexual function. These drugs decrease skeletal muscle tone and block cholinergic synapses at both muscarinic and nicotinic receptors. Various adrenergic impulses may be inhibited as well. Impotence, decreased libido, ejaculation disorders, and prolonged amenorrhea have been reported in individuals taking phenothiazines. Failure to ejaculate has been reported in men treated with thioridazine, although erection and orgasm do not appear to be affected. Thioridazine, which has a significantly greater peripheral alpha adrenergic blocking effect than the other phenothiazines, results in a higher incidence of this side effect. Ejaculation problems have also been reported with the use of chlorprothixene (Taractan) and mesoridazine (Serentil).

Benzodiazepine compounds are commonly prescribed antianxiety medications. Diazepam (Valium) is used for treating anxiety and alcoholism and as a skeletal muscle relaxant. The sedative and relaxing effects of this drug may account for the decreased interest in sexual activity. There have been several reports of anorgasmia in males and females and ejaculation failure (Thompson, 1995). Alternatively, the judicious use of these tranquilizers has been considered of value in the treatment of sexual impotence and other problems involving sexual performance when excessive anxiety was a factor in decreased sexual performance.

Several other types of drugs used in the treatment of psychologic problems depress sexual activity in human beings. Haloperidol (Haldol), an antipsychotic, can adversely affect libido in men. Failure to ejaculate without concomitant alteration of erection or orgasm has been reported in individuals treated with phenoxybenzamine (Dibenzyline), an alpha-adrenergic blocking agent once used to supplement psychiatric therapy. This drug has been referred to as the male contraceptive. Interestingly enough, this product has been used successfully in males with premature ejaculation problems (Ruggiero, 1995).

Antidepressants

Depression is often associated with diminished sexual interest, drive, and activity (see Chapter 19). The drugs used to treat depression often compound these negative effects on sexual function. While antidepressants generally elevate mood and thus increase sexuality, they can cause impotence and influence sexual behavior adversely. The tricyclic antidepressants' effect on sexuality may be related to peripheral anticholinergic effects, such as those produced by some antihypertensives. Examples of these drugs include imipramine (Tofranil) and amitriptyline (Elavil). Although MAO inhibitors may be used as antihypertensives and antidepressants, the impotence that can result may be caused by their tendency to block peripheral ganglionic nerve transmission.

Ethyl Alcohol

Ethyl alcohol is considered for its effects on human sexual function and behavior as a drug of individual and unique notoriety. Revered for centuries as a sexual stimulant and cure of all ills, alcohol is in fact a depressant and is recognized today to have far greater social than therapeutic value. Although a sedative, alcohol in moderate amounts may enhance sexual activity by relieving anxieties and loosening the inhibitions that often shroud sexual behavior.

Beyond a certain limit, however, neither desire nor potency will overcome the depressed physical capability that occurs under its influence. Studies on the pharmacologic action of alcohol show that the central nervous system is more affected by alcohol than is any other system of the body. Electrophysiologic studies suggest that alcohol first depresses the part of the brain responsible for integrating the various activities of the nervous system. The result is that various processes related to thought and motor activities become disrupted.

The first mental processes affected are related to sobriety and self-restraint, producing a less inhibited and less restrained approach to sexual behavior and other activities normally inhibited by previous training or experience. With continued consumption of alcohol, however, the brain becomes narcotized, reflexes become slowed, blood vessels are dilated, and the capacity for sexual function is diminished. In addition, alcohol produces a severe diuretic effect, which may also interfere with sexual function.

Typically, the male alcoholic experiences delayed ejaculation during intoxication and impotence after years of chronic alcoholism. Vascular changes, peripheral neuropathy, and lower testosterone levels because of liver damage are thought to cause the impotence. Body image changes such as testicular atrophy and gynecomastia compound the problem.

Barbiturates

Barbiturates, such as amobarbital (Amytal), pentobarbital (Nembutal), secobarbital (Seconal), and thiopental (Pentothal), are sedative-hypnotic drugs that have general depressant effects on all nervous tissues. As with alcohol, these drugs in prescribed dosage produce relaxation, hypnosis, and sleep with depression of various body functions, including sexual performance and ability. With prolonged use or overdose barbiturates can cause respiratory failure and death. Withdrawal after long-term heavy consumption of barbiturates may result in convulsions. There is no rationale for their use in altering sexual behavior in human beings.

H_2 Receptor Antagonists

H_2 receptor antagonists such as cimetidine (Tagamet) and ranitidine (Zantac) have been reported to cause antiandrogenic effects (impotency, gynecomastia) when administered in high doses for a prolonged time period.

Hormones and Derivatives

Sex hormones act on the central nervous system and other body organs to influence sexual and aggressive behavior, as well as mood and emotional outlook. Thus variations in female hormones may produce the anxiety, irritability, and depression associated with **premenstrual syndrome (PMS)**, whereas male hormones are associated with aggression and increased sexual interest. Evidence indicates that sexual drive may be influenced by sex hormone treatment.

The anabolic steroids are derived from or related to the male sex hormone testosterone. They have been misused by athletes and other postpubertal persons to promote muscle growth and endurance. But when used by normally developed, well-nourished individuals, the effects of these drugs on strength and development are questionable. Considerable evidence indicates these drugs cause virilization, hirsutism, libido changes, and clitoral enlargement in females, and testicular atrophy, impotence, chronic priapism, and oligospermia in males (see Chapter 9).

Additional Medications

A number of other medications have been reported to cause sexual dysfunctions. Ketoconazole (Nizoral), an antifungal agent, may cause oligospermia and decreased libido in males (Cleary et al, 1995). Propranolol (Inderal), a beta-blocking agent, has been associated with decreased libido and erectile dysfunction. Nifedipine (Adalat, Procardia), diltiazem (Cardizem), and verapamil (Calan, Isoptin) are calcium channel blocking agents that may cause erectile dysfunction. Opioids have also been associated with sexual dysfunction (Thompson, 1995).

DRUGS THAT ENHANCE LIBIDO AND SEXUAL GRATIFICATION

Substances to increase sexual potency or drive have been sought throughout history. Inscriptions in the ruins of ancient cultures have described the preparation of "erotic potions," and an endless number of "aphrodisiacs" have been described since then. In contemporary society many drugs and chemicals that modify mood and behavior are claimed to have aphrodisiac properties.

In reality, no known drugs specifically increase libido or sexual performance, and chemicals taken for this purpose without medical advice and especially in combination with other drugs pose the danger of adverse reactions, drug interaction, or overdose. However, many pharmacologically active agents temporarily modify both physiologic responsiveness and subjective perception to enhance the enjoyment, if not the fulfillment, of the sex act. Some of these agents are considered in this section.

cantharis [kan thar is']

Cantharis (cantharidin, Spanish fly), a legendary sexual stimulant, is a powerful irritant and potent systemic poison. It is not an effective sexual stimulant. A powder made from dried beetles (*Cantharis vesicatoria*) found in southern Europe, cantharis can produce severe illness characterized by vomiting, diarrhea, abdominal pain, and shock. When taken internally, it causes irritation and inflammation of the genitourinary tract and dilation of the blood vessels of the penis and clitoris, sometimes producing prolonged erections (priapism) or engorgement, usually without increased sexual desire. Deaths have been reported from the promiscuous use of cantharis as an aphrodisiac. It is currently recognized that cantharis is not an effective sexual stimulant, and it is seldom used in modern medical practice.

yohimbine [yo him been']

Another natural substance with purported aphrodisiac properties is yohimbine, an alkaloid derived from the west African tree *Corynanthe yohimbe*. Yohimbine produces a competitive alpha adrenergic block of limited duration and antidiuresis, probably from the release of antidiuretic hormone. Although yohimbine stimulates the lower spinal nerve centers controlling erection, there is no convincing evidence that it acts as a sexual stimulant. It currently has no therapeutic uses.

opioids and psychoactive agents

The use of drugs such as morphine, heroin, cocaine, marijuana, LSD, and amphetamines as aphrodisiacs has become widespread in contemporary society. These agents can, under certain circumstances, enhance the enjoyment of the sexual experience for some. More commonly, however, sexual behavior decreases. Responsiveness varies because these agents have no particular properties that specifically increase sexual potency, but rather they tend to affect the user according to expectations. Thus the user's state of mind and the amount consumed contribute considerably to the effect achieved. Like alcohol, these drugs act on the central nervous system to weaken inhibitions, which are often the cause of problems involving sexual behavior. Taken in excess or too often, however, these drugs have the opposite effect and inhibit sexual drive and function. Because of these variations, researchers are skeptical of their value.

Marijuana (cannabis), an extract of the *Cannabis sativa* plant, is considered by many to be a sexual stimulant. However, like alcohol, its effect results indirectly from relaxation and release of inhibitions surrounding sexual activity. The active ingredient in marijuana is tetrahydrocannabinol. The pharmacologic effects resulting from smoking marijuana depend on the expectations and personality of the user, the dose, and the prevailing circumstances. Usually the effects of marijuana are time distortion and enhanced suggestibility, producing the illusion that sexual climax is somewhat prolonged. Thus the expectation that marijuana is an aphrodisiac may enhance enjoyment of the sex act. Studies on the properties of marijuana for a specific effect on sexual behavior, however, have shown that it has no such properties. On the contrary, there is evidence that marijuana smokers have a higher incidence of decreased libido and impaired potency than nonusers. In addition, chronic intensive use of marijuana depresses plasma testosterone levels in healthy males and produces gynecomastia in some users. Chromosomal breaks have also occurred.

Lysergic acid diethylamide (LSD) is another drug that, although considered an aphrodisiac by some, has potentially untoward effects on sexual function and behavior. Like marijuana, any alteration of sexual performance produced by LSD is principally subjective. This drug acts almost entirely on the central nervous system. Little response, if any, has been noted in other organ systems that can be attributed to direct effect of LSD, and no biochemical or pharmacologic evidence supports the contention that LSD or similar drugs contain any sex-stimulating properties. On the other hand, the repeated use of LSD may produce serious psychologic problems, which could overall adversely affect sexual interest or activity. Uses of LSD during pregnancy may have a higher rate of malformed babies or stillbirths than nonusers.

Amphetamines such as Dexedrine have also been used to stimulate sexual function. These drugs have a powerful central stimulant action in addition to peripheral alpha and beta sympathomimetic effects. The main effects are wakefulness and alertness, mood elevation, increased motor and speech activity, and often elation and euphoria. Physical performance is usually improved, and fatigue can be prevented or reversed. The effects of amphetamines on sexual performance, however, are inconsistent.

Amphetamines, along with other psychoactive agents, do little to promote the enjoyment of sexual activity and over time may produce adverse psychologic and physical effects that reduce sexual interest and capability.

Drugs That Stimulate Sexual Behavior

Various clinically used or experimental drugs enhance sexual interest or potency as a side effect in both humans and laboratory animals.

levodopa [lee voe doe' pa] (L-dopa)

Levodopa (L-dopa) is a natural intermediate in the biosynthesis of catecholamines in the brain and peripheral adrenergic nerve terminals. In the biologic sequence of events it is converted to dopamine, which in turn serves as a substrate of the neurotransmitter norepinephrine. Levodopa is used successfully in the treatment of Parkinson's syndrome, a disease characterized by dopamine deficiency. When levodopa is administered to an individual with this syndrome, the symptoms are ameliorated, presumably because the drug is converted to dopamine, thereby counteracting the deficiency.

Individuals treated with levodopa, especially elderly men, have been observed to have a sexual rejuvenation. This effect has led to the belief that levodopa stimulates sexual powers. Consequently, studies with younger men complaining of decreased erectile ability have shown that levodopa increases libido and incidence of penile erections. Overall, however, these effects have been short-lived and do not reflect continued satisfactory sexual function and potency. Thus levodopa is not a true aphrodisiac, but the increased sexual activity experienced by parkinsonian clients treated with levodopa may reflect improved well-being and partial recovery of normal sexual functions impaired by Parkinson's disease.

amyl nitrite [am' il]

Amyl nitrite, a drug used in the past to treat angina pectoris, is alleged to enhance sexual activity in humans. As a vasodilator and smooth muscle stimulant, amyl nitrite has been reported to intensify the orgasmic experience for men if inhaled at the moment of orgasm. This effect is probably the result of relaxation of smooth muscles and consequent vasodilation of the genitourinary tract. No effects of amyl nitrite on libido have been reported, but loss of erection or delayed ejaculation may result. Women generally experience negative effects on orgasm when taking this drug.

vitamin E

Much has been said about the positive effects of vitamin E (alpha-tocopherol) on sexual performance and ability in human beings. Unfortunately, little scientific rationale substantiates such claims. The primary reasons for attributing a positive role in sexual performance to vitamin E come from experiments on vitamin E deficiency in laboratory animals. In such experiments the principal manifestation of this deficiency is infertility, although the reasons for this condition differ in males and females. In female rats there is no loss in ability to produce apparently healthy ova or any defect in the placenta or uterus. However, fetal death occurs shortly after the first week of embryonic life, and fetuses are reabsorbed. This situation can be prevented if vitamin E is administered any time up to the fifth or sixth day of embryonic life. In the male rat the earliest observable effect of vitamin E deficiency is immobility of spermatozoa, with subsequent degeneration of the germinal epithelium. However, secondary sex organs are not altered and sexual vigor is not diminished, although vigor may decrease if the deficiency continues.

Because of experimental results such as these, vitamin E has been conjectured to restore potency, or preserve fertility, sexual interest, and endurance in humans. No evidence supports these contentions, but since sexual performance is often influenced by mental attitude, a person who believes vitamin E may improve sexual prowess may actually find improvement. The only established therapeutic use for vitamin E is for the prevention or treatment of vitamin E deficiency, a condition that is rare in humans.

THE NURSE'S ROLE IN HUMAN SEXUALITY

An appreciation of the serious effects of sexual dysfunction on people's lives can produce a special sensitivity to clients' concerns. People often find it easier to confide in and discuss such important personal information with a nurse, male or female, than with anyone else.

High-quality professional nursing therefore should be directed toward achieving the following goals:

- Gaining understanding and acceptance of feelings about one's own sexuality. It takes time and effort to be comfortable enough to be therapeutic with others who are having sexual problems.
- Being open to clients' discussions about sexual concerns.
- Allowing clients to hold any belief or sexual practice they choose that is not overtly harmful.
- Recognizing that it is probably impossible to be truly comfortable with all clients or all related topics. It may be necessary to refer some clients with questions to more adequately prepared personnel. This might be a clinical nurse specialist or a social worker with expertise in dealing with sexual issues.
- Keeping current with the constantly changing data about drugs with potential for causing sexual dysfunction. This becomes more complex with the discovery, for example, that certain drugs in combination elicit unusual sexual responses. Currently, some that are suspect include antihypertensives, antidepressants, antihistamines, sedatives and tranquilizers, ethyl alcohol, barbiturates, steroid hormones and derivatives, opioids and psychoactive drugs, and certain natural substances.
- Being able to identify and interpret client cues about problems dealing with sexuality, such as unexplained noncompliance with medication instructions, certain subjective data from the nursing history, avoidance of the topic, or other subtle cues.
- Discussing clients' medication with them (casual use of drugs and over-the-counter and prescribed drugs), including information about potential adverse reactions.
- Consulting with the prescriber when adverse reactions do appear and suggesting that alternate forms or dosages of drug therapy be sought, if feasible. Such changes may be the route to enhanced compliance.
- Listening with sensitivity to expressed feelings of frustration, anger, anxiety, or fear that may attend body image changes or perceptions of aging and waning sexual attractiveness, which may actually result from drug effects.

SUMMARY

Because drug therapy has many dimensions that affect sexuality and sexual behavior, nurses must be sensitive in their assessment of clients' needs as sexual beings and able to intervene to promote health in this area.

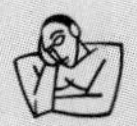

Critical Thinking

1. What are some appropriate assessment questions that will elicit client responses related to diminished libido secondary to a medication?
2. What would be your response if a nonnursing student at your school asked about the sexual effects of cannabis or alcohol?

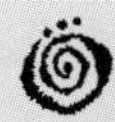

Collaborative Learning Activities

1. Teams will create client situations in which libido and sexual gratification are impaired by a specific drug. Each team will present a role play based on their case study providing "cues" to sexual dysfunction. The class will be challenged to catch the cues and suggest responses to the presenters and offer suggestions for an appropriate client education plan.

BIBLIOGRAPHY

Abramowicz M (Ed.) (1992). Drugs that cause sexual dysfunction: An update, *Med Lett* 34(876):73.

Anderson KN, et al. (Eds.) (1994). *Mosby's medical, nursing, & allied health dictionary* (4th ed.). St Louis: Mosby.

Carpenito LJ (1995). *Nursing diagnosis: Application to clinical practice* (6th ed.). Philadelphia: JB Lippincott.

Cleary JD, Chapman SW, Clark A, & Lucia H (1995). Fungal Infections. In Young LY & Koda-Kimble MA. *Applied therapeutics* (6th ed.). Vancouver: Applied Therapeutics.

Ruggiero RJ (1995). Contraception. In Young LY & Koda-Kimble MA. *Applied therapeutics* (6th ed.). Vancouver: Applied Therapeutics.

Thompson JF (1995). Geriatric urological disorders. In Young LY & Koda-Kimble MA. *Applied therapeutics* (6th ed.). Vancouver: Applied Therapeutics.

Chapter 56

Antineoplastic Chemotherapy

Chapter Focus

Progress in antineoplastic chemotherapy has helped in providing palliation and a greater life expectancy for many persons with a diagnosis of cancer. Unfortunately, though, the cure for most cancers is unknown. Many of the commonly used antineoplastic agents also have undesirable side effects such as fatigue, nausea, vomiting, stomatitis, and bone marrow depression. Nurses not only administer antineoplastic agents as part of their role in many health care agencies but also are primarily responsible for providing care for clients receiving these agents, to promote comfort and minimize the risk for injury associated with them (Box 56-1). The following objectives and key terms are necessary for a good understanding of this chapter.

Key Terms

cancer (p. 855)
combination chemotherapy (p. 857)
dose-limiting effect (p. 858)
Gompertzian growth (p. 856)
metastasis (p. 856)
micrometastases (p. 857)

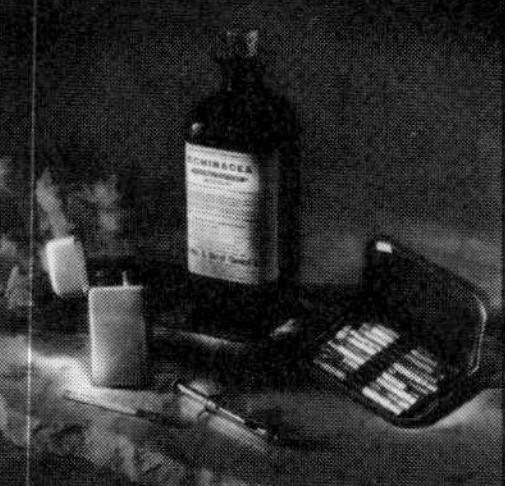

Objectives

1. Identify four major developmental stages of normal and malignant cells.
2. List common antineoplastic drugs and their effects on the cell cycle.
3. Describe the major principles of chemotherapy.
4. Describe the common toxicities of antineoplastic chemotherapy.
5. Discuss age-related considerations for cancer in the elderly and pediatric client.
6. Implement a plan of care using nursing management common to all antineoplastic drug therapy.

Cancer refers to a group of over 300 diseases that is characterized by uncontrolled growth and spread of abnormal cells. It has been estimated that approximately 40% to 45% of Americans will develop cancer during their lifetime (Finley, LaCivita, & Lindley, 1995a). Many people fear cancer, since it is difficult to accept that a small lump or mole that has the potential for rapid growth may lead to serious illness or death. Therefore education and early treatment are imperative to win the battle against cancer, which is second only to cardiovascular disease as a cause of death.

Statistically the chances of developing cancer and dying from cancer are greater now than ever before. In 1996 the number of new cases of cancer in the United States was estimated to be 1,359,150 persons (Parker et al, 1996). This is a vast increase in the reported incidence of cancer compared with past years. While the figures are staggering, the fact that the rise in cancer deaths has not paralleled the rise in cancer incidence indicates that we have made some progress in the war against cancer.

This chapter discusses the principles of antineoplastic chemotherapy and the use of chemotherapeutic drugs in the treatment of cancer. However, to better understand the mechanisms and sites of action of the cancer chemotherapeutic agents, it is important to understand the kinetics of both normal cells and cancer cells.

CELL KINETICS

The reproductive cycles of normal and cancer cells are essentially the same (Figure 56-1). In the presynthesis phase (G_1), RNA and protein synthesis may occur. Also during this phase the decision for cell replication or cell differentiation is determined. The cell progresses to the synthesis phase (S), which is the replication phase; DNA doubles in preparation for cell division. During the postsynthesis or premitotic phase (G_2), DNA synthesis ceases but RNA and protein synthesis continues in order to prepare the cell for mitosis (M), or spindle formation. During the M-phase, cells divide into two completely new cells that may leave the cell cycle to do the following: (1) develop into differentiated cells that perform a specialized function (such as neuron, epithelium, etc.); these cells can no longer undergo cell division; or (2) become either temporarily or permanently nonproliferative (G_0 phase). Cells in the G_0 (or resting) phase may remain in this phase, or may reenter the cell cycle in time, or may mature and die.

BOX 56-1

The Nurse's Role in Administration of Antineoplastic Agents

The role of the nurse is dynamic, increasing in its competencies to meet the needs of the increasing technology and the health care of society. Certainly this evolution of role is being demonstrated in the administration of antineoplastic agents and the monitoring of clients receiving them. Because these types of changes in the responsibilities of the nurse frequently come about by custom and practice rather than law, nurses must ensure that their health care agencies have in place policies and procedures to protect them and their clients. Nursing organizations often provide guidance for health care agencies by indicating their position in relation to the new responsibilities that nurses are to assume. Because there was such a need to identify the knowledge and skills required of the nurse designated to administer and monitor antineoplastic agents, the Intravenous Nursing Society (INS) issued this statement in 1991, authored by C. Rutherford:

Whereas, the administration of antineoplastic agents is established in health care facilities policy and procedure, and

Whereas, written verification of informed consent from the patient or legal guardian is obtained prior to the administration of antineoplastic agents, and

Whereas, the patient is informed and provided instruction regarding all aspects of the therapy which includes but is not limited to potential side effects and complications both physical and psychological associated with this treatment, and

Whereas, the responsibility for administration of these agents includes but is not limited to knowledge of the disease processes, drug classifications, recommended dose and volume to age, height, and weight or body surface area, specific pharmacological indications, drug properties (vesicant and nonvesicant), actions, side effects, adverse reactions, methods of administration, infusion rates, and treatment focus (palliative or curative), and

Whereas, an in-depth knowledge and understanding of the vascular system is a necessary prerequisite for the nurse administering this therapy as well as the ability to identify and preserve venous access, which is crucial for the patient receiving these agents, and

Whereas, selection of appropriate administration equipment is essential to enhance therapy and prevent complications, and

Whereas, the potential complications from these agents must be understood and anticipated and the need for immediate implementation of life-saving interventions recognized, and

Whereas, decreasing the occurrence of antineoplastic agent tissue extravasation and its associative complications requires specific technical expertise in intravenous cannula placement and the skill for accurate and immediate assessment of infiltration, and

Whereas, extravasation protocols for vesicants are established in the facility or agency policy and procedure and when vesicant infiltration occurs are implemented by a nursing professional, skilled in these procedures, to effect the desired outcome,

Therefore, be it resolved that the professional nurse who possesses the necessary knowledge of the disease processes and therapy and has documented clinical competency in intravenous therapy is qualified to administer antineoplastic agents.

Critical thinking questions

- How could a position statement such as this serve to protect the public? How would it serve to protect nurses?
- If you were the nurse manager on an oncology unit, how could you use this position statement?

From Rutherford (1992).

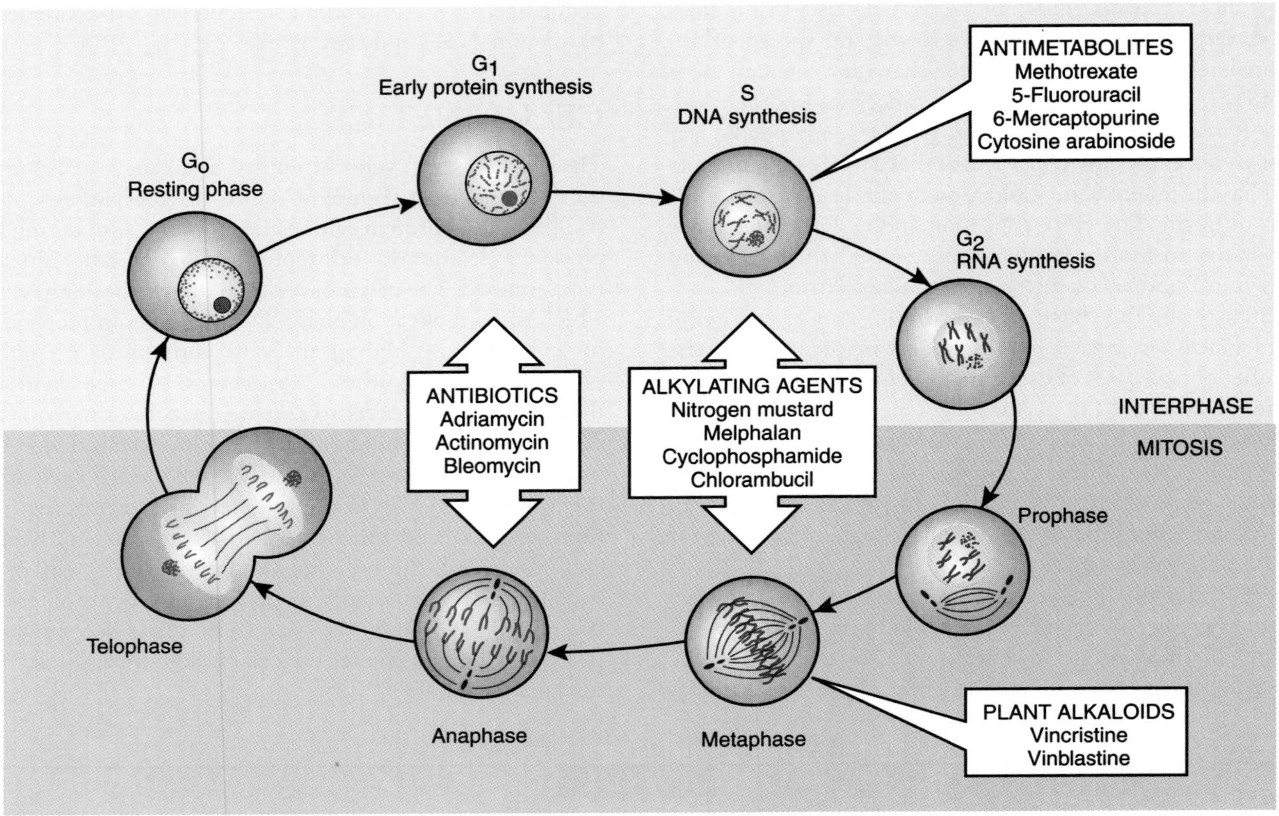

Figure 56-1 Phases of a cell cycle. Drugs are identified by where they exert their effect. (From Beare PG & Myers JL [1994]. *Principles and practice of adult health nursing* [2nd ed.]. St. Louis: Mosby.)

The anticancer agents have different sites of action on the dividing cell cycle. Agents that are most effective in one specific phase are referred to as cell cycle-specific agents. For example, methotrexate is more active in the S-phase of the cell cycle, so it is considered an S-phase cell cycle-specific agent. Antineoplastic agents that are active against both proliferating and resting cells are called cell cycle-nonspecific agents. An example of this group is the alkylating agents (see Table 57-1). Antineoplastic classifications are an important consideration in selecting the appropriate drug(s) for the specific cancerous state. Methotrexate, an agent active predominantly in the S-phase of the cell cycle, would be much less effective in treating large tumor masses, which generally have slowly dividing cancer cells.

Normal cells grow and divide in an orderly fashion. The body process of cell adhesion inhibits the movement of the newly formed cells, and the body's homeostatic mechanisms control the entire cell growth process. Cancer cells may evolve from a hereditary or genetic predisposition plus contact with certain environmental conditions. Generally such neoplastic cells lack the cellular differentiation of the tissues in which they originate and therefore are unable to function like the normal cells around them. Cancer growth is enhanced by an increased rate of cell proliferation that lacks the normal body control system on cellular growth patterns. Cancer cells, because of the genetic differences, lack the cell adhesive property of normal cells, which may lead to **metastasis,** or spread of the cancer.

BOX 56-2

Cancer Cell Growth (Gompertzian)

	Number of cells present	
10^0	1	
10^1	10	
10^2	100	
10^3	1000	Subclinical disease (undetectable by physical examination)
10^4	10,000	
10^5	100,000	
10^6	1,000,000	
10^7	10,000,000	
10^8	100,000,000	
10^9	1,000,000,000	(1 g) Clinical symptoms appear
10^{10}	10,000,000,000	Regional spread
10^{11}	100,000,000,000	
10^{12}	1,000,000,000,000	Metastases
10^{13}	10,000,000,000,000	Lethal

The growth of a cancer is usually rapid in the early stages; but as the tumor enlarges, it nearly outgrows its blood and nutrient supply, and the growth rate pattern decreases or reaches the plateau phase for the tumor. This is referred to as **Gompertzian growth** kinetics (Box 56-2). A cell burden of 10^9 is usually the

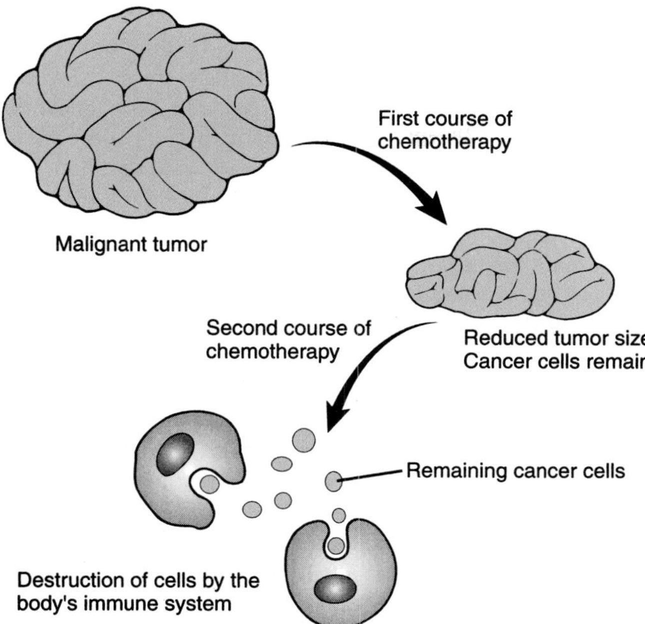

Figure 56-2 Cancer cell response to chemotherapy. (From Beare PG & Myers JL [1994]. *Principles and practice of adult health nursing* [2nd ed.]. St. Louis: Mosby.)

smallest tumor burden (quantitative size) that is physically detectable (palpated). At this point the client has approximately 1 billion cancer cells, which is equal to a tumor about the size of a small grape and weighing 1 g. This is the point at which clinical symptoms usually first appear.

The Papanicolaou (Pap) smear is a cytologic test capable of detecting carcinoma of the cervix and endometrium in the subclinical stages. Early detection and treatment of small cancer lesions that are not detectable by visual examination have dramatically reduced the mortality of cancer of the cervix in the United States and Canada.

Animal studies have shown that chemotherapeutic drugs given in adequate doses to the host will kill a constant fraction of the cancer cells. For example, a drug or drug combination capable of killing 99.9% of the cells would only reduce a 10^{10} cell burden to 10^7 cancer cells. Each course of chemotherapy may reduce cancer cells to eventual levels that may be controlled by the client's immune system (Figure 56-2). This reduction may produce a remission; but if further therapies are not instituted or the immune system is inadequate, the remaining cells may grow into another detectable tumor.

PRINCIPLES OF CHEMOTHERAPY

To obtain optimal therapeutic effects with an antineoplastic agent or with combination cancer chemotherapies, the following principles should be considered:

1. Cancer chemotherapy is most effective against small tumors because they usually have an efficient blood supply and therefore drug delivery to the cancer site is increased. Also, small tumors generally have a higher percentage of proliferating cells so that a higher cell-kill factor is possible.
2. The removal of large, localized tumors by surgery reduces the tumor cell burden and thus contributes to the success of the adjuvant chemotherapy. The major use of adjuvant chemotherapy is to help eradicate the **micrometastases** (the migration of cancer cells via the bloodstream or lymphatic system to grow in organs, bone, or tissues, far from the primary site) of cancer after surgery or radiation.
3. In general, combination cancer chemotherapeutic agents have a higher cancer cell-kill than treatment with a single drug agent.

COMBINATION CHEMOTHERAPY

In the late 1960s **combination chemotherapy,** the use of two or more anticancer drugs at the same time, was initiated for the treatment of acute lymphoblastic leukemia and Hodgkin's disease. When the complete response rates for single agents were compared with the response rates for combination drugs, the results were enlightening. The response rates for the *MOPP* treatment of advanced Hodgkin's disease is a classic illustration, as follows:

Drug	Complete response rates	
M	mustine (Mustargen)	20%
O	vincristine (Oncovin)	<10%
P	procarbazine	<10%
P	prednisone	<5%
	MOPP combination	80%

The following considerations are used to select the drugs for combination chemotherapy:

1. Each drug when used alone should be active against the specific cancer.
2. Each drug should have a different site of action and act at a different point of the cell cycle (specificity).
3. Each drug should have a different organ toxicity or, if the toxic effect is similar, it should occur at different times after drug administration.

When the preceding principles are applied to the MOPP drug therapy, the concept of combination chemotherapy can be understood. First, the previous list illustrates the effectiveness of each drug against Hodgkin's disease. Second, the sites of major activity for each antineoplastic agent are believed to be different.

1. Mustine (Mustargen) is an alkylating agent that can interfere with the replication, transcription, and translation of DNA.
2. Vincristine (Oncovin) inhibits mitosis by interfering with the mitotic spindle.
3. Procarbazine is a weak monoamine oxidase (MAO) inhibitor, and its antineoplastic action is believed to occur during the S-phase. It inhibits the synthesis of DNA, RNA, and protein.
4. Prednisone has lympholytic properties and may produce an antifibrotic effect that would be useful in treating cancer metastases surrounded by fibrous materials. It also improves appetite and general feelings of well-being.

TABLE 56-1 Combination chemotherapeutic regimens

Cancer	Acronym	Drugs
Breast	CMF	cyclophosphamide methotrexate fluorouracil
	CFPT	cyclophosphamide fluorouracil prednisone tamoxifen
Colon	FLe	fluorouracil levamisole
	F-Cl	fluorouracil calcium leucovorin
Lung	CAV	cyclophosphamide doxorubicin (Adriamycin) vincristine
	COPE	cyclophosphamide vincristine (Oncovin) cisplatin (Platinol) etoposide

The third principle, that of different organ toxicity or toxicities that occur at different times, has also been substantiated for the MOPP combinations. The dose-limiting toxicity of bone marrow suppression is a property of both mustine and procarbazine, but the nadir, or the lowest depression point for this effect, occurs approximately 10 days after drug administration for mustine and 21 days after for procarbazine. Thus additive myelosuppressive effects from this combination are essentially avoided. Also, vincristine does not have bone marrow suppression effects but does exhibit a dose-limiting neurotoxicity. Prednisone does not demonstrate bone marrow suppression or neurotoxicity. Therefore the third principle of combination drug therapy is fulfilled.

Oncologists frequently use combination therapy in antineoplastic treatment. Table 56-1 lists other commonly prescribed drug combinations.

TOXIC EFFECTS

Most of the currently available antineoplastic agents appear to act on similar metabolic pathways in both normal and malignant cells. A major limitation of cancer drugs is their lack of tumor specificity. Drug toxicities or side effects may be divided into (1) common side effects, (2) adverse reactions, and (3) specific dose-limiting drug effects. A **dose-limiting effect** is a response to a drug that indicates that the maximum permissible dose has been reached and the drug should be decreased or discontinued.

The *most common side effects* are alopecia (hair loss), nausea, vomiting, anorexia, diarrhea, and stomatitis (inflammation of the mouth). Cancer chemotherapy is most active or effective against dividing cells, but they are not capable of differentiating between cancer cells and normal dividing body cells. Therefore the most rapidly dividing cells in the body, which are in the bone marrow, hair follicles, and gastrointestinal tract, are generally the most affected by the anticancer drugs.

The *most common adverse reactions* that can lead to serious and even life-threatening infections are leukopenia, thrombocytopenia, and anemia. Bone marrow suppression is the major dose-limiting property most frequently encountered in cancer chemotherapy. Nursing assessment and monitoring are critical to improving client care and are reviewed in the nursing management section.

Specific *dose-limiting effects* are adverse reactions that should indicate to the prescriber that the maximum permissible dose has been delivered and the drug needs to be discontinued. Fortunately, this occurs with only certain drugs. For example, drugs that can produce hepatotoxicity include methotrexate (Mexate, Folex), mercaptopurine (Purinethol), lomustine (CCNU, CeeNu), dacarbazine (DTIC-Dome), doxorubicin (Adriamycin), and carmustine (BCNU, BiCU).

Cyclophosphamide (Cytoxan) is associated with hemorrhagic cystitis. (Since dehydration increases the risk factor, adequate fluid intake is important when this agent is administered.) Methotrexate is associated with tubular necrosis, which can be prevented by prehydrating with normal saline and alkalinizing the urine to increase the elimination of the drug. Cisplatin (Platinol) is associated with tubular necrosis. Prehydration with 1 to 2 L of intravenous fluid and adequate fluids after drug administration help to reduce this adverse reaction. Nephrotoxicity, ototoxicity, and peripheral neuropathy have been reported with cisplatin.

Cardiac toxicity is reported with both doxorubicin (Adriamycin) and daunorubicin (Cerubidine). Cardiotoxicity increases in clients who receive more than 550 mg/m^2 of body surface (total accumulated dosage given throughout therapy). Toxicity is also greater in geriatric clients and children under 2 years of age. Since this effect is cumulative if either drug is given, the amount of one drug already received by the client must be considered when planning therapy with the other drug.

Neurologic toxicity may range from tingling of the hands and feet and loss of deep tendon reflexes to ataxia, footdrop, confusion, and personality changes. Drugs reported to produce neurologic effects include vincristine (Oncovin), vinblastine (Velbane, Velsar), and methotrexate (Folex).

AGE-RELATED CONSIDERATIONS

Cancer in the Elderly

Cancer in the elderly is a serious disease and its incidence increases sharply with age. About 50% of all cases of cancer in the United States occur in persons over 65 years old (Patel & Koeller, 1993). When compared with younger cancer victims, the elderly have more concurrent illnesses, which may decrease their ability to withstand the effects of cancer or the antineoplastic therapies. In addition, decreased pulmonary and renal function and decreased bone marrow cellularity may interfere with treatment. Other factors to be considered when managing regimens for elderly persons are the possibility of reduced income and loss of loved ones and family support.

Often compromises in treatment are made because of a person's advanced age; however, data suggest that a dosage reduction of chemotherapy based on age alone is not always appropriate. A treatment approach should be based on the individual cancer and the biologic and physiologic differences noted in the elderly person. More clinical trials are also needed to further examine the relationship between cancer chemotherapy responsiveness and the person's age.

Cancer in Children

While cancer in children is relatively uncommon, in the United States children between the ages of 1 and 14 years most commonly die of cancer. Acute leukemias are the most common pediatric cancer. Carcinomas, which are common in adults, are rare in children, while sarcomas are much more common in children (Finley et al, 1995b). Since tumors in children grow rapidly, childhood cancer is generally more responsive to chemotherapy than is cancer in an adult. Children also tend to tolerate the acute side effects of chemotherapy better than adults. Fifty percent of children with cancer are long-term survivors or are actually cured.

■ Nursing Management

Antineoplastic Chemotherapy

Assessment. Nursing care for clients receiving drug therapy with antineoplastic agents is complex and inseparable from nursing care of the family. The client may be in any state of the disease process and may be facing impending death. In the assessment of the client and family, special considerations should be given to their coping abilities. The approach taken by the nurse should be sensitive and appropriate to the individual needs of the client and family. The client's degree of acceptance of chemotherapy should be assessed, and the nurse may need to help the client deal with mixed emotions about the chemotherapy. The client's and family's knowledge of the chemotherapy and their expectations should also be assessed.

A baseline assessment would include a complete history and physical examination. Diagnostic procedures would be accomplished that are specific to the type of neoplasm and its location.

Nursing diagnosis. For selected nursing diagnoses related to the use of antineoplastic agents, see the Nursing Care Plan on p. 860. Other nursing diagnoses related to chemotherapy might be: altered body nutrition related to anorexia and gastrointestinal distress; impaired gas exchange related to anemia, cardiotoxicity, or pulmonary fibrosis; sensory/perceptual alterations (tactile, auditory) related to neurotoxicity; impaired skin integrity related to extravasation or drug-induced skin pathology; altered cardiopulmonary tissue perfusion related to drug-induced cardiotoxicity; and ineffective individual coping related to the stress of antineoplastic chemotherapy.

Implementation

Monitoring and intervention. The nurse has many responsibilities in dealing with the inevitable side effects of antineoplastic drugs.

The potential for infection is increased because of bone marrow depression. Strict aseptic technique should be used during contact with the hospitalized client, who should also be protected from persons harboring harmful microorganisms. Monitor client's temperature and observe for signs of infection. Frequent blood counts are necessary, and the nurse is often responsible for ensuring that they are taken and the results monitored for early signs of bone marrow depression. A client with an absolute granulocyte count below 100 cells/mm^3 is in danger of infection. Clients with granulocytopenia should maintain scrupulous oral hygiene and receive topical antibiotics for abrasions and scratches. Encourage fluids and avoid indwelling catheters and other invasive procedures. Caution the client to avoid crowds and individuals with infectious diseases (colds, flu, chickenpox, measles, etc.). No one in the client's household should be vaccinated with a live attenuated virus, such as polio. Clients should be instructed to report to the health care provider any signs of infection, such as elevated temperature, sore throat, cough, mouth ulcerations, or burning on urination.

The altered protection occurs for clients with thrombocytopenia when platelet levels fall below 50,000 cells/mm^3. The nurse should avoid taking rectal temperatures and administering suppositories to such clients. Protective care for these clients might include the administration of stool softeners and the use of soft-bristled toothbrushes and electric razors. Soft tissue injury should be avoided, and the use of padded side rails on beds should be considered. Oral preparations of analgesics and other medications should be used to avoid the tissue damage resulting from intramuscular injections. Venipunctures should be done carefully by experienced personnel using strict sterile technique. The client should be instructed to report signs that indicate decreased platelets, such as petechiae, easy bruising, hemorrhage, bleeding from the gums, epistaxis, and blood in the stool and urine.

The kidneys are at risk of injury because of the effectiveness of the antineoplastic agents. Purines are released through cell destruction and converted to uric acid. The possibility of renal failure may result from the precipitation of uric acid crystals in the kidneys. The nurse should monitor the client's intake and output, serum uric acid, blood urea nitrogen, serum creatinine, creatinine clearance, and serum electrolytes. Allopurinol may be prescribed to prevent uric acid accumulation in the kidneys. Fluid intake should be 3 L daily. Cold, clear liquids, such as tea, unsweetened apple juice or other juices, and soft drinks or carbonated beverages such as ginger ale may be well tolerated. Freezing a favorite beverage into ice cubes or popsicles is also recommended.

Nursing Care Plan

Selected Nursing Diagnoses Related to Antineoplastic Agents

Nursing diagnosis	Outcome criteria	Nursing interventions
Alteration in oral mucous membrane related to drug-induced stomatitis or poor oral hygiene	Client will: Demonstrate knowledge of oral hygiene Maintain adequate nutrition and hydration Maintain normal oral mucosa or have decreasing inflammation and/or ulceration	Instruct client to complete all dental work before beginning chemotherapy. Teach optimal oral hygiene to prevent stomatitis. Inspect oral cavity with a tongue blade and light twice daily and before each administration of the antineoplastic drug. Implement appropriate mouth care if inflammation is present. Encourage soothing foods: bland foods, cool liquids, cool foods (popsicles). Instruct client to avoid alcohol and tobacco, spicy or acidic foods, extremes in food temperature, and abrasive foods or those difficult to chew. Consult with prescriber if oral pain relief solution is needed. Instruct client to report any ulcers in or around the mouth.
Risk for infection related to bone marrow depression, leukopenia	Client will: Remain free of infection	Instruct client in reading a thermometer. Teach client to take temperature daily in the afternoon and report any elevation over 101° F. Teach client to avoid being immunized with live virus vaccines and having contact with people with infections. Instruct client to report any signs of infection, such as cough, sore throat, and burning on urination.
Risk for injury related to bone marrow depression, thrombocytopenia	Client will: Exhibit no signs of bleeding or excessive bruising	Avoid performing invasive procedures such as intramuscular injections and rectal temperatures. Inspect intravenous sites, skin, and mucous membranes for signs of bleeding and bruising. Instruct client to report easy bruising, bloody urine, and bleeding from nose or gums. Test urine, emesis, and stool for occult blood. Instruct client to exercise care in oral hygiene and in using safety razors and nail clippers. Teach client to avoid constipation. Encourage the use of caution to prevent falls.
Risk for alterations in bowel elimination, diarrhea, or constipation	Client will: Maintain a normal bowel pattern Have less constipation or diarrhea	Assess client's normal bowel pattern as baseline. If client is constipated, increase fluid intake and roughage in diet. If client has diarrhea, decrease roughage, increase fluids, and give small feedings. Consult with a prescriber if stool softener, laxative, or antidiarrheal is needed. Assess client for fluid and electrolyte status. Monitor bowel movements; record diarrhea as output. Clean and dry the perianal area after each bowel movement. Test stools for occult blood.
Disturbance in self-concept related to alopecia	Client will: Demonstrate progress toward coping with altered body image	Allow client to express apprehensions related to alopecia. Encourage client to obtain cap or hairpiece before treatment begins. Reassure client that hair growth should begin 8 weeks after therapy, but the new growth may be of a different color and texture.
Fluid volume deficit related to nausea and vomiting	Client will: Experience decreased incidence of nausea and vomiting	Administer antiemetic drugs 1-3 hr before the administration of the antineoplastic drugs; or administer antineoplastic therapy before bedtime with an antiemetic and a sedative. Provide the client with frequent, small amounts of liquids of the client's preference (at least 3 L daily).

The client's body image may be disturbed as a result of alopecia. This side effect is extremely distressing to women, even when they have been prepared for it, have cosmetic aids available, and are aware that it is reversible. Clients, even those who have only thinning of the hair, need assurance that the hair will begin to grow back in about 6 to 8 weeks, although it may be a different texture or color. Treatment with hormones may necessitate support for the client in the event of such effects as masculinization in a female client or feminization in a male client. These clients need assistance in coping with body image problems.

Some clients lose their appetite or complain of a bitter or metallic taste in the mouth. Their desire for red meat or other protein foods may be reduced, since these foods are the most commonly perceived as bitter tasting. Because protein is essential for good nutrition, alternative methods of serving proteins should be pursued. Cold cooked turkey, fish, eggs, and dairy products may be suitable substitutes. The biggest meal of the day should be planned for the time the client is usually hungriest, even if that time is early morning or midnight.

Nausea and vomiting that accompany the use of antineoplastic drugs can be relieved by (1) the administration of an antiemetic drug 1 to 3 hours before administration of the antineoplastic drugs or (2) the administration of the antineoplastic drug at night with an antiemetic and a hypnotic, so that the client sleeps all night and experiences fewer side effects. (Box 56-3 describes the emetic potential of chemotherapeutic agents.) The antiemetic can then be continued afterward as necessary. Speeding the passage of food through the stomach is sometimes the solution to the problem of nausea, vomiting, and feelings of fullness. Some quantities of carbohydrates eaten at frequent intervals help achieve this effect. Weigh client to monitor nutritional status.

Liquids should not be drunk at mealtime but instead should be taken frequently throughout the day, up to 30 to 60 minutes before eating. Since hot foods have been reported to contribute to nausea, foods should be served at room temperature or cooler. Resting for 1 to 2 hours after eating is advised because activity can slow the digestive process.

Stomatitis, oral ulcerations, xerostomia (dryness of the mouth), and other oral changes are common side effects of the potent antineoplastic agents and may interfere with the client's nutrition. Good oral hygiene is important to maintain a proper nutritional intake and decrease the possibility of oral infections becoming systemic. The kind of mouthwash solutions used depends on the status of the client's lesions. Small, frequent servings of cold or room-temperature, bland, nonirritating foods are best tolerated by the client. This type of diet also decreases the diarrhea that is a common side effect of cancer chemotherapy. Nystatin oral suspension or other antifungal agent may be prescribed to prevent oral *Candida albicans*.

Diarrhea, as a side effect of antineoplastic drugs, results from the death of the rapidly dividing cells of the bowel mucosa. The nurse should assess the client's bowel status, hydration, and electrolyte levels and record diarrhea as output.

BOX 56-3

Selected Chemotherapeutic Agents: Emetic Potential

High emetic potential

cisplatin
dicarbazine (DTIC)
nitrogen mustard
streptozocin
actinomycin D
doxorubicin
daunorubicin
nitrosoureas (BCNU, CCNU)
procarbazine
cyclophosphamide (IV)
etoposide
mitomycin
methotrexate (high dose)

Low emetic potential

5-FU
vincristine
vinblastine
methotrexate
bleomycin
chlorambucil
melphalan
busulfan
cyclophosphamine (oral)
6-mercaptopurine

From Lane et al (1991).

Clear fluid intake should be encouraged between meals, although intravenous therapy may be needed to replace lost fluids if the diarrhea is severe. Because of the client's frequent defecation, special attention should be given to skin care in the perianal area. Modification of the diet will prevent or decrease diarrhea. The client should be instructed to avoid foods that may cause gas and cramping, such as cabbage, beans, and highly spiced foods. Hot, spicy food should be avoided because it increases peristalsis that reduces nutrition absorption and may cause diarrhea. Reducing high-fiber foods in the diet, such as raw fruits and vegetables, bran, and whole grain cereals and bread, may help to control diarrhea. Foods that are high in potassium (to replace potassium loss through diarrhea) and that usually do not worsen diarrhea include bananas, apricot or pear nectar, red meat, saltwater fish, boiled or mashed potatoes, and orange juice. Test stools for occult blood.

Constipation may also be a problem with some clients. This may be an early symptom of CNS toxicity, impaired intestinal motility from the drug therapy, or may result from eating mostly soft and liquid foods. High-fiber foods and prune juice have a laxative effect; 1 or 2 tablespoons of bran may be added to cooked cereals, casseroles, and homemade baked goods. The client should be encouraged to drink plenty of fluids, preferably 8 to 10 glasses daily. Hot lemon water in the morning usually stimulates bowel activity. The prescriber may order a laxative or stool softener as needed. Avoid enemas because they may injure the intestinal mucosa.

Pain commonly occurs in clients receiving antineoplastic drugs. The treatment of pain associated with cancer, especially chronic pain, requires a careful assessment of the client, consideration of appropriate nursing interventions, and skillful application of pharmacologic agents. Nonpharmacologic techniques for pain relief may assist the client, such as relaxation therapy, guided imagery, aromatherapy, and diversional activities. Chronic pain may progress in a cycle to anxiety or depression, insomnia, fatigue, and increased pain. The factors that modify pain threshold are listed in Figure 14-1.

Nursing interventions may include physical activity to help prevent further deterioration resulting from inactivity. Deep breathing, turning the client, and skin care are some of the actions that reduce complications. In addition to physical and pharmacologic interventions, the client may need psychosocial, intellectual, and spiritual support. The holistic approach of carefully assessing the client's current needs and anticipating and planning for continued care is important in the care of many illnesses but is crucial for a client dying of a progressive illness. A variety of home-care programs are available. In addition, hospice programs have been developed throughout the United States and Canada to help provide the supportive and palliative services necessary for clients with life-threatening illness and their families. The American Cancer Society offers a variety of resources for the client with cancer and the family.

It must be remembered that anticancer drugs are potent drugs that are mutagenic and carcinogenic in animals and may be carcinogenic in humans. Nurses and pharmacists who prepare antineoplastic drugs should institute safety measures such as using proper technique; wearing gloves, mask, and protective clothing; and whenever possible, preparing the solutions in a vertical laminar flow, biologically safe hood. All unused solutions, vials, needles, syringes, gloves, and materials used to clean up spills should be processed as hazardous materials; the waste should be properly incinerated. For further detail, check the policies related to hazardous waste for your health agency.

Although the development of cancer in professionals has not yet been directly related to handling of materials, a relationship between fetal loss and occupational exposure to antineoplastic drugs in nurses has been reported. Governmental regulatory agencies have indicated that it is unacceptable to allow exposure to potential carcinogens to continue until cancer actually occurs. Regulatory agencies should not wait for epidemiologic evidence before taking action to limit exposure to chemicals considered to be carcinogenic.

Education. In addition to the client teaching discussed previously in relation to specific interventions, instruction about drug administration and drug effects may help to ease the client's anxiety. An assessment should reveal the expectations of the client and the family; they may need assistance in accepting a realistic view of the results of chemotherapy. Expectations of total cure may be unrealistic and should not be reinforced, whereas expectations of remission are often appropriate. One of the most important nursing interventions is emotional support to a client who is receiving physically and psychologically distressing therapy. The long periods of therapy, with frequent interruptions and sporadic progress, may compound the client's anxieties.

A client receiving cancer chemotherapy should be cautioned *not* to take any over-the-counter medication before checking with the oncologist. Many over-the-counter preparations contain aspirin, alcohol, or other substances that could interfere with the antineoplastic agents or increase the risk for toxicity. See the Nursing Care Plan on p. 860 for specific areas of client instruction related to selected nursing diagnoses.

Clients commonly return home within 48 hours of receiving chemotherapy, or they receive chemotherapeutic agents at home administered by home health nurses. In addition to learning the technical skills to maintain these therapies at home, the clients and their families need to practice safe handling of cytotoxic drugs and body waste materials at home. The client and family need to know that these chemotherapeutic agents are eliminated from the body through vomitus, urine, and feces. Direct contact with these body waste products can expose a person to the drug during the chemotherapy and for up to 48 hours after the drug has been discontinued. The effects of these drugs may accumulate in the body of the caregiver who is routinely exposed over a period of time if precautions are not taken. For example, this may occur if the caregiver regularly changes and washes the bed linens of a client who is receiving these agents and wets the bed (Blecke, 1989). Soiled bedpans and containers contaminated with vomitus need to be handled with gloves, emptied directly into the toilet, washed with detergent and water without splashing with the rinse water discarded directly into the toilet, and the toilet flushed three times. Hands are always washed after removing the gloves. Skin surfaces contaminated by body wastes or by the drugs themselves should be washed with detergent and water for five minutes. If an eye is involved, wash with water for 10 to 15 minutes and notify the oncologist.

A spill of antineoplastic agents may occur in the home by defective IV fluid bags or IV lines that leak or get disconnected accidentally. Although the client is usually provided a commercially available spill kit that fulfills the Occupational Safety and Health Administration (OSHA) requirements, instruction should be reinforced on the spill kit

Home Health

Home Spill Kit Procedure

A home spill kit that meets OSHA requirements usually contains 2 pairs of unpowdered surgical latex gloves, a disposable gown, chemical splash goggles, a respirator mask, 2 sheets (12 × 12) of disposable material, 2 spill control pillows, a small scoop and brush to collect glass fragments, sharps container, 2 large chemotherapy waste disposal bags, and toxic waste labels. The following suggested procedure will need to be modified for spill kits containing other materials.

- Do not touch the spill with unprotected hands.
- Open the spill kit and put on both pairs of gloves. If the bag or syringe with chemotherapy drugs has been broken or leaking, and you have a catheter or Port-a-Cath in place, first disconnect the catheter from the tubing and rinse and cap according to normal procedure before cleaning the spill.
- Put on the gown (closes in back), splash goggles, respirator.
- Use spill pillows to contain spill; put around puddle to form a V.
- Use the absorbent sheets to blot up as much of the drug as possible.
- Put contaminated cleaning materials directly into the plastic bag contained in the kit. Do not place them on unprotected surfaces.
- Use the scoop and brush to collect any broken glass, sweeping toward the V'ed spill pillows and dispose of the glass in the box of the kit.
- While still wearing the protective gear, wash the area with detergent and warm water using paper towels and put them in the plastic bag with the other waste. Rinse the area with clean water and dispose of the towels in the same plastic bag.
- Remove gloves, goggles, respirator, and gown and place in plastic bag. Put all contaminated materials, including the spill kit box, into the second large plastic bag and label with the hazardous waste label in the kit.
- Wash your hands with soap and water.
- Call the home health nurse, clinic, or prescriber's office promptly to report the spill. Plans need to be made to have the waste material picked up or have you bring it to the hospital for proper disposal.
- If upholstered or carpeted area is contaminated, follow the above procedure—blot as much of the solution as possible with the absorbent sheets, wash the area with detergent, and follow with a clean water rinse. Do not use chemical spot removers or upholstery dry cleaners because they may cause a chemical reaction with the drug.
- If the spill occurs on sheets or clothing, wash in hot water separately from the other wash. Wash clothing or bed linens contaminated with body wastes in the same manner.
- Clients on 24-hour infusions should use a plastic-backed mattress pad to protect the mattress from contamination.

Modified from Blecke (1989).

procedure to prevent undue exposure of the client and caregivers (see the Home Health box above).

Evaluation. Evaluation of drug effects is an integral nursing function in antineoplastic chemotherapy. Often no dosage schedule for antineoplastic agents is universally therapeutic, and the dosage is changed according to the client's response and the toxic effects of the drug. Thus the nurse's evaluation of progress toward therapy goals and communication of both drug toxicity and client response are essential. In evaluating toxic effects, the nurse should be vigilant for early signs, since progression of toxic effects may have severe and irreversible consequences.

SUMMARY

Cancer is a major health issue today. Although many people fear cancer, more people are cured of cancer than ever before. Education for cancer prevention, early detection, and early treatment are essential to combating this disease. For the nurse a knowledge of cell kinetics is essential to understand the mechanisms and sites of action of the cancer chemotherapeutic agents and to appropriately manage the nursing care of clients receiving such agents.

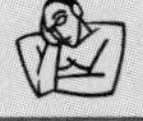

Critical Thinking

1. Mr. Matsui, a 56-year-old client with Hodgkin's disease, is questioning his MOPP therapy. He is concerned about the cost of his health care and wants to know why so many drugs are needed to treat him. What will be your response to Mr. Matsui?
2. Mrs. Hayes has been receiving a course of antineoplastic therapy. Her lab results are returned with her platelet count at 46,000 cells/mm^3 and her absolute granulocyte count at 86 cells/mm^3. What assessments should be obtained? How should she be monitored on a daily basis? What safety precautions will you take with her care?

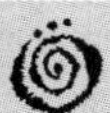

Collaborative Learning Activities

1. Students will discuss experiences of chemotherapy related to them by friends, family, or a particular client that they were assigned within the clinical settings. Were there differences in attitudes before, during, and after therapy? The students will discuss and recognize the uniqueness of each chemotherapy recipient's response.

BIBLIOGRAPHY

Anderson KN, et al. (Eds.) (1994). *Mosby's medical, nursing, & allied health dictionary* (4th ed.). St Louis: Mosby.

Belcher AE (1992). *Cancer nursing*. St Louis: Mosby.

Blecke C (1989). Home chemotherapy safety procedures, *Oncol Nurs Forum 16*(7):719-21, 201.

Carlson PA (1995). Antineoplastic agents, *Crit Care Nurs Q 18*(4):1-15.

Dodd MJ, et al. (1992). Self-care for patients experiencing cancer chemotherapy side effects: A concern for home care nurses, *Home Healthc Nurse 9*(6):21-6.

Dose AM (1995). The symptom experience of mucositis, stomatitis, and xerostomia, *Semin Oncol Nurs 11*(4):248-55.

Finley RS, LaCivita CL, & Lindley CM (1995a). Neoplastic disorders and their treatment: General principles. In Young LY & Koda-Kimble MA (Eds.). *Applied therapeutics* (6th ed.). Vancouver: Applied Therapeutics.

Finley RS, Lindley CL, & Henry DW (1995b). Solid tumors. In Young LY & Koda-Kimble MA (Eds.). *Applied therapeutics* (6th ed.). Vancouver: Applied Therapeutics.

Hedges CB (1994). Recognizing the patient at risk for opportunistic infections, *MEDSURG Nurs 3*(6):445-52.

Lane M, et al. (1991). Dronabinol and prochlorperazine in combination for treatment of cancer chemotherapy-induced nausea and vomiting, *J Pain & Sympt Manag 6*(6):352.

McCance KL & Huether SE (1994). *Pathophysiology: The biological basis for disease in adults and children* (2nd ed.). St Louis: Mosby.

Melmon KL, et al. (1992). *Clinical pharmacology* (3rd ed.). New York: McGraw-Hill.

Parker SL, Tong T, Bolden S, & Wingo PA (1996). Cancer statistics, 1996, *Cancer J Clinicians 46*(1):5-28.

Parker GG (1992). Chemotherapy administration in the home, *Home Healthc Nurs 10*(1):30.

Patel NH & Koeller J (1993). Cancer chemotherapy in the elderly, *Highlights Antineoplas Drugs 11*(4):58-64.

Rhodes VA, Johnson MH, & McDaniel RW (1995). Nausea, vomiting, and retching: The management of the symptom experience, *Semin Oncol Nurs 11*(4):256-65.

Rutherford C (1992). Position paper: Administration of antineoplastic agents, *J Intraven Nurs 15*(1):8-9.

Sansivero GE, et al. (1989). Safe management of chemotherapy at home, *Oncol Nurs Forum 16*(5):711-3.

Chapter 57

Antineoplastic Agents

Chapter Focus

The efficacy of antineoplastic agents as both primary and adjunctive treatment for cancer has greatly increased the use of this therapy. The high level of toxicity associated with these agents requires that the nurse who administers them and monitors the client receiving them possess specialized knowledge and skills. The following objectives and key terms are important for a good understanding of this chapter.

Key Terms

alkylating agents (p. 866)
antibiotic antitumor agents (p. 866)
antimetabolites (p. 866)
leucovorin rescue (p. 874)
mitotic inhibitors (p. 868)
nadir (p. 873)

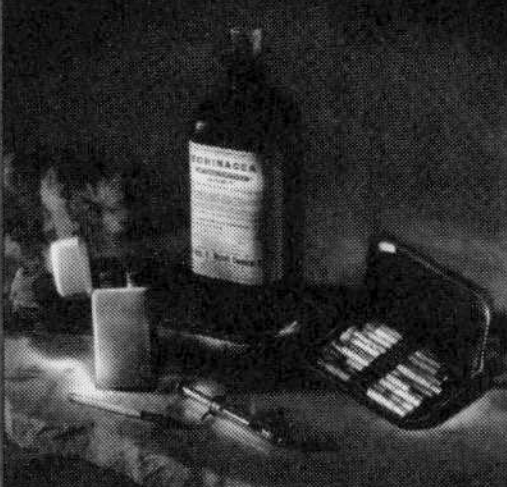

Key Drugs [▲]

cyclophosphamide
methotrexate
doxorubicin
vincristine

Objectives

1. Classify antineoplastic agents based on the major mechanism of action.
2. List common side effects/adverse reactions of antineoplastic drugs.
3. Describe the use of "leucovorin rescue" with methotrexate treatments.
4. Discuss precautions in the preparation and administration of antineoplastic drugs.
5. Implement the nursing management of the care of clients receiving therapy with the various classifications of antineoplastic agents.

The antineoplastic agents do not directly kill tumor cells; they act by interfering with cell reproduction or replication at some point in the cell cycle. (See Chapter 56 for cell cycle discussion.) For cells to proliferate, the genetic material DNA must be replicated once every cell cycle. DNA is the genetic substance in body cells that transfers information resulting in the production of RNA necessary to produce enzymes and protein synthesis (Figure 57-1). The enzymes determine the structure, biochemical activity, growth rate, and functions of the cell. These agents are divided into various classes based on their probable major mechanisms of action (Table 57-1).

The formation of the nucleic acids, DNA and ultimately RNA, requires pyrimidines and purines (nitrogen compounds) as the basic building block materials. **Antimetabolites** have a structure similar to a necessary building block for the formation of DNA. This substance is accepted by the cell as the necessary ingredient for cell growth, but because it is an impostor, it interferes with the normal production of DNA. **Alkylating agents** are drugs that substitute an alkyl chemical structure for a hydrogen atom in DNA. This results in a cross-linking of each strand of DNA, thus preventing cell division. Alkylator-like drugs are chemically different agents that are believed to have an action similar to the alkylating agents.

Antibiotic antitumor agents interfere with DNA functioning by blocking the transcription of new DNA or RNA. In addition, they delay or inhibit mitosis.

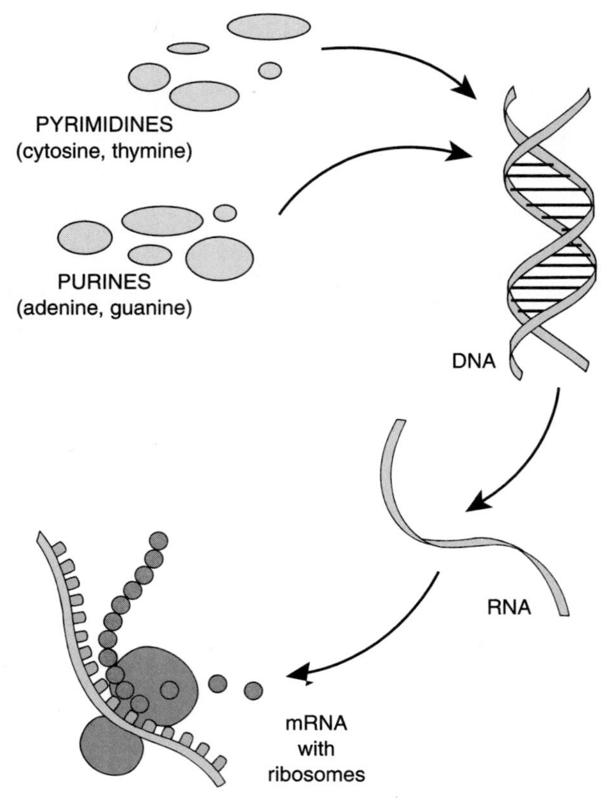

Figure 57-1 Protein synthesis.

TABLE 57-1 Antineoplastic medications

Generic (brand name)	Indications	Major toxicities
Alkylating agents		
Nitrogen mustards		
chlorambucil (Leukeran)	CLL, Hodgkin's & non-Hodgkin's lymphomas	bone marrow suppression
cyclophosphamide* (Cytoxan)	see drug monograph in text	bone marrow suppression, hemorrhagic cystitis
ifosfamide (Ifex)	testicular tumors	bone marrow suppression, nausea, vomiting, encephalopathy
mechlorethamine* (Mustargen)	see drug monograph in text	bone marrow suppression, severe nausea, and vomiting
melphalan (Alkeran)	multiple myeloma, ovarian cancer	bone marrow suppression, allergic reactions
uracil mustard (Uracil Mustard)	CLL, CML, non-Hodgkin's lymphomas, mycosis fungoides	leukopenia, thrombocytopenia
Nitrosureas		
carmustine (BiCNU)	primary brain tumors, multiple myeloma	bone marrow suppression, lung fibrosis, nephrotoxicity

*Drug monograph in text.
ALL, Acute lymphoblastic leukemia; *AML,* acute myelogenous leukemia; *ANLL,* acute nonlymphocytic leukemia; *CLL,* chronic lymphocytic leukemia; *CML,* chronic myelocytic leukemia; *CGL,* chronic granulocytic leukemia.

TABLE 57-1 Antineoplastic medications—cont'd

Generic (brand name)	Indications	Major toxicities
Alkylating agents—cont'd		
Nitrosureas—cont'd		
lomustine* (CeeNu)	see drug monograph in text	bone marrow suppression, anorexia, nausea, vomiting
streptozocin (Zanosar)	pancreatic cancer	nephrotoxicity, nausea, vomiting
Other		
busulfan (Myleran)	CML	bone marrow suppression, hyperpigmentation, gynecomastia
carboplatin (Paraplatin)	ovarian carcinoma	bone marrow suppression, nausea, vomiting, neurotoxicity, neuropathies, ototoxicity
cisplatin* (Platinol)	see drug monograph in text	nephrotoxicity, severe nausea and vomiting, bone marrow suppression
pipobroman (Vercyte)	CGL, polycythemia vera	bone marrow suppression, nausea, vomiting, diarrhea
thiotepa (Thioplex)	breast, ovarian, bladder cancers, lymphomas, malignant effusions	bone marrow suppression
Antimetabolites		
cytarabine (Cytosar-U)	AML, ALL	bone marrow suppression, anorexia, oral and GI ulceration
fluorouracil* (Adrucil)	see drug monograph in text	diarrhea, stomatitis, bone marrow suppression
floxuridine (FUDR)	GI adenocarcinoma with liver metastasis	bone marrow suppression, stomatitis, anaphylaxis
fludarabine (Fludara)	CLL	bone marrow suppression, fever, chills, nausea, vomiting, infection
mercaptopurine (Purinethol)	ALL, AML	bone marrow suppression, anorexia, cholestasis
methotrexate* (Folex)	see drug monograph in text	bone marrow suppression, diarrhea, stomatitis
thioguanine (Thioguanine)	ANLL	bone marrow suppression
Antibiotics		
bleomycin (Blenoxane)	squamous cell carcinoma, lymphomas, testicular cancer	chills, fever, pneumonitis, mucositis, lung fibrosis, hyperpigmentation
dactinomycin (Cosmegen)	Wilms' tumor, Ewing's sarcoma, choriocarcinoma, Rhabdomyosarcoma	bone marrow suppression
daunorubicin liposomal (DaunoXome)	HIV-Kaposi's sarcoma	bone marrow suppression, cardiomyopathy, severe mucositis
doxorubicin* (Adriamycin)	see drug monograph in text	same as daunorubicin
idarubicin (Idamycin)	AML	severe bone marrow suppression, infection, alopecia, nausea, vomiting, hemorrhage
mitomycin (Mutamycin)	disseminated adenocarcinoma of pancreas or stomach	bone marrow suppression
mitoxantrone (Novantrone)	ANLL	cardiotoxicity, severe myelosuppression

Continued

TABLE 57-1 Antineoplastic medications—cont'd

Generic (brand name)	Indications	Major toxicities
Antibiotics—cont'd		
pentostatin (Nipent)	hairy cell leukemia	bone marrow suppression, renal toxicity, rash
plicamycin (Mithracin)	testicular tumors, hypercalcemia	epistaxis, hemorrhage, nausea, bone marrow suppression, stomatitis, vomiting, diarrhea
Mitotic inhibitors		
etoposide (VePesid)	refractory testicular tumors, small cell lung cancer	bone marrow suppression, alopecia
teniposide (Vumon)	ALL	bone marrow suppression, mucositis, alopecia
vinblastine* (Velban)	see drug monograph in text	leukopenia, alopecia, muscle pain, hyperuricemia
vincristine* (Oncovin)	see drug monograph in text	mild to severe paresthesias, jaw pain, ataxia, muscle wasting, constipation
vinorelbine (Navelbine)	non–small cell lung cancer	bone marrow suppression, nausea, vomiting, asthenia

The **mitotic inhibitors,** vinblastine and vincristine, are plant alkaloids that block cell division in metaphase. Vinorelbine (Navelbine) is a semi-synthetic vinca alkaloid that also has antitumor activity in metaphase. They probably have other major sites of action because these agents differ from each other pharmacologically and in therapeutic application. Vinblastine has been used in the treatment of various lymphomas and carcinoma of the breast and testes; vincristine is frequently used to treat acute leukemias and Hodgkin's disease while vinorelbine is indicated for non–small-cell lung cancer.

Hormones, antihormones, corticosteroids, and various other agents are classified in the miscellaneous section of this chapter.

ANTIMETABOLITE DRUGS

The antimetabolite classification contains fluorouracil, floxuridine, fludarabine, methotrexate, cytarabine, mercaptopurine, and thioguanine. Two of the most common agents prescribed, fluorouracil and methotrexate, are reviewed in this section. The antidote leucovorin will also be discussed. See Table 57-1 for additional information on antimetabolite indications and major toxicities.

fluorouracil [flure oh yoor' a sill] (Adrucil, 5-FU)
Fluorouracil is a pyrimidine antagonist that interferes with the synthesis of DNA and RNA. It is a cell-cycle–specific agent that produces its effect in the S-phase of cell division. It is indicated for palliative treatment of carcinomas of the colon, rectum, breast, stomach, and pancreas.

Fluorouracil is metabolized rapidly (within 1 hour) in the tissues to active metabolite floxuridine. Final metabolic degradation occurs in the liver. The drug is distributed throughout the body and also crosses the blood-brain barrier; half-life for alpha phase is 10 to 20 minutes; beta phase is prolonged up to 20 hours because of tissue storage of metabolites. Excretion is primarily respiratory as carbon dioxide (60% to 80%). For major toxicities, see Table 57-1.

A significant drug interaction occurs if fluorouracil is administered with other bone marrow depressants; a dosage reduction of one or both drugs may be necessary. The administration of any live virus vaccine concurrently with fluorouracil should only be done with very close supervision of the oncologist. Fluorouracil will suppress the client's normal defense mechanisms and thus may increase the virus's replication and adverse effects. It is usually recommended that live virus vaccines not be administered until months after chemotherapy has been discontinued. Persons in close contact with the client should not receive immunization with the oral poliovirus vaccine because the live virus is excreted by the person receiving it and can be transmitted to the immunocompromised individual.

The usual adult dose is 7 to 12 mg/kg body weight daily intravenously for 4 days; if no toxicity occurs during the following 3 days, a dosage of 7 to 10 mg/kg body weight is then administered every 3 to 4 days for a total course of 2 weeks. For alternate schedules, see current package insert or drug reference. Maximum dosage for adults is 800 mg/day or 400 mg/day for the high-risk client. Investigational protocols may employ higher dosages than stated in the product's package insert. Review Chapter 2 for legal implications.

Topical fluorouracil preparations (Efudex, Fluoroplex) are used for treatment of skin cancer (basal cell carcinomas) and precancerous skin lesions.

Home Health

Home Administration of Antineoplastic Therapy

Home health care nurses are finding that antineoplastic chemotherapy administration has increased as oncologists have discovered it as a cost-effective means of providing cancer care. However, not all chemotherapeutic agents are appropriate for home administration. Some agents, such as L-asparaginase, have a high prophylactic potential; others, such as cisplatin, require rigorous hydration, which might not be feasible at home. Some chemotherapeutic agents commonly administered at home include bleomycin, doxorubicin, etoposide, fluorouracil, methotrexate, plicamycin, and vincristine.

The nurse should be qualified to administer chemotherapy (see guidelines in Chapter 56) and follow the specific policies established by the home health care agency. The client to receive home chemotherapy should also be carefully selected. A client receiving an antineoplastic agent for the first time, one who is historically noncompliant, and the client who has multiple, chronic, unstable health problems are not good candidates for home chemotherapy. The client's support system and physical environment need to be adequate: a qualified care giver is present should the client experience debilitating side effects and plumbing and telephone services are available. All chemotherapeutic agents should be prepared by a pharmacist using established guidelines and packaged in a leak proof container for transport by the nurse. Supplies need to be available in the home to manage extravasation, anaphylaxis, or a chemical spill. For chemical spill instructions, see Chapter 56.

The nurse should review with the client and family the antineoplastic agent to be administered and the planned treatment schedule, as well as signs and symptoms to report and how to care for the client if they occur. Instruction should be provided about any posttreatment care, such as hydration or medication administration. A 24-hour resource should be available in case the client requires assistance. All of this can be provided in written form to serve as a reference in the home.

An environment conducive to safe administration, without distraction, should be established by the nurse. The client may be comfortably situated in bed or a reclining chair. If the client does not have an implanted venous access device, follow the instruction in Box 57-4 on p. 875. It is recommended that the nurse obtain written orders for the treatment of extravasation at the time the chemotherapy orders are received so that the antidote can be administered without delay.

Nurses should reduce their exposure to these agents as much as possible. Latex gloves are preferred to polyvinyl chloride gloves because they are more resistant to needle punctures. Masks and gowns are not required for administration, but the work surface should be covered by a plastic-backed barrier. All supplies used should be bagged and labeled as toxic waste and returned to the agency or equipment supplier.

Documentation should be done in accordance with agency policy. It is particularly important for the site of the chemotherapy injection and its condition be recorded because the effects of infiltration may not be evident until hours later. If extravasation occurs, record any actions taken to treat the infiltration and the client's response. Record any instructions provided to the client and family to care for the area. If possible, a photograph of the affected area should be obtained to document the degree of tissue damage and provide a guideline for monitoring the site. Recording the client and family response to the therapies will assist in the decision-making regarding whether therapy should be continued in the home or moved to another setting.

Antineoplastic chemotherapy can be provided safely in the home through preparation and knowledge of administration and symptom management for the benefit of clients and their families.

From Jaffe and Skidmore-Roth, 1988; Parker, 1992.

■ Nursing Management

Fluorouracil Therapy

Assessment. Fluorouracil is contraindicated if the client presently has or recently has had chickenpox or herpes zoster, because of the risk of occurrence or exacerbation of these diseases. This contraindication applies to those who have had recent exposure to chickenpox or herpes zoster. See vaccine contraindications above.

Carefully consider use of fluorouracil when the client is pregnant or breastfeeding or has renal or hepatic function impairment, infection, bone marrow depression, or tumor cell infiltration of the bone marrow. If the client has had previous cytotoxic therapy with alkylating drugs or high dose pelvic radiation, a lower dose is recommended. The client should not receive other bone marrow depressants concurrently unless it is part of an antineoplastic combination drug therapy regimen.

Before beginning therapy with fluorouracil, a baseline assessment of the client's overall health status, hematocrit or hemoglobin, total and differential white cell count, platelet count, and renal and hepatic function studies should be obtained. An examination of the client's mouth for ulceration is done with a tongue blade and flashlight before therapy and each dose.

Nursing diagnosis. Clients receiving fluorouracil are at risk for all of the nursing diagnoses discussed in Chapter 56; more commonly occurring are the following: risk for infection related to the drug's immunosuppression action; altered oral mucous membranes (stomatitis); altered comfort related to anorexia, heartburn (esophagopharyngitis), nausea and vomiting, rash (dermatitis), or chest pain related to myocardial ischemia; altered bowel elimination pattern (diarrhea); altered protection related to increased tendency for bleeding related to thrombocytopenia (unusual bleeding or bruising, petechiae, blood in urine or stool); or disturbance in self-concept related to alopecia and darkening of the skin of the soles of the feet and palms of the hands, and the nail beds. In addition, the client is also at risk for complications related to the prolonged use of an arterial catheter to administer the drug, such as thrombosis, embolism, thrombophlebitis, abscesses, and bleeding, leakage, or infection at the catheter site.

Implementation

Monitoring. Monitor leukocyte and platelet counts and watch client for signs of bruising and bleeding, particularly gastrointestinal bleeding. Test stools for occult blood. Lowest levels of leukocyte and platelet counts generally occur 9 to 14 days after the first day of fluorouracil therapy and recover by 30 days.

Monitor BUN, creatinine clearance, and serum uric acid levels. A decrease in creatinine clearance and an increase in the other test values may indicate nephrotoxicity. Fluid intake should be 3000 ml daily.

Monitor temperature and observe for signs of infection, fever, chills, sore throat, low back pain, or painful urination. Observe the client for skin rash and itching. Therapy should be discontinued but may be reinstated at a lower dosage when the side effects have subsided. Check also for oral candidiasis and herpes.

Gastrointestinal disturbances usually occur about the fourth day of therapy and subside 2 or 3 days after the medication is withdrawn. Weakness occurs immediately after the dose is administered and lasts for 12 to 36 hours or longer.

Watch for signs of toxicity and indications for discontinuing the drug, including intractable vomiting, diarrhea, severe stomatitis, WBC below 3500/mm^3, thrombocytopenia (below 10,000/mm^3), and gastrointestinal bleeding. The leukopenia and thrombocytopenia associated with the drug's pharmacologic action are used as measures for the titration of each client's dosage.

Intervention. Dosages are determined by the client's weight. In obese clients or those with edema or ascites, estimated lean body mass is used. Administer antiemetics to reduce nausea and vomiting. If stomatitis occurs, use a topical oral anesthetic to reduce oral discomfort.

The drug may precipitate if exposed to low temperatures. Dissolve the crystals by warming to 140° F (60° C) and allow for cooling before administering. For administration by IV infusion, fluorouracil may be mixed with 5% dextrose injection or 0.9% sodium chloride injection.

Fluorouracil may be administered intraarterially by an infusion pump to ensure a consistent rate of infusion. The nurse should be knowledgeable about and skillful with the specific equipment being used. If the drug is administered intraperitoneally, special nursing management is required (Box 57-1).

Toxicity appears to be reduced by slow intravenous infusion (over 2 to 24 hours); however, bolus injections (over 1 to 2 minutes) may be more effective. Because of the hazards in preparing the doses, consult your institution's guidelines for the handling of antineoplastic agents (Box 57-2).

Take precautions against intravenous infiltration. If extravasation occurs, administration should be stopped immediately and the remaining dose injected into another vein. Cold compresses may reduce local tissue damage. It is not administered intrathecally because of neurotoxicity.

Safety precautions should be taken if the platelet count is low. The precautions include avoidance of invasive procedures or use of extreme care in such procedures; regular examination of skin, mucous membranes, and injection sites for bruising or bleeding; testing of emesis, urine, and stool for signs of occult bleeding; care in the use of grooming implements, toothbrushes, toothpicks, razors, and nail clippers; prevention of constipation; and prevention of physical injury. Platelet transfusions may be required.

Protective isolation should be instituted if WBC falls below 3500/mm^3. Broad-spectrum antibiotics may be administered pending appropriate culture results.

For topical application, wear plastic gloves and wash hands immediately after handling the drug. Avoid occlusive dressings to minimize reactions of normal skin around the affected area. Avoid contact with areas that are easily irritated—the eyes, nasolabial folds, and wrinkles. Be aware that skin sensitivity to the sun may occur. Sun-blocking lotions may be advised. An application of a topical corticosteroid after the completion of the treatment may assist healing.

Education. Clients should be instructed to avoid excessive alcohol and any aspirin intake because of the risk of gastrointestinal bleeding. The client should be cautioned against being immunized with live virus vaccines during fluorouracil therapy, since it may cause rather than prevent the disease. Vaccination is also contraindicated in family members and other persons in close contact with the client. The client should avoid being exposed to infections. Inform the client that alopecia may occur but is reversible and that hair regrowth may be different in texture or color. Instruct the client on safety precautions previously mentioned. See the Home Health Care box on p. 869 for a discussion of working with clients receiving antineoplastics agents at home.

Evaluation. The client will demonstrate signs of clinical improvement without signs and symptoms of infection or bleeding. The client and family will evidence an understanding of fluorouracil therapy.

* ▲ **methotrexate** [meth oh trex' ate] (Mexate, Folex)

Methotrexate is an antimetabolite that is cell-cycle–specific for the S-phase. To synthesize DNA, folic acid must be reduced to tetrahydrofolate by the enzyme dihydrofolate reductase. Methotrexate binds with dihydrofolate reductase, thus inhibiting the synthesis of DNA and RNA. Since malignant cellular growth is usually greater than cell growth of normal tissues, cancer growth may be impaired by methotrexate.

Methotrexate is indicated for the treatment of:

- Breast, head and neck, and lung cancers; trophoblastic tumors; renal, ovarian, bladder and testicular carcinomas; and acute lymphocytic leukemia and non-Hodgkin's lymphomas; and for the prevention and treatment of meningeal leukemia

BOX 57-1

Nursing Management of Intraperitoneal Chemotherapy

During the last 20 years, intraperitoneal (IP) chemotherapy has developed as an accepted modality in ovarian cancer treatment. Sound nursing management of clients receiving IP chemotherapy can minimize complications and thus improve quality of life.

The principles of IP chemotherapy are: (1) tumor size should be small to ensure adequate drug penetration; (2) the drug needs to be mixed in large volumes of solution to allow maximum fluid distribution; and (3) the ratio of plasma drug clearance to peritoneal clearance should be high (i.e., it should clear the peritoneal cavity slowly to have as much tumor exposure as possible but then clear the systemic circulation as quickly as possible).

Ovarian cancer is most suited to IP chemotherapy because it metastasizes by IP seeding, microscopic tumor breaking off, and spreading to the serosal surfaces of the abdominal cavity. It is not until late in its course that it invades organs or spreads outside the peritoneal cavity.

There are three drug delivery systems being used. A temporary, single-use catheter can be placed percutaneously and then removed at the end of each infusion of chemotherapy. However, this can become technically difficult as the number of laparotomies increases causing abdominal adhesions. The Tenckhoff catheter, also used, is a silastic catheter with multiple holes at the distal end. It is placed through the anterior abdominal wall, tunneled subcutaneously, and then enters the peritoneal cavity. The Tenckhoff catheter allows for rapid infusion rates and it can be manipulated to dislodge fibrin deposits that may occur at the end of the catheter. Because it has an external component, it requires daily dressing changes and may decrease the client's acceptance of the catheter related to concept of altered body image.

The Port-A-Cath is totally implantable with a stainless steel port attached to a silastic catheter tunneled the same way as the Tenckhoff catheter. Because the port lies subcutaneously, it needs to be accessed with a noncoring Huber needle each time the catheter is used. Although it has the advantage of lying completely under the skin, it has the disadvantages of decreased infusion rate because of the small lumen of the Huber needle and the requirement of surgical removal of the catheter and port.

Potential complications common to both catheters include decreased drainage owing to sheathlike fibrin deposits that develop around the end of the catheter producing a one-way valve effect, catheter infections, and discomfort on infusion owing to distention of the abdomen and the stretching of adhesions formed from previous therapies.

Most health care facilities use a peritoneal dialysis set with a Y-tubing, with one end going to the client and the other two used for drug administration and drainage. Rapid infusion of the IP chemotherapy is important. Concurrent medications are given to protect specific organs or to prevent systemic toxicities similar to the administration of drugs concurrent with IV chemotherapy.

Nursing management of IP chemotherapy includes daily dressing of the Tenckhoff catheter site or accessing the Port-A-Cath, decreasing the discomfort involved with instillation of the drug, attempting to increase fluid return, and client instruction related to the procedure and catheter used in the institution. Because peritoneal ports are usually placed over the lower edge of the rib cage, placing a pillow under the client on the same side that the port is on assists in access to the port. Because 2 L of fluid are needed to penetrate as much of the peritoneal cavity as possible, the client may experience abdominal pain, shortness of breath, anorexia, nausea, vomiting, diarrhea, constipation, esophageal reflux, and dysuria, which are treated symptomatically. Decreased return from both catheters occurs and the nurse may be required to irrigate the catheter to dislodge fibrin deposits and turn the client to redistribute fluid. Client and family education by the nurse can assist them to decrease their anxiety and to understand what potential problems may arise and how to manage them when they do occur.

From Hoff (1991).

- Advanced cases of mycosis fungoides, osteosarcoma, and for the noncancerous indications of selected cases of severe psoriasis and rheumatoid arthritis that are unresponsive to standard therapies

It is administered orally or parenterally (IM, IV, and intrathecal). The oral preparation reaches peak serum levels within 1 to 2 hours. Limited amounts of methotrexate can cross the blood-brain barrier, but significant quantities pass into the systemic circulation after intrathecal drug administration. It is metabolized intracellularly and in the liver with unchanged drug excreted by the kidneys. For major toxicities, see Table 57-1.

The adult and pediatric methotrexate dosage varies according to the indication and course of treatment. Generally, the antineoplastic adult dosage orally is 15 to 30 mg daily for 5 days, repeated from three to five times with a 7 to 14 day interval between each course. The pediatric oral dosage is 20 to 40 mg/m^2 once a week. For other indications and recommended parenteral doses, see a current package insert or *USP DI* for instructions. See Box 57-3 for gemcitabine, a recently released antimetabolite.

BOX 57-2

Precautions for Handling Antineoplastic Agents

All persons handling cytotoxic (hazardous) drugs, such as antineoplastic agents, should be properly trained in safety procedures and have access to policies and procedures that follow current government and professional practice standards.

Drug preparation and administration

Wash hands thoroughly and wear a disposable gown, surgical latex gloves, and eye protection when preparing or administering cytotoxic drugs.

Whenever possible, it is highly recommended that preparation of injectable antineoplastic agents be performed in the clean-air work station (Hepa filter in BSC or biohazard cabinet).

Use areas for the preparation of drugs only for that purpose. Limit access to that area.

Remove only the required amount of the drug into the syringe. If more is withdrawn accidently, inject the excess back into the vial and dispose of it properly.

Vent vials with a 20-gauge needle to avoid the creation of aerosol particles.

Nurses should not prepare or administer intravenous chemotherapy if they are pregnant because of suspected risk to the fetus from these agents.

Disposal of antineoplastic drugs and equipment

All antineoplastic drugs and all vials, needles, syringes, tubing, and equipment used in their administration need to be discarded with caution. Special leak-proof, puncture-proof, double bagged containers should be used and labeled BIOHAZARD for disposal by incineration.

Needles and syringes should not be broken and/or separated before disposal because leakage of the medication may occur.

Spillage or antineoplastic drug contact with nurse or client

Spillage

Wear two pairs of gloves when cleaning up an antineoplastic drug spill. Wash hands before and after.

Wear a mask and eye protection if the medication is powdered.

Place the spilled substance in a plastic bag. Wipe up the remainder with a damp cloth and also place in the plastic bag.

Seal the bag and place it inside of a second bag, and seal the second bag. Label it BIOHAZARD and send it for disposal by incineration.

Drug contact with nurse or client

Thoroughly wash the affected area with soap and water. If clothing was contaminated. remove clothing immediately.

If eye contact was made, flush the eyes with copious amounts of water, holding the eyelids open during flushing.

Disposal of client excreta

Urine, vomitus, and other body fluids from clients receiving antineoplastic drugs should be handled with caution. Flush excreta down the toilet; wear gloves to avoid contact. Wash containers thoroughly.

▪ Nursing Management

Methotrexate Therapy

Assessment. Methotrexate should not be administered if the client has immunodeficiency. Its use is not recommended when the client is pregnant or breastfeeding because of risk to fetus or infant. Methotrexate is to be used cautiously if the client has ascites, pleural effusion, or renal function impairment since there is increased risk of drug toxicity because excretion is impaired and accumulation may occur. Caution is used, too, if there is bone marrow depression, infection, oral mucositis, peptic ulcer, or ulcerative colitis. With herpes zoster or existing case of or recent exposure to chickenpox, there is the risk of generalized, more severe disease. If there is a history of gout or urate renal stones, the risk of hyperuricemia is increased. Caution should be used in clients with previous cytotoxic drug therapy or radiation therapy. Caution should be used with debilitated, very young, or elderly clients.

Review the client's current medication regimen for significant drug interactions that may occur when methotrexate is given with the drugs listed below.

Drug	Possible effect and management
alcohol or hepatotoxic drugs	**Increases risk of hepatotoxicity. Avoid or a potentially serious drug interaction may occur.**
acyclovir injection	**Neurologic complications may occur with use of intrathecal methotrexate. Avoid or a potentially serious drug interaction may occur.**
asparaginase	**Cell replication is inhibited by asparaginase, thus impairing the therapeutic effects of methotrexate. If asparaginase is administered 9 to 10 days before or within 24 hours after methotrexate, this effect is not reported. The major side effects of methotrexate—gastrointestinal and hematologic (blood components suppression)—may also be reduced in this drug administration schedule. Avoid or a potentially serious drug interaction may occur.**

BOX 57-3

Newly Released Antimetabolite

Gemcitabine (Gemzar) interferes with cell synthesis (S-phase) and also blocks cell progression through the G-1/S part of the cycle. It is indicated for treatment of adenocarcinoma of the pancreas in persons with non-resectable or metastatic pancreatic cancer that have been previously treated with 5-FU.

Side/adverse effects include dyspnea, peripheral edema, flu-like syndrome, nausea, vomiting, diarrhea, rash, paresthesia, and stomatitis. Gemcitabine is administered intravenously; adult dose is 1000 mg/m^2 given over 30 minutes. See current literature for additional information (Olin, 1997).

Drug	Possible effect and management
bone marrow depressants or radiation	Bone marrow depressant effects may be increased. A decrease in drug dosage is usually indicated.
NSAIDs (nonsteroidal anti-inflammatory drugs)	**Concurrent administration may result in severe methotrexate toxicity. Avoid or a potentially serious drug interaction may occur. Refer to manufacturer's recommendations on individual NSAIDs to reduce this possibility.**
probenecid or salicylates	**May interfere with excretion of methotrexate, which results in elevated serum levels. Salicylates may also displace methotrexate from its protein-binding sites, also resulting in increased, and possibly toxic, serum levels. Avoid or a potentially serious drug interaction may occur. If necessary to use in combination, monitor serum methotrexate levels closely. Methotrexate dosage level should be decreased and the client closely monitored for signs of toxicity.**
vaccines, live oral	**May result in a decrease in antibody response along with an increase in side effects/adverse reactions. Avoid or a potentially serious drug interaction may occur.**

Obtain a baseline assessment of the client's general health status, hematocrit or hemoglobin, platelet count, total and differential white cell count, BUN, serum creatinine concentration, serum uric acid levels, and hepatic function studies before the initiation of methotrexate therapy.

Nursing diagnosis. Clients receiving methotrexate should be assessed for the possibility of the following nursing diagnoses; altered protection related to the drug's thrombocytopenic effects (increased tendency to bleed); altered protection related to its immunosuppressive effects; altered mucous membrane (stomatitis); fluid volume deficit (anorexia, nausea and vomiting); body image disturbance related to alopecia; altered comfort related to intrathecal administration (headache, back pain); altered sleep patterns (drowsiness); and the potential complications of dermatologic effects (cutaneous vasculitis or photosensitivity), CNS toxicity after intrathecal administration (confusion, convulsions); nephrotoxicity and hepatotoxicity.

Implementation

Monitoring. Serum methotrexate concentrations are usually monitored every 12 to 24 hours after methotrexate administration until concentrations are less than 5×10^{-8} M to determine leucovorin treatment needed to maintain rescue.

Because of the risk of injury related to nephrotoxicity, monitor BUN, serum creatinine, and uric acid levels and intake and output to ensure that the client is adequately hydrated to prevent hyperuricemia and uric acid nephropathy. Alkalinization of urine (pH greater than 7) will also help prevent renal toxicity.

Monitor AST (SGOT), ALT (SGPT), LDH, and serum bilirubin concentrations and observe the client for signs of hepatotoxicity (yellowing of eyes and skin and dark urine). Monitor CBC and watch for signs of bruising and bleeding, particularly gastrointestinal bleeding. The **nadir,** the lowest cell count, of the platelet count occurs after 7 to 10 days, with recovery about 7 days later.

Because of the risk for infection related to immunosuppression, monitor temperature and observe for signs of infection, fever, chills, or sore throat. The nadir of the leukocyte count occurs after 7 to 10 days, with recovery about 7 days later.

The client's mouth should be examined for altered mucous membranes before the administration of each dose, since stomatitis is a sign of toxicity. Therapy should be discontinued, but it may be reinstated at a lower dosage when the side effects have subsided.

Intervention. Follow the health care agency's policies and procedures for the administration of drugs that have a mutagenic, teratogenic, and carcinogenic risk.

Administer leucovorin calcium within the first 36 to 42 hours of starting methotrexate (or earlier) to block the systemic toxic effects of high-dosage methotrexate (known as "leucovorin rescue"). Leucovorin should be immediately available for administration or high-dosage methotrexate administration should not be initiated.

Reconstitute with sterile, preservative-free sodium chloride for infection for intrathecal use.

Safety precautions should be taken if the platelet count is low. Precautions include avoidance of invasive procedures or use of extreme care in such procedures; regular examination of skin, mucous membranes, and injection sites for bruising or bleeding; testing of emesis, urine, and stool for signs of occult bleeding; care in the use of grooming implements, toothbrushes, toothpicks, razors, and nail clippers; prevention of constipation; and prevention of physical injury.

The client should be maintained on a fluid intake of 3000 ml to ensure an increase in urinary output to prevent nephrotoxicity. If the serum uric acid becomes elevated, allopurinol may be prescribed to reduce it, or sodium bicarbonate may be administered to alkalinize the urine.

Methotrexate should be held and the oncologist consulted if the WBC falls below 1500/mm^3, the neutrophils below 200/mm^3, the creatinine clearance increases by more than 50% from baseline, urine pH below 7.0, or if mouth ulcers or pleural effusion occurs.

Education. Caution the client against being immunized with live virus vaccines during methotrexate therapy, since it may cause the disease rather than prevent it. It is also contraindicated in family members and other persons in close contact with the client. The client should avoid being exposed to infections.

Instruct the client in the importance of continuing the medication despite gastric distress and maintaining adequate fluid intake to prevent nephrotoxicity. Alcohol ingestion should be avoided, since it increases the hepatotoxicity associated with the drug. NSAIDs and salicylate products should be avoided because they increase drug toxicity. Instruct in appropriate safety precautions discussed previously.

The client should be aware that skin sensitivity and photophobia may occur. Sun-blocking lotions and sunglasses may be advised. Inform the client that alopecia may occur but is reversible.

Instruct clients on symptoms of toxicities to report to the prescriber.

Evaluation. The client will demonstrate signs of clinical improvement without signs and symptoms of infection or bleeding. The client and family will evidence an understanding of methotrexate therapy.

leucovorin [loo koe vor' in] (folinic acid, Wellcovorin)
Leucovorin, or folinic acid, is a form of folic acid that does not require dihydrofolate reductase to produce folic acid. Therefore it is used to prevent or treat toxicity induced by folic acid antagonists. It is indicated for the following:

1. Use as an antidote (prophylaxis and treatment) for folic acid antagonists, such as methotrexate, pyrimethamine, and trimethoprim. **Leucovorin rescue** is a term used to describe high-dose methotrexate treatments that use leucovorin to reduce the time that sensitive (normal) cells are exposed to the toxic effects of methotrexate.
2. The treatment of megaloblastic anemia caused by nutritional deficiencies, sprue, or pregnancy and whenever oral folic acid therapy is not appropriate.

Leucovorin is rapidly absorbed orally and converted by the intestinal mucous membrane and liver to 5-methylterahydrofolate, an active metabolite. The onset of action orally is between 20 to 30 minutes; intramuscularly, 10 to 20 minutes; intravenously, less than 5 minutes. Duration of action by all routes is between 3 to 6 hours. It is primarily excreted by the kidneys. For major toxicities, see Table 57-1. No significant drug interactions are reported with leucovorin.

As an antidote to the toxic effect of folic acid antagonists, the adult oral dose is 10 mg/m^2 every 6 hours, until methotrexate blood levels fall to less than 5×10^{-8} M. For additional dosing recommendations, see a current reference or package insert.

■ Nursing Management
Leucovorin Therapy

Leucovorin is administered after methotrexate rather than simultaneously with methotrexate. The first dose is usually administered within 24 to 42 hours of beginning high-dose methotrexate therapy. Such high-dose therapy should not be initiated unless leucovorin is immediately available for administration, since rescue is critical. Leucovorin serves as an antidote that limits the time normal cells are exposed. All nursing management measures for methotrexate administration should be observed.

ALKYLATING DRUGS

Alkylating drugs are frequently used as anticancer agents and are believed to be the first class of medications applied clinically in the modern era of antineoplastic drug therapy. Various groups of alkylating agents are available which include the nitrogen mustards and nitrosoureas. See Table 57-1 for specific drugs in this classification.

This chapter reviews mechlorethamine (Mustargen) and cyclophosphamide (Cytoxan) from the nitrogen mustard category; lomustine (CeeNu) from the nitrosoureas; and cisplatin (Platinol), an alkylator-like drug.

mechlorethamine [me klor eth' a meen] (Mustargen)
The cell-cycle nonspecific agent mechlorethamine is an alkylating agent capable of crosslinking DNA and RNA and also inhibiting protein synthesis. It is indicated for the treatment of lung carcinoma, Hodgkin's and non-Hodgkin's lymphomas, chronic leukemia, malignant effusions, mycosis fungoides, and polycythemia vera. It may be administered intravenously or by intracavitary route (such as intrapleurally or intraperitoneally). A topical preparation is also available to treat cutaneous manifestations of mycosis fungoides.

Mechlorethamine's onset of action is nearly immediate (within seconds or minutes) and it is also rapidly deactivated in body tissues. For major toxicities, see Table 57-1.

The usual adult total dose IV is 0.4 mg/kg in single or divided doses. If clients have previously received drug chemotherapy or radiation, this dosage should not exceed 0.2 to 0.3 mg/kg body weight. For additional dosing recommendations, see a current reference or package insert.

■ Nursing Management
Mechlorethamine Therapy

Assessment. Carefully consider use of mechlorethamine when the client is pregnant or breastfeeding or has bone marrow depression, infection, chickenpox, herpes zoster, tumor cell infiltration of bone marrow, or a history of gout, urate renal stones, or previous cytotoxic drug therapy or radiation therapy.

Review the client's current medication regimen for the risk of significant drug interactions that may occur when mechlorethamine is given with the drugs listed below.

Drug	Possible effect and management
bone marrow depressants or radiation	Increased bone marrow depression may occur. A decrease in drug dosage is usually indicated.
probenecid or sulfinpyrazone	Hyperuricemia and gout may occur. The prescriber may adjust the antigout medications or prescribe allopurinol. The latter is often preferred to prevent drug-induced hyperuricemia.
vaccines, live viral	See methotrexate drug interactions.

A baseline assessment should be obtained for the client's general health status, hematocrit or hemoglobin, platelet count, total and differential white blood cell count, serum uric acid and creatinine levels, liver function studies, and sense of hearing by audiometric testing.

Nursing diagnosis. Over the course of mechlorethamine therapy, the client should be assessed for the occurrence of the following nursing diagnoses: sensory-perceptual alterations related to the drug's ototoxic effects (hearing loss, tinnitus); altered protection related to thrombocytopenia (increased bleeding tendencies), and leukopenia (immunosuppression); altered comfort (headache, rash, pain/redness at injection site, metallic taste); fluid volume deficit related to anorexia, nausea and vomiting; altered mucous membranes (stomatitis); diarrhea; activity intolerance related to weakness; impaired tissue integrity related to extravasation of the drug (Box 57-4); altered sleep pattern (drowsiness); disturbance of self-concept related to alopecia or menstrual irregularities; altered thought processes (confusion); and the potential complications of peripheral neuropathy, allergic reaction, ototoxicity, and uric acid nephropathy.

Implementation

Monitoring. During therapy, continue to monitor lab studies as listed on the baseline assessment. Monitor serum uric acid levels, as well as fluid intake and output. Adequate hydration will help prevent renal complications, although alkalinization of the urine by the administration of sodium bicarbonate may be necessary if serum uric acid levels begin to increase.

Monitor the client's CBC and monitor for the presence of fever, chills, and sore throat. Within 24 hours of the first dose, lymphocytopenia occu rs. Granulocytopenia occurs 6 to 8 days after the dose and lasts 10 days to 3 weeks. Monitor for signs of bleeding such as hematuria, melena, epistaxis, hematemesis, and petechiae. Observe for extravasation during IV administration.

Audiometric testing is required periodically in clients receiving high doses to detect the effects of ototoxicity as early as possible.

Intervention. Do not use if droplets of water appear in the vial before reconstitution. Reconstitute with sterile water for injection or sodium chloride injection fluid only. Reconstitute immediately before or less than 15 minutes before each dose. Discard any unused solution after neutralizing.

Avoid contact with the solution by wearing gloves while preparing and administering it. If contact with the skin, mucous membranes, or eye occurs, irrigate the affected area immediately with large amounts of water for 15 minutes; follow with 2% thiosulfate solution. Neutralize all equipment used in the administration of the drug by soaking for 45 minutes in a solution of equal parts of 5% sodium thiosulfate and 5% sodium bicarbonate. Box 57-5 explains the double syringe method of administration.

When mechlorethamine is given by the intracavitary route, change the client's position (prone to supine to right side to left side) every 10 minutes for an hour to distribute the drug. Administer analgesics before intracavitary administration of mechlorethamine to minimize the discomfort of the therapy. Removal of peritoneal fluid before intracavitary administration of mechlorethamine improves contact of the medication with the cavity lining. Fluid is usually removed from the cavity again 24 to 36 hours after therapy (see Box 57-1).

Caution should be taken against intravenous infiltration. If extravasation occurs, promptly infiltrate the area with sterile isotonic sodium thiosulfate or 1% lidocaine and apply ice compresses for 6 to 12 hours (see Box 57-4).

When applying mechlorethamine topically, follow the specific instructions for application for that client. Usually the client showers, rinses, and dries thoroughly before each treatment and does not shower until treatment the next day.

BOX 57-4

Nursing Management of Extravasation of Vesicant/Irritant Agents

Try to prevent extravasation if at all possible. The best administration site is the forearm. Avoid sites in the hand, wrist, etc., because extravasation at these sites could permanently damage nerves, tendons, and muscles. Dilate veins by wrapping the extremity in warm towels or soaking in warm water rather than using a tourniquet, particularly in elderly or frail clients, because the pressure it creates may rupture the vein wall when you release the tourniquet. Avoid puncturing the same vein more than once; multiple venipunctures promote extravasation if the vein used to administer the drug is distal to the previous site. If unsuccessful in your attempt at venipuncture, select a different vein, preferably in the other arm. If no other vein is available, use an insertion site in the same vein that is proximal to the previous one to prevent extravasation occurring at the so-called upstream venipuncture (Wood & Gullo, 1993).

If extravasation is suspected, stop administration of the chemotherapeutic agent immediately. Leave the IV in place and begin your agency's extravasation procedure. Attempt to aspirate any residual vesicant agent and blood from the IV. Prepare and instill the antidote. Remove the needle. *If you are unable to aspirate residual agent from the IV tubing, do not instill the antidote through the existing IV.* The amount of antidote used will depend on the size of the extravasation and the amount of the drug thought to have been extravasated. Avoid applying direct pressure to the site. Cover lightly with a sterile occlusive dressing. Apply warm or cold compresses as discussed above. Take measurements of the affected area to use as a point of reference during the healing process. Elevate and rest the area. Notify the physician of the extravasation and the actions taken (Studva, 1993). The dose should be completed in another vein.

(*USP DI*, 1996)

BOX 57-5

Double Syringe Method

Some antineoplastic agents have vesicant properties (causing blisters) and require careful handling. The following are common vesicant agents:

dactinomycin	mithramycin
carmustine (BiCNU)	mitomycin C
daunorubicin	vinblastine
doxorubicin	vincristine
mechlorethamine	

These agents should be administered by the double-syringe technique as follows:

1. Select site for administration according to following order of preference: forearm, dorsum of hand, wrist, or antecubital fossa.
2. Use 20- or 21-gauge "butterfly" needle for drug administration. Administer 5 ml normal saline solution and withdraw small amount of blood into tubing to test vein patency. If blood return is poor, select site other than distal location.
3. Administer vesicant agent for a least 3 minutes, drawing blood back into tubing after every 2 to 3 ml solution.
4. Flush with 3 to 5 ml saline solution after administration.
5. If client has pain at site of injection or an unusual sensation during drug administration, extravasation may have occurred, and a new site for drug injection should be selected. The health agency's procedure/protocol for extravasation should be followed.

Use plastic gloves to apply mechlorethamine, avoiding contact with the eyes, nose, and mouth.

The treatment may be continued for months or even years. Safety precautions should be taken regarding invasive procedures and infection avoidance as mentioned previously with antimetabolite drugs.

Nausea and vomiting occur in about 90% of clients, generally within 1 to 3 hours of the dose. Although the vomiting usually lasts only 8 hours, nausea may persist 24 hours. These symptoms may be decreased by the administration of antiemetics before mechlorethamine dosing.

However, if the use of sedatives is also required to control the nausea and vomiting, the mechlorethamine may be administered at night for the convenience of the client.

Avoid invasive procedures such as intramuscular injections when the platelet count is low. The nadir of thrombocytopenia usually occurs within 6 to 8 days, with recovery in 10 days to 3 weeks.

Education. The client should be instructed not to be immunized with live virus vaccines during mechlorethamine therapy and to avoid contact with others receiving immunization during that time.

The female client should be alerted that menstrual periods may become irregular. Hair loss may occur in clients, but they should be told that this effect is usually temporary. Alert the client to the frequency of nausea and vomiting with the administration of this drug, but stress the importance of continuing the medication despite these symptoms.

The client should be instructed in the importance of adequate hydration in the prevention of complications. Allopurinol and/or alkalinization of the urine may also be prescribed to prevent uric acid nephropathy.

For clients receiving high doses, instruction should be provided to report auditory disturbances to their prescriber and/or receive audiometric testing at periodic intervals.

Evaluation. The client will demonstrate signs of clinical improvement without signs and symptoms of infection or bleeding. The client and family will evidence an understanding of mechlorethamine therapy.

▲ **cyclophosphamide** [sye kloe foss' fa mide] (Cytoxan, Procytox♣)

Cyclophosphamide is a cell-cycle–nonspecific agent that cross-links DNA and RNA strands and also inhibits the protein synthesis. It is indicated for:

- Acute and chronic leukemias, carcinomas of the ovary and breast, neuroblastomas, retinoblastomas, Hodgkin's and non-Hodgkin's lymphomas, multiple myeloma, and mycosis fungoides.
- As an immunosuppressant in corticosteroid-resistant nephrotic syndrome.

The drug is well absorbed orally and has limited crossing of the blood-brain barrier. Cyclophosphamide undergoes hepatic metabolism to active and inactive metabolites; has a half-life between 3 to 12 hours; with excretion primarily via the kidneys. For major antineoplastic toxicities, see Table 57-1.

The usual adult antineoplastic dosage is 1 to 5 mg/kg orally daily; intravenous dose is 40 to 50 mg/kg in divided doses over 2 to 5 days. Pediatric intravenous dosage is 2 to 8 mg/kg in divided doses for 6 or more days.

■ Nursing Management

Cyclophosphamide Therapy

Assessment. Carefully consider use of cyclophosphamide when the client is pregnant (see the Pregnancy Safety box p. 877) or breastfeeding or has renal or hepatic function impairment, infection, bone marrow depression, tumor cell infiltration of the bone marrow, or previous cytotoxic drug or radiation therapy. It is not to be used if the client at present has, has recently had, or has been exposed to chickenpox or has herpes zoster because of the risk of exacerbation or increased severity of the disease.

Review the client's current medication regimen for significant drug interactions that may occur when cyclophosphamide is given with the drugs listed below.

Drug	Possible effect and management
bone marrow depressants or radiation	Increased bone marrow depression may occur. A decrease in drug dosage is usually indicated.
cocaine	**Inhibition of cholinesterase activity by cyclophosphamide reduces cocaine metabolism and excretion and may lead to cocaine toxicity. Avoid or a potentially serious drug interaction may occur.**
cytarabine (Cytosar)	**Concurrent use in preparation for bone marrow transplant may result in increased cardiomyopathy with subsequent death. Avoid or a potentially serious drug interaction may occur.**
probenecid (Benemid) or sulfinpyrazone (Anturane)	Hyperuricemia and gout may occur. The prescriber may adjust the antigout medications. Allopurinol is not indicated, since it may increase the bone marrow toxicity of cyclophosphamide. If drugs are given concurrently, monitor closely for toxicity.
immunosuppressant agents including azathioprine (Imuran), chlorambucil (Leukeran), corticosteroids, cyclosporine (Sandimmune), mercaptopurine (Purinethol), and muromonab-CD3 (Orthoclone OKT3)	**Increased risk of infections and further development of neoplasms. Avoid or a potentially serious drug interaction may occur.**
vaccines, live viral	**See methotrexate drug interactions.**

A baseline assessment of the client's general health status, hematocrit or hemoglobin, platelet count, total and differential white blood cell count, serum uric acid and creatinine levels, BUN, and liver function studies should be obtained.

Nursing diagnosis. The nurse should assess the client receiving cyclophosphamide therapy for the following nursing diagnoses related to the drug's effects: altered protection related to leukopenia and an increased tendency for bleeding related to thrombocytopenia; disturbance of self-concept related to gonadal suppression, darkening of skin and nails, or alopecia; activity intolerance related to anemia; altered comfort (headache, rash); fluid volume deficit related to anorexia, nausea, and vomiting; diarrhea; altered mucous membranes related to stomatitis; and the potential complications of allergic reaction; altered cardiac output (cardiotoxicity); hemorrhagic cystitis; nephropathy (a result of hyperuricemia from rapid cell breakdown); pneumonitis; and interstitial pulmonary fibrosis.

Implementation

Monitoring. Monitor BUN, creatinine clearance, serum uric acid level determinations, and exam of urine for microscopic hematuria. A decrease in creatinine clearance and an increase in the other test values may indicate nephrotoxicity.

Pregnancy Safety

Category	Drug
B	amifostine, mesna
C	aldesleukin, anastrozole, asparaginase, dacarbazine, dactinomycin, dexrazoxane, interferon alfa-2a, interferon alfa-2b, levamisole, pegaspargase, testolactone, streptozocin
D	altretamine, busulfan, carboplatin, carmustine, chlorambucil, cladribine, cyclophosphamide, cytarabine, daunorubicin, docetaxel, doxorubicin, etoposide, fludarabine, fluorouracil, flutamide, goserelin, idarubicin, ifosfamide, lomustine, mechlorethamine, mercaptopurine, methotrexate, mitoxantrone, paclitaxel, pentostatin, pipobroman, procarbazine, tamoxifen, teniposide, thioguanine, tretinoin, vinblastine, vincristine, vinorelbine
X	leuprolide, plicamycin

Observe the client for reduced urinary output, weight gain over several days, edema of the feet and lower legs, flank pain, pruritus, urine odor on breath, anorexia, nausea, and vomiting.

Monitor for myelosuppression as evidenced by anemia and leukopenia. Monitor hematocrit, platelet count, and total and differential leukocyte counts. Lowest levels of leukopenia generally occur 7 to 12 days after the first dose. The leukocyte count recovers 17 to 21 days after the last dose. Observe the client for fever of unknown origin, chills, sore throat, unusual bleeding, or bruising.

Monitor vital signs. Observe for cardiotoxicity, such as myopericarditis, as evidenced by tachycardia, fever and chills, shortness of breath. Pneumonitis or other respiratory complications may result in cough and shortness of breath.

Intervention. Reconstituted solutions may be stored for 24 hours at room temperature or 6 days if refrigerated. Antiemetics may be administered concurrently to reduce nausea and vomiting. Maintain the client's fluid intake at 3000 ml daily, unless contraindicated, before treatment and for 72 hours following treatment to ensure frequent voiding, including at least once during the night, thereby minimizing the risk of hemorrhagic cystitis and promoting the excretion of uric acid. Adequate hydration minimizes uric acid nephropathy. Alkalinization of urine or allopurinol administration may also be used to prevent uric acid nephropathy.

Administration of cyclophosphamide is best accomplished early in the day so that most of the drug's metabolites have been excreted before bedtime, preventing continued contact of the metabolites with the bladder mucosa. The drug should be discontinued at the first sign of hemorrhagic cystitis; symptomatic treatment may be instituted through such routes as blood replacement, cryosurgery, or formaldehyde bladder instillation.

Education. Alopecia may occur but is reversible; however, the new hair may be different in color and texture. As with antineoplastic agents previously discussed, instruct the client not to be immunized with live virus vaccines during the course of therapy. Advise the client of the safety precautions mentioned with previous antineoplastic agents.

Advise the client that nausea and vomiting frequently occur with cyclophosphamide therapy, but stress that the medication needs to be taken despite these symptoms.

Evaluation. The client will demonstrate signs of clinical improvement without signs and symptoms of infection or bleeding. The client and family will evidence an understanding of cyclophosphamide therapy.

NITROSUREAS

Nitrosureas are highly lipophilic, alkylating agents that easily cross the blood-brain barrier. These agents are generally, very useful for the treatment of primary brain tumors. See Table 57-1 for antineoplastic drugs and their toxicities.

lomustine [loe mus' teen] (CeeNU)

Lomustine is used to treat primary brain tumors and Hodgkin's lymphomas. It is well absorbed orally; has a half life of approximately 90 minutes (active metabolites half-life is 16 to 48 hours); and is metabolized in the liver and excreted primarily by the kidneys.

Most common side effects include anorexia, nausea, and vomiting. Bone marrow depression is the most severe adverse effect of the nitrosureas. This toxicity is cumulative; thus drug dosage is adjusted regularly, based on the nadir blood count from the previous dose administered. Because of the seriousness of this effect, blood counts are closely monitored. Current reference sources should be reviewed when monitoring a client receiving these agents.

■ Nursing Management

Nitrosurea Therapy

For the nursing management of nitrosurea therapy, see the discussion of the nursing management of cyclophosphamide therapy.

ALKYLATOR-LIKE DRUGS

cisplatin [sis' pla tin] (Platinol)

While the exact mechanism of action of cisplatin is unknown, it is believed to be a cell-cycle–nonspecific agent that has an action similar to the alkylating agents. It cross-links DNA, thus interfering with its function. It is indicated for the treatment of bladder, ovarian, and testicular carcinomas.

Cisplatin (IV) does not significantly cross the blood-brain barrier; half-life is biphasic; alpha is 25 to 49 minutes while beta is 58 to 73 hours. It is metabolized to inactive metabolites that are renally excreted after 5 days, although platinum has been detected in body tissues for 4 months or longer. For major antineoplastic toxicities, see Table 57-1.

Adult dosage varies according to site of cancerous growth; for example, for advanced bladder cancer the dose is 50 to 70 mg/m^2 IV every 3 to 4 weeks. Recommended dosages vary according to cancer, protocol, and also whether therapy is initial or maintenance. Check a current reference for information.

■ Nursing Management

Cisplatin Therapy

Assessment. Carefully consider use of cisplatin when the client is pregnant or breastfeeding or has renal function impairment, infection, hearing impairment, bone marrow depression, or a history of gout, urate renal stones, or previous cytotoxic drug or radiation therapy. Observe cautions for chickenpox, shingles, and live viruses as with other antineoplastic agents.

Review the client's current medication regimen for significant drug interactions that may occur when cisplatin is given with the drugs listed below.

Drug	Possible effect and management
bone marrow depressants or radiation	Increased bone marrow depression may occur. A decrease in drug dosage is usually indicated.
probenecid (Benemid) or sulfinpyrazone (Anturane)	Hyperuricemia and gout may occur. The prescriber may adjust the antigout medications or prescribe allopurinol. The latter is often preferred to prevent drug-induced hyperuricemia.
nephrotoxic or ototoxic drugs	**Concurrent or sequential administration is not recommended. The risk for nephrotoxicity and ototoxicity is increased, especially in clients with renal impairment. Avoid or a potentially serious drug interaction may occur.**
vaccines, live viral	**See methotrexate drug interactions.**

A baseline assessment of the client's underlying condition, including hematocrit or hemoglobin, platelet count, total and differential white blood cell count, serum uric acid and creatinine levels, creatinine clearance, BUN, electrolytes, audiometric testing, and neurologic status should be obtained.

Nursing diagnosis. Clients receiving cisplatin therapy are at risk for the following nursing diagnoses: activity intolerance related to anemia due to myelosuppression; altered protection related to leukopenia and thrombocytopenia; sensory-perceptual alteration related to ototoxicity (hearing loss, tinnitus, loss of balance) or visual disturbances due to optic neuritis or papilledema; altered mucous membranes (stomatitis); altered comfort (pain/redness at injection site); fluid volume deficit related to anorexia, nausea, or vomiting; and the potential complications of anaphylactic reaction, nephrotoxicity/uric acid nephropathy, ototoxicity, optic neuritis, papilledema, and neurotoxicity (loss of reflexes, numbness of fingers and toes, ataxia, seizures).

Implementation

Monitoring. Evaluate for nephrotoxicity, hyperuricemia, and uric acid nephropathy. Nephrotoxicity is cumulative, and the effects may be irreversible with repeated or high dosages. Symptoms are reduced urinary output, weight gain over several days, edema of the feet and lower legs, flank pain, pruritus, urine odor on breath, anorexia, nausea, and vomiting. Metoclopramide (Reglan) is indicated for cisplatin-induced emesis.

Monitor BUN, creatinine clearance, and serum uric acid level. A decrease in creatinine clearance and an increase in the other test values may indicate nephrotoxicity.

Test hearing status before the initial dose and each subsequent dose. Ringing in the ears and difficulty in hearing high frequencies may indicate ototoxicity. Hearing loss is cumulative and may be unilateral.

Monitor for myelosuppression as evidenced by anemia, leukopenia, and thrombocytopenia. Hematocrit, platelet count, and total and differential leukocyte counts should also be monitored. The lowest leukocyte and platelet counts generally occur 18 to 23 days after a dose and recover by 39 days. The client should be observed for fever of unknown origin, chills, sore throat, unusual bleeding, or bruising.

Discontinue administration of cisplatin at the first indication of peripheral neuropathy because it may be irreversible. Symptoms to watch for are numbness or tingling in the fingers, toes, or face and loss of taste. Perform regular neurologic exams.

Do not administer subsequent doses of cisplatin until platelet levels are over 100,000 cells/mm^3, WBC is over 4000 cells/mm^3, creatinine clearance is greater than 90 ml/minute, serum creatinine is less than 1.3 mg/100 ml, or BUN is under 20 mg/100 ml.

Intervention. Follow the health agency's policy for the handling of hazardous materials. Have available drugs and equipment for the treatment of a possible anaphylactic reaction.

Hydrate client with 1 to 2 L of intravenous infusion fluid 8 to 12 hours before a dose, and dilute cisplatin in 2 L of 5% dextrose in one-half or one-third normal saline containing 37.5 g of mannitol. This infusion should be administered over 6 to 8 hours. To reduce nephrotoxicity, adequate hydration of 3000 ml daily should be maintained. Urinary output should be closely monitored. Alkalinization of urine and allopurinol administration may also be used to prevent uric acid nephropathy.

Reduce nausea and vomiting by administering a parenteral antiemetic ½ hour before cisplatin is given. These symptoms usually begin 1 to 4 hours after a dose. Therefore the antiemetic therapy is continued on a schedule as long as necessary. If the nausea and vomiting are severe, cisplatin may be discontinued. As with the nursing management of antineoplastic agents discussed in Chapter 56, observe safety precautions regarding invasive procedures.

Do not use aluminum needles or other equipment containing aluminum. Cisplatin is incompatible with aluminum, which causes a black precipitate and a potency loss.

Education. Instruct client to record intake and output and to report any edema or decrease in urinary output. The client should report any numbness or tingling of the fingers or toes or any ringing in the ears or hearing loss.

As with other antineoplastic agents previously discussed, caution the client against being immunized with live virus vaccines and alert the client to signs and symptoms to report to the prescriber. Instruct in safety measures to be taken while thrombocytopenia exists.

Evaluation. The client will demonstrate signs of clinical improvement without signs and symptoms of infection, bleeding, tinnitus, or hearing loss. Renal function will be adequate. The client and family will evidence an understanding of cyclophosphamide therapy.

ANTIBIOTIC ANTITUMOR DRUGS

The antitumor antibiotics are cytotoxic agents that directly bind DNA, thus inhibiting DNA and RNA synthesis. The early agents in this class cause the clinically limiting adverse effect of irreversible cardiomyopathy. Newer agents are being sought that lack this cardiac toxicity. See Table 57-1 for antineoplastic drugs and their toxicities.

▲ **doxorubicin** [dox oh roo' bi sin] (Adriamycin)

Doxorubicin is an antineoplastic cell-cycle–specific agent for the S-phase of cell division. It is indicated for the treatment of acute leukemia, Wilms' tumor, soft tissue and bone sarcomas, Hodgkin's disease, lymphomas, and breast and various other carcinomas.

Doxorubicin does not cross the blood-brain barrier and is highly tissue bound. It is metabolized in the liver to produce the active metabolite, adriamycinol. The half-life of doxorubicin is biphasic, 0.6 hours and 16.7 hours. The active metabolite has a half-life of 3.3 hours and 31.7 hours. It is metabolized in the liver and excreted primarily in bile. For major toxicities, see Table 57-1.

The usual adult dose is 60 to 75 mg/m^2 intravenously, repeated every 3 weeks. The pediatric dosage is 30 mg/m^2 of body surface daily on 3 consecutive days every month.

■ Nursing Management

Doxorubicin Therapy

Assessment. Carefully consider use of doxorubicin when the client is pregnant or breastfeeding or has bone marrow depression, tumor cell infiltration of the bone marrow, hepatic function impairment, or a history of gout, urate kidney stones, or cytotoxic drug or radiation therapy. If the client has heart disease, the cardiotoxic effects of the drug may occur at lower levels. Caution should be used with elderly clients because of their decreased bone marrow reserves. Observe cautions for chickenpox and shingles as with other antineoplastic agents.

Significant drug interactions are reported with other bone marrow depressant drugs or radiation, probenecid (Benemid) or sulfinpyrazone (Arturane), and with live virus vaccines; see previous comments regarding mechlorethamine drug interactions.

Use of doxorubicin in clients who have received daunorubicin (Cerubidine) increases the risk of inducing cardiotoxicity. Both drugs have cumulative maximum dosing limits that must be followed: a total dose of 550 mg/m^2 from either drug alone or both drugs together. If the client has received previous chest radiation or other cardiotoxic drugs, the maximum dose is reduced to 400 mg/m^2.

The client should have a baseline assessment that includes echocardiography, radionuclide angiography determination of ejection fraction, hematocrit or hemoglobin, platelet count, total and differential white blood cell count, serum uric acid levels, and liver function studies. The client's mouth should be examined for ulceration.

Nursing diagnosis. Assess the client receiving doxorubicin for the possibility of the following nursing diagnoses: altered mucous membranes (stomatitis); altered protection related to immunosuppression (leukopenia) and an increased tendency to bleed due to thrombocytopenia; impaired tissue integrity related to extravasation or cellulitis at the injection site; diarrhea; fluid volume deficit related to anorexia, nausea, and vomiting; disturbance of self-concept related to loss of hair or darkening of skin; and the potential complications of cardiotoxicity (pedal edema, dysrhythmias, shortness of breath), uric acid nephropathy, and allergic response.

Implementation

Monitoring. Monitor serum uric acid levels and intake and output to ensure that the client is adequately hydrated to prevent hyperuricemia. Allopurinol administration and alkalinization of urine may be used to decrease serum uric acid levels.

Monitor the hemoglobin, hematocrit, and platelets, and watch the client for signs of bruising and bleeding, particularly gastrointestinal bleeding.

Monitor the echocardiography and radionuclide angiography for evidence of cardiopathy; observe the client for swelling of the feet and lower legs and shortness of breath. Cardiotoxicity is more common in elderly persons over 70 years of age and in children under 2 years of age. It usually occurs within 1 to 6 months after therapy has begun. Cardiotoxicity may develop suddenly and may be irreversible; it is critical that cardiotoxicity be detected early, when it usually responds to therapy.

Monitor temperature and observe for signs of infection, fever, chills, or sore throat. Monitor the total and differential white cell count. The lowest leukocyte count usually occurs 10 to 14 days after dosage and recovers within 21 days.

Examine the client's mouth for ulcerations before the administration of each dose since stomatitis is a sign of toxicity.

Intervention. Doxorubicin is usually administered slowly, over not less than 3 to 5 minutes, into the tubing of a freely running intravenous solution of 5% dextrose injection or 0.9% sodium chloride injection.

Avoid contact with the solution by wearing gloves while preparing and administering it. If contact with the skin or mucous membranes occurs, wash thoroughly with soap and water. See institutional guidelines for the safe handling of antineoplastic agents.

Take precautions against intravenous extravasation. If extravasation occurs, the intravenous line should be moved to another site for completion of the dose. Ice packs should be applied and the extremity should be elevated to minimize injury. If inflammation is extensive, surgical excision of the area may be required. Do not give intramuscularly or subcutaneously because it will cause tissue necrosis.

As with the nursing management of other antineoplastic agents discussed in Chapter 56, observe safety precautions for invasive procedures.

Education. The client's urine may become reddish for 1 or 2 days after administration of doxorubicin, but it generally clears in 48 hours. Alert the client that a discoloration of the skin and nails may occur, especially in children and blacks.

As with previously discussed antineoplastic agents, discuss with the client the importance of adequate hydration, the possibility of reversible alopecia, and the contraindication of being immunized with live virus vaccines during therapy. Instruct the client to report signs and symptoms of infection (fever, sore throat), bleeding, and congestive heart failure (pedal edema, shortness of breath).

Evaluation. The client will demonstrate signs of clinical improvement without local tissue damage at infusion site or signs and symptoms of cardiotoxicity. The client and family will evidence an understanding of doxorubicin therapy.

MITOTIC INHIBITORS

The primary mitotic inhibitors vinblastine and vincristine (vinca alkaloids derived from a periwinkle plant) are cell-cycle–specific agents that inhibit mitosis during M-phase. Vinorelbine is a semi-synthetic vinca alkaloid. While these agents are similar chemically, they have different therapeutic indications and different side/adverse effects. See Table 57-1 for antineoplastic drugs and their toxicities.

vinblastine [vin blas' teen] (Velban)
▲ **vincristine** [vin kris' teen] (Oncovin)

Vinblastine is used to treat breast and testicular carcinoma, Hodgkin's and non-Hodgkin's lymphomas, Kaposi's sarcoma, and mycosis fungoides. Vincristine is used to treat acute lymphoblastic leukemia, Hodgkin's and non-Hodgkin's lymphomas, rhabdomyosarcoma, neuroblastoma, Wilms' tumor, and various other carcinomas.

Both drugs are administered intravenously and do not cross the blood-brain barrier. They are highly tissue bound with triphasic half-life of 3.7 minutes, 1.6 hours, and 25 hours for vinblastine; 0.07 hour, 2.27 hours, and 85 hours for vincristine. They are metabolized in the liver and excreted primarily in bile.

Neurotoxicity is the major dose-limiting side effect for vincristine while bone marrow suppression is the major undesirable effect for vinblastine. For major antineoplastic toxicities, see Table 57-1.

The adult antineoplastic dosage for vinblastine is 0.1 mg/kg IV weekly, adjusting dosages according to tumor size response and leukocyte counts. Vincristine adult dosage is 0.01 to 0.03

mg/kg as a single dose, weekly. For various dosage schedules, see a current package insert or drug reference.

■ Nursing Management

Vinblastine/Vincristine Therapy

Assessment. Carefully consider use of either drug when the client is pregnant or breastfeeding or has hepatic function impairment, infection, bone marrow depression, tumor cell infiltration of the bone marrow, or a history of gout, urate kidney stones, or cytotoxic drug or radiation therapy. Observe for contraindications for chickenpox and shingles as with other antineoplastic agents. The use of vincristine in clients with neuromuscular disease should be carefully considered.

Review the client's current medication regimen for drug interactions. Both drugs may have significant drug interactions with probenecid (Benemid), bone marrow depressants, sulfinpyrazone (Anturane), and live virus vaccines. For description of the interactions, see the section on mechlorethamine. In addition, these interactions may occur when vincristine is given with the drugs listed below.

Drug	Possible effect and management
asparaginase (Elspar)	When given concurrently with vincristine, an increase in neurotoxicity may result. To reduce the possibility of this interaction, asparaginase should be given only after vincristine is administered, not concurrently or before vincristine.
doxorubicin (Adriamycin)	**If administered with vincristine and prednisone, an increase in bone marrow depressant effects may occur. Avoid or a potentially serious drug interaction may occur.**

The client's baseline assessment should include the status of the underlying condition, bowel and bladder function, muscle tone and reflexes, serum uric acid concentrations, hematocrit, hemoglobin, platelet count, total and differential leukocyte count, and liver function studies.

Nursing diagnosis. Vinblastine or vincristine therapy places the client at risk for the following nursing diagnoses: altered comfort (headache, rash, bloating); fluid volume deficit related to anorexia, nausea, and vomiting; impaired tissue integrity related to extravasation or cellulitis at the infusion site; altered mucous membranes (stomatitis); altered protection related to leukopenia and thrombocytopenia; altered bowel elimination pattern, either diarrhea or constipation; disturbance of self-concept related to alopecia; and the potential complications of hyperuremia or uric acid nephropathy (joint pain, lower back pain) and neurotoxicity (numbness in fingers and toes, blurred vision). With vincristine, altered urinary elimination pattern related to autonomic toxicity evidenced by bed-wetting, increased or decreased urination, painful or difficult urination is also a possibility.

Implementation

Monitoring. Monitor CBC and observe the client for fever, chills, sore throat, bleeding, and bruising to assess risk for infection or physical injury. With vinblastine, the lowest level of leukocytes occurs 5 to 10 days after the last day of administration, and recovery occurs within another 7 to 14 days. With vincristine, leukopenia is usually greatest within 4 days.

Monitor serum uric acid levels and the client's intake and output to ensure adequate hydration for the prevention of uric acid nephropathy and to detect early signs of urine retention.

Monitor the client's neuromuscular status. Watch for ataxia, numbness, tingling, or pain in the fingers or toes, headache, double vision, depression of deep tendon reflexes, and other early signs of neurotoxicity. Monitor the client's bowel status for early signs of autonomic toxicity, such as constipation.

Case Study

The Client with Hodgkin's Disease

Matthew Bennett is a 32-year-old, married salesperson who has been referred to an oncology clinic after a diagnosis of Stage III-A Hodgkin's disease was confirmed by his primary physician. Mr. Bennett first went to his physician after finding a lump in his right axilla that persisted for several months. The oncologist has recommended a program of chemotherapy to include the following drugs:

mechlorethamine (Mustargen)
vincristine (Oncovin)
prednisone (Deltasone)
procarbazine (Matulane)

1. How is each drug classified as a chemotherapeutic agent and what is its effect on the cell cycle?
2. Why is prednisone used as part of the chemotherapy regimen?
3. What measures should the nurse implement before administration of mechlorethamine to reduce nausea and vomiting?
4. What should the nurse do if the intravenous infusion infiltrates during administration of Mustargen or vincristine?
5. During the course of therapy with vincristine Mr. Bennett complains of numbness and tingling in his hands and feet. What is the significance of these symptoms?
6. What precautions should the nurse take when handling the equipment used for drug administration and body fluids?

Monitor the client's nutritional status, weight, and hydration if nausea and vomiting are adverse reactions.

Observe the injection/infusion site for extravasation and cellulitis.

Intervention. Reconstitute with sterile water for injection. Store reconstituted solutions in refrigeration.

Take precautions against intravenous infiltration. If extravasation occurs, stop administration immediately and inject remaining dose into another vein. To alleviate discomfort and inflammation with vincristine extravasation, inject hyaluronidase locally and apply moderate heat or cold compresses.

Administer by intravenous push or inject into the tubing of a running intravenous infusion for 1 minute. Administer only intravenously; intramuscular or subcutaneous administration will cause tissue necrosis; intrathecal administration will cause death.

Intake should be 3000 ml daily. Urine may be alkalinized if serum uric acid levels increase. Use of a laxative or stool softener will help prevent upper colon impaction. Antiemetics are administered as needed.

As with the nursing management of other antineoplastic agents discussed in Chapter 56, observe safety precautions for invasive procedures and avoidance of infections.

Education. Stress the importance of adequate hydration, the possibility of alopecia, and the contraindication of being immunized with live virus vaccines during therapy. See Chapter 56.

Evaluation. The client will demonstrate signs of clinical improvement without local tissue damage at intravenous site, neuropathy, or nephropathy. The client and family will evidence an understanding of vinblastine/vincristine therapy.

MISCELLANEOUS ANTINEOPLASTIC AGENTS

Miscellaneous agents are those that cannot be classified by their mechanism of action into any of the previous groups. In this section, hormones, miscellaneous, cytoprotective and immunomodulator agents are discussed.

Hormonal agents are used in the treatment of neoplasms sensitive to hormonal growth controls in the body. Their exact mechanism of action against neoplasms is unknown, but apparently they interfere with growth-stimulating receptors on target tissues. Such agents are more selective and less toxic than other antineoplastic medications and include corticosteroids, androgens and antiandrogens, estrogens and antiestrogens, progestins, and gonadotropin-releasing hormone.

Since corticosteroids retard lymphocytic proliferations, their greatest value lies in the treatment of lymphocytic leukemias and lymphomas. They are also used in conjunction with radiation therapy to decrease the occurrence of radiation edema in such critical areas as the superior mediastinum, brain, and spinal cord.

Prednisone and dexamethasone are corticosteroids that are often prescribed for clients with cancer. Prednisone has demonstrated a lympholytic and antiinflammatory effect that is useful in the treatment of leukemias, lymphomas, and breast carcinomas. Steroids, especially dexamethasone, are useful in reducing cerebral edema induced by the increasing growth of a brain tumor or from radiation therapy. Individual drugs belonging to this category are discussed in Chapter 49.

Androgens such as testosterone and fluoxymesterone (Halotestin) are used to treat advanced breast carcinoma if surgery, radiation, and other therapies are inappropriate or ineffective.

Tamoxifen [ta mox' i fen] (Nolvadex, Nolvadex-D♣) an antiestrogen preparation, has replaced both androgens and estrogens as the initial approach in breast cancer therapy (Chabner et al, 1996). It blocks the uptake of estradiol and thus is effective for tumors that contain high concentrations of estrogen receptors. The side/adverse effects of tamoxifen include nausea, vomiting, headache; and in females, hot flashes and weight gain; in males, impotency.

Anastrozole [a nahs' troe zole] (Arimidex) and *testolactone* [tes tah lack' tone] (Teslac) inhibit steroid aromatase, thus reducing estrone synthesis in the adrenals, the major source of estrogen in postmenopausal women. They are indicated for palliative therapy of advanced breast cancer in postmenopausal women. Testolactone is also used in premenopausal women with non- or terminated ovarian function.

Estrogens may be used to treat androgen-sensitive prostatic carcinomas or in advanced breast carcinoma in postmenopausal women. For example, estrogens such as *diethylstilbestrol* (DES, Stilphostrol), *polyestradiol* (Estradurin), *ethinyl estradiol* (Estinyl), and *estramustine* (Emcyt) are used to treat advanced prostatic carcinoma. The latter drug is a combination of estradiol and nitrogen mustard that provides both a weak hormone effect and alkylating action. In this combination, estrogen helps to carry the drug into estrogen receptor cells, thus enhancing the nitrogen mustard cytotoxic effects in these cells.

The main precaution in monitoring estramustine is an increased risk of inducing thrombosis, especially in clients with a history of thrombophlebitis or thromboembolic disease.

Avoid immunizations unless specifically ordered by the prescriber. The client and others in the household should avoid immunization with oral poliovirus vaccine.

Estramustine is taken orally (14 mg/kg/day in divided doses), preferably an hour before meals with water. Avoid concurrent consumption of milk, dairy products, or any calcium-containing products.

Bicalutamide [bik ah loot ah mide] (Casodex) competitively inhibits androgens from receptor-binding in target tissues. It is indicated in combination with a luteinizing hormone-releasing hormone, for treatment of advanced prostate cancer. Clinical trials indicate it is comparable to flutamide combination in survival time (Olin, 1996).

Flutamide [floo' ta myde] (Eulexin), an oral antiandrogen product, inhibits the uptake and/or the binding of androgens at the target site. The result is suppression of ovarian and testicular steroidogenesis, thus inducing a medical castration. It is used in combination with *leuprolide* (Lupron), a luteinizing hormone-releasing hormone agonist, to treat metastatic prostate carcinomas. This combination has been reported to prolong survival by at least 25% as compared with leuprolide therapy alone. Side/adverse effects include diarrhea, impotency, and hepatotoxicity.

Goserelin [goe' se rel in] (Zoladex), a palliative agent used in the treatment of advanced prostate carcinoma, is also a luteinizing hormone-releasing hormone. It is a potent inhibitor of pituitary gonadotropins; with long-term administration, the serum levels of testosterone usually drop to the range seen in surgically castrated men within 2 to 4 weeks after initiation of drug therapy. A 3.6 mg dose is implanted subcutaneously in the upper abdominal wall every 28 days. Adverse reactions reported generally are related to the lowered testosterone levels and may include hot flashes, sexual dysfunction, and decreased erections.

Nilutamide (Nilandron) is an antiandrogen used in conjunction with surgery or chemical castration for the treatment of metastatic prostate cancer. It blocks testosterone effects at the androgen receptor in vitro, while in vivo it interacts with the androgen receptor to prevent normal androgen responses. For maximum effect it must be started on the same day as surgical castration (Olin, 1997).

Progestins such as *medroxyprogesterone* (Depo-Provera) and *megestrol* (Megace) are used to treat advanced endometrial cancer. It is primarily a palliative approach that seeks tumor regression and an increase in client's survival time. Megesterol is also indicated for advanced carcinoma of the breast while medroxyprogesterone is also used in clients with advanced renal carcinoma.

Altretamine [al tret' a meen] (Hexalen) is a cytotoxic agent for the palliative treatment of persistent or recurrent ovarian cancer. Its mechanism of action is unknown although chemically it resembles the alkylating agents. Clinically, however, it is effective for ovarian tumors that are resistant to the previously marketed alkylating agents. Side/adverse effects include nausea and vomiting, neurotoxicity, myelosuppression, and CNS changes (ataxia, dizziness, mood alterations). The most significant drug interactions to avoid include cimetidine (increases half-life of altretamine) and monoamine oxidase (MAO) inhibitors (severe hypotension).

Topotecan (Hycamtin), a topoisomerase inhibitor, is indicated for the treatment of relapsed or refractory metastatic carcinoma of the ovary after failure of other therapies. Its action may be due to inhibiting topoisomerase activity in DNA during DNA synthesis. This product should only be administered to women with adequate bone marrow reserves, that is, neutrophils of at least 1500 cells/mm^3 and platelet counts of 100,000/mm^3 or greater. Side/adverse effects include neutropenia (a dose-limiting toxicity), leukopenia, thrombocytopenia, anemia, headache, diarrhea, stomach pain, nausea, vomiting, alopecia, tiredness, dyspnea, and neuromuscular pain. Usual dose is 1.5 mg/m^2 by IV infusion over 30 minutes daily, for 5 days. See a current package insert for detailed information on this product.

Miscellaneous Agents

Asparaginase [a spare' a gi nase] (Elspar, Kidrolase ♣) reduces asparagine to aspartic acid in the body. Asparagine is necessary for cell survival and since normal body cells are capable of synthesizing adequate supplies of asparaginase, they are not affected by an asparaginase deficiency. Certain cancer cells, however, depend on a circulating supply of asparaginase within the blood and when it is decreased, cancer cells will die. Asparaginase is used to treat acute lymphocytic leukemia (ALL). Side/adverse effects are hyperammonemia (headache, anorexia, nausea, vomiting, abdominal cramps), decrease in the blood clotting factors, allergic reactions, liver toxicity, pancreatitis, and anaphylaxis.

Pegaspargase [peg as' per gase] (Oncaspar) is a modification of the L-asparaginase enzyme that is used in combination chemotherapies for use in acute lymphoblastic leukemia in persons unable to take L-asparaginase. Side/adverse effects include hypersensitivity reactions, hepatotoxicity, and coagulopathies.

Cladribine [kla dri been'] (Leustatin) is used to treat hairy cell leukemia. Cladribine enters the cell and is phosphorylated to a deoxyadenosine concentration that accumulates in these cells, interfering with DNA repair and eventually results in cell death. Side/adverse effects include severe anemia, infection, skin rash, bleeding or bruising, anorexia, headache, nausea, vomiting, and fatigue.

Dacarbazine [da kar' ba zeen] (DTIC-Dome) is a cell-cycle–nonspecific agent that inhibits DNA and RNA synthesis and appears to be more active in the late G_2 phase of the cell cycle. It is indicated for the treatment of malignant melanoma and Hodgkin's disease. Side/adverse effects include flu-like syndrome, anorexia, nausea, vomiting, and diarrhea.

Hydroxyurea [hye drox ee yoo ree' ah] (Hydrea) inhibits DNA synthesis without affecting the synthesis of RNA or protein. It is indicated for the treatment of head, neck, and ovarian carcinoma, chronic myelocytic leukemia, and malignant melanoma. Side/adverse effects include bone marrow suppression, diarrhea, anorexia, nausea, vomiting, and drowsiness.

Levamisole [lee vam' i sol] (Ergamisol), a biologic response modifier (immunostimulant), is used in combination with fluorouracil (5-FU) to treat colorectal carcinoma (Dukes C adenocarcinoma). This combination has resulted in an increased survival time (decreased mortality) and decreased risk of cancer recurrence. Significant side/adverse effects of levamisole include bone marrow suppression, nausea, diarrhea, metallic taste, arthralgia, and flulike syndrome.

Mitotane [mye' toe tane] (Lysodren) is an adrenal gland suppressing agent indicated for the treatment of an inoperable carcinoma of the adrenal cortex. Administered orally, it is distributed throughout the body but is mainly stored in fat. Onset of effect is reported within 48 to 72 hours of starting therapy; tumor response is usually within 6 weeks. Significant side/adverse effects of mitotane include adrenal gland insufficiency: dark skin, diarrhea, anorexia, depression, nausea, vomiting, weakness, drowsiness, and lightheadedness.

Irinotecan [i rin' oe tek an] (Captosar) is the first of a new class of oncolytic agents indicated for the treatment of metastatic colorectal cancer or rectal cancer that has occurred or progressed after 5-FU chemotherapy. This product is a topoisomerase 1 inhibitor that binds to the topoisomerase 1-DNA complex, resulting in double-stranded DNA breaks that cause tumor cell death. Irinotecan may cause severe diarrhea, which requires immediate treatment with loperamide (Imodium). Severe myelosuppression, nausea, and vomiting may also occur (Camptosar, 1996).

Paclitaxel [pa kli tax' el] (Taxol) is a natural substance extracted from the yew tree, marketed for the treatment of metastatic ovarian cancer refractory to other drug treatments. It is an antimicrotubule agent that stabilizes microtubule bundles, and therefore interfering with the late G_2 mitotic cell cycle and resulting in inhibition of cell replication. Side/adverse effects of paclitaxel include severe allergic reactions (to prevent, pretreat with a steroid and an H_1 and H_2 antagonist), bone marrow suppression, peripheral neuropathy, muscle pain, alopecia, and gastric distress.

Docetaxel [dok i tax' el] (Taxotere) is also a taxoid that is a semisynthetic product originating from the yew plant. It may produce its effect by binding and stabilizing microtubule bundles thus inhibiting cell mitosis. It is indicated for the treatment of advanced breast cancer. Side/adverse effects of docetaxel include bone marrow suppression, nausea, diarrhea, stomatitis, fever, skin reactions, and myalgia.

Procarbazine [pro kar' ba zeen] (Matulane) is an alkylating agent and a weak monoamine oxidase (MAO) inhibitor that is cell-cycle–specific for the S-phase of cell division. It is believed to inhibit DNA, RNA, and protein synthesis. It is commonly prescribed for the treatment of Hodgkin's disease. Side/adverse effects of procarbazine include bone marrow suppression, pneumonitis, nausea, vomiting, weakness, drowsiness, myalgia, muscle twitching, insomnia, nightmares, and increased nervousness.

Tretinoin [tret' i noyn] (Vesanoid) is a retinoid that appears to enhance maturation of primitive promyelocytes from the leukemic clone, which is followed by reseeding the bone marrow and blood with normal blood cells. It is used to treat acute promyelocytic leukemia. Side/adverse effects of tretinoin include headaches, fever, increased weakness, malaise, shivering, infections, hemorrhage, and peripheral edema.

Cytoprotective Combinations

An antineoplastic drug combination is *ifosfamide* [eye foss' fa mide] (Iflex) with *mesna* [mess' na] (Mesnex). This product is used for the treatment of germ cell testicular tumors. Ifosfamide, an alkylating agent, has been studied since the early 1970s, but its adverse effect of hemorrhagic cystitis (urotoxicity) has limited its usefulness. Mesna has been discovered to be a specific antidote for this type toxicity. Thus using both drugs in combination allows for a more aggressive therapy, while reducing the potential of ifosfamide-induced hematuria and cystitis.

Amifostine [am i fos' teen] (Ethyol) is a cytoprotective agent administered before cisplatin to reduce the potential for renal toxicity. *Dexrazoxane* [dex ra zock' zain] (Zinecard) is a cardioprotective substance used with doxorubicin administration to reduce drug-induced cardiomyopathy. It is an intracellular chelating agent although its mechanism of action is not clearly defined. There are some reports that the use of this product with the 5-FU, doxorubicin (Adriamycin), and cyclosphosphamide (FAC) regimen used to treat breast cancer resulted in a lower response rate to therapy. For this reason, it was recommended that dextrazoxane be used only in individuals that have received the cumulative 300 mg/m^2 dose of doxorubicin and are continuing on this product (Olin, 1996). Side/adverse effects include myelosuppression effects of alopecia, nausea, vomiting, tiredness, anorexia, stomatitis, fever, diarrhea, neurotoxicity, phlebitis, and dysphagia. See a current package insert for detailed dosing and other information.

Immunomodulator Agents

Interferons

Interferon alfa-2a, recombinant (Roferon-A), and *interferon alfa-2b, recombinant* (Intron A), are manufactured by the process of recombinant DNA technology, resulting in highly purified proteins that have an effect similar to the interferon alfa subtypes produced by human leukocytes.

Interferons are released in the body in response to viral infections or substances that induce their release. Interferons have antiviral (inhibit virus replication), antiproliferative (decrease cell proliferation), and immunomodulatory (enhance phagocyte activity and assist the cytotoxicity properties of lymphocytes for target cells) properties. Their mechanism of action as antineoplastic agents is unknown but may be the result of one or more of the three properties identified. For example, in some types of cancer, interferon appears to have a dual effect of both cytotoxic and immune stimulation. Some clients demonstrate an increase in the hematologic factors, granulocytes, platelets, and hemoglobin serum levels.

Interferon alfa-2a and alfa-2b are indicated for the treatment of hairy cell leukemia, genital warts, AIDS-related Kaposi's sarcoma, bladder cancer, and for chronic active hepatitis. Toxicities reported include a flulike syndrome that includes fever, chills, muscle pain, loss of appetite, and lethargy. At higher doses, myelosuppression, nausea, vomiting, neurotoxicity, and cardiotoxicity may occur. For additional information, see the section on drugs affecting the immunologic system.

Aldesleukin [al dess loo' kin] (Proleukin, interleukin-2) is another cytokine biologic product that stimulates immune function and is nearly identical in chemical structure and action to human interleukin-2. It is indicated for the treatment of renal cell carcinoma. This substance appears to stimulate T cell proliferation and is a co-factor in developing cytotoxic T-lymphocyte activity against tumors. Its cytotoxic action may be caused by its enhancing growth of the body's natural killer cells and the lymphokine-activated killer (LAK) cells. Side effects/adverse effects of aldesleukin include edema, anemia, thrombocytopenia, and hypotension.

Granulocyte macrophage-colony stimulating factor (GM-CSF; sargramostim) and *granulocyte colony stimulating factor* (G-CSF; filgrastim, [Neupogen]) are immunomodulator agents with a variety of approved and investigational uses. GM-CSF is used to accelerate myeloid recovery in persons with acute lymphoblastic leukemia (ALL), Hodgkin's disease, and non-Hodgkin's lymphoma undergoing bone marrow transplantation. Complete blood counts are performed to monitor the hematologic response to this drug. Investigationally this drug has been used to increase white blood cell counts in AIDS clients receiving zidovudine (AZT) and to correct neutropenia in aplastic anemia. Closely monitor clients who are receiving lithium or corticosteroids concurrently because the myeloproliferative action of this drug may be increased.

G-CSF (Neupogen) is used to decrease the potential for infection in persons receiving myelosuppressive agents that are associated with severe neutropenia and fever. Neutrophil counts are closely monitored; the drug should be discontinued when the absolute neutrophil count is 10,000/mm^3 or more after the nadir induced by the chemotherapy. The major side/adverse effects of G-CSF include nausea, vomiting, hair loss, diarrhea, fevers, mucositis, anorexia, and fatigue. Bone pain has been reported about 2 to 3 days before the increase in neutrophil count. This pain is usually controlled with nonopioid-type analgesics. Usual starting dose is 5 μg/kg/day by SC or IV injection.

CANCER CHEMOTHERAPY RESEARCH

Cancer chemotherapy research is a priority area of study in the United States and Canada. Many new drugs are being studied with the hope of improving the treatment and survival of cancer and AIDS-induced cancer clients. (AIDS is reviewed in Chapter 64.) The reader is encouraged to monitor professional literature for information on the release of new drugs for the treatment of cancer and for other related research.

Another promising area of study is liposomes as a delivery system to hold lipid-soluble drugs. Drugs encapsulated in a liposome capsule can be distributed differently in the body than free drugs. Liposomes accumulate at sites of inflammation and infection, as well as in some solid tumors. Thus they are under study for the treatment of systemic fungal infections (amphotericin B) and for the treatment of specific cancers. Doxorubicin (Adriamycin), cisplatin (Platinol), and methotrexate (Folex) are just several of the antineoplastic agents currently undergoing clinical testing. Doxorubicin in liposome administration has been reported to deliver the drug more directly to the site of action, resulting in fewer cardiac and other side/adverse effects. Cisplatin in liposomes has been reported to cause much less kidney damage than cisplatin alone. If studies of liposome drug therapy continue to report that, in addition to a decrease in side effects/adverse reactions, therapeutic outcome is also efficacious, then liposomes will have the potential of opening an exciting new avenue of drug delivery in the next few years (Box 57-6; see the Nursing Research box on p. 886).

BOX 57-6

Investigational Drug Classifications

Investigational drugs are agents that have not been released for marketing by the Food and Drug Administration. While responsibility for regulating drugs rests with the FDA, the National Cancer Institute (NCI) is the largest developer of antineoplastic agents in the United States. The NCI has established stringent regulations to monitor the receipt, use, and disposal of investigational drugs. It also requires that investigators report adverse reactions on an established time schedule. For example, anaphylactic reactions to an investigational drug must be reported by phoning a specific branch office that is available on a 24-hour basis. This call must be followed up with a written report within 10 working days.

Investigational drugs are divided into three groups:

	Drug Group	Purpose
Phase I	A	To determine maximum tolerated dosage To detect toxicities associated with various dosage schedules To determine pharmacokinetics and optimum dosing schedule
Phase II	B	To identify antineoplastic activity in specific cancers affecting humans To determine client's response to various drug dosages and schedules
Phase III	C	New agent now compared with previously marketed drugs to ascertain effectiveness, effect on quality of life, mortality, and morbidity

Nursing Research

Chemotherapy, nausea, and vomiting

Chemotherapeutic treatment of cancer has become increasingly more successful in providing greater life expectancy and control of the spread of disease for many persons diagnosed with cancer. However, some persons receiving a protocol of chemotherapy may choose to discontinue treatment based on their inability to tolerate undesirable side effects, of which nausea and vomiting are among the most common and distressing. Pickett (1991) examined the relationship of anticipatory nausea and/or anticipatory vomiting (AN/AV) in adults receiving an initial course of cancer chemotherapy in an outpatient setting with the following set of variables: symptom distress, mood disturbance, stage of disease, sensitivity to conditioning cues, emetic potential of antineoplastic drugs, age, psychosocial stress, and ability to cope.

The setting for the study was seven outpatient chemotherapy clinics in the Northeast, Mid-Atlantic, and Southwest areas. Measures of selected variables were obtained with valid and reliable tools before the administration of chemotherapy on "Day 1" of the first, fourth, and fifth consecutive treatment cycles. Assessment of nausea and vomiting were obtained before administration of chemotherapy. There was a significant difference between subjects who subsequently developed AN/AV and those who did not. Those who developed AN/AV were receiving a drug regimen higher in emetogenic potential, were younger, and had an earlier stage of the disease than those subjects who did not develop AN/AV. This study provided suggestive evidence that it is possible to discriminate between those who will subsequently develop AN and those who will not based on data gathered before the administration of any chemotherapy. Multivariate analysis revealed a high degree of correlation between AN/AV and the following linear composite of variables: emetogenic potential of drug, symptom distress, psychosocial stress, ability to cope, and mood disturbance. This set of predictor variables correctly classified 100% of subjects who subsequently developed AN/AV.

Behavioral interventions strategies for anticipatory symptoms have achieved varying levels of success after the symptoms have become apparent. The findings of this study suggest that it might be possible to identify clients who are at high risk for anticipatory symptoms before clients receive any chemotherapy.

Critical thinking questions

- What would be the implications of these findings for nursing practice?

From Pickett M (1991).

SUMMARY

The antineoplastic agents act by interfering with cell reproduction or replication at some point in the cell cycle. They are classified into various groupings based on their probable mechanisms of action: antimetabolites, alkylating agents, mitotic inhibitors, antibiotic antitumor agents, hormones, cytoprotective and immunomodulator agents, and miscellaneous agents. Because the drugs are nonselective and affect all cells in the body as they replicate, there is always some degree of injury to normal cells. Particularly susceptible are those with a high rate of growth, such as bone marrow, gastrointestinal epithelium, and hair follicles. Bone marrow depression with the resultant anemia, leukocytopenia, and thrombocytopenia is unavoidable, and so the laboratory values for blood counts are used to titrate the individual client's dosage and to determine when the client is most susceptible to infection and hemorrhage. Much of the nursing management of antineoplastic therapy is to prevent injury and infection; promote comfort; provide care for the gastrointestinal effects of stomatitis, nausea, and vomiting and changes in bowel elimination; and assess for the development of nephrotoxicity, neurotoxicity, cardiotoxicity, pulmonary toxicity, and dermatologic effects of these drugs. Although short-term toxicity and side effects occur, the potential for cure or reduction of symptoms is a benefit that most often outweighs the risk and discomfort of the administration.

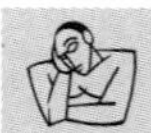

Critical Thinking

1. Mr. Alan Hale, age 48, suddenly develops a high fever and petechiae on his chest and arms. After bone marrow aspiration, his diagnosis is determined to be acute lymphocytic leukemia. The physician puts Mr. Hale on a regimen that contains vincristine (Oncovin). For what nursing diagnoses is Mr. Hale at risk? What lab values should the nurse be monitoring? If Mr. Hale develops a tingling in his fingers and toes, what might be occurring?
2. Mrs. Hextall is returning home after a series of antineoplastic chemotherapies. In discussing her home arrangements for care, she indicates that there should be no problem. Her daughter has moved back in with her, along with her 3-month-old granddaughter, to care for her. Given Mrs. Hextall's altered protection status, what concerns might the nurse have about this arrangement?
3. Given that the antineoplastic agents have a number of potential complications, how would the nurse monitor the client receiving a relevant antineoplastic agent for cardiotoxicity? neurotoxicity? nephrotoxicity?

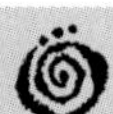

Collaborative Learning Activities

1. Students will prepare before class to present the characteristics of each of the four main classes of antineoplastic agents. A chart on the board will be filled in as the students do their presentations on: (1) indications, (2) mechanisms of action, (3) contraindications, (4) drug interactions, and (5) monitoring and interventions specific to monitoring indicators.

BIBLIOGRAPHY

American Hospital Formulary Service (1996). *AHFS drug information '96*. Bethesda, MD: American Society of Hospital Pharmacists.

Anderson KN, et al. (Eds.) (1994). *Mosby's medical, nursing, & allied health dictionary* (4th ed.). St Louis: Mosby.

Camptosar (1996). Package insert, Pharmacia & Upjohn, #816 907 000.

Chabner BA, Allegra CJ, Curt GA, & Calabresi P (1996). Antineoplastic agents. In Hardman JG & Limbird LE (Eds.). *Goodman & Gilman's the pharmacological basis of therapeutics* (9th ed.). New York: McGraw-Hill.

Hoff ST (1991). Nursing perspectives on intraperitoneal chemotherapy, *J Intrav Nurs* 14(5):309-13.

Jaffee MS & Skidmore-Roth L (1988). *Home health nursing care plans*. St Louis: Mosby.

Olin BR (Ed.) (1996, 1997). *Facts and comparisons*. St Louis: Facts and Comparisons.

Parker GG (1992). Chemotherapy administration in the home, *Home Healthc Nurs* 10(1):30-6.

Patterson W & Perry MC (1993). Chemotherapeutic toxicities: A comprehensive overview, *Contemp Oncol* 3(7):56-64.

Pickett M (1991). Determinants of anticipatory nausea and anticipatory vomiting in adults receiving cancer chemotherapy, *Cancer Nurs* 14(6):334-42.

Studva KV (1993). Programmed instruction: Cancer chemotherapy, *Cancer Nurs* 16(2):145-59.

United States Pharmacopeial Convention (1996). *USP DI: Drug information for the health care professional* (16th ed.). Rockville, MD: The Convention.

Wood LS & Gullo (1993). IV vesicants: How to avoid extravasation, *Amer J Nurs* 93(4):42-6.

Chapter 58

Overview of Infections, Inflammation, and Fever

Chapter Focus

Fever, inflammation, and infection have been a concern to those caring for the ill and injured since ancient times. The majority of clients have experienced these symptoms, not only as a direct result of their injuries or illnesses, but also as the indirect consequence of multiple invasive devices, surgical procedures, and immunosuppression. Nurses have the responsibility of assessment, palliation of symptoms, and evaluation of therapies with these clients. The following objectives and key terms are important for a good understanding of this chapter.

Key Terms

bacteremia (p. 889)
bactericidal agents (p. 893)
bacteriostatic agents (p. 893)
colonization (p. 889)
infection (p. 889)
inflammation (p. 889)
sepsis (p. 889)
septicemia (p. 889)
superinfection (p. 894)

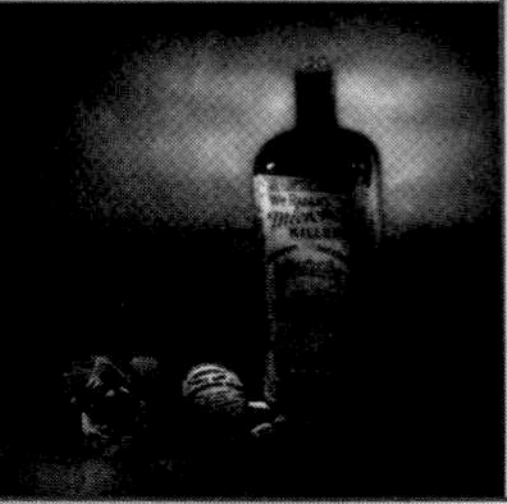

Objectives

1. Describe the mediators of the inflammatory system.
2. Identify different types of fever.
3. Explain the body's set point temperature mechanism.
4. Describe the goal and mechanisms of action of antimicrobial therapy.
5. Identify the general adverse reactions to antimicrobial drugs.
6. Discuss general guidelines for the optimal use of antimicrobial agents.
7. Implement nursing management of a client receiving antimicrobial therapy.

INFECTIONS

Infectious diseases comprise a wide spectrum of illnesses caused by pathogenic microorganisms. Some common pathogens and their most likely sites of infection in the body are listed in Table 58-1. These pathogens cause pneumonia, urinary tract infections, upper respiratory tract infections, gastroenteritis, venereal disease, vaginitis, tuberculosis, and candidiasis.

Infection, the invasion and multiplication of pathogenic microorganisms in body tissues causing disease by local cellular injury, secretion of a toxin, or antigen-antibody reaction in the host, is classified primarily as either local or systemic. A localized infection involving the skin or internal organs, may progress to a systemic infection. A systemic infection involves the whole body rather than a localized area of the body. Several terms describe the degree of local or systemic infection.

Colonization is the localized presence of microorganisms in body tissues or organs, which can be pathogenic or part of the normal flora. Colonization alone is not necessarily an infection but rather it signifies the potential for infection depending on the multiplication of the microorganisms or an alteration in the individual's host defense mechanisms. When flora at its normal colonization site is altered (e.g., by the administration of an antibiotic that affects pathogens and some but not all normal microorganisms), unaffected microorganisms within that environment may grow uninhibited and cause a secondary infection.

Inflammation is a protective mechanism of body tissues in response to invasion or toxins produced by colonizing microorganisms. This reaction consists of cytologic and histologic tissue responses for the localization of phagocytic activity and destruction or removal of injurious material leading to repair and healing.

Bacteremia is the presence of viable bacteria in the circulatory system. **Septicemia** refers to a systemic infection caused by the microorganism multiplication in the circulation. Although bacteremia may lead to septicemia in the immunocompromised host, it is (depending on the pathogen) usually a short-lived, self-limited process. In the immunocompromised host, bacteremia may rapidly produce an overwhelming systemic disease. **Sepsis** is a syndrome involving multiple system organ involvement that is a result of microorganisms or their toxins circulating in the blood.

For nonpathogenic organisms colonizing humans or causing transient bacteremias without tissue invasion, antibiotic therapy is rarely required in the immunocompetent host, whereas prophylactic antibiotic therapy may be required in immunocompromised hosts. In most cases of localized inflammation, such as wound infections, pneumonia, or urinary tract infections, antimicrobials reduce the number of viable pathogens. This permits the immune system to eliminate microorganisms. Antimicrobials are also an essential part of the treatment of septicemia and sepsis.

Microorganisms are divided into several groups: bacteria, mycoplasmas, spirochetes, fungi, and viruses. Bacteria are classified according to their shape, such as bacilli, spirilla, and cocci, and their capacity to be stained. Specific identification of bacteria requires a Gram stain and culture with chemical testing. Gram stain is a sequential procedure that involves crystal violet and iodine solutions followed by alcohol. Gram stain allows the rapid identification of organisms into groups, such as gram-positive or gram-negative rods or cocci. The culture procedures identify specific organisms, but they require 24 to 48 hours for completion.

TABLE 58-1 Primary organisms and common sites of infection

Organism	Infection site
Gram-positive cocci	
Staphylococcus aureus	Burns, skin infections, decubital and surgical wounds, paranasal and middle ear (chronic sinusitis and otitis), lungs, lung abscess, pleura, endocardium, bone (osteomyelitis), and joints
Non-penicillinase producing	
Penicillinase producing	
Staphylococcus epidermidis	
Non-penicillinase producing	
Penicillinase producing	
Methicillin resistant	
Streptococcus pneumoniae	Paranasal and middle ear, lungs, pleura
Streptococcus pyogenes (group A β-hemolytic)	Burns, skin infections, decubitus and surgical wounds, paranasal and middle ear, throat, bone (osteomyelitis), and joints
Streptococcus, viridans group	Endocardium
Gram-positive bacilli	
Clostridium tetani (anaerobe)	Puncture wounds, lacerations, and crush injuries; toxins affecting nervous system
Corynebacterium diphtheriae	Throat, upper part of the respiratory tract
Gram-negative cocci	
Neisseria gonorrhoeae	Urethra, prostate, epididymis and testes, joints
Neisseria meningitidis	Meninges

Continued

TABLE 58-1 Primary organisms and common sites of infection—cont'd

Organism	Infection site
Enteric gram-negative bacilli	
As a group (*Bacteroides, Enterobacter, Escherichia coli, Klebsiella pneumoniae, Proteus mirabilis*, other *Proteus, Salmonella, Serratia, Shigella*)	Peritoneum, biliary tract, kidney and bladder, prostate, decubital and surgical wounds, bone
Bacteroides	Brain abscess, lung abscess, throat, peritoneum
Enterobacter	Peritoneum, biliary tract, kidney and bladder, endocardium
Escherichia coli	Peritoneum, biliary tract, kidney and bladder
Klebsiella pneumoniae	Lungs, lung abscess
Other gram-negative bacilli	
Haemophilus influenzae	Meninges, paranasal and middle ear, lungs, pleura
Pseudomonas aeruginosa	Burns, paranasal and middle ear (chronic otitis media), decubital and surgical wounds, lungs, joints
Acid-fast bacilli	
Mycobacterium tuberculosis	Lungs, pleura, peritoneum, meninges, kidney and bladder, testes, bone, joints
Mycobacterium avium	
Mycoplasmas	
Mycoplasma pneumoniae	Lungs
Spirochetes	
Treponema pallidum (syphilis)	Any tissue or vascular organ of the body
Fungi	
Aspergillus	Paranasal and middle ear, lungs
Candida species	Skin infections, throat, lungs, endocardium, kidney and bladder, vagina
Cryptococcus	
Viruses	
Herpes virus or varicella-zoster virus	Skin infections (herpes simplex or zoster)
Enterovirus, mumps virus, and others	Meninges, epididymis, and testes
Respiratory viruses (including Epstein-Barr virus)	Throat, lungs
Anaerobes	
Gram-positive	Deep wounds, gut
Clostridium difficile	
Clostridium perfringens	
Peptococcus species	
Peptostreptococcus species	
Gram-negative	
Bacteroides fragilis	
Fusobacterium species	

Often the initial or empiric antibiotic selection is based on the prescriber's clinical impression plus the Gram stain procedure; the antibiotic may be changed once culture and sensitivity results are available.

INFLAMMATION

Inflammation is the reaction of body tissues to injury, such as physical trauma, foreign bodies, chemical substances, surgery, radiation, and electricity. The area affected will undergo a series of changes as the body processes attempt to wall off, heal, and/or replace the injured tissue. For example, after an injury occurs, the body will release chemical substances into the tissue that form a wall, called a chemotactic gradient. Fluids and cells will begin to move toward this area.

Blood vessels dilate within 30 minutes of the insult, which provides for an increase in blood flow and exudation of fluid from blood vessels into the injured tissues. The exudate includes protein-rich fluids high in fibrinogen that will attract other substances to the area, such as complement, antibodies, and leukocytes. Fluids collecting in this area will result in edema or swelling. Generally, this occurs within 4 hours of the injury.

During the cellular phase, granulocytes will migrate to the area from the dilated blood vessels at the site. The granulocytes will migrate toward the chemotactic site and accumulate in the area of injury. If the injury is a foreign substance or bacteria, they will engulf and destroy the foreign material (phagocytosis).

Neutrophils, monocytes (macrophages), and lymphocytes (which arrive later) are the granulocytes that affect the injured area. The phagocytosis process tends to localize or wall off the foreign material, to prevent its spread through the tissues. Large numbers of phagocytes lead to pus accumulation and the eventual destruction and removal of the foreign material.

Some pathogens are resistant to destruction and are only walled off, such as tuberculosis bacilli, which can live for many years within the confined cells in the body. Others may transform from a local infection into a systemic infection, thus requiring antimicrobial or antibiotic treatment.

Mediators of the inflammatory system. The complement system is composed of complement components (18 distinct proteins and their cleavage products) present in the blood in the form of inactive proteins called zymogens. Complement is essential in reacting to an acute inflammatory reaction caused by bacteria, some viruses, and immune complex diseases. Complement enhances chemotaxis, increases blood vessel permeability, and eventually causes cell lysis.

Histamine, prostaglandins, arachidonic acid, and leukotrienes are other mediators capable of producing local reactions, smooth muscle contraction, increased chemotaxis, blood vessel vasodilation, and other inflammatory effects. When the foreign agent is destroyed, the resulting debris will be removed by the macrophages and neutrophils, thus resolving the inflammatory reaction.

FEVER

The hypothalamus sets the point at which body temperature is maintained, but body temperature regulation depends on a balance between the heat production and loss. Fever may be the result of infection or an inflammatory process. It may be caused by the release of endogenous pyrogens from the macrophages. These pyrogens, or fever-producing substances, will interfere with the temperature-regulating centers located in the hypothalamus, raising the thermostat set point. The body may respond to the pyrogens by increasing cytokine formation, which in turn increases the synthesis of prostaglandin (PGE_2), which then increases the hypothalamic set point (Insel, 1996). The body will react by conserving heat through vasoconstriction, piloerection (goose flesh), and shivering—all factors that increase the body temperature.

The normal body temperature is 98.6° F (37°C), and the normal range is 97° F to approximately 99° F when measured orally. Rectally, a person's body temperature is 1° F higher than oral. Hyperthermia occurs when the body's temperature rises above normal. When the body temperature reaches 106° F, convulsions may result. If the body's thermoregulatory mechanisms have trouble returning the body temperature to a normal setting, body metabolism may increase so rapidly that the body cannot regulate its own heat production. At 108° F tissue damage occurs and cells begin to die, resulting in irreversible brain damage.

Several types of fever are known. For example, a constant fever that rises or falls only a few degrees above or below a specified point is seen with typhoid fever. An intermittent fever may return to normal once or several times in 24 hours.

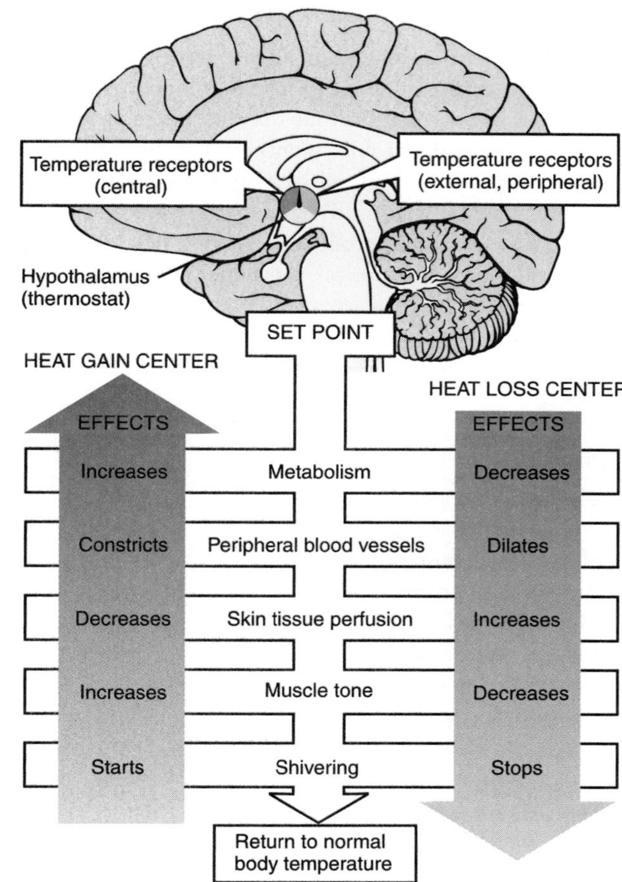

Figure 58-1 Set point temperature mechanism.

This type of fever is associated with pyogenic infections, abscesses, lymphomas, tuberculosis, and drug reactions. A remittent fever fluctuates but does not usually return to normal; this occurs in many viral and bacterial infections. Relapsing fever consists of afebrile episodes of one or more days between fevers, such as in malaria and Hodgkin's disease.

Fever of unknown origin (FUO) has been described as a temperature greater than 103° F recorded daily for more than 2 weeks in a client with an uncertain diagnosis after a week's evaluation in a hospital setting. Most clients with FUO are later found to have an infection, neoplasm, or connective tissue disease.

Body temperature is regulated by nervous system feedback mechanisms through a temperature-regulating center in the hypothalamus. When the hypothalamus is no longer in contact with the pyrogens, it will reset the temperature to the normal set point. Prostaglandins of the E series produced in response to endogenous pyrogens act on the anterior hypothalamus to increase the set point, resulting in fever. Drugs that inhibit the synthesis of E prostaglandins have antipyretic activity (acetaminophen, salicylates). For example, salicylates reduce raised body temperatures by causing the hypothalamic center to reestablish a normal set point. Heat production will not be inhibited, although heat loss will be increased by an increase in cutaneous blood flow and sweating, caused by the lowered thermostat (Figure 58-1). Antibiotics indirectly reduce temperature by destroying the bacteria causing the fever.

ANTIMICROBIAL THERAPY

The treatment of an infectious disease depends on the microorganism group; different groups of antimicrobial agents are used to treat different groups of microorganisms. Table 58-2 lists some antimicrobial agents used in the treatment of infectious diseases. Antimicrobial drugs can help cure or control most infections caused by microorganisms but they alone do not necessarily produce the cure. They are adjuncts to methods such as surgical incision and drainage, pulmonary toilet, and wound debridement for removal of nonviable infected tissue.

The first major antimicrobial agents were the sulfonamides while the second group of antimicrobials were true antibiotics such as penicillin. Antibiotics are natural substances derived from certain organisms (bacteria, fungus, etc.) that are used against infections caused by other organisms. As a result of research, there are now many synthetic and semisynthetic antibiotics. Other antimicrobial agents include the urinary tract

TABLE 58-2 Antimicrobial drugs of choice

Organism	Drug(s)
Gram-positive cocci	
Staphylococcus aureus	
Non-penicillinase producing	penicillin G or V, first generation cephalosporins, vancomycin
Penicillinase producing	first generation cephalosporins, cloxacillin, dicloxacillin, methicillin
Methicillin resistant	vancomycin ± gentamicin ± rifampin
Streptococcus pneumoniae	penicillin G or V
Streptococcus pyogenes (Group A)	penicillin G or V
Streptococcus (Group B)	penicillin G, ampicillin
Streptococcus viridans	penicillin G ± gentamicin
Gram-positive bacilli	
Bacillus anthracis	pencillin G, erythromycin
Corynebacterium diphtheriae	erythromycin
Corynebacterium, JK strain	vancomycin, erythromycin
Listeria monocytogenes	amikacin, gentamicin
Gram-negative cocci	
Neisseria gonorrhoeae	ceftriaxone, cefixime
Neisseria meningitidis	penicillin G, cefotaxime
Gram-negative enteric bacilli	
Escherichia coli	cefotaxime, ceftizoxime
Klebsiella pneumoniae	same as *E. coli*
Proteus mirabilis	ampicillin, cephalosporin
Salmonella species	ceftriaxone, fluoroquinolone
Other bacilli	
Pseudomonas aeruginosa	fluoroquinolone, carbenicillin
Anaerobes	
Gram-positive	
Clostridium difficile	metronidazole
Clostridium perfringens	penicillin G, metronidazole
Clostridium tetani	penicillin G, tetracycline
Gram-negative	
Bacteroides (GI strains)	metronidazole, clindamycin
Mycoplasmas	
Mycoplasma pneumoniae	erythromycin, tetracycline, clarithromycin
Spirochetes	
Treponema pallidum (syphilis)	penicillin G
Fungi	
Asperigillus, *Candida* species	amphotericin B, fluconazole, itraconazole
Viruses	
Herpes simplex	vidarabine, acyclovir

antiseptics and the antimycobacterial, antifungal, and antiviral agents.

Mechanism of action. The goal of antimicrobial therapy is to destroy or to suppress the growth of infecting microorganisms so that normal host defense and other supporting mechanisms can control the infection, resulting in its cure. To exert their effects, antimicrobial agents must first gain access to target sites. Usually this can be accomplished by absorption and distribution of the drug into and by way of the circulatory system. More specific antibiotics or antimicrobial agents are capable of penetrating to the site and having an affinity for the bacterial target proteins. Sometimes, as in the case of infections of the skin and eyes, local application to the infected area may be necessary. Once the drug has reached its site of action, it can have bactericidal or bacteriostatic effects, depending on its mechanisms of action.

Bacteriostatic agents inhibit bacterial growth, allowing host defense mechanisms additional time to remove the invading microorganisms. **Bactericidal agents,** on the other hand, cause bacterial cell death and lysis. Antimicrobial agents may be divided into bacteriostatic and bactericidal categories, with the sulfonamides as an example of the former and the penicillins the latter. Such categorization is not always valid or reliable, however, because the same antimicrobial agent may have either effect depending on the dose administered and the concentration achieved at its site of action. Tetracycline, for example, is generally bacteriostatic but may be bactericidal in high concentrations. Chloramphenicol, which is often listed as a bacteriostatic drug, has bactericidal effects against *S. pneumoniae* and *H. influenzae* in the cerebrospinal fluid.

Antimicrobial agents may exert their bacteriostatic or bactericidal effects in one of four major ways:

1. Inhibit bacteria cell wall synthesis. Unlike host cells, bacteria are not isotonic with body fluids thus their contents are under high osmotic pressure and their viability depends on the integrity of the cell walls. Any compound that inhibits any step in the synthesis of this cell wall causes it to be weakened and the cell to lyse. Antimicrobial agents having this mechanism of action are bactericidal.
2. Disrupt or alter membrane permeability, resulting in leakage of essential bacterial metabolic substrates. Agents causing the effects can be either bacteriostatic or bactericidal.
3. Inhibit protein synthesis. Antimicrobial agents may induce the formation of defective protein molecules; such agents are bactericidal in their action. Antimicrobial agents that inhibit specific steps in protein synthesis are bacteriostatic.
4. Inhibit synthesis of essential metabolites. Antimicrobial agents that work in this manner structurally resemble physiologic compounds and act as competitive inhibitors in a metabolic pathway. Generally, they are bacteriostatic agents. (Box 58-1)

BOX 58-1

Antimicrobials: Classification by Mechanism of Action

Inhibit cell wall synthesis
penicillins
cephalosporins
vancomycin
bacitracin
cycloserine

Alter membrane permeability
amphotericin B
nystatin
polymyxin
colistin

Inhibit protein synthesis
Impede replication of genetic information
nalidixic acid
griseofulvin
novobiocin
rifampin
pyrimethamine

Impair translation of genetic information
chloramphenicol
tetracycline
erythromycin
aminoglycosides
lincomycins

Antimetabolites
sulfonamides
paraaminosalicylic acid (PAS)
isoniazid (INH)
ethambutol

Side/adverse effects. Although the development of antimicrobial agents represents one of the most important advances in drug therapy, these drugs can have adverse and toxic effects. The list of side effects and toxic effects of each specific drug group is long and varied. Table 58-3 identifies some of the major allergic and toxic effects of a few antimicrobial agents. All antimicrobial agents, however, are capable of producing two general types of adverse reactions of which the nurse must be aware.

Allergic or hypersensitivity reactions. Allergic or hypersensitivity reactions may occur with all available antimicrobial agents. Hypersensitivity is a state of altered reactivity in which the body reacts with an exaggerated immune response. Such responses include rash, fever, urticaria with pruritus, chills, a generalized erythema, anaphylaxis, and the Stevens-Johnson syndrome. Stevens-Johnson syndrome is a form of toxic epidermal necrolysis in which the epidermis separates from the dermis, leaving the client with a skin loss similar to a second degree burn.

TABLE 58-3 Antimicrobial drugs: selected allergic and toxic effects

Effect	Drug
Anaphylaxis	penicillin
Hematologic effects	chloramphenicol (low incidence but high mortality)
	sulfonamides (low incidence)
Nephrotoxicity	polymyxins
	aminoglycosides
	sulfonamides (low incidence with newer drugs)
Potential for neuromuscular blockade	polymyxins
	aminoglycosides
Injury to eighth cranial nerve	aminoglycosides

A minor rash may be easily tolerated, but an individual with a generalized rash or erythema accompanied by chills and fever needs medical intervention. For example, an allergic response to a rapid infusion of vancomycin can result in a generalized red skin reaction, fever, and chills; to mitigate this reaction, antihistamines would need to be given. Some rashes fade with continued treatment, as with some individuals receiving ampicillin; however, other symptoms may become more severe, necessitating discontinuing the medication. Respiratory distress (wheezing) or anaphylaxis is a medical emergency requiring immediate attention to prevent a fatal outcome.

Sensitization has occurred through indirect exposure to a drug, such as drinking milk from cows treated with antibiotics or eating poultry or beef from livestock treated with antimicrobials. Previous topical application of antimicrobials may also cause sensitization.

Treatment of allergic reactions includes the use of antihistamines and epinephrine, which block or counteract the effects of the vasoactive mediators of allergy, and the use of corticosteroids, which may reduce tissue injury and edema in the inflammatory response. The use of steroids is controversial in the face of systemic infection because of their prolonged inhibition of normal host defense responses.

Superinfection. **Superinfection** is an infection that occurs during the course of antimicrobial therapy delivered for either therapeutic or prophylactic reasons. Most antibiotics reduce or eradicate the normal microbial flora of the body, which is then replaced by resistant exogenous or endogenous bacteria. If the number of these replacement organisms is large and the host conditions favorable, clinical superinfection can occur.

Approximately 2% of persons treated with antibiotics get superinfections. The risk is greater when large doses of antibiotics are used, when more than one antibiotic is administered concurrently, and when broad-spectrum drugs are employed. The administration of some specific antimicrobials are more commonly associated with superinfection than others. For example, *Pseudomonas* organisms frequently colonize in and infect individuals taking cephalosporins. In a similar manner, clients taking tetracyclines may become infected with *Candida albicans*. Generally, superinfections are caused by microorganisms that are resistant to the drug the client is receiving. In the past penicillinase-producing staphylococci were the most common cause of superinfection. *S. aureus* and *S. epidermidis* superinfections, especially with methicillin-resistant strains, are again on the rise. Gram-negative enteric bacilli and fungi are the most common offenders. The proper management of superinfections includes: (1) discontinue drug being given or replace it with another drug to which the organism is sensitive, (2) culture suspected infected area, and (3) possible administration of an antimicrobial agent effective against the new offending organism.

General guidelines for use. Several important principles guide the judicious and optimal use of the antimicrobial agents. Causes of adverse reactions to antimicrobial agents and therapeutic failures are often related to lack of adherence to the following principles of antimicrobial therapy.

Identification of infecting organism. Because most antimicrobial agents have a specific effect on a limited range of microorganisms, the prescriber must formulate a specific diagnosis about the potential pathogens or organisms most likely causing the infectious process. The drug most likely to be specifically effective against the suspected microorganism can then be selected.

This objective is most reliably accomplished by obtaining specimens from the infected area if possible (e.g., urine, sputum, wound drainage) or by obtaining venous blood specimens and sending them to the laboratory for culture and identification of the causative organism. The recovery of a specific microorganism from appropriate specimens is a significant factor in the determination of antimicrobial therapy. When a significant microorganism has been isolated, laboratory tests for antimicrobial susceptibility to various antimicrobial agents are performed.

It is desirable to receive culture and sensitivity reports before initiating antimicrobial therapy. In some situations, however, it is not practical to wait for these laboratory results. For example, antimicrobial therapy must be initiated without delay in acute, life-threatening situations, such as peritonitis, septicemia, or pneumonia. In such situations the choice of antimicrobial agent for initial use must be based on tentative identification of the pathogen and Gram stain. It is known, for example, that microorganisms commonly isolated in acute adult infections of the lung include pneumococci, *Haemophilus* strain streptococci, and staphylococci. Antimicrobial agents specifically toxic to those organisms may be administered temporarily. The drugs can then be changed, if necessary, after laboratory reports have been received.

When even tentative identification is difficult, either *broad-spectrum* antibiotics, which are effective against a wide range of microorganisms, can be prescribed or several antimicrobial agents may be prescribed for simultaneous administration.

Some infections are most effectively treated with the use of only one antibiotic. In other situations *combined antimicrobial drug therapy* may be indicated. Indications for the simultaneous use of two or more antimicrobial agents include (1) treatment of mixed infections, in which each drug may act on a separate portion of a complex microbial flora; (2) need to delay the rapid emergence of bacteria resistant to one drug; and (3) need to reduce the incidence or intensity of adverse reactions by decreasing the dose of a potentially toxic drug. Indiscriminate use of combined antimicrobial drug therapy should be avoided because of expense, toxicity, and higher incidence of superinfections and resistance.

Sensitivity and resistance of microorganisms. Frequently, a discrepancy exists between the in vitro testing and the activity of the drug within the body. This depends on a number of variables such as affinity for antibiotic active sites and penetration into the bacteria, pH, temperature, and ability of the drug to reach the site of an infection. For example, in the case of meningitis it would be inappropriate to use a drug that does not cross the blood-brain barrier even though the organism tested may be sensitive to the drug.

Resistance refers to the ability of a particular microorganism to resist the effects of a specific antibiotic. Resistance occurs in one of three ways: (1) the antibiotic is unable to reach the potential target site of its action—some organisms, such as *Pseudomonas,* form a protective membrane (a glycocalyx or slime) that prevents the antibiotic from reaching the cell wall; (2) the microorganism may produce an enzyme that acts to reduce or eliminate the toxic effect of the antibiotic to the cell wall. Examples of these enzymes are the beta lactamases that cleave the beta-lactam ring on penicillins and cephalosporins, forming inactive compounds; acylases that acetylate chloramphenicol to yield inactive derivatives and enzymes that inactivate aminoglycosides by phosphorylation, adenylation, and acetylation. (3) The microorganism may also be altered in the individual through several biochemical changes. The changes occur in such a way that the target site for the antibiotic no longer accommodates the drug. In this case a specific organism is said to have "become resistant" to a previously susceptible antibiotic. As a rule, microorganisms resistant to a certain drug will tend to be resistant to other chemically related antimicrobial agents, a phenomenon known as *cross-resistance.* For example, bacteria unresponsive to tetracycline will also be resistant to oxytetracycline and chlortetracycline.

Role of host defense mechanisms. No antimicrobial agent will affect the cure of an infectious process if host defense mechanisms are inadequate. Such drugs act only on the causative organisms of infectious disease and have no effect on the defense mechanisms of the body, which need to be assessed and supported. Many infections do not require drug therapy and are adequately combatted by individual defense mechanisms, including antibody production, phagocytosis, interferon production, fibrosis, or gastrointestinal rejection (vomiting, diarrhea). However, host defense mechanisms may be diminished, as in, for example, diabetes mellitus, neoplastic disease, and immunologic suppression. In addition, the very ill client may require supportive care to ensure adequate oxygenation, fluid and electrolyte balance, and optimal nutrition for antimicrobial therapy to be effective. In some situations surgical intervention is also necessary. In general, in the presence of a substantial amount of pus, necrotic tissue, or a foreign body, the most effective treatment is a combination of an antimicrobial agent and an appropriate surgical procedure.

The status of the host's defense mechanisms will also influence choice of therapy, route of administration, and dosage. If an infection is fulminating, for example, parenteral (preferably intravenous) administration of a bactericidal drug will be selected rather than oral administration of a bacteriostatic drug. Large "loading" doses of antimicrobial agents are often administered at the beginning of treatment of severe infections, to achieve maximum blood concentrations rapidly. However, factors influencing drug dosage are also related to the status of a client's renal function. Because many antimicrobial agents are metabolized and/or excreted by the kidneys, a major management problem exists in regard to individuals with compromised renal function. Drug dosages are then generally reduced in parallel with the client's creatinine clearance levels. Hemodialysis may further alter the therapeutic regimen. In some disease states (such as burns) antibiotic dosage may need to be increased to achieve therapeutic levels. In short, the administration of an antimicrobial agent specifically toxic to the isolated microorganism is not the only important measure in antimicrobial therapy. An additional and very important determinant of the effectiveness of an antimicrobial agent is the functional state of the host's defense mechanisms.

Dosage and duration of therapy. Administering antimicrobial drugs for therapeutic purposes in adequate dosage and for long enough periods of time is an important principle of infectious disease therapy. Fortunately, serum levels of some of the more potent antibiotics can be monitored to prevent or minimize the risk of toxicity, for example, aminoglycosides. The nurse should assess for alterations in renal and hepatic functions, since they both can affect drug dosage, dosing interval, and/or drug toxicity.

Failures in antimicrobial therapy are frequently the result of drug doses being too small or being given for too short a period of time. Generally, antimicrobial therapy should not be discontinued until the client has been afebrile and clinically well for 48 to 72 hours. Follow-up cultures should be obtained to assess the effectiveness of therapy.

Inadequate drug therapy may lead to remissions and exacerbations of the infectious process and may contribute to the development of resistance. When antibiotics are used prophylactically, they usually are given for short periods of time to enhance host defense mechanisms. For example, with perioperative antibiotics a loading dose is given immediately before surgery and continued for 48 hours after surgery.

Antimicrobial agents currently being used are discussed as chemically related groups of drugs. The nurse should be familiar with the general characteristics of each drug group or category and with one or two prototype drugs in each group. Because the dosage for any given antibiotic varies with the type of infection, the site of infection, and the age of the client, only general dosages or dose ranges are given in this text. It is recommended that the manufacturer's package insert or a formulary be consulted for specific dosages.

Nursing Management

Antimicrobial Therapy

Antimicrobial agents destroy or inhibit the growth of microorganisms. Some of these agents are derived from living organisms; others are synthetic and semisynthetic chemical compounds. The goal of antimicrobial therapy for infectious diseases is to destroy or suppress the growth of infecting microorganisms so that normal host defense mechanisms can gain control and eliminate the infecting organisms. Among the microorganisms that can be controlled by these drugs today are most bacteria, many fungi, and a few viruses. For the nurse to safely and effectively manage clients taking antimicrobials, knowledge of host defenses and antimicrobial drugs is necessary.

The primary defense mechanisms against infection in the body are intact skin and mucous membranes, the chemical composition and pH of specific body secretions, phagocytic cells, mechanical movements of certain cells or tissues such as cilia action, coughing, peristalsis, and the inflammatory process. Many factors can impair host defenses and thereby increase the risk for the development of infection by virulent organisms.

Any disruption in the integrity of skin or mucous membranes becomes a portal of entry for disease-producing organisms. In very ill, hospitalized clients or in those who are immunocompromised (e.g., individuals with acquired immunodeficiency syndrome [AIDS] or receiving immunosuppressive therapies), relatively minor breaks in the skin or mucosa can lead to fatal infections. Vigorous teeth cleaning, tube insertions, and injections should be avoided, if possible. Environmental hazards such as furniture obstructions, wet flooring, or the presence of irritating agents should be corrected so that injury is prevented. An impairment of blood supply to body tissues will also reduce host defenses by reducing the overall resistance of the tissues to injury and by preventing the migration of inflammatory cells to the area of injury. Other factors that impair the body's defenses against infection include neutropenia, anemia, protein malnutrition, and autoimmune and antiinflammatory agents such as antineoplastic agents and corticosteroids. Persons with chronic preexisting cardiopulmonary, renal, or metabolic disease and those at the extremes of age are susceptible to the development of infection because of altered organ function. Poor personal hygiene and the suppression of the normal bacterial flora by antibiotics create conditions whereby normal defenses are overwhelmed, resulting in pathogen overgrowth (superinfection).

To exert their effects, antimicrobial agents must first gain access to target sites, usually by absorption of the drug into and distribution through the circulatory system. Then they have bacteriostatic or bactericidal effects, depending on the mechanisms of action. Bacteriostatic agents such as sulfonamides inhibit bacterial growth, allowing host defense mechanisms additional time to remove the invading microorganisms. Bactericidal agents, such as the penicillins, cause bacterial cell death and lysis, superimposing this effect on the effects of host defenses. Antimicrobial agents may exert their bacteriostatic or bactericidal effects by inhibition of cell wall synthesis in bacteria, disruption or alteration of membrane permeability, inhibition of protein synthesis, or synthesis of essential metabolites.

Hundreds of antimicrobial agents are marketed currently, and it is impossible for the nurse to be infinitely knowledgeable about each drug. However, in spite of the numerous and varied drugs available, there are still only a few drug categories to remember. Knowledge of general characteristics of each drug category and of general principles of antimicrobial drug therapy should enable the nurse to function effectively.

In addition to the antibiotics, which include penicillins, cephalosporins, macrolides, lincomycins, vancomycin, aminoglycosides, tetracyclines, chloramphenicol, and polymyxins, major groups of antiinfective drugs include sulfonamides, urinary tract antiseptics, and antimycobacterial, antifungal, and antiviral agents. See Table 58-3 for a brief summary of some major allergic and toxic effects of antimicrobial agents.

Nursing interventions in antimicrobial drug therapy generally relate to (1) assessing the client, (2) assisting in the identification of the infecting organism, (3) actual administration of the drug, (4) monitoring the client's response to the drug, (5) client education, and (5) providing comfort, and prevention and treatment of adverse reactions, including pharmacologic and chemical drug interactions.

Assessment. In the initial assessment of the client, the nurse should document the client's temperature, pulse, respiratory status, and blood pressure to detect fever and systemic responses to fever. Diaphoresis and flushing may also occur. Make note of the client's general behavior; slumped posture, slow and unsteady posture, and careless grooming may indicate fatigue and malaise. Listen to the client's nonspecific symptoms, such as "aching all over," loss of appetite, headache, generalized discomfort, and "not feeling one's self or up-to-snuff." Ask the client about specific indicators: night sweats, pain, dyspnea, or arthalgia. Inspect the skin for heat, erythema, lesions, moistness, and swelling. Inspect and palpate lymph nodes in the area of a suspected localized infection. Examine all the lymph nodes for a generalized infection. In addition, do a history and physical exam with a review of all systems (Grimes, 1991).

If an area of suspected infection is found, cultures are obtained. Obtaining cultures to determine the source and type of infection is frequently the nurse's responsibility. In the event that orders for an antimicrobial agent are given before establishment of an infective source, the nurse should obtain cultures before administering the first dose of the drug ordered.

Specimens obtained for culture should be taken directly to the laboratory and not allowed to stand. Delay may cause the death of fastidious organisms and allow contaminating organisms to overgrow the pathogen. Subsequent culture specimens obtained while the client is receiving antimicrobials should be sent to the laboratory with information regarding the drug(s) being administered. The appropriate selection of laboratory tests for the identification of offending organisms often depends on this knowledge.

Assessment of a client's previous reactions to drugs and to antimicrobial agents in particular is especially important in avoiding allergic reactions to drugs. Careful questioning of the individual regarding drugs previously taken and exact clinical responses to them is an important part of the client's history. Some clients equate common side effects such as nausea and diarrhea with drug allergy. Although these drug responses are important, knowledge of their appearance may not be as sufficient a reason to withhold a specific antibiotic as would a true allergy. Once drug allergies are known, warnings should be prominently displayed on the client's record or hospital chart. As additional precautions, the nurse should (1) ask the client if he or she has drug allergies before administering any medications; (2) tell the client what drug he is receiving; (3) observe the client for at least half an hour after administration of the drug (penicillin in particular), especially if it is administered parenterally and the client has never taken the drug previously; and (4) know what drugs are used for the treatment of allergic responses and where they are kept.

Because the administration of more than one drug to a client is the rule rather than the exception in current hospital practice, the possibility of drug interactions must be taken into account and the client's current medication regimen reviewed for significant interactions if antimicrobial therapy is to be optimally effective. The nurse should be alert to drugs that interact biologically with antimicrobial agents, as well as chemical incompatibilities between antimicrobial drugs and other agents when they are mixed for intravenous administration. The hospital formulary on each unit provides accurate and current information about these interactions.

In addition to the careful history of allergies and other adverse reactions to drugs and the review of the current medication regimen for potential significant drug interactions, the pre-therapy assessment should include the baseline signs and symptoms of the client's infection, as well as WBC, serum electrolytes, and relevant culture and sensitivity.

Nursing diagnosis. Clients receiving antimicrobial therapy have a potential for the following nursing diagnoses: risk for infection and hyperthermia related to ineffectiveness of antimicrobial therapy and/or development of superinfection with another organism; risk for fluid volume deficit related to antimicrobial-induced adverse gastrointestinal reactions or anorexia, nausea and vomiting related to gastric irritation by drug; and the potential complications of allergic reaction, sepsis, and ototoxicity, blood dyscrasias, and nephrotoxicity caused by specific antimicrobial agents.

Implementation

Monitoring. Assess for effectiveness of drug therapy by monitoring the signs and symptoms of the client's infection, including WBC and cultures. In most instances, the client's condition should improve within 48 hrs after the administration of the drug. Be alert for early signs of allergic or other adverse responses to therapy, as well as signs of superinfection such as diarrhea and white patches in the oral cavity and vaginal area (see discussion of the management of adverse responses below). Serum antibiotic concentrations can be monitored through the course of therapy to assess for therapeutic and toxic levels of individual antimicrobials.

In addition to monitoring therapeutic effects of antimicrobials, nurses must monitor the client for the development of common side effects of individual drugs. Fluid and electrolyte imbalances can occur during the course of administering many antibiotics, either from the drug itself, the mode of administration, or side effects such as diarrhea. For example, extracellular volume excess may result from administering multiple intravenous drugs, each of which is diluted in 100 ml of saline. Edema, pulmonary congestion with subsequent shortness of breath, and an increase in body weight all indicate the presence of an extracellular volume excess.

Hypokalemia, resulting from severe diarrhea or the intravenous administration of antibiotic containing large quantities of sodium, produces no obvious clinical signs or symptoms until the potassium deficit is significant. At this point, widespread muscular weakness and cardiac conduction abnormalities appear. In the client whose cardiac function is being monitored, the appearance of U waves may be an earlier indication of low serum potassium. Laboratory demonstration of hypokalemia is frequently the only way to detect this disorder.

Hypernatremia, another commonly seen disorder in clients receiving antimicrobial therapy, is also associated with few early clinical signs or symptoms, with the exception of a high serum sodium value, which occurs frequently because many antimicrobials have a sodium base. In general, when individuals must take prolonged courses of intravenous antimicrobials that can cause fluid and electrolyte imbalances, it may be necessary to obtain serum electrolyte studies periodically.

Intervention. Because the constant and consistent administration of an antimicrobial drug at prescribed dosage intervals is necessary for maintaining therapeutic blood levels of the drug, the nurse should administer such a drug according to prescribed times as accurately as possible. This may mean awakening sleeping clients and ensuring that tests or therapies do not interrupt this schedule.

When antimicrobial agents are administered intravenously, the nurse must observe additional precautions: (1) the drugs should be diluted in neutral solutions (pH 7.0 to 7.2) of isotonic sodium chloride (0.9%) or 5% dextrose in water; (2) the drugs should be administered without the admixture of any other drug to avoid chemical or physical incompatibilities; (3) the drugs should be administered by intermittent intravenous infusions to avoid inactivation (e.g., by temperature) and prolonged vein irritation from high drug concentration; (4) the infusion site must be changed every 48 hours to reduce the risk of chemical phlebitis; and (5) intramuscular antimicrobials should be injected deeply into large muscle masses (such as gluteal), and injection sites should be rotated to prevent tissue irritation.

The establishment of automatic stop and renewal orders in many hospitals is another precaution against adverse reactions and to ensure the effectiveness of a particular drug is evaluated.

Such orders restrict the administration of a prescribed antimicrobial agent to a definite time period (e.g., 7 days); its continued use past that time requires a new prescription.

Education. Clients should be taught principles of antimicrobial therapy clearly enough to understand that these drugs should never be taken without medical supervision and should be taken in strict accordance with their prescriptions. This is especially important because many individuals receiving antimicrobial drugs are not hospitalized and are responsible for self-medication. Clients should be taught, for example:

- not to stop taking these drugs as soon as symptoms abate, because an ineffective course of antimicrobial therapy will allow the opportunity for microbes to mutate and develop resistance to the drug;
- not to share these drugs with family and friends, because they may have allergies and the drug may not be appropriate for their illness;
- and not to take "leftover" antimicrobial drugs for new illnesses, even if symptoms appear similar for many infections may have the same symptoms but be caused by different organisms or by one's that have developed a resistance to the drug. Some drugs become toxic as they degenerate past their expiration date.

Clients who are allergic to an antimicrobial agent should be taught how to protect themselves from future treatment with the drug in question such as by using medical alert wallet cards or tags.

Special administration considerations, expected effects, side effects, and adverse reactions of individual antimicrobials could be appropriately described on "drug sheets" for clients to refer to at home while taking antimicrobial therapy. A telephone number to call when questions arise could also be written on the drug sheets and would convey the message that it was expected and desirable for clients to discuss their concerns about their medications with health care workers.

Occasionally antimicrobials will interfere with the results of home laboratory testing kits, and clients using these must be cautioned. For example, the cephalosporins may produce a false positive reading when individuals with diabetes use commercial chemical testing strips to monitor their urine glucose.

Evaluation. A decrease in the severity or a disappearance of the clinical and laboratory manifestations of infection indicates a positive response to antimicrobial therapy. With local infections redness, heat, edema, and pain should decrease. In the case of a systemic infection, temperature, heart rate, respiratory rate, and white blood cell count should return to normal, and appetite and a sense of well-being should improve. Purulent drainage, if present, should decrease in amount and change to a more normal appearance and consistency. In clients who are seriously ill, an improvement in organ function should accompany other signs of resolution of infection.

Prevention and management of adverse responses

Anaphylaxis. The most serious allergic reaction to antimicrobials is anaphylaxis. This reaction can occur anywhere from a few seconds to 30 minutes after an antibiotic injection. The syndrome associated with this reaction usually begins with diffuse flushing, itching, and a feeling of warmth. Hives may appear on the client's face, neck, and chest. As the syndrome progresses, generalized body edema develops. Massive facial edema signals the possibility of upper airway edema, with impending obstruction and respiratory difficulty from pulmonary involvement. These problems are manifested as a choking sensation, stridor, chest tightness and pain, wheezing, shortness of breath, and restlessness.

The initial step in the emergent management of anaphylaxis is to immediately stop the antibiotic if it is still being infused. If the individual is not in a medical facility, immediate transport to one should be arranged, preferably by a vehicle staffed by paramedics who could establish an artificial airway in the event the client's airway becomes totally obstructed. Reversal of anaphylaxis is accomplished by drug therapy. The antihistamine diphenhydramine (Benadryl) is administered parenterally or orally. Epinephrine 1:1000 can be injected subcutaneously and will reverse the vascular effects of anaphylaxis. Aminophylline or theophylline is administered if bronchospasm persists. If the individual is in anaphylactic shock, vasopressors may be necessary concomitantly with the administration of intravenous fluids for short-term management of hypotension. Corticosteroids (methylprednisolone) may be administered for prevention of protracted symptoms in severe reactions.

Superinfection. The emergence of superinfection may be suspected in the presence of diarrhea or recurrent fever in the client taking antimicrobial drugs. Stomatitis is indicated by the presence of a sore mouth or white patches on the oral mucosa. Monilial vaginitis may produce a vaginal discharge or perineal rash. Localized superinfections may be heralded by increasing redness, heat, edema, pain, and possibly drainage. *C. difficile* as a nosocomial infection may manifest as a pseudomembranous colitis. Children, elderly persons, and others whose normal host defense mechanisms may be weakened should be especially observed for signs of superinfection. In the course of prolonged antimicrobial drug therapy, periodic cultures of the upper respiratory tract and of feces may be indicated to determine changes in bacterial flora that subsequently may be responsible for secondary infection. The nurse should be careful not to introduce new microorganisms and should emphasize asepsis in contacts with clients receiving antimicrobial therapy.

SUMMARY

Infectious disease has been a major health concern of humans even before recorded history and comprises a variety of illnesses caused by pathogenic microorganisms, bacteria, fungi, and viruses. Inflammation is a reaction of the body tissues, not only to infection but also to physical, chemical, and thermal injuries. Fever is a sign of inflammation. All present challenges for nursing care and for antimicrobial therapy.

Antimicrobial agents may be bacteriostatic (inhibiting bacterial growth) or bactericidal (causing bacterial cell death and lysis) or both, depending on the concentration at the site of action. These agents are effective by inhibiting the bacterial cell wall synthesis, altering the membrane permeability, inhibiting protein synthesis, or inhibiting the synthesis of essential metabolites. In general, antimicrobials are well tolerated by humans; however, common to all antimicrobials there may be an allergic or hypersensitive response or a superinfection, an infection that occurs during the course of antimicrobial therapy because of reduction in the normal microbial flora of the body.

The following are guidelines for the use of antimicrobials: identification of the infecting organism, which allows for the selection of the most effective antimicrobial for the specific infecting organism; determination of the ability of a specific antimicrobial to limit the growth of or kill microorganisms in vitro; supportive therapy for the host defense mechanisms; and administration of the agent in an adequate dosage and for long enough periods of time to be effective. Nursing management of antimicrobial therapy includes the assessment of the individual's ability to deal with the stressor of infection, the administration of antimicrobial drugs safely and accurately, the education of the client to do the same with regard to self-administration of the drug, the prevention and management of adverse responses, and the evaluation of the client's response to the drug and progress toward the goal of resolution of the infection.

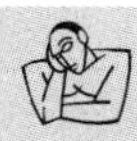

Critical Thinking

1. Susan Brooks is a 71-year-old resident of Laurelmont Nursing Home. She is fond of her early morning cup of coffee to get her day started. One morning she choked while trying to drink her coffee but seemed to recover fully. Some days later, however, you notice that Ms. Brooks has become more restless and agitated than usual and cannot sleep. She has no cough or sputum production, but her temperature is over 102° F. A chest x-ray shows right lower lobe infiltrate, a common finding in aspiration pneumonia. What nursing actions should occur before the initiation of antimicrobial therapy? After 3 days of antibiotic therapy Ms. Brooks develops diarrhea. What do you suspect has occurred? How will you validate your suspicions? How will this change your plan of care for Ms. Brooks? What would be appropriate outcome criteria for her plan of care?
2. Nick Nicholson, a 78-year-old man with Alzheimer's disease, is also a resident of Laurelmont. He has frequent urinary incontinence and wears an external catheter at night. One evening, Mr. Nicholson vomited but otherwise did not seem unwell. The next day, he had a fever of 101° F. He had no cough or sputum production, and his chest x-ray was negative. A urine culture, however, had greater than 100,000 colonies of *E. coli* per millimeter, which indicates that he has a urinary tract infection. What aspects of Ms. Brooks and Mr. Nicholson's plans of care will be the same, and how will they differ? How will you evaluate whether your plan of care for Mr. Nicholson has been effective?

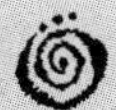

Collaborative Learning Activities

1. A student team will be pre-assigned to respond to critical thinking question number 1. They will develop a plan of care for Ms. Brooks that would be supportive of her body's defense mechanisms to prevent infection in the future.
2. Another student team will respond to the second question. The class will discuss the differences between the two clients and their care.

BIBLIOGRAPHY

Abramowicz M (Ed.) (1994). The choice of antibacterial drugs, *Med Lett* 36(925):53-60.

Anderson KN, et al. (Eds.) (1994). *Mosby's medical, nursing, & allied health dictionary* (4th ed.). St Louis: Mosby.

Balk RA & Parrillo JE (1992). Prognostic factors in sepsis: The cold facts, *Crit Care Med* 20(10):1373-4.

Bone RC (1993). The search for a magic bullet to fight sepsis, *JAMA* 269 (17):2266.

Bruce JL & Grove SK (1992). Fever: Pathology and treatment, *Crit Care Nurs* 12 (1):40-9.

Foster MT (1991). Septicemia, *Hosp Pract* 26(Supplement 5):43-6.

Fraser D (1993). Patient assessment: Infection in the elderly, *J Gerontol Nurs* 19(7):5-11.

Grimes D (1991). *Infectious diseases.* St Louis: Mosby.

Insel PA (1996). Analgesic-antipyretic and antiinflammatory agents and drugs employed in the treatment of gout. In Hardman JC & Limbird LE (Eds.). *Goodman & Gilman's the pharmacological basis of therapeutics* (9th ed.). New York: McGraw-Hill.

McCance KL & Huether SE (1994). *Pathophysiology: The biologic basis for disease in adults and children* (2nd ed.). St Louis: Mosby.

Melmon KL, et al. (1992). *Clinical pharmacology* (3rd ed.). New York: McGraw-Hill.

Miller CA (1993). Infections, resistant microbes, and older adults, *Geriatr Nurs* 14(1):55.

Parent PC (1992). Infection control: Management strategies for adult patients in the critical care environment, *Crit Care Nurs Q* 15(3):1-8.

Schell KH (1993). Current trends in antimicrobial therapy for the critically ill, *Crit Care Nurs Q* 15(4):23-32.

Smeltzer SC & Bare BG (1996). *Brunner and Suddarth's textbook of medical-surgical nursing* (8th ed.). Philadelphia: Lippincott.

Chapter 59 Antibiotics

Chapter Focus

Infectious disease has always held a special threat for humans. There have been eras in which uncontrolled plague and pestilence have shaped the course of mankind. It was not until Edward Jenner made his first public inoculation with smallpox vaccine in 1796 that humans began to have some control over their experience with communicable diseases. The concept of sepsis was gradually accepted over the nineteenth century to help prevent the spread of infection. But not until the advent of the sulfonamides, penicillin, and other antibiotics was there an effective treatment for those with infectious diseases. Today, with the occurrence of drug-resistant strains of microorganisms and the opportunistic bacterial infections that accompany the human immunodeficiency virus (HIV), the importance of disease prevention and the antibiotic agents cannot be overlooked. The following objectives and key terms are important for a good understanding of this chapter.

Key Drugs [▲]

cephalothin
ciprofloxacin
erythromycin
gentamicin
penicillin
trimethoprim-sulfamethoxazole
vancomycin

Key Terms

antibiotic (p. 901)
bactericidal (p. 924)
bacteriostatic (p. 924)
cephalosporin (p. 908)
fluoroquinolones (p. 919)
macrolide antibiotics (p. 911)
penicillins (p. 902)
superinfection (p. 901)
tetracyclines (p. 916)

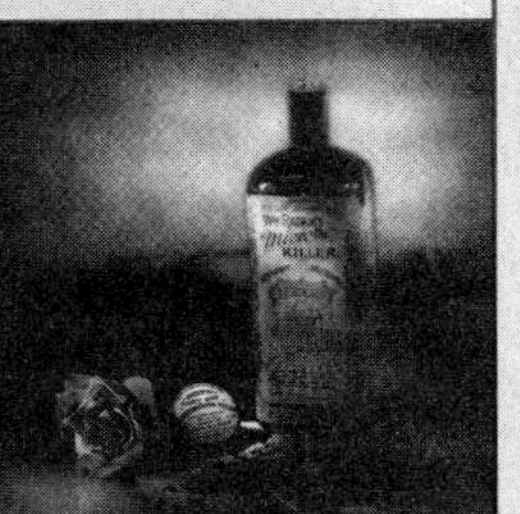

Objectives

1. Discuss the nursing management of antibiotic therapy.
2. Differentiate between peak, trough, and mean serum levels.
3. List four major classifications of antibiotics.
4. Differentiate between different antibiotics within the same general classification.
5. Compare the role of antibiotics, sulfonamides, urinary antiseptics, and urinary tract analgesics in the treatment of urinary tract infections.
6. Implement nursing management of the care of clients receiving antibiotic therapy.

Antibiotics are chemical substances produced from various microorganisms (bacteria, fungus) that kill or suppress the growth of other microorganisms. This term is also used for synthetic antimicrobial agents, such as sulfonamides and quinolones. While hundreds of antibiotics are available that vary in antibacterial spectrum, mechanism of action, potency, toxicity, and pharmacokinetic properties, this chapter is divided into penicillins and related antibiotics, cephalosporins, macrolides, lincomycins, aminoglycosides, tetracyclines, quinolones, miscellaneous antimicrobials and urinary tract antimicrobials. An understanding of the general principles of antibiotic therapy, as discussed in Chapter 58, is essential for the nurse. In addition, before administering an antibiotic, the nurse must be familiar with the specific drug and its actions and effects for the individual client.

Nursing Management

Antibiotic Therapy

Assessment. When an infection is suspected, the nursing assessment is particularly important. Detailed information regarding the client's general health, as well as symptoms indicating an infection, such as elevated temperature, chills, sweats, redness, pain or swelling in an area previously unaffected, fatigue, anorexia, weight loss, cough, change in character or amount of sputum, increased white blood cell count, amount and quality of pus or drainage, should be obtained.

Whenever possible, the infecting organism should be identified before drug therapy begins. The collection of specimens (blood, urine, sputum, wound drainage and discharge) and cultures should be completed before antibiotic therapy starts. Specimens should be carefully obtained following agency guidelines to ensure test accuracy and to protect personnel from exposure to infectious organisms. Prompt treatment is imperative in serious infections, and antimicrobial drugs should not be withheld pending laboratory study and culture results.

Antibiotics, particularly penicillins, have been associated with serious hypersensitivity and allergic reactions. A complete drug history of the client and family helps identify possible hypersensitivity or cross-sensitivity administration of the drugs. Cross-sensitivity often exists between drugs of the same class (e.g., penicillins). Clients intolerant of one antibiotic may be intolerant of similar antibiotics. Information regarding possible contraindications, cautions, potential drug interactions, and drug-taking patterns is also obtained.

Nursing diagnosis. Many antibiotics are administered prophylactically; in such cases, the nursing diagnosis of risk for infection would pertain. Once the client has an infection, then, along with other nursing diagnoses specific to the client, risk for infection transmission is appropriate. See Chapter 58 and the Nursing Care Plan on p. 902 for other selected nursing diagnoses.

Implementation

Monitoring. When an antibiotic is administered for prophylaxis, the client should be monitored for signs indicating the absence or development of infection. When a specific infection is treated, a therapeutic response will be indicated by a decrease in specific signs of infection identified in the baseline assessment (fever, malaise, elevated WBC count, redness, inflammation, drainage, pain, positive cultures). Evaluation of the therapeutic responses is important, since antibiotic therapy may be ineffective for several reasons, including incorrect route of administration, inadequate drainage of abscesses, poor antibiotic penetration of infected tissues, subtherapeutic serum levels, or bacterial resistance to the antibiotic.

Reducing or eliminating normal flora by antibiotic therapy provides an environment conducive to growth of undesirable bacteria, fungus, or yeasts, a condition known as **superinfection.** Examples commonly seen include diarrhea from altered intestinal flora or vaginal yeast infections resulting from a reduction in normal vaginal flora, which suppresses yeast growth.

Adverse reactions vary widely, depending on drug, dose, route of administration, and client-related factors. Refer to nursing management for specific antibiotics for side effects or adverse reactions and specific nursing evaluation related to those drugs.

Allergic reactions are always possible following the first or successive doses. In general it is important to monitor for allergic reactions such as anaphylaxis, skin rashes, urticaria, and bronchospasm. Administration should immediately stop at the first sign of an allergic reaction, and the prescriber should be notified. See Chapter 58 for greater detail.

Intervention. Dosage and routes of administration are highly individualized and are based on the organism or infection being treated, as well as a variety of individual client factors such as age, weight, general health, and preexisting diseases or organ or system dysfunction. Antibiotics are available in various dosage forms for topical, oral, or parenteral use. Dosage adjustments between different forms or routes of administration are necessary because of differences in absorption, distribution, metabolism, or excretion. For example, an oral dose of penicillin G requires five times the parenteral dose to achieve the same serum levels of the drug.

Special attention must be paid to interactions of oral antibiotics with food or other drugs. Some antibiotics should not be administered with food. For example, tetracycline forms a nonabsorbable complex with dairy products, whereas other antibiotics are administered with food to minimize gastric irritation.

The times of antibiotic administration should be spaced as evenly as possible over a 24 hour period to ensure stable and consistent serum levels. Antibiotics ordered four times a day (qid) should be administered every 6 hours. Three times a day (tid) means every 8 hours. It is important to administer antibiotics at the scheduled time to maintain a consistent blood level. Allowable variation differs with specific drugs and institutional policy. As a general rule, antibiotics should be administered within 15 minutes of the scheduled time.

Serum levels of many antibiotics are monitored to determine if the concentration is at the correct (therapeutic) level, high (toxic) level, or low (subtherapeutic) level. Timing of serum determinations is also important. To determine the lowest, or trough, level, the blood is drawn immediately before administering a dose. Mean serum levels are determined at some point between doses, and the highest serum level, or peak level, is determined shortly after dose administration.

Nursing Care Plan

Selected Nursing Diagnoses Related to Antibiotic Therapy

Nursing diagnosis	Outcome criteria	Nursing interventions
Knowledge deficit related to antimicrobial drug therapy	Client will: Express understanding of the purpose, function, and side effects/adverse reactions of drug therapy Demonstrate understanding of proper handling and administration	Assess client's level of knowledge and understanding. Determine education needs of client. Provide information related to: Specific problem being treated with the antimicrobial agent Purpose and function of drug therapy Side effects/adverse reactions of the drug Methods of reducing side effects Answer questions and clarify misconceptions. If drug is to be self-administered, instruct the client in: Proper route and method for administration Proper storage and handling Importance of taking all of the prescribed drug Alert client to possible drug interactions. Instruct the client not to take additional medications without first checking with the prescriber.
Altered nutrition related to gastrointestinal effects of antimicrobial drugs	Client will maintain desired nutritional status	Assess client's normal dietary patterns and intake. Assess normal pattern of bowel function. Emphasize the importance of adequate nutrition. Instruct client to report any gastrointestinal changes (nausea, vomiting, cramping, gas, diarrhea, constipation). Administer in relation to meals and food to minimize side effects (with meals, before or after, depending on specific drug) yet maintain effectiveness of therapy. Encourage intake of active culture yogurt or buttermilk to maintain or restore intestinal flora. Report adverse effects to prescriber.

The desired serum concentration may vary with different drugs and the infecting organism. The exact timing of peak, mean, or trough serum level determinations is determined by each particular drug and route of administration.

Education. Clients should be fully informed about the nature of their condition and the treatment plan. They should understand the medication regimen, including the name of medication (generic and trade names), its general action, purpose, proper handling, dosage, and correct administration. Provide the client with a list of adverse drug reactions, drug-drug interactions, and food-drug interactions, and advise the client of the proper response to take if these interactions occur.

Clients should be instructed to take the medication exactly as prescribed, at evenly spaced intervals, for the full length of time prescribed or until all the drug is gone. Even if the client feels well, the infection may return if the full course of therapy is not completed. Any leftover medication should be appropriately discarded.

A rash, itching, hives, fever, chills, joint pain or swelling, difficulty breathing, or wheezing are signs of an adverse reaction. The drug should be stopped and the prescriber contacted immediately.

Evaluation. If the antibiotic therapy was administered prophylactically, the client will remain free of infectious processes and will demonstrate appropriate practices to prevent infection. If administered therapeutically, the client will maintain or achieve an infection-free state as evidenced by negative cultures, body temperature within normal limits, a WBC within the normal limits for age, and the resolution of any other infection-related symptoms that the client might be experiencing. The client will also effectively manage the therapeutic regimen and demonstrate practices to prevent the spread of infection.

PENICILLINS AND RELATED ANTIBIOTICS

Penicillins are antibiotics derived from a number of strains of common molds often seen on bread or fruit (Figure 59-1). Introduced into clinical practice in the 1940s, penicillin and related antibiotics constitute a large group of antimicrobial

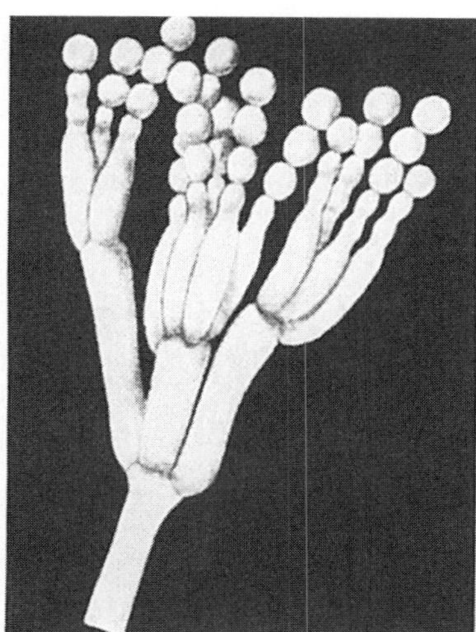

Figure 59-1 Typical penicillus of *Penicillus notatum*, Flemming's strain. (From Raper KB & Alexander DF [1945]. *J Elisha Mitchell Sc Soc* 61:74.)

agents that remain the most effective and least toxic of all available antimicrobial drugs.

Bacteria cell walls are permeable and rigid in order to protect cellular cytoplasm. Penicillins weaken the cell wall by inhibition of transpeptidase enzymes responsible for cross-linking the cell wall strands, which results in cell lysis and death. Therefore penicillins are bactericidal because they inhibit bacterial cell wall synthesis.

Penicillin is not useful in the presence of bacterial enzymes capable of destroying penicillins, such as penicillinase strains of the beta-lactamase enzymes. There are now four different classifications of antibiotics that contain the beta-lactam ring: penicillins, cephalosporins, monobactams and carbapenems. Alteration of the beta-lactam rings (depending on the antibiotic and specific bacteria) has resulted in the formulation of drugs more active against gram-negative cell wall organisms and a decrease in susceptibility to beta-lactamases that inactivate the antibiotic. For example, the beta-lactam altered penicillins, aztreonam and imipenem, are stable in the presence of beta-lactamases while ampicillin and/or amoxicillin must be combined with beta-lactamase inhibitors, such as clavulanate, sulbactam or tazobactam to improve their effectiveness.

Although most penicillins are much more active against gram-positive than gram-negative bacteria; ticarcillin, carbenicillin, aztreonam, imipenem and the combination of penicillins with beta-lactamase inhibitors are more effective against gram-negative bacteria (*E. coli*, *Klebsiella pneumoniae*, and others). Prophylactically, penicillin is indicated for the prevention of diphtheria, bacterial endocarditis, and rheumatic fever. Penicillins are divided into the following:

1. Natural penicillins include penicillin G and penicillin V

   Pencillin G and pencillin V are comparable therapeutically but oral penicillin V is more stable in stomach acid, therefore, it reaches higher serum levels than oral penicillin G.

   Penicillin G is available orally, IM, and IV in various salt formulations, sodium penicillin G, potassium penicillin G, procaine penicillin G, benzathine penicillin G, and a parenteral combination of the latter two formulations. The active substance in all formulations is penicillin G.
2. Penicillinase-resistant pencillins include cloxacillin, dicloxacillin, methicillin, nafcillin, and oxacillin. A chemical alteration of the pencillin structure resulted in penicillins resistant to beta-lactamase inactivation thus they are used to treat penicillinase-producing staphylococcus. These antibiotics though are not effective against methicillin resistant bacteria.
3. Aminopenicillins or broader-spectrum penicillins include amoxicillin, amoxicillin and potassium clavulanate, ampicillin, ampicillin and sulbactam, and bacampicillin. While these antibiotics have the spectrum of activity of pencillin in addition to efficacy against selected gram-negative bacteria, the single agents are usually not very effective against *Staphylococcus aureus* (beta-lactamase producing) bacteria. When combined with beta-lactamase inhibitors, such as potassium clavulanate and sulbactam, the penicillin is protected from inactivation by beta-lactamase enzymes.
4. Extended-spectrum pencillins include carbenicillin, mezlocillin, piperacillin, piperacillin and tazobactam, ticarcillin, and ticarcillin and potassium clavulanate. These antibiotics have a broader spectrum of antimicrobial activity that includes *Pseudomonas aeruginosa*, *Enterobacter*, *Proteus*, and others. Only the combination antibiotics in this category though, are effective against *Staphylococcus aureus* (beta-lactamase producing) bacteria.

Table 59-1 lists pharmacokinetics and usual adult dosages. Side/adverse effects of penicillins include diarrhea, nausea, vomiting, headache, sore mouth or tongue, oral and vaginal candidiasis. Less frequently reported: allergic reactions; anaphylaxis, serum sickness–type reaction (rash, joint pain, fever), hives, and pruritus.

■ Nursing Management

Penicillin Therapy

General nursing management related to antibiotic therapy discussed earlier also applies to the client receiving penicillin therapy.

Assessment. Ascertain sensitivity history to penicillins. Because allergic reactions are a significant problem in the use of penicillins, the nurse must meticulously assess the client's previous drug experiences with special attention to the development of prior drug-related rashes. For infants less than 3 months old, a history of penicillin allergy in the mother should be sought. If at all possible, no penicillin preparation of any kind should be prescribed for or administered to an individual with a history of allergic reaction to the drug. Because of possible cross-sensitization, it also seems wise to avoid the use of cephalosporins in clients with severe or immediate allergic reactions to penicillins. See the Pediatric Implications box on p. 906 on assessing the appropriate antibiotic therapy in children.

TABLE 59-1 Penicillins: pharmacokinetics and usual adult dosing

Classification	Pharmacokinetics			
Drug(s)	Oral absorption (%)	Peak serum (hours)*	Renal excretion (%)†	Usual adult dose
Natural penicillins				
▲ penicillin G				
oral	15-30	1-2	20	200,000-500,000 u q4-6h
IV	—	—	60-90	1-5 mu q4-6h
IM§	—	B-24	60-90	1.2-2.4 mu single dose
		P-4	60-90	600,000 u - 1.2 mu daily
pencillin V				
oral	60-73	0.5-1	20-40	125-500 mg q6-8h
Penicillinase-resistant penicillins				
cloxacillin (Tegopen)				
oral	50	1-2	30-60	250-500 mg q6h
IV ♣	—	E of I	30-60	250-500 mg q6h
dicloxacillin (Dynapen)				
oral	37-50	0.5-1	50-70	125-250 mg q6h
methicillin (Staphcillin)				
IM	—	0.5-1	60-80	1 g q4-6h
IV	—	E of I	60-80	1 g q6h
nafcillin (Unipen)				
oral	erratic	1-2	10-30	250 mg-1 g q4-6h
IM	—	0.5-1	10-30	500 mg q4-6h
IV	—	E of I	10-30	0.5-1.5 g q4h
oxacillin (Prostaphlin)				
oral	30-35	0.5-1	55-60	0.5-1 g q4-6h
IM	—	0.5-1	55-60	250 mg-1 g q4-6h
IV	—	E of I	55-60	250 mg-1 g q4-6h
Aminopenicillins (broader-spectrum)				
amoxicillin (Amoxil)				
oral	75-90	1-2	60-75	250-500 mg q8h
amoxicillin + clavulanate (Augmentin, Clavulin ♣)				
oral	90	1-2	50-78	500 mg q8h
ampicillin (Polycillin)				
oral	35-50	1-1.5	75-90	250-500 mg q6h
IM	—	1	75-90	250-500 mg q6h
IV	—	E of I	75-90	250-500 mg q6h
ampicillin + sulbactam (Unasyn)				
IM	—	—	75-85	1.5-3 g q6h
IV	—	E of I	—	1.5-3 g q6h
bacampicillin (Spectrobid)				
oral	35-50‡	0.5-1‡	70-75‡	400-800 mg q12h
Extended-spectrum penicillins				
carbenicillin (Geocillin)				
oral	30	0.5-1	36	0.5-1 g q6h
IM	—	0.5-1	—	50-83.3 mg/kg q4h
IV	—	E of I	75-95	50-83.3 mg/kg q4h

*Time to peak serum level (hours); †renal excretion of active drug (%, percent excreted unchanged); ‡as ampicillin; *B*, benzathine, and *P*, procaine dosage forms; *mg*, milligram; *g*, gram; *h*, hours; *mu*, million units; *IM*, intramuscularly; *IV*, intravenously; *E of I*, end of infusion. (*USP DI*, 1996).

TABLE 59-1 Penicillins: pharmacokinetics and usual adult dosing—cont'd

Classification	Pharmacokinetics			
Drug(s)	Oral absorption (%)	Peak serum (hours)*	Renal excretion (%/hours)[†]	Usual adult dose
Extended-spectrum penicillins—cont'd				
mezlocillin (Mezlin)				
IM	—	0.5-1	55-60	33.3-58.3 mg/kg q4h
IV	—	E of I	55-60	33.3-58.3 mg/kg q4h
piperacillin (Pipracil)				
IM	—	0.5	60-80	3-4 g q4-6h
IV	—	E of I	60-80	3-4 g q4-6h
piperacillin + tazobactam (Zosyn, Tazocin♣)				
IV	—	E of I	68	3.375-4.5 g q6-8h
ticarcillin (Ticar)				
IM	—	0.5-1	60-80	1 g q6h
IV	—	E of I	60-80	1-4 g q6h
ticarcillin + clavulanate (Timentin)				
IV	—	E of I	60-70	33.3-50 mg q4h

The client's health status should be assessed for conditions for which the administration of penicillin might be contraindicated or need cautious use. Clients with a history of bleeding disorders will require monitoring for bleeding tendencies with the administration of carbenicillin, piperacillin, and ticarcillin because they may cause platelet dysfunction. Clients with a history of gastrointestinal disease, particularly ulcerative colitis and regional enteritis, are more at risk for pseudomembranous colitis as an adverse reaction. The sodium content of high doses of parenteral carbenicillin and ticarcillin should be considered with clients who may be on sodium restrictions, such as those with congestive heart failure and hypertension. Skin rash may occur 43% to 100% in clients with infectious mononucleoses with the administration of ampicillin, bacampicillin, and pivampicillin. Clients with renal function impairment may require lower dosages. See the Pregnancy Safety box on p. 906 for FDA pregnancy categories for the penicillins.

Review the client's medications to determine the possibility of significant drug interactions that may occur, such as the following.

Drug	Possible effect and management
angiotensin-converting enzyme (ACE) inhibitors, potassium-sparing diuretics, potassium-containing drugs, or potassium supplements	If given concurrently with parenteral penicillin G potassium, serum potassium levels may increase, causing hyperkalemia. Monitor closely; dosage adjustments may be necessary.
anticoagulants, oral coumarin or indanedione, heparin or thrombolytic agent	**Increased risk of bleeding when given with high doses of parenteral carbenicillin or ticarcillin, as these drugs inhibit platelet aggregation. Monitor closely for signs of bleeding. Concurrent use of these penicillins with thrombolytic agents also increases the risk for severe bleeding. Avoid or a potentially serious drug interaction may occur.**
antiinflammatory nonsteroidal drugs, platelet aggregation inhibitors (such as salicylates, dextran, dipyridamole (Persantine), valproic acid (Depakote), and sulfinpyrazone (Anturane)	**With high doses of carbenicillin or ticarcillin (parenteral dosage forms), an increased risk for bleeding or hemorrhage exists. These drugs inhibit platelet function and large doses of salicylates may induce hypoprothrombinemia and also gastrointestinal ulcers (from NSAIDs, salicylates, or sulfinpyrazone), all adding to the potential risk of hemorrhage. Avoid or a potentially serious drug interaction may occur.**
cholestyramine (Questran) or colestipol (Colestid)	May decrease absorption of oral penicillin G if given concurrently. Advise clients to take antibiotic first and other medications 3 hours later.
estrogen-containing contraceptives	When used concurrently with ampicillin, amoxicillin, or penicillin V, the effectiveness of the oral contraceptives may be decreased because of increase in estrogen metabolism or reduction in enterohepatic circulation of estrogens. Advise clients to use an alternate method of contraception while taking these antibiotics.
methotrexate (Folex)	Concurrent use with penicillins decreases methotrexate clearance and may result in methotrexate toxicity. Monitor closely. Leucovorin rescue doses may need to be increased and given for a longer period of time.
probenecid (Benemid)	Decreases renal tubular secretion of penicillins, resulting in elevated serum levels and an increase in half-life. It may also increase toxicity. Several combinations of penicillin and probenecid are marketed to take advantage of this effect.

Pediatric Implications

Antibiotic therapy

To assess the appropriateness of antibiotic therapy in children, the following criteria are generally accepted:

1. In choosing empiric therapy, the selected antimicrobial should have documentation of both adequate penetration at the site and proven effectiveness against the common organisms usually isolated from that specific site.
2. If a broad range of possible microorganisms is suspected or if multiple organisms have been isolated from an infection site, then multiple drug therapy may be indicated. Whenever possible though, the minimal number of drugs necessary to treat the infection should be used.
3. If no contraindication is present, the drug of first choice should be selected. The drug dosage regimen should be within the accepted range of current usage for the individual client, taking into account the child's body surface area (height, weight), organ function, and concurrent disease processes.
4. Unless the benefit far outweighs the risk, no antibiotic should be used in clients with prior documentation of an allergic or adverse reaction to the specific medication.
5. Children receiving potent and potentially dangerous drugs, such as gentamicin, amikacin, tobramycin, or vancomycin, for more than 2 days, should have steady-state drug serum concentrations drawn at the appropriate times for evaluation.
6. Whenever possible, cultures should be drawn before initiation of antibiotic therapy. Usual sites cultured include sputum, urine, blood, wound, or non-healing topical sites.
7. Duration of antibiotic therapy should be continued until infection is no longer present. Time periods, though, should not exceed the usual treatment time established for the suspected infection. Prophylactic antibiotic therapy given after uncomplicated surgery is usually discontinued within 48 hours with few exceptions, such as cardiac surgery.

A baseline assessment is necessary as described in Chapter 58.

Nursing diagnosis. Clients receiving penicillin therapy are at risk for the following nursing diagnoses: altered protection related to reduction in normal flora (superinfection) evidenced by darkened tongue (fungal superinfection), white oral plaques, and creamy vaginal discharge (Candida superinfection); altered bowel elimination pattern related to the development of antibiotic-associated pseudomembranous colitis evidenced by watery and severe diarrhea; fluid volume deficit related to nausea, vomiting and/or diarrhea; impaired skin integrity (dermatitis, urticaria [Figure 59-2], rash); and the collaborative problems of allergic response, hepatotoxicity, leukopenia or neutropenia, thrombocytopenia, mental disturbances, seizures, or a cross-sensitivity to cephalosporins, cephamycins, griseofulvin, or penicillamine.

Pregnancy Safety

Category	Drug
B	aztreonam, azithromycin, cephalosporins, metronidazole, nitrofurantoin, penicillins, phenazopyridine
C	cinoxacin, clarithromycin, dirithromycin, fluoroquinolones, gentamicin, imipenam/cilastatin, methenamine, sulfonamides, vancomycin
D	amikacin, kanamycin, netilmicin, streptomycin, tetracyclines, tobramycin
Unclassified	chloramphenicol (not recommended at term or during labor), clindamycin, lincomycin, nalidixic acid (not recommended in pregnancy), spectinomycin, troleandomycin

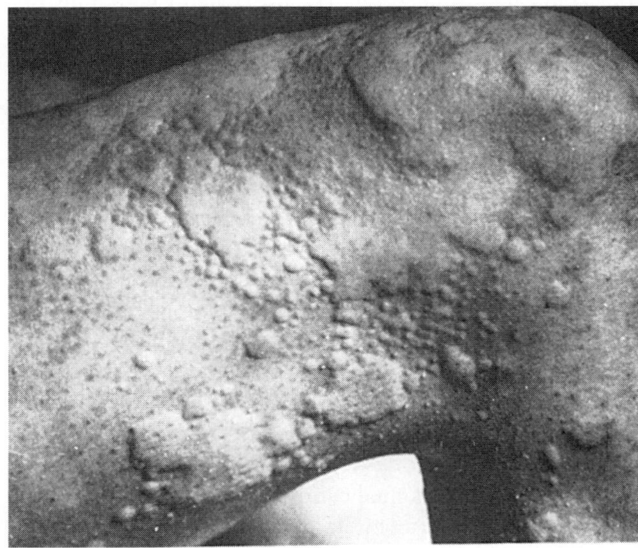

Figure 59-2 Urticaria such as those seen in individuals sensitive to penicillin.

Implementation

Monitoring. Drug interactions with penicillins can increase or decrease the effectiveness of the penicillins and should be monitored. Gentamicin acts synergistically with penicillins against enterococci, as well against *Staphylococcus aureus,* when used with nafcillin or methicillin. On the other hand, acidifying agents such as ammonium chloride, ascorbic acid, methenamine, methionine, and citrus juice destroy oral penicillins, making them less effective. Tetracyclines slow bacterial multiplication and thereby inhibit the penicillins that act against rapidly multiplying bacteria. Erythromycin inhibits the bacteriocidal activity of penicillins against most organisms.

Because of the possibility of bacterial and fungal superinfection, elderly and debilitated clients should be observed carefully for unusual weight loss (pseudomembranous colitis), abdominal cramps and diarrhea, darkened or discolored tongue, and sore mouth. See Box 59-1 for a discussion of antibiotic-associated pseudomembranous colitis (AAPMC).

BOX 59-1

Antibiotic-Associated Pseudomembranous Colitis (AAPMC)

Some clients may develop AAPMC, caused by *Clostridium difficile* toxin, during or after treatment with penicillins, cephalosporins, lincomycins, and imipenem-cilastatin. The condition is characterized by inflammation and necrosis of the mucosal and submucosal layers of the bowel wall evidenced by 2 to 5 semisolid or liquid stools per day in mild cases, and 30 or more watery stools a day in severe disease. Fluid and electrolyte loss, abdominal tenderness, cramping, and fever also occur. It is fatal in 10% to 20% of elderly and debilitated clients. It is called pseudomembranous because the inflammation causes exudative plaques, "pseudomembranes," to form on the mucosal wall.

Two types of clients develop AAPMC: those who are carriers of *C. difficile* and who are given antibiotics; and noncarriers who are given antibiotics and then exposed to the organism through environmental conditions. Spores of the organism have been known to exist for months after an infected client has been discharged (Doughty & Jackson, 1993).

Discontinuation of the causative drug is sufficient therapy for mild cases, but moderate to severe cases may require replacement of fluid, electrolytes, and proteins. In clients nonresponsive to discontinuing the drug and in more severe cases, oral doses of metronidazole, bacitracin, vancomycin, or cholestyramine may be used. The antimicrobials are effective against the organism and the cholestyramine has been shown to bind *C. difficile* toxin in vitro. If the cholestyramine is prescribed concurrently with vancomycin, the drugs should be administered several hours apart since cholestyramine will also bind with oral vancomycin.

Recurrences are not uncommon and are treated with a second round of drugs. Watery diarrhea in AAPMC may occur during therapy and persist for several weeks after therapy. Antidiarrheals are not recommended because they retain the toxin within the bowel prolonging and/or worsening the damage to the colon (*USP DI*, 1996).

Serum electrolytes should be monitored for hyperkalemia and/or hypernatremia when the client is receiving azlocillin, carbenicillin, mezlocillin, penicillin G, piperacillin, and ticarcillin. Renal function studies may be required during prolonged therapy with methicillin, which causes interstitial nephritis in up to 12% of individuals.

The client's vital signs, total and differential white blood cell count and culture results, and stool cytotoxin assays if *C. difficile* colitis occurs, should be monitored. With carbenicillin (parenteral), piperacillin, and ticarcillin, bleeding times (PTT and PT) and serum potassium and sodium should be monitored.

Intervention. In addition to performing nursing measures common to all types of antibiotic drug therapy, as discussed previously in this chapter and Chapter 58, the nurse must be especially cognizant of several factors when penicillins are prescribed.

In administering penicillins, the nurse should remember that oral penicillins are bound to food and are poorly absorbed in acid media. Their administration, therefore, should not be preceded or followed by food for at least 1 hour to minimize binding. Penicillins should not be taken with acidic fruit juices, since juices may facilitate decomposition of penicillins. Box 59-2 lists the effect of food on oral penicillin absorption.

In administering penicillins intravenously, the nurse should note that most penicillins in clinical use are sodium or potassium salts. Significant amounts of cation can be administered when these drugs are given intravenously in massive dosage. For example, 20 million units of potassium penicillin G contains 33 mEq of potassium ion. Fatalities have occurred because of the toxic effect of potassium on the heart following administration of such large doses in the presence of renal insufficiency. Carbenicillin contains 4.7 mEq of sodium per gram and may be administered in doses of 30 to 40 g daily.

BOX 59-2

Effect of Food on Oral Penicillin Absorption*

Drug	Food effect
amoxicillin	None
amoxicillin and clavulanate	None
ampicillin	Decreased
bacampicillin tablet	None
carbenicillin indanyl sodium	Increased
cloxacillin	Decreased
dicloxacillin	Decreased
nafcillin	Decreased
oxacillin	Decreased
penicillin G benzathine	Decreased
pencillin V potassium	Decreased slightly

*Penicillins whose absorption decreases after food intake are generally acid labile; therefore, administer with a full glass of water on an empty stomach 1 hour before or 2 hours after meals.

Case Study
The Client with a Bacterial Infection

Gloria Lawton, a 42-year-old secretary, has come to the clinic complaining of a fever, sore throat, and cough for the past 24 hours. Her posterior pharynx is reddened with patches of purulent exudate. She complains of pain with swallowing. Her cervical lymph nodes are enlarged and tender to touch. Based on the client's symptom history and physical examination the physician suspects a streptococcal infection. After a throat culture is taken, Ms. Lawson is started on amoxicillin 500 mg PO every 8 hours for 10 days.

1. Explain the rationale for getting a throat culture before the first dose of amoxicillin is administered.
2. Before administering the first dose of amoxicillin, what additional assessment data does the nurse need to collect from the client?
3. What should the nurse teach Ms. Lawton about taking the amoxicillin?
4. After the completion of the 10 days of drug therapy Ms. Lawton's upper respiratory symptoms have resolved. However, she is now complaining of intense perineal itching and a vaginal discharge. How should the nurse respond to Ms. Lawton's questions about these symptoms?

Signs and symptoms of hyperkalemia and hypernatremia should be duly noted and reported.

When administering penicillins intravenously, do so intermittently to prevent blood vessel irritation, phlebitis. The intravenous site should be changed at least every 48 hours.

Education. Instruct the client to take the full course of medication, even though feeling better and symptom free. Emphasize the importance of taking evenly spaced doses to maintain therapeutic blood levels. Prescriptions for antibiotics should never be shared with others or saved and taken for a different episode of illness.

Ampicillin, bacampicillin suspension, cloxacillin, dicloxacillin, nafcillin, oxacillin, penicillin G, and the liquid form of bacampicillin should be taken when the stomach is empty.

Amoxicillin, penicillin V, and the tablet form of bacampicillin, however, may be taken with food to decrease gastrointestinal distress.

Women taking penicillins, especially ampicillin, amoxicillin, and penicillin V, should be cautioned to use an alternate form of contraception if they are using estrogen-containing contraceptives.

Clients with diabetes mellitus using copper sulfate urine glucose tests (Clinitest) may have false-positive results while taking amoxicillin, ampicillin, bacampicillin, and penicillin G. Have the client use glucose-enzymatic tests, such as Clinistix or Ketodiastix.

Instruct clients to report failure of their condition to improve in a few days, or the development of severe diarrhea, or rash, fever, or chills, which may indicate a delayed sensitivity reaction.

Evaluation. The client will maintain or achieve an infection free state as evidenced by negative cultures. If administered therapeutically, the client will also evidence a body temperature within normal limits, a WBC within the normal limits for age, and the resolution of any other infection-related symptoms that the client might be having without adverse effects of the drug. For further analysis see the case study above.

CEPHALOSPORINS AND RELATED PRODUCTS

Cephalosporins and related products are chemical modifications of the penicillin structure. These modifications create compounds with different microbiologic and pharmacologic activities. To classify the differences in antimicrobial activity, cephalosporins are divided into four generations. Loracarbef (Lorabid, a carbacephem) a chemically similar drug to second generation cephalosporin is included in this section.

Cephalosporins inhibit cell wall synthesis similar to penicillin and are also, bactericidal. They are effective in numerous situations, but until the third-generation cephalosporins were marketed, the majority were not considered to be drugs of choice for any serious infection. The first generation is primarily active against gram-positive bacteria while the second generation had increased activity against gram-negative microorganisms. The third generation is more active against gram-negative bacteria (ceftazidime and cefoperazone are also effective against *Pseudomonas aeruginosa*) and β-lactamase–producing microbial strains. But the third generation is less effective against gram-positive cocci. Cefepime is a fourth generation cephalosporin that has comparable antimicrobial effects to the third generation and is also more resistant to some β-lactamases (Mandell & Petri, Jr, 1996).

Initially the advantage of cephalosporins over penicillins was their resistance to enzymatic degradation by penicillinase (β-lactamase). But currently, drug resistance has been reported to drugs from all three generations, possibly through four mechanisms: (1) a microorganism lacking an outer cell membrane permeability, causing poor drug penetration in the bacteria; (2) bacteria lacking a receptor for the specific drug; (3) bacteria producing a β-lactamase enzyme that can split the β-lactam ring in the cephalosporins (many such enzymes have been isolated); or (4) development of a type of bacteria tolerance, bacterial strains that are inhibited but not killed by the cephalosporins. The reason for this effect is the lack of, or deficiency in, autolytic enzymes in the bacterial cell wall (Katzung, 1992). Also this class of drugs has been overused; thus reports of bacterial resistance have increased.

Cephalosporin antibiotics are often prescribed for clients allergic to penicillins. The possibility of a cross-reaction is 5% to 15%; however, if the individual reports a serious reaction or anaphylaxis to penicillin, cephalosporins should not be used (Beringer & Middleton, 1995).

Because cephalosporins inhibit cell wall synthesis, cell division, and growth, rapidly dividing bacteria are most affected by them. These agents are indicated for the treatment of a variety of infections and also as presurgery prophylactic agents. Combinations of third generation cephalosporins and aminoglycosides are used synergistically to treat *P. aeruginosa*, *S. marcescens*, and other susceptible organisms.

Cephalosporin side/adverse effects include diarrhea, abdominal cramps or distress, oral and/or vaginal candidiasis, rash, pruritus, redness, or edema. An increase in bleeding episodes and bruising due to hypoprothrombinemia is reported with cefamandole, cefmetazole, cefoperazone and cefotetan. Table 59-2 lists cephalosporin pharmacokinetics and usual adult dose.

■ Nursing Management

Cephalosporin Therapy

General nursing management related to antibiotic therapy discussed earlier also applies to the client receiving cephalosporins.

Assessment. If the client has a history of sensitivity to cephalosporins, penicillin, penicillin derivatives, or penicillamine, the use of cephalosporins is contraindicated. Cephalosporins should be used with caution in clients with a history of bleeding disorders because all may cause hypoprothrombinemia and, potentially, bleeding. As with penicillins, clients with a history of gastrointestinal disease, particularly ulcerative colitis and regional enteritis, are at higher risk for pseudomembranous colitis. It is recommended that clients with renal and hepatic function impairment receive lower dosages. See the Pregnancy Safety box on p. 906 for FDA pregnancy safety categories for cephalosporins.

Review the client's current medications for significant drug interactions that may occur as with the following drugs.

Drug	Possible effect and management
alcohol	**Not recommended with cefamandole, cefmetazole, cefoperazone, or cefotetan. An increase in acetaldehyde in the blood may result, producing a disulfiram [Antabuse]-type reaction such as stomach pain, nausea, vomiting, headaches, low blood pressure, tachycardia, respiratory difficulties, increased sweating, or flushing of the face. Clients should avoid drinking alcohol-containing beverages, medications containing alcohol, or using intravenous alcohol solutions during the administration of these drugs and for 3 days afterward.**
anticoagulants, coumarin or indanedione, heparin, or thrombolytic agents	**Increased risk of bleeding and hemorrhage when given concurrently with cefamandole, cefmetazole, cefoperazone, or cefotetan. These cephalosporins interfere with vitamin K metabolism in the liver, resulting in hypoprothrombinemia. Dosage adjustments of the anticoagulants may be necessary during and after administration of these drugs. Avoid concurrent use of these drugs with thrombolytic agents because of the increased risk of serious bleeding and hemorrhage.**
nonsteroidal antiinflammatory drugs (NSAIDs), especially aspirin, inhibitors, and sulfinpyrazone [Anturane]	**When given with cefamandole, cefoperazone, or cefotetan, an increased risk of hemorrhage exists because of the additive effect on platelet inhibition. Also, high dosages of salicylates and/or the specified antibiotics may induce hypoprothrombinemia, and the GI potential for ulcers or hemorrhage with NSAIDs, salicylates, or sulfinpyrazone may increase when used with the previously mentioned cephalosporins. Avoid or a potentially serious drug interaction may occur.**
probenecid (Benemid)	Probenecid decreases renal tubular secretion of the cephalosporins that are excreted by this mechanism, which can result in increased serum levels, extended half-life, and increased potential for toxicity. Probenecid does not affect the secretion of cefoperazone, ceftazidime, or ceftriaxone. Cephalosporins and probenecid are also used concurrently to treat specific infections such as sexually transmitted diseases, in which a high serum level and prolonged effect are desirable.

A baseline assessment should be accomplished as described in Chapter 58.

Nursing diagnosis. Clients receiving cephalosporins may experience any of the following nursing diagnoses: altered bowel elimination pattern related to antibiotic-associated pseudomembranous colitis; risk for infection (oral or vaginal candidiasis); altered protection related to hypoprothrombinemia and superinfection; impaired tissue integrity (thrombophlebitis); fluid volume deficit related to nausea and vomiting; and the collaborative problems of hypersensitivity (fever, rash), allergic reactions (anaphylaxis, Stevens-Johnson syndrome, renal dysfunction, serum sickness–like reaction), and seizures (high doses or with renal impairment).

Implementation

Monitoring. Because of the possibility of superinfection, observe clients, particularly the elderly and debilitated, for symptoms of bacterial and fungal overgrowth. Bleeding time and prothrombin time should be monitored, since hypoprothrombinemia may occur with these cephalosporins. Many cephalosporins are excreted renally, so most should be monitored by serum drug levels in clients with renal impairment. WBC counts and culture results should be monitored.

Intervention. In addition to performing nursing measures common to all types of antimicrobial drug therapy as

TABLE 59-2 Cephalosporins: pharmacokinetics and usual adult dose

Drug	Pharmacokinetics			Usual adult dose
	Oral absorption (%)	Peak serum (hours)*	Renal excretion (%/hours)†	
First generation				
cefadroxil (Duricef)	95	PO: 1.5-2	93/24	500 mg q12h
cefazolin (Ancef)	—	IM: 1-2 IV: E of I	56-89/6 80-100/24	IM 1 g presurgery IV infusion: 0.25-1.5 g q6-8h
cephalexin (Keflex)	95	PO: 1	80/6 90/8	250-500 mg q6h
▲ cephalothin (Keflin)	—	IM: 0.5 IV: 0.25-0.5	60-70/6	IV infusion: 0.5-2 g q4-6h
cephapirin (Cefadyl)	—	IM: 0.5-1 IV: E of I	70/6	IM/IV: 0.5-1 g q4-6h
cephradine (Velosef, Anspor)	95	PO: 1 IM: 0.8-2 IV: E of I	60-80/6	250-500 mg PO q6h IM/IV: 0.5-1 g q6h
Second generation				
cefaclor (Ceclor)	95	PO: 0.5-1	60-85/8	250-500 mg q8h
cefamandole (Mandol)	—	IM: 0.5-2 IV: E of I	65-85/8	IM/IV: 500 mg q6h
cefmetazole (Zefazone)	—	IV: E of I	71/24	IV: 2 g q6-12h
cefonicid (Monocid)	—	IM: 1 IV: E of I	99/24	IM/IV: 0.5-1 g q24h
cefotetan (Cefotan)	—	IM: 1-3 IV: E of I	50-80/24	IM/IV: 1-2 g q12h
cefoxitin (Mefoxin)	—	IM: 0.3-0.5 IV: E of I	85/6	IV: 1-2 g q6-8h
cefprozil (Cefzil)	95	PO: 1.5	60/8	500 mg q12h
cefuroxine (Zinacef)	pc-52 fasting-37	PO: 2-3.6 IM: 0.75 IV: E of I	32-48/12	250-500 mg q12h IM/IV: 0.75-1.5 g q8h
loracarbef (Lorabid)	90	PO: 0.5-1.2	87-97	200-400 mg q12h
Third generation				
cefixime (Suprax)	40-50	PO: 2-6	50/24	200 mg q12h
cefoperazone (Cefobid)	—	IM: 1-2 IV: E of I	20-30/12‡	IV infusion: 1-2 g q12h
cefotaxime (Claforan)	—	IM: 0.5 IV: E of I	60/6	IV infusion: 1-2 g q4-12h
cefpodoxime (Vantin)	50	PO: 2-3	29-33/12	200 mg q12h
ceftazidime (Fortaz)	—	IM: 1 IV: E of I	80-90/24	IM/IV: 0.5-2 g q8-12h
ceftibuten (Cedax)	—	PO: N/A	56%	400 mg daily
ceftizoxime (Cefizox)	—	IM: 1 IV: E of I	85-95/24	IV: 1-2 g q8-12h
ceftriaxone (Rocephin)	—	IM: 2-3 IV: E of I	33-67/24	IV: 1-2 g q24h
Fourth generation				
cefepime (Maxipime)	—	IM: N/A IV: E of I	N/A	IM/IV: 0.5-1 g q12h

*Time to peak serum level (hours); †renal excretion, percent excreted unchanged/hr; ‡majority excreted unchanged in bile.
IM, Intramuscularly; *IV*, intravenously; *E of I*, end of infusion; *pc*, after meals, *N/A*, not available.
Olin, 1996, *USP DI*, 1996.

discussed in the previous chapter, the nurse must be aware of other factors when cephalosporins are prescribed.

Intramuscular cephalosporins, because they are irritating to tissues and can cause pain, induration, and sterile abscesses following injection, should be given deeply into a large muscle mass.

Perioperative parenteral administration of cephalosporins for prophylaxis is usually discontinued 24 hours after surgery.

Education. Instruct the client to take the full course of medication, even though he or she may feel better and be symptom free. Stress the importance of taking evenly spaced doses to maintain therapeutic blood levels. Cephalosporins may be taken with food if gastric irritation develops.

Clients with diabetes mellitus who are using copper sulfate urine glucose tests (Clinitest) may have false-positive results while taking cephalosporins. Have the client use glucose-enzymatic tests such as Clinistix or Ketodiastix. The client should be cautioned not to drink alcoholic beverages or to take alcohol-containing medications because abdominal cramps, nausea, and vomiting; hypotension, tachycardia, and shortness of breath; and sweating and facial flushing may occur. Instruct clients to read labels, because many cough and cold remedies contain alcohol.

Evaluation. The client will maintain or achieve an infection free state as evidenced by negative cultures. If a cephalosporin is being administered therapeutically, the client will also evidence a body temperature within normal limits, a WBC within the normal limits for age, and the resolution of any other infection-related symptoms that the client might be experiencing without adverse reactions to the drug.

MACROLIDE ANTIBIOTICS

The **macrolide antibiotics** are bacteriostatic, since they inhibit RNA-dependent protein synthesis; but in high concentrations with selected organisms, they may be bactericidal. Currently the macrolide antibiotics include: azithromycin (Zithromax), clarithromycin (Biaxin), erythromycin, dirithromycin (Dynabac) and troleandomycin (Tao). Dirithromycin is a prodrug that is activated during intestinal absorption to an active metabolite, erythromycylamine.

With the exception of troleandomycin, these agents have similar antimicrobial action (against gram-positive and selected gram-negative microorganisms) and are used for respiratory, gastrointestinal tract, skin and soft tissue infections when beta-lactam antibiotics are contraindicated (Olin, 1996). Troleandomycin is only indicated for the treatment of *Streptococcus pneumoniae* and *Streptococcus pyogenes*.

Significant side/adverse effects include:

- azithromycin: stomach pain, nausea, vomiting and diarrhea. Allergic reactions and acute interstitial nephritis are rare adverse effects.
- clarithromycin: anorexia, headache, nausea, vomiting, lethargy, severe anemia, fever, infection, rash.
- erythromycin: abdominal cramps, diarrhea, nausea, vomiting. Hypersensitivity and hepatotoxicity are reported less frequently.
- dirithromycin: stomach pain, headache, nausea and diarrhea.
- troleandomycin: stomach cramps and discomfort.

For macrolide pharmacokinetics and usual adult dose, see Table 59-3.

■ Nursing Management

Erythromycin Therapy

General nursing management related to antibiotic therapy discussed earlier also applies to the client receiving erythromycin.

Assessment. Determine if the client has hepatic impairment, in which case erythromycin is used with caution, particularly with erythromycin estolate. Clients with a history of cardiac arrhythmias may be at risk for a recurrence with high doses of erythromycin.

Review the client's current medications for significant drug interactions that may occur.

TABLE 59-3 Macrolide: pharmacokinetics and usual adult dose

	Pharmacokinetics			
Drug	Oral absorption (%)	Peak serum (hours)*	Renal excretion (%/hours)†	Usual adult dose
azithromycin (Zithromax)	good	2-4	4.5/72‡	500 mg first day then 250 mg daily thereafter
clarithromycin (Biaxin)	good	2-3	20-30/—	250-500 mg q12h
▲ erythromycin	30-65	2-4	2-5/—‡	250 mg q6h IV infusion: 250-500 mg q6h
dirithromycin (Dynabac)	10	—	2/—‡	500 mg daily
troleandomycin (Tao)	—	2	20/—	250-500 mg qid

*Time to peak serum level (hours); †renal excretion, percent excreted unchanged/hr; ‡primarily excreted unchanged in bile; — unavailable.
Olin, 1996; *USP DI*, 1996.

Drug	Possible effect and management
alfentanil (Alfenta)	May increase plasma levels and action of alfentanil. Monitor closely if given in combination.
carbamazepine (Tegretol)	Carbamazepine metabolism may be inhibited, leading to elevated serum levels and, possibly, toxicity. Monitor closely.
chloramphenicol (Chloromycetin) or lincomycins	May antagonize the therapeutic effects of chloramphenicol and lincomycin. Avoid concurrent administration.
cyclosporine (Sandimmune)	Concurrent administration with erythromycin may increase cyclosporine serum levels and increase risk for nephrotoxicity. Monitor closely if given concurrently.
hepatotoxic medications	Increased possibility for liver toxicity; monitor liver function studies closely if given concurrently.
terfenadine (Seldane), astemizole (Hismanal)	**Concurrent drug administrations may increase risk of cardiotoxicity. Avoid or a potentially serious drug interaction may occur.**
warfarin (Coumadin)	May result in decreased warfarin metabolism and excretion leading to an increased risk of bleeding or hemorrhage. Dosage adjustments of coumarin may be necessary during and after treatment with erythromycin. Monitor prothrombin times closely.
xanthines, such as aminophylline, caffeine, oxtriphylline, and theophylline (exception, dyphylline)	An increase in theophylline levels and/or toxicity is reported with this combination of drugs. This effect is usually seen at approximately the sixth day of erythromycin therapy, since it appears to be related to the peak erythromycin serum level. Montor the serum levels of xanthines closely, since dosage adjustments of xanthines may be necessary during and after erythromycin therapy.
zidovudine (AZT)	Concurrent administration with clarithromycin may result in delayed time to peak zidovudine concentrations. Administer doses of these two drugs at least 4 hours apart.

A baseline assessment as discussed in Chapter 58 should be done.

Nursing diagnosis. The client receiving erythromycin may experience the following nursing diagnoses: altered bowel elimination pattern (diarrhea); impaired tissue integrity related to inflammation or phlebitis at injection site; fluid volume deficit related to nausea and vomiting; altered comfort (abdominal cramping); sensory-perceptual disturbance related to hearing loss; altered protection related to the loss of normal flora and development of *C. albicans* (sore mouth or tongue, vaginal itching and discharge); and the collaborative problems of hypersensitivity, hepatotoxicity (dark urine, pale stools, tiredness, and yellowing of sclera and skin), and cardiotoxicity (arrhythmia, bradycardia, fainting, sudden death).

Implementation

Monitoring. Periodic hepatic function studies may be required for those clients receiving high-dose or prolonged intravenous erythromycin gluceptate therapy. Temperature, WBC counts, cultures, and a focal exam of the infection should be done.

Intervention. Macrolide antibiotics should be administered with a full glass of water on an empty stomach (1 hour before or 2 hours after meals) to obtain maximum effect. Enteric-coated tablets, delayed-release capsules, and estolate and ethylsuccinate preparations may be taken with meals and may be used with clients who have a gastrointestinal intolerance to other forms of oral erythromycin. When administering oral suspensions, ensure that they have been refrigerated and shaken well and that the calibrated liquid-measuring device has been used for accurate dosing.

Continuous infusion is preferable to intermittent; however, if intermittent infusion is considered, it should be diluted in 100 to 250 ml of 0.9% sodium chloride injection or 5% dextrose injection and administered over 20 to 60 minutes.

Education. The importance of complying with a full course of therapy, even though the client feels better or is symptom free, should be stressed. This course of therapy should continue at least 10 days in group A beta-hemolytic streptococcal infections to prevent the occurrence of acute rheumatic fever.

If a dose of most medications is missed, it is omitted if close to the next dose; however, with erythromycin the dose is to be taken as soon as possible: if almost time for the next dose and the dosing schedule is 2 doses a day—spacing the missed dose and the next dose 5 to 6 hours apart; or 3+ doses a day—spacing the missed dose 2 to 4 hours apart or doubling the next dose.

Evaluation. The client will maintain or achieve an infection free state as evidenced by negative cultures. If administered therapeutically, the client will also evidence a body temperature within normal limits, a WBC within the normal limits for age, and the resolution of any other infection-related symptoms that the client might be experiencing without adverse effects of the drug.

LINCOMYCINS

clindamycin [klin da mye' sin] (Cleocin, Dalacin C♣)
lincomycin [lin koe mye' sin] (Lincocin)

Lincomycin inhibits protein synthesis by binding to bacterial ribosomes and preventing peptide bond formation. It is primarily bacteriostatic, although it may be bactericidal in high doses with selected organisms. It was used to treat serious streptococci, pneumococci and staphylococci infections but has been replaced by safer and more effective antibiotics.

Clindamycin, which is a semisynthetic derivative of lincomycin, has a similar mechanism of action as lincomycin but it is more effective. It is indicated for the treatment of bone and joint infections, pelvic (female) and intraabdominal infections, bacterial septicemia, pneumonia, and skin and soft tissue infections caused by susceptible bacteria.

Oral clindamycin is well absorbed and should be administered with food or with a full glass (8 oz) of water. It is rapidly distributed to most body fluids and tissues with the exception of cerebrospinal fluid with the highest concentrations noted in bone, bile, and urine. Clindamycin adult half-life is 2 to 3 hours; it reaches peak blood levels within ¾ to 1 hour after oral administration, 1 hour in children, and 3 hours in adults by intramuscular injection and by the end of the infusion by intravenous injection. It is metabolized in the liver and excreted primarily by the kidneys.

The most significant adverse and limiting effect for both drugs is antibiotic-associated pseudomembranous colitis (AAPMC); see Box 59-1 on p. 907.

The usual adult clindamycin dose is 150 to 300 mg (PO, IM, or IV), every 6 hours. In infants 1 month and over, the oral dosage is 2 to 5 mg/kg body weight every 6 hours.

■ Nursing Management
Clindamycin Therapy

General nursing management related to antibiotic therapy discussed earlier also applies to the client receiving clindamycin.

Assessment. Determine whether the client has a history of gastrointestinal disease, particularly ulcerative colitis or regional enteritis, because pseudomembranous colitis may occur with clindamycin therapy. Severe hepatic or renal function impairment will require a reduction in dose.

Review the client's current medication regimen for significant drug interactions that may occur when clindamycin is administered with the following drugs.

Drug	Possible effect and management
anesthetics, such as chloroform, cyclopropane, enflurane (Ethrane), halothane (Fluothane), isoflurane (Forane), methoxyflurane (Penthrane), trichloroethylene, or the neuromuscular blocking agents	**May result in enhanced neuromuscular blockade, skeletal muscle weakness, respiratory depression, or paralysis if this combination is used during or immediately after surgery. Avoid or a potentially serious drug interaction may occur.**
antidiarrheals, adsorbent type (kaolins, attapulgite)	Decreases absorption of oral lincomycins. Avoid concurrent usage or advise client to take the antidiarrheal 2 hours before or 3 to 4 hours after the oral lincomycins.
chloramphenicol (Chloromycetin) or erythromycin	May antagonize the therapeutic effect of lincomycins. Avoid concurrent administration.

A baseline assessment as described in Chapter 58 should be done. A cytotoxin assay of stool may be done for the presence of *C. difficile* before therapy is begun.

Nursing diagnosis. The client receiving clindamycin therapy should be assessed for the following nursing diagnoses: altered bowel elimination pattern (diarrhea) related to the development of antibiotic-associated pseudomembranous colitis; fluid volume deficit related to nausea and vomiting; altered protection related to neutropenia (infection), thrombocytopenia (bleeding), and loss of normal flora (superinfection); and the collaborative problem of hypersensitivity.

Implementation

Monitoring. During therapy, observe the client for abdominal cramps, diarrhea, weight loss, or weakness, which might be indications of pseudomembranous colitis. In addition, monitor the client's temperature, WBC counts, and cultures. Do a focal assessment related to the infection.

Intervention. Administer clindamycin capsules with a full glass of water or with meals to prevent esophageal ulceration.

Education. Stress the importance of complying with a full course of the medication, even though the client feels well and is symptom free. Ten days is considered a minimal course of therapy for streptococcal infections. Instruct the client to take the medication at evenly spaced times to ensure maintenance of serum levels. Alert the client to adverse drug reactions and to report them to the prescriber.

Evaluation. The client will maintain or achieve an infection free state as evidenced by negative cultures. If administered therapeutically, the client will also evidence a body temperature within normal limits, a WBC within the normal limits for age, and the resolution of any other infection-related symptoms that the client might be having without adverse effects of the drug.

▲ vancomycin [van koe mye' sin] (Vancocin)

Vancomycin inhibits bacterial cell walls by binding to a cell wall precursor, a mechanism that differs from penicillin or cephalosporins. This action leads to cell lysis. Vancomycin may also inhibit RNA synthesis. It is bactericidal for many organisms. Vancomycin resistant strains of enterococci though, are documented (*USP DI,* 1996). Oral vancomycin is indicated for the treatment of antibiotic-induced pseudomembranous colitis (*Clostridium difficile*) and the treatment of staphylococcal enterocolitis. Parenteral vancomycin is not recommended for use in antibiotic-associated pseudomembranous colitis. Instead it is indicated for bone and joint infections, bacterial septicemia caused by *Staphylococcus* species and for the prevention and treatment of bacterial endocarditis caused by staphylococcus, including methicillin resistant strains.

Vancomycin's absorption from the intestinal tract is poor. It is excreted mainly in the feces. Parenteral vancomycin has a half-life of 6 hours in adults, about 2 to 3 hours in children. It is primarily excreted by the kidneys. Significant side effects for oral dosing include nausea, vomiting, or taste alterations. Less frequent or rare parenteral adverse effects include ototoxicity and nephrotoxicity. The "red-neck syndrome" is reported after bolus or too rapid drug injection, which results in histamine release and chills, fever, tachycardia, pruritus, rash, or red face, neck, upper body, back and arms (*USP DI,* 1996).

The oral adult dosage of vancomycin for the treatment of *C. difficile* colitis or diarrhea is 125 to 500 mg every 6 hours for 5 to 10 days, repeated if necessary. In children, the dosage is 10 mg/kg (up to 125 mg) every 6 hours for 5 to 10 days, repeated if necessary. By IV infusion the dose is 7.5 mg/kg every 6 hours.

■ Nursing Management
Vancomycin Therapy

General nursing management related to antibiotic therapy discussed earlier also applies to the client receiving erythromycin.

Assessment. Assess the client for hearing loss, since vancomycin has ototoxic properties. Clients with impaired renal function will require reduced dosages, and those with inflammatory intestinal disorders may have increased absorption and therefore a higher risk for toxicity.

Review the client's current medications for significant interactions that may occur when vancomycin is given with the following drugs.

Drug	Possible effect and management
aminoglycosides, amphotericin B parenteral (Fungizone), aspirin, bacitracin, parenteral bumetanide (Bumex), capreomycin (Capastat), cisplatin (Platinol), cyclosporine (Sandimmune), ethacrynate sodium parenteral (Edecrin), furosemide parenteral (Lasix), paromomycin (Humatin), polymyxins, or streptozocin (Zanosar)	**Increases potential for ototoxicity and/or nephrotoxicity. In clients with pseudomembranous colitis or severe kidney impairment, the serum levels of vancomycin may be increased, thus leading to an increased potential for toxicity. Monitor serum levels closely. Avoid or a potentially serious drug interaction may occur.**
cholestyramine (Questran) or colestipol (Colestid)	When given concurrently with the oral dosage form, a reduction in vancomycin antibacterial activity is reported. Avoid this combination if possible. If not, give oral vancomycin several hours apart from the other medications.

In addition to the baseline assessment described in Chapter 58, a stool toxin assay for the presence of *C. difficile* may be required.

Nursing diagnosis. Clients receiving vancomycin therapy should be assessed for the following nursing diagnoses: risk for injury related to histamine release common with bolus or rapid injection (chills, fever, tachycardia, flushing of the face and/or upper body, syncope, tingling, unpleasant taste); fluid volume deficit related to nausea and vomiting; impaired tissue integrity related to extravasation; sensory-perceptual disturbance related to ototoxicity (loss of hearing and tinnitus); and the collaborative problem of nephrotoxicity (blood in urine, greatly increased or decreased frequency of urination and amount of urine).

Implementation

Monitoring. Because oral vancomycin is so poorly absorbed the following monitoring is for the intravenous form of the drug. Renal function studies may be needed before and periodically during high-dose or prolonged therapy. Urinalyses should be monitored for the presence of albumin, casts, and cells in the urine, and decreased specific gravity. Vancomycin serum concentration determinations may be necessary in clients with renal impairment or in clients over 60; peak concentrations should not exceed 25 to 40 µg/ml and trough, 5 to 10 µg/ml. Assess elderly clients for hearing loss over the course of therapy, since they excrete vancomycin more slowly. The IV site should be monitored for extravasation.

Intervention. Administer the oral liquid using the calibrated liquid-measuring device provided by the manufacturer. If the intravenous form is used for oral administration, each vial should be dissolved in 30 ml of water or juice. It may be administered straight or through a nasogastric tube to minimize the unpleasant taste.

Parenteral vancomycin is only to be administered intravenously because it is so irritating to the tissues. Care must be taken to avoid extravasation. To avoid side effects such as hypotension, thrombophlebitis, and "red-neck syndrome," do not administer as a bolus injection. Vancomycin may be administered intermittently in at least 100 ml of 0.9% sodium chloride injection or 5% dextrose injection over 60 minutes. If intermittent IV administration is not feasible, vancomycin may given by continuous IV infusion; 1 to 2 g in sufficient 5% dextrose injection or 0.9% sodium chloride to run over 24 hours. Rotation of the venous sites will help prevent local irritation. Vancomycin is also incompatible with alkaline solutions, heavy metals, and a wide variety of substances. Consult package insert before combining with other drugs or administer alone.

Education. Alert the client to possible side effects or adverse reactions, and instruct him or her to consult with the prescriber should they occur. Instruct the client to take the medication as prescribed and for the full course of therapy.

Evaluation. The client will maintain or achieve an infection free state as evidenced by negative culture results. If administered therapeutically, the client will also evidence a body temperature within normal limits, a WBC within the normal limits for age, and the resolution of any other infection-related symptoms that the client might be experiencing without adverse reactions to the drug.

AMINOGLYCOSIDES

Aminoglycosides are potent bactericidal antibiotics that are usually reserved for serious or life-threatening infections. They are very effective against many bacteria (gram-positive and gram-negative) but are generally reserved for gram-negative infections. Safer and less toxic agents are available to treat the majority of gram-positive infections. Currently available aminoglycosides include:

amikacin [am ih kay' sin] (Amikin)
▲ **gentamicin** [jen ta mye' sin] (Garamycin)
kanamycin [kan ah mye' sin] (Kantrex)
netilmicin [ne til mye' sin] (Netromycin)
streptomycin [strep toe mye' sin]
tobramycin [toe bra mye' sin] (Nebcin)

The mechanism of action for aminoglycosides is to irreversibly bind ribosomes of susceptible bacteria, thus inhibiting with protein synthesis (interferes with the complex between messenger RNA and the bacteria ribosomes), leading to eventual cell death (bactericidal). They are indicated for the treatment of serious or life-threatening infections when other agents are ineffective or contraindicated. They are used with penicillins, cephalosporins, or vancomycin for their synergistic effects and are especially useful for the treatment of gram-negative infections such as those caused by *Pseudomonas* sp., *E. coli*, *Proteus* sp., *Klebsiella* sp., *Serratia* sp., and others.

Aminoglycosides are poorly absorbed from an intact intestinal tract, but are rapidly absorbed intramuscularly. Local topical application or irrigation may lead to absorption from most areas of the body with the exception of the urinary bladder.

The range of therapeutic aminoglycoside serum levels (µg/ml) are as follows:

amikacin	15-25
gentamicin	4-10
kanamycin	15-30
tobramycin	4-10

Significant side/adverse effects of aminoglycosides include nephrotoxicity, neurotoxicity, ototoxicity (auditory and vestibular) and hypersensitivity.

The usual adult dosage of amikacin is 5 mg/kg IM/IV every 8 hours; gentamicin 1 to 1.7 mg/kg IM or by IV infusion every 8 hours; kanamycin is 3.75 mg/kg IM every 6 hours; netilmicin is 1.3 to 2.2 mg/kg IM/IV every 8 hours; streptomycin (tuberculosis adult dose) is 1 g IM daily given in combination with other antimycobacterials; and tobramycin is 0.75 mg to 1.25 mg/kg IM or IV infusion every 6 hours. For additional dosing recommendations, see current package insert or reference.

■ Nursing Management

Aminoglycoside Therapy

General nursing management related to antibiotic therapy discussed earlier also applies to the client receiving aminoglycoside therapy.

Assessment. Infants with botulism and clients with myasthenia gravis and parkinsonism may experience greater muscle weakness because of neuromuscular blockade with the aminoglycosides. Auditory and vestibular toxicity might occur in clients with eighth nerve impairment. Renal function impairment increases the risk of toxicity. A previous history of an allergic response to aminoglycosides would contraindicate the use of another because of cross-sensitivity.

Review the client's current medications for significant drug interactions such as those occurring when aminoglycosides are given concurrently with the following drugs.

Drug	Possible effect and management
other aminoglycosides (two or more concurrently) or capreomycin (Capastat)	**Potential for ototoxicity, nephrotoxicity, and neuromuscular blockade is enhanced. Hearing loss may progress to deafness even after the drug is stopped. In some cases, hearing loss may be reversed. Avoid or a potentially serious drug interaction may occur.**
amphotericin B parenteral (Fungizone), aspirin, bacitracin parenteral, bumetanide parenteral (Bumex), cephalothin (Keflin), cisplatin (Platinol), cyclosporine (Sandimmune), ethacrynate sodium parenteral (Edecrin), furosemide parenteral (Lasix), paromomycin (Humatin), streptozocin (Zanosar), or vancomycin (Vancocin)	Increased potential for ototoxicity and/or nephrotoxicity. Hearing loss may be permanent. If drugs are given concurrently, serial audiometric hearing determinations are suggested. Vancomycin and aminoglycosides may be ordered to prevent bacterial endocarditis or to treat specific infections such as carditis caused by organisms such as streptococci and corynebacteria. In such instances, frequent determinations of drug serum levels and renal function are recommended, since dosage adjustments or other interventions may be necessary.
anesthetics (halogenated hydrocarbon) or citrate-anticoagulated blood by massive transfusions or neuromuscular blocking agents	**May increase neuromuscular blockade. Avoid or a potentially serious drug interaction may occur.**
methoxyflurane (Penthrane) or polymyxins, parenteral	**Increased possibility for nephrotoxicity and/or neuromuscular blockade. Avoid or a potentially serious drug interaction may occur.**

A baseline assessment as described in Chapter 58 should be done. In addition, a urinalysis, audiogram, and renal and vestibular function determination should occur before the start of therapy. With streptomycin, caloric stimulation tests prior to prolonged therapy are to detect a baseline by which to measure the occurrence of vestibular toxicity.

Nursing diagnosis. Clients receiving aminoglycoside therapy should be assessed for the possibility of the following nursing diagnoses: sensory-perceptual alteration related to auditory ototoxicity (loss of hearing and tinnitus), vestibular ototoxicity (dizziness and loss of balance), and peripheral neuritis (tingling of the fingers and toes); and the collaborative problems of hypersensitivity, nephrotoxicity (blood in urine, greatly increased or decreased frequency of urination and amount of urine), or neurotoxicity (muscle twitching, numbness, or seizures). With streptomycin only, there is the potential complication of optic neuritis.

Implementation

Monitoring. Elderly clients are at greater risk of nephrotoxicity and ototoxicity because of reduced renal function, and they generally require smaller daily doses. Loss of hearing, however, may occur in clients with normal renal function. Audiograms, renal function studies, and vestibular function studies should be done periodically during high-dose therapy or therapy over 10 days. Urinalyses should be monitored for the presence of albumin, casts, and cells and decreased specific gravity.

Monitor peak and trough drug levels routinely, since evidence suggests that the incidence of ototoxicity and nephrotoxicity with aminoglycosides correlates with slight elevations of either drug level but particularly with trough levels. The trough concentration is believed to be a more sensitive indicator of renal function than the serum creatinine.

For streptomycin only, caloric stimulation tests, may be required during and after prolonged therapy to detect vestibular toxicity.

Intervention. For intravenous administration, dilute appropriately and administer slowly over a 30 to 60 minute period to prevent neuromuscular blockade as the result of toxic serum levels. Clients should be well hydrated while taking these medications to minimize chemical irritation of the urinary tubules. Intake and output should be monitored. Daily urinalysis may be required during therapy for signs of renal irritation.

For intramuscular forms of the drugs, inject deeply into the upper outer quadrant of the gluteal muscle.

Education. Instruct the client to report any loss of hearing or any ringing or buzzing in the ears that would indicate ototoxicity; any change in urinary pattern or blood in the urine that would indicate nephrotoxicity; dizziness that would indicate vestibular toxicity; or numbness, tingling, or twitching that would indicate neurotoxicity. Stress the importance of taking the full course of medication as prescribed.

Evaluation. The client will maintain or achieve an infection free state as evidenced by negative cultures. If administered therapeutically, the client will also evidence a body temperature within normal limits, a WBC within the normal limits for age, and the resolution of any other infection-related symptoms that the client might be experiencing without adverse effects of the drug.

TETRACYCLINES

Tetracyclines were the first broad-spectrum antibiotics released in the United States. They include a large group of drugs that have a common basic structure and similar chemical activity.

demeclocycline [de me kloe sye' kleen] (Declomycin)
doxycycline [dox i sye' kleen] (Doxychel, Vibramycin)
minocycline [mi noe sye' kleen] (Minocin)
oxytetracycline [ox i tet ra sye' kleen] (Terramycin)
tetracycline [tet ra sye' kleen] (Achromycin V, Novotetra♣)

Tetracyclines are bacteriostatic for many gram-negative and gram-positive organisms; they exhibit cross-sensitivity and cross-resistance. Tetracyclines inhibit protein synthesis by blocking the binding of transfer RNA to the messenger RNA ribosome therefore inhibiting protein synthesis.

Demeclocycline also is used to treat the syndrome of inappropriate diuretic hormone because it inhibits the ADH-induced water reabsorption in the kidneys resulting in diuresis.

The tetracyclines have been commonly used to treat many infections such as acne vulgaris, actinomycosis, anthrax, bacterial urinary tract infections, bronchitis, and numerous systemic bacterial infections sensitive to the tetracyclines.

Oral tetracyclines are fairly well absorbed and distributed to most body fluids. Cerebrospinal fluid levels vary and can range from 10% to 25% of the plasma drug concentration following parenteral administration. Tetracyclines localize in teeth, liver, spleen, tumors, and bone. Doxycycline can reach clinical concentrations in the eye and prostate while minocycline results in high levels in saliva, sputum, and tears. Doxycycline and minocycline are inactivated in the liver, but most tetracyclines are excreted via the kidneys. Table 59-4 lists tetracycline half-life and usual adult dose.

■ Nursing Management

Tetracycline Therapy

In addition to nursing management common to all types of antimicrobial drug therapy, the nurse should observe the following measures when clients are receiving drugs of the tetracycline family.

Assessment. Tetracyclines are contraindicated in pregnant women, breastfeeding women, and children under 8 years of age because they cause permanent mottling and discoloration of the teeth and a decrease in linear skeletal growth rate in the fetus or child.

Clients with a hypersensitivity to one tetracycline may be hypersensitive to the others as well. In addition, clients with hypersensitivities to "caine-type" drugs, such as lidocaine or procaine, may be intolerant of the lidocaine in oxytetracycline injection or the procaine in the tetracycline intramuscular injection.

Use of tetracyclines in clients with renal impairment is not recommended (except for doxycycline and minocycline). Nephrogenic diabetes insipidus may worsen with the administration of demeclocycline.

Review the client's current medications for significant drug interactions that may occur when tetracyclines are given concurrently with the following drugs.

Drug	Possible effect and management
antacids; calcium supplements; choline and magnesium salicylates; iron supplements; magnesium salicylate or magnesium laxatives; foods containing milk and milk products	May result in nonabsorbable complex, thus reducing the absorption and serum levels of the antibiotic. Also, antacids may increase gastric pH, which decreases the absorption of tetracyclines. If given concurrently, advise clients to separate medications by 1-3 hours from the oral tetracyclines.
colestipol (Colestid), cholestyramine (Questran)	May bind oral tetracyclines thus decreasing their absorption. Separate drugs by at least 2 hours.
estrogen-containing oral contraceptives	Concurrent long-term therapy may reduce contraceptive effectiveness; also may result in breakthrough bleeding.

A baseline assessment as described in Chapter 58 should be done.

TABLE 59-4 Tetracycline: half-life and usual adult dose

Drug	Half-life*		Usual adult dose
	Normal	Anuric	
democlocycline (Declomycin)	10-17	40-60	150 mg q6h
doxycycline (Vibramycin)	12-22	12-22	100 mg bid on first day, then 100 to 200 mg daily (PO or IV infusion)
minocycline (Minocin)	11-23	11-23	200 mg initially, then 100 mg q12h (PO or IV infusion)
oxytetracycline (Terramycin)	6-10	47-66	250-500 mg PO q6h or 250-500 mg every 12 hours by IV infusion
tetracycline	6-11	57-108	250-500 mg PO q6h or 150 mg IM q12h

*Half-life in hours. *USP DI,* 1996.

Nursing diagnosis. Clients receiving tetracycline therapy should be assessed for the following nursing diagnoses: altered comfort (heartburn and abdominal cramping); fluid volume deficit related to anorexia, nausea and vomiting; altered bowel elimination (diarrhea); altered protection related to loss of normal flora (fungal overgrowth); and the collaborative problems of hypersensitivity, increased sensitivity of the skin to sunlight, and CNS toxicity (dizziness, syncope), nephrogenic diabetes insipidus, hepatotoxicity, and pancreatitis.

Implementation

Monitoring. Because the risk for superinfection is greater in tetracycline therapy than in therapy with other antimicrobial agents, observe clients carefully for signs and symptoms of secondary infections, especially *Candida* infections. Meticulous oral and perineal hygiene is helpful in preventing *Candida* superinfection.

Monitor the client's temperature, white blood cell count, cultures, and the symptoms of the infection.

Intervention. Tetracyclines should be taken with a full glass of water to prevent esophageal erosion and gastrointestinal irritation. Except for doxycycline and minocycline, they should be taken on an empty stomach (1 hour before or 2 hours after meals) for maximum effectiveness. Avoid administering antacids and laxatives containing aluminum, calcium, or magnesium; iron products; and food, milk, or other dairy products for 1 hour before and 2 hours after tetracycline administration, because they form nonabsorbable complexes with tetracyclines. Administer the oral suspension using the calibrated liquid-measuring device provided by the manufacturer.

Doxycycline may be administered intravenously in concentrations not less than 100 μg/ml or greater than 1 mg/ml, but not intramuscularly or subcutaneously. With oxytetracycline, dilute in at least 100 ml of appropriate IV solution and avoid rapid administration; do not give via IM or SC methods. Tetracycline may be administered via IM method, but not via IV or SC methods; the amount should not exceed 2 ml in each site.

Education. Stress the importance of taking the full course of the medication in evenly spaced doses to maintain serum levels. Photosensitivity may occur and persist for some time after discontinuance of the drug. Instruct the client to avoid direct sunlight and ultraviolet light. If exposure is unavoidable, a sun screen may help prevent a reaction. Alert client to appropriate dosing schedule in relation to food and to drug-drug and drug-food interactions. Instruct the client to discard outdated tetracyclines (show client where expiration date is found), since they become toxic as they decompose.

Evaluation. The client will maintain or achieve an infection free state as evidenced by negative culture results. If administered therapeutically, the client will also evidence a body temperature within normal limits, a WBC within the normal limits for age, and the resolution of any other infection-related symptoms that the client might be experiencing without adverse reactions from the drug.

CHLORAMPHENICOL (CHLOROMYCETIN)

Chloramphenicol, a broad spectrum antibiotic, is a potent inhibitor of protein synthesis. It is a bacteriostatic agent for a wide variety of gram-negative and gram-positive organisms; however, because it is potentially seriously toxic to bone marrow (aplasia leading to aplastic anemia and possibly death), its approved indications are limited.

While chloramphenicol is usually bacteriostatic, in high doses with highly susceptible organisms, it may be bactericidal. It penetrates bacteria cell membranes and reversibly prevents peptide bond formation, thus inhibiting protein synthesis.

It is indicated for the treatment of meningitis (*H. influenzae, S. pneumoniae,* and *N. meningitidis*), paratyphoid fever, Q fever, Rocky Mountain spotted fever, typhoid fever (*Salmonella typhi*), typhus infections, brain abscesses, and bacterial septicemia.

Chloramphenicol has good oral and parenteral bioavailability with highest concentrations reported in the liver and kidneys. Concentrations of up to 50% of serum levels have been noted in cerebrospinal fluid. The palmitate and sodium succinate forms of chloramphenicol are hydrolyzed to free drug in the intestinal tract or the plasma, liver, lungs, and kidneys, respectively. Chloramphenicol is metabolized in the liver to the inactive glucuronide, but in utero and in neonates an immature liver cannot conjugate chloramphenicol, which may result in toxic levels or accumulation of the active drug ("gray syndrome"—blue-gray skin, hypothermia, irregular breathing, coma, cardiovascular collapse).

Half-life of chloramphenicol in an adult is 1.5 to 3.5 hours; in infants (1 to 2 days old) it is 1 to 2 days or more. In infants 10 to 16 days old it is 10 hours. Peak serum levels are reached in 1 to 1.5 hours via the intravenous route or 1 to 3 hours after an oral dose. Chloramphenicol is excreted mainly by the kidneys.

Infrequent side effects of chloramphenicol include diarrhea, nausea, or vomiting. Serious adverse effects include blood dyscrasias, optic neuritis, and possibly, irreversible bone marrow depression that may result in aplastic anemia.

The oral/intravenous adult dosage is 12.5 mg/kg every 6 hours. Pediatric oral/intravenous dosage for premature and full-term infants up to 2 weeks old is 6.25 mg/kg every 6 hours. For infants 2 weeks old and over, it is 12.5 mg/kg every 6 hours. Chloramphenicol is not recommended for use during pregnancy or during breastfeeding.

■ Nursing Management

Chloramphenicol Therapy

The general nursing management for the administration of antibiotic therapy should be applied to chloramphenicol therapy.

Assessment. Consider carefully before using chloramphenicol in clients with bone marrow depression or clients who have had previous cytotoxic drug or radiation therapy because it may cause a dose-related bone marrow depression, aplastic anemia, and other blood dyscrasias. Complete blood counts are necessary for a baseline assessment before therapy. Clients with hepatic and renal function impairment will require a reduction in dose.

Review the client's current medications for significant drug interactions that may occur when chloramphenicol is given concurrently with the following drugs.

Drug	Possible effect and management
alfentanil (Alfenta)	May result in increased alfentanil blood levels, prolonging its effect. Monitor closely.
anticonvulsants, hydantoin; blood dyscrasia-causing drugs, bone marrow depressants; radiation therapy	May result in enhanced bone marrow depressant effects. Dosage reduction may be necessary. Monitor CBCs closely for leukopenia.
antidiabetic oral agents	May inhibit antidiabetic drug metabolism resulting in increased serum levels and hypoglycemic effects of tolbutamide and chlorpropamide. Monitor closely blood glucose levels because dosage adjustment may be necessary.
clindamycin, erythromycin, or lincomycin	Therapeutic action of chloramphenicol and these drugs may be antagonized. Avoid this drug combination.
phenobarbital (Luminal), phenytoin (Dilantin), or warfarin (Coumadin)	Concurrent drug administration may result in elevated drug serum levels and toxicity of these agents. Monitor all drugs metabolized by the liver enzyme system (chloramphenicol inhibits the cytochrome P-450 system) because toxicity may result.

A baseline assessment as described in Chapter 58 should be done.

Nursing diagnosis. Clients receiving chloramphenicol therapy should be assessed for the following nursing diagnoses: fluid volume deficit related to anorexia, nausea and vomiting; altered protection related to dose-related bone marrow depression (leukopenia, thrombocytopenia, anemia); altered bowel elimination (diarrhea); altered thought processes (confusion, delirium) related to neurotoxic reactions; sensory-perceptual disturbances related to optic neuritis (blurred vision, loss of vision, eye pain), and to peripheral neuritis (tingling, numbness, and burning pain of the hands and feet); and the collaborative problems of hypersensitivity (rash, fever, dyspnea) and "gray syndrome" in neonates only.

Implementation

Monitoring. Monitor periodic complete blood counts for dose-related reversible bone marrow depression; reticulocytopenia, leukopenia, thrombocytopenia, decreased RBC. Clinically observe the client for pale skin, sore throat and fever, unusual bruising or bleeding, or unusual fatigue. CBCs are not helpful in predicting drug-related aplastic anemia, which usually occurs after the completion of treatment.

Monitor serum chloramphenicol levels, which should be in the range of 10 to 25 µg/ml, the most effective concentration. Concentrations higher than 30 µg/ml increase the risk of bone marrow depression and gray syndrome.

Intervention. Administer chloramphenicol with a full glass of water on an empty stomach (1 hour before meals or 2 hours after) to maximize effectiveness. When administering the oral suspension, use the calibrated liquid-measuring device provided by the manufacturer. If administered intravenously, the drug should be infused over at least a 1-minute period. Check the intravenous site daily for local irritation.

Education. Because the bone marrow depressant effects of chloramphenicol may increase gingival bleeding and delay healing, instruct the client to delay dental work until blood counts return to normal. Instruct all clients in proper oral hygiene, with cautious use of toothbrushes, dental floss, and toothpicks.

Advise the client to report to prescriber immediately any symptoms of blood dyscrasia, such as sore throat, fever, extreme fatigue, or unusual bleeding or bruising. Alert clients to report activity intolerance and other signs of anemia that may occur weeks or months after therapy because they are indicative of drug-related aplastic anemia.

Caution clients who test their urine with copper sulfate glucose tests (Clinitest tablets) that they may get false-positive reactions. For the course of the antibiotic therapy, recommend the use of Clinistix or Keto-diastix.

Evaluation. The client will maintain or achieve an infection free state as evidenced by negative cultures. If administered therapeutically, the client will also evidence a body temperature within normal limits, a WBC within the normal limits for age, and the resolution of any other infection-related symptoms that the client might be experiencing without adverse effects of the drug.

FLUOROQUINOLONES

Fluoroquinolones are synthetic, broad spectrum agents with bactericidal activity. They alter DNA by interfering with the DNA gyrase, an enzyme necessary for duplication, transcription and repair of bacterial DNA. Examples of quinolones include ▲ ciprofloxacin [sip ro flocks' a sin] (Cipro); enoxacin [a nocks' a sin] (Penetrex); lomefloxacin [lome flocks' a sin] (Maxaquin); norfloxacin [nor flocks' a sin] (Noroxin); and ofloxacin [o flocks' a sin] (Floxin).

The fluoroquinolones are indicated for the treatment of bone and joint, bronchitis, gastroenteritis, gonorrhea, pneumonia, urinary tract, and many other infections caused by susceptible microorganisms. Individual fluoroquinolones may vary in their spectrum of activity, for example, all five drugs are indicated for the treatment of urinary tract infections but only ciprofloxacin is approved to treat bone and joint infections. Therefore the nurse is referred to current references for approved individual drug indications.

The oral bioavailability of fluoroquinolones is good and they are widely distributed in the body with the following half-lives: ciprofloxacin, 4 hours; enoxacin, 3 to 6 hours; lomefloxacin, 7 to 8 hours; norfloxacin, 3 to 4 hours; and ofloxacin, 4 to 7 hours. They are metabolized in the liver (minimally for ofloxacin and lomefloxacin) and excreted primarily by the kidneys.

Significant side effects of fluoroquinolones include dizziness, drowsiness, restlessness, stomach distress, diarrhea, nausea and vomiting. Rare adverse effects include psychosis, confusion, hallucinations, tremors, hypersensitivity, and interstitial nephritis.

The usual adult ciprofloxacin dose is 500 to 750 mg PO, every 12 hours for 1 to 2 weeks; intravenous dose is 400 mg every 12 hours; enoxacin dose is 200 to 400 mg every 12 hours for 1 to 2 weeks; lomefloxacin dose is 400 mg daily for 10 to 14 days; norfloxacin dose is 400 mg every 12 hours for 72 hours; ofloxacin dose is 300 to 400 mg PO or IV, every 12 hours for 10 days. Fluoroquinolones are not recommended for use in infants and children.

■ Nursing Management

Fluoroquinolone Therapy

The general nursing management for the administration of antibiotic therapy should be applied to fluoroquinolone therapy.

Assessment. If a client has had an allergic reaction to any of the fluoroquinolones, they are contraindicated because of cross-sensitivity. Clients with hepatic or renal impairment may require reduced dosages. With CNS disorders such as cerebral arteriosclerosis or epilepsy, or with alcoholism, use the fluoroquinolones with caution because of the risk of CNS toxicity.

Review the client's current medications for significant drug interactions that occur when fluoroquinolones are given concurrently with the following drugs.

Drug	Possible effect and management
antacids, ferrous sulfate or sucralfate	May decrease absorption of ciprofloxacin, reducing drug effectiveness. Administer fluoroquinolones at least 2 hours before these medications.
theophylline and other xanthines	Fluoroquinolones (with the possible exception of lomefloxacin and ofloxacin) may result in increased theophylline plasma levels and toxicity. Monitor theophylline plasma levels closely because dosage adjustments may be necessary.
warfarin	May result in increase anticoagulant effect and potential for bleeding. While not currently reported with all quinolones, it is recommended that prothrombin time (PT) be monitored closely whenever these drugs are administered concurrently.

A baseline assessment as described in Chapter 58 should be done.

Nursing diagnosis. Clients receiving fluoroquinolone therapy should be assessed for the following nursing diagnoses: fluid volume deficit related to anorexia, nausea and vomiting; altered comfort related to arthralgia (joint discomfort, stiffness); impaired tissue integrity related to phlebitis (IV ciprofloxacin and ofloxacin only); altered bowel elimination (diarrhea); altered thought processes related to CNS stimulation (confusion, hallucinations); and the collaborative problems of hypersensitivity (rash, itching, swelling of face), interstitial nephritis (blood in the urine, lower back pain, rash, edema), photosensitivity (increased sensitivity of skin to sunlight), and CNS toxicity (dizziness, headache, insomnia).

Implementation

Monitoring. Monitor the client for signs and symptoms of adverse reactions. Monitor urinary pH because ciprofloxacin becomes more insoluble in an alkaline medium (greater than 7.0), resulting in crystalluria. Monitor client's temperature, WBC counts, cultures, and the symptoms of the infection.

Intervention. Administer drug with a full glass of water. Ensure that the client maintains a urinary output of at least 1200 to 1500 ml daily for adults to minimize the occurrence of crystalluria.

IV ciprofloxacin and ofloxacin should be infused slowly into a large vein over 60 minutes to minimize discomfort and venous irritation.

Education. Stress the importance of taking a full course of therapy, taking all doses as prescribed at evenly spaced intervals to maintain therapeutic serum levels.

Advise the client to report dizziness, lightheadedness, or depression, since these signs indicate CNS toxicity. Visual disturbances such as blurred or double vision and increased light sensitivity should be reported for the same reason.

Avoid taking antacids and fluoroquinolones within 2 hours of each other. With ciprofloxacin, advise the client that photosensitivity is a possible effect of this drug; avoid exposure to sun and sunlamps. However, with norfloxacin photophobia is a concern; advise the client to wear sunglasses and avoid exposure to bright light.

Because visual disturbances, dizziness, lightheadedness, or drowsiness may occur, advise the client to limit activities that require alertness and dexterity until the response to the drug has been determined.

Evaluation. The client will maintain or achieve an infection free state as evidenced by negative cultures. If administered therapeutically, the client will also evidence a body temperature within normal limits, a WBC within the normal limits for age, and the resolution of any other infection-related symptoms that the client might be experiencing without adverse effects of the drug.

MISCELLANEOUS ANTIBIOTICS

This section includes a monobactam, aztreonam; a carbapenem, imipenem-cilastatin; metronidazole; and spectinomycin. Other antibiotics in current use are primarily topical agents, which are discussed in Chapter 66.

aztreonam [az tree' oh nam] (Azactam)

Aztreonam, the first drug in a monobactam class of antibiotics is a synthetic bactericidal antibiotic with activity similar to penicillin. It binds to the penicillin binding protein, resulting in inhibition of bacterial cell wall synthesis, cell lysis, and death. It is active against many gram-negative microorganisms and is used in the treatment of urinary tract, bronchitis, intraabdominal, gynecologic, and skin infections. Most frequently reported side effects include gastric distress, diarrhea, nausea, and vomiting. Less frequently reported effects include hypersensitivity and thrombophlebitis at the site of injection. Administered intravenously, the adult dose is 0.5 to 2 g IV or IM, every 8 to 12 hours.

See penicillins for nursing management of aztreonam, except there are no cautions for significant drug interactions.

imipenem-cilastatin [i mi pen' em-sye la stat' in] (Primaxin IM; Primaxin IV)

Imipenem-cilastatin, a member of a new class of carbapenem antibiotics related to the beta-lactam antibiotics, has a wide spectrum of activity against gram-positive, gram-negative aerobic and anaerobic organisms. Imipenem binds to penicillin-binding proteins thus inhibiting bacterial cell wall synthesis. It is very resistant to degradation by beta-lactamases. Cilastatin inhibits renal dihydropeptidase and blocks the tubular secretion of imipenem thus preventing renal metabolism of this drug. Therefore cilastatin is combined with imipenem to prevent its inactivation by renal dihydropeptidase.

This antibiotic is indicated for the treatment of bone, joint, skin, and soft tissue infections, bacterial endocarditis, intraabdominal bacteria infections, pneumonia, urinary tract and pelvic infections, and bacterial septicemia when caused by susceptible bacterial organisms.

Administered intramuscularly, imipenem time to peak serum level is within 2 hours with a half-life of 2 to 3 hours. Intravenously, the half-life is about 60 minutes. Excretion is primarily by the kidneys. No significant drug interactions have been reported to date with this product.

Significant side/adverse effects of imipenem-cilastatin include gastric distress, diarrhea, nausea, vomiting, allergic type reactions, confusion, lightheadedness, convulsions, and tremors. Pseudomembranous colitis has also been reported with this product.

The usual adult IV infusion dosage is 250 to 500 mg every 6 hours for mild infections to 500 mg every 6 to 8 hours for moderate to severe infections. Maximum dose is 50 mg of imipenem/kg daily. The IM adult dosage is 500 to 750 mg every 12 hours up to a maximum of 1500 mg/day. The dosage for children up to the age of 12 is not determined while older children may receive the adult dose.

The second carbapenem antibiotic released is meropenem (Box 59-3).

■ Nursing Management

Imipenem-Cilastatin Therapy

The general nursing management for the administration of antibiotic therapy should be applied to imipenem-cilastatin therapy.

Assessment. Use with caution with clients with allergy to imipenem, cilastatin or other beta-lactams, such as penicillin and cephalosporins. Clients with CNS disorders, such as history of seizures, are more likely to experience CNS side effects. Clients with renal function impairment require reduced dosages.

Nursing diagnosis. Clients receiving this drug should be assessed for the following nursing diagnoses: risk of injury related to infusion rate reaction due to too rapid an infusion rate (dizziness, diaphoresis, fatigue, nausea and vomiting); altered mucous membranes (glossitis); fluid volume deficit related to nausea, vomiting, and diarrhea; diarrhea; impaired tissue integrity related to thrombophlebitis at infusion site; and the collaborative problems of allergic reactions (rash, hives, fever, dyspnea), CNS toxicity (confusion, dizziness, tremors, seizures), and pseudomembranous colitis (severe abdominal cramps and diarrhea, fever).

Implementation

Monitoring. Monitor for adverse reactions as described above. Monitor clients receiving more than 2 g daily because they are at higher risk for seizures. Observe the client's temperature, WBC counts, cultures and symptoms related to the client's infection.

BOX 59-3

Meropenem (Merrem IV)

Meropenem (Merrem IV) is a bactericidal, broad-spectrum carbapenem antibiotic. It inhibits cell-wall synthesis and is indicated for the treatment of susceptible intraabdominal infections (complicated appendicitis and peritonitis) and bacterial meningitis.

Pseudomembranous colitis, hypersensitivity, and side/adverse effects of diarrhea, nausea, vomiting, headache, and rash have been reported. Adult dose is 1 g IV every 8 hours (Olin, 1997).

Intervention. To minimize the occurrence of imipenem/cilastatin combination infusion rate reaction, doses of 250 to 500 mg of imipenem should be administered over 20 to 30 minutes, 1 g over 40 to 60 minutes; in children, over a 20 to 30 minute period.

Education. Alert the client to report early symptoms of adverse reactions.

Evaluation. The client will maintain or achieve an infection free state as evidenced by negative cultures. If administered therapeutically, the client will also evidence a body temperature within normal limits, a WBC within the normal limits for age, and the resolution of any other infection-related symptoms that the client might be experiencing without adverse effects of the drug.

metronidazole [me troe ni' da zole] (Flagyl, Flagyl I.V.)
Metronidazole is reduced intracellularly to a short-acting, cytotoxic agent that interacts with DNA, thus inhibiting bacteria synthesis resulting in cell death (microbicidal). It is active against many anaerobic bacteria and protozoa.

It is indicated for the treatment of amebiasis (intestinal and extraintestinal), antibiotic-associated pseudomembranous colitis (AAPMC), bone infections, brain abscesses, CNS infections, bacterial endocarditis, genitourinary tract infections, septicemia, trichomoniasis, and other infections caused by organisms susceptible to metronidazole's action.

Oral metronidazole is well absorbed and distributed throughout the body. It reaches peak serum levels within 1 to 2 hours and has a half life of 8 hours. It is metabolized in the liver and primarily excreted in the kidneys.

Significant side effects of metronidazole include dizziness, headache, gastric distress, diarrhea, anorexia, nausea and vomiting. Less frequent and rare adverse effects include peripheral neuropathy, central nervous system toxicity, leukopenia, thrombophlebitis, and vaginal candidiasis.

The usual adult oral dose is 7.5 mg/kg up to maximum of 1 g, every 6 hours for a week or longer. The adult IV infusion dose is 15 mg/kg initially, then 7.5 mg/kg up to a maximum of 1 g, every 6 hours for a week or longer. Maximum daily dose is 4 g.

■ Nursing Management
Metronidazole Therapy

The general nursing management for the administration of antibiotic therapy should be applied to metronidazole therapy.

Assessment. Because metronidazole may cause CNS toxicity, any individual with active organic CNS disease, such as epilepsy, should be carefully evaluated before treatment with the drug. With clients who have their sodium intake restricted, the sodium content of the parenteral dosage forms should be considered. Clients with a history of blood dyscrasias should be monitored carefully because metronidazole may cause leukopenia. Reduced dosages may be required for clients with hepatic dysfunction. To use metronidazole for giardiasis, the organism should be identified.

Review the client's current medications for significant drug interactions such as when metronidazole is given concurrently with the following drugs.

Drug	Possible effect and management
alcohol	**Metronidazole interferes with the metabolism of alcohol, leading to an accumulation of acetaldehyde. This may result in disulfiram (Antabuse)-type effects: flushing, headaches, nausea, vomiting, and abdominal distress. Avoid or a potentially serious drug interaction may occur.**
anticoagulants (coumarin or indanedione)	May enhance anticoagulant effects by inhibiting their metabolism. Monitor closely with prothrombin tests if given concurrently. Dosage adjustments may be necessary.
disulfiram (Antabuse)	**Avoid concurrent use or use within 14 days of disulfiram administration in alcoholic clients. Adverse reactions such as confusion and psychosis have been reported.**

A baseline assessment as described in Chapter 58 should be done.

Nursing diagnosis. The client receiving metronidazole should be assessed for the following nursing diagnoses: altered comfort (headache and unpleasant metallic taste); fluid volume deficit related to anorexia, nausea, vomiting, and diarrhea; impaired tissue integrity related to the development of thrombophlebitis (IV administration only); altered protection related to leukopenia and loss of normal flora (fungal overgrowth); sensory-perceptual disturbances related to peripheral neuropathy (numbness, tingling, and pain in the hands and feet); altered thought processes related to CNS toxicity (confusion, mood changes); and the collaborative problems of hypersensitivity (rash, itching), seizures related to high doses, and pancreatitis (severe abdominal pain, nausea and vomiting).

Implementation

Monitoring. Assess clients periodically for symptoms of peripheral neuropathy such as numbness and tingling of the hands or feet. Mood changes and irritability also indicate CNS toxicity.

Monitor complete blood counts frequently for blood dyscrasia and instruct the client to report immediately to the prescriber any symptoms of sore throat, unusual tiredness or weakness, or unusual bleeding or bruising.

If metronidazole is administered for giardiasis, three stool examinations taken several days apart, beginning 1 to 2 weeks after treatment, should be accomplished to determine the success of therapy. Additional specimens may be required if symptoms persist.

Intervention. Administer oral forms with meals to minimize gastrointestinal irritation. Parenteral metronidazole is to be administered by slow intravenous infusion. It may be administered continuously or intermittently over a 1-hour period. If administered concurrently with a primary IV, the primary IV should be discontinued while the metronidazole is infused. The sodium content of the parenteral forms of the drug should be considered in the sodium intake for clients who have their sodium intake restricted.

Education. Advise the client that the drug may cause an unpleasant taste in the mouth, diminished taste sensation, and a dry mouth. The use of sugar-free candies, ice cubes, and frequent mouth rinses may bring some relief to the client. If therapy is long-term, dry mouth may contribute to dental caries and gum disease, and the client should receive regular dental checkups.

Stress the importance of completing a full course of therapy, even though the client may be feeling well and be symptom free. The doses should be evenly spaced to ensure therapeutic serum levels are maintained.

Advise the client not to ingest alcoholic beverages while taking metronidazole, because a disulfiram-like effect may result (flushing, nausea and vomiting, and abdominal cramping).

If metronidazole is being prescribed for trichomoniasis, the client will need to prevent reinfection from her male partner. He will need concurrent drug therapy and to use a condom until the infection is resolved in both partners.

Advise the client that the urine may turn a darker color, but this change is not medically significant.

Evaluation. The client will maintain or achieve an infection free state as evidenced by negative culture results. If administered therapeutically, the client will also evidence a body temperature within normal limits, a WBC within the normal limits for age, and the resolution of any other infection-related symptoms that the client might be experiencing without adverse effects of the drug.

spectinomycin [spek ti noe mye' sin] (Trobicin)
Spectinomycin's therapeutic indication is the treatment of infections caused by *Neisseria gonorrhoeae*. It is bacteriostatic because it inhibits protein synthesis in the bacteria cell. It is for intramuscular use only and generally is recommended as an alternate regimen for individuals with gonorrhea that have antibiotic resistance or cannot take ceftriaxone.

It is not effective for treating syphilis and should not be used for mixed infections (gonorrhea and syphilis), since it can mask the symptoms of syphilis. Side/adverse effects include chills, fever, nausea, dizziness and urticaria. Usual adult dose is 2 g IM as a single dose, followed by doxycycline or in pregnant women, erythromycin (Olin, 1996).

■ Nursing Management
Spectinomycin Therapy

The general nursing management for the administration of antibiotic therapy should be applied to spectinomycin therapy.

Assessment. Spectinomycin is contraindicated if the client has a hypersensitivity to the drug. This drug was used for the treatment of gonococcal infections in children; however, the diluent to reconstitute spectinomycin contains 0.945% benzyl alcohol, which has been associated with fatal gasping syndrome in infants.

Nursing diagnosis. The client may experience the following during spectinomycin therapy: risk for injury related to dizziness, altered comfort (pain at the site of injection, abdominal cramping); fluid volume deficit related to nausea and vomiting.

Implementation

Monitoring. Observe the client for 45 to 60 minutes after injection because anaphylaxis has been reported. Monitor the client with a gonococcal infection for concurrent syphilis by serologic examination at the beginning of therapy and after 3 months. Obtain cultures of gonococcal infection sites to monitor for the effectiveness of therapy.

Intervention. Spectinomycin is for IM use only. Agitate vial thoroughly to ensure even suspension of the drug. Administer deep IM in the ventrogluteal site or vastus lateralis site. Inject the suspension using a 20-gauge needle, only 5 ml in each site.

Education. Caution the client that dizziness may occur and to plan activities to avoid operating hazardous equipment until the drug's vertigo effects are known. The client should be instructed to use a condom with their partner to prevent infection, and it may be necessary to treat the partner concurrently to prevent reinfection.

Evaluation. Gonococcal infection sites should evidence negative culture results after 3 to 7 days.

URINARY TRACT ANTIMICROBIALS

Urinary tract infections (UTI) are the most common bacterial infections reported in the United States. Between 10% to 20% of women will experience at least one urinary tract infection in their lifetime. The incidence of UTIs increases in institutional settings, up to as much as 35% to 40% of the population in extended stay hospitals (Sahai, 1995). (See Box 59-4 for predisposing risk factors for UTIs.)

Differentiation between an upper UTI (pyelonephritis) and lower UTI (cystitis) infection is usually based on the presenting signs and symptoms. The upper UTI usually causes pain in the lower back, flank, or stomach, plus fever, sweating, nausea, vomiting, weakness, and headache. A lower UTI presents with complaints of a pattern of frequent but small amounts on urination, urgency, dysuria, and perhaps, incontinence. However, in approximately a third of UTIs, the infection may be present both in the upper and lower urinary tract. Urinary tract infections are primarily caused by bacteria.

In community-acquired infections, most UTIs are caused by gram-negative aerobic bacilli from the intestinal tract, such as *Escherichia coli*. It has been reported that *E. coli* may cause up to 90% of all community-acquired, uncomplicated UTIs (Sahai, 1995). Hospital-acquired infections are often complicated and difficult to treat. Organisms involved include *Pseudomonas aeruginosa*, *Serratia*, *Enterobacter* and other gram-negative microorganisms.

BOX 59-4

Predisposing Risk Factors for UTIs

Risk factors	Frequency Reported
urinary tract instrumentation (urethral and ureteral catheterization)*	up to 67%
pregnant women	4%-10%
nonpregnant women	2%-5%

*After a week of indwelling catheterization, up to 100% colonization and bacteriuria (Ahronheim, 1992).

Drug therapies for lower UTIs are often started before culture and sensitivity reports are known. The most probable infecting organism and the antibiotic sensitivity can be predicted from the previous information.

Today with the increasing development of antibiotic resistance, the medications that are most effective for UTIs are the sulfonamides, such as ▲ trimethoprim-sulfamethoxazole (TMP-SMX) and cephalosporins. Alternate medications include the urinary tract antiseptics, aztreonam, and fluoroquinolones whereas phenazopyridine (Pyridium) is used primarily as a urinary tract analgesic.

■ Nursing Management

Urinary Antimicrobial Therapy

Assessment. Initial assessment of the client provides baseline information and includes history of past UTIs and the signs and symptoms of the current UTI. Drug allergies, concurrent drug therapy, or altered function of any body system may affect the drug therapy.

Nursing diagnosis. The client receiving urinary antimicrobial therapy is at risk for the following nursing diagnoses: risk for injury related to a preexisting health condition, drug interaction, or side/adverse effect of the drug; knowledge deficit related to the antimicrobial therapy; and ineffective management of the therapeutic regimen. See the Nursing Care Plan below for other selected nursing diagnosis.

Implementation

Monitoring. Periodic assessment should include the client's health status relating to fever, chills, flank pain, and nausea and vomiting; frequency and urgency of urination; dysuria; costovertebral tenderness; gross hematuria and pyuria; and general well-being. Urinalyses should be monitored for WBCs, RBCs, casts, protein, crystals, and bacteria. Urine culture and sensitivity examinations should indicate the drug's efficacy. CBCs should also be monitored. Serum antibiotic concentrations can be monitored during the course of therapy to assess for therapeutic and toxic levels of specific antimicrobials. In addition to monitoring the therapeutic effects of these antimicrobials, the nurse must assess the client for the development of common side effects/adverse reactions of individual drugs. See discussions of specific drugs for these effects.

Intervention. Nursing interventions relative to antimicrobial drug therapy were discussed in greater detail in Chapter 58. Generally, these interventions relate to (1) assistance in the identification of the infecting organism, (2) actual administration of the drug, (3) assessment of the client's response to the drug, (4) client education, and (5) prevention and treatment of the adverse responses, including pharmacologic and chemical drug-drug interactions. Obtaining urine specimens to determine the causative organism for UTI is frequently the nurse's responsibility. Through client education most clients can obtain a clean-catch urine sample of appropriate quantity and quality for laboratory testing. The health care provider will specify whether a midstream clean-catch or catheterized specimen is required. In either case it is essential that the procedure be done appropriately to ensure the most accurate results. A basic nursing text should be consulted for these procedures. Specimens for culture should be taken directly to the labo-

Nursing Care Plan

Selected Nursing Diagnoses Related to Administration of Urinary Tract Antimicrobials

Nursing diagnosis	Outcome criteria	Nursing interventions
Infection, risk for	Prevention of infection or resolution of symptoms of infection:	
	Temperature remains within the normal range	Monitor and record temperature at least every 4 hours. Report elevations.
	WBC remains within the normal range.	Monitor WBCs. Report significant changes.
	Urine cultures demonstrate no pathogens.	Culture urine as ordered and monitor results.
	Urine is clear and odorless.	Use strict aseptic technique when inserting urinary catheters.
	Fluid intake of 3000 ml/24 hr.	Encourage a fluid intake of at least 3000 ml daily.
Knowledge deficit related to medication regimen	Client will describe underlying conditions and how the drug relates to the condition, how and when to take the medication, common drug interactions, safety precautions, common side effects/adverse reactions, and which of these warrant reporting.	Assess learning needs and learning readiness. Plan with client for the achievement of realistic goals. Provide information to meet outcome criteria. Administer medication with food or milk to decrease GI distress. Alert client that medication may cause a discoloration of the urine.
	Self-administer medication safely and accurately.	Instruct client to take medication as ordered and to consult with the prescriber if no improvement is seen within a few days.

ratory to prevent death of the suspect organisms and to prevent the growth of contaminating ones.

If an antimicrobial agent is ordered before the infecting organism has been identified, it is important that the urine sample for initial culture be obtained before the first dose of the drug is administered. With subsequent specimens for culture, it is important to describe the client's antimicrobial regimen for the laboratory because the selection and interpretation of laboratory tests often depend on this information.

Because around-the-clock administration of antimicrobial drugs at prescribed intervals is required for maintaining therapeutic blood levels of these drugs, it is the nurse's responsibility to see that this is accomplished. This is done by providing the necessary client education, which may entail awakening sleeping clients and ensuring that tests or therapies do not interrupt the dosing schedule.

Education. Clients should be taught the principles of antimicrobial therapy so that these drugs can be self-administered safely. The necessity of adherence to an inconvenient around-the-clock schedule may require special reenforcement. Compliance for the full course of therapy is essential to prevent the possible development of resistant strains of microorganisms. "Leftover" antimicrobial medications should not be used for new bouts of UTI, but disposed of properly. The prescriber should be consulted for any new bouts of infection. For specific instructions for each drug, refer to the text.

Instruct the client to avoid coffee, tea, juices with high citric acid content, cola, alcohol, chocolate, and spices, which often irritate a sensitive bladder. Daily fluid intake for a client with a UTI should be at least 3000 ml, unless contraindicated, to help flush the urinary tract of organisms. The client should be taught health practices that may reduce the chance of developing another UTI (Box 59-5).

Evaluation. Evaluation of the client for therapeutic responses to antimicrobial agents is a primary nursing responsibility. A decrease in the severity or a disappearance of the clinical and laboratory manifestations of the UTI indicates a positive response to antimicrobial therapy (e.g., absence of pathogen on cultures; normothermia; WBC within the normal range; and absence of urgency, frequency, and burning of urination).

BOX 59-5

Client Education to Reduce Occurrence of UTIs

UTIs frequently occur as a result of contamination of the lower urinary tract with perineal bacteria. Preventive measures attempt to reduce perineal bacteria and prevent bacteria from entering the lower urinary tract. Client education should focus on these two measures and include the following instructions:

1. Good perineal hygiene helps reduce bacterial growth.
2. Female clients should always wipe from the front to the back to prevent contamination of the urinary tract with fecal bacteria.
3. Emptying the bladder soon after intercourse helps wash out bacteria that may have entered the urethra.
4. Cotton undergarments (or synthetics with a cotton crotch) that "breathe" are preferred to synthetics that foster bacterial growth.
5. Drinking six to eight glasses of fluids per day and urinating often helps to cleanse the urinary tract of bacteria.

SULFONAMIDES

Sulfonamides (TMP-SMX is most commonly used) are among the most widely used antibacterial agents in the world, particularly for UTI. These agents are primarily **bacteriostatic,** in concentrations that are normally useful in controlling infections in the human being rather than **bactericidal.** All the sulfonamides used therapeutically are synthetically produced and because they are structurally similar to paraaminobenzoic acid (PABA), they inhibit a bacterial enzyme (dihydropteroate synthetase) necessary to incorporate PABA into dihydrofolic acid.

The blocking of dihydrofolic acid synthesis results in a decrease in tetrahydrofolic acid, which interferes with the synthesis of purines, thymidine, and DNA in the microorganism. Therefore, bacteria most sensitive to sulfonamides are those that synthesize their own folic acid. The presence of pus, necrotic tissue, and serum interferes with the activities of the sulfonamides because PABA is present in such materials. Among the microorganisms highly susceptible to sulfonamides are group A beta-hemolytic streptococci, pneumococci, *Neisseria meningitides, N. gonorrhoeae, E. coli, Pasteurella pestis, Bacillus anthracis, Shigella* species, *Haemophilus influenzae,* and *Pneumocystis carinii.*

The absorption of sulfonamides is good, with peak serum levels reached between 2 to 6 hours for the majority of them; and 6 to 12 hours for sulfamethoxazole, the intermediate acting sulfonamide. These agents are acetylated in the liver and excreted primarily by the kidneys.

While the newer sulfonamides, such as sulfisoxazole and sulfacetamide, are quite soluble (even in acid urine), it is recommended that individuals increase their fluid intake in order to maintain a urine output of at least 1200 ml/day (*USP DI,* 1996).

Table 59-5 describes side/adverse effects and usual adult dose range, for urinary tract agents.

■ Nursing Management

Sulfonamide Therapy

In addition to instituting the nursing management common to all types of antimicrobial therapy for UTIs, the nurse should observe the following considerations for individuals receiving sulfonamides.

Assessment. Although cross-sensitization with sulfonamides is not as severe as among penicillins, it is safer to avoid all sulfonamides in clients who develop hypersensitivity to any one agent. Cross-sensitivity also exists with some diuretics, such as acetazolamide and the thiazides, and

TABLE 59-5 Urinary tract agents: Side/adverse effects and usual adult dose

Drug	Usual adult dose	Side/adverse effects
Sulfonamides		*Common:* anorexia, diarrhea, nausea, vomiting, dizziness, headaches, pruritus, rash
sulfadiazine (generic)	2-4 g PO initially, then 1 g q4-6h	
sulfamethizole (Thiosulfil Forte)	0.5-1 g PO q6-8h	*Less common:* muscle & joint pain, fever, sore throat, Stevens-Johnson syndrome, pain on urination, increased bleeding tendencies
sulfamethoxazole (Gantanol)	2 g PO initially, then 1 g q8-12h	
sulfisoxazole (Gantrisin)	2-4 g PO initially, then 0.75 to 1.5 g q4h	
Antiseptics		
cinoxacin (Cinobac)	250 mg PO q hs	*Less common:* nausea, rash, pruritus, diarrhea, anorexia, vomiting, photosensitivity, tinnitus, insomnia
methenamine mandelate (Mandelamine)	1 g PO qid	*Less common:* nausea, rash, stomach distress,
methenamine hippurate (Hiprex)	1 g PO bid	painful urination, low back pain
nalidixic acid (NegGram)	1 g PO q6h	*Common:* diarrhea, nausea, vomiting, rash, pruritus, headache, drowsiness *Less common:* visual disturbances, such as, double or blurred vision, halos or very bright appearance around lights
nitrofurantoin (Furadantin)	50-100 mg PO q6h	*Common:* stomach distress, diarrhea, anorexia, nausea, vomiting, and pneumonitis
Analgesic		
phenazopyridine (Pyridium, Phenazo♣)	200 mg PO tid	*Less common:* stomach cramps or distress, headache *Rare:* hemolytic anemia, renal failure, hepatotoxicity, aseptic meningitis

with sulfonylurea antidiabetic agents, so, as always, the nurse should obtain an accurate history of the client's sensitivities. Avoid sulfonamide use in clients with hepatic and renal dysfunction, blood dyscrasias, glucose-6-phosphate dehydrogenase deficiency, and porphyria. Administration of sulfonamides is contraindicated in neonates. See Pregnancy Safety box on p. 906 for FDA categories of antimicrobials used for UTIs.

The client's current medication regimen should be reviewed for significant drug interactions:

Drug	Possible effect and management
anticoagulants, such as coumarin or indanedione derivatives; anticonvulsants (hydantoin); oral antidiabetic agents, or methotrexate	These agents are highly protein bound; concurrent drug administration may displace them from their protein-binding sites, resulting in increased serum levels and possible toxicity. Metabolism of these agents may also be inhibited by sulfonamides. Monitor closely for signs of toxicity, which indicate need for dosage adjustments.
hemolytics, other	Increased potential for toxicity. Monitor closely.
hepatotoxic medications	Increased risk of inducing liver toxicity. Closely monitor for symptoms, such as yellow eyes or skin.
methenamine (Mandelamine)	Methenamine requires an acid urine to be active and effective. It may precipitate if given with a sulfonamide and result in crystalluria. Do not administer concurrently.

A baseline assessment of the client's symptoms related to the UTI as well as a CBC and urinalysis should be obtained.

Nursing diagnosis. Clients receiving sulfonamide therapy should be assessed for the development of the following nursing diagnoses: altered comfort (dizziness, headache); fluid volume deficit related to anorexia, nausea, vomiting, and diarrhea; diarrhea; and the potential complications of hypersensitivity (rash, fever), photosensitivity (increased sensitivity of skin to sunlight), blood dyscrasias (unusual bruising or bleeding, sore throat, fever, unusual fatigue), hepatitis (yellow eyes or skin), Lyell's syndrome (difficulty in swallowing, blistering of skin), Stevens-Johnson syndrome (aching joints and muscles, weakness, skin changes), goiter, interstitial nephritis, hematuria, or crystalluria.

Implementation

Monitoring. Because renal toxicity is a potentially serious problem, monitor the hospitalized client's urinary output and ensure that it totals at least 1500 ml in 24 hours. Maintenance of urinary output at this level decreases the tendency for crystals to form. The urine should be examined visually for the presence of crystals; in long-term sulfonamide therapy periodic urinalysis should be done to determine if crystals are present. Monitor urinalysis to determine status of UTI and early detection of crystalluria. Carefully observe the client for toxic effects, such as rash, sore throat, or purpura.

In prolonged sulfonamide therapy the client requires periodic blood counts to assess for the occurrence of hematologic side effects (anemia, granulocytopenia, and thrombocytopenia).

Intervention. Administer sulfonamides on an empty stomach with a full glass of water to enhance absorption. However, if the common adverse reaction of nausea and vomiting occurs, administer with food to decrease gastrointestinal distress. Do not administer sulfonamides with antacids because the latter inhibit their action by decreasing absorption.

Education. Clients should be instructed to drink at least 3 quarts of fluids per day unless contraindicated for renal or cardiac conditions. Liquids and vitamins, such as ascorbic acid, that produce acid urine should be avoided. Inform the client of the importance of completing a full course of drug therapy, even though he or she may feel better after several days of therapy. Instruct the client to observe for and report any dermatologic reactions after initiation of the sulfonamide. Fever may occur after 7 to 10 days of therapy, indicating a serum sickness–like reaction. It may be accompanied by joint pain, urticaria, and leukopenia. All these responses are indications for discontinuation of the drug and follow-up referral to the prescriber. Advise the client to avoid direct skin exposure to the sun and sunlamps because skin photosensitivity may be present. Alert clients with diabetes that sulfonamides may cause false-positive urine sugar and urine ketone test results.

Evaluation. The client will experience a decrease in the severity or a disappearance of the clinical and laboratory manifestations of the UTI (e.g., absence of pathogen on cultures, normothermia, WBC within the normal range, absence of urgency, frequency and burning of urination).

URINARY TRACT ANTISEPTICS

Cinoxacin, methenamine mandelate, nalidixic acid, and nitrofurantoin are the primary urinary tract antiseptics. Urinary tract antiseptics are drugs that exert antibacterial activity in the urine but have little or no systemic antibacterial effects. Their usefulness is limited to the treatment of UTIs.

cinoxacin [sin ox' a sin] (Cinobac)
Cinoxacin inhibits replication of bacterial DNA, thus producing bactericidal urinary effects. It is absorbed well orally; its serum levels are usually low, whereas its urinary levels are high. This product does cross the placenta. The time for peak serum levels is between 2 and 3 hours. Cinoxacin is metabolized in the liver and excreted by the kidneys. For urinary tract agents: side/adverse effects and usual adult dose range, see Table 59-5.

methenamine mandelate [meth en' a meen] (Mandelamine)
methenamine hippurate [Hiprex, Urex, Hip-Rex♣]
Methanamine, which is used to treat UTIs, combines the action of methenamine and mandelic acid or hippurate acid salts. Its effectiveness depends on the release of formaldehyde, which requires an acid medium. The acids released from the mandelate or hippurate salts contribute to this acidity. Formaldehyde may be bactericidal or bacteriostatic, and its effects are believed to be the result of denaturation of bacteria protein. It is ineffective in alkaline urine. Because of its fairly wide bacterial spectrum, low toxicity, and low incidence of resistance, methenamine has often been the drug of choice in long-term suppression of infections.

Methenamine is absorbed orally and takes ½ to 2 hours to reach peak urinary formaldehyde levels at a urinary pH of 5.6, while the enteric-coated methenamine mandelate reaches its urinary peak in 3 to 8 hours. Excretion is via the kidneys. For urinary tract agents: side/adverse effects and usual adult dose range, see Table 59-5.

Drug	Possible effect and management
urinary alkalizers, such as antacids (calcium and/or magnesium), carbonic anhydrase inhibitors, citrates, sodium bicarbonate, or thiazide diuretics	May result in an alkaline urine, thus inhibiting methenamine's conversion to formaldehyde and rendering it ineffective. Avoid concurrent drug administration.
sulfamethizole (Thiosulfil Forte)	**In acid urine, the formaldehyde produced may precipitate with certain sulfonamides, which increases the potential for crystalluria. Avoid or a potentially serious drug interaction may occur.**

nalidixic acid [nal i dix' ik] (NegGram)
Nalidixic acid appears to inhibit bacterial DNA synthesis by interfering with the polymerization of DNA. Resistance usually develops rapidly during treatment with this drug. This drug is indicated for the treatment of UTIs caused by the *Proteus, Klebsiella, Enterobacter,* and *E. coli* species.

Nalidixic acid is well absorbed orally, reaches peak serum levels in 1 to 2 hours and peak urine levels in 3 to 4 hours. It is metabolized in the liver with approximately 30% converted to the active metabolite, hydroxynalidixic acid; excretion is via the kidneys. For urinary tract agents: side/adverse effects and usual adult dose, see Table 59-5.

Nalidixic acid when given with oral anticoagulants (e.g., coumarin, dicumarol) may displace the anticoagulants from their protein binding sites, resulting in enhanced anticoagulant action. Dosage adjustments may be necessary, so monitor the client's risk for injury related to an increase in bleeding tendency if concurrent therapy is necessary.

nitrofurantoin [nye tro fyoor' an toyn] (Furadantin, Macrodantin)

Nitrofurantoin is a broad-spectrum bactericidal agent at therapeutic serum levels. It is reduced by bacteria to reactive substances that inactivate or alter bacterial ribosomal proteins. It is indicated for the treatment of urinary tract infections caused by organisms such as *E. coli, S. aureus, Klebsiella, Enterobacter,* and *Proteus* species.

After oral administration nitrofurantoin is absorbed and has a half-life of 20 to 60 minutes. Approximately 65% of the drug is rapidly metabolized and inactivated in the liver and body tissues and excreted by the kidneys. For urinary tract agents: side/adverse effects and usual adult dose, see Table 59-5.

Drug	Possible effect and management
hemolytic agents	Increased possibility of toxic side effects. Monitor blood counts for anemia closely if concurrent therapy is necessary.
neurotoxic medications	Increased risk of inducing neurotoxicity. Monitor closely for dizziness, drowsiness, or headache if concurrent therapy is necessary.
probenecid (Benemid) or sulfinpyrazone (Anturane)	Tubular secretion of nitrofurantoin will be inhibited, leading to increased serum levels and possible toxicity. A decrease in urinary concentrations and effectiveness may also result. Dosage adjustment of probenecid may be required.

Nursing Management
Urinary Antiseptic Therapy

The following nursing measures include general ones for all urinary antiseptics and specific ones for particular antiseptics. Refer to Nursing Management of Urinary Antimicrobial Therapy (p. 923) for general nursing care of these clients.

Assessment. The nurse should ascertain whether the client has preexisting hepatic or renal function impairment because urinary antiseptics are used cautiously in such instances. Use nitrofurantoin cautiously with clients with peripheral neuropathy (because it may be worsened), and also with clients with pulmonary disease (because the drug may cause a pulmonary reaction, including pneumonitis). CNS damage or a history of seizures is an indication to use caution with the administration of nalidixic acid.

Nursing diagnosis. The client receiving urinary tract antiseptic therapy may experience the following nursing diagnosis: risk for injury related to a preexisting health condition, drug interaction, or side/adverse effect of the drug; knowledge deficit; and ineffective management of the therapeutic regimen.

Implementation

Monitoring. The client's progress should be monitored periodically by client reports of decreased symptoms of UTI, urinalysis, CBCs, and hepatic and renal function studies. With nitrofurantoin, pulmonary studies may be indicated.

Intervention. Acidification of the urine inhibits the growth of many urinary tract microorganisms and thereby enhances the effects of several urinary antiseptics. Thus, when clients with UTIs are encouraged to consume large volumes of fluids, fluids that increase urine acidity, such as cranberry juice or prune juice, should be selected (Williams, 1989). Vitamin C will also acidify the urine and can enhance antiinfective therapy.

Methenamine is most effective when the urine pH is 5.5 or less. Urine pH is easily monitored at the bedside and at home with commercially available test strips.

Urinary antiseptics may be given with food or just after meals to prevent gastrointestinal distress. If oral solutions are used, the nurse should ensure that they are shaken well and administered with the calibrated device provided by the manufacturer.

Education. The client should be instructed to complete a full course of therapy even if marked improvement occurs within a few days. If there is not significant improvement in the client's symptoms in the first 3 days of therapy, the prescriber should be notified. Compliance can be increased by suggesting cranberry sauce if the client considers cranberry juice unpalatable. Cranberry juice contains a compound that prevents bacteria from anchoring themselves in the bladder. Eating more protein, plums, or prunes, will also help to make the urine more acid (*USP DI,* 1996). Most fruits, particularly citrus fruits and juices, milk and other dairy products, and other alkalinizing foods should be avoided. Alka-Seltzer and sodium bicarbonate, which alkalinize the urine, should be avoided.

The client should be advised that dizziness and drowsiness may occur with these drugs and that these symptoms should be reported to the prescriber. Driving and other activities requiring alertness should be avoided until there is resolution of symptoms. With nalidixic acid, caution the client to report any visual disturbances to the prescriber.

Photophobia may occur during cinoxacin use. The client should be advised to avoid bright sunlight and to wear sunglasses. A possibility of photosensitivity exists with nalidixic acid during therapy and for up to 3 months after it is discontinued. The client should be cautioned to avoid direct skin exposure to sunlight and sunlamps.

Clients with diabetes should use Clinistix, Diastix, or TesTape to test for glucosuria because nitrofurantoin and nalidixic acid may produce a false-positive result with Clinitest. The client taking nitrofurantoin should be advised that urine may have a brown color. Nitrofurantoin is discolored by alkalis and strong light. The client should not use metal pill boxes unless they are stainless steel or aluminum because the drug decomposes on contact with other metals.

Evaluation. The client will experience an absence of urgency, frequency, and burning on urination and the urine culture will show an absence of pathogen growth.

AZTREONAM AND THE FLUOROQUINOLONES

Aztreonam and fluoroquinolones (ciprofloxacin, norfloxacin, ofloxacin) are potent drugs used in the treatment of UTIs. Aztreonam is effective against many gram-negative bacteria and appears to be a safer agent than aminoglycoside therapy in the seriously ill person. Generally, the fluoroquinolones are preferred agents when antibiotic-resistant bacteria is suspected. Refer to the previous sections for information on these medications.

URINARY TRACT ANALGESIC

phenazopyridine [fen az oh peer' i deen] (Pyridium) Phenazopyridine's exact mechanism of action is unknown, but it appears to have a topical analgesic or local anesthetic effect on the mucosa of the urinary tract. Phenazopyridine is used for urinary tract irritation, such as pain and burning on urination and urinary frequency. It is only indicated for short-term use because the underlying reason for the irritation should be determined and treated appropriately.

Phenazopyridine is metabolized by the liver and other body tissues and is excreted by the kidneys. For urinary tract agents: side/adverse effects and the usual adult dose, see Table 59-5.

▪ Nursing Management

Phenazopyridine Therapy

Assessment. Phenazopyridine is contraindicated in clients with G6PD deficiency, impaired renal or hepatic function.

Nursing diagnosis. The client receiving phenazopyridine therapy has the potential nursing diagnosis of altered comfort (headache, abdominal cramps) and the collaborative problems of hemolytic anemia (fatigue), renal function impairment, methemoglobinemia, allergic dermatitis, and hepatotoxicity (yellow eyes or skin).

Implementation

Monitoring. The client's progress should be monitored periodically by client reports of decreased symptoms of urgency and burning on urination.

Intervention. Phenazopyridine is usually prescribed in conjunction with an antimicrobial or urinary antiseptic. Administer with food to decrease gastrointestinal distress. Phenazopyridine may be discontinued after 2 days if the client's discomfort has resolved.

Education. The client should be told that the urine will become reddish orange and may stain clothing. The client should be instructed to observe for yellowness of the skin and sclera. This may indicate an accumulation of the drug owing to renal impairment. If this occurs, discontinue drug and notify the prescriber. Clients with diabetes should use Clinistix, Diastix, or TesTape to test for glucosuria because Clinitest may give a false-positive result with this drug. Alert the client not to wear soft contact lens during therapy or they may be permanently stained.

Evaluation. The client will experience an absence of urgency, frequency, and burning on urination.

SUMMARY

Antibiotics are chemical substances that kill or suppress the growth of microorganisms. Once the nurse has acquired an understanding of the principles of antibiotic therapy, the particular drugs may be classified by groups, actions, and effects for familiarization. They are generally classified as follows. Penicillins are derived from molds and inhibit the synthesis of bacterial cell walls; they are bactericidal for a wide range of gram-positive and some gram-negative organisms. Cephalosporins, now in their third generation, are chemical modifications of the penicillin structure and are bactericidal by inhibiting cell wall synthesis. Macrolide antibiotics, the most important of which is erythromycin, are bacteriostatic by inhibiting protein synthesis and bactericidal in higher concentrations with selected organisms. Lincomycins, which inhibit protein synthesis in bacteria by binding ribosomes of susceptible organisms, are primarily bacteriostatic, except in higher concentrations with selected organisms, in which case they are bactericidal. Vancomycin is bactericidal for many organisms and bacteriostatic for enterococci by inhibiting RNA synthesis and bacterial cell wall synthesis, causing lysis. Aminoglycosides are potent bactericidal antibiotics that are usually held in reserve for serious or life-threatening infections. Tetracyclines block the binding of transfer RNA complex to the ribosome and so are bacteriostatic for a wide range of gram-positive and gram-negative organisms. Chloramphenicol inhibits protein synthesis and is bacteriostatic for a wide range of organisms; however, because of its toxicity for bone marrow, its use is limited. Fluoroquinolones inhibit bacterial RNA synthesis and are bactericidal. Metronidazole, a short-acting cytotoxic agent that interacts with DNA, is effective against anaerobic bacteria and protozoa.

Urinary tract infections are a common reason for seeking medical care in the community as well as a major result of nosocomial infections in institutions; and their incidence increases with age. Antimicrobial therapy for UTIs includes antibiotics (sulfonamides), urinary tract antiseptics, monobactams and fluoroquinolones, and urinary tract analgesics.

Although a repertoire of antibiotics can be used in the treatment of infections, we cannot become complacent in their use. With the emergence of newly recognized pathogens and drug resistance in known strains of organisms, the use of immunosuppressive agents, and the increase in invasive procedures for diagnosis and treatment, the risk of infection in certain populations has increased.

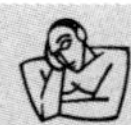

Critical Thinking

1. Why is the assessment stage so important in the nursing process in antibiotic therapy?
2. Kevin Reardon, age 27, has been prescribed oral ampicillin for an otitis media. On the third day of ampicillin therapy, Mr. Reardon telephones the clinic to indicate he has developed diarrhea. What might be occurring with Mr. Reardon's therapy? What action should the nurse take?
3. In many countries where prescription regulations are not as restrictive as in the United States and Canada, many antibiotics are OTC drugs, including chloramphenicol. What might be the consequences of this lack of regulation?
4. Why is it important to monitor urinary output with the administration of the various antimicrobials?
5. Molly Ellis, age 22, has an acute lower urinary tract infection. Her health care provider prescribes the sulfonamide sulfisoxazole for 10 days. What instruction may be required to enable Ms. Ellis to effectively manage her drug therapy? What instruction should be reviewed with the client to assist her to prevent recurrences of the UTI?

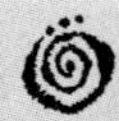

Collaborative Learning Activities

1. Discuss how many in the class have ever taken antibiotics. How many finished their entire prescription. Discuss why they did not complete the prescription. What teaching interventions would they use in anticipating clients might have the same problems with compliance?
2. Student teams will be pre-assigned to represent the various groups of antibiotics. Draw a chart on the board with indications, mechanisms of action, contraindications, specific monitoring and interventions, and client teaching in the left hand margin. Label the vertical columns with the drug groupings. Fill in the chart as the teams make their presentations.
3. The students will create on the board a nursing care plan for sulfonamide therapy for a client with a UTI.

BIBLIOGRAPHY

Ahronheim JC (1992). *Handbook of prescribing medications for geriatric patients.* Boston: Little, Brown.

American Hospital Formulary Service (1996). *AHFS drug information '96.* Bethesda, MD: American Society of Hospital Pharmacists.

Anderson KN, et al. (Eds.) (1994). *Mosby's medical, nursing,& allied health dictionary* (4th ed.). St Louis: Mosby.

Beringer PM & Middleton RK (1995). Anaphylaxis and drug allergies. In Young LY & Koda-Kimble MA (Eds.). *Applied therapeutics: The clinical use of drugs* (6th ed.). Vancouver, WA: Applied Therapeutics.

Cunha BA (1992). The urologic uses of aminoglycosides, *Emerg Med* 24(7):299.

Danziger LH & Itokazu GS (1995). Gastrointestinal infections. In Young LY & Koda-Kimble MA (Eds.). *Applied therapeutics:The clinical use of drugs* (6th ed.). Vancouver, WA: Applied Therapeutics.

Doughty DB & Jackson DB (1993). *Gastrointestinal disorders.* St Louis: Mosby.

Duma RJ (Ed.) (1992). Recognition and management of nursing home infections. Bethesda, MD: National Foundation for Infectious Diseases.

Grimes D (1991). *Infectious disease.* St Louis: Mosby.

Just PM (1994). Overview of the fluoroquinolone antibiotics, *Pharmacother* 13(2,Pt 2):4S.

Katzung BG (1992). *Basic and clinical pharmacology* (5th ed.). Norwalk, CT: Appleton & Lange.

Mandell GL & Petri, Jr WA (1996). Antimicrobial agents. In Hardman JG & Limbird LE (Eds.). *Goodman & Gilman's the pharmacological basis of therapeutics* (9th ed.). New York: McGraw-Hill.

Melmon KL, et al. (1992). *Clinical pharmacology* (3rd ed.). New York: McGraw-Hill.

Mullenix T, et al. (1993). Urinary tract infections and prostatitis. In DiPiro JT, et al. *Pharmacotherapy* (2nd ed.). Norwalk, CT: Appleton & Lange.

Mylotte JM, et al. (1993). Staying on top of hospital infections, *Patient Care* 27(2):116.

Olin BR (Ed.) (1997). *Facts and comparisons.* St Louis: Facts and Comparisons.

Sahai JV (1995). Urinary tract infections. In Young LY & Koda-Kimble MA (Eds.). *Applied therapeutics* (6th ed.). Vancouver: Applied Therapeutics.

Schell KH (1993). Current trends in antimicrobial therapy for the critically ill patient, *Crit Care Nurs Q* 15(4):23-32.

Semla TP, et al. (1993). *Geriatric dosage handbook.* Cleveland: American Pharmaceutical Association & Lexi-Comp.

United States Pharmacopeial Convention (1994). *Advice for the patient: Drug information in lay language* (14th ed.). Rockville, MD: The Convention.

United States Pharmacopeial Convention (1996). *USP DI: Drug information for the health care professional* (16th ed.). Rockville, MD: The Convention.

Williams SR (1995). *Basic nutrition and diet therapy* (10th ed.). St Louis: Mosby.

Chapter 60

Antifungal and Antiviral Drugs

Chapter Focus

Clients receiving broad-spectrum antibiotics for an infection, immunosuppressed clients as the result of a transplant or antineoplastic therapy, and clients with acquired immunodeficiency syndrome (AIDS) are all at risk for the development of superinfection with fungal or viral organisms. Certainly, the growth of the AIDS epidemic has fostered pharmaceutical research for agents to combat diseases caused by these organisms. The last few years have seen the FDA approving these drugs in record time compared to past reviews. The nurse then needs to remain current in the knowledge of old standards and newly approved antifungal and antiviral drugs. The following objectives and key terms are important for a good understanding of this chapter.

Key Terms

candidiasis (p. 931)
chemoprophylactic (p. 937)
fungi (p. 931)
mycoses (p. 931)

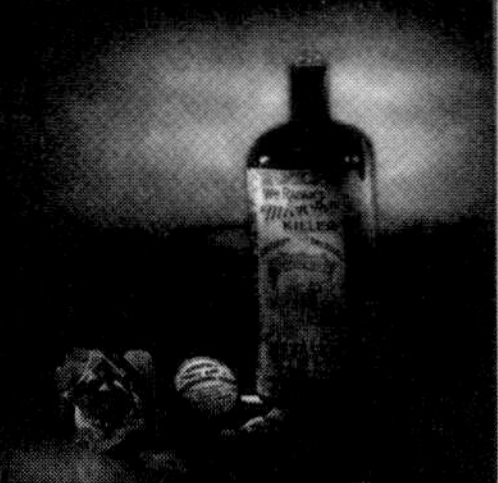

Key Drugs [▲]

amphotericin B
ketoconazole
acyclovir
zidovudine
indinavir

Objectives

1. List four commonly used antifungal agents.
2. Describe five side effects/adverse reactions of antifungal agents.
3. Implement nursing management of the care of clients receiving antifungal agents.
4. State two reasons why effective antiviral drug therapy is more limited than antibacterial and antifungal therapy.
5. List four commonly used systemic antiviral agents.
6. Implement the nursing management of the care of clients receiving antiviral therapy.

ANTIFUNGAL DRUGS

Human infections by **fungi** can be caused by any of about 50 species of plantlike, parasitic microorganisms. These simple, parasitic plants, lacking chlorophyll, are unable to make their own food and so are dependent on other life forms. The infections by fungi, termed **mycoses,** can range from mild and superficial to severe and life threatening. Infecting organisms can be ingested orally or become implanted under the skin after injury or inhaled if the fungal spores are airborne. One species of fungi, *Candida albicans*, is usually part of the normal flora of the skin, mouth, intestines, and vagina; overgrowth and systemic infection from it may result from antibiotic, antineoplastic, and corticosteroid drug therapy. This is referred to as an opportunistic infection. Oral **candidiasis** (thrush) is common in newborn infants and immunocompromised clients, whereas vaginal candidiasis is common in pregnant women, women with diabetes mellitus, or in women who take oral contraceptives. The prevalence of mycoses is increasing as an opportunistic infection in clients with AIDS, as the incidence of AIDS increases. Nonopportunistic fungal infections such as blastomycosis, histoplasmosis and others, are usually rare.

The lag in the development of antifungal chemotherapy is related to the high chemical antifungal concentrations necessary that cannot be tolerated by the human host. Therefore only a few antifungal compounds are available for systemic use. Topical antifungal preparations are discussed in Chapter 66. The following discussions include only systemic agents.

▲ **amphotericin B** [am foe ter' i sin] (Fungizone Intravenous)

Amphotericin B can be fungistatic or fungicidal, depending on the concentrations achieved clinically. This drug does not have a therapeutic effect on bacteria or viruses. Amphotericin B binds to sterols in the fungus cell membrane increasing cell permeability which results, in a loss of potassium and other elements from the cell.

Amphotericin B is effective for treating aspergillosis; blastomycosis; candidiasis (moniliasis); coccidioidomycosis; cryptococcosis; fungal endocarditis; histoplasmosis; cryptococcal meningitis; fungal septicemia; and many other systemic fungal infections.

Administered parenterally, amphotericin B is widely distributed in the body; has a half-life in adults initially of 24 hours while the elimination half-life is approximately 15 days. The site of metabolism is unknown, but excretion is via the kidneys. About 40% of the drug is excreted over 7 days, but it has still been detected in the urine for at least 7 weeks after the drug was discontinued.

Common side/adverse effects with IV infusion of amphotericin B include headache, gastrointestinal distress, anemia, hypokalemia, fever, chills, nausea, vomiting and renal impairment.

The adult dose for systemic fungus infection is usually a 1 mg test dose in 5% dextrose solution administered over 10 to 30 minutes. This is followed by increments of 5 to 10 mg amphotericin B infusion (up to 50 mg/day), administered over 2 to 6 hours, depending on the infection and the individual's tolerance of the medication. The pediatric dose is initially, a 0.25 mg/kg daily in 5% dextrose administered over 6 hours. The dose may be increased gradually (up to 1 mg/kg/day), depending on the infection and the child's tolerance of this medication.

Amphotericin B lipid complex injection (Abelcet) is a liposomal encapsulation of amphotericin used to treat aspergillosis in persons that are refractory to or unable to tolerate standard amphotericin B therapy. The liposome formulation provides a therapeutic effect with significantly less nephrotoxicity than amphotericin B. The most common side/adverse effects include fever, chills, nausea, hypotension, vomiting, dyspnea and respiratory failure.

The usual daily dose for adults and children is 5 mg/kg by single infusion, at a rate of 2.5 mg/kg/hr. See current references for additional information on this product (Abelcet, 1996).

■ Nursing Management

Amphotericin B Therapy

Assessment. Amphotericin B is used with caution if renal function impairment exists. Although it is not renally excreted, amphotericin B is nephrotoxic and can worsen any preexisting renal pathologic condition. It is also administered with caution if there is intolerance to the drug or if the client is receiving other nephrotoxic agents.

The client's current medication regimen should be reviewed for significant drug interactions such as those that may occur when amphotericin B is given with the following drugs:

Drug	Possible effect and management
adrenocorticoids, glucocorticoids, mineralocorticoids, (ACTH)	May result in severe hypokalemia; if given concurrently, frequent serum potassium determinations should be performed. May decrease adrenal cortex response to corticotropin (ACTH).
bone marrow depressants, radiation therapy	May produce increased bone marrow depressant effects; monitor blood cell counts closely because dosage adjustments may be necessary if anemia, leukopenia, or thrombocytopenia become extreme.
digitalis glycosides	Amphotericin B–induced hypokalemia may increase the potential for digitalis toxicity. Monitor closely for arrhythmias, anorexia, nausea, vomiting or other indications of possible toxicity.
nephrotoxic medications, potassium-depleting diuretics	Increased risk of nephrotoxicity; monitor closely for edema and oliguria, since dosage adjustments may be necessary.

A baseline assessment of the client's general health status should be obtained including the underlying condition, weight, BUN, serum creatinine concentrations and electrolyte levels, and complete blood and platelet counts. Appropriate specimens should be obtained before therapy to identify the causative fungi.

Nursing diagnosis. Clients receiving amphotericin B are at risk for the following nursing diagnoses: fluid volume deficit related to anorexia, nausea and vomiting; activity intolerance related to anemia or hypokalemia; hyperthermia; altered protection related to leukopenia and thrombocytopenia; impaired tissue integrity related to extravasation or thrombophlebitis at the infusion site; sensory-perceptual disturbances related to polyneuropathy (numbness, tingling, or burning in hands and feet), hearing loss or change in vision; and the collaborative problems of infusion-related reaction (fever, chills, nausea, vomiting, headache, hypotension), electrolyte imbalances (hypokalemia, hypomagnesemia), hypersensitivity, cardiac arrhythmias, and nephrotoxicity (increased or decreased urinary output).

Implementation

Monitoring. Monitor vital signs and observe the client for adverse reactions (shortness of breath, fever, chills, nausea, and vomiting) during the test dose (1 mg in 50 to 150 ml of dextrose 5% in water and administered over 2 to 4 hours) and the first 1 to 2 hours of each dose. Febrile response usually lasts for less than 4 hours after the infusion.

Blood urea nitrogen (BUN) and serum creatinine values should be determined every other day as the dosage is increased to optimal level, and then weekly once the maintenance dosage is achieved until the drug is discontinued. If BUN levels exceed 40 mg/dl or serum creatinine increases to 3 mg/dl, dosage should be decreased or discontinued until renal function improves. Serum potassium and magnesium levels should be monitored twice a week. Blood counts should be monitored weekly in anticipation of bone marrow suppression.

Pain at the site of infusion may indicate extravasation. Be cautious, since the drug causes local tissue irritation and thrombophlebitis.

Clients receiving the drug intravenously should be assessed for gastrointestinal disturbances such as anorexia, indigestion, nausea and vomiting, and diarrhea. Daily monitoring of weights will determine if these symptoms are associated with weight loss. Monitor fluid intake and output to determine fluid loss and renal status. Observe for signs of hypokalemia such as muscle cramps, irregular pulse, and weakness or lethargy. Monitor for symptoms of bone marrow suppression (fever, sore throat, and unusual bleeding or bruising) and report them to the prescriber.

Intervention. Amphotericin B should not be used if there is any evidence of precipitate or foreign matter in the vial. The package inserts should be read before administration of the drug for major points of safe delivery. Because amphotericin B is incompatible with a wide range of drugs, confirm its compatibility with other drugs before preparing the infusion.

Reconstitute only with the diluents recommended; sodium chloride or bacteriostatic agents such as benzyl alcohol will cause the drug to precipitate. The pH of the dextrose injection should be above 4.2 before the addition of the drug. The manufacturer's package insert provides the aseptic procedure for testing and adjusting the pH if that should be necessary. If in-line intravenous filters are used, they should have at least a 1-μm mean pore diameter, or they may filter out clinically significant amounts of the drug. Gloves should be worn while preparing the drug. Infuse slowly over 3 to 4 hours to minimize adverse cardiovascular reactions. Every half-hour during administration, shake the hanging solution to keep it in suspension.

Administering the drug on alternate days and over a 6 hour period may reduce the incidence of side effects. If therapy is interrupted for more than 7 days, the dosage should be restarted at the lowest level and increased to the appropriate therapeutic level. The duration of the course of amphotericin B should be sufficient to prevent a relapse.

Febrile reactions during administration may be minimized if a small dose of intravenous adrenocorticoid is administered just before the infusion of amphotericin B. Antipyretics and antihistamines are also used. Nephrotoxicity may also be minimized by sodium bicarbonate diuresis or salt loading just before administration of amphotericin B. Heparin may be added to the intravenous infusion of amphotericin B to help prevent thrombophlebitis at the intravenous site. The infusion site should be changed with each dose to minimize the development of thrombophlebitis.

If the client has gastrointestinal symptoms during the administration of amphotericin B, a pleasant and relaxed atmosphere for mealtimes should be provided, small, frequent feedings of high-protein, high-calorie foods of the client's choice should be encouraged, and good oral hygiene maintained. Palliative medication may be necessary if the client is experiencing indigestion, vomiting, or diarrhea.

Education. The client should be advised to complete essential dental work before starting therapy with amphotericin B or to delay it until completing the course of the drug because the bone marrow suppressant effects may cause gingival bleeding and delay healing.

Appropriate oral hygiene should be taught, including gentle use of soft toothbrushes and floss and avoidance of toothpicks. Advise the client to alert the nursing staff at the first indication of pain at the intravenous site.

Alert the client to side effects and adverse reactions of the drug and the need to report these promptly.

Evaluation. The client's infection will be alleviated without evidence of any adverse reactions of amphotericin B.

Azole Antifungals

The azole antifungals include the following:

fluconazole [floo koe' na zole] (Diflucan)
itraconazole [eye trah koe' na zole] (Sporanox)
▲ **ketoconazole** [kee toe koe' na zole] (Nizoral)
miconazole [my kon' a zole] injection (Monistat i.v.)

The azole antifungals may be fungistatic or fungicidal agents, depending on dosage and systemic levels achieved. Ergosterol is the primary sterol in fungus cell membranes and these agents affect the biosynthesis of the fungal sterols by interfering with the cytochrome P-450 enzyme system. The result is impaired or depleted ergosterol biosynthesis, inhibiting fungus growth.

TABLE 60-1 Azole antifungals: pharmacokinetics and usual adult dose

Drug	Pharmacokinetics		Usual adult dose
	Peak serum (hrs)*	Half-life (hrs)†	
fluconazole (Diflucan)	1-2	adults: 30 children: 14-20	100-200 mg PO/IV daily
itraconazole (Sporanox)	3-4	single dose-21 steady state-64	200 mg PO once or twice a day
ketoconazole (Nizoral)	1-4	8	200 to 400 mg PO daily
miconazole (Monistat i.v.)	E of I	20-25	0.2 to 1.2 g/IV infusion

*Time to peak serum concentration. †Half-life for normal renal function. *E of I*, End of infusion. Olin, 1996; *USP DI*, 1996.

Fluconazole and itraconazole have a greater affinity for fungal P-450 activity than for the human liver cytochrome P-450 system. Fluconazole has good penetration in cerebrospinal fluid (CSF); thus it is used for the treatment of cryptococcal meningitis, whereas itraconazole has poor CSF penetration but is widely distributed in the body and is indicated for treatment of aspergillosis, blastomycosis, and histoplasmosis.

Ketoconazole is well distributed in body fluids (saliva, bile, urine, breast milk, and inflamed joint fluid), tendons and other body tissues. It is indicated for the treatment of disseminated and mucocutaneous candidiasis, paracoccidioidomycosis and recalcitrant tinea infections. Miconazole is also widely distributed in body tissues but neither ketoconazole nor miconazole adequately crosses the blood-brain barrier. Miconazole is primarily indicated for the treatment of disseminated and chronic mucocutaneous candidiasis.

Pharmacokinetically, fluconazole, itraconazole and ketoconazole are administered orally, while fluconazole and miconazole may be administered intravenously. Oral administration rates are good if fluconazole is administered in the fasting state while itraconazole and ketoconazole should be administered with food. Ketoconazole requires an acid medium for dissolution and absorption therefore, achlorhydria, hypochlorhydria or an increase in stomach pH caused by medications will impair absorption of ketoconazole. For Azole antifungals: pharmacokinetics and usual adult dose, see Table 60-1.

Side/adverse effects of azole antifungals include nausea, vomiting, stomach distress and diarrhea. Rash is more commonly reported with itraconazole. Ketoconazole although rarely, has caused gynecomastia and impotency due to inhibition of adrenal steroid and testosterone synthesis. Menstrual irregularities have also been reported. Miconazole may cause phlebitis at the injection site and if injected too rapidly nausea, vomiting, and cardiorespiratory arrest have been reported.

■ Nursing Management

Azole Antifungal Therapy

Assessment. The risk of administration of fluconazole should be considered for clients with impaired renal function; doses may need to be decreased or the dosage interval increased for these clients. There is not a renal limitation for itraconazole. However, hypersensitivity to either drug or other azole antifungal agents may be a contraindication for use of the drug. Clients with achlorhydria or hypochlorhydria, as commonly occurs with clients with AIDS, may have reduced absorption of these drugs. Use fluconazole cautiously with clients with alcoholism or hepatic function impairment because these clients are at risk for drug-induced hepatotoxicity. Ketoconazole has been known to cause a disulfiram-like reaction (flushing, rash, peripheral edema, headache, nausea and vomiting) as a response to alcohol ingestion.

The client's current medication regimen should be reviewed for possible significant drug interactions such as may occur when these agents are given with the following drugs:

Drug	Possible effect and management
alcohol or hepatotoxic drugs	Concurrent use increases the risk for hepatotoxicity. Also use of alcohol and ketoconazole is reported to cause a disulfiram-like reaction.
antacids, anticholinergics, histamine H_2 receptor antagonists, omeprazole (Prilosec), sucralfate (Carafate), didanosine (ddI) (Videx, DDL)	These drugs increase gastrointestinal pH thereby reducing the absorption of itraconazole and ketoconazole. Administer the drugs at least 2 hours apart.
antidiabetic agents (oral—chlorpropamide (Diabinese), glyburide (DiaBeta), glipizide (Glucotrol), tolbutamide (Orinase)	May result in increased serum concentrations of these antidiabetic agents, resulting in hypoglycemia. Closely monitor blood glucose levels if drugs are given concurrently because a dosage adjustment of the antidiabetic agents may be necessary.
astemizole (Hismanal) or terfenadine (Seldane)	**Concurrent use results in elevated plasma levels of astemizole or terfenadine by inhibiting their metabolic pathway, which may result in cardiac arrhythmias and death. Avoid or a potentially serious drug interaction may occur.**

Continued

Drug	Possible effect and management
carbamazepine (Tegretol)	Concurrent use decreases itraconazole levels, may lead to treatment failures.
cyclosporine (Sandimmune)	Closely monitor plasma cyclosporine levels; they have been reported to increase in some individuals receiving both drugs concurrently.
digoxin (Lanoxin)	Itraconazole increases serum digoxin levels, leading to digoxin toxicity. Monitor digoxin levels carefully.
phenytoin (Dilantin)	Closely monitor phenytoin levels because increased serum levels are reported in clients receiving both drugs concurrently.
rifampin (Rifadin) or rifabutin (Mycobutin)	Concurrent drug administration may result in increased fluconazole metabolism. Monitor closely; the fluconazole dose may need to be increased.
warfarin (Coumadin)	May result in a decrease in warfarin metabolism, resulting in an increase in prothrombin time (PT). Closely monitor prothrombin times in clients receiving both drugs concurrently.

A baseline assessment of the client's general health status, including the underlying infection, weight, BUN and serum creatinine values, and liver function tests is necessary. Appropriate specimens should be taken to identify the causative fungi before therapy is initiated.

Nursing diagnosis. The client receiving azole antifungal agents should be assessed for the following nursing diagnoses: impaired tissue integrity due to IV administration (phlebitis); altered comfort (headache, photophobia); sexual dysfunction (impotence) (ketoconazole only); disturbance of self-concept in male clients related to gynecomastia or impotence (ketoconazole only); fluid volume deficit related to anorexia, nausea, vomiting, and diarrhea; and the collaborative problems of anemia, agranulocytosis, thrombocytopenia, Stevens-Johnson syndrome (blistering or peeling of skin) and hepatotoxicity.

Implementation

Monitoring. Monitor the site of the infection for improvement since the dosage and length of treatment are determined by this and the individual's general response to therapy. Clients with HIV infection have greater incidence of side effects (21%) than those who are HIV negative (13%) and so require closer management. Blood urea nitrogen (BUN) and serum creatinine values should be determined routinely until the drug is discontinued.

Clients receiving the drug should be assessed for gastrointestinal disturbances such as anorexia, indigestion, nausea and vomiting, and diarrhea. Daily weights will determine if these symptoms are associated with weight loss. Monitor fluid intake and output to determine fluid loss and renal status. Clients receiving itraconazole require periodic serum potassium determination because hypokalemia has occurred, leading to ventricular fibrillation.

The miconazole intravenous site should be monitored periodically for pain and inflammation, which would indicate phlebitis. Monitor complete blood counts for anemia and thrombocytopenia. Monitor serum electrolytes for hyponatremia and blood lipids for increases periodically.

Liver function studies need to be monitored; although a mild, transient increase in transaminases may occur with therapy, it may, on rare occasion, progress to hepatotoxicity. Observe the client for dark urine, jaundice, and right upper quadrant abdominal pain.

Intervention. The oral fluconazole dosage is almost the same as the daily intravenous dosage because it is almost completely bioavailable. If the client is receiving hemodialysis, the fluconazole should be administered after dialysis is performed so that plasma concentrations of the drug are not reduced. There is no change of therapy required for clients on continuous ambulatory peritoneal dialysis (CAPD). Administer oral itraconazole with food to increase bioavailability. Maintenance therapy for both drugs may be required with HIV-infected clients to prevent relapse of their infection. Consult with the prescriber for a prescription for an antiemetic to manage nausea or vomiting or an analgesic if the client develops a drug-induced headache.

For clients with achlorhydria taking ketoconazole tablets, absorption may decrease. To minimize this effect, the prescriber may prescribe that each tablet be dissolved in 4 ml of 0.2N hydrochloric acid. The solution may be further diluted with a small amount of water and administered through a plastic or glass straw to prevent contact with the teeth. Have the client rinse his or her mouth with water and swallow the solution.

With IV fluconazole, administer by continuous infusion, using an infusion pump, not to exceed 200 mg/hour. Do not mix other drugs with fluconazole.

The first dose of miconazole should be a test dose of 200 mg administered by intravenous infusion to determine whether the client is hypersensitive to the drug. Dilute each dose of miconazole in at least 200 ml of 0.9% sodium chloride solution or 5% dextrose injection for intravenous infusion. This solution will be stable at room temperature for 24 hours. If the solution darkens, it should be discarded because it has deteriorated. Do not mix with other medications. Administer intravenous infusions of miconazole over 30 to 60 minutes to prevent dysrhythmias or increases in heart rate that may result from rapid administration. The nausea and vomiting secondary to the administration of miconazole may be minimized by reducing the dosage, slowing the infusion rate, or administering an antiemetic before beginning the infusion. Infusions of the drug should not be administered at mealtimes to help prevent gastrointestinal effects. If pruritus occurs, it may be controlled by diphenhydramine. Intravenous administration of miconazole must be supplemented by bladder irrigation with miconazole solution in mycoses of the bladder and by intrathecal administration of the drug in the case of fungal meningitis, alternating the injections between cervical, lumbar, and cisternal punctures every 3 to 7 days.

Education. Recommend that the client take ketoconazole with meals or food to minimize nausea and enhance absorption. Therapy is usually long term, in some cases months or years. Encourage the client to continue to take the medication for the full course of therapy even if feeling better. Taking the drug at the same time every day increases compliance. Infected areas should be reevaluated periodically.

Caution the client to avoid alcoholic beverages while on ketoconazole therapy. Advise the client to avoid exposure to bright light or to wear sunglasses because of the drug's photophobic effects. Because ketoconazole causes drowsiness, caution the client to avoid activities that require mental alertness until the response to the drug has been determined.

Advise client to complete the full course of medication, to maintain regular visits with the prescriber for monitoring, and to be alert for significant side/adverse effects to report to the provider.

With IV miconazole, instruct the client to alert the nurse if he or she has trouble breathing, skin rash, or fever and chills, which are signs of hypersensitivity. Advise the client that it may take weeks or months for a therapeutic response.

Evaluation. The client's infection will be alleviated without evidence of any adverse reactions to azole antifungal therapy.

flucytosine capsules [floo sye' toe seen] (Ancobon, Ancotil♣)

Flucytosine enters fungus cells, where it is converted to fluorouracil, an antimetabolite. It interferes with pyrimidine metabolism, thus preventing nucleic acid and protein synthesis. It has selective toxicity against susceptible strains of fungi because the body cells do not convert significant quantities of this drug into fluorouracil.

Flucytosine is indicated for the treatment of fungal endocarditis caused by *Candida* species, fungal meningitis (by *Cryptococcus* species), and fungal pneumonia, septicemia or urinary infections caused by *Candida* or *Cryptococcus* species. It is well absorbed orally and widely distributed in the body including cerebrospinal fluid (CSF); the latter being approximately 60% to 90% of serum concentrations. Flucytosine, with a half-life of 2.5 to 6 hours is not significantly metabolized but is excreted via the kidneys, mostly as unchanged drug.

Common side/adverse effects of flucytosine include gastric distress, anemia, hepatitis, hypersensitivity, and bone marrow suppression. The adult and pediatric oral dosage is 12.5 to 37.5 mg/kg every 6 hours.

■ Nursing Management

Flucytosine Therapy

Assessment. Use with caution if a client has preexisting bone marrow suppression, has had or is currently using cytotoxic drug or radiation therapy, or has hepatic or renal function impairment. Renal impairment necessitates a dosage adjustment. The drug is contraindicated if the client is allergic to flucytosine.

Administration of flucytosine concurrently with bone marrow depressants or radiation therapy may enhance bone marrow suppressant effects; monitor CBCs closely, since dosage adjustments may be necessary.

A baseline assessment of the client's general health status, including the underlying infection, weight, complete blood and platelet counts, BUN and serum creatinine values, and liver function values is necessary. Appropriate specimens should be taken to identify the causative fungi before therapy is initiated.

Nursing diagnosis. Clients receiving flucytosine should be assessed for the possibility of the following nursing diagnoses: altered comfort (headache and abdominal cramping); fluid volume deficit related to anorexia, nausea and vomiting; activity intolerance related to anemia; altered protection related to leukopenia or thrombocytopenia; altered thought processes (confusion, hallucinations) related to CNS effects; and the collaborative problems of hypersensitivity and the development of hepatitis.

Implementation

Monitoring. Assess the client's fungal infection for improvement. Monitor intake and output to ensure adequate hydration and to minimize adverse renal reactions. Weigh daily to monitor nutritional status if the client has gastrointestinal side effects. Monitor the client for signs of bone marrow depression such as sore throat and fever and signs of unusual bleeding, bruising, weakness, or tiredness.

Monitor blood counts and renal function studies during the course of therapy, as well as hepatic function studies such as (AST [SGOT]), (ALT [SGPT]), serum alkaline phosphatase, and serum bilirubin concentrations.

The serum level of flucytosine may be measured to ascertain whether it is being maintained in the therapeutic range, 25 to 120 μg/ml. Side effects are more common with serum levels >100 μg/ml. The serum concentrations are also used to assess renal excretion and prevent drug accumulation in clients with renal function impairment (creatinine clearance <40 ml/min).

Intervention. If multiple-dosage units are prescribed as a single dose, administer over 15 minutes to help prevent nausea and vomiting. Treat palliatively with antiemetics if these symptoms occur. Flucytosine is usually administered concurrently with parenteral amphotericin B to prevent the fungal resistance that may develop rapidly if it is used alone.

Education. Encourage the client to comply with the full course of therapy, even if feeling better. Progress should be monitored by regular visits to the health care provider. Advise the client to report any syncope, dizziness, or drowsiness to the health care provider.

As with amphotericin B, advise the client to complete dental work before or delay it until after a course of flucytosine. Recommend the gentle use of soft toothbrushes and dental floss and the avoidance of toothpicks because of the risk of gingival bleeding.

Evaluation. The client's infection will be alleviated without evidence of any adverse reactions to flucytosine.

griseofulvin microsize [gri see oh ful' vin] (Grisactin, Grifulvin V, Fulvicin-U/F, Grisovin-FP♣)

griseofulvin tablets, ultramicrosize (Fulvicin P/G)

Griseofulvin is a fungistatic agent; it inhibits fungus cell mitosis during metaphase. It is also deposited in the keratin precursor cells in skin, hair, and nails, thus inhibiting fungal invasion of the keratin. When infested keratin is shed, healthy keratin will replace it. Griseofulvin is indicated for the treatment of susceptible organisms for onychomycosis, tinea barbae, tinea capitis, tinea corporis, tinea cruris, and tinea pedis.

The oral absorption of microsize griseofulvin varies from 25% to 70% of the oral dose, while the ultramicrosize form is nearly completely absorbed. If griseofulvin is administered with or after a fatty meal, absorption is significantly enhanced. Griseofulvin is distributed in keratin layers in the skin, hair, and nails with very little being distributed in body tissues and fluids. It has a half-life of 24 hours and reaches peak serum levels in about 4 hours. Metabolism is in the liver and is primarily excreted unchanged in feces.

The most commonly reported side effect is headache; less frequently noted is hypersensitivity, confusion, gastric distress, oral thrush, weakness and photosensitivity.

The oral adult microsize dose is 500 mg orally daily or divided in two doses. To treat tinea pedis or onychomycosis, the dose is 500 mg twice daily. The pediatric dosage is 5 mg/kg every 12 hours (*USP DI*, 1996). The ultramicrosize adult dose is 250 to 375 mg daily.

■ Nursing Management

Griseofulvin Therapy

Assessment. If the client has preexisting porphyria, lupus erythematosus, hepatic function impairment, or sensitivity to griseofulvin, administer the drug with caution.

The client's current medication regimen should be reviewed for significant drug interactions such as may occur when griseofulvin is given with the following drugs:

Drug	Possible effect and management
anticoagulants, oral: coumarin or indanedione	Decreased anticoagulant effect may be noted; monitor prothrombin times closely until a stable serum level is achieved. Dosage adjustments may be required during and after griseofulvin administration.
contraceptives, estrogen-containing oral	Chronic, long-term use of griseofulvin may decrease the effectiveness of oral contraceptives. May see intercycle menstrual bleeding, amenorrhea, or pregnancy. Advise client to use an alternate method of contraception when taking griseofulvin.
Other hepatic enzyme-inducing agents	May increase potential for toxicity; monitor closely for dark urine, jaundice, yellow sclera, and changes in hepatic function studies.

The client's baseline assessment should include the underlying condition for which the griseofulvin is prescribed, mental status, a complete blood count, serum creatinine, urinalysis, and hepatic function studies. As with other antiinfectives, obtain specimens for culture before starting griseofulvin therapy.

Nursing diagnosis. The client receiving griseofulvin should be assessed for the possibility of the following nursing diagnoses: altered comfort (headache, abdominal cramping); fluid volume deficit related to anorexia, nausea and vomiting; risk for injury related to dizziness; altered protection related to leukopenia and agranulocytopenia; altered mucous membranes related to oral thrush; altered sleep pattern (insomnia) related to CNS effects; sensory-perceptual disturbances related to peripheral neuritis (numbness and tingling of the hands and feet); altered thought processes (confusion) related to CNS effects; and the collaborative problems of hypersensitivity, photosensitivity, or the development of hepatitis (jaundiced skin and sclera).

Implementation

Monitoring. Monitor blood counts and hepatic and renal function studies periodically during therapy. Therapy is continued until clinical signs or laboratory confirmation indicates the causative organism is eradicated.

Intervention. Administer with meals to help prevent gastrointestinal distress and to enhance absorption. Therapy is even more effective if the meal is fatty. If the client is on a low-fat diet, consult the prescriber. Concurrent use of an appropriate topical agent maximizes the therapeutic effect of griseofulvin and reduces the possibility of relapse. Administer the oral suspension using the calibrated measuring device provided by the manufacturer.

Education. Encourage the client to comply with the full course of therapy, even if feeling better. Regular visits to the prescriber are necessary to check progress.

Frequent shampoos and clipping of the hair and nails will support the therapeutic effect of the drug, as will keeping affected skin areas clean and dry. Advise the client that skin may be more sensitive to sunlight and recommend avoiding direct sunlight and using sun screens.

Advise the client to report any symptoms of fever and sore throat to the prescriber, since they may indicate blood dyscrasias. Because the drug may cause dizziness, the client should avoid tasks that require mental alertness until the response to the drug can be ascertained. Instruct the client about good oral hygiene and to report any soreness or irritation of the mouth, which might indicate a fungal overgrowth, oral thrush. Advise the client not to ingest alcoholic beverages while taking griseofulvin, because it may potentiate the effects of alcohol, causing tachycardia and flushing.

Evaluation. The client's infection will be alleviated without evidence of any adverse reactions of griseofulvin.

nystatin lozenges [nye stat' in] (Mycostatin)
nystatin (Mycostatin, Nilstat, Nadostine♣)

Nystatin is an antibiotic primarily used to treat cutaneous or mucocutaneous infections caused by the monilial organism *Candida albicans*. Nystatin adheres to sterols in the fungal cell membrane altering cell membrane permeability, resulting in loss of essential intercellular contents.

Nystatin is not absorbed from the gastrointestinal tract, producing a local antifungal effect. It is excreted in the feces. Side effects are generally rare; infrequently abdominal distress is reported.

The usual oral adult dose for candidiasis is 200,000 to 400,000 U lozenges dissolved slowly in the mouth 4 or 5 times daily. Oral suspension dose is 400,000 to 600,000 U orally four times daily while the tablet dose is 500,000 to 1,000,000 units orally three times daily.

■ Nursing Management

Nystatin Therapy

Assessment. It should be determined if the client has an intolerance to nystatin. A baseline assessment of the client's underlying condition should be obtained. There are no significant drug interactions.

Nursing diagnosis. The client receiving nystatin should be assessed for the possibility of the following nursing diagnoses: fluid volume deficit related to anorexia, nausea and vomiting; altered comfort (abdominal cramping); and altered bowel elimination pattern (diarrhea).

Implementation

Monitoring. Nystatin is virtually nontoxic and well tolerated by all age groups. Monitor the client's infection throughout the course of therapy. Examine the mouth with a tongue blade and flashlight.

Intervention. Shake oral suspensions thoroughly before measuring dosages. With the prepared oral suspension, use the calibrated dosage-measuring device provided by the manufacturer. When mixing dry powdered nystatin, add the dose to 120 to 240 ml of water; administer immediately since it contains no preservatives. Lozenges or pastilles are used to treat oral candidiasis because they are slow to dissolve and are in contact longer with the buccal mucous membrane. With infants, swab nystatin on the oral mucosa.

Education. Instruct the client to perform oral hygiene before taking each dose of nystatin. Half the dosage is placed in each side of the mouth. The medication is swished and then held in the mouth for as long as possible. Lozenges are to be dissolved slowly in the mouth.

Caution the client to complete the full course of therapy even if feeling better. It should be continued for at least 48 hours after normal culture results are obtained and symptoms have disappeared.

Alert the client to report to the prescriber symptoms of nausea, vomiting, diarrhea, or increased irritation at the site of infection.

Evaluation. The client's infection will be alleviated without the client developing any adverse gastrointestinal effects from the nystatin therapy.

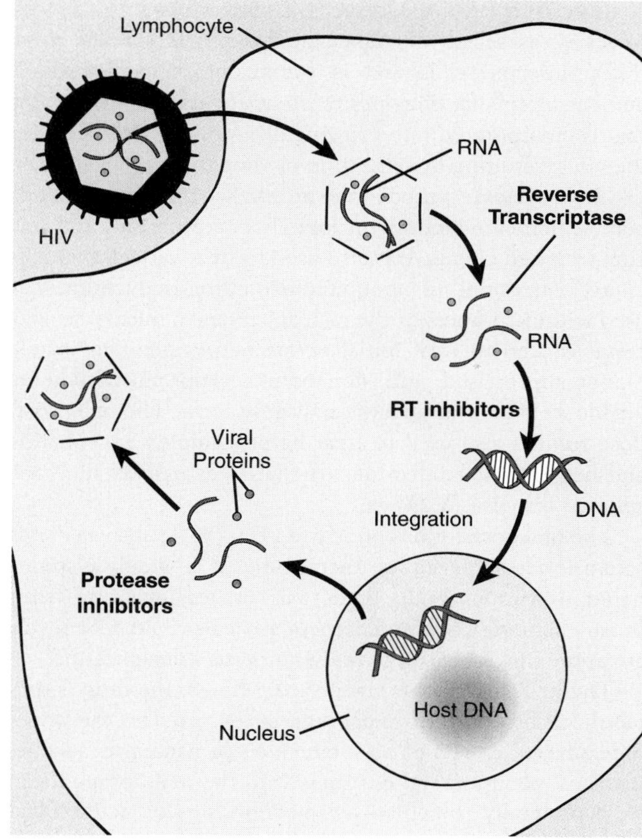

Figure 60-1 Inhibition sites for human immunodeficiency virus (HIV). The HIV genes are composed of RNA, which is translated to DNA by reverse transcriptase (RT) enzyme in order to reproduce. The RT inhibitors interfere with virus production at this site. When integrated DNA becomes part of the cell, the cell produces viral proteins requiring protease enzyme for the production of new HIVs. The protease inhibitors block this enzyme to prevent the release of new viruses into the bloodstream. As a result, combination therapies can reduce the load of new HIV produced in the body.

ANTIVIRAL DRUGS

Chemotherapy for viral diseases has been more limited than chemotherapy for bacterial diseases because development and clinical application of antiviral drugs is difficult. In many viral infections, the replication of the virus in the body reaches its peak before any clinical symptoms appear. By the time signs and symptoms of illness appear, the multiplication of the virus is ending, and the subsequent course of the illness has been determined. Therefore, to be clinically effective, antiviral drugs must be administered in a **chemoprophylactic** manner as preventive agents before disease appears.

A second factor limiting the development of antiviral drugs is that viruses are true parasites; they replicate within the mammalian cell and utilize the host cells' enzyme systems. Thus drugs that would inhibit virus replication would also disturb the host cells and may therefore be too toxic for use.

The protease inhibitors are currently the most potent antiviral agents available. These agents have suppressed viral replication for up to a year in clinical trials and administering them in combination therapies has decreased viral loads and increased CD4 counts (MacDonald & Kazanjian, 1996). Studies of various combinations and their effect on HIV/AIDS complications and disease progression are currently being investigated (Figure 60-1).

The antivirals reviewed here include acyclovir (Zovirax), amantadine (Symmetrel), famciclovir (Famvir), foscarnet (Foscavir), ganciclovir (Cytovene), ribavirin (Virazole), rimantadine (Flumadine), and valacyclovir (Valtrex). In addition, antivirals in current use (alone or in combination) for the treatment of HIV infection are divided into (a) reverse transcriptase inhibitors (nucleoside analogues), (b) protease inhibitors, and (c) nonnucleoside reverse transcriptase inhibitors. The reverse transcriptase inhibitors include didanosine (DDL, Videx), lamivudine (3TC, Epivir), stavudine (D4T, Zerit), zalcitabine (ddC, Hivid), and zidovudine (AZT, Retrovir). Protease inhibitors include indinavir (Crixivan), ritonavir (Norvir), and saquinavir (Invirase). The nonnucleoside reverse transcriptase inhibitor is nevirapine (Viramune).

▲ **acyclovir** [ay sye' kloe ver] (Zovirax)
Acyclovir is selectively taken up by herpes simplex virus (HSV)-infected cells and is eventually converted via a number of cellular enzymes to an active triphosphate form that is incorporated into growing DNA chains produced by the virus, resulting in, inhibition of viral DNA replication.

Oral acyclovir is used in the prophylaxis and treatment of genital herpes infections in immunocompromised and uncompromised clients. It is also used to treat varicella (chickenpox) infections in nonimmunocompromised children if used within 24 hours of the rash appearance. Injectable acyclovir is used to treat initial severe herpes genitalis in immunocompromised and nonimmunocompromised clients unable to take or absorb the oral dose form. The parenteral dose form is also used to treat herpes simplex encephalitis and herpes zoster infections, the latter caused by the varicella-zoster virus (VZV).

The oral dose form is poorly (15% to 30%) absorbed, but serum levels achieved are therapeutic. It is widely disseminated to various body fluids and tissues including cerebrospinal fluid (CSF), and herpetic vesicular fluid. CSF levels are approximately 50% of the serum drug concentration.

The half-life is approximately 2.5 hours; the drug is metabolized by the liver and primarily excreted in the urine. Side/adverse effects of acyclovir include nausea, headache, diarrhea, vomiting and dizziness with the oral dosage form; or parenterally, phlebitis at injection site or acute renal failure with rapid injection.

The usual oral adult dose for herpes genital infection: initially, 200 mg orally every 4 hours during waking hours (five times daily) for 10 days. For chronic suppressant, recurrent infection, the dose is 400 mg orally twice a day. The varicella dose for children 2 to 12 years old is 20 mg/kg up to 800 mg/dose four times daily for 5 days.

The parenteral adult dosage for severe genital herpes is 5 mg/kg every 8 hours for 5 days. For other dosage recommendations, see current package insert.

■ Nursing Management

Acyclovir Therapy

Assessment. If the client has preexisting dehydration or renal function impairment, use acyclovir with caution, since these clients are at greater risk for nephrotoxicity. A history of neurologic abnormalities or a previous neurologic reaction to cytotoxic agents may indicate a tendency for such responses to acyclovir. A hypersensitivity to acyclovir or ganciclovir would require special caution.

Review the client's current medication regimen. When acyclovir is given concurrently with other nephrotoxic drugs, the potential for nephrotoxicity is increased. Monitor renal function closely.

Assess lesions before administering the drug and daily throughout therapy. A baseline BUN and serum creatinine concentration should be determined because precipitation of acyclovir crystals occurring in the renal tubules may result in renal tubular damage progressing to acute renal failure.

Nursing diagnosis. The client receiving acyclovir therapy should be assessed for the possibility of the following nursing diagnoses: impaired tissue integrity related to inflammation or phlebitis at the injection site; altered comfort related (headache); fluid volume deficit related to anorexia, nausea and vomiting; risk for injury related to lightheadedness; altered bowel elimination pattern (diarrhea); and the collaborative problems of acute renal failure (oliguria, thirst, anorexia, nausea, vomiting, fatigue) and encephalopathic effects (coma, confusion, seizures, tremors).

Implementation

Monitoring. Renal function studies, BUN levels, and serum creatinine concentrations should be done during therapy to monitor for the drug's nephrotoxic effects. Fluid intake and output should be monitored, particularly if the client is receiving bolus injections of acyclovir. Monitor the lesions for resolution.

Intervention. The capsules may be administered with meals to minimize gastrointestinal distress. When dispensing the oral suspension, shake it well and use the calibrated measuring device supplied by the manufacturer.

Intravenous acyclovir should be administered via infusion pump at a constant rate for at least 1 hour to prevent precipitation of drug crystals in the renal tubules. The client should also receive hydration during the infusion and for 2 hours afterward to prevent this effect. Avoid rapid or bolus injection of the drug. Rotate infusion sites to prevent phlebitis. The intravenous solution is not to be used topically or orally or administered intramuscularly or subcutaneously.

Education. The client will need accurate information about herpes, its symptoms, transmission, and course of the illness and treatment. Because herpes genitalis is sexually transmitted, misinformation about it abounds. The client should avoid sexual activity if either or any participant has symptoms of herpes. Condom use may help prevent the spread of the infection, but spermicidal jellies or diaphragms probably will not. Acyclovir will not prevent the transmission of the disease or cure it.

The full course of therapy should be taken; however, caution the client not to take the drug longer than prescribed. Six months is generally the limit of long-term therapy. Report to the prescriber if symptoms do not subside.

Medication should be initiated as soon as possible after symptoms appear. The client should be instructed to begin the medication as soon as itching, tingling, or pain develops at the site to minimize the episode of herpes.

Instruct the client regarding comfort measures such as wearing loose-fitting clothing to minimize irritation of the lesions. The infected areas should be kept clean and dry.

Caution female clients to obtain a Pap smear at least annually, since women with genital herpes are at higher risk for cervical cancer than women without genital herpes.

Because dizziness is an adverse effect of this agent, the client should be cautioned against performing tasks that require mental alertness, such as driving, until the response to the drug has been ascertained.

The client should be encouraged to maintain good dental hygiene and visit the dentist regularly for teeth cleaning and to monitor for the development of gingival hyperplasia.

Evaluation. The client's infection will go into remission with a decrease in time to full crusting, and a decrease in vesicles, ulcers, and crusts without the client experiencing any adverse effects of acyclovir therapy.

amantadine [a man' ta deen] (Symmetrel, Symadine) Amantadine appears to block the uncoating of the influenza A virus and the release of viral nucleic acid into host respiratory epithelial cells. It also increases dopamine release and inhibits the reuptake of dopamine and norepinephrine centrally. Therefore, amantadine is indicated for the prevention and treatment of influenza A, for treatment of Parkinson's disease and for the treatment of drug-induced, extrapyramidal reactions.

Amantadine is rapidly absorbed orally and distributed to saliva and nasal secretions and crosses the blood-brain barrier. It has a half-life of 11 to 15 hours reaching a peak serum level within 2 to 4 hours. Its onset of action as an antidyskinetic is usually within 2 days. It is excreted mostly unchanged by the kidneys.

The side/adverse effects of amantadine include CNS toxicity, gastric distress, and with chronic therapy, livedo reticularis (a vasospastic disorder worsened by exposure to cold and is evidenced by a reddish blue mottling of the legs and sometimes, arms). It also may induce anticholinergic side effects and orthostatic hypotension.

The adult oral antiviral dose is 200 mg orally daily or 100 mg every 12 hours. Antidyskinetic dosage is 100 mg PO once or twice a day.

■ Nursing Management
Amantadine Therapy

Assessment. The following health problems would indicate cautious use of amantadine: congestive heart failure and/or peripheral edema, since the drug may worsen the condition; epilepsy, since the drug may increase seizure activity; and renal impairment, since accumulation of the drug increases CNS adverse effects.

Elderly clients are more prone to have confusion and difficulty in urination as frequent effects of amantadine because of its antimuscarinic activity.

Review the client's current drug regimen for significant drug interactions that may occur when amantadine is given with the following drugs:

Drug	Possible effect and management
alcohol	**Increased risk for CNS side effects such as dizziness, fainting episodes, confusion, or circulatory problems reported. Avoid or a potentially serious drug interaction may occur.**
anticholinergics	May result in an increase in anticholinergic side effects, such as hallucinations, dry mouth, blurred vision, confusion, and nightmares. Monitor closely since dosage adjustment of amantadine may be required.
CNS-stimulating agents	**May cause increased CNS stimulation, resulting in insomnia, increased irritability, and nervousness. Cardiac arrhythmias and convulsions may also occur. Avoid or a potentially serious drug interaction may occur. If given concurrently, be sure to monitor pulse rate and neurologic status closely.**

A baseline assessment of the client's infection or neurologic status should be obtained.

Nursing diagnosis. The client receiving amantadine should be assessed for the possibility of the following nursing diagnoses: altered comfort (rash, headache, dry mouth, anorexia, and nausea); altered sleep pattern (insomnia); risk for injury related to the development of orthostatic hypotension; altered thought processes (confusion, hallucinations, severe mental or mood changes) related to CNS toxicity; impaired verbal communication related to CNS effects; altered urinary elimination (retention); altered bowel elimination pattern (constipation); and the collaborative problems of seizures, livedo reticularis, corneal deposits, and congestive heart failure.

Implementation

Monitoring. Closely monitor clients receiving dosages over 200 mg/day for side effects/adverse reactions. Blood pressure and TPR monitoring is indicated, particularly for the first few days after a dosage increase.

If the client is taking amantadine for parkinsonism, dyskinetic symptoms such as tremors, rigidity, and disturbances of gait should be monitored throughout the course of therapy.

Clients in end stage renal disease (ESRD) require plasma concentrations monitored, since a single dose may provide therapeutic levels for 7 to 10 days.

Intervention. If administered as a chemoprophylactic agent, it should be started in anticipation of contact with, or as soon after exposure to, individuals having influenza A infections and continued for at least 10 days after exposure. If given concurrently with the influenza vaccine, continue for 2 to 3 weeks.

Syncope, insomnia, and nausea may be minimized by changing from a once-daily dosage to a twice-daily schedule. Administering the last daily dose several hours before bedtime helps to minimize insomnia.

When administering the syrup form of the drug, use the calibrated measuring device provided by the manufacturer.

Education. Caution the client to avoid alcoholic beverages while taking amantadine, since alcohol increases the risk of CNS effects such as dizziness, syncope, and confusion.

If the client is taking amantadine as an antiviral medication, its course should be started before or as soon as possible after exposure. The client should complete the full course of therapy and should notify the prescriber if viral infection symptoms do not decrease within a few days.

Clients taking the drug as an antidyskinetic medication should complete the course of therapy as prescribed and not take more than the prescribed dosage. The client should be advised that it may require 2 or more weeks to obtain full benefit from the drug. Counsel the client to gradually resume physical activities. The drug dosage should be discontinued gradually.

Mental confusion, hallucinations, and difficulty sleeping are indications of CNS toxicity and should be reported to the prescriber promptly.

Advise clients to change positions from lying to sitting or standing and from sitting to standing with caution because of the orthostatic effects of amantadine.

Clients may decrease the discomfort of mouth dryness with ice, sugarless gum, or candy. Encourage oral hygiene to prevent caries and oral candidiasis.

Alert the client to the possible occurrence of a purplish, red rash, which disappears 2 to 12 weeks after the medication is discontinued.

Because amantadine may cause drowsiness or dizziness, caution the client to avoid tasks such as driving until the response to the drug has been determined.

Evaluation. The client's infection will be eliminated or symptoms of parkinsonism reduced without the client experiencing any adverse effects.

famciclovir [fam sye' kloe veer] (Famvir)
Famciclovir, a prodrug of penciclovir the active antiviral substance, has inhibitory action against herpes simplex viruses (types 1 and 2) and varicella zoster virus. It is indicated for the treatment of genital herpes and acute herpes zoster (Olin, 1996).

Administered orally, famciclovir is well absorbed and converted in the intestinal wall to the active penciclovir. It reaches peak serum level in about 1 hour; half life is 2 to 3 hours; and it is excreted primarily unchanged in urine and feces.

Side/adverse effects of famciclovir include headaches, weakness, gastric distress and fatigue. Usual adult dose is 500 mg PO every 8 hours for 1 week.

▪ Nursing Management
Famciclovir Therapy

Assessment. Famciclovir therapy is contraindicated for clients with a sensitivity to the drug. Elderly clients and those with renal impairment may require dosage reduction and careful monitoring.

Review the client's concurrent medication regimen for potential drug-drug interactions such as with theophylline which decreases renal clearance of famciclovir, and probenecid (Benemid) which increases serum levels of famciclovir.

A baseline assessment of the client's lesions should be documented.

Nursing diagnosis. The client receiving famciclovir therapy may experience the following nursing diagnoses/collaborative problems: fatigue and altered comfort (headache, nausea).

Implementation

Monitoring. Assess the client's lesions during therapy. In addition, monitor for the presence of postherpetic neuralgia pain during and after therapy.

Intervention. Famciclovir therapy should be started as soon as herpes is diagnosed, preferably within 48 hours of onset. It may be administered without regard to food.

Education. Review client education for acyclovir.

Evaluation. The client's lesions will be minimal with decreased time to crusting and a decrease in vesicles, ulcers and crusting without experiencing any adverse effects of famciclovir.

foscarnet [fos car' net] (Foscavir)
Foscarnet is a virostatic agent; that is, it inhibits viral replication of all known herpes viruses in vitro, which includes the cytomegalovirus (CMV), herpes simplex virus types 1 and 2, Epstein-Barr virus, and varicella-zoster virus. It acts by selective inhibition at the pyrophosphate binding site of viral DNA polymerase. If the drug is discontinued, viral replication will resume. It is currently used to treat cytomegalovirus retinitis in clients with acquired immunodeficiency syndrome (AIDS).

This drug is administered by intravenous infusion, has an elimination half-life of 3.3 to 6.8 hours, reaches peak serum level at the end of the infusion, is not metabolized, and is excreted primarily unchanged in the urine.

Common side/adverse effects of foscarnet include nephrotoxicity, gastric distress, and neurotoxicity. It may also cause neurotoxicity, anemia, and leukopenia.

For induction, the usual adult dose by IV infusion is 60 mg/kg every 8 hours for 2 to 3 weeks. Maintenance dosage is 90 to 120 mg/kg daily.

▪ Nursing Management
Foscarnet Therapy

Assessment. If the client has renal impairment, the dosage must be modified based on the client's creatinine clearance. Dehydration will promote renal toxicity. A baseline assessment of the client's underlying infection and renal function should be ascertained.

The client's current drug regimen should be reviewed for significant drug interactions such as may occur when foscarnet is given with the following drugs:

Drug	Possible effect and management
acyclovir (Zovirax), aminoglycosides, amphotericin B (Fungizone), and other nephrotoxic medications	May result in increased risk of renal toxicity. Monitor renal status closely if drugs are administered concurrently.
pentamidine (Pentam 300)	**Concurrent administration of IV pentamidine with foscarnet may result in severe hypocalcemia, hypomagnesemia, and nephrotoxicity. Avoid or a potentially serious drug interaction may occur.**

Nursing diagnosis. The client receiving foscarnet therapy should be assessed for the following nursing diagnoses: altered comfort related to phlebitis (pain at the site of infusion); altered protection related to anemia and leukopenia; fluid volume deficit related to anorexia, nausea, and vomiting; sensory-perceptual alterations related to cytomegalovirus retinitis secondary to the ineffectiveness of the drug; and the collaborative problems of neurotoxicity (anxiety, confusion, dizziness, headache, tremor, seizures, pain or numbness in hands and feet) and nephrotoxicity.

Implementation

Monitoring. Monitor the client's vision status, intake and output, serum electrolytes (calcium, magnesium, phosphate, potassium), BUN, creatinine clearance, and signs and symptoms of the client's infection.

Intervention. The client must be adequately hydrated to prevent renal toxicity. Foscarnet is administered by slow IV infusion using a controlled infusion device over 1 hour for low doses and 2 hours for high doses. Rapid or direct IV injection may cause potentially toxic serum concentrations. It may be administered via a central or peripheral vein, but infusion solution for peripheral infusion must be diluted to 12 mg/ml to minimize local irritation.

Intravitreal injection may be used for the treatment of cytomegalovirus retinitis in clients with an intolerance to acyclovir and advanced renal function impairment.

Education. Alert the client to report any change in urinary elimination pattern or a worsening vision pain in the involved eye(s).

Evaluation. The client's infection will be alleviated with the client experiencing any untoward effects of foscarnet therapy.

ganciclovir [gan sye' kloe vir] (Cytovene, Cytovene-IV)

Ganciclovir is converted intracellularly to the triphosphate form which is the active, antiviral agent. In the presence of the cytomegalovirus, ganciclovir is rapidly phosphorylated to ganciclovir-triphosphate, which then inhibits viral DNA polymerase, suppressing viral DNA synthesis. If ganciclovir is discontinued, viral replication will resume.

Ganciclovir is administered by IV infusion or by intravitreal injection. Serum half-life is 2.5 to 3.6 hours while vitreous fluid half-life is about 13 hours. This drug is primarily excreted unchanged by the kidneys.

The oral ganciclovir is indicated only for maintenance of CMV retinitis in persons that had resolution of active retinitis after induction therapy with parenteral ganciclovir. The oral dosage form has a half-life of 3-5.5 hours and reaches peak serum concentration in 3 hours if administered with food. An intravitreal ganciclovir implant (Vitasert Implant) is in phase III studies and thus far, it has been found to be more effective in delaying the progression of retinitis than IV ganciclovir (Hitchens, 1996).

Common side/adverse effects of ganciclovir include granulocytopenia, thrombocytopenia, and possibly, gastric distress.

The usual adult dose by IV infusion for induction is 5 mg/kg every 12 hours for 2 to 3 weeks. Maintenance dosage is 5 mg/kg daily. The maintenance dose with oral ganciclovir is 1000 mg three times daily with food.

See Box 60-1 for information on cidofovir, a new agent for CMV retinitis.

■ Nursing Management

Ganciclovir Therapy

Assessment. The client should be assessed for any preexisting renal or hepatic function impairment that will require dosage modification. A baseline assessment should also include the client's underlying condition, neurologic status, and CBC. Risk-benefit must be determined for clients with absolute neutrophil count <500 cells/mm^3 or platelet count <25,000/mm^3.

Review the client's current therapeutic regimen for significant drug interactions such as may occur when ganciclovir is given with the following drugs.

BOX 60-1

Cidofovir (Vistide)

Cidofovir (Vistide) approved for treatment of CMV retinitis, has several advantages over other CMV drug therapies. This product is only given IV once every 2 weeks; therefore, the client does not need a surgically implanted catheter, which is often a major source of infections. Cidofovir has been reported to be active against CMV that is resistant to either ganciclovir or foscarnet but it may not be effective against CMV that is resistant to both drugs (Cidofovir Approved, 1996).

Drug	Possible effect and management
bone marrow depressant drugs	Concurrent use may result in increased bone marrow depressant effects. Monitor CBC closely for neutropenia and thrombocytopenia.
zidovudine (AZT)	**May result in severe hematologic toxicity. Avoid or a potentially serious drug interaction may occur. If used concurrently, use extreme caution.**

Nursing diagnosis. The client receiving ganciclovir therapy should be assessed for the following nursing diagnoses: With IV administration: altered protection related to neutropenia and thrombocytopenia; altered thought processes related to CNS toxicity (mood changes, nervousness); fluid volume deficit related to anorexia, nausea and vomiting; altered tissue integrity related to inflammation and phlebitis at the infusion site; and the collaborative problems of seizures and coma. With intravitreal administration: sensory/perceptual alterations (visual) related to bacterial endophthalmitis, retinal detachment, scleral induration, or subconjunctival hemorrhage.

Implementation

Monitoring. The client's infection should be monitored, as well as CBC and platelet counts, BUN, creatinine clearance, and ophthalmic exams.

Intervention. Ganciclovir is administered by slow IV infusion using a controlled infusion device. Rapid or direct IV injection may cause potentially toxic serum concentrations. It may be administered via a central or peripheral vein. Sterile water for injection should be used to reconstitute the drug, *not* bacteriostatic water. Use the same precautions as when handling cytotoxic solutions; consult your institution's procedure manual.

Intravitreal injection is used for clients unresponsive to IV therapy or those with severe mylosuppression due to ganciclovir therapy.

Education. Alert the client to reportable drug-induced signs and symptoms, or if contracting an infection, fever, or chills.

Instruct females of reproductive age on ganciclovir to use effective contraception because the drug has mutagenic and teratogenic potential (see Pregnancy Safety Box on p. 942). Male clients should use barrier contraception during treatment and for at least 90 days after therapy.

Pregnancy Safety

Category	Drug
B	amphotericin B, didanosine, famciclovir, ritonavir, saquinavir, valacyclovir
C	acyclovir, amantadine, fluconazole, flucytosine, foscarnet, ganciclovir, indinavir, itraconazole, ketoconazole, lamivudine, miconazole, nevirapine, rimantadine, stavudine, zalcitabine, zidovudine
X	ribavirin

Pregnancy safety for griseofulvin is not established, although it is recommended not to take this drug during pregnancy because of reported teratogenic effects.

Evaluation. The client's infection will be alleviated without the client experiencing any untoward effects.

ribavirin for inhalation [rye ba vye' rin] (Virazole)
Ribavirin is virustatic with a mechanism of action that is diverse and not completely understood. It rapidly penetrates viral infected cells and is believed to reduce intracellular guanosine triphosphate (GTP) storage; inhibits viral RNA and protein synthesis, thus inhibiting viral duplication, spread to other cells, or both. It is indicated for serious viral pneumonia caused by respiratory syncytial virus (RSV).

Following oral inhalation, it is well absorbed and rapidly distributed to plasma, respiratory tract secretions, and erythrocytes. Half-life is 9.5 hours after oral inhalation and approximately 40 days in erythrocytes. Ribavirin is metabolized in the liver and excreted primarily by the kidneys.

Side/adverse effects are rare but with chronic administration, may include skin rash or irritation.

The adult dosage for ribavirin for inhalation aerosol has not been established. For viral pneumonia in children, administer by oral inhalation via a Viratek small-particle aerosol generator, using a 20 mg/ml ribavirin concentration in the reservoir. Administer over 12 to 18 hours per day for 3 to 7 days.

■ Nursing Management

Nursing Management: Ribavirin Therapy

Assessment. Although not indicated for use in adults, health care workers and visitors who spend time at the bedside may become environmentally exposed. There is risk of teratogenic and/or embryocidal effects for women who are pregnant. No significant drug interactions have been reported.

A baseline assessment should be obtained of the client's infection.

Nursing diagnosis. The child receiving ribavirin is at risk for altered comfort related to direct contact chemical irritation evidenced by conjunctivitis and/or rash. Health care workers in the environment with the client may experience the same effects and headache.

Implementation

Monitoring. Monitor the child's respiratory status before and after administration. If administered to clients receiving ventilation assistance, observe for increased positive-end expiratory pressure and increased positive inspiratory pressure, which occur if ribavirin precipitates within the ventilator apparatus. The equipment should be checked at least every half-hour to prevent fluid accumulation in the tubing. Therapy is generally effective if begun within the first 3 days of respiratory syncytial virus therapy.

Intervention. Therapy with ribavirin may begin before the diagnosis is confirmed by diagnostic tests; however, treatment should not continue if the presence of RSV is not confirmed.

Ribavirin aerosol is to be administered only with the Viratek SPAG Model SPAG-2. See the SPAG-2 manual for exceptions.

To prepare the solution for inhalation, add a measured quantity of sterile water for injection or for inhalation to each 6-g vial, which is adequate to dissolve the drug. Do not use bacteriostatic water. Transfer the solution to a clean, sterilized SPAG-2 reservoir. Dilute the solution with sterile water to a total volume of 300 ml. Ensure that the final solution is free of particulate matter. Always discard the remaining solution when its level gets low and add freshly reconstituted solution to the reservoir. The solution retains its potency at room temperature for 24 hours. Do not administer concurrently with any other medication by aerosolization.

Education. Instruct the parents about the ribavirin therapy, its action, route of administration, equipment involved, frequency of treatments, and adverse effects.

Evaluation. The client's infection will be alleviated without adverse effects.

rimantadine [ri man' ti deen] (Flumadine)
Rimantadine, an analog of amantadine, inhibits viral replication by blocking or reducing the uncoating of viral RNA in host cells. It is indicated for the treatment and prevention of influenza type A respiratory tract infections.

This product is well absorbed orally; reaches peak concentration in 1 to 4 hours; half life of 13 to 38 hours in children (4 to 8 yrs old), 25 to 30 hours in younger adults (22 to 44 years), and 32 hours in the elderly (71 to 79 years). It is metabolized in the liver and primarily excreted by the kidneys.

Rimantadine side effects are uncommon with the elderly having a higher incidence of side effects than younger adults. Side/adverse effects include CNS effects and gastric distress.

For rimantadine prophylaxis and treatment, children over 10 and adults, the dose is 100 mg twice a day. For elderly nursing home clients or persons with severe liver or renal impairment, the recommended dose is 100 mg daily.

■ **Nursing Management**
Rimantadine Therapy

Assessment. It should be determined if the client has a history of epilepsy or other seizure disorder because rimantadine increases the risk of seizures. Clients with hepatic function impairment have a reduced clearance of rimantadine. Hypersensitivity to amantadine or rimantadine precludes the use of the drug.

Nursing diagnosis. The client receiving rimantadine therapy is at risk for the following: fluid volume deficit related to anorexia, nausea, and vomiting; sleep pattern disturbance (insomnia); altered comfort (headache); and risk for injury (dizziness).

Implementation

Monitoring. Monitor for the drug's side effects and for the beginning symptoms of influenza A.

Intervention. Administration should be continued for 10 days following exposure. It may be administered daily for 6 to 8 days during an influenza epidemic. If administered concurrently with influenza A viral vaccine, it should be for a period of 2 to 3 weeks until protective antibodies have developed. But because it is only 70% to 80% effective in this instance, elderly clients and high risk individuals may continue therapy longer.

Education. Stress the importance of taking the drug everyday and around the clock to maintain steady serum levels.

Evaluation. The client will not contract influenza A or will have mild symptoms without experiencing any adverse effects of the rimantadine.

valacyclovir [va la sye' kloe veer] (Valtrex)

Valacyclovir is a prodrug that is converted to acyclovir by first pass intestinal and liver metabolism. It is indicated for the treatment of herpes zoster (shingles) caused by varicella-zoster virus in immunocompetent persons. When compared to acyclovir, valacyclovir was reported to be more significant in reducing the pain and postherpetic neuralgia associated with herpes zoster in persons over 50 years old. Valacyclovir has not been studied in children, immunocompromised individuals or in persons with disseminated zoster (*USP Update*, 1996).

Administered orally, valacyclovir is well absorbed and converted to acyclovir, the active substance. It reaches peak serum levels in 1.6 to 2 hours; half-life is 2.5 to 3.3 hours. Valacyclovir is converted to inactive metabolites by alcohol and aldehyde dehydrogenase and excreted primarily in urine.

No serious adverse effects of valacyclovir have been reported to date. Side effects include nausea, headache, weakness, gastric distress, and dizziness. The usual adult dose is 1 gram 3 times daily for 1 week.

For the nursing management of valacyclovir, see the nursing management of acyclovir.

Reverse Transcriptase Inhibitors

didanosine [dye dah' noe seen] (ddI, Videx)

Didanosine is converted intracellularly to its active form ddA-TP which in turn, inhibits HIV DNA reverse transcriptase. This action results in suppression of HIV replication. Didanosine is indicated for the treatment of acquired immunodeficiency syndrome (AIDS) and advanced human immunodeficiency virus (HIV) in clients exhibiting a decreased response to or clients who are unable to take zidovudine.

This product, which is available in oral dosage forms, is considered to be acid labile. Therefore oral formulations are buffered to increase gastric pH to protect didanosine from gastric acid destruction. Didanosine crosses the blood-brain barrier; has a half-life of 1.5 hours in adults; and reaches peak serum concentration in 30 to 60 minutes. Excretion is primarily via the kidneys.

The common side/adverse effects of didanosine include peripheral neuropathy, CNS toxicity, gastric distress and dry mouth.

The usual adult dosage for clients weighing less than 60 kg is 167 mg orally every 12 hours; for clients more than 60 kg, 250 mg every 12 hours. For pediatric dosing schedule, check current package insert or drug reference for didanosine for buffered oral suspension.

■ **Nursing Management**
Didanosine Therapy

Assessment. It should be determined that the client does not have a history of or actual pancreatitis or peripheral neuropathy or these conditions will recur or worsen. There is a greater risk, too, of acute pancreatitis if the client has AIDS, elevated serum triglycerides, a history of alcohol abuse, or renal or hepatic function impairment. Cautious use is required for clients on sodium restrictions because each 2 tablet dose contains 529 mg of sodium and each single dose packet for powder for oral solution contains 1380 mg of sodium. Baseline assessment of the client's infection and serum amylase, lipase, and triglycerides should be obtained.

The client's current medication regimen should be reviewed for significant drug interactions such as may occur when didanosine is given with the following drugs:

Drug	Possible effect and management
alcohol, asparaginase (Elspar), azathioprine (Imuran), estrogens, furosemide (Lasix), nitrofurantoin (Furadantin), pentamidine IV (Pentam 300), sulfonamides, sulindac (Clinoril), tetracyclines, thiazide diuretics or valproic acid (Depakene), or other drugs associated with pancreatitis	**Concurrent drug use may result in pancreatitis. Avoid or a potentially serious drug interaction may occur. If combination therapy is necessary,use extreme caution.**

Continued

Drug	Possible effect and management
chloramphenicol, (Chloromycetin), cisplatin (Platinol), dapsone (Avlosulfon), ethambutol (Myambutol), ethionamide (Trecator-SC), hydralazine (Apresoline), isoniazid (INH), lithium, metronidazole (Flagyl), nitrofurantoin (Furadantin), nitrous oxide, phenytoin (Dilantin), stavudine (Zerit), vincristine (Oncovin) or zalcitabine (HIVID), or other drugs associated with peripheral neuropathy	**May increase potential for peripheral neuropathy. Avoid or a potentially serious drug interaction may occur. If it must be used, monitor closely for numbness and tingling in the fingers and toes.**
dapsone (Avlosulfon), itraconazole (Sporanox), or ketoconazole (Nizoral)	May result in decreased absorption of dapsone or ketoconazole because they require an acidic media for absorption. Administer these drugs at least 2 hours before didanosine.
fluoroquinolone antibiotics such as ciprofloxacin (Cipro), norfloxacin (Noroxin), and ofloxacin (Floxin) or tetracyclines	Concurrent drug administration may reduce absorption of these antibiotics because didanosine chewable tablets and pediatric powder contain magnesium and aluminum antacids that may chelate the antibiotics, thus reducing absorption. If both drugs are prescribed, give antibiotics at least 2 hours before or 2 hours after these didanosine products. The buffered didanosine powder for oral solution has a citrate buffer that does not interfere with the antibiotics, thus its use would reduce the potential for this interaction (*USP DI*, 1996).

Nursing diagnosis. The client should be assessed for the possibility of the following nursing diagnoses: altered skin integrity related to drug-induced rash; altered comfort (headache, dry mouth); altered protection related to leukopenia, anemia, and granulocytopenia; risk for injury related to dizziness; and the collaborative problems of CNS depression, cardiomyopathy, hepatitis, retinal depigmentation, acute pancreatitis and peripheral neuropathy.

Implementation

Monitoring. Observe the client for abdominal pain and numbness of the fingers and toes. Monitor serum amylase, lipase, and triglycerides over the course of the therapy. Ophthalmic exams should be done in children every 3 to 6 months to detect corneal pigmentation.

Intervention. Didanosine should be administered on an empty stomach, at least 1 hour before or 2 hours after a meal. The tablets should not be swallowed whole but thoroughly chewed, crushed, or dissolved in water before administration. Dissolve in at least 30 ml of water, stir, and have the client swallow it immediately. The powder form for oral solution needs to be dissolved in 120 ml of water, which may take 2 to 3 minutes. Administer immediately after dissolution.

Education. Alert client to report any abdominal discomfort or nausea and vomiting or change of sensation in the fingers or toes to the prescriber. Caution clients with sodium restriction about the high sodium content of the drug.

Evaluation. The client's infection will be alleviated without the client experiencing any adverse effects of the drug.

lamivudine [la mi' vue deen] (3TC, Epivir)

Lamivudine is used in combination with zidovudine for the treatment of HIV infection, based on evidence of disease progression. It is converted in the body to an active metabolite (L-TP) which then inhibits HIV reverse transcription by terminating the viral DNA chain. It also inhibits RNA and DNA-dependent DNA polymerase functions of reverse transcriptase. Clinical trials are underway to evaluate the effects of this combination on the progression of HIV infection (Olin, 1996).

Rapidly absorbed after oral administration, L-TP has an intracellular half-life of 10 to 15 hours and is excreted primarily unchanged, by the kidneys.

Side/adverse effects of lamivudine include headaches, fatigue, fever, nausea, vomiting, diarrhea, gastric pain or distress, anorexia, neuropathy, insomnia, depression, cough, and skeletal muscle pain.

Usual dose of lamivudine for adolescents (12 to 16 years old) and adults is 150 mg PO twice a day.

■ Nursing Management

Lamivudine Therapy

Assessment. Lamivudine therapy is contraindicated for clients with a sensitivity to the drug. Elderly clients and those with renal impairment may require dosage reduction and careful monitoring. Use with pediatric clients with a history of pancreatitis only if there is no alternative and only with extreme caution.

Review the client's current drug regimen for potential drug interactions such as with trimethoprim/sulfamethoxazole (Bactrim, TMP/SMX), which increases the blood levels of lamivudine; and zidovudine (AZT), which has its blood levels increased by lamivudine.

Obtain a baseline assessment of the client's HIV infection. CD4, CBC, serum amylase, and liver function determinations should be obtained before the initiation of lamivudine therapy.

Nursing diagnosis. The client receiving lamivudine therapy has the potential for the following nursing diagnoses/collaborative problems: fatigue; altered comfort (headache, nausea, musculoskeletal pain); altered protection related to neutropenia, anemia, and thrombocytopenia; sleep pattern disturbance (insomnia); altered bowel elimination (diarrhea); ineffective airway clearance (cough); and the potential complications of neuropathy and pancreatitis (children only).

Implementation

Monitoring. Periodically throughout therapy, the client's CD4, CBC with differential and platelets, serum amylase levels, and liver function studies should be monitored. Assess the client for changes in symptoms of HIV infection, opportunistic infections, and peripheral neuropathy (tingling, burning, and weakness of hands and feet). Monitor pediatric clients for symptoms of pancreatitis, such as nausea, vomiting, and abdominal pain.

Intervention. Administer lamivudine without regard to food.

Education. Advise client to take lamivudine as ordered. Emphasize the importance of keeping follow up appointments for blood work and provider visits and not taking other medications, including OTCs, without consulting the prescriber. Caution the client that lamivudine does not cure the disease or prevent its spread to others. Instruct in the use of condoms, avoidance of sexual contact, and avoidance of sharing needles or giving blood to prevent the spread of the disease to others. Encourage the reporting of symptoms of neuropathy or pancreatitis to the prescriber immediately.

Evaluation. The client receiving lamivudine therapy should experience the slowing of the progression of the HIV infection and its sequelae.

stavudine [stav' yoo deen] (d4T, Zerit)

Stavudine is an antiviral agent indicated for the treatment of advanced human immunodeficiency virus (HIV) infection or acquired immunodeficiency syndrome (AIDS) in persons that have not responded or are unable to take zidovudine and proven therapeutic agents. Stavudine is converted to stavudine triphosphate which then competes with deoxythymidine triphosphate resulting in inhibition of HIV replication and DNA synthesis.

Oral stavudine is rapidly absorbed, reaches peak serum level in 0.5 to 1.5 hours; it has a half-life of 1 to 1.6 hours and is primarily excreted unchanged by the kidneys. Side/adverse effects include dose-related, peripheral neuropathy and anemia.

The usual adult oral dose of stavudine is 30 mg every 12 hours for persons weighing <60 kg; 40 mg every 12 hours for persons >60 kg.

■ Nursing Management

Stavudine Therapy

Assessment. Stavudine is contraindicated in clients with a hypersensitivity to this drug, didanosine, zalcitabine, or zidovudine, or in clients with severe peripheral neuropathy. The drug is used with caution with clients with advanced HIV infections, bone marrow suppression, renal and hepatitis disease, folic acid or B_{12} deficiency, or women who are pregnant or lactating. A review of the client's concurrent medication regimen is required. If the client is on a drug with myelosuppressant properties, there is a greater risk of myelosuppression with stavudine.

A baseline assessment of the client should include documentation of the client's symptoms, a neurologic exam, a CBC, and renal and liver function studies.

Nursing diagnosis. The client receiving stavudine is at risk for the following nursing diagnoses: altered protection related to bone marrow suppression (anemia); sensory/perceptual alteration (tactile) related to peripheral neuropathy; and the potential complication of hepatitis.

Implementation

Monitoring. Monitor the client's blood, renal and hepatic studies. Monitor the client's neurologic status, intake and output, and bowel pattern.

Intervention. The drug may be taken with or without food. It should be administered every 4 hours around the clock.

Education. Instruct the client to report symptoms of peripheral neuropathy (tingling, burning or numbness of the extremities). Advise the client to report to the prescriber other signs of infections, such as sore throat, cough, urinary burning, swollen lymph nodes, fever, and malaise.

Caution the client that the drug is not a cure and that he or she is still infectious. Other drugs may be necessary to control symptoms, but consultation with the prescriber is needed before taking any other drugs, including OTCs.

Evaluation. The client should experience less symptoms of the HIV infection, such as decreased diarrhea, fatigue, night sweats, and increased body weight.

zalcitabine [zal sye' ta bean] (ddC, Hivid)

The antiviral agent, zalcitabine, is converted by cellular enzymes to its active form, ddC-TP, which inhibits viral reverse transcriptase, inhibiting viral replication. In vitro studies, zalcitabine has been reported to be approximately 10 times more potent than zidovudine against HIV (*USP DI*, 1996). Zalcitabine is indicated for the treatment of advanced HIV infection and acquired immunodeficiency syndrome (AIDS) in persons that either cannot take zidovudine or in those that have disease progression while taking zidovudine.

Administered orally, zalcitabine is metabolized intracellularly to ddC-TP; it reaches peak serum levels in 1 to 2 hours and has a half-life of 1 to 3 hours. It is excreted primarily via the kidneys. Side/adverse effects include peripheral neuropathy, gastric distress, and headache.

The usual adult oral dosage for is 0.75 mg zalcitabine alone or in combination with 200 mg of zidovudine every 8 hours.

■ Nursing Management

Zalcitabine Therapy

Assessment. Determine if the client has a history of alcohol abuse or of hepatic dysfunction because the risk of drug-induced adverse hepatic effects are greater. If the client has preexisting peripheral nerve dysfunction or advanced HIV disease, there is increased risk for peripheral neuropathy.

A baseline assessment of the client should include neurologic status, AST (SGOT), ALT (SGPT), alkaline phosphatase, CBC, and creatinine clearance. The dosage will be based on the client's creatinine clearance.

Review the client's current medications for significant drug interactions such as may occur when zalcitabine is given with the following drugs:

Drug	Possible effect and management
alcohol, asparaginase (Elspar), azathioprine (Imuran), estrogens, furosemide (Lasix), methyldopa (Aldomet), nitrofurantoin (Furadantin), pentamidine IV (Pentam 300), sulfonamides, sulindac (Clinoril), tetracyclines, thiazide diuretics, or valproic acid (Depakene)	**Concurrent use increases the potential risk of pancreatitis. Avoid or a potentially serious drug interaction may occur. If given, monitor for abdominal pain, anorexia, nausea and vomiting, and serum amylase determinations.**
aminoglycosides parenteral, amphotericin B (Fungizone), foscarnet (Foscavir)	May decrease renal excretion of zalcitabine, which may result in toxicity. If administered, monitor serum levels of the drug closely.
chloramphenicol (Chloromycetin), cisplatin (Platinol), dapsone (Avlosulfon), ethionamide (Trecator-SC), hydralazine (Apresoline), isoniazid (INH), lithium, metronidazole (Flagyl), nitrofurantoin (Furadantin), nitrous oxide, phenytoin (Dilantin), or vincristine (Oncovin)	**Concurrent drug administration may result in increased potential for peripheral neuropathy. Avoid or a potentially serious drug interaction may occur. If administered, monitor client closely for numbness and tingling in the fingers and toes.**

A baseline assessment should include a neurologic exam, liver function studies, and serum amylase, lipase, and triglycerides.

Nursing diagnosis. The client receiving zalcitabine therapy should be assessed for the following nursing diagnoses: sensory-perceptual alterations related to peripheral neuropathy; impaired skin integrity related to rash; fatigue; altered comfort (headache); altered protection related to neutropenia, thrombocytopenia, and anemia; fluid volume deficit related to anorexia, nausea, and vomiting; risk for injury related to dizziness; altered mucous membranes (oral ulcers); and the collaborative problems of neuropathy, hepatic dysfunction, and pancreatitis.

Implementation

Monitoring. The client's underlying infection should be monitored, as well as CBCs, creatinine clearance, and hepatic function studies. Monitor and document the client's peripheral reflexes at least once a day. Observe for signs and symptoms of gastrointestinal distress.

Intervention. Zalcitabine should be administered 1 hour before meals or 2 hours after to enhance absorption. Zalcitabine is frequently administered in conjunction with zidovudine.

Education. Alert the client to the action, purpose, dose, frequency of the dose, and signs and symptoms that should be reported to the prescriber.

Evaluation. The client's infection will be controlled without the client experiencing any adverse effects of zalcitabine therapy.

▲ **zidovudine** [zye doe' vue deen] (AZT, Retrovir)

Zidovudine is an antiviral agent (virustatic) that intracellularly is converted to monophosphate, diphosphate and then zidovudine triphosphate by cellular enzymes. The triphosphate form competes with natural thymidine triphosphate for incorporation in growing chains of viral RNA-dependent DNA polymerase (reverse transcriptase), thus inhibiting viral DNA replication. It has a greater affinity for retroviral reverse transcriptase than for the human alpha-DNA polymerase; thus it selectively inhibits viral replication.

Zidovudine is indicated for the treatment of human immunodeficiency virus (HIV) infection and acquired immunodeficiency syndrome (AIDS) in adults with a CD4 lymphocyte count of 500/mm^3 or less. Zalcitabine may be used in combination with zidovudine, especially when the CD4 count is 300/mm^3 or less.

Administered orally, zidovudine is rapidly absorbed and distributed in plasma and cerebrospinal fluid; reaches a peak serum level in 0.5 to 1.5 hours, and has a half-life of approximately 1 hour (in serum, 3.3 hours intracellularly). It is metabolized in the liver and excreted by the kidneys.

Side/adverse effects of zidovudine include nausea, myalgia, insomnia, severe headaches, and bone marrow depression.

The adult oral dose for treatment of symptomatic HIV infection is 100 mg every 4 hours around the clock (600 mg daily). For asymptomatic HIV infection, the adult dose is 100 mg every 4 hours while awake (500 mg daily). For children 3 months to 12 years old, the oral dose 90 to 180 mg/m^2 every 6 hours.

The parenteral adult dose for symptomatic HIV infection is 1 mg/kg by IV infusion administered over 60 minutes every 4 hours around the clock, until oral therapy can be used. The pediatric dosage is 120 mg/m^2 every 6 hours.

■ Nursing Management

Zidovudine Therapy

Assessment. Assess the client's general health before initiating zidovudine therapy. The following health problems indicate that the drug is to be used with caution:

bone marrow depression, which may result in blood dyscrasias; hepatic and renal function impairment, which may affect elimination of the drug and cause toxicity; folic acid or vitamin B_{12} deficiency, which may result in increased sensitivity to hepatotoxicity and hypersensitivity to zidovudine.

Review the client's current medications for significant drug interactions such as may occur when zidovudine is given with the following drugs:

Drug	Possible effect and management
bone marrow depressants, radiation therapy	May exacerbate bone marrow depression and toxicity. Dosage reductions may be necesary. Monitor CBCs closely for leukopenia and anemia.
clarithromycin (Biaxin)	Concurrent drug administration has been reported to result in a lower peak plasma level of zidovudine. Monitor serum concentrations of the drug closely.
ganciclovir (Cytovene)	**Concurrent use has been reported to result in synergistic myelosuppressive toxicity. Since this is a serious hematologic toxicity, avoid or a potentially serious drug interaction may occur.**
probenecid (Benemid)	May result in decreased liver metabolism of zidovudine resulting in increased serum levels and increased risk of toxicity. There is also a high incidence of rash (*USP DI*, 1996). Monitor serum drug concentrations closely if drugs are administered concurrently.

A baseline assessment of the client should include the underlying condition, CBC with MCV, and liver function tests.

Nursing diagnosis. The client receiving zidovudine is at risk for altered comfort (headache, myalgia); fluid volume deficit related to anorexia, nausea and vomiting; altered sleep patterns (insomnia); altered thought processes (confusion); altered protection related to leukopenia and anemia; anxiety; and the collaborative problems of hepatotoxicity (malaise, anorexia, nausea, abdominal discomfort), myopathy (muscle atrophy, weakness, and discomfort), and neurotoxicity (confusion, seizures).

Implementation

Monitoring. Monitor the client's underlying condition. Monitor the client's CBC, which should be done at least every 2 weeks during therapy. Observe the client for fever, sore throat, unusual bleeding or bruising, or unusual tiredness, all of which are symptoms of bone marrow depression. These symptoms may occur even after the medication is discontinued and should be reported to the health care provider. Liver function tests should also be monitored.

Intervention. Zidovudine should be diluted before administration to no greater than 4 mg/ml in 5% dextrose injection and given IV over 1 hour at a constant rate.

The client may experience changes in taste, swelling of the lips and tongue, and mouth ulcers. These symptoms may affect the client's desire or ability to eat. The client must receive good oral hygiene to prevent infection and promote comfort. Food and fluid intake should be monitored to ensure adequate nutrition. Encourage the client to take small but frequent high-protein meals. Serve meals attractively and offer foods the client prefers. Bland and smooth textured foods may be better tolerated.

Education. Advise the client to take the medication exactly as prescribed and not to take more in the hope that it will be more effective or to discontinue the medication without medical advice in despair that it is not effective. Other medications should not be taken concurrently without the approval of the prescriber. The client should take the medication every 4 hours around the clock. Setting an alarm clock to interrupt sleep and maintain this schedule can ensure therapeutic blood levels.

The client should be advised of the importance of regular supervision by the prescriber to check blood counts. Alert the client that dizziness and syncope are effects of zidovudine and that hazardous activities requiring mental alertness should be avoided until the response to the drug has been determined.

Advise the client to avoid sexual contact or to use condoms to prevent transmission of the AIDS virus to sexual partners and not to share needles with others.

Advise the client to complete essential dental work before starting therapy with zidovudine or to delay it until completing the course of the drug because bone marrow depressant effects may result in gingival bleeding and delayed healing. Teach appropriate oral hygiene, including gentle use of toothbrushes and floss, and avoidance of toothpicks.

Evaluation. The client's infection will be controlled and the client will not experience adverse effects of the drug.

Protease Inhibitors

▲ **indinavir** [in din' a veer] (Crixivan)

Indinavir was released under the Food and Drug Administration's accelerated review for the treatment of HIV infection in adults. While its complete mechanism of action is unknown, indinavir appears to inhibit the replication of retroviruses (HIV type I and 2) by interfering with HIV protease. Indinavir affects the replication cycle of HIV and is active in both acute and chronically infected cells, which are generally not affected by the dideoxynucleoside reverse transcriptase inhibitors, such as, didanosine, lamivudine, stavudine, zalcitabine and zidovudine. Thus this product has a virustatic effect due to its HIV protease inhibitor effects (AHFS, Supp A, 1996).

Administered orally, indinavir reaches a peak serum level in approximately 1 hour; it is metabolized in the liver and excreted primarily by the kidneys.

Side/adverse effects of indinavir include gastric distress, nausea, vomiting, diarrhea, headache, dizziness, fatigue, fever, flu-like syndrome, and chest pain. The usual adult dose is 800 mg every 8 hours.

Except for the cautions related to pancreatitis in pediatric clients, the nursing management for indinavir is as for lamivudine.

ritonavir [ri ton' a veer] (Norvir)
Ritonavir is an inhibitor of HIV-1 and HIV-2 protease that interferes with the production of the HIV virus. Use of this product results in the production of noninfectious, immature HIV substances (Olin, 1996).

Administered orally, ritonavir reaches peak serum levels within 2 or 4 hours (fasting or nonfasting); 5 metabolites have been identified with ritonavir but only the M-2 metabolite has antiviral activity. Most of this drug is excreted in feces.

Side/adverse effects of ritonavir include weakness, nausea, vomiting, diarrhea, stomach distress, taste alterations, peripheral paresthesias, allergic reactions, back or chest pain, chills, facial edema, flu symptoms, and many other potential adverse effects. Check current reference for complete list.

The usual dose is 600 mg twice a day, with meals.

The nursing management of the care of the client receiving ritonavir is as for lamividine with the following exceptions: There are not the cautions in relation to the use of the drug and pediatric pancreatitis. Ritonavir has significant drug interactions. Ritonavir may produce large increases in the serum concentrations of the following drugs: amiodarone (Cardarone), astemizole (Hismanal), bepridil (Vascor), bupropion (Wellbutrin), cisapride (Propulsid), clozapine (Clozaril), flecainide (Tambocor), meperidine (Demerol), piroxicam (Feldene), propafenone (Rhythmol), propoxyphene (Darvon), rifabutin (Mycobutin), and terfenadine (Seldane). These drugs have known risks of cardiac arrhythmias, hematologic abnormalities, CNS toxicity (seizures, and other serious adverse effects; do not administer concurrently with ritonavir. In addition, concurrent administration with highly metabolized sedatives and hypnotics, such as alprazolam (Xanax), clorazepate (Tranxene), diazepam (Valium), estazolam (ProSom), flurazepan (Dalmane), midazolam (Versed), triazolam (Halcion), and zolpidem (Ambien), may result in extreme sedation and respiratory depression; do not coadminister.

saquinavir [sa kwin' a veer] (Invirase)
Saquinavir inhibits HIV protease, preventing the cleavage of viral polyproteins. It is used in combination with the nucleoside analogs to treat advanced HIV infection in selected individuals. For example, it may be prescribed concurrently with zidovudine (AZT) in untreated persons or with ddC in persons that were previously treated with extended AZT therapy. Clinical studies based on disease progression and survival, are underway to determine the clinical benefits of combination therapy.

Administered orally, saquinavir has extensive first-pass metabolism, is highly protein bound, is metabolized in the liver, and is excreted in feces primarily. Side effects are usually mild and include diarrhea, abdominal distress, headache, and weakness. Serious adverse effects are rare and may include confusion, Stevens-Johnson syndrome, seizures, thrombocytopenia, ataxia, anemias, and hepatotoxicity.

The usual dose in combination with a nucleoside analog is 200 mg 3 times a day, administered within 2 hours of a full meal.

■ Nursing Management

Saquinavir Therapy

Assessment. Saquinavir therapy is contraindicated for clients with a sensitivity to the drug. Elderly clients and those with hepatic impairment may require dosage reduction and careful monitoring. Safe use with pediatric clients under the age of 16 years has not been established.

Review the client's current drug regimen for potential drug interactions such as with the following drugs:

Drug	Possible effect and management
rifampin (Rifadin), rifabutin (Mycobutin), carbamazepine (Tegretol), dexamethasone, phenobarbital, phenytoin (Dilantin)	These drugs decrease saquinavir blood levels; concurrent use should be avoided.
terfenadine (Seldane), astemizole (Hismanal)	**Saquinavir may increase blood levels of these drugs and increase the risk of cardiovascular toxicities. Avoid or a potentially serious drug interaction may occur.**
calcium channel blockers, clindamycin (Cleocin), dapsone (Alvosulfon), quinidine, triazolam (Halcion)	Saquinavir may increase blood levels of these drugs. Monitor closely for drug toxicities.
ketoconazole (Nizoral)	This drug increases blood levels of saquinavir. Monitor client closely for adverse effects of saquinavir.

Obtain a baseline assessment of the client's AIDS symptoms and opportunistic infections. CBC and liver function determinations should be obtained before the initiation of saquinavir therapy.

Nursing diagnosis. The client receiving saquinavir therapy has the potential for the following nursing diagnoses/collaborative problems: fatigue; altered comfort (headache, nausea, abdominal discomfort); altered protection related to anemia and thrombocytopenia; altered bowel elimination (diarrhea); and the potential complications of CNS toxicity (confusion, ataxia, seizures) and hepatotoxicity.

Implementation

Monitoring. Periodically throughout therapy, the client's CBC with platelets and liver function studies should be monitored. Assess the client for changes in symptoms of AIDS, opportunistic infections, and CNS toxicity (confusion, ataxia, seizures).

Intervention. Administer saquinavir within 2 hours of a full meal for increased absorption.

Education. Advise client to take saquinavir as ordered. Emphasize the importance of keeping follow up appointments for blood work and provider visits and not taking other medications, including OTCs without consulting the prescriber. Caution the client that saquinavir does not cure the disease or prevent its spread to others. Instruct in the use of condoms, avoidance of sexual contact, and avoidance of sharing needles or giving blood to prevent the spread of the disease to others. Encourage the reporting of symptoms of CNS toxicity and hepatotoxicity to the prescriber immediately.

Evaluation. The client receiving saquinavir therapy should experience the slowing of the progression of the HIV infection and its sequelae.

Non-nucleoside, Reverse Transcriptase Inhibitor

nevirapine (Viramune)

Nevirapine is a nonnucleoside antiviral agent that binds directly to reverse transcriptase to block the RNA-dependent and DNA-dependent DNA polymerase activity. This drug can cause resistant HIV if given alone; therefore it should be administered in combination with at least another antiretroviral agent.

Administered orally, nevirapine is well absorbed; reaches peak serum levels in 4 hours; and is distributed in cerebrospinal fluid (45% or serum concentration). Nevirapine is metabolized in the liver and is also an inducer of hepatic cytochrome P450 metabolic enzymes; thus, auto-induction or an increased clearance and a decrease in drug half-life occurs within 2 to 4 weeks of therapy.

Side/adverse effects include nausea, headache, diarrhea, fever, and life-threatening skin reactions, such as Stevens-Johnson syndrome. Discontinue nevirapine in individuals that develop a severe rash or a rash accompanied with other symptoms such as fever, myalgia, fatigue, oral lesions, and conjunctivitis.

Initial therapy is 200 mg PO daily for 2 weeks; maintenance dose is 200 mg twice daily in combination with another antiretroviral agent.

SUMMARY

Mycoses, infections of humans by fungi, range from very mild to life-threatening conditions, some even the result of overgrowth during antibiotic, antineoplastic, or corticosteroid therapy.

Unfortunately, antifungal therapy is not as developed as antibacterial chemotherapy. Most agents are quite toxic to humans in concentrations that would be effective against most fungi, so most preparations are topical. However, amphotericin B, fluconazole, flucytosine, griseofulvin, itraconazole, ketoconazole, miconazole, and nystatin are effective systemic fungistatic and fungicidal agents used for the treatment of a wide variety of mycotic infections.

Antiviral chemotherapy is even more difficult because by the time symptoms of the illness appear, the multiplication of the virus is ending and the course of the illness is set. Antiviral agents would need to be administered prophylactically to be most effective. In addition, viruses are true parasites and use the host cells' enzyme systems, so any effective therapy would also injure the host and thereby be too toxic for use. Antiviral agents in use are acyclovir, amantadine, didanosine, foscarnet, ganciclovir, nevirapine, ribavirin, rimantadine, ritonavir, stavudine, vidarabine, zalcitabine, and zidovudine. Prevention and management of adverse effects are a major nursing responsibility for both antiviral and antifungal agents.

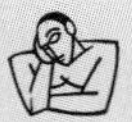

Critical Thinking

1. Why is antiviral therapy more limited than antibacterial or antifungal therapy?
2. Alice Mild, a 20-year-old college student, has been admitted to the hospital with histoplasmosis. The physician has prescribed amphotericin B to be administered 0.25 mg/kg IV. If Alice weighs 154 pounds, how many milligrams will her dose be? What precautions will the prescriber take before the infusion begins to minimize adverse effects of the drug? How will the nurse monitor Alice's health status during the infusion?

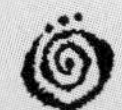

Collaborative Learning Activities

1. Students will be preassigned to write a vignette about a client receiving an antifungal or antiviral. Have them pose questions (and answers) related to the nursing care of the client in their case. These cases and questions will be presented in class. The rest of the class will answer the questions.

BIBLIOGRAPHY

Abelcet (1996). Abelcet package insert. The Liposome Co., Inc. #1-1001-41-US-D.

American Hospital Formulary Service (1996). *AHFS drug information: Current developments, Supplement A.* Washington, DC: American Society of Hospital Pharmacists.

American Hospital Formulary Service (1996). *AHFS drug information '96.* Bethesda, MD: American Society of Hospital Pharmacists.

Anderson KN, et al. (Eds.) (1994). *Mosby's medical, nursing, & allied health dictionary* (4th ed.). St Louis: Mosby.

Cidofovir Approved (1996). *PI Perspective: Project Inform.* San Francisco: San Francisco Project Inform.

Cohen BA & Brady M (1992). Practices surrounding ribavirin administration, *Pediatr Nurs 18*(3):253-7.

Hayden FG (1996). Antimicrobial agents: Antiviral agents. In Hardman JG & Limbird LE (Eds.). *Goodman & Gilman's the pharmacological basis of therapeutics* (9th ed.). New York: McGraw-Hill.

Hitchens K (1996). New eye implant for treating cytomegalovirus, *Hosp Pharm Report 10*(4):20.

Jury DL (1993). More on RSV and ribavirin, *Pediatr Nurs 19*(1):89-91.

MacDonald L & Kazanjian P (1996). Antiretroviral therapy in HIV infection: An update. *Hosp Formul 31*(9):780-804.

Melmon KL et al. (1992). *Clinical pharmacology* (3rd ed.). New York: McGraw-Hill.

Olin BR (Ed.) (1996). *Facts and comparisons.* St Louis: Facts and Comparisons.

Podrasky DL (1989). Amphotericin B: The nurse's role in controlling adverse reactions, *Focus Crit Care 16*(3):194.

Smith DG Jr & Handy CM (1992). A protocol for foscarnet administration, *J Intraven Nurs 15*(5):274-7.

United States Pharmacopeial Convention (1996). *USP DI: Drug information for the health care professional* (16th ed.). Rockville, MD: The Convention.

Chapter 61
Other Antimicrobial Drugs and Antiparasitic Drugs

Chapter Focus

Many of the diseases discussed in this chapter were thought to be eradicable within this century. The teaching of good health practices and the use of effective drugs and insecticides held promise to end these diseases, such as malaria and tuberculosis, endemic in many parts of the world. Although the World Health Organization considered that malaria might be eradicated by 1964 with the combined use of DDT and antimalarial drugs, DDT was found to be harmful and the *Anopheles* mosquito that carries the organism became resistant to the insecticide. In addition, the ability of the pathogens to become drug-resistant in both tuberculosis and malaria has made health officials less optimistic. Tuberculosis is back, with an increase of 18.4% in 1991, as we have seen the growth of ideal environments for the resurgence of TB—the homeless, the drug-addicted, the impoverished, the immunosuppressed, and recent immigrants from countries where the disease is still endemic. These diseases will continue to be a challenge to health care providers for some time. The following objectives and key terms are important for a good understanding of this chapter.

Key Terms

amebiasis (p. 967)
Hansen's disease (p. 975)
helminths (p. 969)
malaria (p. 951)
toxoplasmosis (p. 969)
trichomoniasis (p. 969)
tuberculosis (p. 957)

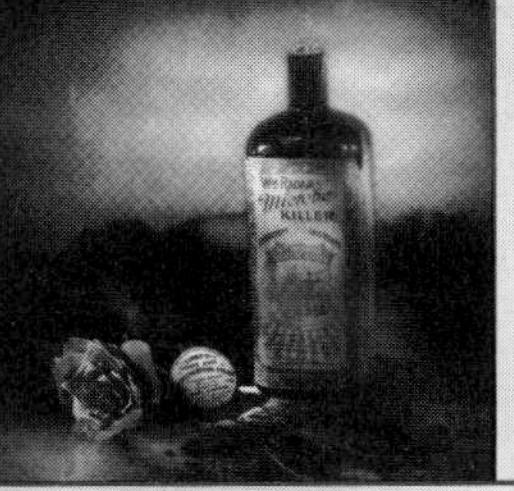

Key Drugs [▲]

chloroquine
isoniazid
rifampin
pyrazinamide

Objectives

1. Discuss the life cycle of the malarial parasite in the human body.
2. Implement nursing management of the care of clients receiving antimalarial drug therapy.
3. Implement nursing management of the care of clients receiving antitubercular drug therapy.
4. Describe the life cycle of the ameba, as well as intestinal and extraintestinal amebiasis in humans.
5. Discuss antiamebiasis agents and their nursing management.
6. Discuss other protozoan diseases and the drugs used in their treatment.

Antimicrobial and antiparasitic agents include antimalarial, antituberculous, amebicidal, anthelmintic, and leprostatic medications. Sulfonamides are reviewed in Chapter 59, Antibiotics.

MALARIA

Malaria has been and still is a prevalent disease in spite of efforts to control the causative parasite and insect vector. While it is endemic to the tropics, in 1988 approximately 1000 cases of malaria were diagnosed in the U.S. and Canada (Anandan, 1995). Four species of the genus *Plasmodium* are responsible for human malaria: *Plasmodium vivax, P. malariae, P. ovale,* and *P. falciparum. P. ovale,* which is found in West Africa, is considered rare. *P. falciparum* malaria is the most lethal form of malaria and is usually resistant to chloroquine.

Malaria is transmitted to humans by the bite of an infected female *Anopheles* mosquito, as well as by blood transfusion (usually *P. malariae*), congenitally, or by contaminated needles commonly used by drug abusers.

Life Cycle of the Malarial Parasite

To understand the chemotherapy of malaria, it is essential to review the life cycle of the malarial parasite, the plasmodium. Figure 61-1 presents the cycle in seven basic steps.

Plasmodia have two interdependent life cycles: the sexual cycle, which takes place in the mosquito, and the asexual cycle, which occurs in the human body.

Sexual cycle. The sexual cycle is noted in step 7 of Figure 61-1. The female *Anopheles* mosquito becomes the carrier of the parasite by drawing blood containing male and female forms from an infected person. These sexual forms of the parasite are known as gametocytes. In the stomach of the mosquito the female gametocytes are fertilized by the males; zygotes form, which result in numerous cell divisions that develop into sporozoites. The formation of sporozoites in the mosquito completes the sexual cycle. Sporozoites then migrate to the salivary glands of the infected mosquito and are injected into the bloodstream of the human by the bite of the female insect (step 1, Figure 61-1).

Asexual cycle. In the human the asexual cycle of the plasmodium consists of the exoerythrocytic phase and the erythrocytic phase.

Exoerythrocytic phase. Shortly after the introduction of the sporozoites into the circulation of the human, they leave the blood and enter fixed tissue cells (reticuloendothelial cells) of the liver, where multiplication and maturation take place (step 2). For a period of time (8 to 42 days), which varies with different plasmodia, the individual exhibits no symptoms, no parasites are found in erythrocytes, and the blood is noninfective. This phase is known as the preerythrocytic stage. The parasites are called primary tissue schizonts, or preerythrocytic forms. After this stage, the young parasites burst from the liver cells as merozoites.

Erythrocytic phase. When merozoites enter the bloodstream, they penetrate the erythrocytes and begin the erythrocytic phase of their existence (step 3a). In the case of *P. vivax* (but not *P. falciparum*) some of the merozoites invade other tissue cells to form secondary exoerythrocytic forms (step 3b). The relapses in *P. vivax* and other forms of malaria are believed to be caused by the successive formations of merozoites produced by various secondary exoerythrocytic forms of the parasite. Drugs affecting malarial parasites in the bloodstream do not always destroy those in the exoerythrocytic, or tissue, stage.

After the merozoites bore into red blood cells, they again multiply, but this time asexually, and erythrocytic schizonts are formed. The erythrocytic phase is completed when the parasitized red blood cells rupture, setting free many more merozoites that are formed from the schizonts. Pyrogenic substances are also liberated, causing a rapid rise in body temperature (step 4). Some of the merozoites may be destroyed in the plasma of the blood by leukocytes and other agents, but some enter other erythrocytes to repeat the cycle (step 5). The recurring chills, fever, and prostration that are prominent clinical symptoms of malaria occur when the red blood cells rupture and release the young parasites with foreign protein and cell products. The erythrocytic phase lasts 48 to 72 hours, depending on the plasmodium involved. After a few cycles, some of the asexual forms of the malarial parasites develop into sexual forms called gametocytes (step 6). When the mosquito bites a person infected with malarial parasites and ingests the sexual forms, the cycle begins again.

P. vivax is the most common form of malaria; this infestation is usually mild, drug-resistance is uncommon and it can easily be suppressed with antimalarial medications. The *P. falciparum* strain of malaria is less common but much more severe than *P. vivax*. Drug-resistant strains of *P. falciparum* are reported and the symptoms with this infestation occurs at irregular intervals and can cause very serious complications. If untreated or treatment is delayed, the disease may progress to irreversible cardiovascular shock and death. While relapses are reported with *P. vivax,* once the *P. falciparum* form is eliminated, no dormant forms are in the liver, therefore no relapses are reported with *P. falciparum*.

Persons who harbor the sexual forms of plasmodia are called carriers, since it is from carriers that mosquitos receive the parasite forms that perpetuate the disease. The asexual forms cause the clinical symptoms of malaria. Carriers should avoid giving blood, since it is possible that the recipient of this blood will contract malaria or become a carrier. An increasing number of malaria cases (some fatal) have occurred from transfusions of infected blood. Some of these infected individuals who donated blood may have once lived in a malarious area. Any person who has had malaria or has been exposed to the disease by visiting a region where it is prevalent must be disqualified as a blood donor.

Antimalarial Medications

The choice of a drug for treatment of malaria is based on the particular malarial strain involved and the stage of the

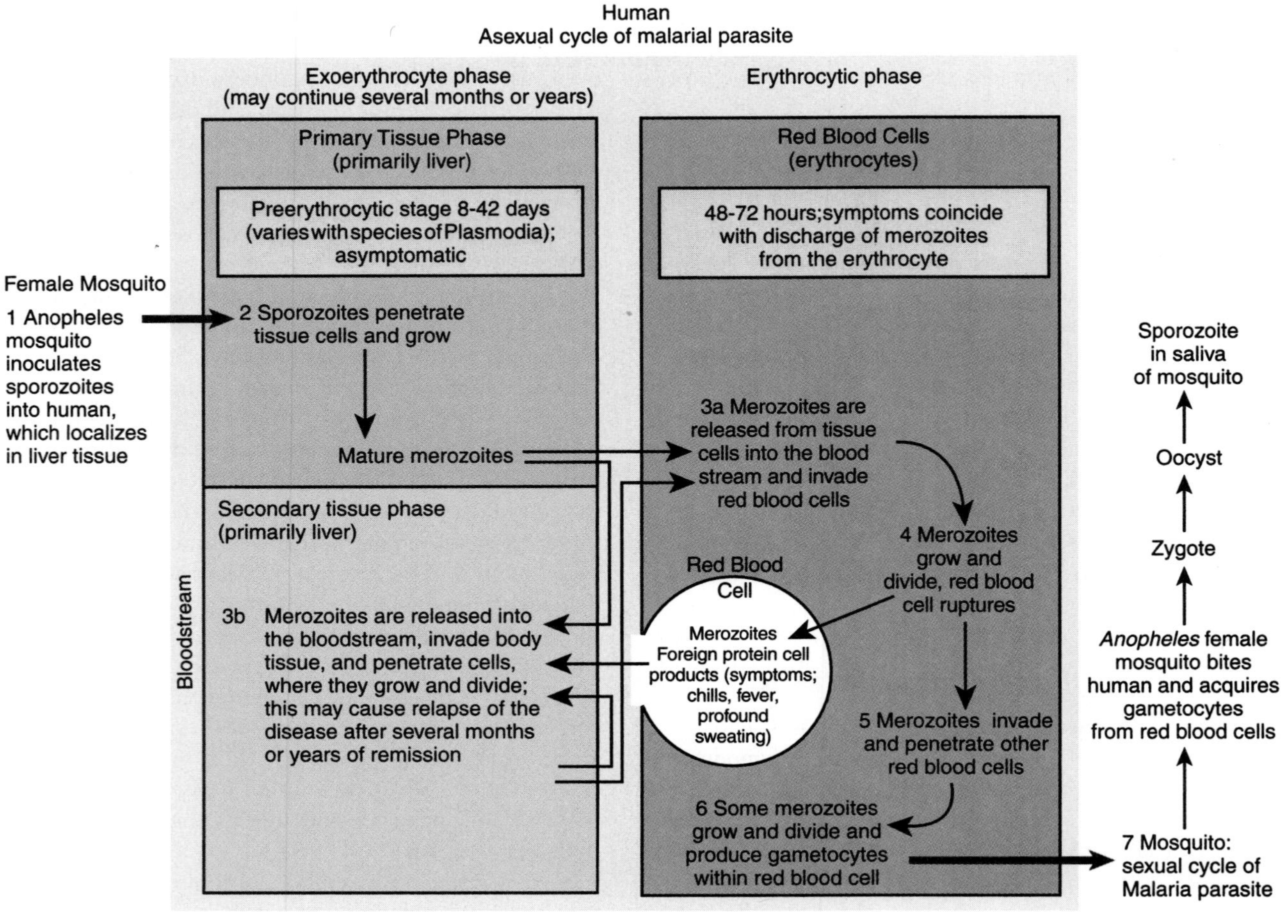

Figure 61-1 Life cycle of the malarial parasite.

Plasmodium life cycle. The drugs (schizonticides), therefore, are classified according to the type of therapy they provide, which is as follows:

1. Travelers to endemic areas should receive malaria chemoprophylaxis. Calling the Centers for Disease Control and Prevention ([404] 332-4555 for computer assisted information) can verify if malaria prophylaxis and also, if chloroquine-resistant *P. falciparum* has been reported in a specific country (Anandan, 1995). Chloroquine, which suppresses the asexual erythrocytic forms, is effective against all species of malaria except the drug-resistant, *P. falciparum*.
2. In chloroquine-resistant, *P. falciparum* areas, mefloquine is used for prophylaxis or, if the person cannot take mefloquine, doxycycline is recommended.
3. Clinical cure of an acute malaria attack occurs when multiplication of the parasites within the erythrocyte is interrupted, thereby terminating the malarial symptoms of the attack. If chloroquine-resistant, *P. falciparum* is present, then combination therapies such as pyrimethamine and a sulfonamide (sulfadoxine) may be necessary.
4. For eradication of latent forms of *P. vivax* that persist and may cause infection relapse, primaquine therapy may be recommended. This drug is usually started after an acute attack or during the last few weeks of chloroquine prophylaxis. To induce a radical cure requires medications that destroy both the exoerythrocytic and erythrocytic parasites to prevent relapsing malaria; therefore, primaquine is given with chloroquine, which suppresses the erythrocytic cycle.

The emergence of drug-resistant strains of malaria, particularly that caused by *P. falciparum*, poses a major public health problem throughout the world. Despite the combined efforts of many countries to eradicate malaria, it remains the most devastating infectious disease in the world because of the many lives lost and the economic burdens it imposes. Fortunately, in the United States and Canada, endemic malaria has been completely eradicated.

It is essential that travelers contemplating a trip to malarious areas of the world be aware of the need to obtain information from their health care provider about measures for reducing exposure to the disease. Malaria exists in Haiti, Mexico, Central and South America, the Middle East, and many other countries.

▲ **chloroquine** [klor' o kwin] (Aralen)
hydroxychloroquine [hye drox ee klor' oh kwin] (Plaquenil)

The mechanisms of action as an antiprotozoal to treat malaria are unknown but may be a result of their ability to bind or alter DNA properties. They increase the pH of acid vesicles, thus interfering with its functions. During suppressive therapy, they inhibit the erythrocytic stage of development of plasmodia while in acute malarial attacks, they interfere with erythrocytic schizogony of parasites.

As the drugs selectively accumulate in parasitized erythrocytes, they have a selective toxicity in the erythrocytic stages of plasmodial infestation.

These agents are indicated for the prevention and treatment of malaria for the four strains of plasmodium. Curing *P. vivax* and *P. ovale* malaria requires primaquine administration also. Hydroxychloroquine is also approved for the treatment of rheumatoid arthritis and for discoid and systemic lupus erythematosus.

The drugs are fairly well absorbed orally, widely distributed in body tissues, and reach peak serum levels in approximately 3 to 3.5 hours. The terminal half-life of chloroquine is 1 to 2 months while the terminal half-life for hydroxychloroquine in blood is approximately 50 days, in plasma 32 days. Both drugs are partially metabolized in the liver, and excreted by the kidneys.

Side/adverse effects for chloroquine are usually mild, dose-related and reversible. Gastric distress, headaches, pruritus, blurred vision, and difficulty in reading are most commonly reported. Hydroxychloroquine in short term use, also has mild and dose-limiting side effects. But in chronic use or high-dose therapy, hydroxychloroquine may cause retinal changes, visual disturbances, irreversible retinal damage, blood dyscrasias and ototoxicity. It is not currently recommended by the CDC for treatment in malaria (CDC, 1996).

The usual oral chloroquine adult dose to suppress malaria is 500 mg daily every 7 days. Pediatric dosage is 8.3 mg/kg PO daily (not exceeding adult dose) every 7 days. The parenteral adult dose is 200 to 250 mg IM repeated in 6 hours if needed. Do not exceed 1000 mg in the first day.

Hydroxychloroquine adult oral dose is 400 mg daily, every 7 days. The pediatric dosage is 6.4 mg/kg PO daily, repeated weekly.

■ Nursing Management

Chloroquine and Hydroxychloroquine Therapy

Assessment. These drugs are used with caution in the presence of hypersensitivity to chloroquine and hydroxychloroquine, retinal or visual field changes, and pregnancy (to prevent retinal damage in the fetus). Long-term therapy in children is also contraindicated. These drugs are also used with caution in individuals with liver disease, which may require reduced dosages, and in individuals with G6PD deficiency and hematologic disorders because they may cause blood dyscrasias. Avoid the use of these drugs in individuals with psoriasis or porphyria, since these conditions may become exacerbated. Clients with severe neurologic disorders may be further compromised by polyneuritis, ototoxicity, seizures, or neuromyopathy from the administration of these two drugs.

There are no drug interactions of clinical significance.

A baseline assessment of the client should include CBC, ophthalmologic examination, and neuromuscular examination including deep tendon reflexes of the knee and ankle reflexes.

Nursing diagnosis. The client receiving therapy with chloroquine and hydroxychloroquine should be assessed for the following nursing diagnoses: altered comfort (headache and itching, particularly in black clients; fluid volume deficit related to anorexia, nausea, vomiting, and diarrhea; altered bowel elimination pattern (diarrhea); altered protection related to blood dyscrasias (agranulocytosis, aplastic anemia, neutropenia, thrombocytopenia); self-concept disturbance related to blue-black discoloration of the skin and fingernails or alopecia; sensory-perceptual disturbances related to ototoxicity (tinnitus and hearing loss) or to ocular toxicity (retinopathy, keratopathy, or cataracts evidenced by blurred vision); altered thought processes related to the development of psychosis (mood and mental changes); and the collaborative problems of cardiovascular toxicity (hypotension, QRS prolongation), neuromyopathy, or seizures.

Implementation

Monitoring. Obtain a baseline and periodic CBC and test for glucose-6-phosphate dehydrogenase (G6PD) deficiency to avoid the occurrence of hemolytic anemia (see Cultural Aspects box below). Signs of blood dyscrasia are fever, sore throat, fatigue, and easy bruising. Perform periodic tests of muscle strength and reflexes, particularly in clients on long-term therapy. Consult with prescriber to discontinue therapy if positive signs occur. Discontinue drugs at first sign of retinal changes and/or visual disturbances and continue to observe client for possible progression even after therapy has been discontinued.

Observe client for drug resistance. Failure to prevent or cure clinical malaria may require treatment with quinine if the person is infected with a resistant strain of the parasite.

Intervention. Administer oral drugs with milk or meals to minimize gastric irritation. If the client is on parenteral therapy, substitute oral administration as soon as possible.

Hydroxychloroquine tablets may be crushed and placed in gelatin capsules or mixed with jam or gelatin to make them easier to swallow.

Education. Initiate suppressive therapy 2 weeks before exposure and continue medication while staying in malarious area. Maintain drug regimen for 4 weeks after leaving the region. Notify a health care provider if fever develops while traveling or within 2 months after leaving the endemic area. In addition to taking this medication to avoid contracting malaria, the client should also be instructed to stay indoors in well-screened areas after sundown, sleep under mosquito

Cultural Aspects **G6PD and Antimalarial Agents**

About 10% of African-Americans and 5% to 10% of Sephardic Jews, Greeks, Iranians, Chinese, Filipinos, and Indonesians have glucose-6-phosphate dehydrogenase (G6PD) deficiency. It is transmitted as an X-linked trait. Without G6PD, red blood cell metabolism is impaired by chloroquine and other antimalarial drugs. Acute intravascular hemolysis may occur if these drugs are given. Treatment is by transfusion. Some blood banks do test for G6PD deficiency in areas where malarial treatment is common.

From Kudzma, 1992.

netting at night, wear trousers and long-sleeved shirts, and use mosquito repellent on exposed skin surfaces.

Instruct the client to take drug for the full course of treatment even if feeling better. This will ensure that the infection is completely eradicated and that the symptoms will not return. To obtain the full effect of the drug, inform the client to follow a regular schedule by taking it the same day each week. Keep drug out of reach of children. Fatalities in children have occurred after ingestion of one 300 mg tablet.

Instruct the client to keep regularly scheduled visits for ophthalmoscopic and audiometric examinations and report to the prescriber any signs of visual and auditory disturbances. This is to prevent irreversible retinopathy, which may occur even after discontinuation of therapy.

Explain to client that the drug may cause a red or brown discoloration of the urine, which is not medically significant.

When drug is administered for rheumatoid arthritis, inform the client that therapeutic benefits usually do not occur until 6 to 12 months after therapy has been initiated.

Caution the client to avoid alcoholic beverages while taking this drug. Since the medication may cause dizziness, advise the client to avoid tasks that require mental alertness until the response to the medication has been determined.

Evaluation. The client will be free of malarial infection.

mefloquine [me' floe kwin] (Lariam)

Mefloquine is a blood schizonticide; it prevents the replication of asexual erythrocytic parasites but has no effect on the gametocytes of *P. falciparum*. Its exact mechanism of action is unknown although it is believed to inhibit protein synthesis (bind DNA), increase intravascular pH of acid vesicles in the parasite, and may have a variety of other actions. However, it is not effective in eliminating the exoerythrocytic or intrahepatic stages of *P. vivax* or *P. ovale* infections.

It is indicated for the prevention and treatment of chloroquine-resistant malaria and multiple drug-resistant strains of *P. falciparum*. It is also used to prevent malaria caused by *P. vivax, P. ovale,* and *P. malariae*.

Mefloquine is well absorbed orally, widely distributed in the body reaching peak serum levels in 7 to 24 hours. It has an elimination half-life of 13 to 33 days, is partially metabolized in the liver, and is excreted primarily in bile and feces.

Side/adverse effects of mefloquine are infrequent and dose-related. They occur more commonly in therapeutic than in prophylaxis drug regimens and include vomiting, headache, dizziness, insomnia, gastric distress and visual disturbances.

The usual adult dose for prophylaxis is 250 mg once a week, beginning 1 week before travel, then weekly during traveling and for 1 month after leaving the endemic areas. Therapeutic dose for chloroquine-resistant *P. falciparum* malaria is 1250 mg orally as a single dose.

■ Nursing Management

Mefloquine Therapy

Except for the following drug interactions, the nursing management of mefloquine therapy is essentially the same as the previously discussed nursing management of chloroquine and hydroxychloroquine, p. 953.

Significant drug interactions may occur when mefloquine is given with the following drugs (also see Box 61-1):

Drug	Possible effect and management
chloroquine (Aralen)	May increase seizure activity. Monitor closely.
divalproex (Depakote) or valproic acid (Depakene)	Decreased serum levels of valproic acid reported with loss of seizure control. Monitor serum levels if concurrent drug therapy is necessary.

primaquine [prim' a kween]

Primaquine's mechanism of action is unknown, but it can bind and alter DNA. It is very effective in the exoerythrocytic stages of *P. vivax* and *P. ovale* malaria and against the primary phase (exoerythrocytic stage) of *P. falciparum* malaria. It is also effective against the sexual forms (gametocytes) of plasmodia (especially *P. falciparum*). It is indicated to prevent malaria relapses (radical cure) caused by *P. vivax* and *P. ovale* and is also effective against gametocytes of *P. falciparum*.

Primaquine is absorbed orally and reaches peak level within 2 to 3 hours. With a half-life of approximately 6 hours it is rapidly metabolized in an unspecified site and a small amount is excreted via the kidneys.

Side/adverse effects of primaquine include gastric distress and hemolytic anemia.

The adult oral dose is 26.3 mg daily for 2 weeks. Pediatric dosage is 680 μg/kg daily for 2 weeks. Primaquine is not recommended for use during pregnancy.

■ Nursing Management

Primaquine Therapy

Assessment. The more serious adverse effects of primaquine involve individuals with a genetically determined glucose-6-phosphate dehydrogenase (G6PD) deficiency, which can cause a lethal hemolysis of red blood cells. This disorder occurs in about 8% of black males and other dark-skinned individuals such as Asians and some Mediterranean peoples. However, there is evidence that the enzyme G6PD in the red blood cells is essential for metabolism in the plasmodia; hence persons with a genetic deficiency of G6PD in their red blood cells are believed to have some natural immunity to malaria.

BOX 61-1

Potentially Life-Threatening Drug Interaction with Mefloquine

Mefloquine, when given concurrently with beta blockers, calcium channel blocking agents, quinidine, or quinine, may result in increased risk of dysrhythmias, cardiac arrest, and seizures (with quinine). If possible, avoid concurrent drug administration. If absolutely necessary to administer drugs concurrently, monitor client closely and also advise him or her to take mefloquine at least 12 hours after the last dose of quinidine or quinine.

Review the client's current medications for significant drug interactions that may occur when primaquine is given with the following drugs:

Drug	Possible Effect and Management
other hemolytic agents	**May increase risk for myelotoxic effects; monitor for muscle weakness and diminished deep tendon reflexes closely. Avoid or a potentially serious drug interaction may occur.**
quinacrine (Atabrine)	**Not recommended; an increase in primaquine toxicity is reported. Avoid or a potentially serious drug interaction may occur.**

A baseline assessment should include CBC, hemoglobin, and glucose-6-phosphate dehydrogenase determination.

Nursing diagnosis. The client receiving primaquine should be assessed for the following nursing diagnoses: fluid volume deficit related to anorexia, nausea and vomiting; altered protection related to leukopenia; and the collaborative problems of hemolytic anemia and methemoglobinemia.

Implementation

Monitoring. Monitor complete blood counts and hemoglobin determinations weekly for a sudden decrease in hemoglobin concentration, erythrocyte count, or leukocyte count; discontinue medication if this occurs. Monitor for the signs of hemolytic anemia, which are fatigue, fever, pallor, anorexia, darkened urine, and back, leg, or abdominal pain. Also monitor for the less frequently occurring methemoglobinemia with cyanosis, dizziness, dyspnea, and fatigue.

Intervention. Gastric irritation can be minimized by administering drug with meals or antacids.

Education. Encourage the client to comply with the full course of medication and to report any symptoms of adverse reactions promptly.

Evaluation. The client will be free of infection, without any adverse effects of primaquine.

quinine [kwye' nine]

Quinine was the first drug used to treat malaria. As a schizontoicidal agent it concentrates in parasitized erythrocytes, which may be why it has selective toxicity during the erythrocytic stages of plasmodial infections. It can also bind to DNA thus inhibiting RNA synthesis and DNA replication.

Quinine sulfate was indicated in combination with other drugs, for the treatment of chloroquine-resistant malaria caused by chloroquine-resistant, *P. falciparum*, but today it is no longer used for malaria because more effective and less toxic drugs are available. Quinine has been reported to cause congenital malformations and stillbirths; therefore, this drug should not be taken by pregnant women (see Pregnancy Safety box above).

■ Nursing Management

Quinine Sulfate Therapy

Assessment. Quinine is to be administered with caution in clients with glucose-6-phosphate dehydrogenase (G6PD) deficiency because it may cause hemolytic anemia (see the Cultural Aspects box on p. 953). Clients with hypoglycemia may have the condition worsen because quinine stimulates the release of insulin from the pancreas. Quinine may exacerbate muscle weakness in clients with myasthenia gravis and may cause thrombocytopenic purpura. Clients with a history of blackwater fever may be disposed to its complications, including anemia and hemolysis with renal failure when administered quinine. Use with caution in clients with cardiac arrhythmias because prolongation of QT may occur with quinine. Note quinine has quinidine-like activity.

Review the client's medications for significant drug interactions. When quinine is given with mefloquine, an increased incidence of convulsions and ECG abnormalities have been reported. Administer mefloquine at least 12 hours after the last dose of quinine. If both drugs must be given concurrently, the client should be hospitalized and closely monitored for cardiac dysrhythmias and seizure activity.

A baseline assessment should include a description of the client's disease symptoms, CBC, and if the client has an existing cardiovascular problem, an ECG.

Nursing diagnosis. The client receiving quinine should be assessed for the following nursing diagnoses: fluid volume deficit related to anorexia, nausea, vomiting, and diarrhea; altered protection related to agranulocytosis, hemolytic anemia, hypoprothrombinemia and thrombocytopenia; sensory-perceptual alterations related to ocular toxicity (visual defects, blindness); and the collaborative problems of altered cardiac output related to cardiovascular toxicity (hypotension, arrhythmias, cardiac arrest), hypersensitivity (rash, fever, dyspnea), cinchonism (blurred vision, headache, ringing in ears), hepatotoxicity, allergic reaction, and CNS toxicity (confusion, seizures, coma).

Implementation

Monitoring. Observe for symptoms of cinchonism (tinnitus, dizziness, altered auditory acuity, visual disturbances, headache, gastrointestinal distress, nausea, and diarrhea).

Pregnancy Safety

Category	Drug
B	rifabutin, niclosamide, praziquantel
C	capreomycin, clofazimine, cycloserine, dapsone, isoniazid, mebendazole, mefloquine, oxamniquine, pyrazinamide, pyrimethamine, rifampin, thiabendazole
D	streptomycin
X	primaquine, quinine
Unclassified*	aminosalicylates, chloroquine, diethylcarbamazine, hydroxychloroquine, ethambutol, ethionamide, iodoquinol, paromomycin, piperazine, pyrantel

*Risk-to-benefit ratio should be carefully evaluated before use.

These symptoms disappear when the drug is discontinued. Monitor serum concentration levels; levels above 10 mg/100 ml may cause symptoms of cinchonism.

Intervention. Since quinine irritates the gastrointestinal mucosa, the capsule should be administered intact with food. Except for its use in chloroquine-resistant falciparum malaria, for which it has been the traditional antimalarial remedy, quinine has been replaced by more effective and less toxic drugs.

Education. Instruct the client to remain compliant to the antimalarial medication regimen for the full course of the prescription. Instruct client to report to the prescriber if any side effects/adverse reactions appear.

Evaluation. The client is free of infection.

■ ■ ■

pyrimethamine tablets [peer i meth' a meen] (Daraprim)

pyrimethamine with sulfadoxine (Fansidar)

Pyrimethamine is an antiprotozoal agent used to treat malaria and toxoplasmosis. It binds to and inhibits the protozoal enzyme dihydrofolate reductase, thus inhibiting the conversion of dihydrofolic acid to tetrahydrofolic acid. This results in a depletion of folate which is essential for nucleic acid synthesis and protein production. Pyrimethamine in combination with mefloquine and sulfadoxine is indicated for the treatment of chloroquine-resistant *P. falciparum* malaria. The drug is also combined with a sulfapyrimidine sulfonamide to treat toxoplasmosis caused by *Toxoplasma gondii*.

Pyrimethamine is orally absorbed and widely distributed in the body, although it concentrates mainly in blood cells, kidneys, liver, and spleen. It reaches peak plasma levels in 3 hours and has a half-life of 80 to 123 hours. It is metabolized in the liver and excreted via the kidneys.

Side/adverse effects of pyrimethamine with high doses include gastric distress, atrophic glossitis, and blood dyscrasias.

The adult oral dose in specific world areas, such as Southeast Asia, East Africa, or the Amazon, is 75 mg of pyrimethamine in combination with 750 mg mefloquine and 1.5 g of sulfadoxine as a single dose. For additional dosing recommendations, see a current package insert or the *USP DI*.

■ Nursing Management

Pyrimethamine Therapy

Assessment. Risk-benefit must be considered in nursing mothers because pyrimethamine may disrupt the folic acid metabolism in the nursing infant.

To prevent possible central nervous system toxicity in individuals with convulsive disorders, use a small initial dose for treatment of toxoplasmosis. Use pyrimethamine with caution for clients with anemia or bone marrow depression because pyrimethamine may cause folic acid deficiency, which results in megaloblastic anemia and blood dyscrasias. Do not use for treatment of resistant form of parasite.

When administered concurrently with other bone marrow depressants, an increase in leukopenia and/or thrombocytopenia may occur. Monitor CBCs closely.

A baseline assessment should include a CBC and platelet count as well as a description of the client's disease symptoms.

Nursing diagnosis. The client receiving pyrimethamine should be assessed for the following nursing diagnoses: fluid volume deficit related to anorexia, nausea, vomiting, and diarrhea; altered protection related to blood dyscrasias (agranulocytosis, megaloblastic anemia, thrombocytopenia); altered oral mucous membranes related to folic acid deficiency (pain and inflammation of the tongue-atrophic glossitis); and the collaborative problems of hypersensitivity (rash), neurotoxicity (excitability, seizures), respiratory depression, and circulatory collapse.

Implementation

Monitoring. The high dosage required for treating toxoplasmosis could approach the toxic level. Monitor CBCs and platelet counts. If folic acid deficiency develops, dosage may be reduced. Clinical symptoms of folic acid deficiency are soreness, redness, or burning of the tongue; pharyngitis; ulcers in the mouth; or diarrhea. Folinic acid (leucovorin) restores the depressed platelet or white blood counts to normal levels.

Intervention. Administer medication with milk or food to minimize gastric irritation. For children, tablets may be crushed to prepare 1% solution in normal saline. Use within 24 hours at room temperature. If mixed with cherry syrup NF, use immediately after preparation.

If taken to prevent malaria, the medication should be taken 2 weeks before entering a malarious area and be continued for 6 weeks after leaving it. Besides building tissue stores of the drug, early administration will allow assessment of the client's tolerance of the drug.

Education. Advise the client to have weekly blood counts and platelet counts during therapy if on high dosage therapy. If taken as a malaria suppressant, instruct the client to follow the dosage schedule as prescribed by taking the drug the same day each week.

Advise the individual to sleep under mosquito netting to avoid being bitten by malaria-carrying mosquitoes while in the endemic areas. Advise the wearing of proper clothing so that arms and legs are covered, especially at dawn and during evening hours, when mosquitoes are out. The use of mosquito repellent on uncovered areas of the skin may help to protect the individual from the bites of infected mosquitoes.

Instruct the client to report to the prescriber any signs of possible blood dyscrasia (fever, sore throat, unusual bleeding or bruising, extreme weakness, and fatigue). Alert the client to use caution in dental hygiene, such as soft toothbrushes, no dental floss or toothpicks. Defer dental work until blood counts are within normal limits.

Fansidar (pyrimethamine with sulfadoxine) should only be used when the traveler is going to areas where chloroquine-resistant malaria is prevalent and is planning to stay longer than 3 weeks because of the risk of severe skin reactions. The drug should be discontinued and a health care provider notified at the first sign of a rash.

Evaluation. The client is free of infection, without any adverse effects of pyrimethamine.

TUBERCULOSIS

Tuberculosis (TB), a chronic granulomatous infection caused by the acid-fast bacillus, *Mycobacterium tuberculosis*, declined in incidence in the United States until 1985 when an increased incidence was noted in native-born Americans. Worldwide, approximately 8 million new TB cases are diagnosed with 2.9 million dying from this disease (Cali, 1995). Nursing home residents account for nearly 25% of the tuberculosis cases in the United States (Yoshikawa, 1995). The increase in tuberculosis is largely attributed to the increasing numbers of individuals with AIDS, to persons living on the street or homeless persons, drug abusers, undernourished or malnourished persons, or those taking immunosuppressant drugs or suffering from cancer. Thus high risk persons are groups living in crowded facilities with less than optimum health care.

Mycobacterium tuberculosis, the bacteria that causes tuberculosis, most commonly affects the lungs, but other body areas can also be infected, such as bones, joints, skin, meninges, or genitourinary tract. This bacteria is an aerobic bacillus that needs a highly oxygenated organ site for growth; thus the lungs, growing ends of bones, and cerebral cortex are ideal sites. Tubercle bacilli may be transmitted by airborne droplets but cannot be transmitted on objects such as dishes, clothing, or sheets and bedding (Figure 61-2). Sharing an enclosed environment with an infected person creates a high risk of developing this infection (Ebert, 1993; Elpern & Girzadas, 1993).

The development of drug-resistant tuberculosis (TB) is a major concern today. It has been estimated that there is approximately a 9% incidence of drug-resistant organisms in the United States (Ward, 1995). Resistance to 2 or more drugs (multi-drug resistant TB or MDR-TB) has resulted in outbreaks in institutional facilities. Between 1990 to 1992, 9 institutions with a reported outbreak of MDR-TB were investigated by the CDC. They were found to have a high prevalence of HIV infection (20% to 100%) and a high mortality rate in persons with MDR-TB (72% to 89%). At least 17 health care or institutional workers at these facilities also developed MDR-TB (CDC, 1993).

Pathogenesis

Tubercle bacilli droplets are transmitted by coughing or sneezing by an infected person. Persons producing sputum generally have many bacilli and are more infectious than the infected person who does not cough. Three types of tubercle bacilli are pathogenic to humans: human to human, bovine to human, and avian to human. Avian TB is rare in the United States and Canada, and with the pasteurization of milk and testing of cows, bovine TB is much less prevalent. Thus the primary source of transmission is human to human.

When the tubercle bacilli enter the lungs, infection can spread to other body organs through the blood and lymph system. Usually, however, the infection may become dormant and be walled off by calcified and fibrous tissues. The bacilli become inactive, perhaps for the lifetime of the host. If host defenses break down, however, or if the host receives an immunosuppressive drug, the bacilli may be reactivated.

Drug Treatment Regimens

Effective drug regimens are available to treat tuberculosis. Drug selection is based on the development of drug-resistant organisms and drug toxicity. General guidelines include:

1. To avoid the development of drug-resistant organisms, all individuals diagnosed with TB (isolated *M. tuberculosis*) should have drug susceptibility tests on their first isolation.
2. In most instances, the result of the in vitro susceptibility test is unknown when drug therapy is started. It is recommended that a four-drug regimen be instituted (especially in areas where primary isoniazid resistance occurs) because this regimen provides an adequate drug regimen that will be at least 95% effective, even in the presence of drug-resistant organisms. The recommended drugs are INH, rifampin, pyrazinamide (PZA), and ethambutol or streptomycin (CDC, 1993; Mandell & Petri, 1996).
3. When drug susceptibility results are available, the drug regimen can be adjusted.
4. Monitor the prescribed therapy regimen closely to support client compliance, to detect side effects or adverse reactions, and to register progress of the treatment program.

■ Nursing Management

Antituberculous Therapy

This general nursing management for antituberculous agents will be supplemented by specific considerations for each agent.

Assessment. Cultures for *Mycobacterium* and tests for the organism's susceptibility to the antitubercular drugs should be obtained before and periodically during the course of drug therapy. Sputum specimens can help confirm active TB and help to estimate the degree of infectiousness. If the client has suspected pulmonary TB, he or she should have at least three sputum specimens examined by smear and culture. The smear test can detect mycobacterial organisms, but culture testing takes much longer, from 2 to 12 weeks (Boutotte, 1993). The client may also exhibit nonspecific symptoms, fatigue, weakness, anorexia, weight loss, night sweats, or low-grade fever. X-ray examinations may show nodular lesions, patchy infiltrates (many in the upper lobes), cavity formation, scar tissue, and calcium deposits.

Nursing diagnosis. The client with tuberculosis will have the nursing diagnosis of risk for infection transmission, at least initially. Also to be considered are the following: ineffective breathing pattern; altered nutrition: less than required; risk of injury related to the ineffectiveness of the antituberculosis drug; knowledge deficit related to unfamiliarity with disease process and treatment methods; ineffective management

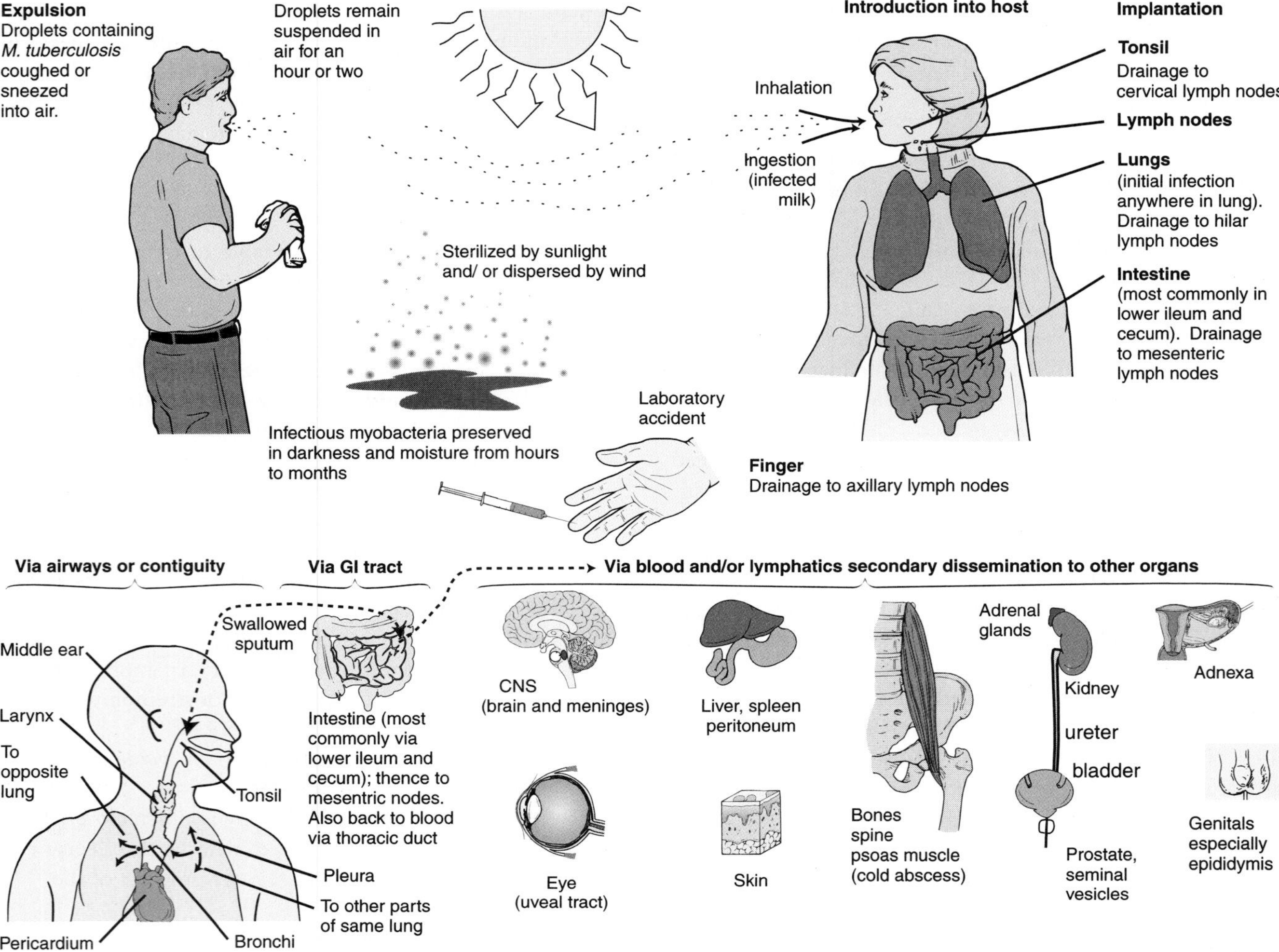

Figure 61-2 Dissemination of tuberculosis.

of the therapeutic regimen; and any collaborative problems that might relate to complications of the disease.

Implementation

Monitoring. Sputum cultures and x-ray examinations are used to monitor the client's status, as well as the general health status of the client. Monitor the client for symptoms that indicate resolution of the infection: diminished cough and sputum production; decreased fever and night sweats; reduction of cavitation on x-ray examination; reduction of anorexia with concomitant weight gain; and decreased acid-fast bacteria (AFB) in sputum specimens. (See the Home Health box at right on medication monitoring in the community.)

Intervention. The nurse should attempt to administer these drugs with consideration for the client's comfort. For example, gastrointestinal disturbances following administration can be reduced by concurrent administration of food or antacids.

Education. The client must take prescribed medications regularly and without interruption for maximum therapeutic effectiveness. A person who is responsible for self-medication should be instructed about the necessity of taking these drugs, two or more concurrently, according to the prescribed regimen and not to discontinue them when feeling better. Alert the client to the adverse effects of the specific drugs and the need to report them immediately. Instruct clients responsible for self-medication about the necessity for periodic medical evaluations to evaluate the effectiveness of therapy.

Remind the client to get sufficient rest. Stress the importance of having a well-balanced diet. Use small, frequent meals if anorexic. Record weight weekly.

When peripheral neuritis appears as a side effect of the antitubercular drugs, teach clients precautionary strategies to avoid injury from burning agents and sharp objects until the alteration in sensation is remedied.

Teach clients measures that minimize disease transmission, such as covering the mouth when coughing and sneezing.

Evaluation. The client's sputum culture result is negative and the client can effectively self-manage the therapeutic regimen.

Home Health

Antitubercular Medication Management in the Community

Nursing management of an antitubercular therapeutic regimen has the following expected outcomes: completion of an effective course of therapy, consisting of at least two drugs to which the organism is susceptible; keeping the course of therapy as short as possible to promote client adherence; and preventing transmission of outbreaks (Boutotte, 1993).

1. Monitor the client's response to therapy. A client with pulmonary TB should have sputum tested at least monthly until culture results are negative. This follow-up sputum testing is necessary to determine how long therapy should last and response to therapy. Once effective anti-TB therapy begins, the number of organisms in the smear tests will decrease and the client's symptoms will improve. If the specimens remain positive after 3 months of therapy, it suggests that the disease is the result of a drug-resistant organism or that the client is not taking medications as prescribed.
2. Ensure client adherence. Instruct the client in the importance of taking the medication for the duration of therapy, even after he or she is feeling better. Assess for adherence at every follow-up visit. Pill counts are helpful. Urine tests are available as a dipstick test that can detect INH in urine 24 to 48 hours after the drugs were taken. Rifampin also turns the urine orange-colored for several hours after a dose.

   The most effective way to ensure client compliance is "directly observed therapy (DOT)." DOT requires that someone actually observe the client take every dose of medication for the entire therapeutic regimen. DOT programs increase adherence in both rural and urban settings. A hospital in New York City reported that only 11% of clients under care for TB reported to an outpatient clinic for further treatment when discharged from the hospital. In contrast, a program in which DOT is routinely used for all clients had a completion rate of 98%. Although expanding use of DOT may require additional resources, intermittent, directly observed regimens are cost-effective (CDC, 1993). DOT can be conducted with regimens given once a day, 2 times/week, or 3 times/week.
3. Monitor for adverse drug reactions.

Because of the long-term nature of drug therapy in tuberculosis, clients may need support in maintaining the therapeutic regimen and in managing side effects of the tuberculosis drugs.

Antituberculous Agents

aminosalicylate [a mee noe sal i' si late] (PAS, Tubasal, Nemasol♣)

Aminosalicylate is a bacteriostatic agent closely related to aminobenzoic acid (PABA); thus it competitively inhibits folic acid formation resulting in suppression of the growth and reproduction of *M. tuberculosis*. In combination with other antituberculars, it is indicated for the treatment of *M. tuberculosis*, pulmonary and extrapulmonary.

Aminosalicylate is well absorbed orally, distributed to various body fluids with high levels accumulating in pleural fluids, kidney, lungs, and liver tissues. Half-life is between 45 and 60 minutes, although clients with impaired renal function may have a half-life of up to 23 hours. Peak serum level is reached within 1 to 2 hours. This drug is metabolized in the liver and excreted by the kidneys.

Side/adverse effects of aminosalicylate therapy include hypersensitivity reaction and gastric distress.

The adult oral dose given in combination with other antimycobacterials is 3.3 to 4 g every 8 hours. Maximum daily dose is 20 g. The pediatric dose in combination with other antimycobacterials is 50 to 75 mg/kg PO every 6 hours.

■ Nursing Management

Aminosalicylate Therapy

In addition to the nursing management discussed in the general section on antitubercular drug therapy, consider the following:

Assessment. A history of allergic reaction to other salicylates and sulfonamides may indicate a cross-intolerance for aminosalicylate, in which case the drug would be contraindicated.

Aminosalicylates should be used with caution if the client has any of the following preexisting conditions: gastric ulcer, because gastric irritation may increase; G6PD deficiency because of a risk of hemolytic anemia; or severe renal or hepatic function impairment, which would require reduced dosages. Congestive heart failure should preclude the use of aminosalicylate because its high concentrations of sodium may lead to fluid volume excess.

The concurrent use of aminobenzoates is not recommended because it may be absorbed by the bacteria in preference to aminosalicylates and so reduce the bacteriostatic properties of the aminosalicylates.

A baseline assessment is to be done as described in the previous section on antitubercular drug therapy.

Nursing diagnosis. The client receiving aminosalicylates should be assessed for the following nursing diagnoses: fluid volume deficit related to anorexia, nausea, vomiting, and diarrhea; activity intolerance related to hemolytic anemia—with G6PD deficiency (pallor, backache, abdominal pain) and myxedema (weight gain; dry, puffy skin, changes in menstrual cycle), or an infectious mononucleosis-like syndrome (fever, headache, rash, sore throat, fatigue); and the collaborative problem of hepatitis (yellow sclera and skin) and crystalluria.

Implementation

Monitoring. Monitor client for adverse reactions to the drug therapy as above. Serum sodium levels should be monitored periodically during drug therapy for hypernatremia and urinalyses for crystals, casts, cells, and decreased specific gravity.

Intervention. Administer with meals or antacids to minimize gastrointestinal distress. When administering the dry powder form of the drug, mix thoroughly with diluent and ensure that the client takes all of liquid to obtain the full dose.

Do not administer aminosalicylates within 6 hours of rifampin or aminosalicylate calcium within 2 or 3 hours of oral tetracyclines.

The client should have a fluid intake of 3000 ml daily, and the urine should be maintained at neutral or alkaline pH to minimize crystalluria.

Education. Therapy may have to continue for 1 to 2 years or longer, so the client's ability to effectively manage the therapeutic regimen is extremely important. Compliance may be difficult because of gastric irritation or hypersensitivity responses.

Clients with diabetes who test their urine with copper sulfate urine glucose tests may have false-positive test results. Clients should instead use Clinistix or Ketodiastix.

Evaluation. The client's sputum culture result is negative and the client can effectively manage the therapeutic regimen.

capreomycin [kap ree oh mye' sin] (Capastat)

Capreomycin is an antimycobacterial agent with an unknown mechanism of action. It is indicated in combination therapy for the treatment of pulmonary tuberculosis caused by *M. tuberculosis* after primary medications (streptomycin, isoniazid, rifampin, pyrazinamide and ethambutol) fail or when these medications cannot be used because of resistant bacilli or drug toxicity.

Administered parenterally, capreomycin has a half-life between 3 to 6 hours and reaches peak serum level is 1 to 2 hours after IM administration. It is excreted by the kidneys, primarily unchanged. Side/adverse effects include nephrotoxicity and hypersensitivity.

The adult dose in combination with other antitubercular agents is 1 g IM daily for 2 to 4 months followed by 1 g two or three times weekly.

■ Nursing Management

Capreomycin Therapy

In addition to the nursing management discussed in the general section on antitubercular drug therapy, consider the following:

Assessment. The health assessment should determine if the client has the following preexisting conditions: dehydration, which increases the risk of toxicity due to increased serum levels of the drug; myasthenia gravis and parkinsonism, in which the neuromuscular deficits may increase; impairment of the eighth cranial nerve, because the drug may cause increased auditory and vestibular toxicity; and renal impairment, which may increase because of the nephrotoxic effects of the drug.

Because of these effects, fluid balance, audiograms, and vestibular and renal function determinations should be assessed before therapy.

The client's medication regimen should be reviewed because there are some drug interactions with capreomycin that are potentially life-threatening, such as those listed below.

Drug	Possible effect and management
When capreomycin is administered with any of the following drugs, very serious reactions may result. Avoid if possible.	
aminoglycosides	**Increased risk for developing ototoxicity, nephrotoxicity, and neuromuscular blockade. Hearing loss may progress to deafness, even after the drug is stopped. This can be a very dangerous combination.** *Avoid.*
amphotericin B parenteral (Fungizone), bacitracin parenteral, bumetanide parenteral (Bumex), cisplatin (Platinol), cyclosporine (Sandimmune), ethacrynic acid (Edecrin) or furosemide parenteral (Lasix), paromomycin (Humatin), streptomycin or vancomycin (Vancocin)	**Concurrent or even sequential use of capreomycin with any of these drugs can increase the risk of ototoxicity and/or nephrotoxicity. Hearing loss may occur and progress to deafness, even if drugs are stopped.** *Avoid if at all possible.*
methoxyflurane (Penthrane) or polymyxins, parenteral	**The potential for nephrotoxicity and/or neuromuscular blockade is increased, which may lead to respiratory depression or paralysis.** *Avoid concurrent or sequential drug administration.*
neuromuscular blocking agents	**May result in increased neuromuscular blocking effects, resulting in respiratory depression or paralysis. Monitor closely, especially during surgery or in the postoperative period.** *If possible, avoid this combination.* **If not, closely monitor and keep anticholinesterase agents or calcium salts on hand to reverse the blockade.**

Nursing diagnosis. The client receiving capreomycin should be assessed for the following nursing diagnoses: impaired tissue integrity related to injection of capreomycin (pain, bleeding, or induration at the injection site); sensory-perceptual alterations related to auditory ototoxicity (tinnitus or hearing loss), or to vestibular ototoxicity (dizziness or unsteadiness); and the collaborative problems of hypersensitivity (rash, swelling, fever), hypokalemia (arrhythmia, anorexia, nausea and vomiting, muscle cramps, fatigue), nephrotoxicity (increased or decreased frequency of urination or amount of urine); and neuromuscular blockade (fatigue, weakness, drowsiness, dyspnea).

Implementation

Monitoring. Weekly renal functions studies should be done; if the BUN is above 30 mg/dl, the medication should be stopped. Fluid intake and output should be monitored throughout therapy. In addition, liver function studies should be done periodically, as well as serum potassium levels. Audiograms and vestibular function determinations should be monitored.

Intervention. To prepare for intramuscular administration, add 2 ml of 0.9% sodium chloride injection or sterile water for injection to the vial. Allow 2 to 3 minutes for dissolution to occur. Reconstituted solutions may darken, but this does not affect their potency. They are stable for 48 hours at room temperature or 14 days if refrigerated.

Administer intramuscularly deep into a large muscle mass to increase absorption and minimize pain and the risk of sterile abscesses.

Education. The client should maintain regular contact with the health care provider to monitor his or her condition. Symptoms of tinnitus, hearing deficit, and/or vertigo should be reported to the prescriber.

Evaluation. The client will be free of infection and able to effectively manage the therapeutic regimen.

cycloserine [sye kloe ser' een] (Seromycin)

This is a broad-spectrum antibiotic that can be bacteriostatic or bactericidal, depending on drug concentration at infection site and organism susceptibility. It is an antimycobacterial agent that interferes with bacterial cell wall synthesis. In combination with other drugs, it is indicated for the treatment of active pulmonary and extrapulmonary tuberculosis after failure of the primary antitubercular medications.

Cycloserine is well absorbed orally and is widely distributed in body tissues and fluids. It reaches peak serum level between 3 and 4 hours, with a half-life of 10 hours. About 35% of cycloserine is metabolized with excretion primarily via the kidneys.

Side/adverse effects of cycloserine include headache and dose-related, CNS toxicity.

The adult oral dose used in combination with other drugs is 250 mg every 12 hours for 2 weeks, then the dose is increased as necessary up to 250 mg every 6 to 8 hours. Maximum daily dose is 1 g. Pediatric dosage is 10 to 20 mg/kg daily, in divided doses.

■ Nursing Management
Cycloserine Therapy

In addition to the nursing management discussed in the general section on antitubercular drug therapy, consider the following:

Assessment. Cycloserine should be used with caution if the client has the following preexisting conditions: severe renal impairment, alcoholism, or seizure disorders because the risk of seizures is greater; or severe anxiety, depression, or psychosis because these conditions may be worsened.

BUN and serum creatinine concentrations should be determined before administering cycloserine. CBC will serve as a baseline since this drug has been associated with vitamin B_{12} and/or folic acid deficiency resulting in anemia.

Review the client's current medications for significant drug interactions that may occur when cycloserine is given with the following drugs:

Drug	Possible effect and management
alcohol	**In chronic alcohol abusers, it may increase the risk of seizures. Avoid or a potentially serious drug interaction may occur.**
ethionamide (Trecator-SC)	May increase CNS side effects such as seizures. Monitor closely, as dosage adjustments may be necessary.

Nursing diagnosis. The client receiving cycloserine should be assessed for the following nursing diagnoses: altered comfort (headache); sensory-perceptual disturbances related to peripheral neuritis (numbness, tingling in fingers and toes); and the collaborative problems of hypersensitivity (rash) and CNS toxicity (anxiety, confusion, dizziness, drowsiness, irritability, depression, nightmares, mood swings, suicidal ideation, seizures).

Implementation

Monitoring. Renal function studies and CBCs may be required periodically. Serum cycloserine levels may also be required; levels should be 25 to 30 μg/ml, levels above 30 μg/ml are to be avoided.

Intervention. If the client experiences gastrointestinal irritation, administer cycloserine after meals. Therapy may be continued for 1 to 2 years or longer.

Education. Caution the client to avoid alcohol while taking this medication, because it increases risks of CNS toxicity such as dizziness, mental disturbances, and seizures.

Advise the client to report immediately to the prescriber any signs of dizziness, drowsiness, numbness or tingling of fingers and toes, or thoughts of suicide.

Evaluation. The client will be free of infection without any adverse effects of cycloserine and will also effectively manage the therapeutic regimen.

ethambutol [e tham' byoo tole] (Myambutol, Etibi♣)

This antitubercular agent is bacteriostatic; it is believed to diffuse into the mycobacteria bacilli and suppress RNA synthesis. It is effective only against actively dividing mycobacteria. It is indicated in combination with other drugs for the treatment of tuberculosis.

Ethambutol is absorbed orally and distributed to most body tissues and fluids with the exception of cerebrospinal fluid. High concentrations are found in the kidneys, lungs, saliva, urine, and erythrocytes. The time to peak serum level is 2 to 4 hours, half-life is between 3 and 4 hours. Ethambutol is metabolized in the liver and excreted by the kidneys.

Side/adverse effects of ethambutol include gastric distress, confusion, disorientation, headache, and optic neuritis.

The adult oral dose in combination with other agents is 15 to 25 mg/kg daily.

■ Nursing Management
Ethambutol Therapy

In addition to the nursing management discussed in the general section on antitubercular drug therapy, consider the following:

Assessment. When the client has preexisting optic neuritis and/or renal impairment, use ethambutol with caution. It may also increase uric acid concentrations, so care must be taken with clients with gout. Weigh client carefully, since dosage is based on weight.

If ethambutol is administered concurrently with other neurotoxic agents, the risk of neurotoxicity, such as optic and peripheral neuritis, occurring is increased. A baseline ophthalmic exam should be done before the initiation of ethambutol therapy.

Nursing diagnosis. The client receiving ethambutol should be assessed for the following nursing diagnoses: altered comfort (headache); altered thought processes (confusion); fluid volume deficit related to anorexia, nausea and vomiting; sensory-perceptual disturbances related to optic neuritis (red-green color blindness, blurred vision, or vision loss); and the collaborative problems of hypersensitivity (rash, fever, arthralgia), hyperuricemia and gout (pain and swelling of joints, particularly the big toe, ankle, and knee), and peripheral neuritis (numbness, tingling of fingers and toes).

Implementation

Monitoring. Ethambutol is known to decrease visual acuity and the ability to see red and green. This presents a safety hazard, especially in driving motor vehicles, and clients should be tested for these visual disturbances frequently during drug therapy. Discontinuation of the drug is usually indicated when visual acuity is disturbed.

Uric acid determinations are required periodically during the course of therapy because elevated levels may result in gout.

Intervention. Administer with food to minimize gastrointestinal distress. Administer ethambutol in a single daily dose; divided doses may not result in therapeutic serum levels. It is administered concurrently with other antitubercular agents because of the tendency for bacterial resistance to occur when it is used alone.

Education. Encourage the client to visit the health care provider regularly to monitor progress. Therapy may have to continue for 1 to 2 years or longer. If no improvement occurs in 2 to 3 weeks, this should be reported to the prescriber. Report promptly signs of optic neuritis (blurred vision, any loss of vision or red-green perception, or eye pain) or peripheral neuritis (numbness, tingling, or weakness in the hands and feet).

Evaluation. The client will be free of infection without any adverse effects of ethambutol and will be able to effectively manage the therapeutic regimen.

ethionamide [e thye on am' ide] (Trecator-SC)

Ethionamide is an antimycobacterial agent indicated for the treatment of tuberculosis after failure of the primary antitubercular agents (streptomycin, isoniazid, rifampin, and ethambutol). Its mechanism of action is unknown, but it is believed to inhibit peptide synthesis.

Ethionamide is well absorbed orally and distributed to most body tissues and fluids, including cerebrospinal fluid. It has a half-life of 2 to 3 hours, and may be metabolized in the liver and excreted primarily by the kidneys.

Side/adverse effects of ethionamide include gastric distress, orthostatic hypotension and peripheral neuritis.

The adult oral dose in combination with other agents is 250 mg every 8 to 12 hours. The pediatric dosage is 4 to 5 mg/kg orally every 8 hours.

▪ Nursing Management

Ethionamide Therapy

In addition to the nursing management discussed in the general section on antitubercular drug therapy, consider the following:

Assessment. Ethionamide is administered cautiously to clients with diabetes mellitus because its administration will make the management of the diabetes more difficult due to drug-related hypoglycemia. Clients with severe hepatic dysfunction have a higher risk of hepatic adverse effects. Clients with an intolerance for niacin, isoniazid, and pyrazinamide may also be intolerant of ethionamide.

Concurrent use of cycloserine will increase the risk for CNS toxicity, especially seizures. Dosage adjustments may be necessary and the client should be monitored closely for CNS toxicity.

A baseline assessment should include cultures, ophthalmologic examination, neurologic exam, and hepatic function determinations.

Nursing diagnosis. The client receiving ethionamide should be assessed for the following nursing diagnoses: altered comfort (rash and metallic taste); fluid volume deficit related to anorexia, nausea and vomiting; risk of injury related to orthostatic hypotension (dizziness upon standing); altered thought processes related to CNS toxicity (confusion, depression, mood and mental changes); self-concept disturbance related to gynecomastia (in males); sensory-perceptual disturbances related to optic neuritis (blurred or loss of vision) or peripheral neuritis (numbness or tingling of the fingers and toes); and the collaborative problems of hepatitis (yellow sclera and skin), hypoglycemia (tachycardia, shakiness, confusion), and goiter/hypothyroidism (weight gain, dry, puffy skin, lethargy, coldness).

Implementation

Monitoring. Although its incidence is rare, optic neuritis (blurred vision, vision loss, and/or eye pain) does occur. The client should have a thorough ophthalmologic examination periodically and at the first indication of symptoms related to vision changes. To monitor for hepatotoxic effects, AST (SGOT) and ALT (SGPT) should be done at least monthly during the course of therapy. Observe the client for jaundice. Cultures should be done periodically throughout therapy to monitor progress.

Intervention. Administer with meals to minimize gastrointestinal distress. If gastrointestinal upset occurs, it may be minimized by a divided dosage schedule or by administration with a rectal suppository. In both cases, however, serum concentrations may not be adequate. Pyridoxine may be prescribed concurrently to prevent peripheral neuritis.

Bacterial resistance develops rapidly if the drug is administered alone, so it is administered in combination with other antimycobacterial drugs.

Education. Advise the client about the importance of complying with the medication regimen, particularly when such a course may be continued for 1 to 2 years or more. Regular visits to the health care provider are necessary to monitor progress and for periodic eye examinations. Any symptoms related to changes in vision should be promptly reported to the prescriber.

Advise the client that because ethionamide may cause dizziness, drowsiness, or weakness, hazardous activities requiring mental alertness such as driving should be avoided until the response to the medication has been ascertained. Alert the client to other potential side effects, such as mental depression or mood changes.

Evaluation. The client will be free of infection without any adverse effects of ethionamide and will be able to effectively manage the therapeutic regimen.

▲ isoniazid [eye soe nye' a zid] (Nydrazid, INH)

Isoniazid is an antimycobacterial (bactericidal) agent that affects mycobacteria in the division phase. Exact mechanism of action is unknown but is believed to inhibit mycolic acid synthesis and cause cell wall disruption in susceptible organisms. Isoniazid is indicated for the treatment and prevention of tuberculosis.

Isoniazid is well absorbed orally and is widely distributed throughout the body. The time to peak serum level is 1 to 2 hours for fast drug acetylators (metabolism) or 4 to 6 hours for slow drug acetylators. Half-life in fast acetylators is 0.5 to 1.6 hours; slow acetylators' half-life is 2 to 5 hours. Isoniazid is metabolized in the liver, primarily by acetylation to inactive metabolites, some of which may be hepatotoxic. The rate of acetylation by the liver is genetically determined; slow acetylators have a decrease in hepatic N-acetyltransferase. (See the Cultural Aspects box below.) Excretion is primarily via the kidneys.

Side/adverse effects of isoniazid include gastric distress, anorexia, nausea, vomiting, weakness, hepatitis, and peripheral neuritis.

The adult oral and parenteral (IM) prophylactic dose of isoniazid is 300 mg daily. The parenteral (IM) treatment dosage when administered in combination with other agents is 5 mg/kg up to 300 mg once daily. The oral treatment dosage when given in combination with other agents to treat tuberculosis is 300 mg daily. The pediatric dosage for prophylaxis orally and parenterally (IM) is 10 mg/kg up to 300 mg daily.

Cultural Aspects — Acetylation Polymorphism

Acetylation polymorphism, a well-known example of a genetic defect in drug metabolism, was first studied when isoniazid therapy was introduced for the treatment of tuberculosis. Individuals were classified as fast or slow eliminators of isoniazid on the basis of a metabolic defect in their ability to metabolize the drug. This polymorphism is especially important in the study of ethnic and racial drug responses because the proportions of rapid acetylators (RA) and slow acetylators (SA) vary dramatically in different ethnic and/or geographic populations (Meyer, 1992). For example, both Caucasian and black populations have approximately equal numbers of SAs and RAs, whereas in Eskimo or Japanese populations the percentage of SAs is particularly low (7% to 22%) and that of RAs is high (Levy, 1993).

Critical thinking question

- How would knowing whether your client was an RA or an SA affect your clinical management of the client's isoniazid therapy?

isoniazid combinations

For ease of drug administration, isoniazid has been combined with rifampin (Rifamate) and in dual packs (Rimactane/INH). See individual headings (isoniazid and rifampin) for additional information.

■ Nursing Management

Isoniazid Therapy

In addition to the nursing management discussed in the general section on antitubercular drug therapy, consider the following:

Assessment. Mycobacterial cultures and sensitivities should be done before therapy. Also included in the baseline assessment should be hepatic function determinations and the status of the underlying tuberculosis.

Isoniazid should be administered cautiously to clients with a history of alcoholism and/or hepatic function impairment because there is increased risk of hepatitis. Clients with an intolerance for niacin, ethionamide, and pyrazinamide may also be intolerant of isoniazid.

Review the client's current medications for significant drug interactions that may occur when isoniazid is given with the following drugs:

Drug	Possible effect and management
alcohol	Daily use of alcohol may result in increased isoniazid metabolism and increased risk of hepatotoxicity. Monitor clients because adjustment may be necessary.
alfentanil (Alfenta)	Isoniazid inhibits liver metabolism, which may decrease the alfentanil metabolism leading to increased alfentanil serum levels and prolonging its duration of action. Monitor serum levels closely.
carbamazepine (Tegretol)	May result in increased carbamazepine serum levels and toxicity. Monitor serum levels closely.
disulfiram (Antabuse)	May increase incidence of CNS side effects such as ataxia, irritability, dizziness, or insomnia. Monitor closely for these symptoms because dosage reduction or even discontinuation of disulfiram may be required.
hepatotoxic drugs	**May increase potential for hepatotoxicity. Avoid or a potentially serious drug interaction may occur.**
ketoconazole (Nizoral), miconazole (Monistat i.v.) (parenteral), or rifampin (Rifadin)	Isoniazid with ketoconazole may decrease serum levels of ketoconazole; if both isoniazid and rifampin are given with ketoconazole, the serum levels of ketoconazole or rifampin have been reported to be undetectable. Therefore combining isoniazid or rifampin together or singly with ketoconazole or parenteral miconazole is not recommended. Rifampin with isoniazid may increase the potential for hepatotoxicity, especially in clients with liver impairment

Continued

Drug	Possible effect and management
ketoconazole (Nizoral), miconazole (Monistat i.v.) parenteral, or rifampin (Rifadin)	and/or in fast acetylators of isoniazid. Monitor closely for hepatotoxicity, especially during the first 90 days of therapy.
phenytoin (Dilantin)	May result in impaired phenytoin metabolism, leading to increased serum levels and toxicity. Phenytoin dose may need to be adjusted. Monitor serum phenytoin closely.

Nursing diagnosis. The client receiving isoniazid should be assessed for the following nursing diagnoses: fluid volume deficit related to anorexia, nausea, vomiting, and diarrhea; sensory-perceptual alterations related to peripheral neuritis (numbness and tingling of the fingers and toes) and optic neuritis (blurred or loss of vision); altered protection related to leukopenia, thrombocytopenia, and anemia (fever, sore throat, fatigue, unusual bruising, or bleeding); impaired tissue integrity related to intramuscular injection (local irritation); and the collaborative problems of hepatitis (yellow skin and sclera), neurotoxicity (depression, psychosis, seizures), and hypersensitivity (fever, rash, arthralgia).

Implementation

Monitoring. To monitor for hepatotoxic effects, AST (SGOT) and ALT (SGPT) should be done at least monthly during the course of therapy. The client should be observed for symptoms of jaundice. Clients over 50 years of age are more prone to the development of hepatitis. At the first signs of hepatotoxicity, isoniazid should be discontinued.

Although its incidence is rare, optic neuritis (blurred vision, vision loss, and/or eye pain) does occur. The client should have an ophthalmologic examination at the first indication of symptoms related to vision changes. Cultures are done periodically throughout therapy to monitor the effectiveness of the drug.

Intervention. Administer with meals or antacids to minimize gastrointestinal distress. If aluminum-containing antacids are required, administer at least 1 hour after isoniazid is given. However, oral absorption may be decreased if the drug is taken with food or antacids.

Pyridoxine may be prescribed concurrently to prevent peripheral neuritis. This may not be required for children if their dietary intake of vitamins is adequate.

There are slow and fast acetylators of isoniazid. Slow acetylators may require lower dosages and are more apt to develop adverse reactions, particularly peripheral neuritis. The highest prevalence of slow acetylators are found in Egyptian, Israeli, Scandinavian, other Caucasian, and black populations; the lowest in Eskimo, Oriental, and Native American populations. (See the Cultural Aspects box on p. 963 on acetylation polymorphism.)

Education. Encourage the client's compliance with the full course of isoniazid therapy. Regular visits to the health care provider are necessary to monitor progress and for periodic eye examinations. Any symptoms related to changes in vision should be promptly reported to the prescriber.

Since alcohol decreases the effects of isoniazid by increasing its metabolism, it should not be used in combination with isoniazid.

Clients with diabetes who test their urine with copper sulfate tests (Clinitest) may obtain false-positive test results. Other tests (Clinistix, Tes-Tape) for urine glucose are unaffected.

Evaluation. The client's sputum culture result is negative without any adverse effects of isoniazid and the client is able to effectively manage the therapeutic regimen.

▲ **pyrazinamide** [peer a zin' a mide]
(pms Pyrazinamide, ♣, Tebrazid ♣)

Pyrazinamide is an antimycobacterial agent with an unknown mechanism of action. Depending on concentration at site of action and susceptibility of the mycobacteria, this drug can be bacteriostatic or bactericidal. It is indicated in combination with other agents for the treatment of tuberculosis.

Pyrazinamide is well absorbed orally and is widely distributed in the body. The time to peak serum level is 1 to 2 hours, elimination half-life is 9 to 10 hours. Pyrazinamide is primarily metabolized in the liver and excreted by the kidneys.

Side/adverse effects of pyrazinamide include arthralgia, related to hyperuricemia.

The adult oral dose when given in combination with other agents is 15 to 30 mg/kg daily, up to a maximum dose of 2 g daily.

■ Nursing Management

Pyrazinamide Therapy

In addition to the nursing management of antitubercular drug therapy previously discussed, consider the following:

Assessment. Specimens for mycobacterial cultures and sensitivity testing should be acquired before therapy. Clients with impaired hepatic function should not receive pyrazinamide unless absolutely essential as it is hepatotoxic. Hepatic function studies should be done before therapy with this agent.

Because pyrazinamide increases serum uric acid concentrations, use with caution with clients with a history of gout. It should be ascertained if the client has an intolerance for ethionamide, niacin, or isoniazid because there may be a cross-intolerance with pyrazinamide.

A baseline assessment as discussed in Chapter 58 should be done.

Nursing diagnosis. The client receiving pyrazinamide should be assessed for the following nursing diagnoses: impaired skin integrity (rash and itching); altered comfort related to hyperuricemia (gouty arthritis—pain and swelling of joints, especially the big toe, ankle, and knee); and the collaborative problem of hepatotoxicity (anorexia, fatigue, yellow skin, and sclera).

Implementation

Monitoring. Cultures should be done periodically throughout therapy to monitor progress, as well as the monitoring of serum uric acid levels to ensure that an acute episode of gout may be prevented. AST (SGOT) and ALT (SGPT), determinations should be done every 2 to 4 weeks to monitor for hepatotoxicity. Observe clients for jaundice and symptoms of acute gouty arthralgia (pain and swelling of joints such as the big toe, knee, and ankle).

Intervention. Pyrazinamide should be administered concurrently with other antitubercular drugs to minimize bacterial resistance. Usually isoniazid, rifampin, pyrazinamide, and streptomycin or ethambutol are given together daily, or 2 or 3 times a week for 16 weeks. When results of susceptibility for these medications are available, the regimen is altered as appropriate. Either all four drugs are taken daily for 2 weeks, followed by twice weekly administration for 6 weeks, then isoniazid and rifampin twice weekly for 16 weeks. The other regimen is the same four medications taken 3 times a week for 16 weeks. All of these doses are taken under the direct observation of a health care provider to ensure compliance.

Education. Encourage the client to remain compliant with the full course of therapy, which is long term. Regular visits to the health care provider are essential for monitoring progress. Clients testing their urine with sodium nitroprusside urine ketone tests may have color interference and should use another test for urine ketones.

Teach clients measures to prevent gout, such as maintaining a fluid intake of 2500 ml daily, adjusting to optimum weight, and limiting intake of alcohol and foods high in purines, such as organ meats (liver, kidneys, hearts, sweetbreads), shellfish, and sardines.

Evaluation. The client will be free of infection without any adverse effects of pyrazinamide and effectively manage the therapeutic regimen.

rifabutin [riff' a byoo tin] (Mycobutin)

Rifabutin is an antimycobacterial indicated for the prophylaxis for disseminated *Mycobacterium avium* complex (MAC) in persons with advanced HIV infection. It inhibits DNA-dependent RNA polymerase in susceptible *E. coli* and *B. subtilis* but its effecting MAC is currently unknown.

It is absorbed from the GI tract, reaches peak serum levels in 2 to 4 hours and has a terminal half-life of 45 hours. Metabolized in the liver, rifabutin is primarily excreted by the kidneys.

Side/adverse effects include nausea, vomiting, and skin rash. The usual adult dose is 300 mg daily.

■ Nursing Management

Rifabutin Therapy

Assessment. It should be determined that the client does not have a hypersensitivity to rifabutin or rifampin. Rifabutin is not administered to clients with active tuberculosis; they are better treated with the therapies described above. If rifabutin is administered to active tuberculosis as a prophylaxis of MAC there is the risk of the tuberculosis becoming resistant to both rifabutin and rifampin.

Nursing diagnosis. The client on rifabutin therapy has a potential for developing the following nursing diagnoses: fluid volume deficit related to nausea and vomiting; altered comfort related to arthralgia (joint pain) and myalgia (muscle pain); impaired skin integrity (rash); altered protection related to neutropenia; and the potential complication of pseudojaundice.

Implementation

Monitoring. Platelet counts and white blood cell counts should be done periodically to monitor for neutropenia, and rarely, thrombocytopenia. Monitor the client for the development of MAC.

Intervention. Rifabutin is absorbed more quickly if administered on an empty stomach; however, if GI distress occurs administer the drug with food. The contents of the capsules may be mixed with applesauce or pudding for clients with difficulty swallowing.

Education. Alert the client that the drug will turn body secretions and excretions (urine, feces, saliva, perspiration, and tears) a reddish orange to reddish brown. Discolored tears may also stain soft contact lens.

Stress the need for regular visits to the prescriber to monitor progress.

Evaluation. The client will not contract MAC and will manage effectively the therapeutic regimen.

▲ **rifampin** [rif' am pin] (Rifadin, Rofact)

Rifampin is a broad-spectrum bactericidal antibiotic (antimycobacterial) that blocks RNA transcription. It is indicated for the treatment of tuberculosis and for asymptomatic meningococcal carriers of *Neisseria meningitidis*. It is well absorbed orally and widely distributed in the body. Rifampin is lipid soluble, thus it may reach and kill intracellular and extracellular susceptible bacteria. Time to reach peak serum level is 1.5 to 4 hours; elimination half-life is up to 5 hours. It is metabolized in the liver and excreted primarily in the feces.

Side/adverse effects of rifampin include gastric distress, hypersensitivity, and a flu-like syndrome.

The rifampin adult oral dose in combination with other agents (for tuberculosis) is 600 mg daily. To treat asymptomatic meningococcal carriers, the dose is 600 mg orally twice daily for 2 days. For children 1 month and older, the dose to treat tuberculosis (with other antituberculars) is 10 to 20 mg/kg daily. For asymptomatic meningococcal carriers, the dose is 5 mg/kg orally every 12 hours for 2 days.

■ Nursing Management

Rifampin Therapy

In addition to the nursing management of antitubercular drug therapy previously discussed, consider the following:

Assessment. Clients with impaired hepatic function and/or active or history of alcoholism should not receive rifampin unless absolutely essential because of the high risk for hepatotoxicity. Specimens for mycobacterial cultures and sensitivity testing and hepatic function studies (ALT [SGPT], AST [SGOT], serum alkaline phosphatase, serum bilirubin levels) should be obtained before therapy.

Review the client's current medications for significant drug interactions that may occur when rifampin is given with the following drugs:

Drug	Possible effect and management
alcohol	Daily use of alcohol may increase the risk of rifampin-induced hepatotoxicity and increase the rate of rifampin metabolism. Monitor hepatic function studies closely, as dosage adjustments may be necessary.
antidiabetic agents (oral)	Concurrent use enhances the metabolism of the antidiabetic drugs; dosage adjustment may be indicated.
corticosteroids, glucocorticoids, and mineralocorticoids, anticoagulants, oral warfarin (Coumadin) or indanedione, digitalis glycosides, disopyramide (Norpace), mexiletine (Mexitil), tocainide (Tonocard), quinidine, azole antifungals, phenytoin (Dilantin) or chloramphenicol (Chloromycetin)	Rifampin increases levels of liver-metabolizing enzymes and therefore may decrease the effectiveness of these medications, which are metabolized by the liver. Monitor serum levels of these drugs closely to ensure therapeutic levels because dosage adjustments may be needed.
estrogen-containing oral contraceptives, estramustine, or estrogens	Decreases effectiveness due to increased liver metabolism of estrogen. May result in menstrual irregularities, spotting, and unplanned pregnancies. Advise clients of the possible effects when these drugs are combined and advise alternative contraception.
hepatotoxic drugs, other	**Increases the risk of hepatotoxicity. Avoid or a potentially serious drug interaction may occur.**
isoniazid (INH) or ketoconazole (Nizoral) oral or miconazole parenteral (Monistat i.v.)	**Increased risk for hepatotoxicity. See comments within the discussion of isoniazid. If possible, avoid concurrent drug administration.**
methadone	May decrease the effectiveness of methadone, and may induce methadone withdrawal in dependent clients. Monitor closely; dosage adjustments may be necessary during and after rifampin therapy.
verapamil, oral	Accelerates the metabolism of oral verapamil, decreasing blood levels and decreasing its cardiovascular effects.
xanthenes, aminophylline, oxtriphylline, theophylline	Increases the metabolism of these drugs increasing drug clearance. Monitor with serum levels of the client's xanthene drug.

Nursing diagnosis. The client receiving rifampin should be assessed for the following nursing diagnoses: altered comfort related to rash (hypersensitivity) and "flu-like" syndrome (chills, fever, headache, generalized discomfort); altered bowel elimination (diarrhea); altered protection related to fungal overgrowth (sore mouth and tongue) and blood dyscrasias; fluid volume deficit related to nausea, vomiting and diarrhea; altered urinary elimination related to interstitial nephritis evidenced by greatly decreased frequency of urination and amount of urine; and the collaborative problem of hepatitis and Redman syndrome (red-orange discoloration of skin, mucous membranes, and sclera).

Implementation

Monitoring. Cultures should be done periodically throughout rifampin therapy to monitor progress. In addition, hepatic function studies are required before and intermittently during therapy as with other antitubercular drugs. The client should be monitored for jaundice, yellow sclera, and dark urine, which may indicate hepatotoxicity.

Intervention. Reduced dosages may be required for clients with impaired hepatic function (not more than 8 mg/kg/day).

Administer rifampin with a full glass of water on an empty stomach for optimal absorption unless the client experiences dyspepsia, in which case it may be given with food. Contents of the capsule may be mixed with applesauce or jam for clients with difficulty swallowing.

Rifampin is administered concurrently with other antitubercular drugs to minimize bacterial resistance and the treatment period may be 6 months to 2 years.

Education. Encourage the client to complete the full course of therapy, which may take years. Regular visits to the health care provider are essential for monitoring progress.

Alert the client that there may be a reddish-brown discoloration of urine, feces, saliva, sputum, sweat, and tears, but this effect is not hazardous. However, clients who wear soft contact lens should be cautioned that this same effect may permanently color the lens.

Women taking oral contraceptives who are also receiving rifampin should be cautioned to use an alternate form of contraception.

Clients should be advised to avoid alcoholic beverages while taking rifampin because it increases the risk of hepatotoxicity.

Evaluation. The client will be free of infection without any adverse effects of rifampin and able to effectively manage the therapeutic regimen.

streptomycin injection [strep toe mye' sin]

Streptomycin is a aminoglycoside antibiotic that is poorly absorbed from the gastrointestinal tract; therefore it is given intramuscularly. It was one of the first effective agents used in the late 1940s to treat tuberculosis, and it still is an important agent in managing severe tuberculosis. Like the other aminoglycosides, its major toxicities include ototoxicity and nephrotoxicity, especially when given to clients with impaired renal function or with other medications with the same toxicities. See Chapter 59 for detailed information on the aminoglycosides and their nursing management.

The adult dose for streptomycin is 1 g IM daily. As soon as possible, reduce dose to 1 g two or three times weekly. For geriatric clients, the dose is 500 to 750 mg daily, in combination with other antitubercular agents. For children, the dose is 20 mg/kg daily, in combination with other antitubercular agents. Maximum daily dose is 1 g.

AMEBIASIS

Amebiasis is an infection of the large intestine produced by a protozoan parasite, *Entamoeba histolytica*. This infestation is found worldwide but is prevalent and severe in tropical areas. It also has been detected in poorly sanitized areas, including some rural communities, Native American reservations, migrant labor farm camps and is also common in homosexual males (Anandan, 1995). Transmission is usually through ingestion of cysts (fecal to oral route) from contaminated food or water or from person-to-person contact. Poor personal hygiene can increase the spread of this parasite.

Life Cycle of Ameba

The protozoan has two stages in its life cycle: (1) the trophozoite (vegetative ameba), which is the active, motile form, and (2) the cyst, or inactive, drug-resistant form that appears in intestinal excretion. The *trophozoite stage* is capable of ameboid motion and sexual activity. Because of its susceptibility to injury, it generally succumbs to an unfavorable environment. However, under certain circumstances, the trophozoite protects itself by entering the *cystic stage*. During this phase the protozoan becomes inactive by surrounding itself with a resistant cell wall within which it can survive for a long time, even in an unsuitable environment.

The complete life cycle of the ameba occurs in humans, the main host. It begins by ingestion of cysts that are present on hands, food, or water contaminated by feces. On reaching the stomach the hydrochloric acid does not destroy the swallowed cysts, but instead they pass unharmed into the small intestine. The digestive juices penetrate the cystic walls, and the trophozoites are released. The motile amoebae later pass into the colon, where they live and multiply for a time, feeding on the bacterial flora of the gut.

The presence of bacteria is essential for their survival. Finally, before excretion, the trophozoites move toward the terminal end of the bowel and again become encysted. After the cysts are eliminated in the feces, they remain viable and infective. Unfortunately, the cycle may begin again when the cysts appearing in fecal excretion are ingested through contamination of food or water.

The parasite causing amebiasis replicates in three major locations: (1) the lumen of the bowel, (2) the intestinal mucosa, and (3) extraintestinal sites. Thus amebiasis is classified according to its primary site of action: intestinal amebiasis, where amebic activity is restricted to the bowel lumen or intestinal mucosa, or extraintestinal amebiasis, where parasitic invasion occurs outside the intestine.

Intestinal amebiasis. Intestinal amebiasis may be manifested as an asymptomatic intestinal infection or a symptomatic intestinal infection that may be mild, moderate, or severe.

Asymptomatic intestinal amebiasis. In asymptomatic intestinal amebiasis the action of the parasite is restricted to the lumen of the bowel. The individual is asymptomatic but becomes a carrier of the disease by passing mature cysts of the parasite in formed stools. Outside the body the cysts can live for several weeks, surviving dry, freezing, or high temperature conditions. By this means the infection is transmitted from person to person by flies or contaminated food or water. Ordinary concentrations of chlorine in water purification do not destroy the cysts. If the carrier fails to follow any drug treatment, serious gastrointestinal pathologic problems eventually develop. Occasionally mild symptoms exist including vague abdominal pain, nausea, flatulence, fatigue, and nervousness.

Symptomatic intestinal amebiasis. Symptomatic amebiasis occurs when the trophozoites in the lumen of the bowel penetrate the mucosal lining of the colon. After they multiply and thrive on bacterial flora, a large infestation occurs, producing diarrhea and abdominal pain. The increased loss of fluid may cause prostration. In addition, ulcerative colitis may result. This state of the disease is called intestinal amebiasis and is usually diagnosed as mild, moderate, or severe according to the intensity of the symptoms and the extent of the disease.

Extraintestinal amebiasis. The term *extraintestinal amebiasis* means the parasites have migrated to other parts of the body, such as the liver or occasionally the spleen, lungs, or brain. When the parasites are in the liver, necrotic foci develop because of the parasites' destructive effect on tissues. When there is liver involvement, the terms *liver abscess* and *hepatic amebiasis* are usually used.

Antiamebiasis Agents

Drugs for the treatment of amebiasis are classified according to the site of the previously described amebic action. Luminal amebicides act primarily in the bowel lumen and are generally ineffective against parasites in the bowel wall or tissues. Tissue amebicides are drugs that act primarily in the bowel wall, liver, and other extraintestinal tissues. No single drug is effective for both types of amebiasis; therefore a luminal and extraluminal (tissue) amebicide or combination therapy is often prescribed. The intestinal amebicide are considered to be: iodoquinol, metronidazole, and paromomycin; the extraintestinal ones: chloroquine and metronidazole.

iodoquinol [eye oh do kwin' ole] (diiodohydroxyquin, Yodoxin)

Iodoquinol is an antiprotozoal with an unknown mechanism of action. It is poorly absorbed from the intestinal tract; thus it produces its effect against the trophozoites of *E. histolytica* at the site of intestinal infestation. It is indicated for the treatment of intestinal amebiasis in asymptomatic carriers of *E. histolytica*.

Following administration and local effect, iodoquinol is excreted in the feces. Side/adverse effects include gastric distress, hypersensitivity, fever, and chills.

The adult oral dose is 650 mg three times a day, after meals for 20 days. The pediatric dosage is 40 mg/kg orally in three divided doses after meals for 20 days.

■ Nursing Management
Iodoquinol Therapy

Assessment. Iodoquinol should be used with caution if the client has the following preexisting conditions: intolerance to iodoquinol, chloroxine, iodine, pentaquine, or primaquine; optic neuropathy; thyroid, hepatic, or renal disease.

Clients should have an ophthalmologic examination before and periodically during iodoquinol therapy.

A baseline assessment as described in Chapter 58 should be done. Stool specimens should be collected and taken directly to the lab for the detection of parasites.

Nursing diagnosis. The client receiving iodoquinol should be assessed for the following nursing diagnoses: altered comfort (rash, itching of rectal area, or headache); fluid volume deficit related to nausea, vomiting, and diarrhea; hyperthermia; altered bowel elimination (diarrhea); sensory-perceptual alterations (visual disturbances) related to optic atrophy, optic neuritis, or subacute myelooptic neuropathy, or (numbness and tingling of the fingers and toes) related to the development of peripheral neuropathy; and the collaborative problem of thyroid enlargement.

Implementation

Monitoring. Intake and output should be documented, as well as frequency and character of stools. Fresh, warm stools should be monitored for the presence of amoebae. Diarrhea may occur the first few days of therapy with iodoquinol. Alert the prescriber if it continues for more than 3 days.

The development of a neurologic disorders such as myelooptic neuropathy, optic atrophy, optic neuritis, and peripheral neuropathy have been implicated in treatment with prolonged high doses.

Iodoquinol may cause thyroid enlargement, and it interferes with certain thyroid function tests by increasing protein-bound serum iodine levels. The drug contains approximately 64% iodine.

In children, the administration of iodoquinol for chronic diarrhea has been responsible for causing optic atrophy and permanent loss of vision. Thus administration of this drug is not advocated for treatment or prophylaxis of "traveler's diarrhea" or for use in chronic nonspecific diarrhea.

Intervention. Administer drug after meals to minimize gastrointestinal irritation. The course of therapy may be repeated if necessary only after a 2 to 3 week rest period.

For ease of administration to children and for clients that may have difficulty swallowing, tablets may be crushed and mixed with applesauce, gelatin dessert, or ice cream.

Education. Clients should be instructed in proper hygiene to prevent reinfection. Inform the client that any results of thyroid function studies completed within 6 months of the discontinuance of iodoquinol may be distorted.

Evaluation. The client will be free of amoebae in stools for 1 year and able to effectively manage the therapeutic regimen.

paromomycin [par oh moe mye' sin] (Humatin)
Paromomycin is both an amebicidal and an antibacterial agent. The drug is an aminoglycoside antibiotic with antibacterial properties similar to that of neomycin. Paromomycin acts directly on intestinal amoebae and on bacteria such as *Salmonella* and *Shigella*. Because the drug is poorly absorbed from the gastrointestinal tract, it exerts no effect on systemic infections such as extraintestinal amebiasis. It is indicated for the treatment of acute and chronic intestinal amebiasis and for adjunct therapy in management of hepatic coma.

Paromomycin is poorly absorbed from the intestinal tract; thus most of the drug is excreted in the feces. Side/adverse effects include nausea, diarrhea and gastric distress. Paromomycin is an aminoglycoside; therefore the drug interactions possible with this family of medications may also occur with paromomycin. See the discussion of aminoglycoside antibiotics in Chapter 59.

The adult and pediatric dosages to treat intestinal amebiasis is 25 to 35 mg/kg daily, in three divided doses given with meals for 5 to 10 days. To manage hepatic coma, the adult dosage is 4 g daily in divided doses at regular intervals for 5 or 6 days.

■ Nursing Management
Paromomycin Therapy

See Chapter 59 for detailed discussion of the nursing management of aminoglycosides.

Assessment. Paromomycin is contraindicated for use in intestinal obstruction and in ulcerative bowel lesions because of possible systemic absorption. It is only to be used for lumenal amebiasis.

Nursing diagnosis. The client receiving paromomycin should be assessed for the following nursing diagnoses: fluid volume deficit related to nausea, vomiting, and diarrhea; altered bowel elimination (diarrhea); activity intolerance related to lightheadedness and dizziness; and auditory disturbances related to tinnitus and hearing loss.

Implementation

Monitoring. Examine fresh, warm stools for the presence of amoebae at weekly intervals for 6 weeks after the end of therapy and monthly for 2 years to indicate that the client is not harboring the parasite. Notify the prescriber if ringing of the ears or dizziness occurs because the drug is ototoxic.

Intervention. Administer after meals to minimize gastrointestinal distress.

Education. Teach the client proper personal hygiene to prevent reinfection.

Evaluation. The client will be free of amoebas in stools for 1 year and able to effectively manage the therapeutic regimen.

Other Drugs

Metronidazole (Flagyl) is an antibacterial, antiprotozoal, and anthelmintic agent. It is used for treatment of extraintestinal and intestinal amebiasis. When used in the treatment of invasive amebiasis, it is recommended that it be administered with a luminal amebicide, such as iodoquinol or paromomycin.

Mechanism of action appears to be due to an interaction between the intracellular reduced metronidazole (which is cytotoxic) and DNA, which results in inhibition of nucleic acid synthesis and cell death. For additional drug information, see Chapter 59.

Chloroquine (Aralen) is used to treat amebic liver abscess, usually in combination with other drugs. See previous drug discussion earlier in this chapter for further information on this drug.

Dehydroemetine (Mebadin) and diloxanide furoate (Furamide) are also antiinfective agents used to treat amebiasis but are available only from the Centers for Disease Control and Prevention (Parasitic Disease Drug Service, Division of Host Factors, Center for Infectious Disease, Atlanta, GA, 30333), because they are considered investigational agents.

OTHER PROTOZOAN DISEASES

Several other protozoan diseases are widespread throughout the world and may be encountered in clinical practice in the United States and Canada. In this section each disease and the primary antiprotozoan agent used in its treatment will be described.

Toxoplasmosis

Toxoplasmosis is caused by an intracellular parasite, *Toxoplasma gondii*. This parasite is found worldwide and infests a variety of animals, including humans. It is often harbored in the host with no evidence of the disease. Toxoplasmosis is contracted by ingesting cysts found in inadequately cooked raw meat or by accidentally ingesting cysts from cat feces.

The most common form of the disease in the United States and Canada is usually subclinical. Symptomatically the individual may experience lymphadenopathy, fever, and occasionally a rash on the palms and soles. The most serious complication of toxoplasmosis is meningoencephalitis. Toxoplasmosis is treated with a combination of sulfadiazine and pyrimethamine, both of which alter the folic acid cycle of the *Toxoplasma* organism, resulting in its death. The oral dosage of pyrimethamine is 25 mg/day for 3 to 4 weeks; the dosage of sulfadiazine is 1 to 4 g/day for 1 to 3 weeks.

Trichomoniasis

Trichomoniasis is a disease of the vagina caused by *Trichomonas vaginalis*. Its characteristic presentation consists of a wet, inflamed vagina, a "strawberry" cervix, and a thin, yellow, frothy malodorous discharge. Usually both sexual partners are infected by this organism, which can be identified microscopically from semen, prostatic fluid, or exudate from the vagina. Infections often recur, which indicates that the protozoans persist in extravaginal foci, male urethra, or the periurethral glands and ducts of both sexes.

Metronidazole (Flagyl) is the drug of choice, and treatment must be given simultaneously to both partners involved for cure.

HELMINTHIASIS

The disease-producing **helminths** are classified as metazoa, or multicellular animal parasites. Unlike the protozoa, they are large organisms that have a complex cellular structure and that feed on host tissue. They may be present in the gastrointestinal tract, but several types also penetrate the tissues, and some undergo developmental changes during which they wander extensively in the host. Because most anthelminthics used today are highly effective against specific parasites, the organism must be accurately identified before treatment is started, usually by finding the parasite ova or larvae in the feces, urine, blood sputum, or tissues of the host.

Parasitic infestations do not necessarily cause clinical manifestations, although they may be injurious for a number of reasons.

1. Worms may cause mechanical injury to the tissues and organs. Roundworms in large numbers may cause obstruction in the intestine; filariae may block lymphatic channels and cause massive edema; and hookworms often cause extensive damage to the wall of the intestine and considerable loss of blood.
2. Toxic substances produced by the parasite may be absorbed by the host.
3. The tissues of the host may be traumatized by the presence of the parasite and made more susceptible to bacterial infections.
4. Heavy infestation with worms will rob the host of food. This is particularly significant in children.

Helminths that are parasitic to humans are classified as (1) Platyhelminthes (flatworms), which include two subclasses: cestodes (tapeworms) and trematodes (flukes), and (2) Nematoda (roundworms).

Platyhelminths (Flatworms)

Cestodes

Cestodes are tapeworms, of which there are four varieties: (1) *Taenia saginata* (beef tapeworm), (2) *T. solium* (pork tapeworm), (3) *Diphyllobrothrium latum* (fish tapeworm), and (4) *Hymenolepis nana* (dwarf tapeworm). As indicated by the name of the worm, the parasite enters the intestine by way of improperly cooked beef, pork, or fish or from contaminated food, as in the case of the dwarf tapeworm.

The cestodes are segmented flatworms with a head or scolex, which has hooks or suckers that are used to attach to tissues, and a number of segments, or proglottids, which in some cases may extend for 20 to 30 feet in the bowel. Drugs affecting the scolex allow expulsion of the organisms from the intestine. Each of the proglottids contains both male and female reproductive units. When filled with fertilized eggs, they are expelled from the worm into the environment. Upon ingestion, the infected larvae develop into adults in the small intestine of the human. The larvae may travel to extraintestinal sites and enter other tissues such as the liver, muscle, and eye. The tapeworms, with the exception of the dwarf tapeworm, spend part of their life cycle in a host other than humans—pigs, fish, or cattle. The dwarf tapeworm does not require an intermediate host.

The tapeworm has no digestive tract; it depends on the nutrients that are intended for the host. Subsequently, the victim suffers by eventually developing nutritional deficiency.

Trematodes. Trematodes, or flukes, are flat, nonsegmented parasites with suckers that attach to and feed on host tissue. The life cycle begins with the egg, which is passed into fresh water following fecal excretion from the body of the human host. The egg containing the embryo forms into a ciliated organism, the *miracidium*. In the presence of water the miracidium escapes from the egg and enters the intermediate host, the freshwater snail, which exists extensively in rice paddies and irrigation ditches. After entry, the fluke forms a cyst in the lungs of the snail. In the cyst, many organisms develop. They can penetrate other parts of the snail and grow into worms called *cercariae*. Eventually, the cercariae are released from the snail into the water, attaching themselves to blades of grass to encyst. A human, the final host, then becomes infected by the parasite.

When encysted organisms in snails or even fish and crabs are swallowed by humans, they develop into adult flukes in different structures of the body. The flukes therefore are classified according to the type of tissues they invade. Following ingestion, the eggs of *Schistosoma haematobium* appear in the urinary bladder and cause inflammation of the urogenital system. This can result in chronic cystitis and hematuria. Infestations with *S. japonicum* and *S. mansoni* produce intestinal disturbance with resultant ulceration and necrosis of the rectum. *S. japonicum* is more concentrated in the veins of the small intestine. If the liver and spleen become infected, the disease is usually fatal. *S. mansoni* prefers the portal veins that drain the large intestine, particularly the sigmoid colon and rectum. Unlike the other parasites, the cercariae of *S. mansoni* are not ingested but burrow through the skin, especially between the toes of the human host who is standing in contaminated water. They then make their way to the portal system, where they mature into adult flukes.

Schistosomiasis (bilharziasis) is endemic to Africa, Asia, South American, and the Caribbean islands. The disease can be controlled largely by eliminating the intermediate host, the snail.

Travelers to these areas must avoid contact with contaminated water for drinking, bathing, or swimming. Unfortunately, the disease has been introduced in the United States and Canada by immigrants or individuals who have traveled to the endemic areas.

Nematoda (Roundworms)

Nematoda are nonsegmented, cylindrical worms that consist of a mouth and complete digestive tract. The adults reside in the human intestinal tract; there is no intermediate host. Two types of nematode infection exist in the human: the egg form and the larval form.

Egg infective form. *Ascaris lumbricoides* is a large nematode (about 30 cm in length) and is known as the "roundworm of humans."

The adult *Ascaris* usually resides in the upper end of the small intestine of the human, where it feeds on semidigested foods. The fertilized egg, when excreted with feces, can survive in the soil for a long time. When inadvertently ingested by another host, the embryos escape from the eggs and mature into adults in the host. To prevent the disease, proper sanitary conditions and meticulous personal habits must be observed.

Infection with *Enterobius vermicularis*, or pinworm, is highly prevalent among children and adults in the United States. Adult pinworms reside in the large intestine. However, the female migrates to the anus, depositing her eggs around the skin of the anal region. This causes intense itching and can be noted especially in children.

Diagnosis is made with the Graham sticky tape method. Ingestion of excreted eggs can infect an individual. In addition, eggs that contaminate clothing, bedding, furniture, and other items may be responsible for continuing the reinfection of an individual and initiating the infection of others.

Larval infective form. *Necator americanus* (New World) or *Ancylostoma duodenale* (Old World) hookworms are somewhat similar in action. They reside in the small intestine of humans. When the eggs are excreted in the feces, the larvae hatch in the soil. The larvae can penetrate the skin of humans, particularly through the soles of the feet, producing dermatitis (ground itch). On entry into the small intestine, they develop into adult worms. During the process they extravasate blood from the intestinal vessels and cause a profound anemia in the victim. The presence of eggs in the feces indicates a positive test for hookworm disease. This infection can be avoided by wearing shoes.

Trichinella spiralis is a small pork roundworm that causes trichinosis. In humans the disease begins by ingestion of insufficiently cooked pork or bear meat. On entry of encysted meat into the small intestine, the larvae are released from the cysts.

Following maturation, the females develop eggs that later form into larvae. They then migrate by the bloodstream and the lymphatic system to the skeletal muscles and encyst. Encapsulation and eventually calcification of the cysts occur. Diagnosis of trichinosis is made by muscle biopsy, whereby microscopic examination reveals the presence of larvae. The disease is prevented by thoroughly cooking pork and bear meat before eating.

Anthelmintic Agents

Anthelmintic drugs are used to rid the body of worms (helminths). Anthelmintics are among the most primitive types of chemotherapy. It has been estimated that one third of the world's population is infested with these parasites.

diethylcarbamazine [dye eth il kar' ba ma zeen] (Hetrazan)

Diethylcarbamazine has a microfilaricidal and a macrofiaricidal effect. The microfilaricidal action is to increase the loss of microfilariae and inhibits the rate of embryogenesis from nematodes. It has no sterilizing effect on adult worms. It is indicated for the treatment of Bancroft's filariasis, loiasis, onchocerciasis, and tropical eosinophilia.

It is absorbed after oral administration and is distributed to nonfatty tissues. Peak serum level is reached in 1 to 2 hours, half-life is 8 hours. Excretion is via the kidneys. The most frequently reported side effects include joint pains, increased weakness, headache, and dizziness. Less often reported are the symptoms of nausea and vomiting. The most frequently reported adverse reactions are facial swelling, especially around the eyes, and pruritus. Less often reported are elevated temperature, rash and painful, tender glands especially in the neck, armpits, or groin area.

The adult dosage is 2 to 3 mg/kg PO three times daily. For tropical eosinophilia the dose is 6 mg/kg PO daily for 4 to 7 days.

■ Nursing Management

Diethylcarbamazine Therapy

Assessment. Treatment of pregnant clients should be deferred until after delivery. Treatment is also contraindicated with ocular onchocerciasis because long-term therapy may cause inflammation and then degenerative changes in the optic disc and retina. Ophthalmologic examinations should be part of the baseline assessment. In addition, if diethylcarbamazine is administered for Bancroft's filariasis and loiasis, microfilarial blood concentrations and skin biopsy for intradermal microfilariae should be obtained before therapy.

Nursing diagnosis. The client receiving diethylcarbamazine should be assessed for the following nursing diagnoses: altered comfort (headache, itching, and swelling of face, rash, lymphadenopathy, and arthralgia); fatigue; hyperthermia; fluid volume deficit related to nausea and vomiting; risk for injury related to lightheadedness and dizziness; and visual disturbances related to night blindness, tunnel vision, and vision loss.

Implementation

Monitoring. If allergic reactions (swelling and itching of skin, fine papular rash, tenderness of lymph nodes, headache, fever, tachycardia, conjunctivitis, uveitis) occur as the result of the substances released when the microfilariae are destroyed, report to the prescriber. Microfilarial blood concentrations are used to monitor this effect. Antihistamine therapy or corticosteroids are usually prescribed to relieve these symptoms. Ophthalmoscopic examinations are performed on clients treated for onchocerciasis. Report immediately any signs of itching or swelling of eyes. Corticosteroid eye drops may be administered for treatment of this condition. Blood and skin samples are obtained periodically to monitor the client's progress.

Intervention. For ease of administration, the tablet may be chewed, swallowed whole, or crushed and mixed with food. No dietary restrictions, laxatives, or posttreatment purging are required. A second course of therapy will be required if the client is not cured in 3 weeks.

Education. Emphasize the importance of following meticulous hygiene: washing hands before eating and after going to toilet, keeping hands or objects from mouth.

For treatment of filariasis, stress the importance of remaining under prescriber's care. Failure to follow drug regimen eventually can obstruct lymph flow, thereby producing hydrocele, elephantiasis of limbs, enlarged scrotum or breasts, and chyluria (milk-like urine).

Evaluation. The client will have 3 negative stool samples after the completion of the therapy. For pinworms, the client will have perianal swabs be negative for 7 days. The client/care giver will be able to effectively manage the therapeutic regimen.

mebendazole [me ben' da zole] (Vermox)

Mebendazole is a vermicidal and may also be ovicidal for most helminths. It causes degeneration of a parasite's cytoplasmic microtubules, which results in blocking glucose uptake in the helminth, leading to death of the parasite. It is indicated for the treatment of *Trichuriasis* (whipworm), *Enterobiasis* (pinworm), *Ascariasis* (roundworm), *Ancylostoma* (common hookworm), and *Necator* (American hookworm), singly or in mixed infestations.

Mebendazole oral absorption is increased if given with fatty foods. It is distributed to serum, cyst fluid, liver, hepatic cysts, and muscle tissues, with a half-life of 2.5 to 5.5 hours. It is metabolized in the liver and excreted primarily in feces. Side effects of mebendazole are uncommon and include gastric distress, diarrhea, nausea, and vomiting.

The adult and pediatric dosage (children 2 years and over) is 100 mg PO twice daily for 3 days. If necessary, this dosage may be repeated in 2 to 3 weeks.

■ Nursing Management

Mebendazole Therapy

Assessment. Clients with Crohn's ileitis and ulcerative colitis may have increased absorption with mebendazole and therefore be at greater risk for toxicity. Those with hepatic function impairment may require lower dosages.

A CBC is required before therapy because mebendazole may cause a leukopenia.

Collect pinworm specimen for a baseline assessment: wrap a transparent strip of cellophane (sticky side out) tape around a tongue blade and press against perianal area. Then place sticky side of tape on a glass slide and send to laboratory. Female worm emerges from the rectum during the night to lay eggs in the perianal area. This causes the client to become restless during sleep. The emerging worms can be seen at night with a flashlight.

For roundworms, whipworms, and capillariasis send a baseline stool sample that is warm to the lab.

Nursing diagnosis. The client receiving mebendazole should be assessed for the following nursing diagnoses: altered comfort (headache); fluid volume deficit related to nausea, vomiting, and diarrhea; altered bowel elimination (diarrhea); altered protection related to neutropenia (sore throat, fever, and fatigue); body image disturbance related to alopecia; risk for injury related to lightheadedness and dizziness; and the collaborative problem of hypersensitivity.

Implementation

Monitoring. Continue to monitor progress with perianal or stool examinations. To collect a stool specimen, collect stool specimen in clean, dry, and properly labeled container and send to laboratory. Do not contaminate specimen with water, urine, or chemicals because parasite may be destroyed. Review CBCs for neutropenia.

Intervention. For ease of administration, tablets may be crushed and mixed with applesauce or other food. No dietary restrictions, laxatives, or posttreatment enemas are necessary.

For pinworm infestation, treat all family members because it is readily transmitted from person to person.

Education. Stress the importance of handwashing and of sanitary disposal of feces. Avoid walking barefoot to prevent hookworm. The larvae hatch in the soil and penetrate through the skin. Instruct client to take frequent showers rather than baths, to change underclothes, nightclothes, bedclothes, and towels daily, and to disinfect toilet facilities daily. Instruct the client to wash the perianal area daily to prevent reinfestation.

For pinworm, instruct the client to wash (not shake) all the bedclothing and nightclothes after treatment.

For hookworm or whipworms, instruct the client to take iron supplements during treatment and for up to 6 months afterward if the client is anemic.

Evaluation. The client will have three negative stool samples after the completion of the therapy. For pinworms, the client will have perianal swabs be negative for 7 days. The client will be able to effectively manage the therapeutic regimen.

niclosamide [ni kloe' sa mide] (Niclocide)

Niclosamide is an anthelmintic that affects the mitochondria of the cestode, inhibiting aerobic and may inhibit anaerobic metabolism, on which many cestodes depend for survival. Contact with the drug results in destruction of the scolex and proximal segments of the organism, the proglottids. The scolex, when loosened from the intestinal wall, is usually digested in the intestine. Consequently, identification of the worm in the feces cannot be made.

Niclosamide is indicated for the treatment of *Taenia saginata* (beef tapeworm), *Diphyllobothrium latum* (fish tapeworm), *Hymenolepis nana* (dwarf tapeworm), *Dipylidium caninum* (dog and cat tapeworm), and *T. solium* (pork tapeworm) infestations.

Because niclosamide is poorly absorbed from the intestinal tract, this drug can exert its effect on intestinal helminths, the site of its action. Excretion is in the feces. The most frequently reported adverse reactions of niclosamide are stomach pain or distress, anorexia, nausea, and vomiting. Infrequent or rare side effects include gastric distress, dizziness, sedation, pruritus of the rectum, rash, and a bad taste in the mouth.

Niclosamide tablets should be thoroughly chewed and taken with water. The adult dosage for fish and beef tapeworms is four tablets (2 g) as single dose; for dwarf tapeworm the dose is four tablets (2 g) daily for 1 week. For additional dosing recommendations, see current package insert or drug reference.

■ Nursing Management
Niclosamide Therapy

Assessment. Niclosamide should not be administered to clients who are hypersensitive to the drug.

Nursing diagnosis. The client receiving niclosamide should be assessed for the following nursing diagnoses: altered comfort (headache, unpleasant taste, rash, and itching of the perianal area); fluid volume deficit related to nausea, vomiting, and diarrhea; altered bowel elimination (diarrhea); and risk for injury related to drowsiness, lightheadedness, and dizziness.

Implementation

Monitoring. Stress the importance of follow up studies; the client is considered cured only if stool examination results are negative for a minimum of 3 months. Stool examination is required 1 month and 3 months following drug regimen.

Intervention. Administer the drug after a light meal such as breakfast. No dietary restrictions are required before or after treatment. Instruct client to chew tablet thoroughly and swallow with a small amount of water. For children crush the tablet to a fine powder and mix with a small amount of water to form paste. If the client is constipated, a mild laxative should be prescribed to ensure a normal bowel movement. Treatment may be administered on an outpatient basis.

Education. Advise client to take the drug for the full course of therapy to prevent return of infection. Stress the importance of reporting progress to the prescriber. If there is no improvement, a second course of therapy may be required. Niclosamide destroys the tapeworm on contact while in the intestine. The killed worms (including the scolex) are passed in the stool and may not be seen.

In the treatment of *T. solium* (pork tapeworm), a saline purge such as magnesium sulfate should be given 1 or 2 hours after the administration of niclosamide to prevent the development of cysticercosis in the intestinal tract. Moreover, the procedure provides a good possibility of expulsion of an intact scolex. Note that niclosamide has no effect on cysticercosis.

Because the drug may cause dizziness, warn individual about driving a motor vehicle or operating dangerous machinery.

Instruct client to observe strict hygiene (both personal and environmental) to prevent reinfection. This observance applies particularly to *H. nana* (dwarf tapeworm).

Evaluation. The client will have three negative stool samples over a period of 3 months after the completion of the therapy.

oxamniquine [ox am' ni kwin] (Vansil)

Oxamniquine is schistosomicidal against both immature and mature worms and it produces its effect by causing worms to shift from the mesenteric veins to the liver, where they are then destroyed. Male schistosomes appear to be more susceptible to this drug than females, but after a successful treatment with this agent, the female schistosomes stop laying eggs. Oxamniquine is indicated for the treatment of schistosomiasis.

It is well absorbed orally with a time to peak serum level of 1 to 1.5 hours. It is metabolized in the liver and excreted by the kidneys. Oxamniquine is usually well tolerated with infrequent side effects including gastric distress, dizziness, sedation, and headaches.

The pediatric and adult oral dose is 15 mg/kg twice a day for 1 or 2 days, depending on the strain of organism.

■ Nursing Management

Oxamniquine Therapy

Assessment. Use oxamniquine with caution in individuals with a history of convulsive disorders because seizures are more apt to occur.

Nursing diagnosis. The client receiving oxamniquine should be assessed for the following nursing diagnoses: altered comfort (headache, rash); fluid volume deficit related to nausea, vomiting, and diarrhea; altered bowel elimination (diarrhea); hyperthermia (particularly in Egyptian clients); risk for injury related to drowsiness, dizziness, and seizures; altered thought processes related to auditory and visual hallucinations; and the collaborative problem of hypersensitivity.

Implementation

Monitoring. Monitor temperature and observe for signs and symptoms of side effects/adverse reactions.

Intervention. Administer after meals to minimize side effects such as dizziness, drowsiness, and gastrointestinal distress. Oxamniquine therapy does not require special preparation such as fasting, dietary restrictions, or enemas.

Caution the client to avoid hazardous tasks requiring mental alertness, such as driving, until the response to the drug has been ascertained.

Advise the client that oxamniquine causes a reddish orange discoloration of the urine that is harmless.

Encourage the client to complete the full course of therapy and to check with the prescriber if there is no improvement after completing a full course of therapy.

Evaluation. The client will be free of infection without any adverse effects of the oxamniquine and able to effectively manage the therapeutic regimen.

piperazine [pi' per a zeen] (Entacyl)

Piperazine is an antihelmintic that affects the worm muscle (paralysis), possibly by blocking the stimulating effects of acetylcholine at the myoneural junction. The muscle paralysis of roundworms makes them unable to maintain their position in the host; they are dislodged and expelled as a result of normal peristalsis.

Piperazine is indicated for treatment of enterobiasis (pinworms) and ascariasis (roundworm). It is absorbed orally, reaching a peak serum level in 2 to 4 hours. It is partially metabolized in the liver and primarily excreted by the kidneys. Side/adverse effects of piperazine include gastric distress and central nervous system side effect (headaches, dizziness, ataxia, trembling).

The adult dose is 3.5 g PO daily for 2 days for ascariasis. For children the dosage is 75 mg/kg (up to 3.5 g) daily for 2 days. For adults and children the dose for enterobiasis is a single daily dose of 65 mg/kg (maximum daily dose is 2.5 g) for 7 consecutive days.

■ Nursing Management

Piperazine Therapy

Assessment. Observe individuals with renal insufficiency for signs of neurologic symptoms. The drug is contraindicated for use in renal or hepatic impairment and in convulsive disorders.

Nursing diagnosis. The client receiving piperazine should be assessed for the following nursing diagnoses: altered comfort (headache); fluid volume deficit related to nausea, vomiting and diarrhea; altered bowel elimination (diarrhea); hyperthermia (hypersensitivity); risk for injury related to drowsiness, dizziness; altered thought processes (memory defect); and the collaborative problems of hypersensitivity and seizures.

Implementation

Monitoring. Continue to monitor progress with perianal or stool examinations.

Intervention. The drug may be taken with food. Some prescribers prefer single-dose therapy with mebendazole or pyrantel pamoate. No dietary restrictions, laxatives, or enemas are required with piperazine.

Education. Stress the importance of handwashing and of sanitary disposal of feces. Instruct the client to wash the perianal area daily to prevent reinfection. Underwear and bed linens should be changed daily to prevent reinfection. Wash (not shake) all bedding and night clothes after treatment to prevent reinfection. All family members should be treated at the same time.

Evaluation. The client will have three negative stool samples after the completion of the therapy. For pinworms, the client will have perianal swabs be negative for 7 days. The client will be able to effectively manage the therapeutic regimen.

praziquantel [pray zi kwon' tel] (Biltricide)

Praziquantel is an anthelmintic that penetrates cell membranes and increases cell permeability in susceptible worms. This results in an increased loss of intracellular calcium, contractions, and muscle paralysis of the worm. The drug also disintegrates the schistosome tegument (covering). Subsequently, phagocytes are attracted to the worm and ultimately, kill it.

Praziquantel is indicated for the treatment of schistosomiasis, opisthorchiasis (liver flukes), and clonorchiasis (Chinese or Oriental liver fluke) infestations. Praziquantel is absorbed orally and reaches peak serum level in 1 to 3 hours. Half-life is 0.8 to 1.5 hours for praziquantel, 4 to 6 hours for its metabolites. It is excreted by the kidneys and is generally well tolerated.

Side/adverse effects of praziquantel include headache, lightheadedness, gastric distress, sweating, and fever. For clonorchiasis, the adult or pediatric dosage for children 4 years and older is 25 mg/kg three times a day for 1 day.

■ Nursing Management

Praziquantel Therapy

Assessment. Praziquantel is contraindicated in clients with ocular cysticercosis because destruction of the parasites in the eye by the medication may cause severe ocular damage. Use with caution with clients with liver disease.

Nursing diagnosis. The client receiving praziquantel should be assessed for the following nursing diagnoses: altered comfort (headache); fluid volume deficit related to nausea, vomiting, and diarrhea; altered bowel elimination (diarrhea); hyperthermia; risk for injury related to lightheadedness, weakness, and dizziness; and the collaborative problem of hypersensitivity (rash).

Implementation

Monitoring. Urine exams for the eggs of *Schistosoma hematobium* are necessary at 1, 3, and 12 months after therapy to provide proof of a cure.

Intervention. No special preparations such as fasting, dietary restrictions, or laxatives are necessary for the administration of praziquantel. However, the tablets should be taken with meals and swallowed whole with a small amount of fluid to avoid the extremely bitter taste. Chewing the tablets may cause gagging and vomiting.

Education. The client should be encouraged to comply with the medication regimen and to visit the prescriber regularly to monitor progress. Because of praziquantel's side effects of dizziness and drowsiness, caution the client to avoid hazardous activities such as driving until the response to the medication has been ascertained.

Evaluation. To monitor the effectiveness of praziquantel, stool examinations are completed at specific intervals, depending on the parasite:

- Intestinal, liver, and blood flukes: 1 week and 1, 6, and 12 months after treatment
- Lung flukes: 1 month after treatment
- Tapeworms: 1 and 3 months after treatment
- For *Schistosoma haematobium* and *S. mekongi*, urine examinations are required at 1, 3, and 6 months to determine proof of cure. A client is not considered cured unless examination results have been negative for several months.

pyrantel [pi ran' tel] (Antiminth, Combantrin ♣)

Pyrantel is an antihelmintic that is a depolarizing neuromuscular blocking agent; it causes contraction and then paralysis of the helminth muscles. The helminths are dislodged and then expelled from the body by peristalsis. Pyrantel is indicated for the treatment of ascariasis, enterobiasis, and helminth infestations.

This product is poorly absorbed from the gastrointestinal tract. Pyrantel reaches peak serum level in 1 to 3 hours and is primarily excreted in the feces. Side/adverse effects include gastric distress and CNS side effects.

The adult and pediatric (2 years and over) dose of pyrantel for ascariasis and enterobiasis is 11 mg/kg PO as a single dose. If necessary, it may be repeated in 2 to 3 weeks.

■ Nursing Management

Pyrantel Therapy

Assessment. Use with caution with clients with a hypersensitivity to pyrantel. Perianal swabs and stool examinations confirm the presence of the helminth. Concurrent use of piperazine is not recommended as it antagonizes the antihelmintic effects of pyrantel.

Nursing diagnosis. The client receiving pyrantel should be assessed for the following nursing diagnoses: altered comfort (headache); fluid volume deficit related to anorexia, nausea, vomiting, and diarrhea; altered bowel elimination (diarrhea); risk for injury related to CNS effects (drowsiness, lightheadedness, and dizziness); and the collaborative problem of hypersensitivity.

Implementation

Monitoring. For pinworms, monitor with cellophane tape swabs of the perianal area, starting 1 week after treatment, every morning before bathing or defecation. For roundworms, stool examinations are checked 2 weeks after therapy.

Intervention. The administration of pyrantel does not require special preparation such as fasting, dietary restrictions, laxatives, or enemas. It may be taken with or without food or at any time of day. Shake well and use the calibrated measuring device provided to accurately measure the dosage.

Education. Encourage the client to take the full course of therapy and visit the prescriber on a regular basis to monitor progress. Alert the client to avoid hazardous tasks requiring mental alertness such as driving until the response has been determined.

For pinworm infestation, it is important to wash, without shaking, all the bed linens and nightclothes to prevent reinfestation. All household members should be treated simultaneously. Stress proper hygiene, both personal and environmental, with the client.

Evaluation. For pinworms, perianal examinations using cellophane tape swabs with negative results for 7 consecutive days indicate cure. For roundworms, stool examination results should be negative for ova, larvae, or worms 2 to 3 weeks after completion of therapy.

thiabendazole [thye a ben' da zole] (Mintezol)

Thiabendazole's mechanism of action is unknown but it has been reported to inhibit specific enzymes (fumarate reductase) in the helminth. It is vermicidal. Thiabendazole is indicated for the treatment of cutaneous and visceral larva migrans (creeping eruption) strongyloidiasis, and trichinosis.

Thiabendazole is rapidly absorbed orally reaching a peak serum level in 1 to 2 hours. Half-life ranges from 0.9 to 2 hours with metabolism in the liver and excretion via the kidneys. Side/adverse effects include gastric distress, neuropsychiatric and central nervous system adverse effects, and dry mouth and eyes.

The adult and pediatric (13.6 kg and over) dose of thiabendazole for cutaneous larva migrans is 25 mg/kg PO twice a day for 2 days. If lesions are still present, the dosage may be repeated 2 days after the completion of the initial treatment. For other dosing recommendations, see a current package insert or *USP DI*.

■ Nursing Management

Thiabendazole Therapy

Assessment. The drug should be used with caution in clients with hepatic or renal dysfunction. When given concurrently with theophylline, theophylline clearance is decreased, which may result in elevated serum levels and toxicity. Monitor theophylline levels.

Nursing diagnosis. The client receiving thiabendazole should be assessed for the following nursing diagnoses: fluid volume deficit related to anorexia, nausea, vomiting, and diarrhea; altered bowel elimination (diarrhea); sensory/perceptual disturbances (visual)—blurred vision, and (tactile)—numbness or tingling in the hands and feet; altered thought processes related to neuropsychiatric toxicity (irritability, disorientation, hallucinations); and the collaborative problems of Stevens-Johnson syndrome, crystalluria, and CNS toxicity (seizures).

Implementation

Monitoring. For strongyloidiasis, sputum examinations will monitor progress; for all other organisms, stool examinations approximately 2 to 3 weeks after therapy. Observe client for hypersensitivity reaction to detect severe erythema multiforme (Stevens-Johnson syndrome).

Intervention. Thiabendazole should be administered after meals to minimize anorexia, nausea and vomiting; no dietary restrictions, laxatives, or enemas are required with this drug. For the oral suspension form, shake well and use the calibrated measuring device provided to ensure accurate dosage. Chew or crush tablet form before swallowing.

Education. Encourage the client to comply with the full course of treatment and to visit the prescriber to monitor progress. Because of the side effects of dizziness and drowsiness, caution the client to avoid hazardous activities such as driving that require alertness. Teach proper hygiene, personal and environmental.

Evaluation. The client will be free of infection and able to effectively manage the therapeutic regimen.

LEPROSY

Leprosy, or **Hansen's disease,** is caused by *Mycobacterium leprae* in humans. Although estimates indicate that nearly 15 million people have leprosy worldwide, in the United States it is more frequently found in Hawaii and areas of Texas, Louisiana, and Florida. Leprosy has also been seen in foreign-born clients, especially those from the Philippines, Mexico, and Vietnam. It is more prevalent in males than females (3 to 1) in some areas.

Although the precise mode of transmission is unknown, the incubation period for leprosy is a few months to decades. Large numbers of leprosy bacilli are generally shed from skin ulcers, nasal secretions, the gastrointestinal tract and, perhaps, biting insects.

M. leprae is a bacillus that in humans first presents as a skin lesion—a large plaque or macule that is erythematous or hypopigmented in the center. More numerous lesions, peripheral nerve trunk involvement, and the common complications of plantar ulceration of the feet, footdrop, loss of hand function, and corneal abrasions may follow.

Most cases can be arrested, if not cured, by appropriate therapy and management. The drugs of choice are dapsone and clofazimine.

dapsone [dap' sone] (DDS, Avlosulfon♣)

Dapsone is an antibacterial (antileprosy) agent that is bacteriostatic with an action similar to that of the sulfonamides. It may also be a dihydrofolate reductase inhibitor. Dapsone is effective against *M. leprae,* the cause of leprosy, therefore it is indicated for the treatment of all types of leprosy and for dermatitis herpetiformis.

Dapsone is absorbed orally, distributed throughout the body, and found in fluids and in all body tissues. Time to peak serum level is 2 to 6 hours; half-life is approximately 30 hours. It is acetylated by N-acetyltransferase in the liver; thus slow acetylators are more apt to develop higher serum levels and adverse reactions than fast acetylators. Excretion is via the kidneys.

Side/adverse effects of dapsone include hypersensitivity, hemolytic anemia, and methemoglobinemia. The adult dapsone antileprosy dose (given in combination with other antileprosy drugs) is 50 to 100 mg orally daily. As a suppressant for dermatitis herpetiformis, the adult dose is 50 mg PO daily initially, increased as necessary until symptoms are controlled. The dosage for children as an antileprosy agent is 1.4 mg/kg PO daily.

■ Nursing Management

Dapsone Therapy

Assessment. Administer dapsone cautiously in clients with anemia, deficiencies of G6PD and methemoglobin reductase because hemolytic anemia may occur. Use caution also with clients with hepatic or renal function impairment. The drug is also contraindicated with clients who are hypersensitive to dapsone and sulfonamides. A CBC and platelet count should be completed before dapsone therapy for a baseline assessment, as well as ALT (SGPT) and AST (SGOT) levels.

Review the client's current medications for significant drug interactions that may occur when dapsone is given with the following drugs:

Drug	Possible effect and management
dideoxyinosine (ddI)	Concurrent drug administration may reduce absorption of dapsone. Dapsone requires an acid media for absorption while dideoxyinosine is given with a buffer to neutralize stomach acid to increase absorption. Administer dapsone a minimum of 2 hours before ddI.
hemolytic agents	**Increase the potential for serious adverse effects. Avoid or a potentially serious drug interaction may occur.**

Nursing diagnosis. The client receiving dapsone should be assessed for the following nursing diagnoses: altered comfort (headache); fluid volume deficit related to anorexia, nausea, and vomiting; altered thought processes (mood and mental changes); altered protection related to leukopenia, thrombocytopenia, and anemia; and the collaborative problems of methemoglobinemia (bluish discoloration of the skin and lips), exfoliative dermatitis, peripheral neuritis (numbness and tingling of the hands and feet), hypersensitivity (rash), and a "sulfone syndrome"—a hypersensitivity reaction that occurs after 6 to 8 weeks of therapy with fever, malaise, lymphadenopathy, exfoliative dermatitis, and anemia.

Implementation

Monitoring. Once therapy has started, a complete blood count should be determined monthly for 3 months, and then semiannually for the remainder of dapsone therapy. The dosage may be reduced or suspended if CBC values are diminished: RBCs, below 2.5 million/mm^3; hemoglobin, below 9 g/dl; WBCs, below 5000/mm^3. In addition, the client should be observed for the development of hemolytic anemia; symptoms are pale skin, fever, and unusual tiredness and weakness.

Hepatic function studies should be done if the client develops anorexia, nausea, vomiting, or jaundice. Peripheral neuritis (numbness and tingling of the hands and feet) and exfoliative dermatitis (itching and scaling of the skin and loss of hair) are also indications for dosage interruption.

Intervention. Because of bacterial resistance, this drug is usually given with other antimycobacterial agents.

Education. Encourage the client to comply with the dapsone regimen and stress that use of the drug is long-term or indefinite. Taking the medication at the same time each day will assist compliance. Stress the importance of regular visits to the prescriber to monitor progress.

Caution the client that dapsone may cause dizziness and drowsiness; hazardous activities requiring mental alertness such as driving should be avoided until the response to the drug has been determined.

Evaluation. The client's infection will be arrested without any adverse effects of dapsone and able to effectively manage the therapeutic regimen.

clofazimine [kloe fa' zi meen] (Lamprene)

Clofazimine's antileprosy mechanism of action is unknown; it has a slow bactericidal effect on *M. leprae*, inhibits mycobacterial growth and tends to bind preferentially to mycobacterial DNA. It is indicated as a secondary drug for the treatment of leprosy, especially in the dapsone-resistant type of leprosy.

Clofazimine has a variable oral absorption and is distributed primarily in fatty tissues and cells. Macrophages take up this drug and further distribute it throughout the body. Half-life is about 2 to 3 months with chronic therapy with time to peak serum level between 1 and 6 hours. It is excreted primarily in feces.

Side/adverse effects of clofazimine include gastric distress, ichthyosis and discoloration of skin, feces, sweat, tears and urine.

The adult dose in dapsone-resistant leprosy, in combination with one or more other agents, is 50 to 100 mg PO daily.

■ Nursing Management

Clofazimine Therapy

Assessment. Clients with gastrointestinal problems are at risk for GI bleeding, bowel obstruction, splenic infarction and enteritis. There are no significant drug interactions with this drug.

Nursing diagnosis. The client receiving clofazimine should be assessed for the following nursing diagnoses: altered comfort (photosensitivity, rash and itching, and change in taste; fluid volume deficit related to anorexia, nausea, and vomiting; altered thought processes (mood and mental changes, especially depression and suicidal thoughts related to skin discoloration); self-concept disturbance related to pink, red, or brownish-black discoloration of the skin and lips; risk for injury related to dizziness and drowsiness, and the potential complications of gastrointestinal bleeding and toxicity, hepatitis.

For further discussion of the nursing management of clofazimine, see the discussion of nursing management for dapsone.

SUMMARY

Malaria is still a prevalent disease despite the World Health Organization's attempts to eradicate it by controlling the insect vector and the causative parasite. Although it is essentially considered a tropical disease, nurses in the United States and Canada may come into contact with imported cases because both countries have populations that travel extensively and provide havens for refugees and immigrants from areas in which the disease is endemic. Chloroquine, hydroxychloroquine, mefloquine, primaquine, quinine, and other drugs are commonly used agents for the prevention and treatment of malaria.

The incidence of tuberculosis is increasing because of the increasing numbers of persons with AIDS, persons living in the street or homeless, drug abusers, malnourished individuals, and those taking immunosuppressant drugs. Generally three or more antituberculous agents are administered concurrently for their additive effect and to minimize the risk of the organism becoming drug resistant. Aminosalicylates, capreomycin, cycloserine, ethambutol, ethionamide, isoniazid, pyrazinamide, rifampin, and streptomycin are commonly used antituberculous agents.

Amebiasis, an infection of the large intestine by *Entamoeba histolytica*, is prevalent in tropical areas, again imported by travel, but it is also found in poorly sanitized areas of Canada and the United States. Transmission is fecal to oral, through the ingestion of cysts from contaminated food and water. Antiamebiasis agents in current use are iodoquinol and paromomycin. Other protozoan diseases of concern are toxoplasmosis and trichomoniasis.

Helminths, worms parasitic to man, may be flatworms (platyhelminths), of which there are two types, tapeworms (cestodes) and flukes (trematodes), or roundworms (nematodes). They cause injury to the host in a variety of ways: by causing damage to and loss of blood from the intestinal wall, producing toxic substances absorbed by the host, traumatizing the host's tissues and making the host more susceptible to infection, and competing with the host for sustenance within the bowel. Anthelmintic agents most commonly used are diethylcarbamazine, mebendazole, niclosamide, oxamniquine, piperazine, praziquantel, pyrantel, and thiabendazole.

Leprosy, or Hansen's disease, caused by *Mycobacterium leprae*, is treated with dapsone and clofazimine.

All of these diseases and the therapeutic agents used in their prevention and treatment are not commonly dealt with by most nurses; however, familiarity with them is necessary to appropriately manage them when they do occur.

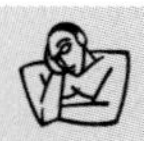

Critical Thinking

1. Why is it necessary to determine whether an antimalarial is being used prophylactically, to suppress symptoms, or for the acute phase of malaria?
2. Why are three or more antituberculous drugs administered concurrently?
3. What advice would you provide for someone who was traveling to a place where malaria was endemic? amebiasis? leprosy?

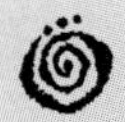

Collaborative Learning Activities

1. Preassigned student teams will draw up nursing care plans for clients receiving antimicrobial and antiparasitic therapy as follows: (1) a returned serviceman who shows signs of malaria; (2) a young female drug addict who has contracted tuberculosis; (3) a 45-year old anthropologist returning from overseas with amebiasis; (4) a child who was found to have a tapeworm; (5) an elderly immigrant from the Philippines who has recently been diagnosed with leprosy.

BIBLIOGRAPHY

American Hospital Formulary Service (1996). *AHFS: drug information '96.* Bethesda, MD: American Society of Hospital Pharmacists.

Anandan JV (1995). Parasitic infections. In Young LY & Koda-Kimble MA (Eds.). *Applied therapeutics: The clinical use of drugs* (6th ed.). Vancouver, WA: Applied Therapeutics.

Anderson KN, et al. (Eds.) (1994). *Mosby's medical, nursing, & allied health dictionary* (4th ed.). St Louis: Mosby.

Boutotte J (1993). TB: The second time around, *Nursing* 23(5):42-9.

Cali TJ (1995). Tuberculosis: Implications for the 1990s and beyond, *Clin Consult* 14(12):1-12.

Centers for Disease Control and Prevention (1996). *Prescription drugs for malaria.* Document No. 221010, Centers for Disease Control and Prevention, pages 1-3.

Centers for Disease Control and Prevention (1993). Initial therapy for tuberculosis of the era of multidrug resistance: Recommendations of the Advisory Council for the Elimination of Tuberculosis, *Mort Morb Wkly Rep* 42(RR-7):1-8.

Centers for Disease Control and Prevention (1994). Guidelines for preventing the transmission of *Mycobacterium tuberculosis* in health-care facilities, *MMWR* 43(RR-13):1-132.

Ebert SC (1993). Tuberculosis. In DiPiro et al. *Pharmacology: A pathophysiological approach* (2nd ed.). Norwalk, CT: Appleton & Lange.

Elpern EH & Girzadas AM (1993). Tuberculosis update: New challenges of an old disease, *MEDSURG Nurs* 2(3):176-83.

Grimes D (1991). *Infectious diseases.* St Louis: Mosby.

Kuzma EC (1992). Drug response: All bodies are not created equal, *Amer J Nurs* 92(12):48.

Levy RA (1993). *Ethnic and racial differences in response to medicines: Preserving individualized therapy in managed pharmaceutical programs.* Reston, VA: National Pharmaceutical Council.

Lordi GM & Reichman LB (1993). Drug-resistant tuberculosis: The new face of an old enemy, *Drug Therapy* (March):17-28.

Malseed RT & Wilson BA (1993). Isoniazid and rifampin therapy for tuberculosis: What patients need to know, *MEDSURG Nursing* 2(3):236-8.

Mandell GL & Petri Jr AW (1996). Drugs used in the chemotherapy of tuberculosis, Mycobacterium avium complex disease, and leprosy. In Hardman JG & Limbird LE (Eds.). *Goodman & Gilman's the pharmacological basis of therapeutics* (9th ed.). New York: McGraw-Hill.

Meyer UA (1992). Drugs in special patient groups: Clinical importance of genetics in drug effects. In Melmon KL, et al. (Eds.). *Clinical pharmacology: Basic principles in therapeutics* (3rd ed.). New York: McGraw-Hill.

Olin BR (Ed.) (1996). *Facts and comparisons.* St Louis: Facts and Comparisons.

United States Department of Health and Human Services (1988). *Health information for international travelers.* Washington, DC: US Dept. HHS.

United States Pharmacopeial Convention (1996). *Drug information for the health care professional* (16th ed.). Rockville, MD: The Convention.

U.S. Public Health Service Task Force on Prophylaxis and Therapy for *Mycobacterium avium* complex (1993). Recommendations on prophylaxis and therapy for disseminated *Mycobacterium avium* complex for adults and adolescents infected with human immunodeficiency virus, *MMWR* 42(42):14-20.

Ward Jr ES (1995). Tuberculosis. In Young LY & Koda-Kimble MA. *Applied therapeutics: The clinical use of drugs* (6th ed.). Vancouver: Applied Therapeutics.

Yoshikawa TT (1995). Tuberculosis in the nursing home, *Nurs Home Med* 3(9):207-213.

Chapter 62

Overview of the Immunologic System

Key Terms

acquired immunity (p. 980)
antibodies (p. 981)
B lymphocytes (B cells) p. 980)
complement system (p. 981)
immunity (p. 981)
passive immunity (p. 982)
T lymphocytes (T cells) (p. 979)

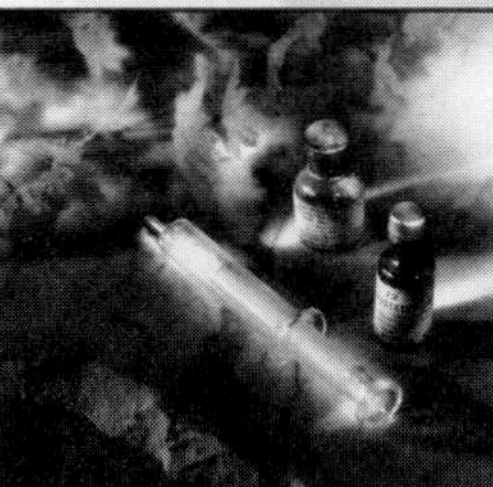

Objectives

1. Identify the lymphoid organs of the immune system.
2. Describe the role of each of the lymphoid organs in the defense of the body against foreign biologic and/or chemical substances.
3. Identify the immunocompetent cells involved in the immune response.
4. Compare and contrast the functions of the three major groups of T cells.
5. Describe the action of B cells in response to foreign antigens.
6. Identify the five classes of antibodies and their functions.
7. Compare and contrast humoral and cell-mediated immunity.
8. Describe the various types of immunity.

The immunologic system is composed of cells and organs that defend the body against invasion by foreign biologic and/or chemical substances. The immunocompetent cells in the body have an inherent ability to distinguish foreign protein substances from the body's own cells. This chapter reviews the organs and tissues of the immune system, the immunocompetent cells, and the types of immunity.

THE IMMUNE SYSTEM

The spleen, tonsils, lymph nodes, and thymus are the lymphoid organs located in the body. The lymphoid tissues are mainly lymphocytes and plasma cells, which travel freely throughout the human system. The two major classes of lymphocytes are T-cell and B-cell lymphocytes, which are discussed in the section Immunocompetent Cells. Figure 62-1 identifies the organs and tissues of the immune system.

Spleen

The spleen, the largest lymphatic organ in the body, is located on the left side in the extreme superior, posterior corner of the abdominal cavity, and performs two main functions. It is: (1) a storage site or reservoir for blood and (2) a processing station for red blood cells (i.e., the RBCs near the end of their life cycle will break down in the spleen). Macrophages lining the pulp and sinuses of the spleen remove cellular debris and process hemoglobin in the red pulp area of the spleen. The white pulp area of the spleen contains lymphocytes and plasma cells that are involved in the immune process. The spleen intercepts foreign matter or antigens that have reached the bloodstream.

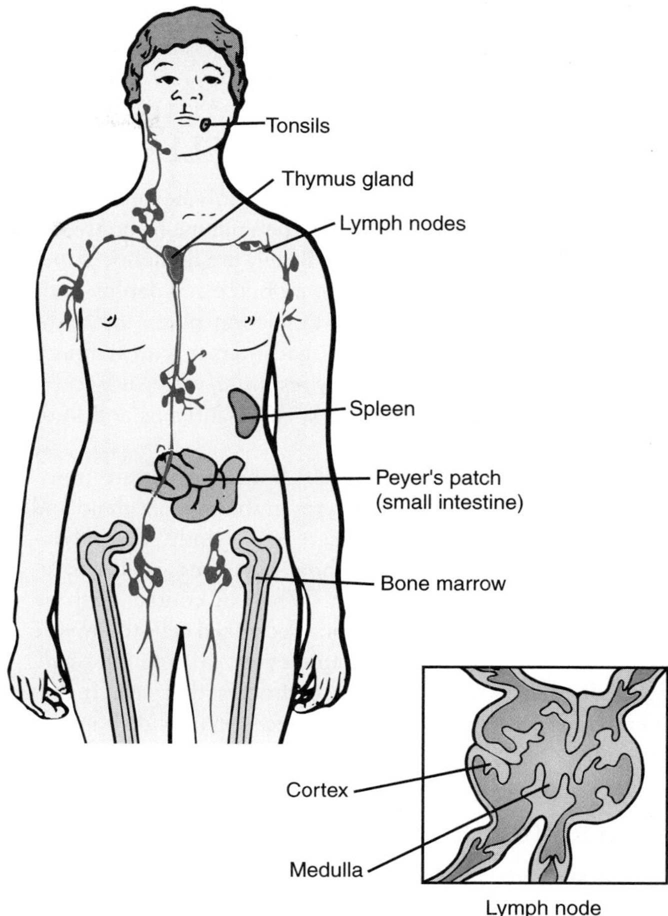

Figure 62-1 Location of organs and tissues of the immune system; insert shows cross-section of lymph node.

Tonsils

The tonsils are an accumulation of lymphoid tissue, named according to their location: lingual, palatine, and pharyngeal tonsils. They intercept foreign bodies or antigens that enter the body by way of the respiratory tract. Similar lymphoid tissue is located in the submucosal areas of the gastrointestinal tract (Peyer's patches) to intercept antigens (bacteria and viruses) entering from the gut. Other lymphoid tissues are located in the bone marrow and help to intercept antigens in the blood and in the lymph nodes.

Lymph Nodes

The lymph nodes are capsulated organs located throughout the body that are involved with lymph circulation. The outer portion of the lymph node is the cortex, and the inner portion is the medulla. The thymus-dependent zone exists in the deep area or middle cortex. This area contains mainly **T lymphocytes,** lymphocytes formed or seeded from the thymus gland, which when exposed to an antigen divide rapidly and produce large numbers of new T cells sensitized to that antigen.

Lymph nodes are essentially a row of in-line filters that screen the lymph flowing through it. Many lymphocytes and macrophages are located throughout the lymph nodes, especially in the cortical, paracortical, and medullary areas. T lymphocytes are located mainly in the paracortical region, whereas plasma cells are found in the medullary sinuses.

Thymus Gland

The thymus gland is located in the mediastinal area. It processes lymphocytes, and in the early years up to puberty, it rapidly produces lymphocytes. The immune system is developed when immature lymphocytes from the bone marrow are processed in the thymus gland and then sent to the spleen, the lymphatic system, and other tissues and organs in the body to mature. The lymphocytes are active against some bacteria and viruses, allergens, fungus infections, and foreign tissue.

At birth, the thymus gland is larger than it is in an adult. By the time a person reaches puberty, the thymus has grown to nearly six times its original size. After puberty this gland undergoes involution, and in the elderly, it is usually a small mass of reticular fibers with some lymphocytes and connective tissue. Although its importance was largely discounted over the years, today it is one of the most important areas for medical research.

Scientists are searching for answers to the many questions about the thymus gland and its relationship to the other tissues and organs in the immune system.

IMMUNOCOMPETENT CELLS

Mononuclear T and B cells and the polymorphonuclear leukocytes (PMLs) are involved in the immune response, although only mononuclear T and B cells are immunocompetent cells, cells with the ability to mobilize and deploy antibodies and other responses to stimulation by an antibody. The PMLs are nonspecific cells that interact with lymphocytes to produce an inflammatory response, whereas B and T cells are capable of recognizing specific antigens and initiating the immune response.

In humans, stem cells from the bone marrow are transformed to T cells or T lymphocytes in the thymus gland and B cells or B lymphocytes elsewhere in the body. The T lymphocytes then migrate to lymphoid tissue and organs as reviewed in the previous section. When in contact with an antigen, T lymphocytes will form specialized cells to provide cellular immunity. The **B lymphocytes,** a type of small, agranulocytic leukocyte, form antibodies that search out, identify, and bind with specific antigens to provide humoral immunity.

T Lymphocytes (T Cells)

T cells are generally long-lived. When they are not in their special areas, they circulate continuously through the body by way of the bloodstream and lymphatic system. They are involved with the B lymphocytes (B cells) in that they can cooperate with them (helper T cells) or inhibit them (suppressor T cells). The B cells do not interact with the thymus. Clones are groups of lymphocytes capable of forming one specific antibody (B cell or T cell) to respond to a specific type of antigen; only the specific antigen can activate the specialized clones.

When the T cells first contact an antigen, the lymphocytes that recognize the foreign substance will proliferate, thus giving rise to larger numbers of cells that have the capacity to recognize and respond to this antigen. Some of the cells will go on to produce antibody or cell-mediated immune-type responses, whereas others will increase the population of antigen-sensitive memory cells. This is called **acquired immunity,** an immunity that is not innate but obtained during life. The second exposure to this antigen will provoke a more powerful response by the specific T cells.

Three major groups of T cells identified in the past few years include: (1) cytotoxic T cells, (2) helper T cells, and (3) suppressor T cells.

Cytotoxic T cells. This type of cell can bind tightly to organisms or cells that contain their binding-specific antigen. Then the T cells release cytotoxic (probably lysosomal) enzymes directly into the cell. Cytotoxic T cells are capable of killing microorganisms, cancer cells, viruses, heart transplant cells, and other cells that are foreign to the person's body. Body tissue that contains viruses or foreign cells may also be attacked by the killer cells.

Helper T cells. These compose the majority of the T cells and help the immune system in many ways. They increase the activation of B cells, cytotoxic T cells, and suppressor T cells by antigens. Helper T cells clones are activated by very small amounts of antigens, quantities that may not activate the previously mentioned B cells, cytotoxic T cells, or suppressor T cells. Once the helper T cells are activated, they secrete lymphokines, which are chemical factors that attract macrophages to the site of infection or inflammation and increase the response of these three lymphoid cells to the antigen.

Helper T cells may also secrete interleukin-2, a lymphokine that is capable of stimulating the action of other T cells, such as cytotoxic T cells and some suppressor T cells.

Helper T cells also secrete macrophage migration inhibition factor, another lymphokine. This substance slows or stops the migration of macrophages into the affected area and will also activate the macrophages present to be more effective phagocytotic agents. The activated macrophages can attack and destroy a vastly increased number of the invading organisms.

Acquired immunodeficiency syndrome (AIDS) is the final outcome of an infection with the human immunodeficiency virus (HIV). This virus binds to protein on the cell membranes of the helper T lymphocytes (T4 cells), monocytes, macrophages, and colorectal cells. The helper T cells are destroyed by the virus, which leads to the immunodeficiency known as AIDS. See additional information on this disease and treatment in Chapter 64.

Suppressor T cells. Less is known about these cells than the others, but it is known that they can suppress the function of both cytotoxic and helper T cells. This suppression may be useful in preventing excessive immune reactions that can cause severe body damage. These cells are often called *regulatory T cells.*

B Lymphocytes (B Cells)

B-lymphocyte clones are dormant in lymphoid tissue until a foreign antigen appears. The macrophages in the lymphoid tissue phagocytize the foreign substance, and the adjacent B lymphocytes and perhaps the T cells are activated. B cells specific for the antigen will enlarge, and some will differentiate to form plasmablasts, a plasma cell precursor, and memory cells. The plasmablasts proliferate and divide, so that in 4 days, approximately 500 plasma cells will be present for each original plasmablast. The plasma cells rapidly produce gamma globulin antibodies that are secreted into the lymph and transported by the blood.

Cells similar to those in the original clone are called memory cells. A second exposure to the same antigen will cause a more rapid and potent antibody response. The first response to an antigen may be slow, weak, and of short duration. The second response will be much more rapid, far more potent and prolonged, and antibodies will be formed for months rather than only for a few weeks. This is the reason why vaccination using several doses given at periods of weeks or months apart is so effective (see Figure 62-2).

ANTIBODIES

Antibodies are gamma globulins (a type of protein), called immunoglobulins, that are specific for particular antigens. They are produced by lymphoid tissue in response to antigens. At the present time, five classes of antibodies have been identified: IgG, IgM, IgA, IgD, and IgE. (The "Ig" stands for immunoglobulin, and the other letters designate the classes.)

IgG is the major immunoglobulin in the blood (about 75% to 80% of the total antibodies in the normal person) and is capable of entering tissue spaces, coating microorganisms, and activating the complement system, thus accelerating phagocytosis. It is the only immunoglobulin capable of crossing the placenta to provide the fetus with passive immunity until the infant can produce its own immune defense system.

IgM is the first immunoglobulin produced during an immune response. It is located primarily in the bloodstream and develops in response to an invasion of bacteria or viruses. IgM activates complement and can destroy foreign invaders during the initial antigen exposure. Its level decreases in approximately 1 week, while IgG levels are progressively increasing.

IgA is located primarily in external body secretions—saliva, sweat, tears, mucus, bile, and colostrum—and it is found in respiratory tract mucosa and in plasma. It helps to provide a defense against antigens on exposed surfaces and antigens that enter the respiratory and gastrointestinal tracts. The plasma cells in the intestinal area secrete IgA and secretory component to defend the body against bacteria and viruses.

The function of IgD is unknown. It is in the plasma and has been located on lymphocyte surfaces together with IgM, so it may be associated with binding antigens to the cell surface. Although levels of IgD are increased in chronic infections, IgD does not appear to have a particular affinity for specialized antigens.

IgE binds to histamine-containing mast cells and basophils. It can mediate the release of histamine in immune response to parasites (helminths) and in some allergic conditions. It is often called the *reaginic antibody* because of its involvement in immediate hypersensitivity reactions. Concentrations of it are low in the serum because the antibody is firmly fixed on tissue surfaces. Once activated by an antigen, it will trigger the release of the mast cell granules, resulting in the signs and symptoms of allergy and anaphylaxis.

IMMUNITY

Links in the chain of the infectious disease may be broken at many points. One link can be broken by attacking the pathogen (human disease-causing organism) with antimicrobial or antiinfective therapy. Another can be broken by augmenting human resistance by using biologic agents such as vaccines and serums, which artificially supply antibodies or catalyze the ability of the immune system to produce its own. An immunologic reaction that destroys or resists foreign cells or their products (antigens) is termed **immunity.** The most successful antigens, or immunogens, are protein or polysaccharide macromolecules that are usually bacterial, viral, fungal, or rickettsial in origin.

The primary types of immunity are humoral immunity and cell-mediated immunity.

Humoral Immunity

Antigens may be recognized by T-helper cells that activate specific B cells, by a strong B-cell response to the invasion of certain antigens (such as large polymers, *E. coli*, dextrans), or by a macrophage intermediary. Macrophage interactions often enhance the antigen recognition by both T and B cells in the body. Humoral response is described as primary or secondary immune response.

Primary response. The foreign antigen in the body will bind to specific B cells to produce specialized antibody-producing plasma cells. Usually within 6 days, antibodies that are specific to the antigen can be found in the blood. Initially the immunoglobulin is IgM, which increases in quantity for up to 2 weeks; then production declines so that very little IgM is present in a few weeks. After the initial IgM evaluation, IgG antibodies start to appear at approximately day 10, peak in several weeks, and maintain high levels for a much longer time period (Figure 62-2).

Secondary response. This response is often called the *memory response,* because the immune system responds so much faster to the second exposure to the same antigen. Both T and B memory cells are involved in beginning immediate production of antibodies in large amounts.

The second part of humoral immunity is activation of the **complement system,** a series of approximately 20 proteins that circulate in the blood in an inactive form. When an antigen-antibody complex triggers complement, each

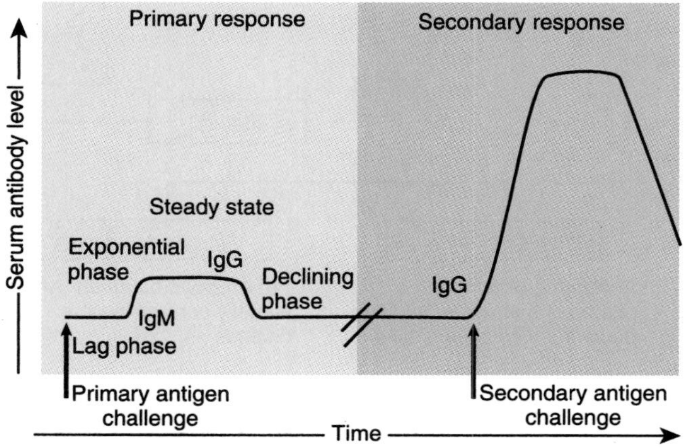

Figure 62-2 Primary and secondary immune responses. (From Mudge-Grout CL [1992]. *Immunologic Disorders.* St. Louis: Mosby.)

component in the cascade is activated in precise order. This reaction causes the mast cell release of substances that produce redness, increased heat, and edema of inflammation. It may also cause bacterial cell death and damage to normal tissue that surrounds the affected area.

Cell-Mediated Immunity

Cell-mediated immunity is the result of contact between T cells and antigens. Receptors on the T-cell surface are capable of recognizing foreign antigens, and antigen destruction may occur through one of two processes: (1) directly, by injecting chemical compounds into the target cell membrane (killer activity by cytotoxic T cells) or (2) by secreting lymphokines. The lymphokines can enhance or suppress the action of other lymphocytes, or they can create a chemotactic gradient in the area that will attract macrophages (and eosinophils, basophils, neutrophils) to the site. Cell-mediated immunity (delayed hypersensitivity) involves only the direct action of T cells without humoral assistance.

Natural and Acquired Immunity

The body has certain inherited and innate abilities to resist encounters with antigens. This ability is known as *natural resistance* or *natural immunity,* which is not to be confused with naturally acquired immunity. Some general defenses inherent to natural resistance come from factors familiar to the focus of nursing; for example, adequate rest, nutrition, exercise, and freedom from undue stress. Physiologic factors, which discourage proliferation of microbes, including the acidity of gastric secretions, respiratory tract cilia, and bactericidal lysozymes in tears. During a lifetime an individual may also acquire further immune capabilities through both natural and artificial means. This type of acquired immunity is conferred by either active or passive action (Figure 62-3).

Unbroken skin is extremely effective in barring entry to microorganisms, but a barrage of defenses is mounted by the inflammatory response if invasion does succeed. The immune system identifies the threatening antigens or allergens and creates specific gamma globulins destructive to the particular species of antigen. These gamma globulins, or antibodies or immunoglobulins (Ig), are proteins that are chemically complementary and specifically configured to lock into the foreign antigen, inactivating it.

Antibodies also activate cellular defenses to phagocytize the invading microorganisms. Custom-made gamma globulins, or antibodies, provide acquired immunity to the specific type of antigen for varying lengths of time. Those antibodies will then gradually disappear from the serum, but the potential for their rapid replication in response to a repeat challenge by that specific antigen continues to exist after the initial exposure. Consequently, the result is known as *naturally acquired immunity,* which is a process of *naturally acquired active immunity* because of the body's active involvement in creating the antibodies. Naturally acquired immunity can also result from a process of **passive immunity** when antibodies made by the mother's body are passively transferred by means of the placenta or by breast milk (especially colostrum, the breast milk produced shortly after delivery) to the fetus or infant.

On the other hand, artificial induction of the immune state, *artificially acquired immunity,* is initiated purposefully for protection of the susceptible individual. It may also be induced either actively or passively. Artificially acquired *active* immunity is evoked by the deliberate administration of antigens, either live partially modified organisms, killed organisms, or their toxins. The parenteral route is the predominant mode of administration. Periodic reactivation of actively acquired artificial immunity against certain organisms by booster doses (e.g., tetanus) is sometimes necessary. Artificially acquired *passive* immunity is conferred by the parenteral administration of antibody-containing immune serum from immune humans or animals (see Figure 62-3).

Artificially acquired active immunity generally secures protection for a longer duration than any kind of passive

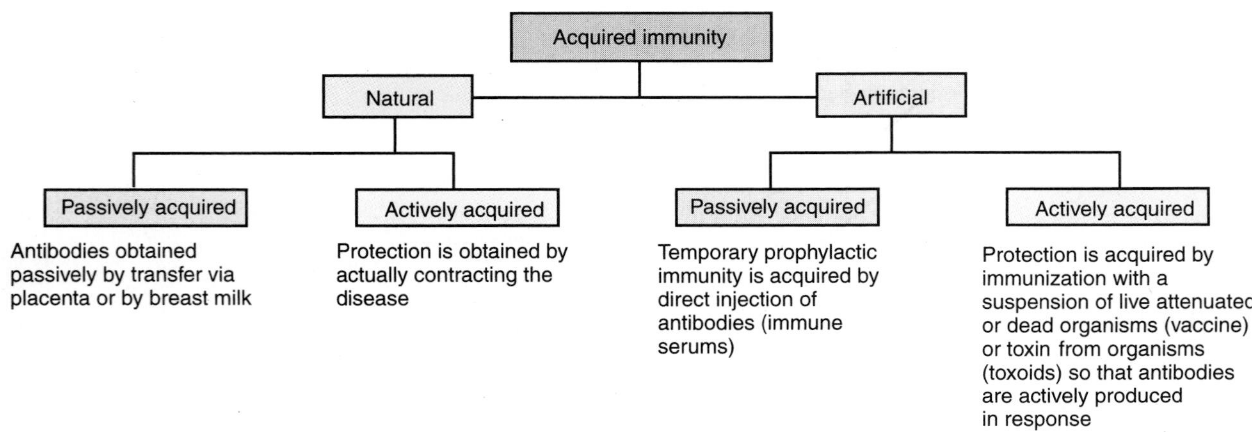

Figure 62-3 The process of acquired immunity.

TABLE 62-1 Comparison of active and passive immunity

	Active immunity	Passive immunity
Source	Individual	Other human or animal
Efficacy	High	Low to moderate
Method	Contracting disease Immunization with vaccines or toxoids	Administer preformed antibody by injection, maternal transplacental transfer or in breast milk
Time to develop	5-21 days	Immediate effect
Duration	Long, up to years	Usually shorter in time
Ease of reactivation	Easy with booster dose	Can be dangerous; anaphylaxis may occur, especially if animal sources are used
Purpose	Prophylaxis	Prophylaxis and therapeutic

immunity and is usually the prophylactic treatment of choice for populations at potential risk. Side effects may include local pain at the injection site and headache with mild to moderate fever. Because of the agents used, *active* immunity results in fewer adverse effects than passive immunity. Artificially acquired *passive* immunity is often chosen for susceptible individuals following a known exposure. A combination of active and passive approaches is also occasionally used. A number of products used in artificial passive immunization have caused adverse reactions because of individual hypersensitivities to animal products, especially horse serum or eggs, to the preservative used in a medication, or to an antibiotic. The products of bacterial metabolism are the agents responsible for other adverse reactions.

Presence of a mild to moderate upper respiratory tract infection or pregnancy does not always prohibit immunization; however, an immunosuppressed state (as a result of cancer chemotherapy or disease) may. Current manufacturers' instructions should always be consulted. Table 62-1 makes a direct comparison of the capabilities and effects of active and passive immunities.

SUMMARY

The immunologic system consists of lymphoid organs, the spleen, tonsils, lymph nodes, and thymus, and immunocompetent cells, known as T lymphocytes (T cells) and B lymphocytes (B cells), all of which defend the body against invasion of foreign biologic and chemical substances. Antibodies are immunoglobulins that are specific for particular antigens. Immunity is the immunologic reaction that destroys or resists foreign cells or their products. It may be natural or artificial and actively or passively acquired. Pharmacologic therapy is usually aimed at strengthening the body's immunologic status for the prevention of disease.

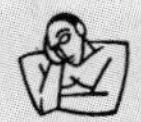

Critical Thinking

1. As a bacterium, entering a human body, what do you anticipate will be your experience encountering T cells? You have invited a friend, a virus, to meet you by entering via the respiratory system. What will be her experience with the various antibodies?
2. What type of immunity do the following have:
   a. A. child recovering from the measles?
   b. A 6-week-old nursing infant?
   c. A first-grader with a DPT and polio vaccine booster?
   d. A nurse who receives hepatitis B immune globulin after exposure to hepatitis B?
3. Suppose you had an additive that could be used with injectable solutions that would delay but not stop the release of the drug from an injection site into the blood. If you injected an antigen in one injection site, and into another an antigen mixed with the additive that would cause delay of absorption for 2 to 3 weeks, which injection would result in the greater response of antibody production? Why? (Seeley and Tate, 1992).

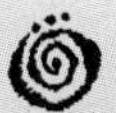

Collaborative Learning Activities

1. Three teams will describe the function of the three major groups of T cells. A fourth team will do the same for B cells. Create a chart on the board so that the action of these cells can be described succinctly.
2. Five more teams will perform the same type of activity with the five specific antibodies.

BIBLIOGRAPHY

Anderson KN, et al. (Eds.) (1994). *Mosby's medical, nursing, & allied health dictionary* (4th ed.). St Louis: Mosby.

Guyton AC (1990). *Textbook of medical physiology* (8th ed.) Philadelphia: WB Saunders.

Klein DM & Witek-Janusek L (1992). Advances in immunotherapy of sepsis, *DCCN 11*(2):75.

McCance KL & Huether SE (1994). *Pathophysiology: The biological basis for disease in adults and children* (2nd ed.). St Louis: Mosby.

McIntyre WJ & Tami JA (1993). Immunology for the consultant pharmacist, *Consult Pharm 8*(4):376.

Mudge-Grout CL (1992). *Immunologic disorders.* St Louis: Mosby.

Seeley RS & Tate P (1995). *Anatomy and physiology* (3rd ed.). St Louis: Mosby.

Thibodeau GA & Patton KT (1996). *Anatomy and physiology* (3rd ed.). St Louis: Mosby.

Van Wynsberghe D, Noback CR, & Carola R (1995). *Human anatomy and physiology* (3rd ed.). New York: McGraw-Hill.

Chapter 63

Serums, Vaccines, and Other Immunizing Agents

Chapter Focus

Edward Jenner's observation, over 200 years ago, that milkmaids who developed cowpox were rarely victims of smallpox prompted him to develop the first vaccine. A modern version of this vaccine led to the eradication of smallpox in 1980, a health success for the world. The development of vaccines against more than 20 infectious diseases has revolutionized the approach to public health. In the last two decades alone, nine new or improved vaccines have become available. Today advances in molecular biology are enabling scientists to develop new vaccines against diseases that continue to plague the world (NIAID, 1992). The following objectives and key terms are important for a good understanding of this chapter.

Key Terms

active immunity (p. 985)

antibody titer (p. 985)

immunoprophylaxis or passive immunization (p. 995)

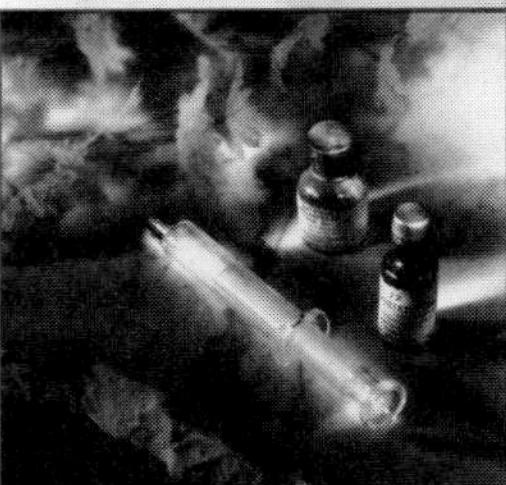

Objectives

1. Discuss the present status of immunization and anticipated future developments.
2. State the appropriate immunization schedule for children until the age of 2 years.
3. Identify immunizations recommended for adults.
4. Describe the recommended use of tetanus toxoid and tetanus immune globulin in wound management.
5. Discuss the nursing management of immunotherapy.
6. List side effects/adverse reactions of immunizations and correlate them with client education.
7. Compare the advantages and disadvantages of live attenuated and inactivated biologic products.

The body's first defense against invasion by potentially lethal microorganisms is intact skin and mucous membranes. The antiinflammatory process and/or a competent immune system are the body's defense against microbes that break this barrier. **Active immunity** exists when the body is capable of producing specific antibodies to combat infections caused by specific antigens or microbes. This immunity may be referred to as *naturally acquired immunity* in that a person who recovers from an infectious disease produces antibodies and memory cells against that specific antigen. The next time the body is in contact with the same antigen, the immune system will be primed to destroy the antigen which is known as *naturally acquired active immunity*.

A passively acquired immunity occurs when antibodies are transferred from a human or animal to a susceptible person. Newborn infants usually have passive acquired immunization that is naturally acquired from their mothers. However, this type of immunity protects only for short periods of time (weeks to several months).

Vaccines and toxoids are available to provide artificially acquired active immunity; vaccines contain whole microbes (dead or attenuated) which are not pathogenic but can induce antibody formation. Toxoids contain detoxified microbe by-products, which are antigenic and also induce antibody production. Sera and antitoxins contain exogenous antibodies and are used to provide artificially acquired passive immunity.

OVERVIEW

The critical age period for immunization is from birth through grade school entry and during the school years (many states now require maintenance of immunizations as a criterion for retention in the school system). Certain groups are found to be at high risk: adolescents, new parents (unimmunized or with waning immunity, exposed to childhood illness or vaccines), debilitated persons and health care providers. Other groups such as migrant workers and recent immigrants to the United States and Canada are predictably at high risk for infectious diseases. See the Cultural Aspects box below for a discussion of risk factors for Hib meningitis.

International political and economic upheavals and the refugee influx to the United States and Canada have illustrated the major problems encountered in other countries: diphtheria, measles, hepatitis B, tuberculosis, and malaria carrier status. Immunization programs that are taken for granted in the United States, Canada, and other countries are not as well funded in developing countries.

As a group, adolescents also seem to be at high risk for preventable infections. Of these, certain subgroups may be particularly in need of immunization, such as athletes, heavy drug users, runaways, foreign travelers, and those isolated from or rejecting traditional health care. Several million children are not immunized against measles, polio, rubella (German measles), mumps, diphtheria, pertussis (whooping cough), and tetanus.

Newspapers and television news coverage have reported the adverse reactions associated with the pertussis and other vaccines, which has served to bias some individuals against vaccination. See the Nursing Research box on p. 986 on the perceptions of vaccine efficacy among inner-city parents. It is important to stress that the vaccines are not without some risks but that the serious risks associated with not being vaccinated and actually contracting the disease are greater still. Diphtheria, tetanus, polio, and the other diseases can cause crippling and death, and most of these diseases are very contagious. Schedules for immunizations for these diseases have been developed as guidelines for the practitioner and for parents to ensure adequate protection for their children (Table 63-1).

A valid history of clinical disease or obtaining an **antibody titer** or the concentration of antibodies in the serum, for some of these diseases is useful in determining disease

Cultural Aspects — Ethnicity as a Risk Factor: Implications for Immunization

In planning for immunization programs, populations are examined for their risk of having the disease. These groups are then targeted for intensive immunization efforts. In the case of *Haemophilus influenzae* type b, inoculation with the Hib vaccine has been demonstrated to provide high immunogenity in all age groups. But what groups should be targeted for immunization?

Reece (1991) reports that in addition to age (i.e., younger than 18 months), day-care placement is an important risk factor. Infants less than a year of age placed in day-care facilities have an attack rate that is 10 times that of infants who do not attend day-care programs. Ethnicity is not generally considered a risk factor in and of itself. However, Reece reports that Native Americans and Eskimos from Alaska are at greater risk for contracting invasive Hib infections. Navajo Indians have an annual Hib-meningitis infection rate of 173 per 100,000 in children under 5 years, and Alaskan Eskimos have a rate of 409 per 100,000. Black and Hispanic children may also be at increased risk. Children who have household contact with an index case of invasive disease are also at substantial risk for infection—585 times the rate of same-age individuals within the general population.

Critical thinking questions

- What other factors besides ethnicity have contributed to the infection rates of the groups mentioned above?
- Given the information above, how would you develop an immunization program if all those groups were found within your community?

From Reece (1991).

Nursing Research

Perceptions of vaccine efficacy, illness, and health among inner-city parents

A resurgence of measles in the past decade has focused attention on the limitations of current immunization programs, particularly for inner-city, low-income populations. As part of a larger study of immunization rates, Keane et al (1993) discussed perceptions of disease severity and vaccine efficacy, as well as the prioritization of the tasks of parenthood, with 40 parents of infants living in inner-city Baltimore to discover their beliefs about immunization. The focus group approach was used. A focus group, usually 4 to 12 people, is a group interview technique that relies on the interaction between group members, rather than between an interviewer and a respondent. All parents/guardians of infants aged 18 to 24 months who attended the Pediatric Ambulatory Center, the community-based health center of the Department of Pediatrics, University of Maryland School of Medicine, were invited by letter to participate in a 2-hour discussion of why parents do or do not use health care services, including immunizations. Forty parents participated in the focus group discussions.

Vaccines were considered only partly successful; susceptibility to chickenpox after vaccination was repeatedly cited as evidence of vaccine failure. Fever was seen as a primary indicator of illness; thus, vaccines were believed to cause, rather than prevent, illness. Immunization was not considered a high-priority parental responsibility. These findings suggest that future interventions should be aimed at changing parental perceptions of vaccines as ineffective and of fever after immunization as an indicator of illness. Educational strategies building on local perceptions may be more likely to be effective than external perceptions. Finally, immunizations should be made easily available, even during clinic visits for a child's illness.

Critical thinking questions

- What misconceptions did the parents in this study have?
- If you were working at the Pediatric Ambulatory Center, how would you conduct an educational program to provide information to parents?

From Keane et al (1993).

TABLE 63-1 Recommended schedule for routine active vaccination of infants and children*

Vaccine	At birth (before hospital discharge)	1-2 months	2 months†	4 months	6 months	6-18 months	12-15 months	15 months	4-6 years (before school entry)
Diphtheria-tetanus-pertussis§			DTP	DTP	DTP			DTaP/DTP¶	DTaP/DTP
Polio, live oral			OPV	OPV	OPV**				OPV
Measles-mumps-rubella							MMR		MMR††
Haemophilus influenzae type b conjugate									
HbOC/PRP-T§,§§			Hib	Hib	Hib		Hib¶¶		
PRP-OMP§§			Hib	Hib			Hib¶¶		
Hepatitis B***									
Option 1	HepB	HepB†††				HepB†††			
Option 2		HepB†††		HepB†††		HepB†††			

*See Table 4 [of original document] for the recommended immunization schedule for infants and children up to their seventh birthday who do not begin the vaccination series at the recommended times or who are >1 month behind in the immunization schedule.

†Can be administered as early as 6 weeks of age.

§Two DTP and Hib combination vaccines are available (DTP/HbOC [TETRAMUNE™]; and PRP-T [ActHIB™, OmniHIB™] which can be reconstituted with DTP vaccine produced by Connaught).

¶This dose of DTP can be administered as early as 12 months of age provided that the interval since the previous dose of DTP is at least 6 months. Diphtheria and tetanus toxoids and acellular pertussis vaccine (DTaP) is currently recommended only for use as the fourth and/or fifth doses of the DTP series among children aged 15 months through 6 years (before the seventh birthday). Some experts prefer to administer these vaccines at 18 months of age.

**The American Academy of Pediatrics (AAP) recommends this dose of vaccine at 6-18 months of age.

††The AAP recommends that two doses of MMR should be administered by 12 years of age with the second dose being administered preferentially at entry to middle school or junior high school.

§§HbOC: [HibTITER®] (Lederie Praxis). PRP-T: [ActHIB™, OmniHIB™] (Pasteur Merieux). PRP-OMP: [PedvaxHIB®] (Merck, Sharp, and Dohme). A DTP/Hib combination vaccine can be used in place of HbOC/PRP-T.

¶¶After the primary infant Hib conjugate vaccine series is completed, any of the licensed Hib conjugate vaccines may be used as a booster dose at age 12-15 months.

***For use among infants born to HBsAg-negative mothers. The first dose should be administered during the newborn period, preferably before hospital discharge, but no later than age 2 months. Premature infants of HBsAg-negative mothers should receive the first dose of the hepatitis B vaccine series at the time of hospital discharge or when the other routine childhood vaccines are initiated. (All infants born to HBsAg-positive mothers should receive immunoprophylaxis for hepatitis B as soon as possible after birth.)

†††Hepatitis B vaccine can be administered simultaneously at the same visit with DTP (or DTaP), OPV, Hib, and/or MMR.

From Centers for Disease Control and Prevention (1994). General Recommendations on Immunization: Recommendations of the Advisory Committee on Immunization Practices (ACIP). *MMWR* 43(No. RR-1):9.

exposure and immunity. However, proven exposure to the disease does not always guarantee immunity. Therefore timely immunizations are even more important if the potential for development of the disease is imminent or increased, as it is for persons traveling to foreign countries where some diseases are endemic, indigenous to a geographic area or population. Required and recommended immunizations for foreign travel are constantly changing and are best obtained before travel from the local department of health.

Any time a traumatic wound (especially a puncture wound) is encountered, the individual's tetanus immunization status must be assessed. If the person has not been fully immunized within the past 10 years, or if the wound is contaminated and an immunization is more than 5 years old, a booster dose of tetanus toxoid may be in order. In adults, tetanus and diphtheria toxoid is recommended because the individual's diphtheria protection will be enhanced by this combination (McCormack & Brown, 1996).

Most new parents today are too young to remember the fear engendered by the very mention of childhood illnesses a few decades ago. For example, measles, the most common childhood disease, can cause pneumonia, encephalopathy, deafness, blindness and seizures in 1 out of every 1000 children with this disease (McCormack & Brown, 1996). If parents are not convinced, outbreaks of diseases (e.g., poliomyelitis) may make the argument for us. Complacency about childhood illnesses and their current and potential threats must be shaken. The initial effects of childhood illnesses can be very serious, and more potential future hazards are currently being discovered (e.g., the possible association of mumps with eventual diabetes and of chickenpox with shingles).

A request for exemption from required immunizations for school entry on medical grounds can be obtained from the child's physician. A model form for exemption on religious grounds can be obtained from the Christian Science Committee on Publications. However, it is *theoretically* possible that the right to exempt certain children could interfere with "herd immunity" by sustaining a continued pool of susceptibles, thereby maintaining a hazard that would be unacceptable to other parents, who might apply legal and other pressures.

Community health nurses, school nurses, teachers, local public health departments, the Department of Health and Human Services, and the World Health Organization need to work together to share expertise in educating the public, in case finding and reporting, in screening, and in mass immunization programs.

CURRENT ISSUES

Refinements and developments in clinical immunology field are advancing with the Center for Disease Control and Prevention (1994) issuing the following general recommendations:

Spacing of Immunizations

When multiple doses of a particular immunization are recommended to achieve an adequate antibody response, the time interval between dosages should be followed. While a time that is longer than the recommended interval is acceptable and does not require starting over, shorter intervals are *not* acceptable because the overall antibody response will be decreased and some persons will have an increased frequency in local or systemic adverse reactions (Centers for Disease Control and Prevention [CDC], 1994). While live vaccines such as the oral polio and yellow fever vaccines can be given at any time with an immune globulin, there is some evidence that high doses of immune globulin can inhibit the immune response to measles vaccine for over a 3-month period. Because there are instances when an inactivated vaccine interferes with other killed or live antigens, see Table 63-2 and 63-3 for the recommended guidelines for spacing the administration of live and killed antigens and immune globulin.

Vaccination in special situations (CDC, 1994):

- premature infants should be vaccinated on the same chronological age schedule as full-term infants with the same recommended vaccine dose.
- there is no contraindication to breastfeeding and vaccinations.
- vaccinations during pregnancy depends on weighing the potential risk of the vaccine to the disease exposure. For example, tetanus and diphtheria toxoids are rou-

TABLE 63-2 Guidelines for spacing the administration of live and killed antigens

Antigen combination	Recommended minimum interval between doses
≥2 Killed antigens	None. May be administered simultaneously or at any interval between doses.*
Killed and live antigens	None. May be administered simultaneously or at any interval between doses.†
≥2 Live antigens	4-week minimum interval if not administered simultaneously.§ However, oral polio vaccine can be administered at any time before, with, or after measles-mumps-rubella, if indicated.

*If possible, vaccines associated with local or systemic side affects (e.g., cholera, parenteral typhoid, and plague vaccines) should be administered on separate occasions to avoid accentuated reactions.

†Cholera vaccine with yellow fever vaccine is the exception. If time permits, these antigens should not be administered simultaneously, and at least 3 weeks should elapse between administration of yellow fever vaccine and cholera vaccine. If the vaccines must be administered simultaneously or within 3 weeks of each other, the antibody response may not be optimal.

§If oral live typhoid vaccine is indicated (e.g., for international travel undertaken on short notice), it can be administered before, simultaneously with, or after OPV.

From Centers for Disease Control and Prevention (1994). General Recommendations on Immunization: Recommendations of the Advisory Committee on Immunization Practices (ACIP). *MMWR* 43(No. RR-1):15.

TABLE 63-3 Guidelines for spacing the administration of immune globulin preparations* and vaccines

Simultaneous administration		Nonsimultaneous administration		
		Immunobiologic administered		
Immunobiologic combination	Recommended minimum interval between doses	First	Second	Recommended minimum interval between doses
Immune globulin and killed antigen	None. May be given simultaneously at different sites or at any time between doses.	Immune globulin Killed antigen	Killed antigen Immune globulin	None None
Immune globulin and live antigen	Should generally not be administered simultaneously.† If simultaneous administration of measles-mumps-rubella (MMR), measles-rubella, and monovalent measles vaccine is unavoidable, administer at different sites and revaccinate or test for seroconversion after the recommended interval (Table 8).	Immune globulin Live antigen	Live antigen Immune globulin	Dose related†,§ 2 weeks

*Blood products containing large amounts of immune globulin (such as serum immune globulin, specific immune globulins [e.g., TIG and HBIG], intravenous immune globulin [IGIV], whole blood, packed red cells, plasma, and platelet products).

†Oral polio virus, yellow fever, and oral typhoid (Ty21a) vaccines are exceptions to these recommendations. These vaccines may be administered at any time before, after, or simultaneously with an immune globulin-containing product without substantially decreasing the antibody response (35).

§The duration of interference of immune globulin preparations with the immune response to the measles component of the MMR, measles-rubella, and monovalent measles vaccine is dose-related (Table 8 of original document).

From Centers for Disease Control and Prevention (1994). General Recommendations on Immunization: Recommendations of the Advisory Committee on Immunization Practices (ACIP). *MMWR* 43(No. RR-1):16.

tinely used for susceptible pregnant women; hepatitis B vaccine, influenza, and pneumococcal vaccines are also recommended for pregnant women at risk for the infection or from complications of the disease.

- contraindications to all vaccines include a history of anaphylaxis to the individual vaccine or a component of it; or the presence of moderate to severe illness with or without a fever. Generally, immunocompromised individuals should not receive any live vaccines. Special exceptions for the immunocompromised person and specific recommendations for their household contacts are available (CDC, 1994).

AIDS Vaccine

Acquired immunodeficiency syndrome (AIDS), which often results in fatal, unusual malignancies and opportunistic infections, has been recognized as an immunodeficiency state that results from an infection with a human retrovirus, the human immunodeficiency virus (HIV). While new drugs have been released to treat AIDS, the search for an HIV vaccine has not been productive (Santiago, 1996).

Two HIV envelope protein gp120 vaccines were tested in HIV-positive persons, but in 1994 the development of infections after administration of the vaccines resulted in cancellation of the major clinical trials (McCann, 1994). While trials with this vaccine are continuing in Thailand, other researchers believe an HIV vaccine such as ALVAC, which stimulates both a cellular and a humoral response, may hold some promise. It is still in phase I trials but it is expected to be approved for phase II trials in the United States in the near future. Some investigators are looking at a completely new vaccine, one that prevents the disease but not the infection itself.

Many viral vaccines work by preventing the acute illness from developing, and not by preventing the infection itself. This method though may be risky with HIV but investigators are looking into this possibility currently by testing in primates (Santiago, 1996). See Chapter 64, Immunosuppressants and Immunomodulators.

SIDE EFFECTS/ADVERSE REACTIONS

As important as protection from debilitating infectious disease is, immunization is not without some risk. *Side effects* (i.e., slight fever, sore injection site, or minor rash) are usually mild and transient; occasionally more *serious effects* (i.e., encephalitis and convulsions) are reported.

Although serious, the incidence of these effects, when weighed against the effects of diseases preventable through immunization, usually tips the balance in favor of immunization, particularly for those at high risk.

Joint pains and malaise may also be seen, especially after certain live and inactivated vaccines. Rarely allergy to the egg protein providing the culture medium for the organism involved, to antiserums or antitoxins, to the mercury preservative, or to contained antibiotics causes a reaction that is usually controllable by antihistamines. When any unusual or severe reaction occurs, the nurse should contact the prescriber and an informational form should be sent to the Centers for Disease Control. Vaccinees should be given a contact's name in case they become sick and should visit a physician, hospital, or clinic within 4 weeks after immunization.

Monitoring any adverse reactions is part of a surveillance system to detect uncommon, severe, previously unrecognized, and rare reactions to vaccination. Past examples are the Guillain-Barré syndrome accompanying a small percentage of influenza vaccinations, encephalitis following measles vaccine, and peripheral neuropathy after rubella vaccinations; these are all *very* rare occurrences.

Even though uncommon, a large number of benign, expected reactions could indicate a "hot" lot of vaccine. Data are collected by the CDC for comparison with national data and are published in the *Quarterly Adverse Reaction Report*.

Minor expected reactions can be treated with acetaminophen (if the prescriber approves) and rest. Severe fevers (more than 103° F) can be treated with acetaminophen and sponge baths to reduce the temperature; occasionally a convulsion may accompany a high temperature, and parents need to be advised. Serum sickness sometimes occurs after repeated serum injections; it consists of rash, urticaria, arthritis, adenopathy, and fever starting hours or even days after the injection. Treatment consists of analgesics, antihistamines, or corticosteroids.

Rare but serious anaphylactic reactions can cause urticaria, dyspnea, cyanosis, shock, or unconsciousness that occurs within minutes of injection. This is not normal; it is an emergency situation. Therefore a nurse or someone responsible should observe any recipient of immunotherapy for up to half an hour after therapy. Treatment for anaphylaxis may require administration of epinephrine. Vasopressors and intermittent positive pressure breathing (IPPB) oxygen, antihistamines, and corticosteroids may help. Immunization therapy may cautiously be resumed after all signs of anaphylaxis are gone.

Nurses often find themselves in charge of vaccination programs and clinics. Because nurses are often the first to be consulted by clients, keeping current on the changes in immunizations is important. A description of biologic agents (active and passive) used for immunization and their secondary effects may be found in Table 63-4. Also see Box 63-1 for information on RespiGam.

Nursing Management

Immunotherapy

Assessment. Before an immunization is given, an interview with the client and family should take place. The individual's age, current physical condition and general resis-

Text continued on p. 994

TABLE 63-4 Biologic agents for active immunization

Active immunization uses either inactivated (K or killed) material or live (L) attenuated agents.
Advantages: Usually higher levels of antibody are induced and it is not necessary to repeat the procedure frequently.
Disadvantages: Adverse effects may occur, such as allergic reactions, that are not usually seen with passive immunization.
See Box 63-2 for advantages and disadvantages of live attenuated and inactivated biologic products.

Product	Route of administration	Primary immunization schedule	Comments	Nursing assessment for contraindications and side effects/implementation
Cholera vaccine	(K) bacteria SC, IM	Two doses, 1-4 wk apart (adult dose)	Provides 50% protection for about 6 mo.	*Assessment.* Contraindications: acute illness; severe reaction or allergic response to previous dose; pregnancy evaluated individually. Precautions: review of hypersensitivity history. Side effects: redness, induration, pain at site; occasionally—malaise, headache, mild to moderate temperature elevations. *Implementation.* Administer IM in the deltoid muscle to adults and children over 3. Have epinephrine 1:1000 on hand.
Hemophilus influenza	IM	See Table 63-1.	Efficacy improved if given to child under 2 years old.	*Assessment.* Contraindicated in immunosuppression, acute illnesses, and febrile states. *Implementation.* Shake vial well. Store in medical refrigerator. May be given at the same time as DPT but at different sites. Reconstitute with diluent provided. Record date on vial. Refrigerate; stable 30 days. Have epinephrine 1:1000 available.

Continued

TABLE 63-4 Biologic agents for active immunization—cont'd

Product	Route of administration	Primary immunization schedule	Comments	Nursing assessment for contraindications and side effects/implementation
Hepatitis B	(K)-IM	See Table 63-1.	Provides >90% protection.	*Assessment.* Contraindications/precautions: hypersensitivity. Safety and efficacy not yet established for children under 3 mo of age and in pregnant or breastfeeding women. Clinical judgement would probably weigh the risk of the disease higher than the potential risks caused by the vaccine's secondary effects. Delay giving vaccine in serious active infection or in presence of severely compromised cardiopulmonary status. Frequent handwashing, gloving (especially if any breaks in skin), and isolation modalities are essential for nurses in particular. Side effects: 50% report various degrees of temporary injection site soreness; occasionally—101° F fevers are reported; infrequently—malaise, headache, nausea, myalgias, arthralgias. *Implementation.* Shake before drawing up suspension; inspect for particles; do not dilute. Store opened and unopened vials in the refrigerator.
Influenza	(K)-IM	One dose. Split doses used in persons under 13 years old (lower incidence of side effects).	Give annually by November.	*Assessement.* Contraindications: hypersensitivity to egg products; individuals who are immunosuppressed; acute febrile illness; do not inject intravenously. Precautions: pregnancy; keep epinephrine on hand; not effective against all possible strains of influenza virus; resterilize jet injection apparatus if contaminated with blood; complete immunizations by November. Toxic drug reactions may occur (especially with phenytoin, warfarin, or theophylline) following viral infection or vaccination. Side effects; local tenderness, redness, induration; fever, malaise, myaglia; rare—allergic skin and respiratory reactions and Guillian-Barré syndrome; vary rare—encephalopathy. *Implementation.* Inject IM into deltoid or lateral mid-thigh or gluteus. Refrigerate. Have epinephrine 1:1000 available.
Measles virus vaccine	(L)-SC	One dose at 12 to 15 mo; earlier if epidemic occurs. See Table 63-1.	If given before 15 mo, may need to reimmunize. Also may prevent disease if given within 72 hr of exposure to measles.	*Assessment.* Contraindications: neomycin or chicken product hypersensitivity; active febrile infection; active untreated TB; immunosuppression or immunodeficiency; bone marrow or lymphatic deficiencies; pregnancy (pregnancy should also be avoided for 3 mo after vaccination). Precautions: give no sooner than 3 mo after transfusion of blood/plasma/human ISG of more than 0.02 ml/lb body weight.

TABLE 63-4 Biologic agents for active immunization—cont'd

Product	Route of administration	Primary immunization schedule	Comments	Nursing assessment for contraindications and side effects/implementation
Measles virus vaccine —cont'd				Give with or after TB skin test. Do not give within 1 mo of immunization by other live virus vaccines except one of the MMR type or combination. Side effects: moderate fever to 102° F, rash (in 5-12 days); rare—fever more than 103° F with convulsions; 1 per million occurrences—encephalitis or subacute sclerosing panencephalitis; previous recipients of killed virus vaccine—local swelling, redness, vesiculation. *Implementation.* A 25-gauge ⅝-inch needle is recommended. Refrigerate before reconstitution and afterward. Use within 8 hr; avoid light at all times. Inject 0.5 ml reconstituted vaccine subcutaneously. Solution may be pink or yellow but must be clear. Discard cloudy solutions. Have epinephrine 1:1000 available.
Meningococcal meningitis vaccine	SC	One dose. If a household disease, antibiotic prophylaxis (rifampin) should be given for several days, since antibody response requires at least 5 days.	Used in epidemics	*Assessment.* Obtain immunization and allergy history. Contraindications: immunosuppression; acute illness. Precautions: pregnancy. Side effects: mild, local erythema. *Implementation.* Administer in a single parenteral dose. Do not give IV. Have epinephrine 1:1000 available.
Mumps vaccine	(L)-SC	One dose	If administered before 1 year old, reimmunization may be necessary.	*Assessment.* Contraindications and precautions: same as for measles vaccine with following exceptions in side effects. Side effects: mild fever (uncommonly more than 103° F); low incidence of parotitis, orchitis, purpura, allergic reactions (urticaria); very rare—encephalitis and other nervous system reactions. *Implementation.* Same as measles vaccine.
Pertussis (in DTP)	(K)-IM	As per DTP (see Table 63-1)	Use only whole cell DTP for first three doses. See Table 63-1.	*Assessment.* Contraindications: acute infection; previous reactions to an initial dose (all 3 antigens or only pertussis may be omitted then) such as fever greater than 103° F (39° C), convulsions, altered consciousness, focal neurologic signs, "screaming fits," shock/collapse, purpura; preexisting neurologic disorder; immunosuppression; older than 6 yr (give Td instead). Precautions: reactions to DTP call for reevaluation and possibly administration of Td only.

Continued

TABLE 63-4 Biologic agents for active immunization—cont'd

Product	Route of administration	Primary immunization schedule	Comments	Nursing assessment for contraindications and side effects/implementation
Pertussis vaccine—cont'd				Side effects: usual—local redness, induration, and possible tenderness; possible abscess; mild to moderate fever. *Implementation.* Administer IM into deltoid or thigh, varying site each time. Shake before using. Refrigerate. Have epinephrine 1:1000 available.
Pneumococci polyvalent vaccine	SC, IM	See current literature	Not used in children under 2 yr old.	*Implementation.* Keep refrigerated. Inject into deltoid or midlateral thigh. Have epinephrine 1:1000 available. *Assessment.* Contraindications: hypersensitivity, revaccination, pregnancy, intradermal administration, and IV administration. Will not protect against specific antigens not included. Within 10 days of start of chemotherapy of Hodgkin's disease, vaccine is contraindicated. Precautions: active infection; under 2 yr of age; immunosuppression; severely compromised cardiac or pulmonary function; history of pneumococcal infection. Keep epinephrine on hand. Side effect: local redness and soreness, induration, fever greater than 100.9° F; rare—anaphylactoid reactions.
Poliomyelitis vaccine	(L)-Oral	See Table 63-1.		*Assessment.* Contraindications: never administered parenterally or in acute illness; advanced, debilitated condition; persistent vomiting or diarrhea; immunodeficient or immunosuppressed states. Precautions: will not modify/prevent existing or incubating disease. Side effect: rarely—paralytic disease after vaccination or after contact with vaccinee (advise unimmunized close contacts of vaccinee to seek immunization as needed). *Implementation.* Store frozen, thaw before use, and agitate before giving 2 drops orally, in chlorine-free water, simple syrup, or milk, or on bread, cake, or cube sugar (usually dropper supplied). See package insert for specific storage advice. Change of color from pink to yellow is not remarkable.
Rabies vaccine Rabies	(K)-IM	Preexposure: two doses a week apart followed by a third dose in between 21-28 days. Postexposure: see current literature for guidelines		*Assessment.* History of hypersensitivity dictates cautious use of rabies vaccine. *Implementation.* Flush and cleanse wound; possible initial prophylaxis with tetanus and antibiotic therapy. Have epinephrine 1:1000 available. Discontinue corticosteroids during immunization.

TABLE 63-4 Biologic agents for active immunization—cont'd

Product	Route of administration	Primary immunization schedule	Comments	Nursing assessment for contraindications and side effects/implementation
Rubella vaccine	(L)-SC	One dose. See Table 63-1.	Give between 12-15 mo of age. Do not give during pregnancy. Woman must not become pregnant for 3 mo after injection. Contraceptive counseling may be needed.	*Assessment.* Contraindications and precautions as for Attenuvax with the following exceptions. Contraindications: postpubertal females with rubella titers of more than 1:8; pregnancy (pregnancy also to be avoided for 3 mo after vaccine). Precautions: theoretical possibility of live virus transmission from nose/throat of vaccinees. Side effects: occasionally—mild symptoms of naturally acquired rubella (lymphadenopathy, urticaria, rash, malaise, sore throat, fever, headache, polyneuritis, arthralgias, local pain, swelling, redness; fever rarely more than 103° F); very rarely—encephalitis. *Implementation.* Same as for measles vaccine.
Tetanus toxoid	IM	Included in DTP (see Table 63-1).	DTP is preferred for children while tetanus and diphtheria (Td) is preferred for adults. Tetanus toxoid is usually used to test cell-mediated immunity.	*Assessment.* Contraindications; not for treatment of an actual tetanus infection; any acute infection; immunosuppression. Precautions: hypersensitivity; keep epinephrine on hand; history of cerebral damage, neurologic disorders, or febrile convulsions should be evaluated individually. Side effects: occasionally—Arthus-type response to high levels of tetanus antibody (antitoxin) in those receiving regular or frequent tetanus toxoid boosters (thus the recommended 10-yr interval between Td booster). Response may include significant local symptoms of redness, edema resembling a giant "hive," axillary lymphadenopathy; systemic symptoms can include low fever, malaise, aches and pains, general urticaria, tachycardia, and hypotension. Prolonged intervals between primary immunizing doses has no effect on eventual immuity status. *Implementation.* Shake well and give deep IM, avoiding blood vessels. Refrigerate, but do not freeze. Have epinephrine 1:1000 available.

BOX 63-1

RespiGam

Respiratory syncytial virus intravenous immune globulin (RespiGam) was approved to prevent the serious lower respiratory tract infection caused by respiratory syncytial virus (RSV) in children under 2 years old that were either born prematurely or have bronchopulmonary dysplasia. This product reduces the incidence and duration of RSV hospitalizations and also the severity of the disease in high-risk infants. It is infused once a month during the RSV period from November through April (Pharmacy News, 1996).

BOX 63-2

Live vs Inactivated Products

The advantages of live attenuated-type immunization are the long-lasting immunity, and the similarity of the resistance that occurs to that which is produced by the natural disease. The disadvantages with the live immunization are an increased risk of inducing disease, plus the fact that a mild disease state is usually needed in order to induce immunity. One also has a higher risk of the vaccine being contaminated, and finally, the product is more labile, requiring special storage.

The inactivated (killed) biologic product is easier to ship and store. It is usually highly purified and has little risk of inducing a disease from infection. The disadvantage is that it provides a short-acting immunity so that the person often needs reimmunization. It may or may not simulate protective type factors, and it may not prevent a reinfection without the actual disease having been present.

tance to disease, history of exposure to infectious diseases (both past and potential), and previous immunizations should be assessed. Providers are required to provide detailed information on the risks and benefits of immunization. A signed consent form must be obtained before immunization. Printed information can be shared at this time to ensure the parent/client is aware of side/adverse effects and how to manage them (Merenstein et al, 1994). A list of the general contraindications to immunization follows:

1. Current acute or febrile illness
2. Immunosuppressive therapy in progress or immunodeficient state
3. Recent immune serum globulin (ISG), plasma, or blood transfusions
4. Pregnancy—"live" vaccines especially may prove to be teratogenic or may cause infection in the fetus and therefore need to be avoided or given with caution. Inactivated vaccines if necessary, may be administered during the second trimester of pregnancy. All women of childbearing age should be immunized against polio, measles, mumps, rubella, tetanus, and diphtheria. If the pregnant woman is not immunized, only tetanus and diphtheria vaccines may be administered during pregnancy (DiPiro et al, 1993).
5. Certain malignancies that leave the individual infection-susceptible (e.g., leukemias, lymphomas)
6. Simultaneous administration of another *single* live virus, unless proved safe
7. Prior unusual or allergic reaction to the same or similar vaccine
8. Allergy to antibiotics in vaccine, thimerosal as a preservative, or other constituents

Minor afebrile infections such as the common cold are not usually contraindications to immunization.

Routinely assess individuals (especially children) for immune status. High-risk groups include adolescents, new parents, individuals not vaccinated with the live measles vaccine, migrant workers, and recent immigrants. Elderly individuals, especially those in nursing homes, as well as those with chronic health problems, are at particular risk for respiratory infections and should be encouraged to obtain annual influenza virus vaccinations.

Individuals who have been exposed or are at risk of exposure to one of the childhood diseases or serious communicable diseases or who have incurred a traumatic wound are also candidates for immunization.

Be aware that a history of hypersensitivity reactions to the biologic agent or to any contained antibiotics or preservatives is a contraindication to immunotherapy. Pregnancy may or may not be a contraindication, depending on clinical judgment and manufacturers' instructions.

Always assess the client's allergy history carefully and test for hypersensitivity before administering animal sera. Keep epinephrine on hand to counter any potentially dangerous event (such as anaphylaxis).

Nursing diagnosis. The client receiving immunotherapy has the potential for the following selected nursing diagnoses: altered comfort (malaise, headache, rash, lymphadenopathy, and pain and tenderness at the injection site); hyperthermia; and the potential complication of allergic reaction and encephalopathy.

Implementation

Monitoring. Because of the risk of anaphylaxis after any immunization, ask clients to remain in the immediate area for up to half an hour for observation of any developing adverse reactions. Be alert for the early symptoms of such a reaction; hives, shock-like appearance, confusion, and hypotension.

Intervention. Immune antisera and globulin are administered intramuscularly unless otherwise noted. **Passive immunization** or **immunoprophylaxis** should always be administered as soon as possible after exposure to the agent.

Almost all immunotherapy is parenteral and must be given by the specified route and with the specified diluent to avoid either local reactions (especially seen when the intracutaneous route is used) or possible anaphylaxis (especially when the intravenous route is used). All needles should be changed after the vaccine is withdrawn from the vial, if possible. Aspiration after insertion is, of course, also necessary to prevent the danger of depositing the dose into the bloodstream.

Be aware that a crying, wriggling baby or child presents a challenging moving target for injection and must be temporarily restrained. This can often be accomplished just as effectively in the warmth and security of another's arms (the mother's, if feasible) rather than on hard table surface. Taking out the needle and syringe and explaining that "this may hurt for only a minute" *just before* the actual injection will lessen the fear of pain.

Record the dates of immunization at the time of administration, and give a copy to the recipient or parents for permanent safekeeping. Explain that this record may be invaluable later when these dates may be required on applications to school, summer camp, college, or visas for travel to other countries.

Be aware that most products will lose potency at temperatures higher than 2° to 8° C (35.6° to 46.4° F) except for TOPV, which must be frozen. Most immunization agents should therefore be stored in a medical refrigerator, where a thermometer is placed nearby, and replaced immediately after use. They should not be stored near a heat source, on a window sill, or on a refrigerator door shelf because of unpredictable temperatures.

Apply and explain appropriate isolation precautions when caring for individuals with known or suspected exposure to the communicable diseases. Assuming that someone else will take this responsibility at the outset is unwise.

Education. Perceptions and misconceptions concerning immunization must be clarified. The relative safety and merits of immunization versus risks of the disease process itself (both short- and long-range) should be discussed, using statistics where appropriate. The client and/or family should be told that a repeat immunization, if records are unclear, is usually not contraindicated; the risk if usually minimal, and future protection is ensured. Unimmunized parents should be identified and probably immunized before their children, especially when oral polio vaccine is administered.

Noncompletion of an immunization series may occasionally be prevented if vaccinees or their parents know that interruption of the series or a prolonged period between phases of immunization makes no difference to eventual antibody levels. A copy of the immunization schedule given to the client or family also enhances compliance with the immunization series.

Complete, written, and accurate documentation of immunizations with dates is rare even in office records. Nonetheless, having access to these data is important. Therefore teaching parents or vaccinees to keep careful written records for each vaccination, especially in view of the high mobility of our population, is crucial. Simple blank forms are available for this purpose and should be given to parents or the vaccinee with an explanation and advice to keep them updated and in a safe place (e.g., with health record files at home or in the family Bible) and to bring them to each child's appointment.

Teach clients or their parents how to recognize and differentiate between anticipated side effects and serious adverse reactions. Acetaminophen may be taken for the not uncommon aches, local pain and swelling, or mild temperature elevations, which may occur within 24 hours. Recipients of immunotherapy should understand whom they are to contact if complications occur later.

Evaluation. The client will receive immunity without experiencing adverse effects of the drug.

■ ■ ■

Sources of information on immunization include primarily the Public Health Service Advisory Committee on Immunization Practices (ACIP), which advises the public health agencies, and the Committee on Control of Infectious Diseases (the Red Book Committee), which is drawn from the members of the American Academy of Pediatrics and advises the private health sector. The ACIP can be contacted through the Centers for Disease Control in Atlanta. Because the two groups maintain a slightly different perspective, minor inconsequential variations in recommendations may occasionally be noted. Other sources include local public health departments and printed package inserts included with the vaccine or serum. Biologic preparations and accompanying inserts are regulated by the Bureau of Biologics of the FDA. The state of the art of immunotherapy is in rapid flux. The only constant in immunization practice is change itself. To read, attend seminars, and consult with experts is to keep pace.

SUMMARY

Immunization is available for a number of diseases whose prevalence has abruptly declined because of availability of vaccines and sera; such diseases include measles, polio, rubella, mumps, diphtheria, and tetanus. Vaccines are also available for yellow fever, hepatitis B, influenza, rabies, cholera, typhoid, plague, and other diseases. Smallpox has been eradicated because of a World Health Organization campaign of near-universal vaccination. Although these preparations are available, nurses must still educate the public to minimize complacency regarding the diseases for which they provide protection and to promote immunization.

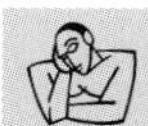

Critical Thinking

1. A teenaged mother brings her infant to the clinic for its first well-baby checkup at 6 weeks. What would you include in your teaching to her regarding her baby's immunizations?
2. As an adult and as a nursing student, what immunizations should you have and why?

 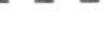

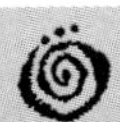

Collaborative Learning Activities

1. A team of students will role play a mother bringing in her baby for its routine immunizations at 6 months. What does the nurse need to assess? What instructions will the mother need before the immunizations? The nurse will instruct the mother on how to hold the baby while the nurse gives the injection.

BIBLIOGRAPHY

Abramowicz M (Ed.) (1990). Routine immunization for adults, *Med Lett* 32(819):54.

Anderson KN, et al. (Eds.) (1994). *Mosby's medical, nursing, & allied health dictionary* (4th ed.). St. Louis: Mosby.

Centers for Disease Control and Prevention (1994). General recommendations on immunization: Recommendations of the Advisory Committee on Immunization Practices (ACIP), *MMWR* 43(RR-1):1-38.

DiPiro JT, et al. (1993). *Pharmacology: A pathophysiological approach* (2nd ed.). Norwalk, CT: Appleton & Lange.

Holt DN (1992). Recommendations, usage and efficacy of immunizations for the elderly, *Nurs Practit* 17(4)51-9.

Keane V, et al. (1993). Perceptions of vaccine efficacy, illness, and health among inner-city parents, *Clin Pediatr* 32(1):2-7.

McCann J (1994). Researchers tout triple therapy for HIV/AIDS, *Hosp Pharm Rep* 8(9):18.

McCormack JP & Brown G (1996). Traumatic skin and soft tissue infections. In Young LY & Koda-Kimble MA (Eds.). *Applied therapeutics* (6th ed.). Vancouver: Applied Therapeutics.

Merenstein GB, Kaplan DW, & Rosenberg AA (1994). *Handbook of pediatrics* (17th ed.) Norwalk, CT: Appleton & Lange.

National Institutes of Allergy and Infectious Diseases (NIAID) (1992). Evolution of vaccine development, *Neonat Netw* 11(4):43-4.

National Institutes of Allergy and Infectious Diseases (NIAID) (1992). Vaccines in clinical trials, *Neonat Netw* 11(4):45-7.

Olin BR (Ed.) (1996). *Facts and comparisons*. St Louis: Facts and Comparisons.

Pharmacy News (1996). Drug updates. *J Am Pharm NS36*(4):225.

Reece SM (1991). New protection against *Haemophilus influenzae* type b infections in infants and young children, *Nurs Practit* 16(11)27.

Santiago L (1996). Slow progress on HIV vaccines. *GMHC Treatment Issues* 10(4):1-4.

Chapter 64

Immunosuppressants and Immunomodulators

Chapter Focus

As client acuity levels increase and treatments become more complex, nurses are increasingly aware of the impact of the immune system on treatment regimens of clients. Because nurses administer treatments that decrease immunity (immunosuppressants) or enhance immune function (immunoglobulin), they need to maintain a working understanding of the immune system, how it relates to the clinical picture of clients, and the agents that affect it. The following objectives and key terms are important for a good understanding of this chapter.

Key Terms

acquired immunodeficiency syndrome (AIDS) (p. 1005)
human immunodeficiency virus (HIV) (p. 1005)
immunocompromised state (p. 998)
immunomodulating agent (p. 1005)
immunosuppressant agents (p. 998)

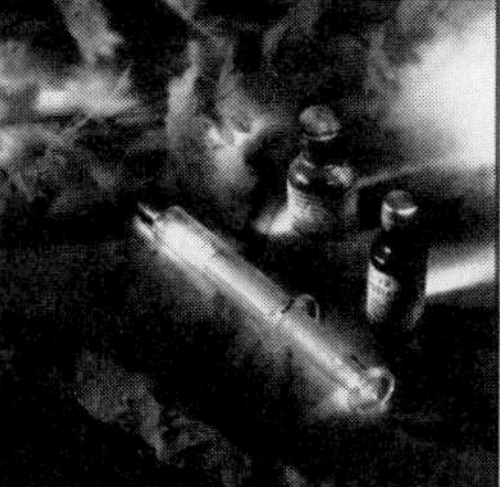

Key Drug [▲]

azathioprine

Objectives

1. Identify the four factors relating to the immune system that can lead to an immunocompromised state.
2. Discuss the general nursing management of the immunosuppressed client.
3. Compare and contrast the nursing management of clients receiving azathioprine, cyclosporine, muromonab-CD3, mycophenolate mofetil, and tacrolimus therapy.
4. Implement the nursing management of the care of clients receiving immunosuppressant and immunomodulator agents.

The rejection of kidney, liver, and heart allogenic transplants has led to the development of **immunosuppressant agents,** or agents that decrease or prevent an immune response. A foreign substance or organ transplant in the body, activates an immune response by the release of macrophages to phagocytize and process the foreign substance. In addition, interleukin-1 production increases, which activates helper T cells containing a surface receptor or CD3. The activated T cell stimulates production of killer or cytotoxic T-lymphocytes and B-lymphocytes in part by producing interleukin-2. T-cells are necessary for cellular immunity (attack the foreign substance directly and with released toxic substances) and the B-lymphocytes are responsible for humoral immunity or the production of antibodies. The primary sites of action of the immunosuppressant agents are noted in Figure 64-1.

Immunodeficiency or immunosuppression may also occur from a genetic or an acquired disorder of the immune system. Although genetic disorders such as agammaglobulinemia or severe combined immune deficiency syndrome (SCIDS) are usually diagnosed shortly after birth, acquired disorders may occur at any time throughout life. Acquired immunodeficiency may be induced by a variety of drugs, such as chemotherapeutic and immunosuppressant agents, radiation therapy, or through viral infections such as acquired immunodeficiency syndrome (AIDS). Because AIDS often has devastating complications and a fatal outcome, much research interest has been directed toward the development of immunomodulating or immunostimulating medications.

An **immunocompromised state** may result from one or more of the following: (1) inhibition of granulocyte formation leading to severe neutropenia; (2) impairment of synthesis and antibody production; (3) loss of mucocutaneous barriers that permit bacteria or microorganisms access to internal organs, which may occur in a variety of therapeutic situations, such as after the use of medical devices (central venous catheters, Foley catheters, endotracheal tubes) or after chemotherapy; (4) impairment of cellular immunity such as macrophages and T-cell lymphocytes (usually seen in clients who receive immunosuppressive agents, i.e., corticosteroids, cyclosporine, etc., certain types of cancer [Hodgkin's lymphoma], or organ transplant recipients).

In the majority of clients, combinations of these defects are common because several immune functions may be affected at the same time. For example, chronic therapy with antineoplastic medications will affect granulocytes and cellular immunity. Chemotherapy may result in the loss of mucocutaneous barriers or the development of mucositis and ulcers in the mouth and gastrointestinal tract. These individuals are at a greater risk for the development of bacterial, fungal, or viral infections. This chapter reviews some of the primary agents that suppress, modify, or stimulate the human immune system.

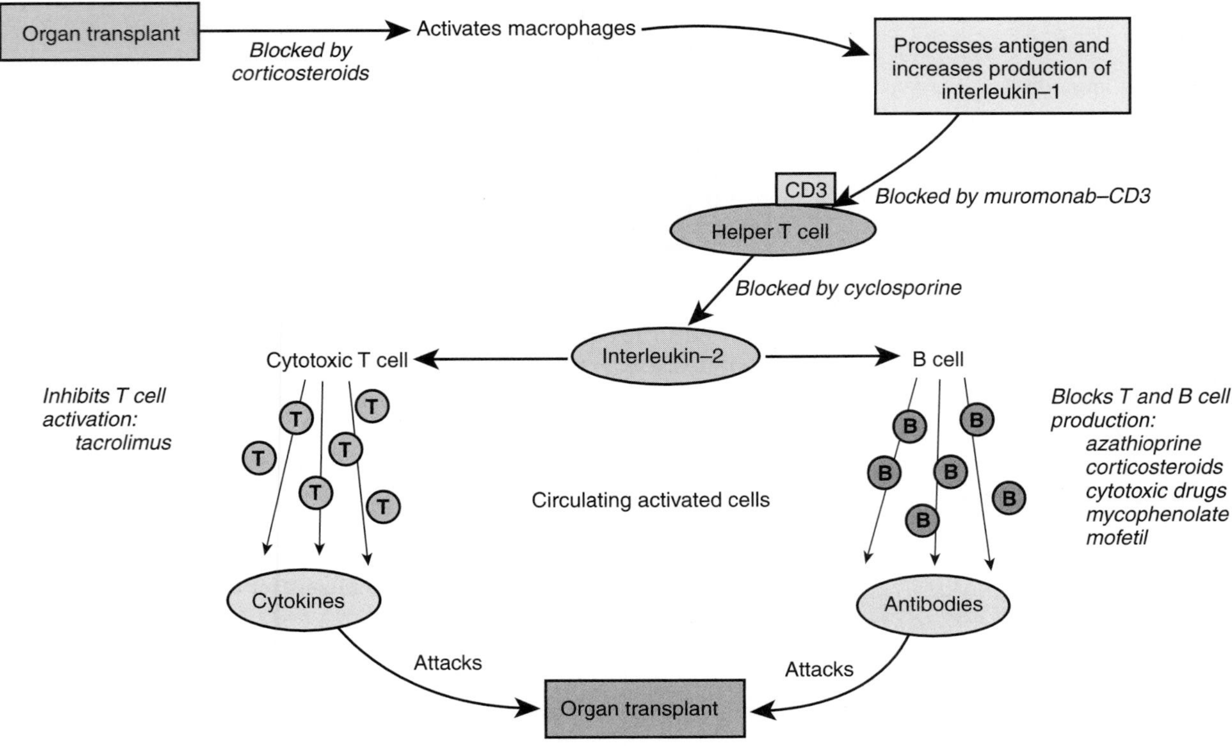

Figure 64-1 Sites of action for immunosuppressive agents.

Nursing Management

The Immunosuppressed Client

The care of the client with a secondary immunodeficiency, which is immunosuppression caused by the therapeutic regimen, focuses on the treatment of the underlying condition and the immunotherapy.

Assessment. The client should be assessed for his or her understanding of the condition and feelings about the illness. The availability of a support system should be considered.

It should be determined that the client does not have, and has not recently had or been exposed to either chickenpox or herpes zoster because of the risk of the occurrence of severe generalized disease when an immunosuppressing drug is administered.

Nutritional status should be assessed, as well as the client's likes and dislikes so that nutritional counseling will be effective, since these clients have usually had some weight loss or require a modified diet. Level of comfort should be determined with regard to activity tolerance and participation in therapies.

Assess the client for opportunistic infections. The head, eyes, ears, neck, and throat should be examined for: white patches on tongue and oral mucosa (thrush); pulling at the ears; tympanic membrane inflammation; impaired hearing; purulent nasal drainage; and tender sinuses. Nutritional, renal, and gastrointestinal assessment would be indicated by decreased weight and height in children; chronic diarrhea; and/or malabsorption. An examination of the mucous membranes of the mouth, vagina, and perianal areas might evidence ulcers, thrush, and/or herpetic lesions. The client's skin and nails may have recurrent infections. The cardiovascular system usually is within normal limits, except for tachycardia with severe infections. The respiratory tract may be unremarkable unless pneumonia is present. Then the findings may be dyspnea, tachypnea, nasal flaring, use of accessory muscles, retractions, decreased breath sounds, rales, and/or green or yellow sputum. Neuromuscular development may be delayed in children. Psychosocially, the client may be irritable, and children may have failure to thrive. Perform an initial age-appropriate developmental screening.

Nursing diagnosis. The administration of immunosuppressive agents increases the client's risk for the following nursing diagnoses: anxiety related to actual or perceived threat to biologic integrity, self-concept, or unfamiliar people or surroundings; altered bowel pattern (diarrhea); activity intolerance related to weakness and fatigue; altered comfort; altered protection related to immunodeficiency; risk for infection related to inadequate immunity; risk for injury related to bleeding/hemorrhage secondary to thrombocytopenia; altered nutrition (less than body requirements) related to decreased intake secondary to anorexia, nausea, vomiting or chronic infection; altered mucous membranes related to drug-induced stomatitis or mycotic superinfection; impaired skin integrity related to cutaneous reactions to drug; diarrhea; ineffective airway clearance related to excessive sputum caused by infection; impaired gas exchange related to alveolar-capillary membrane changes secondary to inflammation; hyperthermia related to infection; risk for altered growth and development related to prolonged illness and hospitalization; social isolation related to altered health status and prolonged hospitalization; and the potential complications of neurologic sequelae and fluid and electrolyte imbalances.

Implementation

Monitoring. Assess for signs of opportunistic infections such as night sweats, fever, fatigue, involuntary weight loss, persistent diarrhea, headache, persistent cough, and presence of green or yellow sputum. Monitor the client's temperature frequently and the results of any cultures. Auscultate lungs for rales, consolidation, and pleural friction rub. Monitor ABGs. Monitor CBCs; WBCs indicate the drug's effectiveness; drug dosage is usually titrated on the leukocyte and platelet counts. Assess nutritional status daily, note weight, fluid intake and output, caloric intake, hematocrit, hemoglobin, and serum protein and albumin values. Monitor for dehydration (decreased urine output, increased specific gravity, poor skin turgor, confusion). Assess stool, urine, emesis, and secretions for the presence of occult blood. Assess and document skin for redness and purulent drainage, and mucous membrane integrity for redness, creamy white patches, black furry tongue. Also monitor skin color and capillary refill. Assess client's tolerance to activity by assessing blood pressure, respiratory rate, and pulse rate before and immediately after activity. Monitor the client for verbal or nonverbal indications of anxiety and social isolation.

Intervention. Careful medical asepsis is a priority with the immunosuppressed client. Thorough handwashing, avoiding other persons with infection, and promoting the client's own resources to prevent infection are essential nursing interventions. Provide meticulous mouth, skin, and perianal care. Proper mouth care with a topical antifungal agent will help to prevent oral candidiasis.

Injections should be avoided when possible; if necessary, the skin should be cleansed with povidone-iodine and allowed to dry for 30 seconds. Clean all cuts and scrapes immediately with antiseptic soap. Avoid unnecessary and invasive procedures (biopsy, barium enemas, etc.); when they are necessary, prophylactic antibiotic coverage is required. Irrigating solutions, vases, and other standing collections of water in which organisms may breed should be avoided.

Administer antipyretics as ordered and monitor response; acetaminophen should be used rather than aspirin for children.

Education. Advise a well-balanced diet and a fluid intake of at least 1500 ml daily to minimize the risk of tissue dehydration and of urinary tract infection associated with low urinary output. Instruct the client to avoid trauma (e.g., breaks in the skin), and to seek medical treatment for wounds that do not heal quickly. Encourage meticulous oral hygiene, including cautious use of toothbrushes, dental floss, and toothpicks, and regular dental care to minimize gingival inflammation and early detection of altered oral mucous membranes. Promote pulmonary toilet by encouraging the client to perform frequent breathing or incentive spirometry exercises.

Encourage ambulation; if client is unable, reposition frequently. Alcohol and aspirin ingestion should be avoided to minimize the risk of gastrointestinal bleeding.

Instruct the client to report any signs and symptoms of infection (sore throat, malaise, headache, fever, dysuria, urinary frequency), bleeding gums, bruising, or signs and symptoms of hepatic dysfunction (abdominal pain, jaundice, pruritus, clay-colored stools). Advise the client to consult the prescriber before taking any OTC medications including aspirin or of receiving any vaccinations while taking immunosuppressant medications. No live viral vaccines should be given to the client and no one in the household should receive oral polio vaccine. Reinforce the importance of health care provider appointments for follow-up care and laboratory examinations.

The client and family should be taught to monitor the client's blood pressure at home. Instruct the client to report any significant changes in blood pressure, hematuria, cloudy urine, decreased urinary output, sudden weight gain, edema of the face or ankles, headache, or unusual fatigue.

If the immunosuppressant is taken to prevent transplant rejection, emphasize the importance of lifelong therapy.

Evaluation. Immunosuppression of the client should occur without the rejection of the transplanted tissue, the presence of infection, or impaired skin integrity. The client/caregiver should also be able to describe methods of preventing infection and the need to maintain optimal nutrition, and other issues to effectively manage the therapeutic regimen.

IMMUNOSUPPRESSANTS

The primary immunosuppressant drugs are azathioprine (Imuran), cyclosporine (Sandimmune), muromonab-CD3 (Orthoclone OKT3), mycophenolate mofetil (CellCept), and tacrolimus (FK506, Prograf).

▲ **azathioprine** [ay za thye' oh preen] (Imuran)
Azathioprine is indicated as an adjunct medication to prevent rejection in renal organ transplants and for severe, active rheumatoid arthritis in persons who have not responded to other therapies. The mechanism of action for azathioprine is unknown but it appears to suppress T and B cell production primarily; that is, it suppresses cell-mediated hypersensitivity and antibody production. In combination with steroids, it appears to have a steroid-conserving effect; a lower dose of steroid may be used to treat chronic inflammatory processes when given with azathioprine.

Azathioprine is available in oral and parenteral dosage forms. Orally it is well absorbed from the intestinal tract, has a half-life of 5 hours, with an onset of action of 6 to 8 weeks in rheumatoid arthritis and perhaps 4 to 8 weeks in other inflammatory disease states. It is metabolized in the liver to active metabolites (6-mercaptopurine and 6-thioinosinic acid) with further metabolism by xanthine oxidase. It is primarily excreted via the biliary system.

The most frequent side effects of azathioprine reported are anorexia and nausea or vomiting. Frequent adverse reactions include leukopenia or infection and megaloblastic anemia. The client is usually asymptomatic but may also have fever, chills, cough, low back or side pain, pain on urination, or increased weakness. The risk of hepatotoxicity is greater when the dosage of azathioprine exceeds 2.5 mg/kg daily.

The pediatric and adult immunosuppressant dose is 3 to 5 mg/kg orally 1 to 3 days before or at the time of surgery, or if given intravenously, before, during, or immediately after surgery. The maintenance dosage is 1 to 2 mg/kg. For rheumatoid arthritis, the adult oral dose is l mg/kg daily, adjusted every 1 to 2 months as necessary.

■ Nursing Management
Azathioprine Therapy

In addition to the general nursing management of the immunosuppressed client (p. 998), clients receiving azathioprine therapy require the following nursing care.

Assessment. It is essential to assess exposure to or presence of infection. Any infection that the client might have may become life-threatening with the administration of azathioprine. Caution should also be used with clients who have had previous cytotoxic drug and radiation therapy. Clients with renal or hepatic function impairment or severe xanthine oxidase deficiency will have reduced metabolism/excretion of the drug with increased risk of azathioprine toxicity; dosages may need to be reduced.

If azathioprine is administered for rheumatoid arthritis, assess the client's range of motion, status of affected joints (swelling, pain, and strength), and ability to accomplish activities of daily living before and periodically during therapy. Hematologic function should be monitored via complete cell counts before therapy is initiated.

Review the client's current medication regimen. Significant drug interactions may occur when azathioprine is given, such as with the following drugs:

Drug	Possible effect and management
allopurinol	**Allopurinol inhibits xanthine oxidase, which may result in increased azathioprine activity and toxicity. Avoid or a potentially serious drug interaction may occur. If it is absolutely necessary to give both drugs concurrently, reduce the dosage of azathioprine to one fourth to one third of the usually prescribed dosage; monitor closely and adjust dosage as needed.**
immunosuppressant agents, other (glucocorticoids, cyclophosphamide, cyclosporine)	**May increase the risk for developing infections and/or neoplasms. Avoid or a potentially serious drug interaction may occur.**
vaccines, live virus	**Immunization with live vaccines should be postponed in persons receiving this drug and also in close family members.** **The use of a live virus vaccine in immunosuppressed clients may result in increased replication of the vaccine virus, may increase side effects/adverse reactions to the vaccine virus, and possibly cause a decrease in the client's antibody response to the vaccine.**

Implementation

Monitoring. Complete blood counts should be done weekly during the first month, twice a month for the next 2 to 3 months, and monthly thereafter. Notify the prescriber if the leukocyte count is less than 3000/mm^3 or if platelets are less than 100,000/mm^3; therapy will be reinstituted at reduced dosages when these counts reach an acceptable level, usually after 7 to 10 days. A decrease in hemoglobin may indicate bone marrow suppression. Renal and hepatic function studies should be monitored with the same frequency. Increased alkaline phosphatase, bilirubin, SGOT (AST), SGPT (ALT), and amylase concentrations may indicate hepatotoxicity.

Intervention. Azathioprine is usually started 1 to 5 days before transplantation and restarted within 24 hours after transplantation. Administer oral doses of azathioprine with or after meals to minimize gastrointestinal distress. Reconstitute each 100 mg for intravenous use by adding 10 ml of sterile water for injection to the vial and swirling to dissolve. It may be administered by intravenous push or further diluted with 0.9% sodium chloride injection or 5% dextrose and 0.9% sodium chloride injection for intravenous infusion. It may be administered over a time period of 5 minutes to 8 hours. Once reconstituted, azathioprine is stable at room temperature for 24 hours.

Education. If azathioprine is being administered for rheumatoid arthritis, the client should be advised to continue physical therapy and other concurrent therapy (salicylates, NSAIDs, glucocorticoids) as prescribed. Because azathioprine has teratogenic effects, advise female clients who are of childbearing age to practice contraception during the course of therapy and for at least 4 months after its completion (see the Pregnancy Safety box below).

Evaluation. Effectiveness for rheumatoid arthritis is evidenced by the client experiencing decreased pain, stiffness, and swelling of the affected joints in 6 to 8 weeks. The client's transplant will not be rejected and the client will be able to effectively manage the therapeutic regimen.

cyclosporine [sye' klow spor een] (Sandimmune)

Cyclosporine is a potent immunosuppressant used for the prevention of organ (renal, hepatic, or cardiac allografts) transplant rejection. It is usually administered in combination with corticosteroids. Its mechanism of action is unknown, but studies indicate it inhibits the formation and release of interleukin II, the substance necessary to induce cytotoxic T-lymphocytes response to an antigenic challenge. It does not cause significant myelosuppression or bone marrow depression.

Pregnancy Safety

Category	Drug
C	cyclosporine, muromonab-CD3, mycophenolate mofetil, tacrolimus
D	azathioprine

Cyclosporine is available in oral and parenteral dosage forms. Orally, its bioavailability is variable (about 30%) which may improve with increasing doses and chronic administration. Absorption may decrease after a liver transplant or in clients with liver impairment or gastrointestinal dysfunction, such as diarrhea or vomiting. It has a half-life of approximately 7 hours in children, and of 19 hours in adults; orally it reaches peak serum levels in 3.5 hours. It is extensively metabolized in the liver and excreted primary in bile and feces.

The most frequently reported side effects are dose related and include hirsutism and tremors. Adverse effects include nephrotoxicity, gingival hyperplasia (bleeding, swollen gums) and severe hypertension, the latter usually associated with 25 to 50 mg/kg doses of cyclosporine. Lymphomas and other lymphoproliferative-type disorders have been reported; some have regressed when the drug is stopped (*USP DI*, 1996). Gingival hyperplasia, a common problem with the use of this drug, is generally reversible about 6 months after cyclosporine is discontinued.

The pediatric and adult oral dose is 12 to 15 mg/kg daily, starting 4 to 12 hours before surgery and continuing for 7 to 14 days afterward. The dose is then decreased weekly until the maintenance dose of 5 to 10 mg/kg daily is reached. Children may need higher or more frequent dosing because they seem to metabolize this drug rapidly. The IV dose is 2 to 6 mg/kg daily until the client can take oral medication.

■ Nursing Management

Cyclosporine Therapy

In addition to the general nursing management of the immunosuppressed client (p. 998), clients receiving cyclosporine therapy require the following nursing care.

Assessment. Monitor the client for signs and symptoms of hypersensitivity (dyspnea, wheezing, hypotension) and have resuscitation equipment near when the drug is administered intravenously.

As with azathioprine therapy, determine that the client does not have and has neither recently had nor been exposed to chickenpox or herpes zoster because of the risk of severe generalized disease. Any infection that the client might have may become life-threatening with the administration of cyclosporine. Clients with renal and hepatic function impairment may require reduced dosage.

Review the client's current medication regimen for potential significant drug interactions that may occur if cyclosporine is given with the following drugs:

Drug	Possible effect and management
androgens, cimetidine (Tagamet), danazol (Danocrine), diltiazem (Cardizem), estrogens, erythromycin, ketoconazole (Nizoral), or miconazole (Monistat i.v.)	May result in increased serum levels of cyclosporine, increasing the potential risk for hepatotoxicity and nephrotoxicity. If drugs must be administered concurrently, use extreme caution and monitor closely.

Continued

Drug	Possible effect and management
diuretics, potassium-sparing (amiloride, spironolactone, or triamterene) or potassium supplements or salt substitutes	May increase the risk of hyperkalemia. Monitor serum levels and signs and symptoms of hyperkalemia (confusion; irregular heart rate; paresthesias of hands, feet, or lips; respiratory difficulties; increased weakness; feeling of weak or heavy legs).
immunosuppressants, other	Increases risk of developing infection or lymphoproliferative-type disorders (lymphomas, etc.). Use extreme caution if given concurrently.
lovastatin (Mevacor)	When used in heart transplant clients, it may increase the risk of developing rhabdomyolysis and acute renal failure. Monitor closely if concurrent therapy is necessary.
vaccines, live virus	See azathioprine.

Renal and hepatic function studies are done before therapy is begun and periodically thereafter. Blood pressure, serum electrolyte determinations and dental exam should be performed.

Nursing diagnosis. In addition to the nursing diagnoses cited earlier in the chapter, the client taking cyclosporine has the potential for: disturbed self image related to gingival hyperplasia; altered cardiac output related to hypertension; and the potential complication of pancreatitis.

Implementation

Monitoring. Serum cyclosporine levels are evaluated periodically during a course of therapy and dosages are adjusted accordingly. Significant changes in renal and hepatic function may necessitate a reduction in dosage or a discontinuation of cyclosporine. Serum potassium and lipid levels may also be increased. Blood pressure is checked periodically to detect hypertension.

Intervention. When administering the oral solution, use the calibrated measuring device supplied by the manufacturer. Because cyclosporine is a mixture of alcohol and vegetable oil and has an unpleasant taste, thoroughly mix it with chocolate milk or orange juice at room temperature and drink at once. Use a glass container to prevent adherence and rinse with additional juice or milk to ensure that the entire dose is taken. Wipe the measuring device dry; do not wash after use.

The intravenous infusion is begun 4 to 12 hours before surgery and continued postoperatively until the client can tolerate an oral dosage form. The drug is prepared for intravenous infusion by diluting each 1 ml in 20 to 100 ml of 0.9% sodium chloride injection or 5% dextrose injection. Glass containers are preferred to prevent the leaching of diethylhexylphthalate (DEHP) from the PVC infusion bags into the cyclosporine solution. However, some agencies will use PVC containers and prepare the drug just before it is given. Significant amounts of the drug are lost when it is administered through PVC tubing. The solution is stable for 24 hours in 5% dextrose injection. In 0.9% sodium chloride injection at room temperature, cyclosporine is stable for 6 hours in a PVC container and for 12 hours in a glass container. Infuse over 2 to 6 hours using an infusion pump, or continuously over 24 hours.

Education. Advise the client about the need for close monitoring by the prescriber. Warn the client to avoid immunizations unless approved by the prescriber and to avoid others who have been immunized with oral poliovirus vaccine. Alert the client to report any signs of infection as soon as noted. Instruct the client of the need to maintain good dental hygiene and to visit a dentist frequently for teeth cleaning to help prevent gingival hyperplasia.

Evaluation. The client will not demonstrate signs of organ rejection and will remain free of hepatotoxicity and nephrotoxicity. The client will also effectively manage the therapeutic regimen.

muromonab-CD3 [myoo roe moe' nab-CD3] (Orthoclone OKT3)

Muromonab-CD3 is a monoclonal antibody that reacts with CD3 receptor on the surface of T-lymphocytes. It blocks the activation and functions of the T cells in response to an antigenic challenge. Thus it functions as an immunosuppressant and does not cause myelosuppression.

Muromonab-CD3 is indicated for the treatment of acute renal organ transplant rejection and is usually given in combination with azathioprine, cyclosporine, and/or corticosteroids. It is also administered to treat acute rejection (steroid-resistant) in cardiac and hepatic transplants. Available parenterally, it acts to reduce activated T cells within minutes after administration. It reaches steady state plasma levels in about 3 days and has a duration of action of about 7 days. In other words, the number of circulating CD3-positive T cells will return to baseline levels within a week after discontinuation of muromonab-CD3.

The most frequent adverse reactions of muromonab-CD3 occur with the first course. The first-dose effect consists of lightheadedness, elevated temperature, chills, nausea, vomiting, diarrhea, headache, dyspnea, chest pain, and tremors and trembling. These effects may be repeated to a lesser degree after the second dose but are rarely encountered with later doses. Fever and chills that occur later may be caused by infection. Anaphylaxis, hypersensitivity, encephalopathy, convulsions, cerebral edema, and aseptic meningitis syndrome are reported, less frequently.

The adult dose is 5 mg daily for 10 to 14 days. Children under 12 years old receive 0.1 mg/kg/day for 10 to 14 days.

■ Nursing Management

Muromonab-CD3 Therapy

In addition to the general nursing management for immunosuppressed clients (p. 998), clients receiving muromonab-CD3 require the following nursing care:

Assessment. The client's temperature should be taken before drug administration. A temperature above 37.8° C (100° F) should be lowered with antipyretics and infection should be ruled out before muromonab-CD3 administration. Fluid volume excess is a contraindication for the drug because of the risk of life-threatening pulmonary edema if this drug is administered.

The most significant drug interactions for which the client's current drug regimen should be reviewed occur with other immunosuppressant agents and live virus vaccines.

See the drug interactions listed for azathioprine for a description of these interactions.

Nursing diagnosis. The client receiving muromonab-CD3 has the potential for the following nursing diagnoses in addition to the ones cited in the general nursing management of immunosuppressed clients: hyperthermia, risk for injury related to first-dose reaction (chest pain, diarrhea, dizziness, fever and chills, nausea and vomiting, tachycardia, dyspnea, tremors); and the potential complication of aseptic meningitis syndrome, pulmonary edema, and encephalopathy.

Implementation

Monitoring. Monitor the client's temperature frequently for several hours after administration, especially with the first two doses. A first-dose reaction may occur evidenced by the symptoms listed above. These symptoms occur in most clients 30 minutes to 6 hours after the first dose and may last several hours. They may occur to a lesser extent after the second dose but rarely occur after that. Fever and chills occurring later in therapy may be caused by infection. The client should be assessed also for headache, stiff neck, and photosensitivity because aseptic meningitis syndrome may occur in the first 3 days of therapy. CBCs should be monitored periodically throughout the course of treatment.

Observe the client for fluid volume excess: auscultate the lungs, check for peripheral edema, monitor daily weights, and monitor fluid intake and output. Monitor vital signs. Observe for signs of infection.

Intervention. Cardiopulmonary resuscitation equipment and medications should be immediately available during the administration of the first dose. Muromonab-CD3 should be administered by intravenous push over a period of less than 1 minute by a health care provider who is experienced in immunosuppressive therapy.

Methylprednisolone may be administered intravenously before the first dose to minimize first-dose reaction. IV methyprednisolone (1 mg/kg of body weight) may be administered before to the first dose. Intravenous hydrocortisone sodium succinate may be given 30 minutes after the first and possibly the second dose for the same reason. Antihistamines may also be used to minimize first-dose reaction. The client's temperature should be maintained below 37.8° C (100° F) with acetaminophen.

Muromonab-CD3 is prepared for intravenous administration by drawing the solution through a low protein-binding 0.2- or 0.22-µm filter, then discarding the filter and attaching the appropriate needle for administration. The drug is not administered by intravenous infusion or with other solutions.

Education. The client should be prepared for the possibility of first-dose reaction and asked to report any of the adverse signs and symptoms of that reaction or of aseptic meningitis syndrome.

Evaluation. The client receiving muromonab-CD3 therapy will not experience organ rejection.

mycophenolate mofetil [mye koe fee' noe late moe' fe tyl] (CellCept)

Mycophenolate used in conjunction with cyclosporine and corticosteroids is indicated for the prophylaxis of renal transplant rejection. Mycophenolate is metabolized to MPA, an active metabolite that inhibits the response of T- and B-lymphocytes to mitogenic and allospecific stimulation. Therefore this drug has a cytostatic effect on lymphocytes. It also suppresses antibody formation by B-lymphocytes and may inhibit the influx of leukocytes into inflammatory and graft rejection sites.

Available orally, it is rapidly metabolized to the active metabolite, MPA and other inactive metabolites. MPA half-life is 18 hours with excretion primarily in the kidneys.

Major side-adverse effects of mycophenolate include diarrhea, vomiting, and respiratory infections (leukopenia, sepsis). Peripheral edema, urinary tract infections, anemia, hypertension, and abdominal pain are also reported.

Oral dose administered within 3 days of transplantation is 1 g twice a day with cyclosporine and corticosteroids.

■ Nursing Management

Mycophenolate Therapy

In addition to the general nursing management of the immunosuppressed client (p. 998), clients receiving mycophenolate therapy require the following nursing care.

Assessment. It is essential to assess exposure to or presence of infection. Any infection that the client might have may become life-threatening with the administration of mycophenolate. The drug is contraindicated in clients with a hypersensitivity to the drug. Caution should also be used with clients with serious pathology of the gastrointestinal tract or history of ulcer disease or GI bleeding. Clients with renal function impairment will have reduced excretion of the drug with increased risk of mycophenolate toxicity; dosages may need to be reduced.

Complete blood cell counts and electrolytes should be determined before therapy is initiated. Baseline renal and hepatic function studies should be obtained.

Review the client's current medication regimen. Significant drug interactions may occur when mycophenolate is given, such as with the following drugs:

Drug	Possible effect and management
immunosuppressant agents, other (azathioprine, glucocorticoids, cyclophosphamide, cyclosporine)	May increase the risk for developing infections and/or neoplasms.
acyclovir (Zovirax), ganciclovir (Cytovene)	**These drugs compete with mycophenolate for renal excretion and may increase each others toxicity. Avoid or a potentially serious drug interaction may occur.**
antacids (magnesium and aluminum hydroxide); cholestyramine (Questran), colestipol (Colestid)	These drugs decrease the absorption of mycophenolate. Administer mycophenolate 1 hour before or 2 hours after antacids and bile acid sequestrants.

Continued

Drug	Possible effect and management
vaccines, live virus	**Immunization with live vaccines should be postponed in persons receiving this drug and also in close family members. The use of a live virus vaccine in immunosuppressed clients may result in increased replication of the vaccine virus, may increase side effects/adverse reactions to the vaccine virus, and possibly cause a decrease in the client's antibody response to the vaccine.**

Nursing diagnosis. Clients receiving mycophenolate may experience the following nursing diagnoses/collaborative problems: altered bowel elimination (diarrhea); altered protection related to leukopenia; risk of infection; and the potential complications of GI bleeding and increased risk of malignancy.

Implementation

Monitoring. Complete blood counts should be done weekly during the first month, twice a month for the next 2 to 3 months, and monthly thereafter. Notify the prescriber if the absolute neutrophil count is less than 100,000/mm^3. Renal and hepatic function studies and electrolytes should be monitored periodically during therapy. Increased alkaline phosphatase, bilirubin, SGOT (AST), SGPT (ALT), and amylase concentrations may indicate hepatotoxicity. Increased serum creatinine may occur, as well as, hyper- or hypocalcemia, hyperuricemia, hypoglycemia, hypoproteinemia, and hyperlipidemia.

Intervention. Mycophenolate is given within 72 hours of transplantation. Administer oral doses on an empty stomach, 1 hour before or 2 hour after meals. Capsules should be swallowed whole, not opened, crushed, or chewed.

Education. Female clients who are of childbearing age need to practice two reliable forms of contraception or abstinence, during the course of therapy and for 6 weeks following the end of therapy.

Instruct the client to take mycophenolate as directed. Stress the need for lifelong therapy to prevent transplant rejection. Emphasize the need to seek medical attention if symptoms of organ rejection occur. Advise avoiding others with infectious diseases. Encourage the client not to take other medications without consulting with the prescriber and to maintain followup appointments for lab work and clinical monitoring.

Evaluation. The client's transplant will not be rejected and the client will be able to effectively manage the therapeutic regimen.

tacrolimus [tak roe lye' mus] (FK506, Prograf)

Tacrolimus in conjunction with corticosteroids, is indicated for the prophylaxis of organ (liver) rejection. It inhibits activation of T-lymphocytes and although its exact mechanism of action is unknown, it is believed to bind to FKBP-12 protein and form complexes that prevent T-lymphocyte activation.

It is available orally and parenterally. Oral absorption is variable reaching a peak blood level in 1.5 to 3.5 hours. It is metabolized in the liver (primarily by the cytochrome P-450 system) to a number of metabolites including several active ones; less than 1% is excreted in the urine.

Major side-adverse effects of tacrolimus include headaches, tremors, diarrhea, hypertension, nausea, and renal dysfunction. Hyperkalemia, hypomagnesemia, and hyperuricemia have also been reported. Hyperglycemia has been reported that has required insulin therapy (Olin, 1996).

By IV infusion, the adult dose is 0.05-1 mg/kg/day, converted to oral as soon as possible, usually in 2 to 3 days of therapy. Initial oral adult dose is 0.15-0.3/mg/kg/day. Adults are usually started at the lower dose range while children need and tolerate a higher dose of this product.

▪ Nursing Management

Tacrolimus Therapy

In addition to the nursing management of the immunosuppressed client (p. 998), the following nursing considerations are recommended.

Assessment. Tacrolimus use is contraindicated with clients with hypersensitivity to the drug or to HCO-60 polyoxyl hydrogenated castor oil (contained in the injection solution). Use the drug cautiously with clients with renal and hepatic impairment.

Review the client's current drug regimen for potential drug interactions, such as:

Drug	Possible effect and management
aminoglycoside antiinfectives, amphotericin B (Fungizone), cisplatin (Platinol), or cyclosporine (Sandimmune)	Concurrent use increases the risk of nephrotoxicity. Allow 24 hrs to pass after discontinuing cyclosporine before starting tacrolimus. Monitor renal function studies carefully.
ACE inhibitors, potassium-sparing diuretics	Concurrent use increases risk of hyperkalemia. Monitor serum potassium levels.
antifungals, bromocriptine (Parlodel), calcium channel blockers, cimetidine (Tagamet), clarithromycin (Biaxin), cyclosporine (Sandimmune), danazol (Danocrine), erythromycin, methylprednisolone, metoclopramide (Reglan)	Concurrent use increases tacrolimus blood levels. Observe client for symptoms of toxicity.
phenobarbital, phenytoin (Dilantin), carbamazepine (Tegretol), rifamycins	Concurrent use decreases tacrolimus blood levels. Monitor tacrolimus blood levels frequently. Dosage adjustments may be necessary.
vaccines, live	**Avoid concurrent use. Other than live vaccines may be less effective if given concurrently.**

A baseline assessment should include serum creatinine, serum electrolytes, CBC, and platelet count. The client's clinical status should be documented.

Nursing diagnosis. The client receiving tacrolimus may experience the following nursing diagnoses/collaborative problems: altered comfort (headache, abdominal pain, generalized aches); impaired skin integrity (rash, pruritus); sleep pattern disturbance (insomnia); fluid volume deficit related to anorexia, nausea and vomiting; altered protection related to anemia, leukopenia, and thrombocytopenia; and the potential problems of nephrotoxicity (hypertension, peripheral edema, ascites), neurotoxicity (paresthesia, tremor, neuropathy, seizures), GI bleeding, lymphoma, and electrolyte imbalances (hyperglycemia, hyperkalemia, hypomagnesemia).

Implementation

Monitoring. Observe client for hypersensitivity response for at least 30 minutes after IV tacrolimus and frequently thereafter. Monitor BP closely during therapy. Monitor CBCs and platelet counts, serum electrolytes, serum creatinine levels, and tacrolimus blood levels. Assess client for symptoms of nursing diagnoses above. Monitor pediatric clients closely because higher doses are necessary to maintain adequate blood levels.

Intervention. Tacrolimus therapy should be initiated no sooner than 6 hours after transplant. Concurrent glucocorticoid therapy may occur. Intravenous administration is by continuous infusion over 24 hours. The client should be changed to oral administration of tacrolimus as soon as possible to reduce the risk of adverse reactions to IV tacrolimus, usually 8 to 12 hours after the last IV dosing.

Education. Instruct the client to take tacrolimus at the same time each day and as directed, emphasizing need for lifelong therapy to prevent rejection. Inform the client of symptoms of organ rejection and the need to seek medical attention at once if they occur. Reinforce the importance of keeping appointments for lab work and followup care. Advise clients of child bearing potential of the risks of taking tacrolimus while pregnant and instruct on contraception as needed.

Evaluation. The client on tacrolimus therapy will not experience transplanted organ rejection.

IMMUNOMODULATING AGENTS

Biotechnology refers to the development of new agents that can either activate the body's immune defenses or modify a biologic response to an unwanted stimulus, such as an antitumor response. These agents are called **immunomodulating agents.** With the advent of recombinant DNA technology in the early 1980s, new agents were made available in larger quantities for clinical trials and investigations. Although still in its infancy, this area of study has the potential for solving some of the mysteries about disease that have eluded researchers for centuries and may also provide pharmaceuticals that control the devastation, pain, and suffering induced by many viral diseases, AIDS, and cancer.

Acquired Immunodeficiency Syndrome

A pathogenic retrovirus known as **human immunodeficiency virus (HIV)** is the etiologic agent in **acquired immunodeficiency syndrome (AIDS)** (Box 64-1). In 1992, HIV infection was the leading cause of death in men and the fourth leading cause of death in women, between the ages of 25 and 44 years old. In AIDS reported deaths between 1981 and 1993, more than 50% were associated with homosexual activity while 24% was secondary to contaminated IV drug paraphernalia.

While the early spread of HIV disease was primarily among homosexual men, IV drug abusers, and in persons receiving contaminated blood products, in the last few years disease progression in these populations has declined while an increased incidence has been reported in heterosexuals, especially females and infants. Most of the pediatric AIDS cases were due to perinatal transmission. Although AIDS can affect all racial groups, current statistics indicate that the epidemiology of pediatric cases is much more common in black and Hispanic children, than in Caucasian (Morse, Shelton, & O'Donnell, 1996).

The HIV virus is transmitted sexually, via blood and blood products, or from a mother with AIDS to her child during birth. Commercial blood transfusion transmission is considered rare today but transmission via IV drug abusers is still very common. Current evidence indicates that the AIDS virus is not transmitted by shaking hands, hugging, social kissing, coughing, sneezing, or sharing meals. It is also not contracted from swimming pools, toilet seats, hot tubs, dishes, or via food prepared by persons infected with the AIDS virus. HIV is transmitted by intimate contact with the body fluids of an infected person, which can occur through sex, sharing of contaminated needles and syringes (drug addicts), blood or blood product transfusions, and from mother to child, before, during, or shortly after birth.

Because health care workers with documented invasive exposure to the HIV virus may test positive for the HIV antibody, the Centers for Disease Control and Prevention (CDC) has issued guidelines for health care workers to follow so as to minimize the possibility of virus exposure and transfer (Tartaglione et al, 1993).

Because there is no known cure for AIDS at this time; teaching should focus on disease prevention.

HIV Life Cycle

Although the pathogenesis of AIDS is not fully understood, HIV is an intracellular infection that primarily infests CD4 T lymphocytes. The virus is a retrovirus that has RNA in its core; therefore after it binds to CD4+ T-lymphocyte receptor cells in the body, it releases its RNA into the cytoplasm. It also has the potential of infecting monocytes and macrophages. Reverse transcriptase, an enzyme carried by HIV, assists in transcribing the HIV RNA into viral DNA strands in the host body. Thereafter, activation of this DNA will result in production of viral substances that infect other CD4+ T-lymphocyte cells leading to the eventual loss of functioning CD4 lymphocytes.

BOX 64-1

AIDS Overview

Human Immunodeficiency Virus (HIV)

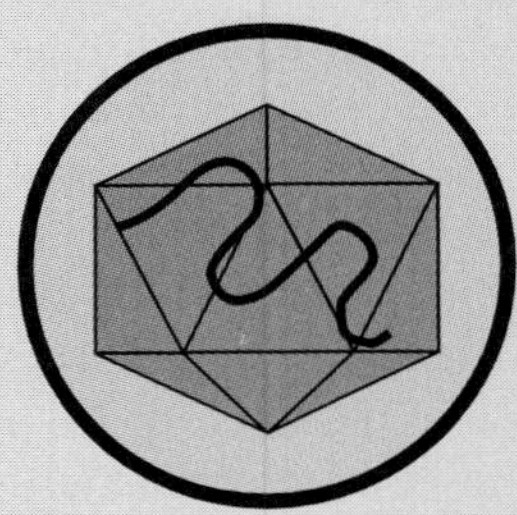

T cell and macrophage infiltration and destruction

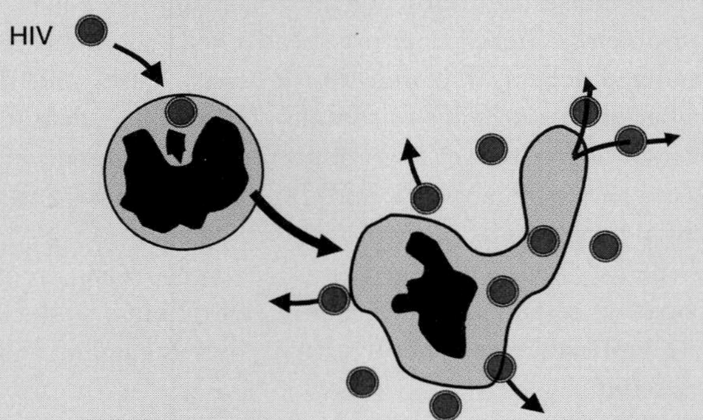

HIV virus enters T cells and macrophages, which, ironically, are the cells the body sent to destroy the virus. By reproduction the virus eventually kills them.

AIDS has no cure. Note that:
- The HIV reproduces faster than any other virus.
- It is present in the bloodstream in very small amounts; thus it is currently hard to target with medications.

AIDS has been diagnosed in:
- All races
- Men, women, and children
- Homosexuals and heterosexuals

AIDS in the Elderly:
- 10% of cases are persons over 50 years old; in 1992, 10,000 were over 60 years old.
- Majority of clients between the ages of from 50 to 59 are homosexual/bisexual; older persons were infected by blood transfusions.
- Older clients diagnosed with AIDS have much shorter lifespans after diagnosis than younger persons.
- Nearly 50% of all elderly clients with AIDS develop symptoms of dementia (personality changes, impaired concentration, apathy, etc. [Cowan, 1993]).

AIDS may be acquired by:
- Intravenous drug use with an infected or contaminated needle.
- Sexual contact with an infected person. The virus is transmitted in blood products, semen, breast milk, and vaginal secretions. A small tear in the rectum lining or in the vagina can provide an entrance for the virus.
- AIDS can be transmitted during birth or during breast feeding, if the mother is AIDS infected.
- HIV-infected persons are not always sick, but they can still transmit the AIDS virus.

Client Counseling:

To reduce the possibility of infection:
- Allow no exchange of body fluids
- Do not share needles
- Recommend use of latex condoms or nonoxynol-9 cream with a condom

Symptoms of HIV infection:
- Fever
- Chills
- Skin rash
- Sore or aching muscles
- Enlarged glands
- Headache
- Weight loss
- Women: chronic vaginal infections; may not present with fever, chills, or loss of weight

The CD4+ helper cells destroyed by the virus, eventually leads to the immunodeficiency disease known as AIDS. The CD4+ cells are needed directly and indirectly for proper functioning of the human immune system. Both the humoral immune response, which involves antibodies produced by B lymphocytes, and the cellular immune response involving stimulation of the cytotoxic T cells (or T8 cells), are mediated by the helper-inducer T cells (Wong, 1993). Therefore a severe decline or destruction of CD4 cells by the HIV is responsible for the multiple symptoms of AIDS—severe suppression of the immune system leading to opportunistic infections and cancers. See Box 64-2 for functions of a T4 helper cell and Figure 64-2 for T-cell effects in the body.

The revised CDC classification for HIV infection emphasizes the importance of the CD4+ T-lymphocyte count. The system includes all symptomatic and asymptomatic persons with a CD4 count <200 CD4+ T-lymphocytes/µl or a CD4+ T-lymphocyte percentage of total lymphocytes of <14. This expanded definition has been estimated to result in an increased number of AIDS cases reported initially, thus allowing for better surveillance and earlier interventions for this devastating disease state. Three clinical conditions, pul-

BOX 64-2

Functions of a T4 Helper Cell

T4 cells are responsible for a variety of immune functions, some of which include:

1. Release of colony-stimulating factors and lymphokines to stimulate production of leukocytes, such as macrophages and eosinophils.
2. Activation of the natural killer cells (cytotoxic NK cells), which are large lymphocytes in the blood that have non-antigen–specific antitumor and antibacterial properties.
3. T4 helper-inducer cells can activate the T8 suppressor cells, which will stop antibody production, or the T4 suppressor-inducers can activate T8 cytotoxic T cells and stimulate B cells to increase production of antibodies.

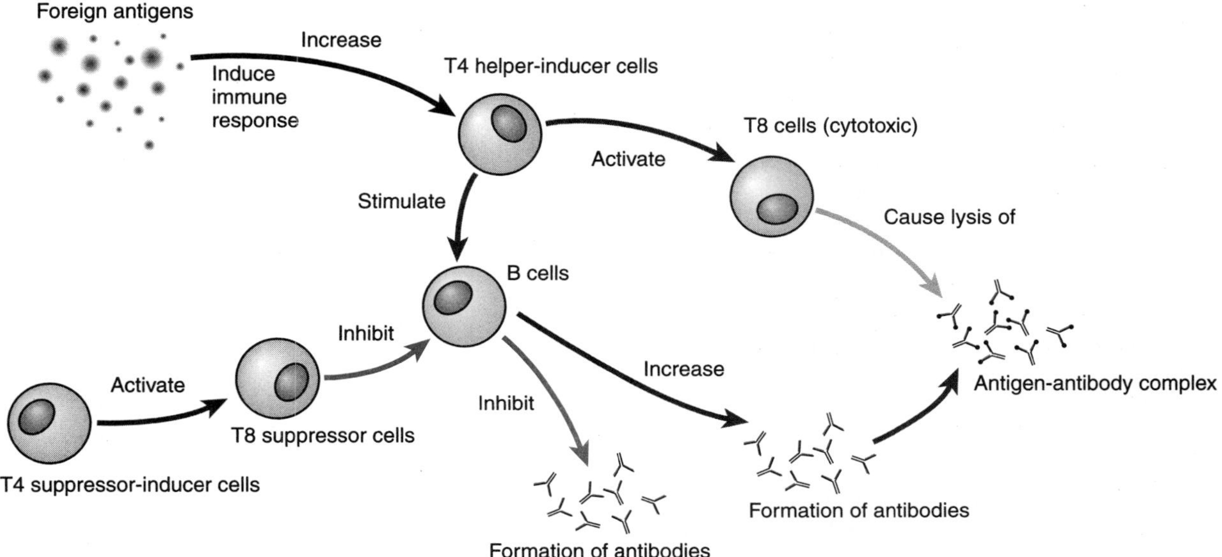

Figure 64-2 T4 cell effects in the body. T4 cells are mainly the helper-inducer type of cells. They increase when antigens are present. T4 suppressor-inducer cells do not respond to antigens. They indirectly act to suppress antibody formation.

monary tuberculosis, recurrent pneumonia, and invasive cervical cancer have also been added to the previous identified AIDS conditions (CDC, 1992) (Table 64-1).

As CD4+ T-lymphocytes decline, the risk and severity of opportunistic infections increases; therefore the utilization of this system helps to identify persons in need of close medical attention. Instituting antiviral therapy and antimicrobial prophylaxis in correlation with HIV immunosuppression levels as measured by the CD4+ T-lymphocytes has slowed the rate of progression from HIV status to AIDS-defined clinical conditions (CDC, 1992). Zidovudine (AZT) was the first antiretroviral agent for treatment of AIDS but mutations of HIV have developed that resulted in resistance to this drug. The second class of antiretrovirals, the protease inhibitors, includes ritonavir (Norvir), indinavir (Crixivan), and saquinavir (Invirase).

Ongoing trials with drug combinations (such as AZT and saquinavir or AZT/ddC and a protease inhibitor) appear to be more effective than the individual drugs alone and may help to delay resistance to the individual agents. The results of the investigational trials are still pending (Henahan, 1995; Gilden, 1996), although difficult questions about individual protease inhibitor's efficacy, when to use, costs, potential adverse effects and drug interactions are still in the discovery phase (Gilden, 1996; Project Inform, 1996).

The prognosis of HIV disease is variable with some persons remaining in a fairly stable state for many years. But in the later stages the breakdown in cellular immunity results in the development of opportunistic infections in the body. (See Table 64-2 for Drugs of Choice for AIDS-related Infections.) In advanced stages of AIDS most clients usually have a very low helper T-cell count and usually, the majority die within a few years. Box 64-3 discusses the most common opportunistic infection, *Pneumocystis carinii* pneumonia (PCP). For further analysis, see the case study on p. 1010.

Immunotherapy

Lymphokines (interleukins 1 and 2), interferons (primarily alpha) and granulocyte or granulocyte-macrophage colony-stimulating factors (G-CSF or filgrastim [Neupogen] or

Text continued on p. 1010

TABLE 64-1 1992 Revised criteria for HIV classification and AIDS surveillance*

Clinical categories	CD4 + T-cell categories ≥500/µl	200-499/µl	<200/µl
A. Asymptomatic HIV infection or persistent generalized lymphadenopathy or acute HIV infection with	A1	A2	A3
B. Symptomatic conditions due to HIV infection not in C, i.e.	B1	B2	B3
Bacillary angiomatosis			
Candidiasis, oropharyngeal			
Candidiasis, vulvovaginal (persistent, responds poorly to treatment)			
Cervical dysplasia			
Fever (38.5° C) or diarrhea lasting > 1 month			
Hairy oral leukoplakia			
Herpes zoster, 2 distinct episodes			
Idiopathic thrombocytopenic purpura			
Listeriosis			
Pelvic inflammatory disease (PID)			
Peripheral neuropathy			
C. AIDS Indicators	C1	C2	C3
Candidiasis of bronchi, trachea, or lungs			
Candidiasis, esophageal			
Cervical cancer, invasive			
Coccidioidomycosis, disseminated or extrapulmonary			
Cryptococcosis, extrapulmonary			
Cryptosporidiosis, chronic, intestinal (>1 month)			
Cytomegalovirus disease (other than liver, spleen, or nodes)			
Cytomegalovirus retinitis (with vision loss)			
Encephalopathy, HIV related			
Herpes simplex: chronic ulcer(s) (>1 month); or bronchitis, pneumonitis or esophagitis			
Histoplasmosis, disseminated or extrapulmonary			
Isosporiasis, chronic intestinal (>1 month)			
Kaposi's sarcoma			
Lymphoma, Burkitt's, immunoblastic, or primary of brain			
Mycobacterium avium complex or *M. kansasii*, disseminated or extrapulmonary			
Mycobacterium tuberculosis, any site			
Mycobacterium other species, disseminated or extrapulmonary			
Pneumocystis carinii pneumonia			
Pneumonia, recurrent			
Progressive multifocal leukoencephalopathy			
Salmonella septicemia, recurrent			
Toxoplasmosis of brain			
Wasting syndrome due to HIV			

**MMWR* (1992) criteria for persons 13 years or older with 2 or more positive tests for HIV antibodies in addition to a specific antibody supplemental test (e.g., Western blot, immunofluorescence assay), virus isolation test, HIV antigen detection, or positive results from any other highly specific licensed HIV test.

The 1993 revised classification system for HIV infection and AIDS surveillance includes the classifications A, B, and C plus numbers 1, 2, or 3. Categories A, B, and C are described under the clinical categories, whereas A3, B3, C1, C2, and C3 are AIDS-indicator conditions. The numbered letters refer to the CD4+ T-cell counts (*MMWR*, 1992).

TABLE 64-2 Drugs of choice for AIDS-related infections

AIDS-related infections	Syndrome	Drugs
Fungal infections		
candidiasis (oral thrush)	presents as white plaque type lesions on sides of tongue; may present as sore throat, difficulty swallowing, and pain near sternum	nystatin suspension, troches or clotrimazole (Mycelex) or ketoconazole (Nizoral)
cryptococcus meningitis	headache, fever, nausea, vomiting, photophobia, stiff neck, seizures, and mental status changes	amphotericin B plus flucytosine
Viral infections		
cytomegalovirus (CMV)	serious infection; can be life-threatening; affects eyes (can cause blindness), CNS, lungs, and GI tract	ganciclovir (Cytovene) and foscarnet (Foscavir)
herpes simplex virus (HSV)	persistent or recurrent disseminated skin ulceration; encephalitis, perioral, and perianal lesions may occur	acyclovir (Zovirax) or vidarabine (Vira-A)
Mycobacterial infections		
mycobacterium avium complex (MAC)	common infection in AIDS; may be asymptomatic or symptomatic with GI symptoms, fever, weight loss, anemia	multi-drug therapy with drugs listed under TB; disseminated form: clarithromycin or in disseminated type infection; azithromycin in combination with other drugs
mycobacterium tuberculosis	pulmonary and extrapulmonary tuberculosis seen in this population	multi-drug therapy with isoniazid, pyrazinamide, rifampin, and ethambutol
Protozoal infections		
Pneumocystis carinii pneumonia (PCP)	see Box 64-3	
toxoplasmosis	encephalitis, brain abscess, focal neurologic problems, seizures, headaches, lethargy	sulfadiazine plus pyrimethamine

BOX 64-3

Pneumocystis carinii pneumonia (PCP)

Pneumocystis carinii pneumonia is a common infection in persons with bone marrow transplants and AIDS. Untreated PCP has a high mortality rate.

Symptoms

Fever; dry, persistent, nonproductive cough; shallow breathing; progressive shortness of breath; weight loss; night sweats.

Treatment

Active infection

TMP-SMX*, IV or PO: 15 to 20 mg TMP/kg/day and 75 to 100 mg/kg/day SMX in 4 divided doses for 2 to 3 weeks.
Pentamidine IV (Pentam 300): 4 mg/kg/day administered over 60 to 90 minutes for 2 to 3 weeks.
Atovaquone (Mepron): 750 mg every 8 hours for 3 weeks.
Trimetrexate (Neutrexin), a dihydrofolate reductase inhibitor: 45 mg/m^2 every 6 hours for 3 weeks. This product may be given with sulfadiazine: 1 g every 6 hours for 3 weeks.

Prophylaxis

TMP-SMX PO: 160 mg TMP with 800 mg SMX daily twice a day or three times a week (Morse, Shelton, & O'-Donnell, 1996).
Pentamidine inhalation (NebuPent): 300 mg once a month (Olin, 1996).

*TMP-SMX, trimethoprim-sulfamethoxazole (Co-Trimoxazole).

Case Study
Home Treatment of the Client with AIDS

Robbie Parks is a 21-year-old construction worker. He has a history of heroin abuse. He had been experiencing fever, weight loss, and diarrhea and has been diagnosed as having AIDS. At this time he has a low-grade fever, severe diarrhea, and a productive cough. He is admitted to the hospital with *Pneumocystis carinii* pneumonia. While he is hospitalized he develops systemic candidiasis. He is treated symptomatically, the symptoms, resolve somewhat, and he is discharged. He is sent home on fluconazole (Diflucan) 400 mg IV qd the first day and then 200 mg IV qd for the following 4 weeks.

1. Describe the postulated mechanism of action for fluconazole.
2. What side effects of the medication should this client be taught to look for?
3. What substance has the potential for interaction with the drug?
4. Robbie's symptoms have completely resolved, and he wonders how much longer he must receive the drug. What should you tell him?

GM-CSF-Leukine, [Leucomax]) are under investigation to help the compromised immune system. Lymphokines are protein substances released by sensitized lymphocytes when in contact with specific antigens to activate macrophages to stimulate humoral and cellular immunity for the host. Interleukins have been called the chemical messengers of immune cell communication. Interleukin-2 is believed to be a T-cell growth factor that promotes the long-term survival and growth of the T lymphocytes, which is necessary for the continuation of the immune response and is also involved in the rejection of transplanted organs. While some persons have been helped with these therapies, to date the data on their effectiveness is conflicting and at least in some instances, required adjuvant therapies (Morse, Shelton, & O'Donnell, 1996).

■ Nursing Management

Colony Stimulating Factors (CSF) Therapy

In addition to the general nursing management of the immunosuppressed client (p. 998), clients receiving filgrastim (as an example of immunomodulator therapy) require the following nursing care:

Assessment. Because CSF therapy is used in clients with serious underlying disease and because many adverse effects that have been reported in clients receiving the drug also occur in clients not receiving the drug, a causal relationship between the drug and the adverse effects is not clear. A complete baseline assessment should be done with the client to facilitate the monitoring of any change in signs and symptoms that may occur.

If the client has excessive leukemic myeloid blasts in the bone marrow or peripheral blood (10% or more) more growth may be stimulated by CSF agents. For filgrastin, sensitivity to *E. coli*-derived proteins must be determined; with sargramostin, sensitivity to yeast-derived proteins.

Nursing diagnosis. The client receiving CSF agents is at risk for the following nursing diagnoses: altered comfort (pain at injection site, headache, arthralgias, myalgias [first-dose reaction for sargramostin]); impaired tissue integrity (thrombophlebitis at infusion site) and the potential complications of allergic reaction, arrhythmias, and pericarditis.

Implementation

Monitoring. CBCs and platelet counts should be performed twice weekly. CSF therapy is usually discontinued if the absolute neutrophil count (ANC) exceeds 10,000/mm^3. Be alert to the development of adult respiratory syndrome. Check the client's blood pressure because a transient hypotension may occur. Monitor the client's general health status to provide for supportive care.

Intervention. If administered to a client receiving chemotherapy, immunomodulator therapy is usually begun at least 24 hours after the last dose of chemotherapy and is discontinued at least 24 hours before the next dose of chemotherapy.

Examine the vial to ensure that the solution is clear and does not contain particulate matter. Do not shake the vial. Keep the medication refrigerated, although it is stable for 24 hours at room temperature.

Education. If it is determined that the client or caregiver can safely and effectively administer the drug in the home, they should be given the client information supplied by the manufacturer. They should also receive instructions on the proper dosage and administration of the drug, including aseptic technique. Instruction should be provided on the proper safe disposal of needles, syringes, and any unused drug.

Evaluation. The client's ANC will exceed 10,000/ mm^3. The client or caregiver will effectively manage the therapeutic regimen.

SUMMARY

Immunosuppressants and immunomodulators are relatively new products that are used to lessen or modify an immune system response. Research is extensive, and many new pharmacologic products are likely to be developed in the next few years. Nursing management centers on careful medical asepsis, proper diet and oral hygiene, and prevention of infection. As new drugs continue to be introduced, the nurse's role in this important new therapy is likely to continue to expand.

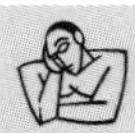

Critical Thinking

1. Susan Goode, age 35, has just received a kidney transplant. Her physician has prescribed cyclosporine 15 mg/kg PO daily. What is the mechanism of action by which cyclosporine prevents transplant rejection? What nursing care is required to support Susan's cyclosporine regimen?
2. Herman Myers, age 45, is receiving cyclic antineoplastic chemotherapy. He has been prescribed filgrastim to combat his chemotherapy-induced neutropenia. What is special about the timing of the administration of the two medications? Why is that timing important?

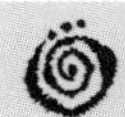

Collaborative Learning Activities

1. Student teams will discuss the nursing management of immunosuppressed clients. Each team will discuss a nursing diagnosis with its associated monitoring, intervention, client education, and evaluation.

BIBLIOGRAPHY

American Hospital Formulary Service (1996). *AHFS drug information '96*. Bethesda, MD: American Society of Hospital Pharmacists.

Anderson KN, et al. (Eds.) (1994). *Mosby's medical, nursing, & allied health dictionary* (4th ed.). St Louis: Mosby.

Centers for Disease Control and Prevention (CDC) (1992). 1993 revised classification for HIV infection and expanded surveillance case definition for AIDS among adolescents and adults, *MMWR* 41(RR-17):1.

Cowan K (1993). AIDS in the elderly, *Geriatr Med Curr* 14(1):4.

Gilden D (1996). Protease inhibitor new math, *GMHC Treat Iss: Newslet Experimen AIDS Therap* 10(5):3-6.

Henahan S (1995). Resistance fighters, *Drug Top* 139(16):32-33.

Jahansouz F & Kriett JM (1993). Transplantation: A review of immunosuppressive agents, *Crit Care Nurs Q* 15(4):13-22.

Morse GD, Shelton MJ, & O'Donnell AM (1996). Human immunodeficiency virus (HIV) infection. In Young LY & Koda-Kimble MA (Eds.). *Applied therapeutics* (6th ed.). Vancouver: Applied Therapeutics.

Mudge-Grout CL (1992). *Immunologic disorders*. St Louis: Mosby.

Olin BR (Ed.) (1996). *Facts and comparisons*. St Louis: Facts and Comparisons.

Project Inform (1996). The new era in AIDS treatment, *PI Perspect* 18:1-8.

Tartaglione TA, et al. (1993). Principles and management of the acquired immunodeficiency syndrome. In DiPiro JT, et al. *Pharmacotherapy* (2nd ed.). Norwalk, CT: Appleton & Lange.

United States Pharmacopeial Convention (1996). *USP DI: drug information for the health care professional* (16th ed.). Rockville, MD: The Convention.

Wong RJ (1993). Treating HIV infection: What pharmacists need to know, *Amer Pharm* NS33(5):57.

Chapter 65

Overview of the Integumentary System

Chapter Focus

The skin is the body's largest organ, forming a protective boundary between the internal environment and external world. Drugs are applied to the skin in the case of impaired skin integrity, and the skin is also being increasingly used for the administration of drugs for systemic purposes. The nurse must know the structure and function of the skin to administer drugs for both purposes. The following objectives and key terms are important for a good understanding of this chapter.

Key Terms

apocrine glands (p. 1013)
dermis (p. 1013)
eccrine glands (p. 1013)
epidermis (p. 1013)
exocrine glands (p. 1013)
melanin (p. 1013)
sebaceous glands (p. 1013)

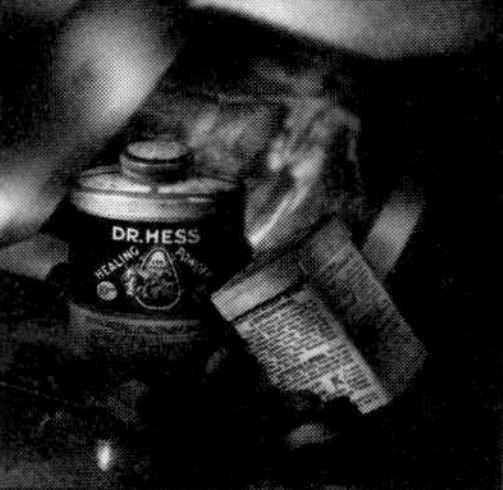

Objectives

1. Describe the two layers of the skin.
2. Differentiate between the three types of exocrine glands.
3. Explain five major functions of the skin.
4. Name three appendages of the skin.

The skin (or integument) has been described as the largest organ in the body. In most disease states, medications are administered at a site that is distant from the target organ, but in dermatology, medications can be directly applied to the target site. Because skin functions are vital to an individual's survival and also quite diverse, this chapter reviews the structure of the skin, functions of the skin, and skin appendages (Figure 65-1).

STRUCTURE OF THE SKIN

The skin is made up of two layers, the epidermis and the dermis. The **epidermis**, or outer skin layer, consists of four strata or layers:

1. Stratum corneum (horny layer)—outer dead cells that have been converted to keratin, a water-repellent protein. This layer forms a protective cover for the body; it will desquamate or shed and be replaced by new cells from the bottom layers.
2. Stratum lucidum or clear layer—this area contains translucent flat cells; keratin is formed here.
3. Stratum granulosum or granular layer—granules are located in the cytoplasm of these cells. Cells die in this layer of skin.
4. Stratum germinativum—this has been divided into two layers in some references; the top layer is the stratum spinosum, and the innermost layer is the stratum basale. The latter two names were devised to describe the cellular structure of the two layers; stratum spinosum contains spinelike cells, whereas stratum basale has column-shaped cells. The cells in the latter area germinate; they undergo cellular mitosis to generate new cells for the skin.

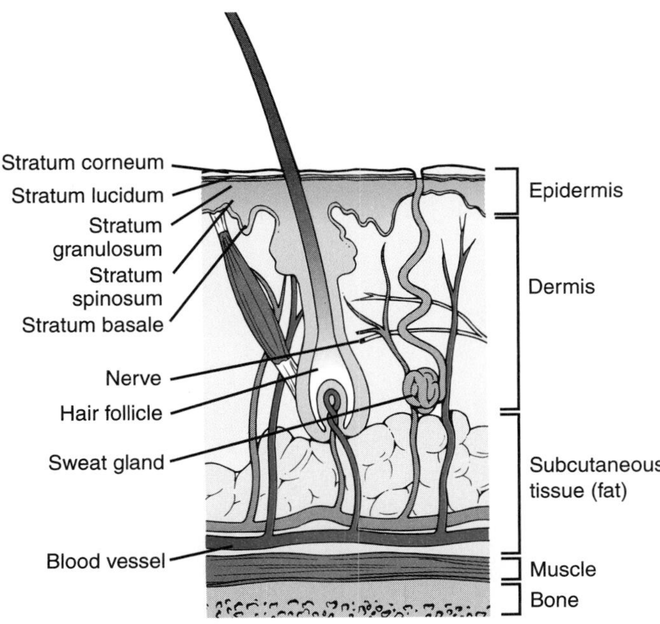

Figure 65-1 Structures of the skin.

Melanocytes, which are responsible for synthesizing **melanin**, a skin color pigment that occurs naturally in the hair and skin, are also located deep in the stratum germinativum. The more melanin that is present, the deeper the brown skin color. Melanin also is a protective agent; it blocks ultraviolet rays, thus preventing injury to underlying dermis and tissues.

The epidermis has no direct blood supply of its own; it is nourished only by diffusion. The **dermis** lies between the epidermis and subcutaneous fat. It is approximately 40 times thicker than the epidermis, and it contains and provides skin support from its blood vessels, nerves, lymphatic tissue, and elastic and connective tissues. The two main divisions of the dermis are the papillary dermis and the reticular dermis. Sweat glands, sebaceous glands, and hair follicles originate in the reticular dermis, and their structures branch out in the papillary dermis.

Below the dermis layer is the hypodermis or subcutaneous layer, which contributes flexibility to the skin. Subcutaneous fat tissue is an area for thermal insulation, nutrition, and cushioning or padding.

The skin contains three types of **exocrine glands**—sebaceous, eccrine, and apocrine. These exocrine glands are multicellular glands that open on the surface of the skin through ducts in the epithelium. **Sebaceous glands** are large, lipid-containing cells that produce sebum, the oil or film layer that covers the epidermis, especially abundant in the scalp, face, anus, and external ear. This protects and lubricates the skin, so it is not only water repellent but also has some antiseptic effects. The sebaceous fluid travels by way of a short duct (sebaceous duct) to the hair follicles in the upper dermis. Thus hair, which is located everywhere on the skin except the palms, soles, and mucous membrane tissues, is lubricated.

The **eccrine glands,** or sweat glands, are also widely distributed on the skin surface, including the soles and palms. These glands help to regulate body temperature by promoting cooling by evaporation of their secretion and also help to prevent excessive skin dryness.

The **apocrine glands** are located mainly in the axillae, genital organs, and breast areas. They are odoriferous and are believed to represent scent or sex glands.

Normal skin pH is 4.5 to 5.5, which is weakly acidic. This acid mantle is a protective mechanism because microorganisms grow best at pH 6 to 7.5. Infected areas of the skin usually have a higher pH.

FUNCTIONS OF THE SKIN

The skin serves many functions in the body. Some of the major functions are listed here:

- Protective function—The skin forms a protective covering for the entire body. It protects the internal organs and their environment from external forces. Thus it is a barrier against microorganism and chemical body invasion.
- Organ of sensation—Nerve endings permit the transfer of stimuli sensations, such as heat, cold, pressure, and pain.

- Body temperature regulator—It maintains a body temperature homeostasis by regulating heat loss or heat conservation. Blood vessels in the dermis area can dilate, and perspiration increases when the body temperature is elevated. If the body temperature is below normal, the skin blood vessels constrict and perspiration is decreased to conserve body heat.

Skin excretes fluid and electrolytes (sweat glands), stores fat, synthesizes vitamin D (when skin is exposed to sunlight or ultraviolet rays, the steroid 7-dehydrocholesterol, which is normally present in the skin, is converted to vitamin D_3), and provides a site for drug absorption. Fat-soluble vitamins (A, D, E, and K), estrogens, corticoid hormones, and some chemicals can be absorbed through skin.

Skin contributes to the concept of body image and a feeling of well-being. A disfiguring skin condition can lead to emotional problems, and a chronic skin condition may also lead to depression.

APPENDAGES OF THE SKIN

The appendages of the skin are the hair, nails, and skin glands. These areas are discussed when drug therapy is specific for these sites.

SUMMARY

The skin, the largest organ of the body, consists of two layers, the epidermis and the dermis. The pharmacologic activity of dermatologic agents occurs at the target site. Skin injuries, lesions, and disorders result in a variety of dermatologic problems for the individual and nursing care issues for the health care provider. Major skin problems are discussed in the next chapter.

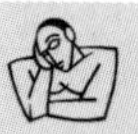

Critical Thinking

1. Johnny, age 10, is outside playing ball on a hot summer's day. How does his skin serve to regulate his body temperature?
2. In what other ways does the skin function to protect the body?

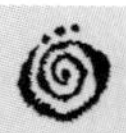

Collaborative Learning Activities

1. Two pairs of students will present the chapter's material. The first pair will illustrate the structure of the skin, and the second pair will relate the function of the structures presented by the first pair.

BIBLIOGRAPHY

Anderson KN, et al. (Eds.) (1994). *Mosby's medical, nursing, & allied health dictionary* (4th ed.). St Louis: Mosby.

DiPiro JT, et al. (1993). *Pharmacology: A pathophysiological approach.* (2nd ed.). Norwalk, CT: Appleton & Lange.

Seeley RR, Stephens TD, & Tate P (1995). *Anatomy and physiology* (3rd ed.). St Louis: Mosby.

Thibodeau GA & Patton KT (1996). *Anatomy and physiology* (3rd ed.). St Louis: Mosby.

Van Wynsberghe D, Nolack CR, & Carola R (1995). *Human anatomy and physiology* (3rd ed.). New York: McGraw-Hill.

Chapter 66

Dermatologic Drugs

Chapter Focus

The integumentary system is the largest organ system in the body. The skin performs a number of vital functions, such as protecting internal structures from mechanical and chemical damage, preventing the entry of infectious agents, providing protection against ultraviolet radiation from the sun, preventing dehydration, regulating temperature, producing vitamin D, and detecting stimuli. In addition, the skin often contributes to our definition of who we are through color, aging processes, scarring, and other conditions. Clients with skin disorders may experience body image disturbance along with their physical conditions. The nurse needs to be not only skilled at various procedures related to treatment of disorders of the skin but also sensitive to the client as a whole. The following objectives and key terms are necessary for a good understanding of this chapter.

Key Terms

ectoparasite (p. 1032)
keratolytic (p. 1027)
sun protection factor (SPF) (p. 1023)

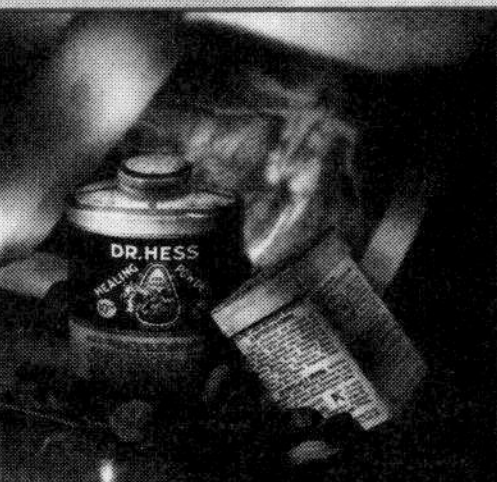

Objectives

1. State the principles of skin absorption.
2. Describe different types of lesions and some of the conditions associated with them.
3. Identify common drug-induced dermatologic conditions.
4. Identify life-threatening drug-induced skin eruptions.
5. Describe the general goals of dermatologic therapy.
6. Describe the general dermatologic preparations and their indications: baths, soaps, solutions, lotions, and cleansers.
7. Implement the nursing management of the care of clients receiving therapy with topical antiinfectives, antiinflammatory corticosteroids, topical anesthetics, and acne and burn products.
8. Discuss ectoparasitic diseases and the use of topical ectoparasiticidal drugs in their treatment.

Many dermatologic preparations are available to treat the numerous, common skin disorders. Often particular ointments, creams, powders, or specific vehicles provide a desired effect without the addition of an active ingredient. For example, for the person with dry, scaly skin found in psoriasis or dry eczema, an ointment with an occlusive emollient effect is desired, such as lanolin, or a synthetic base. The person with a moist or dry skin condition may receive a cooling emollient preparation that is also moisturizing, such as a cream formulation.

The individual with an acute inflammation that is weeping or oozing often needs a drying and soothing lotion, such as a saline solution, aluminum acetate solution, or calamine lotion. A lichenified, oozing skin problem (eczema) may need a protective and drying agent, such as coal tar paste, Lassar's paste, or zinc compound paste. If the skin problem is sore, wet and located on an elbow or knee, then a dusting powder such as talcum or starch may be appropriate to reduce friction and help dry the area.

SKIN DISORDERS

Reactions or disorders of the skin are manifested by symptoms such as itching, pain, or tingling and by signs such as swelling, redness, papules, pustules, blisters, and hives. Some common dermatologic disorders in the United States and Canada include acne vulgaris (cystic acne and acne scars), atopic dermatitis, eczema, folliculitis, fungus infections, herpes simplex, lichen simplex chronicus, psoriasis, seborrheic dermatitis, verruca (warts), and vitiligo.

A reaction of the skin that makes the individual uncomfortable or unsightly may be due to sensitivity to drugs, allergy, infection, emotional conflict, genetic disease (e.g., atopic eczema, psoriasis), hormonal imbalance, or degenerative disease. Sometimes the cause of the skin disorder is unknown and the treatment may be empiric in the hope that the right remedy will be found.

Dermatologic diagnosis includes physical assessment, personal and family medical history, drug history including OTCs, and laboratory tests cytodiagnosis, and biopsy.

When the nature of the lesion has been established, its characteristics should be defined according to size, shape, surface, and color (Box 66-1).

The next step is to discover the distribution of the condition because a diagnosis can at times be made from the distribution alone. However, it should not be inferred that because a disease is not found in its usual pattern of distribution, it can be ruled out as a possible diagnosis. For example, psoriasis is commonly found on the extensors, but occasionally it will be seen as a solitary lesion in the external ear. A basal cell carcinoma is most common on the face, but occasionally it occurs on the trunk. On the other hand, rosacea only attacks those areas of the face that flush.

Box 66-2 is a summary of the vast number of dermatologic reactions to drugs, and their characteristic lesions and sequelae. Some may even be life-threatening. See Table 66-1 for the most common drugs involved in life-threatening drug-induced skin eruptions.

The nurse always needs to be cognizant of a client's drug history and current therapy to relate such lesions and sequelae to the appropriate cause because simply discontinuing a particular drug often resolves a complicated dermatologic problem or sequelae of unknown origin.

1. Eczema and dermatitis are noninfectious inflammatory dermatoses. Contact dermatitis has clinical features that include skin rash with eczema (red, thick, crusty, fissured, suppurating area) in various stages. The causes may be from contact with a primary irritant (acids, oils, soaps) in the environment, home, or work place or from a delayed allergic reaction (as seen with poison ivy contact).
2. Atopic dermatitis appears as a general eczema dermatitis usually on the flexor body surfaces; it has genetic associations with hay fever or asthma.
3. Seborrheic dermatitis often appears on the scalp, eyebrows, ears, or sternum as a brown to red scaly rash.
4. Stasis dermatitis often preceding a venous stasis ulcer is found on the lower legs secondary to venous stasis and poor vascularity and is brown and eczematous in appearance.
5. Papulosquamous eruptions are noninfectious inflammatory dermatoses that include urticaria (hives), psoriasis, pityriasis rosea, lichen planus, and exfoliative dermatitis. The nurse will see acute urticaria as an insidious-appearing, itchy erythematous wheal resulting from an allergen. Chronic urticaria appears as a large hive without the sensation of itch or pruritus and is often accompanied by angioneurotic edema.
6. Psoriasis often appears as erythematous plaques and orange-red-brown lesions covered with silvery scales. Psoriasis is often found on the scalp and extensor surfaces of the limbs and neck. Often the nails become thick and irregular.
7. Pityriasis rosea is a self-limited oval salmon-colored patch that follows the axis of skin cleavage lines. The major patches appear on the trunk, and smaller scales appear on the peripheral areas.
8. Infectious inflammatory dermatoses include viral diseases (verruca [wart], herpes simplex, varicella zoster/chickenpox), bacterial diseases (impetigo, folliculitis, furuncle [boil]), and fungal diseases. Herpes simplex and infectious inflammatory dermatoses appear as vesicles with an inflamed base and have an incubation period of up to 2 weeks in the primary infection. Late antibody development occurs. The herpes virus Type 1 affects skin and the oral cavity while herpes virus Type 2 affects the skin of neonates and genital mucosa. The recurrent infection is a reactivation of the older infection or new infection; antibodies appear early.
9. Fungal diseases, which include tinea or dermatophytosis, appear in the following various clinical

Text continued on p. 1020

BOX 66-1

Different Types of Lesions and Some Conditions Associated with Them

Macule—flat; nonpalpable; circumscribed; less than 1 cm in diameter; brown, red, purple, white, or tan in color
Examples: Freckles; flat moles; rubella; rubeola; drug eruptions

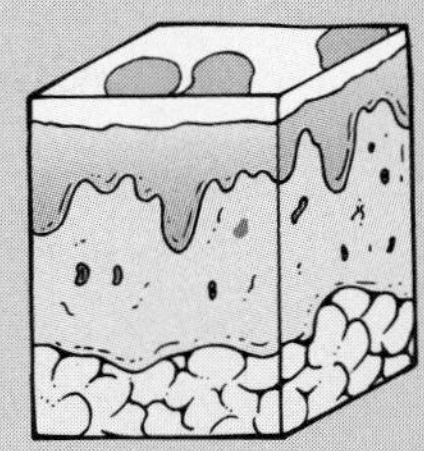

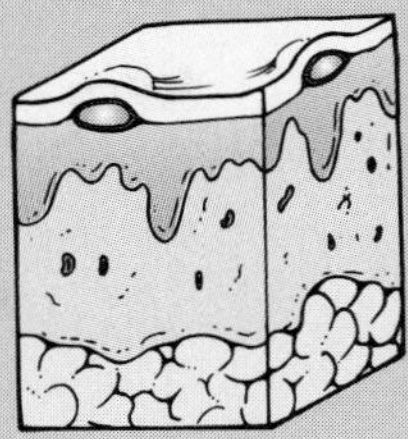

Vesicle—elevated; circumscribed; superficial; filled with serous fluid; less than 1 cm in diameter
Examples: Blister varicella

Papule—elevated; palpable; firm; circumscribed; less than 1 cm in diameter; brown, red, pink, tan, or bluish red in color
Examples: Warts; drug-related eruptions; pigmented nevi; eczema

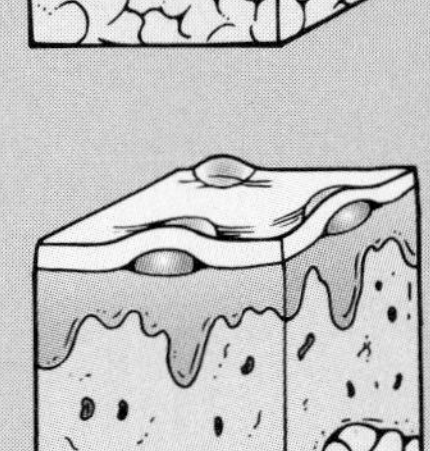

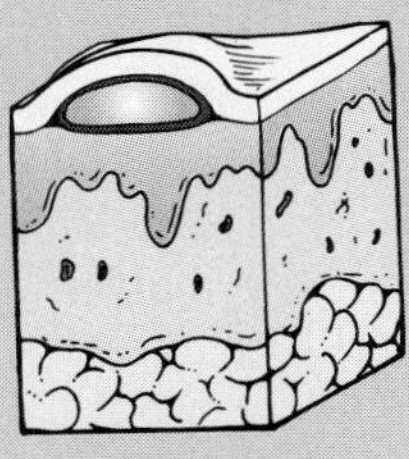

Bulla—vesicle greater than 1 cm in diameter
Examples: Blister; pemphigus vulgaris

Plaque—elevated; flat topped; firm; rough; superficial papule greater than 1 cm in diameter, may be coalesced papules
Example: Psoriasis; seborrheic and actinic keratoses; eczema

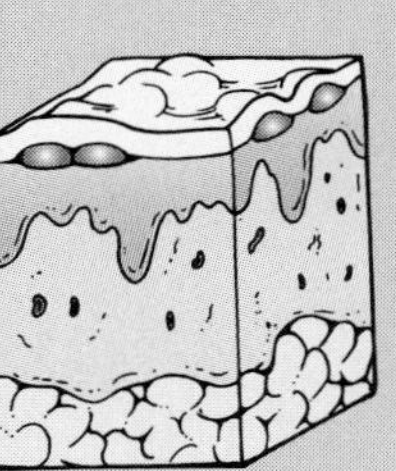

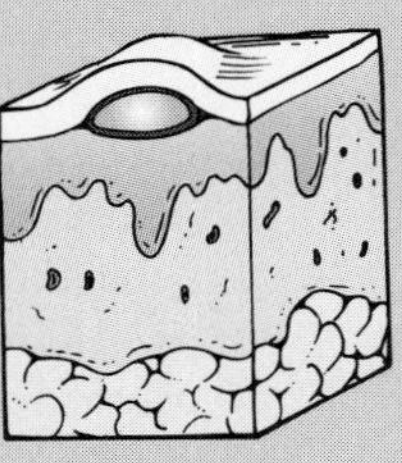

Pustule—elevated; superficial; similar to vesicle but filled with purulent fluid
Examples: Impetigo; acne; variola; herpes zoster

Wheal—elevated, irregular-shaped area of cutaneous edema; solid, transient, changing variable diameter; pale pink in color
Examples: Urticaria; insect bites

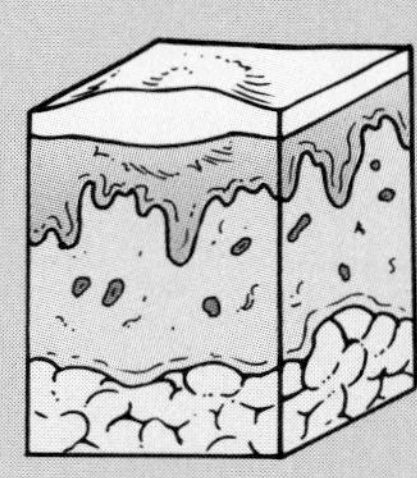

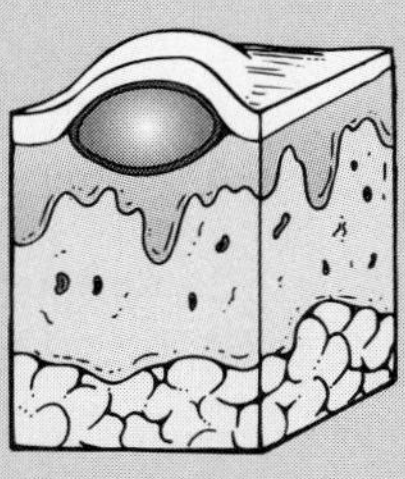

Cyst—elevated; circumscribed; palpable; encapsulated; filled with liquid or semi-solid material
Example: Sebaceous cyst

Nodule—elevated; firm; circumscribed; palpable; deeper in dermis than papule; 1 to 2 cm in diameter
Examples: Erythema nodosum; lipomas

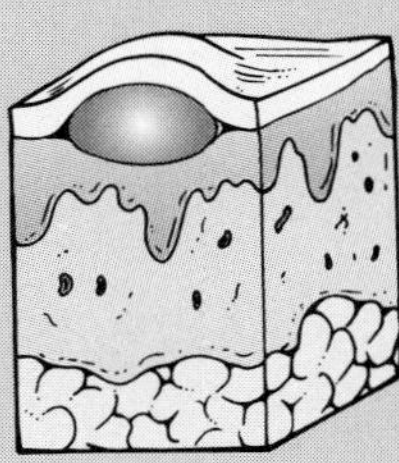

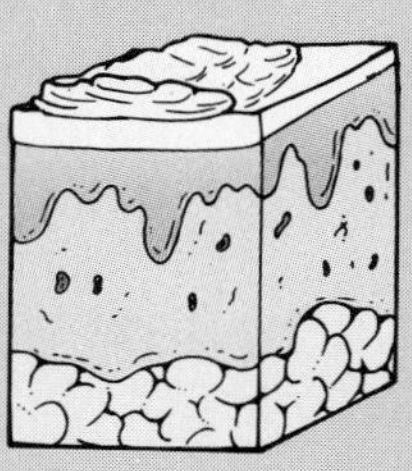

Scale—heaped-up keratinized cells; flaky exfoliation; irregular; thick or thin; dry or oily; varied size; silver, white, or tan in color
Examples: Psoriasis; exfoliative dermatitis

Tumor—elevated; solid; may or may not be clearly demarcated; greater than 2 cm in diameter; may or may not vary from skin color
Example: Neoplasms

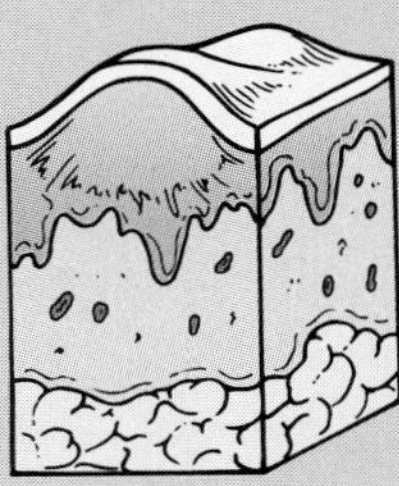

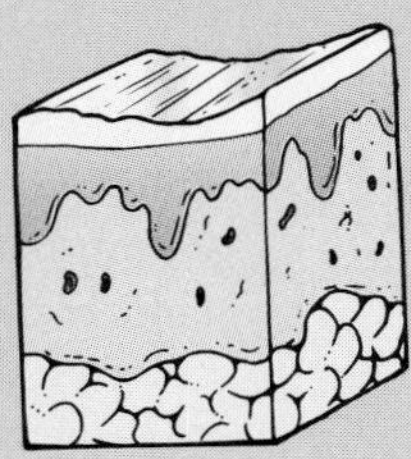

Lichenification—rough, thickened epidermis; accentuated skin markings due to rubbing or irritation; often involves flexor aspect of extremity
Example: Chronic dermatitis

From Beare PG & Myers JL (1998). *Adult health nursing* (3rd ed.) St Louis: Mosby.

BOX 66-2

Common Drug-Induced Dermatologic Conditions

Drugs causing an acneform reaction

ACTH
androgenic hormones
corticosteroids
cyanocobalamin
hydrantoins
iodides
methyltestosterone
oral contraceptives

Drugs causing purpura

ACTH
allopurinol
amitriptyline
anticoagulants
barbiturates
carbamides
chloral hydrate
chlorothiazide
chlorpropamide
chlorpromazine
corticosteroids
digitalis
fluoxymesterone
gold salts
griseofulvin
iodides
meprobamate
penicillin
quinidine
rifampin
sulfonamides
thiazides
trifluoperazine

Drugs causing urticaria

ACTH
amitriptyline
barbiturates
chloramphenicol
dextran
enzymes
erythromycin
griseofulvin
hydantoins
insulin
iodides
meperidine
meprobamate
mercurials
nitrofurantoin
opioids
penicillin
penicillinase
pentazocine
phenolphthalein
phenothiazines
propoxyphene
rifampin
salicylates
serums
streptomycin
sulfonamides
tetracyclines
thiouracil

Drugs causing alopecia

alkylating agents
anticoagulants
antimetabolites
bleomycin
mephenytoin
methimazole
methotrexate
norethindrone acetate
quinacrine
oral contraceptives
warfarin
trimethadione

Drugs causing morbilliform reactions

anticonvulsants
anticholinergics
antihistamines
barbiturates
chloral hydrate
chlordiazepoxide
chlorothiazide
gold salts
griseofulvin
hydantoins
insulin
meprobamate
mercurials
para-aminosalicylic acid
penicillin
phenothiazines
quinacrine
salicylates
serums
streptomycin
sulfonamides
sulfones
tetracyclines
thiouracil

Drugs causing lichenoid reactions

chloroquine
gold salts compounds
para-aminosalicylic acid
quinacrine
quinidine
thiazides

Drugs causing fixed eruptions

acetylsalicylic acid
amphetamine sulfate
anthralin
antipyrine
barbiturates
belladonna
bismuth salts
chloral hydrate
chloroquine
chlorothiazide and sun
chlorpromazine
chlortetracycline
dextroamphetamine
diethylstilbestrol
digitalis
dimenhydrinate
diphenhydramine
disulfiram and alcohol
ephedrine
epinephrine
ergot alkaloids

BOX 66-2

Common Drug-Induced Dermatologic Conditions—cont'd

Drugs causing fixed eruptions—cont'd

erythrocin
eucalyptus oil
gold compounds
griseofulvin
iodine
ipecac
karaya gum
magnesium hydroxide
meprobamate
mercury salts
methenamine
opioids
oxytetracycline
para-aminosalicylic acid
penicillin
phenobarbital
phenolphthalein
phenytoin
potassium chlorate
quinacrine
quinidine
quinine
reserpine
salicylates
saccharin
scopolamine
sodium salicylate
streptomycin
sulfadiazine
sulfapyridine
sulfathiazole
sulfisoxazole
sulfonamides
tetracyclines
tripelennamine
vaccines and immunizing agents

Drugs causing contact dermatitis

antihistamine
atabrine
bacitracin
benzocaine
bleomycin
chloramphenicol
chlorhexidine
chlorphenesin
chlorpromazine
diphenhydramine
ephedrine
formaldehyde
iodine
isoniazid
lanolin
meprobamate
mercurials
neomycin
nitrofurazone
novobiocin
para-aminosalicylic acid
parabens
penicillin
peru balsam
phenindamine
phenol
procaine and other anesthetics
promethazine
quinacrine
quinine
resorcin
streptomycin
sulfonamides
tetracylines
thiamine
thimerosal

Photosensitizers

acetohexamide
aminobenzoic acid
anesthetics (procaine group)
antimalarials
barbiturates
benzene
bergamot (perfume)
carbamazepine
carbinoxamine d-form
carrots, wild
cedar oil
celery
chlorophyll
citrus fruits
clover
coal tar
contraceptives, oral
corticosteroids, topical
cyproheptadine
desipramine
diethylstilbestrol
digalloyl trioleate (sunscreen)
dill
diphenhydramine
disopyramide
dyes (methylene blue, toluidine blue)
estrone
fennel
fluorescein dyes
5-fluorouracil
gold salts
grass (meadow)
griseofulvin
haloperidol
lavender oil
lime oil
9-mercaptopurine
methotrimeprazine
methoxsalen
methoxypsoralen
mustards
nalidixic acid
naphthalene
oral contraceptives
parsley
parsnips
phenolic compounds
phenothiazines
phenytoin
porphyrins
promethazine
pyrazinamide
quinethazone
quinidine
quinine
salicylanilides
salicylates
sandalwood oil (perfume)
silver salts
sulfonamides
sulfonylureas (antidiabetics)
tetracyclines
thiazide diuretics
tolbutamide
toluene
tricyclic antidepressants
tridione
trimethadione
vanillin oils
xylene

TABLE 66-1 Life-threatening drug-induced skin eruptions

Skin eruption	Description	Drugs involved	
Exfoliative dermatitis	Entire surface of skin is red and scaly and will eventually slough off. Hair and nails may also be affected. Eruption may take weeks or months to resolve after causative agent is stopped. If not resolved, it may be fatal.	barbiturates carbamazepine demeclocycline furosemide gold griseofulvin	penicillin phenothiazines phenytoin sulfonamides tetracyclines
Stevens-Johnson syndrome (erythema multiforme)	Severe form that involves widespread eruptions or lesions usually on face, neck, arms, legs, hands, and feet. May also involve mucosa, may produce fever and malaise. Syndrome may last months and is life-threatening.	May result from use of many drugs, especially carbamazepine, penicillin, phenytoin, sulfonamides, tetracyclines	
Lupus erythematosus	Erythematous rash that may be flat or elevated, (butterfly) on cheek (malar), and across nose. Joint swelling and pain, rash, oral ulcers, serositis, renal, hematologic, pulmonary, and other systems may be affected. Reversible when drug is stopped.	hydantoins, hydralazine, isoniazid, procainamide, quinidine, trimethadione	

classifications: tinea capitis (caused by either a *Trichophyton* or *Microsporum* fungal infection in children or adults); tinea corporis (or *Microsporum* in children; *Trichophyton* in adults); tinea cruris (*Epidermophyton* or *Trichophyton*); and tinea pedis; onychomycosis (*Trichophyton*); and tinea versicolor (*Malassezia furfur*). Tinea or dermatophytosis often appears as a scaly erythematous circular lesion. Tinea versicolor appears as a brown discoloration. Breaking of the hair is seen in tinea capitis or barbae, and with onychomycosis the client has thick, discolored nails.

■ Nursing Management

Dermatologic Agent Therapy

Assessment. Both a thorough history and an objective examination of the dermatologic condition are essential for the initial assessment and ongoing evaluation of nursing care. The nurse should elicit information regarding the onset of the problem; changes in the condition since onset; specific cause if known, or if not, recent exposures to new or different activities that might give a clue about cause; client-determined or prescriber-prescribed factors that may have alleviated the condition; and the client's psychologic response to the problem. Direct inspection and observation should be accomplished with a good light source. Palpation may be necessary, particularly in the instance of assessment of dark skin, where erythema may not be noticeable but warmth and edema of the involved area can be determined. Observations should be systematic and thorough, comparing the left side with the right. Descriptions need to be specific, using the metric system for measurement, and recorded. It may be helpful to take a Polaroid photo of the affected area as a baseline observation. Recorded changes determine progress towards achieving the desired outcome of resolution of the dermatologic problem.

Nursing diagnosis. Clients receiving care with dermatologic agents are at risk for the following nursing diagnoses: impaired skin integrity; altered comfort (pain, burning, or itching of the affected areas); risk for infection related to open skin areas; self-care deficits related to the location of the affected areas; knowledge deficit related to new or altered dermatologic therapy; and disturbance in self-concept related to perceived and actual disfigurement of the affected areas.

Implementation

Monitoring. Observation and palpation are essential to evaluate progress of the resolution of the dermatologic condition. The description of the dermatologic condition including its area, body part involvement, depth, surface appearance, color, drainage, sensation, and healing should be monitored and documented along with any systemic effects such as fever.

Documentation should be made as to the prescribed therapy's effectiveness.

Intervention. Manufacturer's instructions should be followed in detail for application of the various preparations used for dermatologic conditions. In addition, some conditions may be severe enough to require supportive therapy that is more systemic in nature. See also Boxes 66-3 and 66-4 on skin absorption principles and general goals of therapy.

Education. If the etiology of the condition is known, unless it is genetic, the nurse should counsel the client on avoidance of exposure to the causative agent to prevent future episodes. Advise the client to maintain good hygiene of the unaffected areas of the body and to cleanse the affected area only in the prescribed fashion. Instruct the client not to touch affected areas and to dress to avoid or minimize contact with the involved area. Apply only prescribed preparations to the area and follow through with therapy even when the improvement may not be immediate. Avoid exposure of the involved areas to direct sunlight unless it is advised as a

BOX 66-3

Principles of Skin Absorption

Keratin in the outer skin layer provides a waterproof barrier. To enhance drug absorption, the epidermis, or keratin skin layer, needs to be hydrated. Therefore some medications are placed under an occlusive dressing (such as plastic wrap) or administered in an occlusive type of ointment (petroleum jelly) because both will trap and prevent water loss (sweat) from the skin, thus increasing epidermis hydration.

Fat- or lipid-soluble drugs are better absorbed through skin than water-soluble drugs.

In specific body areas, the skin is very thin (eyelids, scrotum area, or the skin of a child) or very thick. The palms of the hands or soles of feet are nearly impenetrable by topical agents.

Products with alcohol content may be administered for drying effects.

Steroid products thin the skin and many are contraindicated for the face, groin, and axillae. Fluorinated steroids should not be used for these areas. If a steroid is necessary, hydrocortisone is generally recommended.

BOX 66-4

General Goals of Therapy

Identify and remove the cause of the skin disorder, if possible.

Institute measures to restore and maintain the structure and normal function of the skin.

Relieve symptoms that are produced by the disorder, such as itching, dryness, pain, and infection.

part of therapy. The client should be instructed to report any side effects or adverse reactions to the prescriber.

Evaluation. The lesions should decrease in size and eventually disappear if the treatment is successful.

■ ■ ■

As previously stated, so many dermatologic products are available that it would be difficult to discuss them all in this chapter. For the sake of simplicity, this chapter discusses three selected groups of dermatologic products: general, prophylactic agents, and therapeutic agents. Some general dermatologic products include those previously discussed plus solutions, baths, soaps, wet dressings, and soaks.

Prophylactic agents include sunscreens, protectives, and antiseptics and disinfectants. Therapeutic agents include the antiinfectives, antiinflammatory corticosteroids, keratolytic agents, acne products, stimulants and irritants, topical anesthetics, burn products for second- and third-degree burns, antiaging products, and ectoparasiticidal topical drugs.

GENERAL DERMATOLOGIC PREPARATIONS

This section refers to single and combination formulations used as bath preparations, cleansers, soaps, solutions and lotions, emollients, skin protectants, wet dressings and soaks, and rubs and liniments.

Baths

Baths may be used to cleanse the skin, medicate, or to reduce temperature. The usual method of cleansing the skin is by the use of soap and water, but this may not be tolerated in skin diseases. In some cases even water is not tolerated and inert oils must be substituted. Persons with dry skin should bathe less frequently than those with oily skin. Frequent bathing tends to stimulate oil production, causing oily skin to remain oily. It is possible to keep the skin clean without a daily bath. Nurses are sometimes accused of overbathing hospitalized clients, causing their skin to become dry and itchy. For dry skin, an oily lotion is preferable to alcohol (isopropyl or ethyl).

To render baths soothing in irritative conditions, oatmeal, starch, or gelatin may be added; usually 1 to 2 ounces per gallon of water. Oils such as Alpha-Keri and oilated oatmeal in a proportion of 1 oz to a tub of water decreases the drying effect of water and helps relieve the itching of a sensitive, xerotic skin. Lubricating topical medication or bland emollient should be applied immediately after the bath while skin is still moist because this increases absorption and hydration.

Soaps

Ordinary soap, the sodium salt of palmitic, oleic, or stearic acids alone or in a mixture, is made by saponifying fats or oils with alkalies. The oil used for castile soap is supposed to be olive oil; some soaps are made with coconut oil. The consistency of the soap depends on the major acid and alkali used.

Although all soaps are relatively alkaline, an excess of free alkali or acid is a potential source of skin irritation. Medicated soaps contain antiseptics, but soaps per se are antiseptic only to the degree that they mechanically clean the skin. Many people believe that soap and water are bad for the complexion which is erroneous because a clean skin helps to promote a healthy skin. The soap used in maintaining a clean skin should be mild and contain a minimum of irritating materials. Perfumed or medicated soaps may be harmful if the skin is extra sensitive to soap products, if the soap is not adequately rinsed off the skin, if it stimulates excess production of natural skin oils, or if it dries the skin excessively. Soaps are irritating to mucous membranes, and they are used in enemas mainly because of this action.

Solutions and Lotions

Soothing preparations may be liquids that carry an insoluble powder or suspension, or they may be mild acid or alkaline solutions, such as boric acid solution, limewater, or aluminum acetate used as wet dressings and soaks. The bismuth salts and starch are also commonly used for their soothing effect.

Aluminum acetate solution (Burow's solution, modified Burow's solution). A mild astringent that coagulates bacterial and serum protein. It is diluted with 10 to 40 parts of water before application.

Calamine lotion. Calamine lotion contains calamine, zinc oxide, bentonite magma and glycerin in a calcium hydroxide solution. It is a soothing lotion used for the dermatitis caused by poison ivy, insect bites, prickly heat, etc.

Cleansers

Cleansers are usually free of soap or are modified soap products that are recommended for persons with sensitive, dry, or irritated skin or those who may have had a previous reaction to a soap product. These cleansers are less irritating, may contain an emollient substance, and may also have been adjusted to a slightly acidic or neutral pH. Included in this category are Aveeno Cleansing Bar, Lowila Cake, and others.

Emollients

Emollients are fatty or oily substances that may be used to soften or soothe irritated skin and mucous membrane. An emollient is often used as a vehicle for other medicinal substances. Examples of emollients include lanolin, petroleum jelly (Vaseline), vitamin A and D ointment, vitamin E, and cold cream. Examples of emollient products on the market include Panthoderm; vitamin E topical products; vitamin A and D topicals; Lubriderm; Dermassage; Nivea Skin; and many more.

Skin Protectants

Skin protectants are used to coat minor skin irritations or to protect the person's skin from chemical irritants. Some commercially available products include AeroZoin, Benzoin, Benzoin, and Benzoin Compound.

Wet Dressings and Soaks

Wet dressings and soaks include some of the preparations discussed under solutions and lotions. These liquids are either a wet or an astringent type of dressing used to treat inflammatory skin conditions, such as insect bites and poison ivy. Aluminum acetate solution, Domeboro Powder, and others are available for this use.

Rubs and Liniments

Rubs and liniments are indicated for pain relief for intact skin. Pain caused by muscle aches, neuralgia, rheumatism, arthritis, and sprains are the types of pain that usually respond to these products. The ingredients in the preparations may include a counterirritant (e.g., camphor, oil of cloves, methyl salicylate), an antiseptic (chloroxylenol, eugenol, thymol), local anesthetic (benzocaine), or analgesics (salicylate-containing substances). Examples from this category include Aspercreme, Ben-Gay, and Icy Hot.

For information on capsaicin topical, see Chapter 14, Analgesics.

PROPHYLACTIC AGENTS

Protectives

Protectives are soothing, cooling preparations that form a film on the skin. To be useful they must not macerate the skin, prevent drying of the tissues, and must keep out light, air, and dust. Nonabsorbable powders are usually listed as protectives, but they are not particularly useful because they stick to wet surfaces and have to be scraped off and do not stick to dry surfaces at all. Nonabsorbable powders include zinc stearate, zinc oxide, certain bismuth preparations, talcum powder, and aluminum silicate.

Collodion is a 5% solution of pyroxylin in a mixture of ether and alcohol. When collodion is applied to the skin, the ether and alcohol evaporate, leaving a transparent film that adheres to the skin to protect it. Flexible collodion is a mixture of collodion with 2% camphor and 3% castor oil. The addition of the latter makes the resulting film elastic and more tenacious. Styptic collodion contains 20% tannic acid and therefore is astringent, as well as protective.

Although it is safe to say that no substances known at present can stimulate healing at a more rapid rate than is normal under optimal conditions, preparations that act as bland protectives may help by preventing crusting and trauma. In some instances they may reduce offensive odors.

Sunscreen Preparations

Extended exposure to the sun, whether from sunbathing or as a normal consequence of an outdoor occupation, may lead to sunburn and/or premature aging of the skin (photoaging). Certain chemicals (e.g., tetracyclines, sulfonamides, thiazides, phenothiazines), plants, cosmetics, and soaps may cause photosensitivity or phototoxicity occurs when an ultraviolet wavelength substance (UVA absorbing compound) is present on the skin in sufficient amounts and is also exposed to a particular sunlight wavelength. The substance absorbs the offending wavelength, energy is transferred and the result is it becomes destructive to surrounding tissues. The exposed skin rapidly becomes red, painful, prickling, or burning with peak skin reaction reached within 24 to 48 hours of exposure. This reaction does not involve the immune system.

A photoallergy reaction is different from a phototoxic reaction; it is less common and requires prior exposure to the photosensitizing agent. The immune system is involved and when the photosensitizers react with UVA, a delayed hypersensitivity reaction occurs. The reaction occurs several days after exposure and presents as severe pruritus and a rash that can spread to skin areas that were not exposed to sunlight (Mailloux, 1995).

Excessive exposure to ultraviolet rays (UVR) may result in skin damage that progresses from minor irritations to a precancerous skin condition and, perhaps, to skin cancer later in life. Cutaneous malignant melanoma has been associated with excessive sun exposure, especially during childhood; whereas large cumulative UVR doses over a lifetime appears to increase the incidence of nonmelanoma skin cancers.

Sunscreen preparations are applied either to absorb or reflect the sun's harmful rays. Absorbing agents are chemicals such as aminobenzoic acid (*p*-aminobenzoic acid, or PABA), benzophenones, cinnamates, and anthranilates; reflectors are physical agents such as titanium dioxide and zinc oxide. The latter agents are opaque (i.e., they look like thick paste) and must be applied heavily; thus they are not cosmetically acceptable to most persons.

The spectrum for ultraviolet radiation includes UVA, UVB, and UVC. UVA, or long-wave radiation, has a wavelength of 320 to 400 nm (nanometers) and is the closest to visible light. UVB has also been determined to be responsible for skin cancer induction, although the carcinogenic properties of UVB appear to be augmented by UVA. Approximately 90% of UVB radiation is blocked by the earth's ozone layer, with the balance absorbed by the epidermal skin layer. UVB has a wavelength between 290 and 320 nm which causes erythema and is also associated with vitamin D_3 synthesis. The UVC radiation from the sun does not appear to reach the earth's surface; therefore this type of radiation is usually emitted by artificial ultraviolet sources. UVC can cause some erythema but will not stimulate tanning.

The **sun protection factor** (SPF) is a ratio between the exposures to ultraviolet wavelengths required to cause erythema with and without a sunscreen. This is expressed as MED, or the minimal erythemal dose. Therefore if a person experiences 1 MED with 25 units of UV radiation (in an unprotected state), and if after application of a sunscreen the person requires 250 units of radiation to produce 1 MED, then this product would be given an SPF rating of 10. The higher the SPF, the longer it takes to develop a tan. If a person normally burned with 1 MED within 30 minutes, then applying a sunscreen with an SPF of 6 would allow that person to stay in the sun six times longer, or for nearly 3 hours, before reaching 1 MED. The following is the recommended SPF for various skin types (Mailloux, 1995):

Type	Description	SPF recommended
1	Always burns, never tans, usually very fair complexion with red or blond hair and freckles	≥15
2	Burns easily, tans minimally, usually fair skinned	≥15
3	Sometimes burns but gradually tans	10-15
4	Minimal burning, always tans	6-10
5	Rarely ever burns, always tans	4-6
6	Never burns but tans darkly	unnecessary

The best way to choose a sunscreen agent is according to your skin type, the length of time spent in the sun, the usual intensity of the sun's rays in your geographic area, and the type of preparation or formulation you prefer.

The FDA advisory review panel has established three categories of sunscreens according to the products' active ingredients. Ingredients that absorb 95% or more of the radiation in the UV range of 290 to 320 nm are called sunscreen-sunburn preventive agents. If the active ingredient absorbs at least 85% of the radiation in the UV wavelength from 290 to 320 nm, then it is called a sunscreen-suntanning agent. An opaque agent that reflects or scatters all radiation in the UV range from 290 to 760 nm is a sunscreen-opaque sunblock agent. Most products are a combination of the first two types of agents, and the primary difference between a preventive agent and a suntanning agent might be the concentration of the active ingredient.

The nurse should advise clients appropriately on the selection and use of a sunscreen. Sunscreens should be liberally applied to all exposed body areas (except eyelids) and reapplied as frequently as recommended, in order to achieve the maximum effectiveness.

Reapplication is usually every 2 to 3 hours. Refrain from being in the sun when the sun's rays are most direct and damaging, between 10 AM and 2 PM. Wear sunscreen and limit exposure on overcast or cloudy days. Very little UV radiation is blocked by the cloud cover, although infrared radiation that contributes to the sensation of heat is usually reduced. This heat reduction might give an individual a false sense of security against a sunburn. Be aware of reflective surfaces; the sun's rays can be reflected on skin from water, concrete, snow, and sand. Keep infants out of the sun—sunscreens should always be used on children over 6 months old.

It has been projected that the use of an SPF 15 from 6 months of age through 18 years of age will result in a 78% reduction in the incidence of skin cancer over a person's lifetime (DeSimone, 1993).

See Table 66-2 for examples of sunscreen agents, including their SPFs and waterproof or water-resistant labels, if appropriate.

TABLE 66-2 Selected sunscreen preparations

Name	SPF	Waterproof/water resistant*
Hawaiian Tropic Baby Faces Sunblock	50	waterproof
Coppertone Moisturizing Sunblock	45	waterproof
PreSun Active	30	waterproof
Blistex Ultra Protection	30	water resistant
Coppertone Moisturizing Sunblock	25	waterproof
Coppertone Sport	15	waterproof

**Waterproof,* maintains sunburn protection after water exposure for up to 80 minutes.
Water resistant, maintains sunburn protection after water exposure for up to 40 minutes.

THERAPEUTIC AGENTS

Topical Antiinfectives

Antiinfectives include topical antibiotics, antiviral, and antifungal agents.

Antibiotics

The most frequent causative organisms of skin infections (exodermas) are *Streptococcus pyogenes* and *Staphylococcus aureus.* Folliculitis, impetigo, furuncles, carbuncles, and cellulitis often result from these organisms. These common skin disorders are infections for which topical prophylaxis antibiotics may be applied. Some of these agents are discussed next; other topical antibiotics are discussed in sections on acne products, antifungals, and antivirals.

bacitracin [bass i tray' sin]
Bacitracin is very useful in the local treatment of infectious lesions. The ointment form (Baciguent) is most commonly used, although it has also been used in solution to moisten wet dressings or as a dusting powder. It is odorless and nonstaining, and its use seldom results in sensitizing; however, allergic contact dermatitis has occurred.

neomycin [nee oh mye' sin]
Neomycin has been used successfully in the treatment of infections of skin and mucous membrane. Applied topically, it occasionally irritates the skin, and allergic contact dermatitis is reported, especially when neomycin is used on stasis ulcers. An ointment (Mycitracin), which combines *neomycin, bacitracin,* and *polymixin B,* may be more efficacious in mixed infections than when these agents are used singly.

In conditions where absorption of neomycin may occur (including burns and trophic ulceration), there is the potential for nephrotoxicity, ototoxicity, and neomycin hypersensitivity reactions. This risk is seen more frequently in persons with compromised renal function, in clients with extensive burns, and in clients using other aminoglycoside antibiotics. Sensitization may occur to any of the antibiotic ingredients, and prolonged use may produce superinfection as an overgrowth of nonsusceptible organisms such as fungi. Photosensitivity is reported with topical gentamicin.

■ ■ ■

The possibility of hypersensitivity occurs when chloramphenicol is used topically, as does the additional risk of bone marrow hypoplasia, blood dyscrasias, itching, burning, angioneurotic edema, urticaria, and vesicular and maculopapular dermatitis. Tetracyclines may stain clothing and cause erythema, irritation, and swelling locally. See Table 66-3 for a list of topical antibiotics and their spectrums of activity.

Although erythromycin generally has activity against gram-positive organisms, it is also approved for the treatment of acne vulgaris.

Mupirocin [myoo peer' oh sin] (Bactroban) is a topical antibacterial preparation indicated for the treatment of impetigo caused by *Staphylococcus aureus* and other beta-hemolytic streptococci. It is usually applied to affected areas three times daily.

TABLE 66-3 Spectrums of antimicrobial activity of topical antibiotics

Antibiotic	Spectrum of activity: Gram +	Gram −	Broad spectrum
bacitracin ointment		X	
chlortetracycline ointment			X
chloramphenicol cream			X
erythromycin liquid or ointment	X		
gentamicin cream and ointment			X
neomycin cream and ointment			X

Many topical preparations and antibiotic combinations available over the counter are labeled as first aid products to help prevent infection in minor cuts, burns, or injuries. They cannot be recommended to treat known infections. Prescription antibiotic ointments are generally indicated for the treatment of minor or surface bacterial infections.

Antivirals

acyclovir [ay sye' kloe ver] (Zovirax Ointment 5%)
Acyclovir inhibits the viral enzymes necessary for DNA synthesis. Topical acyclovir is used for the treatment of initial episodes of herpes genitalis and for herpes simplex in immunocompromised clients. However, in many instances systemic acyclovir is much more effective and may be the preferred formulation.

The more frequent side/adverse effects of acyclovir include local pain, pruritus, or stinging. The dosage is adequate covering of the lesions with ointment every 3 hours six times daily for 7 days.

■ Nursing Management

Acyclovir Therapy

In addition to the nursing management of dermatologic agent therapy, the following factors should be considered.

Dose per application will vary depending on lesion area; a ½-inch ribbon of ointment covers approximately 4 inches of surface area. Store ointment at 15° C to 25° C (59° F to 78° F).

Instruct the client to use a finger cot or rubber glove when applying the ointment to prevent autoinoculation to other sites. Avoid contact with eyes. Advise annual or more frequent Pap smears because women with herpes genitalis are more likely to develop cervical cancer. Recommend the wearing of loose clothing and keeping affected areas clean and dry to prevent further irritation. Advise the client to avoid sexual activity if either partner has active lesions. Even if the partner is asymptomatic the disease can still be sexually transmitted; use of a condom may help prevent transmission of herpes depending on the location of the lesion.

TABLE 66-4 Topical antifungal agents

Name	Prescription drug	Over-the-counter	Special comments
amphotericin B (Fungizone)	X		Equivalent to nystatin against *Candida albicans* (Monilia) infections.
ciclopirox olamine (Loprox)	X		Broad-spectrum antifungal. Used for tinea pedis, tinea cruris, tinea corporis, candidiasis caused by *C. albicans*, and tinea versicolor caused by *M. furfur.*
clioquinol (Vioform)		X	Antibacterial and antifungal. May cause staining of clothes, skin, or hair.
clotrimazole (Lotrimin, Mycelex)	X	X	Broad-spectrum antifungal agent.
econazole nitrate (Spectrazole)	X		Broad-spectrum antifungal agent.
haloprogin (Halotex)	X		Synthetic antifungal agent. Broad spectrum.
ketoconazole (Nizoral)	X		Broad-spectrum synthetic antifungal agent.
miconazole (Micatin)		X	Used for tinea pedis (athlete's foot), tinea cruris, tinea corporis, and tinea versicolor.
(Monistat-Derm)	X		Lotion preferred for intertriginous areas.
nystatin (Mycostatin, Nilstat)	X		Antifungal antibiotic with both fungicidal and fungistatic effects.
tolnaftate (Tinactin, Aftate)		X	Used for topical fungus skin infections.
triacetin (Fungoid)	X		Treats athlete's foot and other topical fungus infections.
undecylenic acid (Desenex)		X	Antifungal and antibacterial for athlete's foot and ringworm, with exception of nails and hairy sites. Also used for diaper rash, prickly heat, minor skin irritations, jock itch, excessive perspiration, and skin irritation in the groin area.

Antifungals

There are few fungi that produce keratinolytic enzymes to provide for their existence on skin. Three infectious fungi can cause local fungal infections without systemic effects: *Microsporum, Trichophyton,* and *Epidermophyton*. The possibility of a mixed infection with these fungi must never be overlooked.

Fungi exist in a moist, warm environment, preferably in dark areas such as skin areas covered by shoes and socks (tinea pedis or athlete's foot). Immunologic mechanisms may have an important role in fungal control. The triad for suspicion for fungal infections is an immunologic deficit, a specific fungal involvement, and the skin condition.

The stratum corneum is a layer of dead desquamated cells that are shed normally or are dissolved in sebum. The fungi invade this layer and cause inflammation and induce sensitivity when they penetrate the epidermis and dermis. Because the stratum corneum is shed daily, the ability to spread or transmit the fungi is by contact.

The most commonly reported side effects/adverse reactions with the use of the topical antifungals include local irritation, pruritus, burning sensation, and scaling. Erythema, blistering, stinging, peeling, urticaria, pruritus, and general irritation may occur with products like clotrimazole.

The primary topical antifungal agents include undecylenic acid products (Desenex and others), clioquinol (Vioform), miconazole (Micatin), econazole (Spectazole), ciclopirox (Loprox), clotrimazole (Lotrimin), oxiconazole (Oxistat), triacetin (Fungoid), haloprogin (Halotex), tolnaftate (Tinactin), nystatin, gentian violet, and a variety of antifungal combination ointments, powders, and liquids. See Table 66-4 for the generic name, trade name, status of (OTC or prescription), and comments on the products.

■ Nursing Management

Antifungal Agent Therapy

In addition to the nursing management of dermatologic agent therapy previously discussed, consider these points:

Assessment. Carefully note skin characteristics, symptoms, and predisposing factors such as trauma, suppressed immunity, general health, hygiene practices, or exposure to infecting agent. If laboratory tests, such as cultures of exudate or tissue, are to be obtained they should be obtained before the topical agent is applied.

Implementation

Intervention. Topical substances for antifungal purposes should be applied liberally to a clean, dry, affected skin area. An occlusive dressing should not be applied unless directed by the prescriber. Avoid contact of these substances with the eyes. Store below 85° F (30° C) but do not freeze.

Education. Encourage compliance with the full course of therapy. Fungal infections generally require prolonged therapy. The nurse may encourage the client with a superficial fungal infection to practice adequate hygiene to discourage growth. Some principles of hygiene are the following: (1) the affected area should be dry and aerated, and clothing that is warm or that causes an occlusive environment of moisture should be avoided; (2) the body areas may be kept dry by using powders (with or without antifungal ingredients) to prevent maceration; (3) before applying the antifungal medication the area should be washed with mild soap and water, and dried; (4) friction or trauma of the area may be avoided by not wearing tight-fitting clothing, which causes friction; clothing should be laundered daily. For infants with anogenital lesions, avoid tight diapers, disposable diapers, and plastic pants. For clients with foot infections, advise cotton socks, well-ventilated shoes or sandals.

Evaluation. Use of these agents may lead to skin sensitization and result in symptoms of hypersensitization, increasing redness and swelling, weeping, and itching and burning not present at the beginning of therapy. If no improvement is seen within 4 weeks, the client needs to be reevaluated.

Corticosteroids

Topical corticosteroids are generally indicated for relief of inflammatory and pruritic dermatoses. They also offer the benefit of less systemic side effects and allowing direct contact with the localized lesion.

The effectiveness of the topical corticosteroids is a result of their antiinflammatory, antipruritic, and vasoconstrictor actions. Topical corticosteroids may also stabilize epidermal lysosomes in the skin, and fluorinated steroids are antiproliferative.

Fluorinated topical corticosteroids (fluocinonide, betamethasone and others) are used for the treatment of dermatologic disorders such as psoriasis because of their antiinflammatory, antipruritic, and vasoconstrictive actions, as well as their ability to decrease cell proliferation. They are very potent agents and are less likely to cause sodium retention.

A correlation exists between the potency and the therapeutic efficacy of corticosteroids (Box 66-5). The vehicle (aerosol, cream, gel, lotion, ointment, solution, or tape) in which the corticosteroid is placed may alter the vasoconstrictor property and therapeutic efficacy. Corticosteroid skin penetration is enhanced by the following vehicles (in decreasing order of effectiveness): ointments, gels, creams, and lotions.

Ointment bases and propylene glycol both enhance the penetration of the corticosteroid and its vasoconstrictor effects. As a result of their occlusive nature ointments hydrate the stratum corneum, permitting granular steroid penetration. Lotions are well suited for hairy areas or for lesions that are oozing and wet. Creams and ointments are well suited for dry, scaling, thickened, and pruritic areas. Sprays, lotions, and gels are suited for the scalp or hairy areas. Sprays are aesthetically suitable for acute weeping lesions, are cooling, and have antipruritic effects. All these vehicles influence absorption and therapeutic effect.

The rate of percutaneous penetration after application also influences therapeutic efficacy. Steroid percutaneous penetration increases with its vehicle base solubility. It is limited by three factors: rate of dissolution, rate of passive diffusion, and drug penetration rate (the skin itself is a barrier, and the stratum corneum is a rate-limiting membrane). The skin is selectively permeable by regional variations in absorptive capacity. Because most topical corticosteroids are in suspension vehicles (ointments, creams, lotions), the addition of a solvent (propylene glycol) to the product can enhance drug dissolution, which may improve absorption. The sebum, enzymes, and perspiration of the skin convert topical suspensions partially to solutions needing the inclusion of a solvent, surfactant, or emulsifier in the vehicle to increase the rate of dissolution and distribution. Inflamed skin absorbs topical steroids to a greater degree than thick or lichenified skin.

Side/adverse effects of topical corticosteroids include: acneiform eruptions, allergic contact dermatitis, burning sensations, dryness, itching, hypopigmentation, purpura, hirsutism (usually facial), folliculitis, round and swollen face, alopecia (usually of scalp), overgrowth of bacteria, fungus, and virus, and immunosuppression.

The adult dosage is one or two applications daily as directed. Application frequency depends on site, response of the cutaneous eruption to medication, and application technique.

BOX 66-5

Potencies of Topical Steroid Products

The following list compares relative potencies of the topical corticosteroid products.

Most potent
clobetasol (Temovate 0.05%)
halobetasol (Ultravate 0.05%)

High potency
amcinocide (Cyclocort)
betamethasone dipropionate (Diprosone 0.05%)
desoximetasone (Topicort 0.25%)
fluocinolone (Lidex 0.05%)

Moderate potency
betamethasone (Benisone 0.025%)
betamethasone valerate (Valisone 0.1%)
desoximetasone (Topicort 0.05%)
flurandrenolide (Cordran 0.025%)
triamcinolone (Aristocort)

Less potency
desonide (Tridesilon)
fluocinolone acetonide (Synalar 0.01%)
hydrocortisone 0.25% to 2.5%

■ Nursing Management

Topical Corticosteroid Therapy

In addition to the nursing management of dermatologic agent therapy previously discussed, consider the following:

Assessment. The age of the skin affects absorption of the potent fluorinated corticosteroids; the very young and the very old have skin that is more permeable.

Implementation

Monitoring. If prolonged treatment is required, it is prudent for the prescriber to monitor plasma cortisol levels clinically every month until the steroid is discontinued. Most side effects are temporary and are resolved when the topical steroid is discontinued.

Occlusive dressings may cause folliculitis from bacterial or candida infection, hyperthermia from heat retention, or systemic effects related to increased drug absorption.

Intervention. Taper therapy gradually.

Education. To enhance client compliance the reasons for occlusive dressing procedure should be explained to the client. This technique intensifies percutaneous penetration of the topical steroid and concentrates the medication in the area where it is most needed.

Keratolytics

Keratolytics (keratin dissolvers) are drugs that soften scales and loosen the outer horny layer of the skin. Salicylic acid and resorcinol are drugs of choice. Their action makes the penetration of other medical substances possible by cleaning the involved lesions. Salicylic acid is particularly important for its keratolytic effect in local treatment of scalp conditions, warts, corns, fungous infections, acne, and chronic types of dermatitis. It is used up to 20% in ointments, plasters, or collodion for this purpose.

Acne Products

Acne vulgaris is a skin disease that involves increased sebum production and abnormal keratinization that leads to the formation of a keratin plug at the base of the pilosebaceous follicle; it affects up to 90% of adolescents (Seaton, 1995). The reduction and removal of sebum and bacteria, specifically *Propionibacterium acnes*, are the target of acne vulgaris therapy.

Treatment of acne therapy may include (1) removal of keratin plugs, (2) decreasing the amount of *P. acnes*, (3) lowering the amounts of free fatty acid and formation, (4) decreasing the sebum production, and (5) effectively improving the appearance of the individual for psychosocial benefits.

Of the many treatment modalities in acne therapy, only the topical forms of benzoyl peroxide, tetracycline, erythromycin, clindamycin, tretinoin, and isotretinoin will be discussed here.

benzoyl peroxide

Benzoyl peroxide slowly and continuously liberates active oxygen, producing an antibacterial, keratolytic and drying effect. The release of oxygen into the pilosebaceous and comedone area creates unfavorable growth conditions for *P. acnes* and reduces the release of the fatty acids from sebum. Additionally, the drying vehicle aids in shrinking the papules or pustules but does not have an effect on comedones or cysts. Benzoyl peroxide is used in the treatment of acne vulgaris.

Benzoyl peroxide is absorbed and metabolized in the skin to benzoic acid. Approximately 5% of the benzoic acid is absorbed and excreted in the kidneys. Acne improvement is usually noted in 4 to 6 weeks of therapy. Side/adverse effects are infrequent and include dry or peeling skin, red skin, or sensation of warmth of the skin, severe redness, pruritus, blisters, and burning or swelling of skin caused by an allergic reaction. No significant drug interactions are reported.

In adults and children 12 years and older, benzoyl peroxide lotion (5% or 10%) is applied one to four times daily.

Topical Antibiotics

Topical and systemic antibiotics used in the treatment of acne have an unknown mechanism of action. Acne is not an infection nor is it contagious but *P. acnes* appears to convert comedones to inflamed pustules or papules. The antibiotics may decrease the colonization of *P. acnes* thus decreasing the formation of sebaceous fatty acid byproducts, preventing the formation of new acne lesions. Examples of the antibiotics utilized include clindamycin, erythromycin and tetracycline. Topical erythromycin and clindamycin are most commonly prescribed for mild to moderate acne while oral antibiotics (tetracyclines) are generally reserved for severe acne, for individuals that are intolerant or did not respond to topical agents. Treatment failures have been associated with antibiotic resistance (Seaton, 1995).

clindamycin [klin da mye' sin] (Cleocin T topical solution)

Topical clindamycin may be as effective as low-dose, oral tetracycline therapy for inflammatory acne. Skin phosphatases, by hydrolysis, convert inactive clindamycin phosphate to active clindamycin base, which is excreted by the kidneys.

This is one of the most widely used topical antibiotics indicated in the treatment of acne vulgaris. Side/adverse effects include: dry, scaly and/or peeling skin; stinging or burning sensation, and hypersensitive skin reaction.

■ Nursing Management

Clindamycin Therapy

See general discussion of nursing management of dermatologic agent therapy on p. 1020.

Assessment. Cross-resistance exists with lincomycin and antagonism with erythromycin. Contraindications demonstrated by hypersensitivity to any form of clindamycin or lincomycin may apply to the topical preparation. During the client interviews the nurse should inquire about any previous sensitivity not only to clindamycin but also to other antibiotics or allergens and a history of regional enteritis. Atopic clients should be questioned because some absorption may occur through the skin.

Implementation

Intervention. For adults and children apply a thin film twice daily to affected area.

erythromycin topical solution [er ith roe mye' sin] (A/T/S, EryDerm)

Erythromycin topical solution is also indicated for the treatment of acne vulgaris. Side/adverse effects include: skin reactions such as erythema, desquamation, tenderness, dryness, pruritus, burning, oiliness, and acne.

■ Nursing Management
Erythromycin Topical Solution Therapy

See general discussion of nursing management of dermatologic agent therapy on p. 1020.

Assessment. Hypersensitivity to erythromycin or the other components of the solution (alcohol, propylene glycol, or acetone) is a contraindication to its use. A cumulative irritant effect may occur with concomitant use of peeling, desquamating, or abrasive agents.

Implementation

Intervention. Erythromycin topical solution is applied to affected areas, morning and evening.

Education. Caution the client that erythromycin solution should not be used near the eyes, nose, mouth, and other mucous membranes.

tetracycline topical solution [tet ra sye' kleen] (Topicycline)

Topical tetracycline, which is believed to suppress *P. acnes* growth, is directly applied to the pilosebaceous units (hair follicle and sebaceous gland), which are most numerous on the face, back, chest, and upper arms.

Side/adverse effects include dry, scaly skin, stinging, pain, redness or swelling at site of application.

Low dose, oral tetracycline (usually 250 mg/day) is usually reserved for severe acne as reviewed previously. This dose may be increased for acute acne flare-ups but should be decreased to maintenance dosing within a month or so. While low dose therapy has been continued for years, it has been recommended that the antibiotic be discontinued periodically (Seaton, 1995). This may help reduce the potential for side/adverse effects and possibly drug resistance.

■ Nursing Management
Topical Tetracycline Therapy

See general discussion of nursing management of dermatologic agent therapy on p. 1020.

Implementation

Education. Tetracycline is generously applied twice daily (morning and evening) to affected areas until the skin is wet. Because of the 40% ethanol and other components, the eyes, nose, mouth, and mucous membrane areas should be avoided. Normal use of cosmetics is permitted. (See Chapter 59 for a more complete discussion of tetracycline.) Transient stinging or burning may often occur. The slight yellow superficial coloring of the skin of light-complected clients may be washed off. Under a source of ultraviolet light (sun, sunlamp), the treated areas will fluoresce.

tretinoin [tret' i noyn] (retinoic acid, vitamin A acid, [Retin-A])

Tretinoin is an irritant that stimulates epidermal cell turnover, which causes skin peeling; this reduces the free fatty acids and horny cell adherence within the comedone. Tretinoin is used in the treatment of acne vulgaris in which comedones, pustules, and papules predominate (see the Nursing Research box at right).

Side effects/adverse reactions of tretinoin reported include red and edematous blisters, crusted, stinging or peeling skin, and temporary alterations in skin pigmentation. Concomitant topical use with drying or peeling agents such as benzoyl peroxide, resorcinol, salicylic acid, and sulfur may result in excessive keratolytic and peeling effects. Tretinoin emollient cream (Renova) was released to treat facial wrinkles caused by age or the sun. This product contains 0.05% tretinoin and is the first prescription with this indication (Olin, 1996).

■ Nursing Management
Tretinoin Therapy

See general nursing management of dermatologic agent therapy on p. 1020.

Implementation

Monitoring. Irritation and desquamation are most likely during the first 1 to 3 weeks of treatment.

Intervention. Apply each night by covering the area lightly before the person retires. Some clients require less frequent applications or use a lower-percentage strength, and others may respond to the higher-percentage dosage forms. Application should be done after thorough cleansing of area, allowing a minimum of 30 minutes for it to dry. If tretinoin is applied to wet skin an increased drying effect and redness may occur.

Education. Clients with sunburned skin, skin sensitive to ultraviolet light, or skin exposed to weather extremes must exercise caution and avoid tretinoin until the skin has recovered. The client must avoid medicated or abrasive cleansers, astringents, soaps, and cosmetics that have a drying effect and a high alcohol concentration. The client will be excessively sensitive to sun and should wear SPF sunscreens during therapy.

isotretinoin [eye soe tret' i noyn] (Accutane)

Isotretinoin is an oral and topical product indicated for the treatment of severe recalcitrant cystic acne. This product inhibits sebaceous gland activity thus decreases sebum formation and secretion. It also has antikeratinizing and antiinflammatory effects. It is reserved to treat severe acne and has induced prolonged remissions in severe cystic acne.

Women who are pregnant or are planning to become pregnant should not use this preparation. Many spontaneous abortions have been reported in pregnant women, as well as major abnormalities (hydrocephalus, microcephalus, external ear, and cardiovascular problems) in the fetus at birth.

■ Nursing Management
Isotretinoin Therapy

In addition to the discussion of the general nursing management of dermatologic agents therapy, consider the following:

Nursing Research

The use of topical tretinoin for photoaging

In practice, topical tretinoin is probably used more often to treat aging skin than to treat acne. Ortho has reformulated the agent as 0.05% tretinoin in an emollient cream base (Renova). Although tretinoin has been promoted in the lay media as a cure for wrinkles, the effects of therapy involve the whole range of photodamage. Tretinoin not only cosmetically improves fine and coarse wrinkling, but also decreases skin laxity, roughness, sallowness, and hyperpigmentation. The agent reduces the number of precancerous skin lesions and stimulates new collagen and possibly new elastin production. It increases the thickness of epidermal and granular layers, decreases melanin content, and makes the stratum corneum more compact (Bhawan et al, 1991).

The use of topical tretinoin must be discussed with the client in the context of a complete program of photoprotection. Instruct the client to use sunscreens, wear hats and protective clothing when in the sun, avoid sun exposure between 10 AM and 2 PM (standard time), when the greatest damage can occur. Ensure that the client understands that shade does not offer protection from ultraviolet radiation.

Despite the desirability of some of the positive skin changes, the use of tretinoin to treat photodamaged skin remains highly controversial. Many physicians see the benefits as cosmetic rather than medical. The FDA Advisory Committee shared some of this concern in recommending that the Renova labeling indicate that tretinoin improves the appearance of the skin but does not actually repair sun-damaged skin. On the other hand, many dermatologists advocate a different perspective, that tretinoin is a medical treatment for a serious medical condition. The client has suffered environmental exposure to a harmful substance, which has caused damage and can benefit from therapy. Helping clients look better is as legitimate a goal as reducing cancer risk, and positive psychologic effects have been documented with such therapy (Gupta et al, 1991).

Critical thinking questions

- Do you believe that therapy, such as tretinoin therapy, is beneficial for clients? Is this therapy for cosmetic reasons justifiable in a health system with scarce resources? If the treatment of mildly to moderately photoaged skin with topical tretinoin has a favorable psychosocial effect upon a client, wouldn't this enhance the client's health from a holistic perspective?

From Dicken et al (1992).

Assessment. It should be ascertained that the client is not pregnant by a negative pregnancy test and an appropriate history and physical examination because isotretinoin has been demonstrated to cause fetal abnormalities. The client of child-bearing age should be assessed for her capability to comply with mandatory contraceptive measures; these should be accomplished for at least 1 month before therapy, during therapy, and for 1 month after the end of therapy (see the Pregnancy Safety box at right).

Review the client's medication regimen if the oral form of the drug is used. Isotretinoin is not recommended to be taken concurrently with etretinate, tretinoin, or vitamin A because additive toxic effects may result. Use of tetracyclines with isotretinoin increases the risk for the development of pseudotumor cerebri (a condition characterized by increased intracranial pressure, headache, blurring of the optic disc margins, vomiting, and papilledema without neurologic findings, except palsy of the sixth cranial nerve).

The client should receive a baseline CBC, serum electrolyte profile, blood lipid levels, blood glucose levels, and hepatic function studies. These should also be monitored throughout therapy.

Nursing diagnosis. The client receiving isotretinoin is at risk for the following nursing diagnoses: altered comfort (headache, 5%; inflammation of the eye, 40%; skin rash, <10%; pain, tenderness, stiffness of muscles, bones, or joints, 16%; and dryness of mouth, skin, and eyes, 80%); impaired skin integrity (scaling, redness, inflammation of the lips, 90%); altered thought processes (depression); and the potential complications of nosebleeds, 80%; cataracts, optic neuritis, corneal opacities and pseudotumor cerebri; hepatitis; and inflammatory bowel disease.

Pregnancy Safety

Category	Drug
B	topical clindamycin, erythromycin, meclocycline, and tetracycline; lindane, malathion topical, permethrin, silver sulfadiazine
C	benzoyl peroxide, corticosteroids (topical), crotamiton, mafenide, tretinoin
X	isotretinoin

Implementation

Monitoring. Monitor lab reports as mentioned above as well as the nursing diagnoses and potential complications above.

Education. The client is to receive both oral and written instructions regarding the hazards of pregnancy and indicate her understanding and acceptance of the written warnings.

The client receiving isotretinoin should be alerted not to donate blood during or for 30 days after therapy, because of risk to the fetus of a pregnant woman who may receive the blood. Because isotretinoin may increase plasma triglyceride concentrations, those clients at particular cardiovascular risk should be cautioned: those with a history of high alcohol intake, obesity, or a history or family history of hypertriglyceridemia or diabetes mellitus.

Alert the client to avoid concurrent use of vitamin A, unless prescribed by a physician to minimize additive toxic effects. Avoid the ingestion of alcohol because of possible hypertriglyceridemia and consequent cardiovascular risks. Caution about a decrease in night vision; the client should alert the prescriber if this occurs. The client may also be intolerant of contact lenses because of dryness of the eyes. Wearing contact lenses may need to be discontinued during the course of therapy if an ocular lubricant is not successful in the relief of the dryness. Ice or sugar-free gum or candies may be recommended to correct mouth dryness.

Evaluation. Improvement in the cystic acne should occur after 1 to 2 months, but may require 4 to 5 months of therapy.

Burn Products

Burn injuries range from mild and superficial to very severe with extensive skin loss associated with systemic and metabolic complications. Approximately 12,000 Americans die annually of thermal injury (Mailloux, 1995). The chief cause of death is shock, a fact of considerable significance in any effective plan of treatment.

Burns cause lesions of the skin accompanied by pain. The burn may be caused by heat (thermal burn), chemical cauterizing agents (chemical burns), or electricity (electrical burns). Sources may be friction, lightning, or electromagnetic energy sources (ultraviolet light, x-rays, lasers, or atomic explosion). The types of burns that result from various sources are relatively specific and diagnostic.

Consideration of what takes place in the damaged tissues clarifies many points of treatment. At first capillary permeability is altered in the local injured area; permeability is increased, resulting in a loss of plasma and weeping of the surface tissues. If the burn is at all extensive, considerable amounts of plasma fluid may be lost in a relatively short time.

This depletes the blood volume and causes a decreased cardiac output and diminished blood flow. Unless the situation is rapidly brought under control, irreparable damage may result from rapidly developing tissue anoxia. The lack of sufficient oxygen and accumulation of waste products from inadequate oxidation results in loss of tone in the minute blood vessels. The increased capillary permeability then extends to tissues remote from those suffering the initial injury. Thus a generalized edema often develops, and the vicious cycle once established tends to be self-perpetuating. One of the aims of the treatment of burns is therefore to stop the loss of plasma and to replenish that which is lost as quickly as possible.

Partial- or full-thickness burns must be thought of as open wounds with the accompanying danger of infection. The infection must be prevented or treated. The treatment, however, must be such that it will not cause any further destruction of tissue or of the small islands of remaining epithelium from which growth and regeneration can take place.

Burns are classified by degree, which is determined by the depth of skin involved within a geographic designation. First-degree burns involve only the epidermis, causing erythema with characteristic dry, painful reddening and edema without blistering or vesiculation (e.g., overexposure to sun or flash burn). Second-degree burns involve the epidermis extending into the dermis and may be superficial or involve deep dermal necrosis. Epithelial regeneration may extend from the deep skin appendages such as hair follicles and sebaceous glands that penetrate the dermis. This burn is characterized by a moist, blistered, very painful surface (e.g., flash or scald burns from nonviscous liquids). Third-degree burns involve destruction of the entire dermis and epidermis characterized by white, lustrous, or opaque skin; dry, leathery skin; or coagulated, charred skin without sensation as a result of the destruction of nerve endings (e.g., flame burns or hot viscous liquids). Fourth-degree burns extend into subcutaneous fat, muscle, or bone; appear black and dry in appearance and cause scarring.

The severity of electrical burns depends on the amount of voltage received, the condition of the skin (e.g., cuts, abrasions, and moisture, which lower resistance), and contraction of flexor muscles, which inhibits release from the power source. Electrical burns result in necrosis of more tissue than thermal burns and are of three types. In Type I, the electrical current causes effects on blood vessels such as occlusion, thrombosis, or tissue destruction. In Type II, electrical burns from high-tension currents (e.g., an electrical arc) produce a crater in the skin. Type III electrical burns are similar to flame burns because the arc flame ignites the person's clothes.

Chemical burns occur after contact with acid or alkali; the initial treatment is water irrigation of the affected area followed by neutralization. Chemical burns may occur in the mouth and appear as a white slough owing to necrosis of the epithelium and underlying connective tissues.

First-aid treatment of burns. An important first-aid treatment for minor and major burns regardless of cause (chemical, electric, thermal) is to immediately cool the wound to remove irritants, decrease inflammation, and constrict blood vessels; this reduces the permeability of the blood vessels and checks edema formation. Cold tap water can be used to flush the wound thoroughly and to cool hot clothing. The more quickly the wound is cooled, the less tissue damage there is likely to be, and the more rapid will be the recovery. No greasy ointments, lard, butter, or dressings should be applied, since these agents will inhibit loss of heat from the burn, which will increase both discomfort and tissue damage. The burn may be left exposed to the air, or cold wet compresses may be applied until the person can be transported for medical attention.

Burn victims treated in an emergency room or burn unit will be stabilized with intravenous fluids, given analgesics for pain, and sedated, if necessary. Such individuals are immunized with tetanus toxoid and/or tetanus immunoglobulin, depending on their immunization status. Catheterization may be necessary to measure urinary output, depending on the client's status. Following stabilization, the burn wound is cleaned with a mild soap and water and a sterile, nonadherent gauze dressing with hydrophilic petrolatum is applied to the wound. In some settings, synthetic dressings (Duoderm, Opsite) may be utilized. Topical antiinfective therapy may also be indicated. Silver sulfadiazine is usually preferred because of its broad-spectrum activity and also, this product is easy and painless to apply and remove from the burn. Povidone iodine was commonly used in some centers and it also penetrates eschar. But povidone iodine causes pain on application and when dry, will harden the eschar area (Mailloux, 1995).

silver sulfadiazine [sul fa dye' a zeen] (Silvadene)
Silver sulfadiazine is an antiinfective agent with broad antimicrobial activity against many gram-negative and gram-positive bacteria, similar to mafenide. It acts only on the cell membrane and cell wall to produce its bactericidal effect.

Silver sulfadiazine is used in second- and third-degree burns for the prevention and treatment of sepsis. It softens eschar, facilitating its removal and preparation of the wound for grafting.

Silver sulfadiazine is available as a 1% cream to be applied topically to cleansed, debrided burn wounds once or twice daily. It should be applied with a sterile gloved hand to a thickness of about 1.5 mm. Burn wounds should be continuously covered with the cream. Daily bathing and debriding are important and dressing may or may not be used.

Therapy is usually continued until satisfactory healing has occurred or the wound is ready for grafting. Because silver sulfadiazine inhibits bacterial growth, delayed eschar separation may occur, necessitating escharotomy to prevent contractures. Pain, burning, and itching occur infrequently after application of the silver sulfadiazine cream.

Silver sulfadiazine may cause a hypersensitivity reaction; if this occurs, the drug should be discontinued. Hemolysis may occur in persons with glucose-6-phosphate dehydrogenase deficiency. When silver sulfadiazine is applied to extensive areas of the body, significant amounts of the drug may be absorbed, reaching therapeutic serum levels and producing adverse reactions characteristic of the sulfonamides. Renal function in these clients should be monitored and the urine examined for sulfa crystals.

For nursing management of the client with silver sulfadiazine therapy, consult Chapter 71.

mafenide [ma' fe nide] (Sulfamylon)
Mafenide (sulfonamide), a broad-spectrum, antibacterial (bacteriostatic) topical agent, penetrates eschar even in the presence of pus and serum. It is a carbonic anhydrase inhibitor though, that can alter acid-base balance resulting in metabolic acidosis. In contrast to silver sulfadiazine, it is usually painful on application.

On application, mafenide rapidly diffuses through partial (second-degree) and full-thickness (third-degree) burns and has proved to be an effective means for preventing and retarding bacterial invasion in burn wounds. While relatively nontoxic, burning or pain on application and allergic reactions have been reported. It is rapidly metabolized to a metabolite and eliminated by way of the kidneys.

■ Nursing Management

Mafenide Therapy

In addition to the general discussion of the nursing management of dermatologic agent therapy, consider the following:

Implementation

Monitoring. Because this drug and metabolite are strong carbonic anhydrase inhibitors, acidosis (metabolic) may occur, usually compensated by hyperventilation. The client should be carefully observed for any signs resulting in respiratory alkalosis. If rapid or labored respirations occur, the ointment should be washed off the wound.

Intervention. Therapy can be interrupted for 2 to 3 days without impairing the bacterial control of the wound while continuing fluid therapy and acid-base restoration.

Education. Mafenide may cause some discomfort when first applied (in 1/16-inch layer once or twice daily)—a burning or pain sensation may occur that lasts from a few minutes to as long as an hour. This is a highly stable drug. It remains active for several years and does not need to be refrigerated except in tropical countries.

Topical Antipruritics

Antipruritic agents are given to allay itching of skin and mucous membranes. There is less need for these preparations as the constitutional treatment of persons with skin disorders is better understood. Dilute solutions containing phenol have been widely used. Dressings wet with potassium permanganate 1:4000, aluminum subacetate 1:16, boric acid, or physiologic saline solution may cool and soothe and thus prevent itching. Lotions such as calamine or calamine with phenol (phenolated calamine), and cornstarch or oatmeal baths may also be used to relieve itching.

Local anesthetics such as dibucaine and benzocaine may decrease pruritus, but their use is not recommended because of their high sensitizing and irritating effects. The application of hydrocortisone in a lotion or ointment in a strength of 0.5% to 1% has proved to be one of the best methods of relieving pruritus and decreasing inflammation. An additional advantage is its low sensitizing index.

Topical Ectoparasiticidal Drugs

Ectoparasites are insects that live on the outer surface of the body. Ectoparasiticides are drugs used against those animal parasites. For human use these drugs are more frequently referred to as *pediculicides* and *scabicides (miticides)*, reflecting the parasite treated with each group.

Pediculosis is a parasite infestation of lice on the skin of a human. Lice are transmitted from one person to the next by close contact with infested persons, clothing, combs, and towels. There are three different varieties of infestations: (1) pediculosis pubis, caused by *Phthirus pubis* (pubic or crab louse), (2) pediculosis corporis, caused by *Pediculus humanus corporis* (body louse), and (3) pediculosis capitis, caused by *P. humanus capitis* (head louse) (Figure 66-1). A characteristic finding of pediculosis corporis, except in heavily infested individuals, is that the parasite is absent from the body but inhabits seams of clothing that come in contact with the axillae or that are in the beltline or collar.

Common findings in a person who is infested include pruritus, nits (eggs of louse) on hair shafts, lice on skin or clothes, and, with pubic lice, occasionally sky-blue macules on the inner thighs or lower abdomen. The drug of choice is the pediculicide lindane (gamma-benzene hexachloride).

Scabies is a parasitic infestation caused by the itch mite, *Sarcoptes scabiei*. It is transmitted from one person to the next by close contact, such as sleeping next to an infested individual. It bores into the horny layers of the skin in cracks and folds, causing irritation and pruritus. Itching occurs almost exclusively at night. The adult infestation is usually generalized over the body especially in web spaces between fingers, wrists, elbows, and buttocks. The drug of choice is permethrin cream because it is considered to be more effective than crotamiton and lindane (Anandan, 1995).

■ Nursing Management

Topical Ectoparasiticidal Therapy

Assessment. The first approach to the treatment of both pediculosis and scabies is identification of the source of infestation. Next, decontamination of clothing and personal articles used by the infested person is necessary. This can be done by washing clothing and bedding with hot, soapy water or by dry cleaning items that cannot be washed. Usually all persons involved, such as the whole family, are treated to prevent reinfestation.

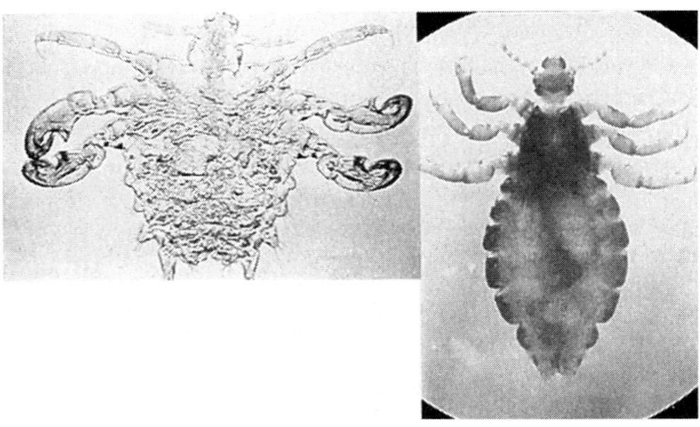

Figure 66-1 Pubic louse (*Phthirus pubis*), *left*, and body louse (*Pediculus humanus*), *right*. Notice that the first pair of legs on the pubic louse are thinner than the second and third pairs. Also, the abdomen is shorter. On the body louse, all legs are approximately the same length and the abdomen is longer.

lindane [lin' dane] (gamma-benzene hexachloride; [Kwell])

Lindane is both a scabicide and a pediculicide because it is effective in the treatment of both lice and mite infestations. It is available in a 1% cream, lotion, and shampoo. For the treatment of pediculosis pubis and infestations of *Pediculus humanus capitis*, the cream or lotion is applied in a sufficient quantity to cover the skin and hair of the infected and surrounding areas, left on for 12 hours and then thoroughly washed. It seldom needs to be applied more than once. The shampoo is worked into the hair and left on for 4 minutes. Then the hair is rinsed and dried, and nits (eggs) are combed from the hair shafts. Retreatment is usually not necessary.

For the treatment of scabies, the cream or lotion is used. If crusted lesions are present, a warm bath preceding the application of lindane is recommended. Lindane is applied over the entire body from the neck down. It is left on for 8 hours and then washed off. Usually one application is sufficient. It is common to have pruritus after application, but this does not indicate a need for reapplication unless live mites can be demonstrated.

Lindane occasionally will cause an eczematous skin rash. It penetrates human skin and has a potential for central nervous system toxicity (seizures, increased irritability, dizziness, etc.), especially in children.

crotamiton [kroe tam' i tonn] (Eurax)

Crotamiton indicated for the treatment of scabies, it is rubbed into the skin from the chin down, particularly in the folds and creases of the body and moist areas, such as underarms and groin. It is reapplied in 24 hours, and 48 hours after the second application it is washed from the body surface. Two applications of crotamiton usually eradicate most infestations. In resistant cases it may be applied again 1 week later.

Crotamiton available as a 10% cream or lotion may cause an occasional skin rash on application.

permethrin [per meth' rin] (Nix)

Permethrin acts on the nerve cell membranes of lice, ticks, mites, and fleas. It disrupts the sodium channel repolarization thus paralyzing the parasites. It has a high cure rate (up to 99%) in treating head lice after only a single application. The most common side effects/adverse reactions include pruritus, mild burning on application, transient erythema, edema, and rash.

malathion [mal' i thye one] (Ovide)

Malathion is an organophosphate cholinesterase inhibitor available for the treatment of head lice and ova. This product is usually effective in lice-infested individuals within 24 hours and is well tolerated. Malathion lotion is rubbed into the scalp and left to air dry. Because the drug is flammable, the individual must be warned to avoid open flames, smoking, and to not use a hairdryer. The hair should be shampooed 8 to 12 hours after application; dead lice are combed out.

SUMMARY

Many dermatologic agents are available and used to treat the numerous skin disorders that occur. Three major groups of preparations were discussed: general, prophylactic, and therapeutic agents. General dermatologic preparations include bath substances, cleansers, soaps, solutions and emollients, skin protectants, wet dressings and soaks, and rubs and liniments. Many are soothing and used to promote comfort of the client who has a dermatologic condition. Prophylactic agents form a film on the skin to keep out sun, light, air, or dust. Therapeutic agents may be antiinfectives (antibiotics, antivirals, and antifungals), corticosteroids, keratolytics, acne products, burn products, antipruritics, and ectoparasiticidal drugs. The nurse must apply these preparations correctly and safely and instruct the client to do likewise if they are to be self-administered. Evaluating the effectiveness of dermatologic agents is based on the diminution of the affected areas without adverse effect.

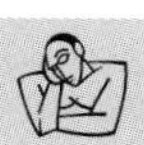

Critical Thinking

1. Ronald Jones, age 48, comes to the clinic with a superficial skin infection as the result of an abrasion he received on the job as a construction worker. The health care provider orders the wound to be cleansed and dressed with bacitracin ointment, 500 units/g, which the client is to continue tid, and a culture and sensitivity. As the nurse, what action will you take and in what sequence of events?
2. What teaching would you provide to a mother who has discovered a pediculosis infestation in one of her children?

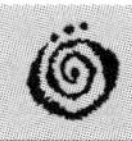

Collaborative Learning Activities

1. One student team will discuss the general nursing management of dermatologic drugs. The second team will describe the differences for agents to treat burns. The third team will cover the nursing management of topical ectoparasiticidal agents.

BIBLIOGRAPHY

Anandan JV (1995). Parasitic infections. In Young LY & Koda-Kimble MA (Eds.). *Applied therapeutics: The clinical use of drugs* (6th ed.). Vancouver: Applied Therapeutics.

Anderson KN, et al. (Eds.) (1994). *Mosby's medical, nursing, & allied health dictionary* (4th ed.). St. Louis: Mosby.

Bhawan, J, et al. (1991). Effects of tretinoin on photodamaged skin: A histologic study, *Arch Dermatol* 127:666.

DeSimone II EM (1993). Sunscreen and suntan products. In Covington TR (Ed.). *Handbook of nonprescription drugs* (10th ed.). Washington, DC: American Pharmaceutical Association.

Dicken CH, et al. (1992). Retinoids: What role in your practice? *Patient Care* 26(10):18-19, 25-8, 31-32,34, 37, 41-5.

Fitzpatrick TB, et al. (1993). *Dermatology in general medicine, vols I & II* (4th ed.). New York: McGraw-Hill.

Gupta MA, et al. (1991). Treatment of mildly to moderately photoaged skin with topical tretinoin has a favorable psychosocial effect: A prospective study, *J Amer Acad Dermatol* 24:780.

Mailloux AT (1995). Photosensitivity and burns. In *Applied therapeutics* (6th ed.). Vancouver: Applied Therapeutics.

Olin BR (Ed.) (1996). *Facts and comparisons.* St Louis: Facts and Comparisons.

Parks BR, et al. (1989). Treatment of head lice and scabies infestations in children, *Pediatr Nurs* 15(5):522.

Seaton TL (1995). Acne. In Young LY & Koda-Kimble MA. (Eds.). *Applied therapeutics* (6th ed.). Vancouver: Applied Therapeutics.

Seeley RR, et al. (1995). *Anatomy and physiology* (3rd ed.). St Louis: Mosby.

United States Pharmacopeial Convention (1996). *USP DI: Drug information for the health professional* (16th ed.). Rockville, MD: The Convention.

Chapter 67

Debriding Agents

Chapter Focus

Nurses have the major responsibility for the assessment of the client's risk for pressure sores and the planning for the care provided to prevent them. When pressure sores do occur, then cleansing, debridement, and dressing of the wounds are necessary. Knowledge of the various debriding agents will allow the nurse to apply the most appropriate agent for the client's pressure sores, given their location, size, presence of eschar, or state of granulation. The following objectives and key terms are necessary for a good understanding of this chapter.

Key Terms

debridement (p. 1035)
eschar (p. 1039)
granulation tissue (p.1039)
proteolytic enzyme (p. 1038)
pressure sore (p. 1035)

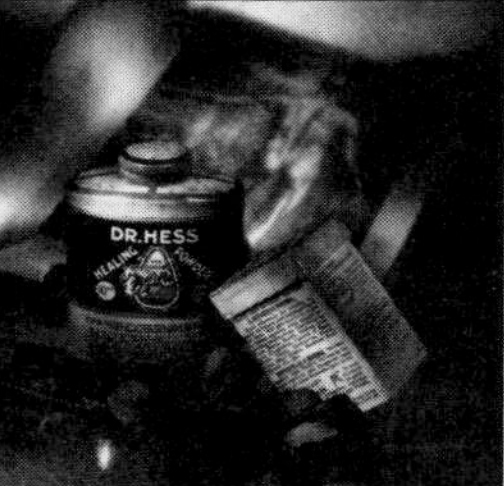

Objectives

1. Use preventive and treatment measures to reduce the occurrence of decubitus ulcers.
2. Describe a classification system for grades of decubitus ulcers.
3. State the purpose of proteolytic enzyme preparations in the treatment of decubitus ulcers.
4. Implement the nursing management of the care of clients receiving topical enzymatic agents.
5. Describe the mechanism of action of nonenzymatic agent therapy for decubitus ulcers.
6. Implement the nursing management of the care of clients receiving nonenzymatic agent therapy for decubitus ulcers.

This chapter covers debriding agents, which are agents used to remove dirt, foreign objects, damaged tissue, and cellular debris from a wound or burn to prevent infection and promote healing. In treatment of a wound, **debridement** is the first step in cleansing it; debridement also allows examination of the extent of the injury.

PRESSURE SORES

The **pressure sore** (bed sore or decubitus ulcer) is a break in the skin and underlying subcutaneous and muscle tissue caused by abnormal, sustained pressure or friction exerted over the bony prominences of the body by the object on which the body part rests. It results in vascular insufficiency and ischemic necrosis, and it most frequently affects debilitated, comatose, immobilized, or paralyzed clients. According to the Agency for Health Care Policy and Research (AHCPR), the prevalence of pressure ulcers ranges from 9.2% in acute care facilities; 33% in critical care patients, and up to 23% in skilled care facilities and nursing homes (Bergstrom et al., 1994). In addition to the human suffering of clients and their families, the total cost of treating such wounds was estimated as exceeding $1.335 billion (Bergstrom et al, 1994).

There are many contributing causes to this condition that must be treated. Among the local and systemic are the following: obesity or malnutrition; debilitation; a pressure and shearing force on the lower body if the head of the bed is raised more than 30 degrees; a loss of sensation of pressure or pain; muscle atrophy and motor paralysis; a reduction in the amount of adipose tissue between skin and underlying bone; emaciation and dehydration; poor nutrition because of an inadequate intake of vitamins, minerals, and trace elements (such as copper and zinc); friction; local anatomic defects; trauma; incontinence; edema; infections; heat and moisture (maceration); hypertension; septicemia; and local circulatory interference.

The bacterial flora of pressure sores (present in stages II, III and IV) are both gram-negative and gram-positive organisms, which include *Staphylococcus aureus, Streptococcus* groups A and D, *Escherichia coli, Clostridium tetani,* and *Bacteroides, Proteus, Pseudomonas, Klebsiella,* and *Citrobacter* organisms. Parenteral antibiotics (adequate levels in granulating wounds are not reached) may be needed in difficult-to-treat infected pressure sores as an adjunct to surgical management just before and at time of surgery.

An individual with a full-thickness loss of skin may be a candidate for surgical intervention either to cover the ulcer area or to stabilize the wound. Surgical decisions include the underlying disease, the ability of the client to withstand surgery, and the condition or prognosis of the pressure sore (especially those in which all soft tissue is destroyed, exposing bone).

■ Nursing Management

Pressure Sore

Assessment. To assess the client's risk of developing pressure sores, the nurse must know the causes of pressure ulcers. Most health care agencies have assessment guides by which to assess the client's risk (Figure 67-1). These assessment guides address common risk factors such as mobility, activity, mental status, medications that affect blood circulation or cognition, incontinence, nutritional status, and other current illnesses. Clients are assessed and given a score; the higher the score, the higher the risk. These assessment guides are usually completed upon admission of the client to the agency, so nurses should continue to monitor the client for the risk of impaired skin integrity over the course of the client's stay with the health care agency.

Nursing diagnosis. The pertinent nursing diagnosis is either risk for impaired skin integrity, given the client's assessment score; or if the client evidences skin changes such as erythema not resolving in 30 minutes, blister, or tissue erosion, an actual impairment of skin integrity. Risk for infection and altered comfort: pain may also occur.

Implementation

Monitoring. Monitor the bony prominences of the ankles, coccyx, elbows, heels, hips, knees, shoulders, and other areas having thin layers of subcutaneous tissue. Continue to assess the client for the presence or worsening of risk factors as discussed above. If a pressure sore occurs, assess the wound on a daily basis for gradual reduction in size; measure and record wound size at its greatest length, width, and depth. Determine the stage of the wound and describe the appearance of the wound as to necrotic debris, eschar, granulation tissue, drainage, color, and odor. Assess for pockets, tracts, and undermining. Observe the wound margins for induration or tenderness.

Intervention. Prevention and treatment of pressure sores are centered around treatment of underlying causes, providing a well-balanced nutritional state, and minimizing or eliminating the pressure or friction causing tissue damage. The following are some preventive and treatment measures that the nurse may use to reduce the occurrence of impaired skin integrity.

1. Change the client's position frequently (every 1 to 2 hours day and night) for pressure relief.
2. Maintain a clean, dry, and wrinkle-free bed. Bed clothes should be smooth rather than coarse and should be changed frequently.
3. Provide active and passive exercise to increase muscle and skin tone and to improve vascularity, or use a whirlpool for hydrotherapy.
4. Position the client with pillows and pads, not exceeding a 30-degree elevation of the head.
5. Use hydrofloat devices, silica gel pads, polystyrene, and convoluted foam pads and heel protectors to reduce pressure. Place them on a mattress in direct contact with the client's skin. The mattress should be free of surface bulges and indentations and have a uniform, flat surface to prevent friction or wrinkles.
6. Use an alternating pressure mattress pad covered with one layer of sheet to promote circulation and reduce the occurrence of tissue ischemia.
7. Provide meticulous skin hygiene with frequent inspections for abnormal alterations. Wash gently with warm water and, if needed, mild nondetergent

SKIN INTEGRITY HIGH RISK FORM

	PARAMETERS	0	1	2	3	4	5	SCORE
1.	General state of health	Good	Fair	Poor	Moribund			
2.	Predisposing diseases	Absent	Slight	Moderate	Severe			
3.	Mental status	Alert	Lethargic	Semicoma	Comatose			
4.	Nutrition	Good	Fair	Poor	None			
5.	Fluid intake	Good	Fair	Poor	None			
6.	Activity	Ambulates	Needs help			Chairfast	Bedfast	
7.	Mobility	Full	Limited			Very limited	Immobile	
8.	Incontinence	None	Occasional			Frequent	Total	
							TOTAL	

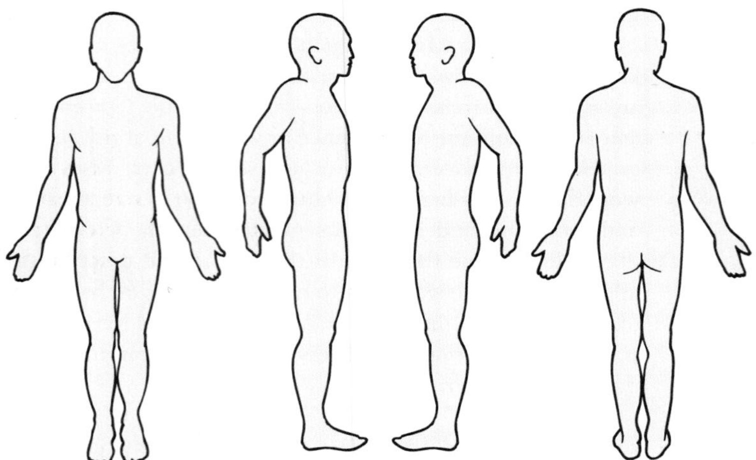

Draw and Number Impairments

	#1
Stage:	
Size:	
Shape:	
Drainage:	
	#2
Stage:	
Size:	
Shape:	
Drainage:	
	#3
Stage:	
Size:	
Shape:	
Drainage:	

Date/Signature: ________________

PARAMETERS:

1. GENERAL STATE OF HEALTH:
   - 0–Good: injury limited to one area, no major health problems
   - 1–Fair: minor surgery or controlled health problems
   - 2–Poor: major surgery or serious health problems
   - 3–Moribund: prognosis fatal, death within 3 months
2. PREDISPOSING DISEASE:
   - 0–Absent: no vascular disease, anemia, diabetes, neuropathies
   - 1–Slight: controlled diabetes, anemia, mild vascular diseases, mild skin disorder
   - 2–Moderate: brittle diabetes, advanced vascular disease, unheaied ulcers, absent peripheral pulses
   - 3–Severe: uncontrolled diabetes/anemia, severe vascular disease manifested by: decreased sensation, edema of ankles and feet, thin atrophic skin, brown pigmentation with stasis dermatitis
3. MENTAL STATUS:
   - 0–Alert: oriented, communicates appropriately
   - 1–Lethargic: listless, sluggishness, slow to respond
   - 2–Semicoma or confused: responds to painful stimuli, unable to cooperate with pressure relief
   - 3–Comatose: no verbal response, no response to pain
4. NUTRITION:
   - 0–Good: weight within normal limits
   - 1–Fair: under or overweight, enternal or parenteral nutrition meeting RDA
   - 2–Poor: losing weight slowly or obese, seldom eats 1/2 served portion, enteral feeding tolerated poor, i.e., high gastric residual, diarrhea
   - 3–None: losing weight rapidly, emaciated, unable to eat, refuses to eat, no nutritional support
5. FLUID INTAKE:
   - 0–Good: 1500 cc, skin warm resilient, normal turgor
   - 1–Fair: 1000-1500 cc, dry skin and flaccid, concentrated urine output
   - 2–Poor: ↓1000 cc, skin dry, cracked and flaky, mouth dry, lips parched, decreased urine output in the absence of renal disease
   - 3–None: no fluid intake
6. ACTIVITY:
   - 0–Ambulates: walks without help
   - 1–Needs help: requires assistance, uses crutch, walker
   - 2–Chairfast: cannot ambulate, confined to chair
   - 3–Bedfast: remains in bed constantly
7. MOBILITY:
   - 0–Full: voluntarily changes position
   - 1–Limited: cannot voluntarily move all extremities, cast on arm or leg, pain with movement
   - 2–Very limited: move only with assistance, severe pain with movement, body cast, paraplegia, hemiparesis
   - 3–Immobile: never voluntarily changes position, contractures prevent movement, quadriplegia
8. INCONTINENCE:
   - 0–None: control of bowel and bladder
   - 1–Occasional: stress incontinence, occasional diarrhea with the continent patient
   - 2–Frequent: usually of urine and/or bowels
   - 3–Total: no control of bowel or bladder

Figure 67-1 Assessment guide. A score of 12 or greater is an indication that the client is at risk for impaired skin integrity. This nursing diagnosis should be included in the client's care plan.

soap; rinse and blot dry with a soft towel. An emollient lubricating lotion may be used after washing to keep the skin soft.

8. Keep the skin of incontinent clients dry and clear of urine and fecal contamination because maceration from moisture promotes tissue breakdown and predisposes patients to infection. Perspiration in the continent client is also a cause of maceration. Trimmed nails prevent self-inflicted injury caused by scratching of the skin.
9. Maintain nutritional support for a positive nitrogen balance, tissue turgor, and adequate fluid intake with 3800 to 4600 cal/24 hours, a diet high in protein, vitamins, minerals, and trace elements. The client's hemoglobin level should be 12 g/100 ml or more, and the serum protein above 6 mg/100 ml.
10. Necrotic pressure sores often require debridement by surgical or drug methods and meticulous wound care.
11. Clients should be offered analgesia before pressure sore care in keeping with the extent of the wound and the client's preferences.
12. Treatment regimens are based on the extent of skin involvement.

Education. The preventive measures should be taught to clients, family members, or other caregivers of bedridden or other clients who are at risk for developing pressure sores. If a pressure sore is present, inform the client that the preparations used are to promote healing and describe the procedure involved in cleansing and dressing the wound. (See the Home Health box at right).

Evaluation. The client's skin will remain warm, without erythema, and intact or if a pressure sore exists, the wound will diminish in size and form a healthy, clean surface.

Home Health

Wound Care at Home

Instruction should be provided for the caregiver if decubitus care is to be done in the home. This should include all the supportive care to the client, such as positioning, nutrition, and hydration discussed in the interventions. Pressure sore dressings should be changed as ordered by the prescriber or when soiled.

Dressing supplies, the debriding agent, gloves, and a bag for disposal of the soiled dressings should be gathered together before the dressing change is begun. The client should be positioned for comfort and for good access to the pressure sore. The decubitus should be assessed each time the dressing is changed; the size and character of the wound is recorded to monitor progress. Any increase in drainage or foul smell should be reported to the nurse.

Expose the pressure sore and drape the client for modesty as much as possible. Glove hands and remove the soiled dressing, pulling the adhesive tape in the direction of the pressure sore. Mineral oil may be used to loosen the adhesive tape. Discard the old dressings in the bag and discard gloves. Glove hands to clean the wound from the center out using one stroke each time until crusting and old drainage are removed. Apply pharmacologic agent as ordered using swabs, a tongue blade, or gloved fingers. Apply outer dressings. Remove gloves and secure dressing with tape. Discard soiled gloves in bag.

PHARMACOLOGIC MANAGEMENT

A treatment plan for pressure sores should take into consideration four basic principles: (1) assessment and interventions to improve the client's general health, which may help to reduce factors contributing to the problem, such as incontinence, anemia, or edema; (2) reducing pressure sites by positioning or the use of padding, special beds, and other items, thus increasing blood flow to the site; (3) maintaining a clean wound site; and (4) use of an appropriate agent for treatment or stimulation of granulation tissue.

The treatment of pressure sores depends on the stage of the ulcer and the condition of the wound bed. In many instances, cleansing and debridement prevents bacterial colonization from progressing to an infection. If a clean ulcer has exudate or does not heal after 2 to 4 weeks of treatment, a 2 week trial with topical antibiotics should be considered. The topical agent should be effective against gram-positive, gram-negative and anaerobic bacteria, such as triple antibiotic or silver sulfadiazine (Bergstrom et al, 1994).

If the ulcerated area does not respond, a tissue biopsy and bacterial culture is recommended in addition to, an evaluation for osteomyelitis. Systemic antibiotics are necessary for sepsis, osteomyelitis, bacteremia, and advancing cellulitis (Bergstrom et al, 1994).

Saline solutions are considered safe and effective in cleaning most pressure sores. Avoid the use of povidone iodine, iodophor, Dakin's solution, acetic acid and hydrogen peroxide because they are reported to be cytotoxic, i.e. toxic to fibroblasts and interfere with the granulation process (Eastman, 1995).

Pressure sores have been classified into four grades or stages (Figure 67-2):

Stage I—A red area that overlies a bony or tendinous (tendons) site that remains even when the pressure is relieved

Stage II—A partial-thickness skin loss involving epidermis and/or dermis

Stage III—Skin ulcer extends into exposed subcutaneous tissue; may include necrotic tissue, sinus tract formation, exudate, and/or infection

Stage IV—Deep skin ulcer that exposes muscle and bone; usually the body enzymes separate the eschar, sloughing of tissue results in an ulcer; may include necrotic tissue, sinus tract formation, exudate, and/or infection

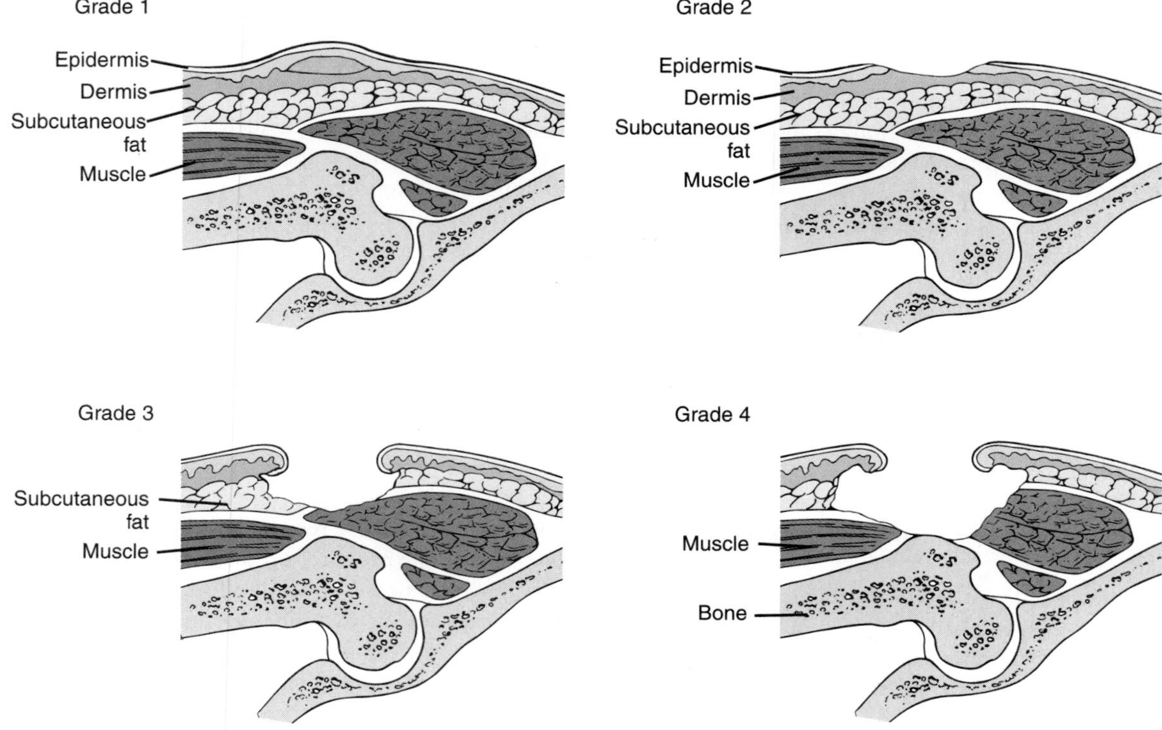

Figure 67-2 The four grades of pressure sores.

In addition to the nursing management previously reviewed, numerous treatment protocols have been applied. Therefore, depending on the evaluation of the wound, the physician, the nurse, and local practice, the treatment approach can vary considerably. Table 67-1 is a recommended treatment protocol based on the previous staging system.

TABLE 67-1 Decubitus ulcers: recommended treatment protocol

Staging	Typical treatment modalities
Stage I or II	Silicone spray, transparent or hydrocolloidal dressing
Stage III	Wet to dry dressings, enzymatic debridement, hydrocolloidal dressing
Stage IV	Wet to dry dressings, enzymatic debridement, surgical debridement

Proteolytic (Debriding) Enzymes

Debridement is used to remove necrotic and sloughing tissue in a pressure ulcer. This tissue delays healing and provides a media for bacterial infestation. Although commonly used for debridement, wet-to-dry saline dressings can be irritating, painful, and disruptive to healthy tissue. Proteolytic enzymes are used for chemical debridement; they digest or liquefy necrotic tissue. The drawback with these preparations is that 2 or 3 days are usually needed to get rid of an eschar. However, their use is appropriate for noninfected necrotic sites and for clients unable to tolerate surgical intervention. If used for infected necrosis tissue, a systemic antibiotic may also be necessary.

The enzyme preparation should be discontinued when granulation tissue is evident, or if bleeding occurs during gentle cleansing (Chamberlain et al, 1992). In very serious ulceration, or if complications are present (osteomyelitis), surgical debridement may be required.

Most enzymes contain the suffix "ase" in their name plus the name of the substrate on which they act. For example, collagenase acts on and degrades collagen; hyaluronidase acts on hyaluronic acid, a ground substance of connective tissue. Enzymes are also grouped according to the reactions they catalyze. For example, **proteolytic enzymes** hasten the hydrolysis of proteins. Because enzymes are proteins, they may be antigenic and cause toxic reactions of an immunologic type.

The enzymes discussed in this chapter are used topically for *medical* or *chemical debridement*—the removal, by enzymatic digestion, of necrotic and injured tissue, clotted blood, purulent exudates, or fibrinous accumulations in wounds. This action cleans the wounds and facilitates healing.

■ Nursing Management

Proteolytic Enzyme Therapy

The following are aspects of care for clients being treated with topically applied enzymatic drugs (not the nonenzymatic agents). These are in addition to the aspects of care previously discussed in nursing management of pressure sores.

Before topical aseptic application of enzymes, the wound should be thoroughly cleansed (flushing away necrotic debris and fibrinous exudates) with a solution that does not inactivate the enzyme (e.g., physiologic saline or sterile distilled water). Healing wounds should be cleansed gently; high-pressure irrigation or aggressive scrubbing with gauze pads should be avoided because tissue will be traumatized and healing delayed. Solutions containing heavy metals, detergents, and antiseptics should be avoided to prevent inactivation of the enzymes. As much necrotic tissue should be removed with forceps and scissors as can be readily removed. All previously applied ointment should be removed before new ointment is applied to the substrate.

Dense, dry, and thick **eschar,** or crust, should be cross-hatched by the physician with a no. 10 or 11 blade for adequate contact of enzyme to the substrate of necrotic debris. Ointment should be applied directly to the wound with a sterile tongue depressor or spatula and then covered with sterile petrolatum gauze or sterile gauze (or other nonadhering dressing), or it can be applied with a sterile gauze pad that is then placed over the wound. A bandage and/or tape should then be used to hold the dressing in place. Ointment or jelly preparations should be confined to the wound. The surrounding healthy tissue (or skin) should be protected from the enzyme (e.g., zinc oxide paste can be used). The treated lesion should be kept moist and protected from drying. The enzyme must be in direct contact with the wound for a sufficient length of time, usually about 4 days. To avoid delayed healing, the enzyme should be discontinued when the wound is cleaned and debrided, and when **granulation tissue** (healthy pink, soft new tissue) is evident. Secondary skin closure or grafting may follow optimal debridement.

Topical enzymes used for debriding may increase the risk of bacteremia in the debilitated individual; this may necessitate monitoring of these clients for systemic bacterial infections. Clients should be observed for allergic or sensitivity reactions (e.g., dermatitis and febrile reactions).

collagenase [kole' a jen aze] (Santyl)

Collagenase an enzymatic debriding agent, is capable of degrading both native and denatured collagen. Other proteolytic enzymes act only on denatured collagen. Thus it is claimed that collagenase produces more effective debridement by acting on collagen at the wound edges, where necrotic slough is anchored. This product is used to debride necrotic lesions and severe burns.

This ointment should be applied only within the area of the lesion, since a transient erythema has been reported as a cutaneous reaction on the wound surface or the area adjacent to the lesion. This reaction may be prevented by applying a protectant (e.g., zinc oxide paste) around the lesion.

■ Nursing Management

Collagenase Therapy

See the previous discussion of general nursing management of pressure sores and debriding agents. Before collagenase is applied, the client's therapies should be reviewed for significant drug interactions that may occur if collagenase is used in conjunction with the following drugs:

Drug	Possible effect and management
Burow's solution and other acidic solutions	Collagenase can be inactivated by irrigating the lesion with acidic solutions such as Burow's (pH 3.6 to 4.4). The optimal pH range for collagenase is 6 to 8; an alteration outside this range will decrease the enzyme's activity.
detergents, soaps, cleansing agents, heavy metal ions (mercury, silver) antiseptics (iodine, hexachlorophene, benzalkonium chloride, etc), boric acid	Activity of collagenase is inhibited.

The area is cleansed of debris by gentle irrigation with sterile normal saline. The ulcer should be patted dry with a sterile gauze pad. If infection is present, a topical antibacterial agent (e.g., neomycin, bacitracin-polymyxin B solution or powder) is applied directly to the ulcer surface before collagenase.

Collagenase should be applied once daily for in-patients and every other day for out-patients. If the wound is deep, collagenase should be applied directly with a wooden tongue depressor or spatula. The application should be repeated if the dressing area is soiled (e.g., because of incontinence).

The average time for complete debridement of dermal ulcers and decubiti with collagenase is about 11 days. This time permits debridement of necrotic tissue and establishment of granulation tissue. Careful observation of the wound bed is indicated. The enzyme should be stopped when granulation tissue is evident. The ointment does not have to be refrigerated; it is stored at room temperature.

fibrinolysin and desoxyribonuclease [fye bri nol' ih sin/des ock see rye bo nu' klee aze] (Elase)

The proteolytic enzymes fibrinolysin and desoxyribonuclease have individual effects; fibrinolysin digests fibrin or blood clots and desoxyribonuclease digests deoxyribonucleic acid (nucleic acids). Because purulent exudates are composed mainly of fibrin and nucleic acids, this product produces its effects on denatured proteins (devitalized tissue) while the protein elements of living cells are unaffected.

An ointment that contains the two enzymes in combination with chloramphenicol is also available. The added antibiotic bacteriostatic properties inhibit bacterial protein synthesis in infected lesions. Systemic antibiotics are also indicated when clinical infection has been verified by positive culture results.

This product is used to debride inflamed and/or infected lesions, including surgical wounds, ulcerative lesions, second- and third-degree burns, and wounds resulting from circumcision or episiotomy. The combination product with antibiotic is preferred for infected lesions. This product is also used for treatment of vaginitis and cervicitis (intravaginal use), and irrigation of infected wounds and superficial hematomas not adjacent to or near fatty tissue.

■ Nursing Management
Fibrinolysin and Desoxyribonuclease Therapy

See the previous discussions for general nursing management of pressure sores and the client on debriding agent therapy.

Obtain the client's sensitivity history because allergic reactions have been observed in persons who are sensitive to bovine source materials, mercury compounds (thimerosal, a mercury derivative, is used as a preservative in the ointment base of Elase), or chloramphenicol.

The preparation is available as an ointment or as a dry powder in vials, in which case it will need to be reconstituted with 10 to 50 ml of 0.9% sodium chloride injection. The solution may then be used as a spray or for a wet dressing. Saturate strips of fine-mesh gauze or unfolded sterile gauze pads in the solution and pack the ulcerated area with the gauze, ensuring that it is in contact with the necrotic substrate. The dressing should be allowed to dry in contact with the tissue, which may take 6 to 8 hours. Remove the gauze 3 or 4 times a day. As the gauze dries, the necrotic tissues slough, become enmeshed in the gauze, and so are removed from the wound. After 2 to 4 days the wound should become clean and begin to evidence granulation tissue. Mix the preparation on a daily basis because it becomes inactive after 24 hours.

sutilains [soo' ti lains] (Travase)

Sutilains is a sterile preparation of proteolytic enzymes that digests necrotic soft tissues and purulent exudates. It aids in the selective removal of only nonviable protein in necrotic soft tissue, and of purulent exudate from open wounds and ulcers resulting from second- and third-degree burns, decubiti, peripheral vascular disease, and wounds (incisions, trauma, pyogens).

Side effects are mild; they include mild, transient pain (managed with a mild analgesic), local paresthesia, bleeding, and transient dermatitis.

■ Nursing Management
Sutilains Therapy

See also the previous discussion of general nursing management of the client with topical enzymatic therapy.

Assessment. Sutilains should not be applied to wounds communicating with major body cavities, wounds with exposed major nerves or nerve tissue, neoplastic ulcers, or wounds in women of child-bearing age. Because its use causes increased fluid and blood loss, it should be used with caution in clients with limited cardiac and pulmonary reserves.

The client's wound therapy should be reviewed for significant drug interactions that may occur if sutilains is used in conjunction with the drug discussed with collagenase therapy.

Implementation

Monitoring. Monitor as described under the general nursing management for pressure sores. If bleeding or dermatitis occurs, the drug should be discontinued. Although systemic allergic reactions have not been reported, the drug is capable of causing an antibody response.

Intervention. Sutilains is prepared as an ointment containing 82,000 casein units/g ointment base (15 g tubes). It must be refrigerated at a temperature between 2° C and 10° C.

The wound should be thoroughly cleansed (including removal of antiseptics) with water or isotonic sodium chloride solution and left moist or wet before a thin layer of sutilains ointment is applied up to ½-inch beyond the area needing debriding. When used for extensive burns, the ointment should only be used on 10% to 15% of the burned skin area at one time. The area should then be covered with loose, wet dressings. The process should be repeated 3 to 4 times daily, although adequate responses have occurred with 1 to 2 changes daily. A moist environment is necessary for this agent's enzymatic activity. In concomitant use with topical antibiotics, apply sutilains first.

This drug must be kept away from the eyes; if contact occurs, the eyes should be rinsed with copious amounts of sterile water.

Evaluation. If dissolution does not occur in 24 to 48 hours, the drug should be discontinued.

Topical Enzyme Combination Products

Trypsin and papain (proteolytic enzymes), balsam Peru (mild antibacterial agent that aids in improving circulation in the wound area by stimulating the capillary bed), castor oil (protective covering, improves epithelialization), urea (emollient and keratolytic), and chlorophyll derivatives (aid in controlling wound odor and healing) have been formulated into various combinations and marketed. For example, Granulex contains trypsin, Balsam Peru, and castor oil, whereas Panafil contains papain, urea, and chlorophyll derivatives.

Such products may be ordered for administration once or twice daily. The wound area should be cleansed by flushing with physiologic saline before application each time. Be aware that hydrogen peroxide solution can inactivate papain activity.

Nonenzymatic Agents

dextranomer [dex tran' oh mer] (Debrisan)

Dextranomers are hydrophilic beads placed in the wound to absorb exudate, bacteria and other matter. It is used for cleansing only a wet or secreting wound (not dry wounds) and the action continues until all the beads are saturated. The assumption of a grayish-yellow color by the beads indicates that they are saturated and ready for removal.

■ Nursing Management
Dextranomer

See the previous discussion of the general nursing management of pressure sores.

Dextranomer is available in 4 g packages and 60 and 120 g containers, and in paste form. The contents of each container should be used for only one person to limit cross-contamination.

To initially prepare the wound it should be irrigated with sterile water or saline and the area should be left moist. A whirlpool bath will assist in removing persistent patches of beads. To apply, the beads should cover the wound surface to a depth of 3 mm to 6 mm (1/8 to 1/4 inch) (e.g., 4 g of beads covers a wound or ulcer 1½ × 1½ inches). A paste mixture is often used for areas that are either irregular body surfaces or are difficult to reach. If the premade paste dosage form is not available (10 g foil packets), the nurse may mix the beads with glycerin (only glycerin) and dress the wound in the usual manner. The beads or paste must be reapplied every 12 hours or more often while reducing the number of applications as the exudate diminishes. If the wound is a cratered pressure sore, allow for expansion of the beads by not packing the wound tightly. Dextranomer should be used only in body areas where complete removal is possible (not deep fistulas or sinus tracts). The nurse should be aware that if the beads are spilled on the floor, the floor becomes slippery, creating a work hazard.

The wound should be lightly bandaged on all four sides to hold the beads in place and prevent maceration from occlusion. The degree of wound secretion determines the number of dressing changes (usually one or two daily profuse secretions may necessitate three or four dressing changes). Changes are done before encrustation or full saturation of the beads (grayish yellow color) to prevent drying and to facilitate bead removal by irrigation (e.g., sterile water, saline). These moisture-reactive dressings for pressure sores and leg ulcers may remain in place for 1 to 7 days, and by interacting with the available skin moisture, a bond is created that keeps them in place. While in place over the wound, the moisture-reactive particles imbedded in a polymer base interact with the wound fluid exudate, creating a soft moist gel over the wound, which eases dressing removal with minimal damage to newly formed regenerating tissues.

During the first few days, as the edema is reduced, the wound itself may appear larger in size than it did before treatment. Therapy should be discontinued when healthy granulation is established. Treatment of an underlying pathologic condition (such as venous or arterial flow or pressure) is concurrent. Clients with diabetes mellitus and immunosuppression may be susceptible to severe infections. A client occasionally may have some minor pain during dressing changes.

flexible hydroactive dressings and granules (Duo-Derm)

The control of wound fluid exudate absorption is a function of the rate at which the dressing interacts with the exudate. These dressings are indicated for necrotic wounds only after the thick eschar at the wound margin is removed. It provides local management of venous stasis ulcers, ulcers secondary to arterial insufficiency, diabetes mellitus, trauma, pressure sores, and superficial wounds. The granule form is for local management of exudating dermal ulcers in association with the dressings.

■ Nursing Management

Flexible Hydroactive Dressings and Granules

See the previous discussion of the general nursing management of pressure sores.

Assessment. Use in the following dermal conditions should be avoided: tissue of muscle, tendon, or bone; ulcers with infection (tuberculosis, syphilis, or deep fungal infections); and active vasculitis (periarteritis nodosa, systemic lupus erythematosus, and cryoglobulinemia).

Implementation

Monitoring. During the initial phase of treatment, the wound increases in size and depth because of the cleaning away of the necrotic debris.

Intervention. The liquefied material left in the wound (seen when the dressing is removed) has the appearance of pus and should be washed away before further wound evaluation proceeds.

Clean the wound site before applying this product. Follow the specific instructions outlined in the package labeling. The characteristic disagreeable dermal ulcer odor, apparent when the dressing is removed or from wound leakage, may be diminished with the use of the granule dosage form during excess exudation periods.

During periods of infection, the dressings or granules should be discontinued and antibiotic treatment started until the infection is completely treated.

Excessive exudate, when present, may necessitate the granule dosage form application into the wound to prevent leakage and allow the dressing to remain in place longer and reduce dressing changes.

metronidazole [me troe ni' da zole] (Flagyl)

Metronidazole is an antiinfective systemic agent used investigationally to treat Grades III and IV anaerobically infested, decubitus ulcers (Olin, 1996). An approved topical metronidazole (MetroGel) is used to treat acne rosacea in adults (*USP DI*, 1996).

SUMMARY

Pressure sores add greatly to the length and cost of a hospital stay. They are best prevented, but when they do occur they are then treated with proteolytic enzyme or nonenzymatic preparations, depending on the cause and extent of the wound.

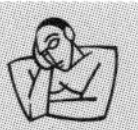

Critical Thinking

1. How do the indications for the use of proteolytic enzyme preparations differ from the uses for flexible hydroactive dressings and granules?
2. How might a nurse determine that it is time to discontinue the use of proteolytic enzyme preparations?

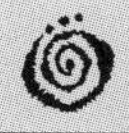

Collaborative Learning Activities

1. Four student teams will each be assigned one of the grades of pressure sores. Each team should describe the grade, nursing care for that grade, and what debriding agents would be appropriate for that stage and why?

BIBLIOGRAPHY

Alterescu V & Alterescu KB (1992). Pressure ulcers: Assessment and treatment, *Ortho Nurs 11*(2):37-49.

Anderson KN, et al. (Eds.) (1994). *Mosby's medical, nursing, & allied health dictionary* (4th ed.). St Louis: Mosby.

Bergstrom N, Bennett MA, Carlson CE, et al. (1994). *Treatment of pressure ulcers: Clinical practice guidelines,* No. 15. Rockville, MD: U.S. Dept of Health and Human Services. Public Health Service, Agency for Health Care Policy and Research. AHCPR Pub 95-0652.

Braun JL, et al. (1992). What really works for pressure sores, *Patient Care 26*(2):63-6, 71-3, 75-8, 81.

Chamberlain TM, et al. (1992). Assessment and management of pressure sores in long-term care facilities, *Consul Pharm* 7(12):1328-40.

Eastman SR (1995). Prevention and treatment of pressure ulcers: Interpretation and practical application of AHCPR guidelines: Part 1. *Clin Consul 14*(10):1-8.

Jaffee MS & Skidmore-Roth L. (1993). *Home health nursing care plans* (2nd ed.). St Louis: Mosby.

Olin BR (Ed.) (1996). *Facts and comparisons*. St Louis: Facts and Comparisons.

United States Pharmacopeial Convention (1996). *USP DI: Drug information for the health care professional* (16th ed.). Rockville, MD: The Convention.

Zanowiak P (1992). Safe and effective management of pressure ulcers, *US Pharm: Skin Care Supp 6*:6.

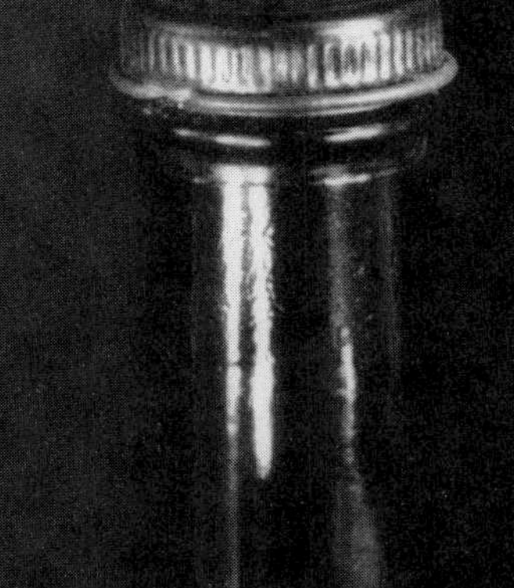

Chapter 68
Vitamins and Minerals

Chapter Focus

Over-the-counter vitamin and mineral preparations are very popular in the United States and Canada. Inappropriately used, though, these dietary supplements possess the capacity for producing toxic reactions. Vitamins and minerals, however, often are not perceived as being drugs by consumers. It is imperative that nurses incorporate vitamin therapy assessment and instruction into their practice to be supportive of appropriate nutrient management for their clients. The following objectives and key terms are important for a good understanding of this chapter.

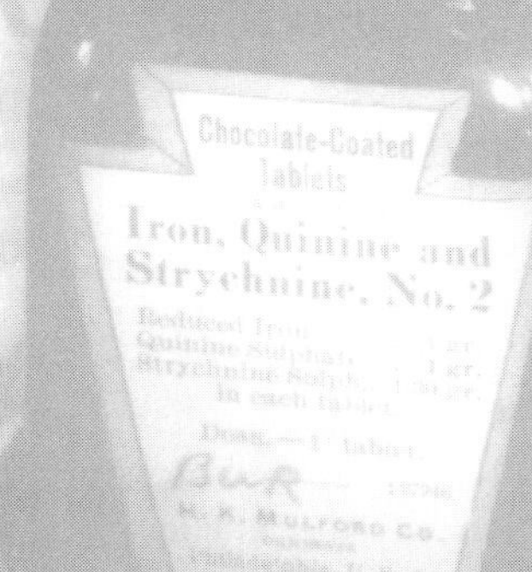

Key Terms

avitaminosis (p. 1044)
fat-soluble vitamins (p. 1044)
hypervitaminosis (p. 1048)
vitamin (p. 1044)
water-soluble vitamins (p. 1044)

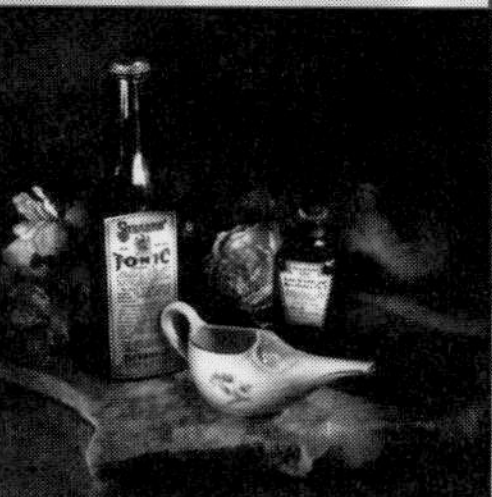

Objectives

1. Review the recommended daily allowances of vitamins and minerals.
2. Discuss factors that might contribute to inadequate intake of vitamins and minerals.
3. Describe the difference between fat-soluble and water- soluble vitamins.
4. Cite the results of a deficiency or excess of each vitamin.
5. Implement the nursing management essential to the care of clients receiving vitamin therapy.
6. Compare the contents of OTC vitamin and mineral preparations with recommended daily allowances.

The nutritional needs of the individual are best met by adequate oral ingestion of fluids and regular, balanced meals. Breast milk or formula meets the normal nutrition needs of the infant; strained and chopped table foods are added to the diet as tolerated by the growing child. Throughout life, challenges to nutrition status can occur that necessitate nutrient, vitamin, mineral, electrolyte, and fluid replacement or supplementation. Debilitation from nutritional deprivation may impair wound healing; reduce collagen, hormone, and enzyme synthesis; and decrease essential protein production, reducing circulating albumin, fibrinogen, and hemoglobin. Malnutrition or mild-to-moderate starvation produces serious cellular biochemical changes, including diminished liver glycogen stores, that start the first day of deprivation. Diminished protein stores are supplemented via gluconeogenesis because amino acids are converted into glucose as an energy source. Tissue proteins are depleted and short-lived in the intestinal mucous membranes, liver, pancreas, and kidney tubular epithelia. Muscle proteins are converted to provide energy, and adipose tissues are metabolized to produce free fatty acids for energy substrates. The byproducts of fatty acid oxidation (ketones) are used as energy for the brain if starvation is prolonged.

Unusual or abnormal circumstances necessitating administration of the various nutritional modalities, such as vitamin replacement and enteral or parenteral feedings, are discussed in the following sections.

VITAMINS

Vitamins are organic compounds that help maintain normal metabolic functions, growth, and tissue repair. Mechanisms of action, specific indications for use, and pharmacokinetics are not well understood for all vitamins, nor have dosages been established for all vitamins. However, vitamin supplement therapy may be essential during periods of nutritional challenge, typically during rapid growth, pregnancy, lactation, or convalescence. Other challenges to nutrition occur with inadequate nutrient ingestion, malabsorption syndromes, and increased nutrient requirement caused by specific disease states, such as celiac sprue and ulcerative colitis. An increase in cellular proliferation in the latter conditions may result in key nutrient depletion, such as of folic acid.

Insufficient dietary intake of vitamins and other essential nutrients occasionally may be traced to impoverished diets resulting from cultural, religious, or personal beliefs; fad diets; alcoholism; poverty; ignorance; or lack of available food. Mild forms of **avitaminosis** (vitamin deficiency), however, are more common in the United States and Canada (often as a result of alcoholism) than the pronounced deficiency states of beriberi, pellagra, rickets, or scurvy. The potential for iatrogenic starvation, however, exists because of ignorance or oversight on the part of the health care personnel who routinely fail to assess their clients' nutrition status or do not know how to correct it when necessary. Many medical procedures, such as nothing by mouth (NPO) orders to prepare the person for various gastrointestinal x-rays and procedures, may also potentiate client malnutrition.

A commonly prescribed intravenous solution of dextrose 5% in water only delivers 170 calories/L—and purely in the form of a carbohydrate. Multiple cleansing enemas or prolonged gastrointestinal suction rob the body of essential electrolytes. Only perfunctory medical assessment may be made of the effects of intraoperative blood losses or of wound drainage on nutrition needs, and surgery always is accompanied by increased nitrogen excretion. Also, common nursing problems that result when the client does not, cannot, or will not eat are often not given adequate medical attention to enable satisfactory nursing care.

Vitamin preparations and other, more aggressive, supportive nutrition therapies are needed for the hospitalized client more often than is recognized because only a few vitamins are synthesized in the body. Vitamin K is formed by bacteria in the gut; vitamin D is produced when skin is exposed to sunlight; and small, insufficient amounts of vitamin B also are made in the gut. Thus most vitamins must either be ingested in food or taken as dietary supplements. There are two schools of thought concerning the consumption of vitamin supplements. Nutrition experts generally believe that the average American diet contains adequate vitamins and that additional supplements are unnecessary. Others, though, refer to surveys that indicate specific segments of our society—the elderly, smokers, nursing home residents, teenagers—who reportedly do not consume the RDA levels of all vitamins and minerals. The most effective approach to correct such deficiencies is through diet, perhaps with the help of a dietitian. However, there are some circumstances in which a vitamin or nutritional supplement is indicated.

Table 68-1 reviews vitamins and recommended daily dietary allowances (RDAs).

Vitamins are classified as being fat soluble or water soluble. The **fat-soluble vitamins** are A, D, E, and K. They are stored in the liver and fatty tissue in large amounts, and a deficiency in these vitamins occurs only after long deprivation from an adequate supply or disorders preventing their absorption. **Water-soluble vitamins** include the B complex group and C. These vitamins are not stored in the body in large amounts, and short periods of inadequate intake can lead to a deficiency. Vitamins are important components of enzyme systems that catalyze the reactions for protein, fat, and carbohydrate metabolism.

Many multivitamin capsules and tablets vary in their contents. "Optional vitamins" (E, B_6, folic acid, pantothenic acid, and B_{12}) may or may not be included as ingredients in OTC multivitamin preparations. However, the most popular OTC multivitamin preparations contain all the vitamins needed by humans. Most OTC vitamin preparations are designed to meet daily body needs completely without regard for the amounts of various vitamins contained in the daily diet.

■ Nursing Management

Vitamin and Mineral Therapy

Good nutrition is essential for good health. The nurse's participation in health promotion includes the provision of

TABLE 68-1 Vitamin review

Vitamin	Sources	Adverse effects*	Deficiency effects	RDA†
Fat soluble				
A	fish-liver oil, liver, butter, yellow fruit, green leafy vegetables, milk	acute: confusion, irritation, diarrhea, dizziness, visual alterations, skin peeling, severe vomiting chronic: bone pain, dry, cracked skin or lips, fever, increased urination, anorexia, loss of hair, seizures, vomiting	night blindness, xerophthalmia, keratomalacia, skin lesions	Infant: 375 μg Child‡: 400-700 μg Male: 1000 μg Female: 800 μg Pregnant: 800 μg
D	fish-liver oil, fortified milk, fish, exposure to sunlight	early with hypercalcemia: constipation (mostly in children), diarrhea, headache, increased thirst and urination, metallic taste, nausea, vomiting late: bone and muscle pain, increase blood pressure, pruritus, lethargy, mood alterations, pancreatitis	bone-muscle pain, pain, weak, softening of bones that may result in fractures	Infant: 7.5-10 μg Child‡: 10 μg Male: 5-10 μg Female: 5-10 μg Pregnant: 10 μg
E	nuts, green leafy vegetables, wheat and rice germ	acute: visual disturbances, headache, nausea, stomach pain, weakness, blurred vision chronic: increased bleeding tendencies in vitamin K deficient clients, alters thyroid metabolism, impairs sexual function	hyporeflexia, ataxia, myopathy, anemia, may increase cancer risk	Infant: 3-4 μg Child‡: 6-7 μg Male: 10 μg Female: 8 μg Pregnant: 10 μg
K	liver, green leafy vegetables	hypersensitivity, (flushing, dyspnea, chest pain), taste alterations	increase bleeding (ecchymoses, hematuria, GI bleeding, etc.)	Infant: 5-10 μg Child‡: 15-30 μg Male: 45-80 μg Female: 45-65 μg Pregnant: 65 μg

Continued

TABLE 68-1 Vitamin review—cont'd

Vitamin	Sources	Adverse effects*	Deficiency effects	RDA[†]
Water soluble				
B_1 (thiamine)	whole grain and enriched cereals, beef, pork, peas, beans, nuts	low oral toxicity	peripheral neuritis, loss of muscle strength, depression, memory loss, anorexia, poor memory, dyspnea	Infant: 0.3-0.4 mg Child[‡]: 0.7-1 mg Male: 1.2-1.5 mg Female: 1 mg Pregnant: 1.5 mg
B_2 (riboflavin)	milk, cheese, eggs, green leafy vegetables, whole grain and enriched cereals and breads, organ meats	low toxicity	sore throat, stomatitis, red, painful or swollen tongue, facial dermatitis, anemia	Infant: 0.4-0.5 mg Child[‡]: 0.8-1.2 mg Male: 1.4-1.8 mg Female: 1.2-1.3 mg Pregnant: 1.6 mg
B_3 (niacin)	meats, eggs, milk, dairy products	flushing, pruritus, feelings of warmth high doses: dizziness, arrhythmias, dry skin, hyperglycemia, myalgia, nausea, vomiting, diarrhea	skin eruptions, stomatitis, diarrhea, enteritis, headache, dizziness, insomnia, memory impairment, dementia	Infant: 5-6 mg Child[‡]: 9-13 mg Male: 15-20 mg Female: 13-15 mg Pregnant: 17 mg
B_6 (pyridoxine)	liver, meats, whole-grain bread/ cereals, soybeans, eggs, vegetables	acute: low toxicity chronic high doses: neurotoxicity- ataxia, numb feet, clumsiness	seborrhea-like skin lesions, stomatitis, seizures, peripheral neuritis	Infant: 0.3-0.6 mg Child[‡]: 1-1.4 mg Male: 1.7-2 mg Female: 1.4-1.6 mg Pregnant: 2.2 mg
B_9 (folic acid)	liver, fresh green vegetables, yeast, some fruits	allergic reaction, red skin, fever, skin rash, pruritus	megaloblastic anemia	Infant: 25-35 μg Child[‡]: 50-100 μg Male: 150-200 μg Female: 150-180 μg Pregnant: 400 μg
B_{12} (cyanocobalamin)	fish, egg yolk, milk, fermented cheeses	no toxicity	irreversible nervous system damage (paresthesia, ataxia), memory loss, confusion, dementia, abnormal hematopoiesis	Infant: 0.3-0.5 μg Child[†]: 0.7-1.4 μg Male: 2 μg Female: 2 μg Pregnant: 2.2 μg
C (ascorbic acid)	citrus fruits, tomatoes, potatoes, strawberries, cabbage	kidney stones, dizziness high doses: diarrhea, red skin, headache, nausea, vomiting	scurvy (loosening of teeth, gingivitis, anemia Infants: irritability, pain if touched	Infant: 30-35 mg Child[‡]: 40-45 mg Male: 50-60 mg Female: 50-60 mg Pregnant: 70 mg

*Adverse *effects* will include acute and chronic or early and late overdose symptoms, when available.
[†]RDA is the recommended daily allowance recommended from dietary sources.
[‡]Child 1 to 10 yrs old.
Allen Jr, 1996; Marcus & Coulston, 1996; *USP DI*, 1996.

Pregnancy Safety

Category	Drug
A	thiamine, pyridoxine, folic acid
C	vitamin D, cyanocobalamin (vitamin B_{12}), ascorbic acid (vitamin C), iron
X	vitamin A
Unclassified	niacin, riboflavin, vitamin K, vitamin E

information regarding all aspects of nutrition. With the many misconceptions regarding vitamins and minerals and their function in health and the prevention of illness prevalent today the nurse has an important role in the provision of accurate dietary counseling with regard to vitamins and minerals.

Assessment. A dietary history for the client will provide the nurse with insights into the client's eating patterns (e.g., in the last 24 hour period). In addition, obtain information related to food source and preparation, living arrangements, financial status, coping patterns, knowledge of nutrition, and physiologic alterations that the client is experiencing as background for client teaching. This will also enable the nurse to be more specific with the client regarding his or her dietary planning. Obtain height and weight. Assess for signs of the specific vitamin or mineral deficiency throughout therapy. (See specific vitamin for relevant nursing management.) Consider that vitamin and mineral requirements may change with age and health status (e.g., in pregnancy). (See the Pregnancy Safety box above for FDA categories for vitamins). Baseline diagnostic studies can be obtained for the specific vitamin or mineral deficiency (e.g., serum folic acid and hemoglobin determinations).

Nursing diagnosis. The general nursing diagnosis for clients with vitamin and mineral deficiencies would be: altered nutrition, less than body requirements. Depending on the type and severity of the deficiency and the nature of the individual client's signs and symptoms, other nursing diagnoses or collaborative problems would be relevant.

Implementation

Monitoring. Food diaries will assist in the monitoring of the client's effective management of the therapeutic regimen. Regression of the client's symptoms should be noted. Weight should be recorded at every visit; with children, the height should also be recorded.

Intervention. Use the calibrated measuring device provided by the manufacturer for accurate dosing. Chewable tablets should be thoroughly chewed or crushed before swallowing. Use caution in administering fat-soluble vitamins to children, since they are more sensitive to high doses.

Education. Discussions with the client regarding vitamins should cover their function in the body, signs of vitamin deficiency, and unproven uses. Diet is the treatment of choice in vitamin deficiencies; vitamins are not a substitute for a balanced diet.

Instruct the client about the food pyramid with its six food groups and, in particular, about specific foods that supply the vitamin in which he or she is deficient. Supplements are only needed if the dietary intake is insufficient to meet body requirements. Megadoses are not recommended, and there is the risk of toxicity with chronic overdoses; the RDA should not be exceeded. However, there is a great deal of research about the prophylactic role for vitamins.

Evaluation. The client will not evidence signs or symptoms of vitamin or mineral deficiency.

Fat-Soluble Vitamins

vitamin A [Aquasol A]

Vitamin A, the fat-soluble, growth-promoting vitamin, is essential for growth in the younger age groups, for normal function of the retina, and for maintenance of health at all ages. Vitamin A (retinol) is derived from animals, whereas the provitamin A carotenoids are found in plants. Beta-carotene, the most active carotenoid from plants, is hydrolyzed in the body to form two molecules of vitamin A. Animal fats, such as those found in butter, milk, eggs, and fish liver, are sources of the carotenoids that were originally derived from plants and stored in animal tissues.

Vitamin A is essential in promoting normal growth and development of bones and teeth and maintaining the health of epithelial tissues of the body. Its function in relation to normal vision and the prevention of night blindness has been studied carefully. Vitamin A actually is part of one of the major retinal pigments, rhodopsin, and thus is required for normal "rod vision" in the retina of human beings and many animals.

Vitamin A has the following indications:

1. It is used to treat or relieve symptoms associated with a deficiency of vitamin A, such as night blindness (nyctalopia), hyperkeratosis, retarded growth, xerophthalmia, keratomalacia, weakness, and increased susceptibility of mucous membranes to infection.
2. Certain analogs are used to treat acne (see Chapter 66).
3. Vitamin requirements increase during pregnancy and during breastfeeding; when possible, these needs are best met with food rather than with drugs. However, prescribers may recommend vitamin supplementation especially in women who may not consume a proper diet or those in a high-risk category, such as heavy cigarette smokers, alcohol or substance abusers, or women pregnant with more than one fetus (see the Nursing Research box on p. 1048). Consuming excessive amounts of vitamins, especially of the fat-soluble vitamins, may be dangerous to both the mother and fetus. Large doses of vitamin A may cause neurologic and skin damage in adults, and excessive doses are known to produce highly toxic effects in rats and in young children.

Nursing Research

Vitamin A supplementation and child mortality

Large doses of vitamin A are clearly lifesaving when given to children with measles, according to a new study conducted by Frederick Mosteller, Ph.D., and his colleagues from the Harvard School of Public Health. Measles is responsible for about 1.5 million deaths worldwide each year, and children in developing countries are particularly susceptible because of problems in obtaining and distributing measles vaccine in these areas. Vitamin A supplements may also benefit children in developed countries. In another recent study, U.S. children with measles had lower blood levels of vitamin A than children who did not have measles.

The Harvard study conducted a meta-analysis of findings from four hospital-based studies and eight community-based studies of children, mainly from developing countries, and found that large doses of vitamin A lowered the risk of death by 60% in hospitalized children and 90% in hospitalized infants, even in populations in which vitamin A deficiency was not a problem. Ordinarily, the risk of measles-related diarrhea was less severe in children who took vitamin A supplements, and there were 70% fewer deaths among children receiving supplements who developed measles-related pneumonia either before or during their hospital stay.

The investigators concluded that vitamin A supplements should be given to all measles patients in developing countries, whether or not they have symptoms of vitamin A deficiency. They call for further research on the effects of vitamin A as a supplement to conventional therapy for other serious childhood diseases, such as diarrhea and lower respiratory infections.

Critical thinking questions

- Given that there is at present only one approved use for vitamin A, that of vitamin A deficiency, how do you explain these findings?
- Which would be more cost effective or have the better risk-benefit ratio, vitamin A therapy or immunization for measles? Under what circumstances?

From Fawzi et al (1993).

Vitamin A and carotene are readily absorbed from the normal gastrointestinal tract. Efficient absorption depends on fat absorption and therefore on the presence of adequate bile salts in the intestine. Certain conditions, such as obstructive jaundice, some infectious diseases, and the presence of mineral oil in the intestine, may result in vitamin A deficiency in spite of the amount ingested being normal.

Vitamin A is stored to a greater extent in the liver than elsewhere. The liver also functions in changing carotene to vitamin A; this function is inhibited in liver diseases and in diabetes. The amount of vitamin A stored depends on the dietary intake. When intake is high or excessive, the stores formed in the liver may be sufficient to last several years. Vitamin A is metabolized by the liver and excreted by the feces and kidneys. For adverse and deficiency effects plus RDA, see Table 68-1.

The vitamin A dosage depends on the age, sex, purpose (prophylaxis or treatment) and condition of the individual. See a current reference for dosing information.

■ Nursing Management

Vitamin A Therapy

In addition to the discussion of general nursing management of vitamin therapy, the following relates specifically to vitamin A.

Assessment. Obtain a baseline of the client's vision, including night blindness, and appearance of the eyes, skin, and mucous membranes. In addition to dry skin and corneal changes, infants may evidence failure to thrive and apathy. Serum vitamin A levels less than 20 µg/dl in adults and 10 µg/dl in children indicate vitamin A deficiency.

The vitamin is contraindicated with clients with hypervitaminosis A and administered cautiously in clients with renal function impairment because serum vitamin A levels are increased.

When vitamin A is given concurrently with etretinate (Tegison) or isotretinoin (Accutane), an increase in toxic side effects may result. Avoid concurrent administration if possible. If not, monitor closely for retinoid toxicity (headache, nausea, vomiting, elevated liver enzymes, hair loss, hepatomegaly, and dry, fissured skin).

Nursing diagnosis. The client with vitamin A deficiency therapy is at risk for the following nursing diagnoses: sensory/perceptual alterations (night blindness), fatigue, impaired skin integrity, and altered mucous membranes. Nursing diagnoses associated with vitamin A use are: altered comfort (headache, bone or joint pain, general feeling of discomfort, irritability); altered mucous membranes (dry mouth, dry or cracking of lips); fluid volume deficit (anorexia, nausea, vomiting); self image disturbance related to loss of hair or yellow-orange patches on palms of hands, soles of feet, or skin around the nose and mouth; hyperthermia; altered elimination of urine (frequency); and fatigue.

Implementation

Monitoring. Monitor the client's diet, signs and symptoms of vitamin A deficiency or hypercarotenemia (orange coloration of the skin and eyes) and **hypervitaminosis** A (see Nursing Diagnosis above), and serum vitamin A levels. Hypervitaminosis is an abnormal condition resulting from intake of toxic amounts of one or more vitamins, especially over a long period of time.

Intervention. Administer oral vitamin A with or after meals.

Education. Provide the client with nutritional counseling. The best sources of dietary vitamin A are fish liver oil, liver, kidney, egg yolk, butter, milk, cream, cheese, and fortified margarine; and its precursor carotene, found in dark green leafy vegetables and yellow and orange fruits and vegetables.

Water-miscible products are available for clients with fat malabsorption. If administered IV, vitamin A is adsorbed by

PVC containers and tubing. Exposure to light causes degradation of vitamin A, so total parenteral solutions containing vitamin A should be protected from the light.

Evaluation. The client will achieve adequate vitamin A serum concentrations, consume adequate dietary vitamin A, and maintain normal vision and intact skin.

vitamin D

The term *vitamin D* is applied to two substances that affect the proper utilization of calcium and phosphorus in the body. Both substances have the ability to prevent or cure rickets. The plant vitamin D is referred to as *vitamin D_2* or *ergocalciferol*; the natural form of vitamin D is produced in the skin by ultraviolet irradiation of 7-dehydrocholesterol and is referred to as *vitamin D_3* or *cholecalciferol*. Although ergocalciferol contains a chemical double bond and an extra methyl group, the difference is not significant physiologically.

Both cholecalciferol and ergocalciferol are metabolized in the liver to calcifediol, which is then transported to the kidney where it is converted to calcitriol, which is believed to be the most active analogue (Marcus, 1996).

Calcitriol appears to bind to a receptor in the intestinal mucosa, is incorporated into the cell nucleus, resulting in the formation of a calcium-binding protein that increases calcium absorption from the intestine. Parathyroid hormone and calcitriol both act to control the transfer of calcium ions from bones into the extracellular fluid; therefore they maintain a calcium homeostasis effect in the extracellular fluid. Although an essential vitamin, vitamin D is found in only a few foods of the average American/Canadian diet (see Table 68-1).

Other vitamin D analogs available include alfacalcidol (One-Alpha♣), calcitriol (Rocaltrol), and dihydrotachysterol (Hytakerol). They are preferred in certain situations such as, for the person in renal failure, as they do not require required conversion for their action. They also have shorter half-lives so any toxic adverse effects would be easier to manage. Calcifediol (Calderol) appears to have some vitamin D activity in addition to its conversion to the active metabolite calcitriol.

Vitamin D is necessary for the absorption and utilization of calcium and phosphorus in the body and for the normal calcification of bone. In the absence of vitamin D (even if the calcium and phosphate intake is adequate) rickets in children and osteomalacia in adults may result. Vitamin D is used to treat and prevent nutritional rickets, osteomalacia, hypoparathyroidism, and osteoporosis (Marcus, 1996).

The incidence of rickets is low in the United States and Canada but it can occur in young children who are restricted to vegetarian diets without milk supplementation, or in infants who are breast fed by mothers who did not take prenatal vitamins nor drink milk. A vitamin D deficiency results in an inadequate intake and perhaps an excessive loss of calcium from the body.

Vitamin D is absorbed from the small intestine (ergocalciferol requires the presence of bile salts for absorption). It is protein bound, stored mainly in fat and in the liver. The serum half-life of calcifediol is about 16 days; of calcitriol from 3 to 6 hours; of ergocalciferol, within 19 to 48 hours, but the latter can be stored in fat sites for longer periods. Onset of hypercalcemic effect for calcitriol within 3 to 6 hours; for dihydrotachysterol, within hours, although maximum effect is seen in 7 to 14 days; for ergocalciferol, within 12 to 24 hours, although therapeutic response may not be seen until 10 to 14 days later.

Duration of effect after oral administration is calcifediol, 15 to 20 days; calcitriol, 3 to 5 days; dihydrotachysterol, up to 9 weeks; and ergocalciferol, up to 6 months. Excretion is via the bile and kidneys. For adverse and deficiency effects plus RDA, see Table 68-1.

The usual adolescent and adult dose for alfacalcidol is 1 µg/day; calcifediol is 50 to 100 µg/day; calcitriol 0.25 mg/day, and dihydrotachysterol 125 µg to 2 mg/day. Dosages are adjusted periodically, as necessary. Pediatric dosages vary. See a current reference for recommendations.

■ Nursing Management
Vitamin D Therapy

See also the nursing management of vitamin therapy.

Assessment. The administration of vitamin D is contraindicated in clients with hypercalcemia, hypervitaminosis D, or renal osteodystrophy with hyperphosphatemia because there is the risk of metabolic calcification. The nurse's assessment should rule out these conditions before initiation of vitamin D therapy. Other conditions for which caution should be used in the administration of vitamin D are arteriosclerosis, hyperphosphatemia, hypersensitivity to vitamin D, and renal or cardiac impairment.

A baseline assessment of the client's skeletal status by x-ray and appearance of bone malformations should be obtained. Serum calcium levels under 7.5 mg/dl, serum inorganic phosphorus levels under 3 mg/dl, serum citrate levels under 2.5 mg/dl, and elevated serum alkaline phosphatase levels indicate vitamin D deficiency.

Review the client's current medication regimen for significant drug interactions, which may occur when vitamin D products are given with the following drugs:

Drug	Possible effect and management
antacids containing magnesium	May result in hypermagnesemia, especially in clients with chronic renal failure. Avoid concurrent administration if possible; if not, monitor closely for diminished reflexes, muscle weakness, drowsiness, confusion, lethargy, bradycardia, and hypotension.
calcium preparations in high doses or thiazide diuretics	Increases risk for hypercalcemia. Monitor closely for drowsiness, lethargy, weakness, muscle flaccidity, hypertension, anorexia, nausea, constipation, polyuria, and flank pain.
vitamin D, other products	**Increased risk of toxicity. Avoid or a potentially serious drug interaction may occur.**

Nursing diagnosis. Clients receiving vitamin D therapy may experience the following nursing diagnoses because of their underlying vitamin D deficiency: altered comfort related to ineffective drug therapy (pain in the legs and lower back), risk for injury related to motor deficits related to skeletal deformities and weakness, and impaired physical mobility related to poorly developed muscles. Nursing diagnoses related to the drug toxicity itself are: altered bowel pattern (constipation or diarrhea); fatigue; fluid volume deficit related to anorexia, nausea, or vomiting; and altered comfort (headache, metallic taste).

Implementation

Monitoring. Along with periodic evaluations of renal function, serum calcium levels should be monitored weekly during early therapy so as to aid establishing the dosage because of the narrow therapeutic range. Serum calcium values should be in the 8 to 9 mg/dl range, and the calcium times phosphorus product (Ca × P in mg/dl) should not be greater than 58. Other examinations may be required according to the client's response to therapy.

Children should have their growth measurements monitored over the course of therapy because growth may be inhibited by prolonged administration of the drug. X-rays are recommended every 3 to 6 months until the client is stable.

Assess for signs of toxicity, see nursing diagnoses above.

Education. Stress the importance of regular visits to the health care provider to monitor progress. Review with the client any instructions for a special diet or for a calcium supplement, if prescribed. Foods high is vitamin D include fish and fish liver oils, egg yolks, as well as vitamin-D–fortified milk. Judicious exposure to sunlight will be helpful.

The client should be cautioned not to use any OTC products that contain calcium, phosphorus, or vitamin D unless approved by the prescriber. Clients taking calcifediol or calcitriol should avoid the use of antacids containing magnesium.

Evaluation. The client will consume adequate dietary vitamin D and remain free of pain. The child or infant will maintain adequate growth.

vitamin E (α-tocopherol)
vitamin E capsules (Aquasol E)

Vitamin E is a fat-soluble vitamin that is present in margarine made from plant oils such as cottonseed oil; and in green, leafy vegetables and whole grains. While a number of compounds have been found to exhibit vitamin E activity, the most active of these is α-tocopherol as it is the substance used to calculate the food content of vitamin E.

Studies have reported a significant decrease in coronary artery disease in persons consuming large doses of vitamin E. The hypothesis is that oxidation of lipoproteins reduces atherogenesis (Steinberg, 1993).

Rimm et al (1993) studied 39,910 male health care professionals in the United States for 4 years and assessed their intake of various nutrients, including vitamin E. They found that males who consumed a high intake of vitamin E had a lower risk of developing coronary artery heart disease. Stampfer et al (1993) followed 87,245 female nurses between the ages of 34 to 59 years for up to 8 years. They reported similar findings in females: middle-aged women using vitamin E supplements for more than 2 years had a reduced risk of developing coronary heart disease. In both studies the participants excluded anyone with a history of cardiovascular disease. Further studies are necessary to evaluate the vitamin E dosages necessary to produce this effect and also the potential risk of toxicity from long-term consumption of large doses of vitamin E.

Vitamin E is an essential nutrient, but its exact function is unknown. It has been reported to have antioxidant properties when used in conjunction with dietary selenium, to prevent the effects of peroxidase on unsaturated bonds in the cell membranes, and to protect red blood cells from hemolysis. It is also known to be a cofactor for several enzyme systems in the body.

The absorption of vitamin E from the GI tract requires the presence of bile salts, dietary fats and normal pancreatic functioning. Vitamin E binds to beta lipoproteins in the blood and is stored in all body tissues, especially in fat depots (which contain up to a 4 year requirement of this vitamin). It is metabolized in the liver and excreted in bile and kidneys. For adverse and deficiency effects, see Table 68-1.

When vitamin E is given concurrently with large doses of iron supplements, vitamin E oxidation increases which increases the daily requirement for vitamin E. If given concurrently, monitor closely to determine an appropriate intervention.

The usual adult dose for vitamin E deficiency is 100 to 400 units daily. Pediatric dosages vary. See a current reference for recommendations.

■ Nursing Management
Vitamin E Therapy

See also the nursing management of vitamin therapy.

Assessment. Before the initiation of vitamin E therapy, it should be ascertained whether the client has hypoprothrombinemia as a result of vitamin K deficiency or iron deficiency anemia because vitamin E in doses over 400 U will aggravate the former and interfere with the hematologic response to iron therapy in the latter.

A baseline assessment should include the presence or absence of edema, condition of the skin, and extent of muscle weakness. A serum α-tocopherol level below 0.5 mg/dl in adults and below 0.2 mg/dl in infants confirms vitamin E deficiency.

Nursing diagnosis. The client with a vitamin E deficiency may experience the following selected nursing diagnoses: fluid volume excess; impaired skin integrity; and impaired physical mobility. Nursing diagnoses associated with vitamin E use are: sensory/perceptual disturbance (visual) (blurred vision); altered bowel patterns (diarrhea), fatigue, altered comfort (headache, nausea or stomach cramps, dizziness); and risk for injury related to increased bleeding tendencies.

Implementation

Monitoring. Monitor the client's dietary intake, regression of symptoms, and serum α-tocopherol levels.

Intervention. Water-miscible forms are more readily absorbed from the gastrointestinal tract, but parenteral administration may be necessary if the malabsorption syndrome is severe. The client taking large doses of vitamin E for prolonged periods of time should be assessed for signs of toxicity: see nursing diagnoses above.

Education. Although vitamin E deficiency is infrequent, dietary instruction for clients may be necessary. Foods high in vitamin E are vegetable oils, wheat germ, whole-grain cereals, egg yolk, and liver.

Evaluation. The client will maintain a diet adequate in vitamin E, experience normal muscle strength, intact skin, and α-tocopherol levels within normal limits.

vitamin K

Vitamin K is a fat-soluble vitamin. (See Chapter 31 for drug monograph and Table 68-1 for vitamin review.)

Water-Soluble Vitamins

The water-soluble vitamins are ascorbic acid (vitamin C) and B vitamins. The B vitamins are often found together in food and referred to as vitamin B complex. They are chemically dissimilar though, and have different metabolic functions. This B grouping is largely based on their having been discovered in sequential order. A sensible and increasingly popular trend promotes discarding such names as *vitamin* B_1 and B_2 and referring to these vitamins as *thiamine* and *riboflavin*. The vitamin B complex includes thiamine, riboflavin, nicotinic acid, pyridoxine, folic acid, pantothenic acid, biotin, choline, inositol, and vitamin B_{12} (cyanocobalamin).

This discussion will be limited to the B vitamins that are associated with deficiency states and for which information on therapeutic application is available: thiamine (vitamin B_1), riboflavin (vitamin B_2), niacin (nicotinic acid), pyridoxine (vitamin B_6), vitamin B_{12} (cyanocobalamin), and folic acid.

thiamine [thye' a min] (vitamin B_1) thiamine (Biamine, Bewon🍁)

Thiamine in combination with adenosine triphosphate (ATP) results in thiamine pyrophosphate coenzyme, substance necessary for carbohydrate metabolism. Thiamine is used to prevent and treat thiamine deficiency, which can result in beriberi or Wernicke's encephalopathy.

Thiamine is well absorbed from the GI tract, except in malabsorption syndrome or in the presence of alcohol, which inhibits absorption. It is metabolized in the liver and excreted by the kidneys. Side effects are usually rare. Skin rash, pruritus, or respiratory difficulties (wheezing) may occur rarely after a large intravenous dose is administered (anaphylactic reaction).

The usual adult dose is determined by the age, sex and degree of vitamin deficiency and ranges from 5 to 30 mg/day. For recommended pediatric dose, see a current reference.

■ Nursing Management
Thiamine Therapy

Also see nursing management of vitamin therapy.

Assessment. Thiamine rarely causes toxicity in individuals with normal renal function. Because a deficiency of a single B vitamin occurs infrequently, the client needs to be assessed for multiple deficiencies.

A baseline assessment of the client should include neurologic and mental status, pulse rate, and blood pressure, and 24-hour urinary thiamine levels. The deficiency levels vary by age; for adults less than 27 μg/dl would indicate deficiency.

Nursing diagnosis. The client with a thiamine deficiency may exhibit the following nursing diagnoses: altered thought processes (confusion, psychosis); decreased cardiac output (tachycardia, palpitations); and sensory-perceptual alterations (neuropathy, ataxia, nystagmus).

The only potential complication with the administration of thiamine is anaphylactic reaction, usually after a large IV dose.

Implementation

Monitoring. Continue to monitor the client with indicators in the baseline assessment.

Intervention. In most instances the vitamin is administered in an oral preparation; however, if this is not acceptable or possible, parenteral forms are available.

Education. Instruction for the client should include sources that are high in thiamine, such as whole grain or enriched cereals and meats, particularly pork, nuts, fish, organ/muscle meat, poultry, rice bran, legumes, and green vegetables.

Evaluation. The client will maintain a diet adequate in thiamine, a normal neurologic and cardiovascular status, and normal levels of urinary thiamine.

riboflavin [rye' boo flay vin] (vitamin B_2)

Riboflavin is converted in the body into two coenzymes: flavin mononucleotide (FMN) and flavin adenine dinucleotide (FAD), substances necessary for normal tissue respiration. Riboflavin is also necessary to activate pyridoxine, to convert tryptophan to niacin, and may also be connected to maintenance of erythrocyte integrity.

Riboflavin is indicated for the prevention and treatment of riboflavin deficiency; usually this deficiency does not occur in healthy persons but may be detected as a result of malnutrition or intestinal malabsorption.

Riboflavin is well absorbed in the GI tract and has a half-life of approximately 1 to 1.5 hours. It is metabolized in the liver and excreted by the kidneys. Side effects are rare. No significant drug interactions have been reported with riboflavin.

The usual adult dose to treat riboflavin deficiency ranges from 5 to 10 mg. See a current reference for additional dosing information.

■ Nursing Management
Riboflavin Therapy

Also see nursing management of vitamin therapy.

Assessment. A baseline assessment of the client with riboflavin deficiency should include examination of the skin and mucous membranes, appearance of the eyes and vision status, and RBC, hemoglobin, and hematocrit. Riboflavin deficiency may be detected by measuring erythrocyte or urinary riboflavin concentrations.

Nursing diagnosis. The client with a deficiency in riboflavin and ineffective riboflavin therapy may experience the following nursing diagnoses: altered mucous membranes (cracking of the lips and corners of the mouth, glossitis); impaired skin integrity (seborrheic dermatitis in nasolabial folds, scrotum, labia; generalized dermatitis); and sensory-perceptual alterations (light sensitivity, burning of the eyes).

Implementation

Monitoring. Vitamins that are water-soluble rarely cause toxicity in individuals with normal kidney function. Monitor indicators within the baseline assessment.

Education. Alert the client that large doses of riboflavin may cause the urine to become yellow in color. The best food sources of riboflavin are milk and dairy products, meats, eggs, fish, poultry, enriched grains/cereals, and green, leafy vegetables (see Table 68-1).

Evaluation. The client will maintain adequate dietary intake of riboflavin, have intact skin and mucous membranes, normal vision, and urinary riboflavin concentration values within the normal range.

niacin [nye' a sin] (nicotinic acid)
niacin extended-release (Nicobid, Slo-Niacin)
niacinamide tablets/injection

Niacin converted to niacinamide in the body, is part of two coenzymes, nicotinamide adenine dinucleotide (NAD) and nicotinamide adenine dinucleotide phosphate (NADP), necessary for glycogenolysis, tissue respiration, and lipid, protein, and purine metabolism. As an antihyperlipidemic agent, niacin lowers serum cholesterol and triglyceride levels by reducing very-low-density lipoprotein (VLDL) synthesis. VLDL is the precursor to low-density lipoprotein, the main carrier of cholesterol in the blood.

Niacin and niacinamide are indicated for the prevention and treatment of vitamin B_3 deficiency conditions. A niacin deficiency may result in pellagra. Only niacin is indicated as a treatment adjunct for hyperlipidemia but its usefulness may be limited by its side effects, especially its vasodilating effects. Niacinamide does not cause direct peripheral vasodilation.

With the exception of the malabsorption syndromes, both niacin and niacinamide are readily absorbed orally and have a half-life of 45 minutes. Whereas onset of action to reduce triglyceride serum levels is several hours, to reduce cholesterol levels takes several days. Niacin is metabolized by the liver and excreted in the kidneys. For side effects/adverse reactions, see Table 68-1. No significant drug interactions are reported with its use.

For antihyperlipidemia, the usual adult dose for niacin is 1 g PO daily, increased every 2 to 4 weeks as necessary. As dose of niacin and niacinamide vary according to age and sex of the individual, check current reference for additional information.

■ Nursing Management

Niacin Therapy

Also consult nursing management of vitamin therapy.

Assessment. Before large doses are administered it should be determined if the client has arterial bleeding, diabetes mellitus (niacin only), peptic ulcer, or hepatic disease, since all these conditions will be aggravated by niacin and niacinamide.

A baseline assessment should include activity tolerance, skin status, bowel status, and neurologic and mental status.

Nursing diagnosis. The client with a niacin deficiency and ineffective niacin therapy may experience the following nursing diagnoses: activity intolerance (fatigue, muscle weakness); altered comfort (headache, indigestion); impaired skin integrity (dermatitis); altered mucous membranes (red and sore mouth, tongue, and lips); altered bowel elimination (diarrhea); and altered thought processes (confusion, disorientation, hallucinations). Clients on niacin therapy may experience: altered comfort (flushing, headache—with niacin only); impaired skin integrity (pruritus); and the potential complication of hepatitis—with long-term use of extended-release niacin).

Implementation

Monitoring. Monitor the client's progress by indicators within the baseline assessment. If individuals are receiving large doses of niacin or niacinamide for prolonged periods, blood glucose and hepatic function should be monitored.

Intervention. Administer with milk or food to help prevent gastrointestinal distress. Oral administration of niacin is preferred. Parenteral niacin is used only when the oral route is not acceptable or possible. If administered intravenously, do not exceed a rate of 2 mg/min.

Education. Alert the client that for the first 2 weeks of therapy to expect a feeling of warmth, a flushing of the skin of the face and neck shortly after taking the tablets. This sensation may be reduced by starting with a low dosage that is gradually increased to the therapeutic level. Niacinamide is preferred because it lacks this blushing effect.

Stress the importance of regular visits to the health care provider to monitor the effectiveness of the medication and the client's progress.

Because one of the adverse effects is dizziness, caution the client to avoid hazardous tasks that require mental alertness until the response to the medication has been determined.

The best food sources of niacin are meats, eggs, whole grain and enriched cereal/bread/flour, milk, and other dairy products (see Table 68-1).

Evaluation. The client will maintain an adequate dietary intake of niacin and not evidence any signs of niacin deficiency.

pyridoxine [peer i dox' een] (vitamin B_6)
pyridoxine extended release (Rodex)

Pyridoxine is taken up by erythrocytes and converted into pyridoxal phosphate, a coenzyme necessary for many metabolic functions that affect proteins, carbohydrates, and lipid utilization in the body. Pyridoxine is also involved with the conversion of tryptophan to niacin or serotonin.

Pyridoxine is indicated to treat or prevent pyridoxine deficiency. A deficiency state can lead to sideroblastic anemia, neurologic disturbances, seborrheic dermatitis, cheilosis, and xanthurenic aciduria.

Oral pyridoxine is well absorbed from the jejunum and converted in erythrocytes to pyridoxal phosphate, which is totally protein bound in the plasma. It has a half-life of 15 to 20 days and is metabolized by the liver and excreted in the kidneys. Side effects and adverse reactions are very rare. Side effects are seen only when dosages of 200 mg/day are given for more than a month, resulting in a dependency-type syndrome. Megadoses can cause problems (see Table 68-1).

The usual pyridoxine dose varies according to age, sex and degree of vitamin deficiency. See a current reference for dosing recommendations.

■ Nursing Management

Pyridoxine Therapy

Also consult the section on nursing management of vitamin therapy.

Assessment. Initial assessment should determine whether the client has Parkinson's disease, which is treated with levodopa. A significant drug interaction occurs when pyridoxine is given with levodopa. Levodopa's antiparkinsonian effects may be reduced or reversed. This effect is not reported with the carbidopa-levodopa combination.

A baseline assessment of the client with a pyridoxine deficiency should include inspection of the skin and mucous membranes and neurologic status. Pyridoxine deficiency is indicated by decreased serum transaminase and RBC levels and reduced urinary excretion of pyridoxic acid.

Nursing diagnosis. The client with a pyridoxine deficiency and ineffective pyridoxine therapy may experience the following nursing diagnoses: impaired skin integrity (dermatitis); fatigue; activity intolerance related to anemia (weakness); risk of injury related to unsteady gait; and disturbed sleep pattern (drowsiness).

Implementation

Monitoring. Observe for improvement of deficiency symptoms. Evaluate for nutritional adequacy.

Intervention. Intravenous pyridoxine may be administered undiluted at a rate of 50 mg/min and may be added to most IV solutions.

Education. Large doses of pyridoxine for a period of several months may result in sensory neuropathy affecting gait and causing numbness of the hands and feet.

Best food sources of pyridoxine are meats, poultry, fish, eggs, bananas, potatoes, sweet potatoes, lima beans, and whole grain cereals.

Evaluation. The client will maintain adequate dietary intake of pyridoxine, intact skin and mucous membranes, and normal neurologic and mental status.

cyanocobalamin [sye an oh koe bal' a min] (vitamin B_{12})
hydroxocobalamin [hye drox oh koe bal' a min] (Alphamin)

Cyanocobalamin is a coenzyme for a variety of metabolic functions that include protein synthesis, and fat and carbohydrate metabolism. It is also needed for growth, cell replication, hematopoiesis, and nucleoprotein and myelin synthesis.

BOX 68-1

Vitamin B_{12} Nasal Spray

Nascobal, a vitamin B_{12} nasal spray, was approved as a maintenance drug for persons in remission after IM therapy for conditions such as pernicious anemia. The dose is usually 500 μg intranasally once a week. A warning on the product states that if the person is not properly maintained on this spray, resumption of intramuscular vitamin B_{12} is necessary.

Side/adverse effects include infection, headache, glossitis, nausea, and rhinitis (FDA News and Product Notes, 1997).

Cyanocobalamin is used to treat pernicious anemia (caused by lack of intrinsic factor) and to prevent and treat vitamin B_{12} deficiency caused by malabsorption or strict vegetarianism. Vitamin B_{12} deficiency can lead to macrocytic megaloblastic anemia and irreversible neurologic damage.

For vitamin B_{12} to be absorbed orally, the intrinsic factor must be present in the intestinal tract. It is highly protein bound with a half-life of 6 days, and reaches peak serum level in 8 to 12 hours. It is metabolized (and stored) by the liver and excreted in bile and urine. After parenteral injection, anaphylactic reactions are possible but rare (see Table 68-1). No significant drug interactions are reported.

The usual dose varies according to age, sex, and degree of vitamin deficiency. See Box 68-1 for information on the nasal spray form of vitamin B_{12}. See a current reference for dosing recommendations.

■ Nursing Management

Cyanocobalamin Therapy

See also the section on nursing management of vitamin therapy.

Assessment. Cyanocobalamin is contraindicated in Leber's disease (a rare type of blindness as the result of as autosomal recessive trait) as optic nerve atrophy has occurred rapidly after its administration because cyanocobalamin levels are already elevated.

Plasma vitamin B_{12} levels should be determined before therapy begins and on about the sixth day of therapy. Diagnosis of vitamin B_{12} deficiency should be confirmed by the lab (serum B_{12} levels under 150 pg/ml) or the initiation of B_{12} therapy will mask pernicious anemia or a folic acid deficiency.

A baseline assessment should include activity tolerance, neurologic status, RBC count, hemoglobin, hematocrit, and serum cobalamin level.

Nursing diagnosis. The client with a cyanocobalamin deficiency and ineffective cyanocobalamin therapy may have the following nursing diagnoses: activity intolerance related to anemia and sensory-perceptual alterations (peripheral neuritis, hyperactive reflexes). Clients with cyanocobalamin therapy may also experience: diarrhea, altered comfort (pruritus), and the potential complication of anaphylaxis.

Implementation

Monitoring. During the first 48 hours of therapy, serum potassium should be monitored closely for the possibility of severe hypokalemia. Hypersensitivity, which occurs rarely, is demonstrated by skin rash and, after parenteral administration, wheezing. Serum B_{12} levels should be taken the fifth and seventh days of therapy.

Intervention. Administer oral forms with meals to enhance absorption. Parenteral cyanocobalamin is administered IM or SC, not IV. Although small amounts are sometimes included in total parenteral nutrition (TPN).

Education. Stress compliance with the medication regimen if the client is on life-long therapy following a gastrectomy or ileal resection, or for pernicious anemia. For these conditions the drug is administered intramuscularly because of the absence of intrinsic factor.

The best food sources of vitamin B_{12} are meats, seafood, poultry, egg yolk, milk, and fermented cheeses.

Evaluation. The client will maintain an adequate dietary intake of B_{12}, normal neurologic status, serum B_{12} levels above 150 pg/ml, and RBCs, hemoglobin, and hematocrit within normal limits.

folic acid (vitamin B_9)
folic acid (Folvite, Apo-Folic♣)

Folic acid is converted to tetrahydrofolic acid in the body, which is necessary for normal erythropoiesis, metabolism of amino acids, and nucleoprotein synthesis.

Folic acid is used to treat and prevent folic acid deficiency. Folic acid should not be administered until pernicious anemia has been ruled out as a potential diagnosis. If administered to clients with undiagnosed pernicious anemia it will correct the hematologic changes and mask pernicious anemia while the underlying neurologic damage progresses.

A folic acid deficiency may result in megaloblastic and macrocytic anemias and glossitis. A deficiency of maternal folic acid is associated with neural tube defects.

Folic acid is absorbed mostly from the upper duodenum; is highly protein bound, metabolized (and stored) in the liver, and excreted by the kidneys. Folic acid in the presence of vitamin C (ascorbic acid) is converted in the liver and serum to its active form, tetrahydrofolic acid, by dihydrofolate reductase.

Side effects/adverse reactions are rare. Allergic reaction (elevated temperature and rash) or yellow discoloration of urine may occur. The usual folic acid dose varies according to age, sex, and degree of vitamin deficiency. See a current reference for dosing recommendations.

■ Nursing Management
Folic Acid Therapy

See also the section on nursing management of vitamin therapy.

Assessment. It should be determined if the client has pernicious anemia because folic acid will reverse hematologic abnormalities, but the neurologic aspects of the disease will continue to progress. No significant drug interactions are reported.

A baseline assessment should include the client's activity tolerance, RBC count, hemoglobin, and hematocrit.

Nursing diagnosis. The client with folic acid deficiency will probably have activity intolerance and altered protection secondary to anemia. Those receiving folic acid may experience the potential complication of anaphylaxis.

Implementation

Monitoring. Monitor the client's progress using the indicators in the baseline assessment.

Intervention. Folic acid is available as oral tablets or it may be administered IV undiluted over 1 minute. It may be added to most IV solutions.

Education. Alert the client that large doses of folic acid may turn the urine yellow. The best food sources of folic acid are yeast, liver, whole grain, bran, fresh leafy vegetables, fruits, nuts, dried beans, and lentils.

Evaluation. The client will maintain an adequate dietary intake of folic acid, a tolerance for desired activities, and RBC count, hemoglobin and hematocrit within normal limits.

ascorbic acid (vitamin C)

Ascorbic acid is necessary for collagen formation in fibrous tissue including bone, and in the development of teeth, blood vessels, and blood cells. It also plays a role in carbohydrate metabolism. It is believed to stimulate the fibroblasts of connective tissue and thus promote tissue repair and the healing of wounds. It also may help maintain the integrity of the intercellular substance in the walls of blood vessels; the capillary fragility associated with scurvy is explained on this basis. It may be necessary for the metabolism of phenylalanine, tyrosine, folic acid, norepinephrine, histamine, and iron.

The effectiveness of ascorbic acid in preventing or relieving cold symptoms, or in the treatment of cancer, infertility, aging, or peptic ulcer is primarily unproven. Studies performed over the years have not substantiated these claims (*USP DI*, 1996).

Ascorbic acid is well absorbed from the GI tract and stored in plasma and cells, with the highest concentration found in glandular sites. It is metabolized in the liver and excreted by the kidneys. (see Table 68-1).

The adult dosage as a nutritional supplement is 50 to 100 mg daily. To treat a vitamin C deficiency the dosage varies according to age and severity of vitamin deficiency.

■ Nursing Management
Ascorbic Acid Therapy

See also nursing management of vitamin therapy.

Assessment. Because of the risk of the formation of urinary stones when large doses of vitamin C are given to persons with the following conditions, it should be determined that the client does not have cystinuria, oxalosis, or a history of gout or urate renal stones. Large doses may also precipitate a crisis in sickle cell anemia. Clients with diabetes mellitus may find interference with glucose testing with large doses of vitamin C.

Concurrent use of ascorbic acid with deferoxamine (Desferal) may enhance tissue iron toxicity, especially in the heart, causing cardiac decompensation. The oral dose of ascorbic acid should be given 1 to 2 hours after the initiation of a deferoxamine infusion when adequate levels of deferoxamine have been achieved.

If the purpose of administering vitamin C is to acidify the urine, urinary pH will need to be monitored to determine effectiveness of the drug.

A baseline assessment of the client should include inspection of the skin and mucous membranes, comfort levels, mental status, and serum ascorbic acid levels. For a child, check the bowel status and temperature. Serum ascorbic acid levels less than 0.2 mg/dl confirm deficiency.

Nursing diagnosis. The client with a vitamin C deficiency and ineffective ascorbic acid therapy may experience the following nursing diagnoses: altered comfort (limb and joint pain); altered mucous membranes (swollen or bleeding gums); altered protection related to capillary fragility (petechiae, ecchymoses); and altered thought processes (irritability, depression, hysteria). Clients receiving ascorbic acid therapy may experience: diarrhea; altered comfort (headache, flushing of skin, stomach cramps); fluid volume deficit related to nausea and vomiting; and the potential complication of oxalate kidney stones.

Implementation

Monitoring. Monitor the client using the indicators in the baseline assessment.

Intervention. IV ascorbic acid can be administered undiluted at a rate not to exceed 100 mg/min. It can also be added to IV solutions and given as a continuous infusion. Too rapid of bolus therapy may cause dizziness and syncope. Ensure that the oral effervescent tablet form is dissolved in water just before administering.

Education. Clients taking more than 600 mg daily may have a small increase in urination; more than 1 g daily, diarrhea; and more than 2 to 3 g daily of prolonged therapy, withdrawal scurvy. The best food sources of vitamin C are citrus fruits, tomatoes, strawberries, cantaloupe, and raw peppers.

Evaluation. The client will maintain adequate intake of dietary vitamin C; healthy skin, mucous membranes, and mental state; and a serum ascorbic acid within the normal limits.

Multiple-Vitamin Preparations

Numerous multivitamin preparations are available in the United States and Canada. Supplemental preparations should provide 100% of the United States RDA to meet the needs of the vast majority of clients. Extra-potency or high-potency vitamins are rarely necessary for routine supplementation. In addition, the nurse should be aware that many preparations contain chemicals that are not yet known to be associated with any known deficiency states.

MINERALS

Although many minerals are available, this discussion is limited to iron, the most commonly prescribed mineral for iron-deficiency anemia. Other minerals are reviewed in other sections of this book.

iron supplements

Iron is an essential mineral for the proper functioning of many biologic systems in the body. It functions as an oxygen carrier in hemoglobin and myoglobin, for tissue respiration, and for many enzyme reactions in the body. It is also stored in various body sites, such as the liver, spleen, and bone marrow. Iron deficiency is the most common nutritional deficiency in the United States resulting in anemia. Young children and women, especially pregnant women, are most frequently affected.

Iron is supplied through diet (lean red meats) and iron supplements. Ingested iron is converted to the ferrous state by gastric juices, which is then more readily absorbed in the body. The absorption of iron will be increased if it is taken with ascorbic acid (vitamin C), orange juice, veal, and other animal tissues. Coffee, tea, milk, eggs, whole grain breads and cereals decrease iron absorption.

Iron is indicated for the treatment of iron-deficiency anemia. In iron deficiency, between 10% to 30% of iron is absorbed while in normal individuals, about 5% to 15% is usually absorbed. Ferrous iron is absorbed better than the ferric dosage form. Iron binds to transferrin and is transported to bone marrow to aid in red blood cell production. Iron is not eliminated physiologically by the body. Excess iron intake can result in accumulation and iron toxicity. Small amounts are lost daily in shedding of skin, nails, hair, breast milk, urine, and menstrual blood. In healthy adults the daily iron loss is approximately 1 mg per day for males and postmenopausal females and 1.5 mg to 2 mg per day in healthy premenopausal females.

Most common side effects of iron therapy include nausea, vomiting, constipation (diarrhea, less frequently reported), and abdominal cramps. For treatment of iron toxicity, see the Management of Drug Overdose Box on p. 1056).

■ Nursing Management

Iron Therapy

See the section on general nursing management of vitamin and mineral therapy.

Assessment. Complete a thorough dietary history and assess the client's nutritional status to ascertain the possible causes of the anemia and the need for client education.

Iron should be administered for iron-deficiency anemias specifically rather than all anemias in general. Some anemic conditions such as thalassemia may actually result in excess deposits of iron in the body.

It should be determined that the client does not have a disorder of iron metabolism such as hemochromatosis, which causes an excess deposition of iron in the tissues, skin pigmentation, cirrhosis of the liver, and decreased carbohydrate tolerance; or hemosiderosis, an increase in tissue iron stores without associated tissue damage.

Some elderly clients may need larger doses of iron than the usual daily adult dose for iron deficiency anemia because the reduction of gastric secretions and achlorhydria that accompanies aging inhibits the ability to absorb iron.

MANAGEMENT OF DRUG OVERDOSE

Iron Supplement

- **Early signs of acute toxicity:** diarrhea that may contain blood, fever, severe abdominal cramps/pain, vomiting.
- **Late signs:** pale, cold skin; convulsions; increased weakness; sedation; blue tinted lips, fingernails, and palms of hands; irregular heart beat; hypotension, metabolic acidosis; cardiovascular collapse.
- **Treatment:** seek medical attention immediately.
  - induce emesis with ipecac syrup or lavage containing sodium bicarbonate, depending on condition of the individual.
  - maintain fluid and electrolyte balance
  - antidote (deferoxamine) is used for severe iron toxicity. Avoid antidote if person has renal failure.
  - monitor laboratory tests (serum iron, hemoglobin, hematocrit, electrolytes, blood gases, blood glucose, total iron-binding capacity, complete blood counts, etc.) closely.
  - if necessary, an exchange transfusion may be utilized.

A baseline assessment of the client should include activity tolerance, hemoglobin, hematocrit, reticulocyte count, and plasma iron values.

Review the client's current medication regimen for significant drug interactions that may occur when iron salts are given concurrently with these drugs:

Drug	Possible effect and management
acetohydroxamic acid (Lithostat)	Iron may be chelated by the acetohydroxamic acid resulting in reduced absorption of both drugs. If iron therapy is necessary for a client receiving acetohydroxamic acid, it is suggested that iron be administered parenterally.
calcium supplements, milk or dairy products, coffee, fiber or selected food products (see previous section)	Decreased iron absorption may result. Schedule iron supplements at least 1 hour before and 2 hours after administration of these substances.
dimercaprol (BAL in oil)	A toxic complex may result if iron and dimercaprol are given concurrently. Postpone daily administration of iron for at least 24 hours after dimercaprol is discontinued. If a severe iron deficiency occurs while client is receiving dimercaprol, a blood transfusion may be indicated.
etidronate (Didronel)	May result in decreased absorption of oral etidronate. Teach clients to avoid consumption of iron products within 2 hours of etidronate.
tetracyclines, oral	Decreases absorption of tetracycline, which may result in reduced antibiotic effectiveness. May impair hematologic effectiveness of the iron supplement. Avoid concurrent administration.
tetracyclines, oral	Reduces absorbability and decreases therapeutic effects of tetracyclines. Administer iron supplements 2 hrs after tetracyclines.
vitamin E	Concurrent administration with iron may reduce the client's hematologic response to iron therapy. If larger iron doses are administered, vitamin E requirements may also need to be increased. Close monitoring is suggested when concurrent therapy is administered.

Nursing diagnosis. The client receiving iron therapy is at risk for the following nursing diagnoses: activity intolerance related to ineffectiveness of the therapy (anemia); altered bowel elimination (constipation or diarrhea); body image disturbance related to stained teeth from liquid forms of iron; fluid volume deficit related to nausea and vomiting; and the potential complications of allergic reaction (backache, chills, dizziness, fever, headache, nausea, tingling of hands or feet) or toxicity (fever, nausea, stomach pain, vomiting, and diarrhea, sometimes with blood).

Implementation

Monitoring. The hemoglobin, hematocrit, reticulocyte count, and plasma iron values should be monitored every 3 weeks during the first 2 months of oral iron therapy or a few days after the initiation of parenteral therapy. It usually takes 1 to 2 months for the hemoglobin concentration of a person with iron deficiency anemia to reach normal levels on oral therapy.

Intervention. The ferrous rather than ferric preparation of iron provides for the most efficient absorption of iron. Iron is best administered on an empty stomach. When taken with food, its absorption may be decreased by as much as a half to a third.

Administer with a full glass of water to prevent staining of the teeth with liquid iron preparations. A drinking straw or a dropper may be used to place the dose well back on the tongue to prevent contact with the teeth. Oral preparations of iron should be discontinued before parenteral iron therapy begins.

Anaphylaxis has been known to occur up to 24 hours after parenteral administration. Epinephrine should be available during injection of iron dextran, particularly in clients with asthma and known allergies. A test dose of 25 mg should be administered, intramuscularly or intravenously, to all clients at least 1 hour or longer before their first therapeutic parenteral dose.

For intravenous administration of iron dextran, do not mix with other medications or add it to parenteral nutrition solutions. It should be administered undiluted and at a rate of not more than 1 ml/min. Flush the intravenous line with normal saline for injection. Maintain the client in a recumbent position for 30 minutes in case orthostatic hypotension should occur.

It is recommended that iron dextran be administered by the Z-track technique (see Chapter 5) using a 2 to 3 inch, 19 or 20 gauge needle, into the muscle mass of the upper outer quadrant of the buttock. It should never be injected into the upper arm or any other exposed area because of the possibility of the preparation staining the skin dark brown. To minimize staining of the flesh, use a separate needle to withdraw the drug from the vial.

Education. The client should be alerted that iron preparations cause black stools, which are medically insignificant.

However, if the client experiences other symptoms of internal blood loss, such as bloody streaks in the stool, abdominal tenderness, cramping, or pain, the prescriber should be notified.

Instruct the client to maintain a diet rich in sources of iron, such as liver, green leafy vegetables, potatoes, dried peas and beans, dried fruit, and enriched flour, bread, and cereals.

Evaluation. The client will maintain adequate dietary intake of iron, tolerate activities as desired, and maintain hemoglobin, hematocrit, reticulocyte count, and plasma iron values within normal limits.

SUMMARY

Nutritional requirements are best met by oral ingestion of adequate fluids and regular, balanced meals. When clients experience altered nutrition, less than the body requires, the nurse may participate in various nutritional modalities, such as vitamin replacement and enteral or parenteral feedings. Vitamins are essential to help maintain normal metabolic functions, growth, and repair of tissue.

Most vitamin deficiencies are not singular but multiple, because of impoverished diets resulting from alcoholism, poverty, fads, or ignorance. Replacement therapy is available for the water-soluble vitamins—C and the B-complex groups—as well as the fat-soluble ones—A, D, E, and K. Water-soluble vitamins are not stored in the body, so deficiencies can appear after short periods of inadequate intake. Fat-soluble vitamins, on the other hand, are stored in the liver and fatty tissue in large amounts, so deficiencies occur only after long deprivation. However, toxic levels then are easier to reach with vitamin supplements. Iron deficiency is the most common nutritional deficiency in the United States and Canada, especially in young children and women. Supplement therapy is practical, but as in all nutritional deficiencies the best remedy is dietary intake.

Critical Thinking

1. How would you plan to incorporate the U.S. RDA requirements for vitamins and minerals into a day's diet for a vegetarian? For a Puerto Rican client? For an edentulous client? For an elderly client on a limited income with only biweekly access to transportation?

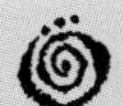

Collaborative Learning Activities

1. Take 10 minutes and write down your diet for the last 24 hours. Using your nutrition books, analyze the diet's vitamin and mineral content. Did you meet the US RDA requirements for vitamins and minerals? How would you modify your diets to do so? What are the barriers to these modifications?

BIBLIOGRAPHY

Allen, Jr LV (1996). Nutritional products. In Covington TR (Ed.). *Handbook of nonprescription drugs* (11th ed.). Washington, DC: American Pharmaceutical Association.

American Hospital Formulary Service (1996). *AHFS: Drug information '96*. Bethesda, MD: American Society of Hospital Pharmacists.

Anderson KN, et al. (Eds.) (1994). *Mosby's medical, nursing, & allied health dictionary* (4th ed.). St Louis: Mosby.

Covington TR (Ed.) (1993). *Handbook of nonprescription drugs* (10th ed.). Washington, DC: American Pharmaceutical Association and The National Professional Society of Pharmacists.

Fawzi WW, et al. (1993). Vitamin A supplementation and child mortality, *JAMA* 269(7):898.

FDA News and Product Notes (1997). New formulations/combinations, *Formulary* 32(1):23-24.

Katzung BG (1992). *Basic and clinical pharmacology* (5th ed.). Norwalk, CT: Appleton & Lange.

Linderborn KM (1993). Independently living seniors and vitamin therapy: What nurses should know, *J Gerontol Nurs* 19(8):10-20.

Marcus R (1996). Agents affecting calcification and bone turnover. In Hardman JF & Limbird LE (Eds.). *Goodman & Gilman's the pharmacological basis of therapeutics* (9th ed.). New York: McGraw-Hill.

Marcus R & Coulston AM (1996). Chapter 62, Water-soluble vitamins and Chapter 63, Fat-soluble vitamins. In Hardman JG & Limbird LE (Eds.). *Goodman & Gilman's the pharmacological basis of therapeutics* (9th ed.). New York: McGraw-Hill.

Rimm EB, et al. (1993). Vitamin E consumption and the risk of coronary heart disease in men, *N Engl J Med* 328(20):1450.

Sharts-Hopko NC (1993). Folic acid in the prevention of neural tube defects. *MCN* 18(4):232.

Stampfer MJ, et al. (1993). Vitamin E consumption and the risk of coronary disease in women, *N Engl J Med* 328(20):1444.

Steinberg D (1993). Antioxidant vitamins and coronary heart disease, *N Engl J Med* 328(20):1487.

United States Pharmacopeial Convention (1996). *USP DI: Drug information for the health care professional* (16th ed.). Rockville, MD: The Convention.

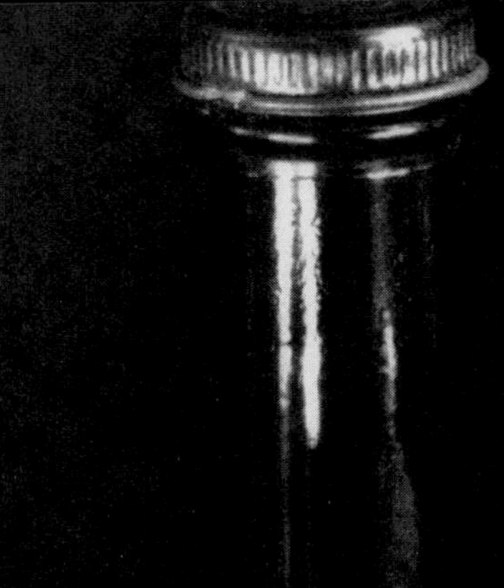

Chapter 69

Fluids and Electrolytes

Chapter Focus

The concept of fluid and electrolyte balance cuts across the nursing care of all clients. It is essential that the nurse have an understanding of the physiology involved to accurately identify clients at risk for specific imbalances so that derangements can be detected early and corrective measures taken. The following objectives and key terms are necessary for a good understanding of this chapter.

Key Terms

dehydration (p. 1059)
extracellular fluid (p. 1059)
intracellular fluid (p. 1059)
milliequivalent (mEq) (p. 1068)
osmosis (p. 1060)
overhydration (p. 1059)

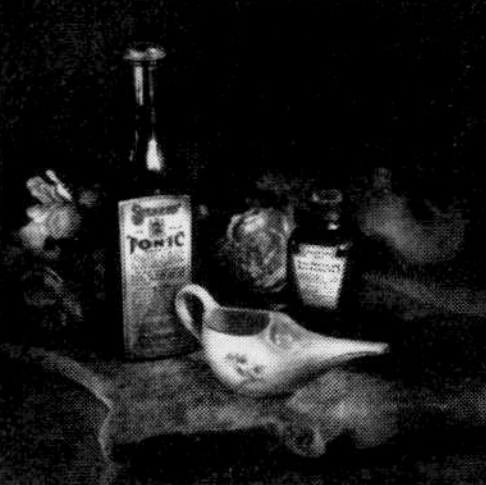

Objectives

1. Identify the various therapeutic reasons for the infusion of intravenous solutions.
2. Describe the role of water in human physiology.
3. Explain water transport in the body.
4. Describe the four categories of parenteral solutions, and give examples of particular solutions in each category.
5. Identify abnormal states of fluid-electrolyte balance.
6. Describe the symptoms of hypertonic dehydration by clinical grading.
7. State the normal requirements, dietary sources, specific functions, and problems associated with an excess or deficiency of sodium, potassium, calcium, and magnesium.
8. Implement nursing management for care of clients receiving intravenous therapy.

The intravenous administration of parenteral fluids has become more prevalent during the past 50 years. Initially the problems associated with the use of unsafe solutions were because of pyrogens. Once this issue was resolved, the advances in the technology of intravenous therapy has resulted in products that have significantly improved patient safety (Box 69-1).

INTRODUCTION

Approximately 50% of all clients in hospitals today receive some type of intravascular therapy (Irvine & Vogt, 1993). There has also been a vast increase in outpatient and home administration of IV medications, hyperalimentation, and fluids. New, sophisticated delivery systems have been developed and different methods of application are constantly being conceived. Intravenous solutions are infused for various therapeutic reasons; some examples are listed here:

- To replace fluids and electrolytes
- To correct acid-base imbalance
- To administer medications
- To maintain ready access to the venous system if any of the first three measures is anticipated
- To measure changes in venous pressure
- To measure the kidneys' excretory capabilities by diagnostic test
- To administer essential nutrients

Blood and its components are transfused intravenously to (1) replace blood volume or plasma fractions; (2) restore the blood's capabilities for oxygen carrying, clotting, or oncotic pressure; or (3) cleanse the plasma of harmful constituents by exchanges. Intravenous hyperalimentation or parenteral nutrition solutions are infused to complement or supplement dietary intake of individuals in deprived nutrition states.

BOX 69-1

Intravenous Therapy: 1930s to Today

Early 1930s

Intravenous injections were reserved for only seriously ill clients.

Only a physician could perform the venipuncture.

1940s

Massachusetts General Hospital became one of the first hospitals to assign a nurse to intravenous therapy.

The job description included administering intravenous solutions and blood transfusions, cleaning the infusion sets for reuse, and cleaning and sharpening needles for reuse.

Primary responsibility was of a technical nature: administering and maintaining the infusions and keeping the equipment clean and functional.

1950s to 1990s

Improvements and innovations in equipment (such as pumps and monitors), needles (Intracaths, and so forth), tubing, development of plastic and disposable equipment, and an increased variety of commercially prepared intravenous fluids increase the safety of intravenous therapy.

The development of intravenous filters prevents particulate matter, bacteria, or fungus from entering the bloodstream.

Intravenous route is used to administer many medications and hyperalimentation fluids, in addition to intravenous fluids.

Intravenous nurse specialists, intravenous departments or teams in the hospital, standards for client care, and professional organizations to promote intravenous therapy as a speciality area in nursing are developed.

FLUIDS

Depending on the amount of adipose tissue present, water comprises from 45% to 75% of the total human body weight. Infants and young children have more water per unit of body weight than adults, and female adults have less water content than male adults. The greatest amount of body water (up to 45% of body weight) is to be found in the **intracellular fluid**; the remainder of body water is located in the **extracellular fluid.** Intracellular fluid is the fluid inside the cells, where the chemical reactions of all metabolism essential to life occur. Extracellular fluid is the fluid surrounding the cells; plasma, interstitial fluid, and lymph, as well as extracellular portions of dense connective tissue, cartilage, and bone. The volume of fluid in the two body fluid compartments varies with age and differs in the sexes. In this fluid, metabolic exchanges between cells and tissues and the external environment occur.

The importance of body water is highlighted by two facts: (1) it is the medium in which all metabolic reactions occur, and (2) precise regulation of volume and composition of body fluid is essential to health. In the healthy individual, body water remains remarkably constant, maintained by a balance between intake and excretion—the water gained each day is equal to the water lost. If the water gained exceeds the water lost, fluid volume excess, or **overhydration,** and edema will occur. If the water lost exceeds the water gained, fluid volume deficit, or **dehydration,** will occur. If 20% to 25% of body water is lost, death usually occurs.

Water, an excellent solvent that permits many substances to be dispersed through it, also has a high dielectric constant that permits ionization of electrolytes. These electrolytes are important in maintaining any physiologic processes and body fluid volume and distribution. They include the cations sodium (Na^+) for extracellular fluid, and potassium (K^+) and magnesium (Mg^{++}) for intracellular fluid; and the anions chloride (Cl^-) and bicarbonate (HCO_3^-) for extracellular fluid, and phosphate (PO_4^{--}) and protein for intracellular fluid.

Intracellular ions also occur in the extracellular fluid but in smaller amounts. Water is also an excellent lubricant between membranes, and it functions well as a heat insulator and heat exchanger.

Daily intake of water in some form is essential to maintain water balance. During starvation, human beings can go several weeks without food but can survive only a few days without water. The average volume of water consumed daily is: 120 to 150 ml/kg body weight in neonates and infants, 120 to 130 ml/kg in children, and 30 ml/kg in adults.

Thirst, the subjective desire to ingest water, helps maintain water balance. Although thirst is complex and not well understood, a decrease in saliva and dryness of the mouth and throat induce it. Dehydration of thirst receptors may lead to their stimulation.

Water intake occurs primarily by (1) drinking fluids, (2) ingesting food containing moisture (most foods contain a high percentage of water), and (3) absorbing water formed by the oxidation of hydrogen in the food during metabolic processes, which produces about 0.5 L of water per day.

Water is lost from the body in five principal ways: (1) by way of the kidneys as urine, (2) through the skin as insensible perspiration and sweat, (3) through expired air as water vapor, (4) through feces, and (5) through the excretion of tears and saliva. Urine excretion accounts for 50% to 60% of the total daily water loss. Urine output, of course, varies with the amount of water ingested.

Water loss by the kidney varies with the solute (molecular ions or particles) load and the antidiuretic hormone (ADH or vasopressin) level. If an increase in solute load occurs (as in diabetes mellitus or following ingestion of excessive amounts of food especially those that generate solutes, such as sodium from salty foods), the kidney excretes sufficient urine to transport the solutes into the bladder. The reabsorption of water in the distal convoluted tubules is controlled by vasopressin, the antidiuretic hormone (ADH). An increase in ADH levels will lead to an increase in water reabsorption, which produces a more concentrated urine. ADH (vasopressin) is secreted by the posterior pituitary gland. This secretion is regulated by osmoreceptors located in the supraoptic nucleus. ADH has an action on specific vasopressin receptors on the medullary tubular cell to stimulate cyclic AMP (cAMP) production in this cell. The cAMP activates an enzyme that alters protein structure in the cell membrane to increase tubular cell permeability to water. This will increase water resorption and increase urine osmolality.

Water Transport in the Body

Water travels from less concentrated areas to areas with higher concentrations of solutes or dissolved substances by **osmosis**. The solutes may be electrolytes, such as potassium chloride or sodium chloride, which, when dissolved in water, yield potassium cations and chloride anions (a chemical balance is maintained) or nonelectrolytes, such as dextrose, urea, or creatinine. Each fluid compartment in the body—intracellular and extracellular compartments—has its own electrolyte composition (Table 69-1). Disturbances in electrolyte composition can be reflected in clinical symptoms in the client.

TABLE 69-1 Normal body electrolyte distribution*

Electrolytes	Extracellular (mEq/L) Plasma	Interstitial	Intracellular (mEq/L)
sodium (Na^+)	142	146	15
potassium (K^+)	5	5	150
calcium (Ca^{++})	5	3	2
magnesium (Mg^{++})	2	1	27
chloride (Cl^-)	103	114	1
bicarbonate (HCO_3^-)	27	30	10

*In addition, phosphates, sulfates, and other substances are located in the extracellular and intracellular fluids.

Osmolality refers to the total solute concentration usually expressed per liter of serum. The osmotic pressure is decided by the number of solutes in solution. For example, if the extracellular fluid contained a large amount of dissolved particles and the intracellular fluid had a small amount of dissolved particles, then the osmotic pressure from the intracellular fluid would force water to pass from the less concentrated area to the more concentrated extracellular area. This would occur until both concentrations were equal. Therefore deciding on the appropriate intravenous therapy for a client would necessitate knowing the electrolyte values. The level of sodium, the principal electrolyte in the extracellular fluid, is essential to know, although potassium levels are also important, along with serum osmolality, current disease state or illnesses, specific laboratory values if appropriate, and the initial signs and symptoms.

Parenteral Solutions

Parenteral solutions generally may be divided into four categories: (1) hydrating solutions, (2) isotonic solutions, (3) maintenance solutions, and (4) hypertonic solutions (Table 69-2).

Hydrating solutions include dextrose 2.5%, 5%, or higher in water or in 0.2% to 0.5% normal saline. (Hypotonic saline—note that full strength normal saline is not included in this category.) Hydrating solutions are used to hydrate or to prevent dehydration. They are often used to assess kidney status before specific electrolytes are ordered as replacement and maintenance therapy and also to help increase diuresis in dehydrated individuals.

Dextrose is a source of calories (1 L of 5% dextrose = approximately 170 calories) that is rapidly metabolized in the body. Dextrose solutions are considered isotonic or more than isotonic in the bottle; but internally, dextrose is metabolized leaving water that decreases the osmotic pressure of the plasma, easily transfers to body cells, and provides water immediately to dehydrated tissues.

TABLE 69-2 Four categories of selected parenteral solutions*

	Na^+	K^+	Mg^{++}	Ca^{++}	Cl^-	Osmolarity
Hydrating solutions						
dextrose 2.5%, 5%, 10%						126,252,505
dextrose 2.5% in 0.45% NaCl injection†	56				56	280
dextrose 5% in 0.45% NaCl injection‡	7				77	405
Isotonic solutions						
normal saline or sodium chloride injection (0.9% NaCl)	154				154	310
Ringer's injection	147	4		4	155	310
lactated Ringer's injection	130	4		3	109	275
Maintenance solutions						
Plasmalyte 56	40	13	3		40	111
Plasmalyte 148 (or Normosol-R, Isolyte S)	140	5		3	98	295
Hypertonic solutions						
sodium chloride, 3% injection	513				513	1025
sodium chloride, 5% injection	855				855	1710

*Normal plasma contains Na^+ (136-145), K^+ (3.5-5), Mg^{++} (1.5-2.5), Ca^{++} (4.3-5.3), Cl^- (100-106), HCO_3^- (27); osmolarity (280-300 mOsm); electrolytes given as mEq/L; osmolarity as mOsm/L.
†Dextrose 2.5% = 25 g dextrose/L or 85 calories.
‡Dextrose 5% = 50 g dextrose/L or 170 calories.

Isotonic solutions are usually prescribed to replace extracellular fluid losses that occur from blood loss, severe vomiting episodes, or any situation in which the chloride loss is equal to or greater than the sodium loss. Isotonic or normal saline is also used before and after a blood transfusion. The reason is that hemolysis of red blood cells, which occurs with dextrose in water, is avoided by using this product.

Isotonic sodium chloride is also used to treat metabolic alkalosis, especially when it occurs in the presence of fluid loss. The increased administration of chloride ions will help to decrease the number of bicarbonate ions in the individual. Other solutions considered isotonic preparations include Ringer's injection and lactated Ringer's injection. A major difference between Ringer's injection and lactated Ringer's injection is the 28 mEq of lactate, a precursor of bicarbonate, in the lactated injection. Thus lactated Ringer's is preferred for individuals with metabolic acidosis perhaps caused by burns or infections. Ringer's injection, however, has more chloride ions; thus it is more useful in treating dehydration from reduced water intake, vomiting, or diarrhea or for clients with hypochloremia.

Maintenance solutions or multiple electrolyte solutions have been formulated to replace daily electrolyte and extracellular needs and water. Such solutions may also be indicated to replace electrolytes and water loss from severe vomiting or diarrhea. With these preparations, the extracellular replacement is usually achieved within 2 days (usually 1 to 3 L/day is administered), and this should be closely monitored by laboratory tests. If maintenance solutions are continued after the client's deficits have been corrected, the excess sodium may lead to circulatory overload, pulmonary edema, and heart failure. Examples of maintenance solutions include PlasmaLyte and Normosol.

Hypertonic solutions are used to treat hypotonic expansion (water intoxication) when the increased body fluid volume is caused by water only. This can happen under several different circumstances: (1) hospitalized clients who receive large amounts of dextrose 5% in water or electrolyte-free solutions to replace fluid and electrolytes lost from vomiting, diarrhea, diuresis, or gastric suction, or (2) most likely in elderly clients during the postoperative period when water is retained in response to stress (endocrine response to stress).

When behavioral changes, such as lethargy, confusion, and perhaps, disorientation occur postoperatively in the elderly person, overhydration or hypotonic expansion should be considered. Central nervous system signs and symptoms such as increased tiredness, muscle twitching, headaches, nausea, vomiting, and even seizures have been noted. Weight gain is always present and the blood pressure may be normal or elevated.

In milder cases, the treatment usually includes withholding all fluids until excess fluids are excreted. In severe cases of hyponatremia, small quantities of hypertonic sodium chloride are administered to (1) increase the osmotic pressure, (2) increase the water flow from body cells to the extracellular compartment, and (3) to enhance excretion of the fluids by the kidneys.

The typical hypertonic saline is a 3% or 5% solution that, when ordered, must be administered slowly with close supervision (to prevent pulmonary edema). Close monitoring of laboratory tests for electrolytes is also required.

Fluid-Electrolyte Balance

A dynamic relationship exists in the body between water and sodium, and abnormal states of hydration can be classified as (1) dehydration (volume depletion), (2) overhydration

TABLE 69-3 Differences among three types of dehydration

	Hypotonic	Isotonic	Hypertonic
Cause	Loss of salt (NaCl)	Blood loss	Water loss or lack of sufficient fluid intake
Effect on ICF and ECF compartments	Volume ICF↑ Volume ECF↓	Decrease in ECF volume	Decrease in ICF and ECF volume
Significant signs:			
Rate of water elimination	Increased	Decreased	Decreased
Thirst			Early warning, because of cell dehydration
Pulse rate	Increased, weak, thready	Regular	Regular in early stages
Behavioral signs	May see vomiting, abdominal cramps		Confusion, irritability, agitation
Late stages	Skin turgor Weak pulse, lethargy, confusion, death owing to circulatory failure	Shock, weak Weak, thready	Skin turgor Dry, furrowed tongue; death
Clinical lab results:			
Hematocrit	Increased	Increased	Increased
Hemoglobin	Increased	Increased	Increased
Sodium levels	Decreased		Increased

(hypervolemia or volume excess), (3) loss of water in excess of sodium (hypernatremia), and (4) loss of sodium in excess of water (hyponatremia). The second abnormal state is overhydration or volume excess, which was reviewed under the description of hypertonic solutions in the preceding section. The other three abnormal states may be viewed as various types of dehydration.

Dehydration

Table 69-3 illustrates the differences between the three types of dehydration. Note that the causes of the three dehydration states are different, as are the effects on fluid compartments in the body and some of the initial signs and laboratory values, especially sodium concentration. This is very important information because it will aid the physician not only in diagnosing the initial condition but also in choosing an appropriate intravenous therapy for the individual client.

Hypertonic dehydration caused by heat exhaustion resulting from water depletion can occur on land or sea. Many cases of boaters lost at sea or refugees fleeing their countries for another country run out of water for days before being rescued or reaching land. Such persons require intensive care for their dehydration, and some may die from this deprivation (Table 69-4).

The nurse should be aware that geriatric clients with decreased renal function will be more vulnerable to dehydration and electrolyte imbalance. As a result of the aging process the additional physiologic changes experienced by the elderly may also make them more susceptible to the adverse effects of fluid and electrolyte administration, such as overhydration or decreased renal excretion of exogenous potassium or magnesium with resultant toxic accumulation in the body.

TABLE 69-4 Hypertonic dehydration symptoms

Clinical grading	Symptoms
Mild or early	Increased thirst. Usually a 2% body weight loss.
Moderate to severe	Very dry mouth, difficulty in swallowing, scant urine output (highly concentrated urine), increased pulse rate and body temperature, poor skin turgor; an approximate 6% body weight loss.
Extreme or very severe	All previous symptoms plus impaired mental and physical capabilities, rectal temperature very high, respiratory difficulties (hyperventilation that may lead to tetany), cyanosis, severe oliguria or anuria, circulatory failure, loss of more than 7% in body weight. Usually coma and death occur when approximately 15% of body weight is lost.

ELECTROLYTES

The major electrolytes in the body are sodium, potassium, calcium, and magnesium. This section will review the normal requirements, sources, specific functions, and problems associated with an excess or deficiency of the electrolyte.

Sodium

Sodium is the major electrolyte in the extracellular fluid; the normal range is from 136 to 145 mEq/L of plasma. The sodium content in the body is regulated by sodium consumption (dietary) and sodium excretion by the kidneys. In the average person with normal renal function, sodium excretion will closely match sodium intake. This aids in keeping sodium content in the body at a constant level even if sodium intake is somewhat varied. Major dietary sources of sodium are table salt (sodium chloride), catsup, mustard, cured meats and fish, cheese, peanut butter, pickles, olives, potato chips, and popcorn. The typical American diet provides between 3 to 6 grams of sodium per day (Johnson & Lalonde, 1993), while the recommended dietary sodium allowance is much less. Sodium is necessary for control of body water; for the electrophysiology of nerve, muscle, and gland cells; and for the regulation of pH and isotonicity.

Hyponatremia

Hyponatremia may be detected when the serum level falls below 135 mEq/L. It may be induced by excessive sweating with replacement of only the water, infusion of large quantities of nonelectrolyte parenteral fluids, and adrenal insufficiency or gastrointestinal suctioning with replacement fluids limited to water by mouth.

Symptoms include lethargy, hypotension, stomach cramps, vomiting, diarrhea, and possibly, seizures. Deficiency states are usually treated with Ringer's solution or normal saline injection.

Hypernatremia

Hypernatremia is seen when the serum sodium levels are higher than normal, usually >150 mEq/L. This excess may be induced by excessive use of saline infusions, inadequate water consumption (as described previously), or excess fluid loss without a corresponding loss of sodium.

Signs and symptoms include edema; hypertonicity; red, flushed skin; dry, sticky mucous membranes; increase in thirst; temperature elevation; and a decrease in or absence of urination. Treatment includes reducing salt intake and using dextrose in water intravenously to promote diuresis and increase the excretion of both salt and water from the blood.

Potassium

Potassium is the major electrolyte in the intracellular fluids. The amount of potassium in the intracellular fluid is approximately 150 mEq/L, whereas the amount in the plasma is between 3.5 and 5 mEq/L. Even though this plasma amount appears to be low, it is of great importance, since serum potassium must be maintained between 3.5 and 5 mEq/L for survival. The diet of most individuals contains from 35 to 100 mEq of potassium daily and normally, any excess potassium is excreted by the kidney in the urine. Potassium plays an important part of (1) muscle contraction, (2) conduction of nerve impulses, (3) enzyme action, and (4) cell membrane function.

Hypokalemia

Hypokalemia or potassium deficit may be caused by chronic administration of intravenous solutions containing little or no potassium; diuretic therapy with potassium-depleting medications; reduced dietary intake (e.g., in persons on "starvation diets"); poor absorption because of steatorrhea, regional enteritis, or short bowel syndrome; loss of gastrointestinal secretions, which are very rich in potassium, due to vomiting, diarrhea, GI suction or fistula drainage; extensive burn conditions; or in the presence of excessive amounts of adrenocortical hormone.

Unlike sodium, which is reabsorbed when the serum sodium level is low, potassium ions continue to be excreted in the urine when the serum potassium level is low. As potassium loss continues, the individual's condition deteriorates unless potassium intake is increased and normal levels are reestablished.

With hypokalemia, impaired skeletal muscle function may cause profound weakness or paralysis, including paralysis of the respiratory muscles, while impaired smooth muscle function may result in ileus. Cardiac effects of hypokalemia include increased sensitivity to digitalis with potential toxicity and ECG changes. Early potassium deficiency may be detected by the use of the electrocardiogram as the T wave tends to flatten when serum potassium levels are below 3.5 mEq/L while it tends to elongate vertically when the serum potassium level is 5.8 mEq/L or higher. Atrioventricular block and cardiac arrest may occur.

Hypokalemia also causes movement of Na^+ and H^+ from extracellular fluid and the excretion of H^+ which may elevate plasma pH resulting in metabolic alkalosis. Other effects are decreased water reabsorption in the renal tubule, resulting in polyuria, and hypochloremia.

Treat hypokalemia by replacing potassium orally or parenterally. Be aware though, that a hazard of parenteral correction is potassium poisoning, or hyperkalemia.

Parenteral or intravenous administration. The dose of potassium supplements depends on the individual requirement and requires close supervision. *Intravenous potassium must always be diluted* and administered slowly. Potassium generally is given only to individuals with a documented adequate urine flow. In dehydrated clients, it is best to give a potassium-free fluid first to hydrate the client and determine urinary output.

It is recommended that parenteral fluids should not contain more than 40 mEq/L of potassium and the rate of administration should not be more than 20 mEq/hour (*AHFS*, 1996). Whenever possible, the oral preparations or consumption of foods high in potassium should replace the intravenous potassium solutions (see Chapter 34, Diuretics).

The parenteral potassium salts are available as acetate, chloride, and phosphate salts. Generally, the potassium chloride is the preferred preparation, since the chloride will help to correct the hypochloremia that often is seen with hypokalemia. In general, the alkalinizing potassium salts (acetate, bicarbonate, citrate, or gluconate) may be necessary to treat hypokalemia associated with metabolic acidosis (a rare situation).

Oral administration. Potassium salts available include acetate, bicarbonate, chloride, citrate, and gluconate alone or in combinations for oral administration. Liquid preparations are generally preferred for oral therapy and most contain 10, 20, or 40 mEq of potassium/15 ml. These preparations must be diluted with fruit juice or water before ingestion and taken after meals with a full glass of water to minimize the gastrointestinal irritation. For powder preparations, closely follow the manufacturer's instructions. The uncoated and enteric-coated (no longer available in the United States) dosage forms of potassium have caused intestinal and gastric ulcers with bleeding episodes (*AHFS*, 1996). Although still available, they are rarely used medically, instead, liquid, effervescent, powders, and extended-release dosage forms (wax matrix, microencapsulated) are currently preferred products. The nurse should be aware that ulceration has also been reported with the extended-release products (although much less frequently than with the other products), and these preparations should be reserved for clients who cannot or will not take the liquid or effervescent potassium.

If the client complains of stomach pain, swelling, or severe vomiting or gastrointestinal bleeding is noted, the extended-release potassium should be stopped immediately and the prescriber should be contacted. Potassium supplements are contraindicated in clients with severe renal impairment, untreated chronic adrenocortical insufficiency (Addison's disease), hyperkalemia, and severe burn conditions or acute dehydration. They should also be avoided or used with extreme caution in persons taking potassium-sparing diuretics or angiotensin-converting enzyme (ACE) inhibitors. Solid dosage forms of potassium should not be administered to clients with esophageal compression caused by an enlarged left atrium or other anatomic variation resulting in increased compression in this area. In such cases, ingestion of potassium-rich foods may also be helpful. (See Box 34-1, Foods Rich in Potassium.)

The dosage of potassium supplements depends on individual requirements. The approximate daily allowance for adults is 40 to 50 mEq; for infants, about 1 to 3 mEq/kg body weight daily.

⚠ MANAGEMENT OF DRUG OVERDOSE

Treatment of Hyperkalemia

- For mild hyperkalemia, remove or treat the cause. For example, if the person is receiving potassium supplements or an ACE inhibitor, stop the medications. If metabolic acidosis is present, treat this condition.
- Moderate to severe hyperkalemia may require infusing hypertonic dextrose solutions with insulin to shift potassium into the cells. Sodium bicarbonate parenteral may be used to correct acidosis and also help shift serum potassium into cells. Calcium gluconate is administered intravenously under constant ECG monitoring for severe cardiac toxicity. Calcium counteracts the adverse effects of potassium on the neuromuscular membranes, so this is a temporary measure only. Lowering of the potassium levels is critical to reversing this situation.
- All the above methods do not remove potassium from the body. Sodium polystyrene sulfonate (Kayexalate), a cation exchange resin can be given orally or rectally to remove potassium from the body.
- Oral adult dose of sodium polystyrene sulfonate is 15 g one to four times daily in water or preferably a 70% sorbitol solution to reduce the possibility of constipation. The rectal (retention enema) adult dose is 25 to 100 g of resin suspended in 100 to 200 ml of sorbitol or 10% dextrose in water. This dose may be administered every 6 hours.
- Laxatives must be used when the drug is given orally. Since its action is considered slow, the previously discussed treatments are indicated if ECG changes indicate severe potassium intoxication. Administration should be discontinued when the serum potassium level falls to 4 or 5 mEq/L.
- Side effects of sodium polystyrene sulfonate treatment include anorexia, nausea, vomiting, constipation, hypokalemia, and hypocalcemia. Fecal impaction has also been reported; it can be prevented with the use of laxatives (*USP DI*, 1996).

Hyperkalemia

Hyperkalemia, or potassium excess, can be caused by acute or chronic renal failure; the release of large amounts of intracellular potassium in burns, crush injuries, or severe infections; overtreatment with potassium salts; or metabolic acidosis, including diabetic ketoacidosis, which causes a shift of potassium from the cells into the extracellular fluids.

Hyperkalemia causes interference with neuromuscular function, which may result in abdominal distention, diarrhea, weakness and paralysis. Cardiac effects caused by hyperkalemia result from impaired conduction. The ECG shows widening and slurring of the QRS complexes, peaked T waves, depressed ST segments, and possibly disappearance of P waves. Ventricular fibrillation and cardiac arrest may occur.

The treatment of hyperkalemia depends on the serum level of potassium and the electrocardiogram (ECG) patterns. Mild hyperkalemia is usually a serum level below 6.5 mEq/L with ECG changes limited to peaking of the T waves. Moderate hyperkalemia is a potassium serum level between 6.5 and 8 mEq/L while severe hyperkalemia is serum levels above 8 mEq/L with an ECG pattern of absent P waves, widened QRS complex, or ventricular dysrhythmias. For treatment of hyperkalemia, see the Management of Drug Overdose Box above.

Calcium

Calcium (Ca^{++}) is essential for growth and bone ossification, neuromuscular transmission, cell membrane permeability, the maintenance of excitability in nerve fibers, hormone secretion and action, muscle contraction, maintenance of cardiac and vascular tone, many enzyme activities, and the normal coagulation of blood.

Almost all of the 1000 to 1200 g calcium in the normal adult is in the skeletal tissue, and only about 1% of the total body calcium is in solution in body fluids. About half the calcium in plasma is bound to complex organic anions (e.g., bicarbonate and phosphate). Nearly all unbound serum calcium is ionized. Normal serum calcium concentration is 4.5 to 5.5 mEq/L or 9 to 11 mg/100 ml.

Recommended dietary allowance of calcium for adults is 0.8 to 1.2 g daily. Pregnant or lactating women need 1.2 g; children 1 to 3 years 0.4 to 0.8 g; and 4 to 10 years 0.8 g. The intake of calcium in a balanced diet is sufficient for normal body needs. Absorption of calcium depends on how well it is kept in solution in the digestive tract; an acid medium favors calcium solubility and absorption in the upper intestinal tract. Absorption is decreased by the presence of alkalis and large amounts of fatty acids. Adequate intake of vitamin D appears to promote calcium absorption. Calcium is excreted in the urine and feces, as well as in perspiration. Estrogen deficiency promotes calcium loss.

Maintenance of normal concentration of serum calcium depends on the interactions of three agents: parathyroid hormone, vitamin D, and calcitonin. Parathyroid hormone and vitamin D mobilize the removal of calcium from bone, the principal source of calcium for extracellular fluids. Parathyroid hormone also promotes renal tubular reabsorption of calcium and a slight increase in intestinal absorption of calcium. Calcitonin synthesized in the thyroid gland moderates or decreases the rate of removal of calcium from the bone.

Hypocalcemia

Hypocalcemia or a decrease in serum calcium, results from (1) hypoparathyroidism, (2) chronic renal insufficiency, (3) hypoalbuminemia, (4) malabsorption syndrome, and (5) deficiency of vitamin D. Hypoparathyroidism may follow thyroidectomy, since several parathyroid glands frequently are removed with this surgery. If the function of the remaining gland(s) is impaired, the result is depressed parathyroid activity.

Individuals who are bedridden tend to develop a negative calcium balance because the ion is lost from bones and excreted. This effect is likely to be serious when long immobilization of the client is necessary.

Hypocalcemia increases excitability of the nerves and the neuromuscular junction, which leads to muscle cramps, muscle twitching, and tetany. Numbness and tingling of the fingers, toes, and lips occurs. Hypertonicity of muscle may cause tonic contractions of the hands and feet (carpopedal spasm) while increased neural excitability may cause convulsions, abnormal behavior, and personality changes. In children, prolonged hypocalcemia has resulted in mental retardation. The ECG shows a prolonged QT interval and an inverted T wave. In prolonged hypocalcemia, defects can occur in the nails, skin, and teeth; cataracts may appear; and calcification of the basal ganglia may occur.

Regardless of the underlying cause, severe hypocalcemia is treated initially with intravenous administration of rapidly available calcium ions. For latent tetany, mild symptoms of hypocalcemia, and maintenance therapy, an oral calcium salt is given. Vitamin D may also be prescribed. Overdosage of calcium may cause hypercalcemia, which results in anorexia, nausea, vomiting, weakness, depression, polyuria, and polydipsia.

Calcium must be administered cautiously to clients undergoing digitalis therapy, since calcium potentiates the effect of digitalis and may precipitate dysrhythmias. ECG monitoring of the client is recommended when parenteral calcium is administered.

Calcium salts are used as a nutritional supplement, particularly during pregnancy and lactation. They are specific in the treatment of hypocalcemic tetany. They have also been used for their antispasmodic effects in cases of abdominal pain, tenesmus, and colic resulting from disease of the gallbladder or painful contractions of the ureters. The basic salts of calcium are also used as antacids. Approximately 1 to 1.5 g calcium per day has been recommended to prevent postmenopausal bone loss or osteoporosis.

The most widely used calcium salt is calcium carbonate which requires an acid medium to form soluble calcium salts, since it is nearly insoluble in water. Absorption of or dissolution of calcium phosphate and calcium sulfate are also pH dependent, whereas calcium lactate, calcium citrate, and calcium gluconate are considered pH independent. In elderly persons and postmenopausal women, impaired stomach acid production is common therefore the high stomach pH or achlorhydric state results in a decreased solubility of the pH-dependent calcium salts.

Since the different calcium salts have different amounts of calcium present, many professionals choose the calcium salt with the highest percentage of calcium per gram because then, a smaller quantity of drug may be administered. For example, if the recommended daily dose of calcium is 1000 mg/day, then it would be necessary to administer nearly 10 g of calcium gluconate to reach this amount, whereas only 2.5 g of calcium carbonate per day would be required. This then requires the consumption of smaller quantities of tablets to obtain the same amount of calcium, assuming of course, the calcium is soluble under the conditions present in the client (Table 69-5).

To improve calcium carbonate tablet solubility, especially in achlorhydric conditions, it is recommended the tablets be taken with meals, when acid secretion is highest. Avoid taking the tablets on an empty stomach or at night because these are times when acid secretions are minimal. Calcium phosphates and tricalcium phosphate have little usefulness in possible achlorhydric states and, perhaps, even in the normal person. Both products have a very poor dissolution rate or pattern, thus reducing the possibility of calcium absorption. Perhaps in clients with known achlorhydric states, the soluble calcium salts (lactate or citrate) might be the appropriate form to use even though it will be necessary to use more tablets to provide sufficient quantities of calcium. Selected food consumption is another source for calcium (Table 69-6).

TABLE 69-5 Calcium content of various calcium salts

	Percent calcium	Amount calcium per tablet	Tablets needed for 1 g calcium
calcium carbonate	40	260 mg/650 mg	4
calcium gluconate	9	45 mg/500 mg	22
calcium lactate	13	42 mg/325 mg	24
calcium phosphate tribasic	39	600 mg/1565 mg	1.66

TABLE 69-6 Foods with high calcium content

Food	Calcium content
Yogurt, lowfat (1 cup)	275-400 mg
Skim milk (1 cup)	300 mg
Cheese, Swiss (1 oz)	272 mg
Cheese, cottage (1 cup)	215 mg
Cheese, cheddar (1 oz)	200 mg
Broccoli, raw (1 cup)	100 mg
Ice cream (½ cup)	100 mg
Ice milk (¾ cup)	132 mg

Hypercalcemia

Hypercalcemia, or elevated serum calcium levels, may be caused by neoplasms with or without bone metastases. Carcinoma of the ovary, kidney, or lung can synthesize and secrete a parathyroid-like hormone, causing hypercalcemia. Other common causes are hyperparathyroidism, thiazide diuretic therapy, multiple myeloma, sarcoidosis, and vitamin D intoxication.

Clinical manifestations of hypercalcemia are highly variable and involve many organ systems because calcium may be deposited in various body tissues. The symptoms may include:

- Gastrointestinal: anorexia, nausea, vomiting, constipation, and abdominal pain.
- Neurologic: weakness, apathy, depression, amnesia, confusion, stupor, and coma may occur.
- Renal: polyuria and nephrocalcinosis may occur, seriously impairing renal function, which may lead to edema, uremia, and hypertension, which may be irreversible.
- Cardiovascular: increased cardiac contractility, ventricular extrasystoles, and heart block. ECG changes include a short QT segment and characteristic signs of heart block.

Treatment is variable and aimed at controlling the underlying disease. In dehydrated persons, restore extracellular fluid volume with normal saline infusions which also, increases calcium excretion. Furosemide may be prescribed to enhance diuresis but thiazide diuretics should be avoided because they block or lower calcium excretion. Chelating (binding) agents, such as disodium edetate has been used in acute hypercalcemia in selected individuals. It increases renal excretion of calcium by forming soluble complexes with the calcium that are not reabsorbed by the renal tubules.

Biphosphonates such as etidronate (Didronel) and pamidronate (Aredia) inhibit bone resorption, which decreases serum calcium. They are used to treat Paget's disease and hypercalcemia of neoplasms; for the latter, though, pamidronate is more potent and usually the preferred agent. An antineoplastic drug, plicamycin (Mithracin), also reduces serum calcium levels (Tang & Lau, 1995; *USP DI*, 1996).

Magnesium

Magnesium (Mg^{++}) is an important ion for the function of many enzyme systems.

Hypomagnesemia

Hypomagnesemia, a deficit of magnesium, may be encountered in chronic alcoholism, severe malabsorption, starvation, diarrhea, prolonged gastrointestinal suction, vigorous diuresis, acute pancreatitis, and primary aldosteronism. Magnesium, the second most abundant intracellular cation, plays an important role in regulating the sodium-potassium ATPase pump function, neuromuscular transmission, cardiovascular function, and mitochondrial and other cellular functions in the body.

Magnesium deficiency may result in additional electrolyte problems (hypokalemia, hypocalcemia), cardiac arrhythmias, and neurotoxicity. It may also cause an increase in neuromuscular irritability and contractility, coarse tremor, muscle spasm, delirium, athetoid movements, nystagmus, and tetany. It also causes tachycardia, hypertension, and vasomotor changes and increases the risk of digitalis toxicity in persons taking cardiac glycosides.

Hypomagnesemia may be treated with intravenous fluids containing magnesium, 10 to 40 mEq/day for severe deficit, followed by 10 mEq/day for maintenance. The use of intravenous fluids containing from 3 to 5 mEq magnesium/L may avert magnesium deficiency that arises from prolonged administration of intravenous solutions that do not contain magnesium.

Hypermagnesemia

Hypermagnesemia occurs primarily in individuals with chronic renal insufficiency. Adverse effects include flushing, sweating, hypothermia, areflexia, paralysis, and depression of cardiac, CNS, and respiratory functions. Decreased muscle cell excitability is caused by blockade of the myoneural junction (inhibition of acetylcholine release). Cardiac depression effects result in an increase in conduction time with the ECG evidencing a lengthened PR segment and a prolonged QRS complex. If the Mg^{++} concentration continues to increase, third-degree atrioventricular block and cardiac arrest may occur.

An excess of Mg^{++} may require dialysis. Since calcium acts as an antagonist to Mg^{++}, calcium salts may be given parenterally. Normal serum concentration is 1.5 to 2.5 mEq/L, with one third bound to protein and two thirds free. A toxic blood level is magnesium greater than 4 mEq/L. Magnesium has physiologic effects on the nervous system similar to those of calcium.

Additional Single-Salt Solutions

In addition to the previously discussed salt preparations, ammonium chloride injection and sodium lactate injection are also available for use.

Ammonium chloride injection is indicated to treat hypochloremia and metabolic alkalosis (not associated with severe liver disease) to prevent tetany or renal damage. Most cases respond to sodium chloride solution, but for the rare, nonresponsive situation, ammonium chloride is available. Ammonium chloride has been used as a urinary acidifier to promote excretion of alkaline substances.

This product is available in 20 ml vials (100 mEq) and the dose selected depends on the individual (usually 1 to 2 vials) in normal saline infused slowly.

Sodium lactate injection available as a 1/6 molar solution contains 167 mEq/L each of sodium and lactate ions. It is used to treat metabolic acidosis when no evidence of an elevated lactic acid level exists. Sodium lactate is converted to sodium bicarbonate in the liver. In persons with lactic acidosis or impaired liver function, sodium bicarbonate is preferred.

■ Nursing Management

Intravenous Therapy

Intravenous fluid and dextrose or electrolyte replacement by infusion continues to be the most common application of intravascular therapy. Although the dosage and choice of solution is tailored to the client's needs by the prescriber according to the disorder and body surface area, monitoring the therapy is the nurse's responsibility. With the increasing prevalence of clients receiving some type of intravascular therapy in hospitals, as well as in home settings, the role of the nurse in intravenous therapy has also grown and developed. See the Home Health box above for additional information on IV therapy in the home.

Consider intravascular therapy a closed-system, sterile procedure. It is invasive, and its effects are relatively irreversible; therefore take care to perform and maintain it precisely.

Assessment. Assessment begins with an understanding of the purpose of the particular client's intravenous therapy and the potential risks to the client. Those clients who are debilitated, have a renal or cardiovascular problem, are prone to infection, or have very sclerotic veins are particularly at risk for complications related to intravenous therapy.

Factors to be considered for site selection include the following: suitable location, purpose of infusion, expected duration of therapy, condition of veins, restrictions imposed by client's current health status and past health history, and dominant extremity (Metheny, 1992). Unless contraindicated, it is most appropriate to use veins in the nondominant upper extremity. When more than one puncture is anticipated, it is better to make the first venipuncture distally and work proximally. Avoid venipuncture in the affected arm of clients with axillary dissection as in radical mastectomy or clients with impaired mobility of the upper extremity as in unilateral paralysis secondary to CVA. In both instances circulation may not be adequate and will affect the flow of the infusion, causing increased edema.

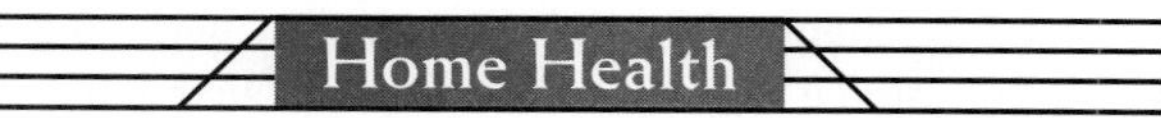

Home IV Therapy Clients

The provision of IV therapy to clients in their homes is growing in practice. It allows the client to remain in a home setting, be more comfortable, and to perform many daily activities. There may also be cost benefits for clients and health care agencies.

Clients should be carefully selected to receive home IV therapy. Instruction should begin in the hospital and be completed before the client is discharged. If the nurse is to provide the IV therapy on a home visit, all of the nursing processes applicable to institutional care will be adapted for the home setting. If the IV therapy is to be self-administered or administered by a caregiver in the home, it should be determined that the client/caregiver is willing and capable of administering the therapy safely. This capability includes the economics and transportation to obtain supplies; fine movement coordination to manipulate the equipment; understanding of asepsis, rationale for therapy, the interventions, potential complications and whom to contact in case of emergency. Instruct the client in any activity limitations; how to check the venipuncture site for any complications; what to do if redness, swelling, or pain occurs, if the dressing becomes soiled, if blood appears in the tubing, or if the alarm on the electronic infusion device goes off. If the client is using a heparin lock, teach the client how and when to flush it. Have the client document a daily check of the venipuncture site. Have the client/caregiver return demonstrations. Develop a number of "what if . . ." scenarios to test the client's understanding and decision-making skills before an urgent situation occurs. Encourage the client/caregiver to contact the health care provider for assistance if required.

Nursing diagnosis. Every individual with an intravenous infusion is at risk for the following nursing diagnoses: impaired tissue integrity related to infiltration, thrombosis, thrombophlebitis, and necrosis; pain at the administration site; and the potential complications of pulmonary edema, pyrogenic reaction, speed shock, and sepsis. Because of their smaller body size, infants and children are especially at risk for overhydration.

Implementation

Monitoring. Continued reassessments of laboratory data reports are essential for clients receiving electrolyte replacement therapy. Serum electrolytes should not exceed the following accepted ranges during intravenous therapy:

Sodium	135 to 145 mEq/L
Chlorides	95 to 108 mEq/L
Potassium	3.5 to 5 mEq/L
Calcium	4.5 to 5.8 mEq/L
Magnesium	1.5 to 2.5 mEq/L

Note that fluctuations in potassium, calcium, and magnesium must be watched carefully during intravenous electrolyte therapy, since even a small deviation in these creates a much greater risk than in those electrolytes with a wider range of normal values. Understanding that milliequivalents (mEq) are not related to milligrams also is important; "mEq" does not reflect a measure of weight.

Milliequivalents measure the number of chemically active ions in solution, which is a more precise measure of the relative potency of an electrolyte solution than weight-by-volume measurements. (See Chapter 5 for equipment and technical aspects of intravenous therapy.)

Remember that ongoing assessment of client response is essential to preventing complications from intravenous therapy. The entire intravenous system should be monitored from fluid container down to the client's infusion site. Such assessments are to be made frequently. Flow rates may change 20% to 40% during an infusion; check the flow rate every hour if not using an infusion pump. Calculating the need for hourly changes in intravenous flow rates based on individual fluid output may be the nurse's responsibility. The nurse may titrate infusion fluid intake according to the amount of hourly urine, gastric, or other outputs over specified periods.

Ongoing assessment of the client receiving intravenous therapy should include observations for the following complications.

Infiltration. Infiltration occurs when the needle is dislodged from the vein, permitting the solution to enter the surrounding tissues, which causes pain and edema. Nurses should check the infusion site frequently for signs of infiltration (painful blanched cool swelling at infusion site without blood return). There may also be a significant decrease in the flow rate, or it may stop altogether if the infiltration is extensive.

To detect infiltration in a questionable IV site, locate the vein in which the parenteral solution is infusing. Place two fingers on the vein, about 3 to 4 inches above the injection, depending on the length of the needle or catheter that is in place. Observe the drip chamber while applying digital pressure. If the flow of solution in the drip chamber stops, it indicates that the needle is in the vein. If there is no alteration of the flow in the drip chamber, the needle is probably in the tissue because flow continues into the tissues even if the vein is occluded (Metheney, 1992). If infiltration is confirmed, stop the infusion.

Thrombosis. An intravascular blood clot occurs when platelets agglutinate and fibrin strands and red and white blood cells adhere to the platelet mass. A thrombus may form any time a blood vessel is injured, including injury by venipuncture. A thrombus may form in or around the needle or catheter, plugging the lumen; if this occurs, the infusion stops.

Thrombophlebitis. Blood clot formation and inflammation of the vein may result from several factors: chemical, due to the pH of the solution or the toxicity of the drug being administered; mechanical, due to injury of the vein by movement of the cannula; and septic, due to contamination. Thrombophlebitis is manifested by pain, heat, swelling, redness along the vein's course, and loss of motion of the affected part.

Pain at administration site. Pain occurs when (1) the needle touches the venous wall, (2) too much tension is put on the needle or tubing, and (3) irritating drugs are administered too rapidly.

Necrosis. Death and sloughing of tissue can occur when irritating drugs or solutions, such as epinephrine or norepinephrine, infiltrate into the tissues.

Pulmonary edema. Pulmonary edema occurs when the circulatory system is overloaded with fluids. Careful monitoring of flow rate and of urinary output is necessary. Central venous pressure monitoring, particularly in clients with cardiac disease, can help to prevent this hazardous complication. The client will exhibit dyspnea on exertion, orthopnea, and coughing. Tachycardia, tachypnea, dependent crackles, neck vein distention, and diastolic (S_3) gallop may be heard. Coughing produces a frothy, bloody sputum. Dysrhythmias may occur. The client becomes cold, clammy, sweaty, and cyanotic; the blood pressure falls and the pulse becomes thready.

Pyrogenic reactions. Pyrogenic reactions occur when pyrogens, or fever-producing substances, are introduced into the circulatory system. Bacterial pyrogens are filtrable, thermostable products of bacterial origin and activity that may accumulate and tend to cause a severe rigor when injected into the body. Pyrogenic reactions are characterized by fever and chills, malaise, headache, backache, nausea, vomiting, and vascular collapse with hypotension, if severe.

Air emboli. Although they rarely occur, air emboli have a 40% to 50% mortality (McConnell, 1986). However, cannulation of central veins is far more likely to be associated with air embolism than is cannulation of the peripheral veins (Thielen, 1990). The occurrence of the following symptoms in a client receiving an infusion may indicate the presence of an air embolism: dyspnea and cyanosis; hypotension; weak, rapid pulse; loud, continuous churning sound over the precordium (not always present); and loss of consciousness.

The assessment for some clients may include whether IV fluids should be used at all (Box 69-2).

BOX 69-2

Should IV Fluids Be Given to the Dying?

Intravenous fluids are often provided to terminally ill clients in the belief that electrolyte imbalance and dehydration are painful, agonizing events. It is also feared that the lack of medical intervention may be interpreted as abandonment, provoking familial condemnation and raising the specter of malpractice (Rousseau, 1992).

However, from a legal standpoint, IV fluids may be withheld or withdrawn in the same manner as other medical treatments with the proviso the client requests such limitations. And a study by Andrews and Levine (1989) reports that dehydration is not painful and may even be beneficial to a dying client. Although the administration of IV fluids may produce a temporary sense of well-being, it often aggravates the client's symptoms. Hydration will increase urinary output, frequently necessitating the insertion of an indwelling catheter and exposing the client to infection. Pulmonary and pharyngeal secretions will increase, precipitating cough, dyspnea, and pulmonary edema; pulmonary symptoms will increase. Increased gastrointestinal secretions will exacerbate nausea and vomiting. Intravenous fluid may also produce peripheral edema and increase the risk of skin breakdown. All of these symptoms will increase the client's discomfort, and the IV fluids may prolong the dying process. On the other hand, fluid deprivation would cause a reduction in these symptoms. The fluid and electrolyte imbalance produced by dehydration may be a natural anesthetic, reducing the discomfort associated with the dying process (Rousseau, 1992).

Once a client decides for terminal dehydration, the nurse's role is to provide scrupulous oral hygiene to reduce inflammation and minimize discomfort and to provide the client and family emotional support.

Critical thinking questions

- As a nurse, what feelings do you have about partcipating in the care of a dying client in which IV rehydration is being withheld?
- How would you respond when asked about the rationale for this approach to the care of the dying client?

From PC Rousseau (1992). Why give IV fluids to the dying? *Patient Care* 26 (10):71.

Intervention. Maintain a steady, even flow at the rate ordered; do not speed up rates to make up for lost time (watch the literature, however, for a resolution of the question about slowed rates being more compatible with basal metabolic rates during the before-dawn hours). Use every aid to facilitate therapy, such as calculating drops to be infused per minute and then time-taping the container. Use of an electronic infusion device (EID) is the standard for practice in many institutions, either a controller that regulates IV flow rates by gravity or a controller that uses positive pressure to maintain flow (Box 69-3). Avoid the use of restraints and the checking of blood pressures on the arm receiving the infusion because the cuff interferes with fluid flow, forces blood back into the needle, and may cause formation of a clot. See Chapter 5 for techniques associated with intravenous therapy.

BOX 69-3

Recognizing a Hazard of Electronic Infusion Devices

Accidental, uncontrolled free flow of medication may occur when an IV administration set is removed from an electronic infusion device (EID). Although EIDs have been on the market for a number of years, only in the last 3 years have incidents of overdosing as the result of free flow begun to be reported anecdotally about this danger. This scarcity of information may be due to health care professionals blaming themselves, rather than considering the overdoses to be the result of an EID design flaw. However, many of the EID manufacturers are recognizing the problem and modifying their equipment to correct the problem. Because the switch to safer equipment takes time, nurses need to be alert to ways to protect their clients from this hazard. Ensure that only health care providers, fully prepared in EID technology, be authorized to set up, adjust, or remove IV administration sets. Some instances of overdose have been attributed to clients, nursing assistants, or x-ray technicians removing a pump to undress or ambulate. Check yourself that the infusion is not running when the pump is removed. Be sure to check or recalculate the infusion rate. Visible labels should be applied to EIDs that do not prevent free flow to alert staff to the possible occurrence of free flow with that equipment. Limit the use of one type of EID to each unit to increase staff familiarity with a particular EID. Use only protected EIDs in critical care units or with critical care drugs (Cohen and Davis, 1993).

Although the technology with which we practice is created to facilitate the provision of more effective nursing care, we need to remain vigilant as we apply it to clinical practice.

However, changes in solutions may require changes in equipment. Be aware of the options available in selecting a filter for the specific intravenous infusion. Several different intravenous filter products are designed for different filtration needs. Filters are available in a range of sizes and in add-on or in-line form:

- A 5 μm filter removes *particulate* material and is designed to filter gross particulate matter. The smallest particle visible to the unaided eye is approximately 30 μm across.

- A 0.5 μm filter is considered a *bacteria-retention* filter, which is designed to prevent passage of most particulate matter and certain fungi and bacteria. A yeast cell is approximately 3 μm in diameter.
- The 0.22 μm filter is called a *sterilizing* filter, since it is designed to prevent passage of virtually all particulate matter and most bacteria for at least 24 hours. Bacteria range in size from 0.2 to 2 μm in diameter. Travenol Laboratories and other manufacturers provide these filters for use with the add-on or in-line systems. Select a 0.22 μm filter for parenteral nutrition solutions.

Tightly secure all connections in the administration setup to prevent air from being drawn in. Do not allow containers to empty completely, since air in the tubing could be driven into the vein when another full container is attached. Throughout all client activities keep containers about 3 feet above the site. If not using an infusion devise, a higher position will cause the solution to infuse too rapidly; if too low, blood may find its way into the needle or tubing and clot there. Avoid using areas of flexion (e.g., the wrist or antecubital fossa), but if use of the site is necessary, use an armboard.

Nurses should take the necessary precautions to prevent thrombophlebitis by doing the following: using sterile aseptic technique with proper cleansing of skin before inserting of the needle; checking solutions for precipitation, debris, sediment, or change in color before and during intravenous therapy; ascertaining that no intravenous bottle or tubing is left in place for more than 24 hours, since some organisms proliferate at room temperature in intravenous fluids; and changing and dating the intravenous setup and site dressings every 24 hours to reduce the possibility of sepsis. In addition, especially with the administration of irritating drugs, use veins with ample blood volume, use a cannula smaller than the vein to provide for greater hemodilution, administer irritating drugs slowly, rotate venipuncture sites every 48 to 72 hours, and avoid injecting intravenous infusions into leg veins or small veins.

If infiltration, thrombus, thrombophlebitis, or necrosis occur, the infusion should be discontinued and restarted at another site. If the IV has infiltrated, elevate the arm and apply heat to promote absorption of the infiltrated solution. Infiltration is especially serious when infusions of vasopressors (e.g., norepinephrine, dopamine) or vesicants (e.g., many antineoplastic agents) are involved; this is usually known as extravasation. If extravasation occurs, the infusion should be stopped *immediately* and the known antidote injected subcutaneously in minute amounts immediately at many sites in the edematous area. Dress the wound, elevate the extremity, and apply heat or cold, depending on the infiltrated agent, to the client's comfort. See Chapter 57 for specific agents and their antidotes.

If a thrombus has occurred, the infusion should be restarted at a new site with a new needle or catheter. Attempts to unplug the needle by forcing a bolus of solution in a syringe through the needle into the vein is unwise and unsafe. Theoretically, the thrombus may become an embolus and lodge in a vital organ, causing more serious complications such as pulmonary embolus. Although most hospital policies discourage irrigating, the practice is widespread, and as there is no confirmed pulmonary embolism reported, it would seem to support the justification for irrigating (Wong, 1995). Again elevate the affected extremity and apply heat to enhance resorption of the thrombus.

When thrombophlebitis occurs, the infusion should be stopped, the needle withdrawn, and the condition reported and recorded immediately. Treatment usually consists of applying moist heat to the affected area and resting the body part; anticoagulant therapy also may be ordered.

If pain occurs at the venipuncture site in the absence of other symptoms, adjust the needle and relieve the tension by readjusting the needle support or relaxing the pull on the tubing, and administer irritating drugs at a slow rate. These actions may alleviate the pain and discomfort.

Pulmonary edema is considered to be a medical emergency and the physician needs to be notified as soon as the client's fluid volume excess is noted. The IV infusion is slowed to a "keep open" (KVO, keep vein open) rate to provide access for emergency medications. Oxygen can be started to improve gas exchange. Monitor vital signs every 15 to 30 minutes. Monitor arterial blood gases, intake and output. A bronchodilator may be ordered to decrease bronchospasm; diuretics to mobilize extravascular fluid; digitalis or pressor agents to increase cardiac contractility; nitroprusside to decrease peripheral vascular resistance, preload, and afterload; and morphine to reduce anxiety and dyspnea. Provide support for the client who will be fearful due to decreased respiratory capacity.

If a pyrogenic reaction is suspected, the infusion should be stopped *at once*. The solution should not be discarded but instead sent to the pharmacist. Pyrogenic reactions are treated symptomatically but must be reported and recorded. The stock number should be noted, since an entire batch of solutions may be contaminated.

Consult agency infusion specialists, such as members of the intravenous therapy team, when available, if you encounter difficulties.

Education. Clients or family members should be informed to notify the nurse if pain or swelling occurs at the infusion site or if any symptoms of the complications previously mentioned occur. Instruct the ambulatory client to ambulate with the involved arm held lightly at the waist and with the unaffected arm guiding the IV pole. Advise the client to avoid actions that elevate the arm with the venipuncture, such as combing hair or shaving with that arm.

Evaluation. The client will receive fluid and electrolyte therapy as ordered, with the serum electrolytes determinations returning to or remaining within the normal limits and without evidencing any adverse effects of IV therapy.

SUMMARY

The administration of intravenous fluids and electrolytes has become commonplace in the experience of hospitalized clients. They are administered for a variety of reasons: to replace fluids and electrolytes, to correct acid-base imbalance, to administer medications, to maintain access to the venous system, to measure changes in the venous pressure, to measure renal function, and to administer essential nutrients. With the increased prevalence of intravascular therapy, the role of nursing management in intravenous therapy has also grown and developed.

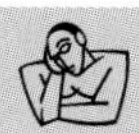

Critical Thinking

1. What role do water, potassium, sodium, calcium, and magnesium contribute to survival?
2. How would you minimize the risk of the various complications of IV therapy?

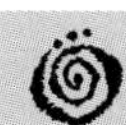

Collaborative Learning Activities

1. Student teams will write a case study relevant to clients with fluid volume excess, fluid volume deficit, hyponatremia, hyperkalemia, and hypokalemia in need of IV therapy. Formulate questions based on your case study related to assessments and interventions that would be necessary in caring for such clients.

BIBLIOGRAPHY

American Hospital Formulary Service (1996). *AHFS drug information '96*. Bethesda, MD: American Society of Hospital Pharmacists.

Anderson KN, et al. (Eds.) (1994). *Mosby's medical, nursing, & allied* health dictionary (4th ed.). St Louis: Mosby.

Brown RG (1993). Disorders of water and sodium balance, *Postgrad Med* 93(4):227-8, 231, 234, 239-40,244, 246.

Brown RO (1993). Hypomagnesemia in critically ill patients: Issues in pharmacotherapy, *ACCP Report* 13(3):6.

Cohen MR & Davis NM (1993). Recognizing the dangers of free flow from an EID, *Nursing* 23(6):56-9.

Johnson JA & Lalonde RL (1993). Congestive Heart Failure. In DiPiro JT, et al. (Eds.). *Pharmacotherapy: A pathophysiological approach* (2nd ed.). Norwalk, CT: Appleton & Lange.

McConnell E (1986). Preventing air embolism in patients with central venous catheters, *Nurs Life* 6:47.

Mendyka BE (1992). Fluid and electrolyte disorders caused by diuretic therapy, *AACN* 3(3):672-80.

Metheny NM (1992). *Fluid and electrolyte balance: Nursing considerations* (2nd ed.). Philadelphia: JB Lippincott.

Meyer I (1993). Sodium polystyrene sulfonate: A cation exchange resin used in treating hyperkalemia, *ANNA J* 20(1):93-5.

Olin BR (Ed.) (1996). *Facts and comparisons*. St Louis: Facts and Comparisons.

Owens MW (1993). Keeping an eye on magnesium, *Amer J Nurs* 93(2):66-7.

Rousseau PC (1992). Why give IV fluids to the dying?, *Patient Care* (July 15):71-4.

Tang I & Lau AH (1995) Fluid and electrolyte disorders. In Young LY & Koda-Kimble MA (Eds.). *Applied therapeutics: The clinical use of drugs* (6th ed.). Vancouver: Applied Therapeutics.

Theilen J (1990). Air emboli: A potentially lethal complication of central venous lines, *Focus Crit Care* 17(5):374.

United States Pharmacopeial Convention (1996). *USP DI: Drug information for the health care professional* (16th ed.). Rockville, MD: The Convention.

Wong DL (1995). *Whaley & Wong's nursing care of infants and children* (5th ed.). St Louis: Mosby.

Wood LS & Gullo SM (1993). IV vesicants: How to avoid extravasation, *Amer J Nurs* 93(4):42-6.

Chapter 70

Enteral and Parenteral Nutrition

Chapter Focus

Enteral and parenteral feedings are commonly used to provide nutritional support for clients who, for some reason, cannot consume adequate nutrients through the normal processes of ingestion. The nursing focus for the nursing diagnosis "altered nutrition" is on assisting the client or family in improving nutritional intake; it should not be used to describe individuals who are prescribed nothing by mouth (NPO) or cannot ingest food (Carpenito, 1992). Because enteral and parenteral nutrition is used most commonly for clients who are NPO or cannot ingest food, the potential complications of electrolyte imbalances and negative nitrogen balance are considered by this chapter. The following objectives and key terms are necessary for a good understanding of this chapter.

Key Terms

amino acid (p. 1079)
enteral nutrition (p. 1073)
essential amino acids (p. 1079)
hyperalimentation (p. 1078)
negative nitrogen balance (p. 1076)
nonessential amino acids (p. 1079)
protein-sparing nutrition (p. 1080)
semiessential amino acids (p. 1080)
total parenteral nutrition (TPN) (p. 1078)

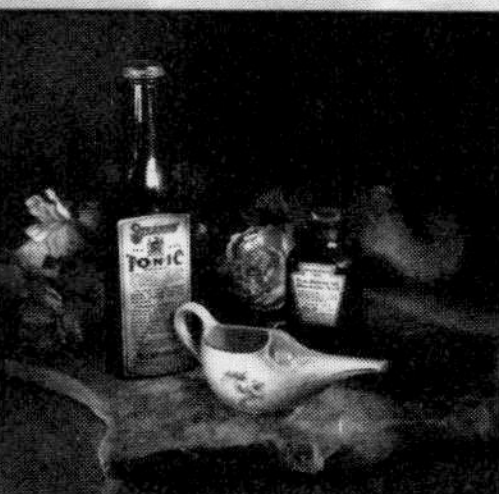

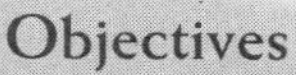

Objectives

1. Describe common techniques used for the delivery of enteral feedings.
2. Distinguish among elemental, polymeric, modular, and altered amino acid formulations for enteral feedings.
3. Identify major drug-food interactions to be aware of when enteral nutrient formulations are being administered.
4. Implement nursing management of the care of clients receiving enteral formulations.
5. Discuss parenteral protein-sparing nutrition, peripheral-vein parenteral nutrition, and central hyperalimentation and the indications for their use.
6. Describe the components of total parenteral nutrition solutions and the function of each element in the attainment of the body's requirement.
7. Cite possible complications of parenteral nutrition therapy.
8. Implement nursing management of the care of clients receiving parenteral nutritional therapy.

To achieve and maintain good health requires a regular intake of sufficient amounts of protein (amino acids), carbohydrates, fats, vitamins, and minerals. While under normal conditions adequate nutrition can be achieved by the ingestion of a balanced diet, there are situations when the nutritional needs of the body will not be met. Such conditions include malnutrition, severe inflammatory bowel disease and other GI diseases, coma, postsurgical complications, major burns, and others. For such persons, nutritional support is necessary. Over the past 30 to 40 years, many advances have been recorded in the fields of both enteral and parenteral nutrition. Clinical nutrition is now a recognized and active entity for improving health care in all settings, including the client's home, long-term care facilities, and hospitals. Today nutritional programs or specific products have been developed for individuals with specific disease states or illnesses. In this chapter, enteral and parenteral nutrition are reviewed, along with selected disease states and criteria for use of the specific nutritional products.

ENTERAL NUTRITION

Malnutrition among hospitalized persons and nursing home residents is associated with complications such as muscle atrophy, slow wound healing, impaired immunocompetence, infection, and death. Other complications include peripheral edema caused by reduced plasma proteins and its resultant decreased oncotic pressure, dry and flaky skin, and hair loss.

Malnutrition is also reflected in reduced total lymphocyte count, serum albumin, and transferrin levels (or iron-binding capacity). An increase in 24-hour urine urea nitrogen concentration reflects the protein catabolism that occurs with malnutrition.

Stress in relation to hospitalization may alter a client's usual eating habits. Unfamiliar foods and general malaise resulting from illness also may cause clients to lose their appetites. An inadequate oral intake may result from oropharyngeal surgery, trauma, neoplasm, paralysis, or esophageal fistula. Fasting before surgery or for a diagnostic workup may also be nutritionally depleting. When sepsis, trauma, major surgery, inflammation, infection, or severe burns supervene, energy needs may be doubled. If the gastrointestinal tract is functional, however, enteral or tube feedings may effectively supply essential nutrition. **Enteral nutrition** is the oral or tube feeding of an individual, usually via a nasogastric, nasoduodenal, gastrostomy, or jejunostomy tube (Figure 70-1). The cost per person for tube feedings is about equal to a regular hospital diet and provides more complete control and assessment of intake. Tube feedings also may be used to supplement inadequate oral intake and parenteral nutrition as it is being tapered.

Enteral feedings may be administered by bolus doses, typically 250 to 400 ml of formula every 4 to 6 hours; by intermittent feedings using a 20 to 30 minute drip; or by continuous gravity or enteral pumps. The continuous method over 16 to 24 hours has had more success because it helps prevent complications such as dumping syndrome and avoids the need for frequent tube irrigations. Dumping syndrome is the result of a sudden influx of feeding and the creation of a high osmotic gradient within the small intestine, which cause a sudden shift of fluid from the vascular compartment to the intestinal lumen. Plasma volume decreases, causing vasomotor responses such as increased pulse rate, hypotension, weakness, pallor, sweating, and dizziness. Rapid distention of the intestine produces a feeling of fullness, cramping, nausea, vomiting, and diarrhea.

Enteral feedings can be administered by the following routes: nasogastric, nasoduodenal, esophagostomy, gastrostomy, and jejunostomy. The last three are more invasive, requiring surgically created stomas, and thus are less preferred routes for short-term enteral feeding. Nasogastric, esophagostomy, and gastrostomy feedings allow for more natural digestion in the stomach. Aspiration is a risk with nasogastric tubes because the incomplete closure of the esophageal sphincter may result in gastric reflux.

Although feedings administered directly into the small intestine reduces the risk of aspiration, gastrointestinal distress and diarrhea may develop because of the sudden influx. Skin excoriation and infection are potential risks in gastrostomies and jejunostomies because the surgical opening penetrates the peritoneum. These complications are avoided in the cervical esophagostomy, a surgically created, skin-lined canal tunneled from the lower neck border and extending to below the cervical esophagus.

The selection of tube feeding formula depends on the client's nutritional needs, concomitant disease states, lactose intolerance, and gastrointestinal competence, as well as on convenience, feasibility, and cost. Nutritional assessment may be based on anthropometric parameters, biochemical data, and physical findings, as well as on medical, diet, drug, and socioeconomic histories. Ideal body weight (IBW) can be obtained from tables or by estimation as follows and can be used instead of actual weight because, if an individual is obese, the adipose tissue would require less energy for maintenance. If the actual weight were used in the calculations, the client would receive excessive calories.

- *Men:* 106 pounds (48 kg) for the first 5 feet (150 cm) plus 6 pounds (2.7 kg) per inch (2.5 cm) over 5 feet (plus or minus 10%)
- *Women:* 100 pounds (45 kg) for the first 5 feet plus 5 pounds (2.2 kg) per inch over 5 feet (plus or minus 10%)

Enteral Formulations

While numerous different enteral formulations are available, they can be broadly divided into oligomeric, polymeric, modular components, and specialized formulations (Rollins, 1996).

1. Oligomeric formulas are chemically defined formulations that require minimum digestion and produce minimal residue in the colon. The two oligomeric subgroups include true elemental formulations that contain free amino acids and peptide-based formulas

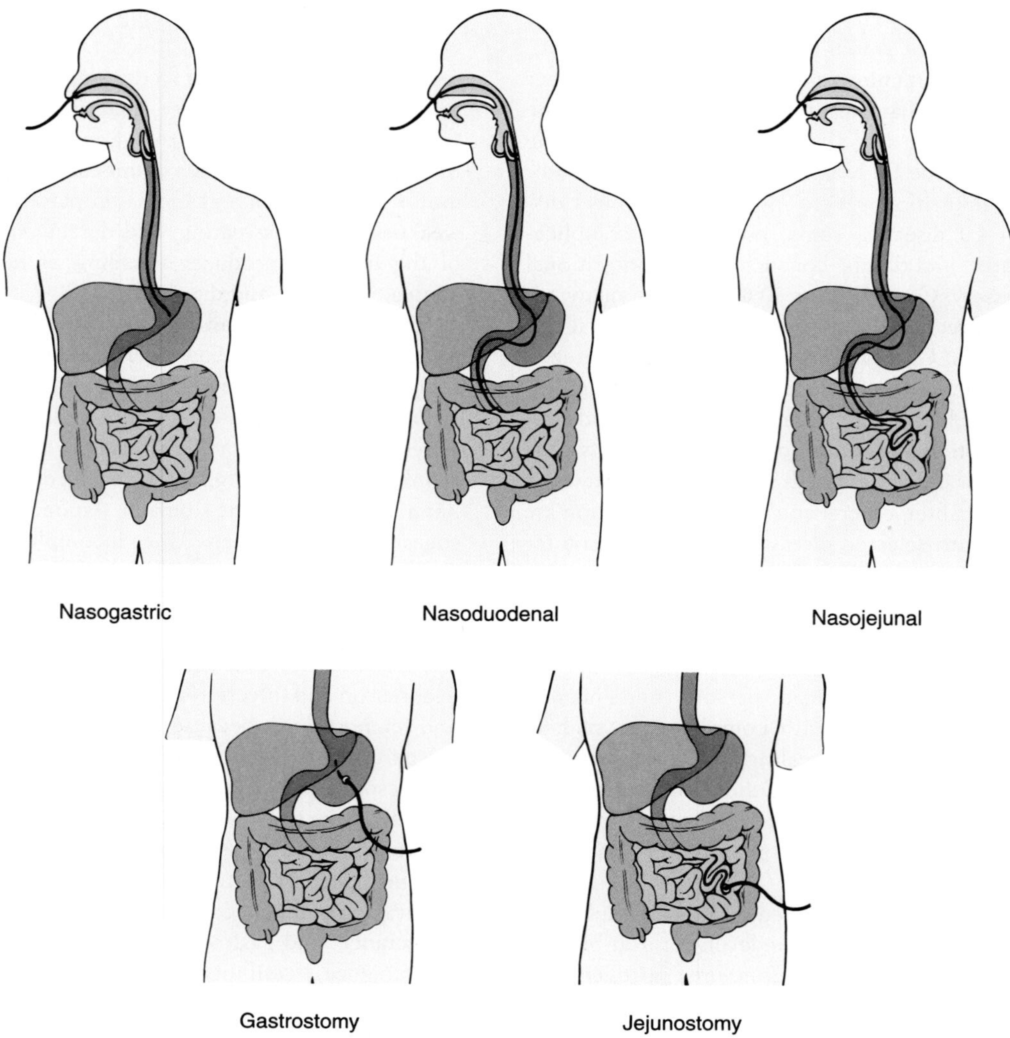

Figure 70-1 Tube feeding routes. (Modified from Beare PG & Myers JL [1997]. *Principles and practice of adult health nursing* [3rd ed.]. St. Louis: Mosby.)

that contain dipeptides and tripeptides and/or crystalline amino acids. These formulations are indicated for persons with partial bowel obstruction, inflammatory bowel disease, radiation enteritis, bowel fistulas, and short bowel syndrome.

2. Polymeric formulations are the most commonly prescribed complete formula, enteral preparations. Such formulas contain complex nutrients: protein (e.g., casein and soy protein); carbohydrate (e.g., corn syrup solid, maltodextrins); and fat (vegetable oil or milk fat) and are preferred for persons that have a fully functional gastrointestinal tract and few or no specialized nutrient requirements. They should not be used in clients with a malabsorption problem. These formulas are preferred because the hyperosmolarity of the oligomeric preparations cause more gastrointestinal problems than the polymeric formulations.
3. Modular formulations are single-nutrient formulas, i.e., protein, carbohydrate, or fat. Such a formula can be added to a monomeric or polymeric formulation to provide a more individual specialized nutrient formulation.
4. Specialized formulations are indicated for individuals with specific disease states such as, genetic errors of metabolism (e.g., phenylketonuria, homocystinuria, maple syrup urine disease), acquired disorders of nitrogen accumulation (e.g., cirrhosis or chronic renal failure), and in persons who are catabolic because of injuries or infection (Table 70-1).

Drug-Food Interactions

A number of drug-enteral nutrient interactions have been identified, but this possibility is often overlooked when enteral nutrient formulations are being administered. Since the interactions can be clinically significant, the major drug interactions with enteral or tube feedings are listed in Table 70-2.

TABLE 70-1 Examples of commercial enteral formulations

Formulations	Comments
Oligomeric	
Elemental	
Vivonex TEN	Contains free amino acids, linoleic acid, vitamins, minerals
Peptide-based	
Peptamen Liquid	Composed of hydrolyzed whey proteins, carbohydrates, fat, vitamins, and minerals
Polymeric	
Nutrient source	
Blenderized	
Compleat Regular	Has beef, fruits, vegetables, nonfat milk, vitamins, and minerals; tube feeding preparation
Milk-based	
Sustacal powder	Composed of nonfat and whole milk, sugars, butter, vitamins, and minerals; contains high protein content and lactose
Lactose-free	
Ensure-Plus	Higher caloric formulation of protein, carbohydrates, fat, vitamins, and minerals that is lactose-free
Modular components	
Carbohydrate	
Polycose	Glucose polymers derived from cornstarch; high source of calories from carbohydrate
Protein	
Amin-Aid	Contains essential amino acids, carbohydrates, and fat; has high caloric formula indicated for acute or chronic renal failure
Fats	
MCT Oil	Medium chain triglycerides that need less bile acid for digestion; does not provide any essential fatty acids
Specialized formulations	
Renal failure	
Amin-Aid	See above
Hepatic failure	
Hepatic-Aid II	Contains amino acids (about 50% protein as branched-chain amino acids or BCAA), carbohydrates, and fat. Hepatic encephalopathy reportedly improved by increased serum levels of BCAA (Rollins, 1996); used for chronic liver disease
Pulmonary disease	
Pulmocare	Composed of calcium and sodium caseinate, amino acids, carbohydrates, fats, vitamins, minerals; has high caloric content; fat in this preparation is primarily from canola oil and corn oil (60%) plus 40% from MCT; persons with respiratory disease that received high fat, low carbohydrate diets demonstrated improvement in respiratory monitoring parameters (Rollins, 1996)

TABLE 70-2 Drug interactions with enteral and tube feedings

Drug	Comments
carbamazepine (Tegretol)	Bioavailability of carbamazepine suspension is affected if given through a polyvinyl NG feeding tube. Serum levels also decreased when administered during enteral feedings. Recommended that suspension be diluted and given as described in phenytoin below.
phenytoin (Dilantin)	Lower serum phenytoin levels reported. Recommended approach is to stop enteral feeding for 2 hours before and after phenytoin administration; flushing tubing with 2 oz of water before giving phenytoin suspension is recommended.
warfarin (Coumadin)	Warfarin resistance reported when drug was administered with an enteral preparation. Interaction may be due to vitamin K in the feeding or due to warfarin binding to protein ingredients in the formulation.

Closely monitor persons receiving the above and any other drugs in combination with enteral formulations. Laboratory tests such as serum drug levels or prothrombin time, when appropriate, may be ordered (Estoup, 1994). For additional information, see Miyagawa, 1993.

Nursing Management

Enteral Nutrition Therapy

Assessment. A baseline assessment of the client should include body weight, history of weight loss, and any clinical manifestations of undernutrition. The nutritional history should include, with cause if possible, inadequate nutrient intake, excessive nutrient losses or failure to absorb nutrients, increased metabolic requirements, or medications that might have a catabolic effect, such as corticosteroids or antineoplastic agents. Baseline laboratory determinations, such as serum albumin, serum electrolytes, serum transferrin, serum prealbumin, urine creatinine clearance, and the total lymphocyte count are indicators of protein nourishment. Hemoglobin, hematocrit, mean corpuscular volume (MCV), mean corpuscular hemoglobin (MCH), mean corpuscular hemoglobin concentration (MCHC), and the various blood levels of specific vitamins and minerals are indicators of vitamin and mineral nourishment.

Enteral feedings generally are contraindicated in individuals who are capable of oral intake or who have adynamic ileus, intestinal obstruction, intractable vomiting, or esophageal fistulas.

Nursing diagnosis. See the Nursing Care Plan below for nursing diagnoses related to a client with enteral tube feedings. In addition, the potential complications of **negative nitrogen balance** (a condition in which more nitrogen is excreted than is taken in, indicating the wasting of tissue) and electrolyte imbalances exist.

Implementation

Monitoring. Monitor the client's nutritional status using the indicators mentioned above in the baseline assessment. Assess client for respiratory distress, frothy sputum, abnormal lung sounds, or new pulmonary infiltrates on x-ray examination. Tinting formula with blue food coloring assists assessment for aspiration.

Assess periodically for residual gastric volume and tube placement, particularly before each feeding or before administering a dose of a medication into the feeding tube. For continuous feedings, simply stop the feeding and measure the residual by aspirating the stomach contents with a syringe. It is not necessary to clamp off the tube and wait for an interval of time because these feedings should move through the system continuously. If the residual is more than the volume of 2 hours of continuous feeding, return the

Nursing Care Plan

Selected Potential Nursing Diagnoses for the Client with Enteral Tube Feedings

Nursing diagnosis	Outcome criteria	Interventions
Altered bowel elimination: diarrhea	The client will have soft, formed stools fewer than 3 times daily.	Record frequency and consistency of stools. Decrease the hypertonicity of the feedings by diluting if it is not contraindicated. Check the client's medication regimen for diarrhea-causing drugs. Assess the hygiene used in the administration of the feedings. Perform a digital examination to ensure the client does not have a fecal impaction. Administer antidiarrheals as prescribed.
Risk for aspiration	The client will not experience aspiration.	Assess client for respiratory distress, frothy sputum, abnormal lung sounds, new infiltrates on x-ray. Tinting formula with blue food coloring assists assessment. Elevate the head of bed at least 30 degrees during and for 1 hour after feeding. Verify placement of feeding NG or NJ tube with air auscultation. Aspirate for residual contents every 4 to 8 hours or before each residual feeding. Hold the feeding and notify the prescriber if residuals are greater than the amount of 2 hours of continuous feeding or 50% the volume of previous intermittent feeding.
Fluid volume deficit	Fluid balance will be maintained. Hematocrit, BUN, and urine specific gravity will be within normal limits.	Assess client for poor skin turgor, dry mucous membranes, and thirst. Monitor fluid intake and output. Monitor lab values for increases in BUN, hematocrit, and urine specific gravity. Provide increased amounts of water through feeding tube.

aspirate, hold the feeding, and consult with the physician. For intermittent administration, measure residual volume halfway between feedings. If the residual is greater than 50% of the previous feeding, return the aspirate, hold the feeding, and notify the physician. In both of these instances, a reduction in the volume of the feeding may be necessary.

Monitor bowel sounds to ensure that the client has good bowel function. Bowel elimination pattern and fluid intake and output should be carefully documented.

Many types of enteral formulas are lactose-free (nonmilk proteins are the base) for clients who lack sufficient lactase in intestinal brush bodies for lactose absorption. Blacks, Asians, American Indians, and Jews are particularly prone to lactase deficiency. Lactose ingestion causes varying degrees of diarrhea, abdominal cramps, bloating, and flatulence. Isotonic formulas may be useful in preventing the dumping syndrome.

Intervention. Although the gastrointestinal tract is the optimal route for nutrient administration, in many ill clients the normal ingestion of food is difficult, if not nearly impossible, to achieve. Enteral nutrient preparations were designed for such persons. These formulations may be given by the nasoenteral route through thin, flexible tubing that is generally well tolerated by the client. These feeding tubes are now made from silicone or polyurethane compounds and have much smaller lumen sizes, No. 5 through 10 French. These are much preferred to the older, thicker rubber or polyvinyl chloride types (Salem pump, Levin tube) that stiffen in contact with digestive juices. Aspiration for residual gastrointestinal contents and irrigation of these small-lumen tubes, however, may be more difficult than with the older, larger types.

Small-diameter feeding tubes also get clogged more easily. To prevent formula residue buildup, some suggest flushing tubes every 4 hours (and each time feeding is interrupted) with 20 ml of cranberry juice followed by 10 ml of water. Acidity of the juice breaks up the formula residue, and the water prevents sugar from crystallizing.

Transnasal tube placement in the intestine requires the use of longer, mercury- or tungsten-weighted feeding tubes that gradually are advanced by peristalsis. This takes about 24 hours, and radiographic confirmation of tube placement must be made.

If tube feedings must be administered for long time periods, then surgical placement of a gastrostomy (G) tube or a jejunostomy (J) tube can be instituted. This will help reduce the need for the frequent flushing and replacement of the nasoenteral tube and is more comfortable for the client. A more common procedure in use today is the placement of a G tube percutaneously by using endoscopic guidance; this is known as the percutaneous endoscopic gastrostomy (PEG).

Initially, the infusion of enteral formulas is begun at half-strength concentrations at a rate of 50 ml/hour. This rate and strength can then be titrated according to the client's tolerance to the formulation. For example, the rate may be increased by 25 ml/hour and the concentration increased to three-quarter strength, which eventually will be increased to the full-strength formulation. The desired calories and total volume ordered will then be administered, assuming the client can tolerate the full-strength preparation. To avoid inducing vomiting or diarrhea, the increases in rate and fluid concentration should not be made simultaneously.

The more rapid the feeding, the more likely complications such as hyperglycemia or dumping syndrome may occur. However, nursing efforts should be maintained to encourage intake because the milk-based formulas, for example, contain 1 kcal/ml, and the client must take 1000 to 2000 ml of formula to achieve their caloric needs and to obtain all the RDAs for the vitamins and minerals. Elevate the head of bed at least 30 degrees during and for 1 hour after feeding. Warm the feeding to room temperature before administering.

The enteral preparation may be given continuously or by cyclic administration. Cyclic feedings are similar to a person's normal feeding cycle and are the preferred method in some settings. If the client cannot or does not drink additional water while on the formulations, additional water may be added to the enteral formulations. In general, enteral formulations that have 1 kcal/ml usually contain approximately 80% water, whereas the formulations with more concentrated kcal per ml have less than 70% water.

If the nurse has slowed the rate of administration, lowered the concentration by diluting the formula, and had the solutions at room temperature, and the client still develops diarrhea, then the prescriber needs to be consulted regarding the osmolality of the formula. Antidiarrheal preparations may also be helpful in controlling the diarrhea.

In the case of accidental aspiration after a tube feeding into the stomach, the tube may be advanced through the pyloric sphincter to prevent future regurgitation. The resultant hyperosmolality in the small intestine, however, potentiates hyperglycemia or the dumping syndrome. Physiologic osmolality is approximately 280 mOsm/L, but some preparations are greater than 400 mOsm/L.

The state of the art of enteral feedings is in rapid evolution. One source for current information is Ross Laboratories, 625 Clinton Ave, Columbus, OH, 43216.

Education. Tube feedings self-administered at home are now possible with the advent of smaller tubes and infusion instrumentation that incorporates improved human engineering features. Necessary preparation of the client and another family member should begin 5 to 7 days before discharge. Individualized instruction with return demonstrations of learning take about 3 to 6 hours, perhaps more if it includes learning insertion and removal of the tube. Incorrect tube placement is signified by coughing, choking, difficulty in speaking, or cyanosis. The concept of correct tube placement cannot be overemphasized. Written and verbal instructions related to possible secondary effects are also necessary (Table 70-3). Resumption of daily activities at home is more inconvenient for the tube-fed ostomy client who must loosen clothing or undress for each feeding.

Clients receiving tube feedings are deprived of the usual personal and social gratifications of the eating act. They may feel

Home Health

TPN in the Home Setting

The client and family/caregiver should have the opportunity to practice the procedures in the hospital under nursing supervision. Review the procedures for the storage of the solution. It should be picked up or delivered every day for the client. Instruct the client to keep the containers refrigerated, but allow it to come to room temperature before administering the solution. Advise the client to check the expiration date, label of contents, and the appearance of the solution.

The dressing is to be changed at least every 2 days. Instruct the family/caregiver to use aseptic technique when changing the dressing. The site should be inspected for swelling, redness, or drainage and reported to the health care provider if found. Demonstrate to the family how to irrigate the catheter. Instruct the client in appropriate pump settings, how the infusion pump works, how to care for the pump, and what to do if the alarm goes off. Also demonstrate how to change the solution bag, tubing, and filter.

Explain that the client should be weighed daily and the client's intake and output monitored. Ask them to observe for edema. Show the client and family how to check urine glucose levels. Review the potential complications of TPN, such as chills, fever, dyspnea, chest pain, and coughing with adverse reaction to lipid infusion; dyspnea, chest pain, and coughing with air embolism; nervousness, faintness, and tachycardia with hypoglycemia; nausea, vomiting, polyuria, polydipsia, and positive urine glucose or acetone with hyperglycemia. Instruct the client to discontinue the infusion if any of these occur and to contact the prescriber. Recommend that the client keep the telephone number of the prescriber, the nursing service, and community emergency services within easy reach.

TABLE 70-3 Most common secondary effects of tube feedings

Condition	Cause	Preventive action
Aspiration	Impaired gag reflex	Put head of bed at 30-60 degrees for feedings and for 1 hour after
	Uncuffed tracheostomy tube	Stop; suction trachea; inflate cuff before feedings
	Decreased gastric motility	Check for residual of feedings and tube placement
	Misplaced tube	Check taping and placement of tube
		Advance tube through pyloric sphincter
		Add blue food coloring to tube feeding to monitor for aspiration
Obstructed tube	Plugged tube end-ports	Flush tubing before and after feedings or instillation of medications
		Shake or mix formula well
Hyperglycemia, dumping syndrome: nausea, vomiting, diaphoresis, cramping	Osmotic intolerance to hyperosmolar load of feeding, rapid rate, or high concentration; ice-cold feeding	Change volume or rate of delivery and dilute feeding temporarily
		Allow feedings to warm slightly

"different" and alienated from others. To some, it may be symbolic of a rapidly deteriorating state of health and a last resort for survival. They especially need to understand the procedure, its rationale, and what to expect from it. Once given the opportunity to discuss its meaning, many can go on to participate actively in their own feedings and to express greater satisfaction.

Evaluation. The client will experience adequate nutrition and maintain or progress to a normal weight for height ratio without diarrhea, aspiration, or fluid volume deficit.

PARENTERAL NUTRITION

Parenteral nutrition is the treatment of choice for selected clients who are unable to tolerate and maintain adequate enteral intake. Often called **hyperalimentation or total parenteral nutrition (TPN)**, it is the intravenous approach to complete nutrition. TPN can supply all the calories, dextrose, amino acids, fats, trace elements, and other essential nutrients needed for growth, weight gain, wound healing, convalescence, immunocompetence, and other health-sustaining functions. TPN provides these components in the ratio of a regular diet. It promotes anabolism by supplying all necessary nutrients in excess of those needed for energy expenditure, and it may be infused through a central vein, a peripheral vein, or both, simultaneously.

Although related nomenclature has not yet been standardized, partial parenteral nutrition has come to denote parenteral nutrition therapy with intravenous solutions that are lacking some essential elements, notably fats. While insulin and heparin (and several other medications) have been added to parenteral nutrition preparations for specific individuals, in general, the addition of medications to TPN solutions should be avoided because of the potential incompatibilities of the medication with the nutrients in the solution (Holcombe, 1996). The major parenteral systems for nutritional support are these:

1. Peripheral vein total parenteral nutrition (PTPN)
2. Central-line venous hyperalimentation

Peripheral Vein Total Parenteral Nutrition

Peripheral vein total parenteral nutrition (PTPN) is prescribed for clients needing nutritional support, for whom insertion of a central venous line for total parenteral nutrition may not be possible or necessary. The individual may be nutritionally healthy or have slight to moderate nutritional deficits without being in a hypermetabolic state. The individual's current health status indicates that a nutritional deficit will probably occur if nutritional therapy is not instituted.

PTPN is considered a temporary measure to provide an appropriate nitrogen balance in clients with mild deficits or ones who are NPO with a slightly elevated metabolic rate. It may be prescribed to precede a procedure that imposes restrictions on oral feedings; for gastrointestinal illnesses that prevent oral food ingestion; for anorexia caused by radiation or chemotherapy in cancer treatment programs; or following surgery, if the individual's nutritional deficits are minimal but oral food consumption will not be instituted for 5 or more days. It is not indicated for nutritionally depleted clients with a hypermetabolic state. If used in such persons, it should be a temporary measure until central vein hyperalimentation can be initiated.

The solution is composed of 3% to 5% isotonic amino acids, mixed with a carbohydrate solution (usually dextrose 5% to 7%), vitamins, minerals, and electrolytes for administration through a peripheral vein. The solution will provide between 500 and 700 calories/day. The major advancement in this therapy is the use of a lipid as a nonprotein source of calories. Dextrose, when administered peripherally, must be limited to a 10% solution to avoid sclerosing of the veins. Some institutions also limit the concentration of electrolytes to be infused for the same reason.

Peripherally administered lipid preparations or intravenous fat emulsions (Liposyn, Intralipid, and others) are a source of additional calories for the individual.

Central Hyperalimentation

In central hyperalimentation, a catheter is placed in a central vein, the subclavian vein most commonly, in order to administer solutions that contain hypertonic glucose and amino acids. Because of its blood flow, the central vein can accept the high-osmolar concentrated solutions. Central hyperalimentation or total parenteral nutrition (TPN) is usually composed of the three major nutrients—dextrose, crystalline amino acids, and lipid emulsions—plus vitamins, minerals, trace elements, electrolytes, and water. The solutions may vary according to the individual's requirements and, in general, according to the supplier of the basic amino acid solution. Special preparations of amino acids are also available for the client with a specific disease state.

Central hyperalimentation is used primarily for persons with nonfunctioning gastrointestinal tracts, those that should not use the oral route for more than 5 to 7 days, or for persons that either have a limited peripheral access or their needs cannot be met by peripheral formulations (Holcombe, 1996). For example, individuals with conditions of short bowel syndrome, acute pancreatitis, enteric or enterocutaneous fistulas, active inflammatory process, gastrointestinal tract obstruction, major trauma, or burns, with whom enteral feedings are not possible, may need central hyperalimentation for survival.

BOX 70-1

Potentially Life-Threatening Drug Interaction

The amount of calcium and phosphorus (or phosphates) in a total parenteral nutrition (TPN) admixture must be closely monitored because life-threatening events and deaths have been reported from calcium phosphate precipitation. The FDA issued warnings concerning this drug interaction that include the following:

- utilize an in-line filter whenever infusing TPN solutions centrally or peripherally.
- start TPN admixtures within 24 hours after mixing or keep at room temperature. If refrigerated, start within 24 hours of rewarming.
- if acute respiratory distress symptoms occur, *stop infusion immediately*.
- special compounding instructions were issued to pharmacists on this safety alert.

Mirtallo, 1994; FDA, 1994.

Solution Formulations

The basic total parenteral solution contains amino acids, carbohydrates (dextrose), lipids, and micronutrients (trace elements, vitamins, etc.).

See Box 70-1 for a potentially life-threatening drug interaction.

Amino Acids

Amino acids are necessary to promote the production of proteins (anabolism), to reduce protein breakdown (catabolism), and to help promote wound healing. Protein is composed of amino acids, which are identified as essential and nonessential. **Essential amino acids** cannot be synthesized by the body while **nonessential amino acids** can be synthesized from a nitrogen source (amino acids, ammonium salts, urea). All natural amino acids are needed for growth and development and must be present concurrently in the proper amounts for protein synthesis to occur. The adult can synthesize all but eight of these amino acids; these eight therefore are considered essential in adults. To the extent that oral intake of amino acids is limited, protein synthesis depends on an exogenous source. The **semiessential amino acids** (histidine, arginine) are not synthesized in adequate amounts during growth periods; thus 10 amino acids are considered essential in infants.

A healthy adult usually minimally requires approximately 0.9 g protein/kg, whereas an infant or child needs from 1.4 to 2.2 g/kg. In undernourished or traumatized persons, this requirement can increase substantially, such as up to sixfold in a traumatized or seriously ill individual, since this person's daily need is approximately 3 g/kg body weight. A nonprotein source of calories must be provided with the amino acids to offset their use as an energy source.

Amino acid solutions contain crystalline amino acid (Aminosyn and many others); solutions are also available with electrolytes. Amino acid crystalline solutions contain synthetic amino acids but not peptides. This is the preferred form of amino acid because most persons are able to tolerate this formulation.

Dextrose usually is administered with these solutions because of the protein-sparing action of carbohydrates. If the protein is administered without adequate calories in the form of carbohydrate, the protein will be used for the body's caloric need rather than for repair and regeneration of tissue.

Protein-sparing nutrition is usually reserved for the client who has minimal protein deficiencies and sufficient fat stores. A 3% to 5% isotonic amino acid is mixed with carbohydrate-free fluids, vitamins, minerals, and electrolytes that are administered by peripheral vein. The solution will provide approximately 400 to 600 calories/day. The individual will meet many energy requirements by using the free fatty acids and ketones derived from their endogenous adipose tissue, thereby preserving their protein compartment in the body. This type usually is used for short-term periods for clients who are not nutritionally compromised and are not in a hypermetabolic state.

Carbohydrates

Carbohydrates and lipids are used as the primary source of calories for the individual. One gram of D-glucose provides 3.4 calories, whereas fat supplies 9 calories/g and protein supplies 4 calories/g. Concentrations of dextrose solutions above 10% are hyperosmolar and too irritating to be given continuously peripherally; thus they should be administered through central venous catheters. Centrally, the concentration of dextrose solutions infused is usually between 25% and 35%.

When dextrose is administered without lipids as the primary source of calories, hyperglycemia usually occurs. Since dextrose requires insulin for utilization, using a combination of caloric sources, dextrose and lipids, will help decrease the potential for hyperglycemia and extra need for insulin in some individuals. Dextrose alone also increases the rate of metabolism and production of carbon dioxide, which may increase the client's respiratory demands. Administering a combination caloric preparation of dextrose and lipids will reduce the increase in respiratory demands.

Other sources of calories available, although not as prevalent in usage, include alcohol in dextrose solution and invert sugar and electrolytes solution (Olin, 1996).

The dextrose used in formulations is derived from corn sugar; however, a very small portion of the population may be sensitive to corn derivatives. For such persons, invert sugar derived from cane or beet sugar is an alternative.

Alcohol is another substrate providing 7 kcal/g, and it does not require insulin for peripheral utilization. Providing enough calories would necessitate a quantity of alcohol that would produce a potential for intoxication and hepatotoxicity. Since dextrose is inexpensive and readily available, it is almost always the preferred product for administration.

Fats

lipid emulsions (Intralipid; Liposyn)

Fat constitutes 40% to 50% of the total calories supplied in the average North American diet. Fat emulsions are derived from either soybean or safflower oil, which provides a mixture of neutral triglycerides and unsaturated fatty acids. The two functions of intravenous fat emulsions in parenteral nutrition are to supply essential fatty acids and to be a source of energy or calories (9 calories/g).

Linoleic, linolenic, and arachidonic acids are essential in humans. Linoleic acid cannot be synthesized in the body, and it is the precursor to both linolenic and arachidonic acid. If linoleic acid is either unavailable or deficient, the enzyme system will act on oleic acid to synthesize eicosatrienoic acid, which is incapable of functioning like arachidonic acid. Essential fatty acid deficiency (EFAD) is noted with clinical signs of hair loss, scaly dermatitis, growth retardation, reduced wound healing, decreased platelets, and fatty liver. This necessitates the intravenous administration of a fat emulsion to correct the biochemical alteration.

The fat emulsions currently available are either safflower oil (Liposyn) or soybean oil (Intralipid) or a combination of both (Liposyn II). Fat emulsion particles are thought to be metabolized from the bloodstream in a manner similar to that of the chylomicrons, which appear in the blood postprandially. Fat emulsions may minimize hyperglycemia, hyperinsulinemia, and hyperosmolar syndrome, which often occurs in clients given dextrose as the only source of parenteral caloric nutrition. Fat emulsions pose some dangers for persons with severe liver disease, pulmonary disease, anemia, or blood coagulation disorders and for acutely ill clients with elevated serum concentrations of C-reactive protein. Fat emboli and accumulation of intravascular fat may occur in lungs of premature, preterm, or low-birth-weight infants (infusion rate not to exceed 1 g/kg in 4 hours). A normal diet should be 40% fat, 40% protein, and 20% carbohydrate.

Trace Elements and Electrolytes

Although some of the commercial parenteral nutrition solutions contain trace elements, or minerals, persons placed on long-term administration should be evaluated for trace element deficiencies. Trace element solutions are available

TABLE 70-4 Trace elements

Elements	Dose*	Deficiency symptoms
copper	0.5-1.5 mg	decrease in red and white blood cells; hair and skeletal abnormalities; defective tissue growth
chromium	10-15 μg	neuropathy, confusion, impaired glucose tolerance, ataxia
manganese	150-800 μg	defective growth, nausea, vomiting, weight loss, skin rash, CNS alterations (ataxia, seizures)
selenium	40-80 μg	muscle aches, pain or tenderness, cardiomyopathy, kwashiorkor
zinc	2.5-4 mg	nausea, vomiting, diarrhea, weakness, anorexia, growth retardation, anemia, hypogeusia, rash, depression, eye lesions, defective wound healing, and hepatosplenomegaly

*Recommended daily adult dose.

individually (zinc, copper, manganese, chromium, and selenium) and in combination formulations (MTE formulations and others). Several trace metal formulations are also available in combination with electrolytes [Tracelyte and others].

Examples of the signs and symptoms of trace element deficiency, normal serum levels, and primary excretion sites are noted in Table 70-4. It is also critical to monitor serum electrolyte levels, especially the cations sodium, potassium, calcium, and magnesium and the anions of chloride, phosphate, bicarbonate, and acetate. Generally, serum levels of trace elements are not routinely monitored.

If iron replacement is necessary, oral replacement is the preferred route of administration. If it cannot be administered orally, then it can be given by intramuscular Z-track injection or by intravenous injection or infusion. Do not mix iron with other drugs or add it to parenteral nutrition solutions. For additional information on iron [Iron Dextran], the reader is referred to a current package insert or current drug reference book.

Vitamins

The client receiving parenteral feedings will also need additional vitamins. Usually a combination of multivitamin infusion (MVI) and, perhaps, additional vitamins will be given on alternate days to meet the client's needs for fat-soluble vitamins A and D and the water-soluble vitamins (B and C). Such preparations, if prescribed, can be added to the parenteral nutrition solution. Vitamin K is usually administered weekly by IM or SC injection. The specific dosage and frequency for vitamin regimens depend primarily on the individual client's needs and the usual protocols of the prescriber.

Special Formulations or Administration

Specially formulated amino acid preparations are available for clients in special disease conditions; such as renal failure, those with high metabolic stress, encephalopathy, and those in liver failure. For example formulas, such as HepatAmine, are used for hepatic failure, and Nephramine and others for renal failure.

Parenteral nutrition is often administered in a home setting, usually in one single container per day. Whenever possible, all the necessary nutrients are combined and administered on a cycling basis, depending on the individual. Cyclic therapy is the infusion of the feeding over less than 24 hours, to free the individual from constant therapy. Often such preparations are administered during the evening and night hours (Holcombe, 1996)

Nursing Management

Parental Nutrition Therapy

Assessment. A baseline assessment of the client should include body weight, history of weight loss, and any clinical manifestations of undernutrition. The nutritional history should include, with cause if possible, inadequate nutrient intake, excessive nutrient losses or failure to absorb nutrients, increased metabolic requirements, or medications that might have a catabolic effect, such as corticosteroids or antineoplastic agents. Baseline laboratory determinations, such as serum albumin, serum electrolytes, serum transferrin, serum prealbumin, urine creatinine clearance, and the total lymphocyte count are indicators of protein nourishment. Hemoglobin, hematocrit, mean corpuscular volume (MCV), mean corpuscular hemoglobin (MCH), mean corpuscular hemoglobin concentration (MCHC), and the various blood levels of specific vitamins and minerals are indicators of vitamin and mineral nourishment.

Nursing diagnosis. The client receiving parenteral nutrition therapy may experience the following nursing diagnoses: risk for infection; fluid volume deficit; fluid volume excess; and the potential complications of negative nitrogen balance related to the underlying condition, hyperglycemia/hypoglycemia, depressed levels of the electrolytes potassium, phosphate, calcium or magnesium, trace element deficiencies (Box 70-2), and essential fatty acid deficiency (EFAD), caused by prolonged fat-free hyperalimentation therapy.

Implementation

Monitoring. Close, ongoing reassessment of clients' responses to this complex therapy is essential. In particular, the development of circulatory fluid overload or electrolyte imbalance should be monitored for, by assessments of vital signs, fluid intake and output, and electrolyte studies. A uniform infusion rate should be maintained at all times as prescribed by the prescriber. Infusion instrumentation does not eliminate the need for alert nursing care, since it has the same potential for malfunction as all equipment does.

Some level of glucosuria may occur, particularly at initiation of therapy, since insulin response is challenged by the glucose load. The urine may be tested at 6-hour intervals for glucose, acetone, and protein. The client should be weighed

BOX 70-2

Complications of Parenteral Nutrition

Complications arising from infection and sepsis
- Catheter seeding from bloodborne or distant infection
- Contamination of catheter entrance site during insertion or long-term catheter placement
- Solution contamination

Complications that are metabolic in origin
- Azotemia
- Cholelithiasis
- Dehydration from osmotic diuresis
- Electrolyte imbalance
- Hyperammonemia
- Hyperosmolar, hyperglycemic, nonketotic coma (HHNC)
- Hyperphosphatemia and hypophosphatemia
- Hypocalcemia
- Hypomagnesemia
- Rebound hypoglycemia or sudden cessation of parenteral nutrition
- Trace element deficiencies

Complications arising from subclavian catheterization
- Air embolism
- Arteriovenous fistula
- Brachial plexus injury
- Cardiac perforation, tamponade
- Catheter embolism
- Catheter misplacement
- Central vein thrombophlebitis
- Endocarditis
- Hemothorax
- Hydromediastinum
- Hydrothorax
- Pneumothorax
- Subclavian artery injury
- Subclavian hematoma
- Subcutaneous emphysema
- Tension pneumothorax
- Thoracic duct injury

on a daily basis at the same time of day, wearing the same type of clothing, and on the same scale, preferably the first thing in the morning after voiding. Blood urea nitrogen (BUN) is tested daily for 3 to 5 days, then every other day as needed. A sequential multichannel autoanalyzer (SMA) 12/60 procedure should be done weekly, as well as tests for protein, partial thromboplastin time (PTT), and complete blood count (CBC). Serum electrolytes should be monitored daily. With lipid formulations, monitor serum triglycerides closely. There is less aggressive monitoring of the long-term stable client receiving TPN.

Monitor clients with diabetes mellitus carefully; insulin may be required to control hyperglycemia. Clients with cardiac insufficiency need to be watched closely for fluid volume excess. Observe the infusion site regularly for inflammation and infection and peripheral infusion lines for phlebitis.

Daily recording of the following data and communication of abnormal values to the prescriber are critical. These data include blood glucose in excess of 200 mg/100 ml; weight loss; and change in pulse and blood pressure; sweating; elevated temperature; swelling and edema over the puncture site or on the head, neck, or face; abnormal serum electrolytes; distended veins in the neck, arms, and hands; convulsions; coma; or other radical changes in the client's condition.

Intervention. Because these balanced nutritional solutions provide an excellent medium for growth of microorganisms, strict asepsis must be employed when preparing solutions (usually done by pharmacists, ideally under a laminar flow hood) and when handling solutions or the insertion site.

Hickman or Broviac catheters are two central venous catheters that can be used for intermittent infusions of drugs, parenteral feedings, and other adjunctive therapies. These catheters are designed so that the ends may be capped between infusions. Heparinized saline is instilled at the completion of infusions, and the tube is recapped. Except during lipid infusions, in-line filters may be used to trap air and bacteria. Parenteral lines are reserved for hyperalimentation.

The fat emulsions may be administered either peripherally or centrally. If fat emulsions are coinfused from separate containers that flow into the same vein as the dextrose and amino acid solutions, use a Y connector positioned just in front of the infusion site. The lipid infusion line should be at least 6 inches higher than the dextrose-amino acid line because the lipid emulsion has a lower specific gravity. If it is not administered in this order, the lipid emulsion may flow backward into the amino acid-dextrose line.

Parenteral nutrition intake may begin at a rate less than 1 L/12 hours for the first 2 days. If tolerated, the rate may be increased gradually during the first 5 days to the final goal rate. Ideally, the rate of parenteral nutrition solutions should be regulated by infusion pump to maintain a steady flow.

Peripheral infusions are limited to 2.5% amino acids and dextrose 10%.

Do not shake lipid emulsion infusions that have separated in solution to mix them; instead discard them based on agency policy. Fats in these lipid emulsions have been found to leach out the plasticizer DEHP in polyvinyl chloride tubing. Since the toxic potential for DEHP is not known, it is wise to use the administration sets provided by the manufacturer with fat emulsions in parenteral nutrition therapy.

Dressings should be changed if they become wet or dislodged; they are designed to be air-occlusive. Specific protocols for dressing changes can be found in selected references. Report any elevation of the client's temperature to the physician. Cultures (fungal, bacterial) should be taken of the insertion site, tubing, parenteral solutions, and the client's blood. Peripheral vein sites are generally changed routinely every 10 to 12 hours.

Air embolism is a potential hazard with central venous lines because of the low pressure in the venous system. Tubing connections must be kept taped to prevent their separation. When necessary, tubing should be changed quickly with the client in a supine position and executing Valsalva's maneuver (forced exhalation against a closed glottis). Central line insertions should be accomplished in Trendelenburg's position.

Education. Parenteral nutrition can now be continued at home for indefinite periods of time for those who need ongoing nutritional support and who meet the criteria. Education of the client and family is essential with regard to the purposes and techniques of the following: preventing infection, care of the solution and flow rate regulation, daily weights, recording of intake and output, urine monitoring for glycosuria, and the need for close contact with community health nurses and other personnel. The client and family/caregiver must understand infusion pump monitoring before taking on full responsibility for this technology. Every attempt should be made to resume the usual activities of daily living and to integrate this therapy into the client's life-style. See the Home Health box for nursing care of client who is receiving TPN in the home, p. 1078.

Evaluation. The client's nutritional status will be improved. Weight increases of 2 to 3 pounds a week can be expected if therapy is successful, until the client's weight is within normal limits for height and age. The client should also evidence improved strength and activity tolerance and healthy gums and oral mucous membranes. Laboratory values should be within normal limits for BUN and serum albumin, protein, hematocrit, hemoglobin, vitamin B_{12}, folic acid, cholesterol, and lymphocyte and transferrin levels.

SUMMARY

Nutrition in the form of enteral or parenteral solutions plays a vital role in the treatment of clients. Enteral nutrition bypasses the upper gastrointestinal tract, introducing liquid enteral formula or pureed foods directly into the stomach or small intestine by way of a feeding tube. Enteral feeding is indicated for clients who have a functional GI tract but cannot take sufficient food by mouth. Complications of enteral nutrition may be mechanical or metabolic. Parenteral nutrition refers to the intravenous administration of a solution containing dextrose, proteins, electrolytes, vitamins, and trace elements in amounts that exceed the client's energy needs. It is used in instances where enteral feeding is contraindicated or ineffective. In both enteral and parenteral nutrition, the nurse has an important role to ensure that clients are adequately nourished in a safe manner.

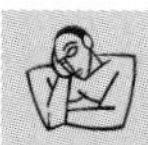

Critical Thinking

1. Jean Sims, age 76, was admitted to the hospital because of several chronic ailments, including asthma and emphysema, and esophageal motility problems. She had been losing weight rapidly because she was having trouble swallowing and was working so hard to breathe that she wasn't getting enough to eat. The physician has inserted a gastrostomy tube percutaneously rather than insert a nasogastric tube. What are the advantages for this client of the PEG compared to a nasogastric tube?
2. Would TPN have any advantages for Mrs. Sims? Why or why not?

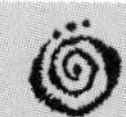

Collaborative Learning Activities

1. Present the complications of nasogastric tube feeding. How would you prevent these from occurring? What intervention should be taken if each of these complications occurred?

BIBLIOGRAPHY

American Hospital Formulary Service (1996). *AHFS drug information '96*. Bethesda, MD: American Society of Hospital Pharmacists.

Anderson KN, et al. (Eds.) (1994). *Mosby's medical, nursing, & allied health dictionary* (4th ed.). St Louis: Mosby.

Beare PG & Myers JL (Eds.) (1994). *Principles and practices of adult health nursing*. St Louis: Mosby.

Beizer J (1992). Enteral feeding in the LTC setting, *Long Term Care Forum* 2 (2):8.

Bockus S. (1993). When your patient needs tube feedings: Making the right decisions, *Nursing* 23 (7):34-42.

Carpenito LJ (1995). *Nursing diagnosis: Application to clinical practice* (6th ed.).Philadelphia: JB Lippincott.

Estoup M (1994). Approaches and limitations of medication delivery in patients with enteral feeding tubes, *Crit Care Nurse* 14 (2):68-78.

Food and Drug Administration (1994). Safety alert: Hazards of precipitation associated with parenteral nutrition, *Amer J Hosp Pharm* 51 (6):1427-8.

Holcombe BJ (1996). Adult parenteral nutrition. In Young LY & Koda-Kimble MA. (Eds.) *Applied therapeutics: The clinical use of drugs* (6th ed.). Vancouver: Applied Therapeutics.

Lipman TO (1993). Total parenteral nutrition: Indications for hospitalized adults, *Drug Ther* (January), p. 67-73.

McCloskey JC & Bulechek (Eds.). *Nursing interventions classification (NIC)* (2nd ed.). St Louis: Mosby.

Metheney N (1993). Minimizing respiratory complications of nasoenteric tube feedings: State of the science, *Heart Lung* 22 (3):213-22.

Mirtallo JM (1994). The complexity of mixing calcium and phosphate, *Amer J Hosp Pharm* 51 (6):1535-6.

Miyagawa CI (1993). Drug-nutrient interactions in critically ill patients, *Crit Care Nurse* 13 (10):69-90.

Olin BR (Ed.) (1996). *Facts and comparisons*. St Louis: Facts and Comparisons.

Rollins CJ (1996). Adult enteral nutrition. In Young LY & Koda-Kimble MA (Eds.). *Applied therapeutics: The clinical use of drugs* (6th ed.). Vancouver: Applied Therapeutics.

United States Pharmacopeial Convention (1996). *USP DI: Drug information the health professional* (16th ed.). Rockville, MD: The Convention.

Chapter 71

Antiseptics, Disinfectants, and Sterilant Agents

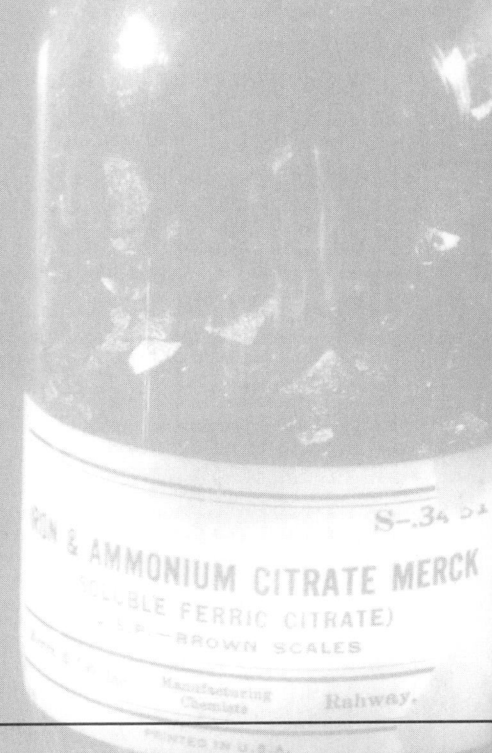

Chapter Focus

Most infectious diseases are transmitted in one of four ways: airborne transmission (inhalation of contaminated, evaporated droplets); vector-borne transmission of an organism by an intermediate carrier, such as a mosquito); contact transmission (direct or indirect contact with the source); and enteric transmission (oral-fecal transmission through direct or indirect contact with feces or objects heavily contaminated by feces). Nurses both practice and teach good aseptic and sterile technique to inhibit the transmission of infection. But in the last two transmission methods, contact and enteric transmission, nurses work to break the cycle by using antiseptics, disinfectants, and sterilant agents to decontaminate surfaces and equipment to prevent the spread of infection. The following objectives and key terms are important for a good understanding of this chapter.

Key Terms

antiseptic (p. 1085)
bactericidal (p. 1085)
bacteriostatic (p. 1085)
disinfectant (p. 1085)
medical asepsis (p. 1085)
nosocomial infection (p. 1085)
sterilization (p. 1085)
surgical asepsis (p. 1085)

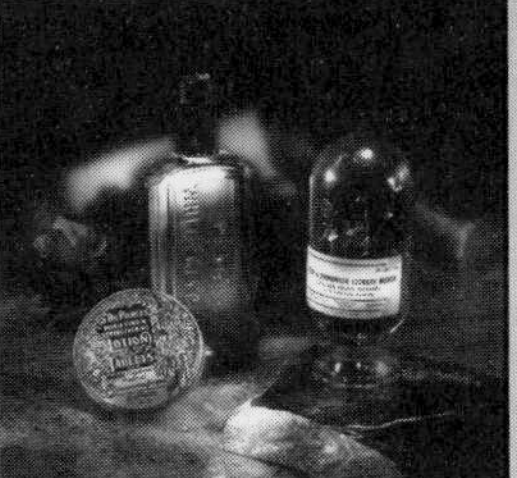

Objectives

1. Compare nosocomial infections and community- or home-acquired infections.
2. Differentiate between medical asepsis and surgical asepsis.
3. Describe the characteristics of an ideal antiseptic/disinfectant.
4. Discuss the mechanisms of action of antiseptics and disinfectants.
5. List the indications for use of common antiseptics and disinfectants.
6. Discuss the uses and limitations of silver nitrate and silver sulfadiazine.
7. Describe the effectiveness of iodine compounds and iodophors.
8. Explain the mechanism of action of oxidizing agents.
9. Discuss the current uses of sterilants.
10. Implement nursing management for the safe and effective use of antiseptics, disinfectants, and sterilants.

Infections and infectious diseases, although differing in type and character, occur in people in all settings—hospitals, institutions, the community at large, and the home.

Community-acquired infections in usually healthy individuals, are often benign, and are relatively responsive to treatment. *Streptococcus pneumoniae* or *M. pneumoniae* infections are common in this population. **Nosocomial infections** are those that are acquired in a hospital and most frequently are due to gram-negative (*Pseudomonas, Proteus, Serratia, Providencia,* and others) infections (Bailey & Powderly, 1992). Nosocomial infections have been called one of the most significant current ecologic problems in North America. They are occasionally caused by virulent microorganisms resistant to antibiotics.

Urinary tract infections and postoperative wound infections account for the majority (approximately 70% or more) of the nosocomial infections detected in a hospital setting. The high-risk areas, such as critical care units, burn units, and dialysis units, usually have the highest incidence of infection outbreaks and of antibiotic resistance in the hospital. Nurses must be aware of the problem and of methods used to reduce the incidence of nosocomial infections in their practice.

MEDICAL AND SURGICAL ASEPSIS

Medical asepsis (absence of pathogenic organisms) and **surgical asepsis** (absence of all microorganisms) are used in health care to reduce the number and spread of organisms. These approaches presume the presence of pathogens (organisms capable of inducing disease or infection in human beings) or potential pathogens in the immediate environment and seek to limit their transmission.

Methods in surgical asepsis destroy *all* microorganisms, including spores; in medical asepsis, only *pathogens* are destroyed or inhibited. The focus in surgical asepsis is to keep all organisms out of a designated area (e.g., fresh wound), but in medical asepsis it is to remove or destroy the pathogens in the area and to contain the remaining nonpathogens there by conscious efforts. The former uses "sterile technique" (use of sterile equipment or sterile fields) and the latter uses "clean technique" (such as hygienic measures, cleaning agents, antiseptics, disinfectants, and barrier fields). Which is applied in any given situation depends largely on the susceptibility of the host, the organism's virulence, and other factors in the infectious cycle.

Sterilization

An object is sterile if it is free of all forms and types of life. **Sterilization** is a process that destroys all forms of life on an instrument or utensil, in a liquid, or within a substance. Living tissue (of clients, nurses, or surgeons) cannot be sterilized by any known means without damage to that tissue; therefore the process known as sterilization is applied only to objects. It is also important to grasp the concept put forth by the Council on Pharmacy and Chemistry that the terms *sterile, sterilizer,* and *sterilization* can be used only in the absolute sense; there is no acceptable concept of relative sterility. However, just because a piece of equipment is labeled "sterilizer" does not mean that it is totally and permanently effective for sterilizing. Nor does the term *sterilized* testify to an object's current condition of purity.

Several acceptable and practicable sterilization methods now exist. Steam under pressure (autoclaving) is preferred as the most effective. Ethylene oxide is a gas sterilant used for heat-labile materials, for sharp-edged instruments that could be dulled by steam, for electrical and anesthesia equipment, and for bedding. Hot air ovens are used to sterilize glassware. Chemical sterilants are also employed when necessary.

ANTISEPTICS AND DISINFECTANTS

Antiseptics and disinfectants are often chemical agents used to kill many of the pathogens within a given population of microorganisms. Their mechanisms of action are generally not very effective against spores of bacteria and fungi, many viruses, and some very resistant bacterial strains. As a group, the effects of disinfectants and antiseptics differ from sterilization largely in the degree and type of organisms destroyed. Disinfectants and antiseptics kill only pathogens, but sterilizing kills all types of organisms.

Although some of the literature uses the terms *disinfectant* and *antiseptic* interchangeably, this is erroneous and confusing. **Disinfectants** differ from **antiseptics** in the matter on which they are used and in their ability to destroy organisms. Disinfectants are used only on nonliving objects; they are toxic to living tissue. Antiseptics are chemicals typically applied only to living tissue, so they must be less potent or made more dilute to prevent cell damage. Such lessening of potency, although crucial to viable tissue, decreases effectiveness accordingly. Some definitions of antiseptics emphasize their inhibiting rather than destructive effects. The narrow range of tolerance by tissues to antiinfective topical preparations tends to limit the variety and number of acceptable antiseptic agents available. Therefore antiseptics may differ markedly from disinfectants in chemical composition or may simply be a dilute version of a disinfectant for use on intact tissue. Thus some chemical substances may be used either as an antiseptic or as a disinfectant, depending on concentration.

Antiseptics and disinfectants are further categorized as **bacteriostatic** or **bactericidal** in character. Antiseptics are most often bacteriostatic; they retard the growth and replication of bacteria but do not kill off the entire bacteria population. Disinfectants, as bactericides, actually kill bacteria but perhaps not all types (depending on the disinfectant, its specificity, and so on) and often not fungi, viruses, or spores. Other disinfectants—fungicides, virucides, and sporicides—act specifically on these organisms. Germicides is an all-encompassing term for agents that work against many types of "germs"—bacteria, fungi, viruses, and spores.

Organisms vary in sensitivity to disinfectants and antiseptics in general (Box 71-1). However, factors such as the dormant and impervious spore forms of some bacteria, the waxy

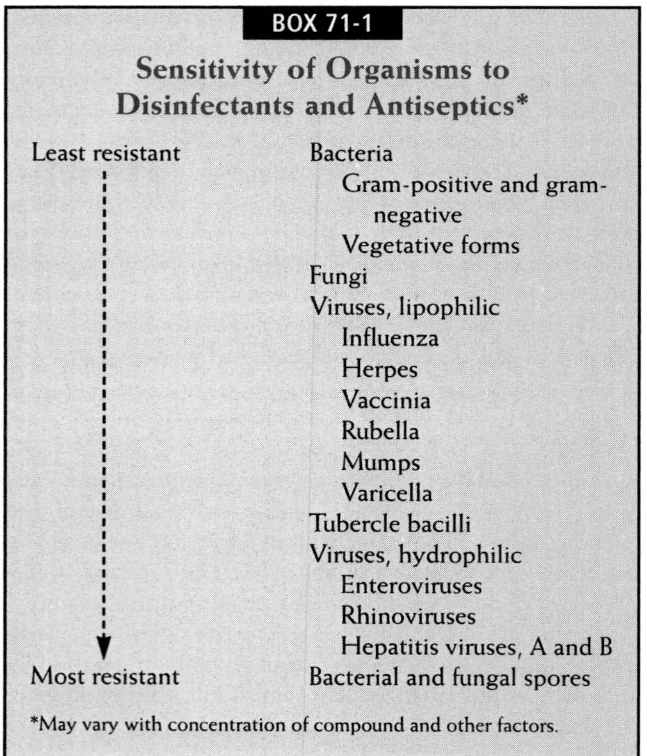

BOX 71-1

Sensitivity of Organisms to Disinfectants and Antiseptics*

Least resistant
- Bacteria
  - Gram-positive and gram-negative
  - Vegetative forms
- Fungi
- Viruses, lipophilic
  - Influenza
  - Herpes
  - Vaccinia
  - Rubella
  - Mumps
  - Varicella
- Tubercle bacilli
- Viruses, hydrophilic
  - Enteroviruses
  - Rhinoviruses
  - Hepatitis viruses, A and B
- Bacterial and fungal spores

Most resistant

*May vary with concentration of compound and other factors.

envelopes of the tubercle bacilli, certain properties of some types of gram-positive bacteria (staphylococci and enterococci), some gram-negative bacteria (*Salmonella* and *Pseudomonas* species), and hepatitis viruses make them highly refractory to many forms of disinfectants or antiseptics.

The ideal all-around antiseptic/disinfectant does not yet exist. Such an ideal agent would have to do the following:

- Be destructive to all forms of microorganisms without being toxic to human cells
- Have a low incidence of hypersensitivity
- Be active in the presence of organic matter and soaps
- Be stable, noncorrosive, nonstaining, and inexpensive

The current criteria for an effective disinfectant, however, includes the ability to destroy within 10 minutes all vegetative bacteria (not spores) and fungi, tubercle bacilli, animal parasites, and viruses (not hepatitis viruses). Many variables affect the relative efficiency of a product. These include the ingredients' ability to dissolve, mix, and work in the presence of organic matter such as blood or other exudate, and also, penetrate into recesses. Other properties include chemical composition, concentration, pH, ionization, surface tension, temperature, and length of time required for action. Thus in actual clinical use, there may be extreme variability in the effectiveness of any given product, depending on the specific application and the situation. Although several standard tests for efficacy of these products are available, the results are subject to the same variables and may also be difficult to administer.

Currently, there are few established guidelines for specific approved use of any particular disinfectant: a disinfectant is considered a disinfectant whether it is to be used on corridor floors or on surgical instruments. This method of classifying permits widespread practices such as the common use of iodophor solutions as disinfectants when they have earned FDA approval as antiseptics. Antiseptics are not required to be as potent as disinfectants. Relative usefulness of various antiseptics can be compared based on their therapeutic index. This index is the relationship between the specific antiseptic concentration proved to be effective against microorganisms without irritating tissues or interfering with healing. Other decisive factors are the potential for causing hypersensitivity reactions or systemic absorption. *Thorough handwashing still predominates as the most effective measure for controlling the spread of infection.*

To place the concepts of sterilization, disinfection, and antisepsis in perspective, it should be clear that these processes differ in the degree to which they destroy organisms. Thus anything that is sterile can also be considered both disinfected and antiseptic. (The converse is, of course, not true.) All of these processes correctly begin with handwashing, even when gloves are worn. It has been repeatedly demonstrated that clean, washed hands are crucial deterrents to microorganism growth, reproduction, and transmission in any environment.

Antiseptics and disinfectants may act in three ways.

1. They may bring about a change in the structure of the protein of the microbial cell (denaturation), which often proceeds to coagulation of protein with increased concentration of the chemical agent.
2. They may lower the surface tension of the aqueous medium of the parasitic cell, which increases plasma membrane permeability. This results in lysis or destruction of cellular constituents. (The surface-active agents are thought to act this way.)
3. They may alter a metabolic process in the microbial cells, which interferes with the cell's ability to survive and multiply.

Phenols

Phenol was used for over 100 years as an antiseptic and disinfectant but today it may be used in some facilities as a disinfectant. All phenols are deadly poisons if taken internally or applied topically to abraded skin. They are also corrosive to equipment.

■ Nursing Management

Phenol Use

Phenol and phenolic compounds are intended for disinfectant use only. These disinfectants should not come in contact with the skin in concentrations stronger than 2%; they should never come in contact with broken skin. If accidental skin contact is made or if a burning sensation is noted, the area should be washed with copious amounts of water. When used to clean bassinets and mattresses in poorly ventilated nurseries, phenolic disinfectants have produced epidemics of neonatal hyperbilirubinemia and fatalities have been documented in infants. Since phenol in concentrations above 5% has been implicated in the promotion of tumor growth, studies are underway to determine the carcinogenic, mutagenic, and teratogenic safety of this agent.

hexachlorophene [heks' a klo roe feen] (pHisoHex, Septisol)

Hexachlorophene is a bacteriostatic agent that was incorporated into detergent creams, soaps, lotions, shampoos, and other topical products to reduce the incidence of pathogenic bacteria on the skin. Because of its toxicity, especially in infants, it is currently available only by prescription for surgical scrub purposes and as a bacteriostatic skin cleanser against staphylococci and other gram-positive bacteria. It is used as a surgical scrub and bacteriostatic skin cleansing agent, although other antiseptics such as chlorhexidine, are more effective and safer agents.

Although single skin washing is no more effective than soap in reducing the number of bacteria, this product has a cumulative antibacterial property and with repeated use will steadily decrease bacterial flora. However, cleansing with alcohol and repeated washing with soap removes its antibacterial residue.

Hexachlorophene is a toxic agent that can be absorbed through the skin causing gastric symptoms and CNS toxicity. Daily topical use on newborns or application several times daily to the skin or vagina in adults has resulted in confusion, diplopia, lethargy, convulsions, respiratory arrest, and death. Hexachlorophene is usually not routinely used or recommended for bathing infants. It also should not be used on mucous membranes or burned or denuded skin or for any prolonged skin contact without rinsing. Dermatitis and photosensitivity are also reported.

■ Nursing Management

Hexachlorophene Use

Most authoritative sources recommend against the use of pHisoHex for bathing infants or in pregnant or hypersensitive persons.

There is a potential for poisoning because if there is accidental excessive exposure to or ingestion of these agents a resultant CNS toxicity may occur. Observe clients with prolonged exposure for signs of CNS toxicity: change in sensorium, double vision, lethargy, and seizures.

These products are highly toxic if ingested and easily absorbed even through intact skin if not thoroughly rinsed. Do not leave in contact with skin or mucous membranes, as in occlusive dressings, wet packs, lotions, or vaginal packs. Avoid contact with the eyes. Use should be discontinued if gastric or central nervous system signs appear.

PHisoHex is most effective for handwashing when no other antiseptic or solvent follows the rinse, since its antibacterial effects are progressive and cumulative with repeated use. If used for a preoperative preparation, scrub the operative site and surrounding areas every day for 3 days for optimal effectiveness. PHisoHex may turn brown when exposed to light, but this does not affect its action. Dispensers should be cleaned every 1 to 2 weeks.

hexylresorcinol [hex ill re sore' sin ole]

Hexylresorcinol is a stainless and odorless antiseptic. Although quite irritating to body tissues, diluted solutions of hexylresorcinol are used to cleanse skin wounds and are also used in mouthwashes or pharyngeal antiseptic preparations. Occasionally a marked hypersensitivity reaction may occur.

■ Nursing Management

Hexylresorcinol Therapy

Watch for and advise discontinuation of this product if there are signs of inflammation or irritation, which may indicate hypersensitivity rather than simple dermal irritation.

Dyes

Rosaniline dyes are a group of basic dyes used only occasionally today as antibacterial and antifungal agents. Most of these dyes (gentian violet, methyl violet, and others) have been removed from the market or have been replaced by other topical products.

Mercury Compounds

thimerosal (Mersol)

Organic mercurial agents (e.g., thimerosal) are more bacteriostatic, less irritating, and less toxic than the inorganic mercurials, yet they have a relatively low therapeutic index. The mercurial antiseptics probably act by inhibiting bacterial sulfhydryl enzymes, however, they inhibit tissue enzymes as well, which reduces their usefulness. Mercurial antiseptics are relatively slow acting, and organisms may revive if they come into contact with open wounds or body fluids. Bacterial spores will resume activity even after prolonged application of a mercurial antiseptic. Tissue and fluid proteins may compete for the mercury, leaving less free mercury for activity against microorganisms.

Thimerosal is available in solution, tincture (Merthiolate) and as an antiseptic spray.

Skin irritations and hypersensitivity have been reported with the use of mercury compounds.

Triclosan (Septisol) is a disinfectant, bacteriostatic agent with activity against gram-positive and gram-negative microorganisms. Health care personnel use is as a skin cleanser, handwash and shampoo. It should not be used as a surgical scrub.

■ Nursing Management

Mercury Compounds

Before using, assess if client has a history of hypersensitivity to mercury compounds. These products should not be used with infants or young children.

The client is at risk for sensitivity to mercury compounds evidenced by irritation that was not present before the start of therapy and for poisoning (mercury) related to accidental or excessive exposure to these agents evidenced by cloudy urine, dizziness, headache, soreness of the gums, nausea, and skin rash.

Observe client for signs of toxicity and the site of application for contact allergy dermatitis. Cleanse wound thoroughly before applying agent. Let dry before dressing wound. Thimerosal will sting when applied. Do not apply to large areas of abrasions, since the mercury may be absorbed systemically and cause toxicity. Avoid contact with the eyes. For the ointment, apply enough to cover affected areas and gently rub it in.

Make consumers aware of the very limited value of these products as antiseptics and disinfectants in comparison to their potential risks as poisons and allergens. There may be unwarranted reliance on them in the home, since they are relatively inexpensive. Children especially seem to like the pretty red stain left on the skin as evidence of germicidal effectiveness. These products should be stored out of reach of children.

Silver Compounds

silver nitrate; silver protein, mild; silver sulfadiazine (Silvadene)

Locally applied, many inorganic silver compounds have antiseptic qualities. Those silver salts that are highly ionizable and soluble produce astringent or caustic actions. Free silver ions precipitate bacterial cellular proteins, resulting in bactericidal effects. Effectiveness of these agents is directly proportional to their concentration and duration of contact time. An immediate bactericidal effect occurs when silver solutions are applied to tissue. The silver proteinate that is formed slowly liberates small amounts of ionic silver, which provides continued bacteriostatic action. An unexplained strongly bactericidal quality resides in distilled water when it is in contact with metallic silver. Silver nitrate reacts with soluble chloride, iodides, and bromides to form insoluble salts, stopping the action of silver nitrate. Thus its action can be halted if necessary by irrigation of the area with sodium chloride solutions. This chemical characteristic explains why solutions of silver salts penetrate tissues slowly; apparently chlorides precipitate the silver ions and inactivate them.

Silver nitrate 1% solution is used to prevent gonorrheal ophthalmia neonatorum. *Silver protein, mild (Argyrol S.S. 10%)* is used to treat local mild inflammation in the eye, nose, and throat. Finally, *silver sulfadiazine (Silvadene)* is bactericidal for many gram-positive and gram-negative organisms and yeast, and it also inhibits bacteria resistant to other agents. It is used to prevent and treat infections in second and third degree burns.

Side effects/adverse reactions. With silver nitrate 1% solution, eye redness or irritation is the primary adverse reaction; with other silver nitrate preparations, it is skin irritation. With long-term use, it can cause permanent discoloration of the skin because of the deposit of reduced silver (argyria). Prolonged use of mild silver protein can result in permanent skin discoloration and conjunctival argyria. With silver sulfadiazine (Silvadene), allergic skin reactions may occur. Other adverse effects are difficult to attribute directly to silver sulfadiazine, since other therapeutic drugs are usually being administered concurrently. Leukopenia and perhaps systemic sulfonamide adverse reactions may occur.

Dosage and administration. With silver nitrate 1% solution, 2 drops of this solution are instilled and allowed to remain in the eyes for no longer than 30 seconds. The American Academy of Pediatrics endorsed a recommendation to eliminate eye irrigation after instillation of the silver nitrate (Olin, 1996). In many hospitals, topical erythromycin or tetracycline ophthalmic ointments have replaced silver nitrate because they are effective against chlamydia and gonococcus eye infections (DiPiro, 1993).

For infections, instill 1 to 3 drops of silver protein, mild (Argyrol S.S.) in eye(s) every 3 to 4 hours for several days; for preoperative use, place 2 or 3 drops in eye(s), then rinse with a sterile irrigating solution.

Silver sulfadiazine (Silvadene) is applied with a sterile gloved hand once or twice daily to a 1/16 inch thickness. Keep burn areas covered with this product at all times.

■ Nursing Management

Silver Compound Therapy

Assessment. Question client about hypersensitivity to silver (or sulfonamides in Silvadene Cream), blood dyscrasias, porphyria, or a glucose-6-phosphate dehydrogenase deficiency; these conditions may preclude treatment with these compounds. The effects in children and in pregnant or breastfeeding women are not known.

Concurrent use of silver sulfadiazine with proteolytic enzymes, such as collagenase, papain, or sutilains, is contraindicated since the heavy metal salts may inactivate the enzymes.

Nursing diagnosis. The client receiving silver compound therapy may be at risk for altered comfort (an itching or burning feeling on treated areas).

Implementation

Monitoring. Evaluate affected skin areas daily and note any changes. Perform ongoing evaluation of clients treated with these compounds to limit adverse effects related to hypersensitivities, crystalluria, blood dyscrasias, or electrolyte imbalances because of absorbed drug components. If silver sulfadiazine is used in the treatment of extensive burns, monitor clients for serum sulfa concentrations, crystalluria, and renal function.

Intervention. Store silver nitrate solutions at temperatures between 15° and 30° C (59° to 86° F) and protected from light. Do not use Silvadene Cream if its white color has darkened. Use only the appropriate concentrations of antiseptic purposes to avoid irritation and burns to tissue. Sodium chloride can be used to flood the area should this occur accidentally.

Store silver nitrate solutions out of reach of children and never take internally. Since sulfadiazine may be absorbed from Silvadene Cream, clients should increase their fluid intake to prevent crystalluria.

Although application of silver sulfadiazine is not painful, application of silver nitrate in solution may be quite painful, especially when applied to burns. Therefore give clients analgesics before dressing changes.

Cleanse wounds before treatment to remove exudate, debris, and blood; this will prevent premature inactivation of these products. Wearing a sterile glove apply a thin layer to affected areas, keeping the affected areas covered with silver sulfadiazine at all times. Reapply if the cream is washed or worn off. Dressings may be applied but are not necessary over silver sulfadiazine.

Take care with silver solutions to keep spills and stains to a minimum. Gloves are advised when working with silver solutions. Most tissue stains caused by Silvadene gradually disappear. Stains may be removed from linens, clothing, and shoes by applying household chlorine bleach.

Education. Alert the client that rarely the skin may stain a brownish black. Instruct in the proper application technique.

Evaluation. The client's wound evidences granulation and healing by primary intention or split-thickness skin grafting within an appropriate time frame.

See also Nursing Management: Silver Sulfadiazine in Chapter 66, Dermatologic Drugs.

Halogens

Chlorine Compounds

Although chlorine can be bactericidal (it is ineffective against acid-fast bacteria), sporicidal, viricidal, and amebicidal, the elemental form of chlorine itself has limited usefulness as a disinfectant because the gas is difficult to handle. The antibacterial action of chlorine is said to be caused by the formation of hypochlorous acids, which results when chlorine reacts with water. Therefore chlorine containing products that can release hypochlorous acid are in use today.

1. *Sodium hypochlorite solution, 1%* is used to sterilize equipment while the 0.5% solution is used as an antiseptic for wound irrigation. This solution is of limited usefulness for wound irrigations, except for debridement purposes, because they are irritating to the skin and delay the clotting process. Common household bleaches are usually 5% solutions of sodium hypochlorite. Therapeutic solutions are unstable and must be freshly prepared before use. See the Nursing Research box below for the use of hypochlorite solutions for preventing the spread of AIDS among IV drug users.
2. Oxychlorosene (Clorpactin) is a combination product that contains hypochlorous acid, which when released is effective (bactericidal) against both gram-negative and gram-positive organisms, fungi, yeast, viruses, molds, and spores. It is indicated for the treatment of localized infections, especially if caused by resistant organisms; to cleanse and irrigate necrotic debris, wounds, sinus tract, and empyemas. Dilutions of this product are also used in urology and ophthalmology.

■ Nursing Management

Chlorine Compounds

Dakin's solution, a diluted 0.5% sodium hypochlorite solution adjusted to a neutral pH with sodium bicarbonate, was

Nursing Research

Bleach programs for preventing AIDS among IV drug users: modeling the impact of HIV prevalence

Intravenous drug users (IVDUs) risk HIV infection from sexual contact and from sharing injection equipment—needles, syringes, or other items—with infected individuals. While protective changes in behavior have been reported among homosexuals, most IVDUs continue to place themselves at risk. The growing importance of drug use as a mode of HIV transmission has led to increased attention to AIDs prevention among intravenous drug users.

This study examines the effectiveness of bleach distribution, a program to prevent HIV transmission via shared needles. Bleach programs employ outreach workers to distribute small bottles of bleach, which IVDUs use to disinfect their injection equipment. An important argument for the implementation of bleach programs has been that they are more politically feasible than needle exchange programs.

Siegel and others (1991) examined whether and to what extent initial HIV prevalence among IVDUs influences program effectiveness. Because the difficulty of conducting longitudinal surveys of transient IVDU populations prevents studies of existing programs, modeling provides a practical means for studying the conditions that determine the success of bleach programs.

The investigators used a Markov model to assess the role of the initial HIV prevalence among drug users. The model incorporates survey data on risk behaviors and published information describing HIV incubation and mortality. It predicts life expectancy for cohorts of IVDUs with and without a bleach program to estimate program effectiveness.

Siegel and others found that bleach programs can produce the greatest life year savings in areas of low HIV prevalence. In the lowest prevalence scenario (0.02 initial prevalence), initiation of the program resulted in a projected savings of 2.3 life years per HIV-negative drug user, compared with 1.7 and 1.3 years under medium (0.25) and high (0.60) prevalence, respectively.

The investigators concluded that while bleach programs are beneficial to all groups of IVDUs, these results highlight the advantages of introducing bleach programs early when prevalence is still comparatively low in a drug-user population.

Critical thinking questions

- Because HIV prevalence among drug users can increase rapidly, what do you think the opportunities are for early intervention with bleach programs?
- In your own community, what types of programs are available for IVDUs to prevent the spread of HIV? If a bleach program is not available, how would you go about instituting one?

From Siegel JE et al (1991).

once widely used to treat suppurating wounds, but its solvent action delays clotting.

Store chlorine products in marked containers out of the reach of children. If a chlorine agent is swallowed, a poison control center should be contacted and emergency treatment sought. Store these products away from light and in airtight containers, if possible. Avoid spills on skin or delicate tissues because it will cause irritation. Avoid spills on clothing or contact with hair because of its bleaching properties. Rinse thoroughly with clear water if a spill occurs.

Iodine and Iodophors

iodine tincture; povidone-iodine solution

(Betadine)

Iodine is slightly soluble in water but is soluble in alcohol and in aqueous solutions of sodium and potassium iodide. Iodine is volatile, and solutions should not be exposed to air except during use. In its elemental or free form, iodine is very rapidly bactericidal, viricidal, fungicidal, and lethal to protozoa; it is less effective against spores. It is one of the most efficient chemical disinfectants and antiseptics currently in use.

Some iodine compounds are believed to be superior to other antiseptics because all types of bacteria may be destroyed with a single concentration of iodine, effective over a wide pH range. Organic matter interferes with the potency of iodine only when it is first applied; later, effectiveness increases because of diffusion as the iodine complexes dissociate. This initial delayed effect in the presence of organic material may also be offset by the increased strengths of the solution concentrations now on the market.

Iodine solution is used for the treatment of minor wounds, abrasions, and infected wounds while iodine tincture is preferred for intact skin procedures, such as skin preparation before invasive procedures, Hickman catheter and parenteral nutrition dressing changes, and intravenous needle insertions. Aqueous solutions are thought to be as effective as tincture of iodine for similar therapeutic purposes but because they are less irritating, they are used for abraded skin areas.

An aqueous solution of 5% iodine and 10 potassium iodide (Lugol's solution) can also be given orally in the treatment of goiter (see Chapter 48). The various iodine compounds marketed for antisepsis and disinfection include Iodine Topical and Iodine tincture (the most commonly used iodine antiseptic). While they both contain 2% iodine and 2.4% sodium iodide, the solution is in water while the tincture has 47% alcohol.

Iodophor: Povidone-iodine (Betadine, Operand)

Iodophors have become widely used as *antiseptics*. This is the only purpose for which they have been approved by the FDA, although in practice they continue to be used for disinfection of certain equipment. Iodophors are a group of iodine compounds combined with povidone (carrier), which increases the water solubility of iodine and provides a slow release of iodine. It has the same germicidal action of iodine without producing irritation to skin and mucous membranes. Povidone-iodines are available in many formulations, such as solution, 2% scrub, spray, foam, vaginal gel and suppositories, ointment, mouthwash, or perineal wash.

Side effects/adverse reactions. Iodine is toxic if taken internally. It is locally corrosive to gastrointestinal tissues but is inactivated by gastrointestinal contents. Iodine tincture may be transiently quite painful when applied to open skin areas, but the aqueous solution form stings only slightly. These agents may be absorbed through the skin and in chronic use, may affect thyroid function. Neonates have developed hypothyroidism following topical application of povidone-iodine. Marked hypersensitivity reactions do occur occasionally even with topical application. These are manifested by severe systemic reactions of fever and generalized skin eruptions.

■ Nursing Management

Iodine Compounds and Iodophors

Assessment. Before iodine compounds and iodophors are applied, ask client about any past allergic reactions to iodine, shellfish, or iodine-containing diagnostic agents. If there is doubt substitute another product. Do not use povidone-iodine as a vaginal douche during pregnancy.

Nursing diagnosis. The client is at risk for impaired skin integrity related to hypersensitivity or local irritation, and altered comfort with iodine tincture related to pain and stinging on application of the agent.

Implementation

Monitoring. Observe the area for irritation not present at the initiation of therapy. Monitor the lesions on a periodic basis for healing.

Intervention. These products are exceptionally valuable because of their efficiency, low toxicity, and low cost.

Do not bandage or tape areas treated with tincture of iodine; if treated with povidone-iodine, a cover dressing may be applied if necessary. If irritation develops, wash the skin.

Artificially elevated blood glucose determinations have been noted when povidone-iodine swabs were used for skin preparation. Soap and water cleansing of fingertips before skin puncture for blood glucose monitoring by some reagent strips is recommended.

Iodophors will stain only starched linen or clothing. Tinctures and solutions of iodine may stain more freely.

Education. Advise the client to purchase iodine preparations in very small quantities and discard routinely after a short time, since evaporation of the solvent or vehicle will leave concentrated iodine preparation that may burn tissues on application.

Evaluation. The client will demonstrate signs of wound healing within an appropriate time frame. If the agent is used as an antiseptic to prepare for a procedure, there will be no evidence of sepsis following the procedure.

Oxidizing Agents

hydrogen peroxide

Hydrogen peroxide is a weak antiseptic that when in contact with a tissue enzyme (catalase), is converted to effervescent oxygen to produce an antibacterial action and cleansing effect on the wound. The presence of blood and pus though, will decrease the efficacy of hydrogen peroxide (McEvoy, 1996). The antiseptic action of hydrogen peroxide is fairly fast acting and short-lived; it acts as an antibacterial only as long as the bubbling action continues.

Oxygen that is released is particularly suited for destroying aerobic microorganisms in wounds, but as an antibacterial it is weak and slow. Its effervescence action, though, provides a mechanical effect to aid in removing foreign tissue debris. Several products containing hydrogen peroxide are marketed.

Hydrogen peroxide topical solution is available in a 3% solution in water and used to irrigate suppurating wounds and some extensive traumatic wounds. It should be used in areas where the oxygen can escape, therefore it should not be instilled into closed body spaces or abscesses (McEvoy, 1996). It is not recommended for use in pressure ulcers because it and many other antiseptic agents are considered to be cytotoxic to normal tissues (Bergstrom et al, 1994).

The official hydrogen peroxide solution has been further diluted with water into a 1/2 or 1/4 strength for most applications. The mouthrinse or mouth wash (Peroxyl) is a 1.5% solution.

Side effects/adverse reactions. If small amounts of diluted hydrogen peroxide solutions are swallowed, it rapidly decomposes in the stomach into relatively harmless molecular oxygen and water. Repeated use as a mouthwash may cause hypertrophied papillae of the tongue ("hairy tongue"), a reversible condition. The concentrated solutions used for hair bleaching may cause skin irritation and contact dermatitis.

■ Nursing Management

Oxidizing Agents

To delay deterioration of the contents, store solutions in tightly capped, amber containers to protect from light and air. Solutions in containers should be discarded frequently, and fresh solutions should be used. The rapidity and vigor with which bubbling occurs may be used as a general guide to the freshness of the solution. The bubbling action makes hydrogen peroxide useful for removing mucus secretions from equipment (i.e., inner cannulae of tracheostomy tubes).

Do not leave paper cups containing hydrogen peroxide where clients can reach them. Because the solution looks like water, clients have mistakenly drunk it despite the unusual taste. Although very small amounts will not be harmful, large amounts in the stomach could be harmful because of resultant effervescence in the stomach, a closed cavity. These compounds, like all medications, should be kept secured and out of children's reach.

Biguanides

chlorhexidine [klor hex' i deen] (Hibiclens)

Chlorhexidine is a biguanide with antiseptic action against both gram-positive and gram-negative bacteria, such as *Pseudomonas aeruginosa.* Chlorhexidine acts by disrupting the bacterial cell's plasma membrane (particularly gram-positive organisms).

A bactericidal skin cleansing solution containing chlorhexidine (Hibiclens) is useful as a surgical scrub, a handwashing agent for personnel, and a skin wound cleanser. Chlorhexidine oral rinse (Peridex, PerioGard) is also used as an antibacterial dental product to treat gingivitis between dental visits.

Side effects/adverse reactions. Chlorhexidine is a relatively safe antiseptic. There have been reports of deafness occurring when these products came into contact with the middle ear through a perforated eardrum. Rare secondary effects include dermatitis, photosensitivity, and irritation of mucosal tissue. Physiochemical properties of these agents suggest that absorption through the skin is minimal.

As a handwash, Hibiclens is applied, water added, and friction applied for 15 seconds. Skin wounds should be washed gently with Hibiclens and rinsed. For surgical scrubs hands and forearms are scrubbed with approximately 5 ml Hibiclens for 3 minutes without water, while using a brush or sponge. After hands and forearms are rinsed, washing is repeated for 3 more minutes.

■ Nursing Management

Chlorhexidine

Use judgment when diluting these agents, since their effectiveness may be greatly reduced in proportion to the dilution. Certain solutions less than 4% may actually support bacterial growth. Chlorhexidine-treated areas should not be wiped with alcohol, which will neutralize the intended residual action. Do not use chlorhexidine on delicate tissues such as eyes and mucous membranes. The area should be rinsed promptly if this occurs. Advise clients not to swallow chlorhexidine compounds (especially when used for mouth care).

Surface-Active Agents

benzalkonium chloride (Zephiran Chloride)

As wetting agents, emulsifiers, or detergents, surface-acting agents are considered superior to soaps because they can be used in hard water, are stable in acid or alkaline solutions, decrease surface tension more effectively, and are less irritating to the skin.

Benzalkonium chloride is a cationic (has a positive electric charge on the active portion of the agent) quaternary ammonium compound used in solution as a topical antiseptic or as a disinfectant. It is generally believed that benzalkonium chloride is not very reliable in either role. As an antiseptic it has a limited antibacterial spectrum, it lacks fast action and has a potential for inducing toxicity. As a disinfectant, the solution has to be changed regularly to maintain concentration and effectiveness. It is also inactivated by anionic substances, such as soap and organic materials.

The mechanism of action is not known for certain, but it may be due to bacteria enzyme inactivation.

Side/adverse reactions. Chemical burns may occur if benzalkonium chloride is allowed to stay in contact with tissues, as in wet packs or occlusive dressings. Delicate tissues may be injured if specified dilution recommendations are not used. Ingestion only rarely causes toxicity. Hypersensitivity reactions can occur. The tincture and the spray formulations are flammable.

This agent is slow acting in comparison to iodine. Therapeutic effects are thought to be in direct relation to the concentration of the solution used. Depending on the purpose and tissues or equipment to be treated, recommended dilutions range from 1:750 (tincture or aqueous solutions) on intact skin, minor wounds, and abrasions, to 1:5000 or 1:10,000 (aqueous solution) for mucous membranes and broken or diseased skin. A variety of gram-positive and gram-negative organisms and many fungi and viruses (not hepatitis) are said to be susceptible. Tap water that contains metallic ions, organic matter, or resin-deionized water may reduce its effectiveness.

■ Nursing Management
Benzalkonium Chloride

If any of these compounds have been used, continue to monitor the area or utensil critically for contamination. In view of the highly questionable efficacy of surface-active agents, especially benzalkonium chloride, question an order or a suggestion to use them as antiseptics or disinfectants. Suggest the substitution of an iodophor, alcohol, or other compound. Use only the concentration recommended for each specified area. Do not use with occlusive dressings.

Do not apply these compounds to areas previously treated with soaps or anionic agents. Do not apply to delicate tissues. Flood the area with water if these agents are accidentally introduced. Do not reuse solutions after soaking cotton balls, dressings, or instruments.

Avoid using Zephiran to disinfect thermometers. If it must be used, use not less than the recommended 1:750 concentration. Do not use the tincture of spray formulation near an open flame.

Miscellaneous Agents

nitrofurazone (Furacin)

Nitrofurazone is a broad antibacterial topical agent active against many bacteria that cause local infections, including *Staphylococcus aureus, Streptococcus, E. coli,* and others. It is indicated as adjunct therapy to clients with second and third degree burns when bacterial resistance to other agents is a problem; and also used during skin grafting when bacterial contamination may result in graft rejection or a donor site infection.

Side effects/adverse reactions. Rash, itching, local edema (dermatitis), and allergic reactions have been reported. Hypersensitivity occurs early in the treatment of a few individuals. Bacterial and fungal superinfections may occur. Furacin is not absorbed significantly through mucosal or burned tissues, and systemic toxicity is rare. However, its prophylethylene glycol base may be absorbed and challenge the client with renal dysfunction.

The 0.2% cream, ointment or solution may be applied directly on the area or to a gauze dressing for application. Efficacy is reduced in the presence of heavy microbial contamination, plasma, or blood. Resistance seldom develops.

■ Nursing Management
Nitrofurazone Therapy

Assessment. Determine that the client has not had a previous sensitivity reaction to the drug. Pregnant women should avoid use of this product unless the potential benefits outweigh the possible risks to the fetus. Judgment should be used in treating individuals who have renal disorders with these preparations, which include polyethylene glycol because it may produce adverse effects. Geriatric clients are at higher risk for allergic responses to nitrofurazone.

Nursing diagnosis. The client is at risk for impaired skin integrity, which occurs in approximately 1% of those treated, related to allergic contact dermatitis (erythema, pruritus, and burning).

Implementation

Monitoring. Evaluate affected areas daily. If areas do not seem to be responding to treatment by Furacin, consider the possibility of overgrowth by nonsusceptible organisms such as fungi and *Pseudomonas* or an allergic response. Watch for dermatitis or other manifestations of hypersensitivity to this product.

Intervention. Cleanse the affected area before each dressing change. Treatment by Furacin may be suggested in instances of burn or wound infections resistant to other medications. As a solution, nitrofurazone may be sprayed directly on the wound. If the solution is cloudy, it may be warmed to restore clarity. To apply the ointment, use sterile gloves and cover the affected areas with a thin layer. Meticulous sterile technique is essential during dressing changes and when opening and withdrawing Furacin-saturated dressings from their sterile packets. Nitrofurazone darkens on exposure to light, the discoloration does not affect the potency of the drug.

Severe skin reactions to nitrofurazone may require topically applied steroids or short-term administration of systemic corticosteroids.

Education. Clients should be instructed to apply nitrofurazone correctly and alerted to its adverse reactions.

Evaluation. The client's wound will evidence granulation and healing by primary intention or split-thickness skin grafting within an acceptable time frame.

Alcohols

ethanol [eth' a nole] (ethyl alcohol)
isopropanol [eye soe proe' pa nole] (isopropyl alcohol)

A 70% alcohol solution is antiseptic. The 70% aqueous solution is more effective in reducing the surface tension of bacterial cells than absolute alcohol, which precipitates protoplasm at the periphery of the cell and thus tends to inhibit penetration of the agent. Alcohol also inhibits growth of bacteria, so it is often used as a preservative of biologic specimens and in some prepackaged injectables and medications. Alcohols may precipitate cellular proteins. They are potent viricidal agents.

Alcohol is used topically as a bactericidal; to prepare skin for minor invasive procedures (using commercially packaged skin wipes); for disinfection of heat-labile instruments, polyethylene tubing, catheters, implants, prostheses, smooth hard-surfaced objects, hinged instruments, and inhalation and anesthesia equipment. Because of their rapid evaporation rate, dilute solutions of alcohols are still occasionally used as sponge baths to reduce fever, although systemic absorption may be especially harmful to neonates and children. Alcohols are also used as preservatives in solutions, diluents or to dissolve other drugs, and in combination with many other drugs for over-the-counter purchase (often without rationale). Ethyl alcohol is also ingested purposefully as an intoxicating beverage.

Toxicity. Essentially, all of the alcohols are poisonous drugs when taken internally, depending on the dose. Isopropyl alcohol is inherently highly poisonous; ethyl alcohol, pure alcohol made from vegetables, fruits, canes, and grains, is used in alcoholic beverages. The degree to which fractional distillation is carried out determines the resultant concentration.

Side effects/adverse reactions. When continuously inhaled or absorbed through the skin, alcohols can cause intoxication. Ethyl alcohol is irritating if left in contact with skin for prolonged periods. If ethyl alcohol is applied to open skin, a film that can harbor microorganisms develops. Isopropyl alcohol causes subcutaneous vasodilation, which can cause needle sites and incisions to bleed somewhat more freely.

Ethyl alcohol is slightly less effective as an antiseptic than isopropyl alcohol. Efficacy may depend on the concentration used and the amount of mechanical friction applied. The most effective solutions of ethyl alcohol are concentrations of 50% to 70%; stronger solutions are less effective. At concentrations of 70%, almost 90% of the bacteria on skin are killed within 2 minutes if the wet surface is allowed to dry naturally. Inadequate disinfection may occasionally result even if friction is conscientiously applied to surfaces.

Isopropyl alcohol is employed in aqueous solutions of 70% concentration or undiluted as 99% concentration (isopropyl rubbing alcohol). It may be combined with other disinfectants such as iodine and formaldehyde to improve efficiency.

■ Nursing Management

Ethanol and Isopropanol

Assessment. Alcohols should not be used to disinfect wounds because they cause tissue irritation with painful burning and stinging, and they precipitate protein in which bacteria may grow. Use with caution as a rub with children as the inhalation of fumes may be intoxicating.

Nursing diagnosis. For children and debilitated clients there exists the potential for poisoning because the individual is at risk of accidental exposure to or ingestion of these agents.

Implementation

Monitoring. If alcohol is externally applied to reduce fever, the client's temperature should be monitored regularly.

Intervention. The antiseptic action of alcohols can be enhanced by mechanical cleansing of the skin with water and a detergent before their application, by gentle rubbing with a sterile gauze during application, and allowing the area to dry for 2 minutes without fanning. Be prepared to apply more pressure and possibly a small pressure dressing after given an injection or discontinuing an intravenous infusion if alcohol has been applied to the site, because evaporate of the alcohol may cause localized, surface vasodilation. If the individual is also receiving anticoagulant therapy, the bleeding may be extensive.

If used in a home setting to disinfect thermometers, cleanse thermometers with detergent and tepid water before placing them to soak in an alcohol solution, because any adherent organic matter will inhibit the solution's action. Alcohol solutions themselves may harbor organisms and may rust instruments; therefore they are often not the best solution for disinfecting or for sterile storage of equipment.

After an alcohol rub, the application of an emollient alleviates the dry feeling of the skin.

Education. Alert personnel, clients, and parents that all alcohols are inherently or potentially poisonous and that intoxications or dangerous poisoning can occur as a result of their absorption, inhalation, or ingestion. Keep alcohols secured and out of the reach of children.

Evaluation. If used for fever reduction, the client's temperature will be within normal limits.

Acids

acetic acid (vinegar); benzoic acid; lactic acid; boric acid

Various acids have been used as antiseptics or cauterizing agents and of these, vinegar is the most commonly used, especially in community health nursing, because of its practicality, availability, and low cost. Other acids that are employed as antiseptics include benzoic acid (0.1%), which prevents bacterial and fungous growth; lactic acid, which is used primarily as a component of spermatocides in the United States and boric acid, which is so mild that it is used in eye and ear preparations. Of these other acids, most have lost credibility as effective antiseptics, such as, the implication of boric acid in cases of serious systemic intoxication by absorption.

Acetic acid provides an acid medium that inhibits the growth of organisms dependent on a neutral or alkaline medium. In a 5% concentration, acetic acid is germicidal to many organisms while it is bacteriostatic at lower concentrations. A mild vinegar solution is often recommended as a vaginal douche for antisepsis in the prevention or suppression of vaginal infections. Acetic acid may also be used as a mild antiseptic-deodorant for many other applications, such as bladder irrigation (0.25% concentration), and diaper soaks.

■ Nursing Management

Acetic Acid

A mildly effective, soothing vaginal douche can be prepared by adding 1 to 2 tablespoons of white household vinegar

(5%) to 1 quart of warm water. Stronger concentrations are no more effective and may irritate mucosal tissues. The residual pungent odor of acetic acid may be a deterrent to its use.

The use of aseptic technique is essential when irrigating solutions are used for urethal catheters. The solution should not be used unless it is clear and the container is undamaged with the seal intact. After the container is opened, the solution is to be used promptly to minimize bacterial growth. Unused portions of the solutions should be discarded. Antiseptics instilled in urinary collection bags should be of concentrations that are not injurious to bladder mucosa in case the bag is inadvertently raised so that contents reflux into the bladder.

STERILANTS

Aldehydes

formaldehyde solution

Formaldehyde solution is a 37% concentration of formalin (by weight). It is a clear, colorless disinfectant liquid that, on exposure to air, liberates a pungent, irritating gas. In a concentration of 1% to 10%, it kills microorganisms and spores in between 1 to 6 hours. It is effective against bacteria, fungi, and viruses and acts by combining with them to precipitate protein. It has been widely used as a disinfectant for instruments.

glutaraldehyde (Cidex)

Glutaraldehyde (Cidex), 2% alkaline solution, is a liquid disinfectant used as a germicidal agent to disinfect and sterilize some rigid optical instruments and prosthetic equipment. It kills some microorganisms in 10 minutes, spores in 10 hours. However, the solution is unstable and contact with skin should be avoided.

SUMMARY

Medical asepsis and surgical asepsis are used in health care settings to reduce the number and spread of organisms. Although thorough handwashing is still the best method for accomplishing this reduction, antiseptics, disinfectants, and sterilants need to be used. Antiseptics are chemicals typically applied to living tissue to decrease the microbial population, whereas disinfectants are used only on nonliving objects, since they are caustic to living tissue. Antiseptics and disinfectants may be either bacteriostatic or bactericidal, or they may be both, depending on the concentrations employed. Sterilants free objects of all forms and types of life. Although these substances are used for therapeutic purposes, they still are caustic and so require careful handling to prevent irritation and injury.

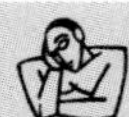

Critical Thinking

1. Given the criteria for the ideal antiseptic/disinfectant, which of the agents in this chapter would be closest to the ideal? Why?
2. Mrs. Taylor, age 24, was prescribed pHisoHex for her preoperative facial scrubs for the rhinoplasty she was having as a day stay case. When she comes to the clinic for a postoperative follow-up visit, she asks about using the pHisoHex she has left over from her scrubs for her baby's diaper rash. What will you respond?

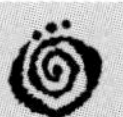

Collaborative Learning Activities

1. The students will record what antiseptics and/disinfectants that they use at home. Tabulate the findings and then discuss why that agent is used (family tradition or research finding). Discuss the merits and disadvantages of each of the agents.

BIBLIOGRAPHY

American Hospital Formulary Service (1996). *AHFS drug information '96.* Bethesda, MD: American Society of Health-System Pharmacists.

Anderson KN, et al. (Eds.) (1994). *Mosby's medical, nursing, & allied health dictionary* (4th ed.). St Louis: Mosby.

Bailey TC & Powderly WG (1992). Treatment of infectious disease. In Woodley M & Whelan A. *The Washington manual: Manual of medical therapeutics* (27th ed.). Boston: Little, Brown.

Bergstrom N, Bennett MA, & Carlson CE, et al. (1994). *Treatment of pressure sores: Clinical practice guideline,* No. 15. Rockville, MD: US Department of Health and Human Services. Public Health Service. Agency for Health Care Policy and Research. AHCPR Publication No. 95-0652.

DiPiro JT, et al. (Eds.) (1993). *Pharmacotherapy: A pathophysiologic approach* (2nd ed.). New York: Elsevier.

Katzung BG (1992). *Basic and clinical pharmacology* (5th ed.). Norwalk, CT: Appleton & Lange.

Olin BR (Ed.) (1996). *Facts and comparisons.* St Louis: Facts and Comparisons.

Siegel JE, et al. (1991). Bleach programs for preventing AIDS among IV users: Modeling the impact of HIV prevalence, *Amer J Publ Health 81* (10):1273-9.

United States Pharmacopeial Convention (1996). *USP DI: Drug information for the health care professional* (16th ed.). Rockville, MD: The Convention.

Chapter 72

Diagnostic Agents

Chapter Focus

Diagnostic and laboratory tests are one more source of information for the nurse in the assessment and ongoing monitoring of clients. The nurse is also responsible for the preparation of the client for diagnostic studies and for coordination of the completion of these tests. Many of these examinations require diagnostic agents with which the nurse needs to be knowledgeable to appropriately instruct and care for clients undergoing diagnostic testing. The following objectives and key terms are important for a good understanding of this chapter.

Key Terms

computed tomography (CT) (p. 1100)
nuclear magnetic resonance imaging (MRI) (p. 1100)
ultrasonography (p. 1100)

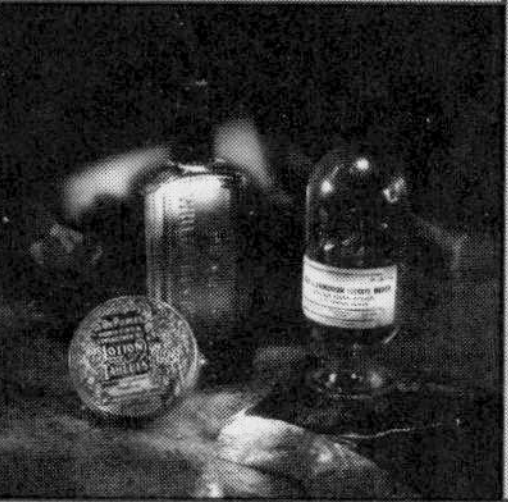

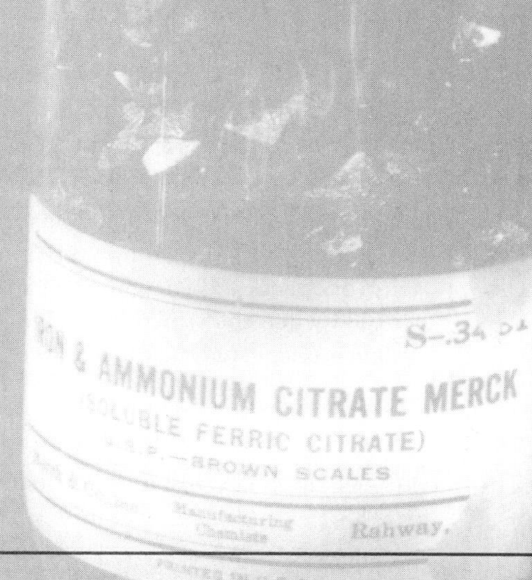

Objectives

1. Describe the mechanism of action of radiopaque contrast medium.
2. State of method of absorption, metabolism, and excretion of barium sulfate and iodinated contrast media.
3. Discuss the nursing assessments necessary to detect side effects/adverse reactions from the administration of iodinated contrast medium and the appropriate nursing interventions to manage the initial symptoms.
4. Explain the pharmacokinetics of diagnostic agents used as radioactive tracers and imaging agents.
5. State the indications, secondary effects, and nursing management of common nonradioactive agents used for evaluating organ function and challenging glandular response.
6. Discuss common tests used for screening for selected health conditions.

Diagnostic agents are chemical substances used to diagnose or monitor a client's condition or disease. As diagnostic agents, certain secondary chemical characteristics are used to confirm a diagnosis or prognosis or to guide therapy. For example, one type of diagnostic agent may interact with a bodily fluid specimen as a reagent to produce a color as an indicator, or it may induce an inflammatory response or an enhancement of a particular gland's functioning.

Other agents may act by contrasting and enhancing visibility on x-ray film of the lumens or cavities of internal body structures. Some, because of a special affinity and uptake by certain organs, permit critical assessment of organ function. Diagnostic agents may also have side effects and adverse reactions, just like any drug. Thus it is necessary that the nurse know the agent used, its mechanism of action, and indications for use. Secondary effects are equally important, since many agents have a somewhat narrow range of safety. In some instances, nurses are responsible for correctly collecting and testing specimens and interpreting the results. Specialized training and professional education are necessary to administer some kinds of agents; others are packaged in simple kit form for over-the-counter sale. Because the field of diagnostics and its products is burgeoning, manufacturers' instructions should always be consulted to be assured of current information.

RADIOPAQUE AGENTS FOR VISUALIZING ORGAN STRUCTURE

When injected or instilled, radiopaque contrast agents make the body cavity or compartment more radiographically dense or opaque than neighboring anatomic structures. They are used when the structural integrity of a soft-tissue organ system is under study. Ordinary x-ray examinations are useful only for studies of dense materials such as bone. Radiopaque contrast media may also permit visualization of organs' functional dynamics as part of associated diagnostic tests.

Many of these agents contain molecular iodine in the radiopaque contrast medium to provide the opacity necessary for outlining internal organ cavities, lumens, or ducts that would otherwise be invisible by x-ray examination or fluoroscopy.

Barium contrast media consist of barium sulfate powder and a vehicle such as hydrosol gum for mixing with prescribed volume of water to provide a suspension for oral or rectal administration. Iodinated radiopaque agents consist of substituted, triiodinated, benzoic acid derivatives or water-soluble, triiodinated, benzoic acid salts. Check manufacturers' instructions for ingredients.

The prescriber should be consulted when a client reports a history of idiosyncratic response or hypersensitivity to iodine, shellfish, or contrast media, or a history of multiple radiographic or radionuclide studies. The most common radiopaque contrast agents are barium sulfate suspensions and iodinated contrast materials. Table 72-1 lists Medications, Iodine Content, and Indications.

Indications

1. Barium-containing preparations are typically used to opacify the gastrointestinal (GI) tract which is generally performed when ulcers, inflammatory bowel disease, or cancer is suspected. One of the most common uses of barium contrast media is in "double-contrast" studies for gastrointestinal tract evaluation. "Double contrast" is a method of making an x-ray image by using two contrast agents, usually a gaseous medium and a water-soluble radiopaque agent.
2. The most frequent clinical use of iodinated contrast media include intravenous urography and angiography.

TABLE 72-1 Medications, iodine content, and indications

Medication	Indications	Iodine content
Contrast media		
diatrizoate sodium injection (Hypaque Sodium)	cerebral angiography aortography cholangiography	150 mg/ml (25% solution) 300 mg/ml (50% solution)
iocetamic acid (Cholebrine)	oral cholecystography	465 mg/750 mg tablet
iopanoic acid (Telepaque)	oral cholecystography	333 mg/500 mg tablet
ipodate (Oragrafin)	oral cholecystography	3 grams contains 61.7% iodine
tyropanoate (Bilopaque)	oral cholecystography	430 mg/750 mg capsule
Other agents		
amiodarone (Cordarone)	antiarrhythmic	74 mg/200 mg tablet
iodoquinol (Yodoxin)	antiprotozoal	134-416 mg/tablet
echothiophate iodide ophthalmic (Phospholine Iodide)	antiglaucoma cyclostimulant diagnostic aid	5-41 μg/drop
idoxuridine ophthalmic (Herplex, Stoxil)	antiviral	18 μg/drop

Modified from Farwell & Braverman, 1996; *USP DI*, 1996.

Iodinated contrast media are often used during computed tomography (CT) of the head and body to visualize vascular structures and to detect tumors.

Pharmacokinetics. Radiopaque agents may be administered by the oral, vaginal, rectal, intravenous, intraarterial routes or they may be instilled into other body cavities. Orally administered iodinated agents for visualization of the gallbladder are absorbed across the GI mucosa and enter the systemic circulation through the portal venous system. Orally or rectally administered iodinated media for delineation of the GI tract are absorbed only minimally, but enough so that the renal tract may also be visualized. Barium sulfate preparations are not absorbed. They are metabolized by the liver and gallbladder and excreted by the kidneys.

Side effects/adverse reactions. Radiopaque agents are not without risk. Effects are diverse, mild to moderate in severity, and usually occur within 1 to 3 minutes. However, delayed reactions may occur up to 1 hour after injection. Anaphylaxis and hypersensitivity reactions are also reported.

Intravenous cholangiography has caused the highest number of reactions and has therefore been largely replaced by radionuclide diagnostics and retrograde duodenal examination. Excretory urography is performed frequently with only rare serious reactions. Milder reactions result from administration of oral cholecystographic agents. Certain agents are more likely to cause secondary effects than others; manufacturers' information should be consulted.

A history of allergy puts the client at twice the risk of reaction to contrast media, although, paradoxically, these are not true hypersensitivity reactions. Clients with a previous anaphylactoid reaction to contrast media may have an increased risk of tenfold or more (Olin, 1996).

Barium sulfate preparations, since they are not absorbed internally, are only potentially hazardous when administered to persons with bowel perforations or fistulas. If allowed to remain in the colon, barium sulfate may cause constipation. Hospitalization and close observation during the procedures are recommended for persons who have high potential for reactions or complications.

The most common side effects reported are nausea or flushing, with feelings of warmth over the abdomen and chest. Severely dehydrated clients, the elderly, infants, and the seriously ill tolerate these hemodynamic and hyperosmolar changes less well than others do.

Rare adverse reactions include cerebral hematomas, hemodynamic alterations, sinus bradycardia, transient ECG changes, ventricular fibrillation, and petechiae.

Diazoate salts inhibit blood coagulation, which may result in a severe thromboembolic event (McEvoy, 1996). Platelet aggregation is inhibited by several of the agents. Exacerbations of sickle cell disease may result from intravascular injections of contrast media.

Renal system involvement may be manifested by nephrosis of proximal tubular cells in excretory urography, which may proceed to renal failure. Altered respiratory status may include rhinitis, cough, dyspnea, bronchospasm, asthma, laryngeal or pulmonary edema, and subclinical pulmonary emboli.

The senses may be impaired, such as distorted taste sensations, or irritated, itching, tearing eyes, or conjunctivitis. Hypersensitivity reactions and anaphylaxis may occur. History of allergy predisposes to reactions to contrast media.

■ Nursing Management

Radiopaque Agents

Assessment. Radiographic examinations are not without hazard to the client or to personnel. Risk-benefit ratios must be established on an individual basis. Reactions may arise from either physical or chemical properties of the compounds used. Almost any organ system may be affected. (See Side effects/adverse reactions.) Conduct a careful history related to kidney, thyroid, or liver disease. Take an allergy history paying particular attention to previous reactions to contrast media or iodine-containing foods, such as shellfish or iodized table salt. Pretreatment with prednisone, diphenhydramine (Benadryl), and ephedrine for clients with a history of iodine hypersensitivity and those with a generally positive allergy history may minimize but not prevent hypersensitivity reactions. This pretreatment regimen reduced the incidence of adverse reactions in one study from 35% to 3%. Do not mix these pretreatment medications for concurrent administration with the contrast media; they are incompatible.

It is recommended that radiography, fluoroscopy, or computed tomography not be performed in a female client who is pregnant or after the first 10 days after menses.

Review the client's current medication regimen for significant drug interactions which may occur when the oral cholecystographic agents are given with the drugs listed below.

Drug	Possible effect and management
cholestyramine (Questran)	The cholestyramine will absorb the cholecystographic agents, thus interfering with the test. Avoid concurrent administration for at least 8 hours or more when tests involving these agents are scheduled.
iodipamide meglumine IV	Prior administration of the oral agents may block liver metabolism and excretion of this drug. Administration of both drugs within 24 hours is not recommended.
urographic agents	Renal toxicity has been reported in clients with abnormal liver function when tests involving these agents were done following the oral urographic agents. Avoid concurrent administration.

The following interactions may occur when the radiopaque parenteral agents are given with the drugs listed below.

Drug	Possible effect and management
aspirin, nonsteroidal anti-inflammatory drugs, and other antiplatelet agents	May enhance the antiplatelet effect, since high levels of iodipamide meglumine, diatrizoate sodium, and diatrizoate meglumine all inhibit platelet aggregation. Monitor the client for bleeding and the platelet count.
inotropic agents	May result in a paradoxic cardiac depressant effect, which is dangerous if client has an ischemic myocardium. Monitor closely if agents must be administered concurrently.

Assist in making the decision to administer anesthesia to restless or agitated clients, especially children. Closely monitor the condition of anesthetized clients; they are at higher risk for adverse reactions than unanesthetized clients.

Have a baseline assessment of the client's vital signs, mental status, and level of consciousness before testing.

Nursing diagnosis. The client receiving radiopaque agents for diagnostic testing should be assessed for the following nursing diagnoses: altered comfort (flushing of the skin, nausea); altered tissue integrity related to irritation or extravasation at the injection site; altered protection related to leukopenia, thrombocytopenia, and anemia; altered bowel elimination (constipation); and the collaborative problems of hypersensitivity to the agent, nephrotoxicity, adverse cardiovascular and CNS effects of the agent.

Implementation

Monitoring. Monitor levels of consciousness and vital signs during the procedure as feasible and afterward for at least 1 hour. Monitor for flushing of the skin, nausea, and other untoward effects of the agents.

Intervention. Prepare clients appropriately for their examinations using protocols from the radiology department. A repeat preparation and examination may be necessary if visualization was sufficiently impaired. This impairment may be the result of inadequate bowel preparation, tablets not taken as directed, or foods and fluids other than water were not withheld. Manufacturers' instructions for dose preparation and administration should be followed. Iodinated radiopaque agents may be administered orally (tablets, paste, granules, or suspensions), rectally (enema), parenterally, or instilled. The tablet form of the agent may require four to six of the tablets taken over a short interval the morning before the test, with the client ingesting nothing else but water after their administration. Barium sulfate compounds are noniodinated, and most are prepared from powders for suspensions to be taken orally or instilled rectally. The volume of orally administered reconstituted agents is about 8 ounces; the enema volume may range from 500 to 1500 ml. Intravenous injection volumes vary according to the agent, from 20 to 300 ml. Direct injection of certain high concentrations of iothalamate solutions should never be made into carotid or vertebral arteries. Elderly clients should be hydrated before barium tests to help prevent post-test constipation.

Nurses should ask for lead shielding devices and client-supporting devices before participating in radiographic examinations. If the nurse is frequently involved, individual cumulative exposure should be monitored by wearing a film badge that is checked monthly or quarterly. Wear it outside any shields; obtain reports. Along with the client going to the radiology department, transport a bedpan, an emesis basin, tissues, and a warm blanket (room temperature and equipment in radiologic units are often noted to be cold).

Have drugs, equipment, and medical assistance readily available in case of an emergency such as cardiac arrest.

Obtain an order for enemas until clear or laxatives as necessary after a barium enema or similarly instruct the client.

Education. Apprise clients and all those working in an environment of ionizing radiation that therapy may be current and long-term effects of radiation and of the fact that these effects are cumulative. Since there is no established safe dosage, single or cumulative, keep exposure to a minimum. The risks and benefits of each procedure should be weighed carefully by the clinician and the informed client.

Instruct the client, as appropriate, to prepare for the specific examination. This may require taking the agent with water the night before the procedure, the administration of enemas, or not ingesting anything but water until the test is completed. Explain as appropriate that the procedure may include the administration of about 8 ounces of a fairly thick oral suspension or a retention enema and that position changes may be necessary during the procedure.

Evaluation. The client will complete the diagnostic procedure without any adverse effects of the agents.

AGENTS FOR EVALUATING ORGAN FUNCTION

Some diagnostic agents can be used to track and visualize the functional processes of organ systems. Inferences can be made about organ function by measurement of the degree or rate at which the agent is distributed, taken up, sequestered, secreted, or excreted from the target organ system or by measurement of the volume or flow rates. Some of these diagnostic agents are radionuclides (a species of radioactive atom characterized by higher atomic number than bodily tissues) whose gamma-ray emissions can be tracked or whose residues can be sampled. Other nonradioactive agents are dyes, polysaccharides, or other substances whose dissemination may be traced by color changes or chemical analysis.

Radioactive Agents

A *radionuclide* is an unstable form of a chemical element. Radiopharmaceutical agents are those in which one of the nonradioactive atoms has been replaced by a radioactive atom. They are either of natural origin or are produced by particle accelerators or generators. The process of neutron activation used in nuclear medicine to produce radionuclides describes the capture of a slow neutron into a stable nucleus with the subsequent emission of a gamma ray. Transmutation is a similar operation, using instead a fast neutron. After injection or ingestion of the resultant nuclide, its pharmacokinesis can be followed by a gamma-ray detector combined with either a rectilinear scanner, scintillation camera, Bender-Blau camera, or other radiation-display device. Some substances such as glucose, ^{14}C, air, blood, lymph, spinal fluids, urine, or biopsy specimens may be collected and the residual radioactivity analyzed or counted as it is excreted. These data are used to make inferences about organ disorders and the body's ability to absorb, metabolize, or excrete substances.

Ionizing radiation. Much can be learned through the use of radiation that could not otherwise be discovered or diagnosed. Like any other diagnostic technique, a risk-benefit ratio must be determined. Ionizing radiation has the ability to knock electrons out of atoms, creating electrically charged ions. This radiation may be defined as electromagnetic radiation (x-rays and gamma rays) or particulate radiation (electrons, occasionally beta particles, protons, neutrons, or atomic nuclei with kinetic energy).

Impact by emitted radiation energy may disrupt bonds between atoms in such crucial biologic molecules as DNA. Disruption can lead to cell death, mutations, or defective mitosis. Energy that is absorbed by tissues can lead to acute effects (as in radiotherapy or radiation accidents) or chronic effects (as from multiple low radiation doses). Effects (like cataracts) may appear only after long periods or in subsequent generations.

The amount of radiation absorbed by tissues during radiologic tests is determined by the dose administered, the half-life of the radionuclide, the energy, the mode of decay, and the length of time the agent dwells within the body. There is no known safe dosage of ionizing radiation despite limits set by the Nuclear Regulatory Commission and the National Council on Radiation, Protection and Measurements.

Estimations of the amount of radiation emitted, the effect, and the dose absorbed may be denoted by the following terms. A *roentgen* is the amount of gamma or x radiation that creates 1 electrostatic unit of ions in 1 ml of air at 0° C. A *rem* is the predicted effect on the human body of a 1-roentgen dose. A *rad* is a unit of measurement of absorbed ionizing radiation energy. One rad = 100 ergs of radiation energy per gram of matter.

Although arbitrary, annual limits for radiation for the general population and for any single gestational period have been set at 0.5 rem (for x-rays, 1 rem is equal to 1 rad) and for closely monitored occupational workers at about 3 rem/year. Most nurses, physicians, and other health personnel are not routinely monitored for radiation exposure unless assigned to an area with high potential for exposure. Their risk for cumulative exposure is nonetheless higher than that of the general population. (See the Nursing Research box at right.)

Very little is known about the full effects of radiation. Certain increased risks are associated, however, as follows: infertility, birth defects, potential for certain malignant neoplasms, and manifestations of aging. Exposure to low-level ionizing radiation, such as that from radiographic examinations, and agents containing radionuclides add to the individual's total radiation history. Effects may be insidious, perhaps manifesting themselves in crucial enzyme defects many years after exposure. There is some evidence of the body's ability to repair chromosomal damage, but the scope of this ability is unknown.

"Excessive radiation exposure" is any unnecessary exposure above natural background levels. Although natural background radiation adds to the cumulative risk, medical and dental therapies account for the largest proportion of artificially generated exposure.

Indications. Most radionuclides in use today in radiology are for imaging of organs, evaluating organ function, or detecting or treating cancer. The role of nuclear imaging is gradually diminishing because of increased reliance on computed tomography, ultrasound, and magnetic resonance imaging.

Nursing Research

Radiation hazard in the health care environment

The potential hazard of ionizing radiation exposure to health care workers who routinely stabilize the necks of trauma patients during cervical spine radiography was studied by Singer et al. Using an artificial torso, they placed a radiation monitor where a health worker's fingers, hands, arms, and thyroid gland would be, and standard cervical spine radiographs were taken. If the simulated exposures were indicative of actual patient situations, a health care worker who holds the head of a trauma patient four times each week with unshielded hands would receive more than twice the maximum allowable annual occupational radiation exposure to the extremities recommended by the National Council of Radiation Protection and Measurements. It was concluded that health workers who routinely stabilize the necks of trauma patients during cervical spine radiography may incur a radiation risk and that 0.5-mm lead-equivalent gloves provide an effective barrier to ionizing radiation (Singer, 1989).

Rules and regulations of federal agencies and state radiation protection programs provide the bases for hospital policy regarding radiation safety for nurses. Each agency with radiology services has a radiation safety officer to ensure that radiation exposures to health care personnel will be as low as reasonably achievable and that special consideration will be given to pregnant nurses (Janowski, 1992).

Critical thinking questions

- Why is it particularly important that pregnant women be protected from radiation?
- Janowski (1992) indicated that many nurses and other health care providers have a strong fear—almost a phobia—of radiation. Why might that be so? What could be done to minimize this fear?

From Singer et al (1989); Janowski (1992).

Radionuclides are used as tracers to evaluate physiologic and biochemical functioning of organ systems. By imaging methods, extremely sensitive radioactivity sensing devices make it possible to detect, count, visualize, and analyze minute amounts of radionuclides. Uniquely useful applications of nuclear imagery include the following:

1. Thyroid enlargement or disease. Agents currently used include ^{131}I and ^{123}I. They are iodine isotopes that emit a type of radiation that can be mapped externally. Usually a 24 hour uptake study is employed to determine the extent and areas of thyroid activity. A scan is then performed to evaluate any thyroid mass or enlargement. "Cold" tumors have a 20% to 25% probability of representing a thyroid cancer. Tumors that localize the radionuclide well are usually benign.

2. Screening individuals with diagnosed malignancies for metastases. Many clients treated for breast cancer, colon cancer, malignant melanoma, lymphoma, prostate cancer, and lung cancer, among others, are often successfully evaluated periodically by scintigrams of the liver, spleen, and skeletal system. A scintigraph is a photographic recording showing the distribution and intensity of radioactivity in various tissues and organs following the administration of a radiopharmaceutical. The risk-benefit ratio is very high, and information about new or recurrent disease can help the oncologist and the client make crucial decisions about goals, management, prognosis, and so forth.
3. Evaluation of heart disease is a primary application of nuclear imagery. Computers are used to analyze data from the images to detect the extent of myocardial damage and wall motion abnormalities and to estimate the ejection fraction of the ventricles. Underlying coronary artery disease can also be estimated by the use of radionuclides before catheterization or other invasive procedures.
4. Tracking physiologic substances and assessment of the status of an organ (e.g., renal function, biliary excretion, etc). In addition to diagnostic uses, some radiopharmaceuticals may be administered therapeutically to deliver radiation to internal body tissues (e.g., ^{131}I for destruction of thyroid tissue in hyperthyroidism). Radioactive tracer substances may also be incorporated into a nonradioactive drug to track the second drug's pharmacokinetics for research purposes.

Computed tomography (CT) scans body parts in a series of contiguous slices with pencil-thin x-ray beams, which, after passing through the body, produce data from detectors positioned diametrically across from the beam source. Huge amounts of data are integrated and displayed by computer as a video image. CT presents a series of two-dimensional images representing a reconstructed "slice" in the axial plane. By viewing a series of these images, one can perceive the anatomy in a three-dimensional sense. CT therefore often conveys more information than other modalities about lesion density, location, and size.

CT has largely replaced older techniques such as pneumoencephalography and angiography in the diagnosis of intracranial disease, though angiography is still used in this application. CT may eliminate the need for other x-ray examinations, but it is not considered a first-line, or screening, technique. Radionuclide scans continue to be used for initial diagnostic screening and for specific tests where their results are more fruitful. Radiation exposure from CT varies depending on the equipment used and the frequency of testing, but it is said to be equal to or sometimes considerably higher than ordinary x-ray techniques or radionuclides. Although CT is considered to be a noninvasive procedure, intravenous contrast material is frequently injected to enhance structures for differential diagnosis. This is referred to as CT with infusion.

Ultrasonography is a nonradioactive diagnostic modality with cardiovascular, abdominal, obstetric, and other applications. It is used with anatomic and physiologic information obtained by other nuclear medicine techniques. Ultrasound examinations yield data about organ contours and tissue consistency or, in the case of Doppler scanning, blood flow patterns. Results can be distorted in the presence of bone or gases in the body. The secondary effects of high-frequency sound waves on cellular structures and functions are not fully known, though such tests are considered to be noninvasive and innocuous by many in the field.

Nuclear magnetic resonance imaging (MRI) is a diagnostic modality that uses radio waves and a magnet, not radiation, drugs, biopsy specimens, or body fluids. Like CT, MRI provides sectioned imagery but gives more than the gross anatomic information gained by CT scanning. MRI supplies extremely detailed images of internal heart and brain structures, for example, and is capable of imaging areas of the spine, abdomen, and extremities. It can differentiate between lesions and normal tissue. Persons ineligible for diagnostics by MRI include those with metal prostheses or pacemakers, because the strong magnetic field surrounding the client may move some metallic devices, or a metallic object may result in a distorted test image.

Pharmacokinetics. Each type of radionuclide emits alpha or beta particles or gamma rays, or a combination of these. This spontaneous emission of charged particles is termed radioactive decay and eventually results in disintegration of the nucleus. The time it takes for the original radioactivity to decay to one half its original value is known as the physical or radioactive *half-life* of the particular radionuclide. Like a drug, the rate at which a tracer substance is excreted from the body also influences its effects, both valuable and undesirable.

Dosage and administration. Manufacturers' current directions should be reviewed. Dosages are not detailed here because they vary with individual needs.

The major considerations in radionuclide dosing are the amount of radioactivity that is administered to produce effective readings and the secondary radionuclide effects. While the radioactive material is in the body, it is irradiating even after the study has been completed, whereas x-rays irradiate from an external source and do so only while the body is exposed during the examination. The radionuclide dosage unit for imaging or nonimaging doses of radionuclide is a *microcurie* (one millionth of a curie). A *curie* is a specified measure of radioactivity associated with a specific amount of a radioactive substance, e.g., a radionuclide. Recommended dosages are spelled out in manufacturers' literature. The client's absorbed dose of each radionuclide has been predicted for each procedure with the following three factors being considered: (a) the biologic parameters that describe the uptake, distribution, retention, and release of the radiopharmaceutical in the body; (b) the energy released by the radionuclide and whether it is penetrating or nonpenetrating; and (c) the fraction of the emitted energy that is absorbed by the target.

The ultimate radiation dose to both the target organ and the whole body is somewhat less in radionuclide nonimaging procedures than in imaging procedures. It is considerably more in radiation therapy (not discussed here).

Shielding is a practical method to prevent or reduce excess radiation exposure of staff or clients during certain diagnostic examinations. Shielding reduces radiation intensity to acceptable limits in body areas not intended for exposure during the radiologic examination. Alpha and beta radiation require very little shielding. An alpha particle can be blocked by the thickness of a sheet of paper, a beta particle by an inch of wood, but several feet of concrete or several inches of lead are necessary to stop gamma or x radiation. Half-value layer is the term describing the thickness of any material required to reduce the intensity of an x-ray or gamma-ray beam to half its original value. Because of its characteristic density, lead is the material typically used in radiation shielding equipment and coverings such as aprons and gloves.

■ Nursing Management

Radioactive Agents

In addition to the nursing management of clients receiving radiopaque contrast media, consider the following:

Implementation

Intervention. The basic principles of radiation exposure safety are relative to the source of radiation: *time* spent in the radioactive field, *distance* from the source, and *shielding*. The amount of radiation absorbed is directly proportional to the time spent in a radioactive field and inversely related to the distance from the source of radioactive emission. Thus quality nursing care requires careful planning so that limitations on time spent in the radioactive field do not reduce the quality of client care.

Wear rubber or plastic gloves when handling bedpans, urine specimens, or continuous drainage bags of clients within a day or two after nuclear medicine procedures. Wherever radionuclides are used, one person, designated the radiation safety officer, has the responsibility for safety in case of spills or accidents with radioactive materials. This officer should be consulted if there is a break in safety procedures or if, for example, linen has been contaminated by vomitus or excreta within 24 hours of administration of a radiopharmaceutical. Although it may be determined that unusual precautions are not needed, it is wise to seek consultation as needed.

Follow instructions by radiopharmaceutical manufacturers about radionuclide storage (some require refrigeration), dosage, and technique. Errors in technique must not be tolerated, especially with regard to the handling of radiopharmaceuticals, disposal of contaminated equipment, and proper shielding of all present for radiologic and imaging procedures. Monitoring badges should be worn by those regularly participating in these procedures. Protection should be assured for those who are unfamiliar with these procedures. Women of child-bearing age who are more than 10 days after menses or who are pregnant should not assist. (*Radiation therapy* requires other precautions.)

Education. Clients' anxieties may be heightened by the uncertainty of unknown diagnosis, fear of radiation, and cold or unfamiliar surroundings. Clients may be introduced to the personnel, surroundings, and the large equipment some time before scheduled examinations and given opportunity for questions and explanations.

Clients should be taught that there may be some discomfort at the site of injection, taste alterations, or a feeling of warmth or discomfort in various parts of the body if the administered agent contains an iodine preparation. If a counter or rectilinear scanner is used, clients should be advised that it may typically emit irregular clicks as it collects data; it does not emit radiation. Since clients may be required to maintain a single position on a hard surface for extended periods or may be briefly restrained, supply foam wedge supports and coverings as necessary. Explain that personnel may wear strange-looking gray or green apparel to shield them from excess radiation and that clients too will be protected by protocols that have been established. Then adhere to them.

Give clients written instructions, especially about the specific time they should return for the examination after the nuclide dose. Explain that the test must be performed at a very specific time after the medication is administered (at the point of a specific half-life).

Follow your health care agencies policies related to length, frequency, and duration of exposure to clients in the post-test period. Provide instructions too on care for the client at home.

Nonradioactive Agents

Nonradioactive Agents for Evaluating Organ Function via Volumes and Flows

These relatively biologically inert and nonradioactive substances are commonly used to measure flow rates, fluid volumes, diffusion, concentration ability, and organ function. These compounds are mostly dyes, polysaccharides, or other substances that can be assayed chemically or detected by characteristic colors after administration. Many of the dye tests determine the rate of plasma clearance of the dye by the organ under study. The ability to measure certain parameters against known normal values at defined points in the procedure makes these compounds useful as diagnostic aids. They are used variously for evaluation of cardiac output, liver or kidney function or blood flows, circulation time, intestinal absorption, and so forth (Box 72-1).

These compounds are administered primarily by the intravenous or intramuscular routes. They are rapidly absorbed by the organ system under examination and are usually excreted by that system. These drugs are relatively pharmacologically inert and are used to measure specific physiologic functions without themselves significantly altering those functions (Table 72-2).

Nonradioactive Agents for Challenging Glandular Response

Certain compounds are used diagnostically to challenge a particular system, often glandular, to produce measurable responses. Secretory responses indicate whether there is functional integrity within the secreting gland or system. Many of these testing agents are protein substances that mimic the action of naturally occurring bodily chemicals such as secretagogues for exocrine gland response and stimulants for

BOX 72-1

Selected Multiple Urine Tests

Measures	Chemstrip GP	Combistix	HemaCombistix	Uristix-4	Keto-Diastix	Chemstrip 6	Labstix	BiliLabstix	Multistix SG*	Multistix 7	Multistix 10 SG*	Chemstrip 9	Multistix 9	Chemstrip 2LN	Multistix 2
glucose	X	X	X	X	X	X	X	X	X	X	X	X	X		
protein	X	X	X	X		X	X	X	X	X	X	X	X		
pH		X	X			X	X	X	X	X	X	X	X		
blood		X	X			X	X	X	X	X	X	X	X		
ketones					X	X	X	X	X	X	X	X	X		
bilirubin								X	X		X	X	X		
urobilinogen									X		X	X	X		
nitrite				X						X	X	X	X	X	X
leukocytes				X		X				X	X	X	X	X	X

Modified and adapted from Olin, 1996.
*Also measures specific gravity.

TABLE 72-2 Selected nonradioactive agents for evaluation of organ function

Agent	Indication(s)	Secondary effects	Nursing management
aminohippurate sodium	measure renal plasma flow and tubular secretory mechanism	nausea, vomiting, cramping, flushing, and tingling	give IV at constant rate; caution with clients with low cardiac reserve, may precipitate congestive heart failure
D-xylose (Xylo-Pfan)	evaluates intestinal absorption	infrequent: nausea, vomiting, cramps, and diarrhea	there are a number of medical conditions that give false positives with this test; check the literature
indocyanine green (Cardio-Green)	measures cardiac output, hepatic function, and used for ophthalmic angiography	low incidence of side effects	caution with clients who have a history of iodide allergy; IV
inulin	diagnostic for renal function	minimal side effects	intravenous injection
mannitol (Osmitrol)	diuretic, antiglaucoma, antihemolytic	dry mouth, thirst, headache, acidosis, dehydration. Contraindicated in anuria, intracranial bleeding, severe dehydration, and pulmonary edema	IV infusion; monitor vital signs and urinary output closely

Modified from AHFS, 1996; *USP DI*, 1996.

endocrine secretion. Since most of these agents are administered IM or IV, they move rapidly to the site of action. Degradation of these agents is equally rapid.

Nonradioactive agents are used to evaluate or enhance capabilities such as thyroid secretion, gallbladder contraction, insulin response, and gastric acid secretory function. These testing agents act on the targeted gland or site as releasing factors. Thus secondary effects may be as widespread and disruptive to bodily chemical balance as a large dose of the secretion or hormone itself (Table 72-3).

Epinephrine, antihistamines, corticoids, and a tourniquet should be readily available for all tests in case of severe reactions. Analgesics, nasogastric suction equipment, vasodilators (for histamine agents), intravenous glucose solutions

TABLE 72-3 Common nonradioactive agents for evaluating body response

Agent	Indications/secondary effects	Nursing management
edrophonium (Tensilon)	Diagnostic: myasthenia gravis; cholinergic. Secondary effects: severe cholinergic reaction; bradycardia or cardiac standstill; dysrhythmias.	Have IV atropine 1 mg, available to relieve the adverse muscarinic effects of edrophonium. Monitor vital signs carefully. Have facilities available for CPR, cardiac monitoring, and respiratory assistance. A placebo may be administered first as if it were the test dose to evaluate baseline muscular capabilities. A number of drugs may be withheld for at least 8 hrs; check with prescriber.
histamine	Diagnostic: gastric function. Secondary effects: flushing, dizziness, headache, dyspnea, asthma, urticaria, hypotension or hypertension, tachycardia, GI distress, convulsions.	Withhold food for 12 hr and fluids and smoking for 8 hr before test. Withhold medications: antacids, anticholinergics, alcohol, histamine, histamine receptor antagonists, insulin, parasympathomimetics, adrenergic blockers, corticosteriods. Keep epinephrine available for severe hypotension.
pentagastrin (Peptavlon)	Diagnostic: gastric function in pernicious anemia, Zollinger-Ellison and other GI conditions. Secondary effects: hypersensitivity, stimulates pancreatic secretion, GI distress or bleeding.	Drug of choice for gastric secretion testing. Withhold food, liquids, and smoking after midnight before test. Inform client a nasogastric tube will be passed. Withhold medications as above with histamine. After test, observe for GI distress. Resume usual diet and medications.
protirelin (Thypinone)	Diagnostic: thyroid function. Secondary effects: blood pressure alterations, breast enlargement, nausea, increased urination, dizziness, dry mouth, headache.	Have client urinate and assume a supine position. Drug is administered as a bolus over 15-30 seconds. Take BP frequently over the first 15 minutes. Increases in BP (less than 30 mm Hg) are more common than decreases. Use caution in clients with whom rapid changes in BP would be dangerous.
sincalide (Kinevac)	Diagnostic: gallbladder and pancreatic function. Secondary effects: hypersensitivity, nausea, cramps, dizziness, flushing.	Administered IV. Adverse effects usually occur immediately after the injection and last for a few minutes.
tolbutamide (Orinase Diagnostic)	Diagnostic: pancreatic islet cell function. Secondary effects: severe hypoglycemia.	Instruct client to adhere to a 150-300 g/day carbohydrate diet for 3 days before test and to fast overnight. Avoid smoking during fast and the test. Tolbutamide not administered to clients with known sensitivities to the drug or other sulfonylurea drugs. Withhold medications: salicylates and other drugs known to potentiate the hypoglycemic action of tolbutamide for 3 days before the exam (see Chapter 50). If severe hypoglycemia occurs during the test, administer 12.5-25 g of glucose in a 25%-50% IV.

(for tolbutamide), and atropine (for edrophonium) should also be kept available. Manufacturers' instructions should be followed very closely because nearly all these compounds are administered parenterally and in very small doses.

AGENTS FOR SCREENING AND MONITORING DISORDERS AND IMMUNE STATUS

Screening and monitoring agents may be extracts of common allergens (ragweed, grasses, trees, molds, animal dander, and foods) or purified derivatives or concentrates of microbial antigens, hormones, or animal cellular antigens, or they may be chemical reagents. Many chemical reagents for common diagnostic purposes are packaged in simple kit form for over-the-counter or prescribed purchase; they may also be used routinely in institutions and primary health care settings.

Mechanism of action, pharmacokinetics. Antigens applied topically or intradermally cause antigen-antibody reactions, which may be manifested by a local inflammatory response at the test site. The test site is assessed after a prescribed time interval. A positive response is indicated by the presence of erythema and induration (a firm lump under the skin). In the case of microbial antigen challenge, this positive response may merely indicate a previous exposure to the microbe or its products, but not necessarily the presence of an active disease process. False negative results may also occur, and further investigation may be necessary. The size of the erythematous area or induration may be measured to estimate the degree of the person's sensitivity or immune response. These responses may be short lived or of lifelong duration. (See also Chapter 63.)

Persons who are immunosuppressed because of cancer chemotherapy or radiation treatments, malnutrition, debilitation, or congenital or acquired immunodeficiency syndrome (AIDS) may demonstrate no response (anergy) when tested with a prescribed battery of antigen challenges. These persons are extremely vulnerable to infection and may need metabolic support and precautions to avoid infection. Test results may not be reliable in those who have viral infections, are febrile or uremic, or have recently received live viral vaccinations.

Indications. Some diagnostic agents measure a person's physiologic response or hypersensitivity to the agent as a specific chemical challenge. These agents are typically used in simple baseline screening procedures as part of an initial diagnostic workup. Some are used in skin tests by patch, prick, scratch, or intradermal injection to assess hypersensitivity (allergy), anergy (congenital or acquired inability to develop a cell-mediated reaction), cellular immunity, or antibody response (Table 72-4). Others are used as reagents in specimens of blood, urine, and bodily discharges for detection of the levels of certain components to facilitate diagnosis or to monitor known conditions (Table 72-5; see Box 72-1).

TABLE 72-4 Biologic agents for diagnostic tests

Biologic product*	Indication/adult dose
Tuberculin (purified protein derivative, PPD, Mantoux Test) (Aplitest, Tuberculin Tine Test)	Diagnostic: tuberculosis Adult dose; 5 U.S. units, intradermal. Special instructions for application of Tine test should be followed.
Tuberculin (PPD) (Aplisol, Tubersol)	Diagnostic: tuberculosis Adult dose: 5 U.S. units, intradermal following specific instructions as noted by manufacturer or *USP DI*.
Allergenic extracts	Several hundred individual purified fluid allergens available for diagnosis and hyposensitization of allergies: pollens, poison ivy, foods, dusts, yeast and other allergens. Treatment: periodic subcutaneous injection of gradually increasing potent dilutions of specific allergen.

*See nursing management for each of these agents.

Side effects/adverse reactions. Local reactions to skin tests do not usually cause discomfort. Occasionally a highly positive reaction will result in vesiculation and necrosis of overlying skin; corticosteroids may be ordered. Transient tachycardia, malaise, or low-grade fever may occur separately from a local reaction. Occasionally, a person may report systemic allergic reactions of urticaria, sneezing, or dyspnea. Rarely an overwhelming antigen-antibody response may occur, an anaphylactic response, calling for emergency measures such as the administration of epinephrine and respiratory and circulatory support. All these secondary effects are more likely to occur if hyposensitization therapy is begun, since this includes a well-controlled program of increasing dosages of the allergen in question.

Dosage and administration. For certain standardized tests such as that for coccidioidomycosis, the dosage is fixed (0.1 ml of a 1:100 dilution). Dosages for allergy testing are also very small (0.02 to 0.05 ml) but may be individualized. Manufacturers' instructions for all these diagnostic agents should be followed carefully.

■ Nursing Management

Screening Agents

Assessment. Administer these preparations with care because of their propensity to trigger allergic reactions. Question the client regarding any previous reactions to skin testing. If the client responds positively, dilute test doses of less than one tenth the usual concentration may then be administered.

TABLE 72-5 Common tests for screening selected conditions

Identifies/detects	Test(s)	Available	Identifies/detects	Test(s)	Available
ketones in blood or urine	Acetone tests: Acetest, Ketostix	tablets, strips	human immunodeficiency virus (HIV) tests	HIV-1 LA Recombigen, HIV-1 Latex Agglutination test, HIVAB HIV-1 EIA, others	kits
protein in urine	Albumin tests: Albustix	strips	meningitis	Bactigen N Meningitidis	slide tests
nitrate, uropathogens, bacteria	Microstix-3, Uricult	culture paddle, strips	mononucleosis	Mono-Diff, Mono-Latex, others	kits
bilirubin in urine	Ictotest	tablets	occult blood screening	ColoCare, Colo-Screen, others	kits
urea nitrogen in blood	Azostix	strips	ovulation tests	Answer Ovulation, Clearplan Easy, Ovu-Quick Self-Test, others	kits
Candida albicans, vaginal	Isocult for Candida, CandidaSure	culture paddle reagent slides	human chorionic gonadotropin pregnancy tests	Advance, Answer Plus, Answer Quick & Simple, Fact Plus, others	kits
Chlamydia trachomatis	Chlamydiazyme, Sure Cell Chlamydia	kits	rheumatoid factor	Rheumatex, Rheumaton	slide tests
cholesterol	Advanced Care Cholesterol Test-for home use	kit	hemoglobin S sickle cell test	Sickledex	kit
cryptococcal neoformans in CSF and serum	Crypto-LA	slide tests	*Staphylococcus aureus*	Isocult for Staphylococcus	culture paddles
gastrointestinal duodenal fluid stomach acid	Entero-Test Gastro-Test	string capsules string capsules	streptococci tests	Sure Cell Streptococci, Bactigen Strep B, others	kits
glucose in blood	Chemstrip bG, Dextrostix, Diascan, Glucometer Encore, and others	strips	virus tests, miscellaneous	Human T-Lymphotropic Virus Type, Sure Cell Herpes, Rubazyme for Rubella, others	kits
glucose in urine	Clinitest, Chemstrip bG, Clinistix, Tes-Tape	tablets, strips			
gonorrhea	Biocult-GC, Gonozyme Diagnostic, others	kits			

Implementation

Monitoring. Be prepared for major allergic manifestations such as angioedema, urticaria, serum sickness, or anaphylactic shock, which can occur. Have the person wait for 30 minutes to observe for development of an allergic reaction.

Intervention. Inspect the liquid extract of the antigen for clarity; do not use it if particles are seen. As appropriate, use one of the following methods for administering these diagnostic test agents.

A sterile needle or other instrument may be used to prick or scratch the skin after a drop of the extract is placed on the skin. Depending on the approach used, the results may be read directly or after the testing patch has been removed.

Intradermal injections are commonly done on the ventral surface of the forearm. Use a tuberculin syringe with a 25 to 27 gauge needle. Inject intradermally with the needle nearly parallel to the skin surface, making certain that the needle does not penetrate deeper, into subcutaneous tissue.

This intradermal insertion will increase the precision with which the results may be interpreted; in tuberculin tests it will also prevent febrile reactions.

Stop inserting the needle as soon as the tip of the needle, with its bevel up, has entered the skin but is still visible. Then inject the antigen with steady pressure. A correctly administered intradermal injection will immediately raise a small, colorless bleb or lump.

Have medications available for emergency administration: antihistamines such as diphenhydramine and epinephrine, 0.2 ml for subcutaneous use. Equipment for full circulatory and respiratory support should also be available.

Evaluation. After the injection, there is a prescribed wait, often 20 minutes or several days (depending on the antigen), before the local reaction should be assessed for erythema and induration. A positive reaction to some antigens is determined by the presence of induration alone; erythema is not always a criterion. *Erythema* (redness) is categorized as follows:

(trace)	Faint discoloration
+ (one plus)	Pink
++	Red
+++	Purplish red
++++	Vesiculation or necrosis

Measure the single largest *induration* (area of hardness) or the largest coalesced induration. Induration can be measured with precision in the following way: Placing your index, middle, and ring fingers together, stroke the test site to determine the presence of induration. To delimit the indurated area, using a ball-point pen, draw a line *toward* the indurated area in four directions. Edges of the induration can easily be perceived as the ball-point tip touches them. Stop each marking when the edge is perceived. Then measure the diameter of the remaining unmarked indurated area in millimeters. Or use the following criteria for indurations:

(trace)	Barely palpable
+	Palpable, but not visible
++	Easily palpable and visible; indurated area buckles when squeezed gently
+++	Easily palpable and visible; does not buckle when squeezed gently
++++	Vesiculation or necrosis

Criteria used to categorize Mantoux tuberculin test results according to induration diameter are as follows: less than 5 mm is a negative result; 5 to 9 mm is a questionable result, retesting by another method may be necessary; and more than 9 mm is a positive result.

Indurations resulting from multiple puncture tuberculin testing devices are interpreted as positive if more than 2 mm in diameter. Results are considered less reliable than results of Mantoux tests.

SUMMARY

Diagnostic agents are chemical substances used to diagnose or monitor a condition or disease. Just like other drugs, they may also have side effects and adverse reactions. Radiopaque agents are used for visualizing organ structure. Examinations used for evaluating organ function involve radioactive agents, computed tomography, ultrasonography, and nuclear magnetic resonance imaging. Nonradioactive agents may be used for evaluating organ function via volumes and flows and challenging glandular response. Other agents are available for screening and monitoring the immune status and disorders. It is essential then that the nurse know the agent used, its mechanism of action, and indications, and how to prevent or minimize any adverse effects.

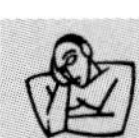

Critical Thinking

1. Bobby Brown, age 24, a newly hired teacher, is required by the school board to have a medical history and physical examination including diagnostic skin testing with tuberculin, the PPD test, completed before his employment is finalized. Why would the PPD be included? What would constitute a positive response for a PPD? What would a positive response indicate? Suppose Mr. Brown tells the nurse who is about to administer his PPD that he has had a positive response to the test in the past. What action should the nurse take?
2. Sally Grey, age 54, has been advised by her health care provider to get a mammogram every year. She confesses to you that she is concerned about excessive radiation exposure. How will you respond?

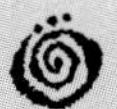

Collaborative Learning Activities

1. Five teams will develop a case study, hopefully based on a client you have cared for in a clinical setting, involving administration of (1) a radiopaque agent; (2) a nonradiopaque agent: (3) a nonradioactive agent for evaluating organ function; (4) a nonreactive agent for challenging glandular response; or (5) a screening agent.

   Each team should identify: (1) type of diagnostic agent; (2) actions and important properties of the agent; (3) precautions, indications, desired effects, and secondary or adverse effects with their case. You should also prepare appropriate nursing interventions, and analysis and evaluation of the nursing interventions in their specific case. However, before you present the final part on nursing interventions, question your classmates on the analysis and nursing interventions.

BIBLIOGRAPHY

American Hospital Formulary Service (1996). *AHFS drug information '96*. Bethesda, MD: American Society of Hospital Pharmacists.

Anderson KN, et al. (Eds.) (1994). *Mosby's medical, nursing, & allied health dictionary* (4th ed.). St Louis: Mosby.

DiPiro JT, et al. (Eds.) (1993). *Pharmacotherapy*. (2nd ed.). Norwalk, CT: Appleton & Lange.

Early PJ & Sodee DB (1991). *Principles and practice of nuclear medicine* (2nd ed.). St Louis: Mosby.

Farwell AP & Braverman LE (1996). Thyroid and antithyroid drugs. In Hardman JG & Limbird LE (Eds.). *Goodman & Gilman's the pharmacological basis of therapeutics* (9th ed.). New York: McGraw-Hill.

Haaga JR & Alfidi RJ (1988). *Computed tomography of the whole body* (2nd ed.). St Louis: Mosby.

Jankowski CB (1992). Radiation protection for nurses: Regulations and guidelines, JONA 17(2):30-4.

Olin BR (Ed.) (1996). *Facts and comparisons.* St Louis: Facts and Comparisons.

Pagana KD & Pagana TJ (1997). *Mosby's diagnostic and laboratory test reference* (3rd ed.). St Louis: Mosby.

Singer CM, et al. (1989). Exposure of emergency medicine personnel to ionizing radiation during cervical spine radiography, *Ann Emerg Med* 18(8):822.

United States Pharmacopeial Convention (1996). *USP DI: Drug information for the health care professional* (16th ed.).Rockville, MD: The Convention.

Watson J & Jaffee MS (1995). *Nurse's manual of laboratory and diagnostic tests* (2nd ed.). Philadelphia: FA Davis.

Chapter 73

Poisons and Antidotes

Chapter Focus

As with most critical illnesses, assessment followed by appropriate interventions will influence the ultimate outcome for the client with poisoning. The role of the nurse is important not only in the treatment of such clients, but also for the teaching of safety promotion and accident prevention to keep poisonings from occurring. The following objectives and key terms are important for a good understanding of this chapter.

Key Terms

acute poisoning (p. 1109)
chronic poisoning (p. 1109)
gastric lavage (p. 1115)
poison (p. 1109)
toxicology (p. 1109)
toxidromes (p. 1110)

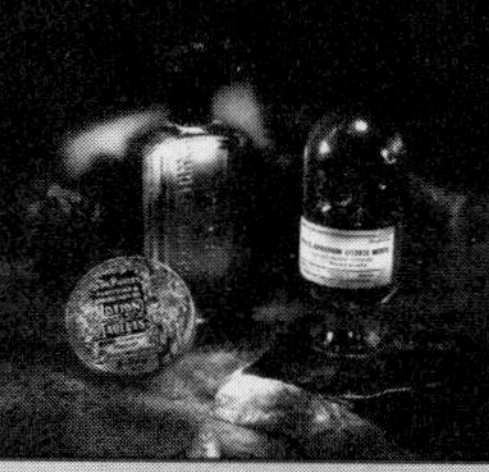

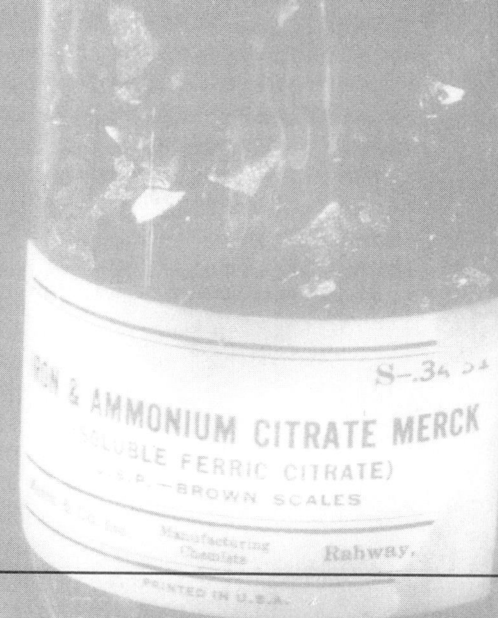

Objectives

1. Discuss the major causes of poisoning in children of various ages.
2. List at least five objective and/or subjective nursing assessments of a client presenting with a suspected poisoning.
3. Describe the four grades of drug overdose-induced coma.
4. Discuss the major drugs causing organ or tissue damage resulting from chemical poisoning.
5. Implement nursing management of the care of a client with suspected poisoning.
6. Implement the nursing management of the pharmacologic treatment of acetaminophen, cyanide, iron, and insecticide overdose.

Regional poison control centers reported 1.8 million calls concerning drug or chemical exposures in the United States during 1991. Approximately 25% of this number required professional treatment with 764 deaths reported (Watson, 1996). While the incidence of children's poisoning is high, mortality rate in this population is usually low. The majority of children's ingestion cases are accidental as compared to most adult drug overdoses which are intentional, the result of a suicide attempt or drug abuse. The latter drug overdoses are reviewed in Chapter 9, Substance Misuse and Abuse.

An unusual type of poisoning has resulted from the proliferation of battery-operated games, cameras, hearing aids, calculators, and watches. An estimated 500 to 600 miniature button or disk batteries are swallowed each year by persons of all ages. Their major component is aqueous potassium hydroxide, which also is used to unclog pipes. Children can mistake small batteries for candy; adults may mistake them for medication tablets. Batteries that lodge in the esophagus, cecum, or other areas of the gastrointestinal tract present two problems: (1) they are locally corrosive to mucosa, causing ulceration or perforation in 1 to 2 hours; and (2) they may cause mercury poisoning when certain battery contents leak. Endoscopic or surgical removal is necessary if the battery remains in the stomach for more than 24 hours, if gastric or peritoneal irritation develops, if radiologic evidence shows the battery lodging or leaking in the gastrointestinal tract, or if the particular type of battery is prone to leakage.

See the Cultural Aspects box below for a discussion of poisoning associated with ethnic remedies.

DETECTION OF POISONS

Toxicology is the study of poisons, their action and effects, methods of detection, and diagnosis and treatment of poisoning. A **poison** can be defined as any substance that in relatively small amounts can cause death or serious bodily harm. All drugs are potential poisons when used improperly or in excess dosage. Poisoning may be acute or chronic. In **acute poisoning** the effects are immediate while in **chronic poisoning** the effects are insidious because of cumulative effects of small amounts of poison absorbed over a prolonged period. Chronic poisoning causes chronic illness, which may or may not be reversible.

Nurses may be confronted with a suspected poisoning in many ways. A mother may call, upset that her small child has

Cultural Aspects Poisoning Associated with Use of Traditional Ethnic Remedies

Traditional herbal products are widely available in the United States and Canada. The consumption of these traditional ethnic remedies can have adverse health effects. However, because they are not marketed as a drug, these products have not been subjected to standard tests for safety and effectiveness.

Kwan and others (1992) reported a case of digitalis toxicity in a 90-year-old Chinese man after he had taken a nonprescription Chinese medication, Yixin Wan, which contained several ingredients including toad venom, ginseng, pearl, and musk. According to the package, it has been shown to be helpful to the client with coronary artery disease and congestive heart failure. Cardiac glycosides are present in a large number of plant extracts and in the venom of toads, and the clinical toxicity of toad venom has been described.

As the result of publicly funded childhood blood lead screening tests in California, Flattery and others (1993) reported 40 cases of elevated blood lead levels in children who had received traditional ethnic remedies. For 36 of the 40 cases, the traditional remedies reported were the Hispanic remedies used for digestive problems, azarcon or greta. Other remedies were paylooah (Southeast Asia) used for rash or fever, surma (India) used to improve eyesight, and an unnamed ayurvedic substance from Tibet used to improve slow development. In many cases, family members initially denied remedy use but reported such use with subsequent case follow-up efforts. The reluctance of family members to report the use of traditional ethnic remedies during initial interviews may reflect factors such as uncertainty about the legality of using such medicines, belief in the effectiveness of these remedies, and concerns regarding responsibility for the child's illness. Also, some persons may not consider these substances to be "remedies" or "medicines"; health care providers should ask about the use of these substances by their common names (USPHS, US Dept of Health and Human Services, 1993).

Horowitz and others (1993) report life-threatening bradycardia with rapid onset and central nervous system and respiratory depression that developed in three unrelated children in Colorado following ingestion of Jin Bu Huan tablets, a Chinese herbal medicine used for relieving pain. On analysis the active ingredient was determined to be levo-tetrahydropalmatine (L-THP), a naloxone resistant substance that results in sedation, analgesia, neuromuscular blockade, and dopamine receptor antagonism. The hazard of this particular substance was a combination of factors, the extreme potency of L-THP, the misidentification of the source plant, the false and potentially leading medical claims, the availability of the product, and the lack of childproof packaging.

To prevent cases of unintentional poisoning associated with herbal and other botanical products, such products should be sold in childproof packaging and kept in childproof containers, and parents should be informed about the potential toxicity of these products. In addition, accurate labeling of the active ingredient is critical to enable prompt and proper medical treatment for unintentional poisoning (USPHS, US Dept of Health and Human Services, 1993).

The use of traditional ethnic remedies in the United States and Canada is quite common. The elderly of ethnic populations and the newly arrived immigrants have a strong cultural belief in traditional medicines and less confidence in "modern" medicine. These traditional remedies are easily obtained in ethnic stores and pharmacies. With a rapidly growing, culturally diverse population, health care providers must be alert for the potential toxicity of nonstandard therapies that these individuals may be taking.

Critical thinking questions

- In your own community, how could you increase your skill in taking drug histories to identify traditional ethnic remedies?
- How could you work within your community to help prevent the poisonings described above?

taken one of her contraceptive pills; a nursing home resident may accidentally drink the glass of peroxide mixture intended as a mouthwash; or a teenager who cannot be aroused may be brought into the emergency room.

Cues that typically point to poisoning include sudden, violent symptoms of severe nausea, vomiting, diarrhea, collapse, or convulsions. If possible, it is important to find out what poison has been taken and how much. Additional information that might prove helpful to the physician in making a diagnosis includes answers to questions or reports of observed phenomena, with the nurse noting the following:

- Any reports of poison contact by the victim
- Poisoning in the "at-risk" age group of children 1 to 5 years old
- Report of a history of previous poisonings or ingestion of foreign substances
- Diverse symptoms or signs referable to multiple organ system involvement that defy diagnosis
- A history of suicidal intent or thought
- Symptoms appearing suddenly in an otherwise healthy individual or a number of persons becoming ill about the same time, as might occur in food poisoning
- Anything unusual about the person, the clothing, or the surroundings; evidence of burns about the lips and mouth; discolored gums; needle (hypodermic) pricks, pustules, or scars on the exposed and accessible surface of the body or dilated or constricted pupils, as may be seen in drug addicts; any skin rash or discoloration
- The odor of the breath, the rate of respiration, any difficulty in respiration, and cyanosis
- The quality and rate of the pulse
- Appearance and odor of vomitus, if any, as well as accompanying diarrhea or abdominal pain
- Any abnormalities of stool and urine, any change in color or the presence of blood
- For signs of involvement of the nervous system, the presence of excitement, muscular twitching, delirium, difficulty in speech, stupor, coma, constriction or dilation of the pupils, and elevated or subnormal temperature

Coma caused by drug overdose is characterized by the following categories:

Grade I—individual asleep but easily aroused, reacts to painful stimuli, deep tendon reflexes present, pupils normal and reactive, ocular movements present, and vital signs stable

Grade II—pain response absent, deep tendon reflexes depressed, pupils slightly dilated but reactive, and vital signs stable

Grade III—deep tendon and pupillary reflexes absent and vital signs stable

Grade IV—respiration and circulation depressed

The nurse should *refrigerate in a covered container all specimens* of vomitus, urine, or stool for examination and possible submission to the proper authority for analysis. This is of particular importance not only in making or confirming a diagnosis, but also in the event that the case has medicolegal significance.

Any of the signs listed earlier should be noted carefully for report to the position control center or physician in charge. However, full reliance on signs and symptoms for clear-cut diagnosis and poison identification is fraught with danger, since these incidents may occur concurrently with an episode of acute disease, especially in children (e.g., aspirin intoxication), and symptoms may be similar or otherwise confusing. Also, more than one substance may be responsible for the signs of poisoning observed.

Not all substances commonly ingested accidentally are toxic if small amounts are taken only once. Poison control centers define a small amount as the quantity of a substance contained in "a taste," "one bite," or "a small piece," as opposed to "a mouthful." Although subjective, this is typical of data received when taking a poisoning history. A list of some frequently ingested products that are usually systematically nontoxic if taken in small amounts follows:

- Abrasives, bleaches (sodium hypochlorite, less than 5%)
- Chalk
- Cigarettes, cigarette ash, cigars
- Cosmetics, perfume, cologne, deodorants
- Crayons (if labelled C.P., A.P., or C.S., – 130-46)
- Glues, rubber cement
- Hydrogen peroxide (medicinal, 3%)
- Indelible pen or magic markers
- Ink in full cartridge of a ballpoint pen
- Paint (latex)
- Pencil (graphite or coloring)
- Saccharin and cyclamates
- Safety matches (ingestion of less than 20 books of matches)
- Soaps, liquid shampoos, household detergents (except dishwasher detergents)
- Toothpaste (unless heavy ingestion of fluorides)
- Vitamins (in amounts usually available for a single overdose, unless containing iron)

Ingestion of small amounts of these nonedible substances may produce mild gastric irritation but not systemic poisoning. However, contact with a poison control center or physician is important (essential, if symptoms exist), since no product or drug is entirely safe for ingestion, and hypersensitivity reactions can occur.

In assisting with poisoning diagnosis and toxic substance identification, nurses (especially emergency room nurses and nurse practitioners) should familiarize themselves with certain clusters of signs associated with common drug poisonings or overdoses. These have been called **toxidromes** and are listed in the Box 73-1. Other common single signs and their associated causative toxins are listed in Table 73-1.

BOX 73-1

Toxidromes*

atropine, scopolamine, anticholinergics: dry skin, tachycardia, beet-red skin color, agitation, dilated pupils, delirium, hyperthermia, hallucinations, coma

barbiturates, sedative-hypnotics, tranquilizers: ataxia, drowsiness, slurred speech (without an alcohol breath odor), respiratory depression, hypotension

cholinergics (such as organophosphates), **mushrooms** (*Amanita or Galerina*): salivation, lacrimation, involuntary urination and defecation, miosis, pulmonary congestion, seizures

opioids: miosis, respiratory depression, hypotension, slow respiration, coma

salicylates: fever, vomiting, hyperglycemia, mixed respiratory alkalosis and metabolic acidosis, hyperpnea

tricyclic antidepressants: anticholinergic signs and symptoms, plus dysrhythmias (prolonged QRS duration on ECG report), convulsions, coma

*The drugs or drug types in bold are followed by clusters of signs of poisonings.

TABLE 73-1 Single signs that suggest presence of certain toxins

Sign	Inference
Abdominal colic	black widow spider bite heavy metals withdrawal from narcotic depressant
Ataxia	alcohol barbiturates bromides carbon monoxide hallucinogens heavy metals organic solvents phenytoin (Dilantin) tranquilizers
Coma and drowsiness	alcohol (ethyl) antihistamines barbiturates, other hypnotics carbon monoxide opiates salicylates tranquilizers
Convulsions or muscle twitching	alcohol amphetamines antihistamines boric acid camphor chlorinated hydrocarbon insecticides (DDT) cyanide lead organophosphate insecticides plants (azalea, iris, lily-of-the-valley, water hemlock) salicylates strychnine
Convulsions or muscle twitching—cont'd	withdrawal from drugs: barbiturates, benzodiazepines (Valium, Librium), meprobamate
Paralysis	botulism heavy metals plants (poison hemlock, etc.) triorthocresyl phosphate (plasticizer)
Oliguria/anuria	carbon tetrachloride ethylene glycol (antifreeze) heavy metals hemolysis caused by naphthalene, plants, and so on methanol mushrooms oxylates petroleum distillates solvents
Oral signs	
Breath odors	
Acetone	acetone alcohol (methyl or isopropyl) phenol salicylates
Alcohol	ethyl alcohol
Bitter almonds	cyanide
Coal gas	carbon monoxide
Garlic	arsenic dimethyl sulfoxide (DMSO) phosphorus organophosphate insecticides thallium

Continued

TABLE 73-1 Single signs that suggest presence of certain toxins—cont'd

Sign	Inference
Salivation	arsenic
	corrosive substances
	mercury
	mushrooms
	organophosphate insecticides
	thallium
Pupillary changes	
Dilated	amphetamines
	antihistamines
	atropine
	barbiturates (when combined with coma)
	cocaine
	ephedrine
	LSD (occasionally)
	methanol
	withdrawal from narcotic depressants (occasionally)
Constricted, pinpoint pupils	mushrooms (muscarinic)
	opiates
	organophosphate insecticides
Nystagmus on lateral gaze	barbiturates
	minor tranquilizers (meprobamate, benzodiazepines), phenytoin (Dilantin)
Respiratory alterations	
Increased	amphetamines
	barbiturates (early sign)
	carbon monoxide
	methanol
	petroleum distillates
Paralysis	salicylates
	botulism
Slowed or depressed	organophosphate insecticides
	alcohol (late sign)
	barbiturates (late sign)
	opiates
	tranquilizers
Wheezing/pulmonary edema	mushrooms (muscarinic)
	opiates
	organophosphate insecticides
	petroleum distillates
Skin color changes	
Jaundice	aniline dyes/coal tar colors
	arsenic
	carbon tetrachloride
	castor bean
	fava bean
	mushroom
	naphthalene (moth repellent/insecticide)
Red flush	yellow phosphorus
	alcohol
	antihistamines
	atropine
	boric acid
	carbon monoxide
	nitrites
Cyanosis	tricyclic antidepressants
	aniline dyes
	carbon monoxide
	cyanide
	nitrites
	strychnine
Violent emesis (with or without hematemesis)	aminophylline
	bacterial food poisoning
	boric acid
	corrosives
	fluoride
	heavy metals
	phenol
	salicylates

POISON CONTROL CENTERS

There are approximately 600 poison control centers in the United States, the majority located near hospitals or in emergency rooms of large community hospitals. Their telephone numbers are listed in the local telephone book or may be obtained from a pharmacist. The *Physician's Desk Reference* (PDR) includes a list of certified poison control centers that are open 24 hours a day and are staffed to answer specific questions from the public or from professionals about identification of ingredients in trade-named products, estimate their toxicity, and suggest specific treatment for poisonings.

CLASSIFICATION OF ACTION OF POISONS

The classification of poisons is as broad as the classification of drugs, since any drug is a potential poison when used in excess. Poisons may be classified in various ways such as: grouped according to chemical classifications as organic and inorganic poisons; as alkaloids, glycosides, and resins; or as acids, alkalis, heavy metals, oxidizing agents, halogenated hydrocarbons, and so on. Poisons also may be classified according to the organ or tissue of the body in which the most damaging effects are produced. Some poisons injure all cells they contact; they are sometimes called protoplasmic poisons or cytotoxins. Others have more effect on the kidney (nephrotoxins), the liver (hepatotoxins), or the blood-forming organs.

Poisons that affect chiefly the nervous system are called neurotoxin poisons. They must be studied separately because different symptoms characterize each one. Symptoms of toxicity are mentioned with each of these drugs in previous chapters. Although symptoms of this group of poisons are to some extent specific, certain symptoms are encountered repeatedly and are associated with many poisons. Drowsiness, dizziness, headache, delirium, coma, and convulsive seizures always indicate central nervous system involvement. On the other hand, dry mouth, dilated pupils, and difficulty swallowing are associated with overdosage of atropine or one of the atropine-like drugs; ringing in the ears, excessive perspiration, and gastric upset may be associated with salicylate overdosage.

Many times the precise mechanism of action is not known; death may be caused by respiratory failure, but exactly what happens to cause depression of the respiratory center may not be known. The human body depends on a constant supply of oxygen if various physiologic functions are to proceed satisfactorily. Anything that interferes with the use of oxygen by the cells or with the transportation of oxygen will produce damaging effects faster in some cells than in others. Carbon monoxide from automobile engines and unvented gas heaters is one of the most widely distributed toxic agents. It poisons by producing hypoxia and finally asphyxia. Carbon monoxide has a great affinity for hemoglobin and forms carboxyhemoglobin. Thus the production of oxyhemoglobin and the free transport of oxygen is interfered with; oxygen deficiency soon develops in the cells. Unless exposure to the carbon monoxide is terminated before 40% of hemoglobin has been changed to carboxyhemoglobin, anoxia may produce serious brain damage. Death occurs when 60% of the hemoglobin has been changed to carboxyhemoglobin.

The cyanides act somewhat similarly in that they bring about cellular anoxia, but they do so differently. They inactivate certain tissue enzymes so that cells are unable to utilize oxygen. Death may occur very rapidly. Curare and the curariform drugs in toxic amounts bring about paralysis of the diaphragm, and again the victim dies from lack of oxygen.

Certain drugs have a direct effect on muscle tissue from the body, such as that of the myocardium, or the smooth muscle of the blood vessels. Death results from the failure of circulation or cardiac arrest. The nitrites, potassium salts, and digitalis drugs may exert such toxic effects. Strong acids and alkalis denature and destroy cellular proteins. Examples of corrosive acids are hydrochloric, nitric, and sulfuric acids. Sodium, potassium, and ammonium hydroxides are examples of strong and caustic alkalis. Locally, these substances cause destruction of tissue, and death may result from hemorrhage, perforation, or shock. Corrosive poisons may also cause death by altering the pH of the blood or other body fluids, or they may produce marked degenerative changes on vital organs such as the liver or kidney.

SPECIFIC POISONS, SYMPTOMS, AND SUGGESTED EMERGENCY TREATMENT

Since the emphasis is on *prompt* treatment, health care may be best served by quick action by informed bystanders at the scene who apply first-aid measures while help is sought from the poison control center and while transportation to a hospital or other health care setting is arranged. A first-aid chart that offers instruction for various poisoning emergencies is included in Box 73-2.

The caller to the poison control center should have the following information, if available:

1. Physical appearance of the substance
2. Odor, color, and texture; distinguishing characteristics of the substance
3. Trade name or chemical name, if known
4. Purpose or how the substance was meant to be used
5. Label statements relating to "poison" content or flammability

After the events of the suspected poisoning have been assessed, prompt medical interventions must be instituted. Nursing management will therefore be guided by the four major goals.

1. Vital functions (respirations, circulation, and others) will be maintained, supported, or restored.
2. The toxic substance will be removed or eliminated from the system as soon as possible.
3. The action of certain specific poisons may be counteracted, reversed, or antagonized by specific antidotes.
4. Recurrences will be reduced or prevented.

Support of Vital Functions

Basic to the treatment of poisoning is intensive supportive therapy, good nursing care, and minimal dangerous invasive interventions. Nursing care of the poisoned client should focus on restoration, support, and maintenance of such vital functions as ventilation, circulation, and acid-base and fluid-electrolyte balance. Emotional support for the client and others involved in this crisis is crucial.

A general assessment and history should be performed quickly and competently to determine the extent of any impairments of body systems or particular susceptibilities. Expert nursing care is essential to observe the following for information indicating impending complications:

1. Level of consciousness
2. Vital signs. Temperature may be elevated with certain central nervous system (CNS) stimulants and salicylates and depressed with others. Transient cardiac dysrhythmias may occur; anticipate obtaining an electrocardiogram. Pulmonary congestion, airway obstruction, or apnea is common; aspiration of vomitus can occur.

Implemented plans may include:

1. Turning, deep breathing, coughing, and suctioning

BOX 73-2

First Aid for Possible Poisoning

Remember: any nonfood substance may be poisonous.

1. Keep all potential poisons—household products and medicines—out of children's reach.
2. Use "safety caps" (child-resistant containers) to avoid accidents.
3. Have 1 ounce of ipecac syrup in your home and in your first-aid kit for camping, travel, and so on.
4. Keep your poison center's and your physician's phone number handy.

If you think an accidental ingestion has occurred:

1. Keep calm. Do not wait for symptoms—call for help promptly.
2. Find out if the substance is toxic; your poison control center or your physician can tell you if a risk exists and what you should do.
3. Have the product's container or label with you at the phone.
   a. If a poison is on the skin:
      Immediately remove affected clothing.
      Flood involved parts of body with water, wash with soap or detergent, and rinse thoroughly.
   b. If a poison is in the eye:
      Immediately flush the eye with water for up to 20 minutes.
   c. If a poison is inhaled:
      Immediately get the victim to fresh air. Give mouth-to-mouth resuscitation if necessary.
   d. If vomiting has been recommended:
      Give appropriate dose of ipecac syrup as instructed, followed by at least one glass (8 ounces) of clear liquid. If the patient does not vomit within 15 to 20 minutes, give 1 more tablespoon of ipecac and more water. Do *not* use salt water.

Never induce vomiting if:

1. The victim is in a *coma* (unconscious).
2. The victim is *convulsing* (having a seizure).
3. The victim has swallowed a caustic or corrosive (e.g., lye).

For reemphasis:

1. Always call to be certain of possible toxicity before undertaking treatment.
2. Never induce vomiting until you are instructed to do so.
3. Do not rely on the label's antidote information, since it may be out of date. Call instead.
4. If you have to go to an emergency room, take the tablets, capsules, capsules, container, and/or label with you.
5. Do not hesitate to call your poison center or your physician a second time if the victim seems to be getting worse.

From Covington, 1993; Schauben, 1990.

2. Auscultation to demonstrate a need for chest x-ray examination, suctioning, tracheostomy, endotracheal intubation, blood gas determinations, supplemental oxygen, and a respirator/ventilator

It is also essential that the victim be positioned to prevent aspiration of vomitus and that mouth care be attended to promptly after emesis. Moderate amounts of plain water by mouth (if a gag or swallow reflex is present) may be all that is needed to dilute or effectively inactivate many ingested poisons. Close attention to developing problems and responsive intervention can often fend off the need for more aggressive medical therapies that tax the already tenuous condition of the poisoned individual.

Removal or Elimination of Poison

Careful evaluation of the individual who has been affected by a toxic substance is essential to determine which of the foregoing steps take priority and by which route the poison should be removed or eliminated, if necessary. The route is largely determined by the manner of the poisoning. Removal of ingested substances can be attempted in several ways: (1) by directly removing it from the stomach, if the poisoning is discovered early; (2) by increasing the rate of transit of the poison through the colon, even though little or no absorption occurs there and thus may not be effective; or (3) if the substance has probably already been assimilated into the system or was injected, by attempting to remove or filter it from the bloodstream. Contact poisons may be flushed from the skin, eyes, and other external areas by copious volumes of plain, flowing water from a pitcher or other container. Inhaled toxins are treated by removing the patient to fresh air and administering artificial respiration or oxygen and other supportive measures as necessary.

Various methods exist for the removal or elimination of poisons from the gastrointestinal tract or systemic circulation: emesis, gastric lavage, cathartics, diuretics, dialysis, or occasionally blood exchange transfusions or hemoperfusion through charcoal or exchange resins.

Emesis

Generally, if more than 4 hours have elapsed since a poison ingestion, emptying the stomach will be ineffective. Exceptions are poisonings by anticholinergic drugs, which slow gastric motility, and by salicylates, which promote pyloric spasm. Some drugs, such as ethanol, are absorbed too rapidly to be recovered after 1 hour. However, when situations have warranted emptying the stomach, whole tablets have occasionally been recovered even a day later. Because of this, some recommend emptying the stomach even after a delay.

The most effective method for removing ingested toxins is usually the most natural one—emesis, done as soon as possible. In some instances, however, emesis is contraindicated (Box 73-3). If vomiting does not or cannot occur naturally, ipecac syrup is usually administered. Apomorphine is no longer recommended for emesis because ipecac syrup is safer and a more convenient product to use (*USP DI*, 1996). However, neither emetic may be effective if the ingested substance is a sedative-hypnotic, a phenothiazine, or a tricyclic antidepressant, all of which have antiemetic properties.

ipecac syrup [ip' e kak]

The most commonly used emetic is ipecac syrup which acts both centrally and locally by stimulating the vomiting center and by irritating the gastric mucosa. The usual dose for adults is 15 to 30 ml, followed immediately by 240 ml of water. Four to eight ounces of water is given with the following dosages: children 6 months to 1 year, a 5 to 10 ml dose (under special circumstances only); children 1 to 12 years old, a 15 ml dose. Vomiting usually occurs in 15 to 30 minutes. The dose may be repeated once after 20 minutes if the first dose is not effective.

If vomiting does not occur within 30 minutes, gastric lavage should be performed. Ipecac is cardiotoxic if absorbed and may cause conduction disturbances, atrial fibrillation, or myocarditis. Ipecac syrup is available without a prescription in 1 ounce (30 ml) bottles bearing the following instructions:

1. For emergency use to cause vomiting in poisoning. Before using, call physician, poison control center, or hospital emergency room immediately for advice.
2. Warning—Keep out of reach of children. Do not use if strychnine, corrosives such as alkalis (lye) and strong acids, or petroleum distillates such as kerosene, gasoline, fuel oil, coal oil, paint thinner, or cleaning fluid have been ingested.

Gastric Lavage

If the person is conscious, drug-induced vomiting is usually preferable to gastric lavage, particularly in children, since aspiration of vomitus is less likely to occur. Nurses should employ the necessary measures to reduce the likelihood of aspiration of vomitus (e.g., proper positioning of client). Occasionally, induction of vomiting may be facilitated by stimulating the pharynx, but time should not be wasted in repeated futile attempts.

If emesis cannot be induced, **gastric lavage** should be begun *except* under most of the same contraindicating conditions (e.g., untreated convulsions, absent reflexes, corrosives). Gastric lavage is the washing out of the stomach with sterile water or a saline solution. Lavage *may* be preferred treatment for pregnant women and for individuals who have ingested more than 2 ml/kg body weight of a petroleum distillate and who should have endotracheal intubation to protect the airway. Lavage may be contraindicated in the presence of cardiac dysrhythmias.

BOX 73-3

Contraindications for Induced Emesis in Poisonings

Infants up to 1 year of age
Comatose or convulsing patient
Absent gag and cough reflexes
Ingestion of:
- Convulsion-inducing substances
- Sharp objects (e.g., glass, nails) along with toxic substance
- Central nervous system (CNS) poisons (e.g., camphor, strychnine), which must be removed more quickly by lavage

Acids, alkalis, or petroleum distillates, such as kerosene, gasoline, or paint thinner, etc.
Presence of hematemesis

From Schauben, et al. 1990; Wuest, et al, 1992.

An Ewald orogastric tube, no. 16 to 30 French, may be used to lavage children; tube sizes for adult lavage range from no. 34 to 42. The newer, clear-plastic Levacuator tube also may be used. A standard nasogastric tube is too narrow for extraction of particulate matter such as intact tablets (Figure 73-1). Stomach contents should be aspirated first and saved for toxicologic analysis if necessary.

Several liters of half-strength saline solution may be used in increments of 50 to 100 ml for children and 150 to 200 ml for adults during repeated lavages until return flows are clear. (Remember that dead space in the tube itself accounts for 20 to 25 ml of the fluid instilled.) Neither emesis nor lavage is guaranteed to empty the stomach completely.

Activated Charcoal

Following emesis or lavage, activated charcoal prepared as a aqueous slurry, may be administered to act as an absorbent. Activated charcoal should be given as soon after poison ingestion as feasible, but not after ipecac and emesis, since it will adsorb the ipecac. Activated charcoal adsorbs many substances, thus it is used as an adjunct in the treatment of oral poisonings with heavy metals, mercuric chloride, strychnine, phenol, atropine, phenolphthalein, oxalic acid, poisonous mushrooms, aspirin, and most drugs. It is not effective for poisoning with ethanol, methanol, caustic alkalis, ferrous sulfate, boric acid, gas, kerosene, lithium and mineral acids. The charcoal mixture need not be removed from the stomach afterward because no known adverse effects exist. Activated charcoal can also serve as a stool marker to indicate when further gastrointestinal absorption of the ingested poison has ended. Tablets or capsules of charcoal should not be used for treatment of poisoning, since they are less effective than the powder.

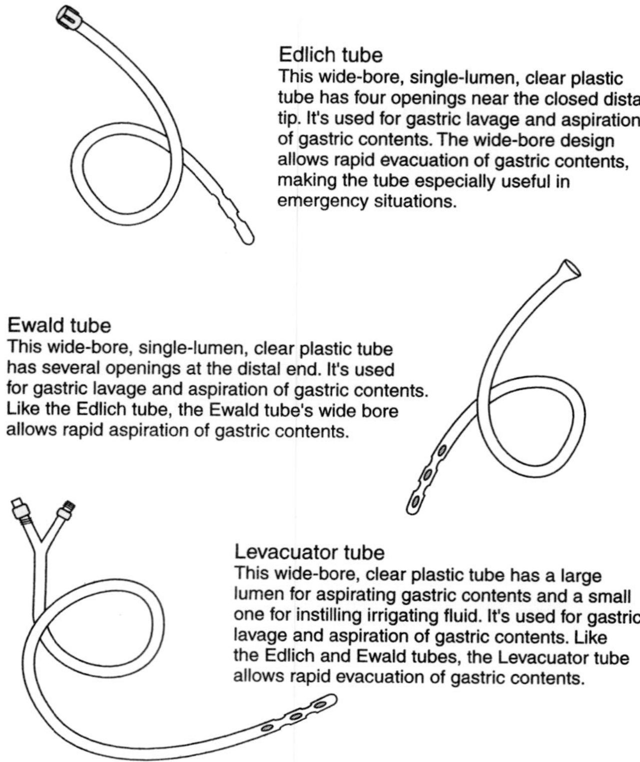

Figure 73-1 Various tubes used for lavage techniques.

Other Treatments

Other ways used to block or eliminate toxins from the system include forced diuresis, cathartics and enemas, dialysis, hemoperfusion, and exchange transfusions. These methods should be reserved as treatment under certain conditions and for specific poisons because they are not universally effective and are much less commonly used than emesis or lavage.

Changing the pH of the urine by alkalinization (sodium bicarbonate) may enhance excretion of certain drugs, such as salicylates and possibly, tricyclic antidepressants. Forced acid diuresis is probably more potentially hazardous but is often recommended for poisoning with amphetamines and fenfluramine (Pondimin).

Clearance of poisons directly from the bloodstream by peritoneal dialysis or hemodialysis, hemoperfusion, or transfusion is occasionally done to augment other measures previously discussed. Peritoneal dialysis is less effective than hemodialysis or hemoperfusion. The degree to which they may be useful depends in part on the properties of the substance (i.e., whether it freely circulates or whether it is bound to plasma proteins or to tissues). Various lists of substances amenable to dialysis exist; some substances for which hemodialysis has *not* proved useful are as follows (*USP DI*, 1996; Aweeka, 1996): cefixime (Suprax), clindamycin (Cleocin), diazepam (Valium), cyclosporine, digoxin (Lanoxin), phenytoin (Dilantin), propranolol (Inderal), and zidovudine (Retrovir).

PREVENTION OF POISONING

The focus of nursing on primary care and its corollary, prevention, applies readily to poisonings. Prevention has always been emphasized by the nursing profession, and now other disciplines are beginning to take part. Combined efforts with drug information centers and other health professionals and creative approaches have already had an impact on the frequency of certain categories of drug poisoning, notably aspirin poisoning.

Various creative graphic symbols appear on labels of poisonous substances to alert the adult and/or nonreading child to the potential hazard contained therein. "Mr Yuk," an ugly, green-faced, scowling image, is one of these. Tricky-to-open caps appear to delay if not totally prevent children's indiscriminate use of medicines. Others who have no need for these caps can request medication in the familiar easy-to-open caps.

There is much to learn about toxins in our environment, both apparent and potential, and therefore much to do in the way of poison prevention, but concerted, thoughtful efforts have already had a positive effect on statistics.

ANTIDOTES

The number of antidotes for specific toxins is minimal; no widely accepted "universal antidote" exists. Nevertheless, some general statements can be made about antidotes. Antidotes are more effective after the stomach is empty. The correct dose to reverse toxicity depends on the specific drug involved, its half-life, and the severity of toxicity shown. Antidotes work by any of the following mechanisms: (1) antagonizing or stimulating receptor sites that have been rendered hyperfunctional or dysfunctional by the poison; (2) interfering with enzyme inhibition; (3) administering the product of metabolism that has been interfered with; (4) inhibiting the biotransformation of a substance to a poisonous metabolite; (5) giving an agent that inactivates the toxic product; (6) chelation (forming highly stable complexes, tying up the substance—usually a heavy metal such as iron); and (7) producing immunotherapy—the use of antidrug antibodies to bind and inactivate drugs (e.g., there is a report of severe digoxin poisoning reversed with sheep digoxin-specific antibodies).

■ Nursing Management

Care of the Client with Poisoning

Assessment. An assessment should be done quickly to determine what substance is involved so that immediate action can be taken to prevent or minimize its effects. Symptoms may include, depending on the causative agent, nausea and vomiting, abdominal cramping, convulsions, change in the level of consciousness, and decreased rates of pulse and respiration. Assess cardiopulmonary and respiratory function. Poisoning should be suspected in any unconscious person with no history of diabetes, seizure disorders, or trauma.

To assist in the determination of the agent, the lips and mouth are checked for excessive salivation, burns, or difficulty swallowing. The breath should be assessed for its odor. Some petroleum and cleaning products have distinctive smells which can be identified.

The pupils should be checked for dilation or constriction, which may also help to indicate the substance.

If the person is conscious, he or she should be questioned about what substance and what quantity were taken. With the unconscious person, identification of the substance is facilitated by clues in the environment. Empty containers, open bottles or medication containers, or syringes should be gathered and taken to the hospital with the person. Often the containers will list the ingredients of the substance to assist the health care providers in the choice of treatment or antidote.

Toxicologic studies, which include drug screens, can determine poison levels in the mouth, vomitus, urine, feces, or blood or on the person's hands and clothing and confirm the diagnosis. In inhalation poisoning, chest x-rays might show pulmonary infiltrates or edema.

Implementation

Monitoring. Carefully monitor vital signs and level of consciousness. Observe the client for nausea, vomiting, diarrhea, and abdominal cramping. The client's vomitus, stool, and urine should be observed for abnormalities such as the presence of blood. These body substances need to be retained for analysis for medical and legal reasons.

Intervention. Immediate action is required in the case of poisoning to prevent the absorption of the substance. If the person is unconscious, he should be transported as soon as possible to a hospital. If the individual is conscious, a physician and/or the poison control center should be contacted immediately. The telephone number of the nearest poison control center is usually listed in the front of the telephone directory with other emergency numbers for the community.

If the poison has been inhaled, such as a toxic gas or carbon monoxide, the individual should be removed from the source to the fresh air and oxygen administered if available. Cardiopulmonary resuscitation should be started if indicated. Call 911; the victim will need to be transported to the hospital.

If the substance is a contact poison, absorbed through the skin and mucous membranes, the individual should be rinsed off immediately with copious amounts of water. The clothing should then be removed and the skin rinsed again. A shower would then be the best method of removal of the agent from the skin.

If the poison is ingested, the objective is to prevent absorption of the substance either by inducing vomiting or by lavage to remove the agent or by administering an agent to inactivate the poisonous substance. The most recommended method of inducing vomiting is to have the patient take 15 ml of syrup of ipecac followed by a full glass of water. This procedure may be repeated in 20 minutes if necessary. If lavage is attempted and the person is unconscious, it should be done while a cuffed endotracheal tube is in place to prevent aspiration. Vomiting or lavage should not be attempted with the ingestion of caustic substances or hydrocarbons, found in petroleum products. Care for the ingestion of these substances is to give nothing by mouth and urgently seek medical assistance.

If the substance has a known antidote, it will be administered by the physician.

Other nursing interventions relate to the supportive care of the acutely ill client. Monitor vital signs and report changes immediately. If respirations are depressed, administer oxygen and suction. Maintain intravenous fluids as ordered. Keep the client warm and turn frequently to promote drainage from the respiratory tract.

If the poisoning was intentional, as a suicide attempt, safety precautions should be instituted to protect the client from further self-destructive behavior and a psychiatric referral should be considered.

Education. To prevent accidental poisoning, families should be assisted to evaluate environmental hazards in the home. All medications should be clearly labeled with type, dosage, and storage requirements, and the client's ability to safely self-medicate should be assessed before there is an expectation for self-medication.

Clients should be cautioned that toxic substances are not to be stored in food containers, containers that are not properly labeled, or stored in a place that is accessible to children. Medication should not be stored beyond the date of expiration. Poisonous plants should not be kept in households where there are small children.

Syrup of ipecac is a necessary ingredient in a household first aid container, as well as the appropriate directions for its use.

In interactions with clients, nurses should be alert to the presence of anger, depression, withdrawal, and faulty judgment that might precede intentional or unintentional poisoning.

Evaluation. Regression of the client's symptoms would indicate the successful elimination and inactivation of the poison.

COMMON POISONS

Alcohols (ethanol, isopropyl, and methyl) are reviewed in Chapter 9, Substance Misuse and Abuse, and acetaminophen is covered in Chapters 11 and 14, OTC Medications and Analgesics. Carbon monoxide, iron, and organophosphate insecticides are reviewed here.

Carbon Monoxide

Carbon monoxide (CO) is an odorless gas produced by the incomplete combustion of carbon or carbonaceous materials. Sources of the gas include improperly maintained heating systems, improperly ventilated charcoal cookers or fireplaces, and industrial furnaces such as those in steel mills. Automobile exhaust contains 3% to 7% CO. No other poison causes as many deaths in the United States and Canada as does CO. Inhalation of automobile exhaust is a common method of suicide while accidental home and industrial exposure to CO is much more common than generally appreciated.

Poisoning by CO results from pulmonary absorption of the gas which readily combines with hemoglobin to form carboxyhemoglobin. The oxygen in hemoglobin is replaced thus lowering available oxygen carried by the blood to the body tissues. With the addition of each CO molecule the oxygen molecules remaining on the hemoglobin become so tightly bound that they are not readily released to the oxygen starved tissues. CO is measured in blood as the percent carboxyhemoglobin (%HbCO). Additionally, CO gas dissolved in blood but not bound to hemoglobin diffuses into the body tissues and poisons cytochrome enzymes necessary for cellular utilization of oxygen.

The symptoms of CO poisoning are generally related to %HbCO. Clinically, only mild if any symptoms occur at 10% HbCO and cigarette smokers may have CO up to this level. The initial signs of poisoning usually occur at 10% to 30% HbCO; these signs include throbbing headache, nausea, vomiting, dizziness, weakness, and visual disturbances. These early symptoms of intoxication are nonspecific and may be attributed to a number of other causes unless a history of CO is available or laboratory tests demonstrate elevated %HbCO. At 40% to 50% HbCO, syncope, tachycardia, tightness in the chest, and tachypnea occur. HbCO has a cherry pink color rather than the red color of oxyhemoglobin; therefore the patient may have a cherry pink coloration of the skin. Percent HbCO in excess of 50% causes life-threatening convulsions, coma, dangerously compromised cardiopulmonary function, and possible death. Fatalities from suicide or victims of fires often have %HbCO of 60% to 80%.

Treatment for CO poisoning is based on the client's symptoms and %HbCO. Hyperbaric oxygen is the antidote of choice because oxygen under pressure is capable of replacing CO from hemoglobin and the iron containing respiratory cytochrome enzymes in the tissues.

Ninety-five percent of absorbed CO is excreted by the lungs; however, once removed from the source of exposure, the half-life of CO in normal ambient air is 4 hours. If 100% oxygen is administered, the half-life ($t^{1}/_{2}$) decreases to 40 minutes. Hyperbaric oxygen at 3 atm decreases the $t^{1}/_{2}$ of CO to only 23 minutes. In severe poisoning, cardiopulmonary support is maintained throughout therapy. Additional drug therapy to control dysrhythmias, cerebral edema, and convulsions may be indicated.

■ Nursing Management

Carbon Monoxide Poisoning

See the general nursing management for poisoning.

Iron

Iron supplements are a leading cause of pediatric poisoning deaths in the United States; 11 children died from a reported 5,144 accidental ingestions of iron preparations (The White Sheet, 1993). Iron overdoses have also been noted to result in profound mental retardation; thus such products should be dispensed in child resistant containers and stored in an area that is not readily accessible to small children.

Iron deficiency is a primary cause of anemia in both infants and adults. Thus iron is often added to infant formulas and foods and is available in over 100 commercial products for adults, including multiple and prenatal vitamins. Available products use a number of forms of iron, various salts and chelates. The toxic effects of iron are caused by its elemental form; therefore the relative toxicity of iron salts is related to the percent of elemental iron. For example, ferrous fumarate (33% iron) is more toxic on a weight basis than ferrous gluconate (12% iron).

On ingestion, large amounts of iron cause local corrosive actions on the gastric and duodenal mucosa and upper gastrointestinal tract. Initial symptoms of iron poisoning include nausea, vomiting, upper abdominal pain, and bloody diarrhea. The corrosive action destroys the normal mucosal barrier to iron absorption, allowing rapid absorption of large amounts of iron into the general circulation. These overdose concentrations of iron exceed the binding capacity of transferrin, the iron-carrying protein of the blood. The excess free iron readily diffuses into various tissues and binds to the sulfhydryl (SH) radicals of numerous enzymes and structural proteins. This binding of iron to compounds necessary for normal cellular function poisons the tissue cells.

Six to twentyfour hours after ingestion symptoms of systemic intoxication—cyanosis, pulmonary edema, and possible cardiovascular collapse—start to occur. Within a few days, coagulation defects, hepatic necrosis, and renal failure may develop. As with adults, the initial symptoms of pediatric iron poisoning are characterized by repeated vomiting, abdominal pain, and diarrhea. However, frequently a latent phase occurs when the initial symptoms abate and the child appears well for a 6 to 12 hour period, which is followed by rapid illness and the development of shock. The determination of serum iron will indicate the severity of the intoxication and prevent the possible dangerous misinterpretation of this latency period.

Additionally, serum iron values indicate the necessity of the initiation of antidotal therapy. Serum iron concentrations of 350 μg/dl or less are rarely associated with clinical illness. Concentrations between 350 and 500 μg/dl call for observation of the client for the development of clinical signs of intoxication. For concentrations above 500 μg/dl, deferoxamine (an iron chelating agent) therapy is recommended.

The treatment for iron poisoning includes general supportive measures, and a specific antidote to bind the ingested iron. Emesis may be induced to expel unabsorbed iron tablets in the stomach; also, sodium bicarbonate lavage is indicated, since bicarbonate converts ferrous iron to ferrous carbonate, which is poorly absorbed. After lavage, 200 to 300 ml of the bicarbonate solution should be left in the stomach. When indicated by toxic serum iron concentrations (+500 mg/dl), deferoxamine, a chelating agent, should be administered.

Deferoxamine is a specific chelator that binds free serum iron and iron associated with hepatic and splenic stores. Deferoxamine does not bind with zinc, copper, or other trace metals. The deferoxamine-iron complex is nontoxic and freely excreted by the kidneys.

■ Nursing Management

Iron Poisoning

Refer to the section on nursing management of the care of the client with poisoning on p. 1116. The following information is specific to iron poisoning.

Assessment. Take careful history to elicit possibility of pregnancy. Advise against the use of deferoxamine if client is pregnant, or may have severe renal impairment.

Implementation

Intervention. Institute emesis or gastric lavage as soon as possible. Initiate supportive measures, including maintenance of clear airway and interventions related to presence of shock and to acidosis. Administer deferoxamine using long needle and Z-track method; may add 0.2 to 0.3 ml of air to medication in syringe to prevent pain and induration at site of injections. Carefully controlled, slow intravenous infusion rates may be equally effective in preventing infusion pain.

Education. Tell client to expect reddish brown coloration of urine and stools.

Organophosphate Insecticides

Organophosphate compounds are highly effective insecticides. Their chemical structure is unstable, resulting in their disintegration into nontoxic radicals within days after their application. Therefore they do not persist or accumulate in the environment or animal tissues as do the chlorinated insecticides such as DDT. This accounts for their addition to numerous commercial products from flea collars, bug bombs, and flypapers to most home and commercial insect sprays. This popularity accounts for the high potential for accidental poisoning by organophosphates.

Organophosphate compounds are powerful inhibitors of the enzyme acetylcholinesterase (ACHE), which breaks down the neurotransmitter acetylcholine (ACh) (see Chapter 21). Organophosphates are generally rapidly absorbed in the body by all routes, although individual organophosphates display a wide variation in their ability to penetrate the skin, in oral absorption, and thus in their toxicity. For example, malathion does not penetrate the skin well and its oral toxicity is low, making it a popular insecticide for use in home products.

The signs and symptoms of organophosphate insecticide poisoning are related to inhibition of ACHE, which results in an accumulation of ACh in the parasympathetic nervous system. Hence, all organs affected by ACh are overstimulated. The expected results of organophosphate poisoning are as follows: bradycardia, hypotension, dyspnea, wheezing, miosis, blurred vision, convulsions, muscular fasciculations, and profuse sweating. A common mnemonic for symptoms of organophosphate intoxication is SLUDGE: *s*alivation, *l*acrimation, *u*rination, *d*efecation, *g*astrointestinal distress, and *e*mesis. The usual mode of death is respiratory arrest caused by bronchospasm, decreased pulmonary muscle strength, and finally depression of central nervous system control of respiration. The sequence in which specific systems develop is related to the route of exposure. Respiratory tract effects appear first after inhalation, whereas gastrointestinal effects appear initially after ingestion. Skin absorption results in immediate profuse sweating and muscle weakness.

Therapy for organophosphate poisoning involves the support of cardiopulmonary function, clearance of respiratory tract secretions to maintain a clear airway, and the use of appropriate antidotes, atropine and 2-PAM (Pralidoxamine, Protopam). Atropine competitively antagonizes the action of ACh at muscarinic receptors on organs innervated by postganglionic parasympathetic nerves and cholinergic sympathetic nerves (Chapter 21).

Atropine is effective in blocking muscarinic symptoms of bradycardia, bronchoconstriction, and excess secretions; however, muscular fasciculations are refractory to this antidote. These involuntary contractions and twitchings and respiratory paralysis are best treated with 2-PAM, a cholinesterase reactivator that removes organophosphates bound to AChE. This then frees AChE to break down the accumulated ACh, thereby resuming normal activity at the neuromuscular junction. 2-PAM also directly detoxifies certain organophosphates. Side effects of 2-PAM include dizziness, nausea, headache, and tachycardia.

■ Nursing Management

Organophosphate Poisoning

In addition to the management of care of the client with poisoning on p. 1116, consider the following:

Assessment. If there is cyanosis, establish and maintain an airway first. Document the extent of SLUDGE symptoms.

Implementation

Monitoring. Closely monitor both respiratory status and secretion production, since doses of atropine may be predicated on this information. Plan to monitor client's status closely for 72 hours.

Intervention. Copious secretions may necessitate nearly continuous suctioning at first; anticipate supplemental oxygen therapy. Induce vomiting or perform gastric lavage if poison was ingested. Cleanse skin of any insecticide contaminant if present. If signs of excessive atropinization appear, plan for treatment with physostigmine to antagonize atropine. Anticipate need to administer pralidoxime [Protopam] if poisoning is severe.

SUMMARY

Poisoning, accidental or intentional, is a commonplace reason for admission to a hospital emergency room. Children make up the majority of the accidental poisoning population, whereas intentional poisoning is more likely to be the result of a suicide attempt or an abused substance overdose.

No matter how poisonings are classified, the care provided focuses on prompt treatment, the identification of the substance, if possible, the support of vital functions, the removal or elimination of the poison, and the prevention of future occurrences.

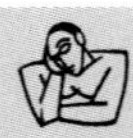

Critical Thinking

1. In what poisoning situations would the following be the most appropriate therapy: emesis? gastric lavage? refraining from induced vomiting?
2. Two-year-old Samantha Rogers has been brought to the emergency room by her mother after she found Samantha in the bathroom with a container of toilet bowl cleaner (alkali base) in her hands. She is crying and her lips are swollen and excoriated. Mrs. Rogers believes that Samantha has ingested some of the liquid. What sequence of actions should the nurse take?

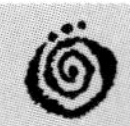

Collaborative Learning Activities

1. Three teams will present: (1) general first aid for poisoning; (2) the location of emergency equipment in the basic science labs, and why and how this would be used; and (3) where in the clinical setting is the equipment for emergency eye care, and why and how this material would be used.

BIBLIOGRAPHY

Anderson KN, et al. (Eds.) (1994). *Mosby's medical, nursing, & allied health dictionary* (4th ed.). St Louis: Mosby.

Aweeka FT (1996). Dosing of drugs in renal failure. In Young LY & Koda-Kimble MA (Eds.). *Applied therapeutics: The clinical use of drugs* (6th ed.). Vancouver: Applied Therapeutics.

Kwan T, et al. (1992). Digitalis toxicity caused by toad venom, *Chest* 102(3):949-50.

Lammon CA & Adams MH (1992). Organophosphate overdose: Nursing strategies, *DCCN* 11(6):310-7.

Melmon KL, et al. (1992). *Clinical pharmacology* (3rd ed.). New York: McGraw-Hill.

Oderda GA & Jennings JC (1996). Emetic and antiemetic products. In Covington TR (Ed.). *Handbook of nonprescription drugs* (11th ed.). Washington, DC: American Pharmaceutical Association.

Olin BR (Ed.) (1996). *Facts and comparisons.* St Louis: Facts and Comparisons.

PDR (1996). *Physician's desk reference* (50th ed.). Oradell, NJ: Medical Economics.

Public Health Service, US Department of Health and Human Services (1993). Jin bu huan toxicity in children—Colorado, *MMWR* 42(33):633-6.

Public Health Service, US Department of Health and Human Services (1993). Lead poisoning associated with use of traditional ethnic remedies—California, 1991-1992, *MMWR* 42(27):521-4.

United States Pharmacopeial Convention (1996). *USP DI: Drug information for the health professional* (16th ed.). Rockville, MD: The Convention.

Watson WA (1996). Clinical toxicology. In Young LY & Koda-Kimble MA (Eds.). *Applied therapeutics: The clinical use of drugs* (6th ed.). Vancouver: Applied Therapeutics.

Wong DL (1995). *Whaley's & Wong's nursing care of infants and children* (5th ed.). St Louis: Mosby.

Wuest JR & Gossel TA (1992). A primer for pharmacists on treatment of poisoning, *Fla Pharm Today* 56(3):22.

Appendix A
Sugar-Free Products*

The following is a selection of sugar-free products by therapeutic categories. Check labels, though, because some of these medications may contain sorbitol, alcohol, or other sources of carbohydrate.

ANTACIDS

Alka-Seltzer Original
Alka-Seltzer, Lemon-Lime
Aluminum Hydroxide Gel
Gaviscon Liquid
Gelusil Liquid
Maalox
Maalox HRF
Riopan
Riopan Plus
Titralac
Titralac Plus

ANALGESICS

Acetaminophen Oral solution, USP, Cherry
Arthritis Pain Formula
Aspirin, Delayed-Release
Bayer Aspirin
Bufferin Arthritis Strength
Bufferin Extra Strength
Excedrin Aspirin Free
Feverall Sprinkle Caps
Motrin IB
Nuprin
Panadol
Tempra Tylenol

COUGH, COLD, AND ANTIHISTAMINES

Benadryl Dye-Free
Benylin Adult Cough Formula
Benylin Expectorant Cough Formula
Cheracol Sore Throat
Diabetic Tussin Allergy Relief
Diabetic Tussin DM
Guaifenesin CF
Guaifenesin DM
Naldecon DX, Adult
Naldecon DX, Children's
Naldecon EX, Children's
Naldecon EX, Pediatric
Naldecon Senior DX
Naldecon Senior EX
Robitussin Pediatric Cough
Tussar-SF

FOOD SUPPLEMENTS

Criticare HN
Fibersource
Fibersource HN
Impact
Impact with Fiber
Isocal
MCT Oil
Vivonex T.E.N.

LAXATIVES

Doxidan
Dulcolax
Fiberall, Natural
Haley's M-O
Konsyl
Metamucil Sugar Free
Milk of Magnesia
Surfak

*Check label ingredients because manufacturers may alter or reformulate their products.

Appendix B
Alcohol-Free Products*

ANALGESICS

Acetaminophen Oral Solution USP
Liquiprin, Infants'
Panadol, Children's
Panadol, Infants'
Tempra 1
Tempra 2
Tylenol, Children's Cherry Flavor
Tylenol, Children's Liquid
Tylenol, Infants'

ANTIASTHMATIC PRODUCTS

Alupent Syrup
Dilor G Liquid
Metaprel Syrup
Slo-Phyllin GG Syrup
Theolair Liquid

COUGH, COLD, AND ANTIHISTAMINES

Actifed
Benadryl
Benadryl Decongestant
Benylin Adult Cough Formula
Benylin Expectorant Cough Formula
Chlor-Trimeton Allergy
Demazin
Diabetic Tussin Allergy Relief
Diabetic Tussin DM
Diabetic Tussin EX
Dimetapp
Dimetapp Decongestant, DM
Dimetapp Decongestant, Pediatric
Drixoral Cough Liquid Caps
Guaifenesin DM
Naldecon DX, Adult
Naldecon DX, Children's
Naldecon DX Pediatric
Naldecon EX
Naldecon Senior DX
NyQuil Children's Cold/Cough
PediaCare Cough-Cold
Robitussin
Robitussin Night Relief
Robitussin PE
Sudafed Plus
Sudafed, Children's
Triaminic AM Cough & Decongestant Formula
Triaminic AM Decongestant Formula
Triaminic Expectorant
Tussar-DM
Tylenol Children's Cold Multi-Symptom
Vicks 44d Pediatric
Vicks DayQuil

GARGLE/MOUTHWASHES

Chloraseptic Gly-Oxide Liquid
Orabase-O
Orabase Plain
Oral-B Anti-Cavity Rinse

PSYCHOTROPICS

Haldol Concentrate
Stelazine Concentrate
Thorazine Syrup

*Check label ingredients because manufacturers may alter or reformulate their products.

Appendix C
Drugs That Cause Body Organ Damage

The following are examples of drugs that may cause hepatotoxicity, nephrotoxicity, neurotoxicity, and ototoxicity.

HEPATOTOXICITY

acetaminophen (Tylenol, others) with chronic, high-dose therapy or in an acute overdose situation.
alcohol
amiodarone (Cordarone)
anabolic steroids
ACE inhibitors
iron overdose
nonsteroidal antiinflammatory drugs (NSAIDs)
asparaginase (Elspar)
carbamazepine (Tegretol)
carmustine (BCNU, BiCNU)
dantrolene (Dantrium)
dapsone
daunorubicin (Cerubidine)
disulfiram (Antabuse)
erthyromycins
estrogens
felbamate (Felbatol)
fluconazole (Diflucan)
flutamide (Eulexin)
gold compounds
halothane
HMG-CoA reductase inhibitors
isoniazid (INH)
itraconazole (Sporanox)
ketoconazole (Nizoral)
labetalol (Normodyne)
mercaptopurine (Purinethol)
methotrexate (Mexate)
methyldopa (Aldomet)
naltrexone (ReVia; in chronic use, high dosages)
niacin (high dosages, controlled release)
nitrofurans (Furadantin, Macrodantin)
phenothiazines
phenytoin (Dilantin)
rifampin (Rifadin)
sulfamethoxazole and trimethoprim (Bactrim, Septra)
sulfonamides
valproic acid (Depakene)
vitamin A (chronic high dose usage or overdose)
zidovudine (AZT, Retrovir)

NEPHROTOXICITY

acetaminophen (acute, high doses)
acyclovir, parenteral (Zovirax)
aldesleukin (Proleukin)
aminoglycosides
amphotericin B, parenteral (Fungizone)
analgesic combinations that contain acetaminophen, aspirin or other salicylates used in high dosages, chronically.
nonsteroidal antiinflammatory drugs (NSAIDs)
ciprofloxacin
cisplatin (Platinol)
cyclosporine (Sandimmune)
deferoxamine (Desferal; chronic use)
edetate calcium disodium (Versenate; high dosages)
edetate disodium (high dosages)
foscarnet (Foscavir)
gold compounds
ifosfamide (IFEX)
lithium
methotrexate (high dose therapy)
methoxyflurane (Penthrane)
pamidronate (APD)
penicillamine (Cuprimine)
pentamidine (Pentam)
plicamycin (Mithracin)
polymyxins, parenteral
rifampin
streptozocin (Zanosar)
sulfamethoxazole and trimethoprim
sulfonamides
tetracyclines (exceptions are doxycycline and minocycline)
tiopronin (Capen)
vancomycin, parenteral (Vancocin)

NEUROTOXICITY

altretamine (Hexalen)
aminoglycosides (parenteral and topical irrigation)
asparaginase (Elspar)
capreomycin (Capastat)
carbamazepine (Tegretol)
carboplatin (Paraplatin)
chloramphenicol, systemic (Chloromycetin)
ciprofloxacin (Cipro)
cisplatin (Platinol)
cycloserine (Seromycin)
cytarabine (Cytosar)
didanosine (Videx)
disulfiram (Antabuse)
ethambutol (Myambutol)
ethionamide (Trecator-SC)
fludarabine (Fludara)
imipenem
interferon, alpha and gamma
isoniazid (INH)
lincomycin (Lincocin)
lindane, topical (Kwell)
lithium (Lithane)
methotrexate, intrathecal
metronidazole (Flagyl)
mexiletine (Mexitil)
nitrofurantoin (Furadantin, Macrodantin)
pemoline (Cylert)
penicillins, parenteral
polymixins, parenteral
pyridoxine (chronic, high dose use)
quinacrine (Atabrine)
quinidine
quinine
stavudine (d4T, Zerif)
tetracyclines
vincristine (Oncovin)
zalcitabine (ddC, HIVID)

OTOTOXICITY

aminoglycosides (parenteral and topical irrigation)
nonsteroidal antiinflammatory drugs (NSAIDs)
bumetanide, parenteral (Bumex)
capreomycin
carboplatin
chloroquine (Aralen)
cisplatin
deferoxamine (chronic, high-dose usage)
erythromycin (high dosages and renal impairment)
ethacrynic acid (Edecrin)
furosemide (Lasix)
hydroxychloroquine (Plaquenil)
quinidine
quinine
salicylates (chronic high dose use; overdoses)
vancomycin, parenteral (high dosages and renal impairment)

Appendix D
Food-Drug Interactions

Drug category/medication	Foods to avoid	Rationale
Antacids		
calcium carbonate (Tums)	Avoid large amounts of dairy products	Milk or cream may increase acid secretion.
	If used as a calcium supplement, avoid concurrent administration of bran and whole grain breads or cereals.	Reduces absorption of calcium
Antibiotics		
erythromycin, penicillins*	Meals, acidic fruit juices, citrus fruits, or acidic beverages, such as cola drinks	The antibiotics are acid labile (reduced absorption). Take medication 1 hour before meals or apart from acidic foods or 2 hours after meals.
tetracyclines	Calcium-containing foods: milk, ice cream, yogurt, cheeses, and others	Calcium may complex with tetracycline, resulting in reduced absorption of the antibiotic. Most tetracyclines, with the exception of doxycycline and minocycline, should be administered 1 hour before or 2 hours after meals.
Anticoagulants		
warfarin (Coumadin), dicumarol, heparin	Beef liver and green leafy vegetables contain vitamin K (spinach, cabbage, brussels sprouts)	Vitamin K can counteract therapeutic action of anticoagulants. A normal, balanced diet will not interfere with this medication. Fad or extreme diets with foods high in vitamin K can affect anticoagulant activity.
Laxative		
mineral oil (Agoral plain, Mineral Oil)	Take 2 hours apart from food.	May decrease absorption of vitamins A, D, E, and K. Also reduces absorption of calcium.
	Do not administer at bedtime.	Aspiration of mineral oil may induce lipid pneumonitis.
MAO inhibitors		
phenelzine (Nardil), tranylcypromine (Parnate)	Foods with high tyramine content, such as aged cheese (brie, cheddar, processed American, camembert, and others), aged meat, sour cream, yogurt, pickled herring, chicken liver, canned figs, raisins, bananas, avocados, soy sauce, yeast extract, meat tenderizers, alcoholic beverages such as beer and wine (chianti, sherry, or hearty red wines), sausages, chocolate, anchovies	Concurrent use may result in severe headache, nosebleed, chest pain, eyes sensitive to light, or severe hypertension which may result in a hypertensive crisis.

*Erythromycin base (E-Mycin, Ery-Tab, E-Mycin Eryc) or stearates (Erypar, Erythrocin Stearate, Ethril, Wyamycin S) are best absorbed in the fasting state. Erythromycin ethylsuccinate (E.E.S.), estolate (Ilosone), and enteric-coated erythromycin may be given before or with meals. Penicillin, such as penicillin G, ampicillin, cloxacillin, cyclacillin, dicloxacillin, nafcillin, and oxacillin may have decreased absorption if given with food or acidic-type products.

Appendix E Drugs That Change Urine or Stool Color

Medications that may alter urine color

Drug	Possible color changes
amitriptyline (Elavil)	Blue-green
anticoagulants (coumarin and others)	Pink, red, or dark brown (indicative of systemic bleeding)
cascara sagrada	In acid urine, brown; basic urine, yellow to pink; on standing, black
iron salts, dextran, and others	Brown to black
laxatives (danthron, senna)	Pink to red or brown
laxatives (phenolphthalein)	Pink to red
levodopa (Laradopa, Dopar)	May cause dark urine and sweat
methyldopa (Aldomet, Dopamet🍁)	Pink, amber to dark urine
metronidazole (Flagyl)	Dark urine
nitrofurantoins (Furadantin, Macrodantin)	Yellow to rusty brown urine
phenazopyridine (Pyridium, Phenazo🍁)	Orange red urine; may stain clothing
phenytoin (Dilantin)	Red-brown or darkening of urine
phenothiazines (chlorpromazine, or Thorazine, and others)	Pink, red, or orange urine
rifampin (Rifadin, Rofact🍁)	Red, orange, or brown urine, stool, saliva, sweat, and tears

Medications that may alter stool color

Drug	Possible color changes
antacids with aluminum salts (Maalox, Mylanta, and others)	White specks or discoloration of stools
anticoagulants (coumarin and others)	Red, orange, to black because of internal bleeding
bismuth or iron salts	Black
laxative (phenolphthalein)	Red
laxative (senna)	Yellow, orange to brown
phenazopyridine (Pyridium and others)	Orange, red

Appendix F
Time to Draw Blood for Specific Medications

Serum drug levels are used to aid the prescriber in (1) determining dosage adjustments for drugs with a narrow range between therapeutic effect and toxicity and (2) providing information to evaluate a suspected toxicity or noncompliance.

Blood samples are usually drawn according to the pharmacokinetics of the individual drug. For example, to obtain a steady state serum level, the blood sample should be drawn at approximately 5 drug half-lives after therapy was instituted.

Gentamicin (Garamycin) has a short half-life; therefore peak and trough levels are usually ordered to ensure adequate therapy. The peak serum level (P) is usually obtained 15 to 30 minutes after an intravenous dose or 1 hour after an intramuscular dose. The trough (Tr) serum level should be drawn just before the next scheduled dose. Trough serum levels are used to predict the risk of adverse reactions; a rising trough level or levels above 2 μg/ml have been associated with increased toxicity.

Therapeutic ranges of serum drug concentrations

	Serum concentration		
Drug	Ther (μg/ml)	Tr (μg/ml)	Time for blood sampling (hours after last dose)*
Antibiotics			
amikacin (Amikin)	15-25	5	See previous discussion on gentamicin
gentamicin (Garamycin)	4-10	2	See previous discussion on gentamicin
netilmicin (Netromycin)	6-10	2	See previous discussion on gentamicin
tobramycin (Nebcin)	4-10	2	See previous discussion on gentamicin
Anticonvulsants			
carbamazepine (Tegretol)	4-12		SS 1-2 wk. Before morning dose (Tr).
phenobarbital	10-40		SS 10-30 days. Before morning dose (Tr.)
phenytoin (Dilantin)	10-20		SS 1-4 wk. Oral (Tr). before next dose; IV, 2-4 hr after loading dose.
primidone (Mysoline)	5-12		SS 2-3 days for primidone; phenobarbital as above. Before next dose (Tr).
valproic acid (Depakene, Depakote)	50-100		SS 2-3 days. Before next dose (Tr).
Cardiovascular drugs			
digoxin (Lanoxin)	0.8-2 ng/ml		SS 1 wk. Before next dose (Tr). at least 6 hr after last dose to allow for drug distribution in the body.
lidocaine (Xylocaine)	1.5-5		SS 7-12 hr. Anytime during IV infusion.
procainamide (Pronestyl)	4-10 mg/ml		SS 12-24 hr. Before next dose (Tr.)
quinidine (various drugs)	3-6		SS 30 hr. Before next dose (Tr.)
Respiratory drugs			
theophylline (various drugs)	asthma 10-20		SS 1-2 days in adults, up to 1 week in neonates. IV infusion, anytime; oral, before next dose (Tr.)

**SS*, Time to reach drug steady state. The SS time is noted first, then the suggested appropriate time of blood sampling for the specific drug. *Tr*, Trough.

Appendix G
Additional Drug Product Information

Generic (brand name)	Drug category	Indication	Usual adult dose	Comments
acitretin (Soriatane)	retinoid	severe recalcitrant psoriasis	N/A	N/A
adapalene (Differin)	retinoid	acne vulgaris	Apply daily at hs to affected areas	Avoid sunlight and application to eyes, lips, and mucous membranes
alprostadil (Caverject, Muse)	prostaglandin E_1	impotency	Intracavernosal and intraurethral	See current literature for information
amlexanox (Aphthasol)	topical	aphthous ulcers	Apply to ulcer 4 times daily	Institute good oral hygiene and apply after meals and at bedtime
amsacrine (Amsidyl)	antineoplastic	acute leukemia and lymphoma	N/A	Most common side effects include nausea, vomiting, diarrhea, alopecia, bone marrow depression, and hypersensitivity reactions
anagrelide (Agrylin)	antiplatelet	essential thrombocythemia	0.5 mg PO qid	Monitor platelet counts every 2 days during first week then at least weekly thereafter
atorvastatin (Lipitor)	HMG-CoA reductase inhibitor	hypercholesterolemia mixed dyslipidemia	10-80 mg PO daily	Monitor liver function tests before and during therapy Advise client to report unexplained muscle pain, malaise, or fever to the prescriber (myopathy)
azelastine (Astelin)	histamine (H_1) antagonist	allergic rhinitis	2 sprays in each nostril bid	Bitter taste, nasal burning, somnolence, sore throat, and dry mouth reported
beclomethasone (Vanceril Double Strength)	steroid	asthma	One inhalation (84 μg) twice a day	This product is double the strength of Vanceril
bentoquatam (IvyBlock)	topical lotion	rash preventative	Topical lotion	Used to prevent poison ivy, oak, or sumac rash
brimonidine (Alphagan)	alpha$_2$ adrenergic agonist	glaucoma or ocular hypertension	1 drop in affected eye tid	Advise clients using soft contact lenses to wait 15 min after drug administration before inserting the lenses
butenafine (Mentax)	antifungal	tinea pedis, tinea corporis, tinea cruris	Apply once daily	Very effective agent, can cure tinea pedis with one month of treatment

NIDDM, non–insulin-dependent diabetes mellitus; N/A, not available.

Olin, BR (1997). *Facts and Comparisons.* St. Louis: Facts and Comparisons; FDA Updates (1997). Drug News, *Pharmacy Today* 3(5):17; Drug News (1997). FDA Updates, *Pharmacy Today* 3(6):14; Special Report (1997). New Drug Parade-Part 1. *Hospital Pharmacist Report* 11(2):58-60; *USP DI Update* (1997). Volume I and II, Rockville, MD: The United States Pharmacopeial Convention.

Generic (brand name)	Drug category	Indication	Usual adult dose	Comments
cabergoline (Dostinex)	synthetic ergot	hyperprolactemia	0.25 mg PO twice weekly	Used to treat hyperprolactemic disorders caused by idiopathic or pituitary adenomas; advise client to avoid pregnancy
danaparoid (Orgaran)	antithrombotic	prophylaxis for deep venous thrombosis or pulmonary thromboembolism after surgery	750 anti-factor X units SC twice a day	Must be administered subcutaneously only in abdominal wall skin fold; see current reference
delavirdine (Rescriptor)	reverse transcriptase inhibitor	HIV infection	400 mg PO tid	Tablets need to be mixed in water before administration
enalapril & felodipine ER (Lexxel)	ACE inhibitor & calcium channel blocking agent	antihypertensive	N/A	N/A
flucloxacillin (Fluclox🍁)	penicillin	antibacterial	250-500 mg every 6 hours	Increased risk of cholestatic jaundice; monitor closely
fluticasone (Flonase)	corticosteroid	rhinitis, allergic	Spray each nostril once daily	Contact prescriber if signs of respiratory infection occur during therapy
fluvoxamine (Luvox)	serotonin reuptake inhibitor	obsessive-compulsive disorder	50 mg PO qhs, titrated every 4 to 7 days as needed	Maximum daily dose is 300 mg Inhibits cytochrome P_{450} isoenzymes; many potentially serious drug interactions may occur; check current reference
fosfomycin (Monurol)	antibiotic	urinary tract infection	Take one packet in 4 oz of water	May be taken with or without food; symptoms usually improve 2 or 3 days after dose
glatiramer (Copaxone)	immune modifier	relapsing, remitting multiple sclerosis	20 mg SC daily	Transient chest pain reported; alternate injection sites as recommended in insert
glimepiride (Amaryl)	sulfonylurea	diabetes mellitus (NIDDM)	1-4 mg PO daily	Take with breakfast
imiquimod (Aldara)	topical	external genital & perianal warts	Apply 3 times weekly, qhs	Leave on skin for 6-10 hrs; may cause erythema at site
Invermectin (Stromectol)	antihelmintic	intestinal parasites	Dosed by weight; see current package literature	Take with glass of water; repeat stool examinations are recommended
levofloxacin (Levaquin)	fluoroquinolone	antibiotic	500 mg PO daily	Space medication 2 hr before or after antacids containing magnesium or aluminum, sucralfate, iron, and zinc preparations
Levonorgestrel/ 20 µg ethinyl estradiol (Alesse)	hormones	oral contraceptive	one tablet daily	Low dose birth control pill available in 21 and 28 day regimens
midodrine (ProAmatine)	$alpha_1$ adrenergic agonist	severe orthostatic hypotension	10 mg PO tid	Side effects include paresthesias, pruritus, piloerection, supine hypertension, and urinary retention
miglitol (Glyset)	antidiabetic agent	diabetes mellitus (NIDDM)	25 mg PO tid	Drug delays digestion of carbohydrates, therefore it is taken with first bite of each major meal

Continued

Generic (brand name)	Drug category	Indication	Usual adult dose	Comments
Morphine SR (Kadian)	opioid	analgesic	20 mg-100 mg PO daily or every 12 hr	Extended release morphine; see chapter 14 for additional information
nalmefene (Revex)	opioid antagonist	opioid overdose	0.5 mg/70 kg IV initially; if needed, second dose of 1 mg/ 70 kg may be given 2-5 min after	Duration of action is longer than most opioids and anesthetics May cause nausea, vomiting, hypertension and tachycardia; see literature for detailed instructions May cause skin photosensitivity reaction; see literature for detailed instructions
nelfinavir (Viracept)	antiviral	HIV infection	740 mg PO tid with food	Most common side effect is diarrhea, which may be controlled with loperamide; advise women taking oral contraceptives to use alternate contraceptive measures
nicotine inhaler (Nicotrol)	—	smoking cessation	Dose: one spray in each nostril/hr (maximum 5 doses/hr or 40 doses/day)	Should not be used longer than 3 months
olopatadine (Patanol)	ophthlamic antihistamine	allergic conjunctivitis	1-2 drops in affected eyes bid (at 6-8 hr interval)	May cause headache, burning or stinging, dry eye or pruritus
penciclovir (Denavir)	topical antiviral	herpes labialis, recurrent	Apply to lesions every 2 hrs during waking hours for 4 days	Apply to lips and face only
pivampicillin (Pondocillin🍁)	penicillin	antibacterial	525-1050 mg PO twice daily	Avoid in infants under 3 months as it decreases plasma carnitine levels
Pivmecillinam (Selexid🍁)	penicillin	antibacterial	200 mg 2-4 times daily for 3 days	Same as pivampicillin
polifeprosan 20 with carmustine implant (Gliadel Wafer)	antineoplastic	recurrent glioblastoma multiforme	Wafers are placed in resection cavity	Early studies indicate extended survival rates
progesterone vaginal gel (Crinone 8%)	natural progesterone	progesterone replacement	Applicatorful (90 mg) twice daily	First product that delivers progesterone directly to uterus, used to assist infertile women that have a progesterone deficiency
quinupristin/ Dalfopristin (Synercid)	streptogramin	antibiotic	N/A	New class of antibiotics; used in treatment of gram-positive infections resistant to other antibiotics
ropivacaine (Naropin)	local anesthetic	anesthesia for surgery, postoperative pain management	See current literature	Long-acting local anesthetic
sodium phenylbutyrate (Buphenyl)	antihyperammonia agent	urea cycle disorders	9.9 to 13 gms/m^2 PO in divided doses daily	Mix with food or liquids before administration; do not mix with acid liquids such as coffee or tea
sparfloxacin (Zanaflex)	fluroquinolone	antibiotic	200 mg PO daily	May be administered with or without food
tamsulosin (Flomax)	$alpha_1$ receptor antagonist	benign prostatic hyperplasia (BPH)	0.4 mg PO daily	Side effects include postural hypotension, dizziness, and abnormal ejaculation

Generic (brand name)	Drug category	Indication	Usual adult dose	Comments
tazarotene (Tazorac)	topical	psoriasis, acne	Applied once daily	Can be used on up to 20% of body surface area; may cause local irritation
terfenadine (Seldane)	antihistamine	This was removed from the text because the Food and Drug Administration has decided to remove it from the market. Safer antihistamines are available and are reviewed in chapter 39.		
tiludronate (Skelid)	biphosphonate	Paget's disease	400 mg PO daily for 3 months	Take with 8 oz of water; do not take with food, antacids, or indomethacin (allow 2 hr between)
tizanidine (Zanaflex)	alpha$_2$ adrenergic agonist	spasticity (spinal cord injuries or multiple sclerosis)	N/A	Side effects include dry mouth, sedation, weakness, and hypotension
topiramate (Topamax)	miscellaneous	anticonvulsant (adjunct therapy)	200 mg PO bid	Advise client to maintain adequate fluid intake to reduce risk of renal stone formation; do not crush or break tablets (bitter taste)
valproate sodium (Depacon)	anticonvulsant	parenteral	Administered as an hour infusion; dose is equivalent to oral valproate	IV infusion—do not exceed 20 mg/ml
valsartan (Diovan)	angiotension II antagonist	antihypertensive	80 mg PO daily, titrate as necessary	Reported side effects are mild and transient; antihypertensive response occurs within 14 days; maximum effect noted after 30 days

Disorders Index

T

U

V

W

X-Y-Z

General Index

E

F

J

K

M

N

O

U

CULTURAL ASPECTS

CASE STUDY